GOMELLA'S

NEONATOLOGY

Management, Procedures, On-Call Problems, Diseases, and Drugs

EIGHTH EDITION

Editor

TRICIA LACY GOMELLA, MD
Assistant Professor of Pediatrics, Part-Time
Johns Hopkins University School of Medicine
Baltimore, Maryland

Senior Associate Editor
FABIEN G. EYAL, MD
Professor of Pediatrics
University of South Alabama Health System
Chief, Division of Neonatology
USA Children's and Women's Hospital
Mobile, Alabama

Associate Editor
FAYEZ BANY-MOHAMMED, MD, FAAP
Clinical Professor of Pediatrics
Program Director
Neonatal-Perinatal Medicine Fellowship Program
University of California, Irvine School of Medicine
UC Irvine Medical Center
Orange, California

New York   Chicago   San Francisco   Athens   London   Madrid   Mexico City
Milan   New Delhi   Singapore   Sydney   Toronto

ISBN 978-1-259-64481-8
MHID 1-259-64481-2
ISSN 0697-6295

This book was set in Minion Pro by Cenveo® Publisher Services.
The editors were Andrew Moyer and Christie Naglieri.
The production supervisor was Catherine H. Saggese.
Project management was provided by Tania Andrabi, Cenveo Publisher Services.

This book is printed on acid free paper.

Section Editors

PROCEDURES

Brooke D. Vergales, MD
Associate Professor of Pediatrics
Division of Neonatology
University of Virginia School of Medicine
Program Director, Neonatal Perinatal Fellowship Program
University of Virginia Health System
Charlottesville, Virginia

PHARMACOLOGY

Kristin K. Bohannon, PharmD
Clinical Pharmacist
Pediatric Pulmonary Clinic
Cook Children's Medical Center
Fort Worth, Texas

Pui-Man (Julia) Ho, PharmD, BCPPS
Clinical Staff Pharmacist–Pediatrics
Kentucky Children's Hospital
UK HealthCare, Pharmacy Services
Lexington, Kentucky

Valerie D. Nolt, PharmD, BCPPS
General Pediatrics Clinical Pharmacist Specialist
Department of Pharmacy
C.S. Mott Children's Hospital and Von Voigtlander Women's Hospital
Michigan Medicine
University of Michigan
Ann Arbor, Michigan

International Editorial Board

To my twin sons, Leonard and Patrick, and singletons Andrew and Michael.

Contents

SECTION VII. Infectious Diseases

Contributors

Zubair H. Aghai, MD, FAAP
Professor of Pediatrics
Director of Neonatology Fellowship Program
Director of Neonatology Research at Jefferson
Sidney Kimmel Medical College–Thomas
    Jefferson University
Attending Neonatologist
Nemours at Thomas Jefferson University
Philadelphia, Pennsylvania
The Golden Hour

Irfan Ahmad, MD, FAAP
Associate Clinical Professor of Pediatrics
University of California Irvine
Director, Surgical Neonatal Intensive
    Care Unit
Children's Hospital of Orange County
    (CHOC) Children's Hospital
Orange, California
*Necrotizing Enterocolitis; Spontaneous
    Intestinal Perforation*

Noorjahan Ali, MD, MS
Assistant Professor of Pediatrics
Division of Neonatal-Perinatal Medicine
University of Texas Southwestern Medical
    Center
Dallas, Texas
Resuscitation of the Newborn

Captain Mutaz Aljader, MD
Department of Surgery
King Hussein Medical City
Royal Medical Services
Amman, Jordan
Hematuria

Marilee C. Allen, MD
Professor of Pediatrics
The Johns Hopkins School of Medicine
Department of Pediatrics, Division of
    Neonatology
The Johns Hopkins Charlotte Bloomberg
    Children's Center
Co-Director, Infant Neurodevelopmental Clinic,
    The Kennedy Krieger Institute
Baltimore, Maryland
*Counseling Parents Before High-Risk
    Delivery; Follow-Up of High-Risk Infants*

Gad Alpan, MD, MBA
Clinical Professor of Pediatrics
New York Medical College
Regional Neonatal Center, Maria Fareri
    Children's Hospital
Valhalla, New York
*Infant of a Mother with Substance Use
    Disorder; Patent Ductus Arteriosus;
    Persistent Pulmonary Hypertension of
    the Newborn*

Stephanie Attarian, MD, IBCLC
Assistant Professor of Clinical Pediatrics
Vanderbilt University School of Medicine
Mildred Stahlman Division of Neonatology
Monroe Carell Jr. Children's Hospital at
    Vanderbilt
Nashville, Tennessee
Nutritional Management

Fayez Bany-Mohammed, MD, FAAP
Clinical Professor of Pediatrics
Program Director
Neonatal/Perinatal Medicine Fellowship
    Program
University of California, Irvine School of
    Medicine
University of California, Irvine Medical
    Center
Orange, California
*Chlamydial Infection; Cytomegalovirus;
    Gonorrhea; Hepatitis; Herpes Simplex
    Viruses; Human Immunodeficiency
    Virus; Meningitis; Methicillin-Resistant
    Staphylococcus aureus Infections;
    Parvovirus B19 Infection; Rubella;
    Sepsis; Respiratory Syncytial Virus;
    Syphilis; TORCH (TORCHZ) Infections;
    Toxoplasmosis; Ureaplasma Infection;
    Varicella-Zoster Infections*

Daniel A. Beals, MD, FACS, FAAP
Professor, Surgery and Pediatrics
Chief, Division of Pediatric Surgery
Marshall University
Hoops Family Children's Hospital
Huntington, West Virginia
Neonatal Bioethics

Vincenzo Berghella, MD
Director of Division of Maternal-Fetal
  Medicine
Director of Maternal-Fetal Medicine
  Fellowship Program
Sidney Kimmel Medical College
Thomas Jefferson University Hospital
Philadelphia, Pennsylvania
Fetal Assessment

Marianne Besnard, MD
Pediatrician
Department of Neonatology
Centre Hospitalier de la Polynésie Française
Taaone Hospital
Pirae, Tahiti
French Polynesia, France
Dengue Infection, Neonatal

Ramachandra Bhat, MD
Associate Professor
Department of Pediatrics
University of South Alabama Health System
USA Children's and Women's Hospital
Mobile, Alabama
Polycythemia and Hyperviscosity

Dilip R. Bhatt, MD, FAAP, FACC, FACMQ
Neonatologist and Pediatric Cardiologist
Kaiser Permanente Fontana Medical Center
Fontana, California
Associate Clinical Professor
Loma Linda University
Loma Linda, California
Isolation Guidelines

Kristin Bohannon, PharmD
Clinical Pharmacist
Pediatric Pulmonary Clinic
Cook Children's Medical Center
Fort Worth, Texas
*Effects of Drugs and Substances on
  Lactation and Infants; Medications Used
  in the Neonatal Intensive Care Unit;
  Cover Tables "Emergency Medications
  and Therapies for Neonates"; Aerosol
  Therapy in Neonates; Medications for
  Neonatal Seizures; Hyperkalemia
  Management in Neonates; Medications
  for Neonatal Hypotension; Medications
  for Neonatal Hypertension*

Andrew C. Bowe, DO, FAAP
Neonatologist
Pediatrix Medical Group
Assistant Professor of Pediatrics
Mercer University School of Medicine
Macon, Georgia
*Immunization Guidelines; Rash and
  Dermatologic Problems; Figures 80–1,
  80–20, and 80–21*

Vera Joanna Burton, MD, PhD
Assistant Professor of Neurology and
  Developmental Medicine
Kennedy Krieger Institute
Johns Hopkins School of Medicine
Baltimore, Maryland
*Counseling Parents Before High-Risk
  Delivery; Follow-Up of High-Risk Infants*

Glenn Canares, DDS, MSD
Clinical Assistant Professor
Clinical Director of Pediatric Dentistry
Department of Orthodontics and Pediatric
  Dentistry
University of Maryland School of Dentistry
Baltimore, Maryland
*Dental Section Update of Newborn Physical
  Examination*

Gary E. Carnahan, MD, PhD
Medical Director of Transfusion Medicine,
  Coagulation, and Chemistry
  Laboratories
USA Health Hospitals
Assistant Professor of Pathology
University of South Alabama Health System
Director of Pathology and Clinical
  Laboratories
USA Health Children's and Women's Hospital
Mobile, Alabama
Blood Component Therapy

Leslie Castelo-Soccio, MD, PhD
Assistant Professor of Pediatrics and
  Dermatology
University of Pennsylvania School of
  Medicine
Philadelphia, Pennsylvania
*Figures 7–2, 80–2, 80–3, 80–4, 80–5,
  80–6, 80–7, 80–8, 80–9, 80–10,
  80–11, 80–12, 80–13, 80–14, 80–15,
  80–17, 80–18, 80–19, 93–1*

Pik-Kwan Chow, NNP, MSN
Neonatal Nurse Practitioner
Christiana Care Health System
Newark, Delaware
Laryngeal Mask Airway

Jermaine T. Clayborne, BSN, CCRN, CFRN, FP-C
Nurse Manager
Medical Transport Network
University of Virginia Health System
Charlottesville, Virginia
Neonatal Transport

Carol M. Cottrill, MD (deceased)
Former Pediatric Cardiologist
UK HealthCare
Department of Pediatrics
University of Kentucky
Lexington, Kentucky
Arrhythmia; Congenital Heart Disease; Defibrillation and Cardioversion

Kristin Lee Crisci, MD
Chief, Sections of Pediatric Radiology and Diagnostic Radiology
Senior Radiologist
Abington Hospital, Jefferson Health
Abington, Pennsylvania
Imaging Studies

Lesley N. Davidson, MD
Neonatologist
Pediatrix Medical Group of Kentucky
Baptist Health Lexington
Lexington, Kentucky
Pain in the Neonate

Nirmala S. Desai, MBBS, FAAP
Professor of Pediatrics
Department of Pediatrics, Division of Neonatology
Kentucky Children's Hospital
UK HealthCare
University of Kentucky
Lexington, Kentucky
Ostomy Care; Pain in the Neonate

Rebecca A. Dorner, MD, MHS
Neonatology Fellow
Department of Pediatrics
Division of Neonatology
The Johns Hopkins Charlotte R. Bloomberg Children's Center
The Johns Hopkins Hospital
Baltimore, Maryland
Counseling Parents Before High-Risk Delivery; Follow-Up of High-Risk Infants

John M. Draus, Jr, MD
Associate Professor of Surgery and Pediatrics
Kentucky Children's Hospital
UK HealthCare
University of Kentucky
Lexington, Kentucky
Surgical Diseases of the Newborn: Abdominal Masses; Surgical Diseases of the Newborn: Abdominal Wall Defects; Surgical Diseases of the Newborn: Alimentary Tract Obstruction; Surgical Diseases of the Newborn: Diseases of the Airway, Tracheobronchial Tree, and Lungs; Surgical Diseases of the Newborn: Retroperitoneal Tumors; Figures 123–1, 123–2, 123–3, 126–2

Kevin C. Dysart, MD
Associate Medical Director
Newborn/Infant Intensive Care Unit
Children's Hospital of Philadelphia
Professor of Clinical Pediatrics
Perelman School of Medicine, University of Pennsylvania
Philadelphia, Pennsylvania
Infant of a Diabetic Mother

Fabien G. Eyal, MD
Professor of Pediatrics
University of South Alabama Health System
Chief of Division of Neonatology
USA Children's and Women's Hospital
Mobile, Alabama
Temperature Regulation; Sedation and Analgesia; Anemia; Coagulation Disorders; Respiratory Management; Hydrocephalus and Ventriculomegaly; Fluid and Electrolytes; Air Leak Syndromes

Maria A. Giraldo-Isaza, MD
Maternal-Fetal Medicine Specialist
Florida Perinatal Associates
Obstetrix Medical Group
Tampa, Florida
Fetal Assessment

W. Christopher Golden, MD
Assistant Professor of Pediatrics
Division of Neonatology
Johns Hopkins University School of Medicine
Neonatologist and Medical Director,
 Newborn Nursery
The Johns Hopkins Hospital
Baltimore, Maryland
Zika Virus (Congenital Zika Syndrome)

Michael Gomella, BS
University of Maryland
School of Dentistry
Class of 2021
University of Maryland, Baltimore
Baltimore, Maryland
Dental Section
Update of Newborn Physical Examination

Tricia Lacy Gomella, MD
Part-Time Assistant Professor of Pediatrics
Department of Pediatrics
Johns Hopkins University School of Medicine
Baltimore, Maryland
*Gestational Age and Birthweight Classification;
 Newborn Physical Examination; Point-
 of-Care Ultrasound; Abnormal Blood
 Gas; Apnea and Bradycardia (A's and
 B's): On Call; Bloody Stool; Cyanosis;
 Death of an Infant; Eye Discharge and
 Conjunctivitis; Gastric Residuals;
 Gastrointestinal Bleeding from the Upper
 Tract; Hyperglycemia; Hyperkalemia;
 Hypokalemia; Hyponatremia; No Stool in
 48 Hours; No Urine Output in 24 Hours;
 Pneumoperitoneum; Pneumothorax;
 Poor Perfusion; Pulmonary Hemorrhage;
 Traumatic Delivery; Vasospasms and
 Thromboembolism; Abbreviations; Apgar
 Scoring; Temperature Conversion Table;
 Weight Conversion Table; Chartwork*

Carolyn P. Graeber, MD
Assistant Professor of Ophthalmology
New York Medical College
Boston Children's Ophthalmology
Valhalla, New York
*Eye Disorders of the Newborn; Retinopathy
 of Prematurity*

Olga E. Guzman, RN, BSN, CIC
Director of Infection Prevention and Control
Kaiser Permanente San Bernardino
 Service Area
Fontana/Ontario, California
Isolation Guidelines

Wayne E. Hachey, DO, MPH
Medical Director
NA Medical
Sanofi Pasteur
Swiftwater, Pennsylvania
Meconium Aspiration

Janell F. Hacker, MSN, APRN, NNP-BC
Neonatal Nurse Practitioner
Department of Pediatrics
Division of Neonatology
University of Kentucky College of Nursing
Kentucky Children's Hospital
UK HealthCare
Lexington, Kentucky
Ostomy Care

Pip Hidestrand, MD, FACC
Section Head of Pediatric Cardiology
Eastern Maine Medical Center
University of New England College of
 Osteopathic Medicine
Bangor, Maine
*Defibrillation and Cardioversion; Congenital
 Heart Disease*

Pui-Man (Julia) Ho, PharmD, BCPPS
Clinical Staff Pharmacist – Pediatrics
Kentucky Children's Hospital
UK HealthCare, Pharmacy Services
Lexington, Kentucky
*Effects of Drugs and Substances on
Lactation and Infants; Medications Used
in the Neonatal Intensive Care Unit;
Cover Tables "Emergency Medications
and Therapies for Neonates"; Aerosol
Therapy in Neonates; Medications for
Neonatal Seizures; Hyperkalemia
Management in Neonates; Medications
for Neonatal Hypotension; Medications
for Neonatal Hypertension*

H. Jane Huffnagle, DO, FAOCA
Clinical Professor of Anesthesiology and
Obstetrics and Gynecology
Sidney Kimmel Medical College, Thomas
Jefferson University
Director of Obstetric Anesthesia
Department of Anesthesiology
Thomas Jefferson University Hospital
Philadelphia, Pennsylvania
Obstetric Anesthesia and the Neonate

Musaddaq Inayat, MBBS, FAAP
Consultant Neonatologist
Department of Neonatology
Danat Al Emarat Hospital
Abu Dhabi, United Arab Emirates
*Calcium Disorders (Hypocalcemia,
Hypercalcemia); Magnesium Disorders
(Hypomagnesemia, Hypermagnesemia)*

Jamieson Jones, MD
Director
Division of Neonatology
Desert Care Network
Palm Springs, California
*Complementary and Integrative Medical
Therapies in Neonatology*

Genine Jordan, MSN, APRN
Neonatal Nurse Practitioner
Kentucky Children's Hospital
UK HealthCare
Lexington, Kentucky
*Management of the Extremely Low
Birthweight Infant During the
First Week of Life*

David E. Kanter, MD
Neonatologist
Herman and Walter Samuelson Children's
Hospital at Sinai
Sinai Hospital of Baltimore
Baltimore, Maryland
Is the Infant Ready for Discharge?

Kaitlin M. Kenaley, MD
Attending Neonatologist
Christiana Care Health System
Newark, Delaware
Management of the Late Preterm Infant

Neelima Kharidehal, MD, MRCPCH
Consultant Neonatologist
Rainbow Children's Hospital
Hyderabad, Telangana
India
Seizure Activity: On Call; Seizures

Omar El Khateeb, MD
Consultant Neonatologist
King Fahad Medical City
Riyadh, Saudi Arabia
Intracranial Hemorrhage

Brian Christopher King, MD
Postdoctoral Fellow
Baylor College of Medicine
Texas Children's Hospital – Newborn Center
Houston, Texas
Postdelivery Antibiotics

Amy Kogon, MD, MPH
Assistant Professor of Pediatrics
Perelman School of Medicine
Department of Pediatrics
University of Pennsylvania
Children's Hospital of Philadelphia
Philadelphia, Pennsylvania
Acute Kidney Injury

Margaret A. Lafferty, MD, FAAP
Attending Neonatologist
Nemours at Thomas Jefferson University
Hospital
Clinical Assistant Professor of Pediatrics
Sidney Kimmel Medical College–Thomas
Jefferson University
Philadelphia, Pennsylvania
The Golden Hour

William G. Mackenzie, MD, FRCSC, FACS
The Shands and MacEwen Endowed Chair
of Orthopedics
Chairman Department of Orthopedic
Surgery
Nemours/Alfred I. duPont Hospital for
Children
Wilmington, Delaware
Professor of Orthopedic Surgery
Sidney Kimmel Medical College, Thomas
Jefferson University
Philadelphia, Pennsylvania
Orthopedic and Musculoskeletal Problems

George T. Mandy, MD
Associate Professor of Pediatrics
Baylor College of Medicine
Texas Children's Hospital
Section of Neonatology
Houston, Texas
Hypoglycemia

Angela Michaels, MD
Attending Neonatologist
Henrico Doctors' Hospital
Richmond, Virginia
Pediatric Instructor
University of Virginia Children's Hospital
Charlottesville, Virginia
*Peripheral Intravenous Extravasation and
Infiltration: Initial Management;
Heelstick (Capillary Blood Sampling);
Lumbar Puncture (Spinal Tap);
Paracentesis (Abdominal);
Pericardiocentesis; Transillumination
and Point-of-Care Ultrasound;
Venous Access: Umbilical Vein
Catheterization; Venous Access:
Venipuncture (Phlebotomy)*

Prasanthi Koduru Mishra, MD
Neonatologist
Southern California Permanente Medical
Group
Kaiser Permanente
Anaheim, California
*Neonatal Encephalopathy; Pertussis;
Tuberculosis*

Shaun Mohan, MD, MPH
Assistant Professor of Pediatrics
Kentucky Children's Hospital
UK HealthCare—Joint Pediatric Heart
Care Program
University of Kentucky
Lexington, Kentucky
Arrhythmia

Yona Nicolau, MD, FAAP
Associate Professor, School of Medicine
Department of Pediatrics, Division of
Neonatology
University of California Irvine, Irvine School
of Medicine
Orange, California
*Enteroviruses and Parechoviruses;
Lyme Disease*

Valerie D. Nolt, PharmD
General Pediatrics Clinical Pharmacist
Specialist
Department of Pharmacy
C.S. Mott Children's Hospital and
Von Voigtlander Women's Hospital
Michigan Medicine
University of Michigan
Ann Arbor, Michigan
*Effects of Drugs and Substances in
Lactation and Infants; Medications Used
in the Neonatal Intensive Care Unit;
Cover Tables "Emergency Medications
and Therapies for Neonates"; Aerosol
Therapy in Neonates; Medications
for Neonatal Seizures; Hyperkalemia
Management in Neonates; Medications
for Neonatal Hypotension; Medications
for Neonatal Hypertension*

Julius Oatts, MD
Assistant Professor
Department of Ophthalmology
University of California, San Francisco
San Francisco, California
*Retinopathy of Prematurity Table; Neonatal
Ophthalmology Tables*

Namrita Jain Odackal, DO
Attending Neonatologist
Department of Neonatology
St. Vincent Hospital
Billings, Montana
Abdominal Distension; Illustrator Figure 50–1

Alix Paget-Brown, MD
Associate Professor of Pediatrics/Neonatology
Associate Director of the Medical Transport
    Network
Director of the Newborn Emergency
    Transport System
University of Virginia Medical Transport
    Network
University of Virginia Health Science Center
Charlottesville, Virginia
Neonatal Transport

Murali Reddy Palla, MD
Assistant Professor of Pediatrics
Division of Neonatology
Kentucky Children's Hospital
UK HealthCare
University of Kentucky
Lexington, Kentucky
Apnea; Exchange Transfusion

Arjan te Pas, MD, PhD
Professor of Neonatology
Division of Neonatology
Leiden University Medical Center
Leiden, Netherlands
Transient Tachypnea of the Newborn

Monika S. Patil, MD
Assistant Professor of Pediatrics
Section of Neonatology
Baylor College of Medicine
Texas Children's Hospital
Houston, Texas
Polycythemia: On Call

David A. Paul, MD
Clinical Leader, Women and Children's
    Service Line
Chair, Department of Pediatrics, Christiana
    Care Health System
Newark, Delaware
Professor of Pediatrics
Sidney Kimmel Medical College, Thomas
    Jefferson University
Philadelphia, Pennsylvania
Multiple Gestation

Françoise Pawlotsky, MD
Pediatrician
Department of Neonatology
Centre Hospitalier de la Polynésie Française
Taaone Hospital
Pirae, Tahiti
French Polynesia, France
Dengue Infection, Neonatal

Stephen A. Pearlman, MD, MSHQS
Quality and Safety Officer, Event
    Management and Women and
    Children's Services
Christiana Care Health System
Newark, Delaware
Clinical Professor of Pediatrics
Sidney Kimmel Medical College, Thomas
    Jefferson University
Philadelphia, Pennsylvania
Management of the Late Preterm Infant

Keith J. Peevy, MD
Professor of Pediatrics and Neonatal-
    Perinatal Medicine
University of South Alabama Health System
USA Children's and Women's Hospital
Mobile, Alabama
Polycythemia and Hyperviscosity

Valerie D. Phebus, PA-C
Physician Assistant (PA-C)
Envision Healthcare at Joe DiMaggio
    Children's Hospital
Memorial Healthcare System
Hollywood, Florida
*Management of the Extremely Low
    Birthweight Infant During the
    First Week of Life*

Jacek J. Pietrzyk, MD, PhD
Department of Pediatrics
Jagiellonian University Medical College
Krakow, Poland
Figure 80–16

Caleb John Podraza, MD, MBA
Assistant Professor of Pediatrics
Uniformed Services University of the Health
    Sciences
Bethesda, Maryland
Director of Neonatology
Naval Medical Center Camp Lejeune
Camp Lejeune, North Carolina
Myasthenia Gravis (Transient Neonatal)

Nina Powell-Hamilton, MD, FAAP, FACMG
Medical Geneticist
Nemours/Alfred I. duPont Hospital for Children
Wilmington, Delaware
Clinical Assistant Professor of Pediatrics
Sidney Kimmel Medical College, Thomas Jefferson University
Philadelphia, Pennsylvania
Common Multiple Congenital Anomalies: Syndromes, Sequences, and Associations; Genetic and Genomic Testing in the Newborn Period; Newborn Screening

Puneeta Ramachandra, MD
Assistant Professor of Urology and Pediatrics
Thomas Jefferson University Hospital, Philadelphia, Pennsylvania
Attending Pediatric Urologist
Nemours/Alfred I. duPont Hospital for Children
Wilmington, Delaware
Surgical Diseases of the Newborn: Urologic Disorders; Urinary Tract Infection

Rakesh Rao, MD
Associate Professor of Pediatrics
Washington University School of Medicine in St. Louis
Division of Newborn-Medicine
Assistant Medical Director
St. Louis Children's Hospital Neonatal Intensive Care Unit
St. Louis, Missouri
Intrauterine (Fetal) Growth Restriction; Nutritional Management; Osteopenia of Prematurity (Metabolic Bone Disease)

Ana Ruzic, MD
Assistant Professor of Surgery and Pediatrics
Kentucky Children's Hospital
UK HealthCare
University of Kentucky
Lexington, Kentucky
Surgical Diseases of the Newborn: Abdominal Masses; Surgical Diseases of the Newborn: Abdominal Wall Defects; Surgical Diseases of the Newborn: Alimentary Tract Obstruction; Surgical Diseases of the Newborn: Diseases of the Airway, Tracheobronchial Tree, and Lungs; Surgical Diseases of the Newborn: Retroperitoneal Tumors; Figures 123–1, 123–2, 123–3, 126–2

Lauren Sanlorenzo, MD, MPH
Assistant Professor of Pediatrics
Mildred Stahlman Division of Neonatology
Monroe Carell Jr. Children's Hospital at Vanderbilt
Vanderbilt University School of Medical
Nashville, Tennessee
Studies for Neurologic Evaluation

Taylor Sawyer, DO, MEd, CHSE-A
Associate Professor of Pediatrics
University of Washington School of Medicine
Director of Medical Simulation
Director, Neonatal-Perinatal Medicine Fellowship
Seattle Children's Hospital
Seattle, Washington
Resuscitation of the Newborn

Rajasri Rao Seethamraju, DCH, FRCPCH, CCT (Neonatology)
Consultant Neonatologist
Rainbow Children's Hospital, Hyder Nagar
Hyderabad, Telangana
India
Seizures

Rita Shah, MD
Assistant Professor
Section of Neonatology
Baylor College of Medicine
Texas Children's Hospital
Houston, Texas
Hypotension and Shock

Jeanne S. Sheffield, MD
Professor, Gynecology and Obstetrics
Director, Division of Maternal-Fetal
    Medicine
Johns Hopkins University School of
    Medicine
The Johns Hopkins Hospital
Baltimore, Maryland
Zika Virus (Congenital Zika Syndrome)

Karuna Shekdar, MD
Assistant Professor of Clinical Radiology
Perelman School of Medicine
University of Pennsylvania
Department of Radiology, Neuroradiology
    Division
Children's Hospital of Philadelphia
Philadelphia, Pennsylvania
MRI Images 12–7, 12–8, 12–9

Katie Victory Shreve, RN, BSN, MA
Former Registered Nurse
Department of Pediatrics
Division of Neonatology
UK HealthCare
University of Kentucky
Lexington, Kentucky
Pain in the Neonate

Anna Sick-Samuels, MD, MPH
Instructor of Pediatrics
Division of Pediatric Infectious Diseases
Johns Hopkins University School of
    Medicine
Baltimore, Maryland
Zika Virus (Congenital Zika Syndrome)

Jack Sills, MD
Clinical Professor of Pediatrics
University of California, Irvine School of
    Medicine
Pediatric Subspecialty Faculty
Children's Hospital of Orange County
Orange, California
Neonatal Encephalopathy

Kendra Smith, MD
Clinical Professor of Pediatrics
Division of Neonatology
University of Washington School of Medicine
Seattle Children's Hospital
Seattle, Washington
Extracorporeal Life Support in the Neonate

Ganesh Srinivasan, MD
Program Director
Neonatal-Perinatal Medicine Subspecialty
    Residency Program
The Children's Hospital of Winnipeg
University of Manitoba, Winnipeg
Manitoba, Canada
Thyroid Disorders

Theodora Stavroudis, MD
Associate Professor of Pediatrics
The University of Southern California Keck
    School of Medicine
Section Head, Education
Fetal and Neonatal Institute
Division of Neonatology
Children's Hospital Los Angeles
Los Angeles, California
Studies for Neurologic Evaluation

Wendy J. Sturtz, MD
Assistant Professor of Pediatrics
Sidney Kimmel Medical College,
    Thomas Jefferson University
Philadelphia, Pennsylvania
Attending Neonatologist
Christiana Care Health System
Newark, Delaware
Neonatal Palliative Care

Nathan C. Sundgren, MD, PhD
Assistant Professor of Pediatrics
Baylor College of Medicine
Texas Children's Hospital
Houston, Texas
Hypertension

Gautham Suresh, MD, DM, MS, FAAP
Professor of Pediatrics
Baylor College of Medicine
Section Head and Service Chief of
    Neonatology
Texas Children's Hospital
Houston, Texas
*Hypertension; Hypoglycemia; Hypotension
    and Shock; Polycythemia: On Call;
    Postdelivery Antibiotics*

Jonathan R. Swanson, MD, MSc
Associate Professor of Pediatrics
Chief Quality Officer for Children's Services
Neonatal Intensive Care Unit Medical Director
University of Virginia Children's Hospital
Charlottesville, Virginia
Abdominal Distension

Outi Tammela, MD, PhD
Docent in Neonatology
Head of Division of Neonatology
Department of Pediatrics
Pirkanmaa Hospital District
Tampere University Hospital
Tampere, Finland
Respiratory Distress Syndrome

Aimee M. Telsey, MD
Assistant Clinical Professor of Pediatrics
Icahn School of Medicine at Mount Sinai
Director of Neonatal Research
Louis Armstrong Center for Music and
    Medicine
Mount Sinai Beth Israel
New York, New York
*Complementary and Integrative Medical
    Therapies in Neonatology*

Ahmed Thabet, MD, PhD
Assistant Professor
Department of Orthopedics
El Paso Children's Hospital
Texas Tech University Health Science Center
El Paso, Texas
Orthopedic and Musculoskeletal Problems

Christiane Theda, FRACP, MD, PhD, MBA
Associate Professor
University of Melbourne
Royal Women's Hospital Melbourne
PIPER Newborn Transport at the Royal
    Children's Hospital
Murdoch Children's Research Institute
Melbourne, Australia
*Disorders of Sex Development; Inborn
    Errors of Metabolism with Acute
    Neonatal Onset; Neural Tube Defects*

Hong Truong, MS, MD
Chief Senior Resident
Department of Urology
Thomas Jefferson University Hospital
Philadelphia, Pennsylvania
Acute Kidney Injury

Cherry Uy, MD
Chief, Division of Neonatology
Medical Director, Neonatal Intensive
    Care Unit
UC Irvine Medical Center
Clinical Professor of Pediatrics
UC Irvine Medical Center
Orange, California
*Hyperbilirubinemia: Conjugated;
    Hyperbilirubinemia: Unconjugated
    Therapeutic Hypothermia;
    Hyperbilirubinemia: Conjugated,
    On Call; Hyperbilirubinemia:
    Unconjugated, On Call*

Akshaya Vachharajani, MD
Professor of Pediatrics
Department of Child Health
University of Missouri
Columbia, Missouri
*Osteopenia of Prematurity (Metabolic Bone
    Disease)*

Brooke D. Vergales, MD
Associate Professor of Pediatrics
Division of Neonatology
University of Virginia School of Medicine
Program Director, Neonatal Perinatal
    Fellowship Program
University of Virginia Health System
Charlottesville, Virginia
*Principles of Neonatal Procedures;
    Arterial Access: Arterial Puncture;
    Arterial Access: Percutaneous Arterial
    Catheterization; Arterial Access: Umbilical
    Artery Catheterization; Bladder Aspiration
    (Suprapubic Urine Collection); Bladder
    Catheterization; Chest Tube Placement;
    Endotracheal Intubation and Extubation;
    Gastric and Postpyloric Tube Placement;
    Venous Access: Intraosseous Infusion;
    Venous Access: Peripheral Intravenous
    Catheterization*

Richard M. Whitehurst, Jr, MD
Professor of Pediatrics
University of South Alabama Health System
USA Children's and Women's Hospital
Mobile, Alabama
ABO Incompatibility; Rh Incompatibility

Jean M. Wolf, NNP
Advanced Practice Nurse 2
Neonatal Intensive Care Unit
University of Virginia Children's Hospital
Charlottesville, Virginia
*Venous Access: Peripherally Inserted
    Central Catheter*

Michael Zayek, MD
Professor of Pediatrics
Division of Neonatology
University of South Alabama Health System
USA Children's and Women's Hospital
Mobile, Alabama
*Bronchopulmonary Dysplasia/Chronic Lung
    Disease; Thrombocytopenia and Platelet
    Dysfunction*

PAST CONTRIBUTOR ACKNOWLEDGMENT

This edition of our book is based on a strong foundation of many contributors from previous editions. The editors of the current edition would like to express our appreciation and thanks in particular to the contributors of the 7th edition:

Hubert Ballard, MD; Michael Bober, MD, PhD; Doug Cunningham, MD; Jennifer Das, MD; Steve Docimo, MD; Cathy Finnegan, MS, NNP-BC; Janet Graber, MD; George Gross, MD; Jose Hamm, Jr, MD; Joseph Iocono, MD; Kathy Isaacs, MSN, RNC-NIC; Shamin Jivabhai, MD; Jamieson Jones, MD; Kathy Keen, MSN, NNP-BC; Chris Lehman, MD; Barbara McKinney, PharmD; Solomonia Nino, MD; Paul Noh, MD; Ambadas Pathak, MD; Judith Polak, DNP, NNP-BC; Thomas Strandjord, MD; Christopher Tomlinson, MD; Deborah Tuttle, MD; and Tiffany Wright, MD.

In Honor of Dr. M. Douglas Cunningham

The editor and publisher are pleased to dedicate this edition of *The Lange Clinical Manual of Neonatology* commemorating Dr. Doug Cunningham's career in neonatology and his years of editorial service and leadership on this book.

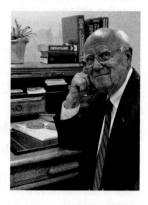

Dr. Cunningham's interest in the care of preterm infants began during his rotation as an intern in the Premature Infant Nursery of San Francisco General Hospital (SFGH; 1965–1966). His attending physician was Dr. June Brady. With much appreciation, he often recalls her great patience and commitment to teaching and her wealth of information for newborn physiology. He passed his first umbilical vein and artery catheters under her watchful eye and guidance.

His internship year coincided with the earliest efforts for intubating and mechanically ventilating preterm infants with ventilators adapted from adult design. Clearly, Dr. Cunningham's premature infant nursery experience at SFGH ignited his career-long fascination with neonatal pulmonology and mechanical ventilation for sick newborn infants.

His interest in neonatology continued throughout his pediatric residency and service at the US Naval Hospital, San Diego (1967–1972). Upon completion of his residency and military service, he entered the newly formed fellowship in neonatology at the University of California, San Diego, under the mentorship of Dr. Louis Gluck (1970–1972). Those were years of clinical advancement with newly designed infant-specific mechanical ventilators, continuous positive airway pressure support, and improved oxygen monitoring. Arterial blood gas studies became routine, and antenatal amniotic fluid studies for fetal lung maturity became a new focal point of collaboration between neonatologists and obstetricians.

Following his fellowship, he received an academic appointment at the University of Kentucky in the Department of Pediatrics with Dr. Jacqueline Noonan as chairperson. She, as the newly appointed chair of pediatrics, was seeking to develop a division of neonatology and to expand newborn care for sick and preterm infants, a service that would reach many underserved communities of the Appalachian counties of eastern Kentucky. Dr. Nirmala Desai, a recent neonatology fellowship graduate from Boston Children's Hospital, joined him. Coupling Dr. Cunningham's University of California, San Diego, experience with that of Dr. Desai's Harvard Boston background, they became a perfect match for advancing neonatal care with Dr. Noonan's support and guidance. In rapid progression over the next 7 years, a neonatology fellowship program was begun. An expansion of the unit for preterm infants from 24 incubators to a new 50-bed capacity neonatal intensive care unit (NICU) was completed, and ambulance and helicopter sick infant transport was inaugurated. Likewise, preterm infant care took on a completely new look as human milk banking came into service, hyperalimentation was used for supplemented nutrition, and mechanical ventilators designed specifically for newborn infants came into regular use.

In 1988, Dr. Cunningham returned to California as a clinical professor with his former mentor Dr. Louis Gluck, then at the University of California, Irvine (UCI). He participated in the expansion of the UCI neonatology program into a multihospital perinatal regional program for 11 neonatal special care units, spanning 5 southern California counties. Throughout his career in the UCI program, Dr. Cunningham was noted for his teaching efforts. He devoted many hours to teaching rounds with medical students, pediatric house staff, and neonatology fellows.

Nearing retirement in 2011, Dr. Cunningham returned to Lexington, Kentucky, and accepted an invitation to also return to the University of Kentucky neonatology program as professor of pediatrics and interim chief of neonatology. An extensive expansion of the program was underway, requiring recruitment of a permanent chief and expanded faculty, fellowship, and support staff—all to accommodate an under-construction 77-bed NICU and regional perinatal program for the eastern counties of the state.

Today, Dr. Cunningham remains as a University of Kentucky professor of pediatrics (part time) and serves as a consultant, lecturer, and mentor for the neonatology fellowship program. He participates regularly as a lecturer for medical students during their pediatric experience. He also serves as a consultant and advisor for the University of Kentucky neonatology residency program for training physician assistants as advanced practice providers in the NICU.

DR. CUNNINGHAM'S REPLY UPON LEARNING THAT THE 8TH EDITION WAS DEDICATED IN HIS HONOR

It has been a personal pleasure for me to see Tricia's success as the originator and longtime editor of this manual. First published in 1988 and now in its 8th edition, it has had unprecedented worldwide success as a clinical guide for the care of sick newborn infants.

I recall the very humble beginnings of the manual that began with Tricia's insistence that it would be the work product of her fellowship in neonatology at the University of Kentucky, rather than an assigned research project. I challenged her to think otherwise, but she remained insistent that she could bring about a publishable manual based on the practical aspects of daily infant care rounds at the University of Kentucky. The culmination of the challenge began when she presented me with a set of drafted chapters. I recall reading them with great interest and congratulated her on their concise text and considerably logical format. The concept of creating "On Call Problems" for the new trainees entering the NICU for the first time was a novel concept that has now been widely embraced in the field of medicine since she first promoted the concept as a teaching tool. It remains a core element in this book's wide appeal. But I countered Tricia with yet another challenge: Could a publisher be found? I was more than a bit taken aback by her quick reply, "I have one, Appleton and Lange. It will be a good fit in the Lange Clinical Manual series." Admittedly, I was smitten by her pluck and success. The future of the manual was conceived on the spot. I recall the pleasure of being asked to write some of the early chapters and to join the project as one of the co-editors.

Recently, a mutual friend asked for a retrospective of what most defined my career. I noted 2 opportunities: first, to have been a part of the beginning of neonatal intensive care for sick newborn infants and the expansion of neonatology as a medical discipline, and second, to have been an associate editor in the development and ongoing success of *The Lange Clinical Manual of Neonatology*.

I often point out to others, with considerable pride, Dr. Tricia Gomella's accomplishments with the manual, which has achieved worldwide distribution and been translated into 12 languages. I have enjoyed the task of helping to identify authors and editing manuscripts from the many contributors of the editions that have followed. In closing, I wish to express my appreciation for your consideration to dedicate the 8th edition of the manual in recognition of my career. My sincerest thank you.

M. Douglas Cunningham, MD
Professor of Pediatrics (part time)
University of Kentucky College of Medicine
Kentucky Children's Hospital
Lexington, Kentucky

Preface

I am pleased to present the 8th edition of *Neonatology*. The first edition was published in 1988 and was started during my neonatology fellowship at University of Kentucky Medical Center in Lexington. The origins of the manual were fairly simple and started as a series of handouts designed to help students and residents make it through their neonatal intensive care unit rotation. Because of a complicated twin pregnancy during my fellowship, I had to delay my training and complete my required neonatology fellowship time at Johns Hopkins University.

While the roots of this manual can be traced back to the University of Kentucky during my fellowship with Dr. Doug Cunningham, it was ultimately completed while I was a fellow at Johns Hopkins University and working at the newly established Bayview campus in Baltimore under Dr. Fabien Eyal. This has made the book somewhat unique because it was originally written from the perspective of a trainee in 2 different neonatology programs. This simple fact, along with the addition of other authors from around the United States and the world, has brought together a diverse group of contributors. I hope you will agree that this approach provides a comprehensive overview of the field of neonatology.

Dr. Doug Cunningham has worked as associate editor on this manual since its inception 7 editions ago. For this, our 8th edition, he has passed the baton to Dr. Fayez Bany-Mohammed from the University of California, Irvine School of Medicine. Dr. Mohammed has been involved with the manual since the 5th edition and has established himself as one of our most outstanding authors. He has previously contributed multiple chapters with a concise writing style that made him a perfect fit to fill Dr. Cunningham's shoes. I also want to publicly express my thanks to Dr. Cunningham. If it was not for his mentorship, this manual would not be in existence. He gave me special permission to develop the earliest versions of the manual during my dedicated fellowship research time. In a most fitting tribute to his contributions to the field of neonatology and his major longstanding contributions to this manual, we have dedicated this edition to Dr. Doug Cunningham.

In this 8th edition, the table of contents was reformatted to make it more user friendly and hopefully more logical. Section I includes essential prenatal and postnatal topics such as "Fetal Assessment," "Obstetric Anesthesia and the Neonate," "Resuscitation of the Newborn," and "Neonatal Transport." Section II encompasses basic assessment and management of a newborn with a new chapter addressing "The Golden Hour." Section III includes advanced management topics such as the evolving areas of complementary and integrative therapies and 2 new chapters: "Genetic and Genomic Testing in the Newborn Period" and "Neonatal Palliative Care." Section IV includes all the basic and advanced bedside procedures commonly used in neonatology. We have added an entire new section on point-of-care ultrasound in Chapter 44. We have also included point-of-care ultrasound information on pertinent procedures. One of the most popular sections of the book, the "On-Call Problems" section, now includes a total of 35 common neonatal problems with 1 new problem added: "Abdominal Distension." Section VI, "Diseases and Disorders," covers all the common and a few not so common, but clinically important, diseases of the neonate. We have added a new subsection on "Infectious Diseases" to encompass the growing literature on infectious diseases that may be present in a neonate. Two new chapters were added in this section addressing dengue infection and Zika virus. The section on neonatal pharmacology includes significant updates of medications commonly used in neonates. Since there are relatively few medications formally approved for use in neonates, the medication information has been carefully curated by our outstanding group of neonatal PharmDs. We believe it to be the most comprehensive list of medications found in a manual such as ours. The "Effects of Drugs and Substances on Lactation and Infants" chapter has been revised to include the most common medications that might be used by a breast-feeding mother. The appendices include other useful reference tables and information. A hallmark of our book has been noting areas that are "controversial," and this edition continues that tradition.

Another exciting and evolving aspect of this manual is its global reach. As our readership has grown worldwide, we have added to our international editorial board. These board members are from many countries: Poland, Jordan, United Arab Emirates, Costa Rica, Saudi Arabia, Peru, French Polynesia, the Netherlands, the Philippines, Finland, India, Israel, Bahamas, Canada, and Australia. These physicians, along with our many international contributors, help to make the manual a useful reference worldwide. The manual has been previously translated into 12 different languages over the past 25 years. These translations include Russian, Spanish, Portuguese, Polish, Chinese (short and long form), Turkish, Greek, Yugoslavian (now Serbian), Italian, Hungarian, and Korean.

I would like to personally thank Dr. Fabien Eyal, my senior associate editor and my fellowship mentor at Johns Hopkins, and Dr. Fayez Bany-Mohammed, my associate editor, for assigning, composing, and reviewing many sections of the manual and for their willingness to always be available for questions. I also want to thank my section editors. Dr. Brooke Vergales, the procedure section editor, spearheaded the procedure chapter updates. I had 3 wonderful PharmDs—Pui-Man (Julia) Ho, Kristin Bohannon, and Valerie Nolt—who worked tirelessly to update the pharmacology and breast-feeding sections, along with their new medication tables, which will enhance several chapters. In addition to their long-term commitment to this manual, the associate editors have brought together outstanding authors from all over the United States and the international community.

I also express appreciation to Louise Bierig, Andrew Moyer, and the editorial and production staff at McGraw-Hill and their colleagues abroad (especially Tania Andrabi) for their extensive assistance during the 2-year journey to complete this new edition. A special thanks to my loving husband Lenny, who helped me extensively concerning matters of editorial content, and my awesome children Patrick, Andrew, Leonard, and Michael (the **PALM team**), who helped troubleshoot computer issues and tolerated many sacrifices while I worked on this and many previous editions of the book over the past 30 years. I owe a debt of gratitude to all of my mother's caregivers (Edie Brewer, Lynn Finney, Skylar Finney, Meryle Voytilla, Calia Broaddus, Anick Biatchon, Veronica Messina, Lillian Colon, and Maria Romero) who took excellent care of my wonderful elderly mother, Nancy Murray Lacy, so I could have the time to work on this edition and to Maisie, our emotional support Bearded Collie, who provided me with humor and love.

Please visit our website, www.neonatologybook.com, for additional information on this manual and for links to enhanced online content for supplemental images, indicated by the symbol [✿] that appears in several chapters. References for each chapter can be accessed from **http://mhprofessional.com/GomellasNeonatology**.

Your suggestions and comments about this manual are always welcome. Readers' comments have helped shape the content of our manual over the previous 7 editions.

Tricia Lacy Gomella, MD
neonatologyeditor@gmail.com

Prenatal, Labor, Delivery, and Transport Management

1 Fetal Assessment

PRENATAL DIAGNOSIS

Prenatal diagnosis refers to those testing modalities used during pregnancy to screen and diagnose fetal aneuploidies and anomalies. Counseling is recommended, ideally in the first trimester, prior to pursuing any type of prenatal screening or diagnostic testing. Screening tests provide risk assessment and determine whether the individual is at increased risk for having a fetus with a genetic condition. Diagnostic testing determines if the fetus is affected by a chromosomal or genetic abnormality by analyzing the fetal DNA through invasive testing. Evolving technology has made the use, interpretation, and choice of appropriate test for each individual challenging for both patients and providers.

FETAL SCREENING TESTS

I. **Nuchal translucency (NT).** An ultrasound measurement of the amount of fluid behind the neck of the fetus, done between 10 0/7 and 13 6/7 weeks[1] when the crown-rump length (CRL) measures 38 to 45 and 84 mm, respectively. An increased NT is defined as a numerical value of $\geq$3 mm or greater than the 95th to 99th percentile for gestational age. An increase in the NT correlates with an elevated risk for chromosomal abnormalities such as trisomy 21, trisomy 18, and Turner syndrome and other genetic diseases such as Noonan syndrome. In addition, gestations with increased NT have an elevated risk of adverse pregnancy outcomes, including fetal cardiac defects and intrauterine fetal demise, even when karyotype is normal. A measurement of NT alone has a low detection rate for trisomy 21 (64%–70%); therefore, it is not recommended as a sole screening test for aneuploidy.

II. **Combined first-trimester screening.** NT combined with a measurement of the maternal serum markers, free β-human chorionic gonadotropin (β-hCG) and pregnancy-associated plasma protein A (PAPP-A), is used to calculate the risk for trisomies 18 and 21. It is performed between 10 3/7 and 13 6/7 weeks' gestation. It is an effective screening tool, with a detection rate of 82% to 87% for trisomy 21 at a 5% false-positive screen rate. Free β-hCG is elevated and PAPP-A is decreased in a pregnancy affected by Down syndrome. A Cochrane review comparing the performance of first-trimester ultrasound markers with or without serum markers for Down syndrome screening found that the combination of maternal age, NT, and serum markers (PAPP-A and free β-hCG) performs better than the use of ultrasound markers alone (except nasal bone) with or without maternal age.

III. **Second-trimester screening.** The **quadruple screen (or quad screen)** involves analyzing levels of 4 maternal circulating factors: maternal serum α-fetoprotein (MSAFP), total hCG, unconjugated estriol, and inhibin A between 15 and 22 6/7 weeks' gestation. The quad screen is used to calculate the risk for trisomies 18 and 21 and open neural tubes defects. For patients who present after 13 6/7 weeks or choose not to undergo first-trimester screening, the quad screen is an option. In a pregnancy affected by Down syndrome, both MSAFP and unconjugated estriol are low and hCG and inhibin A are

---

[1]This nomenclature refers to the number of weeks and the number of days in an incomplete week of gestation.

elevated. The quad screen has a detection rate of approximately 80% for Down syndrome at a 5% false-positive rate. The **penta screen** analyzes the hyperglycosylated hCG plus the 4 quad screen markers and is an alternative for second-trimester screening.

Like first-trimester screening, the quad screen and penta screen require an invasive test to confirm the diagnosis of a chromosomal abnormality (ie, amniocentesis or chorionic villous sampling [CVS]). For patients who chose to undergo first-trimester screening and/or CVS, neural tube defect screening in the form of a second-trimester MSAFP level should be offered. MSAFP is elevated in the presence of an open neural tube defect. Evidence exists that focused ultrasound during the second trimester is an effective tool for detecting an open neural tube defect.

IV. Integrated screening and sequential screening (independent, stepwise, and contingent). These options involve a combination of first- and second-trimester screening.

   A. **Integrated screen.** The NT and maternal serum levels of PAPP-A are obtained in the first trimester, and the quad screen is obtained in the second trimester. When the test does not include an NT measurement, it is called **serum integrated**. With both full-integrated screening and serum screening, the results are reported when all the tests are completed, yielding detection rates for Down syndrome of 94% and 87%, respectively, at a 5% false-positive rate.

   B. **Sequential screening.** NT, PAPP-A, and free β-hCG are measured in the first trimester followed by a quad screen in the second trimester. With the **independent approach**, results are given after the first trimester, and women with an increased risk are offered noninvasive prenatal testing (NIPT) or invasive testing. If there is a low risk, a second-trimester screening is completed and interpreted independently of first-trimester results with a high false-positive rate of 11% at a detection rate of 94%. With the **stepwise approach**, patients determined to be at high risk after the first-trimester screenings are offered NIPT or invasive testing. Otherwise, the second-trimester portion is completed, and the results are given and combined with those from the first trimester. The detection rate is 95% at a 5% false-positive rate. The **contingent approach** begins with the first-trimester portion of the sequential testing and follows with the quad screen when an intermediate risk is noted. Those at high risk are offered NIPT or invasive testing by CVS or amniocentesis. However, those at low risk do not undergo further testing. **The contingent sequential screening has an excellent detection rate and a low false-positive rate, and it is the most cost-effective screening tool for trisomy 21.** A Cochrane review comparing the performance of first- and second-trimester Down syndrome screening suggests that maternal age combined with first-trimester NT and first- and second-trimester serum markers performs better than testing modalities that do not include first-trimester ultrasound or those that include only second-trimester biochemical markers without first-trimester serum markers.

V. **Cell-free fetal DNA screening.** Cell-free fetal DNA (cffDNA) screening is also known as noninvasive prenatal screening, NIPT, or genomic noninvasive prenatal testing. Fetal cell DNA in maternal blood is analyzed to screen for some chromosomal or genetic abnormalities including trisomies 21 (Down syndrome), 18 (Edwards syndrome), and 13 (Patau syndrome) and sex chromosome abnormalities. The detection rate for trisomy 21 is estimated to be as high as 98% to 99% with a <1% false-positive rate. The American College of Medical Genetics and Genomics (ACMG) states that cell-free DNA screening is the most sensitive screening option for Down syndrome and should be available to all pregnant women. The American College of Obstetricians and Gynecologists (ACOG) and the Society for Maternal-Fetal Medicine recommend the test to women at increased risk for fetal aneuploidy, including women with previous pregnancy with a trisomy, advanced maternal age (age 35 years or older), a positive first- or second-trimester maternal screening test, a fetal ultrasound that indicates an increased risk of chromosome abnormality, or a known balanced chromosome translocation in the mother or father. In patients considered to be at low risk for aneuploidy, there is a higher false-positive rate and lower positive predictive value because the prevalence of aneuploidy is also lower. Like other screening modalities, a positive test requires an invasive test to confirm the diagnosis of a chromosomal abnormality. It can be performed from 10 weeks' gestation to term. Nonreportable testing can be the result of low fetal fraction and high body mass index. However, literature also suggests there is an increased risk for chromosomal abnormalities associated with a low fetal fraction. Patients with a nonreportable result can be offered repeat cell-free fetal DNA test or invasive testing. The test does not provide risk assessment for open neural tube defects, and MSAFP screening should be offered between 16 and 18 weeks' gestation. Cell-free DNA can also be used to determine fetal gender and fetal Rh status in pregnancies at risk for isoimmunization. Some laboratories provide risk assessment for some microdeletions by cell-free DNA (such as 22q11 deletion syndrome). However, its clinical utility remains controversial considering the lack of validation in clinical studies, higher false-positive and false-negative rates, and lower positive predictive value when compared to aneuploidy screening.

DIAGNOSTIC TESTING

I. **Chorionic villus sampling.** CVS is usually performed between 10 and 13 weeks' gestation. Chorionic villi are withdrawn from the placenta, either through a needle inserted through the abdomen or through a transcervical catheter, and the cells obtained are grown and analyzed for prenatal diagnosis of karyotypic abnormalities or genetic disorders for which testing is available. Pregnancy loss rates after CVS are similar to those for amniocentesis but are highly operator dependent. CVS is not recommended prior to 10 weeks' gestation due to the increased rate of limb anomalies reported.

II. **Amniocentesis.** Amniotic fluid removed under ultrasound guidance can be analyzed for prenatal diagnosis of karyotypic abnormalities, genetic disorders (for which testing is available), fetal blood type and hemoglobinopathies, and fetal lung maturity; for monitoring the degree of isoimmunization by measurement of the content of bilirubin in the fluid; and for the diagnosis of chorioamnionitis. Testing for karyotypic abnormalities is usually done at 15 to 20 weeks' gestation. The pregnancy loss rate related to amniocentesis is estimated to be 1 in 300 to 1 in 900. Early amniocentesis (before 15 weeks) is generally not recommended because it is associated with a significantly higher rate of fetal loss, preterm premature rupture of membranes, and failed amniotic fluid cultures. Indications for amniocentesis include women at an increased risk of aneuploidy or genetic abnormalities (either by history or abnormal first- or second-trimester screening tests) and fetal structural abnormalities identified on ultrasound.

III. **Chromosomal microarray.** This test allows the identification of small gains and losses in the DNA in addition to the chromosomal aneuploidies identified by standard karyotype analyses. Microarray does not detect balanced translocations or inversions or low-level mosaicism. Studies indicate that the test would detect 1% to 2% of clinically significant genetic abnormalities not detected by karyotype in fetuses without structural abnormalities and 6% of clinically significant genetic abnormalities in fetuses with structural anomalies detected by ultrasound. Diagnostic testing (by CVS or amniocentesis) with microarray analyses should be offered to women carrying a fetus with a structural anomaly detected by ultrasound and in cases of fetal demise. Counseling is important prior to performing a microarray because it can also detect copy variants of unknown clinical significance in 3.4% of patients (with 1.8% of those being likely benign and 1.6% likely pathogenic), adult-onset disease, nonpaternity, and consanguinity. Mothers undergoing diagnostic testing in whom the fetus has no known structural anomaly can choose between standard karyotype and microarray analysis.

IV. **Next-generation sequencing (NGS).** NGS is a high-throughput method to accurately determine the nucleotide sequence of a partial or entire genome of an individual. Whole genome sequencing (WGS) evaluates the entire genome including introns (noncoding DNA regions, likely of no clinical significance) and exons (protein coding regions), whereas whole exome sequencing (WES) focuses on the exon regions of the genome considered to be clinically relevant. NGS is complex, time consuming, and expensive, although costs and sample requirements have all become more reasonable. Prenatal diagnosis by NGS is reserved for clinical research or very selected cases of fetal abnormalities in which a karyotype and microarray have been normal and is only performed after expert genetic counseling.

CARRIER SCREENING

Carrier screening refers to the genetic testing done in asymptomatic patients to determine the presence of a mutation or abnormal gene causing a specific condition, in order to identify couples at risk for passing on such conditions to their offspring.

I. **Ethnic-specific screening.** Ethnic-specific screening is done based on the ethnic background of the individual. This has become more challenging due to multiracial societies and the difficulty in determining a patient's ancestry.

II. **Pan-ethnic screening.** Pan-ethnic screening offers carrier screening for multiple disorders regardless of ethnic background, with each condition being assessed by an individual test.

III. **Expanded carrier screening.** Expanded carrier screening also offers screening for multiple disorders regardless of ethnic background using a single screening panel that detects multiple conditions simultaneously.

Patients should be counseled regarding the availability of prenatal or, ideally, preconceptional ethnic-specific, pan-ethnic, and/or expanded carrier screening. Pretest, posttest, and residual risk counseling and reproductive partner testing in identified carrier individuals should be provided to all patients. Society guidelines have been published regarding recommendations for carrier screening. **See Table 1-1 for some of the most common society guidelines recommendations.** Regarding expanded carrier screening, ACOG recommends that conditions evaluated meet some specific criteria, including a carrier frequency of ≥1 in 100, well-defined karyotype, decreased quality of life, early onset in life, need for medical or surgical therapy, available prenatal diagnosis, and opportunity to improve outcome. ACMG has also published criteria similar to ACOG. However, ACMG indicates optional testing for conditions with mild phenotype, variable expressivity, or incomplete penetrance and for adult-onset diseases.

PRENATAL ULTRASOUND

Prenatal ultrasound examination is used in the following circumstances.

I. **Determination of pregnancy viability.** Once the mean gestational sac diameter is ≥25 mm, an embryo should be seen by transvaginal ultrasound. Once the **CRL** is ≥7 mm, fetal heart motion should be seen by transvaginal ultrasound. Ultrasound is also used in the case of a suspected fetal demise later in pregnancy.

II. **Calculation of gestational age.** Measurement of the **CRL up to and including 13 6/7 weeks' gestation allows for the most accurate assessment of gestational age in the first trimester.** The pregnancy should be re-dated if there is a difference between the last menstrual period (LMP) and the CRL of >5 days prior to 8 6/7 weeks' gestation and >7 days between 9 0/7 and 13 6/7 weeks' gestation. After the first trimester, a combination of biparietal diameter, head circumference, abdominal circumference, and femur length is used to estimate gestational age and fetal weight. The pregnancy should be redated if there is a difference between the LMP and the 4 combined measurements of >7 days between 14 0/7 and 15 6/7 weeks' gestation, >10 days between 16 0/7 and 21 6/7 weeks' gestation, >14 days between 22 0/7 and 27 0/6/7 weeks' gestation, and >21 days after 28 0/7 weeks' gestation.

III. **Diagnosis of multiple pregnancy and determination of chorionicity and amnionicity.** The determination of chorionicity and amnionicity is made by ultrasound examination of the fetal membranes and is best done as early as possible in the first trimester but

Table 1–1. CARRIER SCREENING

Test/Condition	ACOG	ACMG
Cystic fibrosis	Offer to all women	Same as ACOG
Spinal muscular atrophy	Offer to all women	Same as ACOG
Hemoglobinopathies	All women should have a complete blood count (CBC) with red blood cell (RBC) indices If the mean corpuscular volume (MCV) is low, then hemoglobin electrophoresis (Rule/out β-thalassemia trait) and measurement of serum ferritin (R/O iron deficiency) should be done. If MV low, no evidence of iron deficiency anemia, and β-thalassemia are ruled out, DNA based testing is recommended to rule out α-thalassemia. CBC and hemoglobin electrophoresis in African, Middle Eastern, Mediterranean, Southeast Asian, or West Indian descent	No current guideline
Ashkenazi Jewish	Offer Canavan disease, familial dysautonomy, Tay Sachs disease, and cystic fibrosis. Consider also Bloom syndrome, Fanconi anemia, Gaucher disease, mucolipidosis type IV, Niemann-Pick disease, familial hyperinsulinemia, glycogen storage disease type 1, Joubert syndrome, maple syrup urine disease, and Usher syndrome	Same as ACOG
Fragile X syndrome	Offer to women with unexplained ovarian failure or insufficiency, elevated FSH at <40 years old, or family history of fragile X or intellectual disability	Offer to women with family history of intellectual disability
Expanded carrier screening	Offer to all women for selected conditions Expert counseling	Offer to all women for selected counseling Expert counseling

ACMG, American College of Medical Genetics and Genomics; ACOG, American College of Obstetricians and Gynecologists; CBC, complete blood count; FSH, follicle-stimulating hormone; MCV, mean corpuscular volume; RBC, red blood cell.

after 6 weeks' and prior to 14 weeks' gestation. (Chorionicity refers to determining in a multiple pregnancy if the fetuses share a common placenta. In the setting of twins, they can be dichorionic [each fetus has a separate placenta and is in a separate chorion] or monochorionic, where the fetuses share a placenta and chorion [signifying identical twins]. In multiple pregnancies, amnionicity refers to the assessment of the amnion to determine if the fetuses share a common amniotic sac as well as a placenta and chorion. Although the latter sharing situation is rare. it represents a high-risk situation.)

IV. **Anatomic survey.** A routine ultrasound, ideally between 18 and 22 weeks' gestation, is recommended to evaluate fetal anatomy. A large number of congenital anomalies can be diagnosed reliably by ultrasonography, including anencephaly, hydrocephalus, congenital heart defects, gastroschisis, omphalocele, spina bifida, renal anomalies, diaphragmatic hernia, cleft lip and palate, and skeletal dysplasia. Identification of these anomalies before birth can help determine the safest method of delivery and the support personnel needed at delivery. Ultrasonography can also aid in determining fetal gender for patients in whom this determination impacts the likelihood of a known X-linked genetic disorder.

V. **Visual guidance.** Ultrasound is used for guidance during procedures such as amniocentesis, CVS, percutaneous umbilical blood sampling (PUBS), and some fetal surgeries (eg, placement of bladder or chest shunts).

VI. **Assessment of growth and fetal weight.** Ultrasonography is useful to detect and monitor both fetal growth restriction (FGR; defined as an estimated fetal weight <10%) and fetal macrosomia (estimated fetal weight >4000 g or >90%). Evaluation of fetal growth is usually recommended every 3 to 4 weeks. Evidence is accumulating that maternal physical size and race should be considered in customizing the fetal weight for determination of FGR. Estimation of fetal weight is also important in counseling patients regarding expectations after delivering a premature infant. Ultrasound assessment for fetal weight by an experienced sonographer is accurate within 10% to 20% of actual weight.

VII. **Assessment of amniotic fluid volume.** Amniotic fluid volume may be assessed objectively with ultrasound by measuring the **maximum vertical pocket (MVP)**. **The MVP is preferred to the amniotic fluid index** (AFI: total of cord-free deepest vertical pockets in 4 quadrants in centimeters).

A. **Oligohydramnios.** Oligohydramnios is defined as MVP <2 cm. MVP is currently the method of choice compared to AFI methods because it is associated with fewer unnecessary interventions (eg, induction) without an increase in adverse outcomes. Oligohydramnios is associated with increased fetal morbidity and mortality. Spontaneous rupture of membranes is the most common cause. Other causes include placental insufficiency, chronic hypertension, postdate gestation, and fetal anomalies such as renal agenesis, bladder outlet obstruction, cardiac disease, and karyotypic abnormalities.

B. **Polyhydramnios.** Polyhydramnios is defined as MVP ≥8 cm. Causes of polyhydramnios include diabetes, multiple gestations with twin-twin transfusion syndrome, nonimmune hydrops, and fetal anomalies such as open neural tube defects, cardiac diseases, and gastrointestinal obstruction. Most cases of polyhydramnios are idiopathic; however, the risk for fetal anomalies increases with the severity of the polyhydramnios.

VIII. **Ultrasound assessment of placental location and presence of retroplacental hemorrhage.** This is useful in suspected cases of placenta previa or accreta. Most cases of abruptio placentae are not diagnosed by ultrasonography because abruption is an emergent clinical diagnosis.

IX. **Assessment of fetal well-being**

A. **Biophysical profile (BPP).** Ultrasonography is used to assess fetal movements, fetal breathing, fetal tone, and amniotic fluid volume. See BPP under antepartum tests of fetal well-being (Table 1–2).

B. **Doppler ultrasonography.** Doppler ultrasonography of fetal vessels, particularly the **umbilical artery**, is a useful adjunct in the management of high-risk pregnancies, especially those complicated by FGR. Changes in the vascular Doppler pattern (ie, increased systolic/diastolic ratios and absent or reversed end-diastolic flow in the umbilical artery) signal elevations in placental vascular resistance. These abnormalities correlate with an increased risk for perinatal morbidity and mortality. In

Table 1–2. BIOPHYSICAL PROFILE

Variable	Normal Response (2 points)
Fetal breathing	≥1 episode of continuous breathing movement of at least 30 seconds
Fetal gross body movements	≥3 body or limb movements
Fetal tone	≥1 extension of fetal extremity or spine with return to flexion, or opening of fetal hand
Amniotic fluid	≥1 pocket of amniotic fluid of >2 cm in 2 perpendicular planes
Nonstress test	Reactive

high-risk pregnancies, assessment of the **middle cerebral artery** is useful for evaluating for the presence of fetal anemia. The overall use of Doppler ultrasonography has been associated with a 29% decrease in perinatal mortality and fewer inductions of labor and cesarean deliveries in high-risk pregnancies; however, no benefit in using this technique has been demonstrated in screening a low-risk population.

X. **Percutaneous umbilical blood (PUBS).** Under ultrasound guidance, a needle is placed transabdominally into the fetal umbilical artery or vein. Samples of fetal blood can be obtained for karyotype, viral studies, fetal blood type, hematocrit, or platelet count. This also provides a route for in utero transfusion of red blood cells or platelets. PUBS is most often used in cases of severe hemolytic disease of the fetus with or without hydrops, such as that due to Rh or atypical antibody isoimmunization.

ANTEPARTUM TESTS OF FETAL WELL-BEING

Antepartum testing refers to those testing modalities used during pregnancy to assess fetal health and identify fetuses at risk for poor pregnancy outcome.

I. **Nonstress test (NST).** The NST is a simple noninvasive test used to check fetal well-being by measuring the heart rate in response to fetal movements, preferably with the mother lying in a semi-Fowler's position (lying supine on the bed, which is inclined at an angle from 30–45 degrees). Fetal well-being is confirmed if the baseline heart rate is normal and there are periodic accelerations in the fetal heart rate. The following guidelines can be used, although there may be variations between institutions.

A. **Reactive NST.** In a 20-minute monitoring period, there are ≥2 accelerations of the fetal heart rate 15 beats/min above the baseline, each lasting at least 15 seconds. In a fetus <32 weeks' gestation, the accelerations must reach 10 beats/min above the baseline and last at least 10 seconds. The perinatal mortality within 1 week after a reactive NST is ~1.9 per 1000.

B. **Nonreactive NST.** Fetal heart rate does not meet the established criteria during a prolonged period of monitoring (usually at least 40 minutes). There are many causes of a nonreactive NST besides fetal compromise, including fetal sleep cycle, chronic maternal smoking, and exposure to medications such as central nervous system depressants and propranolol. Because of this low specificity (the false-positive rate is ~75%–90%), a nonreactive NST should be followed by more definitive testing such as a BPP or a contraction stress test.

II. **Biophysical profile.** The BPP involves performing an NST to assess fetal heart rate and ultrasound over 30 minutes to assess fetal breathing movements, gross body movements, tone, and amniotic fluid volume. Two points are given for each variable if present and 0 points if absent during the observation period (see Table 1–2). A score of 8 to 10 is considered normal, 6 is equivocal and warrants a repeat BPP in 24 hours, and 0 to 4 is abnormal with delivery usually indicated. Changes in the BPP parameters are due to fetal hypoxemia. Caution is needed since the BPP can also be affected by other factors such as gestational age, medications, and improper technique. The BPP is widely used among institutions to monitor high-risk pregnancies. However, evidence from randomized clinical trials does not support its use to monitor complicated pregnancies. Institutional variation exists regarding gestational age for performance of BPP, starting as low as 24 weeks, even when its utility has only been studied at higher gestational ages.

    A. **Modified biophysical profile.** The BPP scoring system has been modified to shorten testing time. The most common combination includes an evaluation of only an NST and amniotic fluid volume. In some cases, the modified BPP is used as an initial test, and if abnormal, it is followed by additional testing including a full BPP. The stillbirth rate within 1 week of a normal BPP or a modified BPP is the same, at 0.8 per 1000.

III. Contraction stress test (CST). The CST is used to assess a fetus at risk for uteroplacental insufficiency (UPI). The fetal heart rate and uterine contractions are continuously monitored. An adequate test consists of three 40-second contractions within a period of 10 minutes. If sufficient contractions do not occur spontaneously, oxytocin or nipple stimulation may be used. If late decelerations occur during or after contractions, UPI may be present. The CST may be contraindicated in patients with placenta previa, those who have had a previous cesarean section with a vertical incision, and those with high-risk factors for preterm delivery (eg, premature rupture of membranes or cervical insufficiency). CST results are interpreted as follows:

    A. **Negative (normal) test.** No late or significant variable decelerations occur. This result is associated with a very low perinatal mortality rate of 0.3 per 1000 in the week following the test.

    B. **Positive (abnormal) test.** Late decelerations occur with at least 50% of the contractions. This result is associated with an increased risk of perinatal morbidity or mortality and indicates that delivery is usually warranted.

    C. **Equivocal (suspicious) test.** Late or significant variable decelerations occur but with <50% of the contractions. Prolonged fetal monitoring is usually recommended, and the CST should be repeated in 24 hours.

    D. **Equivocal.** Deceleration occurs in the presence of tachysystole (contractions >2 minutes apart lasting >90 seconds).

    E. **Unsatisfactory.** Unsatisfactory indicates there are <3 contractions in 10 minutes or inability to interpret tracing.

IV. Doppler studies. Antepartum Doppler studies are discussed under the earlier prenatal diagnosis section.

V. Fetal movement counting. Maternal perception of fetal movement has been proposed as a tool to evaluate fetal well-being. Different methods have been evaluated including "the count to 10," which involves counting 10 fetal movements over 2 hours during maternal rest. The utility of maternal kick counts to predict stillbirth is **controversial** in the literature. Maternal reports of abnormal fetal counting warrant further evaluation.

INTRAPARTUM TESTS OF FETAL WELL-BEING

Intrapartum testing refers to those testing modalities used during labor to identify fetuses at risk for acidosis, adverse neonatal outcome, or death.

    I. **Electronic fetal heart rate monitoring (EFM).** Although EFM has become widely used, its benefits over intermittent auscultation of the fetal heart rate have been **controversial**. It was not until recently that EFM was associated with a decrease in early infant and neonatal mortality, a decreased risk for Apgar scores <4 at 5 minutes, and a decreased risk of neonatal seizures. EFM is associated with an increase in the rates of both cesarean sections and operative vaginal deliveries. Fetal heart rate monitoring may be **internal**, with an electrode attached to the fetal scalp, or **external**, with a monitor attached to the maternal abdomen. The nomenclature and interpretation of EFM are based on the 2008 National Institute of Child Health and Human Development (NICHD) workshop report and are as follows:

A. **Baseline fetal heart rate (FHR).** Baseline FHR is the rate maintained for at least 2 minutes apart from periodic variations, rounded to the nearest 5 beats/min over a 10-minute period. The normal FHR is 110 to 160 beats/min. Fetal tachycardia is present at >160 beats/min and fetal bradycardia at <110 beats/min. Causes of fetal tachycardia include maternal or fetal infection, fetal hypoxia, thyrotoxicosis, and maternal use of drugs such as parasympathetic blockers or α-mimetic agents. Causes of fetal bradycardia include hypoxia, complete heart block, and maternal use of drugs such as β-blockers.

B. **Variability.** In the normal mature fetus, there are rapid fluctuations in the baseline FHR. This variability indicates a functioning sympathetic–parasympathetic nervous system interaction and is the most sensitive indicator of fetal well-being.
   1. **Moderate variability.** An amplitude range from peak to trough of 6 to 25 beats/min indicates moderate variability and suggests the absence of fetal hypoxia. Marked variability occurs when >25 beats/min is noted.
   2. **Minimal variability.** Minimal variability is quantified as <5 beats/min.
   3. **Absent variability.** Absent variability refers to an amplitude range that is undetectable.
   4. **Decreased variability.** Decreased variability may be caused by severe hypoxia, anencephaly and other fetal neurologic abnormalities, complete heart block, and maternal use of drugs such as narcotics or magnesium sulfate. In addition, variability is decreased during normal fetal sleep cycles.

C. **Accelerations.** Accelerations are often associated with fetal movement and are an indication of fetal well-being. The presence of accelerations suggests the absence of any acidosis.

D. **Decelerations.** There are 3 types of decelerations (Figure 1–1).
   1. **Early decelerations.** Early decelerations result from physiologic head compression and occur secondary to an intact vagal reflex tone, which follows minor, transient fetal hypoxic episodes. These are benign and are not associated with fetal compromise. They appear as mirror images of the contraction pattern.
   2. **Late decelerations.** Late decelerations are a result of UPI and indicate the presence of fetal hypoxia. Potential causes include maternal hypotension, sometimes as a result of supine positioning or regional anesthesia, as well as uterine hypertonicity. More chronic causes of UPI, such as hypertension, postdate gestation, and preeclampsia may predispose a fetus to the development of late decelerations. Although by themselves they reflect only a decreased oxygen tension for the fetus, their persistence may lead to the development of fetal acidemia and eventual compromise. The nadir occurs after the contraction peaks, with the shape demonstrating a gradual decrease and slow return to baseline.
   3. **Variable decelerations.** Variable decelerations result from abrupt compression of the umbilical cord. They can also be seen as a consequence of cord stretch, as in phases of rapid fetal descent, and with a cord prolapse. Variable decelerations tend to increase in the setting of oligohydramnios. The majority of these decelerations are benign and not predictive of an acidemic fetus. However, severe variable decelerations (those lasting >60 seconds), especially in the setting of decreased variability and/or tachycardia, may portend a compromised fetus. They have a "V" or "W" nonuniform shape with a rapid descent and return to baseline: time from baseline to the nadir of the deceleration is 30 seconds.

E. **Interpretation of electronic fetal monitoring.** FHR patterns can be classified in 1 of 3 categories: I (normal), II (indeterminate), or III (abnormal).
   1. **Category I FHR pattern.** This pattern has 4 characteristics: normal baseline rate (110–160 beats/min), moderate variability (6–25 beats/min), absence of late or

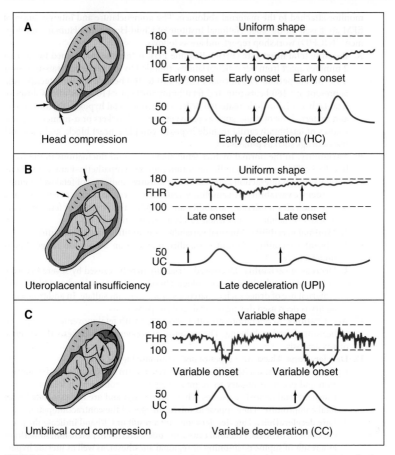

FIGURE 1–1. Examples of fetal heart rate monitoring. CC, cord compression; FHR, fetal heart rate (beats/min); HC, head compression; UC, uterine contraction (mm Hg); UPI, uteroplacental insufficiency. (*Modified with permission from McCrann DJ Jr, Schifrin BS: Fetal monitoring in high-risk pregnancy,* Clin Perinatol. *1974 Sep;1(2):229-252.*)

variable decelerations, and absence or presence of early decelerations or accelerations. In the setting of these findings, there is a high likelihood of a normally oxygenated fetus. Category I FHR is considered normal, and no intervention is needed.

2. **Category II FHR pattern.** Comprises all FHR patterns not in category I or III. Category II tracings are not predictive of abnormal fetal acid-base status. When a category II tracing is identified, a fetal scalp stimulation test may help identify fetuses in which acid-base status is normal. FHR category II pattern requires evaluation, in utero resuscitation with management of possible underlying cause (if identified), and reevaluation. If persistent or progression to category III occurs, urgent delivery should be considered.

3. **Category III FHR pattern.** Category III FHR pattern is abnormal and requires prompt evaluation and initiation of in utero resuscitation while in preparation

for prompt delivery, if the condition does not improve. There are 4 FHR patterns predictive of abnormal fetal acid-base status grouped in category III.

    a. **Sinusoidal pattern.** These include a sinusoidal heart rate, defined as a pattern of regular variability resembling a sine wave, with fixed periodicity of 3 to 5 cycles/min and amplitude of 5 to 40 beats/min. A sinusoidal pattern may indicate fetal anemia caused by fetomaternal hemorrhage or alloimmunization.

    b. **Baseline FHR variability is absent.** The other 3 abnormal FHR patterns in category III are diagnosed when baseline FHR variability is absent and any 1 of the following is present:

        i. **Recurrent late decelerations**

        ii. **Recurrent variable decelerations**

        iii. **Bradycardia**

II. **Fetal scalp blood sampling (FBS).** FBS had been used during labor to determine the fetal acid-base status when the FHR tracing was nonreassuring or equivocal. The test requires that there is rupture of membranes and the cervix is at least 3 cm dilated. Expedited delivery is recommended if the scalp pH is <7.2 or lactate is >4.8 mmol/L. A Cochrane review indicates that "fetal scalp blood lactate estimation is more likely to be successfully undertaken (requires a smaller amount of blood) than pH estimation. Data is controversial in the literature regarding the utility and benefit of fetal blood sampling. Some studies have suggested a decrease in the need for operative delivery with no improved neonatal outcome, while others suggested an increased in instrumental deliveries but less neonatal acidosis." Noninvasive methods (vibroacoustic and fetal scalp stimulation) provide similar reassurance, FBS has been associated with some complications, and evidence to support its use is limited. Therefore, it is not commonly used in clinical care.

III. **Scalp stimulation/vibroacoustic stimulation.** An acceleration in FHR in response to either manual stimulation of the fetal presenting part or vibroacoustic stimulation through the maternal abdomen has been associated with a fetal pH of >7.20. These tests are often used in labor to determine fetal well-being; however, a lack of fetal response to stimulation is not predictive of acidemia.

IV. **Fetal pulse oximetry.** This technique was designed as an adjunct to FHR monitoring in labor and involves the placement of a fetal pulse oximeter transcervically next to the fetal cheek. Normal fetal oxygen saturation as measured by pulse oximetry (SpO_2) is 30% to 70%. Due to the lack of clinical significance in the trials in which it was studied, it is currently not recommended.

TESTS OF FETAL LUNG MATURITY

Fetal lung maturity (FLM) testing is rarely used in current clinical practice because patients are managed based on clinical criteria. The statement by the joint workshop between the Eunice Kennedy Shriver National Institute of Child Health and Human Development and the Society for Maternal-Fetal Medicine states: "The rationale that if significant maternal or fetal risks exist, delivery should occur regardless of biochemical maturity and if delivery could be deferred owing to absence of pulmonary maturity there is not a stringent indication for prompt delivery." FLM is discouraged if delivery is clinically indicated for maternal or fetal reasons because delaying delivery due to an immature result will place the mother and/or fetus at risk. However, a mature result does not reflect maturity in the other organs and can still be associated with adverse neonatal outcome at <39 weeks. ACOG states that when considering delivery in a woman with a suboptimally dated pregnancy, late-term delivery is indicated at 41 weeks' gestation when the gestational age is not known. Some disorders are associated with delayed lung maturation, including diabetes mellitus and Rh isoimmunization complicated by fetal hydrops. Acceleration of FLM is seen in sickle cell disease, maternal narcotic addiction, prolonged rupture of membranes, chronic maternal hypertension, FGR, and smoking. Differences may also occur in various racial groups. FLM is mentioned here for historic purposes only. Different testing modalities for FLM are available (Table 1–3).

Table 1–3. FETAL LUNG MATURITY TESTS

Test	Results Predicting Maturity	Test Considerations
Lecithin-sphingomyelin (L-S) ratio	≥2	Affected by blood or meconium Testing from vaginal pool not possible Costly, difficult to perform, time consuming
Phosphatidylglycerol (PG)	Present (indicates low risk of RDS)	Not affected by blood, meconium, or vaginal infection Testing from vaginal pool possible
Surfactant-albumin ratio (TDx FLM II)	≥55 mg/g	Affected by blood and meconium Testing from vaginal pool not possible Product recently withdrawn from market
Lamellar body count (LBC)	>30,000–50,000/μL	Affected by blood Testing from vaginal pool not possible
Quantus FLM	Low risk or high risk for neonatal respiratory morbidity	Ultrasound cardiac 4-chamber view of the fetal thorax and web-based analysis

RDS, respiratory distress syndrome.

   I. **Lecithin-sphingomyelin (L-S) ratio.** The L-S ratio compares levels of lecithin (principal active component of surfactant), which gradually increase after 28 weeks, to levels of sphingomyelin, which remain constant. **An L-S ratio ≥2:0 is considered mature.**
  II. **Phosphatidylglycerol (PG).** PG appears in amniotic fluid at ~35 weeks, and levels increase at 37 to 40 weeks. This substance is a useful marker for lung maturation late in pregnancy because it is the last surfactant to appear in the fetal lung. It is reported as either **present or absent**, and its presence is a strong marker that respiratory distress syndrome will not occur.
 III. **Surfactant-albumin ratio by TDx fetal lung maturity (TDx FLM II).** This test (Abbott Laboratories, Abbott Park, IL) measures the relative concentrations of surfactant and albumin (milligrams of surfactant per gram of albumin) in amniotic fluid, which increases with increasing lung maturity. This test has been discontinued by the manufacturer.
  IV. **Lamellar body count (LBC).** After its secretion by type II pneumocytes, surfactant is packaged into storage granules called lamellar bodies. This test uses a standard hematologic cell counter to count these lamellar bodies. A count of >50,000/μL suggests lung maturity. However, the optimal cutoff is controversial, with data in the literature ranging from >30,000 to 50,000/μL.
   V. **Quantus FLM (Transmural Biotech, Barcelona, Spain).** This test is the first noninvasive FLM test based on the analysis of an ultrasound images of the fetal lung. A conventional semilateral axial ultrasound section at the level of the cardiac 4-chamber view of the fetal thorax in Digital Imaging and Communications in Medicine (DICOM) format is obtained and uploaded to a web application. The published results are comparable to those of current tests on amniotic fluid (sensitivity 86%, specificity 86%, positive predictive value 62%, negative predictive value 96%.) This test categorizes the risk of developing neonatal respiratory morbidity into 2 levels (high risk or low risk).

CORD BLOOD BANKING

Stem cells from the umbilical cord are collected after the baby is born and are stored by private or public cord blood banks. The family is given a collection kit to bring on the day of delivery. The delivering provider typically collects the blood after the baby is delivered.

After the umbilical cord has been clamped, the blood is drawn with a needle that transfers the blood into a bag that is sealed after the collection is completed. The sample is then taken to the cord blood bank. Parents can opt for cord blood banking, understanding the benefits and limitations; however, it is not universally recommended. Private cord blood banking should be considered when there is a family member with a known condition that can be treated with a hematopoietic transplant. The cells can potentially be used to treat some diseases with an estimated chance of an individual using his or her own cells of 1 in 2700. However, some diseases, including inborn errors of metabolism and genetic diseases, cannot be treated in the same individual because the cells contain the mutation.

2 Obstetric Anesthesia and the Neonate

During birth, the fetal status can be influenced by obstetric analgesia and anesthesia. Care in choosing analgesic and anesthetic agents can often prevent complications such as respiratory depression in the newborn.

I. **Placental transfer of drugs.** Drugs administered to the mother may affect the fetus via placental transfer or may cause a maternal disorder that affects the fetus (eg, maternal drug-induced hypotension producing fetal hypoxia). All anesthetic and analgesic drugs cross the placenta to some degree, usually through flow-dependent passive diffusion. Most anesthetic and analgesic drugs have a high degree of lipid solubility, low molecular weight (<500), and variable protein-binding and ionization capabilities. These characteristics lead to rapid placental transfer.

II. **Analgesia in labor**

A. **Inhalation analgesia.** Inhalation analgesia is not commonly used in the United States because neuraxial (regional) analgesia is widely available. Although not as effective, a mixture of 50% oxygen and 50% nitrous oxide, either premixed (Entonox in Europe) or administered with a blender device (Nitronox in the United States), can be used to lessen the perception of pain. Although placental transfer is rapid, there is no evidence of neonatal respiratory depression or altered neurobehavioral scores. Several problems with inhalational anesthesia limit its routine use:

1. **The need for specialized vaporizers**
2. **Concern for environmental pollution**
3. **Incomplete analgesia**
4. **Maternal childbirth amnesia**
5. **Possible loss of maternal protective airway reflexes**

B. **Pudendal block and paracervical block.** Paracervical blocks are rarely used today because they may precipitate severe fetal bradycardia from reduced uteroplacental and/or fetoplacental perfusion. This occurs because of an increase in uterine activity and/or a direct vasoconstrictive effect of the local anesthetic. If a paracervical block is performed, the fetal heart rate (FHR) must be monitored continuously. Paracervical blocks are effective in the first stage of labor, and pudendal blocks are effective during the second stage. Pudendal blocks have little direct effect on the fetus.

C. **Opioids.** All intravenously (IV) administered opioids are rapidly transferred to the fetus, resulting in dose-related respiratory depression and alterations in Apgar and neurobehavioral scores.

1. **Meperidine.** Meperidine can cause severe neonatal depression including respiratory acidosis, low oxygen saturation, decreased minute ventilation, and increased time to sustained respiration. The risk is least if administered intramuscularly

(IM) within 1 hour of delivery and greatest if given 3 to 5 hours before delivery. Fetal normeperidine, a long-acting meperidine metabolite and significant respiratory depressant, accumulates after multiple doses or a prolonged dose-delivery interval.

2. **Morphine.** Morphine has a delayed onset of action and may generate greater neonatal respiratory depression than meperidine.
3. **Butorphanol and nalbuphine.** These are mixed agonist-antagonist opioid agents that may be safer than morphine because they demonstrate a ceiling effect for respiratory depression with increasing doses. Unlike butorphanol, maternal administration of nalbuphine can result in decreased FHR variability and, rarely, a sinusoidal FHR pattern.
4. **Fentanyl and remifentanil.** These are synthetic opioids, best administered via patient-controlled analgesia. Both are short acting and have no active metabolites. Fentanyl may cause low 1-minute Apgar scores, but neonatal neurobehavioral scores are normal. Remifentanil requires careful monitoring and 1-on-1 nursing care because maternal sedation and respiratory depression are very common.

D. **Opioid antagonist (naloxone).** For respiratory depression after maternal opiate exposure for pain in the laboring mother, positive pressure ventilation is recommended. For prolonged apnea, insertion of an endotracheal tube or laryngeal mask may be necessary. Naloxone is not recommended in this setting as there is concern for complications (seizures, pulmonary edema, and cardiac arrest).

E. **Sedatives and tranquilizers**
1. **Barbiturates.** Barbiturates cross the placenta rapidly and can have pronounced neonatal effects (eg, somnolence, flaccidity, hypoventilation, failure to feed) that may last for days. Effects are intensified if opioids are given simultaneously. Barbiturates rapidly redistribute into maternal tissues before placental transfer; after transfer, they are preferentially uptaken by the fetal liver.
2. **Benzodiazepines (diazepam, lorazepam, midazolam).** These agents promptly cross the placenta and equilibrate within minutes after IV administration. Diazepam accumulates in the fetus; large doses (>10 mg) may persist for days and can result in hypotonia, lethargy, poor feeding, impaired thermoregulation, and an abnormal stress response. Benzodiazepines may also induce maternal childbirth amnesia.
3. **Phenothiazines.** Phenothiazines are rarely used today because they may cause hypotension via central α-blockade and unwanted extrapyramidal movements; they are sometimes combined with a narcotic (neuroleptanalgesia).
4. **Ketamine.** Ketamine induces dissociative analgesia. Doses >1 mg/kg may cause uterine hypertonia, neonatal depression, and abnormal neonatal muscle tone. Doses used in labor (0.1–0.2 mg/kg) produce minimal maternal or neonatal effects.

F. **Lumbar epidural analgesia.** Lumbar epidural analgesia is the most frequently used neuraxial analgesic technique for childbirth. In fact, early epidural placement is encouraged in the most recent American Society of Anesthesiologists (ASA) Practice Guidelines for Obstetric Anesthesia when the service is available. Local anesthetic (eg, bupivacaine, ropivacaine) with or without an opioid is injected incrementally or continuously through an epidural catheter placed in a lumbar (L2–3, L3–4, L4–5) interspace to block the T10 to L1 and S2 to S4 spinal cord segments. Maternal pain and catecholamine levels are reduced, decreasing maternal hyperventilation and improving fetal oxygen delivery. A dilute concentration of local anesthetic plus opioid may lower the amount of local anesthetic needed, enhance the quality of analgesia, and minimize motor block. Infusion of the local anesthetic–opioid combination via a patient-controlled approach (patient-controlled epidural analgesia) rather than at a fixed rate may reduce the dosage of local anesthetic further. Drug accumulation and subsequent neonatal respiratory depression are rare. Maternal hypotension from sympathetic blockade is easily treated with fluid administration and IV ephedrine or preferentially phenylephrine because of improved fetal acid-base status. Unfortunately, labor epidural analgesia is associated with a gradual increase in maternal temperature of up to 1°C. The etiology appears to be inflammatory, not infectious, but may lead to unnecessary neonatal sepsis evaluations. Efforts to lower maternal temperature are prudent because fever, whatever the cause, may be detrimental to the fetal brain.

G. **Intrathecal opioid analgesia/combined spinal epidural (CSE).** Intrathecal opioids (sufentanil or fentanyl ± morphine) provide rapid labor analgesia with minimal motor and sympathetic blockade. They are usually administered in combination with an epidural (CSE) via a "needle-through-needle" technique (spinal needle through epidural needle, opioid injected, epidural catheter placed). When intrathecal analgesia recedes, epidural analgesia takes over. Indications include early first-stage labor (opioid alone), if labor is advanced and progressing rapidly (opioid + bupivacaine), or if there is a reasonable possibility of operative delivery. Transient FHR bradycardia occurs in approximately 10% to 15% of cases, possibly from a rapid decrease in maternal catecholamines and an unopposed oxytocin effect. This may lead to uterine hypertonus or tachysystole and lower fetal perfusion. Therefore, the ASA Practice Guidelines for Obstetric Anesthesia strongly agree that the FHR should be monitored before and after administration of neuraxial analgesia.

H. **Caudal epidural analgesia.** Caudal epidural analgesia blocks the sacral nerve roots and provides excellent pain relief in the second stage of labor. Use is limited during the first stage because the larger doses of local anesthetic needed increase pelvic muscle relaxation and impair fetal head rotation. Fetal intracranial local anesthetic injection can occur also.

I. **Continuous spinal analgesia.** A catheter is placed directly into the subarachnoid (spinal) space either through or over the top of an introducer needle. Usually the introducer is large, making the incidence of spinal headache unacceptably high. An infusion of opioid (fentanyl or sufentanil) with or without bupivacaine is maintained throughout labor.

J. **Local anesthetics.** All of the neuraxial anesthetic/analgesic techniques and local blocks use local anesthetic agents.
   1. **Lidocaine.** Placental transfer of lidocaine is significant, but Apgar scores are not affected in healthy neonates. Acidotic fetuses accumulate larger amounts of lidocaine through pH-induced ion trapping.
   2. **Bupivacaine.** Bupivacaine is theoretically less harmful for the fetus because the higher degree of ionization and protein binding limits placental transfer. Maternal toxicity leading to convulsions and cardiac arrest has been reported after inadvertent intravascular injection. Bupivacaine, in low concentrations, is the most commonly used local anesthetic agent for continuous labor analgesia because it provides excellent sensory analgesia with minimal motor blockade.
   3. **2-Chloroprocaine.** After systemic absorption, 2-chloroprocaine is rapidly broken down by pseudocholinesterase, so very little reaches the placenta or fetus. However, because of its short duration and significant motor blockade, 2-chloroprocaine is not useful for continuous labor analgesia.
   4. **Ropivacaine** is similar to bupivacaine but produces less motor block and less maternal cardiotoxicity. Neurobehavioral scores are slightly better in infants whose mothers received epidural ropivacaine compared with bupivacaine.
   5. **Levobupivacaine** is the purified levorotary isomer (S-enantiomer) of racemic bupivacaine. Like ropivacaine, it has less potential for cardiotoxicity.

K. **Psychoprophylaxis.** The **Lamaze technique** of prepared childbirth involves class instruction for prospective parents. The process of childbirth is explained, and exercises, breathing skills, and relaxation techniques are taught to help relieve labor pain. However, the assumption that the neonate benefits if the mother receives no drugs during childbirth is questionable. Approximately 50% to 70% of women who have learned the Lamaze method request IV/IM pain medication or a neuraxial analgesic during labor. Other techniques include transcutaneous electrical nerve stimulation (TENS), hypnosis, and acupuncture.

III. **Anesthesia for cesarean delivery.** Aortocaval compression may decrease placental perfusion if the mother is positioned supine, so a wedge is placed under the right hip to attain a tilt of 15 to 30 degrees. Neuraxial techniques are chosen in preference to general anesthesia for most cesarean deliveries because it is usually safer for mother and baby. However, if emergent delivery is indicated, general anesthesia has the shortest induction time.

A. **Spinal anesthesia.** Spinal anesthesia (injection of local anesthetic ± opioid directly into the cerebrospinal fluid) requires one-tenth of the drug needed for epidural anesthesia. Maternal and fetal drug levels are extremely low. Hypotension occurs rapidly but can be attenuated by administering 1.5 to 2.0 L of a balanced salt solution IV (preload or co-load) and/or treating with IV ephedrine or phenylephrine. Better quality anesthesia, more rapid placement, and faster onset make spinal anesthesia preferred over epidural anesthesia. In addition, fewer abnormalities in neonatal neurobehavioral scores occur after spinal anesthesia compared with general anesthesia.

B. **Lumbar epidural anesthesia.** Epidural anesthesia is less profound than spinal anesthesia, and a larger dose of local anesthetic is required. Consequently, placental transfer occurs to a small degree, although drug effects can only be detected by neurobehavioral testing. Maternal hypotension occurs more slowly and is less significant because the epidural is dosed incrementally.

C. **Combined spinal epidural.** If a cesarean delivery of prolonged duration is anticipated, a CSE is used. Rapid, intense spinal anesthesia is obtained with the ability to initiate epidural anesthesia when the spinal anesthesia wanes.

D. **General anesthesia.** General anesthesia is used in the following circumstances: strong patient preference, emergency delivery, and contraindications to neuraxial anesthesia. After induction, anesthesia is maintained with a combination of nitrous oxide in oxygen and low doses of inhaled halogenated agents or IV medications.

1. **Agents used for general anesthesia**

   a. **Premedication.** Administration of medications that reduce gastric acid secretion and volume (H_2 receptor antagonists), increase gastric pH (sodium citrate), and speed gastric emptying (metoclopramide) are recommended (ASA Practice Guidelines for Obstetric Anesthesia) to help prevent aspiration. The neonate is not affected by these agents.

   b. **Thiopental.** Thiopental (4–5 mg/kg), a common induction agent, is no longer available in the United States. Rapid redistribution into maternal tissues and preferential uptake by the fetal liver confer low fetal brain concentration and minimal neonatal depression.

   c. **Propofol.** Propofol (2–2.5 mg/kg), although not approved during pregnancy (there are no well-controlled human studies), is the most widespread induction agent in the United States. It rapidly crosses the placenta and distributes into the fetus. Propofol causes more maternal hypotension than thiopental, which may lead to decreased uteroplacental blood flow, but most investigators have reported no difference in neonatal neurobehavioral scores.

   d. **Ketamine.** Ketamine (1 mg/kg) is mainly reserved for induction in severe asthmatics (bronchodilator properties) and in patients with mild to moderate hypovolemia (sympathomimetic properties) when cesarean delivery is emergent. Neonatal neurobehavioral scores are similar to those with thiopental.

   e. **Etomidate.** Etomidate (0.2–0.3 mg/kg) is used to induce parturients who are hemodynamically unstable because it produces minimal effects on cardiorespiratory function. A transient decrease in maternal and neonatal cortisol production may occur after administration.

   f. **Muscle relaxants.** Muscle relaxants are highly ionized, cross the placenta only in small amounts, and have little effect on the neonate.

      i. **Succinylcholine (1–1.5 mg/kg).** In twice-normal doses, succinylcholine is detectable in the fetus, but no respiratory effects are seen until the dose is 5 times normal or both mother and fetus have abnormal pseudocholinesterase levels or activity.

    ii. Rocuronium (1 mg/kg), atracurium, cisatracurium, vecuronium. These are medium-duration nondepolarizing muscle relaxants. In clinical doses, they do not affect the neonate.

  g. Nitrous oxide. Nitrous oxide undergoes rapid placental transfer. Prolonged administration of high (>50%) concentrations can result in low Apgar scores because of neonatal anesthesia and diffusion hypoxia. Concentrations of up to 50% are safe, but neonates may need supplemental oxygen after delivery.

  h. Halogenated anesthetic agents (isoflurane, enflurane, sevoflurane, desflurane, halothane). These agents are used to maintain general anesthesia. Beneficial effects include decreased maternal catecholamines, increased uterine blood flow, and improved maternal anesthesia compared with nitrous oxide alone. Low concentrations rarely cause neonatal anesthesia and are readily exhaled. High concentrations may decrease uterine contractility. The lowest effective concentration is chosen, and the agent is usually discontinued after delivery.

  i. Opioids. All opioids readily cross the placenta and are commonly avoided until after delivery.

2. Neonatal effects of general anesthesia. Maternal hypoxia resulting from aspiration or failed endotracheal intubation can cause fetal hypoxia. Maternal hyperventilation ($PaCO_2$ <20 mm Hg) decreases placental blood flow and shifts the maternal oxyhemoglobin dissociation curve to the left, which can also lead to fetal hypoxia and acidosis.

3. Interval between incision of the uterus and delivery. Incision and manipulation of the uterus produce reflex uterine vasoconstriction and may result in fetal acidosis or asphyxia. A long interval between uterine incision and delivery (>90 seconds) is associated with significantly lower Apgar scores, especially if >180 seconds, and is more important when general anesthesia is employed. Neuraxial anesthesia decreases reflex vasoconstriction, so the interval is less significant.

4. Neuraxial versus general anesthesia

  a. Apgar scores. Early studies showed that neonates had higher Apgar scores at 1 and 5 minutes when neuraxial anesthesia was used. However, newer general anesthetic techniques lower Apgar scores at 1 minute only. This represents transient sedation, not asphyxia. If the interval between induction and delivery is short, the difference in Apgar scores is smaller. Nevertheless, low Apgar scores from sedation do not have the negative prognostic value that those from asphyxia do, provided the neonate is adequately resuscitated.

  b. Acid-base status. The differences in acid-base status are minimal and probably not significant. Infants of diabetic mothers may be less acidotic with general anesthesia because neuraxial anesthesia-induced hypotension may exacerbate any existing uteroplacental insufficiency.

  c. Neurobehavioral examinations. These tests are performed to examine the relationship between motor, neurologic, and behavioral functioning; to detect early central nervous system dysfunction; to predict future outcomes; to evaluate longitudinal development; and to determine the impact of interventions. Detecting atypical development is essential to target early interventions for those most at risk, but also to prevent unnecessary intervention for those who are unlikely to have neurodevelopmental impairment. However, it is important not to administer the tests too early. Xu and colleagues recommend 20 hours after delivery as the earliest appropriate time to obtain results that are not influenced by the acute effects of labor and delivery and thus most accurately represent newborn neurobehavior. Eight assessments appropriate for preterm infants up to 4 months of corrected age are listed in Table 2–1. They include observation of antigravity postures, quality of spontaneous movements, infant motor patterns, reflexes, muscle tone, attention, visual or auditory responses, color, vital signs, and irritability or consolability.

Table 2–1. NEWBORN NEUROBEHAVIORAL ASSESSMENTS

Tool	Age Range	Purposes	Components Tested
APIB (Assessment of Preterm Infants' Behavior)	28 weeks to 1 month	Documentation of the spectrum of preterm/term infants' neurobehavioral functioning/competence	Autonomic, motor, state, attention/interaction, self-regulation
Dubowitz (Dubowitz Neurological Assessment of the Preterm and Full-Term Newborn Infant)	30 weeks to 4 months	Detailed profile of neurologic status; identifies infants with neurologic abnormalities	Posture and tone, reflexes, movements, neurobehavioral responses
GMs (Prechtl's Assessment of General Movements)	Preterm to 4 months	Records spontaneous movements to identify early central nervous system dysfunction	Movement patterns
NAPI (Neurobehavioral Assessment of the Preterm Infant)	32 weeks until term	Measurement of the progression of neurobehavioral performance	Motor development and vigor, scarf sign, popliteal angle, attention/orientation, % asleep, irritability, vigor of cry
NBAS (Brazelton Neonatal Behavioral Assessment Scale)	36 weeks until 6 weeks post term	Identifies individual neurobehavioral functioning and identifies areas of difficulty	Autonomic, motor and reflexes, state, social/attentional
NMBA (Neuromotor Behavioral Assessment)	30 to 36 weeks	Identifies preterm infants who may be developmentally at risk	Neurologic (eg, tone, reflexes), behavioral, autonomic, motor functions
NNNS (Neonatal Intensive Care Network Neurobehavioral Scale)	30 weeks up to 4 months (46/48 weeks post term)	Assesses at-risk infants (eg, substance exposed); documents neurologic integrity and behavioral functioning	Neurologic (tone, reflexes), behavioral, stress/abstinence items
TIMP (Test of Infant Motor Performance)	32 weeks to 4 months	Assesses motor control and organization of posture and movement for functional activities	Orientation of the infant's head in space, auditory and visual stimuli responses, body alignment, limb movements

Note. For clinical purposes, the neurobehavioral assessments GMs, Dubowitz, NAPI, NBAS, and TIMP are suitable, but for research purposes the APIB and NNNS are the assessments of choice. The GMs and TIMP can be used across both settings, having both excellent utility and psychometric properties; they show the strongest associations with neurodevelopmental outcome.

Reproduced with permission from Noble Y, Boyd R: Neonatal assessments for the preterm infant up to 4 months corrected age: a systematic review, *Dev Med Child Neurol.* 2012 Feb;54(2):129-139.

3 Resuscitation of the Newborn

Approximately 10% of all newborns need help with breathing at the time of birth, and 1 in 1000 newborns require resuscitation with chest compressions and cardiac medications. Given the high frequency of newborn resuscitation, it is vital that all neonatal healthcare workers are trained and competent to provide resuscitation to babies in need. Newborn resuscitation cannot always be anticipated in time to transfer the mother before delivery to a facility with specialized neonatal support. Therefore, every hospital with a delivery suite should have a skilled resuscitation team (see Chapter 4, "Neonatal Transport") and appropriate equipment available (Table 3–1).

I. **Normal physiologic events at birth.** Normal transition at birth begins with lung expansion, generally requiring large negative intrathoracic pressures, followed by a cry (expiration against a partially closed glottis). Umbilical cord clamping is accompanied by a rise in systemic blood pressure and stimulation of the sympathetic nervous system. With the onset of respiration and lung expansion, pulmonary vascular resistance decreases, followed by a gradual transition (over minutes to hours) from fetal to adult circulation, with the closure of the foramen ovale and ductus arteriosus.

II. **Abnormal physiologic events at birth.** The asphyxiated newborn undergoes an abnormal fetal to neonatal transition. With asphyxiation, the fetus develops *primary apnea*, during which spontaneous respirations can be induced by appropriate sensory stimuli such as drying. If the asphyxial insult persists, the fetus develops deep gasping, followed by a period of *secondary apnea*, during which spontaneous respirations cannot be induced by sensory stimuli. Death occurs if secondary apnea is not reversed by ventilatory support within several minutes. Because one can never be certain whether an apneic newborn has primary or secondary apnea, resuscitative efforts should proceed as though secondary apnea is present.

III. **Preparation for high-risk delivery.** Preparation for a high-risk delivery is the key to a successful outcome. Cooperation between the obstetric, anesthesia, and pediatric staff is important. As noted in Figure 3–1, each resuscitation should begin with a team briefing and equipment check. Knowledge of potential high-risk situations and appropriate interventions is essential (Table 3–2). It is useful to have an estimation of weight and gestational age (Table 3–3) for calculating drug dosages and equipment size. The team briefing prior to delivery is used for assigning team member roles and reviewing expected resuscitation measures in order to establish a shared mental model within the resuscitation team. Antenatal counseling should be provided to the parents prior to the birth, especially when the fetus is at the limit of viability or when life-threatening anomalies are anticipated.

IV. **Assessment of the need for resuscitation. The Apgar score is assigned at 1, 5, and, occasionally, 10 to 20 minutes after delivery.** It gives a fairly objective idea of how much resuscitation was required at birth and the infant's response to resuscitative efforts. It is, however, not useful during resuscitation. During resuscitation, simultaneous assessment of respiratory activity and heart rate provides the quickest and most accurate evaluation of the need for continuing resuscitation.

A. **Respiratory activity.** Respiratory activity is assessed by observing for chest movement. If there is no respiratory effort or the effort is poor, the infant needs respiratory assistance with positive-pressure ventilation (PPV).

B. **Heart rate.** The heart rate is best evaluated initially by auscultation. Palpation of the umbilical cord is less accurate. The evaluator should tap out each beat so that all team members can hear it or verbally call out the heart rate. If the heart rate is difficult to detect, then a pulse oximetry that displays a heart rate or a 3-lead electrocardiogram (ECG) should be used. A 3-lead ECG may be more reliable than a pulse oximeter in cases of poor systemic perfusion.

Table 3–1. NEWBORN RESUSCITATION EQUIPMENT CHECKLIST

Warm	☐ Preheated warmer
	☐ Warm towels or blankets
	☐ Temperature sensor
	☐ Plastic wrap or bag (<32 weeks)
	☐ Chemical warming blanket (<32 weeks)
	☐ Hat
Clear airway	☐ Bulb syringe
	☐ 10F or 12F suction catheter with 80–100 mm Hg wall suction
	☐ Meconium aspirator
Auscultate/electrocardiogram (ECG)	☐ Stethoscope
	☐ Electronic cardiac monitor (ECG) and ECG leads
Ventilate	☐ Flowmeter set at 10 L/min
	☐ Oxygen blender set at 21% if >35 weeks, 21%–30% if <35 weeks
	☐ Positive-pressure device connected to a blender (positive end-expiratory pressure and peak inspiratory pressure set)
	☐ Term and preterm masks
	☐ 8F feeding tube and syringe
	☐ Oral airway
Oxygenate	☐ Equipment to give free-flow oxygen
	☐ Pulse oximeter probe sensor and monitor
	☐ Target oxygen saturation table
Intubate	☐ Laryngoscope, size 0 and 1straight blades with bright light (size 00 optional)
	☐ Stylet (optional)
	☐ Endotracheal tubes (2.5, 3.0, and 3.5)
	☐ End-tidal carbon dioxide detector
	☐ Measuring tape and/or endotracheal tube insertion depth table
	☐ Endotracheal tube securing device or waterproof tape and scissors
	☐ Laryngeal mask airway, size 1, with 5-mL syringe
Medicate	Access to:
	☐ 1 mg/10 mL (0.1 mg/mL) epinephrine
	☐ Normal saline
	☐ Code sheet for documentation
	☐ Supplies for placing an emergency umbilical vein catheter and giving medications
	☐ Intraosseous supplies (optional)

Data from American Academy of Pediatrics, American Heart Association, Weiner GM, et al: *Textbook of Neonatal Resuscitation*, 7th ed. Chicago, IL: American Heart Association and American Academy of Pediatrics Chicago; 2016.

V. **Neonatal resuscitation at the time of birth.** The American Heart Association (AHA) and American Academy of Pediatrics' (AAP) *Textbook of Neonatal Resuscitation* (7th edition) and the Neonatal Resuscitation Program (NRP) course provide the standard of care for the resuscitation of newborns in the United States and many other countries (see Figure 3–1).

A. **Initial steps of newborn care.** In vigorous term and preterm newborns with intact placental circulation, delaying umbilical cord clamping for 30 to 60 seconds is recommended. In nonvigorous term and preterm newborns with intact placental circulation, it is unclear whether or not there is a benefit from delayed cord clamping. Delayed cord clamping is not recommended in cases where placental circulation is

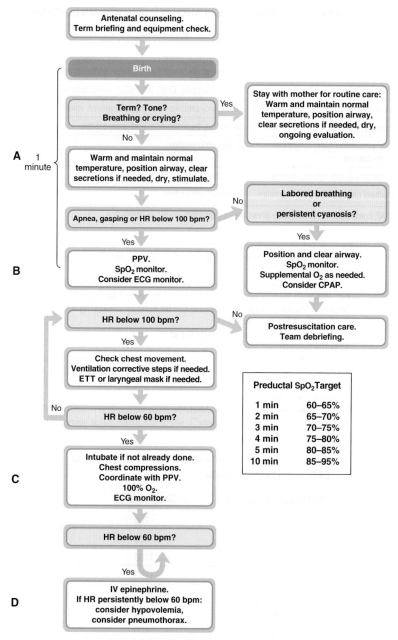

FIGURE 3–1. The 2015 Neonatal Resuscitation Program (NRP) neonatal resuscitation flow diagram. CPAP, continuous positive airway pressure; ECG, electrocardiogram; ETT, endotracheal tube; HR, heart rate; IV, intravenous; PPV, positive-pressure ventilation. (*Reproduced with permission from American Academy of Pediatrics, American Heart Association, Weiner GM, et al:* Textbook of Neonatal Resuscitation, *7th ed. Chicago, IL: American Heart Association and American Academy of Pediatrics Chicago; 2016.*)

Table 3–2. **SOME HIGH-RISK SITUATIONS IN WHICH RESUSCITATION CAN BE ANTICIPATED**

High-Risk Situation	Possible Intervention Needed
Perinatal asphyxia	PPV, intubation, chest compressions, emergency umbilical catheter placement, epinephrine administration
Preterm delivery	Thermal support, CPAP, intubation, surfactant administration
Acute fetal or placental hemorrhage	Emergency umbilical catheter placement, volume expansion
Hydrops fetalis	Intubation, thoracentesis, and paracentesis
Polyhydramnios: gastrointestinal obstruction	Nasogastric suction
Congenital diaphragmatic hernia	Intubation, nasogastric suctioning
Tracheal obstruction with meconium	Endotracheal suction

CPAP, continuous positive airway pressure; PPV, positive-pressure ventilation.

not intact such as cord avulsion, placental abruption, and bleeding placenta previa or vasa previa.

After birth, the newborn should be rapidly evaluated to determine if he/she can stay with its mother or if he/she should be moved to the radiant warmer for further evaluation. A rapid evaluation can be done by answering 3 key questions:
1. **Does the baby look term?**
2. **Does the baby have good muscle tone?**
3. **Is the baby breathing or crying?**

If the answer to all 3 questions is yes, the newborn can stay with its mother to continue the newborn transition. If the answer to any of the questions is no, the newborn should be moved to the radiant warmer for further evaluation by the neonatal resuscitation team.

The following interventions should be done within approximately 60 seconds after birth (eg, **"the golden minute"**): warm the infant, clear secretions, dry and

Table 3–3. **EXPECTED BIRTHWEIGHT (50TH PERCENTILE) AT 24 TO 38 WEEKS' GESTATION**

Gestational Age (weeks)	Birthweight (g)
24	700
26	900
28	1100
30	1350
32	1650
34	2100
36	2600
38	3000

Data from Battaglia FC, Lubchenco LO: A practical classification of newborn infants by weight and gestational age, *J Pediatr.* 1967 Aug;71(2):159-163.

stimulate, and provide assisted ventilation if the infant is apneic, gasping, or has a heart rate <100 beats/min.

B. **Temperature regulation.** The goal temperature for a newborn undergoing resuscitation is between 36.5°C and 37.5°C. Thermal regulation is especially important in the preterm infant. In cases where there is a concern for hypoxic-ischemic encephalopathy, normothermia should be maintained during resuscitation in order to optimize the effect of epinephrine and avoid hypothermia-induced bradycardia. **Therapeutic hypothermia should only start after the resuscitation** if clinically indicated.

Heat loss during resuscitation may be prevented by the following measures:
1. **Dry the infant thoroughly immediately after birth.**
2. **Maintain a warm delivery room.** For preterm newborns, ≤32 weeks' gestation, the temperature in the delivery room should be between 74°F and 77°F (23°C–25°C).
3. **Place the infant under a prewarmed radiant warmer.**
4. **Swaddle the infant in a warm cloth and place in skin-to-skin contact with the mother (eg, "kangaroo care").**
5. **For preterm infants born at <32 weeks, place a thermal mattress under the newborn, cover the newborn with plastic wrap or in a clean food-grade plastic bag up to the level of the neck, and place a hat on the newborn's head.** Warmed humidified resuscitation gases also should be used. Using a temperature sensor and a warmer with a servo-control mechanism can avoid overheating.
6. **The temperature at the time of admission to the nursery or neonatal intensive care unit (NICU) should be recorded in all newborns.**

C. **Ventilatory resuscitation**
1. **General measures**
    a. **Suctioning.** Oropharyngeal and nasal suctioning using either a bulb syringe or a suction catheter should be performed if the infant is not breathing, is gasping, has poor tone, has signs of airway obstruction, or is having difficulty clearing the secretions or if PPV is anticipated. The mouth should be suctioned before the nose to ensure the newborn does not aspirate something in the mouth if it gasps during nasal suctioning. **Deep suctioning of the airway with a suction catheter should be avoided.** Deep suctioning can result in reflex bradycardia due to vagal nerve stimulation.
    b. **Positive-pressure ventilation. Ventilation of the lungs is the most critical action in neonatal resuscitation.** PPV is indicated in newborns who are apneic, gasping, or have a heart rate <100 beats/min. Most infants can be adequately ventilated with a bag and mask provided that the mask is the correct size with a good seal around the mouth and nose and there is an appropriate flow of gas (Figure 3–2). The positioning of the head and neck to open the airway is critical to successful PPV. The correct position of the head and neck is called the "sniffing position," which involves 35 degrees of flexion of the neck and 15 degrees of extension of the head. A T-piece resuscitator is an alternative method to provide PPV that controls peak inspiratory pressure (PIP) and positive end-expiratory pressure (PEEP) and can deliver continuous positive airway pressure (CPAP) (Figure 3–3). When giving PPV, an initial PIP of 20 to 25 cm H_2O and PEEP of 5 cm H_2O are recommended. **During PPV, a rate of 40 to 60 breaths/min should be used to mimic the normal respiratory rate of a newborn.**

    Chest wall movement is the best method to confirm effective ventilation of the lungs. The pneumonic **MR. SOPA** is used by the NRP to highlight the airway corrective steps to take when chest movement is not initially achieved with PPV. The 6 airway corrective steps of MR. SOPA include: (1) **M**ask reapplication, (2) **R**eposition the head, (3) **S**uction the airway, (4) **O**pen the mouth, (5) increase the **P**IP, and (6) place an **A**dvanced airway. In most cases,

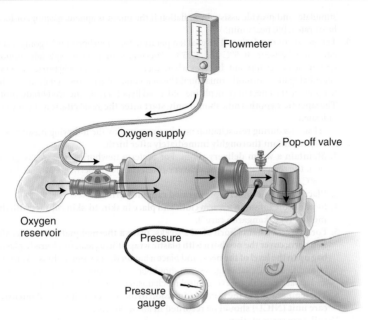

FIGURE 3–2. Bag-and-mask ventilation of the neonate.

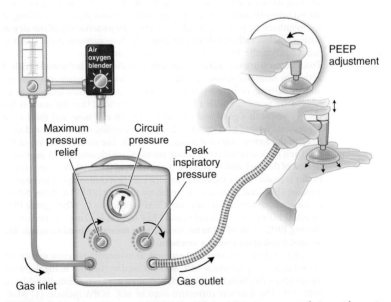

FIGURE 3–3. T-piece resuscitator used to provide positive-pressure ventilation with consistent peak inspiratory pressure and positive end-expiratory pressure (PEEP).

chest movement with PPV can be achieved with the completion of the first 2 steps of the pneumonic MR.SOPA.

c. **Supplemental oxygen.** Oxygen should be used appropriately during neonatal resuscitation. Supplemental oxygen should be titrated to keep preductal (right hand) oxygen saturation in the target range (see Figure 3–1). In newborns born at ≥35 weeks' gestation, PPV should start with 21% oxygen. In newborns born earlier than 35 weeks' gestation, PPV can begin with 21% to 30% oxygen, depending on local practice. Supplemental oxygen can be started at 30%, and titrated as needed, in newborns who are breathing but not maintaining oxygen saturations within the target range. Oxygen should be increased to 100% with the start of chest compressions to maximize systemic oxygen delivery.

d. **Pulse oximetry.** Pulse oximetry should be used to guide treatment when resuscitation is anticipated, to confirm cyanosis, if supplemental oxygen is given, and if PPV is required. **The pulse oximeter probe should be placed on the right hand or wrist of the newborn** in order to measure preductal oxygen saturations. The sensor must be oriented so that it detects the transmitted red light. When applied appropriately, the pulse oximeter will accurately detect the heart rate and oxygen saturations within 1 to 2 minutes. It may be helpful to shield the pulse oximetry probe from the light or adjust the probe location if it is not providing a consistent reading.

e. **Continuous positive airway pressure.** CPAP is a type of respiratory support used to keep the airways open with continuous pressure. In the delivery room, CPAP is applied via a face mask using either a T-piece resuscitator or a flow-inflating bag. **CPAP cannot be given with a self-inflating bag.** CPAP is used in newborns who are spontaneously breathing with a heart rate of >100 beats/min who have either respiratory distress or low oxygen saturations. Resuscitation of a premature infant with respiratory distress syndrome is a common indication for CPAP in the delivery room.

f. **Endotracheal tube intubation and laryngeal mask airway.** Placement of an endotracheal tube (ETT) or laryngeal mask airway (LMA) is indicated in newborns with persistent apnea, gasping, or a heart rate ≤60 beats/min despite effective PPV via a face mask or when face mask ventilation is unsuccessful after completion of the MR. SOPA steps. As seen in Figure 3–1, **ETT or LMA is recommended before starting chest compressions during neonatal resuscitation.** This is because in some cases ventilation through the ETT or LMA can result in a rise in heart rate, thus avoiding the need for chest compressions.

   i. **Endotracheal tube intubation.** The steps involved in placing an ETT are outlined in Chapter 33. Once the endotracheal tube is placed, auscultation of breath sounds and a carbon dioxide (CO_2) detector should be used to confirm tube placement in the trachea. Correct ETT depth can be found in Table 33–3 or by measuring the newborn's nasal-tragus length and adding 1 cm.

   ii. **Laryngeal mask airway.** Placement of an LMA is indicated when tracheal intubation is not feasible due to lack of trained personnel or not successful after a few attempts. LMAs are recommended for the resuscitation of newborns ≥34 weeks' gestation and weighing ≥2000 g. LMAs have not been evaluated during chest compressions or the administration of emergency medications. However, it is reasonable to start compressions with the LMA in place if intubation is not feasible or has been unsuccessful after several attempts. See Chapter 37 for details on LMA placement.

2. **Specific resuscitation circumstances**

a. **Preparation of the parents for resuscitation.** Initial resuscitation usually occurs in the delivery room with 1 or both parents present. It is helpful to prepare the parents in advance, if possible. Describe what will be done, who will be present, who will explain what is happening, where the resuscitation will take place, where the father should stand, why crying may not be heard, and where the infant will be taken after stabilization. Details on the process of counseling parents before a high-risk delivery takes place are outlined in Chapter 55.

    b. **Meconium-stained amniotic fluid (MSAF).** Infants born with MSAF may aspirate meconium in utero, during delivery, or immediately after birth. The sickest of these infants have usually aspirated in utero and generally also have reactive pulmonary vasoconstriction. In the past, the AAP and the AHA recommended endotracheal suctioning in cases of MSAF when the infant was not vigorous at birth. However, due to insufficient evidence, **routine endotracheal suctioning of nonvigorous newborns with MSAF is no longer recommended.** Management depends on whether the infant is vigorous or nonvigorous.

      i. **Vigorous. If the infant is vigorous (good respiratory effort and muscle tone), simply use a bulb syringe to clear meconium-stained secretions from the mouth (first) and nose.** The infant can stay with the mother to receive newborn care.

      ii. **Nonvigorous. If the infant is nonvigorous (depressed respirations and poor muscle tone), take the infant to the radiant warmer. Use a bulb syringe to clear meconium-stained secretions from the mouth (first) and the nose. If the infant is apneic, gasping, or has a heart rate <100 beats/ min, begin PPV.** Routine endotracheal intubation is not recommended for tracheal suction. Endotracheal suctioning should be considered in infants born through MSAF if there is a concern for **tracheal obstruction** with meconium. Meconium aspiration is discussed in detail in Chapter 106.

D. **Perinatal asphyxia.** If the infant is nonvigorous (poor tone and not crying), a brief period of tactile stimulation by rubbing the back and/or tapping the soles of the feet can be used, followed immediately by evaluating respirations and heart rate. **A term infant with a heart rate of <100 beats/min or no spontaneous respiratory activity requires PPV.** PPV should be initiated at 40 to 60 breaths/min, and chest wall movement should be used to confirm effective ventilation of the lungs. If mask ventilation is ineffective at moving the chest, the MR. SOPA steps should be completed. If mask ventilation remains ineffective or prolonged PPV is necessary, endotracheal intubation or placement of an LMA is indicated (see Chapters 33 and 37).

E. **Preterm newborn.** Preterm infants often require immediate lung expansion in the delivery room. Although high PIP may initially be needed to expand the lungs, as soon as the lungs "open up," the pressure should be decreased if the clinical course permits. CPAP administered with a T-piece resuscitator or a flow-inflating bag-and-mask system, providing a pressure of 4 to 6 cm H_2O, may be sufficient to expand the lungs of a preterm infant and improve ventilation. Because many preterm infants can be supported with CPAP alone and do not require intubation or mechanical ventilation, routine use of **prophylactic surfactant for respiratory distress syndrome is not recommended** (see Chapters 9 and 117).

F. **In extremely premature infants** who require intubation at delivery because of severe respiratory distress syndrome, surfactant should be given after initial stabilization. Surfactant administration is not a component of the initial resuscitation and should be delayed until the newborn has a stable heart rate. The surfactant is administered via the ETT and distributed into the lungs using PPV breaths. Prior to giving surfactant, appropriate ETT location should be confirmation by auscultation of equal bilateral breath sounds or chest x-ray. In some cases, the ETT can be removed immediately after surfactant is given using a technique called **INSURE** (**IN**tubate, **SUR**factant, and **E**xtubate). After the extubation, these infants should be placed on CPAP for continued respiratory support. In premature infants initially maintained on CPAP, surfactant can be given if the infant fails CPAP (see Chapters 13 and 117).

G. **Opioid-exposed newborn.** Newborns of mothers who have recently received opioid analgesics or who have used elicit opioids may have respiratory depression and apnea at birth. **The narcotic antagonist naloxone is not recommended to treat apnea in opioid-exposed newborns.** Some studies have linked naloxone use in newborns to seizures, pulmonary edema, and cardiac arrest. The treatment for a newborn with respiratory depression from opioids is respiratory support with PPV and possible LMA placement or endotracheal intubation if the apnea is prolonged.

H. **Air leak or pleural effusion.** A collection of air or fluid in the chest cavity of a newborn can result in severe respiratory distress and persistent bradycardia. Rapid identification of a pneumothorax or pleural effusions is key to effective treatment. In most cases of pneumothorax, there is no time to obtain a chest x-ray to confirm the diagnosis. Therefore, clinical exam findings such as auscultation of decreased breath sounds and transillumination are the primary means of diagnosis. In most cases of pleural effusion, the issue has been identified prior to birth by prenatal ultrasound. In these cases, the delivery team should be prepared to perform needle thoracentesis for emergency air or fluid evacuation. (See Chapter 31 and 75.)

I. **Airway obstruction.** Obstruction of the airway with meconium, vernix, mucus, or other materials can make it impossible to provide effective mask ventilation. Airway obstruction should be suspected in newborns who do not have chest wall movement with PPV after completing the first 5 steps of MR. SOPA. Clearance of the airway can be performed by placing an ETT in the trachea and using a meconium aspirator to suction the airway. This is often more effective than attempting to suction the airway with a bulb syringe or suction catheter (8–10F) since the ETT diameter is larger and more suction pressure can be provided. A negative pressure of 80 to 100 mm Hg is recommended in such cases. (See Chapters 33 and 106.)

J. **Hypovolemic shock.** Hypovolemic shock at birth can result from a variety of peripartum and intrapartum causes including fetal-maternal hemorrhage, bleeding vasa previa, placental laceration, umbilical cord prolapse, tight nuchal cord, and umbilical cord avulsion. Newborns with hypovolemic shock may have a persistent low heart rate that does not improve with resuscitative efforts. Clinical signs of hypovolemic shock include pale skin, delayed capillary refill, and weak pulses. Treatment of hypovolemic shock in the delivery room is placement of an emergency umbilical catheter and volume expansion with 0.9% NaCl (normal saline) or emergency, non–cross-matched, type-O, Rh-negative packed red blood cells in aliquots of 10 mL/kg given over 5 to 10 minutes. (See Chapter 70.)

VI. **Cardiac resuscitation.** During delivery room resuscitation, efforts should be directed first to assisting ventilation because in the vast majority of cases that is all that is needed.

A. **Chest compressions. If the heart rate continues to be <60 beats/min after 30 seconds of effective positive-pressure ventilation that moves the chest, chest compression should be initiated.** During neonatal chest compressions, the thumbs are placed on the lower third of the sternum, between the xiphoid and the line drawn between the nipples (Figure 3–4). The sternum is compressed a third of the anteroposterior diameter of the chest at a regular rate of 90 compressions/min while ventilating the infant at 30 breaths/min, synchronized such that every 3 compressions are followed by 1 breath. Chest compression should be synchronized with ventilations in a 3:1 ratio, regardless of the presence of an advanced airway. The compressor can administer chest compressions from the head of the newborn in order to allow another provider space to place an emergency umbilical catheter. The preferred method for assessing heart rate after chest compressions

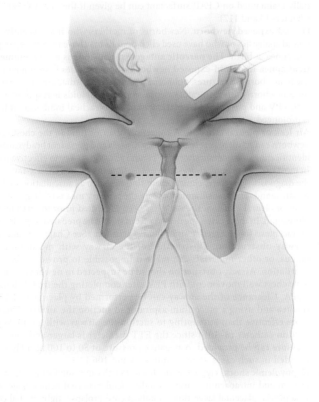

FIGURE 3–4. Technique for chest compressions in the neonate. Note the position of the thumbs on the lower third of the sternum, between the xiphoid and the line drawn between the nipples.

have started is a 3-lead ECG. **The heart rate should be checked every 60 seconds during chest compressions.** Chest compression should be discontinued when the heart rate is >60 beats/min.

B. **Stopping resuscitation. An infant with no heart rate at birth who does not respond to resuscitation efforts may be considered stillborn.** Prolonged resuscitative efforts are a matter for ethical consideration. The AAP and AHA state that **if there is no heart rate after 10 minutes of adequate resuscitation efforts, discontinuation of resuscitation efforts may be reasonable.** However, the decision to continue or discontinue resultative efforts must be individualized.

VII. **Drugs used in resuscitation.** (See also Emergency Medications and Therapy for Neonates, inside the front and back covers, and Chapter 155 for more details.) According to the NRP, 2 medications can be used during neonatal resuscitation: epinephrine and normal saline. Epinephrine is recommended if the heart rate remains <60 beats/min despite adequate ventilation and chest compressions for a minimum of 30 seconds. Volume expansion is recommended if there is a concern for acute hypovolemia or hypovolemic shock.

A. **Route of administration**
   1. **The umbilical vein** is the preferred route for drug administration in the delivery room. A 3.5F or 5F umbilical catheter should be inserted until blood is easily withdrawn (usually 2–4 cm); this shallow placement avoids inadvertent placement in the hepatic or portal vein. Umbilical vein catheterization is discussed in Chapter 48.
   2. **The endotracheal tube** is an alternative route for administration of epinephrine in the delivery room and can be used while vascular access is being obtained. Absorption of medication via the endotracheal route is variable. If the first dose of epinephrine is given through the ETT, a repeat intravenous dose should be given immediately after vascular access is established.
   3. **Alternate routes** of administration include **intraosseous needle** (see Chapter 45) and **peripheral venous catheter** (see Chapter 47).
B. **Medications used in neonatal resuscitation**
   1. **Epinephrine.** Epinephrine may be necessary during resuscitation when adequate ventilation, oxygenation, and chest compression have failed and the heart rate is still <60 beats/min. The primary mechanism of action of epinephrine during cardiac arrest is thought to be via peripheral vasoconstriction resulting in increased afterload to the heart and retrograde filling of the coronary arteries. **The dose of epinephrine is 0.01 to 0.03 mg/kg (0.1–0.3 mL/kg) of 1:10,000 (0.1 mg/mL) solution given intravenously, or 0.05 to 0.1 mg/kg (0.5–1 mL/kg) given by the ETT.** This may be repeated every 3 to 5 minutes.
   2. **Volume expanders.** Hypovolemia should be suspected in an infant requiring resuscitation when there is evidence of acute blood loss with pallor, poor peripheral pulses, long capillary refill times, or poor response to resuscitative efforts. **Appropriate volume expanders include normal saline or uncrossmatched type O–negative packed red blood cells.** Volume expanders are given in 10-mL/kg doses over 5 to 10 minutes.
   3. **Sodium bicarbonate is no longer part of the NRP treatment algorithm.** This is due to a concern that CO_2 is produced when sodium bicarbonate mixes with acid in the blood and that the excess CO_2 may worsen acidosis in infants with impaired ventilation. In addition, rapid administration of sodium bicarbonate has been linked to intraventricular hemorrhage in preterm newborns. **Sodium bicarbonate is still part of the European and UK neonatal resuscitation guidelines** because there is some evidence that using alkali to reverse intracardiac acidosis may sometimes restore the heart rate when all else fails.
VIII. **Newborn resuscitation ethics.** A consistent and coordinated approach by the obstetric and neonatal teams with the prenatal involvement of parents is important in making decisions regarding potentially withholding resuscitation efforts. Neonatal resuscitation is not ethical and should not be offered in cases where there is no chance for survival. Examples of such cases include birth at <22 weeks' gestation and some congenital malformations and chromosomal anomalies. Neonatal resuscitation may be offered in cases where there is a high risk of morbidity and survival is uncertain. In these cases, prenatal counseling regarding resuscitation should include the parents, and the parents' desires should determine the resuscitation plan. Examples of such cases include birth between 22 and 24 weeks' gestation and some chromosomal anomalies and congenital malformations. (See Chapter 23.)
IX. **Neonatal resuscitation after the time of birth.** Neonatal resuscitation guidelines taught in the NRP course (see Figure 3–1) apply to newborns at the time of birth and can also be used during the initial hospital stay in the NICU. Neonates in the NICU, however, have a variety of complex medical conditions that place them at risk for cardiopulmonary arrest from a variety of etiologies not commonly encountered in the delivery room. This has prompted some to question whether Pediatric Advanced Life Support (PALS) guidelines from the AHA should be followed in the NICU in

some cases. One of the key differences between neonatal and pediatric resuscitation guidelines is the chest compression-to-ventilation ratio (neonatal guidelines = 3:1 coordinated compressions to ventilations, versus pediatric guidelines = 15:2 coordinated compressions to ventilations during 2-person resuscitation without an advanced airway, and continuous chest compressions at 100–120 compressions per minute without pausing for ventilations when an advanced airway is present). Because there are no scientific data to resolve this issue, according to the AHA, the resuscitation approach and compression-to-ventilation ratio most commonly used in a provider's practice environment should be used for intubated term or near-term newborns within the first month of life. PALS compression-to-ventilation ratio should be used for intubated newborns who require resuscitation in nonneonatal settings (eg, prehospital, emergency department, and pediatric intensive care unit [PICU]) and those with a cardiac etiology of arrest, regardless of location. Investigations of resuscitation practices in the NICU, PICU, and cardiac intensive care unit (CICU) indicate that the resuscitation guidelines used are primarily determined by patient location rather than age or arrest etiology, with NRP guidelines followed in the NICU and PALS guidelines in the PICU and CICU. Some authors have proposed the creation of advanced neonatal resuscitation guidelines that apply to the special resuscitation needs of newborns in the NICU.

X. **Postresuscitation debriefing.** Postresuscitation debriefing is a facilitated discussion of a clinical event focused on learning and performance improvement. Debriefing enhances communication and teamwork and reduces the frequency of equipment-related problems. Both the AHA and NRP recommend postresuscitation debriefing as standard practice. The structure of the debriefing conversation typically follows the **Gather, Analyze, Summarize** approach, with the discussion focusing on the key behavioral skills of neonatal resuscitation. Using this structure, the facilitator starts the conversation with a team member or the team leader, giving a summary of the clinical event in order to establish a shared mental model of what happened (**gather**). The team then self-examines their performance (**analyze**). During the analysis phase, actual performance is compared to ideal performance using the **plus-delta technique**, which focuses on what went well (plus) and what could be improved (delta). The debriefing ends with a summary of what should be done differently in the future and identification of issues that require further follow-up (**summarize**). Developing a culture that supports postresuscitation debriefing is essential for neonatal care teams to improve neonatal resuscitation performance and clinical outcomes.

XI. **Postresuscitation care.** Infants who require resuscitation at birth should be admitted to the NICU for postresuscitation care. Two important considerations during this period are glucose control and therapeutic hypothermia.

A. **Glucose regulation.** Glucose levels should be maintained within an acceptable range following resuscitation. To prevent hypoglycemia, intravenous glucose administration with dextrose 10% in water or parenteral nutrition should be started as soon as possible after the resuscitation. Glucose levels should be checked frequently following resuscitation to monitor for hypo- and hyperglycemia. For additional information on glucose control, see Chapters 64 and 67.

B. **Therapeutic hypothermia.** Therapeutic hypothermia should be started after resuscitation in newborns >36 weeks' gestation with clinical and laboratory evidence of moderate to severe hypoxic ischemic encephalopathy (HIE). In resource-limited areas, this may require transport of the infant to another center. **When initiating therapeutic hypothermia for HIE, it is critical to wait to start cooling until after the resuscitation is complete.** Starting hypothermia during the resuscitation is counterproductive. Hypothermia induces bradycardia and will make it more difficult to achieve a normal heart rate and return of spontaneous circulation. For additional information on therapeutic hypothermia, see Chapter 43.

4 Neonatal Transport

Many infants are born in a location where definitive care is not available for their condition. These infants subsequently require transportation to a higher level of care. The conditions requiring transport range from prematurity or hyperbilirubinemia to surgical emergencies, need for extracorporeal membrane oxygenation, or therapeutic hypothermia for hypoxic ischemic encephalopathy. The transport of neonates requires specialized providers and equipment in defined neonatal teams (NNTs). There are many different configurations for transport teams. Of 956 neonatal intensive care units (NICUs) identified by Karlsen et al, 398 offered neonatal transport services. Of 335 respondents in this study, 68% were unit-based teams, and the remainder were dedicated teams, either stand alone or hospital affiliated.

I. **Resource mobilization.** Regardless of team type or configuration, efforts should be made to streamline the dispatch process and improve ease of use for referring facilities and physicians. A single contact number for referring facilities or physicians to arrange for transport of ill neonates as well as to obtain consultation when necessary allows open communication as well as rapid mobilization of the NNT.

Timing of NNT mobilization is an important factor to consider. Research has demonstrated that effective resuscitation and stabilization of critically ill neonates is most successful when performed by specially trained retrieval teams. Rapid mobilization of the NNT for high-risk deliveries may not only impact neonatal morbidity and mortality, but also allow for continuous quality improvement and education of local hospital staff through active involvement in the resuscitation and stabilization. Regardless of team type, many variables have to be considered.

A. **Team composition.**
1. **Teams usually have 2 to 4 providers.**
2. **State neonatal transport team requirements can vary.** As an example, the state of Maryland requires 2 licensed providers (physicians, nurse practitioners, nurses, respiratory therapists, paramedics) and 1 emergency medical technician to operate the vehicle.
3. **Neonatal teams are most often an interdisciplinary collaborative practice comprised of a registered nurse working with another nurse, respiratory care provider, or paramedic.** Some teams incorporate physicians (eg, pediatric residents, neonatal fellows, or neonatologists) or advanced practice nurses (eg, neonatal nurse practitioners [NNPs]) routinely or based on the perceived acuity of the infant being transported. Studies have found no difference in mortality or long-term outcomes between physician-nurse and nurse-only teams and have shown that nonphysician personnel can be trained to provide equally safe care and similar outcomes.

B. **Supervision and standard of care.** Medical oversight of emergency medical services (EMS) and interfacility transport is contingent upon federal, state, and local regulations. A transport services typically must have a medical director who is responsible for the overall care provided by the team. Because neonatal transport is a specialized form of interfacility transport, typically service medical directors work closely with a neonatologist to ensure quality care. Specialty care physicians may provide indirect (offline) medical consultation in the form of protocol development and quality case reviews as well as direct (online) consultation in the form of telephone or radio orders.

NNTs should have standing orders in the form of protocols or guidelines to facilitate the provision of care until online medical control can be established. Protocols for the management of emergencies (eg, airway compromise or respiratory failure, shock) should be established. Following emergent stabilization, NNTs traditionally established online medical control to discuss the birth history, hospital course, recent results, assessment findings, and their plan of care. Medical command physicians may ask and answer questions and help establish an ongoing plan of care. The receiving hospital team is often provided an updated estimated time of arrival and apprised of any changes in the neonate's needs (eg, drips/ventilator requirements).

  C. **Team member training.**

    1. **Transport team members have various required certifications.** The most commonly required certifications are Basic Life Support (BLS) and Neonatal Resuscitation (NRP), followed by the S.T.A.B.L.E. program. Providers of transport services usually require some, but not always all, of the following:

      a. **Basic Life Support**

      b. **Neonatal Resuscitation**

      c. **The S.T.A.B.L.E. program.**

        i. **S.T.A.B.L.E. is a widely implemented education program** that focuses exclusively on the postresuscitation/pretransport stabilization care of sick infants.

        ii. **Based on a mnemonic to optimize learning, retention, and recall of information,** S.T.A.B.L.E. stands for **S**ugar, **T**emperature, **A**irway, **B**lood pressure, **L**ab work, and **E**motional support. A seventh module, Quality Improvement, stresses the responsibility of improving and evaluating care provided to sick infants (https://stableprogram.org/).

      d. **Pediatric Advanced life Support (PALS)**

      e. **Advanced Cardiac Life Support (ACLS)**

    2. **Scope of practice.**

      a. **After receiving specialized training and release, transport team members often provide care outside the traditional in-patient scope of practice.** NNT team member scope of practice is defined by the medical director within the constraints of federal, state, and local regulations.

      b. **Transport team members must be able to provide safe and effective care in the field.** A method for establishing initial and ongoing clinical and procedural competency is essential. Training typically includes clinical experiences in the NICU as well as skills labs and clinical simulation sessions.

    3. **Quality improvement.** All transports have to have individuals responsible for quality improvement. Some institutions and teams adhere to publicly available metrics; others develop their own.

  D. **Mode of transportation.**

    1. **This may include ground (ambulance) transportation,** helicopters, or fixed-wing aircraft.

    2. **Mode of transportation may be decided by distance, severity of illness,** regional differences, and availability.

      a. **Dedicated teams are more likely to use all 3 modes.**

      b. **Ground transport is more likely to be used for transports <100 miles;** helicopters are more likely used for 1-way transports of 100 to 200 miles.

II. **Care of the infant and family.** It is optimal for the transport team to have a pretransport briefing prior to departure or while in transit to the referring hospital to establish a plan of care based on known information and ensure that the correct equipment is brought for the transport if it does not regularly reside in the ambulance. It is important for those involved to remember that situations may change and the infant may present differently once on scene.

    The transport teams must be self-sufficient, with all medications and equipment required for the initiation of definitive care for the infant's condition. Although neonatal transport does not follow the traditional "swoop and scoop" transport methodology of adult EMS services and initial stabilization of the neonate is expected, care should be taken not to excessively prolong scene time because this increases the time interval to definitive care for the neonate.

It is important for the transport team to communicate with the family regarding the transport, the hospital they are going to transport the neonate to, and the neonate's current condition. It is very important to provide emotional support for parents and families during this stressful time. It is also important for the transport team to allow parents to see and touch their infant prior to departure and allow pictures as conditions allow. On arrival after transport, the transport team should notify parents of their arrival. Transport team members should refrain from stating definitive outcomes, plans of care, consults, or procedures that will occur once at the tertiary care center because this may result in unrealistic expectations in families.

III. **Treatment and transport consent.** Consent for transport is typically obtained by the referring hospital when the referring physician informs the family of the need to transfer their infant. NNTs should ideally obtain written consent for treatment during the actual transport as well as permission to disclose obtained health information. Transport should not be delayed to obtain firsthand consent if the infant requires emergent care.

IV. **Care of the neonate.**

A. **On arrival,** the team should make the decision as to whether the patient requires any emergency treatment (eg, ongoing cardiopulmonary resuscitation) and tend to these needs.

B. **If no emergency treatment is needed,** the team should obtain a thorough history from the personnel (usually the physician or NNP) at the referring facility.

C. **Proceed to examination of the neonate;** obtain vital signs (temperature, respiratory rate, heart rate, blood pressure, oxygen saturation [SpO_2]), weight, and gestational age, and determine the plan of care.

D. **Check any pertinent laboratory tests** (blood glucose, hematocrit, arterial blood gas levels, any other tests).

E. **Check ventilation and oxygenation** after accessing pulse oximetry and arterial blood gases.

F. **Make sure the infant has a line** (intravenous, umbilical venous, or arterial) for fluids or possible emergency medications.

G. **Once the infant is stable and almost ready to go,** discuss the infant's condition with the parents, answer any questions, obtain signed permits, and reassure parents.

H. **Obtain copies of the mother's and infant's charts,** any radiographs, and any other copies of studies.

I. **It is helpful to have protocols in place to aid in decision making and care provision** that are consistent with that of the tertiary care center to which the neonate will be transported. The transport team should contact their medical command physician to give a report and for any help in decision making or planning care that may be needed, as well as notify the receiving hospital of estimated arrival time and any drip or ventilator requirements or other needs that may be needed on arrival.

J. **Once the infant is in the transport incubator,** efforts should be made to limit opening the incubator on transport due to potential for temperature loss.

V. **Management of some common neonatal transport diagnoses**

A. **Choanal atresia**

1. **Being obligate nasal breathers, newborns with choanal atresia will require some intervention.**

2. **Begin with placing an oral airway.** Consider endotracheal intubation if the oral airway is not sufficient to maintain saturations and respiratory status when calm.

B. **Pierre-Robin sequence**

1. **Infants present with varying degrees of retro-/micrognathia.**

2. **Prone positioning is the first therapy.** Oral airway may be needed.

3. **If intubation is required because previously mentioned therapies have failed,** this would be considered a difficult airway and would be a good use of a laryngeal mask airway.

C. **Esophageal atresia/intestinal obstruction**
1. **Place sump catheter** to suction in proximal esophageal pouch if esophageal atresia or in stomach if more distal obstruction.
2. **Do not place regular feeding tube** to suction due to the risk of this tubing getting attached to gastric or esophageal mucosa and forming an ulcer, erosion, or perforation.
D. **Persistent pulmonary hypertension (PPHN)**
1. PPHN is associated with hypoxemic ischemic encephalopathy, meconium aspiration syndrome, sepsis, congenital diaphragmatic hernia, premature ductal closure, pulmonary hypoplasia, and acidosis.
2. **Obtain pre- and postductal oxygen saturations.** A >10% split with lower postductal saturations is consistent with PPHN.
3. **Optimize ventilation and oxygenation.**
4. **Follow medical command** for individual NICU protocols and oxygenation/blood gas and blood pressure goals.
5. **Be prepared to start inhaled nitric oxide (iNO).**
E. **Congenital diaphragmatic hernia**
1. **Mask ventilation of these infants should be avoided** because this will distend the bowels within the chest cavity.
2. **Infants should be intubated,** ideally prior to arrival of the transport team.
3. **Attempt to place a catheter** to suction in stomach and to decompress bowels.
4. **These infants are at high risk for persistent pulmonary hypertension and pneumothorax.** Be prepared to initiate iNO or needle decompression/chest tube placement.
F. **Open lesions such as gastroschisis or myelomeningocele.** These should be kept moist and wrapped per protocol of the receiving institution to minimize insensible fluid losses, but contamination from fecal matter should be avoided.
VI. **Initiation of definitive therapies on transport.** Some conditions for which a neonate is being transported to a higher level of care are amenable to treatment prior to and during transport, in this way accelerating the provision of definitive care.
A. **Pneumothorax**
1. **The providers at the referring facility will probably have already needle decompressed a tension pneumothorax.** If there is reaccumulation, the team must be prepared to insert a chest tube.
2. **A nontension pneumothorax in an otherwise stable neonate may be followed clinically if the patient is being transported by ground.** However, if the neonate is being flown, flight physiology must be taken into account.
3. **A chest tube may be required in a patient with a clinically insignificant pneumothorax** because the volume of the pneumothorax increases by an estimated 12% to 16% for every 500-ft change in altitude. Many programs use a 20% to 30% pneumothorax volume as a cutoff for requiring decompression prior to flight, and medical command should be consulted in these cases.
B. **Sepsis**
1. **Antibiotics should be part of the medication pack of any neonatal transport team.**
2. **After cultures are drawn, antibiotics should be started** in any cases of suspected infection. Time to administration of antibiotics is significantly shorter in this case than when antibiotics are administered on return, thereby improving outcomes.
C. **Respiratory distress syndrome**
1. **Premature infants with respiratory distress syndrome benefit from earlier** surfactant administration.
2. **Neonatal transport teams should carry surfactant** and be prepared to administer it per recommended dose.

3. **If the infant is already intubated, correct placement of an endotracheal tube should be verified** to avoid 1-sided delivery of surfactant, and if the transport team intubates the infant, a chest x-ray should be obtained prior to surfactant administration.
4. **Ventilator pressures and settings may need to be weaned quickly** after surfactant administration to accommodate improved compliance.

D. **Prostaglandin E$_1$ (PGE$_1$) administration for ductal-dependent congenital heart disease**
  1. **The team must be able to initiate or continue PGE$_1$ on transport.**
  2. **If the team initiates PGE$_1$, one of the side effects is apnea.** This is most likely to occur in premature infants, when PGEs are started at a large dose, and within the first 30 minutes of initiation.
  3. It is *no longer* recommended to intubate an infant on PGE$_1$ only for transport or for PGE$_1$-associated apnea. Current recommendations are to give a bolus dose of caffeine 20 mg/kg intravenously (IV) if apnea is a concern or if the infant is to be transported immediately after initiation of PGE$_1$.
  4. **A second access point must be in place before departure if PGE$_1$ is being administered via peripheral IV.**

E. **Hyperbilirubinemia**
  1. **A biliblanket should be available to the transport team** if it is not owned by the team and kept on the ambulance, and it should be brought on all transports for hyperbilirubinemia.
  2. **Research has shown that phototherapy started on transport,** even for a relatively short duration, decreases need for exchange transfusion.
  3. **Maintenance IV fluids should be used in conjunction with phototherapy.**

F. **Therapeutic hypothermia**
  1. **Once it is determined that a neonate qualifies for therapeutic hypothermia,** referring physicians can be encouraged to start passive cooling, but caution must be used and temperatures closely monitored because there is a risk of overcooling even with passive cooling (ie, turning off temperature support, not surrounding infants with ice packs).
  2. **Once the transport team has arrived, active cooling can begin, or the team can continue passive cooling.** This decision should be institution or team based.
  3. **Benefits of active cooling are many,** whether with servo-controlled cooling equipment or manipulation of transport incubator temperatures with continuous temperature measurements. Neonates with active cooling on transport were more likely to reach the destination at the correct temperature for therapeutic hypothermia, and the temperature range at which they arrived was narrower. As therapeutic hypothermia within 6 hours is the goal, starting cooling on transport increases the likelihood that the correct temperature is reached within the time interval, especially in more rural areas where both distances and time to definitive care are greater than in more urban settings.

G. **Hypoglycemia.** If >12.5% dextrose is anticipated, the patient should have central access, or the team should be prepared to insert an umbilical vein catheter due to the risk of electrolyte disturbances if an increased infusion rate is used instead of a higher dextrose concentration.

VII. **Special neonatal transport considerations**
A. **Care must be taken to secure the neonate in the transport incubator,** using commercial securing devices so that the infant is not injured during the transport.
B. **The greatest cerebral pressure changes can be seen with acceleration and deceleration.** Care must be taken with all infants, but especially with all preterm infants and infants with extremely low birthweight. Exertional forces are greatest in takeoff and landing during rotor transport, but otherwise remain stable and low, whereas exertional forces occur with all decelerations and accelerations in ground transport, which may impact choice of mode.

C. **Temperature must be carefully maintained, and excessive insensitive losses should be avoided.** It is helpful to wrap neonates <1000 g in clear plastic film, exposing only those areas (mouth/nose/IV access) required for care. Incubator temperature should be set appropriately for the weight of the baby, and hyperthermia should be avoided at all costs.

D. **Rotor wing transport is generally considered faster.** However, it can potentially limit the provision of emergency care or procedures during flight due to space and safety concerns.

E. **Mixed modal transport can be considered if the greatest imperative is providing needed equipment and skills to a bedside.** In these cases, transport the team via rotor wing to speed stabilization of the neonate. Then the team and patient may be able to safely return by ground, allowing greater flexibility for care and procedures in route.

F. **Chemical warming mattresses are designed to be started at normal room temperature.** If the mattresses are being kept in a cold environment, they will not achieve optimal temperature and will actually lead to heat loss in the infant, whereas thermal burns can occur if they are stored in a warmer or hot environment and subsequently overheat when started.

G. **When using helicopter or fixed-wing transport, it is important to provide ear protection** because noise levels can exceed 85 dB.

H. **Special consideration must be given to decompressing and venting the stomach,** with placement of nasogastric or orogastric tube prior to departure.

I. **The transport mode should be discussed** in neonates with conditions with contained air, including but not limited to pneumothorax, pneumoperitoneum, anal atresia without fistula, and tracheoesophageal fistula with anal atresia, due to pressure changes in flight because aircraft (rotor and fixed) are not pressurized to sea level, and trapped air could expand and compromise the neonate. Also consider the hypoxemic patient or those with significant oxygen needs because FiO_2 may need to be increased to compensate for altitude.

VIII. **Hand-off of care**

A. **If there is no emergency to move the patient on arrival to the NICU,** a complete set of vital signs including temperature should be performed prior to moving the patient, and a thorough hand-off of care should be given to the receiving team.

B. **The team should be using the same hand-off procedures, medication concentrations, and equipment** as their base NICU to minimize errors.

C. **The team should call the parents** to notify them of the safe arrival of their neonate.

5 The Golden Hour

First described in the field of emergency medicine, the "golden hour" refers to the first 60 minutes following an injury. It was discovered that the sooner trauma patients received definitive care, the better their outcomes. In neonatology, the term "golden hour" refers to the initial 60 minutes of an infant's life following delivery when a critical transition period of adaptation takes place. Particularly for high-risk neonates, optimizing thermoregulation, glycemic control, cardiorespiratory support, and nutrition during this time is critical to achieving successful long-term outcomes. The golden hour provides opportunity for an evidence-based standardized approach to achieve these goals. Evidence shows that implementation of a golden hour protocol decreases mortality as well was the incidence of hypothermia, chronic lung disease, intraventricular hemorrhage, and retinopathy of prematurity.

I. Golden hour for the term infant
   A. The golden hour protocol for a term newborn is composed of delayed cord clamping, maintaining thermoregulation, and the initiation of early breast feeding.
   B. Counseling/team briefing
      1. If there is risk a term newborn will require interventions immediately after birth, the parents should be counseled and the management plan explained prior to delivery.
      2. As with all neonatal resuscitations, clear roles and responsibilities should be established among the team members and all resuscitation equipment prepared.
      3. For an anticipated admission to the neonatal intensive care unit (NICU), staff should be notified.
   C. Delayed cord clamping (DCC)
      1. Per American College of Obstetricians and Gynecologists (ACOG) and Neonatal Resuscitation Program (NRP), clamping of the umbilical cord should be done after at least 30 to 60 seconds. World Health Organization (WHO) guidelines are 1 to 3 minutes after birth.
      2. Delayed clamping for 1 minute leads to a transfer of approximately 80 mL of extra blood to the term neonate.
      3. NRP recommends using DCC for all term infants who do not require resuscitation after birth.
      4. Benefits include higher hemoglobin at 2 to 12 months of age and an increase in total body iron during the first year of life.
      5. DCC may increase the risk for jaundice and need for phototherapy.
      6. Umbilical cord milking is an alternative to DCC but currently not recommended by the NRP.
   D. Preventing hypothermia
      1. Normal temperature in a newborn is between 36.5°C and 37.5°C.
      2. Neonatal hypothermia has been shown to increase neonatal mortality.
      3. The highest risk of neonatal hypothermia is immediately after birth due to the difference in in utero and environmental temperature.
      4. Interventions to prevent hypothermia include raising the temperature of the delivery room, using a radiant warmer, and early initiation of skin-to-skin contact.
         a. The newborn should be received in warm blankets and skin-to-skin contact should be started immediately if no resuscitation is required.
         b. The delivery room temperature should be kept between 23°C and 26°C (74°F and 77°F).

E. Respiratory support
   1. Oxygen support and pulse oximeter
      a. When resuscitation is needed, a pulse oximeter should be placed on the right upper hand or wrist.
      b. Resuscitation of a term newborn should start in room air (21% oxygen) and be titrated to achieve the targeted saturation range per NRP.
      c. If positive pressure is needed, use a T-piece resuscitator to provide consistent peak inspiratory pressure (PIP) and positive end-expiratory pressure (PEEP).
      d. Confirm endotracheal tube placement by a carbon dioxide (CO_2) detector.
F. Initiation of breast feeding
   1. Well term newborns should initiate breast feeding as soon as possible.
   2. The Baby Friendly Hospital Initiative recommends immediate skin-to-skin contact and breast-feeding initiation within the first half hour after birth.
   3. Skin-to-skin contact is associated with increased breast-feeding rates and duration.
G. Preventing hypoglycemia
   1. Newborns at greatest risk for hypoglycemia after birth include large for gestational age infants, infants of diabetic mothers, small for gestational age infants, and infants with intrauterine growth restriction.
   2. These infants should be monitored for hypoglycemia with regular blood sugar measurement for the first 12 to 24 hours.
H. Therapeutic hypothermia for asphyxia (see Chapter 43)
   1. This is a standard of care for asphyxiated term and near-term newborns with moderate to severe neonatal encephalopathy.
   2. Should be started within 6 hours of birth and continued for 72 hours followed by gradual rewarming.
   3. Therapeutic hypothermia reduces mortality and improves neurodevelopmental outcomes.
   4. Turn off radiant warmer and monitor temperature closely for neonates who potentially need therapeutic hypothermia.

II. Golden hour for the preterm infant
   A. Counseling/team briefing
      1. Plan of management and expected complications should be explained to the parents prior to the birth of a preterm neonate.
      2. The chance that a preterm infant will require resuscitation is significantly higher than that of a full-term infant. An experienced and skilled resuscitation team should be present for the delivery of very low birth weight (VLBW) and extremely low birth weight (ELBW) infants. Roles should be assigned to the members of the resuscitation team by the team leader. Equipment should be prepared. The use of preresuscitation check lists that include all the necessary equipment simplifies and streamlines preparation.
   B. Delayed cord clamping (DCC)
      1. ACOG and NRP recommend clamping of the umbilical cord after at least 30 to 60 seconds. WHO guidelines are 1 to 3 minutes after birth.
      2. NRP recommends using DCC for all preterm infants who do not require resuscitation after birth.
      3. DCC is associated with less need for vasopressors, lower blood transfusions for anemia, less intraventricular hemorrhage (IVH), and lower risk of necrotizing enterocolitis and sepsis.
      4. Umbilical cord milking may be an alternative to DCC, but the current NRP guidelines do not support its use.
   C. Preventing hypothermia
      1. Hypothermia in the neonate refers to temperature <36.5°C.
      2. VLBW infants are prone to hypothermia given their large body surface area, poorly developed skin barrier, and thin layer of subcutaneous fat compared to that of term infants.

3. Admission temperature is a strong predictor of neonatal mortality.
   a. Hypothermia leads to increase in mortality, IVH, late-onset sepsis, hypoglycemia, and respiratory distress.
   b. Every 1°C below 36°C on admission temperature is associated with a 28% increase in mortality risk.
4. The delivery room temperature should be kept between 23°C and 25°C (74°F and 77°F).
5. Preheat the radiant warmer well before the baby is born.
6. Polyethylene wrap
   a. Immediately after birth, the neonate should be covered without drying.
   b. Keep the baby fully covered during resuscitation and stabilization.
   c. If umbilical venous catheter is required, cut a small hole in the plastic and pull the umbilical cord. Do not uncover the baby to place umbilical lines.
   d. The wrap should be removed once the infant is stabilized in the nursery.
7. Thermal mattress
   a. A thermal mattress releases heat when a chemical gel inside the mattress is activated to form crystals.
   b. Squeeze the pad to activate the gel at least 5 minutes before the baby is born.
   c. Cover the thermal mattress with a blanket to prevent burns.
   d. It is equally as effective as polyethylene wrap or vinyl bag.
   e. It maintains body temperature during transport of a VLBW neonate.
8. The combined use of a polythene wrap and thermal mattress is more effective in extreme premature infants (<32 weeks' gestation). The temperature should be monitored more closely if the combination is used because this may increase risk for hyperthermia.
9. Covering heads with hats is effective in reducing heat losses.
10. A servo-controlled radiant warmer and a temperature sensor probe should be present in the delivery room.
11. Heated humidified gases with a blender for respiratory support.
12. Use an incubator for transport and upon arrival to the nursery.
    a. Incubator should be rewarmed and double-walled, with humidity.
    b. Incubator minimizes heat loss by conduction, convection, evaporation, and radiation.

D. Respiratory support
   1. Immediate goals are to achieve early functional residual capacity, achieve appropriate minute ventilation, and avoid invasive ventilation when possible. If the baby is breathing spontaneously and the heart rate is >100 beats/min, positive-pressure ventilation is not required. If the baby has respiratory distress or oxygen saturation remains below the target range, continuous positive airway pressure (CPAP) may be helpful.
   2. Sustained inflation
      a. Positive-pressure inflation (15–25 cm H_2O) from 5 to 15 seconds.
      b. Establishes functional residual capacity (FRC), achieves better lung recruitment, helps move fluid from the alveoli to the interstitium, and improves lung expansion.
      c. Sustained inflation has been shown to reduce the need for mechanical ventilation in the first 3 days of postnatal life in preterm infants. However, the use of sustained inflation in the delivery room is controversial and not a part of NRP.
   3. Targeted oxygen saturation
      a. NRP recommends pulse oximetry be used when resuscitation is anticipated, during positive-pressure ventilation (PPV), when supplementary oxygen is administered, or when central cyanosis persists beyond the first 5 to 10 minutes of life.

    b. **Resuscitation of preterm newborns (<35 weeks' gestation) should be initiated with 21% to 30% oxygen,** and this should be titrated to achieve the minute-by-minute saturation goals.
       i. **1 minute, 60% to 65%**
      ii. **2 minutes, 65% to 70%**
     iii. **3 minutes, 70% to 75%**
     iv. **4 minutes, 75% to 80%**
      v. **5 minutes, 80% to 85%**
     vi. **10 minutes, 85% to 95%**
    c. **Preductal oxygen levels should be targeted,** so the pulse oximeter should be placed on the right hand or wrist.
    d. **Oxygen saturation should also be monitored** and maintained within the target range using blended oxygen while transporting neonates to the NICU.

4. **CPAP**
    a. **Since the initial respiratory care given to VLBW and ELBW infants contributes to their long-term respiratory outcomes, maximizing noninvasive ventilation is critical.**
    b. **Seventy percent of VLBW and ELBW infants** can be managed by CPAP in the delivery room.
    c. **The goal of initial respiratory support** is to establish FRC quickly and efficiently with minimal lung trauma.
    d. **CPAP may be given in the delivery room** by flow-inflating bags and T-piece resuscitators.
       i. **Early initiation of CPAP in the delivery room** may reduce the need for intubation and surfactant administration and the total number of ventilator days.
      ii. **Use of CPAP compared to invasive ventilation in the delivery room** reduces bronchopulmonary dysplasia and death at 36 weeks' postmenstrual age.

5. **Invasive ventilation**
    a. **Preterm infants may require invasive ventilation** due to poor respiratory drive or severe respiratory distress.
    b. **If PPV is required,** use the lowest PIP to achieve and maintain the heart rate >100 beats/min. An initial PIP of 20 to 25 cm H_2O is adequate for most preterm infants. While using face-mask ventilation, limit PIP to 30 cm H_2O.
    c. **Intubation should be performed** by a person who is experienced in performing intubations of VLBW and ELBW infants.
    d. **No more than 2 attempts per intubator should be attempted.**
    e. **Intubation should be completed by 30 seconds.**
    f. **Endotracheal tube placement should be confirmed by a CO_2 detector.**
    g. **Caution should be used to avoid giving high tidal volumes,** since this may lead to decreased action of exogenous surfactant and overall greater lung injury with thickened alveolar septa.
    h. **T-piece resuscitator should be used** to provide consistent PIP, PEEP, and tidal volume.

6. **Surfactant**
    a. **Surfactant deficiency in preterm newborns results in increased surface tension and atelectasis,** which ultimately results in lung injury.
    b. **Incidence of respiratory distress syndrome (RDS)**
       i. **<5% after 34 weeks' gestation**
      ii. **30% between 28 and 34 weeks' gestation**
     iii. **60% prior to 28 weeks' gestation**
    c. **Although there is no benefit to prophylactic surfactant administration,** surfactant given within 2 hours of life may be beneficial, since surfactant works synergistically with CPAP to establish and maintain FRC.

        d. **Surfactant administration is not a component of initial resuscitation** and should be delayed until there is a stable heart rate.

        e. **INSURE (INtubation, SURfactant, Extubation) technique**

           i. **For preterm neonates on CPAP, this technique involves early surfactant administration** followed by extubation.

           ii. **This technique allows for avoidance of continuous mechanical ventilation.**

           iii. **Preterm infants who develop RDS should be given surfactant within the golden hour via the INSURE technique** and then continued on CPAP support.

E. Cardiovascular support

   1. **Immediately assess the heart rate.**

   2. **An electrocardiogram monitor with 3 chest leads or limb leads** provides a rapid and reliable method of monitoring heart rate.

   3. **Maintain normal perfusion and blood pressure.**

   4. **Per NRP guidelines, chest compressions should be avoided** until adequate ventilation is achieved.

   5. **Causes of hypotension in the delivery room**

      a. **Asphyxia**

      b. **Sepsis**

      c. **Air leak syndrome**

      d. **Maternal anesthesia**

      e. **Fetal arrhythmias**

      f. **Fetal blood loss (hemorrhage, twin-twin transfusion syndrome)**

   6. **During the golden hour, the goal is to detect shock early in order to begin early management** including intravenous access and use of fluid resuscitation and vasopressors if needed.

F. Prevention of neurologic injury

   1. **Preterm infants (<32 weeks' gestation) are prone to IVH due to a fragile network of blood vessels in their brain.** Obstruction of venous drainage from the head or rapid changes in blood pressure, blood volume, or $PaCO_2$ may increase the risk of IVH in extremely premature infants. Consider the following precautions while managing extremely premature infants during the golden hour:

      a. **Gently handle the baby.**

      b. **Do not position the baby's head lower than the legs.**

      c. **Our institutional practice is to keep the head of the baby in midline position** to prevent obstruction of venous drainage from the brain.

      d. **Avoid high PIP and PEEP during PPV or CPAP.** Excessive PIP or PEEP can increase intrathoracic pressure and decrease venous return from the head.

      e. **Avoid rapid changes in $PaCO_2$.** Rapid fluctuation in CO_2 levels can alter cerebral blood flow and increase risk of IVH.

      f. **Avoid rapid infusion of intravenous fluids.** If volume expansion is required, infuse over 5 to 10 minutes.

G. Early initiation of nutrition

   1. **Total parenteral nutrition (TPN) and enteral nutrition**

      a. **Early nutritional support leads to better growth and neurodevelopmental outcomes,** and providing this nutrition should be a priority in the golden hour.

      b. **Initiation of TPN during the golden hour** helps to support nitrogen balance, growth, and overall health.

      c. **Early administration of parenteral amino acids** prevents protein catabolism and metabolic shock and buffers against hyperglycemia by initiating endogenous insulin secretion.

          d. **Stable preterm infants may be started on enteral feeds,** preferably with maternal breast milk.
2. **Preventing hypoglycemia**
    a. **Preterm infants <1000 g** have a primary failure to produce or store glycogen.
    b. **The goal during golden hour management is to measure the serum glucose within 1 hour** and start an infusion of dextrose immediately once access by peripheral intravenous line or central umbilical line is secured.

H. **Infection prevention**
  1. **Preterm infants are at risk for neonatal sepsis.**
  2. **If a neonate will be treated for suspected sepsis, a blood culture should be obtained and the first dose of antibiotics should be administered within the golden hour.**

I. **Laboratory tests**
  1. **The necessary tests** (blood culture, glucose, blood gas, and chest x-ray) should be done during the golden hour to minimize handling later on.

J. **Monitoring/timing**
  1. **The timing of the above interventions should be recorded** including documentation of resuscitation, birth weight, and temperature upon admission to the nursery; timing of surfactant administration; timing of umbilical catheter placement; and timing of antibiotic administration.

K. **Communication with parents**
  1. **The parents should be informed about the condition of the neonate,** chances of survival, expected morbidities, duration of stay, and further management plan.

6 Gestational Age and Birthweight Classification

Gestation is the period of fetal development from the time of conception to birth. **Gestational age** (or menstrual age), as defined by the American Academy of Pediatrics (AAP), is the "time elapsed between the first day of the last menstrual period (LMP) and the day of delivery." It is expressed in completed weeks (26-week and 4-day-old fetus is expressed as a 26-week fetus). Gestational age is important information for the obstetrician to provide obstetric care. It is critical information for the neonatologist for evaluation of the infant and to anticipate high-risk infants and complications. Gestational age and birthweight classification help the neonatologist to categorize infants, guide treatment, and assess risks for morbidity and mortality. Neonates can be classified based on **gestational age** (eg. preterm, late preterm, early term, full or late term, post term), **birthweight** (eg, extremely low birthweight, very low birthweight, low birthweight), and **gestational age and birthweight combined** (small for gestational age [SGA], appropriate for gestational age [AGA], large for gestational age [LGA]). **The AAP recommends that all newborns be classified by birthweight and gestational age.**

    I. **Gestational age assessment.** Gestational age can be determined prenatally in the fetus and postnatally in the newborn. Gestational age is determined by the "best obstetric estimate," which is based on 4 parameters: first day of LMP, physical examination of the mother, prenatal ultrasound, and history of assisted reproduction. The American College of Obstetricians and Gynecologists, the American Institute of Ultrasound in Medicine, and the Society for Maternal-Fetal Medicine indicate that **antenatal first-trimester**

ultrasonography is the most accurate method to establish gestational age in a pregnancy not achieved through assisted reproductive technologies. The methods they recommend in the first trimester (ultrasound, LMP data) represent the best obstetric estimate for clinical care, and this date should be recorded on the birth certificate. Some feel that the most accurate estimation of gestational age is based on the prenatal estimation (using ultrasound and LMP) in combination with the postnatal assessment using physical and neurologic maturity. Gestational age can also be determined postanally using various examinations including assessment of physical and neuromuscular maturity. It is done if the best obstetric estimate is inaccurate. Postnatal gestational assessment is important, especially in cases where there is no prenatal care, LMP is unknown, and no ultrasounds were done.

A. **Prenatal gestational age assessment.** Determined by a combination of date of the LMP and prenatal ultrasound examination. Based on these, the obstetrician is able to give his or her "best estimate" of gestational age, since variability up to 2 weeks can occur. Use of quickening and physical examination of the mother are not very accurate and are not used if ultrasound is available.

1. **Maternal history**
    a. **First day of the last menstrual period (LMP).** This clinical estimate is very reliable if dates are remembered but depends on an accurate menstrual history and normal maternal physiology. The first day of the LMP is about 2 weeks before ovulation and about 3 weeks before blastocyst implantation. This method can be inaccurate if the incorrect date is reported, with recent use of contraceptives that may affect ovulation, after conception spotting misinterpreted as a period, with variability in ovulation timing, and if the menstrual cycle length is not regular. Studies indicate that using the LMP usually overestimates the gestational age at term. If the **menstrual dates are uncertain**, gestational age is based on the first-trimester ultrasound. If the **menstrual dates are known**, then the LMP can be used for the gestational age and the ultrasound can be done at 18 to 20 weeks to confirm the date when performing an anatomic survey.
    b. **Assisted reproductive technology (ART).** If pregnancy resulted from ART, the ART-derived gestational age should be used to assign the estimated due date. In vitro fertilization pregnancies have a known date of conception, and the gestational age can accurately be predicted within 1 day. If pregnancy was achieved using ART, the gestational age is calculated by adding 2 weeks to the chronologic age (time elapsed from birth). Intrauterine insemination may have a few days' delay.
    c. **Perception of fetal movement by the mother (termed *quickening*).** Date of first reported fetal activity by the mother (18–20 weeks for a primigravida, 16–18 weeks for a multigravida).
    d. **As soon as data from the LMP, the first accurate ultrasound, or both are obtained,** the gestational age and estimated due date should be determined.

2. **Clinical examination**
    a. **Pelvic examination.** Uterine size by bimanual examination in the first trimester can be accurate within 2 weeks. At 6 to 8 weeks, the uterus is the size of a plum; at 8 to 10 weeks, the size of an orange; and at 10 to 12 weeks, the size of a grapefruit.
    b. **Symphysis–fundal height (SFH), fundal height, or McDonald's rule.** This is a measure of the size of the uterus, which corresponds to the gestational age in weeks between 12 and 36 weeks for a vertex fetus. Palpate the superior edge of the pubis symphysis to the palpable top of the uterus to obtain the fundal height. This measurement can be incorrect if there are uterine fibroids, a full bladder, multiple pregnancy, oligo-/polyhydramnios, SGA/LGA infant, or breech position. In resource-poor countries, gestational age can be estimated from serial measurements of pubis symphysis pubis fundal height. It

is only accurate within 4 weeks. Cochrane review states there is insufficient evidence to evaluate the use of SFH measurements during antenatal care and to determine whether SFH measurement is effective in detecting problems with fetal growth (intrauterine growth restriction [IUGR]). **McDonald's rule** (fundal height) relies on the height of the fundus to calculate the duration of pregnancy in weeks or months. To calculate in months: fundal height measurement (in cm) × 2 /7 = duration of pregnancy in months. To calculate in weeks: fundal height measurement (in cm) × 8/7 = duration of pregnancy in weeks.

   i. **12 weeks:** uterine fundus at the pubic symphysis
   ii. **16 weeks:** uterine fundus between the umbilicus and pubis symphysis
   iii. **20 weeks:** uterine fundus at the umbilicus
   iv. **20–34 weeks:** the fundal height in centimeters equals the gestational age in weeks
   v. **36 weeks:** uterine fundus at the xiphoid process of sternum

 c. **Ultrasound examinations. Listed below are the most commonly used ultrasound assessments.** Less common parameters used are binocular distance, transverse cerebellar diameter, fetal foot length, clavicle length, cranial ultrasound assessment, fetal scapular length, corpus callosum measurements, head and midarm circumference, and epiphyseal ossification centers.

   i. **First fetal heart tones by Doppler ultrasound** heard as early as 8 to 12 weeks.
   ii. **Fetal heart motion/beat by ultrasound.** Cardiac activity on ultrasound is detectable at 5.5 to 6.5 weeks by vaginal ultrasound and at 6.5 to 7 weeks by fetal ultrasound.
   iii. **First-trimester examination** (up to and including 13 6/7 weeks' gestation) by ultrasound measurement of the fetus is the most accurate method to establish gestational age. Cochrane review found that early ultrasound (before 24 weeks) may result in fewer inductions for postmaturity because of improved gestational dating.

       (a) **Crown-rump length (CRL) is the most reliable measurement of gestational age up to and including 13 6/7 weeks' gestation,** is accurate within 5 to 7 days, and is most accurate if performed early in the first trimester. It measures the embryo at the tip of the cephalic pole to the tip of the caudal pole. Three measurements should be obtained. Accuracy of gestational age assessment decreases if the CRL measurement is >84 mm (approximately 14 0/7 weeks).
       (b) **Mean sac diameter (MSD)** is no longer recommended for estimating the due date.

   iv. **Second-trimester examination (between 14 0/7 and 27 6/7 weeks' gestation).** Ultrasound measurement of the fetus in the second trimester is based on formulas that use biparietal diameter (BPD), head circumference, abdominal circumference, and femur length.

       (a) **Ultrasound done between 14 0/7 and 22 6/7 weeks:** gestational age accuracy of 7 to 10 days.
       (b) **Ultrasound done between 22 0/7 and 27 6/7 weeks:** gestational age accuracy of 10 to 14 days.

   v. **Third-trimester examination (28 0/7 weeks' gestation and beyond)** is the least reliable measurement of gestational age. The same parameters are used as in the second trimester. Accuracy is within 21 to 30 days.

3. **Laboratory data.** There are multiple biochemical parameters that can aid in the estimation of gestational age and fetal maturity. These include amniotic fluid creatinine concentration, lecithin-to-sphingomyelin ratio, total protein, uric acid, bilirubin, and fetal fat staining cells. The 2 best parameters are amniotic creatinine

(fetal kidney maturity) and lecithin (fetal lung maturity). There are multiple risks of obtaining amniotic fluid by amniocentesis including infection, hemorrhage, and fetal loss.

B. **Postnatal gestational age assessment.** Clinicians usually perform a postnatal gestational assessment on every infant. It is important to perform this assessment, because some prenatal estimates of LMP are incorrect, and an ultrasound (especially first trimester) may not have been done. Another benefit is that it can confirm the obstetrician's date and may provide additional information relevant to the developmental stage. There are many methods to assess gestational age, including rapid assessment of gestational age at delivery, direct ophthalmoscopy of the lens of the eye, and various examinations including assessment of physical and neuromuscular maturity. Metabolic gestational age dating has been studied using newborn screening metabolic profile measurements for use in resource-poor countries.

1. **Rapid assessment of gestational age in the delivery room.** There are multiple methods for rapid assessment of gestational age. Most include some of the following physical characteristics: skin texture, skin color, skin opacity, edema, lanugo hair, skull hardness, ear form, ear firmness, genitalia, breast size, nipple formation, and plantar skin creases. One method for rapid gestational age assessment includes the **most useful clinical signs in differentiating among premature, borderline mature, and full-term infants, which are as follows (in order of utility):** creases in the sole of the foot, size of the breast nodule, nature of the scalp hair, cartilaginous development of the earlobe, scrotal rugae, and testicular descent in males. These signs and findings are listed in Table 6–1.

2. **Direct ophthalmoscopy of the lens is another method for determination of gestational age at 27 to 34 weeks only.** It is based on the normal embryologic process of the gradual disappearance of the anterior lens capsule vascularity between 27 and 34 weeks of gestation. Before 27 weeks, the cornea is too opaque to allow visualization; after 34 weeks, atrophy of the vessels of the lens occurs. This method is reliable to ±2 weeks. The pupil must be dilated under the supervision of an

Table 6–1. **CRITERIA FOR RAPID GESTATIONAL ASSESSMENT AT DELIVERY**

Feature	36 Weeks and Earlier	37–38 Weeks	39 Weeks and Beyond
Creases in soles of feet	1 or 2 transverse creases; posterior three-fourths of sole smooth	Multiple creases; anterior two-thirds of heel smooth	Entire sole, including heel, covered with creases
Breast nodule[a]	2 mm	4 mm	7 mm
Scalp hair	Fine and woolly; fuzzy	Fine and woolly; fuzzy	Coarse and silky; each hair single stranded
Earlobe	No cartilage	Moderate amount of cartilage	Stiff earlobe with thick cartilage
Testes and scrotum	Testes partially descended; scrotum small, with few rugae	?	Testes fully descended; scrotum normal size with prominent rugae

[a]The breast nodule is not palpable before 33 weeks. Underweight full-term infants may have retarded breast development.
Reproduced with permission from Usher R, McLean F, Scott KE: Judgment of fetal age. II. Clinical significance of gestational age and an objective method for its assessment, *Pediatr Clin North Am.* 1966 Aug;13(3):835-862.

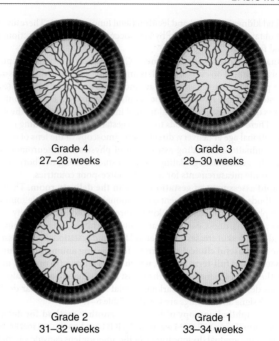

Grade 4
27–28 weeks

Grade 3
29–30 weeks

Grade 2
31–32 weeks

Grade 1
33–34 weeks

FIGURE 6–1. Grading system for assessment of gestational age by examination of the anterior vascular capsule of the lens. (*Reproduced with permission from Hittner HM, Hirsch NJ, Rudolph AJ: Assessment of gestational age by examination of the anterior vascular capsule of the lens,* J Pediatr. *1977 Sep;91(3):455-458.*)

ophthalmologist, and the assessment must be performed within 48 hours of birth before the vessels atrophy. This method is highly accurate and is not affected by alert states or neurologic deficits. The following grading system is used, as shown in Figure 6–1.

　　a. **Grade 4 (27–28 weeks).** Vessels cover the entire anterior surface of the lens, or the vessels meet in the center of the lens.

　　b. **Grade 3 (29–30 weeks).** Vessels do not meet in the center but are close. Central portion of the lens is not covered by vessels.

　　c. **Grade 2 (31–32 weeks).** Vessels reach only to the middle-outer part of the lens. The central clear portion of the lens is larger.

　　d. **Grade 1 (33–34 weeks).** Vessels are seen only at the periphery of the lens.

3. **Examinations based on physical and neuromuscular maturity.** These include the **Dubowitz method, Ballard maturational score, and new Ballard score.** These approaches have used physical and neuromuscular maturity to assess gestational age. Physical criteria alone are more accurate than neurologic criteria alone, with the combination providing the best estimate of gestational age. It is important to note that, in recent studies, gestational assessment in the community in low-resource areas had poor diagnostic accuracy and neonatal anthropometrics were poor for classifying preterm infants in areas with high rates of fetal growth restriction.

　　a. **Dubowitz method.** Dubowitz et al. (1970) originally described a method that included a total of 21 physical and neurologic assessments. The test was widely used but became difficult and time consuming (up to 7 minutes) in performing the assessment, especially on extremely premature and sick infants, and the method overestimated gestational age in premature infants.

   b. **Ballard maturational score.** The Ballard method (1979) shortened the Dubowitz method (now only 3.5 minutes) and had only 6 physical and 6 neurologic criteria. This method was considered inaccurate at assessing gestational age in preterm neonates and postterm and small for gestational age infants.

   c. **New Ballard score.** Ballard et al. (1991) later refined and expanded their test to include the assessment of extremely premature infants (20 weeks). **This is the most commonly used scoring system for assessing gestational age.**

   i. **New Ballard score.** The score spans from 10 (correlating with 20 weeks' gestation) to 50 (correlating with 44 weeks' gestation). It is best performed at <12 hours of age if the infant is <26 weeks' gestation. If the infant is >26 weeks' gestation, there is no optimal age of examination up to 96 hours.

   (a) **Accuracy.** The examination is accurate whether the infant is sick or well to within 2 weeks of gestational age. It overestimates gestational age by 1.3 to 3.3 weeks in infants who are 22 to 28 weeks' gestation. It overestimates gestational age by 2 to 4 days in infants between 32 and 37 weeks' gestation.

   (b) **Criteria.** The score consists of 6 neuromuscular and 6 physical criteria. The neuromuscular criteria are based on the understanding that passive tone is more useful than active tone in indicating gestational age.

   (c) **Procedure.** The examination is administered twice by 2 different examiners to ensure objectivity, and the data are entered on the chart (Figure 6–2). This form is available in most nurseries and online sites. The examination consists of 2 parts: neuromuscular maturity and physical maturity. The 12 scores are totaled, and the **maturity rating** is expressed in weeks of gestation (**gestational age**), estimated by using the chart provided on the form.

   (d) **Neuromuscular maturity**

   (i) **Posture.** Score 0 if the arms and legs are extended, and score +1 if the infant has beginning flexion of the knees and hips, with arms extended; determine other scores based on the diagram.

   (ii) **Square window.** Flex the hand on the forearm between the thumb and index finger of the examiner. Apply sufficient pressure to achieve as much flexion as possible. Visually measure the angle between the hypothenar eminence and the ventral aspect of the forearm. Determine the score based on the diagram.

   (iii) **Arm recoil.** Flex the forearms for 5 seconds and then grasp the hand and fully extend the arm and release. If the arm returns to full flexion, give a score of +4. For lesser degrees of flexion, score as noted in the diagram.

   (iv) **Popliteal angle.** Hold the thigh in the knee-chest position with the left index finger and the thumb supporting the knee. Then extend the leg by gentle pressure from the right index finger behind the ankle. Measure the angle at the popliteal space and score accordingly.

   (v) **Scarf sign.** Take the infant's hand and try to put it around the neck posteriorly as far as possible over the opposite shoulder, and score according to the diagram.

   (vi) **Heel to ear.** Keeping the pelvis flat on the table, take the infant's foot and try to put it as close to the head as possible without forcing it. Grade according to the diagram.

   (e) **Physical maturity.** These characteristics are scored as shown in Figure 6–2.

Name	Date/Time of birth	Sex
Hospital No.	Date/Time of exam	Birthweight
Race	Age when examined	Length
Apgar score: 1 minute ___ 5 minutes ___ 10 minutes		Head circ.
		Examiner

SCORE
Neuromuscular ___
Physical ___
Total ___

Maturity rating

Score	Weeks
−10	20
−5	22
0	24
5	26
10	28
15	30
20	32
25	34
30	36
35	38
40	40
45	42
50	44

Neuromuscular maturity

Neuromuscular maturity sign	−1	0	1	2	3	4	5	Record score here
Posture								
Square window (wrist)	>90°	90°	60°	45°	30°	0°		
Arm recoil		180°	140° to 180°	110° to 140°	90° to 110°	<90°		
Popliteal angle	180°	160°	140°	120°	100°	90°	<90°	
Scarf sign								
Heel to ear								
							Total neuromuscular maturity score	

FIGURE 6–2. Maturational assessment of gestational age (new Ballard score). (*Reproduced with permission from Ballard JL, Khoury JC, Wedig K, et al: New Ballard Score, expanded to include extremely premature infants, J Pediatr. 1991 Sep;119(3):417-423.*)

48

Physical maturity

Physical maturity sign	Score							Record score here
	−1	0	1	2	3	4	5	
Skin	sticky friable transparent	gelatinous red translucent	smooth pink visible veins	superficial peeling &/or rash, few veins	cracking pale areas rare veins	parchment deep cracking no vessels	leathery cracked wrinkled	
Lanugo	none	sparse	abundant	thinning	bald areas	mostly bald		
Plantar surface	heel-toe 40–50 mm: −1 <40 mm: −2	>50 mm no crease	faint red marks	anterior transverse crease only	creases ant. 2/3	creases over entire sole		
Breast	imperceptible	barely perceptible	flat areola no bud	stippled areola 1–2 mm bud	raised areola 3–4 mm bud	full areola 5–10 mm bud		
Eye/ear	lids fused loosely: −1 tightly: −2	lids open pinna flat stays folded	sl. curved pinna; soft slow recoil	well curved pinna; soft but ready recoil	formed and firm, instant recoil	thick cartilage ear stiff		
Genitals (male)	scrotum flat, smooth	scrotum empty, faint rugae	testes in upper canal rare rugae	testes descending few rugae	testes down good rugae	testes pendulous deep rugae		
Genitals (female)	clitoris prominent & labia flat	prominent clitoris & small labia minora	prominent clitoris & enlarging minora	majora & minora equally prominent	majora large minora small	majora cover clitoris & minora		
							Total physical maturity score	

Gestational age (weeks)

By dates _____

By ultrasound _____

By exam _____

FIGURE 6–2. (*Continued*)

49

    (i) **Skin.** Carefully look at the skin, and grade according to the diagram. Extremely premature infants have sticky, transparent skin and receive a score of +1.

    (ii) **Lanugo hair.** Examine the infant's back and between and over the scapulae.

    (iii) **Plantar surface.** Measure foot length from the tip of the great toe to the back of the heel. If the result is <40 mm, give a score of –2. If it is between 40 and 50 mm, assign a score of –1. If the measurement is >50 mm and no creases are seen on the plantar surface, give a score of 0. If there are creases, score accordingly.

    (iv) **Breast.** Palpate any breast tissue and score.

    (v) **Eye and ear.** This section has been expanded to include criteria that apply to the extremely premature infant. Loosely fused eyelids are defined as closed, but gentle traction opens them (score as –1). Tightly fused eyelids are defined as inseparable by gentle traction. Base the rest of the score on open lids and the examination of the ear.

    (vi) **Genitalia.** Score according to the diagram.

  4. **Metabolic gestational age dating.** Prediction models have been developed using newborn metabolic profile, hemoglobin levels, and analyte data from the newborn metabolic screening profiles. The results were very favorable, and one study predicted gestational age within 1 week of the actual gestational age in two-thirds of the infants. This method is accurate and may be useful in resource-poor countries where ultrasound is not readily available. DNA methylation on cord blood and blood spot samples has also been studied and accurately estimates gestational age.

  C. **Newborn classification based on gestational age.** Infants can be classified based on their gestational age. The major classification categorizes the infant as **preterm, term, or postterm.** It is based on the weeks of gestation, completed weeks of gestation, or days. (See Table 6–2 for a full description.) Both **preterm and term** have been further subclassified. **Preterm** has been categorized into **extremely preterm, very preterm, or moderate to late preterm (moderately preterm and late preterm).** Note that the recommendations from the Defining "Term" Pregnancy Workgroup have redefined the **definition of term** pregnancy and recommend subcategorization of the 6-week period from 37 to 42 weeks (**early term, full term, and late term**). They did this because maternal and neonatal outcomes are very different across this 6-week gestational period. They discourage the use of the word "term." (See Table 6–2 for a full description.)

II. **Birthweight classification.** Infants can be classified by birthweight; some of the common terminology classifications used are as follows:

  A. **Micro preemie.** <800 g or 1 lb 12 oz.

  B. **Extremely low birthweight (ELBW).** <1000 g or 2 lb 3 oz.

  C. **Very low birthweight (VLBW).** <1500 g or 3 lb 5 oz.

  D. **Low birthweight (LBW).** <2500 g or 5.5 lb.

  E. **Normal birthweight (NBW).** From 2500 g (5 lb 8 oz.) to 3999 g (8 lb 13 oz.).

  F. **High birthweight (HBW).** From 4000 g (8 lb 13.1 oz.) to 4500 g (9 lb 14 oz.).

  G. **Very high birthweight (VHBW).** >4500 g (9 lb 14 oz.).

III. **Classification by birthweight and gestational age combined.** Newborns can be classified by assessing their gestational age and obtaining their birthweight and plotting these against standardized intrauterine growth charts. This allows categorization as SGA (small for gestational age), AGA (appropriate for gestational age), or LGA (large for gestational age). These refer to the size of the infant at birth and not fetal growth.

  A. **How to decide whether the infant is SGA, AGA, or LGA.** Plot gestational age assessment against weight, length, and head circumference on an intrauterine growth chart to determine whether the infant is SGA, AGA, or LGA. There are multiple intrauterine growth charts available based on different populations, including those by

Table 6–2. **DEFINITIONS OF POSTNATAL GESTATIONAL AGE**

	Weeks of Gestation (number of weeks after the first day of the mother's last menstrual period)	Completed Weeks (number of 7-day intervals after the first day of the mother's last menstrual period)	Days (common medical terminology)
Extremely preterm	<28 weeks	On or before the end of the last day of the 28th week	<197 days
Very preterm	28 0/7 to 31 6/7weeks	On or after the first day of the 29th week through the last day of the 32nd week	197–224 days
Moderately preterm	32 0/7 to 33 6/7 weeks	On or after the first day of the 33 weeks through the last day of the 34th week	225–238 days
Preterm	<37 weeks	On or before the end of the last day of the 37th week	<260 days
Late preterm	34 0/7 to 36 6/7 weeks	On or after the first day of the 35th week through the end of the last day of the 37th week	239–259 days
Early term	37 0/7 to 38 6/7 weeks	On or after the first day of the 38th week through the end of the last day of the 39th week	260–273 days
Full term	39 0/7 to 40 6/7 weeks	On or after the first day of the 40th week through the end of the last day of the 41st week	274–287 days
Late term	41 0/7 to 41 6/7 weeks	On or after the first day of the 42nd week through the end of the day of the 42nd week	288–294 days
Post term	42 0/7 weeks or more	On or after first day of the 43rd week	≥295 days

Definitions of postnatal gestational age are based on **conventional medical definitions** (day of birth counted as day 1) by the American Academy of Pediatrics, the American College of Obstetricians and Gynecologists, and the World Health Organization.

Data from Engle WA, Tomashek KM, Wallman C, et al: "Late-preterm" infants: a population at risk, *Pediatrics.* 2007 Dec;120(6):1390-1401; Spong CY: Defining "term" pregnancy: recommendations from the Defining "Term" Pregnancy Workgroup, *JAMA.* 2013 Jun 19;309(23):2445-2446.

Battaglia and Lubchenco (United States, 1966, 1967), Usher and McLean (Canada, 1969), Beeby (South Wales, 1996), Niklasson (Sweden, 1991), Fenton (South Wales, Sweden, Canada, 2003, revised 2013), Olsen (United States, 2010), and now Boghossian (United States, 2016).

Which chart to use? The original charts were the Battaglia and Lubchenco charts (Figure 6–3). The first Fenton chart (2003) was the Babson and Benda's chart updated with a new format and new data. The revised Fenton Chart (2013) includes the World Health Organization growth standard and reflects actual age to improve preterm infant growth monitoring (Figure 6–4). The Olsen charts are gender-specific intrauterine growth charts that include more infant sizes and new preterm infant growth curves, and they more accurately represent the current ethnically diverse US population (Figure 6–5). Boghossian et al. (2016) have published new sex-specific weight and head circumference for gestational age charts for infants born between 22 and 29 weeks' gestation using data from >156,000 infants from the Vermont Oxford Network database (Figure 6–6). Deciding which chart to use usually depends on the preference of the neonatal intensive care unit.

B. **Definitions and characteristics of AGA, SGA, and LGA**

1. **Appropriate for gestational age (AGA).** Defined as a birthweight between the 10th and 90th percentiles for the infant's gestational age.

2. **Small for gestational age (SGA).** Defined as birthweight 2 standard deviations below the mean weight for gestational age or below the 10th percentile for gestational age. SGA refers to the size of the infant at birth and not fetal growth. SGA is typically associated with **maternal factors** (eg, chronic disease, malnutrition, multiple gestation, high altitude, or conditions affecting the blood flow and oxygenation in the placenta [hypertension, preeclampsia, smoking]), **placental factors** (eg, infarction, previa, abruption, anatomic malformations), **fetal factors** (usually symmetric; birthweight, length, and head circumference all depressed the same), congenital infections (eg, TORCH [toxoplasmosis, other, rubella, cytomegalovirus, herpes simplex virus]; see Chapter 148), chromosomal abnormalities, and congenital malformations (eg, dysmorphic syndromes and other congenital anomalies, fetal diabetes mellitus, familial causes, multiple gestation, constitutional). **IUGR** and **constitutionally small fetus** should be included when discussing SGA infants.

   a. **Intrauterine growth restriction (fetal growth restriction).** (See Chapter 104.) IUGR is a reduction in the expected fetal growth of an infant. The failure to obtain optimal intrauterine growth is due to an in utero insult. There is no standard definition, but a fetus at <10th percentile weight for age or with a ponderal index <10% is sometimes used to classify an infant as IUGR. (**Note:** SGA and IUGR are related but not synonymous. All infants born SGA may not be small as a result of IUGR. All infants born IUGR may not be SGA. SGA is a clinical finding, and IUGR is an ultrasound finding.)

   b. **Constitutionally small infants.** Includes 70% of infants with a birthweight below the 10th percentile. They have no increased obstetrical or neonatal risks. They are constitutionally small, anatomically normal, well proportioned, and have normal development. They grow parallel to the lower percentiles throughout pregnancy. Mothers are usually slim, petite women. The infants are small because of constitutional reasons: maternal ethnicity, female sex, body mass index, and others.

3. **Large for gestational age (LGA).** Defined as birthweight 2 standard deviations above the mean weight for gestational age or above the 90th percentile for gestational age. LGA can be seen in infants of diabetic mothers (maternal or gestational), infants with Beckwith-Wiedemann syndrome or other syndromes, constitutionally large infants with large parents, postmature infants (gestational age >42 weeks), and infants with hydrops fetalis. LGA infants are also associated with increased maternal weight gain in pregnancy, multiparity, male sex,

Name _____
Hospital No. _____
Race _____
Date of birth _____

Date of exam _____
Sex _____
Birthweight _____

Length _____
Head circ. _____
Gestational age _____

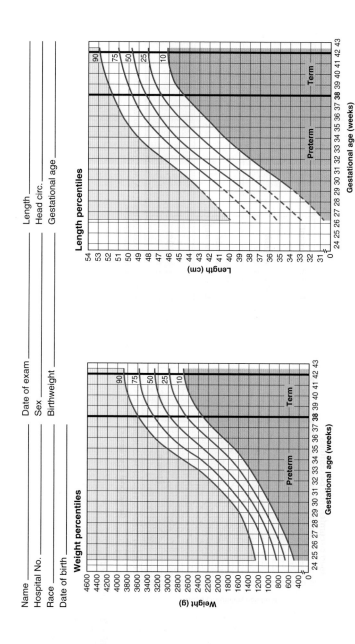

FIGURE 6-3. Classification of newborns (both sexes) by intrauterine growth and gestational age. *(Data from Battaglia FC, Lubchenco IO. A practical classification for newborn infants by weight and gestational age. J Pediatr. 1967;71:159; Lubchenco LO, Hansman C, Boyd E. Intrauterine growth in length and head circumference as estimated from live births at gestational ages from to 42 weeks. Pediatrics. 1966;37:403. Used with permission from Abbott Laboratories, Columbus, Ohio.)*

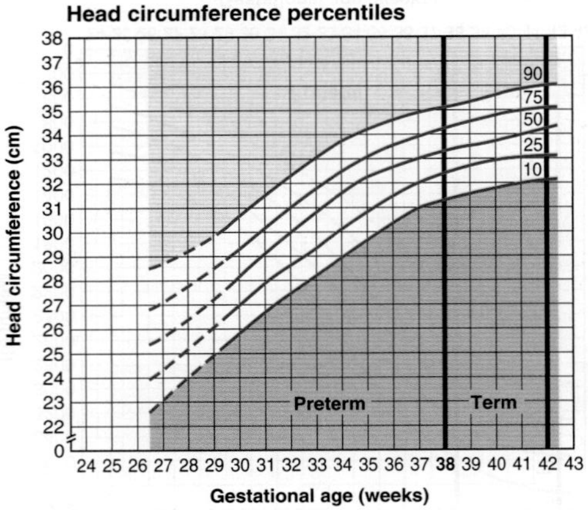

Head circumference percentiles

Head circumference (cm) — y-axis: 22, 23, 24, 25, 26, 27, 28, 29, 30, 31, 32, 33, 34, 35, 36, 37, 38

Gestational age (weeks) — x-axis: 24 25 26 27 28 29 30 31 32 33 34 35 36 37 38 39 40 41 42 43

Percentile curves: 90, 75, 50, 25, 10

Preterm | Term

Classification of infant*	Weight	Length	Head circ.
Large for gestational age (LGA) (>90th percentile)			
Appropriate for gestational age (AGA) (10th to 90th percentile)			
Small for gestational age (SGA) (<10th percentile)			

*Place an "X" in the appropriate box (LGA, AGA, or SGA) for weight, for length, and for head circumference.

FIGURE 6–3. (*Continued*)

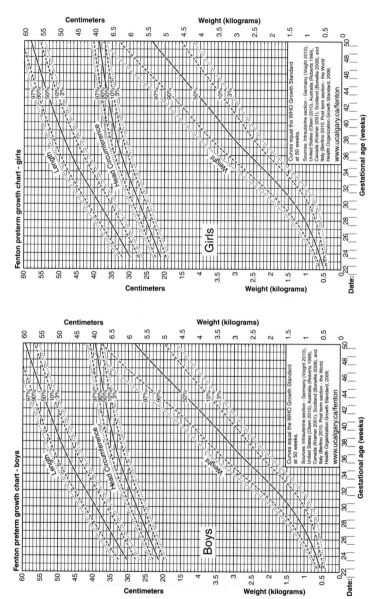

FIGURE 6–4. Growth chart for preterm infants. (*Reproduced with permission from Fenton TR, Kim JH: A systematic review and meta-analysis to revise the Fenton growth chart for preterm infants, BMC Pediatr. 2013 Apr 20;13:59.*)

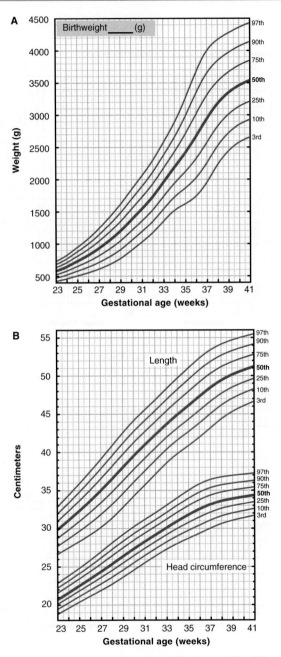

FIGURE 6–5. Intrauterine growth curves for males and females including (**A**) girls weight for age, (**B**) girls length and head circumference (HC) for age, (**C**) boys weight for age, and (**D**) boys length and HC for age. (*Data from Olsen IE, Groveman SA, Lawson ML, et al: New intrauterine growth curves based on United States data,* Pediatrics. *2010 Feb;125(2):e214-e224.*)

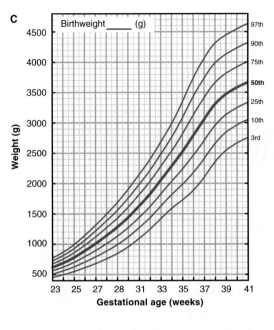

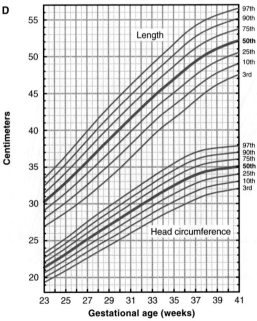

FIGURE 6–5. (*Continued*)

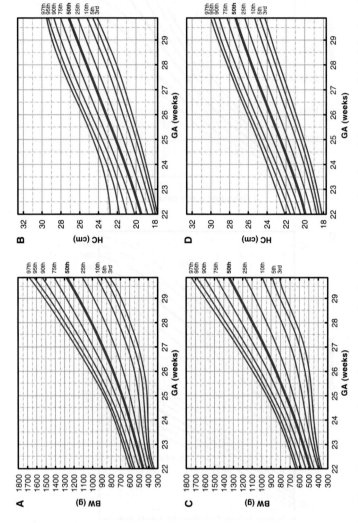

FIGURE 6–6. Birth weight and head circumference for preterm infants born between 22 and 29 6/7 weeks' gestation. (**A**) Girls birthweight and gestational age, (**B**) girls head circumference and gestational age, (**C**) boys birthweight and gestational age, and (**D**) boys head circumference and gestational age. BW, birthweight in grams; GA, gestational age in weeks; HC, head circumference in centimeters. (*Data from Boghossian NS, Geraci M, Edwards EM, et al: Anthropometric Charts for Infants Born Between 22 and 29 Weeks' Gestation, Pediatrics. 2016 Dec;138(6).*)

congenital heart disease, especially transposition of the great arteries ("happy chubby blue male infant"), islet cell dysplasias, and certain ethnicities (Hispanic). LGA infants are sometimes referred to as infants with macrosomia.

    a. **Macrosomia** means "large body." Hispanic women have a higher risk of fetal macrosomia when compared to Asian, African American, and white women. Because males weigh more at birth, it is also more common in males. It is associated with diabetes (gestational and maternal), maternal obesity, and a longer duration of gestation. Macrosomia has multiple definitions in the literature.

        i. **Birthweight >4000 g or >4500 g** regardless of gestational age.

        ii. **Large for gestational age (LGA).** Birthweight ≥90% for gestational age.

        iii. **Weight is above a defined limit** at any gestational age.

IV. **Other age terminology** (recommended terms by the AAP) used to describe the age and gestation of an infant:

  A. **Chronologic age (or postnatal age).** The time elapsed since birth expressed in days, weeks, months, or years.

  B. **Postmenstrual age.** Gestational age plus chronologic age. It is expressed in weeks and is the preferred term to describe premature infants in the perinatal period while the infant is in the hospital.

  C. **Corrected age (or adjusted age; only used in children born preterm <3 years old).** Corrected age is the chronologic age minus the number of weeks born before 40 weeks' gestation and is the preferred term to describe the age of preterm infants after the perinatal period. It is expressed in weeks or months.

  D. **Conceptional age is the time elapsed between the day of conception and the day of delivery.** If pregnancy was achieved by assisted reproductive technology (ART), then a precise conceptional age can be calculated. Typically when the date of conception is known, gestational age is calculated by adding 2 weeks to the conceptional age. Gestational age is the preferred term to be used in clinical pediatrics and conceptional and postconceptional age are no longer recommended terms. Conceptual age and postconceptual age are incorrect terms and should never be used.

7 Newborn Physical Examination

Newborns are examined immediately after birth to quickly assess their respiratory effort, circulation, and temperature; to identify any major congenital abnormalities; and to check for any infectious or metabolic disease that requires immediate treatment. This exam is critical to ensure the transition to extrauterine life proceeds without difficulty. The infant should then undergo a complete physical examination within 24 hours of birth and again at discharge. Specific findings in an infant who has experienced a traumatic birth are reviewed in detail in Chapter 83.

It is best to perform a routine newborn physical exam under a radiant warmer with the lights on. Before even touching the infant, observe and assess color, activity, posture, maturity, and respirations. Perform the examinations that cause the least amount of disturbance first. It is easier to listen to the heart and lungs first and feel the pulses when the infant is quiet. Warming the hands and stethoscope before use decreases the likelihood of making the infant cry.

In addition to examination of the infant, the complete maternal history, including prenatal, perinatal, labor and delivery, family, and social history, should be reviewed. (See Appendix D, "Chartwork.")

I. **Vital signs**
   A. **Temperature.** Indicate whether the temperature is rectal (which is usually 1° higher than oral), oral, or axillary (which is usually 1° lower than oral). Axillary temperature is usually measured in the neonate, with rectal temperature done if the axillary temperature is abnormal. Normal axillary temperature in a newborn ranges from 97.5°F to 99.3°F (36.5–37.4°C).
   B. **Respirations.** The normal respiratory rate in a newborn is 30 to 60 breaths/min. Periodic breathing (≥3 apneic episodes lasting >3 seconds within a 20-second period of otherwise normal respirations) is considered normal and common in newborns.
   C. **Blood pressure.** Blood pressure correlates directly with gestational age, postnatal age of the infant, and birthweight. (For normal blood pressure values, see Table 70–1, Figure 70–1 and Appendix C.)
   D. **Heart rate.** The normal heart rate is 70 to 190 beats/min in the newborn (usually 120–160 beats/min when awake, >170 beats/min with activity or crying, and decreasing to 70–90 beats/min when asleep). In the healthy infant, the heart rate increases with stimulation. See Table 53–1, page 460.
   E. **Pulse oximetry.** Pulse oximetry in the neonatal intensive care unit (NICU) has become standard of care and is sometimes referred to as the "fifth vital sign." (**Note:** Pain assessment has also been referred to as the "fifth vital sign" by some.) It is a simple, painless noninvasive tool used to measure arterial oxygen saturation by measuring the absorption of light in tissue beds. It is commonly used in the NICU as a monitoring tool during oxygen supplementation, during sedation for procedures, perioperatively, in high-risk infants, in the delivery room, and during transport. Pulse oximetry is also used diagnostically in persistent pulmonary hypertension and to screen for critical congenital heart disease (CCHD). Screening pulse oximetry for critical cyanotic heart disease is recommended for all infants before discharge.
      1. **Screening pulse oximetry for critical congenital cyanotic heart disease.** Congenital heart disease is a common birth defect, occurring in approximately 1% of all newborns. CCHD, occurring in approximately 18 in 10,000 infants, is a life-threatening condition with significant morbidity and mortality in the newborn period. These conditions may require heart surgery or catheter-based intervention within the first year of life to prevent end-organ damage or death. As of 2011, universal pulse oximetry screening is recommended for all newborns because low blood oxygen saturation may detect CCHD. This screening has been endorsed by the American College of Cardiology Foundation, March of Dimes, Newborn Foundation, American Heart Association, and American Academy of Pediatrics (AAP). An expert panel was convened again in 2015 to rereview practices and identify areas of improvement. Infants who test positive (up to 79%) can have CCHD or another non-CCHD cause of hypoxemia. Most states in the United States have followed this AAP-endorsed protocol, with New Jersey and Tennessee adopting different algorithms. See Figure 7–1 for the AAP-endorsed CCHD pulse oximetry screening algorithm from the Centers for Disease Control and Prevention (CDC).
         a. **Twelve heart conditions that are detected by screening for CCHD with pulse oximetry include the following:**
            i. **Core/primary targets for CCHD screening (7 most common critical lesions that present with hypoxemia):** Hypoplastic left heart syndrome, pulmonary atresia with intact ventricular septum, tetralogy of Fallot, total anomalous pulmonary venous return, transposition of the great arteries, tricuspid atresia, and truncus arteriosus.
            ii. **Additional/secondary targets for CCHD screening (5 critical lesions that either are less common but present with hypoxia or are more**

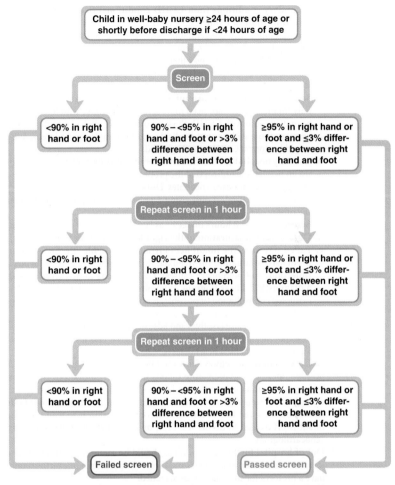

FIGURE 7–1. Screening algorithm for critical congenital heart disease using pulse oximetry. (*Reproduced with permission from Kemper AR, Mahle WT, Martin GR, et al: Strategies for implementing screening for critical congenital heart disease,* Pediatrics. *2011 Nov;128(5):e1259-e1267.*)

common and do not present with hypoxia): Coarctation of the aorta with patent ductus arteriosus (PDA), double outlet right ventricle, Ebstein anomaly, interrupted aortic arch/aortic atresia, and single ventricle physiology.
   b. **Three heart conditions that are potentially screenable by pulse oximetry:** Pulmonary stenosis, aortic stenosis with PDA, and complete atrioventricular canal.
   c. **Heart conditions that are not screenable by pulse oximetry:** Aortic stenosis without PDA, Ebstein anomaly without right to left shunt, coarctation of the aorta without a PDA, and any other left to right shunting lesions.

   d. **Secondary conditions (non-CCHD conditions) that are detected by screening by pulse oximetry:** Hypothermia, infections (including sepsis), hemoglobinopathy, congenital or acquired lung disease, persistent pulmonary hypertension, transient tachypnea of the newborn, a noncritical congenital heart defect, and other hypoxemic conditions.

2. **Newborn nursery/intermediate nursery pulse oximetry screening guidelines**

   a. **Screen all healthy newborn infants.** It is best to screen when alert. The only infants who do not need to be screened are those who have already been diagnosed with CCHD, those who have already had an echocardiogram, or those with serious medical conditions in whom no intervention would be done if CCHD was diagnosed.

   b. **Use only hospital-grade, motion-tolerant pulse oximeters** designed for use in neonates. Confirm that the probes are correct for the machine and are appropriate for use in neonates. Disposable or reusable pulse oximetry probes may be used. If only using 1 pulse oximeter, test one right after the other.

   c. **Screen at 24 to 48 hours of age** or as late as possible for early discharge.

   d. **Obtain oxygen saturation in the right hand and either foot.**

   e. **Failed screen. Is the infant hemodynamically stable? Perform a comprehensive evaluation for hypoxia.** Rule out other reasons for hypoxia (infectious and pulmonary causes). **CCHD needs to be excluded with a diagnostic echocardiogram.** If no obvious cause is found, a pediatric cardiology consultation (if possible) is obtained prior to obtaining a diagnostic echocardiogram.

   f. **Passed screen.** False positives and false negatives may occur. A passed test does not mean the infant does not have CCHD. This test does not detect all cases of congenital heart defects.

3. **NICU screening guidelines.** Screening in the NICU can give higher false-positive rates because premature infants have lower saturations than term infants. Many units follow the standard AAP protocol, some modify it, and some do not screen at all. As noted earlier, it **is recommended that all infants should be screened for CCHD.** One recommendation is to wait until the infant is off oxygen to do the test or, if on oxygen at discharge, obtain an echocardiogram.

4. **Out of hospital births.** All newborns should be screened regardless of the location of birth. Birthing centers and those who perform home births should have a protocol for the infant to be screened.

5. **High altitude.** Infants at a higher altitude have a lower oxygen saturation than those at sea level. Therefore, oxygen saturation thresholds for a positive screening may vary at high altitudes. Adapting the protocol for hospitals at elevations >6800 feet include obtaining an echocardiogram and repeating the pulse oximetry test every 4 hours until the echocardiogram results are obtained, placing the infant in an oxygen hood to replicate sea level, and testing at 30 hours to allow a transition time.

II. **Head circumference, length, weight, chest circumference, abdominal circumference, and gestational age.** (For intrauterine growth charts, see Chapter 6). For standard infant/child growth charts based on CDC and World Health Organization (WHO) data from birth to 36 months, see http://www.cdc.gov/growthcharts/.

   A. **Head circumference and percentile.** Determine the occipital-frontal circumference by placing the measuring tape around the front of the head (above the brow [the frontal area]) and the occipital area. The tape should be above the ears. This is normally 32 to 37 cm at term; percentile is determined by the CDC/WHO table.

B. **Length and percentile.** Normal length is 48 to 52 cm, with the percentile determined by the CDC/WHO table.

C. **Chest circumference.** With the infant supine, measure the circumference of the chest at the level of the nipples during normal breathing. This is a good indicator of low birthweight. Normal is 30 to 35 cm (head circumference is typically 2 cm larger than chest circumference).

D. **Abdominal circumference** is usually not measured unless there is abdominal distension, but a baseline can be valuable because if there is a question of a change in abdominal distension, a measurement is available to compare. Measure the distance 1 cm above the umbilicus in the supine position, not at or below the umbilicus (a full bladder may interfere with the measurement). Multiple variables can affect the measurement: birthweight, time of last feeding and time of last stool, resistance of the abdominal wall, phase of breathing, and amount of abdominal fat. Increases of abdominal circumference of <1.5 cm occur normally and should not be a cause of concern, especially if there are no other abnormal clinical signs. An increase in abdominal girth >2 cm may be considered abnormal, but studies have shown that abdominal circumference may vary by 3.5 cm in one feeding cycle in normal premature infants.

E. **Gestational age and birthweight classification.** See Chapter 6. The AAP recommends all newborns be classified by both birthweight and gestational age. Assess gestational age by using the new Ballard examination and classify as preterm, late preterm, etc. Classify by birthweight, if extremely low birth weight (ELBW), low birth weight (LBW), etc. Determine if small, appropriate, or large for gestational age based on weight and gestational age.

III. **General appearance.** Observe the infant and record the general appearance (eg, activity, skin color, respirations, posture, obvious congenital abnormalities). Much of the newborn examination is done through observation. **The normal resting posture of a term newborn is in flexion; the normal posture of a preterm baby is in extension at rest.** For an infant born in breech presentation, the infant may have fully flexed hips and knees, feet may be near the mouth, or legs and feet may be to the side of the baby. Note if the general movements are normal, note the skin color, look at chest and note respirations and see if breathing is normal or labored, and look for any obvious major congenital anomalies. Are there any signs or symptoms of infection (fever, lethargy, hypothermia, rashes, tachypnea, abdominal distension, irritability, vomiting) or metabolic disease (growth restriction, rash, jaundice, seizures, hepatosplenomegaly, microcephaly, failure to thrive, anomalies)?

IV. **Abnormal odor.** Does the infant have an abnormal odor? Abnormal odors suggest an inborn error of metabolism or infection.

A. **Odor of maple syrup or burnt sugar, sweet odor of the urine:** Maple syrup urine disease.

B. **Odor of sweaty feet:** Isovaleric acidemia, glutaric acidemia type II.

C. **Odor of cat urine:** 3-Hydroxy-3-methylglutaryl–coenzyme A (HMG-CoA) lyase deficiency.

D. **Odor of cabbage:** Tyrosinemia type 1.

E. **Odor of rotten or decaying fish:** Primary trimethylaminuria (seen in preterm neonates fed a choline-containing formula).

F. **Odor of unpleasant musty smell or mousy body odor:** Phenylketonuria (PKU; due to phenylacetic acid in the urine and stool).

G. **Fruity breath smell:** Diabetic ketoacidosis.

H. **Odor of rotten egg:** Smell of hydrogen sulfide, suspect neonatal sulfhemoglobinemia either from drugs or intestinal microbiota.

I. **Foul/stinky urine:** The smell can be from intestinal bacteria that have entered the urine or bacteria producing ammonia, and it may be a symptom of urinary tract infection (especially in an infant with a fever).

V. **Skin.** See also Chapter 80.

A. **Color.** Regardless of race, skin color is normally reddish-purple and changes to a pinkish red in about 24 hours after birth.

1. **Plethora (deep, rosy red [ruddy] color).** Plethora beyond 24 hours after birth is more common in infants with polycythemia but can be seen in an overoxygenated or overheated infant. It is best to obtain a central hematocrit on any plethoric infant.

2. **Jaundice (yellowish color if secondary to indirect hyperbilirubinemia; greenish color if secondary to direct hyperbilirubinemia).** With jaundice, bilirubin levels are usually >5 mg/dL. This condition is abnormal in infants <24 hours of age and may signify Rh incompatibility, sepsis, and TORCH (toxoplasmosis, other, rubella, cytomegalovirus, and herpes simplex virus) infections. After 24 hours, it may result either from these diseases or from such common causes as ABO incompatibility or physiologic causes.

3. **Pallor (washed-out, whitish appearance).** Pallor reflects poor perfusion. It may be secondary to anemia, birth asphyxia, shock, sepsis, or PDA. *Ductal pallor* is the term sometimes used to denote pallor associated with PDA.

4. **Poor perfusion.** Some descriptors include "infant doesn't look good" or "looks mottled." Poor perfusion is inadequate blood flow to the skin tissues. Check capillary refill time by pressing on the sternum for 5 seconds with a finger and noting the time needed for the color to return. See Chapter 77.

5. **Excessive pigmentation.** Infants with more melanin can have increased pigment in the following places: in the axilla, over the scrotum or labia, over the helices of the ear, at the base of the nails, and around the umbilicus. The skin color of the parents and maternal hormones in utero will affect the pigmentation of the infant. The **linea nigra** (dark line down the middle of the abdomen) is from exposure to maternal hormones, is more common in females, and usually resolves spontaneously.

6. **Cyanosis** (desaturation of >3–5 g/dL of hemoglobin is usually necessary for one to note a bluish color)

    a. **Central cyanosis (bluish skin, including the tongue, mucosal membranes, and lips). Low partial pressure of oxygen (PaO_2) and low arterial oxygen saturation (SaO_2).** Caused by low oxygen saturation in the blood. Rule out cardiac, lung, central nervous system (CNS), metabolic, or hematologic diseases.

    b. **Peripheral cyanosis (bluish skin, especially distal extremities with pink lips, mucous membranes, and tongue). Normal oxygen saturation (normal PaO_2).** It is secondary to an increase in deoxygenated blood on the venous side because of increased oxygen extraction by the tissues. It is best noted in the nail beds and can be associated with all the common causes of central cyanosis. Causes of peripheral cyanosis include vasomotor instability, venous obstruction (venous thrombosis), polycythemia, low cardiac output, shock, sepsis, vasoconstriction secondary to cold exposure, and elevated venous pressure.

    c. **Acrocyanosis (bluish hands and feet only). Normal oxygen saturation (normal PaO_2).** Peripheral cyanosis of the extremities. This may be normal immediately after birth or within the first few hours after birth or with cold stress. Spasm of smaller arterioles can cause this (up to 24–48 hours of life). In a normothermic older infant, consider hypovolemia.

    d. **Perioral cyanosis (bluish color around the lips and philtrum [nose to upper lip]). Normal oxygen saturation.** Common after birth, due to the close proximity of the blood vessels to the skin (infants have a superficial perioral venous plexus). It is not a sign of peripheral or central cyanosis and usually resolves after 48 hours.

    e. **Traumatic cyanosis. Normal oxygen saturation (normal PaO_2).** This is cyanosis of the head and face, usually with petechiae, that results from venous congestion. It occurs due to a birth face presentation or an umbilical cord around the neck.

    f. **Pseudocyanosis. Normal oxygen saturation (normal PaO$_2$).** Bluish color of the skin without hypoxemia, hemoglobin abnormality, or peripheral vasoconstriction. The mucous membranes of the mouth are pink. Pressure on the skin fails to blanch. This can mimic peripheral cyanosis except there is no blanching of the skin when pressure is applied. In neonates, it is commonly caused by fluorescent lighting. It can also be due to drug exposure (amiodarone).

    g. **Differential cyanosis.** The upper part of the body is pink, and the lower body is cyanotic, or vice versa.

        i. **Differential cyanosis (most common).** Occurs in infants with a PDA with a right to left shunt. The preductal part of the body (upper) is pink, and the postductal body part (lower) is cyanotic. Oxygen saturation in the right hand is greater than in the foot. Seen in severe coarctation of aorta or interrupted aortic arch or in a newborn with a structurally normal heart, it can occur with severe persistent pulmonary hypertension with right to left shunting through the ductus arteriosus.

        ii. **Reverse differential cyanosis.** This is a **newborn cardiac emergency**. The preductal part of the body (upper part) is cyanotic (blue), and the postductal part (lower part) is pink. This occurs when oxygen saturation is lower in the upper extremity (right hand) than in the lower extremity (foot). This occurs with complete transposition of the great arteries with PDA and persistent pulmonary hypertension or in transposition of the great arteries with PDA and preductal coarctation or aortic arch interruption and supracardiac total anomalous pulmonary venous connection. The ductus allows saturated blood to perfuse the lower body.

    h. **Cyanosis with asphyxia stages after birth (historical degrees of severity)**

        i. **Asphyxia livida (early stage).** The phase during asphyxia when primary apnea occurs (heart rate decreases, respiratory efforts may be present, blood pressure rises then drops, arterial partial pressure of carbon dioxide [PaCO$_2$] and pH increase). The infant is **cyanotic**, has some muscle tone, and has adequate circulation.

        ii. **Asphyxia pallida (late stage).** The phase during asphyxia when secondary apnea occurs (heart rate and blood pressure drop, circulatory collapse, shock, low PaO$_2$, increased PaCO$_2$, low pH). The infant has **pale gray/white skin** and is limp; reflexes are absent, and respiratory efforts are absent.

    i. **Cyanosis in stages of shock**

        i. **Warm shock (early stage of shock).** Extremities are warm, with loss of vascular tone, peripheral vasodilation, tachycardia, bounding peripheral pulses, increase in systemic blood flow, and a decrease in blood pressure.

        ii. **Cold shock (late stage of shock).** Extremities are cold and mottled, with a prolonged capillary refill time (>3 seconds), decreased peripheral pulses, increase in vascular tone, vasoconstriction, decrease in systemic blood flow, and decrease in blood pressure.

  7. **Extensive bruising (ecchymoses) may be confused with cyanosis.** May be associated with a prolonged and difficult delivery and may result in early jaundice. Facial bruising can occur with a tight nuchal cord or difficult delivery. This can be confused with cyanosis. **Petechiae (pinpoint hemorrhages)** can be limited to 1 area and are usually of no concern. If they are

widespread and progressive, then they are of concern, and a workup for coagulopathy should be considered. Upper body petechiae can be seen in pertussis.

8. **"Blue on pink" or "pink on blue."** Whereas some infants are pink and well perfused and others are clearly cyanotic, some do not fit in either of these categories. They may appear bluish with pink undertones or pink with bluish undertones. This coloration may be secondary to poor perfusion, inadequate oxygenation, inadequate ventilation, or polycythemia.

9. **Harlequin sign/coloration.** A clear line of demarcation between an area of redness and an area of normal coloration. This is a vascular phenomenon, and the cause is usually unknown, but it may be due to immaturity of the hypothalamic center that controls the dilation of peripheral blood vessels. The coloration can be benign and transient (a few seconds to <30 minutes) or can be indicative of shunting of blood (persistent pulmonary hypertension or coarctation of the aorta). There can be varying degrees of redness and perfusion. The demarcating line may run from the head to the belly, dividing the body into right and left halves, or it may develop in the dependent half of the body when the newborn is lying on one side. The dependent half is usually deep red, and the upper half is pale. This occurs most commonly in lower birthweight infants. It can also occur in 10% of healthy newborns and usually occurs on the second to fifth day of life. It has been noted after an abdominal paracentesis in an infant with neonatal hemochromatosis. (**Note:** This is not **harlequin fetus,** see page 68).

10. **Cutis marmorata.** Reticular mottling, lacy red pattern of the skin, marbled, purplish skin discoloration.
    a. **Physiologic cutis marmorata.** May be seen in healthy infants and in those with cold stress, hypovolemia, shock, or sepsis. It can be caused by an instability or immaturity of the nerve supply to the superficial capillary blood vessels in the skin. Physiologic dilatation of capillaries and venules occurs in response to cold stimulus. In hypovolemia, shock, and sepsis, it occurs because of insufficient perfusion of the skin, and mottling can occur. It is usually in a symmetric pattern and can be seen on the extremities but also on the trunk. It is most pronounced when the skin is cooled. It disappears with rewarming.
    b. **Persistent cutis marmorata.** Occurs in infants with Down syndrome, Cornelia de Lange syndrome, homocystinuria, Menkes disease, familial dysautonomia, trisomy 13, trisomy 18, Divry-Van Bogaert syndrome, and in hypothyroidism, cardiovascular hypertension, and CNS dysfunction.
    c. **Cutis marmorata telangiectatica congenita.** A rare congenital cutaneous vascular malformation. The marbling is persistent, and 20% to 80% have another congenital abnormality with skin atrophy and ulceration. Asymmetry of the lower extremities is the most common extracutaneous finding. The mottling does not disappear with warming. It can be associated with body asymmetry, glaucoma, retinal detachment, neurologic anomalies, and other vascular anomalies. (See Figure 7–2.)

B. **Hair characteristics of the newborn** can vary and can indicate a serious condition, be part of a syndrome, or be normal and isolated. Look at not only the color of the hair but also the amount of hair. Does the infant have hair whorls, which are patches of hair growing in a circular direction with a center point (may indicate intellectual disability and abnormal brain growth)? Does the infant have dry, coarse brittle hair (hypothyroidism)? Does the infant have normal hair mixed with hypopigmented hair (oculocerebral syndrome with hypopigmentation, Cross syndrome)?

1. **Lanugo.** Downy fine unpigmented hair that acts as a protectant in the womb that is seen in infants on surfaces such as the face, back, or ears; more common

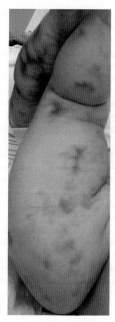

FIGURE 7–2. Cutis marmorata telangiectatica congenita (CMTC). (*Used with permission from Leslie Castelo-Soccio, MD, PhD, Children's Hospital of Philadelphia Division of Dermatology.*)

in premature infants but can be seen in term infants. By the time they are term and born, most infants have lost their lanugo.

2. **Neonatal alopecia (hair loss in the neonate).** Causes include telogen effluvium (hair loss in the first 6 months of life from hormone level drop, high fever, or stress), perinatal trauma causing pressure-induced alopecia (halo ring of hair loss associated with caput succedaneum), birth trauma causing occipital alopecia, pressure over the bony occipital prominence causing occipital hair loss, congenital nevi, aplasia cutis congenita, congenital triangular alopecia, underlying cystic/meningocele lesion, complex developmental disorders (Kabuki syndrome—circumscribed congenital alopecia with severe developmental delay and malformations), hypothyroidism, hypopituitarism, tinea capitis, and rare conditions of total or near total hair loss (atrichia with papular lesions and vitamin D–resistant rickets).

3. **Alopecia areata causes partial (patchy) or total nonscarring hair loss and is very rare in neonates.** Associated with an increased prevalence of human leukocyte antigen alleles DQB1 03 and DRB1 1104. It may be an autoimmune disease or an indicator of severe disease (alopecia totalis/alopecia universalis).

4. **White patch or forelock of hair on the scalp can be is seen in Waardenburg syndrome or tuberous sclerosis.**

5. **Albinism** is autosomal recessive; is characterized by a generalized hypopigmentation of the eyes, skin, and hair (snow white hair, pink eyes, hypopigmented skin); and is seen in all races. Infants with fair skin can have PKU.

6. **Hypopigmented scalp hair can be seen in the following syndromes:** Prader-Willi syndrome, Chédiak-Higashi syndrome, ectrodactyly ectodermal dysplasia clefting syndrome, and piebaldism. Light-colored hair can be seen in

inborn errors of metabolism (PKU) and homocystinuria or can indicate a nutritional deficiency.

7. **Hypertrichosis** ("Werewolf syndrome") is an excessive amount of hair growth for the age, sex, and race of the infant. It can be normal or associated with the following syndromes: trisomy 18, Cornelia de Lange, Coffin-Siris, Barber-Say, Cantu, Hurler, leprechaunism, and others. **Drug-induced hypertrichosis** is seen with fetal hydantoin syndrome and occasionally with fetal alcohol syndrome and postnatal use of diazoxide and corticosteroids. It can also be an indication of congenital adrenal hyperplasia.

8. **Hypotrichosis** can be seen with homocystinuria, ichthyoses, and ectodermal dysplasia.

9. **Hair collar sign** is a ring or collar of long coarser hair that surrounds a bald nodule of skin on the midline of the newborn's scalp. It is a marker of cranial dysraphism, and one needs to rule out meningocele, encephalocele, dermoid cyst, Dandy-Walker malformation, heterotopic brain tissue, or agenesis of the corpus callosum.

C. **Other skin conditions**

1. **Vernix caseosa.** This greasy white substance covers the skin until the 38th week of gestation. Its purpose is to provide a moisture barrier and is completely normal.

2. **Collodion infant.** The skin is covered in a membrane that resembles parchment, and there can be some restriction in growth of the nose and ears. This is usually due to abnormal desquamation, and although sometimes normal, the condition is usually associated with congenital ichthyosis or other rare conditions.

3. **Dry skin.** Infants can have a dry flaky skin, and postdate or postmature infants can exhibit excessive peeling and cracking of the skin. Congenital syphilis and candidiasis can present with peeling skin at birth.

4. **Harlequin fetus.** The most severe form of congenital ichthyosis. Affected infants have thickening of the keratin layer of skin that causes thick scales. Survival of these infants has improved with supportive care. (This condition is different than harlequin sign/coloration.)

5. **Aplasia cutis congenita.** Absence of some or all the layers of the skin. Most common is a solitary area on the scalp (70%). The prognosis is excellent, but if the area is large, surgical repair may be necessary (see Figure 80-1).

6. **Subcutaneous fat necrosis.** A reddish lesion with a firm nodule in the subcutaneous tissue that is freely mobile. It is more common in difficult deliveries, perinatal asphyxia, and cold stress. These lesions are usually benign unless there are extensive lesions, in which case calcium levels should be monitored (see Figure 80-7).

7. **Abnormal fat distribution.** Seen with congenital disorders of glycosylation.

8. **Constriction rings around digits, arms, legs.** Occurs in amniotic band syndrome (see Figure 93-1).

9. **Decreased pigmentation.** Seen in PKU.

D. **Rashes** (rashes are also discussed in Chapter 80)

1. **Milia.** A rash in which tiny sebaceous retention (of keratin) cysts are seen. The whitish yellow pinhead-size concretions are usually on the chin, nose, forehead, and cheeks without erythema (see Figure 80-4). These are seen in approximately 33% of infants, and these benign cysts disappear within a few weeks after birth. **Miliaria** occurs from sweat retention from incomplete closure of the eccrine structures. **Miliaria crystallina** lesions are usually are on the head, neck, and trunk and are from superficial eccrine duct closure. **Miliaria rubra** (heat rash) involves a deeper area of sweat gland obstruction. **Pearls** are large single milia or inclusion cysts that can occur on the newborn's palate (**Epstein pearls**), on buccal or lingual mucosa (**Bohn nodules**), or

dental lamina cysts (on crests of alveolar ridges), genitalia (**penile pearls**), and areola.

2. Sebaceous hyperplasia. In contrast to milia, these raised lesions are more yellow and are sometimes referred to as "miniature puberty of the newborn." The cause is maternal androgen exposure in utero; they are benign and resolve spontaneously within a couple of weeks.

3. Erythema toxicum (erythema neonatorum toxicum). Consists of numerous small areas of red skin with a yellow-white papule in the center. Lesions are most noticeable 48 hours after birth but may appear as late as 7 to 10 days. Wright staining of the papule reveals eosinophils. This benign rash, which is the most common rash in the newborn, resolves spontaneously. If suspected in an infant <34 weeks' gestation, rule out other causes because this rash is more common in term infants (see Figure 80–2).

4. *Candida albicans* rash ("diaper rash"). Appears as erythematous plaques with sharply demarcated edges. Satellite bodies (pustules on contiguous areas of skin) are also seen. Usually the skin folds are involved. Gram stain of a smear or 10% potassium hydroxide prep of the lesion reveals budding yeast spores, which are easily treated with nystatin ointment or cream applied to the rash 4 times daily for 7 to 10 days.

5. Transient neonatal pustular melanosis. A benign, self-limiting condition that requires no specific therapy. The rash starts in utero and is characterized by 3 stages of lesions, which may appear over the entire body: pustules, ruptured vesicopustules with scaling/typical halo appearance, and hyperpigmented macules. These remain after the pustules have resolved (see Figure 80–3).

6. Infantile seborrheic dermatitis. A common rash usually occurring on the scalp "cradle cap," face, neck, and diaper area that is erythematous and with greasy scales. A self-limiting condition that is likely due to maternal hormones.

7. Acne neonatorum (neonatal acne). Lesions are typically seen over the cheeks, chin, and forehead and consist of comedones and papules. The condition is usually benign and requires no therapy; however, severe cases may require treatment with mild keratolytic agents (see Figure 80–6).

8. Herpes simplex. Seen as pustular vesicular rash, vesicles, bullae, or denuded skin. The rash is most commonly seen at the fetal scalp monitor site, occiput, or buttocks (presentation site at time of delivery) (see Figure 80–10).

9. Sucking blisters. Solitary lesions that can be intact blisters or can appear as flat, scabbed areas on the hand or forearm. They are only in areas accessible by the mouth, are benign, and resolve spontaneously.

E. Nevi (moles) can be pigmented, brown or black to bluish, or vascular and may be present at birth (see also Chapter 80).

1. Nevus simplex (fading macular stain; "stork bites," "angel kiss," "salmon patch"). A macular stain is a common capillary malformation normally seen on the occipital area, eyelids, and glabella. They are called "angel kisses" when located on the forehead or eyelids and "stork bites" when on the back of the neck. The lesions disappear spontaneously within the first year of life. Occasionally lesions on the nape of the neck may persist as a medial telangiectatic nevus.

2. Port-wine stain (nevus flammeus). Usually seen at birth, does not blanch with pressure, and does not disappear with time. If the lesion appears over the forehead and upper lip, then **Sturge-Weber syndrome** (port-wine stain over the forehead and upper lip, glaucoma, and contralateral Jacksonian seizures) must be ruled out (see Figure 80–17).

3. Congenital dermal melanocytosis (previously called Mongolian spots) is the most common birthmark. These are slate grey, dark blue, or purple

bruise-like macular spots usually located over the sacrum. Most common in babies of African, Indian, Asian and Hispanic descent, but can occur in <10% of fair-skinned infants. Usually disappear by 5 years of age. (See Figure 80–8.) May be associated with inborn errors of metabolism. Documentation is important because it can be confused with bruising after discharge (child abuse).

4. **Cavernous hemangioma.** Usually appears as a large, red, cyst-like, firm, ill-defined mass and may be found anywhere on the body. Most of these lesions regress with age, but some require corticosteroid therapy. In more severe cases, surgical resection may be necessary. If associated with thrombocytopenia, **Kasabach-Merritt syndrome** (thrombocytopenia associated with a rapidly expanding hemangioma) should be considered.

5. **Strawberry hemangioma (macular hemangioma).** Strawberry hemangiomas are flat, bright red, sharply demarcated lesions that are most commonly found on the face. Spontaneous regression usually occurs (70% disappearance by 7 years of age).

VI. **Head.** Note the general shape of the head. Some amount of molding is normal in all infants and may be more pronounced in infants who are delivered vaginally compared to cesarean section. Inspect for any cuts or bruises secondary to forceps or fetal monitor leads. Check for microcephaly or macrocephaly. Transillumination can be done for severe hydrocephalus and hydranencephaly. Bruising of the vertex of the head is common after birth. Look for unusual hair growth (**hair whorls** are patches of hair growing in a circular direction). Multiple hair whorls or hair whorls in unusual locations can signify abnormal brain growth. **Abnormal hair** can also be seen in some inborn errors of metabolism, including argininosuccinic acidemia, lysinuric protein intolerance, or Menkes kinky hair syndrome. Swelling may represent **caput succedaneum, a cephalohematoma, or a subgaleal hemorrhage.** Examine the occipital, parietal, and frontal bones and the suture lines. The fontanelles should be soft when palpated.

A. **Macrocephaly.** Occipitofrontal circumference is >90th percentile. May be normal or secondary to hydrocephaly, hydranencephaly, or a neuroendocrine or chromosomal disorder.

B. **Microcephaly.** Is a rare neonatal malformation where the infant's head is much smaller compared to babies of the same sex and age. Occipitofrontal circumference is <10th percentile, and brain atrophy or decreased brain size can occur. Causes include infections (rubella, chickenpox, toxoplasmosis, cytomegalovirus, Zika), genetic mutations, malnutrition, exposure to toxins or prescription medications, untreated PKU, or alcohol and substance abuse.

C. **Anterior and posterior fontanelles.** The anterior fontanelle usually closes by 24 months (median age ~13 months) and the posterior fontanelle by 2 months. Normal size of anterior fontanelle is 0.6 to 3.6 cm (African American: 1.4–4.7 cm). Posterior fontanelle size is 0.5 cm (African American: 0.7 cm). A **large anterior fontanelle** can be a normal variation or can be seen in congenital hypothyroidism and may also be found in infants with skeletal disorders such as achondroplasia, osteogenesis imperfecta, or hypophosphatasia, and chromosomal abnormalities such as Down syndrome and in those with intrauterine growth restriction. A **bulging fontanelle** may be associated with increased intracranial pressure, meningitis, or hydrocephalus. **Depressed (sunken) fontanelles** are seen in newborns with dehydration. A **small anterior fontanelle** may be associated with hyperthyroidism, microcephaly, or craniosynostosis.

D. **Cephalic molding.** A temporary asymmetry of the skull resulting from the birth process. Most often seen with prolonged labor and vaginal deliveries, it can be seen in cesarean deliveries if the mother had a prolonged course of labor before delivery. A normal head shape is usually regained within 1 week. Rarely it may be associated with other abnormalities. If it persists, intracranial hypertension can occur.

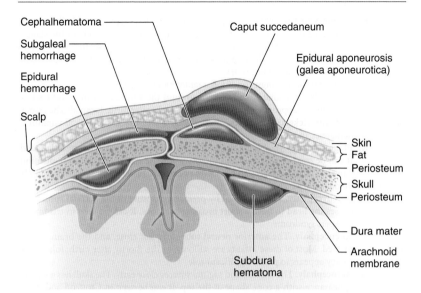

FIGURE 7–3. Types of extradural fluid collections seen in newborn infants. (*Modified from Volpe JJ. Neurology of the Newborn. 4th ed. Philadelphia, PA: WB Saunders; 2001.*)

E. **Caput succedaneum.** A diffuse edematous swelling of the soft tissues of the scalp that **may extend across the suture lines** but usually is unilateral. It does not increase after birth. It is secondary to the pressure of the uterus or vaginal wall on areas of the fetal head bordering the caput. Elicit the characteristic pitting edema by putting firm constant pressure in one area. Usually, it resolves within several days (Figure 7–3).

F. **Cephalhematoma.** A subperiosteal hemorrhage that **never extends across the suture line** and can be secondary to a traumatic delivery or forceps delivery. It increases after birth. Radiographs or computed tomography scans of the head should be obtained if an underlying skull fracture is suspected (<5% of all cephalhematomas). Hematocrit and bilirubin levels should be monitored. Most cephalhematomas resolve in 2 to 3 weeks. Aspiration of the hematoma is rarely necessary (see Figure 7–3).

G. **Subgaleal hematoma/hemorrhage.** The subgaleal area is the area between the scalp and the skull and is a very large space. Hemorrhage occurs between the epicranial aponeurosis and the periosteum, and when pressure is placed, a fluid wave can be seen. It can cross over the suture line and onto the neck or ear. It progresses after birth. It may be necessary to replace blood volume lost and correct coagulopathy if present, and hemorrhage can be life threatening. It can be caused by asphyxia, vacuum extraction, forceps delivery, or coagulopathy (see Figure 7–3).

H. **Increased intracranial pressure.** The increased pressure may be secondary to hydrocephalus, hypoxic-ischemic brain injury, intracranial hemorrhage, or subdural hematoma. The following signs are evident in an infant with increased intracranial pressure:
   1. Bulging anterior fontanelle
   2. Separated sutures
   3. Paralysis of upward gaze ("setting-sun sign")
   4. Prominent veins of the scalp
   5. Increasing macrocephaly

    I. **Craniosynostosis.** The premature closure of ≥1 sutures of the skull; must be considered in any infant with an asymmetric skull. On palpation of the skull, a bony ridge over the suture line may be felt, and inability to move the cranial bones freely may occur. Radiographs of the head should be performed, and surgical consultation may be necessary.

    J. **Craniotabes.** A benign condition, craniotabes is a congenital softening or thinness of the skull that usually occurs around the suture lines (top and back of head) and disappears within days to a few weeks after birth. It can also be associated with rickets, osteogenesis imperfecta, syphilis, and subclinical vitamin D deficiency in utero.

    K. **Plagiocephaly.** An oblique shape of a head, which is asymmetric and flattened. It can be seen in preemies and infants whose heads stay in the same position. Anterior plagiocephaly can be due to premature fusion of the coronal or lambdoidal sutures.

    L. **Brachycephaly.** This is caused by premature closure of the coronal suture and causes the head to have a short broad appearance. It can be seen in trisomy 21 or Apert syndrome.

    M. **Anencephaly.** The anterior neural tube does not close, and the brain is malformed. Most of these infants are stillborn or die shortly after birth; folate deficiency appears to play a significant role.

    N. **Acrocephaly.** The coronal and sagittal sutures close early. The skull has a narrow appearance with a cone shape at the top. It can be seen in Crouzon and Apert syndromes.

    O. **Dolichocephaly/scaphocephaly.** The sagittal suture closes prematurely, and there is a restriction of lateral growth of the skull, resulting in a long, narrow head.

    P. **Skull fracture.** Most commonly occurs secondary to birth trauma from the pressure of the mother's pelvic bones against the skull during labor. Fracture typically involves either a linear (break but no displacement) or depressed ("ping pong" inner buckling of the calvarium) skull fracture. Linear skull fractures usually present with a subgaleal hematoma. Depressed skull fractures may be associated with intracranial bleeding or cephalhematoma and may need further workup.

  VII. **Neck.** Eliciting the rooting reflex (see page 90) causes the infant to turn the head and allows easier examination of the neck. Palpate the sternocleidomastoid for a hematoma and the thyroid for enlargement, and check for thyroglossal duct cysts.

    A. **Short neck.** Seen in Turner, Noonan, Down, and Klippel-Feil syndromes.

    B. **Webbed neck (with redundant skin).** Seen in Turner, Noonan, Down, and Klippel-Feil syndromes.

    C. **Brachial cleft cysts.** Firm, <1-cm cysts that can be on the lateral aspects of the neck, along the anterior margin of the sternomastoid muscle. If dimples are seen here, they are brachial cleft sinuses.

    D. **Cystic hygroma.** The most common neck mass. It is a fluctuant mass that can be transilluminated and is usually found laterally or over the clavicles. Due to lymphatic blockage, it may be associated with chromosomal abnormalities.

    E. **Goiter.** May be a result of maternal thyroid disorders or neonatal hyperthyroidism.

    F. **Thyroglossal duct cyst.** Rarely seen in neonates. They are subcutaneous structures in the midline of the anterior neck at the level of the larynx.

    G. **Torticollis ("wry neck").** A shortening of the sternocleidomastoid muscle that causes the head to go toward the affected side. Treated initially with physical therapy.

 VIII. **Face.** Observe for obvious facial abnormalities such as symmetry of the face. Is there asymmetry of the face with crying? Note the general shape of the nose, mouth, and chin. Look for unequal movement of the mouth and lips. **Coarse facies** (can be seen in acromegaly or inborn errors of metabolism) includes features such as large lips and tongue, saddle-like nose, and large bulging head with prominent scalp veins.

Flat facial profile can be seen in Down syndrome. The presence of **hypertelorism** (eyes widely separated) or **low-set ears** should be noted. If delivered by **forceps, a forceps mark** may be present. It is usually a semicircular mark on the cheek that will resolve spontaneously. **Micrognathia** is a small lower jaw that can interfere with feeding. It is most commonly seen in Pierre Robin sequence but can also be seen in other genetic syndromes.

A. **Low-set ears (melotia).** See Section IX below on ear disorders.

B. **Micrognathia.** A small lower jaw that can interfere with feeding. It is most commonly seen in Pierre Robin sequence but can also be seen in other genetic syndromes.

C. **Hypertelorism (wide-set eyes with extra bone between the eyes).** See page 75.

D. **Asymmetric crying face (ACF),** also called **congenital unilateral lower lip palsy (CULLP).** The face is symmetric at rest and asymmetric during crying, and the mouth is pulled down on one side and not moving on the other side. In ACF, all the other functions of the facial muscles are normal (eg, forehead wrinkling, closure of eyelids, normal sucking, no drooling). Incidence is 1 in 160 live births (usually term, less frequent in preterm) with a male predominance. Major and minor malformations and deformations can be associated with ACF (risk of anomalies is 3.5 times higher, and most common are cardiovascular system and cervicofacial region). It can be caused by nerve compression, agenesis or hypoplasia of the depressor anguli oris muscle (DAOM), or hypoplasia of the depressor labii inferioris muscle (DLIM).

   1. **Nerve compression of one of the branches of the facial nerve** during delivery (mandibular branch of the seventh cranial nerve that innervates the DAOM and DLIM is superficial and is easily compressed). Electromyography shows abnormal values of the mandibular branch of the facial nerve.

   2. **Agenesis or hypoplasia of the depressor anguli oris muscle (DAOM).** Usually on the left side. This muscle controls the downward motion of the lip. The eye and forehead muscles are unaffected with ACF. Ultrasound shows hypoplasia or agenesis of the DAOM.

   3. **Hypoplasia of the depressor labii inferioris muscle (DLIM)** may be associated with other malformations.

E. **Congenital facial nerve paralysis.** This is caused by either trauma (most common) or developmental deformities of the facial nerve (cranial nerve VII).

   1. **Trauma.** The most common cause is birth trauma. Risk factors include an injury from forceps, a large baby, and primiparity. On physical examination, there is facial asymmetry with crying, the corner of the mouth droops, there is drooling on the side of the paresis, the nasolabial fold is absent in the paralyzed side, and there is partial closing of the eye (ptosis). Most symptoms disappear within the first week of life, but sometimes it may take several months. If the palsy persists, absence of the nerve should be ruled out.

   2. **Agenesis of the facial nerve nucleus** (Moebius syndrome) is a rare congenital neurologic disorder that is due to the underdevelopment of cranial nerves VI (lateral eye movement) and VII (facial expression). Infants have facial paralysis, are unable to move their eyes from side to side, and have difficulty swallowing.

IX. **Ears.** Evaluate for an unusual shape or an abnormal position. Confirm that structures of the ear are all present: helix, antihelix, tragus, antitragus, scaphoid/triangular fossa, and external auditory canal. Genetic syndromes are frequently associated with abnormal ear shapes. Assess gross hearing with an infant blinking in response to loud noises. The normal position of ears is determined by drawing an imaginary horizontal line from the inner and outer canthi of the eye across the face, perpendicular to the vertical axis of the head. If the helix of the ear lies below this horizontal line, the ears are designated as **low set.** An otoscopic examination is usually not done on the first examination because the ear canal is usually full of amniotic debris.

A. **Low-set ears (melotia).** Seen with many congenital anomalies, most commonly Treacher-Collins, Down, triploidy, and trisomy 9 and 18 syndromes, fetal aminopterin effects, and trisomy 13 and 21.

B. **Preauricular skin tags (papillomas).** Benign, fairly common, and usually inherited.

C. **Ear pits (preauricular pits).** May be unilateral or bilateral and are usually located at the superior attachment of the pinna. They are more common in the Asian population (~10%).

D. **Hairy ears.** Lanugo hair or can be more prominent in infants of diabetic mothers.

E. **Complete absence of the pinna of the ear (anotia)** is associated with thalidomide and retinoic acid embryopathy. Bilateral anotia is sometimes seen in infants of consanguineous parents.

F. **Small ears (microtia).** Used to describe small pinnae, it is a misshaped dysplastic ear that can be associated with other abnormalities such as middle ear abnormalities. Approximately 50% of infants with microtia will have an underlying congenital syndrome. Pediatric ear, nose, and throat (ENT) evaluation and hearing evaluation are required. A hypoplastic ear may be an indicator of internal ear abnormalities. Renal ultrasound is also recommended. Small ears are seen in trisomy 21, as well as trisomy 18 and 13 triploidy and thalidomide and retinoic acid embryopathy.

G. **Large ears (macrotia).** The auricle is large, and the scaphoid fossa is the most exaggerated part. It is usually bilateral and symmetric. It can be autosomal dominant and can also be associated with Marfan syndrome, fragile X syndrome, De Lange type 2 syndrome, and others.

H. **Lop ear (folded down superior edge of the helix) and cup ear or prominent ear (ear stands away from the head).** Plastic surgery consultation can be obtained.

I. **Satyr ear ("Spock ear").** Characterized by a flattened scaphoid fossa and a flat helix at the superior pole and a third crus into the helix. This is only a cosmetic concern, and molding in the first week of life can be done. Plastic surgery consultation is recommended.

J. **Floppy ears with no cartilage** are associated with bilateral renal agenesis, which is uniformly fatal.

X. **Eyes.** Most infants have some degree of eyelid edema after birth, which usually resolves after the first few days of life. The eyes can still be gently opened and examined. The sclera, which is normally white, can have a bluish tint if the infant is premature because the sclera is thinner in these infants than in term infants. Check for the following: **scleral hemorrhages, exudates** (suggest **conjunctivitis**), and **yellow sclera (icterus)**, which is indicative of hyperbilirubinemia. Check the pupil size bilaterally and verify pupil reactivity; if not the same size, rule out tumor or vascular abnormality. Evaluate eye movements. Is there a **cherry red spot** in the macula of the eye (lipidosis, or occlusion of the central retinal artery)? Check the red reflex with an ophthalmoscope. If a red reflex cannot be obtained or if the pupil is white or cloudy, immediate evaluation by a pediatric ophthalmologist is required. See also Chapter 96.

A. **Leukocoria (opacification of the lens).** A white pupil with loss of a red light reflex. Opacity behind the pupil is sometimes seen without an ophthalmoscope. Evaluate further for:

1. **Congenital cataracts.** If suspected, emergency referral of a pediatric ophthalmologist is necessary for early intervention and to preserve sight. Infants with congenital cataracts should be evaluated for an underlying metabolic, genetic, or infectious cause, and 20% will have an identifiable cause. This can be seen in galactosemia and Zellweger syndrome. An **oil drop cataract** can be seen with galactosemia, and on retinoscopy, one sees a classic "oil droplet" against a red reflex due to accumulation of dulcitol within the lens.

2. **Congenital glaucoma** can present with corneal opacities.

3. **Retinoblastoma.** Tumor requires emergency ophthalmology consultation.
4. **Retinal detachment** is most commonly due to retinopathy of prematurity.
5. **Peters anomaly.** Abnormal cleavage of the anterior chamber occurs from anterior segment dysgenesis. There is a central, paracentral, or complete corneal opacity.

B. **Osteogenesis imperfecta.** Sclera is deep blue.
C. **Small eye (microphthalmia)** is often associated with coloboma.
D. **Colobomas** are missing pieces of tissue in structures of the eye. A key-shaped defect in the iris, eyelid, or other eye structures can be seen, and numerous syndromic and chromosomal abnormalities are associated.
E. **Brushfield spots.** Salt-and-pepper speckling of the iris or white or yellow spots on the iris. Often seen with Down syndrome or may be normal.
F. **Subconjunctival hemorrhage.** Occurs in 5% of newborns as a result of rupture of small conjunctival capillaries and can occur normally but is more common after a traumatic delivery. Petechiae on the forehead may be associated. It is asymptomatic and resolves in a few days.
G. **Conjunctivitis.** Suspected with hyperemia and if a discharge is present. (See Chapter 58.)
H. **Epicanthal folds.** May be normal or may occur in infants with Down syndrome. This is a skin fold of the upper eyelid covering the inner corner of the eye.
I. **Dacryocystoceles.** Obstructions of both the superior and inferior ends of the nasolacrimal duct. Presents as bluish nodules inferior to the medial canthi of both eyes. If bilateral, ENT consult should be obtained to evaluate nasal obstruction.
J. **Dacryostenosis.** The nasolacrimal ducts are too narrow to drain tears properly. Tears may pool on the eyelids and eyelashes. Usually resolves within the first week of life in approximately 50% of infants. In others, it resolves in several weeks to a few months.
K. **Hypertelorism (widely spaced eyes).** The interorbital distance is greater than normal. Normal interorbital distance is 20 mm at birth. This can occur alone or with other congenital deformities.
L. **Nystagmus.** This is an involuntary usually rapid eye movement that can be horizontal, vertical, or mixed. Can be normal if occasional, but if persistent, it needs to be evaluated.
M. **Ptosis.** A drooping of an upper eyelid caused by cranial nerve III paralysis or weakness in the levator muscle. Ptosis and ophthalmoparesis can be seen in transient neonatal myasthenia gravis.
N. **Dysconjugate eye movements.** During the first months of life, infants will have dysconjugate eye movements, where eyes appear to move independently of each other. They may even appear crossed. Transient movements are normal, especially if this occurs when the infant falls asleep or awakes. If the movement is fixed, a consult with a pediatric ophthalmologist should be obtained.

XI. **Nose.** Note the appearance of the nose. Sometimes due to a positional deformity, the nose will be asymmetric. If unilateral or bilateral **choanal atresia** is suspected, verify the patency of the nostrils with gentle passage of a nasogastric tube. **Infants are obligate nose breathers**; therefore, if they have **bilateral choanal atresia,** they will have cyanosis and severe respiratory distress at rest.

A. **Nasal flaring.** Indicative of respiratory distress.
B. **Sniffling/snuffles and discharge.** Typical of congenital syphilis.
C. **Sneezing.** This can be a response to bright light or drug withdrawal.
D. **Dislocated nasal septum.** Incidence of around 4%. The vertical axis of the nose is deviated, and the septum is not straight. Immediate pediatric ENT evaluation is needed, as correction in the first few days of life can prevent a permanent deformity.

XII. **Mouth.** Examine the hard and soft palates for evidence of a cleft palate including submucosal and partial clefts that can be easily missed.

A. **Cleft lip/palate.** Secondary to midline fusion failure. Unilateral clefts are usually an isolated finding; midline clefts are often associated with midline defects in the brain. May interfere with feeding, and ENT consultation is indicated.

B. **Bifid uvula.** The uvula is larger than normal and has 2 halves and may be associated with a submucous palatal cleft.

C. **Positional deformity of the jaw.** Causes asymmetry of the chin, and gums are not parallel to each other, usually due to utero molding. Resolution occurs without treatment.

D. **Epstein pearl.** A small white papule usually in the midline of the palate. Common and benign, it is secondary to epithelial tissue that is trapped during palatal fusion.

E. **Gingival cysts (dental lamina cysts).** Transient oral mucosal cysts located on the alveolar ridge.

F. **Teeth.** Primary teeth usually begin to erupt at 6 to 8 months of age. **Natal teeth** are teeth that are present at birth. **Neonatal teeth** are teeth that erupt during the first 30 days after birth. **Infancy teeth** are teeth that erupt after 30 days. **Supernumerary teeth** are teeth that are not part of the normal dentition and should be extracted. Teeth in newborns are uncommon (prevalence 1:1000 to 1:30,000). Etiology is unknown, but the most common accepted theory is based on hereditary factors. There is conflicting information on sex predilection. The most common area involved is the mandibular region of the central incisors in 85% of cases. Other causes include infection (congenital syphilis has varying effect because some erupt early and some erupt late), endocrine disturbances (excessive secretion by the pituitary, thyroid, or gonads), malnutrition (hypovitaminosis), maternal fever (accelerates eruption), hormonal stimulation, environmental factors (polychlorinated biphenyls [PCBs] and dibenzofuran both increase the occurrence of natal teeth), and position of the tooth germ. The most acceptable theory is hereditary factors causing the superficial localization of the dental follicles. Radiographs are sometimes needed to differentiate whether the teeth are supernumerary or part of the normal deciduous dentition. Clinically, teeth can be classified as mature or immature. Complications include aspiration of the tooth, difficulty in feeding, ulceration to the nipple of the mother, and ulceration to the ventral surface of the tongue (Riga-Fede disease). Pediatric dentistry consultation is recommended to decide treatment (early intervention or no treatment).

1. **Natal teeth (more common).** Erupt most commonly in pairs and are usually poorly attached to the bony structure and can have a poorly developed root system. They are associated with Ellis-van Creveld syndrome, pachyonychia congenita, Rubinstein-Taybi syndrome, steatocystoma multiplex, cyclopia, Pallister-Hall syndrome, short rib polydactyly type II, Wiedemann-Rautenstrauch syndrome, cleft lip and palate, Pfeiffer syndrome, ectodermal dysplasia, craniofacial dysostosis, multiple osteocystomas, adrenogenital, epidermolysis bullosa simplex, Jadassohn-Lewandowski syndrome, Hallermann-Streiff syndrome, Sotos syndrome, and Pierre Robin syndrome. It is best to leave these teeth in the mouth to avoid future space management issues unless symptomatic (highly mobile (risk of aspiration), cause maternal pain during breast feeding, or cause irritation and injury to infant's tongue); then they can be extracted after birth. If loose, it is important to remove the teeth to decrease the risk of aspiration.

2. **Neonatal teeth (less common than natal teeth).** These often have a firm root structure and are typically more securely anchored. If mature and of normal dentition, the tooth should be preserved and maintained in a healthy condition. Pediatric dentistry should be involved with periodic follow-up.

3. **Supernumerary teeth** Evaluate the infant for risk of hemorrhage due to hypoprothrombinemia present in newborns prior to the extraction.

4. **Hutchinson teeth** are an abnormality seen with congenital syphilis. The teeth are smaller, more widely spaced, and have notches on their biting surface. Upper central incisors are the most affected.

G. **Bohn nodules.** Appear as white bumps on the gum (may look like teeth) or periphery of the palate and are secondary from heterotrophic salivary glands or from remnants of the dental lamina. Benign and will resolve without treatment.

H. **Ranula.** Cystic swelling in the floor of the mouth. Many resolve spontaneously, but excision may be indicated in some cases.

I. **Mucocele.** This small lesion on the oral mucosa is secondary to trauma to the salivary gland ducts. Often are benign and resolve spontaneously, but excision may be indicated.

J. **Macroglossia.** Enlargement of the tongue can be congenital or acquired. Localized macroglossia is usually secondary to congenital hemangiomas. Macroglossia can be seen in **Beckwith syndrome** (macroglossia, gigantism, omphalocele, and severe hypoglycemia), **Pompe disease** (type II glycogen storage disease), and **hypothyroidism.**

K. **Glossoptosis.** Downward displacement or retraction of the tongue that is seen in Pierre Robin sequence and Down syndrome.

L. **Ankyloglossia (short lingual frenulum, "tongue tied").** Occurs in 4% to 10% of newborns. Often a frenotomy will be indicated if tongue mobility and feeding are an issue.

M. **Frothy or copious saliva** is commonly seen in infants with an esophageal atresia with tracheoesophageal fistula.

N. **Thrush.** Oral thrush, common in newborns, is a sign of overgrowth of *C albicans*.

O. **Micrognathia (small jaw).** An underdeveloped jaw that is seen in **Pierre Robin syndrome;** other genetic syndromes should be considered.

XIII. **Chest**

A. **Observation.** Note the shape and symmetry of the chest. An asymmetric chest may signify a space- or air-occupying lesion such as tension pneumothorax. Look for tachypnea (increased respiratory rate), retractions (upper and lower chest), xiphoid and sternal subcostal and intercostal retractions, nasal flaring and dilatation, and grunting on expiration. *Note:* **Grunting, nasal flaring, and intercostal or subcostal retractions indicate increased work of breathing.**

1. **Grunting.** Occurs when the glottis is closed during expiration. This improves oxygenation by increasing the end expiratory pressure in the lungs. Occasional grunting is acceptable; grunting with every breath is abnormal. Grunting respirations usually occur in the first few hours of life. In one study, **prolonged or persistent grunting** (lasting >2 hours after birth) in term and near-term infants occurred in 1.2% of newborns. Causes included poor adaptation to extrauterine life (most common cause), transient tachypnea, respiratory distress syndrome, and infection (sepsis and pneumonia). Less common causes included birth trauma, pneumomediastinum, hypoxic ischemic encephalopathy, polycythemia, anemia, meconium aspiration, congenital heart defect, congenital diaphragmatic hernia, malformation of the nose, and immature teratoma of the thymus.

2. **Nasal flaring.** Widening of the nostrils on inspiration; occurs with respiratory distress.

3. **Retractions.** Can be subcostal or intercostal and represent muscles sucked in between the ribs to increase air flow. One sees a shadow at the lower margin of the rib cage with subcostal retractions ("rib shadows"). Mild retractions, usually subcostal, may be normal.

4. **Phonatory abnormalities.** Depend on the level of abnormality or obstruction. Phonation is a primary function of the larynx, and an abnormality of this causes no cry or a weak cry. Laryngeal obstruction can be supraglottic, glottic, or subglottic. A **muffled cry and inspiratory stridor** occur with supraglottic obstruction; a **high-pitched or absent cry** is associated with glottic abnormalities (laryngeal web or atresia). Subglottic stenosis can present with **hoarse or weak cry, stridor,** and obstructive breathing.

a. **Stridor.** A high-pitched sound on inspiration heard without a stethoscope. It can be normal if it occurs occasionally and there are no other signs of respiratory distress. If stridor is persistent, **laryngomalacia is the most common cause.** Other causes include congenital subglottic stenosis, vocal cord paresis, double aortic arch, and other congenital anomalies. **Inspiratory stridor with cyanotic attacks with feeding with aspiration** and pulmonary infections that reoccur can occur with laryngeal and laryngotracheoesophageal clefts.

b. **Intermittent hoarseness, dyspnea, weak cry, or aphonia** can be seen in saccular cysts (a mucus-filled dilatation of the laryngeal saccule).

c. **High-pitched inspiratory stridor and inspiratory cry.** Bilateral vocal cord paralysis.

d. **Weak cry, usually no serious airway obstruction, occasional breathy, feeding problems.** Unilateral vocal cord paralysis.

e. **Mild hoarseness, little airway obstruction.** Thin anterior laryngeal web.

f. **Weaker voice, increased airway obstruction.** Thicker laryngeal webs (>75% glottic involvement) cause aphonia and severe airway obstruction.

g. **Muffled or absent cry.** Laryngeal web or pharyngeal obstruction.

h. **Weak cry, weak sucking, aphonia, and lethargy** can be seen from medications in pregnancy (selective serotonin reuptake inhibitor–induced neonatal abstinence syndrome).

i. **Weak but high-pitched cry resembling a cat.** Cri du chat (5p deletion) syndrome.

j. **Whistling noise** can occur with a blockage in the nostril.

k. **Weak cry.** Hypoglycemia.

l. **Weak cry, mild respiratory distress.** Transient neonatal myasthenia gravis.

m. **High-pitched cry.** Neonatal abstinence syndrome or hypoglycemia.

n. **Hiccups.** Nonketotic hyperglycinemia.

o. **Hoarse cry.** Hypothyroidism.

p. **Aphonia in a newborn.** Laryngeal web, vocal cord paralysis, tracheal agenesis (respiratory distress and impossible to intubate).

B. **Breath sounds.** Listen for the presence and equality of breath sounds. A good place to listen is in the right and left axillae. Absent or unequal sounds may indicate pneumothorax or atelectasis. Absent breath sounds with the presence of bowel sounds plus a scaphoid abdomen (flat abdomen relative to the chest) suggest diaphragmatic hernia; an immediate radiograph and emergency surgical consultation are recommended.

C. **Fractured clavicle.** Palpate both clavicles; if they cannot be palpated easily and crepitus is felt over the clavicle, the infant may have a fractured clavicle. No treatment is necessary. Note that a healed clavicle fracture will have a firm lump (as new bone develops) in the area.

D. **Rib fractures.** Posterior rib fractures are very rare and can result from birth trauma. Risk factors include high birth weight and shoulder dystocia. Other causes include osteogenesis imperfecta, rickets, or fragile bones secondary to prematurity.

E. **Pectus excavatum (funnel chest)** is a sternum that is depressed in shape. Usually, this condition is of no clinical concern but may be associated with Marfan and Noonan syndromes.

F. **Pectus carinatum (pigeon chest).** Caused by a protuberant sternum. May be associated with Marfan and Noonan syndromes.

G. **Prominence of the xiphoid process.** A firm lump at the end of the sternum; it is a benign finding.

H. **Barrel chest.** Occurs when there is an increased anteroposterior diameter of the chest. It can be secondary to mechanical ventilation, pneumothorax, pneumonia, or space-occupying lesions.

I. **Breasts in a newborn.** Usually 1 cm in diameter in term male and female infants and may be abnormally enlarged (3–4 cm) secondary to the effects of maternal estrogens. This maternal effect, which lasts <1 week, is of no clinical concern. A usually white discharge (galactorrhea of the newborn), commonly referred to as **"neonatal milk"** or **"witch's milk,"** may be present and is normal and seen in approximately 5% of term or near-term neonates. It is often seen in infants with larger than average breast nodules and may continue for up to 2 months of age. It is caused by the effects of maternal hormones before birth. The term "witch's milk" is from the ancient folklore that the milk leaking from a newborn's nipple was nourishment for witches or familiar spirits. It is not recommended to remove the milk by massage, as this can cause a neonatal mastitis or breast abscess. **Supernumerary nipples (polythelia)** are extra nipples along the mammary line ("milk line") and occur as a normal variant; their association with renal disorders is *controversial*. They can occur singularly or be multiple and be unilateral or bilateral. Skin tags on the nipple area are usually small and should not be confused with polythelia. **Bloody nipple discharge is rare** in an infant and can be seen in breast-fed and formula-fed infants. Causes can include benign mammary ductal ectasia (most common), ductal hyperplasia caused by maternal hormonal stimulation (usually not bloody), temporarily increased progesterone levels, mastitis (bacterial infection), possible herbal medication use by the mother, and pituitary tumor.

XIV. **Heart.** Observe for heart rate (normal 110–160 beats/min awake, may drop to 80 beats/min during sleep), rhythm, quality of heart sounds, precordium activity, and presence of a murmur. The position of the heart may be determined by auscultation. Physical examination alone can miss up to 50% of cyanotic CCHD, supporting the pulse oximetry screening. (See page 61.) Abnormal situs syndromes and other physical manifestations of congenital heart disease are discussed in Chapter 94.

A. **Murmurs.** May be associated with the following conditions:

1. **Ventricular septal defect.** The most common heart defect, this accounts for approximately 25% of congenital heart disease. Typically, a loud, harsh, blowing, pansystolic murmur is heard (best heard over the lower left sternal border). It is not heard at birth but often on day 2 or day 3 of life. Symptoms such as congestive heart failure usually do not begin until after 2 weeks of age and typically are present from 6 weeks to 4 months. Most of these defects close spontaneously by the end of the first year of life.

2. **Patent ductus arteriosus (PDA).** A harsh, continuous, machinery-type, "washing machine–like," or "rolling thunder" murmur that usually presents on the second or third day of life, localized to the second left intercostal space. It may radiate to the left clavicle or down the left sternal border. It can be heard loudest along the left sternal border. A hyperactive precordium is also seen. Clinical signs include wide pulse pressure and bounding pulses.

3. **Coarctation of the aorta.** A systolic ejection murmur that radiates down the sternum to the apex and to the interscapular area. It is often loudest in the back.

4. **Peripheral pulmonic stenosis.** A systolic murmur is heard bilaterally in the anterior chest, in both axillae, and across the back. It is secondary to the turbulence caused by disturbed blood flow because the main pulmonary artery is larger than the peripheral pulmonary arteries. This usually benign murmur may persist up to 3 months of age. It may also be associated with rubella syndrome.

5. **Hypoplastic left heart syndrome.** A short midsystolic murmur usually presents anywhere from day 1 to 21. A gallop is usually heard.

6. **Tetralogy of Fallot.** Typically, a loud, harsh systolic or pansystolic murmur best heard at the left sternal border. The second heart sound is single.

7. **Pulmonary atresia**
   a. **With ventricular septal defect.** An absent or soft systolic murmur with the first heart sound is followed by an ejection click. The second heart sound is loud and single.
   b. **With intact intraventricular septum.** Most frequently, there is no murmur, and a single second heart sound is heard.
8. **Tricuspid atresia.** A pansystolic murmur along the left sternal border with a single second heart sound is typically heard.
9. **Transposition of the great vessels.** More common in males than females.
   a. **Isolated (simple).** Cardiac examination is often normal, but cyanosis and tachypnea are present along with a normal chest radiograph and electrocardiogram.
   b. **With ventricular septal defect.** The murmur is loud and pansystolic and is best heard at the lower left sternal border. The infant typically has congestive heart failure at 3 to 6 weeks of life.
10. **Ebstein disease.** A long systolic murmur is heard over the anterior portion of the left chest. A diastolic murmur and gallop may be present.
11. **Truncus arteriosus.** A systolic ejection murmur, often with a thrill, is heard at the left sternal border. The second heart sound is loud and single.
12. **Single ventricle.** A loud systolic ejection murmur with a loud single second heart sound is heard.
13. **Atrial septal defects**
    a. **Ostium secundum defect.** Rarely presents with congestive heart failure in infancy. A soft systolic ejection murmur is best heard at the upper left sternal border.
    b. **Ostium primum defect.** Rarely occurs in infancy. A pulmonary ejection murmur and early systolic murmur are heard at the lower left sternal border. A split second heart sound is heard.
    c. **Common atrioventricular canal.** Presents with congestive heart failure in infancy. A harsh systolic murmur is heard all over the chest. The second heart sound is split if pulmonary flow is increased.
14. **Anomalous pulmonary venous return**
    a. **Partial anomalous pulmonary venous return.** Findings are similar to those for ostium secundum defect.
    b. **Total anomalous pulmonary venous return.** With a severe obstruction, no murmur may be detected on examination. With a moderate degree of obstruction, a systolic murmur is heard along the left sternal border, and a gallop murmur is heard occasionally. A continuous murmur along the left upper sternal border over the pulmonary area may also be audible.
15. **Congenital aortic stenosis.** A coarse systolic murmur with a thrill is heard at the upper right sternal border and can radiate to the neck and down the left sternal border. If left ventricular failure is severe, the murmur is of low intensity. Symptoms that occur in infants only when the stenosis is severe are pulmonary edema and congestive heart failure.
16. **Pulmonary stenosis (with intact ventricular septum).** If the stenosis is severe, a loud systolic ejection murmur is audible over the pulmonary area and radiates over the entire precordium. Right ventricular failure and cyanosis may be present. If the stenosis is mild, a short pulmonary systolic ejection murmur is heard over the pulmonic area along with a split second heart sound.

B. **Palpate the pulses (femoral, pedal, radial, and brachial).** Bounding pulses can be seen with PDA. Absent or delayed femoral pulses are associated with coarctation of the aorta.

C. **Check for signs of congestive heart failure.** Signs may include hepatomegaly, gallop, tachypnea, wheezes and rales, tachycardia, and abnormal pulses.

XV. **Abdomen.** See also Chapters 122, 123, and 124.
   A. **Observation.** Obvious birth defects may include an **omphalocele (see Figure 123-3)**, in which organs (usually stomach, intestines, liver) covered by peritoneum protrude out of an opening in the center of the abdomen in the area of the umbilical cord; **gastroschisis (see Figure 123-1), a defect in the abdominal wall to the right of the umbilicus** in which typically the large and small intestines (or other organs) not covered by peritoneum protrude out; or **exstrophy of the bladder (see Figure 127-1)**, in which the bladder protrudes outward through an absent abdominal wall segment.
   B. **Auscultation.** Listen for bowel sounds.
   C. **Palpation.** Check the abdomen for distention, tenderness, or masses. The abdomen is most easily palpated when the infant is quiet or during feeding. In normal circumstances, the liver can be palpated 1 to 2 cm below the costal margin and the spleen tip at the costal margin. Hepatomegaly can be seen with congestive heart failure, hepatitis, some inborn errors of metabolism (storage disorders, urea cycle defects), or sepsis. Splenomegaly is found with cytomegalovirus or rubella infections or sepsis. The lower pole of both kidneys can often be palpated. Kidney size may be increased with polycystic disease, renal vein thrombosis, or hydronephrosis. Abdominal masses are more commonly related to the urinary tract.
   D. **Abdominal circumference.** See page 63.
   E. **Linea nigra.** See page 64.
   F. **Diastasis rectus abdominis.** A protrusion (vertical bulge) from the xiphoid to the umbilicus because of the weakness of the fascia between the 2 rectus abdominis muscles, which causes a separation of the muscles. It can be seen when intraabdominal pressure increases and is typically a benign finding in newborns and will resolve with time.
   G. **Scaphoid abdomen.** A sunken abdomen is associated with congenital diaphragmatic hernia. The abdomen looks flat relative to the chest.
   H. **Prune belly syndrome (Eagle-Barrett syndrome).** Usually seen in males (97%) and of unknown genetic origin, it consists of a large, thin, wrinkled abdominal wall; genitourinary malformations; and cryptorchidism. Surgery may be required, and survival rate has improved.
XVI. **Umbilicus.** Normally, the umbilicus has 2 arteries and 1 vein. The absence of 1 artery occurs in 5 to 10 of 1000 singleton births and in 35 to 70 of 1000 twin births. The presence of **only 2 vessels** (1 artery and 1 vein) could indicate renal or genetic problems (commonly trisomy 18). If there is a **single umbilical artery**, there is an increased prevalence of congenital anomalies (40%) and intrauterine growth restriction and a higher rate of perinatal mortality. If it occurs without any other abnormalities, it is usually benign. **If the umbilicus is abnormal, ultrasonography of the abdomen is recommended.** In addition, inspect for any discharge, redness, or edema around the base of the cord that may signify a **patent urachus or omphalitis.** Some amount of periumbilical erythema is considered normal with separation of the cord. The cord should be translucent; a **greenish yellow color** suggests meconium staining, usually secondary to fetal distress. **Dark stripes** in the cord are intravascular clots and are a normal finding. A normal umbilical cord stump sloughs off at approximately 7 to 10 days of age. (See also Chapter 123, which discusses ophthalmocele and gastroschisis.)
   A. **Omphalitis** is an infection of the cord. This is a very serious condition, can be fatal, and requires immediate treatment. Therefore, any redness of the cord with or without purulent drainage should be promptly evaluated. (See Chapter 80.)
   B. **Patent urachus** is a communication between the bladder and the umbilicus, resulting in urine coming from the umbilicus. Pediatric urology workup is needed to rule out lower urinary tract obstruction. Other urachal abnormalities include urachal cysts and sinuses.

C. **Umbilical hernia.** Results from a weakness in the muscle of the abdominal wall or umbilical ring and usually resolve during the first year of life without treatment. Can be seen in hypothyroidism.

D. **Umbilical hematoma.** From rupture of the umbilical vessels, usually the vein, from birth or trauma or a spontaneous occurrence. Risk factors include traction on the cord, chorioamnionitis, cord prolapse cord torsion, velamentous insertion, short cord, or thinning of the cord from a postdate delivery. They are rare (1:5000) and usually resolve with no treatment.

E. **Umbilical hemangioma.** Rare benign tumor but can be very serious. Complementary studies are needed to evaluate associated anomalies, including cutaneous and systemic hemangiomas and other malformations.

F. **Wharton jelly cyst (umbilical cord pseudocyst).** This is a benign condition in which there is a single or multiple fluid-filled spaces within the umbilical cord where liquefaction of the jelly has occurred. The cord appears translucent and cystic, and 20% of infants will have other abnormalities.

G. **Patent omphalomesenteric (vitelline) duct** is a communication between the ileum and the umbilicus. It presents with drainage of enteric contents, often with a prolapse of the duct and adjacent ileum from the umbilicus.

H. **Umbilical polyp** is a bright red nodule representing intestinal or gastric mucosa remnant.

XVII. **Genitalia.** Any infant with a disorder of sex development (presence of genitalia that do not fit into a male or female classification; formerly called "ambiguous genitalia") should not undergo gender assignment until a formal endocrinology and urologic evaluation has been performed (see Chapter 95). *Note:* **A male with any question of a penile abnormality should not be circumcised until he is evaluated by a pediatric urologist or pediatric surgeon.**

A. **Male genital examination.** Observe the color of the scrotum. Pigment in the scrotum varies depending on the ethnicity and hormonal influence. It can also be hyperpigmented from adrenogenital syndromes. A **bluish color** may suggest testicular torsion or trauma and requires immediate urologic/surgical consultation. Infants will have well-developed scrotal rugae at term; a smooth scrotum suggests prematurity. **Examine the penis**; newborn males always have a marked **phimosis** and the foreskin may not be easily retracted. Verify that the testicles are in the scrotum and examine for groin hernias and masses. If born breech by vaginal delivery, the infant can have bruised and swollen genitals from pressure on the cervix.

1. **Determine the site of the meatus.** Hypospadias is an abnormal location of the urethral meatus on the ventral surface of the penis, **epispadias** is abnormal location of the urethral meatus on the dorsal surface of the penis, **dorsal hood** (foreskin that is incompletely formed that covers the dorsal or top of the penis) is associated with hypospadias, and **chordee** is a dorsal or ventral curvature of the penis. **Megalourethra** is congenital dilation of the urethra usually caused by abnormal development of the corpus spongiosum and will require surgical correction.

2. **Check the size of the penis.** It is important to measure the penile size appropriately. In a supine position, using a rigid ruler pressed firmly against the pubic symphysis, grasp the penis with the other hand and carefully stretch it measuring from the tip of the glans to the base of the penis. The average range of stretched penile length is:

   a. **Newborn 30 weeks' gestation: 2.1–2.9 cm**
   b. **Newborn 34 weeks' gestation: 2.6–3.4 cm**
   c. **Term newborn: 3.1–3.9 cm**

   A **micropenis** is defined as a penis that is 2.5 standard deviations below the mean for a given age, without any hypospadic abnormalities. This corresponds to ≤1.5 cm at 30 weeks' gestation, ≤2.0 cm at 34 weeks' gestation, and ≤2.5 cm in a term newborn.

3. **Palpate and check the size of the testicles.** Normal testicles should be similar in size (normal testicular size at birth: width 1.0 cm, length 1.5 cm, volume 1.0 ± 0.14 cm^3).

4. **Priapism.** Persistent erection of the penis is an abnormal finding and can be seen in polycythemia, but the most common neonatal reason is idiopathic.

5. **Webbed penis.** Penoscrotal web can occur and is a contraindication for circumcision.

6. **Buried penis.** Rare congenital penile deformity where the penis appears buried in the tissues surrounding it. Do not circumcise.

7. **Penile pearls.** Similar to Epstein pearls on palate; can be present on the tip of the foreskin and will resolve with time.

8. **Penile torsion.** Check to see position of the penis and if it is toward the midline. If it is facing the thigh, torsion may be present. Also check the position of the median raphe. It should start and end at the midline of the scrotum and the tip of the penis. Mild torsion of <60 degrees is normal. High degrees of torsion will need to be surgically corrected.

9. **Hypoplastic urethra.** Infants will have thinning of the foreskin on the ventral side and a penile raphe that is not straight. If a feeding tube through the urethra is visible through the skin, then a hypoplastic urethra is present and circumcision is contraindicated. A pediatric urology consult should be obtained.

10. **Undescended testicles.** More common in premature infants. Sometimes term infants will have 1 testicle that has not descended from the abdomen to the scrotum. Palpation of the inguinal canal will verify that the testicle is there. **A unilateral undescended testicle is common** and should be followed by routine physical examinations over time. **Bilateral undescended testicles are considered a disorder of sex development.** An ectopic testicle passes through the inguinal ring and then goes off in another location (perineum, femoral canal, superficial inguinal pouch, or the other hemiscrotum).

11. **Hydroceles.** Hydroceles are common, especially in premature infants, and are collections of fluid in the scrotum. They usually disappear by 1 year of age unless associated with an inguinal hernia. If there is a patent processus vaginalis, the fluid is coming from the peritoneal cavity and it is called a **communicating hydrocele.** Palpation or transillumination will assist in the diagnosis.

12. **Neonatal testicular torsion** accounts for 10% of all testicular torsions, and the majority are extravaginal. The testis twists around its vascular pedicle and compromises arterial, venous, and lymphatic flow, which can result in ischemia, infarction, and necrosis. Infants present with an acute scrotal color change (usually bluish) with no signs of pain (in contrast to older patients). The torsed testicle is smaller in size, and this is a surgical emergency to prevent loss of the organ.

13. **Antenatal testicular torsion.** Usually the scrotal appearance is normal. The torsed testicle can be larger in size and feel more mass-like in texture. A Doppler ultrasound should be done to verify blood flow. The torsed testicle must be removed and the opposite side fixed to prevent torsion since it is at an increased risk.

14. **Inguinal hernia** is common in males. The bowel enters the scrotal sac through the patent processus vaginalis. Presents as a fullness in the inguinal area. Premature infants have a higher risk for inguinal hernias (~3%–5% in term infants and 13% in infants born at <33 weeks of gestational age).

15. **Supernumerary testicle** is very rare and is the presence of >2 testes. The most common type is triorchidism, and it is most often left sided. It can be associated with cryptorchidism, indirect inguinal hernia, torsion, and malignancy.

16. **Scrotal hematoma** is a masslike area of the scrotum secondary to blood products from birth trauma, hypoxia, sepsis, or bleeding diathesis. Rule out hemorrhage from abdomen or retroperitoneum and traumatic testicular rupture.

B. **Female genital examination**

1. **Examine the labia majora and minora and clitoris.** Labia majora of term infants are enlarged and frequently reddish in color secondary to maternal hormones. If the labia are fused and the clitoris is enlarged, adrenal hyperplasia should be suspected. The labia minora decrease in size near term.

2. **Clitoromegaly (a large clitoris).** This can be normal in a premature infant or can be associated with maternal drug ingestion (excess androgens during fetal life) or a disorder of sex development such as congenital adrenal hyperplasia. Normal newborn clitoral length is <7 mm, and mean length is 4 mm. Suspect androgen excess if clitoromegaly and hyperpigmentation (ie, congenital adrenal hyperplasia) are present.

3. **Mucosal/vaginal tag.** Commonly attached to the wall of the vagina and is of no clinical significance.

4. **Discharge from the vagina.** Common and is often clear, thick, and whitish or blood tinged. It is secondary to maternal hormones and only lasts a few days. If bloody discharge (pseudo-menses), this can be normal and secondary to maternal estrogen withdrawal.

5. **Vaginal mass. Benign or malignant neoplasms of the vagina are not very common.** The vaginal mass often can be seen with crying or from increased abdominal pressure. Imaging studies are required. The differential of a vaginal mass in a newborn include: most common (hymenal cysts or paraurethral gland cysts); others are prolapsed urethra, vagina, or uterus; ectopic ureterocele; Gartner's duct cyst; Skene's gland cyst; hydrometrocolpos caused by an imperforate hymen; and rhabdomyosarcoma of the vagina.

6. **Paraurethral cyst (rare).** Interlabial spherical cystic mass that is yellowish in color and can cover both urethral meatus and orifice of the vagina. Surgery is usually not necessary because many resolve spontaneously.

7. **Perineal groove (failure of midline fusion).** Rare. This has 3 major features: moist perineal cleft between the anus and the posterior fourchette, hypertrophy of the labial tails, and normal vagina and urethra. Check anus, as some may have an ectopically placed anus. Conservative management is recommended.

8. **Prolapsed ureterocele.** This is a urologic emergency.

XVIII. **Anus and rectum.** Make sure the infant does not have a fistula. Meconium should pass within 48 hours of birth for term infants. Premature infants are usually delayed in passing meconium. Check for patency of the anus to rule out **imperforate anus** (absence of a normal anal opening). Insert a small feeding tube not >1 cm or observe for passage of meconium. Check the position of the anus using the anal position index (API), and if out of range, consult pediatric surgery.

A. **Anal position index (API).**

1. **API in females.** Measure the distance in centimeters from the posterior fourchette (thin fold of skin at the back of the vulva) to the center of the anus divided by the distance between the fourchette and the lowermost point of coccyx. The mean API in term females is 0.45 ± 0.08. Mean ± 2 standard deviations is considered normal.

2. **API in males.** Measure ratio of the distance between the center of the anus and the first scrotal fold to the distance between the first scrotal fold and the lowermost point of the coccyx. Mean API in males is 0.54 ± 0.07 . Mean ± 2 standard deviations is considered normal.

XIX. **Lymph nodes.** Palpable lymph nodes, usually in the inguinal and cervical areas, are found in approximately 33% of normal neonates.

XX. **Extremities.** Examine the arms and legs, check for lack of movement or pain response upon palpation (fracture). Pay close attention to the digits and palmar creases. (See also Chapter 112.) Most infants have 2 major creases on the palm. A single transverse palmar crease is associated with Down syndrome. Edematous hands and feet can be associated with Turner syndrome. Was the infant born breech? If the infant was born frank breech (baby buttocks aimed at birth canal with legs sticking straight up in front with feet near the head), the legs may maintain this position for days after birth.

A. **Syndactyly.** Abnormal fusion of the digits; most commonly involves the third and fourth fingers and the second and third toes. A strong family history exists. Surgery is performed when the neonates are older. Severe syndactyly can involve all 4 digits being fused together.

B. **Polydactyly.** Supernumerary digits on the hands or the feet. The most common is postaxial polydactyly. This condition is associated with a strong family history. Preaxial polydactyly is less common and may have an underlying medical condition. A radiograph of the extremity is usually obtained to verify whether any bony structures are present in the digit. If there are no bony structures, a suture can be tied around the digit until it falls off. If bony structures are present, surgical removal is necessary. Axial extra digits are associated with heart anomalies. **Polysyndactyly** involves more than a normal amount of digits with fusion of some of them.

C. **Brachydactyly.** This is a shortening of ≥1 digits. It is usually benign if an isolated trait.

D. **Camptodactyly.** This usually involves the little finger and is a flexion deformity that causes it to be bent.

E. **Arachnodactyly.** This is spiderlike fingers that can be seen in Marfan syndrome and homocystinuria.

F. **Clinodactyly.** This usually involves the little finger, is usually benign, and is usually a slight medial incurvation, a radial or ulnar deviation. Can be associated with Down syndrome and other genetic disorders.

G. **Finger or toe hypoplasia.** Nail hypoplasia usually accompanies this. This can be seen in association with maternal teratogens, chorionic villus sampling, chromosome abnormalities, and malformation syndromes, or there can be no cause.

H. **Digit or thumb aplasia.** Amniotic bands can cause missing digits. A workup for genetic and chromosomal causes should be done.

I. **Overlapping toes.** Usually a positional deformity that has no significance if an isolated finding. If other abnormal physical findings are seen, a genetic workup may need to be done.

J. **Nail deformities.** Hypoplastic nails can be seen in Turner syndrome, Edward syndrome (with overlapping digits), nail-patella syndrome, and fetal phenytoin exposure. Hyperconvex nails can be seen in Patau syndrome. The fingernails and toenails may be thickened and abnormally colored or shaped in pachyonychia congenita. It is associated with autosomal dominant inheritance related to an abnormal keratin gene.

K. **Arthrogryposis multiplex congenita.** A persistent contracture of the joints of the fingers that can be associated with oligohydramnios.

L. **Positional deformities of the feet.** Positional deformities of the foot are usually from in utero position, and there is resolution without treatment.

M. **Simian crease.** A single transverse palmar crease is most commonly seen in Down syndrome but is occasionally a normal variant seen in 5% of newborns.

N. **Clubfoot (talipes equinovarus).** More common in males, the foot is turned downward and inward, and the sole is directed medially. If this problem can be corrected with gentle force, it will resolve spontaneously. If not, orthopedic treatment and follow-up are necessary.

O. **Metatarsus varus.** A defect in which the forefoot rotates inward (adduction). This condition usually corrects spontaneously.

P. **Metatarsus valgus** is a defect in which the forefoot rotates outward.

Q. **Rocker bottom feet.** Usually seen with trisomy 13 and 18, it involves an arch abnormality that causes a prominent calcaneus with a rounded bottom of the sole.

R. **Tibial torsion.** This is an inward twisting of the tibia bone that causes the feet to turn in. It is most commonly caused by the position in the uterus and resolves spontaneously.

S. **Genu recurvatum.** The knee is able to be bent backward. This abnormal hyperextensibility can be secondary to joint laxity or trauma and is found in Marfan and Ehlers-Danlos syndromes.

T. **Congenital amputation of arms, legs, digits.** Think amniotic band syndrome or maternal substance use.

U. **Extremity fractures.** Incidence is 0.23 to 0.67 in 1000 live births. The majority are caused by birth trauma from vaginal and cesarean breech deliveries and are easily diagnosed by radiography or ultrasonography. Breech delivery remains the most common factor in long bone fractures. General symptoms include swelling around the broken bone, obvious pain, and constant crying. The **humerus** is the second most commonly fractured bone associated with birth trauma. Humerus fracture occurs from rotation or hyperextension of the upper extremity during delivery. Symptoms include decreased movement, pain with palpation and movement of the affected arm, swelling around the broken bone, and obvious constant crying. If the fracture is near the epiphysis, ultrasound or magnetic resonance imaging is better for diagnosis. **Femur fractures** from birth trauma are rare (0.13 in 1000 live births), are usually secondary to torsional injury leading to a spiral fracture, and usually occur in the proximal half of the femur. Infant may present with no symptoms.

XXI. **Trunk and spine.** Check for any gross defects of the spine. An increased amount of hair on the lower back can be normal in infants who have an increase in pigmentation. Any abnormal pigmentation, swelling, or hairy patches over the lower back should increase the suspicion that an underlying vertebral or spinal abnormality exists. A sacral or pilonidal dimple may indicate a small meningocele or other anomaly. Congenital midline vascular lesions may raise suspicion about occult spinal dysraphism (eg, spinal bifida occulta), and if the lesions appear with other abnormal findings, then imaging studies should be done.

A. **Sacral dimples below the line of the natal cleft are benign** (within 2.5 cm of the anus) and have a visible base and no other abnormalities on physical examination. These require no further evaluation. If they are above the natal cleft, an ultrasound is indicated to check for a track to the spinal cord.

B. **Coccygeal pits.** A simple dimple in which the base cannot be seen. These are benign.

C. **Sacral skin tags.** Require spinal ultrasound examination to rule out spinal dysraphism. They may also represent a residual tail.

D. **Meningomyelocele.** A neural tube defect in which there is incomplete closure of the posterior spine; the lumbar spine is the most common location.

XXII. **Hips.** (See also Chapter 112.) When examining the hips, the most important clinical aspect is to **screen for developmental dysplasia of the hip (DDH).** This is a very controversial topic regarding definition, screening, and treatment. The majority of physicians agree that screening is important because the earlier DDH is detected, the simpler and more effective is the treatment. **The AAP published a policy statement in 2000 and an updated clinical report in 2016.** The AAP indicates that screening is beneficial to prevent the late presentation after 6 months of age with hip dislocation or subluxation.

There is no uniform definition of DDH, as the exact definition is controversial. It includes a spectrum of hip disorders, including mild instability of the femoral head, frank dislocation (head of femur is completely out of the acetabulum [hip socket]), partial dislocation, dysplastic hips (spectrum of femoral head or acetabulum dysgenesis that can often be seen radiologically that may or may not cause clinical instability), and subluxated (head of the femur is simply loose in the socket and moves to the edge but not out of the hip socket) or malformed acetabula.

It is difficult to differentiate what developmental variation is versus true disease. The majority of physicians agree it is a condition in which the femoral head has an abnormal relationship to the acetabulum.

A. **Controversy regarding screening and treatment.** Screening is *controversial*, as most mild cases of DDH (neonatal hip instability and dysplasia) resolve spontaneously. Note that no screening program has been shown to completely eliminate the risk of a late presentation of a dislocated hip. The following are the various screening guidelines from the US Preventive Services Task Force (USPSTF), Cochrane review, AAP, American Academy of Orthopedic Surgeons (AAOS), Pediatric Orthopedic Society of North America (POSNA), and Canadian Task Force on DDH:

1. **US Preventive Services Task Force.** "Based on insufficient evidence, the USPSTF does not recommend routine screening for developmental dysplasia of the hip (DDH) as a means to prevent adverse outcomes." This statement only applies to infants who do not have obvious hip dislocations or other abnormalities evident without screening.

2. **Cochrane review.** "There is insufficient evidence to give clear recommendations for practice on screening programs for developmental dysplasia of the hip. There is evidence that delaying treatment for infants with unstable but not dislocated hips, or infants who on ultrasound have mild hip dysplasia by 2 to 8 weeks decreases the need for treatment without a huge increase in late diagnosed dysplasia or surgery."

3. **AAP.** " The AAP recommends that all newborn infants be screened for DDH by physical examination. They also recommend frequent follow up at scheduled well infant visits up to 6 to 9 months of age. For preterm infants they feel that despite the medical urgencies the infant has, it is critical to do a complete physical examination as DDH may go unrecognized in premature infants."

4. **AAOS, POSNA, and Canadian Task Force on DDH.** Each group recommends newborn and periodic screening for DDH.

B. **Incidence. Clinical instability of the hips occurs in approximately 1% to 2% of full-term infants.** The incidence of developmental dislocation of the hip is approximately 1 in 1000 live births. Up to 15% of infants have hip instability or hip immaturity seen on imaging.

1. **Risk factors for DDH.** The majority of infants with DDH do not have any risk factors. Risk factors are additive.

   a. **Breech presentation in the third trimester for both males and females** is probably the **single most important risk factor,** with an incidence of 2% to 27% of boys and girls presenting in breech position. The highest risk is in a female presenting frank breech (sacral presentation, hips flexed, knees extended). Breech position near the end of pregnancy contributes to DDH more than just the breech delivery. Risk may be decreased with cesarean delivery. Breech-associated DDH is milder and has a more rapid spontaneous normalization.

   b. **Female sex with no other risk factors** accounts for 75% of DDH. More common in white females (9:1), this condition is more likely to be unilateral and to involve the left hip. It may be increased in females because of the hormone relaxin, which males are protected from. It makes ligaments stretchier and bones more likely to move out of position.

    c. **Positive family history.** When a first-degree relative is affected, the infant has a 12-fold increased risk of DDH compared with controls. The left hip is more likely to be involved. **Genetics may play** a bigger role than previously thought. If a monozygotic twin has DDH, the risk is 40% to the other twin; if a dizygotic twin has DDH, the risk is 3%.

    d. **Incorrect/improper lower extremity swaddling.** Traditional swaddling puts the hips in an extended and adducted position, which increases the risk of DDH. Traditional swaddling occurs in Navajo Indian, Turkish, and Japanese infants, in whom an increase in DDH is seen.

C. **Recommendations and best practices from the AAP, POSNA, AAOS, and Canadian DDH Task Force.** The goal for the physician is to be able to diagnose hip subluxation or dislocation by 6 months of age. This is done by periodic physical examination and selective ultrasound or radiography, with consultation by orthopedics or a pediatric radiologist.

    1. **Screen all newborns (even premature infants) by physical examination for DDH.** This is the **most important primary screening tool.** Remember, most DDH occurs in infants without risk factors.

        a. **Evaluate for asymmetric thigh or buttock gluteal creases.** Normal inguinal folds do not extend beyond the anus. This is better to observe when the infant is prone.

        b. **Determine if there is limb length discrepancy.** Shortening of the affected leg is a warning sign.

        c. **Test for limited or asymmetric abduction.** Restricted movement can be a significant sign. Normal findings include abduction to 75 degrees and adduction to 30 degrees in a supine infant with stable pelvis. Best to perform after 3 months of age when it is generally positive.

        d. **Perform the Ortolani test.** Perform the Ortolani test (preferred) with or without the Barlow test. Best to perform before 3 months of age, at which point the dislocated hip becomes fixed, making these tests not useful. The Barlow test can be performed but has no proven predictive value for hip dislocation.

           i. **The Ortolani test for stability** (a reductive maneuver) is "where a subluxated or dislocated femoral head is reduced into the acetabulum with gentle hip abduction." This is the most important clinical test for detecting newborn dysplasia. **Do this test gently.** Place the infant in the frog-leg position. Abduct the hips by using the middle finger to apply gentle inward and upward pressure over the greater trochanter. A "clunk sensation" is a palpable and sometimes audible sound that corresponds to the femoral head being dislocated or reduced on exam. It is a significant finding and denotes a true positive test. A hip click is a benign or palpable sound that is caused by benign soft tissue movement and is not associated with the movement of the femoral head, is not predictive of DDH, and, therefore, is clinically insignificant.

          ii. **The Barlow maneuver can be performed but has less clinical significance when compared to the Ortolani maneuver. It has no proven predictive value for future hip dislocation.** It is a test with flexion, adduction, and posterior pressure that tests for laxity. It is "where a reduced femoral head is gently adducted until it becomes dislocated or subluxated." The significance of the Barlow test has been questioned, and some feel there is no value in performing it. In addition, if performed too forcefully or too many times, it could cause instability by stretching the capsule unnecessarily. **AAP recommends that if it is performed that one should gently adduct** the hip while palpating for the head falling out the back of the acetabulum. There should be no posterior directed force applied. A palpable

"clunk" during the Barlow maneuver indicates positive instability with a positive test.
2. **Imaging. Ultrasound or radiography** can be used at any age between 4 and 6 months ("watershed period"). Most sources agree that universal ultrasound imaging is not recommended. The **AAP Choosing Wisely campaign** states "when an infant exhibits no risk factors or physical findings, a screening hip ultrasound to rule out developmental hip dysplasia or developmental hip location should not be ordered." **Selective imaging** is recommended, which includes:
    a. **Hip ultrasonography** should be performed and interpreted using the American College of Radiology and American Institute of Ultrasound in Medicine guidelines by experienced examiners.
      i. **AAP recommends** that one can consider selective hip ultrasound from 6 weeks to 6 months of age in high-risk infants without positive findings. High-risk factors include male or female breech presentation, positive family history, concerned parents, suspicious but inconclusive periodic examination, history of a previous positive instability, and history of tight lower extremity swaddling.
      ii. **AAOS states that moderate evidence** supports performing an imaging study on all infants <6 months old if they have 1 of the following risk factors: breech presentation, family history, or clinical instability.
    b. **Radiography (anteroposterior and frog pelvis plain radiographs). Historically used to diagnose an infant with DDH.** Plain radiography is not recommended before 4 to 6 months of age since the femoral head is composed of cartilage and will not be readily seen. If used, it is recommended after 4 to 6 months of age when the ossification center develops in the femoral head. Because the position can affect the results, make sure the pelvis is not rotated or the gonadal shield is not covering the hip joint. Hip asymmetry, subluxation, and dislocation can be seen on a radiograph when the infant has dysplasia. There is controversy on whether minor variability on the radiograph constitutes actual disease.
      i. **AAP** notes that radiography can be considered for diagnosis in any infant without physical findings >4 months old with risk factors or any infant with an abnormal examination (positive clinical findings).
      ii. **AAOS states there is limited evidence** to use an anteroposterior pelvic radiograph instead of ultrasound at 4 months of age to assess DDH.
3. **Orthopedic referral for suspected hip abnormalities**
    a. **Obtain an orthopedic referral** for a positive Ortolani test, a dislocated hip on a physical examination, or any infant >4 weeks of age who has limited or asymmetric hip abduction.
    b. **Possible indications for an orthopedic referral** include any infant with risk factors for DDH, questionable physical examination, or concern of pediatrician or parents.
XXIII. **Nervous system.** Observe the infant for any abnormal movement (eg, seizure activity, bicycling, and jitteriness) or excessive irritability. **Jitteriness** can be stopped if the extremity is held (unlike **seizures,** which cannot be stopped) and can be normal or be secondary to hypoglycemia (most common), hypocalcemia, or drug withdrawal. Remember, neurologic symptoms of hypotonia, lethargy, poor sucking, seizures, and coma can be seen with some inborn errors of metabolism, which are discussed in Chapter 100. Then evaluate the following parameters:
  A. **Muscle tone**
    1. **Hypotonia.** Observe the posture and activity of the infant. Pick the infant up and see that the arms fall back and almost feel like a ragdoll. In ventral

suspension, the head drops very low, and there is an exaggerated convex curvature of the spine. Floppiness and head lag are seen.

2. **Hypertonia.** Increased resistance is apparent when the arms and legs are extended. Hyperextension of the back and tightly clenched fists are often seen.

B. **Reflexes.** The following reflexes are considered normal for a newborn infant. These primary reflexes reflect normal brainstem activity. CNS depression/injury should be suspected if these reflexes cannot be elicited, and their persistence beyond a certain age can suggest damage of cortical functioning.

1. **Protective reflex.** If the nose and eyes are covered with something, the infant will arch and make efforts to move the item away.

2. **Rooting reflex.** Stroke the lip and the corner of the cheek with a finger and the infant will turn in that direction and open the mouth. This helps the infant find the breast to initiate breast feeding, and this reflex disappears at 4 months.

3. **Babkin reflex.** If both thumbs are pressed equally against the palms, there is a reflex opening of the mouth and a twist of the head on the vertical axis until the median line, and at the same time, the head is bowed forward. This reflex is normal in the first 10 weeks of life; persistence after 12 weeks suggests spastic-motor development disorder.

4. **Glabellar reflex (blink reflex).** Tap gently over the forehead and the eyes will blink.

5. **Sucking reflex.** Touch roof of baby's mouth with finger, pacifier, breast, or bottle nipple and the infant begins to suck. This reflex begins after 32 weeks of pregnancy and is fully developed at 36 weeks. Preterm infants may have a weak sucking ability.

6. **Grasp reflex (palmar grasp).** Place a finger or object in the palm of the infant's hand and the infant will grasp the finger (flexion of the fingers will occur). This reflex is also present in the feet of a newborn. Stroke up the middle of the foot and the toes will curl under as if to grasp the examiner. It is present until 2 to 3 months of age.

7. **Galant reflex.** Suspend the infant in a prone position. Stroke the back in a cephalocaudal direction. The infant should respond by moving the hips toward the stimulated side.

8. **Neck-righting reflex.** Turn the infant's head to the right or left, and movement of the contralateral shoulder should be obtained in the same direction.

9. **Asymmetric tonic neck reflex (fencing reflex).** With the infant in a supine position, turn the infant's head to one side, and the arm and leg on the side of the head that is turned will extend outward, and there will be flexion of the limbs on the opposite side. This is the fencing position.

10. **Moro reflex (startle reflex).** Support the infant behind the upper back with 1 hand, and then drop the infant back ≥1 cm to, but not on, the mattress. This should cause symmetrical abduction of both arms and extension of the fingers followed by flexion and adduction of the arms. Asymmetry may signify a fractured clavicle, hemiparesis, or brachial plexus injury. An absent Moro reflex is of concern and may signify CNS pathology. This reflex normally disappears at 4 to 5 months.

11. **Plantar grasp.** When one strokes the ball of the foot, the toes will curl.

12. **Placing reflex.** Hold the infant upright and place the dorsum of the foot by the edge of the bed; the infant places the foot on the surface. This reflex disappears by 5 months of age.

13. **Stepping/walking reflex.** Hold the infant upright under his or her arms while supporting the infant's head and have the infant's feet touch a flat surface. The infant will appear to take a step and walk.

14. **Positive support reflex.** Hold the infant under the arms with head support, have the feet bounce on a flat surface, and the infant will extend the legs for 20 seconds and then flex the legs into a sitting position.

15. **Swimming reflex.** Place an infant abdomen down in a pool of water and the infant will paddle and kick in a swimming motion up to 6 months of age.

C. **Cranial nerves.** Note the presence of gross nystagmus, the reaction of the pupils, and the ability of the infant to follow moving objects with his or her eyes.

D. **Movement.** Check for spontaneous movement of the limbs, trunk, face, and neck. A fine tremor is usually normal. Clonic movements are not normal and may be seen with seizures.

E. **Peripheral nerves**

1. **Brachial plexus injuries.** These involve damage to the spinal nerves that supply the arm, forearm, and hand. Etiology is multifactorial.

a. **Erb-Duchenne paralysis (upper arm paralysis).** Involves injury to the fifth and sixth cervical nerves and is the most common brachial plexus injury. There is adduction and internal rotation of the arm. The forearm is in pronation, the power of extension is retained, the wrist is flexed, and the Moro reflex is absent. This condition can be associated with diaphragm paralysis.

b. **Klumpke paralysis (lower arm paralysis).** Involves the seventh and eighth cervical nerves and the first thoracic nerve. The hand is flaccid with little or no control. If the sympathetic fibers of the first thoracic root are injured, ipsilateral ptosis, enophthalmos, and miosis (**Horner syndrome**) can rarely occur.

c. **Paralysis of the entire arm.** The entire arm is limp and cannot move. The reflexes are absent.

2. **Facial nerve palsy.** Intrauterine position or forceps can cause compression of the seventh cranial nerve. This results in ptosis, unequal nasolabial folds, and asymmetry of facial movement. Differentiate it from **asymmetric crying facies,** which can be caused by nerve compression, or agenesis or hypoplasia of the depressor anguli oris muscle or hypoplasia of the depressor labii inferioris muscle, which controls the downward motion of the lip. The eye and forehead muscles are not affected in this condition. Asymmetric crying facies can be associated with major and minor deformations or 22q11 deletion.

3. **Phrenic nerve injury.** This can occur secondary to a brachial plexus injury. It causes paralysis of the diaphragm, leading to respiratory distress.

F. **General signs associated with neurologic disorders**

1. **Symptoms of increased intracranial pressure.** Bulging anterior fontanelle, dilated scalp veins, separated sutures, and setting sun sign. (See page 71.)

2. **Hypotonia or hypertonia.**

3. **Irritability or hyperexcitability.**

4. **Poor sucking and swallowing reflexes.**

5. **Shallow, irregular respirations.**

6. **Apnea.**

7. **Apathy.**

8. **Staring.**

9. **Seizure activity.** Sucking or chewing of the tongue, blinking of the eyelids, eye rolling, and hiccups.

10. **Absent, depressed, or exaggerated reflexes.**

11. **Asymmetric reflexes.**

8 Temperature Regulation

The chance of survival of neonates is markedly enhanced by the successful prevention of excessive heat loss. The newborn infant must be kept under a **neutral thermal environment**. This is defined as the external temperature range within which metabolic rate and hence oxygen consumption are at a minimum while the infant maintains a normal body temperature (Figures 8–1 and 8–2 and Table 8–1). The **normal skin temperature** in the neonate is 36.0°C to 36.5°C (96.8–97.7°F), and the **normal core (rectal) temperature is** 36.5°C to 37.5°C (97.7–99.5°F). **Axillary temperature** may be 0.5°C to 1.0°C lower (95.9–98.6°F). A normal body temperature implies only a balance between heat production and heat loss and should not be interpreted as the equivalent of an optimal and minimal metabolic rate and oxygen consumption.

I. **Hypothermia and excessive heat loss.** Preterm infants are predisposed to heat loss because they have a high ratio of surface area to body weight (3–5 times more than the adult), little insulating subcutaneous fat, and reduced glycogen and brown fat stores. In addition, their hypotonic ("frog") posture limits their ability to curl up to reduce the skin area exposed to the colder environment.

A. **Mechanisms of heat loss in the newborn include the following:**

1. **Radiation.** Heat loss from the infant (warm object) to a colder nearby (not in contact) object. It is the major source of daily heat loss (40% or more without clothing/blanket and low room air movement and room air temperature of 24–26°C).

2. **Conduction.** Direct heat loss from the infant to the surface with which he or she is in direct contact such as lying on a cold table or under an x-ray plate.

3. **Convection.** Heat loss from the infant to the surrounding air proportional to the surrounding air temperature and movement velocity.

4. **Evaporation.** Heat loss by water evaporation from the skin of the infant. Immediately after delivery, evaporative heat loss may contribute to >50% of all heat loss. Thereafter, its magnitude is inversely proportional to the degree of immaturity. The underdeveloped stratum corneum results in higher skin permeability for the extremely low birthweight infant (<1000 g body weight). Transepidermal water loss as high as 6 to 8 mL/kg/h may be seen in the most immature infants during the first weeks of life.

B. **Consequences of excessive heat loss.** In contrast to adults, the newborn is unable to compensate for heat loss by increasing production through shivering and increased muscular activity. Heat production is thus performed through a nonshivering process (nonshivering thermogenesis) that involves oxidation of fatty acids from brown fat. Brown adipocytes are found in a discrete location in the cervical-supraclavicular area (the most common) and in perirenal/adrenal and paravertebral regions around the major vessels. They contain a large number of mitochondria, hence their brown coloration. Temperature receptors sensing a low temperature stimulate increased sympathetic output from the central nervous system, resulting in norepinephrine release, which in turn stimulates β-adrenergic receptors in brown fat, increasing cyclic adenosine monophosphate production. The release of cytoplasmic stores of triglycerides and fatty acids increases metabolism, resulting in increased oxygen consumption and heat production. This compensatory augmentation in heat production through the increase in metabolic rate includes the following:

1. **Insufficient oxygen supply and hypoxia** from increased oxygen consumption that can be 2 or 3 times as high as the normal resting value.

2. **Hypoglycemia secondary** to depletion of glycogen stores.

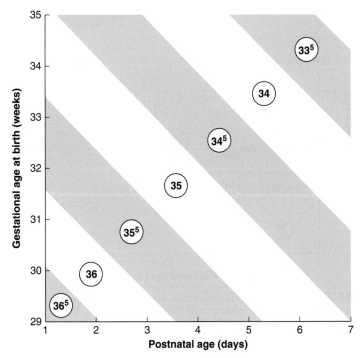

FIGURE 8–1. Neutral thermal environment during the first week of life (in degrees Celsius), based on gestational age. (*Reproduced with permission from Sauer PJ, Dane HJ, Visser HK: New standards for neutral thermal environment of healthy very low birthweight infants in week one of life,* Arch Dis Child. *1984 Jan;59(1):18-22.*)

    3. **Metabolic acidosis** caused by hypoxia and peripheral vasoconstriction.
    4. **Decreased growth.**
    5. **Apnea.**
    6. **Pulmonary hypertension** as a result of acidosis and hypoxia.
  C. **Consequences of hypothermia.** As the capacity to compensate for the excessive heat loss is overwhelmed, hypothermia will ensue.
    1. **Clotting disorders** such as disseminated intravascular coagulation and pulmonary hemorrhage can accompany severe hypothermia.
    2. **Shock** with resulting decreases in systemic arterial pressure, plasma volume, and cardiac output.
    3. **Intraventricular hemorrhage.**
    4. **Severe sinus bradycardia.**
    5. **Increased neonatal mortality.**
  D. **Treatment of hypothermia.** Rapid versus slow rewarming continues to be **controversial**, although the trend is toward more rapid rewarming. Rewarming may induce apnea, hypotension, and rapid electrolyte shifts (Ca^{2+}, K^+); therefore, the hypothermic infant should be continuously and closely monitored regardless of the rewarming method. One recommendation is to rewarm at a rate of 1°C/h unless the infant weighs <1200 g, the gestational age is <28 weeks, or the temperature is <32.0°C (89.6°F) and the infant can be rewarmed more slowly (with a rate not to exceed 0.5°C/h). Another

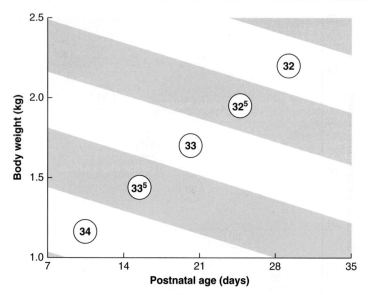

FIGURE 8–2. Neutral thermal environment from days 7 to 35 (in degrees Celsius), based on body weight. (*Reproduced with permission from Sauer PJ, Dane HJ, Visser HK: New standards for neutral thermal environment of healthy very low birthweight infants in week one of life,* Arch Dis Child. *1984 Jan;59(1):18-22.*)

recommendation is that, during rewarming, the skin temperature not be >1°C warmer than the coexisting rectal temperature.

1. **Equipment and techniques**
   a. **Closed incubators.** Usually used for infants who weigh <1800 g. Closed incubators are convectively heated (heated airflow); therefore, they do not prevent radiant heat loss unless they are provided with double-layered walls. Similarly,

Table 8–1. APPROXIMATE NEUTRAL THERMAL ENVIRONMENT IN INFANTS WHO WEIGH >2500 G OR ARE >36 WEEKS' GESTATION[a]

Age	Temperature (°C)
0–24 hours	31.0–33.8[b]
24–48 hours	30.5–33.5
48–72 hours	30.1–33.2
72–96 hours	29.8–32.8
4–14 days	29.0–32.6
>2 weeks	Data not established[b]

[a]For infants <2500 g or <36 weeks, see Figures 8–1 and 8–2.
[b]In general, the smaller the infant, the higher the temperature.
Data from Scopes JW, Ahmed I: Range of critical temperatures in sick and premature newborn babies, *Arch Dis Child.* 1966 Aug;41(218):417-419.

evaporation loss is compensated for only when additional humidity is added to the incubator. One disadvantage of incubators is that they make it difficult to closely observe a sick infant or to perform any type of procedure. Body temperature changes associated with sepsis may be masked by the automatic temperature control system of closed incubators. Such changes will hence be expressed in the variations in the incubator's environmental temperature. An infant can be weaned from the incubator when his or her body temperature can be maintained at an environmental temperature of <30.0°C (usually when the body weight reaches 1600–1800 g). Enclosed incubators maintain a neutral thermal environment by using one of the following devices:

i. **Servo-controlled skin probe attached to the abdomen of the infant.** If the temperature falls, additional heat is delivered. As the target skin temperature (36.0–36.5°C) is reached, the heating unit turns off automatically. A potential disadvantage is that overheating may occur if the skin sensor is detached from the skin or the reverse if the infant is lying on the probe-attached side.

ii. **Air temperature control device.** The temperature of the air in the incubator is increased or decreased depending on the measured temperature of the infant. Use of this mode requires constant attention from a nurse, and it is usually used in older infants.

iii. **Air temperature probe.** This probe hangs in the incubator near the infant and maintains a constant air temperature. There is less temperature fluctuation with this kind of probe.

b. **Radiant warmer.** Typically used for very unstable infants or during the performance of medical procedures. Heating is provided by radiation and therefore does not prevent convective and evaporative heat loss. The temperature can be maintained in the "servo mode" (ie, by means of a skin probe) or the "nonservo mode" (also called the "manual mode"), which maintains a constant radiant energy output regardless of the infant's temperature. Serious overheating can result from mechanical failure of the controls, from dislodgment of the sensor probe, or from manual operation without careful monitoring. Deaths are associated with hyperthermia-induced radiant warmers. On manual mode, such as in the delivery room, they should be used only for a limited period. Insensible water loss may be extremely large in the very low birthweight (VLBW) infant (up to 8 mL/kg/h). Covering of the skin with semipermeable dressing or the use of a water-based ointment (eg, Aquaphor) may help reduce insensible transepidermal water loss. Improved thermal stability can be provided by the addition of a heating mattress.

c. **Hybrid incubator.** More recent development of a hybrid incubator allows the intermittent use of a vertically adjustable radiant heater as well as drop-down incubator walls to improve access while allowing for better control of environmental humidity. Lesser incidence of bronchopulmonary dysplasia and better fluid balance and growth velocity have been reported with the use of these new types of incubators.

d. **Kangaroo mother care.** The infant is placed skin-to-skin in a vertical position between the mother's breasts and under her clothes. This technique was initially advocated as an effective way for mothers to keep their full-term babies warm while breastfeeding and as an alternative method of caring for low-birthweight babies in resource-limited countries. More recently, intermittent kangaroo care skin-to-skin contact (SSC), provided by the mother or father, has been introduced in resource-rich countries for babies requiring neonatal intensive care—even extremely premature infants and those on ventilators. Conduction of heat from parent to infant is sufficiently high to compensate for the increase in evaporative and convective heat loss seen during SSC. Enhanced parental bonding, facilitation of breast feeding, better sleep patterns, and procedural pain relief are some of its purported benefits.

2. **Temperature regulation in the healthy term infant (weight >2500 g).** Studies have shown that a healthy term infant can be wrapped in warm blankets and placed directly into the mother's arms without any significant heat loss.
   a. Place the infant under a preheated radiant warmer immediately after delivery.
   b. Dry the infant completely to prevent evaporative heat loss.
   c. Cover the infant's head with a cap.
   d. Place the infant, wrapped in blankets, in a crib.
3. **Temperature regulation in the sick term infant.** Follow the same procedure as that for the healthy term infant, except place the infant under a radiant or hybrid warmer with temperature servoregulation.
4. **Temperature regulation in the premature infant (weight 1000–2500 g).**
   a. For an infant who weighs 1800 to 2500 g with no medical problems, use of a crib, cap, and blankets is usually sufficient.
   b. For an infant who weighs 1000 to 1800 g:
      i. A well infant should be placed in a closed incubator with servo-control.
      ii. A sick infant should be placed under a radiant or hybrid warmer with servo-control.
5. **Temperature regulation in the extremely low birthweight (ELBW) infant (weight <1000 g).** See Chapter 13.
   a. **In the delivery room.** Considerable evaporative heat loss occurs immediately after birth. Consequently, speedy drying of the infant has been emphasized as a very important aspect of the management of the ELBW infant. A more efficient and different approach has been advocated whereby the infant is placed in a plastic bag from feet to shoulders, without drying, immediately at birth.
   b. **In the nursery.** Either the radiant warmer or the incubator can be used, depending on the institutional preference. **Hybrid devices** offer the combined features of radiant warmer and closed incubator with controllable humidity in a single device, allowing for seamless conversion between modes as deemed clinically necessary.
      i. Radiant warmer
         (a) Use servo-control with the temperature for abdominal skin set at 36.0°C to 36.5°C.
         (b) Cover the infant's head with a cap.
         (c) To reduce convective heat loss, place plastic wrap (eg, Saran Wrap) loosely over the infant. Prevent this wrap from directly contacting the infant's skin. Avoid placing the warmer in a drafty area.
         (d) Maintain an inspired air temperature of the hood or ventilator of ≥34.0°C to 35.0°C.
         (e) Place under the infant a heating pad (K-pad) that has an adjustable temperature between 35.0°C and 38.0°C. To maintain thermal protection, it can be set between 35.0°C and 36.0°C. If the infant is hypothermic, the temperature can be increased to 37.0°C to 38.0°C (*controversial*).
         (f) If the temperature cannot be stabilized, move the infant to a closed incubator (in some institutions).
      ii. Closed incubator. Excessive humidity and dampness of the clothing and incubator can lead to excessive heat loss or accumulation of fluid and possible infections.
         (a) Use servo-control, with the temperature for abdominal skin set at 36.0°C to 36.5°C.
         (b) Use a double-walled incubator if possible.
         (c) Cover the infant's head with a cap.
         (d) Keep the humidity level at ≥40% to 50% (as high as 89% if needed).
         (e) Keep the temperature of the ventilator at ≥34.0°C to 35.0°C.
         (f) Place under the infant a heated mattress (K-pad) that has an adjustable temperature between 35.0°C and 38.0°C. For thermal protection,

the temperature can be set between 35.0°C and 36.0°C. For warming a hypothermic infant, it can be set as high as 37.0°C to 38.0°C.

(g) **If the temperature is difficult to maintain,** try increasing the humidity level or use a radiant warmer (in some institutions).

II. **Hyperthermia.** Defined as a temperature that is greater than the normal core temperature of 37.5°C.

A. **Differential diagnosis**

1. **Environmental causes.** Some causes include excessive environmental temperature, overbundling of the infant, placement of the incubator in sunlight, a loose skin temperature probe with an incubator or radiant heater in servo-control mode, or a servo-controlled temperature set too high.

2. **Infection.** Bacterial or viral infections (eg, herpes).

3. **Dehydration.**

4. **Maternal fever in labor.**

5. **Maternal epidural analgesia during labor.**

6. **Drug withdrawal.**

7. **Unusual causes**

a. **Hyperthyroid crisis or storm**

b. **Drug effect** (eg, prostaglandin E_1)

c. **Riley-Day syndrome** (periodic high temperatures secondary to defective temperature regulation)

B. **Consequences of hyperthermia.** Hyperthermia, like cold stress, increases metabolic rate and oxygen consumption, resulting in tachycardia, tachypnea, irritability, apnea, and periodic breathing. If severe, it may lead to dehydration, acidosis, brain damage, and death. The risk of neurologic injury after asphyxia has been shown to be enhanced in the presence of elevated infant's body temperature.

C. **Treatment**

1. **Defining the cause of the elevated body temperature is the most important initial issue.** Determine whether the elevated temperature is the result of a hot environment or increased endogenous production, such as is seen with infections. In the former case, one may find a loose temperature probe, an elevated incubator air temperature, and the temperature of the extremities of the infant as high as the rest of the body. In the case of "true fever," one expects a low incubator air temperature as well as cold extremities secondary to peripheral vasoconstriction.

2. **Other measures.** Turn down any heat source and remove any excessive clothing.

3. **Additional measures for older infants with significant temperature elevation:**

a. **A tepid water sponge bath.**

b. **Acetaminophen** (5–10 mg/kg per dose, orally or rectally, every 4 hours).

c. **Water-filled cooling blanket** such as the Kool-Kit Neonate and Blanketrol III (Cincinnati Sub-Zero, Cincinnati, OH; see Figure 43–1).

9 Respiratory Management

The management of infants with respiratory distress has long been a basic function of neonatal intensive care. Today, death from acute respiratory failure is uncommon, even among the extremely premature, but significant morbidity from mechanical ventilation persists. Current trends in neonatal ventilation focus on reducing ventilator-induced lung injury, and noninvasive support is preferred. When mechanical ventilation is needed, new ventilators cede as much control as possible to the patient. Optimal treatment continues to be difficult to define, and considerable variability exists in assessing the risk–benefit ratio of various management strategies. This chapter provides an overview of current techniques used for neonatal respiratory support.

I. **Assessing and monitoring respiratory status**

    A. **Physical examination.** The presence of the following signs may be useful in recognizing respiratory distress and evaluating the response to treatment. The absence of signs may be secondary to neurologic depression rather than absence of pulmonary disease.

        1. **Nasal flaring.** One of the earliest signs of respiratory distress, nasal flaring may be present in intubated, ventilated patients as well.

        2. **Grunting.** Commonly seen early in respiratory distress syndrome (RDS) and transient tachypnea, grunting is a physiologic response (partial closure of the glottis during expiration) to prevent end-expiratory alveolar collapse. Grunting helps maintain functional residual capacity (FRC) and therefore oxygenation.

        3. **Retractions.** Intercostal, subcostal, and sternal retractions are present in conditions of decreased lung compliance or increased airway resistance and may persist during mechanical ventilation if support is inadequate.

        4. **Tachypnea.** A respiratory rate >60 breaths/min implies the inability to generate an adequate tidal volume and may persist during mechanical ventilation.

        5. **Cyanosis.** Central cyanosis indicates hypoxemia. Cyanosis is difficult to appreciate in the presence of anemia. Acrocyanosis is common shortly after birth and is not a reflection of hypoxemia.

        6. **Abnormal breath sounds.** Inspiratory stridor, expiratory wheezing, and rales should be appreciable. Unfortunately, unilateral pneumothorax may escape detection on auscultation.

    B. **Blood gases.** Management of ventilation, oxygenation, and changes of acid-base status is most accurately determined by **arterial blood gas studies.**

        1. **Arterial blood gas studies.** The most standardized and accepted measure of respiratory status, especially for the oxygenation of low-birthweight infants. They are considered invasive monitoring and require arterial puncture or an indwelling arterial line. Access is now considered routine by the umbilical artery or peripherally in the radial or posterior tibial artery.

        2. **Normal arterial blood gas values.** May not be the same as target values for particular patients, nor acceptable values. Table 9–1 lists examples of normal values for infants.

        3. **Calculated arterial blood gas indexes.** For determining progression of respiratory distress and are as follows:

            a. **Alveolar-to-arterial oxygen gradient ($AaDO_2$).** Greater than 600 mm Hg for successive blood gases over 6 hours is associated with high mortality in most

Table 9–1. NORMAL RANGE OF ARTERIAL BLOOD GAS VALUES FOR TERM AND PRETERM INFANTS AT NORMAL BODY TEMPERATURE AND ASSUMING NORMAL BLOOD HEMOGLOBIN CONTENT[a]

Gestational Age	PaO_2 (mm Hg)	$PaCO_2$ (mm Hg)	pH	HCO_3 (mEq/L)	BE/BD
Term	80–95	35–45	7.32–7.38	24–26	±3.0
Preterm (30–36 weeks' gestation)	60–80	35–45	7.30–7.35	22–25	±3.0
Preterm (<30 weeks' gestation)	45–60	38–50	7.27–7.32	19–22	±4.0

HCO_3, bicarbonate; BE, base excess; BD, base deficit.
[a]Values for PaO_2, $PaCO_2$, and pH are measured directly by electrodes. HCO_3 and BE/BD values are calculated from nomograms of measured values at normal (14.8–15.5 mg/dL) hemoglobin content and body temperature (37°C) and assuming hemoglobin saturation of ≥88%.

infants if treatment and ventilation do not become effective. The formula for **AaDO$_2$** is

$$A - aDO_2 = \left[(FiO_2)(Pb - 47) - \frac{PaCO_2}{R} \right] - PaO_2$$

where Pb = barometric pressure (760 mm Hg at sea level), 47 = water vapor pressure, $PaCO_2$ is assumed to be equal to alveolar PCO_2, and R = respiratory quotient (usually assumed to be 1 in neonates).

b. **Arterial-to-alveolar oxygen ratio (a/A ratio).** Also an index for effective respiration. The a/A ratio is the most often used index for evaluation of response to surfactant therapy and is used as an indicator for inhaled nitric oxide therapy for pulmonary hypertension. The formula for the a/A ratio is

$$a/A = PaO_2 \Big/ \left[(FiO_2)(Pb - 47) - \frac{PaCO_2}{R} \right]$$

4. **Venous blood gases.** Determination of values is the same as for arterial blood gases, but the interpretation is different. The pH values are slightly lower, and $PvCO_2$ values are slightly higher, whereas PvO_2 values are of no value in assessing oxygenation.

5. **Capillary blood gases.** Arterializing of capillary blood is done by warming the infant's heel just before sampling. The pH value is usually slightly lower, and the PCO_2 is usually slightly higher than arterial values, but this may vary considerably depending on the sampling technique. PO_2 data are of no value.

C. **Noninvasive blood gas monitoring.** Use of these technologies is strongly encouraged. They allow for continuous monitoring and can dramatically reduce the frequency of blood gas sampling, reducing iatrogenic blood loss and decreasing cost. Blood gas sampling is still necessary for calibrating noninvasive measures, determining acid-base status, and detecting hyperoxia.

1. **Pulse oximetry.** The pulse oximeter measures the relative absorption of light by saturated and unsaturated hemoglobin, which absorbs light at different frequencies. The ratio changes in response to the rapid influx of arterial blood during the upstroke of the pulse. Through the detection of the peak of the ratio, the oximeter is able to determine the pulse rate and the percentage of arterial oxygen saturation. SaO_2 is arterial oxygen saturation by direct measurement; SpO_2 is arterial oxygen saturation by pulse oximetry.

a. **Limitations.** Include poor correlation of SaO_2 to PaO_2 at upper and lower PaO_2 values. SaO_2 of 88% to 93% corresponds to PaO_2 of 40 to 80 mm Hg. For infants with high or low saturations, arterial blood gas correlation is needed.

b. **Advantages.** Include minimal damage to the skin and no required manual calibration. SaO_2 by pulse oximetry is less affected by skin temperature and perfusion than transcutaneous oxygen ($tcPO_2$).

c. **Disadvantages.** Include the tendency of patient movement and excessive external lighting to interfere with readings and the lack of correction for abnormal hemoglobin (eg, methemoglobin).

2. **Transcutaneous oxygen ($tcPO_2$) monitoring.** Measures the partial pressure of oxygen from the skin surface by an electrochemical sensor. Contact is maintained through a conducting electrolyte solution and an oxygen-permeable membrane.

a. **Limitations.** Include the need for daily recalibration, relocation to different skin sites every 4 to 6 hours, and irritation or injury to a premature infant's skin secondary to adhesive rings and thermal burns. Poor skin perfusion caused by shock, acidosis, hypoxia, hypothermia, edema, or anemia may prevent accurate measurements.

b. **Advantages.** $tcPO_2$ is noninvasive and *may* provide indication of excessively high PaO_2 (>100 mm Hg).

3. **Near-infrared spectroscopy (NIRS).** The light-absorbing characteristics of oxygenated and deoxygenated hemoglobin are used for this technique. NIRS relies on this differential absorption of light and also on the relatively transparent nature of tissue to infrared light to give an estimation of tissue oxygenation. NIRS represents a weighted average of arterial and venous saturation, which varies from tissue to tissue and over time.

4. **Transcutaneous carbon dioxide monitoring (tcPCO$_2$).** Usually accomplished simultaneously by a single lead enclosed with a tcPo$_2$ electrode.

5. **End-tidal carbon dioxide (CO$_2$) monitoring (ETCO$_2$ or PetCO$_2$).** Expired breath analysis by infrared spectroscopy for CO$_2$ content gives close correlation to PaCO$_2$. This technique is increasingly available for neonates. It gives rapid information about changes in CO$_2$, unlike the slow response time of tcPCO$_2$.

   a. **Limitations.** An adapter to the endotracheal tube is required, which may significantly increase the dead space of the patient's circuit. Accuracy is limited when the respiratory rate is >60 breaths/min or if the humidity of inspired air is excessive. Current devices are of limited use for premature infants.

   b. **Advantages.** It is a noninvasive technique that may correlate well with arterial PaCO$_2$.

D. **Monitoring mechanical ventilation.** Modern mechanical ventilators measure and display many variables.

1. **Inspired oxygen.** Fraction of inspired oxygen (FiO$_2$) is a percentage of oxygen available for inspiration. It is expressed either as a percentage (21%–100%) or as a decimal (0.21–1.00).

2. **Airway pressure.** Measured either at the endotracheal tube connector or within the ventilator, depending on the specific machine. The ventilator may display set and/or measured pressures for mechanical and/or spontaneous breaths. Pressures of common interest are:

   a. **Peak inspiratory pressure (PIP).** The maximum pressure reached during inspiration. The need for high PIP reflects poor pulmonary compliance or the use of excessively large tidal volume.

   b. **Positive end-expiratory pressure (PEEP).** The pressure maintained between breaths. A PEEP of 3 to 4 cm H$_2$O is considered physiologic. Lung compliance is often improved by increasing PEEP to 5 to 6 cm H$_2$O in RDS.

   c. **Mean airway pressure (Paw).** Average of the proximal pressure applied to the airway throughout the entire respiratory cycle (Figure 9–1).

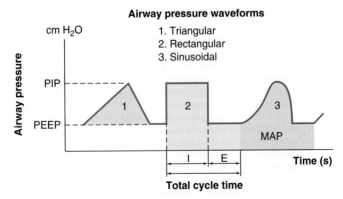

FIGURE 9–1. Graphic representation of ventilator airway pressure waveforms and other ventilator terminology. See Glossary (page 116) for explanations.

    i. $\overline{Paw}$ correlates well with mean lung volume for a given mode and strategy of mechanical ventilation.

    ii. $\overline{Paw}$ >10 to 15 cm H_2O during conventional ventilation is associated with an increased risk of air leaks (pneumothorax or pulmonary interstitial emphysema).

    iii. $\overline{Paw}$ of high-frequency ventilation is *not* strictly comparable with the $\overline{Paw}$ of conventional mechanical ventilation.

3. **Tidal volume (V_T).** A function of PIP during mechanical ventilation, V_T is integrated from flow (mL/s) and measured as milliliters per breath. By convention, V_T is expressed as breath volume adjusted to body weight as milliliters per kilogram. Newer infant ventilators allow setting desired V_T and will adjust PIP automatically in certain modes.

4. **Minute volume (MV).** The respiratory rate and V_T combine to give MV as

$$MV = Rate \times V_T$$
Example: 40 breaths/min × 6.5 mL/kg = 260 mL/kg/min.

5. **Pressure-volume (P-V) and flow-volume (F-V) loops.** A visualization of breath-to-breath dynamics. Flow, volume, and pressure signals combine to give P-V and F-V loops. Loops give inspiratory and expiratory limits of the breath cycle. F-V loops provide information regarding airway resistance, especially restricted expiratory breath flow. P-V loops illustrate changing lung dynamic compliance.

6. **Compliance (C_L).** Values of <1.0 cm H_2O/mL are consistent with interstitial or alveolar lung disease such as RDS. Lung compliance of 1.0 to 2.0 mL/cm H_2O reflects recovery, as in after surfactant therapy.

7. **Resistance (R_L).** Value of >100 cm H_2O/L/s is suggestive of airway disease with restricted airflow such as in bronchopulmonary dysplasia or the need for airway suctioning.

8. **Time constant (K_T).** The product of $C_L \times R_L$ (in seconds). Normal values are 0.12 to 0.15 seconds. K_T is a measure of how long it takes for alveolar and proximal airway pressures to equilibrate. At the end of 3 time constants, 95% of the V_T has entered (during inspiration) or left (during expiration) the alveoli. To avoid gas trapping, the measured expiratory time should be >3 times K_T (0.36–0.45 seconds).

E. **Chest radiographs.** Chest radiographs (see Chapter 12) are essential to the diagnosis of lung disease, in the management of respiratory support, and in the investigation of any acute change in respiratory status.

II. **Types of respiratory support.** Infants with respiratory distress may need only supplemental oxygen, whereas those with respiratory failure and apnea require mechanical ventilatory support. This section reviews the spectrum of available means for ventilatory support, with the exception of high-frequency ventilation (see Section V below). Mechanical ventilatory support offers great benefits but also incurs significant risks. There continues to be considerable ***controversy*** concerning the proper use of any mode or strategy of assisted ventilation. Current practice uses the capabilities of ventilators to automatically coordinate support with patient effort with the goal of maintaining consistent ventilation with minimal risk for mechanical lung injury.

A. **Oxygen supplementation without mechanical ventilation.** Hypoxic infants able to maintain adequate minute ventilation are assisted with free-flow oxygen or air-oxygen mixtures. Continuous pulse oximetry is useful to monitor adequate oxygenation.

1. **Oxygen hoods.** Provide an enclosure for blended air-oxygen supply, humidification, and continuous oxygen concentration monitoring. Hoods are easy to use and provide access to and visibility of the infant.

2. **Mask oxygen.** Usually not as well tolerated or controlled as nasal cannula oxygen delivery.

Table 9–2. **NASAL CANNULA CONVERSION TABLE**

	FiO$_2$			
Flow Rate (L/min)	100%	80%	60%	40%
0.25	34%	31%	26%	22%
0.50	44%	37%	31%	24%
0.75	60%	42%	35%	25%
1.00	66%	49%	38%	27%

General guideline only; numbers are not exact.

3. **Nasal cannula.** Well suited for infants needing low concentrations of oxygen. Delivery can be controlled by flow meters delivering as little as 0.025 L/min. Flow rates of >1 L/min impart distending airway pressure. Table 9–2 gives approximate percentages of nasal cannula oxygen based on flow rates of 0.25 to 1.0 L/min at blended FiO$_2$ settings of 40% to 100%.

B. **Continuous positive airway pressure (CPAP).** A nasal mask, nasal prongs, or an endotracheal tube can be used to apply CPAP to improve PaO$_2$ by stabilizing the airway and allowing alveolar recruitment. CO$_2$ retention may result from excessive distending airway pressure.

1. **CPAP devices** can be broadly divided into 2 types according to their use of flow for CPAP delivery: **continuous or variable flow.**

   a. **Continuous-flow CPAP devices**

      i. **Bubble CPAP.** A warmed humidified gas is continuously provided through the inspiratory limb using a blender and a flow meter. CPAP is created by submersing the expiratory limb of the respiratory tubing into a water chamber to the depth of the desired cm H$_2$O CPAP level. A sufficient flow of gas through the system creates continuous bubbling in the water chamber. Benefits to gas exchange and lung recruitment due to the high-frequency oscillatory content of the bubbling have been hypothesized and disputed. The bubbly bottle CPAP pressure-generating system has the advantage that the adequacy of flow can be seen and heard. However, the pressure at the nares is often higher than the predicted positive pressure based on the set immersion depth. The advantages of bubble CPAP lie mostly in its ease of application and its low cost. Few clinical data are available to infer its superiority over other CPAP devices. Its resurgence in popularity relates to the report of a remarkably low incidence of bronchopulmonary dysplasia (BPD) in a single medical center using this form of CPAP.

      ii. **Ventilator-derived CPAP.** Infant ventilators are used to provide a continuous flow of a blended gas. CPAP is modulated by varying the ventilator's expiratory orifice size. The expiratory valve works in conjunction with other controls, such has flow control and pressure transducers, to maintain the CPAP at the desired level. It is thus less likely than bubble CPAP to be influenced by the presence of a variable leak from the intermittent opening of the oral cavity. It also allows for rapid and simple transition to noninvasive positive-pressure ventilation when required.

   b. **Variable flow CPAP.** These devices (such as Infant Flow SiPAP System) use a dedicated driver and generator with unique fluidic mechanics that adjust and redirect gas flow throughout the respiratory cycle. The expiratory limb of the device is open to the atmosphere. Such devices may assist spontaneous

breathing and reduce the work of breathing by reducing expiratory resistance and maintaining a stable airway pressure throughout respiration. It requires specially designed nasal prongs.
2. **CPAP modes of delivery**
   a. **Nasal mask CPAP.** Requires the proper size mask and a good seal on the face to be effective. Although more cumbersome than nasal prongs, a mask reduces risk of injury to the nasal septum.
   b. **Nasal CPAP (nCPAP).** Because newborn are "obligatory" nose breathers, nasal prongs are the most commonly applied means of delivering CPAP and are used for respiratory assistance in an infant with mild RDS. The prongs are also used after extubation to maintain airway and alveolar expansion in the process of weaning from mechanical ventilation and recovery from respiratory diseases. This treatment maintains upper airway patency and, as such, is useful in infants with apnea of infancy. nCPAP may range from 2 to 8 cm H_2O, although 2 to 6 cm H_2O is most often used. Overdistention of the bronchioles and alveoli can lead to excessive CO_2 retention or air leak (pneumothorax). Gastric distention may be a complication of nCPAP, and an orogastric tube for decompression should be used. Infants can be fed by nasogastric tube during nasal CPAP therapy with close monitoring of abdominal girth.
   c. **Nasopharyngeal CPAP.** An alternative to nasal prongs. An endotracheal tube or long binasal prongs are passed nasally and advanced to the nasopharynx. A ventilator or CPAP device is used to deliver continuous distending pressure as with nasal prongs. This approach is slightly more secure in active infants and may cause less trauma to the nasal septum.
   d. **Endotracheal tube CPAP.** Rarely used or indicated in neonates.
C. **Heated humidified high flow nasal cannula (HHHFNC).** This recent development in neonatal noninvasive respiratory support is gaining popularity and is increasingly being used in clinical practice worldwide. A number of differently branded HHH-FNC devices exist, including the Vapotherm 2000i (Vapotherm Inc. Stevensville, MD, USA) and the Fisher & Paykel Healthcare (Auckland, New Zealand, and Irvine, CA, USA) devices.
   Three main features are common to the high flow (4-L min) delivery devices:
1. **A respiratory circuit** with a means to maintain the temperature and, by extension, the humidity of the continuously delivered gas (of variable FiO_2) until the distal end of the circuit.
2. **A humidifier** to effectively warm and humidify the respiratory gases
3. **Short binasal prongs** with adapter that connects to the delivery circuit and allow little or no excess tubing between the end of the delivery circuit and the actual nasal prongs, minimizing gas cooling and precipitation.
   HHHFNC generates ends expiratory positive airway pressures that is not measured but "estimated" to vary generally between 2 and 10 cm H_2O. This level of pressure is influenced by flow rate (4–8 L/min), nasal cannula size (not to exceed 30%–50% of the nares width), mouth position (oral leak will decrease generated pressures by 50%), and infant size.
   In addition to generating PEEP, HHHFNC may also reduce minute ventilation demand by overcoming increased airway resistance and flushing extrathoracic dead space, thereby reducing rebreathed exhaled CO_2.
   Most meta-analysis suggest a statistically significant difference only for nasal trauma leading to a change of treatment, favoring HHHFNC over NCPAP. Supporting preterm infants on HHHFNC was equivalent in efficacy as any other form of NIV (NIPPV or nCPAP). This efficacy was mainly observed in the moderate to late preterm infants (>28 weeks' gestation at birth), and after extubation from IPPV. There were no statistically significant differences in the odds of death or air leaks or chronic lung disease.

The greater ease of use of HHHFNC devices compared with NCPAP allows both practitioners and family members to handle and care for infants (ELBWIs). Its efficacy compared to CPAP has not been established in particular among infants with a gestation at birth <26 weeks.

The same level of monitoring and nursing observations should be adopted as would be in place for a baby receiving nCPAP. Any patient with nasal trauma from nCPAP should be considered a candidate for rescue with HHHFNC.

D. **Noninvasive ventilation.** This refers to any technique that uses constant or variable pressure to provide ventilatory support, but without tracheal intubation. Sometimes this term includes CPAP techniques described previously. Common examples are **nasal intermittent positive-pressure ventilation (NIPPV)** that combines nCPAP with superimposed ventilator breaths, which may be **synchronized NIPPV (SNIPPV)** with patient breathing movements. (CPAP [PEEP] ranges from 3 to 6 cm H_2O, whereas PIP is set at 10 cm H_2O above CPAP. Inspiratory time ranges from 0.3 to 0.5 seconds and respiratory rate from 10 to 60 breaths/min.) It may be assumed that the pressure delivered is variable and frequently lower than the set PIP, mostly because of leakage at the nose and mouth. For SNIPPV, a technically unsolved problem is the reliable identification of spontaneous breathing efforts in preterm infants to synchronize the noninvasive ventilation. **NIPPV** may be used as a primary mode of respiratory support in preterm infants with RDS but is more often used as a method to decrease the risk of postextubation failure or need for reintubation. Nasal ventilation seems to be particularly helpful in managing apnea. NIPPV may lead to abdominal distension and possibly gastrointestinal perforation. Nasal trauma and leak around the prongs are commonly seen; therefore, careful selection of prong size and monitoring of position are important.

E. **Mechanical ventilation.** The decision to initiate mechanical ventilation is complex. The severity of respiratory distress, severity of blood gas abnormalities, natural history of the specific lung disease, and degree of cardiovascular and other physiologic instabilities are all factors to be considered. **Because mechanical ventilation may result in serious complications, the decision to intubate and ventilate should not be taken lightly.**

1. **Bag-and-mask or bag-to-endotracheal tube handheld assemblies.** These allow for emergency ventilatory support. Portable manometers are always required for monitoring peak airway pressures during hand-bag ventilation. Bags may be self-inflating or flow-dependent, anesthesia-type bags. All handheld assemblies must have pop-off valves to avoid excessive pressures to the infant's airway (see Figure 3–2).

2. **Conventional infant ventilators.** Conventional mechanical ventilation delivers physiologic tidal volumes at physiologic rates via an endotracheal tube. Modern microprocessor-controlled ventilators provide numerous modes of ventilation, which vary in the degree to which patient effort controls the ventilator. These modes are critically dependent on the function of flow and/or pressure sensors for accurate performance.

   a. **Ventilator settings.** Various modes of mechanical ventilation are determined by the parameters that are set by the clinician to determine the characteristics of the mechanical breath and the circumstances under which it is delivered. Not all modes are available on every ventilator, and subtle differences between the same modes may exist between different manufacturers. The characteristics of each breath are as follows:

      i. **Length of breath (T_i).** Either set by the clinician and machine controlled or patient controlled.

         (a) **Time cycled.** Each mechanical breath lasts for a machine-controlled set time: 0.2 to 0.3 seconds for extremely low birthweight (ELBW), up to 0.5 to 0.6 seconds for term.

(b) **Flow cycled.** Each mechanical breath lasts until inspiratory flow falls below a threshold (when the patient reaches end inspiration). The T_i will vary, usually in response to changes in patient effort.

ii. **Size of breath (VT)**

(a) **Volume limited.** Each mechanical breath is the same volume; the pressure used may vary in response to patient effort.

(b) **Pressure limited.** A set pressure is reached with each mechanical breath.

(c) **Volume assurance/guarantee.** The clinician sets both a maximum PIP and a desired VT (target volume) for mechanical breaths. Once the target VT is reached, the ventilator cuts the inspiration short. Some ventilators will decrease PIP for a breath if previous breaths have been cut short. If subsequent breaths are below target VT, the ventilator increases PIP until the set maximum PIP is reached. Ideally, volume assurance/guarantee delivers consistent VT, even with varying patient effort and/or variable lung pulmonary mechanical characteristics.

iii. **Frequency of mechanical breaths**

(a) **Intermittent mandatory ventilation (IMV).** Breaths are delivered at set "mandatory" intervals without regard to patient spontaneous breathing effort.

(b) **SIMV (synchronized IMV).** Breaths are provided a preset number of times, as in standard IMV, but these are synchronized with the infant's spontaneous respiratory effort. During expiration, there is a brief refractory period so that triggering of the mechanical breath can occur only within a trigger window to prevent a mandatory breath to be started during a spontaneous expiratory effort. If no spontaneous effort is detected during a trigger window, a mandatory inflation will be given. Spontaneous breaths in excess of the set ventilator rate are not supported. The minimum and maximum ventilator rates are equal.

(c) **A/C (assist/control).** Each patient initial respiratory effort triggers a ventilator breath. If no effort is sensed, a minimum set rate is delivered. Maximum rate may be much higher than minimum. Excessive trigger sensitivity may lead to auto cycling and much greater rates than needed.

(d) **Pressure support ventilation.** Each patient respiratory effort triggers a concomitant partial assisted mechanical inflation that results in a breath. There is no mandatory backup rate.

iv. **Patient triggers.** The advanced patient-regulated ventilation modes available with modern microprocessor-controlled ventilators depend on reliable detection of patient initial respiratory effort. In the smallest premature infants, it is difficult to separate flow or pressure changes due to inspiratory effort from those due to measurement error or leaks.

(a) **Flow determinations by a pneumotachometer or mass airflow sensors.** Sensors at the patient airway are often more reliable.

(b) **Pressure.** Pressure triggers may be confused by ringing within the circuit, especially with rainout in the tubing.

(c) **Neural.** Using a bipolar esophageal lead placed at the level of the diaphragm, phrenic nerve impulses to the diaphragm can be detected and used to trigger mechanical breaths. Flow and pressure sensors trigger during a breath. Neural sensors potentially allow for the onset of a mechanical breath to match onset of the spontaneous effort. This promising technology has yet to be fully evaluated in neonates.

v. **The preceding sets of parameters are often combined to yield the following modes.** *Note:* Volume assurance/guarantee may be added to pressure-limited modes.

(a) **IMV.** Refers to nontriggered, usually pressure-limited, time-cycled ventilation. **Use:** In absence of reliable patient trigger.

(b) **SIMV.** May be either volume or pressure limited, time cycled. Synchronized pressure-limited, time-cycled ventilation (**PLV**) has been the standard mode of ventilation. **Use:** Prevents the risk of ineffective ventilation and generation of excessive intrapulmonary pressure when a spontaneous exhalation occurs during a "mandatory" mechanical breath. Provides no support for patient breathing above the set rate.

    (i) **SIMV + pressure support.** Patient breaths above the SIMV is provided by the ventilator and is called pressure support breath. The pressure of the triggered assisted breath is usually set well below the SIMV PIP and is called pressure support. **Use:** Decrease the work of breathing. May facilitate weaning.

    (ii) **Volume-targeted SIMV.** Rapidly being adopted as the new standard mode. Expected benefits are decreased variability in delivered breath size resulting in more stable PCO_2 and less chance for intermittent overdistention. Limitations include poor sensor function from air leaks, condensation in the ventilator tubing, or extremely small flows/pressure in ELBW infants.

(c) **Pressure control.** Pressure-limited (usually with a decreasing flow rate during inspiration), time-cycled, A/C. May be volume targeted. **Use:** Provides well-tolerated support in patients with easily sensed respiratory effort.

(d) **Volume control.** Volume-limited, time-cycled, A/C. **Use:** As in pressure control, but may result in more consistent VT.

(e) **Pressure support.** Pressure-limited, flow-cycled support. May be volume targeted. **Use:** In addition to SIMV, especially during weaning.

III. **Pharmacologic respiratory support and surfactant.** Numerous medications are available for improvement of respiration. They represent a broad range of therapeutics, of which the bronchodilators and anti-inflammatory drugs are the oldest and most common. The use of mixtures of inhaled gases such as helium and nitric oxide is a recent form of treatment. Sedatives and paralyzing agents remain *controversial* in neonatal respiratory management. Finally, surfactant replacement therapy has rapidly become a major adjunct in the care of preterm infants, and its use has expanded to disease states other than RDS (hyaline membrane disease), for which it was originally intended. All medications are discussed with regard to dosage and side effects in Table 9–3, but they are briefly reviewed here for the purpose of incorporating their use into respiratory management strategies.

A. **Bronchodilators (inhaled agents).** Most of these drugs are sympathomimetic agents that stimulate β_1-, β_2-, or α-adrenergic receptors. They have both inotropic and chronotropic effects and provide bronchial smooth muscle and vascular relaxation. Albuterol is probably the most commonly used aerosolized bronchodilator. Other bronchodilators are presented in Table 9–3. Two anticholinergic agents (atropine and ipratropium) are also used as inhaled bronchodilators for inhibition of acetylcholine at lung receptor sites and bronchial smooth muscle relaxation. All are used to minimize airway resistance and allow decreased P̄aw needed for mechanical ventilation.

B. **Bronchodilators (systemic).** Aminophylline (parenteral) and theophylline (enteral) are methylxanthines with considerable bronchial dilating action. Neonatal use includes bronchodilation and, more often, stimulation of respiratory efforts.

C. **Anti-inflammatory agents**

    1. **Steroid therapy.** This has been used to treat or prevent chronic lung disease. Although steroid therapy results in significant short-term improvement in pulmonary function, long-term benefit remains unproved. The substantial adverse effects of steroid therapy with dexamethasone have led the **American Academy of Pediatrics (AAP) and the Canadian Pediatric Society to issue a joint recommendation against the routine use of steroid therapy.** Hydrocortisone may provide similar pulmonary benefits without the adverse neurodevelopmental effects of dexamethasone.

Table 9–3. AEROSOL THERAPY IN NEONATES

Drug	Receptors	Side Effects
Albuterol (Salbutamol, Ventolin): 1.25–2.5 mg per dose Dilute with NS to 3 mL Dose: every 4–6 hours	β_2: Long lasting (duration, 3–8 hours) Fewer side effects than metaproterenol	Tachycardia (potentiated by methylxanthines) Hypertension Hyperglycemia Tremor
Atropine: 0.025–0.05 mg/kg per dose (maximum dose 2.5 mg) Dilute IV solution with NS to 2.5 mL Dose: every 6–8 hours	Vagolytic	Tachycardia Arrhythmia Hypotension Ileus, airway dryness If thick secretions, suggest use in combination with albuterol
Budesonide inhalation suspension (Pulmicort Respules): 0.25–0.5 mg per dose Dose: every 12–24 hours	Anti-inflammatory	Side effects: Oral candidiasis, stridor, respiratory infection, adrenocortical insufficiency, growth suppression
Epinephrine, racemic: Dose: 0.05-0.1mL/kg diluted in 2-3 mL of NS. Maximum dose is 0.5mL **Epenephrine:** 1mg/mL injectable Dose: 0.5mL/kg (Maximum dose 5mL)	α-Receptor	Tachycardia Tremor Hypertension
Ilpratropium (Atrovent): Neonates: 25 µg/kg per dose Infants: 125–250 µg per dose Dilute with NS to 3 mL Dose: every 8 hours	Antagonizes acetylcholine at parasympathetic sites	Dizziness Nausea, blurred vision Cough, palpitations Rash, urinary difficulties
Levalbuterol (Xopenex): 0.31–1.25 mg every 4–6 hours as needed for bronchospasm (NHLBI 2007 asthma guidelines)	β_2: R(-)enantiomer of racemic albuterol: little effect on heart rate	Nervousness, tremor, tachycardia, hypertension, hypokalemia. Paradoxical bronchospasm may occur, especially with first use.
Terbutaline (Brethine): 0.01–0.02 mg/kg per dose Dilute IV solution with NS to 3 mL Dose: every 4–6 hours Minimum dose: 0.1 mg	β_2: Peripheral dilation	Hypertension Hyperglycemia Tachycardia

NHLBI, National Heart, Lung, and Blood Institute; NS, normal saline.
Neonate, birth to 28 days postnatal age; **infant**, >28 days to 1 year of age.

2. **Cromolyn.** Prevents mast cells from releasing histamine and leukotriene-like substances. Its actions are slow but progressive over 2 to 4 weeks. Indications for its use in neonates have not been established.
   D. **Inhaled gas mixtures**
      1. **Heliox (helium, 78%–80%; oxygen, 20%–22%).** Produces an inspired gas less dense than nitrogen-oxygen mixtures or oxygen alone. Use of heliox reduces the

increased resistive load of breathing, improves distribution of ventilation, and creates less turbulence in narrow airways. Limited neonatal use has indicated that heliox is associated with lower inspired oxygen requirements and shorter duration of mechanical ventilatory support.

2. **Inhaled nitric oxide (iNO).** A potent gaseous vasodilator produced by endothelial cells. Nitric oxide (NO) is rapidly bound by hemoglobin, limiting its action to the site of production or administration. Delivered in the ventilatory gas, iNO produces vasodilation only in the vascular bed of well-ventilated regions of the lung, thereby reducing intrapulmonary shunt as well as pulmonary vascular resistance. Furthermore, there is no systemic effect.

   a. **Actions.** iNO diffuses rapidly across alveolar cells to vascular smooth muscle, where it causes an increase in cyclic guanosine monophosphate (GMP), resulting in smooth muscle relaxation.

   b. **Dosage.** iNO is administered at low concentration, 2 to 20 parts per million (ppm). The dose is titrated to effect (improved oxygenation being the most common). Rarely do concentrations >20 to 40 ppm yield additional benefit.

   c. **Administration.** iNO is blended into the ventilatory gases, preferably close to the patient connector to avoid excessive dwell time with high oxygen concentrations, which may result in excessive NO_2 concentrations. Inline sensors are used to measure delivered NO and NO_2 concentrations. Techniques for use with high-frequency ventilators have also been developed. **Co-oximetry measurement of methemoglobin is required.** The iNO dose should be decreased if methemoglobin is >4% or if the NO_2 concentration is >1 to 2 ppm.

   d. **Indications for use.** iNO is indicated for hypoxic respiratory failure of term and near-term newborns. Recommendations have been made by the AAP for care and referral of these infants. It is currently under investigation for use in a variety of lung diseases in which inappropriate pulmonary vascular constriction adversely affects oxygenation. The resultant vasodilation may decrease pulmonary vascular resistance in general, thereby reducing right-to-left shunting, or may result in less intrapulmonary shunt, or both. Use in cases of severe respiratory failure suggests that iNO may reduce the need for extracorporeal membrane oxygenation (ECMO) in 30% to 45% of eligible patients. Use of inhaled NO in premature infants with RDS is controversial and is generally used when respiratory failure is associated with pulmonary hypertension associated to hypoplastic lungs.

   e. **Adverse effects.** Systemic vascular effects are *not* seen with iNO use. NO_2 poisoning and methemoglobinemia are the most likely complications.

E. **Other medications**

   1. **Sildenafil.** An oral phosphodiesterase-5 inhibitor, sildenafil reduces pulmonary vascular resistance and is approved in adults for pulmonary hypertension. Its use is attractive in patients with BPD, with further study required before use in newborns.

   2. **Prostacyclin (PGI_2).** A potent pulmonary vasodilator given as an aerosol or intravenous drip. Hypotension may develop. Use with iNO has been reported.

   3. **Bosentan.** An oral endothelin 1 receptor blocker, bosentan reduces pulmonary vascular resistance. Its use in neonates is undefined.

F. **Sedatives and paralyzing agents.** Agitation is a common problem for infant mechanical ventilation. Infants may have interrupted respiratory cycles and respond by "bucking" or "fighting" the ventilator breaths. The agitation that results is often associated with hypoxic episodes. Sedation or muscle relaxation by paralysis may be required. It should be noted, however, that with the use of ventilators with either flow-sensed or patient-triggered synchronized ventilation (SIMV), much less sedation is required, and paralysis is rarely needed. "Fighting" the respirator may indicate inadequate respiratory support because of changes in lung compliance/airway resistance. Careful assessment for possible remedial causes for those changes (eg, obstructed or malpositioned endotracheal tube, pneumothorax) needs to be performed before any pharmacologic intervention.

1. **Sedatives.** Include lorazepam, phenobarbital, fentanyl, or morphine. Each agent has advantages and side effects. (See Chapter 81.)

2. **Paralyzing agents.** Include rocuronium and vecuronium. Prolonged muscle relaxation by paralysis results in considerable body fluid accumulation with the development of pulmonary and skin edema.

G. **Surfactant replacement therapy.** The availability of surfactant treatment has dramatically changed the care of infants with RDS (formally known as hyaline membrane disease). Surfactant administration early in the course of RDS restores pulmonary function and prevents tissue injury that otherwise results from ventilation of surfactant-deficient lungs. As a result, mortality from RDS has decreased dramatically.

1. **Composition.** Currently available surfactants are all of animal origin. Beractant (Survanta) and calfactant (Infasurf) are derived from bovine lung and lung lavage, respectively. Poractant alfa (Curosurf) is derived from porcine lung. All contain the hydrophobic surfactant proteins, SpB and SpC, although at different concentrations. Calfactant and poractant alfa contain surfactant phospholipids. In beractant, additional phospholipid is added to the minced lung extract to increase the ratio of surfactant to membrane phospholipids. Synthetic surfactants that equal the in vivo actions of the natural surfactants have been on the horizon for several years.

2. **Actions.** All surfactant preparations are intended to replace the missing or inactivated natural surfactant of the infant. Surface tension reduction and stabilization of the alveolar air–water interface are the basic functions of surfactant compounds. Air–water interface stability imparts lower alveolar surface tension and prevents atelectasis or alternating areas of atelectasis and hyperinflation.

3. **Dosage and administration.** Each preparation has specific dosage and dosing procedures. Direct tracheal instillation is involved in all preparations. The possibility to effectively administer surfactant through noninvasive nebulization is presently being investigated. Surfactants are given both by continuous infusion via side port on the endotracheal tube adapter and mostly by aliquots via a catheter placed through the endotracheal tube. Changes in body position during dosing aid in more uniform delivery of surfactant. The relative advantages of these methods of administration are currently being studied (see Chapter 117 for detailed information on each medication).

   a. **Prophylactic dosing at birth.** This form of treatment is used less often and only when resuscitation and surfactant administration can be safely pursued simultaneously. Current practice prefers use of CPAP in the delivery room.

   b. **Administration of surfactant preparations after respiratory distress is established.** Currently, surfactant therapy occurs once the patient has been stabilized and the diagnosis of RDS has been established.

   c. **Repeat dosing.** May follow at 6- to 12-hour intervals. Repeat doses should follow loss of response after initial improvement has been seen. Repeat dosing after the second dose is *controversial*.

   d. **Airway obstruction.** May occur during surfactant administration because of the viscosity of the surfactant preparations. Increased mechanical support may be required until the surfactant is spread from the airways to the alveoli.

   e. **Lesser invasive methods of pulmonary administration of surfactant** through methods such as **LISA** (surfactant via thin diameter tubes under direct vision using laryngoscopes) or **INSURE** (intubation and surfactant administration followed by immediate extubation) both in conjunction with CPAP have been described. (See Chapter 90.)

4. **Efficacy.** Efficacy of surfactant treatment can be observed for both immediate and long-term clinical conditions.

      a. Early effects. Include a reduction of FiO_2 need and improved PaO_2, $PaCO_2$, and a/A ratio. Likewise, improved VT and compliance should be noted with improved lung function and decreased ventilator PIPs.

      b. Long-term effects. Should result in decreased necessity for mechanical ventilation and less severe chronic lung disease of infancy. Complications of patent ductus arteriosus, necrotizing enterocolitis, and intraventricular hemorrhage have not been significantly influenced by surfactant therapy to date.

    5. **Side effects**

      a. Small risk of pulmonary hemorrhage.

      b. Secondary pulmonary infections.

      c. Air leak (pneumothorax) following bolus administration of surfactant compounds. Rapid changes in VT require immediate reduction of PIPs. Failure to do so while also decreasing FiO_2 may lead to air leaks.

    6. **Surfactant therapy for diseases other than RDS.** Encouraging preliminary reports of surfactant therapy have been noted in cases of pneumonia, meconium aspiration syndrome, persistent pulmonary hypertension, pulmonary hemorrhage, and acute respiratory distress syndrome (ARDS), but no protocols for treatment are available at this time.

IV. Strategies of neonatal respiratory support

    A. General approach. Although use of the tools and techniques discussed in this section are essential to neonatal intensive care, their use is not without peril. One general approach is to provide the minimal support necessary for adequate gas exchange, unless a more aggressive intervention may change the course of the pulmonary disease, such as early intubation for the delivery of surfactant in RDS. Noninvasive nasal CPAP or ventilation is preferable to intubation and mechanical ventilation. Patient-triggered ventilation modes are usually better tolerated by patients and may result in less need for support. Meta-analysis of volume-targeted ventilation in neonates reveals a decrease in death and BPD/chronic lung disease (CLD) as compared with classic PLV. The optimal use of the myriad modes of assisted ventilation has yet to be determined, but the trend is to use ventilator modes that allow the patient more control. The decision to initiate or escalate ventilatory support should always take into account the risk of ventilator-induced lung injury and systemic effects of poorly controlled ventilation.

      1. **Mechanisms of lung injury**

        a. **Oxygen toxicity.** Risk factor for BPD/CLD and retinopathy of prematurity (ROP) and may be reduced by careful monitoring and the setting of gestational age–appropriate SpO_2 targets.

        b. **Inflammation and infection.** Result from intubation. Use of noninvasive ventilation and early extubation are desired.

        c. **Barotrauma/volutrauma.** Results from overinflation of the lung or stress from repeated reopening of collapsed lung units or from shear between adjacent lung units. Maintenance of FRC using appropriate PEEP and the use of small VT to prevent overdistention help limit injury.

      2. **Adverse effects of poorly controlled ventilation**

        a. **Hyperoxia (high PO_2)** is associated with an increased risk for ROP.

        b. **Hypoxemia (low PO_2)** has been recently associated with increased risk of mortality.

        c. **Overventilation (low PCO_2)** causes a decrease in cerebral blood flow that increases the risk for periventricular white matter injury and cerebral palsy.

        d. **Hypercapnia (high PCO_2)** may increase the risk for intraventricular hemorrhage and poor neurodevelopmental outcome.

        e. **Overinflation** may impair venous return and cardiac output to the point of systemic hypotension.

    B. Initiation of mechanical ventilation for respiratory distress. See Chapter 51, Table 51–1, and below for more detail on management of ventilators.

1. Indications
   a. Failure to maintain adequate PO_2 and PCO_2 with supplemental oxygen and nasal CPAP or nasal ventilation.
   b. Worsening RDS is an indication for early intubation for surfactant administration with subsequent mechanical ventilation.
2. **Ventilator settings.** *Note:* Refer to the operating manual for your specific ventilator to understand the specific modes available.
   a. **Classic pressure-limited ventilation (PLV).** Preferably with synchronization and V_T measurement.
      i. PEEP 4 to 5 cm H_2O.
      ii. T_i 0.3 seconds.
      iii. PIP to yield V_T of 4 to 5 mL/kg. If V_T measurement is unavailable, limit PIP so that chest rise is barely perceptible on breaths without patient effort.
      iv. Rate 30 to 40 per minute SIMV. Higher rates and/or A/C ventilation may result in initial hyperventilation.
      v. Trigger sensitivity setting requires specific machine knowledge. Refer to ventilator manual.
      vi. Evaluate response with clinical examination, noninvasive monitors, and blood gases and chest radiograph as necessary. Adjust PIP and rate as required. See later for managing ventilation.
   b. **Volume-targeted ventilation (VTV)**
      i. PEEP 4 to 5 cm H_2O.
      ii. T_i 0.3 seconds.
      iii. Set volume target to 4 to 5 mL/kg. Set PIP limit high enough for ventilator to meet target.
      iv. Rate 30 to 40 per minute SIMV. Higher rates and/or A/C ventilation may result in initial hyperventilation.
      v. Evaluate response with clinical examination, noninvasive monitors, blood gases, and chest radiograph as necessary. Adjust PIP and rate as required. See later for managing ventilation.
      vi. Large air leaks around the endotracheal tube interfere with volume-targeted ventilator modes. In such cases, either switch to PLV or reintubate with a larger tube.
C. **Fine-tuning mechanical ventilation.** (See also Chapter 51.) Adequate gas exchange must be determined for each patient because goals vary depending on diagnosis, patient's gestational age, and level of support required.
   1. **Low PO_2.** Usually caused by poor matching of ventilation and perfusion (low V/Q ratio). Support beyond the use of supplemental oxygen is directed either at improving aeration in the lung or influencing the distribution of perfusion. To improve oxygenation:
      a. **Maintain lung expansion.** Maintain lung expansion at end expiration by the use of PEEP and the use of surfactant in RDS. Preventing collapse also reduces lung injury from reopening alveoli.
      b. **Recruit collapsed lung by the use of adequate V_T and PIP.**
      c. **iNO selectively decreases vascular resistance in well-ventilated regions of the lung, improving oxygenation.** Extrapulmonary shunt due to persistent pulmonary hypertension may respond to prostacyclin in addition to iNO.
      d. **Consider the use of high-frequency oscillation.** To maintain high mean lung volume in cases of severe, uniform alveolar disease (RDS, ARDS).
   2. **High PCO_2.** Results from inadequate minute volume.
      a. **$PaCO_2$ is decreased by increasing MV.** If V_T is adequate (5–6 mL/kg), an increase in rate is preferable. Special attention is required when adjusting patient-triggered ventilation modes to ensure that a real increase in rate results from an increase in the ventilator set rate.

b. **Increasing Vт requires increasing PIP.** Although a high PIP itself does not necessarily produce lung injury, high-frequency ventilation should be considered if a PIP >20 to 25 cm H_2O is required in a premature infant or >30 cm H_2O in a term infant.

c. **When using patient-triggered ventilation modes,** set the ventilator rate high enough to prevent hypoventilation should the patient become apneic.

3. **Neonatal lung disease.** Rarely static, necessitating frequent adjustments to ventilator parameters.

D. **Weaning from mechanical ventilation and extubation.** As lung function improves with disease resolution, mechanical support should be decreased as quickly as tolerated. Most patients do not need to be "weaned" from mechanical support; they need support decreased to match their need. Continuous monitoring with pulse oximetry and $tcPCO_2$ aids in weaning and limits the need for blood gas sampling. A reduced oxygen requirement and improved compliance (decrease in PIP to maintain Vт) usually herald the weaning phase. **Pretreatment of infants with caffeine may enhance infant response to progressive weaning efforts.** Disease state, gestational age, and caloric support influence response to the weaning process.

1. **PIP.** Usually weaned first because overinflation injury is more deleterious than providing a greater rate than necessary. Volume-targeted ventilation modes may adequately decrease PIP as the lungs heal and provide a somewhat automatic wean.

2. **FiO_2.** Weaned whenever possible as determined by pulse oximetry or blood gases. Decreases in PIP decrease $\overline{Paw}$ and may transiently increase oxygen requirements during weaning.

3. **Progressive rate wean (does not apply to assist/control modes).** Rate settings should be decreased frequently. Infants ready to be weaned tolerate the rate wean and do not require more FiO_2. An infant should be able to maintain adequate minute ventilation without developing hypercarbia or apnea. When the ventilator rate is <15 to 20 breaths/min, the infant should be extubated. Some infants may require several hours to wean, whereas others need several days to a week or more.

4. **Weaning A/C ventilation.** Because all spontaneous breaths are mechanically supported by this mode of ventilation, reduction of the rate below the patient's spontaneous rate has no effect on the level of support. Weaning is accomplished by successive decreases in PIP. When adequate ventilation is maintained with minimal PIP (12–16 cm H_2O), extubation may be attempted.

E. **Care after extubation.** Continued monitoring of blood gases, respiratory effort, and vital signs is required. Additional oxygen support is often needed in the immediate postextubation period.

1. **Supplemental oxygen.** May be given by hood or by nasal cannula. The oxygen concentration may be increased by >5% over the last oxygen level obtained while the infant was on the ventilator.

2. **Nasal CPAP.** May be especially helpful in preventing reintubation secondary to postextubation atelectasis.

3. **Chest radiograph.** If the infant has had an increasing oxygen requirement or has clinically deteriorated, a chest radiograph should be obtained at 6 hours postextubation to monitor for atelectasis.

V. **Overview of high-frequency ventilation.** High-frequency ventilation refers to a variety of ventilatory strategies and devices designed to provide ventilation at rapid rates and very low Vтs. The ability to provide adequate ventilation despite reduced Vт (equal to or less than dead space) may reduce the risk of barotrauma. Rates during high-frequency ventilation are often expressed in hertz (Hz). A rate of 1 Hz (1 cycle/s) is equivalent to 60 breaths/min. All methods of high-frequency ventilation should be administered with the assistance of well-trained respiratory therapists and after comprehensive education of the nursing staff. Furthermore, because rapid changes in ventilation or oxygenation may occur, continuous monitoring is highly recommended. Optimal use of these ventilators is evolving, and different strategies may be indicated for a particular lung disease.

A. **Definitive indications for high-frequency ventilation support**
1. **Pulmonary interstitial emphysema (PIE).** A multicenter trial has demonstrated high-frequency jet ventilator (HFJV) to be superior to conventional ventilation in early PIE as well as in neonates who fail to respond to conventional ventilation.
2. **Severe bronchopleural fistula.** In severe bronchopleural fistula not responsive to thoracostomy tube evacuation and conventional ventilation, HFJV may provide adequate ventilation and decrease fistula flow.
3. **Respiratory distress syndrome (RDS).** High-frequency ventilation has been used with success. It is usually implemented at the point of severe respiratory failure with maximal conventional ventilation (a rescue treatment). Earlier treatment has been advocated. No advantages have yet been demonstrated for a very early intervention (in the first hours of life) when infants are pretreated with surfactant.
4. **Patients qualifying for ECLS (extracorporeal life support).** Pulmonary hypertension with or without associated parenchymal lung disease (eg, meconium aspiration, pneumonia, hypoplastic lung, or diaphragmatic hernia) can result in intractable respiratory failure and high mortality unless the patient is treated by ECLS. The prior use of high-frequency ventilation among ECLS candidates has been successful and eliminated the need for ECLS in 25% to 45% of cases.

B. **Possible indications.** High-frequency ventilation has been used with success in infants with other disease processes. Further study is needed to develop clear indications and appropriate ventilatory strategies before this treatment can be recommended for routine use in infants with these diseases.
1. **Pulmonary hypertension**
2. **Meconium aspiration syndrome**
3. **Diaphragmatic hernia with pulmonary hypoplasia**
4. **Postoperative Fontan procedures**

C. **High-frequency ventilators, techniques, and equipment.** Two types of high-frequency ventilators in the United States are the HFJV and the high-frequency oscillatory ventilator (HFOV).
1. **High-frequency jet ventilator.** The HFJV injects a high-velocity stream of gas into the endotracheal tube, usually at frequencies between 240 and 600 breaths/min and VTs equal to or slightly greater than dead space. During HFJV, expiration is passive. The only HFJV approved by the US Food and Drug Administration is the Life Pulse (Bunnell, Inc., Salt Lake City, UT) ventilator, discussed here.
   a. **Indications.** Mostly used for PIE, the Life Pulse HFJV has been used for the other indications described for all types of high-frequency ventilation.
   b. **Equipment**
      i. **Bunnell Life Pulse ventilator.** The inspiratory pressure (PIP), jet valve "on time," and respiratory frequency are entered into a digital control panel on the jet. PIPs are servo-controlled by the Life Pulse from the pressure port. The ventilator has an elaborate alarm system to ensure safety and to help detect changes in pulmonary function. It also has a special humidification system.
      ii. **Conventional ventilator.** A conventional ventilator is needed to generate PEEP and sigh breaths. PEEP and background ventilation are controlled with the conventional ventilator.

   c. **Procedure**

     i. **Initiation.** Close observation is required at all times, especially during initiation.

      (a) **Replace the endotracheal tube adapter with a jet adapter**

      (b) **Settings on the jet ventilator**

        (i) **Default jet valve "on time."** 0.020 seconds.

        (ii) **Frequency of jet.** 420 per minute.

        (iii) **PIP on the jet.** 2 to 3 cm H_2O below what was on the conventional ventilator. Frequently, infants require considerably less PIP during HFJV.

      (c) **Settings on the conventional ventilator**

        (i) **PEEP.** Maintain at 3 to 5 cm H_2O.

        (ii) **Rate.** As the jet ventilator comes up to pressure, the rate is decreased to 5 to 10 breaths/min.

        (iii) **PIP.** Once at pressure, the PIP is adjusted to a level at least 1 to 3 cm H_2O below that on the jet (low enough not to interrupt the jet ventilator).

   d. **Management.** Management of HFJV is based on the clinical course and radiographic findings.

     i. **Elimination of CO_2.** Alveolar ventilation is much more sensitive to changes in VT than in respiratory frequency during high-frequency ventilation. As a result, the **delta pressure** (PIP minus PEEP) is adjusted to attain adequate elimination of CO_2, whereas jet valve "on time" and respiratory frequency are usually not readjusted during HFJV.

     ii. **Oxygenation.** Oxygenation is often better during HFJV than during conventional mechanical ventilation in neonates with PIE. However, if oxygenation is inadequate and if the infant is already on 100% oxygen, an increase in P̄aw usually results in improved oxygenation. It can be accomplished by:

      (a) **Increasing PEEP.**

      (b) **Increasing PIP.**

      (c) **Increasing jet valve "on time."** 0.022 to 0.026 seconds.

      (d) **Increasing background conventional ventilator** (either rates or pressure).

     iii. **Positioning of infants.** Positioning infants with the affected side down may speed resolution of PIE. In bilateral air leak, alternating placement on dependent sides may be effective. Diligent observation and frequent radiographs are necessary to avoid hyperinflation of the nondependent side.

   e. **Weaning.** When weaning, the following guidelines are used.

     i. **PIP is reduced as soon as possible ($PaCO_2$ <35–40 mm Hg).** Because elimination of CO_2 is very sensitive to changes in VT, PIP is weaned 1 cm H_2O at a time.

     ii. **Oxygen concentration.** Weaned if oxygenation remains good (PaO_2 >70–80 mm Hg).

     iii. **Jet valve "on time" and frequency.** Usually kept constant.

     iv. **Constant attention is paid to the infant's clinical condition and radiographs** to detect early atelectasis or hyperinflation.

     v. **Air leaks are resolved.** Continuation of HFJV occurs until the air leak has been resolved for 24 to 48 hours, which often corresponds to a dramatic drop in ventilator pressures and oxygen requirement.

     vi. **In case of no improvement in the condition.** A trial of conventional ventilation is used after 6 to 24 hours on jet ventilation.

   f. **Special considerations**

     i. **Airway obstruction.** This problem can usually be recognized quickly. Chest wall movement is decreased, although breath sounds may be adequate. The servo pressure (driving pressure) is usually very low.

      ii. Inadvertent PEEP (air trapping). In larger infants, the flow of jet gases may result in inadvertent PEEP. Decreasing the background flow on the conventional ventilator may correct the problem, or it may be necessary to decrease the respiratory frequency to allow more time for expiration.

  2. High-frequency oscillatory ventilator. The HFOV generates V_T less than or equal to dead space by means of an oscillating piston or diaphragm. This mechanism creates active exhalation as well as inspiration. The SensorMedics 3100B HFOV (CareFusion Corporation, San Diego, CA) is currently approved by the US Food and Drug Administration for use in neonates.

    a. Indications. High-frequency oscillatory ventilation is indicated when conventional ventilation used for respiratory failure does not result in adequate oxygenation or ventilation or requires the use of very high airway pressures. Like other forms of high-frequency ventilation, success is more likely when increased airway resistance is not the dominant pulmonary pathophysiology. Best results are seen when parenchymal disease is homogeneous. Some clinicians advocate high-frequency oscillatory ventilation as the primary method of assisted ventilation in premature infants with RDS.

    b. Equipment. HFOV is used without a conventional ventilator. The user-defined parameters are frequency, $\overline{Paw}$, and power applied for piston displacement.

    c. Procedure

      i. Initiation

        (a) Conventional ventilator is discontinued.

        (b) Settings

          (i) Frequency. Usually set at 15 Hz for premature infants with RDS. Larger infants, or those with a significant component of increased airway resistance (meconium aspiration), should be started at 5 to 10 Hz.

          (ii) $\overline{Paw}$. Set higher (2–5 cm H_2O) than on the previous conventional ventilation. If overdistention or air leaks were present before initiation of HFOV, a lower $\overline{Paw}$ should be considered.

          (iii) Amplitude. Analogous to PIP on conventional ventilation and is regulated by the power of displacement of the piston. This power is increased until there is visible chest wall vibration.

        (c) After high-frequency oscillatory ventilation has been initiated, careful and frequent assessment of lung expansion and adequate gas exchange are necessary. Air trapping is a continuous potential threat in this form of treatment. Signs of overdistention, such as descended and flat diaphragms and small heart shadow, are monitored with frequent chest radiographs.

    d. Management

      i. Low PaO_2. An increase in $\overline{Paw}$ may be necessary. Chest radiographs may be helpful in determining the adequacy of lung expansion.

      ii. High $PaCO_2$

        (a) Oxygenation is also poor. The $\overline{Paw}$ may be too high or too low, resulting in either hyperinflation or widespread collapse, respectively. Again, chest radiographs are necessary to differentiate between these 2 conditions.

        (b) Oxygenation is adequate. The amplitude (power) should be increased. Decreasing the rate may be an alternative if hypercapnia is associated with evidence of lung hyperinflation.

    e. Weaning

      i. In the absence of hyperinflation. FiO_2 is weaned before $\overline{Paw}$ for adequate PaO_2. Below 40% FiO_2, wean $\overline{Paw}$ exclusively.

      ii. $\overline{Paw}$. Should be weaned as the lung disease improves with the goal of maintaining optimal lung expansion. Excessively aggressive early weaning of $\overline{Paw}$ may result in widespread atelectasis and the need for significant increases in $\overline{Paw}$ and FiO_2.

   iii. **Amplitude.** Should be weaned for acceptable $PaCO_2$.

   iv. **Frequency.** Usually not adjusted during weaning. A decrease in frequency is necessary when signs of lung overdistention cannot be eliminated by a reduction in $\overline{Paw}$.

   v. **The neonate may be switched to conventional ventilation** at a low level of support or may be extubated directly from HFOV.

  f. **Complications.** Hyperinflation with compromise of cardiac output. Frequent evaluation with chest radiography is advised.

GLOSSARY OF TERMS USED IN RESPIRATORY MANAGEMENT

ARTERIAL-TO-ALVEOLAR RATIO (A/A RATIO). See Section I.B.3.b.

ASSIST. A setting at which the infant initiates the mechanical breath, triggering the ventilator to deliver a preset V_T or pressure.

ASSIST/CONTROL. The same as assist, except that if the infant becomes apneic, the ventilator delivers the number of mechanical breaths per minute set on the rate control.

CONTINUOUS POSITIVE AIRWAY PRESSURE (CPAP). A spontaneous mode in which the ambient intrapulmonary pressure that is maintained throughout the respiratory cycle is increased.

CONTROL. A setting at which a certain number of mechanical breaths per minute is delivered. The infant is unable to breathe spontaneously between mechanical breaths.

END-TIDAL CO₂ (ETCO₂ OR PETCO₂). A measure of the PCO_2 of end expiration.

EXPIRATORY TIME (ET). The amount of time set for the expiratory phase of each mechanical breath.

FLOW RATE. The amount of gas per minute passing through the ventilator. It must be sufficient to prevent rebreathing (ie, 3 times the minute volume) and to achieve the PIP during T_i. Changes in the flow rate may be necessary if changes in the airway waveform are desired. The normal range is 6 to 10 L/min; 8 L/min is commonly used.

FRACTION OF INSPIRED OXYGEN (FiO₂). The percentage of oxygen concentration of inspired gas expressed as decimals (room air = 0.21).

I:E RATIO. Ratio of inspiratory time to expiratory time. The normal values are 1:1, 1:1.5, or 1:2.

INSPIRATORY TIME (T₁). The amount of time set for the inspiratory phase of each mechanical breath.

INTERMITTENT MECHANICAL VENTILATION. Mechanical breaths are delivered at intervals. The infant breathes spontaneously between mechanical breaths.

MINUTE VENTILATION. V_T (proportional to PIP) multiplied by rate.

OXYGEN INDEX (OI). Mean airway pressure (MAP) $\times FiO_2 \times 100/PaO_2$.

OXYHEMOGLOBIN DISSOCIATION CURVE. A curve showing the amount of oxygen that combines with hemoglobin as a function of PaO_2 and $PaCO_2$. The curve shifts to the right when oxygen take-up by the blood is less than normal at a given PO_2, and it shifts to the left when oxygen take-up is greater than normal.

PAO₂. Partial pressure of arterial oxygen.

PAP. The total airway pressure. In the Siemens Servo 900-C, it is the PIP plus the PEEP.

$\overline{Paw}$. The average proximal pressure applied to the airway throughout the entire respiratory cycle.

PCO₂. Carbon dioxide partial pressure.

PEAK INSPIRATORY PRESSURE (PIP). The highest pressure reached within the proximal airway with each mechanical breath. *Note:* In the Siemens Servo 900-C, the PIP is defined as the inspiratory pressure above the PEEP.

PO₂. Oxygen partial pressure.

POSITIVE END-EXPIRATORY PRESSURE (PEEP). The pressure in the airway above ambient pressure during the expiratory phase of mechanical ventilation.

RATE. Number of mechanical breaths per minute delivered by the ventilator.

SaO₂. Oxygen saturation of arterial blood measured by direct measurement (arterial blood gas).

TIDAL VOLUME (VT). The volume of gas inspired or expired during each respiratory cycle.

10 Fluid and Electrolytes

An assessment of body water metabolism and electrolyte balance plays an important role in the early medical management of preterm infants and sick term infants coming to neonatal intensive care. Intravenous or intra-arterial fluids given during the first several days of life are a major factor in the development, or prevention, of morbidities such as intraventricular hemorrhage, necrotizing enterocolitis (NEC), patent ductus arteriosus, and bronchopulmonary dysplasia. Clinicians must pay close attention to the details of maintaining and monitoring body water and serum electrolytes and the management of fluid infusion therapies.

Bodily fluid balance is a function of the distribution of water in the body, water intake, and water losses. Body water distribution gradually changes with increasing gestational age of the fetus. At birth, these gestational changes in body water are reflected in the developing maturity of renal function, transepidermal insensible water losses, and neuroendocrine adaptations. One must account for these variables when deciding the amount of infusion fluids to administer to an infant.

I. **Body water**
   A. **Total body water (TBW).** Water accounts for nearly 75% of the body weight in term infants and as much as 85% to 90% of body weight of preterm infants. TBW is divided into 2 basic body water compartments: intracellular water (ICW) and extracellular water (ECW). ECW is composed of intravascular and interstitial water. For the fetus, there is a gradual decrease in ECW from two-thirds of TBW at 16 weeks' gestation to 53% of the TBW at 32 weeks' gestation. Thereafter, the proportions remain fairly constant until 38 weeks of gestation when increasing body mass of protein and fat stores reduces ECW further by approximately 5%.

   At birth, there begins a further contraction of the ECW as a function of the normal transition from intrauterine to extrauterine life. A diuresis occurs that reduces body weight proportionally to gestational age. For the very low birthweight preterm infant body, weight losses of 10% to 15% can be expected, whereas full-term infants usually lose 5% to 10% of body weight. Intrauterine growth-restricted neonates have a smaller initial weight loss and more rapidly regain their birth weight than their normally grown counterparts.

   B. **TBW balance in the newborn**
      1. **Renal.** Fetal urine flow steadily increases from 2 to 5 mL/h to 10 to 20 mL/h at 30 weeks' gestation. At term, fetal urine flow reaches 25 to 50 mL/h and then drops to 8 to 16 mL/h (1–3 mL/kg/h). These volume changes illustrate the large exchange of body water during fetal life and the abrupt changes forcing physiologic adaptation at birth. Despite marked fetal urine flow in utero, glomerular filtration rates (GFRs) are low. At birth, GFR remains low but steadily increases in the newborn period under the influence of increasing systolic blood pressure, increasing renal blood flow, and increasing glomerular permeability. Infant kidneys are able to produce dilute urine within limits dependent on GFR. The low GFR of preterm infants is the result of low renal blood flow but increases considerably after 34 weeks' postconceptional age. Term infants can concentrate urine up to 800 mOsm/L, compared to the 1500 mOsm/L of older children and adults. The preterm infant kidney is less able to concentrate urine secondary to a relatively low interstitial urea concentration, an anatomically shorter loop of Henle, and a distal tubular and collecting system that is less responsive to antidiuretic hormone (ADH). In extreme prematurity, urine osmolarity can be as low as 70 mOsm/L. Although limitations exist, healthy preterm infants with constant sodium intake but variable fluid infusion between 90 and 200 mL/kg/d are able to concentrate or dilute urine to maintain a balance of body water.

Against the backdrop of changing GFR and variable urine concentrating ability, all infants undergo a diuresis and a natriuresis in the days immediately following birth. Newborn diuresis is a contraction of the ECW and the initiation of body water conservation as the adaptation from an aquatic intrauterine existence to the less humidity and free water-dependent newborn state. The diuresis is facilitated by limited ADH responsiveness but is diminished by increasing serum osmolality (>285 mOsm/kg) and decreasing intravascular volume. Natriuresis is the result of increasing levels of atrial natriuretic peptide and decreased renal sodium absorption; infant kidneys also have decreased secretion of bicarbonate, potassium, and hydrogen ion.

2. **Insensible water loss (IWL).** Evaporation of body water occurs largely through the skin and mucous membranes (two-thirds) and the respiratory tract (one-third). A most important variable influencing IWL is the maturity of the infant's skin. The greater IWL in preterm infants results from body water evaporation through an immature epithelial layer. The stratum corneum is not well developed until 34 weeks' gestation. Throughout the third trimester, the stratum corneum and epidermis thicken. Keratinization of the stratum corneum forms the principal barrier to water loss. Keratinization begins early in the second trimester and continues throughout the third trimester. In addition, IWL is related to a larger skin surface area–to–body weight ratio in preterm infants and relatively greater skin vascularity.

IWL through the respiratory tract is related to the respiratory rate and the water content of the inspired air or air-oxygen mix (humidification). Table 10–1 lists other factors for IWL in newborn infants.

In general, for healthy premature infants weighing 800 to 2000 g cared for in double-walled incubators, IWL increases linearly as body weight decreases (Table 10–2).

However, for sick infants of similar weight cared for under a radiant warmer and undergoing ventilator respiratory support, IWL increases exponentially as body weight decreases.

Phototherapy may increase IWL by way of increasing body temperature and increasing peripheral blood flow. Generally, recommended fluid increases for preterm infants have been 10 to 20 mL/kg/d. This may not be necessary with newer phototherapy lights using light-emitting diodes (LEDs) because they generate very little heat. Moreover, term infants receiving adequate fluid intake and with no other

Table 10–1. FACTORS IN THE NICU ENVIRONMENT THAT AFFECT INSENSIBLE WATER LOSS

Body weight	Inversely proportional to maturity
Radiant warmer use during procedures	IWL increases by 50%–100% over incubator care (see also Chapter 13)
Phototherapy	IWL *controversial*; may be minimal for term infants, but appreciable for preterm infants (up to 25%)
Ambient humidity and temperature in double-walled humidified incubators	High ambient humidity and a thermal neutral environment conserve TBW
High body temperature	May increase loss by 30%–50%
Tachypnea	Variable depending on respiratory support
Skin breakdown	Most often from removal of adhesives denuding skin
Congenital absence of normal skin covering	Large omphaloceles, neural tube defects, or skin losses as in epidermolysis bullosa

IWL, insensible water loss; NICU, neonatal intensive care unit; TBW, total body water.

Table 10–2. **ESTIMATES OF INSENSIBLE WATER LOSS IN PRETERM INFANTS DURING FIRST WEEK OF LIFE IN A THERMAL NEUTRAL ENVIRONMENT**

Birthweight (g)	Insensible Water Loss (mL/kg/d)
<750	100–200
750–1000	60–70
1001–1250	50–60
1251–1500	30–40
1501–2000	20–30
>2000	15–20

Adapted from Martin RJ, Fanaroff AA, Walsh MC: Fanaroff and Martin's Neonatal-Perinatal Medicine: *Diseases of the Fetus and Infant,* 8th ed. Philadelphia, PA: Mosby Elsevier; 2006.

increased body water loss may not need added fluid intake. Occasionally, photo-therapy induces loose stools, and IWL would need to be reconsidered.

3. **Neuroendocrine.** TBW balance is also influenced by hypothalamic osmorecep-tors and carotid baroreceptors. Serum osmolarity >285 mOsm/kg stimulates the hypothalamus, and ADH is released to affect free water retention. In addition, volume diminution affects carotid bodies and baroreceptors to further stimulate ADH secretion to retain free water at the level of the collecting ducts of the distal nephrons. Collectively the osmoreceptors and the baroreceptors seek to maintain TBW with adequate intravascular volume at normal serum osmolarity. In the neonate, hypoxia with acidemia and hypercarbia are potent stimulators of ADH. An excessive secretion of ADH can follow 1 or more insults such as intracranial hemorrhage, sepsis, and/or hypotension. Conversely, excessive ADH secretion can occur in the absence of hyperosmolarity or volume depletion. Thus, a phenomenon known as the **syndrome of inappropriate ADH secretion (SIADH)** can occur. It is manifested as hyponatremia, hypo-osmolar serum, nondilute urine, and low blood urea nitrogen. Because ADH secretion begins early in fetal development, SIADH can occur as readily in preterm infants as in term infants.

C. **Monitoring TBW balance**

1. **Body weight.** Using in-bed scales, body weight should be recorded daily for all infants undergoing intensive care and twice daily for very low birthweight and extremely low birthweight infants. **Expected weight loss** during the first 3 to 5 days of life is 5% to 10% of birthweight for term infants and 10% to 15% of birthweight for preterm infants. A loss of >15% of birthweight during the first week of life should be considered excessive and body water balance carefully reevaluated. If weight loss is <2% in the first week of life, maintenance infusion fluid administra-tion may be excessive.

2. **Physical examination.** Edema or loss of skin turgor, moist or dry mucous mem-branes, sunken or puffy periorbital tissues, and full or sunken anterior fontanel have been time-honored sites to examine for dehydration or overhydration. They may be helpful when observing newborn infants but are unreliable in low birth-weight infants. They must be observed within the context of all other TBW points of monitoring.

3. **Vital signs**

   a. **Blood pressure** can be an indicator of altered intravascular volume, but usually is a later sign rather than earlier sign. Pressure changes and trends are needed in the overall assessment of TBW balance.

   b. **Pulse volumes,** decreased in dehydration in association with tachycardia, are somewhat sensitive indicators of early intravascular volume loss.
   c. **Tachypnea** can be an early sign of metabolic acidosis accompanying inadequate intravascular volume.
   d. **Capillary refill time (CRT)** has been a reliable and time-honored observation. CRT of >3 seconds in term infants is suspect for decreased intravascular volume, whereas a CRT of barely 3 seconds in a preterm infant should be equally suspected.
4. **Hematocrit (Hct).** Increases or decreases of central Hct (venous or arterial) from accepted normal values suggest changes in intravascular volume as it relates to TBW. Apart from obvious hemorrhage, changes in Hct may reflect overhydration or dehydration and must be considered in the assessment of TBW for fluid therapy in the first week of life.
5. **Serum chemistries**
   a. **Sodium values** of 135 to 140 mEq/L are indicative of TBW and sodium balance. Values above or below are suggestive of hyper- or hypo-osmolarity. A sodium value of ≤130 mEq/L frequently suggest overhydration in the first days of life. Excessive sodium deficit or SIADH needs to be considered in its differential diagnosis in conjunction with associated pathology such as gastroenteritis, NEC, renal failure, or preceding severe hypoxemic events. One needs to be aware that a measurement of Na^+ level from a hemolyzed blood sample may result in an inaccurate diagnosis of hyponatremia.
   b. **Serum osmolarity** of 285 mOsm/L (±3 mOsm) is the standard for TBW balance; values above or below must be considered indicative of over or underhydration.
6. **Acid-base status**
   a. **Hydrogen ion (pH).** A less than normal pH (7.28–7.35) can be indicative of metabolic acidosis and will be accompanied by other factors, suggesting a contracted intravascular volume and hyperosmolarity.
   b. **Base deficit.** An increasing base deficit (ie, metabolic acidosis with deficit >5.0) with decreased urine output, decreased blood pressure, and a prolonged CRT strongly suggests hypovolemia.
   c. **Chloride ion, carbon dioxide (CO_2) content, and bicarbonate (HCO_3).** These determinations are important for calculating anion gap and overall acid-base status.
   d. **Anion gap.** The anion gap is a unifying determination for identifying metabolic acidosis in the face of dehydration. It is the sum of the serum sodium and potassium ions *minus* the sum of the serum chloride and bicarbonate ions. The normal range for anion gap is 8 to 16. Values for an anion gap >16 are indicative of an organic acidemia. In the face of dehydration with decreased intravascular volume, lactic acidemia follows poor tissue perfusion and is reflected as a widening anion gap. See Chapter 51.
7. **Urine**
   a. **Urine output should be 1 to 3 mL/kg/h by the third day of life in all newborn infants with normal kidneys.** Preterm infants have limited urine formation on day 1 of life but should begin to increase urine production throughout day 2.
   b. **Urine specific gravity** of 1.005 to 1.012 is consistent with adequate with TBW balance.
   c. **Urine electrolytes and urine osmolarity** offer additional information as to renal concentrating ability. Term infants can concentrate urine to 800 mOsm/kg, whereas preterm infants are limited to 600 mOsm/kg.
D. **Maintenance of TBW.** Infusion fluid therapy for newborn infants (term and preterm) must be calculated to allow for normal ECW losses and body weight losses while avoiding dehydration from excessive IWL. The consequences of dehydration are hypotension, hypernatremia, and acidosis. Conversely, excessive infusion fluid therapy is

associated with clinically significant patent ductus arteriosus and may aggravate respiratory distress. Given careful monitoring for TBW as detailed earlier, the following infusion fluid therapy guidelines are offered for maintenance of TBW balance in term and preterm infants (with the exception of infusion fluid therapy for extremely low birthweight infants; see Chapter 13).

1. **Term infants in need of infusion fluid therapy**
   a. **Day 1.** Give dextrose 10% in water (D10W) at a rate of 60 to 80 mL/kg/d. This provides 6 to 7 mg/kg/min of glucose in support of energy needs while providing limited hydration during the immediate postnatal adaptation period. Neither sodium nor potassium supplementation are needed unless unusual body fluid losses are known.
   b. **Days 2 to 7.** Once tolerance of infusion fluid therapy has been established and confirmed by TBW monitoring (eg, urine output of 1–2 mL/kg/h), the rate and composition of fluid therapy can be modified. The goals of infusion fluid therapy include expected weight loss of 5% body weight, confirmed normal serum electrolyte values, and continued urine output of 2 to 3 mL/kg/h. Specifics of fluid therapy are as follows:
      i. **Infusion fluid volume** 80 to 120 mL/kg/d. May increase to 120 to 160 mL/kg/d by week's end as tolerated or to meet needs per monitoring.
      ii. **Glucose** to be provided to maintain serum glucose values >60 mg/dL; may increase to 8 to 9 mg/kg/min infusion as D10W or D12.5W.
      iii. **Sodium requirement daily** is 2 to 4 mEq/kg/d per monitoring of serum (target values, 135–140 mEq/L).
      iv. **Potassium daily requirements** are 1 to 2 mEq/kg/d per monitoring of serum (target values, 4.0–5.0 mEq/L). Potassium supplementation is not begun until the second or third day and only when normal renal function is confirmed by adequate urine output and normal serum electrolyte values have been established.
      v. **Nutrition.** Infusion fluid glucose does not meet all energy needs for basal metabolism, growth, and activity. Enteral feeds must be started as soon as possible; however, if the infant is unable to take formula by mouth or only in limited amount, then total parenteral nutrition (TPN) becomes necessary. As enteral feeds increase, infusion fluids or TPN can be progressively decreased, but keeping total volume intake at 120 to 160 mL/kg/d.

2. **Preterm infants**
   a. **Day 1.** During the immediate postnatal period, critically ill premature infants may require volume resuscitation for shock or acidosis. Fluids administered during stabilization should be considered when planning subsequent fluid management.
   b. **Days 1 to 3.** Infusion fluid therapy is aimed at allowing a 10% to 15% body weight loss through the first week while maintaining TBW balance and electrolyte balance.
      i. **Infusion fluid volumes.** Preterm low birthweight infants (>1500 g) require 60 to 80 mL/kg/d. Preterm very low birthweight infants (1000–1500 g) require 80 to 100 mL/kg/d. Preterm extremely low birthweight infants (<1000 g) require a range of fluid volumes from 50 to 80 mL/kg/d if cared for in double-walled humidified (80%) closed incubators or in a hybrid humidified incubators. If cared for under a radiant warmer or in incubators without humidity, fluid requirements may be 100 to 200 mL/kg/d (see Table 13–1 for breakdown into 100-g birthweight increments).
      ii. **Glucose supplementation.** Best achieved by D5W or D7.5W infusion fluids to avoid hyperglycemia. Because of the high fluid requirements in the smallest infants, glucose utilization may not be sufficient to prevent buildup of serum glucose and a hyperosmolar state secondary to hyperglycemia.

If allowable, reduced glucose maintenance is preferred, but extremes of hyperglycemia (>150 mg/dL) may require insulin therapy or intragastric sterile water supplementation (controversial).

iii. **Sodium.** During the first week of life, fluid therapy should be managed by increments or decrements of 20 to 40/mL/kg/d depending on weight changes and serum sodium values, while attempting to keep serum sodium at 135 to 140 mEq/L. Sodium supplementation is not usually required in the first 2 to 3 days of life. Sodium supplementation is begun based on body weight losses (postnatal isotonic contraction of ECW compartment, a physiologic diuresis). Usually by day 3 to 5, weight loss and a slight serum sodium decrease from baseline dictate the need to start sodium supplementation by way of the infusion fluids. Judicious restriction of sodium intake during the first 3 to 5 days of life facilitates a trend for normal serum osmolarity throughout the first week of life for preterm infants.

iv. **Potassium.** Supplementation follows that of term infants, meaning that well-established renal function with good urine output is required before supplementation at 1 to 2 mEq/kg/d.

v. **Nutrition.** Caloric needs to provide for the relative hypermetabolic state of low birthweight infants can be met through TPN fluid therapy. Initiation of TPN after the first 24 hours of life is desirable (see Chapters 11 and 13).

c. **Days 3 to 7.** Infusion fluid and electrolyte management is dictated by the monitoring parameters as already given. Infusion fluids should be advanced or decreased as the transition period progresses. Excessive weight loss suggests increased IWL losses and the threat of dehydration. Likewise, edema and minimal or no weight loss suggests excessive fluid administration or decreasing renal function and decreased urine output. All preterm infants should be cared for whenever possible in double-walled incubators for a more stable humidity control and less IWL.

3. **Other infusion fluid calculations and considerations**
   a. **Environmental**
      i. **Radiant warmers.** Infusion fluid volume recommendations as outlined earlier are for assumed double-walled incubator care. If radiant warmer exposure is to be maintained, fluid therapy must be increased by 50% to 100%. Plastic sheeting limits increased needs to 30% to 50%.
      ii. **Phototherapy.** If infant is full term, increased fluid therapy may not be needed. If infant is low birthweight, most likely 10 to 20 mL/kg/d will be needed to minimize IWL while phototherapy lights are in use.
   b. **Glucose.** The normal glucose requirement is 6 to 8 mg/kg/min, and intake can be slowly increased to 10 to 12 mg/kg/min as needed, but with careful monitoring for hyperglycemia and glycosuria to avoid an osmotic diuresis. Calculations for glucose supplementation are:

$$\text{Glucose requirements (mg/kg/min)} = \frac{(\text{Percentage of glucose} \times \text{Rate[mL/h]} \times 0.167)}{\text{Weight (kg)}}$$

An alternate method is

$$\text{Glucose requirements (mg/kg/min)} = \frac{(\text{Amount of glucose/mL [from Table 10-3]} \times \text{Total fluids})}{\text{Weight (kg)}/(60 \text{ min})}$$

Table 10–3. **GLUCOSE CONCENTRATION IN COMMONLY USED INTRAVENOUS INFUSION FLUIDS**

Solution	Glucose Concentration (mg/mL)
Dextrose 5% water	50
Dextrose 7.5% water	75
Dextrose 10% water	100
Dextrose 12.5% water	125
Dextrose 15% water	150

c. **Sodium.** The normal sodium requirement for infants is 2 to 3 mEq/kg/d. The following calculations can be used to determine the amount of sodium (Na^+) per day that an infant will receive from a given saline infusion fluid:

$$\text{Amt of } Na^+/mL \text{ (from Table 10–4)} \times \text{Total fluids/d} = \text{Amt of } Na^+/d$$

$$\frac{\text{Amt of } Na^+/d}{\text{Weight (kg)}} = \text{Amt of } Na^+ \text{ (kg/d)}$$

d. **Potassium.** The normal potassium requirement for infants is 1 to 2 mEq/kg/d. Potassium supplementation should not begin until adequate urine output is established.

II. **Electrolyte disturbances**
   A. **Sodium.** Serum values of 135 to 145 mEq/L represent homeostatic sodium balance. The wide range of 131 to 149 mEq/L is the lower and upper limit for sodium (Na^+) balance. Values above or below are clinical indicators of either hyper- or hyponatremia.
   1. **Hypernatremia**
      a. **Decreased ECW with Na^+ of $\geq$150 mEq/L**
         i. **Causes.** Include increased renal free water losses and/or increased IWL, primarily through skin, especially very low birthweight and extremely low birthweight infants.
         ii. **Clinical findings.** Weight loss, low blood pressure, tachycardia, decreased or absent urine output, and increased urine specific gravity.
         iii. **Treatment.** Requires careful infusion fluid management. **Replacing free water is the first goal, and maintaining Na^+ balance is the second goal.** Both goals need to be accomplished without precipitating rapid ICW and ECW shifts of water or sodium, especially within the central nervous system (CNS). **Excessively rapid correction of hypernatremia can result in**

Table 10–4. **SODIUM CONTENT OF COMMONLY USED INFUSION FLUIDS**

Solution	Sodium Concentration (mEq/mL)
3% normal saline	0.500
Normal saline	0.154
0.50% normal saline	0.075
0.25% normal saline	0.037
0.125% normal saline	0.019

seizures. Hypernatremic dehydration does not represent a deficit of body sodium. Infusion therapy should be guided to reduce serum Na^+ by not more than 0.5 mEq/L/kg/h, or less, with a target of total correction time of 24 to 48 hours. Consider using D5W 0.25 normal saline (NS) as an initial infusion fluid for correction.

  b. **Increased ECW and hypernatremia**

   i. **Causes.** Include excessive administration of normal saline or sodium bicarbonate as in resuscitation efforts or postresuscitation treatment for perinatal asphyxia with metabolic acidosis and hypotension.

   ii. **Clinical findings.** Increased weight gain and edema. If cardiac output has been compromised, findings of edema and weight gain increase. Depending on cardiac status, heart rate, blood pressure, and urine output will be within normal limits or decreased.

   iii. **Treatment.** Involves identification of cardiac status. Identify infusion fluid excesses and establish maintenance infusion fluid limits; thereafter, restrict sodium until serum Na^+ values return to normal range.

2. **Hyponatremia.** See also Chapter 69.

  a. **Increased ECW as increased intravascular water and increased third space interstitial water**

   i. **Causes.** Increased ECW with serum Na^+ <130 mEq/L, which most likely represents excessive infusion fluid administration, and increased third space (interstitial) water secondary to sepsis, shock, and capillary leakage. It may also be secondary to cardiac failure or pharmacologic neuromuscular paralysis during mechanical ventilation. It may occur with fluid retention associated to oliguric renal failure (such as acute tubular necrosis associated with perinatal asphyxia) or in newborn infants developing SIADH following CNS trauma, intracranial hemorrhage, meningitis, perinatal asphyxia, or pneumothorax.

   ii. **Clinical findings.** Result from inadvertent excessive infusion fluid administration: body weight is increased with edema, serum Na^+ is decreased, and urine output is increased with decreased urine osmolarity and specific gravity. Conversely, if SIADH is the root cause of increased ECW and hyponatremia, the clinical findings reveal increased body weight, variable presence of edema, decreased serum Na^+, decreased urine output, and increased urine specific gravity, whereas oliguric renal failure is associated with isosthenuria (neither concentrated nor diluted urine).

   iii. **Treatment.** In both situations, treatment is free water restriction allowing serum Na^+ to concentrate to normal levels. If serum Na^+ is <120 mEq/L and neurologic symptoms are present, consider titrating with infusion of 3% saline solution boluses. Consultation with a nephrologist is recommended.

  b. **Decreased ECW with hyponatremia**

   i. **Causes.** Include excessive diuretic therapy, glycosuria with an osmotic diuresis, vomiting, diarrhea, and third space fluid with NEC.

   ii. **Clinical findings.** Include decreased body weight, signs of dehydration with sunken fontanel, loss of skin turgor, dry mucous membranes, increased blood urea nitrogen, metabolic acidosis, decreased urine output, and increased urine specific gravity.

   iii. **Treatment.** Involves replacing sodium and water while minimizing any ongoing sodium losses (See Chapter 69 for management details.)

  c. **Isotonic losses may occur and present as hyponatremia.** Such losses may be cerebrospinal fluid from drainage procedures, thoracic as in chylothorax, nasogastric drainage, or peritoneal fluid (ascites). Normal saline for fluid replacement usually suffices, or normal saline plus colloid as fresh-frozen plasma or human albumin may facilitate intravascular volume and restore serum saline.

B. **Potassium**
  1. **Hyperkalemia.** Represented by serum K$^+$ values >5.5 mEq/L. Some infants do not manifest symptoms until serum levels reach 7 to 8 mEq/L. Hyperkalemia can be caused by or related to renal failure, hemolysis, massive blood transfusions, exchange transfusions, or inadvertent excessive administration of a potassium solution (eg, KCl). Cardiac conduction is the most immediate concern, and electrocardiographic monitoring is essential until treatment corrects serum K$^+$ levels. For a detailed discussion of hyperkalemia and treatment, see Chapter 65.
  2. **Hypokalemia.** Potassium levels <4.0 mEq/L suggest impending hypokalemia, and values <3.5 mEq/L require treatment to correct. Meanwhile, cardiac conduction abnormalities may occur, and monitoring electrocardiographically, as in hyperkalemia, is essential until hypokalemia is corrected. For a detailed discussion of hypokalemia and treatment, see Chapter 68.
C. **Chloride.** See also Chapter 51, section on metabolic alkalosis.
  1. **Hypochloremia.** Serum values of 97 to 110 mEq/L are taken as normal in most newborn infants. Serum values <97 mEq/L are indicative of low chloride and suggest either inadequate supplementation during infusion fluid therapy or, more commonly, chloride ion losses. Typically, chloride ion accompanies Na$^+$ and K$^+$ as NaCl or KCl solutions in maintenance infusion solutions. Chloride losses independent of Na$^+$ or K$^+$ occur usually from excessive gastrointestinal fluid losses, particularly gastric hydrochloric acid losses. Chloride losses lead to increased bicarbonate reabsorption and metabolic alkalosis.
  2. **Hyperchloremia.** Uncommon in the newborn period but may be found when inadvertent concentrations of Cl$^-$ ion are given in parenteral nutrition solutions. Occasionally increased Cl$^-$ ion is reflective of excessive renal conservation of Cl$^-$ during correction of alkalosis when forming alkaline urine.

11 Nutritional Management

GROWTH ASSESSMENT

I. **Anthropometrics.** Serial measurements of weight, length, and head circumference allow for evaluation of growth patterns.
  A. **Weight.** Birthweight (BW) is reflective of maternal, placental, and fetal environment. Both term and preterm neonates experience weight loss after birth (approximately 10%, or higher in preterm infants) due to loss of extracellular free water. Term infants regain birth weight by 7 to 10 days, whereas preterm infants may take 10 to 15 days to regain birth weight (or even longer in extremely low BW [ELBW] infants). Once BW is reached, average daily weight gain should be 14 to 20 g/kg/d for preterm infants and 20 to 30 g/d for term infants.
  B. **Length.** Length is a better indicator of lean body mass and long-term growth and is not influenced by fluid status. Weekly assessment is recommended using a neonatal length board. Average length gain is 1.4 cm/wk in preterm infants and 0.7 cm/wk in term infants.
  C. **Head circumference.** Occipitofrontal circumference (OFC) reflects brain growth and correlates with long-term neurodevelopment. Weekly assessment is recommended. Preterm infants grow at a rate of 0.9 cm/wk and term infants at 0.33 cm/wk. Premature infants exhibit catch-up growth in head circumference that may exceed normal growth rate, but an increase in head circumference >1.25 cm/wk

may be abnormal and should prompt evaluation for hydrocephalus or intraventricular hemorrhage. Poor head circumference growth may reflect underlying poor nutritional status or medical condition and may be associated with motor and cognitive delays.

D. **Weight for length.** This reflects symmetry of growth. Current weight expressed as a percentage of ideal weight for length can identify infants at risk for under- or overnutrition. Catch-up growth occurs faster if only weight is lagging compared with length and head circumference. Weight gain is slower in large for gestational age infants.

E. **Z-scores.** Z-scores express anthropometric data as a function of standard deviation from the mean or median value and can be used to compare weight for age, weight for height, and height for age across various ages; they are useful for comparing populations.

F. **Body composition.** Body mass index (BMI) for gestational age reference curves allow assessment of proportionality of weight and length growth. BMI and weight for length show high agreement. Body mass composition curves for healthy preterm infants at birth assess patterns of fetal body composition variation and can identify infants at risk for metabolic syndrome.

G. **Growth velocity.** Growth velocity is higher at earlier gestational age; at <27 weeks, it is approximately 20 g/kg/d; at 33 weeks, approximately 14 g/kg/d; and at term, approximately 10 g/kg/d. Fetal growth velocity approximates 1% to 3% of body weight per day.

II. **Classification**

A. **Measurements.** Weight, length, and head circumference are plotted on growth charts to facilitate comparison with established norms.

B. **Growth charts.** Growth can be monitored longitudinally on standard growth charts. For term infants, the World Health Organization (WHO) growth charts (2006) based on data from different ethnicities reflect *growth standards* of healthy breast-fed infants and should be used until 2 years of age. The Centers for Disease Control and Prevention (CDC) growth charts (2000) are a *reference* for anthropometric growth parameters at any given time and should be used to monitor growth after 2 years of age (https://www.cdc.gov/growthcharts/who_charts.htm). The two charts are now merged; the WHO centiles are used before 2 years and the CDC after 2 years (www.who.int/childgrowth/standards/en).

Growth patterns of term infants differ based on diet, with breast-fed infants experiencing rapid early weight gain in the first 6 months and slower weight gain thereafter compared to formula-fed infants, but linear growth remains similar. Breast-fed infants, compared to formula-fed infants, also drop down the centiles between 6 and 18 months with decreases in weight and weight for length.

Two types of **growth charts exist for very low birthweight (VLBW) infants**: those based on fetal (intrauterine growth) and those based on postnatal growth. Intrauterine growth charts provide **fetal reference standards**. Assessment of postnatal growth failure is better reflected on postnatal growth charts, but these are limited because they do not show the "catch-up growth" or the growth velocity relative to the fetus.

Normal growth customarily falls between the 10th and 90th percentiles when adjusted for gestational age. Population-specific customized growth charts have been developed to determine term optimal BW and to identify fetal growth restriction (www.gestation.net). Growth charts from different regions around the world allow monitoring postnatal growth of infants born preterm.

1. The INTERGROWTH-21st study followed intrauterine, newborn, and postnatal growth in 8 diverse geographic regions (Brazil, China, India, Italy, Kenya, Oman, United Kingdom, and United States) and provide growth charts up to 64 weeks after birth (https://intergrowth21.tghn.org); these curves were published in late 2014 and are expected to be used more often in the future.

2. Two commonly used growth charts for preterm infants are the Olsen and Fenton growth charts. The **2010 Olsen growth charts** (https://www.aap.org/en-us/Documents/GrowthCurves.pdf) are based on intrauterine growth of 257,855 singleton infants who were born in the United States between 22 and 42 weeks' postmenstrual age (PMA) and survived. The charts incorporate data from the WHO charts for the period of 39 to 50 weeks' PMA. The **2013 Fenton growth charts** (www.ucalgary.ca/fenton/2013chart) are based on anthropometric measurements from 3 intrauterine growth datasets; BW for gestation data on approximately 676,000 Canadian infants from 22 to 40 weeks' gestation, and length and OFC data from 376,000 Swedish infants from 28 to 40 weeks' gestation and from approximately 27,000 Australian infants from 22 to 40 weeks' gestation. The curves include data to 50 weeks PMA based on the WHO 2006 data. The charts reflect the actual age instead of completed weeks. Both charts (Olson and Fenton) are widely used and easily accessible and are reproduced in Chapter 6.

NUTRITIONAL REQUIREMENTS

I. **Calories.** The energy provided by dietary intake contributes to basal resting metabolism, thermoregulation, physical activity, and growth. In term infants, optimal weight gain is 20 to 30 g/d and usually achieved with a caloric intake between 100 and 120 kcal/kg/d. Preterm infants may require 120 to 140 kcal/kg/d for optimal weight gain that matches or exceeds the fetal growth rate of approximately 14 to 20 g/kg/d. Acutely ill infants become relatively insulin resistant with increased levels of stress hormones, leading to tissue catabolism, and may need higher caloric intake for adequate growth. Examples of states of altered nutritional needs include acute respiratory disease, chronic respiratory disease, sepsis, surgery, and congenital heart disease.

II. **Carbohydrates.** Approximately 10 g/kg/d (12–14 g/kg/d in preterm) are needed to provide 40% to 50% of total calories.

III. **Proteins.** In the term infant, adequate protein intake has been estimated at 1.5 to 2.2 g/kg/d (7%–16% of total calories). Preterm infants require 3.5 to 4.4 g/kg/d.

IV. **Lipids.** In the term infant, fat requirements are estimated at 3.3 to 6 g/kg/d (40%–55% of total calories). Preterm infants require 4 to 7 g/kg/d to account for decreased intestinal fat digestion and absorption.

V. **Long-chain polyunsaturated fatty acids (LCPUFA).** To meet essential fatty acid requirements, preterm infants should receive 385 to 1540 mg/kg/d of linoleic acid and >55 mg/kg/d of linolenic acid. Linoleic and linolenic acids are precursors for arachidonic acid (ARA) and docosahexaenoic acid (DHA), which are important in neural and retinal maturation. LCPUFAs are transferred predominantly through the placenta in the third trimester, which places preterm infants at risk of deficiency. Additionally, concentrations of LCPUFAs in human milk varies (0.1%–1.4%) across regions. Although human milk intake meets the LCPUFA requirements of term infants but not preterm infants, preterm neonates fed LCPUFA-enriched feeds have failed to show benefits in retinal sensitivity and visual acuity. It is not clear if maternal supplementation of DHA would be beneficial for their VLBW offspring.

VI. **Vitamins and minerals.** Guidelines for vitamin and mineral requirements for preterm infants, although not clearly established, are provided in Tables 11-1 and 11-2 for low BW infants. Caution is required with vitamin supplementation because toxicity may occur with both water- and fat-soluble vitamins as a result of immature renal and hepatic function. Vitamin supplementation may be needed with certain types of infant formulas and human milk fortifiers.

A. **Vitamin A.** May be useful in attenuating chronic lung disease in VLBW infants at a dose of 5000 IU intramuscularly 3 times per week for 12 doses.

B. **For infants with osteopenia of prematurity.** Various amounts of calcium, phosphorus, and vitamin D may need to be supplemented. See Chapter 113.

Table 11–1. DAILY ENTERAL VITAMIN AND MINERAL REQUIREMENTS FOR TERM AND
STABLE PRETERM LOW BIRTHWEIGHT INFANTS

Nutrient	Term Infant (per day)	Stable Very Low Birthweight Infant (dose/kg)
Vitamins		
Vitamin A (with lung disease)	400 mcg	700–1500 IU
Vitamin D	400 IU	150-400 IU
Vitamin E	7 IU	6–12 IU
Vitamin K	200 mcg	8–10 mcg
Vitamin C	80 mg	18–24 mg
Thiamine	1.2 mg	180–240 mcg
Riboflavin	1.4 mg	250–360 mcg
Niacin	17 mg	3.6–4.8 mg
Pyridoxine	1.0 mg	150–210 mcg
Vitamin B12	1.0 mcg	0.3 mcg
Folic acid	140 mcg	25–50 mcg
Biotin	20 mcg	3.6–6.0 mcg
Pantothenate	5 mg	1.2–1.7 mg
Choline	125 mg	14.4–28 mg
Minerals		
Calcium	250 mg	150–220 mg
Phosphorus	150 mg	75–140 mg
Magnesium	20 mg	7.9–15 mg
Sodium	1–2 mEq/kg	69–115 mg
Potassium	2–3 mEq/kg	78–195 mg
Iron	1 mg/kg	2–3 mg
Copper	20 mcg/kg	100–230 mcg
Zinc	2.5–5.0 mg/d	1000 mcg
Manganese	5 mcg/100 kcal	0.75–7.5 mcg
Molybdenum	0.75–7.5 mcg	0.3 mcg
Selenium	2 mcg/kg	5–10 mcg
Chromium	0.20 mcg/kg	0.1–2.25 mcg
Iodine	1 mcg/kg	10–55 mcg
Linoleic acid	4.4 g	385–1540 mg
Linolenic acid	0.5 g	>55 mg
Docosahexaenoic acid (DHA)		>18 mg
Arachidonic acid (ARA)		>24 mg

Table 11–2. DAILY PARENTERAL REQUIREMENTS FOR VITAMINS AND MINERALS IN TERM, PRETERM, AND STABLE PRETERM INFANTS

Nutrient	Term Infant (per day)	Stable Very Low Birth Weight Infant (dose/kg)
Vitamins		
Vitamin A (with lung disease)	700 mcg	700–1500 IU
Vitamin D	400 IU	40–160 IU
Vitamin E	7 mg	2.8–3.5 mg
Vitamin K	200 mcg	10 mcg
Vitamin C	80 mg	15–25 mg
Thiamine	1.2 mg	200–350 mcg
Riboflavin	1.4 mg	150–200 mcg
Niacin	17 mg	4–6.8 mg
Pyridoxine	1.0 mg	150–200 mg
Vitamin B12	1.0 mcg	0.3 mcg
Folic acid	140 mcg	56 mcg
Biotin	20 mcg	5–8 mcg
Pantothenate	5 mg	1.2 mg
Minerals		
Calcium		60–80 mg
Phosphorus		45–60 mg
Magnesium		4.3–7.2 mg
Sodium	1–2 mEq/kg	69–115 mg
Potassium	2–3 mEq/kg	78–117 mg
Iron[a]		100–200 mcg
Copper[b]	20 mcg/kg	20 mcg
Zinc	250 mcg/kg	400 mcg
Manganese	1 mcg/kg	1 mcg
Molybdenum	0.25 mcg	0.25 mcg
Selenium[c]	2 mcg/kg	1.5–4.5 mcg
Chromium	0.20 mcg/kg	0.05–0.3 mcg
Iodine	1 mcg/kg	1 mcg

[a]Start supplementation at 6 to 8 weeks.
[b]Omit in cholestatic jaundice.
[c]Start supplementation at 2 to 4 weeks. Omit in renal dysfunction.

   C. **Iron deficiency.** Iron deficiency anemia is associated with short-term and long-term neurodevelopmental deficits, delayed maturation of the auditory brainstem responses, and abnormalities of memory and behavior. Iron supplementation of term infants at risk of iron deficiency is associated with improved neurodevelopmental outcomes. Preterm infants are more susceptible to iron deficiency due to small iron stores at birth, high growth velocity, and phlebotomy losses. Furthermore, anemia may be associated with increased rates of necrotizing enterocolitis (NEC) in this population. Blood transfusions provide a rich source of iron; 1 mL of packed red blood cells provides 0.5 to 1.0 mg of iron, and iron overload may be a risk with multiple transfusions. Delayed cord clamping improves iron stores in both term and preterm infants. **Stable preterm infants without recent blood transfusions** should receive iron supplementation (2–4 mg/kg/d; maximum 15 mg/d) starting at 2 to 4 weeks of age and continued until 12 months. **Formula-fed infants** require less iron supplementation than human milk–fed infants, although iron is more bioavailable in human milk. A rising reticulocyte count may indicate the need for starting iron supplementation. **Term breast-fed infants (but not formula-fed infants)** should receive iron supplementation at 1 mg/kg starting at 4 months until age-appropriate diet is established.

   D. **Recombinant human erythropoietin therapy (rhEPO).** Additional iron supplementation is necessary for infants receiving rhEPO. Recommended dose is 6 mg/kg/d added to enteral feedings or 3 mg/kg/wk (iron dextran) added to parenteral nutrition. For infants receiving high doses of iron, monitoring for hemolytic anemia is important, and vitamin E supplementation (15–25 IU/d) may be required. Administration of rhEPO reduces the number of transfusions in VLBW infants but may have limited efficacy in decreasing the number of blood donors to which the infant is exposed. rhEPO is being currently investigated as a neuroprotective agent. Its use is variable among neonatal intensive care units (NICUs), and it is controversial whether early rhEPO is associated with increased risk of retinopathy of prematurity (ROP).

VII. **Fluids.** See Chapter 10 for fluid requirements.

VIII. **Parenteral nutrition.** (See section on parenteral nutrition, page 155.)

PRINCIPLES OF ENTERAL FEEDING

I. **Term infants.** Term healthy infants should be breast fed within the first hour after birth or as soon as medically stable. Once tolerated, feeding should be advanced to ad libitum. In sick infants, gavage feeds should be started as soon as the infant is clinically stable and milk is available.

II. **Preterm infants.** Enteral feedings with human milk should be initiated as soon as clinically possible, ideally within 24 to 48 hours (see also discussion of trophic feeds later in this chapter). Preterm infants are at risk of postnatal growth and nutritional failure as they are deprived of in utero transfer of nutrients, particularly proteins, fats, and minerals. Early enteral feedings are associated with better endocrine adaptation, enhanced immune functions and gut maturation, decreased time to attain full feeds, and earlier discharge without an increase in risk of NEC. Although the intake of proteins (both enteral and parenteral) and a shorter time to regain BW positively influence neurodevelopmental outcomes, aggressive feeding and rapid weight gain predominantly as fat deposition increase the risks of subsequent metabolic syndrome. In preterm infants, parenteral nutrition should be initiated to provide adequate protein and caloric intake and improve weight gain (see further discussion in section on parenteral nutrition).

III. **Feeding guidelines**
   A. **Type of feeds.** Breast feeding and human milk intake are the biological norm for infant feeding in both the term and preterm infant. Pasteurized donor human milk and commercial formulas are available if maternal milk is unavailable.
   B. **Mode of feeding.** Feeds can be provided orally or via gavage. Oral feeds are the preferred method of delivery if the infant is clinically stable and has a mature feeding pattern; otherwise, gavage feeds can be used. Oromotor coordination (sucking, swallowing, and breathing) is not mature in preterm infants and usually precludes

oral feeds. Limited studies suggest that preterm neonates on noninvasive support (continuous positive airway pressure or high flow) are capable of maintaining airway during feeds, but caution should be exercised with oral feeds. Some institutions allow the infant to attempt nuzzling at breast while on noninvasive respiratory support. This may increase the mother's milk supply and encourage bonding of the mother–infant dyad. Preterm and sick neonates are also at risk for oral aversion.

C. **Contraindications to enteral feeds** Oral feeds are a contraindication in neonates with: a risk for aspiration, such as in intubated patients, and tachypnea (respiratory rate >70 breaths/min); neurologic injury; and in infants with bilious emesis, abdominal distension, or excessive oral secretions. Gavage feeds may be used instead.

Feeding caution should be exercised in the presence of perinatal asphyxia, hemodynamic instability, sepsis, absent or reversed end-diastolic (A/REDF) umbilical arterial flow in utero, severe intrauterine growth restriction (IUGR), indomethacin or ibuprofen therapy, hemodynamically significant patent ductus arteriosus (PDA), polycythemia, severe anemia, and packed red cell transfusion. This caution stems from concerns, in many institutions, for NEC in ELBW and VLBW infants. However, there is increasing evidence that it is safe to provide feeding (at least trophic) for infants exposed to absent or reversed end-diastolic umbilical arterial flow, indomethacin or ibuprofen therapy, and PDA.

D. **Oral care.** Oropharyngeal administration of maternal colostrum or milk exposes infants to the benefits of the mother's own milk. Administration of colostrum directly to the buccal mucosa may mimic the protective effects of amniotic fluid, accelerate intestinal maturation, and improve time to oral feeding.

E. **Minimal enteral feedings.** Minimal enteral or trophic feeds are subnutritional quantities of milk feeds (maternal or donor milk) given during the first few days of life to stimulate the development of the immature gastrointestinal (GI) tract of the preterm infant. This practice, also called hypocaloric, trophic, trickle feedings, low-volume enteral substrate, or GI priming, is characterized by a small-volume feeding to supplement parenteral nutrition. Most institutions consider approximately up to 24 mL/kg/d as trophic feeds. Trophic feeds are usually given for 3 to 7 days prior to advancing feeding volume. Potential benefits include improved feeding tolerance, improved gastric emptying, prevention of GI atrophy, and facilitation of GI tract maturation leading to faster attainment of full enteral feedings. Other benefits may include decreased incidence of cholestasis, nosocomial infections, and metabolic bone disease and decreased hospital stay without an increase in the incidence of NEC.

F. **Feeding advancement.** While advancement protocols vary among institutions, a standardized approach (agreed upon among various NICU providers and implemented consistently) in preterm infants can lead to improved feeding-related outcomes, including less time to full feeds, better weight gain, decreased costs, and decreased incidence of NEC. For stable VLBW infants (between 1000 and 1500 g), rapid advancement (35 mL/kg/d) of enteral feeds versus slower advancement (15–20 mL/kg/d) does not increase the risk of NEC or death and decreases the risk of invasive infection. Most institutions would provide trophic feeds for a period of 5 to 7 days in ELBW infants at 10 to 15 mL/kg/d divided every 2 to 3 hours. At our institution, for example, for infants <1000 g, we start feeds at 15 mL/kg/d divided every 3 hours and advance by 15 mL/kg/d daily as tolerated. For infants >1000 g, we start feeds at 25 to 35 mL/kg/d divided every 3 hours and advance by 25 to 35 mL/kg/d daily as tolerated. Caution should be exercised in infants at high risk of NEC, particularly growth restricted infants with absent or reversed end-diastolic flow and on formula feeds.

G. **Feeding intolerance.** If feeding is initiated but not tolerated, a complete abdominal examination should be performed. Preterm infants <32 weeks may not establish antegrade peristalsis. In the absence of other clinical signs, bilious aspirate by itself is not a contraindication for feedings in VLBW infants. It is questionable whether checking gastric residuals prior to feeds, although routine in most NICUs, can improve feeding intolerance or prevent NEC. When studied, the color and volume of aspirates have not been shown to predict NEC. In addition, aspiration can damage friable gastric mucosa, lead to discarding of nutrients and enzymes that help mature the GI system, and delay time to full feeds. Some institutions have shown that abandoning the practice of checking residuals is safe and allows reaching full feeds early with less exposure to central venous access. In clinically stable infants, increasing feeding volume or continuing feeding (in the face of residuals) may be helpful in improving feeding tolerance due to possible increase in gastric emptying and stimulation of the gastrocolic reflex. Presence of bilious or bloody emesis, blood in stool, abdominal distension, or other systemic signs such as apnea and bradycardia should prompt evaluation for infections and NEC (see Chapter 54 on bloody stool and Chapter 109 on NEC).

H. **Continuous feeds.** Infants with short gut syndromes, feeding intolerance, or gastroesophageal reflux may tolerate continuous feeds better than bolus feeds. However, there is no clear evidence that continuous feeding is better than bolus feeding. Of importance when on continuous feeds, substantial amounts of fat and nutrients from human milk can adhere to the feeding bag, syringe, and tubing and may not be delivered to the infant, resulting in suboptimal growth. The infusion syringe should be placed upward at a 45-degree angle to promote even distribution of human milk fat and fortifier.

FORMS OF ENTERAL NUTRITION: HUMAN MILK (TABLE 11–3)

Breast feeding and human milk are the biological standard for feeding term, preterm, and sick infants. Breast feeding is recommended as the sole source of nutrition for the first 4 to 6 months of age and then as complementary feeds thereafter as long as desired.

I. **Effectiveness of breast feeding and human milk**

A. **Infants.** Breastfeeding provides immunologic protection against bacterial and viral infections (particularly upper respiratory tract infections, otitis media, and GI infections). Risk of sudden infant death is decreased by 36% for infants with any amount of breast feeding >1 month. Breast-fed infants have lower risks of obesity, type 1 diabetes mellitus, celiac and inflammatory bowel disease, and acute lymphocytic leukemia. Breast feeding may improve neurodevelopmental outcomes.

B. **Human milk in the preterm infant**

1. **Effectiveness of human milk in the NICU.** Human milk feeding in preterm infants is associated with less feeding intolerance, less time to reach full feeds, decreased risk of NEC (formula-fed infants have a 6- to 10-fold higher risk), and higher intelligence quotient (IQ) at the age of 8 years. Breast milk may protect against NEC by lowering gastric pH, decreasing intestinal epithelial permeability, improving motility, and altering bacterial flora. Maternal milk feedings are associated with decreased rates of ROP and larger white matter and total brain volumes and have beneficial effects on visual, cognitive, psychomotor, and neurodevelopmental outcomes that persist into childhood. A dose-response relationship between amount of human milk and decreased incidences of feeding intolerance, nosocomial infection, NEC, bronchopulmonary dysplasia (BPD), and ROP has been demonstrated, with benefits seen even with partial human milk feeds (>50 mL/kg) in preterm infants. The volume of human milk intake during an infant's stay in the NICU may directly impact later neurodevelopmental scores.

2. **Postdischarge.** Postdischarge rates of hospital readmission are lower in infants who have ever received human milk even if not receiving human milk at the

Table 11–3. ENTERAL FEEDINGS INDICATIONS AND USES

Formula	Indications	Vitamin and Mineral Supplement[a]
Human milk	All infants	Vitamin D 400 IU/d; iron at 4 months
Breast milk fortifiers	Preterm infant (<1800 g and <34 weeks)	Vitamin D 400 IU/d; iron; MV
Cow milk–based formulas		
Enfamil Infant Similac Advance Similac Organic	Full-term infants: as supplement to breast milk	MV if <32 oz./d (~1 L/d)
Enfamil Gentlease/Similac Sensitive	Term infants: to reduce fussiness or gas	
Gerber Good Start	Term infants: whey protein; moderate mineral content; may be more palatable	
Enfamil Added Rice	Rice starch added for thickening after ingestion (pH sensitive). Used for simple reflux. Not indicated for preterm infants	
Preterm formulas		
Enfamil Premature 20, 24, and 30 Similac Special Care 20, 24, and 30	Preterm infants: for infants on fluid restriction or who cannot handle required volumes of 20-calorie formula to grow. Calcium and phosphorus content to mimic intrauterine accretion rates	
Enfamil Premature 24 High Protein Similac Special Care 24 High Protein	Approximately 10% more protein than above formulas at same caloric density	
Enfamil EnfaCare Similac NeoSure	Preterm infants preparing for discharge; increased protein, calcium, phosphorous, vitamins A and D; promotes better mineralization. Use up to 6–9 months corrected age	
Soy formulas (*Note:* Soy formulas not recommended in infants <1800 g)		
Enfamil ProSobee (lactose and sucrose free) Gerber Good Start Soy Similac Soy Isomil (lactose free)	Term infants: milk sensitivity, galactosemia, carbohydrate intolerance, desire for vegetarian diet. Term infants; hydrolyzed soy proteins *Do not use soy formulas in preterm infants. Phytates can bind calcium and cause rickets*	MV if <32 oz./d (~1 L/d)

(Continued)

Table 11–3. ENTERAL FEEDINGS INDICATIONS AND USES (*CONTINUED*)

Formula	Indications	Vitamin and Mineral Supplement[a]
Protein hydrolysate formulas (casein predominant)		
Nutramigen with Enflora LGG (Probiotic LGG)	Term infants: hypoallergenic, hydrolyzed casein with lactose, galactose, and sucrose free for gut sensitivity to proteins, galactosemia, multiple food allergies, persistent diarrhea, colic due to cow milk allergy	MV if <32 oz./d (~1 L/d)
Pregestimil	Preterm and term infants: disaccharides deficiency, fat malabsorption, diarrhea, GI defects, cystic fibrosis, food allergy, celiac disease, transition from TPN to oral feeding	
Similac Alimentum	Term infants: lactose-free formula; protein sensitivity, pancreatic insufficiency, diarrhea, severe food allergies, colic, carbohydrate, and fat malabsorption	
Free amino acid elemental formulas		
Neocate	Term infants: severe cow milk protein allergies; contains 100% free amino acids (elemental formula)	
EleCare for Infants	Elemental formula containing amino acids indicated for malabsorption, protein malabsorption, short bowel syndromes	
Special formulas		
Similac PM 60/40	Preterm and term infants: problem feeders on standard formula; infants with renal, cardiovascular, or digestive diseases that require decreased protein and mineral levels; breast-feeding supplement; initial feeding	MV and Fe if standard formula weight >1500 g
Enfaport	For infants with chylothorax and LCHAD deficiency	
Metabolic formulas	Special metabolic formulas are available for infants with inherited metabolic disorders www.meadjohnson.com www.abottnutrition.com	

Fe, iron; GI, gastrointestinal; LCHAD, long-chain 3-hydroxyacyl-CoA dehydrogenase; MV, multivitamin; TPN, total parenteral nutrition.
[a]Such as Poly-Vi-Sol (Mead Johnson).

time of discharge. In adolescents who were former preterm infants, lower rates of metabolic syndrome including lower blood pressure and better insulin metabolism have been observed.

C. **Maternal outcomes.** Breast feeding improves maternal and infant bonding and is associated with decreased rates of maternal blood loss, breast cancer, ovarian cancer, postpartum depression, type 2 diabetes, cardiovascular disease, hypertension, and rheumatoid arthritis. Breast feeding also leads to faster return to prepregnancy weight and can help optimize pregnancy spacing.

D. **Immunologic benefits.** Breast milk contains several bioactive factors that protect against bacteria and viruses. Extracellular vesicles deliver proteins, lipids, and long noncoding RNA to affect immune functions. Exosomes in breast milk regulate cellular communication, and microRNA may alter gene expression. Other immunologic benefits of breast milk include:

1. **Anti-infectious and immune properties.** Lactoferrin, lysozyme, lactadherin, defensins, maternal leukocytes, and immunoglobulins are a few of the immune components of human milk that provide protection for the infant. The dose-dependent protection of human milk against NEC and sepsis may be secondary to a decrease in intestinal permeability and bacterial translocation as well as the maturational effects of breast milk on the intestine.

2. **Cytokines and chemokines.** Cytokines in human milk promote maturation of the infant immune and GI systems and decrease excessive inflammatory responses. Chemokines aid infants by providing immune protection, promoting host defense against infection, and decreasing inflammation. Human milk contains the enzyme acetylhydrolase, which antagonizes platelet-activating factor, a major trigger for NEC in premature infants.

3. **Growth factors and oligosaccharides.** Growth factors such as epidermal growth factor and insulin-like growth factor promote GI and immune system maturation. Oligosaccharides act as prebiotics, have antiadhesive activity to deter pathogens from sticking to host mucosa, and modulate cell responses to promote normal gut development.

4. **Hormones.** Breast feeding promotes oxytocin release in both members of the breast-feeding dyad, which encourages bonding and provides maternal empowerment to participate in her infant's care.

E. **Economics.** Breast feeding can reduce costs and improve productivity and morale in the workplace.

II. **Contraindications to breast milk feeding.** Temporary problems in the mother, such as sore or cracked nipples, mastitis, and the presence of "discolored milk" do not preclude nursing. The following are true contraindications to breast feeding.

A. **Infections**

1. **Active tuberculosis.** Breast feeding can resume after 2 weeks of treatment and documentation that the mother is no longer infectious.

2. **Human T-cell lymphotropic virus (HTLV).**

3. **Human immunodeficiency virus (HIV).** This only applies to developed countries with safe alternative forms of infant nutrition. For specific recommendations, see Appendix F. Issues in HIV-infected mothers are discussed in Chapter 138.

4. **Untreated brucellosis.**

5. **Active herpes simplex lesions on the breast.** No direct breast feeding until the lesions have resolved but appropriate to give expressed maternal milk.

6. **Varicella.** Mothers with active varicella that develops 5 days before and 2 days after delivery should be separated from their infants but can provide expressed maternal milk safely.

B. **Metabolic. Galactosemia** is a contraindication to breast feeding. With other inborn errors of metabolism, often a combination of human milk and other metabolic formulas can be used.

C. **Medications, anesthesia, and radiologic studies.** Breast feeding is safe with most medications and after most surgical and most radiologic procedures. Maternal medications should be evaluated for their effect on lactation and milk supply (see Chapter 156).

D. **Breast feeding in mothers with substance use disorders.** Breast feeding can be considered in infants with in utero exposure to illicit substances if mothers are enrolled and compliant in treatment programs, abstinent from illicit drug use for 90 days before delivery, and have negative toxicology screen at delivery. Methadone treatment alone is not a contraindication for breast feeding. The effect of buprenorphine treatment on breast feeding is not clear but appears to be safe.

III. **Support for breast feeding mothers in the NICU.** The benefits of breast feeding or expressed milk feeding should be reviewed with mothers during pregnancy and after birth. Expression and storage of colostrum, skin-to-skin contact, lactation support, rooming in, and nonnutritive feeding should be encouraged. Transition to direct breast feeding should be encouraged when developmentally appropriate.

IV. **Storage.** Human milk can be stored at room temperature for 3 to 4 hours and likely up to 6 hours, in the refrigerator for 72 hours (up to 8 days may be acceptable), frozen at –18°C for up to 6 months, and frozen in a deep freezer at –20°C for up to 12 months.

V. **Donor human milk (DHM).** Maternal milk is the preferred nutritional substrate in infants. However, DHM should be pasteurized (pDHM) and is an acceptable alternative or supplement until maternal milk is available.

A. **Indications for use.** pDHM can be used as a bridge until the mother's own milk is available, and its use can be prioritized for VLBW infants (<1500 g) to decrease the risks of NEC and in medically complex infants (eg, gastroschisis, cyanotic heart disease) who do not tolerate specialized formula. In babies <1500 g, pDHM is used until approximately 34 weeks' gestation to reduce the risks of NEC. Recent trends are showing pDHM being used in term infants delivered directly to families outside of hospital settings. In preterm and low BW infants, formula-fed infants, compared to pDHM-fed infants, have better short-term growth but an almost 3-fold higher risk of NEC.

B. **Safety.** pDHM is available currently in the United States from 3 sources: the Human Milk Banking Association of North America (HMBANA), Medolac (Portland, OR), and Prolacta Biosciences (Minerva, CA); the latter 2 sources are commercial companies. Each source uses a unique method of recruitment of lactating, donating mothers and varied operational processes. Concerns for infections have been addressed; pDHM is considered safe and effective with formalized donor screening and serologic testing, collection and handling protocols, and pasteurization of the milk. Parental counseling should still be carried out prior to use. There have been no reported cases of HIV or hepatitis transmission via pDHM in the United States to date. Short-term heat activation eliminates cytomegalovirus (CMV) effectively.

C. **Limitations**

1. **Growth.** As most donated milk is more mature, the protein and caloric content is lower than that of preterm milk. Since donor milk is pooled, fat content, LCPUFA, DHA, and AHA vary from batch to batch. Early use of pDHM was associated with poor growth, but more recent data suggest that infant growth is not significantly lagging when **fortification** (see later discussion) is added to pDHM.

2. **Cost.** Reimbursement for pDHM by insurance is variable from state to state with no clear guidelines regarding billing procedures.

3. **Effects of heat treatment, storage, and handling.** Heat treatment with either Holder pasteurization or high-temperature short-time pasteurization is used to reduce the risk of bacterial and viral diseases to the milk recipients (see previous discussion). Heat treatment also results in loss of beneficial probiotic bacteria; decreased fat, caloric, and protein content; and decreased lactoferrin

and immunoglobulins but has little effect on micronutrients and vitamins A, D, and E. Human milk oligosaccharides and LCPUFAs remain intact with pasteurization.

4. **Supply.** The supply of pDHM is currently limited. There are 26 milk banks in the United States and Canada that form HMBANA. As noted earlier, there are at least 2 commercial (for-profit) companies that sell human milk or products derived from human milk. The practice of selling human milk openly on the Internet and through social media outlets is increasing, which may further limit the human milk available for donation (see later discussion). The scarcity of this precious resource raises questions about how to increase the supply and equitably allocate it to infants who need it most. On a positive note, the California Perinatal Quality Care Collaborative has shown recently that the availability of pDHM has increased over time (2007–2013) and has been associated with positive changes, including increased breast milk feeding at NICU discharge and decreased NEC rates.

D. **Nonpasteurized DHM.** Nonpasteurized DHM increases the risks of transmission of viral diseases (eg, CMV, hepatitis, HIV) and bacterial contamination to the recipients and, as such, is not recommended. Donor exposure to medications, herbal supplements, and drugs may contaminate donated milk. However, programs are available in some countries (eg, Sweden) where donors are carefully screened for infectious diseases and live unpasteurized milk is used for feeding. There has been a rapid, virtual explosion of milk sharing through groups on the Internet and Facebook; this prompted the US Food and Drug Administration (FDA) to issue a warning against feeding babies breast milk acquired directly from individuals due to potential risks associated with the practice.

VI. **Human milk fortifiers.** Human milk is the preferred substrate for preterm nutrition. However, fortification of the milk is necessary to meet the demands of rapidly growing premature infants despite being higher in protein and energy content compared to mature milk. Use of human milk beyond the second week in preterm infants provides insufficient amounts of protein, calcium, phosphorus, and possibly copper, zinc, and sodium, especially in VLBW infants. Previous older formulations when added to preterm mother's milk resulted in nitrogen retention and increased blood urea levels but with increased somatic and linear growth. One study in low BW infants comparing unfortified human milk versus fortified human milk up to 4 months after discharge noted no differences in growth parameters at 1 year of age. Table 11–4 shows nutrient composition of some of the fortifiers currently available in the United States.

A. **Indications.** The addition of multinutrient fortifiers to either a mother's own milk or DHM increases nutrient content by 10% to 20% and decreases rates of in-hospital postnatal growth failure, metabolic bone disease, and vitamin deficiencies. Fortification of human milk can also help keep feeding volumes lower for infants who are fluid sensitive. Criteria for use of human milk fortifiers include <34 weeks' gestation and/or <1800 g at birth. Fortification (usually with cow milk–based fortifiers after 34 weeks' PMA) is recommended until infants reach approximately 3600 g or at hospital discharge. Postdischarge fortification of human milk is usually not recommended.

Both human milk–based and bovine milk–based fortifiers are available in powder and liquid forms in the United States. Sterile liquid fortifiers are recommended due to the risks of bacterial contamination with powdered fortifiers. A recent analysis of available fortifiers and preterm formula found that, although most fortifiers provide macronutrients within the recommended range, significant variations exist in micronutrient contents. Both excesses and deficiencies of some micronutrients were seen, most notably in the human milk–based fortifier (see following sections), where even additional vitamin supplementation may not be adequate. Fortification of fresh expressed breast milk is not associated with an increase in bacterial growth for up to 6 hours.

Table 11–4. COMPOSITION OF PRETERM HUMAN MILK[a] AND COMMERCIALLY AVAILABLE HUMAN MILK FORTIFIERS (HMF)

Variable	Preterm Human Milk[a]	Prolacta +4 H²MF[b]	Similac HMF Hydrolyzed Liquid[c]	Similac HMF Liquid[c]	Enfamil HMF Acidified Liquid[d]
Volume	100 mL	20 mL: 80 mL = 100 mL	4 packets/ 100 mL = 120 mL	4 packets/ 100 mL = 120 mL	4 vials (5 mL)/ 100 mL = 120 mL
Total calories	67	82	79	79	30
Osmolality (mOsm/kg H$_2$O)	290	<390	450	385	+36
Osmolarity	255				
Protein (g)	1.4	2.3	2.84	2.34	2.2
Fat (g)	3.9	4.9	3.94	4.14	2.3
Linoleic acid (mg)	480		368	311	230
Linolenic acid (mg)	30				
Carbohydrates (g)	6.6	7.1	8.04	8.24	<1.2
Minerals/100 mL					
Calcium (mg)	24.8	123	121	137	116
mEq	1.24	6.14	6	7	5.8
Chloride (mg)	55	73	89	89	45
mEq	1.6	2.06	2.6	2.6	1.27
Copper (mcg)	64.4	115	104	104	60
Iron (mg)	0.12	0.2	0.47	0.47	1.76
Magnesium (mg)	3.1	7.2	9.6	9.9	1.84
Phosphorus (mg)	12.8	64	67	77	63
Potassium (mg)	57	96	118	118	45
mEq	1.5	2.46	2.9	3	1.15
Sodium (mg)	24.8	57	37	37	27
mEq	1.1	2.47	1.6	1.7	1.17
Zinc (mg)	0.34	0.97	1.322	1.3	0.96
Iodine (mcg)	10.7		10	11	
Manganese (mcg)	0.6	<13	7.8	7.5	10
Selenium (mcg)	1.0		2	2	
Vitamins/100 mL					
Vitamin A (IU)	389	373	982	982	1160
Vitamin B1 (mcg)	20.8	20.6	177	177	184
Vitamin B2 (mcg)	48.3	53.6	287	450	260

(*Continued*)

Table 11–4. COMPOSITION OF PRETERM HUMAN MILK[a] AND COMMERCIALLY AVAILABLE HUMAN MILK FORTIFIERS (HMF) (*CONTINUED*)

Variable	Preterm Human Milk[a]	Prolacta +4 H²MF[b]	Similac HMF Hydrolyzed Liquid[c]	Similac HMF Liquid[c]	Enfamil HMF Acidified Liquid[d]
Vitamin B6 (mcg)	14.8	15.9	179	176	140
Vitamin B12 (mcg)	0.04	0.09	0.47	0.31	0.64
Vitamin C (mg)	10.7	8.7	34.6	34.6	15.2
Vitamin D (IU)	2	27.6	118	118	188
Vitamin E (IU)	1.1	1.3	4.2	4.2	5.6
Vitamin K (mcg)	0.2	0.3	8.2	8.2	5.7
Folic acid (mcg)	3.3	8	26.1	26.1	31
Niacin (mcg)	150.3	172.6	3392	3592	3700
Pantothenic acid (mcg)	180.5	219.2	1184	1180	920
Biotin (mcg)	0.4		19.7	25.7	3.4
Choline (mg)	9.4		3.3	10.8	
Inositol (mg)	14.7		5.4	18	

[a]Represents mature preterm human milk.
[b]Prolacta+4 H²MF: 20 mL fortifier to 80 mL preterm milk provides 100 mL of 24 kcal/oz. Other Prolacta H²MF products available.
[c]Similac HMF Hydrolyzed Protein Concentrated Liquid and Similac HMF Concentrated Liquid: 4 packets per 100 mL human milk provide 24 kcal/oz. with 120 mL of total volume.
[d]Enfamil HMF Acidified Liquid: 4 vials (5 mL each) per 100 mL human milk provides 24 kcal/oz. with 120 mL of total volume. Table includes nutrition information for fortifier alone.

The use of fortifiers is associated with in-hospital growth including weight gain, length, and head circumference without increasing morbidities such as NEC or BPD. No significant differences in outcomes have been found with early or late fortification (at 40 mL/kg/d vs 100 mL/kg/d) with regard to feeding tolerance and weight gain. At our institution, we fortify human milk at enteral volumes of 60 mL/kg/d. The details of some of the fortifiers are discussed below.

1. **Similac Human Milk Fortifier Hydrolyzed Protein Concentrated Liquid (commercially sterile)**
   a. **Composition.** The protein is hydrolyzed casein hydrolysate. The carbohydrate is maltodextrin and modified cornstarch. The fat is medium-chain triglycerides (MCTs) from soy and coconut oil. Additional iron and vitamin supplementation is recommended while using this product.
   b. **Calories.** The fortifier provides 24 kcal/fl oz., when added in the ratio of 1 packet/25 mL of human milk. Each packet (5 mL) provides 7 calories, 0.5 g protein, 0.75 g carbohydrate, and 0.21 g fat. Each packet provides 30 mg calcium and 17 mg phosphorous.

2. **Similac Human Milk Fortifier Concentrated Liquid (commercially sterile)**
   a. **Composition.** The protein is from whey protein concentrate. The carbohydrate is corn syrup solids. The fat is predominantly MCTs. Additional iron and vitamin supplementation is recommended while using this product.

      b. Calories. The fortifier provides 24 kcal/fl oz., when added in the ratio of 1 packet/25 mL of human milk. Each packet (5 mL) provides 7 calories, 0.35 g protein, 0.81 g carbohydrate, and 0.27 g fat. Each packet provides 35 mg calcium and 20 mg phosphorous.

      c. Not intended for use in preterm infants once they reach a weight of 3600 g.

  3. Enfamil Human Milk Fortifier–Acidified Liquid (commercially sterile)

      a. Composition. Whey protein hydrolysate, MCT oil, soy oil, ARA, and DHA. The carbohydrate is from citrates and pectin. Additional iron and vitamin supplementation is recommended while using this product.

      b. Calories. The fortifier provides 24 kcal/fl oz., when added in the ratio of 1 packet/25 mL of human milk. Each packet (5 mL) provides 7.5 calories, 0.55 g protein, 0.3 g carbohydrate, and 0.58 g fat. Each packet provides 29 mg calcium and 15.8 mg phosphorous.

      c. Use of >20 vials/d can result in hypervitaminosis A and D.

  4. Prolacta H²MF products

      a. Composition. Commercial human milk–based human milk fortifier made from pasteurized/processed DHM. Additional iron and vitamin supplementation is recommended with its use, and it is available in different calories per ounce.

      b. Calories. The fortifier (Prolact+4 H²MF) provides 24 kcal/fl oz., when added in the ratio of 20 mL fortifier/80 mL of human milk. Each bottle of fortifier provides an additional 28 calories, 1.2 g protein, 1.8 g carbohydrate, and 1.8 g fat. Each bottle of Prolact+4 H²MF provides 103 mg calcium and 53.8 mg phosphorous.

      c. Additional products. Prolacta products are available to add an additional 6, 8, and 10 calories per ounce. Prolacta cream is available as a supplement once goal protein is reached with the addition of Prolacta fortifier to human milk. It adds an additional 2.5 calories per milliliter using mostly fat.

      d. Limitation. With increasing fortification, the volume of maternal (or donor) human milk delivered to the infant is decreased. Additionally, the product is expensive; cost-effective analysis may not justify using it except for the most immature infants. In our institution (Washington University), we use Prolacta for infants with BW <1000 g and continue until 34 weeks' PMA.

 B. Human milk analyzers. There is a trend toward increased use of human milk analyzers for bedside analysis of macronutrient content of human milk in order to customize human milk fortification. However, data are limited to show that customized fortification provides any additional growth or long-term advantage.

 C. Inpatient transition. Transition from fortified human milk feeds to unfortified human milk or to preterm formula varies between institutions; the decision could be based on a specific length of time the patient has received fortification, IUGR status, target weight achieved, or PMA reached. In infants transitioning from donor milk to preterm formula, transition may be considered by 32 to 34 weeks' PMA or approximately 1500 to 1800 g. In infants receiving fortified maternal milk feeds, fortifier should be discontinued and adequate weight gain ensured a few days prior to discharge. In our institution, we transition infants 3 to 5 days before anticipated discharge date (when nippling 75% of their feeds) or at 36 to 38 weeks' PMA.

VII. Other supplements. Previously, the use of supplements or single modulars such as MCT oil, corn oil or corn starch, or protein powders was routine for infants with growth faltering in the NICU. Because these modulars alter the ratio of macronutrients and osmolality of the milk, they are no longer routinely recommended for use.

VIII. Probiotics and prebiotics. Meta-analyses of probiotics show benefits of supplementing milk with probiotics in decreasing the risk of NEC, nosocomial infections, and mortality in VLBW infants. Other benefits reported include decreasing intestinal permeability, improvements in growth and head circumference, and improved feeding tolerance. However, the optimal doses, organisms, and timing of supplementation and the long-term benefits remain unclear. Concerns exist regarding probiotic use and risks of sepsis due to probiotic translocation. (See Chapter 109 on NEC.)

Prebiotics and human milk oligosaccharides such as inulin, galactose, and fructose enhance the growth of beneficial bacteria in the intestinal microbiome such as *Bifidobacterium* and potentially decrease risks of NEC and nosocomial infections. Despite formula supplemented with nonhuman milk oligosaccharides showing improved enteral feed tolerance, these formulas do not affect intestinal permeability. Long-term benefits are not yet known.

IX. **Postnatal growth failure.** Postnatal extrauterine growth restriction (EUGR) occurs in 28% to 75% of preterm births globally. EUGR is defined as growth values <10th percentile or <2 standard deviations (SD) from the mean expected intrauterine growth. Some define EUGR as a change in Z-score >1 SD or >2 SD from birth to discharge. The latter is more predictive of neurodevelopmental outcomes. Better nutritional support is associated with improved growth and neurodevelopmental outcome and EUGR.

X. **Discharge.** Routine fortification is not recommended at discharge of preterm infants, and human milk fortifiers are not available outside the hospital setting. Some have attempted to fortify human milk with preterm powder formula, but there is a risk of infection (*Cronobacter* spp.). Moreover, healthy preterm infants fed fortified maternal milk and unfortified milk after discharge show no significant differences in growth parameters, lean body mass, bone mineral density, or neurodevelopmental outcomes at 18 months of corrected age. In some high-risk neonates, breast feeding can be supplemented with 2 to 3 bottles of a transitional formula to improve protein accretion and bone mineralization.

Formula-fed preterm infants (BW <1500 g or birth gestational age <32 weeks) should continue on a transitional formula (see following section on commercial formula) until 6 to 9 months after term to improve bone mineralization.

FORMS OF ENTERAL NUTRITION: COMMERCIAL FORMULA

When human milk is unavailable, commercial formula may be used for feeding term and preterm infants. Approximately 80% of infants are fed infant formula by the time they reach the age of 1 year old. No special considerations regarding the type of formula apply to healthy, full-term newborn infants for routine feeding. Preterm infants may require more careful planning. Many different, highly specialized formulas are available. Table 11–3 outlines indications for various formulas. The compositions of commonly used infant formulas and breast milk can be found in Table 11–5. Because the nutritional composition of formula changes frequently, the most up-to-date information can be found on the manufacturer's website.

I. **Types of formula**
   A. **Intact cow milk protein-based formulas.** This is the most common human milk substitute. Macronutrient sources and ratios vary widely among brands and different formulations. Iron-fortified formulas reduce the risk of iron deficiency anemia. Some formulas are now fortified with oligosaccharides and nucleotides and with probiotics. Formulas are available as ready-to-feed liquids or as powders that can be reconstituted before feeding, although the latter has been associated with risk of infection.
   B. **Preterm formulas.** Preterm formulas were developed to meet the rapid growth of preterm infants and are fortified with extra calories, protein, minerals, and vitamins. Additionally, fat blends of oils have been optimized to account for the poor absorption in the preterm neonate. The majority of infant formulas (preterm and term) are iso-osmolar or mildly hypoosmolar to improve tolerance and decrease risk of NEC in preterm infants. Only sterile products should be used in the preterm population.
   C. **Soy formulas.** Soy formulas are used in infants who have primary or secondary lactose intolerance or *galactosemia*, or desire for vegetarian diet. Some infants with

Table 11–5. COMPOSITION OF SELECTED INFANT FORMULAS

Characteristics	Mature Human Breast Milk	Enfamil Infant	Similac Advance	Similac Advance Organic (Organic Infant Formula with Iron)	Similac Special Care 20 (with Iron)
Calories/100 mL	68	67	67.6	67.6	67.6
Osmolality (mOsm/kg H$_2$O)	290	300	310	225	235
Protein					
Grams/100 mL	1.05	1.41	1.4	1.4	2.02
% total calories	6	8.5	8	8	12
Source		Nonfat milk, whey (whey:casein = 60:40)	Nonfat milk, whey protein	Organic nonfat dry milk	Nonfat milk, whey concentrate
Fat					
Grams/100 mL	3.9	3.55	3.65	3.65	3.67
% total calories	52	48	49	49	47
Source[a]		Palm olein, soy, coconut, high-oleic sunflower, DHA- and ARA-rich oil blend	High-oleic safflower, soy, and coconut oils (0.15% DHA, 0.40% ARA)	Organic high-oleic sunflower, soy, and coconut oils (0.15% DHA, 0.40% ARA)	MCTs, soy, and coconut oils, (0.25% DHA, 0.40% ARA)
Oil ratio		44:19.5:19.5:14.5:2.5	40:30:29	40:30:29	50:30:18
Linoleic acid (mg)	374	573.3	675.7	581.6	473
DHA (mg)	0.32% ± 0.22%	11.3 (*Crypthecodinium cohnii* oil)	*Crypthecodinium cohnii* oil	*Crypthecodinium cohnii* oil	*Crypthecodinium cohnii* oil
ARA (mg)		22.7 (*Mortierella alpina* oil)	*Mortierella alpina* oil	*Mortierella alpina* oil	*Mortierella alpina* oil

Carbohydrates

Grams/100 mL	7.2	7.4	7.57	7.37	6.97
% total calories	42	43.5	43	43	41
Source	Lactose	Lactose	Lactose, galacto-oligosaccharides	Organic maltodextrin, lactose, sugar, FOS (44:27:27)	Lactose, corn syrup solids (50:50)

Minerals/100 mL

Calcium (mg)	28	52.0	52.8	52.8	121.7
Phosphorus (mg)	14	28.6	28.4	28.4	67.6
Iodine (mcg)	11	10.0	4.1	4.1	4.1
Iron (mg)	0.03	1.20	1.2	1.22	1.2
Magnesium (mg)	3.5	5.3	4.1	4.1	8.1
Sodium (mg)	18	18	16.2	16.2 (7.1)	29.1
Potassium (mg)	52	72.0	71 (1.82)	71 (1.81)	87.2 (2.23)
Chloride (mg)	42	42.0	44 (1.24)	43.9 (1.24)	54.8 (1.55)
Zinc (mg)	0.12	0.66	0.51	0.51	1.01
Copper (mcg)	25	50.0	60.9	60.9	169.1
Manganese (mcg)	0.3	10	3.4	3.4	8.1
Selenium (mcg)	1.5	1.87	1.4	1.4	1.4

Vitamins/100 mL

Vitamin A (IU)	223	200	202	202	845
Vitamin D (IU)	2	50	50.7	40.6	101

(Continued)

Table 11–5. COMPOSITION OF SELECTED INFANT FORMULAS (*CONTINUED*)

Characteristics	Mature Human Breast Milk	Enfamil Infant	Similac Advance	Similac Advance Organic (Organic Infant Formula with Iron)	Similac Special Care 20 (with Iron)
Vitamin E (IU)	0.3	1.3	1.0	1.0	2.7
Vitamin K (mcg)	0.2	6.0	5.4	5.4	8.1
Thiamine/B1 (mcg)	21	53.3	67.6	67.6	169
Riboflavin/B2 (mcg)	35	93.3	101.4	101.4	419
Niacin/B3 (mcg)	180	666.6	710.1	710.1	3381
Vitamin B6 (mcg)	20	40	40.6	40.6	169
Vitamin B12 (mcg)	0.03	0.20	0.17	0.17	0.37
Folic acid (mcg)	5	10.7	10.1	10.1	25
Vitamin C (mg)	4.1	8.0	9	6.1	25
Pantothenic acid (mcg)	180	333.3	304.3	304.3	1285
Biotin (mcg)	0.5	2.0	2.9	2.9	25
Choline (mg)	9.2	16	10.8	10.8	6.8
Inositol (mg)	15	4.0	3.2	3.2	27
Carnitine (mg)		1.34			
Taurine (mg)		4.0			
Prebiotic		Galacto-oligosaccharides, polydextrose	Galacto-oligosaccharide	FOS	
Nucleotides	++	++	++	++	++
Potential renal solute load (mOsm/L)	97.6	125	126.7	126.8	188.2

Characteristics	Enfamil Premature 20 (with Iron)	Similac Special Care 24 (with iron)	Enfamil Premature 24 (with Iron)	Enfamil Premature 24 High Protein (HP) (with Iron)	Enfamil Premature 30 (with Iron)
Calories/100 mL	68	81.2	81	81	101
Osmolality (mOsm/kg H$_2$O)	260	280	320	300	320
Protein					
Grams/100 mL	2.2	2.43	2.7	2.9	3.3
% total calories	13	12	13	14	13
Source	Nonfat milk, whey concentrate	Nonfat milk, whey concentrate	Nonfat milk, whey concentrate	Nonfat milk, whey concentrate	Nonfat milk, whey concentrate
Fat					
Grams/100 mL	3.4	4.40	4.1	4.1	5.1
% total calories	44	47	44	44	44++
Source[a]	MCTs, soy, high-oleic sunflower oils, single-cell oil blend rich in DHA and ARA	MCTs, soy, and coconut oils (0.25% DHA, 0.40% ARA)	MCTs, soy, high-oleic sunflower oils, single-cell oil blend rich in DHA and ARA	MCTs, soy, high-oleic sunflower oils, single-cell oil blend rich in DHA and ARA	MCTs, soy, high-oleic sunflower oils, single-cell oil blend rich in DHA and ARA
Oil ratio		50:30:18	40:30.5:27:2.5	40:30.5:27:2.5	40:30.5:27:2.5
Linoleic acid (mcg)	550	568.1	660	660	820
ARA (mg)	23		34	34	34
DHA (mg)	11.5		17	17	17

(Continued)

Table 11–5. COMPOSITION OF SELECTED INFANT FORMULAS (*CONTINUED*)

Characteristics	Enfamil Premature 20 (with Iron)	Similac Special Care 24 (with iron)	Enfamil Premature 24 (with Iron)	Enfamil Premature 24 High Protein (HP) (with Iron)	Enfamil Premature 30 (with Iron)
Carbohydrates					
Grams/100 mL	7.3	8.36	8.8	8.5	10.9
% total calories	43	41	43	44	43
Source	Lactose, corn syrup solids	Lactose, corn syrup solids (50:50)	Lactose, corn syrup solids (41:59)	Lactose, corn syrup solids (40:60)	Lactose, maltodextrin (15:85)
Minerals/100 mL					
Calcium (mg) (mEq)	112	146.1 (7.3)	134	134	167
Phosphorus (mg)	61	81.2	73	73	91
Iodine (mcg)	16.9	4.9	20	20	25
Iron (mg)	1.22	1.46	1.46	1.46	1.83
Magnesium (mg)	6.1	9.7	7.3	7.3	9.1
Sodium (mg) (mEq)	47	34.9 (1.52)	57	57	71
Potassium (mg) (mEq)	66	104.7 (2.7)	80	80	99
Chloride (mg) (mEq)	72	65.7 (1.8)	86	86	107
Zinc (mg)	1.0	1.21	1.22	1.22	1.52
Copper (mcg)	81	202.9	97	97	122
Manganese (mcg)	4.3	9.7	5.1	5.1	6.4
Selenium (mcg)	3.4	1.6	4.1	4.1	5.1

Vitamins/100 mL

Vitamin A (IU)	910	1014	1100	1100	1100	1370
Vitamin D (IU)	200	121.7	240	240	240	300
Vitamin E (IU)	4.3	3.25	5.1	5.1	5.1	6.4
Vitamin K (mcg)	6.1	9.74	7.3	7.3	7.3	9.1
Thiamine/B1 (mcg)	135	202.9	162	162	162	200
Riboflavin/B2 (mcg)	200	503.2	240	240	240	300
Niacin/B3 (mcg)	2700	4057.8	3200	3200	3200	4100
Vitamin B6 (mcg)	101	202.9	122	122	122	152
Vitamin B12 (mcg)	0.17	0.45	0.20	0.20	0.20	0.25
Folic acid (mcg)	27	30	32	32	32	41
Vitamin C (mg)	13.5	30	16.2	16.2	16.2	20
Pantothenic acid (mcg)	810	1541.9	970	970	970	1220
Biotin (mcg)	2.7	30	3.2	3.2	3.2	4.1
Choline (mg)	16.2	8.1	19.5	19.5	19.5	24
Inositol (mg)	30	32.5	36	36	36	45
Potential renal solute load (mOsm/L)	200	225.8	250	260	260	300
Nucleotides	++	++	++	++	++	++

(Continued)

Table 11–5. COMPOSITION OF SELECTED INFANT FORMULAS (CONTINUED)

Characteristics	Enfamil ProSobee 20 cal/oz.	Enfamil Gentlease 20 cal/oz.	Similac Expert Care NeoSure 22	EnfaCare[c] 22 cal/oz.	Similac PM 60/40	EleCare for Infants[d]
Calories/100 mL	68	68	74.4	74	67.6	67.6
Osmolality (mOsm/kg H₂0)	200	230	250	230 (liquid); 310 (powder)	280	350
Osmolarity (mOsm/L)	180	210	187	220 (liquid); 280 (powder)		
Protein						
Grams/100 mL	1.69	1.55	2.08	2.15	1.5	2.1
% total calories	10	9	11	11	9	15
Source	Soy protein isolates (14%)	Partially hydrolyzed nonfat milk and whey protein solids (soy)	Nonfat milk, whey concentrate	Nonfat milk, whey concentrate	Whey, sodium caseinate	Free L-amino acids
Fat						
Grams/100 mL	3.6	3.5	4.1	3.9	3.79	3.2
% total calories	48	48	49	47	50	42
Source[a]	Palm olein, soy, coconut, and high-oleic sunflower oils, single-cell oil blend rich in DHA and ARA	Palm olein, soy, coconut, and high-oleic sunflower oils, single-cell oil blend rich in DHA and ARA	Soy, coconut, MCT oils (0.25% DHA, 0.40% ARA)	MCT, high-oleic vegetable, soy coconut, single-cell oil blend rich in DHA and ARA	High-oleic safflower, soy, and coconut oils	High-oleic safflower oil, MCTs, soy oil
Oil ratio			45:29:25	20:34:29:14:2.5	41:30:29	39:33:28

H_2O reference: Osmolality (mOsm/kg H_2O)

	573.3	581	557.9	860–950	676.3	568.3
Linoleic acid (mcg)	573.3	581	557.9	860–950	676.3	568.3
ARA (mg)	34	34		34		
DHA (mg)	17	17		17		
Carbohydrates						
Grams/100 mL	7.2	7.2	7.51	7.7	6.9	7.2
% total calories	42	43	40	42	41	42
Source	Corn syrup solids (54%)	Corn syrup solids	Lactose, corn syrup solids (50:50)	Maltodextrin, lactose, corn syrup solids	Lactose	Corn syrup solids
Minerals/100 mL						
Calcium (mg) (mEq)	70	54.6	78.1 (3.9)	89	37.9 (1.89)	78.1 (3.9)
Phosphorus (mg)	46	31	46.1	49	18.9	57
Iodine (mcg)	10.0	10.0	11.2	15.6	4.1	60
Iron (mg)	1.2	1.2	1.34	1.33	0.47	1.22
Magnesium (mg)	7.4	5.3	6.7	5.9	4.06	5.6
Sodium (mg) (mEq)	24	24	24.5 (1.07)	27	16.2 (7.1)	30.5 (1.3)
Potassium (mg) (mEq)	80	73	105.6 (2.7)	78	54.1 (1.38)	101 (2.6)
Chloride (mg) (mEq)	54	42	5.58 (1.57)	58	39.9 (1.13)	40.6 (1.2)
Zinc (mg)	0.80	0.67	0.89	0.74	0.51	0.78
Copper (mcg)	50	50	89.3	67	60.9	85.2
Manganese (mcg)	16.7	10	7.4	11.1	3.4	56.8
Selenium (mcg)	1.89	1.89	1.7	2.1	1.4	1.76

(Continued)

Table 11–5. COMPOSITION OF SELECTED INFANT FORMULAS (*CONTINUED*)

Characteristics	Enfamil ProSobee 20 cal/oz.	Enfamil Gentlease 20 cal/oz.	Similac Expert Care NeoSure 22	EnfaCare[c] 22 cal/oz.	Similac PM 60/40	EleCare for Infants[d]
Vitamins/100 mL						
Vitamin A (IU)	200	200	260.4	330	202.9	184.7
Vitamin D (IU)	40	40	52.1	56	40.6	40.6
Vitamin E (IU)	1.4	1.3	2.68	3	1.01	1.4
Vitamin K (mcg)	5.4	6	8.18	6.7	5.4	8.8
Thiamine/B1 (mcg)	53.3	53.3	130.2	133	67.6	142.0
Riboflavin/B2 (mcg)	60	93.3	111.6	148	101.4	71.0
Niacin/B3 (mcg)	666.7	666.7	1450.6	740–1450	710	1136.6
Vitamin B6 (mcg)	40	40	74.4	50	40.6	57
Vitamin B12 (mcg)	0.2	0.2	0.29	0.22	0.17	0.27
Folic acid (mcg)	10.7	10.7	18.6	19.2	10.1	20
Vitamin C (mg)	8.0	8.0	11.2	11.9	6.1	6.1
Pantothenic acid (mcg)	333.3	333.3	595.1	630	304.3	284.8
Biotin (mcg)	2	2	6.7	4.4	3.0	2.8
Choline (mg)	16.0	16.0	11.9	17.8	8.1	10.1
Inositol (mg)	4.0	4.0	26.0	22	16.2	3.5
Potential renal solute load (mOsm/L)	156	140	187.4	184	124.1	187.0

Characteristics	Similac Alimentum	Enfamil A.R.	Gerber Good Start 20 cal/oz.	Enfamil Nutramigen with AA/Enflora LGG 20 cal/oz.	Pregestimil 20 cal/oz.	Pregestimil 24 cal/oz.
Calories/100 mL	67.6	68	67	68	68	81
Osmolality (mOsm/kg H$_2$O)	370	240 (liquid); 230 (powder)		270 (liquid); 300 (powder)	290 (liquid); 320 (powder)	330
Osmolarity (mOsm/L)		220 (liquid); 210 (powder)		240 (liquid); 270 (powder)	260 (liquid); 280 (powder)	290
Protein						
Grams/100 mL	1.86	1.69	1.48	1.89	1.89	2.3
% total calories	11	10		11	11	11
Source	Casein hydrolysate, L-cysteine, L-tyrosine, L-tryptophan	Nonfat milk	Whey protein concentrate	Casein hydrolysate (17%), amino acids	Casein hydrolysate, amino acid	Casein hydrolysate, amino acids
Fat						
Grams/100 mL	3.75	3.4	3.4	3.5	3.8	4.5
% total calories	48	46		48	49	48
Source[a]	Safflower oil, MCTs, soy oil (0.15% DHA, 0.40% ARA)	Palm olein, soy, coconut, and high-oleic sunflower oils, single-cell blend rich in DHA and ARA	Palm olein, soy, high-oleic safflower or high oleic sunflower, coconut	Palm olein, soy, coconut, and high-oleic sunflower oils, single-cell blend rich in DHA and ARA	MCT, soy, and high-oleic safflower oils	MCT, soy, and high-oleic safflower oils

(Continued)

151

Table 11–5. COMPOSITION OF SELECTED INFANT FORMULAS (*CONTINUED*)

Characteristics	Similac Alimentum	Enfamil A.R.	Gerber Good Start 20 cal/oz.	Enfamil Nutramigen with AA/Enflora LGG 20 cal/oz.	Pregestimil 20 cal/oz.	Pregestimil 24 cal/oz.
Oil ratio	38:33:28				55:35:7.5 and 2.5% oil rich in DHA and ARA (liquid)	
Linoleic acid (mg)	1285	527	600	581	635	746.0 (95.2)
ARA (mg)		34		34	34	26.8
DHA (mg)		17		17	17	13.4
Carbohydrates						
Grams/100 mL	6.9	7.6	7.5	6.9	6.9	8.3
% total calories	41	44		41	41	41
Source	Sugar, modified tapioca starch (70:30)	Lactose, rice starch, maltodextrin	Lactose, corn maltodextrin	Corn syrup solids (45%), modified corn starch (7%)	Corn syrup solids, modified corn starch	Corn syrup solids, modified corn starch
Minerals/100 mL						
Calcium (mg) (mEq)	71 (3.54)	52	45.3	62.7	62.6	74.6
Phosphorus (mg)	50.7	35.3	25.6	34.6	34.6	41.2
Iodine (mcg)	10.1	10.1	8.0	10.0	10.0	11.9
Iron (mg)	1.2	1.2	1.0	1.2	1.2	1.42
Magnesium (mg)	5.1	5.4	4.7	5.3	5.3	8.7

Sodium (mg) (mEq)	29.8 (1.29)	27	18.2	31.3	31.3	37.3
Potassium (mg) (mEq)	79.8 (2.03)	72	72.0	73.3	73.3	87.3
Chloride (mg) (mEq)	54.1 (1.55)	50	43.3	57.3	57.3	68.2
Zinc (mg)	0.5	0.67	0.54	0.67	0.67	0.89
Copper (mcg)	50.7	50	54	50	50	59.5
Manganese (mcg)	5.4	10.0	10.0	16.6	16.7	19.8
Selenium (mcg)	1.4	1.87	2.0	1.89	1.89	2.2
Vitamins/100 mL						
Vitamin A (IU)	202.9	200	200	200	233.3	301
Vitamin D (IU)	30.4	40	50	33.3	33.3	39.6
Vitamin E (IU)	2.03	1.33	1.35	1.3	2.7	3.2
Vitamin K (mcg)	10.1	6	5.4	6	8.0	9.52
Thiamine/B1 (mcg)	40.6	53.3	66.7	54	53.3	63.5
Riboflavin/B2 (mcg)	60.9	93.3	93.3	60	60	71.4
Niacin/B3 (mcg)	913	666.7	700	666.7	666.7	793.6
Vitamin B6 (mcg)	40.6	40	50.0	40	40	47.6
Vitamin B12 (mcg)	0.30	0.2	0.22	0.2	0.2	0.24
Folic acid (mcg)	10.1	10.7	10.0	10.7	10.7	12.7
Vitamin C (mg)	6.1	8.0	6.7	8.0	8.0	9.5
Pantothenic acid (mcg)	507.2	333.3	300	333.3	333.3	396.8
Biotin (mcg)	3.0	2	2.95	2	2	2.4

(Continued)

Table 11-5. COMPOSITION OF SELECTED INFANT FORMULAS (*CONTINUED*)

Characteristics	Similac Alimentum	Enfamil A.R.	Gerber Good Start 20 cal/oz.	Enfamil Nutramigen with AA/Enflora LGG 20 cal/oz.	Pregestimil 20 cal/oz.	Pregestimil 24 cal/oz.
Choline (mg)	8.1	16.0	16.0	16	16	19.0
Inositol (mg)	3.4	4.0	4.0	11.3	11.3	13.4
Potential renal solute load (mOsm/L)	171.3	153		169	169	200
Probiotic			*Bifidobacterium lactis*	*Lactobacillus rhamnosus GG*		
Nucleotides[b]			++			

ARA, arachidonic acid; DHA, docosahexaenoic acid; FOS, fructo-oligosaccharide; MCT, medium-chain triglyceride.

[a]Similac and Enfamil products: *C cohnii* oil, source of DHA; *M alpina* oil, source of ARA.

[b]Nucleotides: Adenosine 5'-monophosphate, cytidine 5'-monophosphate, disodium guanosine 5'-monophosphate, disodium uridine 5'-monophosphate.

[c]Concentration of some nutrients vary depending on powder or liquid concentrate.

[d]Contains molybdenum and chromium.

[e]Corn oil.

milk protein allergy (up to 60%) have a cross reactivity with soy. **Soy formulas increase risk of osteopenia in preterm infants and should be avoided**. Protein concentrations are slightly higher in soy than in cow milk–based formula. The American Academy of Pediatrics does not recommend routine use of soy formula for colic.

D. **Protein hydrolysate.** Formulas with extensively hydrolyzed proteins are used in infants who are severely intolerant (allergic) to cow milk and soy protein. They are also useful in infants at risk for malnutrition including those with cystic fibrosis, short gut syndrome, biliary atresia, and protracted diarrhea. However, these formulas are usually hyperosmolar and more expensive.

E. **Free amino acid formulas.** Amino acid–based formulas are designed for infants with extreme protein hypersensitivity who do not tolerate hydrolyzed formulas. They are expensive, less palatable than hydrolyzed formulas, and difficult to obtain. Additionally, hypophosphatemia and osteopenia have been reported recently as significant complications of their use.

F. **Other formulas.** Other formulas exist made for specific metabolic disease states. Please see manufacturers' websites.

G. **Transitional formulas.** Preterm infants continue to need nutritional supplementation after discharge. Transitional formulas have higher caloric, protein, and mineral content than term formulas. Infants discharged on special formulas (eg, NeoSure, EnfaCare; see Table 11–5) have better somatic growth, weight gain, and bone mineralization.

H. **Organic formulas.** Several organic milk formulas, including soy based, are available that are produced without the use of pesticides, antibiotics, or growth hormones. Concerns have been raised about the presence of high sugar content in some of these formulas and the risk for later childhood obesity and for injury to developing tooth enamel. The increased costs of organic formulas are also considerable. There are no randomized controlled trials comparing the benefits, or lack of benefits, of organic formulas versus proprietary infant formulas.

II. **Preparation, storage, and handling**

A. **Preparation.** There are 3 preparations of formula: ready to feed or use (RTU), concentrated liquid, and powder with comparable nutritional content. RTU can be fed as-is from the container. Concentrated liquid formula must be diluted with equal amounts of water. Powdered formula must be mixed with potable water from a safe source according to manufacturer's instructions. Powdered formula is not sterile and has recently been associated with *Cronobacter sakazakii* contamination. The CDC provides guidelines for preparation of powder formula and recommends the water temperature be greater than 158°F to mix the powder and then be allowed to cool prior to feeding to the infant.

B. **Storage and handling.** RTU and powder-prepared formula should be discarded 1 hour after serving it to an infant. Twenty-four-hour batches are acceptable to make if that particular aliquot has not been exposed to the infant. It should be discarded after 48 hours of refrigeration even when unused. Open cans of powder are good for use for 4 weeks.

TOTAL PARENTERAL NUTRITION

Total parenteral nutrition (TPN) is **the intravenous administration of all nutrients** (fats, carbohydrates, proteins, vitamins, and minerals) necessary for metabolic requirements and growth. **Parenteral nutrition (PN)** is **supplemental intravenous administration of nutrients**. **Enteral nutrition (EN)** refers to oral or gavage feedings.

I. **Indications.** PN is used as a supplement to enteral feedings or as a complete substitution (TPN) when adequate nourishment cannot be achieved by the enteral route. Common indications in infants include extreme prematurity, congenital malformation of the GI tract such as gastroschisis and omphalocele, short bowel syndrome following NEC, congenital heart disease, sepsis, and malabsorption. Most institutions initiate PN while establishing full enteral feeds for infants <34 weeks' gestational age and/or <1800 g. PN should be started on the first day of life and as soon as possible in preterm or sick infants to decrease catabolism and to optimize postnatal growth. Early PN is associated with better weight gain and neurodevelopmental outcomes in the VLBW population.

II. **Methods of PN administration**
A. **Central PN.** Central PN is used when infants have central access such as umbilical lines or for those infants requiring long-term parenteral support. PN involves infusion of a hypertonic nutrient solution (12.5%–25% dextrose, 5%–6% amino acids) into a suitable vessel with rapid flow through an indwelling catheter. Two methods are commonly used for long-term infusion of PN.
   1. **Percutaneously inserted central catheter.** Positioned in the antecubital, temporal, external jugular, or saphenous vein and advanced into a large vessel outside the heart (eg, superior or inferior vena cava; see Chapter 46).
   2. **Tunneled central catheter (Broviac).** Placed surgically in the internal or external jugular, subclavian, or femoral vein.
B. **Peripheral PN (PPN).** PPN can be infused via peripheral veins, but the concentrations of the amino acids and dextrose solution that can be infused are limited by the fragility of veins. The mOsm/L limit for PPN is <900 to 1100 mOsm/L, which limits dextrose to 12.5% and amino acid concentration to 3%; mOsm/L can be calculated with the following equation:

$$\text{mOsm/L} = [\text{amino acids (g/L)} \times 8] + [\text{glucose (g/L)} \times 7]$$
$$+ [\text{Na (mEq/L)} \times 2] + [\text{phosphorus (mg/L)} \times 0.2] - 50$$

Peripheral infusion of PN carries higher risks of infiltration and phlebitis.
C. **Umbilical catheters.** PN can be given through an **umbilical venous catheter** (and occasionally through an **umbilical artery catheter** in some institutions) after ensuring the catheter is central and not in the liver. Hyperosmolar infusion in the hepatic vessels is associated with portal venous thrombosis and portal hypertension. Low-lying umbilical venous catheters should be used only temporarily and treated as peripheral vessels and, therefore, limited to concentrations similar to PPN.

III. **Caloric requirements and densities.** Goal caloric intake (including protein calories) for PN remains around 80 to 90 kcal/kg/d. The optimal amount of energy intake differs for each infant and may be higher for sick and ELBW infants. Caloric densities of various energy sources are as follows:
A. **Dextrose (anhydrous).** 3.4 kcal/g.
B. **Protein.** 4 kcal/g.
C. **Fat.** 9 kcal/g.

IV. **Composition of PN solutions**
A. **Fluids.** Goal fluid parenteral requirements after the first few days of life range from 120 to 150 mL/kg/d for term infants and from 130 to 160 mL/kg/d for preterm infants. These can vary based on clinical status. See Chapter 10 for fluid requirements.
B. **Carbohydrates.** Dextrose is the only commercially available form of glucose, with concentrations of 5.0% to 12.5% dextrose used in peripheral PN and up to 25% dextrose in central PN. **Glucose infusion rates (GIR)** should be calculated as milligrams per kilograms per minute (see Table 11–8 for calculations). Infants should be started on a GIR of 5 to 8 mg/kg/min to allow for appropriate response of endogenous insulin. Infusion rates can then be increased by 0.5 to 2 mg/kg/min each day as tolerated with the goal of maintaining blood glucose concentrations between 50 and 150 mg/dL. For most infants, GIR of 12 to 13 mg/kg/min will provide adequate caloric intake in the presence of stable blood glucose levels.

Excess glucose can lead to glucosuria and osmotic diuresis. Excess glucose is also converted into lipid via lipogenesis, which is an inefficient process that increases energy expenditure.

Endogenous gluconeogenesis in preterm ELBW infants may be independent of glucose infusion, and therefore, this population frequently experiences hyperglycemia. Other factors contributing to hyperglycemia include elevated birth-related catecholamines, use of inotropic drugs, and decreased production of and sensitivity to insulin. In the presence of hyperglycemia, glucose infusion rate should not be reduced below a basal rate of 4 mg/kg/min. Insulin may be required to maintain adequate blood glucose concentrations but is not recommended for routine use. Hyperglycemia in preterm infants is associated with worse outcomes.

Peripheral uptake and utilization of glucose are improved with simultaneous amino acid infusion because it increases endogenous insulin production. Providing glucose alone in the absence of proteins results in negative nitrogen balance that can be reversed by providing 1.1 to 2.5 g/kg/d of protein with energy intake as low as 30 kcal/kg/d. Providing 25 to 30 kcal of nonprotein energy per gram of protein optimizes protein deposition.

C. **Proteins.** In preterm ELBW and VLBW infants, amino acids should be started on day 1 and is associated with better linear growth and neurodevelopmental outcomes. Term infants who are likely to have delayed initiation of EN should also be started as early as possible. Inadequate protein intake may result in failure to thrive, hypoalbuminemia, and edema. Excessive protein can cause hyperammonemia, serum amino acid imbalance, metabolic acidosis, and cholestatic jaundice. Early addition of amino acids to PN may also stimulate endogenous insulin secretion. Postnatal protein loss is inversely proportional to gestational age. Low BW infants lose 1% of endogenous protein daily unless supplemented.

1. **Crystalline amino acid solutions.** The standard solutions originally designed for adults are not ideal because they contain high concentrations of amino acids (eg, glycine, methionine, and phenylalanine) that are potentially neurotoxic in premature infants. Pediatric crystalline amino acid solutions (eg, TrophAmine, Aminosyn PF) contain less of those potentially neurotoxic amino acids as well as additional tyrosine, cystine, and taurine. The lower pH also allows for the addition of sufficient quantities of calcium (2 mEq/dL) and phosphorus (1–2 mg/dL) to meet daily requirements. Furthermore, newer crystalline amino acid solutions are associated with less azotemia, hyperammonemia, and metabolic acidosis than previous formulations. Conditionally essential amino acids are arginine, tyrosine, cysteine, glutamine, glycine, and proline.

2. **Amino acids.** Early protein intake of up to 3 g/kg/d within the first 24 hours is safely tolerated in VLBW infants and improves nitrogen balance, increases ability to synthesize protein, and decreases protein catabolism. Early amino acid supplementation may decrease hyperglycemia and hyperkalemia in ELBW infants by promoting insulin secretion. In term infants, the starting rate should be at least 1 to 2 g/kg/d, with increases of 1 g/kg/d to a goal of 3 g/kg/d. For preterm infants, begin at 3 g/kg/d and advance by 0.5 to 1 g/kg/d to a goal of 3.5 to 4 g/kg/d.

3. **Cysteine hydrochloride.** Cysteine is often added separately to TPN solutions because it is unstable over time and is omitted from preformulated amino acid solutions. The premature infant lacks the ability to convert methionine to cysteine; thus, it is conditionally essential. Cysteine is also converted to cystine and to glutathione, an antioxidant that is important in maintaining calcium homeostasis. Addition of cysteine to TPN lowers the pH of the solution, thereby improving the solubility of calcium and phosphorus. Cysteine may also decrease hepatic cholestasis. The recommended dose is 30 to 40 mg of cysteine per gram of protein (72–85 mg/kg/d). It should be held or used cautiously in infants with metabolic acidosis.

4. **Glutamine.** Glutamine has been identified as a key amino acid, as respiratory fuel for rapidly proliferating cells such as enterocytes and lymphocytes, as a factor in acid-base balance, and as a nucleotide precursor. Glutamine may play a role in maintaining gut integrity and may decrease the incidence of sepsis. Despite all these theoretical benefits, randomized trials show that glutamine supplementation does not have significant effect on mortality or neonatal morbidities including invasive infection, NEC, time to achieve full EN, or duration of hospital stay. There is no commercially available amino acid solution that contains glutamine.

D. **Fats.** Fats are essential for normal body growth and development, in cell structure and function, and in retinal and brain development. Because of their high caloric density, intravenous lipids provide a significant portion of daily caloric needs. Most lipid solutions are derived from soybean, but newer combination oils with olive oil, MCT, and fish oil are now available (eg, Intralipid, Liposyn II, Nutrilipid, Soyacal, Omegavan, Lipoplus, and SMOF lipid). Omegavan is made exclusively from fish oil and is rich in omega-3 fatty acids. SMOF (a third-generation emulsion containing soybean oil, MCT, and fish and olive oil) has an altered ratio of omega-6 to omega-3 fatty acids that may decrease the risks of PN-associated liver disease (PNALD; see discussion of PNALD later in this chapter). Most intravenous fat solutions are isotonic (270–300 mOsm/L). Lipid emulsions contain linoleic and α-linolenic acid; the latter can be converted into DHA. DHA is accumulated in the third trimester, and preterm infants have limited capacity to convert α-linolenic acid to DHA, which plays a critical role in brain development. Delay in initiating lipids can result in biochemical and clinical evidence of essential fatty acid deficiency within 3 days and increase susceptibility to oxidant injury. Intravenous lipids at 0.5 to 1 g/kg/d are needed to prevent essential fatty acid deficiency.

1. **Concentrations.** Lipid emulsions are usually supplied as 20% solutions providing 20 g of triglyceride per 100 mL. Starting lipids at 1 to 2 g/kg/d within 24 hours of birth is well tolerated. Advance by 0.5 to 1.0 g/kg/d as tolerated up to 3.0 g/kg/d. The infusion is given continuously over 20 to 24 hours, and the rate should not exceed 0.12 to 0.15 g/kg/h. To maintain calcium and phosphorous solubility, lipids should be administered separately from proteins because amino acid solutions are acidic. Adding lipids to protein solutions increases the pH and precipitates calcium and phosphorus (see discussion of photoprotection later in this chapter).

2. **Carnitine supplementation.** Carnitine synthesis and storage are not well developed in infants <34 weeks' gestation. Carnitine is a carrier molecule necessary for oxidation of long-chain fatty acids. An exogenous source of carnitine is available from human milk and infant formulas; however, studies have shown that preterm infants on TPN become deficient in 6 to 10 days. Carnitine supplementation of 2 to 10 mg/kg/d is recommended for infants on TPN for >4 weeks. Some institutions use carnitine whenever lipid emulsions are used. Carnitine-deficient infants may experience hypotonic, nonketotic hypoglycemia, cardiomyopathy, encephalopathy, and recurrent infections. Newborn screening programs now test for carnitine deficiency.

E. **Minerals.** More than 80% of bone mineralization occurs in the third trimester. Therefore, preterm infants are at increased risk of metabolic bone disease and require supplementation of calcium and phosphorus. Delays in reaching full enteral feeds, medications such as diuretics and steroids, and risks of precipitation can limit calcium and phosphorus intake and increase risk of osteopenia of prematurity.

1. **Calcium.** Calcium supplementation is typically provided in PN as calcium gluconate. Start at 2 mEq/kg and keep ratio of calcium to phosphorus at 2:1 to help prevent precipitation. Consider an increase if hypocalcemia or development of metabolic bone disease occurs.

2. **Phosphorus.** Phosphorus is typically supplemented in PN as sodium phosphate in the United States. It can be contaminated with aluminum. Start at 1 mEq/kg and keep ratio of calcium to phosphorus at 2:1 to help prevent precipitation. Additional supplements may be needed with hypophosphatemia or metabolic bone disease.

F. **Vitamins.** Multivitamins are added to intravenous solutions in the form of a pediatric multivitamin suspension (MVI Pediatric). Preterm infants are especially prone to vitamin deficiencies due to their compromised stores and rapid growth. The dose of parenteral vitamins for preterm infants with normal organ function should be 1.5 to 5 mL (1.5 mL when patient weight is <1000 g, 3.25 mL when patient weight is 1000–3000 g, and 5 mL when patient weight is >3000 g). The 5-mL reconstituted MVI Pediatric sterile lyophilized powder contains: 2300 IU vitamin A; 400 IU vitamin D; 7 IU vitamin E; 200 µg vitamin K; 80 mg ascorbic acid; 1.2 mg thiamine; 1.4 mg riboflavin; 17 mg niacin; 5 mg pantothenic acid; 1 mg pyridoxine; 1 µg cyanocobalamin; 20 µg biotin; and 140 µg folic acid. Vitamin A delivery can be hampered by binding to plastic tubing.

G. **Trace elements.** Supplementation with zinc, copper, manganese, chromium, selenium, and molybdenum is currently recommended in neonatal PN, and deficiencies may occur if these elements are not added when infants are on long-term PN. Trace elements are added to the solution based on weight and total volume, with both single-agent and combination products commercially available. Increased amounts of zinc (1–2 mg/d) are often given to help promote healing in patients who require GI surgery. For recommended doses of trace elements, see Table 11–6.

H. **Electrolytes.** Electrolytes can be added according to specific needs (see Chapter 10).

I. **Heparin.** Heparin should be added to PN (unfractionated heparin 0.5 U/mL TPN) to maintain catheter patency. In addition, there is a decreased risk for phlebitis and an increase in lipid clearance as a result of release of lipoprotein lipase with use of heparin.

V. **Monitoring of PN.** Hyperalimentation can cause many alterations in biochemical function. Thus, frequent and consistent anthropometric and laboratory monitoring is

Table 11–6. **RECOMMENDATIONS FOR TRACE ELEMENT SUPPLEMENTATION IN TOTAL PARENTERAL NUTRITION (TPN) SOLUTIONS FOR INFANTS**

Element (mcg/kg/d)	Full Term	Premature
Zinc	100–250	400
Copper[a]	20	20
Chromium[b, c]	0.2	0.2
Manganese[a,b]	1	1
Iodide	1	1
Molybdenum[b,c]	0.25	0.25–1
Selenium[c]	2	2–3

[a]Should not be given to infants with cholestasis.
[b]For TPN >4 weeks.
[c]Should not be given to infants with chronic renal failure.

Table 11–7. SUGGESTED MONITORING SCHEDULE FOR INFANTS RECEIVING
PARENTERAL NUTRITION

Measurement	Baseline Study	Frequency of Measurement
Anthropometric		
Weight	Yes	Daily
Length	Yes	Weekly
Head circumference	Yes	Weekly
Intake and output	Daily	Daily
Metabolic		
Glucose	Yes	2–3 times per day initially; then as needed
Calcium, phosphorus, and magnesium	Yes	2–3 times per week initially; then every 1–2 weeks
Electrolytes (Na, Cl, K, CO_2)	Yes	Daily initially, then 2–3 times per week. More frequently in ELBW infants <1000 g
Hematocrit[a]	Yes	Every other day for 1 week; then weekly
BUN and creatinine	Yes	2–3 per week; then every 1–2 weeks
Bilirubin (direct/total)	Yes	Weekly
Total protein and albumin	Yes	Every 2–3 weeks
AST/ALT	Yes	Every 2–3 weeks
Triglycerides	Yes	When at 2 g/kg, monitor until stable (<200 mg/dL) and PRN
Vitamins and trace minerals		As indicated
Urine		
Specific gravity and glucose	Yes	1–3 times per day initially; then as needed (*controversial*)

ALT, alanine aminotransferase; AST, aspartate aminotransferase; BUN, blood urea nitrogen; ELBW,
extremely low birthweight; PRN, as needed.
[a]Due to frequent phlebotomy losses.

recommended for all patients, especially ELBW infants. Recommendations are given
in Table 11–7.

VI. **Complications of PN.** Approximately 70% of infants admitted to the NICU receive
some form of PN, with catheter infiltration and infections as the most common complications. Early initiation and rapid advancement of enteral feeds can limit the complications associated with PN.

A. **Metabolic**

1. **Hyperglycemia.** Hyperglycemia can result from excessive glucose intake or
change in metabolic rate, such as with infection or glucocorticoid administration. Routine insulin infusion to prevent hyperglycemia is not recommended
and is associated with increased risks of mortality, hypoglycemia, and ROP.
Insulin drip may be considered if blood glucose is >200 to 250 mg/dL despite
GIR of <5 mg/kg/min.

2. **Hypoglycemia.** Hypoglycemia can result from sudden cessation of infusion, likely secondary to mechanical issues such as intravenous infiltration. Hypoglycemia may occur with insulin administration.
3. **Azotemia.** Azotemia can result from excessive protein (nitrogen) uptake; however, aggressive protein intake is safe (see earlier discussion), and this issue is less likely with current amino acid formulations. Elevated blood urea nitrogen may actually indicate better amino acid utilization rather than excessive protein intake.
4. **Hyperammonemia.** Currently available amino acid mixtures contain adequate arginine (>0.05 mmol/kg/d). Therefore, if there is an increase in blood ammonia secondary to PN, symptomatic hyperammonemia does not occur.
5. **Abnormal serum and tissue amino acid pattern.** Infants on TPN may have falsely abnormal newborn metabolic screening results due to multiple minor amino acid abnormalities; a protocol of interrupting TPN for 3 hours and replacing the infusion with dextrose 10% in water before newborn screening collection can result in a 74% reduction in false-positive results.
6. **Mild metabolic acidosis.** Metabolic acidosis in preterm infants is more likely a result of lack of urinary acidification and severity of illness leading to hypotension and poor perfusion than a result of PN itself (low pH). Acidosis can be buffered by titrating acetate concentrations in daily PN.

B. **Systemic**
1. **Parenteral Nutrition Associated Liver Disease (PNALD).** With prolonged administration of intravenous lipids, dextrose, and protein in the absence of enteral feeding, cholestasis usually occurs as evidenced by a direct hyperbilirubinemia. Even in the presence of normal bilirubin levels, evidence of liver disease such as fibrosis may be apparent by histopathologic examination after administration of PN. The incidence ranges from as high as 80% in VLBW infants receiving TPN for >30 days (with no enteral feeding) to ≤15% in infants weighing >1500 g receiving TPN for >14 days. Monitoring for abnormalities in liver function and the development of direct hyperbilirubinemia is important in long-term TPN. IUGR infants and those with congenital GI diagnoses are at high risk of developing cholestasis. Fish oil–based lipid emulsions (Omegavan) and combination emulsions (SMOFLipid) have been used in prevention and treatment of TPN-induced cholestasis. Omegavan is available in Europe but can be used in the United States in research settings or in situations of compassionate use. SMOFLipid is an FDA-approved product in adults that has been occasionally used in the NICU; however, there is limited research on its use in neonates. Fish oil–based lipid emulsions may also decrease the risk of ROP. Starting with even minimal amounts of enteral feeds, decreasing lipid dose to 1 g/kg, and cycling lipid infusions (over 12–18 hours) help to decrease PNALD. Copper and manganese should be withheld in the presence of hepatic dysfunction. See Chapters 62 and 98.
2. **Complications of fat administration.** Hypertriglyceridemia may occur; periodic determination of blood triglyceride levels is recommended to maintain plasma triglyceride levels <200 mg/dL. Lipid infusion should be decreased or stopped when these levels are exceeded. Lipid infusion can be associated with platelet dysfunction, acute allergic reactions, deposition of pigment in the liver, and lipid deposition in the blood vessels of the lung. Most metabolic problems apparently occur with rapid rates of infusion and are not seen at infusion rates of <0.12 g/kg/h. Exposure of lipids to light, especially phototherapy, may cause increased production of toxic hydroperoxides. The addition of multivitamins and use of protective or dark delivery tubing decrease peroxide formation and limit vitamins loss. Steroids cause elevated triglyceride levels, whereas sepsis decreases peripheral utilization of lipids, resulting in

hypertriglyceridemia. Free fatty acids (FFA) produced from lipid breakdown compete with bilirubin for binding with albumin, resulting in elevated free bilirubin. The FFA-to-albumin ratio should be kept at <6; lipid infusion should not exceed 1 g/kg/d with plasma bilirubin >10 mg/dL and albumin levels of 2.5 to 3.0 g/dL. Additional complications include thrombocytopenia, increased risk of sepsis, alteration in pulmonary functions, hypoxemia, and increased pulmonary vascular resistance.

3. **Deficiency of essential fatty acids (EFAs).** EFA deficiency can occur within 72 hours in preterm infants if exogenous fatty acids are not supplemented. EFA deficiency is associated with decreased platelet aggregation (thromboxane A_2 deficiency), poor weight gain, scaling rash, sparse hair growth, and thrombocytopenia. Use of only safflower oil to provide lipid emulsions may result in deficiency of omega-3 LCPUFAs. EFAs are essential to the developing eyes and brain of infants.

4. **Photoprotection of parenteral nutrition.** Photoprotection helps decrease vitamin loss and oxidative damage to amino acids and decreases generation of hydrogen peroxides and free radicals. Photoprotection limits alterations in vasomotor tone via generation of lipid peroxides, decreases nitric oxide production, and improves tolerance to minimal EN. Additionally, it has been found to decrease risk of death and chronic lung disease due to lower triglyceride levels. Vitamins, trace elements, and iron should *not* be added together in the parenteral solution to decrease the risks of lipid peroxidation. Increased lipid peroxidation products may adversely influence neurodevelopment.

5. **Mineral deficiency.** Most minerals are transferred to the fetus during the last trimester of pregnancy. The following problems may occur if not adequately supplemented.

   a. **Osteopenia, metabolic bone disease, and pathologic fractures.** See Chapter 113 and the earlier section in this chapter on PN minerals.

   b. **Zinc deficiency.** Zinc deficiency can occur if zinc is not added to TPN after 4 weeks. Cysteine and histidine in PN solution increase urinary losses. Zinc deficiency results in poor growth, diarrhea, alopecia, increased susceptibility to infection, and skin desquamation surrounding the mouth and anus (acrodermatitis enteropathica). Zinc losses are increased in patients with an ileostomy or colostomy.

   c. **Copper deficiency.** Long-term PN puts infants for copper deficiency, which can result in osteoporosis, hemolytic anemia, neutropenia, and depigmentation of the skin.

   d. **Manganese, selenium, molybdenum, and iodine deficiency.** Trace element deficiency may occur if not supplemented after 4 weeks.

   e. **Iron.** Adding iron to PN should be considered for infants on long-term PN who have not received recent blood transfusions, with rhEPO administration, and if ferritin levels fall below 100 ng/mL. Dose is 3 mg/kg/wk given once per week, preferably without vitamins and other trace elements for that day.

C. **Mechanical.** Complications associated with placement of central catheters occur in approximately 4% to 9% of patients and include pneumothorax, pneumomediastinum, hemorrhage, and chylothorax (caused by injury to the thoracic duct). Thrombosis of the vein adjacent to the catheter tip, resulting in superior vena cava syndrome (edema of the face, neck, and eyes), may be seen. Pulmonary thromboembolism may occur. Malpositioned catheters can result in pleural or pericardial effusion and ascites as well cardiac arrhythmias and tamponade. Initial x-ray should show the tip outside the heart, and periodic x-rays may be required to identify catheters at risk of migration. Additionally, infiltration and phlebitis can occur more easily and frequently in infants due to the size and fragility of their vessels.

Table 11–8. **TOTAL PARENTERAL NUTRITION (TPN) CALCULATIONS**

Amino acids:	$\% \text{ Amino acid} = \dfrac{\text{Wt (kg)} \times \text{(g/kg/d)} \times 100}{\text{Vol in 24 h}}$
Dextrose: glucose utilization rate (mg/kg/min):	$\dfrac{\text{Rate (mL/h)} \times \% \text{ Dextose}}{\text{Wt (kg)} \times 6}$
Lipids:	$\text{Rate (mL/h):} \dfrac{\text{g/kg/d} \times 5 \times \text{Wt (kg)}}{24}$

D. **Infectious.** Sepsis can occur in infants receiving central PN. The most common organisms include coagulase-positive and coagulase-negative *Staphylococcus, Streptococcus viridans, Escherichia coli, Pseudomonas* spp., *Klebsiella* spp., and *Candida albicans.* Infection may exacerbate cholestatic liver disease, leading to further morbidities. Standardizing procedures and bundled care of central lines can decrease catheter-related bloodstream infections (ie, central line–associated bloodstream infection [CLABSI]).

E. **Cost.** The costs of PN should be weighed against its risks, particularly when the anticipated need for PN is short term (<5 days). Complications such as CLABSI greatly increase the morbidity, mortality, and length of stay for infants in the NICU. Feeding protocols that encourage initiation and advancement of enteral feeds can help limit the morbidities associated with PN.

VII. **Transitioning to enteral feeds.** As enteral feeding volumes are increasing and volume of PN is decreasing, PN may need to be concentrated to prevent a decrease in caloric intake at the same fluid intake. Condensing PN to 80 to 90 mL/kg/d when enteral feeds reach 60 mL/kg/d helps maintain appropriate caloric intake at goal fluid volumes of 140 to 150 mL/kg/d. This can be accomplished by decreasing lipids to 1 g/kg/d, continuing full goal protein, and leaving dextrose concentrations the same. PN can be discontinued when enteral feeds reach 100 to 120 mL/kg/d.

CALORIC CALCULATIONS

Enterally fed healthy term infants should receive 100 to 120 kcal/kg/d for growth (70–90 kcal/kg/d if receiving TPN only). Some hypermetabolic infants may require >120 kcal/kg/d, and preterm infants can require up to 140 to 150 kcal/kg/d. Approximately 80 to 90 kcal/kg/d of nonprotein calories are required to maintain a positive nitrogen balance (nonprotein calories of 25–30 kcal/1 g of protein). Equations for calculating the caloric intake for EN and TPN follow (Table 11–8).

I. **Enteral nutrition.** Human milk (HM) caloric values can range from 14 to 26 kcal/oz. However, most standard calculations use 20 kcal/oz. Most standard infant formulas are 20 kcal/oz. (Similac uses 19 kcal/oz.) and contain 0.67 kcal/mL. Specific caloric concentrations of formulas are given in Table 11–4. To calculate total daily calories, use the following equation:

$$\text{kcal/kg/d} = \frac{\text{Total mL of HM or formula} \times \text{kcal/mL}}{\text{Wt (kg)}}$$

II. **Carbohydrates.** If only dextrose infusion is given, the total daily caloric intake is calculated as follows. (For caloric concentration of common solutions, see Table 11–9.)

$$\text{kcal/kg/d} = \frac{\text{mL of solution/h} \times 24\text{h} \times \text{kcal in solution}}{\text{Wt (kg)}}$$

Table 11–9. CALORIC CONCENTRATIONS OF VARIOUS PARENTERAL SOLUTIONS

	% Concentration	Caloric Concentration (kcal/mL)
Dextrose Solutions (anhydrous)		
D_5	5	0.17
$D_{7.5}$	7.5	0.255
D_{10}	10	0.34
$D_{12.5}$	12.5	0.425
D_{15}	15	0.51
D_{20}	20	0.68
D_{25}	25	0.85
Protein Solutions (g/d)		
0.5	0.5	0.02
1.0	1	0.04
1.5	1.5	0.06
2.0	2.0	0.08
2.5	2.5	0.10
3.0	3.0	0.12

A 0.5% solution, if given at 100 mL/d = 0.5 g of protein/d.

III. **Proteins.** Use the prior formula given for carbohydrates and the caloric concentrations given in Table 11–9.

IV. **Fat emulsions.** A 20% fat emulsion (Intralipid) contains 2 kcal/mL. Use the following formula to calculate daily caloric intake supplied by Intralipid 20%.

$$\text{kcal/kg/d} = \frac{\text{Total mL/d of solution} \times 2 \text{ kcal/mL}}{\text{Wt (kg)}}$$

MATERNAL NUTRITIONAL STATUS AND FETAL AND POSTNATAL GROWTH

Maternal nutritional status affects fetal and postnatal growth. Maternal BMI and prepregnancy weight, as well as excessive weight gain during pregnancy, increase the risk of fetal adiposity and subsequent obesity. Conversely, increased weight loss in the prepregnancy period in healthy mothers (normal BMI) increases the risk of small for gestational age infants.

Maternal diet supplemented with LCPUFAs, particularly omega-3 fatty acids, may improve BW, length, and length of gestation. Antenatal maternal micronutrient (eg, iron, folic acid) supplementation may influence fetal growth, fetal weight, and length of gestation and decrease infant morbidity. Cord blood vitamin D status is inversely correlated with respiratory infections and childhood wheezing.

Rapid weight gain in neonates starting as early as 6 weeks of age may increase risk of obesity. Accelerated weight gain in IUGR infants increases the risks of "adiposity rebound" and risk of subsequent cardiovascular and metabolic diseases.

GUT MICROBIOTA

Microbial colonization of the neonatal gut is necessary for intestinal development and homeostasis and has increasingly been identified as a key determinant of later health. Gut microbiota colonization and diversity are influenced by maternal diet, gestational age, mode of delivery, use of antibiotics, and type of neonatal feeds. Microbiome colonization patterns over time show strong association with weight Z-scores. For example, predominant staphylococci and *Enterococcus* spp. compared to *Lactobacillus* spp. were associated with poor weight gain in preterm infants. Enterobacteriaceae, streptococci, and *Bacteroides fragilis* have been associated with higher weight gain and BMI Z-scores. Oligosaccharides present in human milk may influence gut microbiome–dependent increase in body mass.

Advanced Management

12 Imaging Studies

Imaging a neonate requires the coordination of several medical professionals including nurses, respiratory therapists, radiology technologists, neonatologists, and radiologists. Effective and ongoing communication among all members of the team is required to ensure the appropriate modality is chosen according to the ALARA principle (**as low as reasonably achievable**) and to allow correct diagnosis. Imaging in the absence of clinical context is fraught with many complications including misdiagnosis. This chapter is a general outline of imaging studies that are commonly used to evaluate the neonate. Your choice in any clinical situation will depend on your institution and available resources.

I. **Common radiologic studies.** The need for radiographs must always be weighed against the risks of exposure of the neonate to radiation (eg, 3–5 mrem per chest radiographic view). The infant's gonads should be shielded as much as possible, and any person holding the infant during the x-ray procedure should also wear a protective shield. For the usual radiographic exposure, personnel need to be only 1 ft outside the zone of exposure.

A. **Chest radiographs**

1. **Anteroposterior (AP) view (supine position).** The single best view for identification of heart or lung disease, verification of endotracheal tube and other line positions, and identification of air leak complications of mechanical ventilation, such as pneumothorax.

2. **Cross-table lateral view (side view of infant lying on the back).** Of limited diagnostic value except to determine whether a chest tube is positioned anteriorly (best for drainage of a pneumothorax) or posteriorly (best for drainage of a pleural fluid collection). Also may visualize the tip of a high umbilical vein catheter and its relationship to the right atrium.

3. **Lateral decubitus view (left lateral decubitus is infant lying on left side down against the film, right lateral decubitus is infant lying on right side down against the film).** Referred to as the "problem-solving film" since it can be used to differentiate a pneumothorax from a pneumomediastinum, or to detect a pleural effusion. Best to visualize a small pneumothorax or a small pleural fluid collection, as either can be difficult to identify on the AP view. **If a pneumothorax is suspected,** a contralateral decubitus view (with the side of interest up) of the chest should be obtained. An air collection between lung and chest wall will be visible on the side on which the pneumothorax is present. For pleural fluid identification, the ipsilateral decubitus view (side of interest should be down). The lateral decubitus view may not be safely obtainable in unstable infants.

B. **Abdominal radiographs**

1. **AP view.** The single best view for diagnosing abdominal disorders such as intestinal obstruction and checking placement of support lines such as umbilical arterial and venous catheters and intestinal tubes. Small bowel cannot be differentiated from large bowel on a plain radiograph because of nondeveloped haustrae in large bowel. It is recommended as the initial radiographic study to determine further workup in a neonate with bilious vomiting up to 1 week of age.

2. **Left lateral decubitus abdominal view (infant placed left side down).** Best for the diagnosis of intestinal perforation. Free intra-abdominal air resulting from bowel perforation will be visible as an air collection between the liver and right lateral abdominal wall.

C. **Chest and abdomen AP view ("babygram" is a colloquial term).** A radiograph that includes the whole body or just the chest and abdomen on a single image. It is most commonly ordered for line placement.

II. **Common radiologic studies with contrast**

A. **Enteric contrast.** Enteric contrast are contrast agents that are used in the GI tract and may be given orally or rectally. Barium sulfate and low-osmolality water-soluble agents are essentially interchangeable with a few exceptions outlined below.

1. **Barium.** Barium sulfate, an inert compound, coats the lining of the gastrointestinal (GI) tract after it is swallowed or introduced per rectum. It is not absorbed from the GI tract and results in no fluid shift. This is the contrast agent of choice in most routine upper GI (UGI) and contrast enema examinations without a suspicion of bowel perforation. **Barium contrast studies are not recommended** in infants with **suspected abdominal perforation or if the destination of the administered contrast is unknown** because barium is irritating to the peritoneum and can result in "barium peritonitis."

2. **Low-osmolality water-soluble contrast agents.** These agents are interchangeable with barium and have replaced high-osmolality contrast agents in neonatal imaging. **Iohexol (Omnipaque)** is the only agent in this category with US Food and Drug Administration (FDA) approval for enteral administration in adults and children. **Omnipaque 180** (180 denotes amount of mg of organic iodine per mL) and **Omnipaque 240** may be used in premature and newborn infants. The off-label use of other contrast agents such as **iodixanol (Visipaque)** is common. **Omnipaque 180, Omnipaque 240, and Visipaque** do not require dilution prior to administration.

a. **Advantages**

i. **If bowel perforation is present,** these substances are nontoxic to the peritoneal cavity. In addition, they do not damage the bowel mucosa.

ii. **If aspirated,** there is limited irritation (if any) to the lungs.

iii. **They have limited absorption from the normal intestinal tract** and thus maintain good opacification throughout the intestinal tract on delayed imaging.

b. **Disadvantages.** None other than a higher cost than barium.

3. **Indications:**

a. **Any UGI or contrast enema in neonate.**

b. **Suspected H-type tracheoesophageal fistula.**

c. **Suspected esophageal or bowel perforation.**

d. **Unexplained pneumoperitoneum.**

e. **Evaluation of "gasless abdomen" in a neonate >12 hours old.**

B. **Neonatal fluoroscopy.** Fluoroscopy is an imaging technique that uses real time x-ray to capture a moving image of an organ usually with contrast. Rapid pulsed fluoroscopy is used to decrease radiation dose. It is most commonly used in neonates to image the gastrointestinal and genitourinary tracts.

1. **Contrast enema.** Used to investigate causes of lower intestinal obstruction such as meconium ileus, small left colon syndrome, ileal atresia, colonic atresia, Hirschsprung disease, anorectal malformation, and colonic stricture following necrotizing enterocolitis (NEC). It can be not only diagnostic but also therapeutic for certain conditions, such as small left colon syndrome and meconium ileus.

2. **Upper gastrointestinal imaging (UGI) imaging.** Diagnose intestinal malrotation, midgut volvulus, gastric outlet obstruction.

a. **Bilious vomiting.** An emergent UGI series is indicated in the workup of a neonate with bilious vomiting. Direct communication with the radiologist is suggested to ensure visualization of ligament of Treitz. Full small bowel study is not required.

b. **Nonbilious vomiting.** Consider delayed gastric emptying, gastroesophageal reflux (GER), and hypertrophic pyloric stenosis. Nonemergent UGI is used in a neonate with nonbilious vomiting and infant <3 months of age with new-onset nonbilious vomiting if targeted ultrasound of the pylorus is not available.

c. **Suspected gastroesophageal reflux (GER).** The pH probe examination and the reflux nuclear scan more reliably identify and quantitate GER than the UGI series.

3. **Esophagram.** Infant is fed contrast material or administered contrast by nasogastric tube, and imaging is done. Used for tracheoesophageal fistula, esophageal stenosis or obstruction, perforation, unexplained pneumomediastinum, to investigate causes of stridor and dysphagia, and for great vessel anomalies.

4. **Small bowel follow-through.** High dose of radiation with combination of pulsed fluoroscopy and x-rays of abdomen. Used to diagnose stricture in a premature infant with feeding intolerance following NEC.

5. **Voiding cystourethrography (VCUG).** A fluoroscopic study of the lower urinary tract with contrast done in the neonate for congenital anomalies of the urinary tract, postoperative evaluation of the urinary tract, bladder outlet obstruction, hematuria, trauma, hydronephrosis/hydroureter, neurogenic bladder, or febrile urinary tract infection.

III. **Radionuclide studies.** Radionuclide studies provide more physiologic than anatomic information and usually involve a lower radiation dose to the patient compared with radiographic examinations.

A. **Reflux scintiscan.** Used for documenting and quantitating GER and is comparable to the pH probe examination and superior to the UGI series. Technetium-99m–sulfur colloid is a radioactive diagnostic agent that is instilled into the stomach with formula, and the tracer is not absorbed. The patient is then scanned in the supine position for 1 to 2 hours with a gamma camera.

B. **Radionuclide cystogram.** Used for documenting and quantitating vesicoureteral reflux. Advantages over the radiographic VCUG include a much lower radiation dose (reduced by 50- to 100-fold) and a longer monitoring period (1–2 hours). A disadvantage is much poorer anatomic detail; bladder diverticula, posterior urethral valves, or mild reflux cannot be reliably identified. This technique should not be the initial examination for evaluation of the lower urinary tract, especially in boys.

C. **Radionuclide bone scan.** Used for evaluation of possible osteomyelitis. This procedure involves a 3-phase study (blood flow, blood pool, and bone uptake) after intravenous injection of technetium-99m–labeled methylene diphosphonate.

1. **Advantages.** Sensitivity to bony changes earlier than with the radiograph.

2. **Disadvantages.** Magnetic resonance imaging (MRI) is preferred if available due to its lack of radiation. A bone scan may not identify the acute phase of osteomyelitis (ie, the first 24–48 hours). Bone scan and MRI require absence of patient motion by immobilization or sedation.

D. **Hepatoiminodiacetic acid (HIDA; hepatobiliary) scan.** Used in certain types of neonatal jaundice to assist in differentiating biliary atresia (surgical disorder) from neonatal hepatitis (medical disorder). Oral phenobarbital (5 mg/kg/d) is given for 5 days prior to the examination (enhances bile flow in the liver).

IV. **Ultrasonography.** Ultrasound should be considered for the first line imaging modality for many indications in a neonate. Common ultrasounds obtained in the neonate include imaging the head, heart (echocardiography), hips for dysplasia, and abdomen/kidneys/bladder. Advantages include that it is noninvasive, it involves no ionizing radiation, imaging can be done in the NICU, and it is a real-time dynamic imaging modality. Disadvantages include the need for specific training, imaging is highly operator dependent, and inability to image through bowel gas and ossified bone.

A. **Ultrasonography of the head.** This is the first imaging study in a full-term infant with seizures. It is also performed in preterm infants to rule out intraventricular hemorrhage (IVH), ischemic change (periventricular leukomalacia [PVL]), hydrocephalus, and developmental anomalies. It can also be used to predict long-term neurodevelopmental outcome (eg, grade III and IV IVH, periventricu-lar cystic lesions, and moderate and severe ventriculomegaly are associated with adverse outcome). It can be performed in the NICU with a portable ultrasound unit. No special preparation is needed. The American Academy of Pediatrics (AAP) recommends that routine screening cranial ultrasound be performed on all infants <30 weeks' gestation once between 7 and 14 days of age and be repeated between 36 and 40 weeks' postmenstrual age. The classification of IVH based on ultrasonographic findings is demonstrated in Figures 12–1 through 12–4.

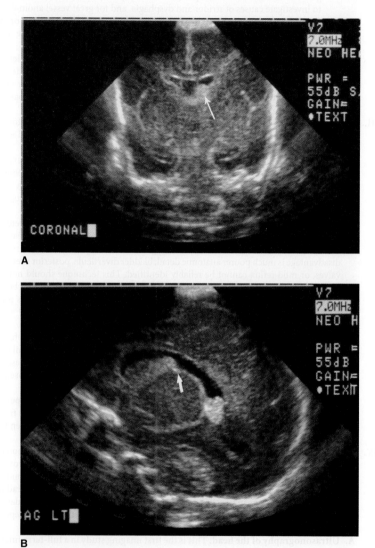

FIGURE 12–1. Ultrasonogram of the brain. Coronal (**A**) and left sagittal (**B**) views show a left germinal matrix hemorrhage (grade I or subependymal) at arrow.

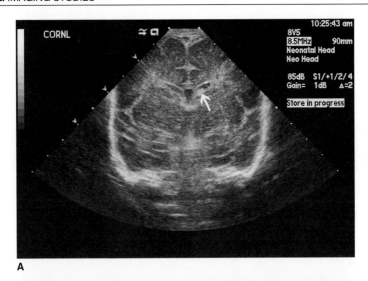

A

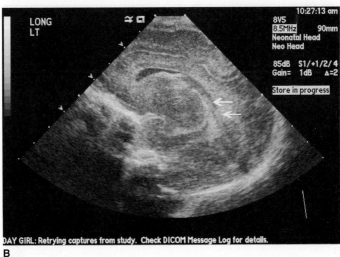

B

FIGURE 12–2. Ultrasonogram of the brain. Coronal (**A**) and left sagittal (**B**) views show a limited intraventricular hemorrhage (IVH) without ventricular enlargement at arrows (grade II IVH).

Figure 12–5 shows a posterior fossa hemorrhage, and Figure 12–6 demonstrates ischemic changes of PVL.
 1. **Grading of IVH** in the neonate by sonography is as follows (based on Papile et al., 1978):
    a. **Grade I.** Subependymal, germinal matrix hemorrhage.
    b. **Grade II.** IVH without ventricular dilatation.
    c. **Grade III.** IVH with ventricular dilatation.
    d. **Grade IV.** IVH with intraparenchymal hemorrhage.

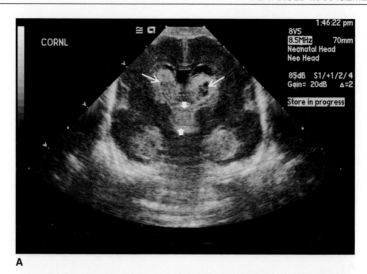

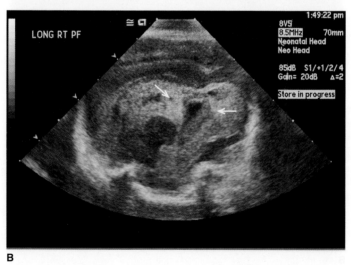

FIGURE 12–3. Ultrasonogram of the brain. Coronal (**A**) and right parasagittal (**B**) views demonstrate severe dilatation of both lateral (small arrows) as well as the third (large arrows) ventricles, which are filled with clots (grade III intraventricular hemorrhage).

  B. Abdominal ultrasonography. Useful in the evaluation of intraabdominal pathology such as abdominal distention, gallbladder disease, biliary obstruction, intraperitoneal fluid, abdominal masses, abscesses, pyloric stenosis, malrotation, and possible causes of renal failure. Ultrasound may be used to diagnose malrotation, but UGI is still the gold standard according to the Society for Pediatric Radiology. The addition of duplex and color Doppler evaluation of vessels can identify portal hypertension and complications of catheter placement such as renal vein thrombosis. In premature infants with NEC who develop a gasless abdomen, ultrasound

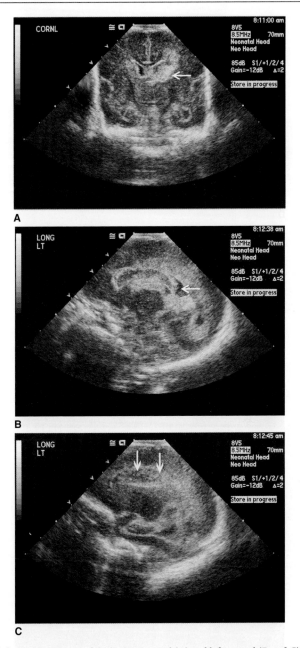

FIGURE 12–4. Ultrasonogram of the brain. Coronal (**A**) and left sagittal (**B and C**) views demonstrate left intraventricular hemorrhage (IVH) with ventricular dilatation and localized left intraparenchymal hemorrhage (grade IV IVH) (arrows). Follow-up sonogram 3 months later (coronal view [**D**] and left sagittal [**E and F**] views) shows resolution of clot, residual mild ventriculomegaly, and focal porencephaly (arrow) at the site of previous parenchymal hemorrhage.

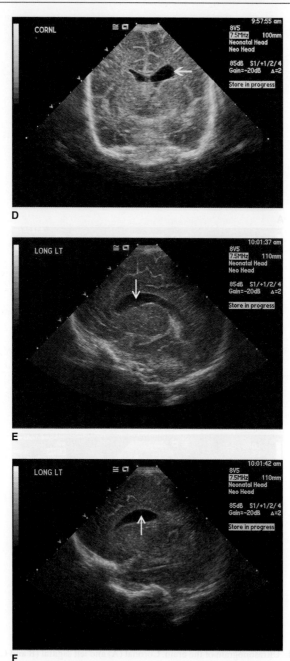

FIGURE 12–4. (*Continued*)

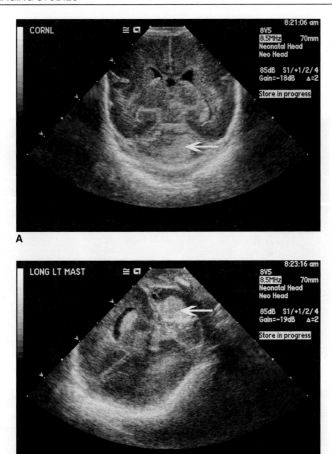

FIGURE 12–5. Ultrasonogram of the brain. Coronal (**A**) and mastoid (**B**) views demonstrate focal hemorrhage into the left cerebellar hemisphere (posterior fossa hemorrhage, arrow).

can evaluate bowel peristalsis, wall thickness, vascularity, and bowel ischemia and may visualize abscess formation and bowel perforation.

C. **Ultrasound of the kidneys and bladder.** First line imaging for urinary tract pathology. Used for any infant with the first febrile urinary tract infection, with decreased urinary output/suspected bladder outlet obstruction, and in the initial evaluation of congenital anomalies of the genitourinary system.

D. **Ultrasound of the hips** is the preferred procedure for ruling out developmental dysplasia of the hip. It is best to do this between 4 and 6 weeks of age because of the high risk of false-positive results. AAP recommends ultrasound of hip to clarify suspicious or equivocal findings on physical examination or to detect a clinically silent developmental dysplasia of the hip (DDH) in a high-risk infant with a normal exam. Risk factors include breech in third trimester, family history of DDH, history of improper swaddling, and history of abnormal hip physical examination in the neonatal period that normalizes.

E. **Ultrasonography of the spinal cord** visualizes the entire spinal cord prior to ossification of the posterior elements without radiation or sedation. It is useful when there are cutaneous manifestations associated with spinal dysraphism including

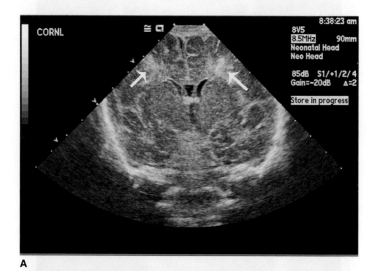

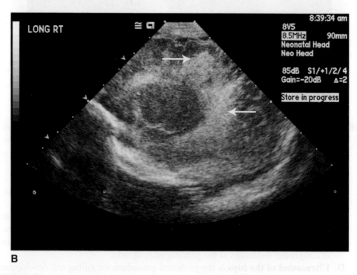

FIGURE 12–6. Ultrasonogram of the brain. Periventricular leukomalacia (PVL). Coronal (**A**) and right sagittal (**B**) views demonstrate increased periventricular echogenicity, suggesting ischemic white matter disease (arrows). Follow-up sonography of the brain 1 month later (coronal [**C**] and sagittal [**D**] views) shows extensive periventricular cystic change reflecting PVL.

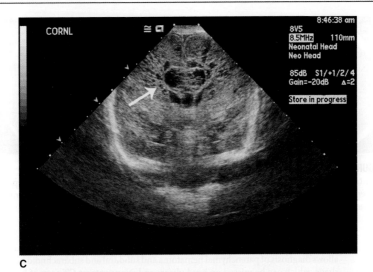

C

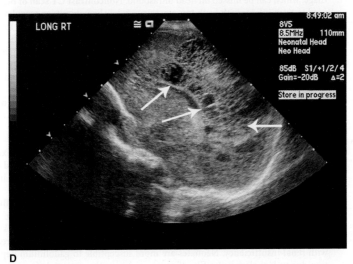

D

FIGURE 12–6. (*Continued*)

midline mass hair tuft, skin discoloration, skin tags, or deep sacral dimple located 2.5 cm above anus. Ultrasound of simple coccygeal dimples without cutaneous findings of spinal dysraphism and <2.5 cm above the anus is of extremely low diagnostic yield and not recommended.

    F. Point-of-care ultrasound (POCUS) in neonatology is the use of a portable ultrasound by a nonradiologist (eg, a neonatologist) and is performed at the bedside of an infant in the NICU or newborn nursery. See Chapter 44.

V. Computed tomography (CT) scanning

    A. CT scan of the head. The use of CT must balance the risk of radiation to the newborn. CT scanning provides more global information than ultrasonography of

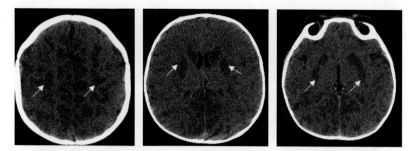

FIGURE 12–7. Noncontrast computed tomography of the brain. Abnormal low density (white arrows) in basal ganglia, subcortical white matter, and cortex consistent with hypoxic ischemic injury. (*Used with permission from Karuna Shekdar, MD, The Children's Hospital of Philadelphia.*)

the head, particularly the periphery of the brain, extra-axial space, and cranium. It allows diagnosis of parenchymal hematoma and subdural and subarachnoid hemorrhage, which can be missed on head ultrasound. **Noncontrast CT scan of brain** is used in term infants with birth trauma, seizures, low hematocrit, or coagulopathy to rule out hemorrhage. CT may be used in patients with encephalopathy following a hypoxic or ischemic event. See Figure 12–7 for an example of hypoxic ischemic encephalopathy (HIE). **Contrast-enhanced CT of the brain** may help in the detection of intracranial vascular anomalies or evaluation of central nervous system (CNS) tumors. Other modalities without radiation, such as cranial ultrasound with Doppler and MRI, are preferred.

B. CT imaging of the neck, chest, abdomen, pelvis, and extremities in the neonate is infrequently performed. Radiography, ultrasound, and MRI are used more commonly.

VI. Magnetic resonance imaging (MRI)

A. Magnetic resonance imaging without contrast. MRI without contrast is an exceptional mode of imaging in the neonate due to its superb anatomic detail and lack of ionizing radiation. It is better than CT to evaluate CNS white matter changes and infarction.

B. MRI with gadolinium-based contrast agents (GBCAs). MRI with GBCAs and their use in the neonatal, pediatric, and adult population are evolving. The deposition of gadolinium utilizing GBCAs has been detected in the bones and brains of adult patients. Gadolinium deposition is dose dependent and increases with renal insufficiency. Neonates are more susceptible to gadolinium deposition due to low glomerular filtration rate and have the potential for numerous contrast-enhanced MRIs over their lifetime. Long-term effects and their clinical significance are not known. According to the most recent FDA drug safety announcement issued May 22, 2017, "[The] FDA identifies no harmful effects to date with brain retention of gadolinium-based contrast agents for MRIs; and will continue to review." The FDA recommends that "health care professionals should consider limiting GBCA use to clinical circumstances in which the additional information provided by the contrast is necessary." Direct communication with the radiologist is required to determine if nonenhanced MRI will answer the clinical question.

C. Common indications for MRI

1. MRI of the brain. Indications include determination of etiology of seizures; determination of hypoxic ischemic injury, congenital malformations, focal cerebral injury (arterial or venous stroke), intracerebral hemorrhage, bilirubin encephalopathy, significant birth trauma, metabolic disorders, history of encephalopathy, or acute encephalopathy; and evaluation of neonatal meningitis. It may have a role in the following: predicting neurodevelopmental outcomes, pre- and postoperative evaluation in neonates with congenital heart disease, and detection of brain insult in extracorporeal membrane oxygenation infants with neurologic signs. See Figure 12–8. MRI of brain is used in preterm infants with profound HIE.

   2. **MRI of the body.** Indications include evaluation of masses/neoplasms, hemangiomas/vascular malformations, congenital cystic masses of the head and neck, mediastinal vascular anomalies, and congenital pelvic GI/genitourinary anomalies.

   3. **MRI of the spine.** Used to further characterize anomalies depicted on ultrasound and can give anatomic details of the malformations of the spine. See Figure 12–9.

   4. **Specific MRI modalities**

      a. **Magnetic resonance arteriography and magnetic resonance venography** are used to define vascular anatomy and flow. The need for intravenous contrast-enhanced magnetic resonance arteriography and venography should be discussed with the radiologist.

Diffusion

ADC maps

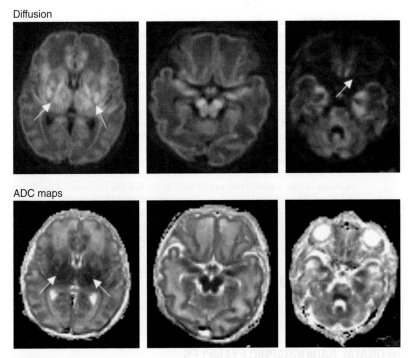

FIGURE 12–8. Magnetic resonance imaging of the brain in preterm infant. Bilateral symmetric restricted diffusion (white arrows) in thalamus, basal ganglia, midbrain, and pons consistent with profound hypoxic ischemic encephalopathy. (*Used with permission from Karuna Shekdar, MD, The Children's Hospital of Philadelphia.*)

T2 sag   **T1 sag**   **T1 axial**   **T2 axial**

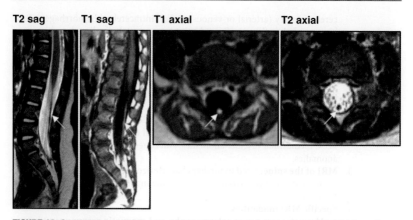

FIGURE 12–9. Magnetic resonance imaging of spine. Low-lying conus at L3. Thickened filum with T1 hyperintense, T2 hypointense signal (white arrows) consistent with tethered cord and fatty filum. (*Used with permission from Karuna Shekdar, MD, The Children's Hospital of Philadelphia.*)

      b. MRI spectroscopy and diffusion-weighted imaging (DWI)/diffusion tensor imaging (DTI) can help with disease prognostication. MRI spectroscopy provides information about biochemical composition of imaged tissue such as in HIE or inherited metabolic diseases. DWI provides an image based on differences in the magnitude of diffusion of water molecules in the brain, and DTI analyzes the 3-dimensional shape of the diffusion. Diseases can be identified earlier (cerebral ischemia), allowing one to monitor treatment and predict outcome.

  D. Disadvantages of MRI include the potential need for sedation. Usually, infants are fed immediately prior to MRI and placed in an MRI-compatible infant immobilizer to avoid sedation; some neonatal units try swaddling with an optional pacifier with or without oral sucrose (feed and wrap/feed and bundle). Transportation of ill neonates outside of the NICU is a second disadvantage. An MRI compatible incubator is now available that can be used to provide safe transport of the infant and allows thermal regulation during transport and the MRI exam. A few centers have infant-sized MRI units in the NICU. In 2017, the FDA approved an infant-sized MRI unit for imaging the neonatal head that can be housed in the NICU (Embrace Neonatal MRI System). Researchers hope to provide advanced imaging to critically ill neonates with minimal disruption in care.

COMMON RADIOLOGIC PREPARATIONS

See Table 12–1 for guidelines for common radiographic studies. Institutional guidelines may vary from these.

NEONATAL RADIOGRAPHIC EXAMPLES

Invasive life support and monitoring techniques depend on proper positioning of the device being used. **Caution is necessary when identifying ribs and correlating vertebrae** in the newborn as a means for determining the proper position of a catheter or tube. Infants often have a noncalcified 12th rib; thus, the 11th rib is mistaken for the 12th rib, and an incorrect

Table 12–1. PREPARATORY PROCEDURES FOR PREMATURE AND NEWBORN INFANT RADIOLOGIC STUDIES[a]

Neonatal Study	Preparation
Upper GI series	NPO for 2 hours for newborns and infants up to 4 months of age
Contrast enema	No preparation needed for evaluation of bowel obstruction or to rule out Hirschsprung disease
Renal sonography	No preparation
Abdominal sonography	NPO for 1 hour for filling of gallbladder
HIDA (hepatobiliary) scan	Oral phenobarbital (5 mg/kg/d) for 5 days prior to the examination
CT of abdomen/pelvis	Oral contrast beginning 2 hours prior to scanning
Voiding cystourethrogram	No preparation required

CT, computed tomography; GI, gastrointestinal; HIDA, hepatoiminodiacetic acid; NPO, nothing by mouth.
[a]Review institution-specific recommendations before ordering.

vertebral count may occur. Infants can also have an abnormal number of ribs. In 5% to 8% of normal individuals, there are only 11 ribs. Eleven ribs also occur in approximately 33% of infants with trisomy 21 syndrome and in campomelic dysplasia and cleidocranial dysplasia. An increased number of ribs can occur in VATER (vertebral anomalies, anal atresia, tracheoesophageal fistula, and radial or renal dysplasia)/VACTERL (vertebral defects, anal atresia, cardiac defects, tracheoesophageal fistula, renal and radial abnormalities, and limb abnormalities) association.

  I. **Endotracheal intubation**
   A. **The preferred location of the endotracheal tube (ETT) tip** is halfway between the thoracic inlet (the medial ends of the clavicles) and the carina. Ideally, it should be 1 cm above the carina, but this may not be possible in infants with severe intrauterine growth restriction and premature infants weighing <1000 g. Correct tube placement is shown in Figure 12–10.
   B. **If the ETT is placed too low,** the tip usually enters the right main bronchus, because it is easier to enter since it is not only a shallower angle but a straighter line than with the left main bronchus. If the ETT is in the right mainstem bronchus, one can see overdistention/hyperinflation of the right middle and lower lungs and underventilation and/or atelectasis of the remaining lungs. The chest film may show asymmetric aeration with both hyperinflation and atelectasis. If the tube extends below the carina or does not match the tracheal air column in position, suspect esophageal intubation. Dilatation of the esophagus and stomach with air and increased proximal intestinal air may also reflect esophageal intubation.
   C. **An ETT placed too high** has the tip above the clavicle, and the x-ray film may show diffuse atelectasis.
  II. **Nasogastric/orogastric tube.** The nasogastric/orogastric tube tip should be in the mid-stomach. It should not be at or above the gastroesophageal junction. Correct placement is shown in Figure 12–11.
 III. **Transpyloric tube.** The weighted feeding tube is ideally placed in the mid to distal duodenum. Correct placement is shown in Figure 12–12.
 IV. **Umbilical vein catheterization (UVC).** The catheter tip should be at the junction of the inferior vena cava and right atrium, projecting just above the diaphragm on the AP chest radiograph. Degree and direction of patient rotation affect how the UVC appears positioned on the radiograph. Due to its more anterior location, the UVC deviates more

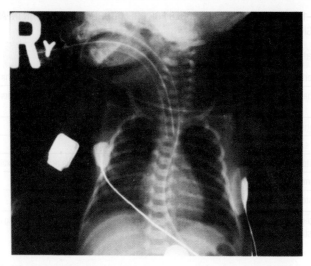

FIGURE 12–10. Chest radiograph showing proper placement of an endotracheal tube.

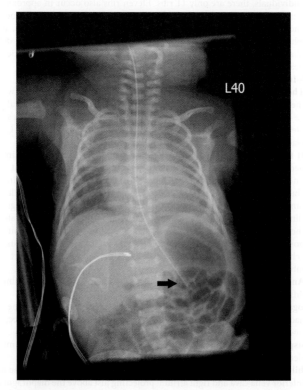

FIGURE 12–11. Chest abdomen film showing the nasogastric tube tip in the mid-stomach (arrow at distal tube).

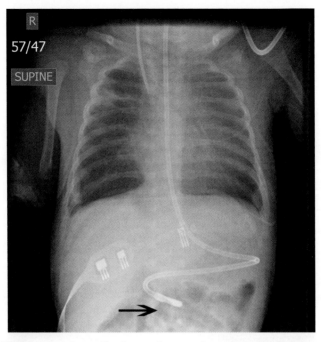

FIGURE 12–12. Chest abdomen film showing the transpyloric tube (weighted feeding tube tip) in the mid to distal duodenum (arrow at distal tube).

from the midline with patient rotation than will the UAC. Figure 12–13 shows correct UVC tip placement.

V. **Umbilical artery catheterization (UAC).** Cochrane review indicates that high catheters should be used exclusively. In certain instances, a catheter may have to be placed in the low position. The use of high versus low UAC placement used to depend on institutional preference. High catheters were once thought to be associated with a higher risk of vascular complications, but a recent analysis showed a decreased risk of vascular complications and no increased risk of hypertension, NEC, IVH, or hematuria. Low catheters are associated with an increased risk of vasospasms.

   A. **If high UAC placement** is desired, the tip should be between thoracic vertebrae 6 and 9 (above the diaphragm, which is above the celiac axis at T12, the superior mesenteric artery at T12–L1, and the renal arteries [L1]) (Figure 12–14).

   B. **For low UAC placement**, the tip should be below the third lumbar vertebra, optimally between L3 and L4 (above the aortic bifurcation, which is at L4–5) (Figure 12–15). A catheter placed below L5 usually does not function well and carries a risk of severe vasospasm in small arteries. Note that the catheter turns downward and then upward on an abdominal x-ray film. The upward turn is the point at which the catheter passes through the internal iliac artery (hypogastric artery).

   Note: If both a UAC and a UVC are positioned and an x-ray study is performed, it is necessary to differentiate the 2 so that line placement can be properly assessed. The UAC turns downward and then upward on the x-ray film, whereas the UVC takes only an upward or cephalad direction.

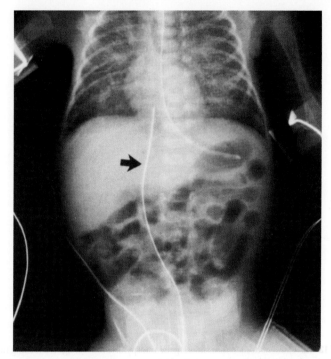

FIGURE 12–13. Radiograph showing correct placement of an umbilical venous catheter (arrow). The tip of the nasogastric tube is properly positioned in the stomach.

VI. **Extracorporeal life support.** ECLS external life support using a membrane oxygenator is described in detail in Chapter 20. See the veno-arterial ECLS cannulae placement and veno-venous ECLS cannulae placement radiographs (Figures 20–3 and 20–4, respectively).

RADIOGRAPHIC PEARLS

I. **Pulmonary diseases.** The neonatal chest radiograph is one of the first and most frequently performed diagnostic examinations performed in the NICU. It plays a significant role in helping the clinician with the etiology and diagnosis of respiratory distress in the newborn.

A. **Respiratory distress syndrome (RDS).** A fine, diffuse reticulogranular pattern is seen secondary to microatelectasis of the alveoli. The chest radiograph reveals radiolucent areas known as air bronchograms, produced by air in the major airways and contrasted with the opacified, collapsed alveoli (Figure 12–16).

B. **Meconium aspiration syndrome.** Bilateral, patchy, coarse infiltrates and hyperinflation of the lungs are present (Figure 12–17). There is an increased incidence of pneumothorax.

C. **Pneumonia.** Diffuse alveolar or interstitial disease that is usually asymmetric and localized. Group B streptococcal pneumonia can appear similar to RDS. Pneumatoceles (air-filled lung cysts) can occur with staphylococcal pneumonia. Pleural effusions or empyema may occur with any bacterial pneumonia (Figure 12–18).

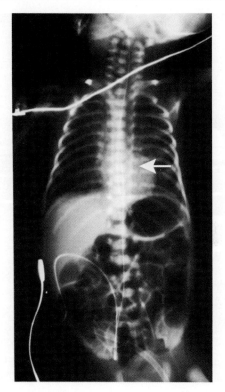

FIGURE 12–14. Radiograph showing correct positioning of a high umbilical artery catheter.

    D. Transient tachypnea of the newborn (TTN). Hyperaeration with symmetric peri-hilar and interstitial streaky infiltrates are typical. Heart may be normal or mildly enlarged. Pleural fluid may occur as well, appearing as widening of the pleural space or as prominence of the minor fissure (Figure 12–19). Radiographs cannot reliably differentiate TTN from neonatal pneumonia. TTN is a diagnosis of exclusion; radiographic findings completely resolve in 24 to 48 hours. Radiographs of neonatal pneumonia may normalize in 1 to 2 weeks.

    E. Bronchopulmonary dysplasia, now referred to as chronic lung disease (CLD). The radiographic appearance is highly variable, from a fine, hazy appearance of the lungs to mildly coarsened lung markings to a coarse, cystic lung pattern (Figure 12–20). Typically occurring in ventilated premature neonates, CLD usually requires a minimum of 7 to 10 days to develop. Many centers no longer rely on the following grading system for this condition, but it is included for historical purposes.

        1. Grade I. X-ray findings are similar to those of severe RDS.

        2. Grade II. Dense parenchymal opacification is seen.

        3. Grade III. A bubbly, fibrocystic pattern is evident.

        4. Grade IV. Hyperinflation is present with multiple fine, lacy densities spreading to the periphery and with areas of lucency similar to bullae of the lung.

    F. Air leak syndromes

        1. Pneumopericardium. Air surrounds the heart, including the inferior border (Figure 12–21). Cardiac tamponade may result.

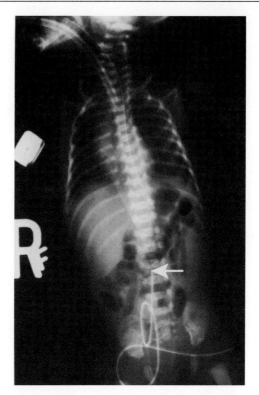

FIGURE 12–15. Radiograph showing correct positioning of a low umbilical artery catheter.

2. **Pneumomediastinum**
   a. **AP view.** A hyperlucent rim of air is present lateral to the cardiac border and beneath the thymus, displacing the thymus superiorly away from the cardiac silhouette ("angel wing sign") (Figure 12–22, left panel).
   b. **Lateral view.** An air collection is seen either substernally (anterior pneumomediastinum) or in the retrocardiac area (posterior pneumomediastinum) (Figure 12–22, right panel).
3. **Pneumothorax.** The lung is typically displaced away from the lateral chest wall by a radiolucent zone of air. The adjacent lung may be collapsed with larger pneumothoraces (as in Figure 12–23). The small pneumothorax may be very difficult to identify, with only a subtle zone of air peripherally, a diffusely hyperlucent hemithorax, unusually sharply defined cardiothymic margins, or a combination of these.
4. **Tension pneumothorax.** The diaphragm on the affected side is depressed, the mediastinum is shifted to the contralateral hemithorax, and collapse of the ipsilateral lobes is evident (Figure 12–23).
5. **Pulmonary interstitial emphysema (PIE).** Single or multiple circular radiolucencies with well-demarcated walls are seen in a localized or diffuse pattern. The volume of the involved portion of the lung is usually increased, often markedly so (Figure 12–24). PIE usually occurs in ventilated preemies with RDS within the initial few days of life.

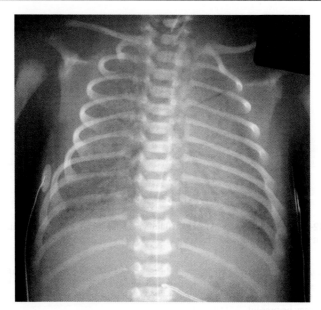

FIGURE 12–16. Chest radiograph showing diffuse granular opacification of the lungs with air bronchograms. In the premature neonate, this would almost always represent respiratory distress syndrome.

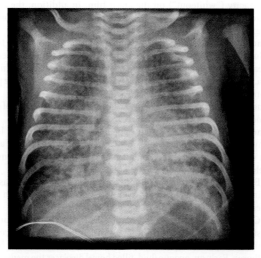

FIGURE 12–17. Chest radiograph showing diffuse coarse increase in lung markings accompanied by hyperinflation, typical for meconium aspiration syndrome.

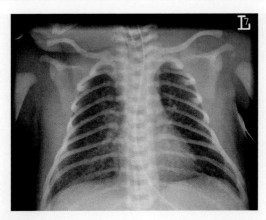

FIGURE 12–18. Diffuse increase in interstitial lung markings is typical with neonatal pneumonia but could also be produced by transient tachypnea of newborn.

G. **Atelectasis.** A decrease in lung volume or collapse of part or all of a lung is apparent, appearing as areas of increased opacity. The mediastinum may be shifted toward the side of collapse. Compensatory hyperinflation of the opposite lung may be present.
  1. **Microatelectasis.** Nonobstructive atelectasis associated with RDS.
  2. **Generalized atelectasis.** Diffuse increase in opacity ("whiteout") of the lungs is visible on the chest film. It may be seen in severe RDS, in airway obstruction, if the ETT is not in the trachea, and in hypoventilation.
  3. **Lobar atelectasis.** Lobar atelectasis is atelectasis of one lobe. The most common site is the right upper lobe, which appears as an area of dense opacity ("whiteout") on the chest film. In addition, the right minor fissure is usually elevated. This pattern of atelectasis commonly occurs after extubation.
H. **Pulmonary hypoplasia.** Small lung volumes and a bell-shaped thorax are seen. The lungs usually appear radiolucent. In unilateral hypoplasia, there is small lung, decreased vascularity, and heart is displaced to hypoplastic side. In bilateral hypoplasia, there is a bell-shaped thorax, low lung volumes, and possible pneumothorax/pneumomediastinum.
I. **Pulmonary edema.** The lungs appear diffusely hazy with an area of greatest density around the hilum of each lung. Heart size is usually increased.
J. **Pulmonary hemorrhage.** Variable appearance with symmetric homogenous to patchy heterogenous shadowing or "whiteout." Quick resolution of airspace disease, often within hours, helps to differentiate this from neonatal pneumonia.
K. **Developmental abnormalities**
  1. **Esophageal atresia.** Dilated upper esophageal pouch. Nasogastric tube coiled in proximal esophagus. Air in the stomach consistent with distal tracheoesophageal fistula (TEF).
  2. **Congenital diaphragmatic hernia (CDH).** Visible aerated lung on ipsilateral side to hernia indicates good prognosis; pneumothorax on contralateral side indicates poor prognosis. In left-sided CDH, stomach and bowel enter the thorax. Early on, opaque fluid-filled bowel displaces the mediastinum. Eventually, cystic radiolucencies deviate the mediastinum. In right-sided CDH, the liver herniates into thorax.
  3. **Congenital pulmonary airway malformation, CPAM, formerly known as cystic adenomatoid malformation.** Appearance on x-ray depends upon the

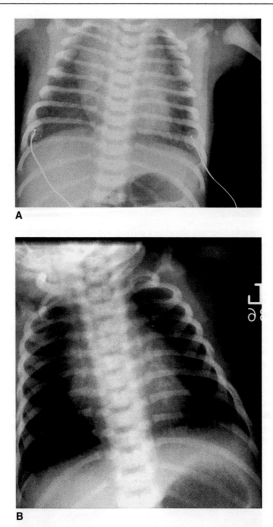

FIGURE 12–19. Chest radiograph (**A**) showing diffuse, mild increase in interstitial lung markings, consistent with transient tachypnea of newborn. The findings had typically resolved by the following day (**B**).

subtype of CPAM. Can see a variety of lesions (multicystic air filled, solid, or with air-fluid levels) or large lesions causing a mediastinal shift. Small lesions may have a normal x-ray.

4. **Pulmonary sequestration.** Normal or increased basal opacity, mediastinal shift if segment is large. If basal opacity fails to clear over 1 or several months, consider sequestration.

5. **Upper airway obstruction.** Severe overinflation of lungs.

6. **Congenital lobar emphysema.** Initially the lobe is fluid filled and opaque on chest radiograph. Affected lobe becomes overaerated, and there is marked decreased in vascularity. Normal lung is compressed.

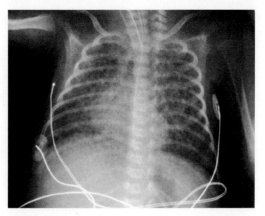

FIGURE 12–20. Chest radiograph showing a diffuse, moderately coarse increase in lung density, which in a 2-month-old ventilated ex-preemie is most consistent with bronchopulmonary dysplasia/chronic lung disease.

II. **Cardiac diseases.** Evaluate the cardiac size and shape, the aorta size, the pulmonary artery size, the presence of increased or decreased pulmonary vasculature, evidence of pulmonary edema (obstruction of blood flow), the position of the heart, and abdominal viscera. The cardiothoracic ratio, which normally should be <0.6, is the width of the base of the heart divided by the width of the lower thorax. An index >0.6 suggests **cardiomegaly.** Lateral chest radiograph will show deviation of the posterior heart border toward the spine with cardiomegaly. The pulmonary vascularity is increased if the diameter of the descending branch of the right pulmonary artery exceeds that of the trachea.

   A. **Cardiac dextroversion.** The cardiac apex is on the right, and the aortic arch and stomach bubble are on the left. The incidence of congenital heart disease associated with this finding is high (>90%).

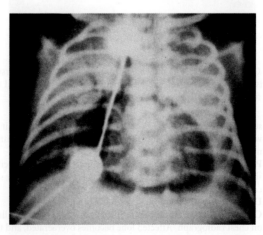

FIGURE 12–21. Chest radiograph showing pneumopericardium in a 2-day-old infant.

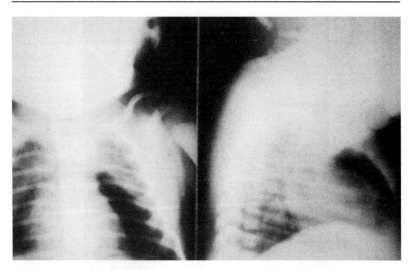

FIGURE 12–22. Pneumomediastinum on anteroposterior (left panel) and cross-table lateral (right panel) radiographs, demonstrating central chest air and elevation of the lobes of the thymus.

    B. Congestive heart failure. Cardiomegaly, pulmonary venous congestion (engorgement and increased diameter of the pulmonary veins), diffuse opacification in the perihilar regions, and pleural effusions (sometimes) are seen.

    C. Patent ductus arteriosus. Diagnosis is made on clinical basis. Cardiomegaly, pulmonary edema, ductal haze (pulmonary edema with a patent ductus arteriosus), and increased pulmonary vascular markings are evident usually after auscultation of heart murmur.

    D. Ventricular septal defect. Findings include cardiomegaly, an increase in pulmonary vascular density, enlargement of the left ventricle and left atrium, and enlargement of the main pulmonary artery.

    E. Coarctation of the aorta
        1. Preductal coarctation. Generalized cardiomegaly, with normal pulmonary vascularity, is seen.
        2. Postductal coarctation. An enlarged left ventricle and left atrium and a dilated ascending aorta are present.

    F. Tetralogy of Fallot. The heart is boot shaped. A normal left atrium and left ventricle is associated with an enlarged, hypertrophied right ventricle and small or absent main pulmonary artery. There is decreased pulmonary vascularity. A right aortic arch occurs in 25% of patients.

    G. Transposition of the great arteries. The chest film may show cardiomegaly, with an enlarged right atrium and right ventricle, narrow mediastinum, and increased pulmonary vascular markings, but in most cases, the chest film appears normal.

    H. Total anomalous pulmonary venous return (TAPVR). Pulmonary venous markings are increased. Cardiomegaly is minimal or absent. Congestive heart failure and pulmonary edema may be present, especially with type 3 (subdiaphragmatic) TAPVR.

    I. Hypoplastic left heart syndrome. The chest film can be normal at first but then may show cardiomegaly and pulmonary vascular congestion, with an enlarged right atrium and ventricle.

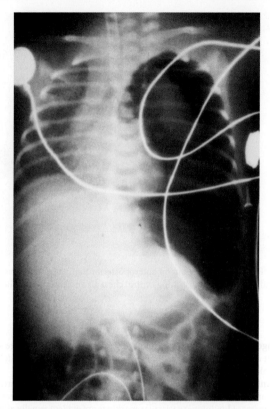

FIGURE 12–23. Left tension pneumothorax as shown on an anteroposterior chest radiograph in a ventilated infant on day 2 of life. Note the accompanying collapse of the left lung, depression of the left diaphragm, and contralateral shift of mediastinal structures, all signs of increased pressure within a pneumothorax.

    J. Tricuspid atresia. Heart size is usually normal or small, the main pulmonary artery is concave, and pulmonary vascularity is decreased.

    K. Truncus arteriosus. Characteristic findings include cardiomegaly, increased pulmonary vascularity, and enlargement of the left atrium. A right aortic arch occurs in 30% of patients.

    L. Atrial septal defect. Varying degrees of enlargement of the right atrium and ventricle are seen. The aorta and the left ventricle are small, and the pulmonary artery is large. Increased pulmonary vascularity is also evident.

    M. Ebstein anomaly. Gross cardiomegaly and decreased pulmonary vascularity are apparent. The right heart border is prominent as a result of right atrial enlargement.

    N. Valvular pulmonic stenosis. Heart size and pulmonary blood flow are usually normal unless the stenosis is severe. Dilatation of the main pulmonary artery is the typical chest film finding.

III. Abdominal disorders. An abdominal film is usually obtained in a neonate with abdominal distension, unexplained emesis or feeding intolerance, suspected obstruction, or acute abdomen. It is important to look for the normal progression of air in the bowel, any dilatation, number of dilated bowel loops, pneumatosis intestinalis, air in the rectum,

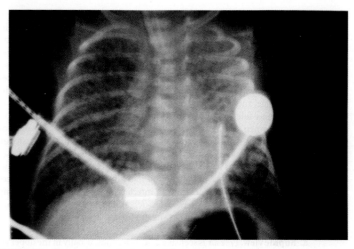

FIGURE 12–24. Chest radiograph showing bilateral pulmonary interstitial emphysema in a 7-day-old ventilated infant.

free air, and ascites. Abdominal and retroperitoneal masses may also require evaluation with imaging.

A. Normal neonatal bowel gas pattern

1. **Normal mosaic bowel gas pattern.** All gas-filled loops are similar in caliber, fitting together like a puzzle.

2. **Normal progression of air in bowel**
   a. **Air in the stomach.** Should occur within 30 minutes after delivery.
   b. **Air in proximal bowel loops.** Should be seen by 3 to 4 hours of age.
   c. **Air in distal bowel loops and rectum.** Should be seen in distal bowel by 6 to 8 hours of age and in rectum by 12 hours. Air in the rectum may not be seen on a radiograph obtained in the supine position because of its dependent location.

3. **Neonatal colon does not have developed haustra.** As a result, it is not possible to differentiate small bowel and colon on abdominal radiograph.

B. Abnormal abdominal findings that deviate from the mosaic pattern

1. **Dilated loops of bowel.** It is usually evident when bowel is dilated since the normal mosaic pattern is lost. As a general guideline, if the loop measures more than the interpedicular width of L2, it is considered dilated. Dilated loops can be seen with continuous positive airway pressure, ileus, ischemia, NEC, and obstruction.
   a. **Neonatal obstruction** is classified as **proximal or distal** according to the number of dilated loops. The presence of ≤3 loops is considered a proximal obstruction; the presence of ≥4 is a distal obstruction. The differential diagnosis for **proximal obstruction** includes gastric atresia, duodenal atresia, duodenal stenosis with anular pancreas, malrotation with Ladd band, proximal jejunal stenosis, and atresia. **Distal obstruction** includes distal jejunal atresia, ileal atresia, meconium ileus, functional immaturity of the colon or small left colon syndrome, Hirschsprung disease, colonic atresia, anal atresia, and anorectal malformations.
   b. **Malrotation with midgut volvulus** is a great masquerader. In an infant with bilious vomiting and this condition, the radiograph may be normal or look like a proximal or distal obstruction.

2. **Calcifications in the neonatal abdomen** is most often seen secondary to in utero bowel perforation. Meconium peritonitis may cause calcifications in the abdomen and in the scrotum in males. Calcifications can occur secondary to enterolithiasis from rectourinary fistula, small bowel obstruction (jejunoileal atresia), total colonic Hirschsprung disease, or rarely, secondary to hepatic calcifications. Calcifications in the infant abdomen may be seen with neuroblastoma, hepatoblastoma, teratoma, calcification of the adrenals after adrenal hemorrhage, and very rarely neonatal Wilms tumor.

3. **Ascites.** Gas-filled loops of bowel, if present, are located in the central portion of the abdomen. The abdomen may be distended, with relatively small amounts of gas ("ground-glass" appearance). A uniform increase in the density of the abdomen, particularly in the flank areas, may be evident.

4. **Air-fluid bowel gas levels.** Seen only on horizontal beam radiographs such as left lateral decubitus or upright abdominal films. Intraluminal fluid becomes dependent and air rises, creating an interface or line. Their presence implies either an abnormal bowel peristalsis such as ileus or bowel obstruction. Air-fluid levels occur proximal to the site of obstruction.

5. **Pneumoperitoneum**
   a. **Supine view.** Free air is seen as a central lucency, usually in the upper abdomen (Figure 12–25).
   b. **Upright view.** Free air is present in a subdiaphragmatic location.
   c. **Left lateral decubitus view.** Air collects over the lateral border of the liver, separating it from the adjacent abdominal wall.

6. **Pneumatosis intestinalis.** Intraluminal gas in the bowel wall (produced by bacteria that have invaded the bowel wall) may appear as a string or cluster of bubbles (submucosal) or a curvilinear lucency (subserosal). It is most

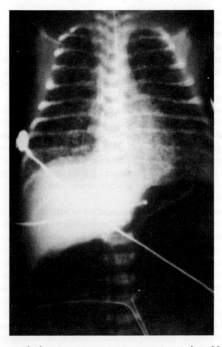

FIGURE 12–25. Radiograph showing pneumoperitoneum in a 3-day-old infant.

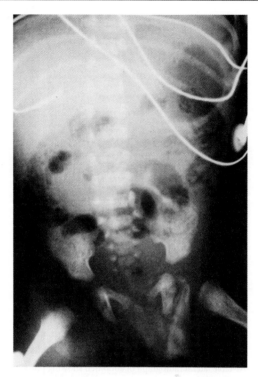

FIGURE 12–26. Abdominal radiograph showing pneumatosis intestinalis.

frequently seen in infants with NEC (Figure 12–26) but can be seen in intestinal obstruction with ischemia (malrotation with midgut volvulus and ischemia).

7. **"Soap bubble" appearance of bowel loops** is present in meconium ileus because of air mixed with meconium. A clue to the diagnosis of meconium ileus is the lack or paucity of air-fluid levels in comparison to the number of dilated bowel loops. The soap bubble appearance, or **Neuhauser sign**, can also be seen in ileal atresia, NEC, and Hirschsprung disease.

8. **Situs inversus (complete).** The stomach, aortic arch, and cardiac apex all are right sided. There is only a limited increased incidence of congenital heart disease.

9. **Ileus.** Distended loops of bowel are present. Air-fluid levels may be seen on the upright or cross-table lateral abdominal film.

10. **Absence of gas in the abdomen.** Absence of gas in the abdomen may be seen in neonates on sedative or muscle-paralyzing medications (eg, pancuronium) because they do not swallow air. It may also be evident in infants with esophageal atresia without tracheoesophageal fistula and in cases of severe cerebral anoxia resulting in CNS depression and absence of swallowing. It has also been seen in long-term persistent nasogastric suction, giant cystic meconium peritonitis, massive gangrene of the small bowel, massive ascites, massive intraabdominal tumors, massive duplication cyst, and omental cyst. The bubble sign in a gasless abdomen is a clue to the diagnosis of UGI obstruction. **Single bubble sign** suggests gastric outlet obstruction (ie, pyloric atresia). **Double bubble sign** suggests duodenal atresia. **Triple bubble sign** suggests proximal jejunal atresia.

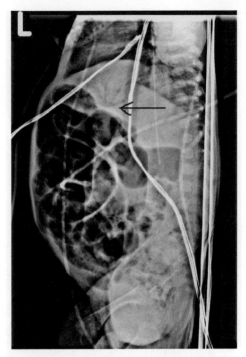

FIGURE 12–27. Cross-table lateral radiograph of abdomen showing portal venous gas at arrow.

11. **Portal venous air (Figure 12–27).** Air is demonstrated in the portal veins (right upper quadrant on supine AP radiograph), often best seen on lateral view. This finding may indicate bowel necrosis (advanced degree of NEC) or intestinal infarction secondary to mesenteric vessel occlusion or iatrogenically introduced gas into the portal vein, which can occur during UVC or exchange transfusion.

13 Management of the Extremely Low Birthweight Infant During the First Week of Life

This chapter addresses the initial care of premature infants of <1000 g birthweight. Many aspects of the care of extremely low birthweight (ELBW) infants are *controversial*, and each institution must develop its own philosophy and techniques for management. It is of utmost importance to follow the practices of your own institution. This chapter offers guidelines that the authors have found useful for stabilizing and caring for extremely small infants.

I. **Delivery room management**
   A. **Ethics/consult.** The neonatologist and other healthcare team members should make every effort to meet with the family before delivery to discuss treatment options for the ELBW infant. Counseling should include discussions with the parents regarding survival rate and both short- and long-term complications based on institutional statistics and the National Institute of Child Health and Human Development (NICHD) Neonatal Research Network calculator. Communication regarding treatment options for the 22- to 24-week gestation infant is crucial. Neonatal bioethics are discussed in detail in Chapter 23. The consult should also include recommendations to the obstetrician (OB) for antenatal steroids (Chapter 117) and magnesium for neuroprotection.
   B. **Resuscitation**
      1. **Delayed cord clamping.** Ask the OB for 30 to 60 seconds of delayed cord clamping unless there are maternal or neonatal contraindications, or cord milking may be considered (American Academy of Pediatrics and American College of Obstetricians and Gynecologists recommendations).
      2. **Thermoregulation.** Consider increasing the ambient temperature of the room to 25°C to 26°C. A polyethylene wrap or bag used immediately after birth prevents heat loss at delivery. In addition, an underlying thermal mattress placed under warmed blankets and a hat provide extra warmth and help stabilize the infant for transport. The wrap is removed and the infant is dried after being placed in a neutral thermal environment in the neonatal intensive care unit (NICU) with stabilization of the infant's temperature.
      3. **Respiratory support.** Oxygen (O_2) use in resuscitation has been challenged in recent years. It takes 7 to 10 minutes for oxyhemoglobin saturations to rise to 90% after delivery. The Neonatal Resuscitation Program recommends availability of pulse oximetry and blended O_2 for resuscitation, starting at 30% fraction of inspired O_2 (FiO_2), and low saturation protocol. For infants who require intubation, surfactant is recommended; however, for infants breathing spontaneously, it remains **controversial**. If the infant is breathing spontaneously and has a heart rate >100 beats/min, continuous positive airway pressure (CPAP) of 4 to 6 cm H_2O should be initiated to prevent atelectasis. CPAP cannot be delivered with a self-inflating bag.
      4. **Transport.** As soon as possible, the infant should be transported to the NICU. Transport must be in a prewarmed portable incubator equipped with blended O_2 and CPAP availability. Infants transported from referring hospitals should be handled in a similar manner.
II. **Temperature and humidity control.** Because the tiny infant has a relatively large skin surface area and minimal energy reserves, a constant **neutral thermal environment** (environmental temperature that minimizes heat loss without increasing O_2 consumption or incurring metabolic stress) is essential. To maintain minimal evaporative heat loss, it is best if the environmental humidity is 80%. Lower ambient humidity requires higher ambient temperatures to maintain infant skin temperature.
   A. **Incubators and hybrid incubators.** ELBW infants should be admitted into prewarmed **double-walled incubators.** Previously, only **radiant warmers** allowed accessibility to the infant; however, they caused large evaporative heat with water losses and somewhat higher basal metabolic rates. As a result, the development and exclusive use of hybrid humidified incubators have become the standard.
   B. **Humidification.** ELBW infants have increased insensible water loss secondary to large body surface area and a greater proportion of body water to body mass. Transcutaneous water loss is enhanced by their thin epidermis and underdeveloped stratum corneum. Increased environmental humidity can minimize these losses. **Warm humidification within the incubator is recommended.** Double-walled incubators provide the best control for monitoring humidity levels.
      1. **Use a respiratory care humidification unit.** Humidification and warming of administered ventilator gases are important to minimize insensible fluid losses

and hypothermia. Infants receiving mechanical ventilation as well as noninvasive respiratory assistance require humidification. In-line warming of ventilator gas circuits minimizes "rainout" of the humidified air and O_2 and maintains airway temperature as close as possible to 35°C. The fluids used for humidification in these systems should be changed every 24 hours.

2. **Minimize nosocomial infection in humidified environments.** Do not allow nonmedical items inside the incubator and change linens regularly if the infant's condition is stable. Change bed every 7 to 10 days per manufacturer's recommendation.

C. **Monitoring and maintenance of body temperature.** Infants weighing <1000 g have poor mechanisms for regulation of temperature and depend on environmental support.

1. **Maintain axillary skin temperature of 36.0°C to 36.5°C.** If skin temperature is outside the range, you may need to change from servo-control to manual control for warming the smallest infants. Use extreme caution while in the manual temperature mode because of the danger of hyperthermia. Rectal thermometers are not to be used for tiny infants; electronic thermometers have become standard.

2. **Record skin temperature.** Using a servo-control skin probe, record skin temperature and environmental temperature every hour until the skin temperature is stable (36.0–36.5°C) and thereafter with recordings at 2-hour intervals.

3. **Record the incubator humidity.** Record every hour until it is stable and then every 2 hours for maintenance.

4. **Weigh low birthweight infants for management of fluids and electrolytes after the third day of life.** The incubator should be equipped with an in-bed scale for continuous weighing of the infant to minimize handling and loss of the thermal-controlled environment.

5. **Other heat-conserving practices.** These include the use of knit hats, fetal positioning, and air boost curtains on incubators.

6. **Accessory items for infant care must be prewarmed.** These items include intravenous (IV) fluids, stethoscope, saline lavages, and any other items that come in direct contact with the infant. Placement of these items in the infant's incubator 30 minutes before use warms them to avoid heat loss by conduction from the infant.

D. **Slow warming or cooling of infants.** Infants who become hypothermic must be gradually rewarmed.

1. **Warming.** If the infant's temperature is <36.0°C, set the warmer temperature 0.4°C higher than the infant's temperature. Continue this procedure until the desired temperature is achieved. Frequent observations of environmental and skin temperatures are essential to evaluate warming efforts. **Do not rewarm faster than 1°C/h.** When skin temperature of 36.5°C is achieved, rewarming efforts should be gradually discontinued, and temperature maintenance by servo-control should be monitored. Rapid rewarming of ELBW infants must be avoided because core body temperatures >37.5°C cause increased insensible water losses, increased O_2 consumption, apneic episodes, increased incidence of intraventricular hemorrhage (IVH), deviations in vital signs, and a detrimental effect on neurodevelopment.

2. **Hyperthermia (skin temperature >37.0°C).** In case of hyperthermia, set the warmer temperature control to 0.4°C lower than the infant's skin temperature. Continue to reduce the warmer temperature until desired temperature is achieved. If increased temperature persists, consider evaluation for pathologic conditions such as sepsis, IVH, or mechanical overheating by exterior lamps. Do not turn off the warmer, as this may cause a sudden decrease in the infant's temperature.

III. **Fluids and electrolytes.** Because of increased insensible water loss and immature renal function, these infants have greater fluid requirements, necessitating IV fluid therapy (see Chapter 10).

 A. **Intravenous fluid therapy**

  1. **Insensible water loss.** Insensible water loss increases with the use of radiant warmers and low ambient humidity. Under these circumstances in which increased insensible fluid loss can occur, additional fluid supplementation is required. However, excessive fluid intake may contribute to the development of a hemodynamically significant patent ductus arteriosus (PDA).

  2. **First day of life.** Table 13–1 gives suggested guidelines for total fluids per kilogram of body weight for the first day of life for infants in humidified incubators/omnibeds and on radiant warmers.

  3. **Second and subsequent days of life.** Fluid management on the second and subsequent days depends on changes in renal function (blood urea nitrogen, creatinine, urine output), serum electrolyte concentrations (see Chapter 10), and body weight (measured after third day of life).

  4. **Additional fluid may be required if phototherapy is used.** The fluid volume should be increased by 10 to 20 mL/kg/d.

   a. **Incubators/omnibeds.** Fluid rates are based on 80% or higher humidity; fluids should be increased incrementally with decreasing environmental humidity.

 B. **Infusion of fluids.** Confirm appropriate line placement and document before infusion (see specific procedure chapter).

  1. **Umbilical artery catheter.** Use only for laboratory and hemodynamic monitoring if other IV access is available. Infuse 0.5 normal saline (NS) + 0.5 U heparin/mL or 0.5 sodium acetate + 0.5 U heparin/mL (sodium acetate aids in acid-base balance).

  2. **Umbilical venous catheter.** Fluids containing glucose and amino acids add 0.5 U heparin/mL to maintenance fluids. Consider use of double-lumen catheters for additional fluid and drug administration.

  3. **Broviac, Hickman, or percutaneous central venous catheters.** Add 0.5 U heparin/mL to maintenance fluids. Avoid placement in first 3 days of life, if possible, to minimize stress.

  4. **Radial arterial line/posterior tibial arterial line.** Add 2 U heparin/mL to 0.5 NS.

 C. **For catheter flushes, use the same fluids as those infused as IV fluids.** Avoid NS as a flush solution because of excessive sodium. In addition, avoid hypotonic solutions (<0.45 NS or <5% dextrose) as these solutions may cause red blood cell hemolysis.

Table 13–1. ADMINISTRATION RATES FOR THE FIRST DAY OF LIFE FOR INFANTS IN HUMIDIFIED INCUBATORS/OMNIBEDS AND RADIANT WARMERS

Birthweight (g)	Gestational Age (wks)	Fluid Rate (mL/kg/d)	
		Incubators[a]	Radiant Warmers[b]
500–600	23	60–80	140–200
601–800	24	60–80	120–150
801–1000	25–27	50–70	100–120

[a]Fluid rates based on 80% or higher humidity; fluids should be increased incrementally with decreasing environmental humidity.
[b]Fluid rates may be decreased with the addition of a humidity tent.

D. Monitoring of fluid therapy. The infant's fluid status should be evaluated at least twice daily during the first few days of life and the fluid intake adjusted accordingly. Fluid status is monitored via measurement of body weight, urine output, blood pressure measurements, serum sodium, hematocrit, and physical examination.

1. **Body weight.** This is the most important method of monitoring fluid therapy. If an in-bed scale is used, weigh the infant daily after the first 3 days of life (to minimize stress). If unavailable, weighing may be delayed to every 48 hours, depending on the stability of the tiny infant, to prevent excessive handling and cold stress. A weight loss of up to 15% of birthweight may be experienced by the end of the first week of life. If weight loss is excessive, environmental controls for insensible fluid losses and fluid management must be carefully reviewed.

2. **Urine output.** This is the second most important method of monitoring fluid therapy. For greatest accuracy, diapers should be weighed before use and immediately after urination.

   a. **First 12 hours.** Any amount of urine output is acceptable.

   b. **12–24 hours.** The minimum acceptable urine output is 0.5 mL/kg/h.

   c. **Day 2 and beyond.** Normal urine output for the second day is 1 to 2 mL/kg/h. After the second day of life and during a diuretic phase, urine output may increase to 3.0 to 5.0 mL/kg/h; values outside this range warrant reevaluation of fluid management.

3. **Hemodynamic monitoring.** This is a valuable tool in assessing fluid status in the infant.

   a. **Heart rate.** The accelerated heart rate of the tiny infant averages 140 to 160 beats/min and is generally considered within normal limits. Tachycardia, with a heart rate >160 beats/min, may be a sign of hypovolemia, pain, inadequate ventilation, anemia, sepsis, or hyperthermia. Low heart rate (<100 beats/min) may be related to hypoxia or medication.

   b. **Arterial blood pressure.** This is most accurately measured via an indwelling arterial catheter and transducer. Cuff pressures are difficult to obtain because of the infant's small size and lower systemic pressures. A recognized standard is to maintain the infant's mean arterial pressure at or equal to the gestational age during the first 48 hours. Thereafter, mean blood pressure increases with chronological age. It is important to evaluate the infant's perfusion, urine output, and acid-base balance in conjunction with blood pressure monitoring.

4. **Electrolyte values.** Serum electrolyte levels should be monitored at least twice daily or every 8 hours for the most immature infants. Sodium and potassium are added as diuresis begins.

   a. **Sodium.** Initially, tiny infants have a sufficient sodium level (132–138 mEq/L), and if there are no ongoing fluid losses, they will not require additional sodium. Serum sodium level may begin to decrease in the postdiuretic phase (usually third to fifth days of life). Subsequently, sodium chloride should be added to the IV fluids (3–8 mEq/kg/d of sodium). **Hyponatremia in the prediuretic phase usually indicates fluid overload, and hypernatremia during the same period usually indicates dehydration, often due to excessive insensible water loss.** For subsequent monitoring of the serum sodium levels:

      i. **Hypernatremia: Na^+ >150 mEq/L.** Differential diagnosis is (a) premature addition of sodium in the pre-diuretic phase, or (b) dehydration, or (c) excessive Na^+ intake.

      ii. **Hyponatremia: Na^+ <130 mEq/L.** Differential diagnosis is (a) fluid overload, or (b) inadequate Na^+ intake, or (c) excessive Na^+ loss.

   b. **Potassium**

      i. **During the first 48 hours after birth.** During this time, tiny infants are prone to increased serum potassium levels of ≥5 mEq/L (range,

4.0–8.0 mEq/L). Most clinicians recommend that no potassium be given during the prediuretic phase. The increase is mostly a result of the following:
- (a) Relative hypoaldosteronism
- (b) Shift of intracellular potassium to the extracellular space due to an immature Na^+/K^+-ATPase pump
- (c) Immature renal tubular function
- (d) Lack of arginine, a precursor to insulin

ii. **K^+ >6 mEq/L mandates close electrocardiogram (ECG) monitoring of T-wave changes and rhythm disturbances along with electrolyte trends, acid-base status, and urine output.** Acidosis should be aggressively treated because this tends to cause intracellular potassium to leak out. Use of Kayexalate enemas is *controversial* in this age group and best avoided if possible. Albuterol metered-dose inhaler (4 puffs every 2 hours; 1 puff = 90 μg) can reduce high levels. Serum K^+ >7 mEq/L can also be treated with insulin, sodium bicarbonate, and calcium gluconate (see Chapter 65).

iii. **3–6 days after birth.** Usually by this time, the initially elevated K^+ level begins to decrease. When K^+ levels approach 4 mEq/L, add supplemental K^+ to IV fluids. Begin with 1 to 2 mEq/kg/d. Measure serum K^+ every 6 to 12 hours until the level is stabilized.

IV. **Blood glucose.** ELBW infants should be supported with 4 to 6 mg/kg/min glucose infusion; start with a 5% to 10% dextrose solution, depending on glucose needs. Amino acid used immediately after birth along with glucose solutions achieves better glucose homeostasis. Bedside glucose levels should be monitored frequently until a blood glucose level of 50 to 90 mg/dL has been established. Abnormal values should be confirmed with serum glucose.

A. **Hypoglycemia is <40 mg/dL for first 48 hours; thereafter <50 mg/dL.** It may occur because of an inadequate glucose infusion rate or a physiologic lack of glycogen stores. In addition, pathologic states such as sepsis, cold stress, or hyperinsulinemia need to be considered.

B. **Hyperglycemia >150 mg/dL.** This can cause osmotic glycosuria, resulting in excessive fluid loss. Hyperglycemia may be secondary to increased glucose infusion rate or pathologic causes such as sepsis, necrotizing enterocolitis (NEC), IVH, or a stress response. Determine the underlying etiology and recalculate glucose administration. Treatment with insulin infusion is *controversial*. An alternative is to decrease the glucose infusion rate (GIR); maintaining glucose infusion as low as 3 mg/kg/min has been demonstrated to provide adequate glucose for cerebral metabolism while not affecting proteolysis and protein turnover.

V. **Calcium.** Serum calcium should be monitored daily. Hypocalcemia in preterm infants is a serum calcium <6 mg/dL. Some institutions also evaluate ionized calcium. In our institution, we provide daily maintenance calcium along with total parenteral nutrition soon after birth (eg, 2 mg of calcium gluconate/mL IV solution). Asymptomatic hypocalcemia is not treated with additional calcium because it resolves with time. Symptomatic hypocalcemia is treated with calcium salts (for dosage, see Chapter 155). This decrease usually happens on the second day of life.

VI. **Nutrition for the metabolically stable infant**

A. **Parenteral nutrition** can be started on admission and continued until the infant is receiving sufficient enteral feeding to promote growth. Along with an adequate GIR of 4 to 6 mg/kg/min, amino acids are started at 2.5 g/kg/d and increased by 0.5 g/kg/d to a maximum of 3.5 to 4 g/kg/d.

B. **Intravenous lipids (20%)** should be started by 24 hours of age; start with 1 to 2 g/kg/d and increase to 3 g/kg/d in 24 hours if triglyceride level is <200 mg/dL. Septic and thrombocytopenic infants require caution before advancing lipids. A generally acceptable safe triglyceride level is <200 mg/dL.

    C. Early feeds of small amounts of breast milk (10–20 mL/kg/d) can promote gut development, characterized by increased gut growth, villous hypertrophy, digestive enzyme secretion, and enhanced motility. This approach is called **trophic feedings.** The decision to either advance or maintain trophic feedings at a constant level should take into account the clinical status of the infant. Initial swabs of colostrum 0.1 mL to each cheek every 6 hours for the first 3 days, as available, should be considered. Trophic feeds should be started with maternal or donor breast milk. The incidence of infection, NEC, and retinopathy of prematurity is decreased when breast milk is used. Mothers should be provided information regarding the benefits of breast milk and should be encouraged to pump their breasts regularly. Once feedings are established, the breast milk can be fortified with supplements. If breast milk is not available, donor breast milk should be used. Use of probiotics is a consideration but *controversial.*

    D. *Controversy* exists with regard to feeding infants while undergoing pharmacologic treatment for PDA closure and during blood transfusions.

VII. Respiratory support. ELBW infants have underdeveloped muscles of ventilation. Many of these infants initially require support by mechanical ventilation; however, others, if vigorous, may be supported with CPAP or noninvasive positive pressure ventilation (NIPPV).

    A. Endotracheal intubation

        1. Type of endotracheal tube (ETT). When possible, use an ETT with 1-cm markings on the side. The internal diameter (ID) of the tube should routinely be 2.5 or 3.0 mm, according to body weight:

            a. <500 to 1000 g. 2.5 mm ID.

            b. 1000 to 1250 g. 3.0-mm ID.

        2. ETT placement. Described in detail in Chapter 33. Confirm proper placement by a chest radiograph study, performed with the infant's head in the midline position, noting the marking at the gum. *Note:* In ELBW infants, the carina tends to be slightly higher than T4. As a means of subsequently checking proper tube position, on every shift, the nurse responsible for the infant should check and record the numbers or letters at the gum line.

    B. Mechanical ventilation. With the advancement of ventilation technology, various modes are available, including volume ventilation, pressure support, and high-frequency ventilation. Ventilation applied appropriately assists the clinician in avoiding overexpansion of the lung or atelectasis.

        1. Conventional ventilation. Tiny infants respond to a wide range of ventilator settings. Some do relatively well on 20 to 30 cycles/min; others require 50 to 60 cycles/min with inspiratory times ranging from 0.25 to 0.35 seconds. The goal is to use minimal pressure and tidal volume for optimal expansion of the lung, avoiding volutrauma and atelectasis. Seek to maintain mechanical breath tidal volumes of 4 to 6 mL/kg; this often may be achieved with as little as 8 to 12 cm of inspiratory pressure and 3 to 5 cm of positive end-expiratory pressure. Pressures can be kept to a minimum by allowing permissive hypercapnia (pH 7.25–7.32, PCO_2 45–60 mm Hg). The following conventional ventilator support guidelines are offered for the initiation of respiratory care. Each tiny infant requires frequent reassessment and revision of settings and parameters. Recommended initial settings for pressure-limited time-cycled ventilators in tiny infants are as follows (see also Chapter 9):

            a. Rate. 20 to 60 (usually 30) breaths/min.

            b. Inspiratory time. 0.25 to 0.35 seconds.

            c. Peak inspiratory pressure (PIP). Select PIP allowing optimal expansion of lungs.

            d. FiO_2. As required to maintain O_2 saturation of 88% to 92%.

            e. Flow rate. 6 to 8 L/min.

    f. Synchronized intermittent mandatory ventilation and volume/pressure control ventilators. These have internal controls that adjust flow delivery. Current ventilators have incorporated enhancements for pressure support, resulting in increased triggering sensitivity, shortened response times, reduced flow acceleration, and improved breath termination parameters.

  2. High-frequency ventilation. Uses small (less than dead space) tidal volumes and extremely rapid rates. The advantage of delivering small tidal volumes is that it can be done at relatively low pressures, reducing the risk of barotrauma. A slight disadvantage is that infant positioning is restricted.

  3. Nasal CPAP (nCPAP). Some ELBW infants may not require mechanical ventilation, whereas others may require ventilation for a short period of time for surfactant replacement. nCPAP has become a mainstay of respiratory management in these infants, initiating soon after birth. Infants requiring intubation and mechanical ventilation should be transitioned to nCPAP as clinical condition allows. nCPAP helps maintain lung expansion and improves oxygenation without significant barotrauma. Care should be taken to use nasal prongs appropriately to prevent nasal injuries and septal breakdown. A gel form of normal saline can help keep nasal passages moist and prevent such injuries.

  4. High-flow nasal cannula. Nasal flows >1 L using blended gases are used as an alternative to nCPAP in the management of respiratory distress and apnea of prematurity. There are insufficient data to establish its safety and efficacy; thus, caution should be used for this population, and it should be reserved for stable infants. Use has become more *controversial*.

C. Monitoring respiratory status

  1. Oxygenation

    a. Blood gas sampling. Arterial catheterization (see Chapter 27 for percutaneous arterial catheterization or Chapter 28 for umbilical arterial catheterization) should be performed for frequent blood gas sampling. As the infant becomes clinically stable, frequency of laboratory testing should be decreased to minimize blood loss and the need for blood transfusions.

      i. Desirable arterial blood gas values in the extremely low birthweight infant:

        (a) PaO_2. 45 to 60 mm Hg.

        (b) $PaCO_2$. 45 to 60 mm Hg.

        (c) pH. 7.25 to 7.32 is acceptable.

      ii. Abnormal blood gas values. Indicate the need for assessment including ETT placement, chest wall movement, effectiveness of ventilation, ventilator malfunction, assessment for pneumothorax, and need for suction. Actions may include immediate chest radiographs, chest wall transillumination (see Chapters 12 and 44), and repeat blood gas determinations.

    b. Continuous O_2 monitoring. Should also be performed, preferably by pulse oximetry. To prevent skin breakdown, pulse oximetry sites should be changed every 8 hours and a protective barrier placed under the probe site. The O_2 mixture should be adjusted to maintain the pulse oximeter reading between 88% and 92% hemoglobin O_2 saturation. Excess oxygenation must be avoided in this group of infants. Failure to closely regulate the administration of O_2 can contribute to the development of retinopathy of prematurity and bronchopulmonary dysplasia.

  2. Chest radiograph

    a. Indications

      i. Abnormal change in blood gas values

      ii. Adjustment of the ETT (to confirm proper positioning)

      iii. Sudden change in the infant's status

      iv. Significant increase in O_2 requirement or frequent desaturations

    b. Technique. A chest radiograph should be taken with the infant's head in the midline position to check for ETT placement.

    c. Radiograph evaluation. Check the chest radiograph for expansion of the lung, chest wall, and diaphragm. Overexpansion (exhibited by hyperlucent lungs and diaphragm below the ninth rib) and underventilation (exhibited by hazy, white lung field—atelectasis) must be avoided. If overexpansion is present, differentiate between volutrauma and air trapping based on the age of the infant and underlying disease process. Consider decreasing the peak airway pressure if volutrauma is suspected. Underexpansion can be treated with the use of CPAP or increasing pressures (peak airway pressure or positive end-expiratory pressure) via the ventilator.

D. Suctioning. Should be done on an as-needed basis. The need for suctioning can be determined with the use of flow-volume loop monitoring, which can illustrate restricted airflow caused by secretions.

    1. Assessment of the need for suctioning. The nurse or physician should consider the following:

        a. Breath sounds. Wet or diminished breath sounds may indicate secretions obstructing the airways and the need for suctioning.

        b. Blood gas values. If significant increase in $PaCO_2$, consider ETT malposition, secretions blocking the airway passages, inadequate ventilation, prior bicarbonate/acetate administration, or pain. Suctioning should be considered to clear the airways and avoid the "ball-valve" effect of thick secretions.

        c. Airway monitoring. By using airflow sensors and continuous computer graphic screen displays, abnormal waveforms indicative of accumulating secretions or airway blockage can be easily seen, and immediate steps can be taken to clear the airway.

        d. Visible secretions in the ETT

        e. Loss of chest wall movement

    2. Suctioning technique

        a. In-line suctioning is recommended to minimize airway contamination. Suctioning should be done only to the depth of the ETT. Use a suctioning guide or a marked (1-cm increments) suction catheter.

        b. Suctioning without lavage solution is recommended. An exception is the use of warm sterile normal saline lavage for thick secretions.

        c. Suction should be regulated. 80 to 100 mm Hg for in-line suction (closed system) and 60 to 80 mm Hg for open system.

E. Extubation

    1. Prior to extubation. Consider use of caffeine citrate loading as it improves respiratory drive and reduces length of time on mechanical ventilation. Recent reports also indicate caffeine to have neuroprotective effects when started at birth.

    2. Indications. When an ELBW infant has been weaned to a mean airway pressure of 6 cm H_2O and a low (30%) FiO_2, extubation should be considered. Most infants >26 weeks and 700 g birthweight can be extubated in the first 72 hours. These are the other parameters to be met for extubation:

        a. Ventilator rate ≤20 breaths/min

        b. Regular spontaneous respiratory rate

    3. Postextubation care. Frequent observation of breathing patterns, respiratory effort, auscultation of the chest, monitoring of vital signs, and blood gas analysis are necessary. After extubation, the infant is placed on CPAP or NIPPV.

F. Vitamin A as a mode of therapy for decreasing chronic lung disease in ELBW infants is well established in clinical trials. Dosing should begin the first week of life (5000 IU intramuscularly [IM] 3 times per week for 4 weeks). Some institutions are reluctant to use this therapy because of the frequency of IM injections. Vitamin A delivery via IV fluids is not effective because it binds to the tubing.

VIII. Surfactant. Some literature supports early administration of surfactant during the first 4 hours of life to decrease chronic lung disease. Recent research supports early CPAP in the delivery room over prophylactic surfactant. Several preparations of surfactant are available; some have the advantage of smaller volume and dosing intervals. It should be administered according to the manufacturer's recommendations. Administration criteria for surfactant include absence of antenatal steroids, increased oxygen demand >30%, and a radiograph consistent with surfactant deficiency (see Figure 12–16).

IX. PDA. Incidence of persistent PDA is inversely proportional to gestational age. Infants should be monitored clinically for signs and symptoms of PDA. An echocardiogram is recommended to rule out other structural heart defects and for confirmation of PDA when concerned. Efforts should be made to minimize the risk of PDA. **Overhydration must be avoided.** Up to 30% of PDAs spontaneously close. Currently it is unclear whether a conservative, pharmacologic, or surgical approach is advantageous. If the decision is made to treat a hemodynamically significant PDA, indomethacin or ibuprofen is generally accepted (see Chapter 114). Acetaminophen may also be considered. Renal and gastrointestinal adverse effects are less common with administration of ibuprofen or with slower infusion rates of indomethacin. Indomethacin can also be considered for IVH prophylaxis, especially in high-risk populations, although its safety and benefit remain *controversial*. Concurrent administration of indomethacin and steroids should be avoided because of the associated risk for spontaneous intestinal perforation.

X. Transfusion. ELBW infants usually have low red blood cell volume, with a hematocrit <40%, and they are subjected to frequent phlebotomies. Most centers keep the hematocrit between 35% and 40%. Lower values may be acceptable if the infant is asymptomatic. Each institution should have transfusion guidelines established to minimize donor exposure and the number of transfusions.

XI. Skin care. Maintenance of intact skin is the tiny infant's most effective barrier against infection, insensible fluid loss, protein loss, and blood loss and provides for more effective body temperature control. Minimal use of tape is recommended because the infant's skin is fragile, and tears often result with removal. **Zinc-based tape** can be used. Alternatives to tape include the use of a **hydrogel adhesive**, which removes easily with water. Hydrogel adhesive products also include electrodes, temperature probe covers, and masks. In addition, the very thin skin of the tiny infant allows absorption of many substances. Skin care must focus on maintaining skin integrity and minimizing exposure to topical agents. Transparent adhesive dressings can be used over areas of bone prominence, such as the knees or elbows, to prevent skin friction breakdown and breakdown under adhesive monitoring devices that are frequently moved. Use of humidity helps maintain skin integrity until skin is mature (2–3 weeks). Humidity can be weaned as tolerated after 2 weeks. *Note:* **When the skin appears dry, thickened, and no longer shiny or translucent (usually in 10–14 days), these skin care recommendations and procedures may be modified or discontinued.**

   A. **Use a hydrogel skin probe, or cut servo-control skin probe covers to the smallest size possible (try a 2-cm diameter circle).** This will help to reduce skin damage resulting from the adhesive.

   B. **Monitoring of O_2 therapy is best accomplished by use of a pulse oximeter.** The probe must be placed carefully to prevent pressure sores. The site should be rotated a minimum of every 8 hours. Alternative means of O_2 monitoring include umbilical catheter blood sampling.

   C. **Urine bags and blood pressure cuffs.** These **should not be used routinely** because of adhesives and sharp plastic edge cuts. Bladder aspirations should be avoided.

   D. **Eye ointment for gonococcal prophylaxis.** Should be applied per routine admission plan. If the eyelids are fused, apply along the lash line.

E. **Cleansing for required procedures (eg, umbilical artery or chest tube).** Use minimal povidone-iodine solution to cleanse the area. After the procedure is completed, the solution should be sponged off immediately with warm sterile water. The use of chlorhexidine in the ELBW infant is *controversial* and should be used per institution guidelines.

F. **Attach ECG electrodes using as little adhesive as possible.** Options include the following:
   1. **Consider using limb electrodes.**
   2. **Consider water-activated gel electrodes.**
   3. **Use electrodes that have been trimmed down and secured with a flexible dressing material.**

G. **An initial bath is not necessary,** but if HIV is a consideration, those infants should receive a mild soap bath when the infant's temperature has stabilized. Warm sterile water baths are given only when needed during the next 2 weeks of life.

H. **Avoid the use of anything that dries out the skin (eg, soaps and alcohol).** Bonding agents should be avoided.

I. **Sterile water-soaked cotton balls.** Helpful for removing adhesive tape, probe covers, and electrode covers.

J. **Environmental.** Use of mattress covers or blankets in humidified environments helps prevent skin breakdown.

K. **Treatment of skin breakdown**
   1. **Clean skin breakdown/excoriated area with warm sterile water, leaving open to air.**
   2. **Apply topical antibiotic over broken-down infected areas, leaving open to air.**
   3. **Apply transparent dressings over excoriated areas.**
   4. **Administer IV antibiotics if necessary.**

XII. **Other special considerations for the ELBW infant**
A. **Infection**
   1. **Cultures.** If the infant is delivered from an infected environment, blood and cerebrospinal fluid should be cultured. Spinal fluid may be deferred if unstable. Surveillance skin cultures may be necessary on admission if methicillin-resistant *Staphylococcus aureus* strains are a threat.
   2. **Antibiotics.** If the infant has a septic risk after obtaining cultures, consider starting empiric **ampicillin** and **gentamicin**. Drug levels must be monitored if using aminoglycosides and the dose adjusted accordingly (see Chapter 155).
   3. **Nosocomial infection.** The ELBW infant is at higher risk for nosocomial infection because of immature immune system, poor skin integrity, and extended hospitalization. Hand hygiene is extremely important in the prevention and containment of infection. All caregivers/visitors should be instructed in appropriate hand hygiene. Consider removal of all jewelry, use of short sleeves, no use of lab coats, and no cell phone use in the NICU. Nosocomial infections should be contained by a cohort of infants and the use of dedicated equipment and staff.
   4. **Chemoprophylaxis with fluconazole.** ELBW infants in NICUs with moderate (5%–10%) or high (>10%) rates of invasive candidiasis should receive prophylaxis with **fluconazole**. Dosage: Start 48 to 72 hours after birth and give 3 mg/kg IV twice a week for 4 to 6 weeks or until IV access is no longer necessary.

B. **Central nervous system hemorrhage.** Cranial ultrasonography may be indicated during the first 7 days for possible intracranial hemorrhage.

C. **Hyperbilirubinemia**
   1. **Risk.** Efforts should be made to keep the serum bilirubin <10 mg/dL. Serum bilirubin may need to be monitored twice daily. An exchange transfusion should be considered when the bilirubin approaches or exceeds 12 mg/dL (see Chapter 34).

    2. **Phototherapy.** To reduce the serum bilirubin level, phototherapy may be needed and can be used to minimize the need for exchange transfusion. Some centers start phototherapy immediately after birth; others when approaching 5 mg/dL. If the infant is treated with phototherapy, reassess fluid needs.

D. Pain. Even the smallest of infants have shown response to painful stimuli. Several multidimensional pain assessment tools are available that include both physiologic (heart rate, O_2 saturation, respiratory rate, and blood pressure) and behavioral indicators (facial expression, vocalization, and motor activity). ELBW pain assessment is very difficult, and none of these tools have been standardized. Our unit uses a pain assessment tool that allows for gestational age adjustment. Pain should be assessed as the fifth vital sign and more often as indicated by pain scores (see Chapter 15).

E. Social problems. Many families have great difficulty in coping with the issues related to their infant's extreme prematurity. Parents should be invited to participate in the infant's care from the beginning. Parent–infant bonding should be promoted, and parents should be encouraged to assist in caring for their child. A social service consultation should be mandatory. Participation in a parent-to-parent support group appears to improve maternal–infant relationships. Experienced nurses and the use of a **primary nurse** together with ongoing communication from the medical team can decrease the parents' stress and keep them up to date on their infant's medical problems. Parent conferences involving the physician, social worker, and primary nurse help the family understand the complex extended care of their infant. Additional discussions may include quality of life, death, dying, withholding and withdrawal of support, and parental religious or spiritual beliefs.

F. Developmental issues

    1. **Minimal stimulation.** These infants do not tolerate handling and medically necessary procedures well. Other stressors include noise, light, and activity such as moving the incubator. Routine tasks should be clustered to allow the infant undisturbed and prolonged periods of rest; each task should have a time limit as well. Consider minimizing hands-on care to every 6 hours, avoiding heel sticks, and limiting ultrasounds/x-rays for the first 3 days of life.

    2. **Positioning.** The fetus is maintained in a flexed position with head midline. Care should be taken to simulate this positioning in the extremely premature infant. For the initial 3 to 7 days, consider keeping the head elevated and midline and body supine, and avoid lifting legs above the head to minimize IVH. A flexed side-lying or prone posture with supportive boundaries is preferred. A change in position is recommended every 4 hours or at the infant's cue after the third day of life. Many positioning aids are available and should be used per institution guidelines.

    3. **Kangaroo care.** This has been defined as "intrahospital maternal–infant skin-to-skin contact" (see Chapters 15 and 22). It promotes behavioral state organization, increased parental attachment/confidence, and nurturing behaviors that support growth and development. Temperature, heart rate, respiratory rate, and O_2 saturation remain within normal limits during kangaroo care. It can be a safe practice for infants with ETTs and central catheters in place if experienced NICU nurses participate closely with cooperative and well-informed parents.

    4. **Environmental issues.** Infants are unable to control their own environment, so efforts must be made to decrease ambient noise to <50 dB and provide cyclic lighting to support their circadian rhythms.

    5. **Parental education.** Family-centered care should be encouraged on admission. Parents should be educated about behavioral cues that invite interaction or signal overstimulation. Parents should be instructed on containment techniques and calming interactions.

14 Management of the Late Preterm Infant

I. **Introduction.** The most commonly agreed upon definition of a late preterm infant is an infant born between 34 0/7 and 36 6/7 weeks' gestation. Older literature refers to these infants as *near term*, suggesting that they are equivalent to term infants. Approximately 10 years ago, the term *late preterm* was introduced into the medical literature to convey an appropriate sense of these infants' vulnerability and increased risk for both short- and long-term complications. Since 2007, >500 articles about late preterm infants have been published, underscoring the increased risk of morbidity and mortality compared to term infants.

   Late preterm births represent approximately 74% of all preterm births. Between 1992 and 2007, the incidence of late preterm births increased from 7.3% to 10.4% of all births. More recently, the rate of late preterm births has decreased to 9.6% in 2014, representing an 8% drop from 2007. This is likely related to an improved understanding of the increased risk of poor neonatal outcomes in this population.

II. **Potential etiologies.** Improvements in obstetrical surveillance over time may contribute to an increased incidence of medically indicated premature deliveries. Recent recommendations from the American College of Obstetricians and Gynecologists that discourage induction or scheduled repeat cesarean deliveries before 39 weeks, as well as specific guidelines for criteria for elective preterm delivery, likely contributed to the decreased rate of late preterm births seen over the past several years. However, not all late preterm deliveries are preventable, and potential etiologies include the following:

   A. **Preeclampsia**
   B. **Spontaneous preterm labor and preterm premature rupture of membranes**
   C. **Multifetal gestations**
   D. **Antepartum bleeding**
   E. **Fetal growth restriction**

III. **Complications of late preterm birth**

   A. **Mortality.** A systematic review investigating the outcomes of >2 million late preterm infants found that these infants were 5.9 times more likely to die within the first 28 days of life as compared to term infants. While the absolute number of deaths of late preterm infants is low, the relative risk is high.

   B. **Respiratory morbidity.** A large systematic review showed that late preterm infants are 17.3 times more likely to develop respiratory distress syndrome than term neonates. This is secondary to immature lung architecture, surfactant deficiency, and deprivation of normal hormonal changes occurring at term that promote the clearance of lung fluid. The risk of respiratory distress increases with decreasing gestational age (relative risk [RR] of 10.9 in 36-week infants, 28.6 in 35-week infants, and 48.4 in 34-week infants). Late preterm infants are also 4.9 times more likely to require intubation and mechanical ventilation, 9.8 times more likely to need CPAP, and 24.4 times more likely to require nasal oxygen compared to term infants. In one review, 11% of late preterm infants with respiratory failure developed chronic lung disease and 5% died, emphasizing the serious long-term consequences of respiratory complications in this population.

   C. **Length of stay.** Studies show that late preterm infants have a similar median length of initial hospital stay as term infants but with wider variability. The most common causes of delayed discharge are jaundice and poor feeding. Late preterm delivery triples the cost of the infant's initial hospital stay.

   D. **Jaundice.** Late preterm infants are at increased risk of hyperbilirubinemia secondary to hepatic immaturity as well as difficulty establishing feeding. A large systematic review showed that late preterm infants are 5 times more likely to have prolonged jaundice requiring treatment compared to term infants. Late preterm infants also may have an increased risk of bilirubin-induced neurologic dysfunction due to immaturity of the blood–brain barrier and decreased bilirubin binding, as evidenced by the 25% of babies in the Kernicterus Registry who were born late preterm. Hyperbilirubinemia is the most common reason for hospital readmission of late preterm infants.

E. **Poor feeding.** Late preterm infants are 6.5 times more likely to have feeding difficulties as compared to term infants. Many late preterm infants with poor feeding require a prolonged initial hospitalization and may require gavage feeds. Suck-swallow coordination and intestinal motility remain immature, which impacts their feeding ability. Late preterm infants may also lack the feeding skills to latch properly and the stamina to take sufficient volumes of breastmilk, resulting in delayed milk production and increased risk of lactation failure. At times, spoon feeding or formula supplementation may be necessary. Breast-feeding protocols for this population that are evidence based have been developed by the California Perinatal Quality Care Collaborative (https://www.cpqcc.org/content/care-and-management-late-preterm-infant-0) and the Academy of Breastfeeding Medicine (https://www.bfmed.org/protocols). Problems with adequacy of breast feeding may persist until these babies reach term equivalent age. Even babies being formula fed may require a nutrient-enriched approach in order to ensure adequate caloric intake.

F. **Temperature instability.** Hypothermia is 10.8 times more common in late preterm infants compared to term infants due to an immature epidermal barrier, higher surface area–to–body weight ratios, decreased amount of brown adipose tissue, and more frequent delivery room interventions.

G. **Hypoglycemia.** Late preterm infants are 7.4 times more likely to experience hypoglycemia compared to term infants. This is secondary to delay in the activity of hepatic glucose phosphate, which is needed in the final step of gluconeogenesis. Hypoglycemia in late preterm infants is further exacerbated by poor feeding, decreased body weight, and low glycogen stores at birth.

H. **Infectious morbidity.** According to a large systematic review, late preterm infants have an increased risk of culture-proven sepsis (RR, 5.6), pneumonia (RR, 3.5), meningitis (RR, 21), and necrotizing enterocolitis (RR, 7.5) compared to term infants.

I. **Sudden infant death syndrome (SIDS) and apnea.** Immaturity of the autonomic nervous system in late preterm infants increases the risk of apnea and bradycardia of prematurity. Infants born between 33 and 36 weeks are twice as likely to die from SIDS as those born ≥37 weeks.

J. **Readmission.** Late preterm infants are almost twice as likely to require readmission after initial hospital discharge. Several studies have demonstrated that early follow-up visits after hospital discharge or home nursing visits were effective at reducing rates of readmission.

K. **Respiratory syncytial virus (RSV) infection.** Late preterm infants have an increased susceptibility to RSV infection due to incomplete lung development, immature immune function, and the relative lack of passively acquired maternal antibodies. The risk of RSV bronchiolitis in infants born between 32 and 36 weeks is similar to those born before 32 weeks. The risk of hospitalization due to RSV infection is twice as high in late preterm infants compared to term infants. According to current American Academy of Pediatrics (AAP) guidelines, late preterm infants do not qualify for palivizumab prophylaxis unless they have additional risk factors such as hemodynamically significant congenital heart disease. Precautions such as decreased contact with sick individuals and good hand hygiene by those handing these infants may be effective risk reduction strategies.

L. **Long-term outcomes.** Multiple studies have shown that late preterm infants are at increased risk for long-term adverse neurodevelopmental and psychosocial outcomes. A systematic review showed that late preterm infants are 3 times more likely to develop cerebral palsy and 1.5 times more likely to develop mental retardation compared to term infants. Late preterm infants are also more likely to have poor school performance, a learning disability, or attention deficit hyperactivity disorder and have a lower likelihood of completing high school. Late preterm infants have increased healthcare utilization during the first year of life and are more likely to have special healthcare needs or a chronic medical condition as compared to term infants.

IV. **Recommendations for management.** Iatrogenic prematurity should be prevented by prolonging pregnancy whenever medically feasible. Specific guidelines from the American College of Obstetricians and Gynecologists regarding indications for preterm delivery can help prevent unnecessary late preterm births. There is recent evidence to suggest that antenatal betamethasone administered to women at risk for late preterm delivery may decrease short-term respiratory morbidities in this population. Additional evidence is necessary before this intervention can be recommended for all women with threated late preterm delivery due to the unknown long-term risks of fetal exposure to corticosteroids, a large number needed to treat to prevent a negative outcome, and a higher rate of neonatal hypoglycemia in the steroid-treated group.

Because late preterm infants are at risk for neonatal complications, as discussed earlier, specific management strategies should be developed for both their initial management after birth as well as their care after discharge home. Early monitoring of respiratory status, temperature, feeding ability, and bilirubin and glucose levels is critical. The AAP has published guidelines for screening and management of hypoglycemia in the late preterm infant. The AAP has also provided specific recommendations for discharge criteria for late preterm infants. In addition to fulfilling discharge criteria for term infants, the late preterm infant requires:

A. **Accurate gestational age assessment**
B. **Absence of medical condition requiring further hospitalization** (ie, hyperbilirubinemia, respiratory distress).
C. **Demonstration of physiologic stability**
   1. **Maintaining normal cardiorespiratory control** with stable vital signs for at least 12 hours prior to discharge.
   2. **Maintaining thermoregulation** with axillary temperature of 36.5°C to 37.4°C (97.7–99.3°F) in an open crib.
   3. **At least 24 hours of successful feeding** in the absence of excessive weight loss.
   4. **Formalized evaluation of breast feeding** when applicable.
   5. **Passing at least 1 stool spontaneously.**
   6. **Successful completion of a car seat safety study** to observe for apnea, bradycardia, and oxygen desaturation.
D. **Screening for hyperbilirubinemia** with arrangement of appropriate follow-up
E. **Assessment of family and home environment risk factors**
F. **Individualized timing of discharge** based on the infant's condition
G. **Follow-up visit with an identified primary care provider** 24 to 48 hours after discharge

In summary, late preterm infants represent a unique patient population with increased risk for both short- and long-term adverse health outcomes. Close monitoring of health status after birth as well as specialized management strategies in the first several days to weeks of life are needed to ensure optimal outcomes for these vulnerable infants.

V. **Late and moderately preterm (LMPT) infants.** There is emerging literature investigating the differences in long-term outcomes of infants born late and moderately preterm (32 0/7–36 6/7 weeks' gestation) compared to both infants born at term as well as infants born very preterm (<32 weeks' gestation). Risk of adverse neurodevelopmental outcomes is well documented in the very preterm population, but the risk for LMPT infants is just beginning to be understood. One study showed that LMPT infants were 3.6 times more likely to have a positive Modified Checklist for Autism in Toddlers (M-CHAT) autism screen compared to term infants. Another study demonstrated that LMPT infants are more likely than term infants to have oral motor problems and picky eating, particularly in those LMPT infants requiring prolonged nasogastric feedings or with behavioral problems. A recent survey of parents in the United Kingdom whose children were 6, 12, and 24 months old found that parents with LMPT children were more likely to report overall poorer health, increased minor respiratory symptoms and need for prescribed inhalers, increased incidence of mild neurosensory impairment, increased frequency of cognitive difficulties, and increased incidence of socioemotional developmental delay compared to parents of children born at term. The pattern of abnormal development and cognitive impairment seen in children born LMPT appears to be milder and of unclear clinical significance compared to that observed in children born very preterm. These recent studies indicate that close monitoring of the long-term health and neurodevelopmental progress of former LMPT infants is imperative, and continued research may lead to better long-term outcomes in this population.

15 Pain in the Neonate

Before the 1980s, it was a common belief that preterm infants lacked the neurodevelopmental capacity to feel pain. This resulted in severe undertreatment of pain in the neonate during hospitalization. It is now known that infants have the required neuroanatomical connections to feel pain, and actually experience a higher degree of sensitivity to pain as compared to children and adults. Neonates are subject to many painful procedures, especially the most immature infant. Although neonatology has made strides in the past 20 years to understand pain, it remains a challenge to effectively assess and treat the various types of pain experienced in the neonatal intensive care unit (NICU). A recent study revealed that there is a worldwide trend of undertreatment of neonatal pain and that more attention should be given to pain prevention, assessment, and treatment. Countries with nationally accepted guidelines for pain management (such as France, Sweden, and the Netherlands) do a better job in treating neonatal pain than those countries without guidelines. The American Academy of Pediatrics (AAP) recently updated the recommendations for managing procedural pain in neonates. These recommendations include the following:

1. Every institution caring for neonates should implement a pain prevention program that includes written guidelines for a stepwise pain prevention and a treatment plan.
2. Validated neonatal pain assessment tools should be used consistently before, during, and after painful procedures.
3. Nonpharmacologic strategies decrease pain scores during short-term mild to moderately painful procedures and should be used. These include facilitated tucking, breast feeding or providing expressed human milk, nonnutritive sucking, sensorial stimulation, and others.
4. Oral sucrose/glucose solutions are effective with mild to moderately painful procedures, either alone or combined with other pain-relief strategies. If used, these solutions need to be tracked as medications.
5. Healthcare providers need to weigh actual benefits and burdens when using pharmacologic treatment methods. It is important to remember that some of the medications can potentiate the hypotension and respiratory depression that can occur with opioid use. Use caution when using newer medications that do not have data in neonates.
6. All providers should receive continuing education on the recognition, assessment, and management of pain.
7. More research needs to be done in this area.

Some have suggested that pain assessment should be considered the fifth vital sign, so with each vital sign determination, pain assessment should be done and recorded.

I. **Physiology of pain in the neonate**
   A. **Definition.** Pain has been defined by the International Association for the Study of Pain as "an unpleasant sensory and emotional experience associated with actual or potential tissue damage or described in such terms of such damage." An infant's response to pain involves a collection of biochemical, physiologic, and behavioral reactions. There are many different layers of an infant's response that can be understood by gestational age and development. Noxious stimuli lead to tissue damage, causing the release of sensitizing substances such as prostaglandins, bradykinin, serotonin, substance P, and histamine. These chemicals produce an impulse that is then transmitted to the nociceptive pathways. Nociception refers to the reflex movement occurring with exposure to noxious stimuli that does not require cortical involvement or the ability to perceive pain.
   B. **Developmental considerations.** Development of sensory nerve endings begins very early in the process of nociception. Cutaneous sensory receptors and spinal reflexes that respond to noxious stimuli develop as early as 7.5 and 8 weeks, respectively. Conscious perception of pain can be felt as early as 25 weeks' gestation.
   C. **Repeated exposure to noxious stimuli.** This can cause physiologic and behavioral disorganization, leading to changes in the neurodevelopmental system of the infant and may change the pain pathway system. This may cause the infant to develop an inability to respond to pain or an exaggerated physiologic response to painful stimuli in the future.

II. **Types of pain in the neonate**
   A. **Birth trauma.** Neonatal pain associated with birth trauma is typically a result of vacuum-assisted births. Some babies may show signs of bruising on the face or head simply as a result of the trauma of passing through the birth canal. Forceps deliveries can leave temporary marks or bruises on the baby's face and head. Cephalohematomas are more common with forceps delivery or vacuum extraction. Acetaminophen may be used for the treatment of associated pain. Clavicular fractures are the most common birth-related fracture. If the fracture is painful, limiting movement of the arm or shoulder may be helpful.
   B. **Acute procedural pain.** The frequency of painful procedures in the NICU can range from 5 to 15 per day. The most optimal method of pain control is to minimize the amount of painful procedures. Painful procedures performed in the NICU include endotracheal tube (ETT) suctioning, intubation, mechanical ventilation, chest tube insertion, retinopathy of prematurity (ROP) examinations, central line placement, intravenous (IV) placement, heel sticks, lumbar puncture, circumcision, patent ductus arteriosus (PDA) ligation, and peritoneal drain placement. (See each procedure chapter for specific recommendations for pain management.)
   C. **Acute postoperative pain.** Postsurgical pain remains an issue in the NICU. The largest risk with postsurgical pain is undertreating. Postoperative pain protocols help standardize practice between healthcare professionals. Routine pain assessment should be performed using scales specific to postoperative or prolonged pain. It is important to alternate pain medications for maximum pain control with minimal toxicity. Opioids are the medications of choice and can be given by continuous infusion or bolus.
   D. **Chronic pain.** Chronic pain remains to be well defined within neonatology. Some view chronic pain as the extension of uncontrolled acute pain. Pain assessment tools should include validated measurement for chronic pain. Research needs to continue in this critical area of study.

III. **Assessment of pain in the neonate.** One of the most challenging aspects of neonatal pain is recognition of the signs, of which people are becoming more aware. Careful assessment is critical when evaluating preterm infants for signs of pain. Assessment must include physiologic as well as behavioral changes since the infant is unable to report his or her own pain.

A. **Common signs of pain in the neonate.** Commonly assessed signs of pain include increased heart rate, changes in respiratory rate, and fluctuations in blood pressure, as well as changes in facial expression such as brow bulge, eyes squeezed shut, nasolabial furrow, crying, palmar sweating, and increased movement.

B. **Physiologic changes due to pain.** These include increased oxygen consumption, ventilation-perfusion mismatch, increased gastric acidity, and disturbance of sleep-wake cycle. Infants experiencing prolonged pain may exhibit decreased heart rate, decreased respiratory rate, decreased oxygen consumption, lethargy, decreased perfusion, and cool extremities.

C. **Metabolic and hormonal changes related to pain.** Reported studies include increased plasma renin (after venipuncture in term infants); increased plasma epinephrine and norepinephrine (after chest physiotherapy (PT) and ETT suctioning in preterm infants); increased plasma cortisol levels (after circumcision without anesthesia); release of growth hormone, glucagon, cortisol, and aldosterone; and decreased insulin secretion (preterm and term infants undergoing surgery with minimal anesthesia).

D. **Perception of pain.** Compared to adults, the neonatal stress responses are 3 to 5 times greater. Functional magnetic resonance imaging (MRI) and near-infrared spectroscopy studies have shown that babies respond to weaker stimuli than adults. Preterm neonates are more sensitive to pain, showing increased excitability to sensory pathways and delayed maturation of descending inhibitory pathways and the endogenous opioid system.

E. **Pain versus discomfort.** Differentiating between infant pain and discomfort can be challenging for healthcare professionals. Premature infants can exhibit minimal response to pain, especially if they are septic or physiologically stressed. Older infants who have experienced multiple incidents or prolonged pain may over- or underreact to pain. Lack of pain response can also be observed in infants with neurologic impairment or those who have been chemically paralyzed.

F. **Pain assessment scales.** There are many pain scales that exist in neonatology. They can be broadly divided into the type of pain they are assessing (acute, prolonged, or postoperative) and by whether they are used for term or preterm infants. There is not one single pain assessment scale that can be applied to all infants. Early neonatal pain scales were designed for healthy babies. Newer scales have been designed for sick infants in the NICU setting. Gestational age and behavioral state have been added to some assessment tools as they may play a major role in pain assessment. The 4 most commonly used pain scales are the **Premature Infant Pain Profile-Revised (PIPP-R), CRIES Neonatal Pain Assessment Tool, Neonatal Infant Pain Scale (NIPS), and Neonatal Pain, Agitation, and Sedation Scale (N-PASS).** There are only 5 scales out of all the pain scales that have undergone rigorous psychometric testing and these include the **Neonatal Facial Coding System, Premature Infant Pain Profile, Neonatal Pain and Sedation Scale, Behavioral Infant Pain Profile, and Douleur Aiguë du Nouveau-né.** These and the other commonly used pain scales are compared in Table 15–1.

IV. **Short- and long-term effects of pain.** Pain can worsen hypoxia, acidosis, hypercarbia, respiratory distress, and hyperglycemia. Untreated pain in the neonate can cause increased catabolism and hypermetabolism. This can also increase susceptibility to infection and increase morbidity and suboptimal outcomes. Eventually, untreated neonatal pain can lead to altered pain sensitivity (either an inability to respond to pain or an exaggerated physiologic response to pain) with permanent neuroanatomic and behavior outcomes. Long-term effects include emotional and behavioral abnormalities, along with learning disabilities. Studies have shown hyperalgesic responses and reduction in pain thresholds, increased incidence of intraventricular hemorrhage and periventricular leukomalacia, and increased somatization.

V. **Pain intervention.** Pain management for neonates is ideally approached from multiple levels as described from a foundation of simply avoiding painful procedures to a top tier

Table 15–1. COMPARISON OF COMMONLY USED PAIN SCALES

Pain Scale	Facial Expression	Cry	Extremities	Vocal Expression	Oxygen Saturation	Vital Signs	Behavioral State	Term Infants	Preterm Infants	Type of Pain
PIPP-R	X				X	X	X	X	X	Acute
CRIES		X		X	X	X	X	X	X	Prolonged postop
NIPS	X	X	X			X	X	X	X	Acute postop
N-PASS	X	X	X		X	X	X	X	X	Acute prolonged level of sedation Postop, ventilated
NFCS	X								X	Acute prolonged postop
COMFORTneo	X	X	X			X	X	X	X	Persistent prolonged, developed for sedation, level of sedation Postoperative pain
EDIN	X		X				X		X	Prolonged
DAN	X	X	X	X					X	Procedural
BPSN	X	X				X	X	X	X	Acute
BIIP	X		X				X	X	X	Acute
FANS		X	X	X	X	X			X	Acute
COVERS	X	X	X		X	X	X	X	X	Acute
PAIN	X	X	X		X	X	X	X	X	Acute
PAT		X	X	X	X	X	X	X	X	Prolonged
SUN	X		X		X	X	X	X	X	Acute

BIIP, Behavioral Indicators of Infant Pain; BPSN, Bernese Pain Scale for Neonates; COVERS, COVERS Neonatal Pain Scale; CRIES, Crying, requires increased oxygen administration, increased vital signs, expression, sleeplessness; DAN, Douleur Aiguë du Nouveau-né; EDIN, Echelle Douleur Aiguë du Nouveau-né; FANS, Faceless Acute Neonatal Pain Scale; NFCS, Neonatal Facial Coding System; NIPS, Neonatal Infant Pain Scale; N-PASS, Neonatal Pain, Agitation, and Sedation Scale; PAIN, Pain Assessment in Neonates; PAT, Pain Assessment Tool; PIPP-R, Premature Infant Pain Profile–Revised; SUN, Scale for Use in Newborns.

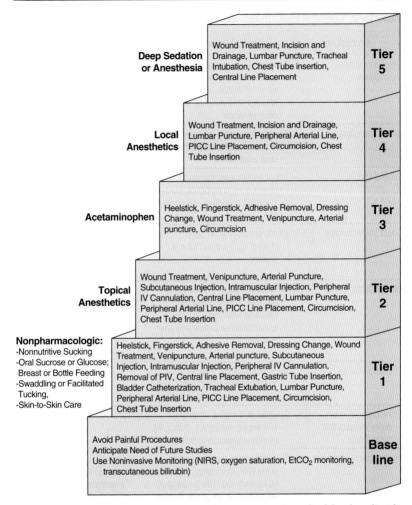

Deep Sedation or Anesthesia	Wound Treatment, Incision and Drainage, Lumbar Puncture, Tracheal Intubation, Chest Tube insertion, Central Line Placement	**Tier 5**
Local Anesthetics	Wound Treatment, Incision and Drainage, Lumbar Puncture, Peripheral Arterial Line, PICC Line Placement, Circumcision, Chest Tube Insertion	**Tier 4**
Acetaminophen	Heelstick, Fingerstick, Adhesive Removal, Dressing Change, Wound Treatment, Venipuncture, Arterial puncture, Circumcision	**Tier 3**
Topical Anesthetics	Wound Treatment, Venipuncture, Arterial Puncture, Subcutaneous Injection, Intramuscular Injection, Peripheral IV Cannulation, Central Line Placement, Lumbar Puncture, Peripheral Arterial Line, PICC Line Placement, Circumcision, Chest Tube Insertion	**Tier 2**
Nonpharmacologic: -Nonnutritive Sucking -Oral Sucrose or Glucose; Breast or Bottle Feeding -Swaddling or Facilitated Tucking, -Skin-to-Skin Care	Heelstick, Fingerstick, Adhesive Removal, Dressing Change, Wound Treatment, Venipuncture, Arterial puncture, Subcutaneous Injection, Intramuscular Injection, Peripheral IV Cannulation, Removal of PIV, Central line Placement, Gastric Tube Insertion, Bladder Catheterization, Tracheal Extubation, Lumbar Puncture, Peripheral Arterial Line, PICC Line Placement, Circumcision, Chest Tube Insertion	**Tier 1**
	Avoid Painful Procedures Anticipate Need of Future Studies Use Noninvasive Monitoring (NIRS, oxygen saturation, EtCO$_2$ monitoring, transcutaneous bilirubin)	**Base line**

FIGURE 15–1. Tiered approach to analgesia in the neonate. EtCO$_2$, end-tidal carbon dioxide; NIRS, near-infrared spectroscopy; IV, intravenous; PICC, percutaneous inserted central catheter; PIV, peripheral intravenous line. (*Reproduced with permission from Witt N, Coynor S, Edwards C: A Guide to Pain Assessment and Management in the Neonate,* Curr Emerg Hosp Med Rep. *2016;4:1-10.*)

of providing deep sedation or anesthesia. There are multiple recommendations for pain relief in the neonate. Witt and colleagues (Figure 15–1) proposed a "tiered" approach to analgesia in the neonate. Hall and Anand have provided guidance on specific procedures summarized in Table 15–2.

A. Nonpharmacologic. This approach is preferable for mild procedural pain due to the short-term efficacy and absence of side effects. It is most effective when combined with a reduction in lighting and sound. It is not to be used in place of pharmacologic therapy with severe and chronic pain. Cochrane review indicates the following: "There is evidence that different nonpharmacological interventions can be used

Table 15–2. COMMON PROCEDURES AND PAIN RELIEF RECOMMENDATIONS

Procedures	Proposed Pain Management	Notes
Arterial or venous cutdown	Nonpharmacologic interventions[a] and topical local anesthetic, lidocaine infiltration, intravenous (IV) fentanyl (1–2 mcg/kg), consider deep sedation	
Arterial puncture	Nonpharmacologic interventions,[a] use topical and subcutaneous local anesthetics	More painful than venipuncture
Central line	Nonpharmacologic interventions,[a] topical local anesthetics, consider low-dose opioids or deep sedation if needed	
Chest physiotherapy	Gentle positioning, fentanyl (1 mcg/kg) if a chest tube is present	Avoid areas of injured or inflamed skin and areas with indwelling drains or catheters
Circumcision	Nonpharmacologic interventions[a] and topical local anesthetic, lidocaine infiltration, IV/oral (PO) acetaminophen before and after procedure	Lidocaine infiltration for distal, ring, or dorsal penile nerve blocks (DPNB); liposomal lidocaine is more effective than DPNB; *never use with epinephrine*
Dressing change	Nonpharmacologic interventions[a] and topical local anesthetic, consider deep sedation if extensive	
Extracorporeal membrane oxygenation cannulation	Propofol 2–4 mg/kg, ketamine 1–2 mg/kg, fentanyl 1–3 mcg/kg, muscle relaxant as needed	
Endotracheal intubation	Give fentanyl (1 mcg/kg) or morphine (10–30 mcg/kg), with midazolam (50–100 mcg/kg) or ketamine (1 mg/kg), use muscle relaxant only if experienced clinician, consider atropine	Superiority of one drug regimen over another has not been investigated
Gastric tube insertion	Nonpharmacologic interventions,[a] consider local anesthetic gel	Perform rapidly, use lubricant, avoid injury
Heel stick	Use nonpharmacologic interventions[a] and automated lance; squeezing the heel is the most painful phase	Venipuncture is more efficient, less painful; local anesthetics, acetaminophen, heel warming will not reduce heel stick pain
Intramuscular injection	Avoid if possible, use nonpharmacologic interventions[a] and topical local anesthetics if procedure cannot be avoided	

(Continued)

Table 15-2. COMMON PROCEDURES AND PAIN RELIEF RECOMMENDATIONS (*CONTINUED*)

Procedures	Proposed Pain Management	Notes
Lumbar puncture	Nonpharmacologic interventions[a] and topical local anesthetic, lidocaine infiltration, careful positioning	Use IV analgesia/sedation, if patient is intubated and ventilated
Peripheral arterial line	Nonpharmacologic interventions[a] and topical local anesthetic, lidocaine infiltration, consider IV opioids	
Peripheral IV catheterization	Nonpharmacologic interventions,[a] topical local anesthetics	
Peripherally inserted central catheter	Nonpharmacologic interventions[a] and topical local anesthetic, lidocaine infiltration, consider IV fentanyl (1 mcg/kg) or IV ketamine (1 mg/kg)	Some centers prefer using deep sedation or general anesthesia
Subcutaneous injection	Avoid if possible, use nonpharmacologic interventions[a] and topical local anesthetics if procedure cannot be avoided	
Suprapubic bladder aspiration	Nonpharmacologic interventions and topical local anesthetic, lidocaine infiltration, consider IV fentanyl (0.5–1 mcg/kg)	
Tracheal extubation	Solvent swab for tape, consider nonpharmacologic interventions	
Umbilical vein catheterization	Nonpharmacologic interventions,[a] IV acetaminophen (10 mg/kg), avoid sutures to the skin	Cord tissue is not innervated; skin injury
Venipuncture	Nonpharmacologic interventions,[a] use topical local anesthetics	Less time, less repeat sampling, and less painful than heel stick

[a]Nonpharmacologic interventions include pacifier, oral sucrose, swaddling, and skin-to-skin contact with mother.
Adapted with permission from Hall RW, Anand KJ: Pain management in newborns, *Clin Perinatol.* 2014 Dec;41(4):895-924.

with preterms and neonates to significantly manage pain behaviors associated with acutely painful procedures."

1. **Kangaroo care or skin-to-skin care.** Kangaroo mother care is a method of skin-to-skin care whereby the mother, father, or caregiver holds the infant upright, flexed, and prone wearing only a diaper next to the caregiver's chest (similar to how kangaroo mothers carry their young in their pouch) (Figure 15–2). Research supports its use to decrease the pain response in both preterm and term infants. It is effective for use in decreasing pain (reduced grimacing, reduced heart rate, improved pain scores, decreased stress and crying time) with heel sticks. A Cochrane review (2017) indicates that kangaroo care appears

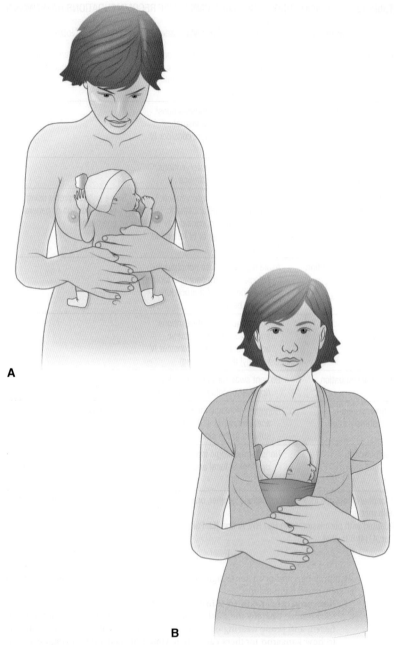

FIGURE 15–2. (**A**) Positioning the baby for kangaroo care. (**B**) Baby in Kangaroo care binder position. (*Reproduced with permission from* Kangaroo Mother Care: A Practical Guide. *World Health Organization, Dept. of Reproductive Health and Research, Geneva Switzerland.* [http://www.who.int/maternal_child_adolescent/documents/9241590351/en. *Accessed January 31, 2019.*])

to be safe and to reduce the pain response to and improve recovery from a single painful procedure (eg, heel stick, venous puncture, intramuscular injections, tape removal).

2. **Breast feeding and breast milk.** These can be used to alleviate procedural pain in neonates undergoing a single painful procedure or ROP examination. Cochrane review states that breast feeding or breast milk should be used to alleviate procedural pain in neonates undergoing a single painful procedure rather than placebo, positioning, or no intervention. Giving glucose/sucrose had similar effectiveness as breast feeding. Supplemental human milk (via a syringe or pacifier) is just as effective as giving sucrose or glucose for treating pain in term infants.

3. **Nonnutritive suck (NNS).** The type of suck associated with a pacifier without breast milk or formula. It seems to increase endogenous endorphins. When used in combination with oral sucrose (24%), it is effective in reducing the pain associated with heel sticks and peripheral IV catheter (PIV) placement. Cochrane review supports that NNS can be used to decrease pain immediately after a procedure and pain 30 seconds after a procedure in preterm and term infants (with low-quality evidence).

4. **Swaddling.** This involves wrapping an infant securely in a blanket. The arms are immobilized to prevent the Moro reflex. Swaddling can cause a decrease in heart rate, an increase in oxygen saturation, and an increase in ability to organize behaviors. It is good to use with heel sticks, PIV starts, ROP examinations, and ETT suctioning. It can also be recommended as a complementary therapy during painful procedures. A Cochrane review states that swaddling in a preterm infant can reduce both pain immediately after a procedure and 30 seconds after; in a neonate, swaddling can reduce pain immediately after a procedure (low-quality evidence).

5. **Facilitated tuck position.** This position brings the body to the middle and is achieved by holding the infant's arms flexed and close to the trunk and legs gently in a flexed position close to the midline of the torso and can be done in the supine, lateral, or prone position. The caregiver uses his or her hands on both the head and lower limbs to maintain the position. It is effective with PIV starts, heel sticks, ROP examinations, and ETT suctioning in decreasing heart rate and recovery time. A Cochrane review states that facilitated tucking in a preterm infant can reduce pain both immediately and 30 seconds after a procedure. In a neonate, facilitated tucking can reduce pain immediately after a procedure.

6. **Positioning.** A prone position can improve breathing effort and decrease the infant's oxygen requirement.

7. **Music.** Music is effective in infants >31 weeks' gestation. It assists with the regulation and reduction of heart rate as well as increase in oxygen saturation. In mature stable infants, music with sucrose was better than music or sucrose alone for heel stick.

8. **Massage.** Massage therapy involves skin manipulation of the soft tissue that includes brushing of the skin, light compression, and gliding and kneading strokes. It enhances vagal activity and modulates insulin and insulin-like growth factor-1. It also decreases cortisol and epinephrine levels. It has been shown to decrease NIPS scores, increase weight gain, and improve neurodevelopmental outcomes in very low birthweight infants. Some small studies suggest that massage therapy had positive effects on the immune system, decreased stress behavior, improved tolerance to pain, improved developmental scores, and resulted in earlier discharge of infants. A Cochrane review states that touch or massage is effective for decreasing pain immediately after a painful procedure in a preterm infant (low-quality evidence).

9. **Acupuncture.** Acupuncture works by stimulating the endorphin system via mechanical or electrical means at acupuncture points, but data are limited in

neonates. A pilot study using magnetic noninvasive acupuncture showed that auricular noninvasive magnetic acupuncture is feasible in neonates and may decrease PIPP-R scores when performing heel sticks.

10. **Applied mechanical vibration.** Infants had lower pain scores and more stable heart rates during heel stick and 2 minutes after heel lance in a pilot randomized controlled trial.

11. **Sensorial stimulation (SS).** SS gently stimulates the tactile, gustatory, auditory, and visual systems. It has been shown to decrease pain during minor procedures. SS includes looking at and gently talking to the neonate, while simultaneously stroking or massaging the face or back as well as administering an oral sucrose or glucose solution prior to a procedure. Using all elements of SS was found to be more effective than sucrose alone in a review of multiple studies.

12. **Familiar odor.** Maternal milk odor has been found to have an analgesic effect on preterm neonates. A Cochrane review indicates that a familiar odor was found to decrease pain during the regulatory phase after needle stick in neonates.

13. **Rocking/holding.** This has not been found to decrease pain after a painful procedure, but helps an infant recover from painful stimuli. Sucking related and rocking/holding were beneficial for term infants during heel lance and IV catheter insertion.

B. **Pharmacologic treatment.** Most often, light pain and moderate pain of short duration are best dealt with using nonpharmacologic pain measures. However, when pain assessment scores indicate moderate to severe pain, pairing pharmacologic pain measures with comfort measures is strongly suggested. Procedures that require the use of pharmacologic pain intervention include nonemergency intubations, mechanical ventilation (with the selective use of opioids), chest tube insertion, central line placement, lumbar puncture, circumcision, PDA ligation, and placement of peritoneal drains and ROP examinations. The most common pharmacologic medication used in newborns with persistent pain is opioids, specifically morphine and fentanyl.

1. **Sucrose.** Oral sucrose is an effective and safe analgesic for decreasing procedural pain from a single event in infants from 25 to 44 weeks' gestational age. The mechanism of action is unknown in neonates, but it is believed the sweet taste may activate the opiate, endorphin, dopamine, or adrenocorticotropic hormone pathway, as it does in animal studies. When combined with NNS, it is shown to be very efficacious with heel sticks. Facilities should adopt a specific protocol to standardize the use of oral sucrose. The optimal dose is not known, but the range is 0.012 to 0.12 g or 0.05 to 0.5 mL of a 24% solution. Recommended dosage is 0.1 to 1 mL (0.2 to 0.5 mL/kg) of 24% sucrose 2 minutes before the procedure. It lasts approximately 4 minutes. Sucrose is effective in infants >27 weeks' gestation; however, it is not approved by the US Food and Drug Administration. Infants who received sucrose were shown to have decreased behavioral pain scores, but there was no difference in their electroencephalograms. Caution should be taken when administering multiple doses of sucrose (worse neurodevelopmental scores in preterm infants getting >10 doses over 24 hours), and administration should be limited to the management of acute procedural pain. It is best if sucrose is treated as a medication, whereby doses are recorded and tracked. A Cochrane review (2016) concluded that sucrose is effective for reducing procedural pain from single events such as heel lance, venipuncture, and intramuscular injection in both preterm and term infants. Optimal dose could not be identified. It was not effective for circumcision, and the effects were inconclusive for arterial puncture, subcutaneous injection, insertion of nasogastric or orogastric tubes, bladder catheterization, eye examinations, and echocardiography exams.

2. **Glucose.** Can be used as an alternative to sucrose. It was found that 20% to 30% glucose solutions decreased pain scores and crying times during

venipuncture and heel sticks. There is no recommendation for dose or timing of administration.

3. **Commonly used pain relief medications in neonates are as follows** (see Chapter 155 for specific dosing information):

   a. **Topical anesthetic agents.** Topical anesthetics include EMLA (eutectic mixture of 2.5% lidocaine and 2.5% prilocaine) cream (most commonly used and studied), 4% tetracaine gel, 4% liposomal lidocaine (shorter onset of action), and S-Caine Peel (7% lidocaine and 7% tetracaine cream). These topical agents decrease pain during venipuncture, percutaneous central venous catheter insertion, and peripheral arterial puncture. EMLA does not work for heel sticks but may work for lumbar punctures when combined with oral sucrose/glucose. Topical agents can cause methemoglobinemia, transient skin rashes, and toxicity in premature infants. A Cochrane review states the following: "The evidence regarding the effectiveness or safety of topical anesthesia for needle-related pain in preterm and term newborns is inadequate to support clinical recommendations."

   b. **Subcutaneous infiltration with lidocaine (0.5–1% lidocaine).** Lidocaine blocks voltage-dependent sodium channels, which blocks low- and high-threshold axons that contribute to painful sensations. It has been used for penile blocks for circumcision (ring block) and for certain skin-breaking procedures (lumbar punctures, chest tube insertion). Buffered lidocaine (lidocaine is acidic and by adding 8.4% sodium bicarbonate solution it decreases the acidity and thereby decreases the pain) can be used.

   c. **Systemic medications for pain in the neonate** are recommended for most invasive procedures. The AAP states that they are recommended for procedures such as circumcision, chest tube insertion and removal, and nonemergency intubations. Pain relief for mechanical ventilation is controversial. The AAP does not routinely recommend routine opioids for all mechanically ventilated infants and a Cochrane review states that opioids should be used selectively in term and preterm infants on mechanical ventilation.

      i. **Medications that provide systemic analgesia include the following:**

         (a) **Opioids.** Opioids are the most common pharmacologic agent used for pain relief in newborns. These provide potent pain relief but are associated with respiratory depression. Careful monitoring is recommended.

            (i) **Morphine sulfate is the most commonly used opioid in neonates.** Side effects include respiratory and CNS depression, arterial hypotension, urinary retention, tolerance, dependence, and constipation.

            (ii) **Fentanyl** is also commonly used and is faster acting than morphine. It has less hypotension, less sedation, and decreased effects on gastrointestinal motility and urinary retention when compared to morphine. It causes chest wall rigidity, and tolerance occurs more rapidly than with morphine. It is the most effective option for ROP exams and intubation.

            (iii) **Alfentanil, sufentanil, and remifentanil** are short-acting medications and are being used for shorter procedures. Remifentanil may be preferred since it is not metabolized by the liver, but there are no studies on long-term use.

         (b) **Acetaminophen** is known for its analgesic effects. It is typically used for mild or moderate pain relief. It has commonly been used for postoperative pain control. IV formulation (Ofirmev) has been approved by the US Food and Drug Administration (FDA) and has decreased the amount of opioids needed after surgery.

    (c) **Nonsteroidal anti-inflammatory drugs (NSAIDs).** These have commonly been used for closure of the PDA in infants. The use of NSAIDs for pain control in newborns has not been recommended because of too many side effects (pulmonary hypertension and renal insufficiency and platelet dysfunction).

    (d) **Medications that have been suggested and used but not well studied in neonates** include the following:

        (i) **Methadone** has satisfactory analgesic effects, but dosing recommendations have not been developed.

        (ii) **Propofol** is a nonbarbiturate anesthetic used for short-term procedural sedation and anesthesia. Side effects in neonates include prolonged hypotension, bradycardia, desaturations and significant variablility in pharmokinetics.

        (iii) **Gabapentin** has been used for refractory pain and agitation and was associated with decreases in pain scores.

        (iv) **Dexmedetomidine** is a selective α_2-adrenergic agonist that produces sedation and analgesia with minimal respiratory depression. It has been used in neonates with congenital heart disease. It is not FDA approved in children but has been used in preterm and full-term neonates with a favorable safety profile over 24 hours.

        (v) **Ketamine** is an N-methyl-D-aspartate receptor antagonist that provides potent sedation, analgesia, and amnesia and is used for anesthesia and analgesia in neonates. There is concern about possible neurotoxicity.

  ii. **Medications that do not provide systemic analgesia but provide sedation** can be used for pain-related agitation and are used along with pain medication. Remember that sedative agents do not have an analgesic effect and should not be used alone to relieve pain. Sedative-hypnotics (most commonly benzodiazepines) are the most widely used because they provide sedation, muscle relaxation, and anxiolysis. Benzodiazepines can also potentiate respiratory depression and hypotension when used with opioids.

    (a) **Benzodiazepines**

        (i) **Midazolam** is the most common benzodiazepine used in the NICU. It has a rapid onset of action. It has been used for computed tomography (CT) scans and procedural sedation. Caution should be exercised as its use has been associated with neurotoxicity (abnormal hippocampal growth and neurodevelopmental outcomes) and adverse short-term effects in the NOPAIN trial.

        (ii) **Lorazepam** has a longer duration of action.

    (b) **Chloral hydrate is not available in the United States** but is used elsewhere for short-term sedation, such as for CT and MRI.

  iii. **Medications that are recommended for nonemergency intubation.** Premedication can decrease pain and discomfort of a nonemergent intubation. See Chapter 33 and Table 33–2 for a list of recommended medications.

VI. Potentially improved pain management practices, as identified by the Vermont Oxford Network Neonatal Intensive Care Quality Improvement Collaborative, include the following (A to F):

A. Reduce the frequency of avoidable painful procedures.

B. Develop a protocol for standardization of sucrose administration.

C. Perform frequent pain assessment.

D. Implement strategies to manage pain during the following: heel sticks, peripheral vascular procedures, circumcision, nonemergent intubation, and mechanical ventilation.

E. **Implement strategies to manage pain during the postoperative period.**
F. **Implement strategies to wean neonates effectively and safely from opiates.**
G. **Other approaches.** Put peripheral arterial or central venous catheters in infants who require multiple blood drawings or heel sticks and cluster care (try to limit disruptions by performing many tasks at once; eg, physical exam, diaper change, suctioning). If possible, use handheld devices that can analyze multiple tests with one blood sample. Try to use noninvasive monitoring as much as possible.

VII. **Conclusion.** Pain continues to be an emerging field of study within the discipline of neonatology. More research is needed regarding the ongoing assessment and treatment of neonatal pain. Healthcare professionals need to diligently document pain assessment and follow-up scores after intervention to ensure proper pain management. Clinical practice guidelines need to be developed for the neonatal community at large for standardization of this practice. Research is evolving to support accurate assessment of pain in the neonate. Monitoring skin conduction scores during painful procedures and measuring the impact of pain on the infant's brain are areas of active investigation. Measurements would include values during the experience of noxious stimuli and the long-term impact on the neurodevelopment of the infant. Other technologies to measure pain response that are being studied include near infrared spectroscopy, amplitude integrated EEG, functional MRI, and heart rate variability. It is through continuous research and commitment to reducing the experience of pain for the neonate that we will fully understand and effectively treat the neonate while supporting their viability.

16 Newborn Screening

I. **Definition.** Newborn screening is the **testing of all newborns in the first few days of life for certain congenital disorders or diseases** that can cause severe lifelong intellectual and physical disabilities, chronic disease, and possibly death if not detected early and treated as soon as possible. The purpose of newborn screening is to identify these conditions and provide treatment as early as possible. **It involves a blood test that screens for multiple congenital conditions, a pulse oximetry test to rule out critical congenital heart disease, and a hearing test to rule out congenital deafness.** This is a population-based system that is mandated in every state. The American Academy of Pediatrics (AAP) and American College of Medical Genetics and Genomics (ACMG) support offering newborn screening to all children. They recommend education and counseling about its benefits, its risks, and what to do if there is a positive result.

II. **Components of newborn screening.** Once thought of as just a newborn screening test, the AAP states it is now a complex system that encompasses 5 very important components:
A. **Testing of all newborns.** involves the following:
1. **A blood test** that screens for certain metabolic or genetic conditions.
2. **A pulse oximetry test** to test for a critical congenital heart defect that requires either a catheter-based intervention or heart surgery.
3. **A routine hearing test** to rule out congenital deafness. Treatment needs to begin before 6 months of age so communication skills can develop.
B. **Timely follow-up** of abnormal screening results. Some disorders can cause severe disabilities and some are fatal if not treated early.
C. **Diagnostic testing** to verify results of the initial screening blood test. The initial blood test does not provide a definitive result to diagnose the infant; it only identifies newborns who need further diagnostic testing.

    D. Management of the disease which usually involves a multidisciplinary approach.
    E. Ongoing evaluation of the newborn screening system.
III. What congenital disorders or diseases should be screened for?
    A. Recommended Uniform Screening Panel (RUSP) is a standardized list of disorders recommended by the secretary of the Department of Health and Human Services and supported by the Advisory Committee on Heritable Disorders in newborns and children from which states select conditions to screen for as part of their universal newborn screening program. Most states screen for the majority of the disorders on RUSP, and some even screen for additional disorders.
    B. Core and secondary conditions of RUSP
        1. Core conditions are disorders that are recommended in every US newborn screening program. There are 35 core conditions on the newborn screening panel. See Table 16–1. **Criteria for conditions to be added to RUSP include:**
            a. It is a clearly defined disorder.
            b. States are able to screen for the disorder.
            c. There is a diagnostic confirmatory test to detect the disorder.
            d. There is available treatment that is effective and evidence to support improved outcome in the presymptomatic or early symptomatic period.
            e. It is beneficial to screen in neonates because it can affect future reproductive decisions of the family.
        2. Secondary conditions are conditions that do not meet all the inclusion criteria but are believed to be clinically significant and are identified when screening for the core conditions. There are 26 secondary conditions. See Table 16–2.
    C. Non-RUSP conditions are additional newborn screening tests that are not on the RUSP list. They have been nominated but, after formal review, are found to be deficient in 1 or more of the criteria to be added to RUSP. This does not mean they should not be screened for. Each state makes choices on what conditions they recommend for screening. Non-RUSP conditions include 5-oxoprolinuria (pyroglutamic aciduria), ethylmalonic encephalopathy, HIV, nonketotic hyperglycinemia, glucose-6-phosphate dehydrogenase deficiency, prolinemia, carbamoylphosphate synthetase deficiency, hyperammonemia/ornithinemia/citrullinemia (ornithine transporter defect), mucopolysaccharidosis type II, toxoplasmosis, Krabbe disease, and Niemann-Pick disease.
    D. State-mandated testing. In the United States, this screening is mandated in every state, but the disorders on the screening panels vary. Screening is done for approximately 4.1 million infants each year, with >12,500 newborns being diagnosed with a detectable and treatable disorder. A list of the screening tests provided by each state can be found on the National Newborn Screening and Genetics Resource Center website at http://genes-r-us.uthscsa.edu.
    E. Genomic testing for newborn screening. The majority of newborn screening is done by tandem mass spectrometry in addition to other forms of testing. Applying genomic technology can help with diagnosing metabolic or nonmetabolic genetic disorders in an infant. This is a useful tool for diagnosing infants with potentially treatable conditions that result from genetic mutations including early-onset seizure disorders, cardiomyopathies, liver and kidney diseases, and others. Difficulties in implementing genetic testing, besides the obvious ethical, legal, and social implications, involve the high cost of testing and cost effectiveness, clinical utility, question of parental consent, the time it takes to get the results (weeks), interpretation of the results, what to do with incidental findings, and ownership and appropriate storage of data. Recommendations in using genomic testing include the following: consider as an add on to current newborn screening, use targeted panels, and limit genomic testing to diseases that manifest and can be treated in the newborn period. Genetic and genomic testing is discussed in detail in Chapter 17.
IV. Newborn screening test
    A. Blood test

Table 16–1. RECOMMENDED UNIFORM SCREENING PANEL OF THE 35 CORE CONDITIONS AND ESTIMATED INCIDENCE (RECOMMENDED BY THE US SECRETARY OF THE DEPARTMENT OF HEALTH AND HUMAN SERVICES)

Condition or Disorder	Estimated Incidence
Amino acid disorders	
Classic phenylketonuria (PKU)	1:19,000–1:13,500
Argininosuccinic aciduria (ASA)	1:70,000
Tyrosinemia type 1 (TYR 1)	1:12,000–1:100,000
Citrullinemia (CIT) type 1	1:157,000
Maple syrup urine disease (MSUD)	1:185,000
Homocystinuria (HCY)	1:300,000
Organic acid condition	
Glutaric acidemia type I (GA I)	1:30,000–1:40,000
Methylmalonic acidemia (methylmalonyl-CoA mutase)	1:5000–1:100,000
3-Methylcrotonyl-CoA carboxylase (3MCC) deficiency	1:36,000
Propionic (PROP) acidemia	1:100,000
β-Ketothiolase (BKT) deficiency	<1:1,000,000
3-Hydroxy-3-methylglutaric (HMG) aciduria	<1:100,000
Isovaleric acidemia (IVA)	<1:250,000
Methylmalonic acidemia (cobalamin disorders)	<1:50,000–1:100,000
Holocarboxylase synthase deficiency	<1:87,000
Fatty acid oxidation disorders	
Medium-chain acyl-CoA dehydrogenase (MCAD) deficiency	1:6400–1:46,000
Long-chain L-3 hydroxyacyl-CoA dehydrogenase (LCHAD) deficiency	1:60,000
Very-long-chain acyl-CoA dehydrogenase (VLCAD) deficiency	1:4000–1:20,000
Trifunctional protein (TFP) deficiency	Unknown
Carnitine uptake defect (CUD)/carnitine transport defect	1:40,000
Hemoglobin disorders	
Sickle cell disease (sickle cell anemia) (Hb SS)	1:200,000
Hb S/C disease	>1:25,000
Hb S/β-thalassemia (Hbs/βTh)	>1:50,000
Endocrine disorders	
Primary congenital hypothyroidism (CH)	1:3000–1:4000
Congenital adrenal hyperplasia (CAH)	1:15,981
Other disorders	
Hearing loss (HEAR)	1:1000
Cystic fibrosis (CF)	1:3500

(Continued)

Table 16–1. RECOMMENDED UNIFORM SCREENING PANEL OF THE 35 CORE CONDITIONS AND ESTIMATED INCIDENCE (RECOMMENDED BY THE US SECRETARY OF THE DEPARTMENT OF HEALTH AND HUMAN SERVICES) (*CONTINUED*)

Condition or Disorder	Estimated Incidence
Classical galactosemia (GALT)	1:47,000
Biotinidase (BIOT) deficiency	1:112,000–1:129,000
Critical congenital heart disease (CCHD)	1:8000–1:10,000
Severe combined immunodeficiencies (SCID)	1:58,000
Glycogen storage disease type II (Pompe)	1:40,000
Mucopolysaccharidosis type I (MPS I) (Hurler)	1:100,000
X-linked adrenoleukodystrophy (X-ALD)	1:20,000
Spinal muscular atrophy due to homozygous deletion of exon 7 in *SMN1*	1:6000–1:10,000

Data from Newborn screening: toward a uniform screening panel and system, *Genet Med.* 2006 May; 8 Suppl 1:1S-252S and Sweetman L, Millington DS, Therrell BL, et al: Naming and counting disorders (conditions) included in newborn screening panels, *Pediatrics.* 2006 May;117(5 Pt 2): S308-S314.

1. **Initial blood specimen.** A heel stick is done between 24 and 72 hours after birth (close to discharge). The blood from the heel is put onto a filter paper card, completely filling each circle, which is sent to the laboratory at the newborn screening and molecular biology branch of the Centers for Disease Control and Prevention,(CDC) ideally within 24 hours of collection, and screened for certain core conditions.

2. **Factors that can influence the results of the blood test.** Factors that can influence the results of the screening blood test include sample timing, diet, gestational age, preterm birth, transfusions (platelets, fresh-frozen plasma [FFP], whole/packed, exchange transfusions), total parenteral nutrition (TPN), antibiotics, and certain nipple creams.

   a. **Sample timing**
      i. **Increase in false positives** if test is done in the first 24 hours: cystic fibrosis and congenital adrenal hyperplasia.
      ii. **Increase in false positives** if test is done in the first 48 hours: thyrotropin method of testing for congenital hypothyroidism.
      iii. **Homocystinuria.** Must test at >24 hours and advisable to repeat at 2 to 4 weeks of age.
      iv. **Medium chain acyl-CoA dehydrogenase (MCAD) deficiency.** Test before 8 days of age.

   b. **Diet.** There needs to be adequate protein intake for the test to be valid for tyrosinemia, phenylketonuria (PKU), and homocystinuria. For galactosemia screening, the infant needs to be on a galactose-containing formula.

   c. **Gestational age**
      i. **Extreme preterm birth.** Increase in false negatives in sickle cell disease and other hemoglobinopathies.
      ii. **Preterm birth**
         (a) **Increase in false positives.** Congenital adrenal hyperplasia (due to normal increase in 17-hydroxyprogesterone); severe combined immunodeficiency screening using the T-cell receptor excision circles (TREC) assay.

Table 16–2. SECONDARY CONDITIONS THAT ARE IDENTIFIABLE WHEN SCREENING FOR THE CORE CONDITIONS LISTED IN TABLE 16–1

| | Metabolic Disorder | | | | |
Secondary Condition	Organic Acid Condition	Fatty Acid Oxidation Disorders	Amino Acid Disorders	Hemoglobin Disorder	Other Disorder
Methylmalonic acidemia with homocystinuria	X				
Malonic acidemia	X				
Isobutyrylglycinuria	X				
2-Methylbutyrylglycinuria	X				
3-Methylglutaconic aciduria	X				
2-Methyl-3-hydroxybutyric aciduria	X				
Short-chain acyl-CoA dehydrogenase deficiency		X			
Medium/short-chain L-3-hydroxyacyl-CoA dehydrogenase deficiency		X			
Glutaric acidemia type II		X			
Medium-chain ketoacyl-CoA thiolase deficiency		X			
2,4 Dienoyl-CoA reductase deficiency		X			
Carnitine palmitoyltransferase type I deficiency		X			
Carnitine palmitoyltransferase type II deficiency		X			
Carnitine acylcarnitine translocase deficiency		X			
Argininemia			X		
Citrullinemia, type II			X		
Hypermethioninemia			X		
Benign hyperphenylalaninemia			X		
Biopterin defect in cofactor biosynthesis			X		
Biopterin defect in cofactor regeneration			X		
Tyrosinemia, type II			X		

(*Continued*)

Table 16–2. SECONDARY CONDITIONS THAT ARE IDENTIFIABLE WHEN SCREENING FOR THE CORE CONDITIONS LISTED IN TABLE 16–1 (*CONTINUED*)

Secondary Condition	Metabolic Disorder				
	Organic Acid Condition	Fatty Acid Oxidation Disorders	Amino Acid Disorders	Hemoglobin Disorder	Other Disorder
Tyrosinemia, type III			X		
Various other hemoglobinopathies				X	
Galactoepimerase deficiency (GALE)					X
Galactokinase deficiency (GALK)					X
T-cell related lymphocyte deficiencies					X

Reproduced with permission from Recommended Uniform Screening Panel. U.S. Department of Health and Human Services. (https://www.hrsa.gov/advisory-committees/heritable-disorders/rusp/index.html. Accessed January 31, 2019.)

      (b) **Increase in false positives and false negatives.** Thyroxine method of testing for congenital hypothyroidism.

      (c) **Increased likelihood** of neonatal tyrosinemia.

   d. **Transfusion** (includes blood [whole or packed], platelets, FFP, exchange transfusions)

      i. **Do the test a few hours after transfusion:** Congenital adrenal hyperplasia.

      ii. **Do the test >90 days after transfusion.** Sickle cell diseases and other hemoglobinopathies, galactose-1-phosphate uridylyltransferase (GALT) deficiency galactosemia, and biotinidase deficiency.

      iii. **Do the test 3 to 6 weeks after transfusion.** Cystic fibrosis.

   e. **Total parenteral nutrition. If the infant is on TPN:**

      i. **False positive:** Homocystinuria, maple syrup urine disease, MCAD deficiency, PKU, tyrosinemia.

      ii. **False negative:** Galactose method of testing for galactosemia.

   f. **Antibiotics.** Use of pivalate-containing antibiotics (pivampicillin, cefditoren) during pregnancy may cause false-positive results when screening for isovaleric acidemia.

   g. **Use of nipple creams containing neopentanoate by nursing mothers** can cause false-positive results when screening for isovaleric acidemia.

  3. **Follow-up** is of utmost importance because certain conditions can be fatal (galactosemia, maple syrup urine disease, congenital adrenal hyperplasia), whereas others can cause severe disabilities if not treated as early as possible. Early detection facilitates timely treatment to prevent lifelong health problems.

   a. **Positive results for time-critical conditions** need to be communicated to healthcare provider within the first 5 days of life.

   b. **Positive results for non–time-critical conditions** need to be communicated to healthcare provider within 7 days of life.

   c. **Invalid, equivocal, or positive results** need to be repeated as soon as possible.

B. Screening for critical congenital heart disease by pulse oximetry is done at 24 to 48 hours of age or as late as possible for early discharge. See Chapter 7.

C. Screening for hearing loss is done before discharge from the hospital. See Chapter 71.

V. Selected disorders included in the newborn screening panels that specifically have AAP fact sheets. The AAP Committee on Genetics has published newborn screening fact sheets that address appropriate testing methods, diagnostic testing if the screen is positive, and follow-up for 12 disorders.

A. Amino acid metabolism disorders

1. **PKU.** A high level of the amino acid **phenylalanine (Phe)** (>20 mg/dL) causes an accumulation of phenylketones. Incidence is 1 in 9000 to 13,500 and higher in those with northern European ancestry and American Indians/Alaska natives.

   a. **Manifestations** include developmental delay, intellectual disability, microcephaly, seizures, eczema, and delayed speech.

   b. **Screening.** Make sure infant is on adequate protein intake before screening. If on TPN, there can be false positives. Three screening methods are Guthrie bacterial inhibition assay (BIA; more false positives), fluorometric analysis, and tandem mass spectrometry (MS/MS). Cutoff values are 2 to 6 mg/dL. Repeat test if screened within the first 24 hours.

   c. **Follow-up.** If positive, check plasma Phe and tyrosine levels; if Phe increased, perform additional studies to see if the infant has a synthesis or recycling abnormality of tetrahydrobiopterin.

   d. **Lifelong dietary treatment** with special medical diets low in Phe. No consensus on optimal level of Phe. Breast feeding is allowed with the addition of Phe-free formula with guidance of metabolic dietician. Tetrahydrobiopterin treatment may also be recommended in some cases.

2. **Maple syrup urine disease (branched-chain ketoaciduria).** Deficiency of the branched-chain α-keto acid dehydrogenase complex, which causes an increase in branched-chain amino acids (BCAAs). There are 5 phenotypes of disease; classic is most common and most severe. Incidence is 1 in 185,000. Incidence is 1 in 176 in Mennonites in certain counties in Pennsylvania (founder effect).

   a. **Manifestations.** Occur between 4 to 7 days and 2 weeks: lethargy, poor sucking, weight loss, abnormal neurologic signs, characteristic odor of urine (maple syrup), seizures, coma, and death.

   b. **Screening.** If the infant is on TPN, a false-positive result may occur. Screening done by MS/MS and a diagnostic peak of leucine, isoleucine, and alloisoleucine.

   c. **Follow-up.** Check blood leucine level. If >3 to 4 mg/dL in the first 24 hours of life or >4 mg/dL at >24 hours, do a plasma amino acid analysis. Concern for disease if increased BCAA and low alanine and alloisoleucine are present. Molecular genetic testing is recommended to confirm the diagnosis. Metabolic team (physician, nutritionist) recommended to follow the infant.

   d. **Long-term treatment** consists of a strict regulated diet for life, BCAA-free supplementation, and trial of thiamine supplementation (50–300 mg/d for 3 weeks). **Treatment during crisis** includes dialysis (peritoneal, continuous venovenous hemofiltration), TPN, and high glucose with insulin.

3. **Homocystinuria.** A biochemical abnormality (of enzymatic defect) resulting in an elevated level of serum homocysteine and methionine.

   a. **Manifestations.** Recurrent thromboemboli, arterial/venous thromboses, developmental delay, intellectual disability, seizures, marfanoid habitus, ocular abnormalities (lens dislocation and progressive myopia), and death. Incidence is 1 in 300,000.

   b. **Screening.** Make sure the infant is on adequate protein before screening. If the infant is on TPN, a false-positive result may occur. Test should be done after 24 hours, with repeat recommended in 2 to 4 weeks. Screen using BIA test (increased blood methionine) or MS/MS (direct methionine assay).

c. **Follow-up.** Do quantitative serum or plasma amino acid determination: increased methionine and homocysteine levels and decreased cysteine levels. Perform urine organic acid profile with MS/MS and gas chromatography: presence or absence methylmalonic acid.

d. **Treatment.** Pyridoxine supplementation (if found to be pyridoxine responsive), methionine-restricted cysteine-supplemented diet (if found to be nonresponsive), folic acid, betaine therapy, aspirin, and dipyridamole (decrease thromboembolism).

4. **Tyrosinemia.** Increased serum tyrosine caused by deficiency of enzyme fumarylacetoacetate hydrolase (FAH; type I) or caused by deficiency of tyrosine aminotransferase (type II) or neonatal tyrosinemia (more common in preterm infants; most common cause of abnormal PKU and tyrosinemia results). Incidence only known for type I (1 in 12,000 to 100,000).

   a. **Manifestations.** Type I: failure to thrive (FTT), vomiting, diarrhea, cabbage odor, fever, hepatomegaly, jaundice, edema, liver disease, death from liver failure. Type II: oculocutaneous syndrome. Neonatal: nonspecific, prolonged jaundice, lethargic, impaired motor activity.

   b. **Screening.** Make sure infant is on adequate protein before screening. In preterm births, there is an increased likelihood of neonatal tyrosinemia (transient). If the infant is on TPN, there is a risk of a false-positive test. It is best to do the test 48 to 72 hours after milk feeding. Use BIA test (abnormal level of tyrosine) or MS/MS (direct measurement).

   c. **Follow-up.** An increased tyrosine level can be seen with other diseases (eg, infections, hemochromatosis, giant cell hepatitis, fructose/galactose enzyme deficiencies), and additional testing is required. Type I: increased urine succinylacetone, nonspecific aminoaciduria, tissue analysis for FAH activity. Type II: increased tyrosine in blood and urine. Neonatal: increased tyrosine and Phe.

   d. **Treatment.** Type I: dietary, liver transplantation, nitisinone. Type II: diet low in tyrosine and Phe. Neonatal: usually transient, decrease protein intake and breast feeding. Possible ascorbic acid supplements.

B. **Fatty acid oxidation disorders**

1. **Medium chain acyl-CoA dehydrogenase (MCAD) deficiency.** Disorder of fatty acid oxidation. Previously implicated in some cases of sudden infant death syndrome (SIDS). Incidence in United States is 1 in 17,000.

   a. **Manifestations.** Vomiting, lethargy, coma, seizures, or death in some cases after 8 to 16 hours of fasting, during illness, or after surgery. Some infants who die are misdiagnosed as having SIDS.

   b. **Screening.** Best to perform test in the first 8 days of life. Best test is MS/MS measuring octanoylcarnitine on filter blood spot.

   c. **Follow-up.** Octanoylcarnitine >1.0 μmol/L needs further testing (plasma acylcarnitine analysis and urinary organic acid analysis to confirm diagnosis, molecular testing).

   d. **Treatment.** Avoid fasting, decrease intake of dietary fat, and provide carnitine supplementation in proven deficiency. If the infant is ill, admit for intravenous glucose and carnitine.

C. **Hemoglobinopathies**

1. **Sickle cell disease.** Group of genetic disorders caused by abnormal hemoglobin, resulting in distorted cells, hemolysis, vascular occlusion, and severe pain. Incidence is 1 in 200,000 in the United States and highest in African Americans (1 in 365 births) and Hispanic Americans (1 in 16,300 births).

   a. **Manifestations.** Later in infancy: painful crises involving the abdominal and musculoskeletal systems, splenic sequestration, priapism, bacterial sepsis/meningitis, stroke, pulmonary hypertension.

   b. **Screening.** Increase in false negatives in extreme preterm birth. Screen before blood transfusion; if the infant had a blood transfusion, do the test >90 days after the transfusion. Screen with isoelectric focusing, high-performance liquid chromatography (HPLC), or cellulose acetate electrophoresis. For retesting, use hemoglobin electrophoresis, HPLC, immunologic tests, and molecular genetic testing.

    c. Follow-up. For abnormal screen, do a second blood sample at <2 months of age. Do isoelectric focusing, HPLC, hemoglobin electrophoresis, and/or DNA analysis.

    d. Treatment. Specialized multidisciplinary care. Prophylactic penicillin (started at 2 months of age), immunizations (pneumococcal), urgent care of acute illness. Some may benefit from hydroxyurea therapy or stem cell therapy.

D. Other newborn screening tests

    1. Congenital hypothyroidism. Inadequate production of thyroid hormone. Incidence is 1 in 2000 to 4000 newborns. It is more common in Asian, Native American, and Hispanic infants. It is 28 times more common among infants with Down syndrome (1 in 100) than in the general population (see also Chapter 129).

        a. Manifestations. Normal at birth (maternal thyroid hormone protective); large fontanels, macroglossia, distended abdomen, umbilical hernia, mottling of skin, wide sutures, constipated, lethargic, increased sleepiness, cool to touch, prolonged jaundice (immature hepatic glucuronyl transferase), deafness, and others.

        b. Screening. Blood spot thyroid-stimulating hormone (TSH) or thyroxine (T_4) or both used. If screening with the T_4 test in a preterm infant, it can be false positive; if screening with the TSH test in a preterm infant, it can be false negative. If testing at <48 hours with the thyrotropin method, false positives can occur. Screen by measuring T_4 first; if low (<10%), then measure thyrotropin. Some measure thyrotropin first.

        c. Follow-up. If screening is abnormal, measure serum T_4; some measure free T_4, TSH, and thyroid-binding proteins. Once diagnosis is made, additional testing may be done to determine etiology (optional), including thyroid ultrasound, thyroid uptake, and scan. If maternal autoimmune thyroid disease is present, measure thyrotropin-binding inhibitor immunoglobulin in mom and baby (to rule out transient hypothyroidism).

        d. Treatment. Levothyroxine (tablet form; 10–15 μg/kg/d) is started as soon as possible after initial blood tests confirm the diagnosis. Pediatric endocrinologist should be involved, and close monitoring is recommended the first 2 to 3 years.

    2. Cystic fibrosis (CF). An autosomal recessive genetic disorder caused by the defect in the *CFTR* gene that affects the secretory glands that make mucus. Incidence is 1 in 3500.

        a. Manifestations. Meconium ileus occurs in 17% of infants with CF. Other manifestations include progressive lung disease with multiple chronic endobronchial infections, nutritional deficits (protein malnutrition) leading to edema, dysfunction of the pancreas, liver disease, and others.

        b. Screening. Do the immunoreactive trypsinogen (IRT) test after the first 24 hours, due to false positives in the first 24 hours. Repeat the test if the infant had a blood transfusion in 3 to 6 weeks. IRT concentration on the initial blood test is the first-tier test. If high, either do a CF mutation analysis from the blood or repeat the test in 2 to 3 weeks to see if there is a persistent elevation of IRT.

        c. Follow-up. Sweat chloride testing (>40 mmol/L to diagnose CF) is recommended after repeat IRT testing and after mutation analysis if 2 disease-causing variants are identified. Sweat chloride testing can be done in term infants at 1 week of age. Mutation analysis is recommended in preterm infants due to poor test validity.

        d. Treatment. Nutrition is of utmost importance. Testing for fecal elastase may help to determine the need for pancreatic enzyme supplements. Fat-soluble vitamins, salt supplements, and pancreatic enzymes are recommended as soon as possible. Respiratory management includes inhalers, chest physiotherapy, and hospitalizations for pulmonary exacerbations.

3. **Biotinidase deficiency** is a condition where the infant is unable to process (reuse and recycle) the vitamin biotin, which is essential for breaking down fats, proteins, and carbohydrates.

   a. **Manifestations.** Seizures, hypotonia, conjunctivitis, apnea, eczematoid rash, developmental delay, sensorineural deafness, optic atrophy. Incidence of profound deficiency is 1 in 112,000; incidence of partial deficiency is 1 in 129,000.

   b. **Screening.** Screen before blood transfusion; otherwise, do the test >90 days after transfusion. Filter paper spotted with whole blood is assessed for biotinidase activity by a semiquantitative colorimetric method. Up to 20% of patients with symptomatic biotinidase deficiency can be missed if screened with MS/MS, so this method should not be used.

   c. **Follow-up.** A serum specimen for quantitative measurement of biotinidase activity should be obtained if the screening results were positive.

   d. **Treatment.** Many symptoms are reversible with treatment; others, such as optic atrophy and deafness, are not. **Profound deficiency:** High-dose biotin therapy (only free form; 5–20 mg/d). **Partial deficiency:** Lower doses of biotin (1–5 mg/d) daily or during stress.

4. **Galactosemia.** An accumulation of galactose in the blood caused by 1 of 3 enzyme deficiencies (GALT deficiency [classic and most common], galactokinase [GALK] deficiency, or galactose epimerase [GALE] deficiency). It can be fatal if not treated early. Incidence is 1 in 47,000 for GALT deficiency and 1 in 40,000 for GALK deficiency; GALE deficiency is extremely rare.

   a. **Manifestations.** Classical GALT deficiency presents within the first few weeks after birth with vomiting, diarrhea, lethargy, hypotonia, prolonged bleeding after venipuncture, hepatomegaly, feeding intolerance, jaundice, and cataracts. GALK deficiency usually presents in a more subtle manner, and bilateral cataracts is the often the only feature seen.

   b. **Screening.** If using the GALT method of testing, screen before blood transfusion; otherwise, do the test >90 days after the transfusion. False negatives can be seen for infants on TPN. If using the galactose method, the infant needs to be on a galactose-containing formula. Screening tests vary by state and measure galactose, galactose-1-phosphate plus galactose, and/or GALT enzyme levels, which can be done using MS/MS. The GALT enzyme test is performed using red blood cells and is diagnostic only for classic galactosemia.

   c. **Follow-up.** All infants with a positive screening result should be seen by a physician as soon as possible and placed on a galactose-restricted diet pending definitive diagnostic testing. Testing for classic galactosemia includes quantitative analysis of GALT and red blood cell galactose-1-phosphate. If normal, quantitative analysis for GALK and GALE is done to rule out these disorders.

   d. **Treatment.** Lifelong galactose restriction is indicated for GALT deficiency, GALK deficiency, and the generalized form of GALE deficiency. Breast feeding is not allowed in these infants. Some suggest that an elemental galactose-free formula is preferred over a soy formula.

5. **Congenital adrenal hyperplasia (CAH).** Group of disorders of the adrenal cortex that affect production of 1 or more of the following: cortisol, aldosterone, or mineralocorticoids. Screening focuses on the most common **21-hydroxylase deficiency** (>90%), which results in impaired conversion of 17-hydroxyprogesterone (17-OHP) to 11-deoxycortisol. Variants in the *CYP21A2* gene result in decreased production of cortisol and aldosterone, causing excess adrenocorticotropic hormone (ACTH) secretion. Incidence is 1 in 15,981 in North America.

   a. **Manifestations.** Depend on subtype. Salt-wasting form (70% of infants affected) can present with adrenal crisis from 1 to 4 weeks of age with vomiting, diarrhea, FTT, lethargy, dehydration, and poor feeding. Circulatory shock and death can occur. Females with the disease may have ambiguous genitalia. The mild form of the disease usually manifests no symptoms as a newborn but later on can present with excessive acne, hirsutism, infertility, and premature axillary and pubic hair.

   b. **Screening benefits.** May prevent a life-threatening acute adrenal crisis, male sex assignment in virilized female newborns, and excess adrenal androgens that affect both males and females. Do the test at >24 hours of age to prevent false positives, before 5 to 7 days, and a few hours after a transfusion. False-positive results are increased in preterm infants. Screening is nonspecific and is done by measuring 17-OHP concentration on the dried blood sample with either radioimmunoassay or dissociation-enhanced lanthanide fluorescence immunoassay.

   c. **Follow-up.** With an abnormal screen, check serum 17-OHP and electrolytes as soon as possible. Other indication for these tests include any newborn with a disorder of sex development. An ACTH stimulation test is useful for ruling out nonclassic CAH in infants with mild elevations of 17-OHP levels.

   d. **Treatment.** Chronic treatment involves supplementation (eg, hydrocortisone 10–25 mg/m^2/d in 2–3 divided daily doses). In infants with salt-wasting CAH, add mineralocorticoid (fludrocortisone [Florinef] 0.05–0.2 mg) and consider supplementation with sodium chloride (2–5 g/d). In times of stress, more specialized treatment is necessary. Infants with CAH should be followed by a pediatric endocrinologist and pediatric urologist. Corrective surgery in severely virilized females may be necessary.

6. **Congenital hearing loss.** Hearing loss that is permanent and is >30 dB in the frequency region for speech recognition. It may be unilateral or bilateral and is either sensorineural or conductive. Causes include variants, ototoxic drug exposure (aminoglycosides), or bacterial or viral infections (cytomegalovirus [CMV], rubella).

   a. **Manifestations.** Seventy percent of cases are nonsyndromic (not associated with a recognized syndrome). Infant will not startle or wake up to loud noises, music, or voices.

   b. **Screening.** Universal screening should be done before initial discharge from the hospital or no later than 1 month of age. Although **automated auditory brainstem response (ABR) and otoacoustic emission (OAE)** are the primary methods used, ABR is the recommended screening tool for infants with neonatal intensive care unit (NICU) stays >5 days because of the high risk of neural hearing loss. If the infant in the newborn nursery does not pass the initial screening test, the infant is usually rescreened before discharge.

   c. **Follow-up.**

      i. **Follow-up testing by an audiologist** should be performed prior to 3 months of age for all infants who do not pass the initial 2 screening tests in the newborn nursery or the initial screening test in the NICU. Rescreening of both ears is recommended.

      ii. **Infants who have 1 or more risk factors** should have ongoing developmentally appropriate hearing screening and have at least 1 diagnostic assessment by an audiologist no later than 24 to 30 months of age regardless of initial screening results. **Risk factors include the following:** family history of permanent or sensorineural hearing loss, in utero infections (CMV, herpes, rubella, syphilis, toxoplasmosis), physical findings such as white forelock (Waardenburg syndrome), craniofacial anomalies, hyperbilirubinemia necessitating exchange transfusion, assisted ventilation, ototoxic medications (gentamicin and tobramycin), loop diuretics (furosemide) including chemotherapy, treatment with extracorporeal membrane oxygenation, culture-positive postnatal infections associated with sensorineural hearing loss (bacterial and viral meningitis, herpes, varicella), mechanical ventilation, neurodegenerative disorders, syndromes known to include hearing loss (neurofibromatosis, osteopetrosis, or Usher, Alport, Pendred, Jervell, Lange-Nielson syndromes), caregiver concern, NICU stay >5 days, or trauma.

E. **Treatment.** A comprehensive approach to the management of infants diagnosed with congenital hearing loss is recommended, which includes a full genetic, pediatric, otolaryngology, dysmorphology, and audiologic evaluation. Referral to an early intervention program or state-run program is recommended as early as possible.

17 Genetic and Genomic Testing in the Newborn Period

Genetic testing is not a new concept in neonatology. Newborn metabolic screening is the largest utilization of universal genetic testing in medicine and has been used in neonatology since 1960. It was then that Dr. Robert Guthrie developed a blood test to screen infants for phenylketonuria. It is estimated that birth defects are detected in 3% to 6% of live births and that congenital malformations, deformations, and chromosomal abnormalities are the cause of approximately 20% of deaths before 1 year of age. Many genetic conditions present in the perinatal period. Understanding of the available technology and the ability to manage all the steps involved in genomic testing have become essential tools for nongenetic specialists, including neonatologists and pediatricians. The study of genetics and genomics overlaps in the DNA analysis of specific genes, with the majority of diseases having complex genetic signatures. Genomics is a relatively new field, arising with the completion of the Human Genome Project in 2003, which mapped over 3 billion nucleotides in the 23 pairs chromosomes. Genomic technology advances have had a major impact on the care of newborns, especially those who are critically ill. Consequently, genomic testing is used more frequently, and as a result, pediatric providers need to be knowledgeable about the wide variety of tools that are becoming available. Information in this chapter is applicable to the newborn screening and congenital abnormalities discussed in Chapters 16 and 93.

I. **Definitions**

A. **Genetics versus genomics.** These terms are commonly used interchangeably but are not strictly the same thing.

1. **Genetics** refers to the study of a single or limited number of genes and their role in heredity.

2. **Genomics** is a broader term and involves the study of the individual's complete DNA sequence (genome). It can encompass the approximately 20,000 genes the genome contains and their interaction with each other and the environment in health and disease.

B. **Exons** are parts of the DNA sequence that code for proteins, whereas **introns** are considered to be noncoding, intergenic regions, which are thought to contain regulatory elements.

C. **Exome** is the total of all the exons (whole-exome sequencing [WES]).

D. **Genome** is the complete DNA sequence, which includes the introns and exons (whole-genome sequencing [WGS]).

E. **Neome** is a term coined to include approximately 1000 genes associated with diseases often presenting in the newborn period.

F. **Genetic sequence variation.** The American College of Medical Genetics and Genomics (ACMG) has classified genetic variants on a 5-tier scale. Pathogenic, likely pathogenic, and variant of uncertain significance (VUS) are included in the clinical report; likely benign and benign variants are not usually included. Variant classification is based on available data, which is why it can change categories with time, going between pathogenic, likely pathogenic, benign, and so on.

1. **Pathogenic variant (previously called a mutation).** A variant in a gene sequence known to cause a disorder or problem.
2. **Likely pathogenic variant.** It is a variant in the gene strongly suspected to cause a disorder or problem, but supporting data may be somewhat limited.
3. **Variant of uncertain significance.** It does not fit the criteria for benign or pathogenic. Testing may detect a variant that has not yet been clearly classified as either disease causing or normal in the general population.
4. **Likely benign variant.** Studies suggest no damaging effect of the variant.
5. **Benign variant (also called polymorphisms).** Available data show that it does not cause disease and occurs commonly in the population.

G. **Single nucleotide polymorphism.** A single nucleotide polymorphism (SNP; pronounced "snip") is a specific variation in a single nucleotide in DNA. SNP microarray analysis can detect polymorphisms as well regions of homozygosity in the setting of uniparental disomy (UPD) as well as parental consanguinity or common ancestry.

H. **Autosomal dominant.** Only 1 pathogenic variant on 1 allele (specific version of a gene on each copy of the chromosome) needs to be present to cause the disease.

I. **Autosomal recessive.** Two pathogenic variants, 1 on each allele, are needed to cause the disease.

J. **Sanger sequencing.** The first DNA sequencing analytic technique, which is time consuming and expensive. However, it is considered the gold standard for its accuracy. Often used clinically for next-generation sequencing (NGS) confirmatory testing.

K. **Next-generation sequencing or deep sequencing.** This describes a high-throughput DNA sequencing technology that is rapid, affordable, and accurate and a standard in most testing laboratories. Usually relies on an automated gene chip microarray analyzer. It is used for genetic (single-gene and gene panel tests) and genomic testing (WES and WGS).

II. **Benefits of early identification of an underlying genetic or genomic disorder**
   A. **Improved patient care.**
   B. **Avoid unnecessary additional diagnostic tests.**
   C. **Avoid nonbeneficial treatment.**
   D. **Family counseling and reproductive planning.**
   E. **Aids in the decision regarding palliative care.**
   F. **Confirms the clinical diagnosis.**
   G. **May give information that is relevant to making a medical decision.**
   H. **Aids in specific drug treatment** (genotypic drugs or pharmacogenomics) or treatment modification or management.
      1. **Vitamin therapy** (identification of *STXBP1* mutation led to the diagnosis of Ohtahara syndrome, which requires folinic acid treatment).
      2. **Ivacaftor (Kalydeco)** for some patients with cystic fibrosis.
      3. **Identification of a gene for focal familial hyperinsulinism** in an infant with refractory hypoglycemia allows planning surgery.
      4. **Cost effectiveness.** Genomic testing may save money by preventing the use of prolonged and expensive diagnostic testing and treatments.

III. **Limitations in the use of genetic or genomic testing**
   A. **Positive results not predictive of clinical course.**
   B. **May lead to an incorrect diagnosis.**
   C. **Incidental findings may reveal genetic mutations that predispose to cancer or neurodegeneration,** or a variant that you were not testing for may be found. Recommendations on how to address these "accidental" discoveries are being debated.
   D. **Cost of testing.** Genomic assays can cost US $1000 to $10,000.

E. **Genetic privacy issues may impact the individuals.** The Genetic Information Non-discrimination Act (GINA) of 2008 protects Americans from discrimination based on their genetic information in both health insurance and employment.

IV. **Common findings that raise suspicion of a genetic or genomic disorder in a newborn**

A. **A critically ill infant with metabolic abnormalities** such as severe lactic acidemia or hyperammonemia.

B. **An isolated major anomaly or multiple congenital anomalies (see Chapter 93).**

C. **Dysmorphic features.**

D. **Growth delay.**

E. **Neurologic problems including hypotonia and seizures.**

F. **Family history of known genetic disorder.**

G. **Abnormal prenatal genetic testing and/or screening.**

V. **Steps in incorporating genetic or genomic testing for diagnosis**

A. **Obtain a detailed history and physical examination.** The physical exam helps to define the **phenotype** (description of physical characteristics) of the infant. The history with the phenotype may help narrow the differential diagnosis and guide specific testing (eg, an infant with physical characteristics suggestive of Down syndrome enables the clinician to just order 1 test, a karyotype to diagnose trisomy 21).

1. **Family history.** Minimum of 3 generation pedigrees. Document known genetic conditions, birth defects, learning and developmental problems, autism, miscarriages, stillbirths, infant or childhood deaths, or consanguinity.

2. **Maternal history.** Medications, drugs, alcohol, toxins, chronic maternal diseases, maternal infections during pregnancy.

3. **Physical examination.** Perform a detailed examination with close attention to congenital anomalies (major and minor). Anthropomorphic measurements need to be done. See examples of physical findings of chromosomal syndromes, sequences, and teratogenic malformation syndromes in Chapter 93.

B. **Testing.** It is often difficult to decide which test to order because frequently there is no one perfect test. Some tests are better for diagnosing specific conditions. Consultation with a geneticist or genetic counselor can help identify the most appropriate test.

1. **Genomic testing approaches**

a. **Targeted diagnostic testing** is the use of a specific genomic test in an infant with a suspected but unconfirmed condition, with the hope that identifying the correct genetic diagnosis will ensure appropriate management. This also facilitates recurrence risk counseling and testing for relatives. It can be helpful for infants with a suspected metabolic condition that is not detectable on newborn screening tests (mitochondrial disorders, Smith-Lemli-Opitz syndrome). Examples of targeted diagnostic testing include multigene panel for Noonan syndrome, fluorescence in situ hybridization (FISH) for Williams syndrome, or *FBN1* sequencing for Marfan syndrome.

b. **Rapid diagnostic broad genomic testing.** This is usually done in critically ill newborns in whom a clinical workup and targeted genetic testing did not diagnose any specific condition. Evidence supports an impact on direct care. In one study, WGS done in 23 critically ill patients who had a nondiagnostic clinical workup revealed compound heterozygous mutations in 30%.

2. **Types of genetic testing and when to order the test.** Genetic testing is already used widely in the neonatal intensive care unit.

a. **American Academy of Pediatrics (AAP) and American College of Medical Genetics and Genomics recommendations for genetic testing in children**

i. **Genetic testing and screening should be offered in the context with genetic counseling** and only if it is in the best interest of the child.

ii. **If genetic testing is recommended for diagnostic testing,** the parents should give permission after hearing the benefits and risks. Pharmacogenomics testing is acceptable with permission of parents.

     iii. **American Academy of Pediatrics and American College of Medical Genetics and Genomics** support mandatory newborn screening to all children. Parents have the option of refusing the screening after education and counseling occur.

     iv. **American Academy of Pediatrics and American College of Medical Genetics and Genomics** do not support routine carrier testing in minors when the testing does not provide health benefits to the child.

     v. **Parents may allow predictive genetic testing for asymptomatic children who are at risk for a disease that occurs in childhood.** It is not recommended for adult-onset conditions unless an intervention is recommended in childhood. It is best to be cautious when providing this test to minors without parental involvement.

     vi. **The same rules of genetic testing in biologic families should apply for adopted children.** In cases of a child having a known genetic risk, prospective parents should be aware, and in rare cases, predictive genetic testing may be considered to ensure the family is willing to accept the challenges.

     vii. **Tissue compatibility testing of all minors is allowed.**

     viii. **Parents/legal guardians should inform the child** of the genetic test results at an appropriate age.

     ix. **American Academy of Pediatrics and American College of Medical Genetics and Genomics** strongly discourage direct to consumer home genetic kits.

C. Genetic test types

  1. Karyotype. Identifies and evaluates the size, shape, and number of chromosomes. Ideal for detecting aneuploidy, such as trisomies and monosomy. Detects large deletions/duplications and translocations. Covers the whole genome but has limited ability to detect smaller deletions and duplications. **Recommended diagnostic test for infants with suspected aneuploidy** (eg, Down syndrome, Turner syndrome, trisomy 18 or trisomy 13), as well as large deletion syndromes (eg, cat eye syndrome or cri du chat syndrome).

  2. Fluorescence in situ hybridization. Rapid analysis test with a quick turnaround that evaluates specific regions of the DNA sequence on a chromosome. Can detect large as well as small deletions; more difficult to detect duplications. Useful for detecting trisomies, microdeletions, and sex chromosome anomalies relatively quickly.

  3. Chromosomal microarray analysis/array comparative genomic hybridization. Detects large and small (micro) deletions or duplications in part of or a whole chromosome. Does not detect a balanced chromosomal rearrangement, triplet repeat expansions, or sequence variations. **First-line test for multiple congenital anomalies and developmental disabilities, especially for patients with a specific recognizable diagnosis.** Useful for some conditions such as 22q11.2 deletion (DiGeorge/velocardiofacial syndrome), Williams syndrome (microdeletion 7q11.23), and 1p36 deletion.

  4. Single-gene sequencing and multigene panel assays. Sequencing involves checking the DNA for sequence alterations or "spelling errors." Targeted sequencing is preferred in the setting of a recognizable phenotype with a high suspicion for a specific diagnosis. Advantages include better coverage of the gene or genes under consideration, compared to WES or WGS, and a lower chance of unclear results. **Order single-gene sequence analysis** on an infant with suspected Marfan syndrome and a multigene panel for an infant with suspected Noonan syndrome.

  5. Epigenetic/methylation analysis. DNA methylation abnormalities can result in inappropriate expression or silencing of some genes. **This test is used in disorders** associated with methylation abnormalities (Beckwith-Wiedemann, Prader-Willi, and Angelman syndromes). These disorders are also associated with other genetic abnormalities, but methylation analysis is the first-tier testing recommended if there is a clinical suspicion in the newborn.

6. **Targeted deletion/duplication analysis.** Order this, for example, on an infant with suspected spinal muscular atrophy.

7. **Targeted/directed mutation analysis.** Order this on a newborn who you suspect may have achondroplasia.

8. **Mitochondrial genetic testing.** Mitochondria are the energy generators of the cell and have their own small genome. Mitochondrial diseases are extremely variable and are transmitted by several modes of inheritance. Findings in the newborn period that may suggest a mitochondrial disorder include hypotonia, feeding problems, need for respiratory support, seizures, lactic acidemia, liver disease, deafness, and ocular disease. Clinical diagnosis can be very difficult because of the overlap with numerous other diseases. Testing for mitochondrial diseases involves analyzing not only the mitochondrial genome but also some specific nuclear genes.

9. **Genomic testing.** Genomic medicine uses the application of WES and WGS data to classify human health and disease.

   a. **When to recommend genomic testing.** ACMG recommends WES and WGS for the following 3 situations:

      i. **Infant's presentation is strongly suggestive of a genetic etiology** but not specific enough for a targeted test.

      ii. **Infant's presentation is consistent with a disorder** that can be caused by many different genes.

      iii. **Infant's presentation suggests a specific condition,** but targeted testing was unsuccessful in making a diagnosis.

   b. **Before ordering whole-exome or whole-genome sequencing, it is recommended the following be done:**

      i. **Formal consultation with a medical geneticist/genetic counselor** for parents or legal guardians.

      ii. **Discuss limitations of the test,** describe possible results, and discuss possibility of VUS, incidental, and secondary findings.

      iii. **Discuss that the parents** have the option of getting or deferring the secondary/incidental findings.

      iv. **Test the infant with parent samples** as a reference to improve the diagnostic yield of WES and WGS.

   c. **Whole-exome sequencing analyzes most, but not all, of the protein-coding regions of the genes.** Useful test for nonspecific phenotypes and when all other tests are negative. WES has limited ability to detect copy number variations, large deletions, triplet repeat expansion, complex rearrangements, epigenetic (imprinting) disorders, and regulatory or deep intronic variants. One example is a newborn with epileptic encephalopathy who had a negative epilepsy panel. WES can be used for patients with features suggestive of a specific condition, such as congenital disorders of glycosylation, Noonan syndrome, or CHARGE (coloboma, central nervous system abnormalities, heart defects, atresia of the choanae, restricted growth and/or development, genital abnormalities, and ear anomalies) syndrome, where targeted testing is unrevealing.

   d. **Whole-genome sequencing is the broadest test available. It analyzes the majority of the DNA sequence of an individual.** WGS has been designed to identify not only variations in single nucleotides but also large genomic rearrangements. It is thought to have the potential to replace current genetic tests, including chromosomal microarray analysis (CMA), multigene panel testing, and WES; however, there are still several limitations, similar to those described for exome sequencing. WGS is expected to become the preferred clinical practice, with a yield estimated at approximately 100 times more data than WES. At present, it is not being used clinically and is currently only considered when previous testing including microarray analysis and WES does not reveal a diagnosis. One example is a newborn with epileptic encephalopathy who has a negative microarray analysis and WES.

18 Studies for Neurologic Evaluation

Although continued improvements in neuroimaging and neuromonitoring have added insight into the developing brain and have helped the clinician to identify infants at risk for poor neurologic outcome, available techniques continue to have limited accuracy in predicting neurodevelopmental outcomes. Moreover, given the enormous plasticity of the neonate's brain, even significant detectable defects may result in "normal" neurodevelopmental outcomes. Nevertheless, imaging and monitoring modalities hold future promise in assisting clinicians to better identify and refer patients at risk for neurodevelopmental sequelae.

I. **Neuroimaging**
   A. **Ultrasonography**
      1. **Definition.** Using the bone window of a fontanelle, sound waves are directed into the brain and reflected according to the echodensity of the underlying structures. The reflected waves are used to create 2- and 3-dimensional images.
      2. **Indication.** Ultrasonography is preferred for identification and observation of germinal matrix/intraventricular hemorrhage and hydrocephalus. Ultrasound is valuable in detecting midline structural abnormalities, hypoxic ischemic injury, periventricular leukomalacia, subdural and posterior fossa hemorrhage, ventriculitis, periventricular calcifications, tumors, cysts, and vascular abnormalities.
      3. **Method.** A transducer is placed over the anterior fontanelle, and images are obtained in coronal and parasagittal planes. The posterior or mastoid fontanelle is the preferred acoustic window for the imaging of the infratentorium, including the fourth ventricle, brainstem, and cerebellum. Ultrasonography's advantages include high resolution, portability, safety (no sedation, contrast material, or radiation), noninvasiveness, and low cost. Disadvantages include the lack of visualization of non-midline structures, especially in the parietal regions, and the lack of differentiation between gray and white matter.
      4. **Results.** The integrity of the following structures may be evaluated with ultrasonography: all ventricles, the choroid plexus, caudate nuclei, thalamus, septum pellucidum, and corpus callosum.
   B. **Doppler ultrasonography**
      1. **Definition.** Doppler ultrasonography also uses a bone window to direct sound waves into the brain. The sound waves from the transducer are reflected by red blood cells in the vessel, and their frequency travels proportionally to the velocity of the circulating red blood cells. These changes are measured and expressed as the **pulsatility index and resistance index (RI)**. The angle of the probe in relation to the flow affects the Doppler shift and requires exact standards for serial measurements.
      2. **Indication.** Doppler ultrasonography of the anterior cerebral artery is a sensitive and specific tool for measuring **cerebral blood flow (CBF)** and resistance in the neonatal period.

$$\text{CBF (cm}^3/\text{time)} = \text{CBF velocity (cm/time)} \times \text{area (cm}^2).$$

Doppler ultrasonography is of clinical value in states of cessation of CBF (eg, brain death or cerebrovascular occlusion), states of altered vascular resistance (eg, hypoxic ischemic encephalopathy, hydrocephalus, or arteriovenous [AV] malformation), and ductal steal syndrome.
      3. **Method.** Combined with conventional ultrasonography to identify the blood vessel, Doppler ultrasonography produces a color image indicating flow (red = toward the transducer; blue = away from the transducer). CBF velocity is measured as

the area under the curve of velocity waveforms. Small body weight and low gestational ages negatively influence the success rate in visualizing intracranial vasculature. Contrast-enhanced ultrasound is a novel technique, whereby intravenously injected gas-filled microbubbles (smaller than red cells) generate an increased signal, from acoustic impedance mismatch, allowing for enhanced visualization of blood vessels. This has been used for improved characterization of perfusion abnormalities in neonates with hypoxic ischemic injury.

4. **Results.** Doppler ultrasonography measurements can be compared with age-adjusted norm values for systolic, end-diastolic, and mean flow velocity. Elevated RI suggests vasoconstriction and diminished blood flow velocity. Conversely, diminished RI suggests vasodilation with increased blood flow velocity. Serial measurement of CBF and RI may be helpful in following lesions associated with increased cerebral pressure (eg, determining the need for a ventriculoperitoneal shunt in progressive hydrocephalus).

C. **Computed tomography**

1. **Definition.** Using computerized image reconstruction, computed tomography (CT) produces 2- and 3-dimensional images of patients exposed to ionizing radiation.

2. **Indication.** CT is the preferred tool for evaluation of the posterior fossa and non-midline disorders (eg, blood or fluid collection in the subdural or subarachnoid space). It is also helpful in the diagnosis of skull fractures. CT is used less often in neonatal units given the risks of exposure to ionizing radiation in infancy, which has been linked to development of future malignancies.

3. **Method.** The patient is advanced in small increments in a scanner, and images (cuts) are obtained. Cerebral white matter (more fatty tissue in myelin sheaths around the nerves) and inflammation appear less dense (blacker) than gray matter. Calcifications and hemorrhages appear white. If a patient receives contrast material, blood vessels and vascular structures (eg, falx cerebri and choroid plexus) appear white. Spaces containing cerebrospinal fluid are clearly shown in black, making it easy to identify diseases that alter their size and shape. Bones also appear white but are poorly defined, and details are better evaluated in a "bone window." Disadvantages include radiation exposure, the need for transportation, hypothermia, and the potential need for sedation during the procedure.

4. **Results.** CT provides detailed information on brain structures not accessible by ultrasonography and is superior to magnetic resonance imaging in the diagnosis of intracranial calcifications.

D. **Magnetic resonance imaging**

1. **Definition.** Inside a strong magnetic field, atomic nuclei with magnetic properties (hydrogen protons being most common) align themselves and emit an electromagnetic signal when the field is terminated and the nuclei return to their natural state. Computers reconstruct the signal into 2-dimensional image cuts. A variety of contrasts can be obtained in magnetic resonance imaging (MRI) including T1- and T2-weighted imaging (reflecting 2 relaxation time constraints, longitudinal and transverse, respectively), diffusion-weighted imaging (DWI), blood-oxygen-level-dependent (BOLD) imaging, and proton-density weighted imaging. In functional MRIs (fMRI), such as BOLD and DWI, underlying brain physiology is reflected in the created images.

2. **Indication.** MRI is the preferred tool for a number of brain disorders in the neonate that are difficult to visualize by CT, such as disorders of myelination or neural migration, ischemic or hemorrhagic lesions, agenesis of the corpus callosum, AV malformations, and lesions in the posterior fossa and the spinal cord. Diffusion-based MRI is the most sensitive to acute brain injury in the first week after injury. Conventional T1- and T2-weighted MRI is preferred after 1 week following the injury. Conventional MRI has been used at term equivalent or at the time of discharge from the hospital to predict neurologic outcome.

3. **Method.** The patient is advanced in small increments in a scanner, and images (cuts) are obtained. Gray matter appears gray and white matter, white. Cerebrospinal fluid and bones appear black; however, the fat content in the bone marrow and the scalp appear white. In T1 and T2 MRI, fluid may appear dark or bright, depending on the type of weighted image. Advantages of MRI include the ability to identify normal and pathologic anatomy without ionizing radiation and insight into neurologic prognosis. Disadvantages include the need for transportation and sedation, need for a ferromagnetic-free environment, the potential for hypothermia, and difficulties in monitoring during the procedure. Ventilated infants pose a special problem, and ferromagnetic-free MRI incubators have been developed and used to help prevent motion artifact, provide improved cardiorespiratory monitoring, maintain temperature and fluid status, and improve image quality by using built-in head coils. Ferromagnetic-free tracheostomy tubes are a necessary consideration for infants with tracheostomy tubes.

4. **Results.** MRI provides high-resolution images of the brain with exquisite anatomic detail and allows diagnosis of a number of illnesses easily missed by CT. The temporal development of the prenatal brain, including the emergence of sulci and gyri and the myelination process, has been described, allowing for a more meaningful interpretation of MRI in premature infants. Quantitative volumetric MRI has been used to demonstrate the effects of postnatal dexamethasone on cortical gray matter volume and to help provide long-term prognosis for neurologic outcome. Diffusion-weighted signal abnormalities appear early after a hypoxic ischemic event, and restricted diffusion on DWI is an early predictor of outcome. The volume of restricted diffusivity has been shown to provide a measure of the severity of acute brain injury in the setting of hypoxic ischemic injury. fMRI promises new insights into the functional reorganization of the brain after injury. Newer magnetic resonance spectroscopy allows the study of metabolic mechanisms through quantitative measurements of certain metabolites.

E. **Near-infrared spectroscopy**

1. **Definition.** Light in the near-infrared range can easily pass through skin, thin bone, and other tissues of the neonate. At selected wavelengths, light absorption depends on oxygenated and deoxygenated hemoglobin as well as oxidized cytochrome *aa* 3, allowing for qualitative measurements of oxygen delivery, cerebral blood volume, and brain oxygen availability and consumption.

2. **Indication.** Although use of near-infrared spectroscopy (NIRS) is not generalized, it has potential as a bedside tool to follow cerebral oxygen delivery or CBF including in cardiac patients. It is a useful technique to assess the effects of diseases such as congenital heart disease and new treatments and common interventions (eg, endotracheal suction, continuous positive airway pressure) on cerebral perfusion and oxygenation.

3. **Method.** A fiberoptic bundle applied to the scalp transmits laser light. Another fiberoptic bundle collects light and transmits it to a photon counter.

4. **Results.** NIRS allows qualitative determination of oxygen delivery, cerebral blood volume, and oxygen consumption. In intubated infants, NIRS has been used to identify pressure-passive cerebral circulation, a condition associated with a 4-fold increase in periventricular leukomalacia and severe intraventricular hemorrhage.

II. **Electrographic studies**

A. **Basic conventional electroencephalogram**

1. **Definition.** An electroencephalogram (EEG) captures the electrical activity between reference electrodes on the scalp. In the neonatal period, cerebral maturation and development result in significant EEG changes during different gestational ages that must be considered when interpreting results. The minimum duration for basic EEG is 1 hour, which allows for capture of sleep-wake cycle; the average duration of basic EEG is 1 to 8 hours.

    2. **Indication.** Basic EEG monitoring is indicated in infants thought to be at low risk for seizure activity and should not be used for infants who are at high risk for acute brain injury or seizure, as these infants require long-term continuous conventional EEG. Infants at low risk would include non–critically ill term infants without asphyxia, encephalopathy, or metabolic disorders and infants known to have normal central nervous system (CNS) anatomy. Basic EEG is helpful for differentiating seizure activity from paroxysmal nonepileptic events and avoidance of unnecessary medications.

    3. **Method.** Several electrodes are attached to the infant's scalp, and the electrical activity is amplified and measured. Recordings can be traced on paper or can be saved electronically. EEG waves are classified into different frequencies: delta (1–3/s), theta (4–7/s), alpha (8–12/s), and beta (13–20/s).

    4. **Results.** EEGs are sensitive to a number of external factors, including acute and ongoing illness, medications or drugs, position of the electrodes, and state of arousal. Obtaining a basic EEG for at least 1 hour allows for interpretation of the full sleep cycle, including active sleep, quite sleep, and intermediate sleep. EEG assesses for continuity versus discontinuity, synchrony, and age-appropriate electrographic landmarks. A number of abnormal findings can be documented on the EEG of the term and preterm infant, including the following:

      a. Abnormal pattern of development.

      b. Depression or lack of differentiation.

      c. Electrocerebral silence ("flat" EEG).

      d. Burst suppression pattern (depressed background activity alternating with short periods of paroxysmal bursts). Burst suppression patterns are associated with especially high morbidity and mortality and poor prognosis.

      e. Persistent voltage asymmetry.

      f. Sharp waves (multifocal or central).

      g. Periodic discharges.

      h. Rhythmic α-frequency activity.

B. Continuous conventional electroencephalogram

    1. **Definition.** Continuous conventional electroencephalogram (cEEG) captures the electrical activity between reference electrodes on the scalp over a prolonged period of time, ≥24 hours.

    2. **Indication.** Indications for cEEG includes infants with documented or high suspicion for seizure activity, acute neonatal encephalopathy, active CNS infections, CNS malformations, metabolic disorders, perinatal stroke or sinovenous thrombosis, and CNS trauma. Additionally, cEEG allows for refinement in seizure management by accurately diagnosing electrographic seizure activity and modifying treatment accordingly.

    3. **Method.** Methodology for cEEG is identical to basic EEG; however, the testing period is longer, a minimum of 24 hours in duration.

    4. **Results.** cEEG interpretation is the same as basic EEG with greater volumes of data, which allows for evolving assessment over time.

C. Polygraphic video electroencephalogram

    1. **Definition.** Polygraphic video electroencephalogram (VEEG) adds synchronized video monitoring of the infant, whereas the EEG captures the neuronal electrical activity. Synchronized video allows for the characterization of clinical events and is helpful in assessing artifacts that may mimic electrographic seizures. Short-term VEEG lasts on average 2 to 8 hours, and long-term VEEG is done for >24 hours.

    2. **Indication.** Infants with neonatal encephalopathy, paroxysmal events concerning for seizure, or the presence of high-risk diagnoses or interventions, including hypoxic ischemic encephalopathy, ischemic stroke, acute toxic metabolic processes, and occasionally extracorporeal membrane oxygenation, are ideal candidates for continuous VEEG.

3. **Method.** An electrode cap is placed on the patient's scalp, and mounted video cameras provide continuous video, audio, and brainwave monitoring. This network can be linked to a central server and be displayed for online remote observation. A bedside observer who can mark key clinical events in a written log or electronically is recommended. Key clinical events include suspected seizure activity, initiation of cooling protocol, and administration of neuroactive drugs. Duration of VEEG is dependent on indication for testing. Ideally, VEEG should be continued until multiple "typical" events are captured. If seizure activity is captured, it is recommended that VEEG monitoring continue until the patient has been seizure-free for at least 24 hours.

4. **Results.** The EEG reading and reporting are the same as in cEEG with the advantage of utilizing video to inform the interpretation process. Assessment of background activity and specific waves and patterns indicative of brain development holds promise.

D. **Amplitude-integrated electroencephalogram**

1. **Definition.** Amplitude-integrated electroencephalogram (aEEG) is a method for continuous long-term monitoring of overall brain activity utilizing a single EEG lead. Cerebral function monitor (CFM) refers to the specific monitor, which produces the aEEG output. The CFM filters and compresses the detected neurologic activity and provides information on the general level of electrical activity occurring throughout the brain. The aEEG output can be interpreted by neonatal staff without full knowledge of EEG to quickly determine overall neurologic status.

2. **Indication.** aEEG is sensitive for early prediction of outcome in asphyxiated term newborns. aEEG is used for assistance in the identification of clinical and subclinical seizure activity. In addition, it has been used to select patients for neuroprotective measures such as head or total-body cooling and has been useful in providing information on neurodevelopmental outcome in cases of hypoxic ischemic encephalopathy and intraventricular hemorrhages. The aEEG has also been used under other conditions including metabolic disorders, congenital anomalies, extracorporeal membrane oxygenation, and postoperative monitoring.

3. **Method.** aEEG uses a single lead, consisting of 3 wires placed over the biparietal or frontal region. The signal processing attenuates activity below 2 Hz and above 15 Hz, and the bandwidth reflects variations in minimum and maximum EEG amplitude. The aEEG recording is digitally displayed on screen of the CFM. Ideally, infants monitored with aEEG also have at least 1 standard EEG to obtain additional electrocortical information.

4. **Results.** The aEEG provides information on the background pattern of electrical activity of the brain (Table 18–1), the presence or absence of the sleep-wake cycle (SWC), and/or the presence of epileptiform activity and other examples of neonatal aEEG patterns (Figure 18–1). After asphyxia, the occurrence of a moderately or severely abnormal aEEG trace has a positive predictive value >70% for abnormal neurologic outcome. Burst suppression, low voltage, and flat trace in the first 12 to 24 hours after injury are associated with a poor prognosis. SWC returning before 36 hours is associated with a good outcome, and SWC returning after 36 hours is associated with a bad outcome. The sensitivity of aEEG for neonatal seizure detection is limited; however, compared to management based on clinical seizure detection alone, use of aEEG has been shown to reduce the total seizure duration in neonates.

E. **Peripheral nerve conduction velocity**

1. **Definition.** Nerve conduction velocity allows the diagnosis of a peripheral nerve disorder by measuring the transmission speed of an electrical stimulus along a peripheral (median, ulnar, peroneal) nerve. Because of smaller nerve fiber diameters affecting the nerve transmission speed, neonates have a lower nerve conduction velocity than adults.

Table 18–1. SUMMARY OF NORMAL SINGLE-CHANNEL AMPLITUDE-INTEGRATED ELECTROENCEPHALOGRAPHY FEATURES IN NEWBORNS AT DIFFERENT GESTATIONAL/ POSTCONCEPTIONAL AGES

Gestational or Postconceptional Age (wk)	Dominating Background Pattern	SWC	Minimum Amplitude (mcV)	Maximum Amplitude (mcV)	Burst/h
24–25	DC	(+)	2–5	25–50 (to 100)	>100
26–27	DC	(+)	2–5	25–50 (to 100)	>100
28–29	DC/(C)	(+)/+	2–5	25–30	>100
30–31	C/(DC)	+	2–6	20–30	>100
32–33	C/DC in QS	+	2–6	20–30	>100
34–35	C/DC in QS	+	3–7	15–25	>100
36–37	C/DC in QS	+	4–8	17–35	>100
38 +	C/DC in QS	+	7–8	15–25	>100

C, continuous; DC, discontinuous background pattern; QS, quiet/deep sleep; SWC, sleep-wake cycling; SWC (+), imminent/immature; SWC +, developed SWC.
Reproduced with permission from Hellström-Westas L, Rosén I, de Vries LS, et al: Amplitude-integrated EEG Classification and Interpretation in Preterm and Term Infants, *NeoReviews.* 2006 Feb;7(2):e76-e87.

2. **Indication.** In the weak and hypotonic neonate, nerve conduction velocity is an important tool in diagnosing a peripheral nerve disorder.
3. **Method.** A peripheral nerve is stimulated with a skin electrode, and the corresponding muscle action potential is recorded with another skin electrode. To determine the nerve conduction alone (as opposed to nerve conduction, synaptic transmission, and muscle reaction), the nerve is stimulated at 2 points, and the resulting muscle response times are subtracted. The distance between the 2 points of stimulation divided by the time difference equals the nerve conduction velocity.
4. **Results.** Nerve conduction velocities are prolonged in disorders of myelination and in axon abnormalities and may have potential clinical value in combination with other tests (eg, muscle biopsy or electromyogram) in these disorders. Initially, infants with anterior horn cell disorders (eg, Werdnig-Hoffmann paralysis) have normal nerve conduction but may demonstrate decreased velocity later in the course. Neuromuscular junction and muscle disorders do not alter nerve conduction velocity. This test is also used for gestational age assessment.
F. **Evoked potentials.** An evoked potential is an electrical response by the CNS to a specific stimulus. Evoked potentials are used to evaluate the intactness and maturity of *ascending* sensory pathways of the nervous system and are relatively unaffected by state, drug, or metabolic effects.
   1. **Auditory evoked potential**
      a. **Definition.** An auditory evoked potential (AEP) is an electrical response by the CNS to an auditory stimulus.
      b. **Indication.** Brainstem AEPs may be used to detect abnormalities in threshold sensitivities, conduction time, amplitudes, and shape and may be useful as a hearing screen in high-risk infants.

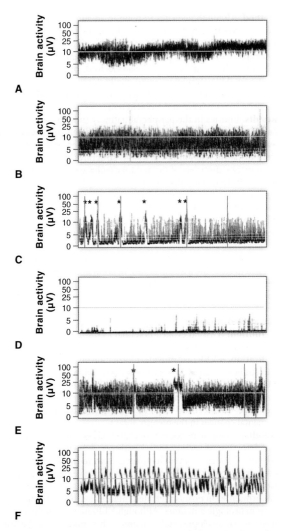

FIGURE 18–1. Sample amplitude-integrated electroencephalography (aEEG) patterns. The patterns are classified as follows: (**A**) **Continuous normal voltage** (normal background pattern for term infants characterized by continuous activity with lower amplitude at [5]-7-10 μV and maximum amplitudes at 10-25-[50] μV). (**B**) **Discontinuous normal voltage** (mildly abnormal in term infants, can be normal in some preterm infants depending on the postmenstrual age at the time of monitoring; characterized by discontinuous activity with some variability in the minimum amplitude, but mainly <5 μV and maximum amplitude >10 μV). (**C**) **Burst suppression** (abnormal background pattern characterized by minimum amplitude without variability at 0-2 μV intermixed with bursts of high-voltage activity >25 μV) with 7 short seizures (asterisks). (**D**) **Isoelectric or flat trace** (severely abnormal background pattern with inactive background corresponding with electrocerebral inactivity). (**E**) **Two seizures** (asterisks) can be identified by a rise in the upper and lower margins against a discontinuous normal voltage background. (**F**) **Saw-tooth pattern** of status epilepticus. (*Reproduced with permission from Bonifacio SL, Glass HC, Peloquin S, et al: A new neurological focus in neonatal intensive care,* Nat Rev Neurol. *2011 Aug 2;7(9):485-494.*)

    c. Method. Although neonates respond to an auditory stimulus with brainstem as well as cortical evoked responses, the latter are variable, depending on the state of arousal, and thus are difficult to interpret. As a result, AEPs (generated by a rapid sequence of clicks or puretones) traveling along the eighth nerve to the diencephalon are recorded by an electrode over the mastoid and vertex as brainstem AEPs, amplified, and digitally stored. The shape (a series of waves) and latency of brainstem AEPs depend on gestational age. This technique is sensitive to movement and ambient noise.

    d. Results. Injuries in the peripheral pathway (middle ear, cochlea, and eighth nerve) result in an increased sound threshold and an increase in latency of all waves, whereas central lesions cause only increased latency of waves originating from distal (in relation to the lesion) structures. Brainstem AEPs are used to demonstrate disorders of the auditory pathways caused by hypoxia-ischemia, hyperbilirubinemia, infections (eg, cytomegalovirus or bacterial meningitis), intracranial hemorrhage, trauma, systemic illnesses, or drugs (eg, aminoglycoside or furosemide). In low birthweight infants, brainstem AEPs have a high false-positive rate secondary to known gestational differences (longer latency, decreased amplitude, and increased threshold in preterm infants). Up to 20% to 25% of infants in the neonatal intensive care unit have abnormal (failed) tests, and most have normal tests at 2 to 4 months. In asphyxiated infants, abnormal brainstem AEPs are associated with neuromotor impairments. Because infants with congenital infection and persistent pulmonary hypertension may experience progressive hearing loss, they require serial hearing evaluations even if results are normal.

 2. Visual evoked potential

    a. Definition. A visual evoked potential (VEP) is an electrical response by the CNS to a visual stimulus.

    b. Indication. A VEP may provide information on disorders of the visual pathway and has been used as an indicator for cerebral malfunctioning (eg, hypoxia).

    c. Method. An electrical response to a visual stimulus (eg, light flash in neonates or checkerboard pattern reversal in older children) is measured via a surface electrode. The electrical response is complex and undergoes significant developmental changes in the preterm infant.

    d. Results. When corrected for conceptional age, visual evoked responses allow the detection of various visual pathway abnormalities. Although generalized insults such as severe hypoxemia may result in temporary loss of visual evoked responses, local abnormalities may have similar results (eg, compression of the pathway in hydrocephalus). Persistent visual evoked response abnormalities in postasphyxiated infants have been strongly correlated with poor neurologic outcomes. Although VEPs may aid in the prognosis of long-term neurodevelopmental outcomes, they may not be helpful in predicting blindness or loss of vision. Improvements in visual evoked responses have also been applied to determine the success of interventions such as a ventricular-peritoneal shunt. The prognostic value in preterm infants is *controversial*.

 3. Somatosensory evoked potential

    a. Definition. A somatosensory evoked potential (SEP) is an electrical response by the CNS to a peripheral sensory stimulus.

    b. Indication. SEPs allow insight into disorders of the sensory pathway (peripheral nerve, plexus, dorsal root, posterior column, contralateral nucleus, medial lemniscus, thalamus, and parietal cortex).

    c. Method. SEPs have been recorded over the contralateral parietal scalp after providing an electric stimulus to the median or the posterior tibial nerve. SEPs are technically more difficult to obtain than auditory brainstem evoked potentials and are age dependent with significant changes occurring in the first months of life.

    d. Results. SEPs may allow evaluation of peripheral lesions such as spinal cord trauma and myelodysplasia as well as cerebral abnormalities such as hypoxia, ischemia, hemorrhage, hydrocephalus, hypoglycemia, and hypothyroidism. SEP abnormalities in term infants have a high positive predictive value for neurologic sequelae and abnormal neurodevelopmental outcome. The significance of SEP remains *controversial* in the preterm infant.

III. Clinical neurodevelopmental examination

    A. Definition. The clinical neurodevelopmental examination combines the assessment of posture, movement, extremity and axial muscle tone, deep tendon reflexes, pathologic reflexes (eg, Babinski sign), primitive (or primary) reflexes, cranial nerve and oromotor function, sensory responses, and behavior by an *experienced* clinician.

    B. Indication. All infants should undergo a brief neurologic examination, including tone and reflex assessment, as part of their initial physical examination. A more detailed neurodevelopmental examination should be performed on high-risk infants. Important risk factors include prematurity, hypoxic ischemic encephalopathy, congenital infection, meningitis, significant abnormalities on neuroimaging studies (eg, intraventricular hemorrhage, ventricular dilatation, intraparenchymal hemorrhage, infarct, or cysts), and feeding difficulties.

    C. Method. The experienced clinician should examine the infant when stable, preferably during the recovery phase. However, the examination may also be quite useful when performed serially, as with hypoxic ischemic encephalopathy. The infant's state of alertness may affect many responses, including sensory response, behavior, tone, and reflexes. Normal findings change according to age (actual and postconceptional).

        1. The full-term neonate. The normal full-term neonate has flexor hypertonia, hip adductor tone, hyperreflexia (may have unsustained clonus), symmetric tone and reflexes, good trunk tone on ventral suspension, some degree of head lag on pulling to a sitting from a supine position with modulation of forward head movement, presence of pathologic (eg, Babinski sign) and primitive reflexes (eg, Moro, grasp, and asymmetric tonic neck reflexes), alerting to sound, visual fixation, and a fixed focal length of 8 in.

        2. The preterm neonate. Before 30 weeks' postconceptional age, the infant is markedly hypotonic. Extremity flexor and axial tone and the reflexes emerge in a caudocephalad (ie, lower to upper extremity) and centripetal (ie, distal to proximal) manner. Visual attention and acuity improve with postconceptional age. The extremely preterm infant can suck and swallow, but coordination of suck with swallow occurs at approximately 32 to 34 weeks' postconceptional age. Flexor tone peaks at term and then becomes decreased in a caudocephalad manner. In comparison with full-term neonates, preterm infants at term have less flexor hypertonia, more extensor tone, more asymmetries, and mild differences in behavior.

    D. Results. Abnormalities on neurodevelopmental examination include asymmetries of posture or reflexes (especially significant if marked or persistent), decreased flexor or extremity tone or axial tone for postconceptional age, cranial nerve or oromotor dysfunction, abnormal sensory responses, abnormal behavior (eg, lethargy, irritability, or jitteriness), and extensor neck, trunk, or extremity tone. A normal neonatal neurodevelopmental examination is reassuring, but an abnormal examination cannot be used to diagnose disability in the neonatal period. The more abnormalities that are found on examination and the greater the degree of abnormality (eg, marked neck extensor hypertonia), the higher the incidence of later disability, including cerebral palsy and intellectual disability.

19 Blood Component Therapy

I. **Blood banking procedures**
   A. **Type and screen.** Whenever possible, serum or plasma samples from both mother and infant should be obtained for initial ABO group and Rh(D) type determinations.
      1. **Investigations of the maternal sample should include:**
         a. **ABO group and Rh(D) type.**
         b. **Screen for unexpected red cell antibodies** by an indirect antiglobulin technique (IAT).
            i. **Unexpected (or atypical) red cell antibodies** are clinically significant allogeneic antibodies (alloantibodies) other than the isohemagglutinins, anti-A and/or anti-B, whose presence may be expected depending on the ABO group.
            ii. **If possible, review maternal antenatal records** regarding antibody evaluations.
      2. **Investigations of the infant (or umbilical cord) sample should include:**
         a. **ABO group and Rh(D) type.**
         b. **Direct antiglobulin test** (DAT) performed on neonatal red cells.
         c. **In the absence of maternal serum or plasma,** the infant's serum or plasma is screened for unexpected antibodies by an IAT.
            i. **Infants very rarely make alloantibodies during the first 4 months of life,** but they may have maternal alloantibodies acquired transplacentally.
            ii. **Repeat ABO group and Rh(D) type determinations may be omitted** throughout the remainder of the neonate's hospital admission or until age 4 months is attained, whichever occurs sooner.
         d. **If a non–group-O neonate is to be transfused with non–group-O erythrocytes,** which are incompatible with the maternal ABO group, then the neonate's serum or plasma must be tested for anti-A and anti-B using an IAT. If either antibody is detected, then donor erythrocytes that lack the corresponding antigen must be chosen for transfusion.
   B. **Type and cross-match red blood cells**
      1. **Perform an initial screen** for unexpected (or atypical) red blood cell (RBC) antibodies.
         a. **Test donor candidate red blood cells against infant's serum or plasma** (from umbilical cord [preferred] or venous blood) and inspect for agglutination and/or hemolysis after incubation at 37°C (98.6°F).
         b. **Alternatively, if mother and neonate are ABO compatible,** then maternal serum or plasma may be used (to limit neonatal venipunctures).
         c. **If this initial screen for red cell antibodies is negative,** then there is no need to perform cross-matching during the remainder of the neonate's hospital admission or until age 4 months is attained, whichever occurs sooner. **If the initial screen for RBC antibodies is positive, then additional testing must be done.**
      2. **Perform tests to determine the specificity** of any antibodies identified.
         a. **Using an indirect antiglobulin technique, test maternal or infant serum or plasma** against a panel of group O reagent erythrocytes of known antigenic phenotype.
      3. **Transfused red cells** used typically must lack the corresponding antigen(s) and be compatible by antiglobulin phase cross-match with maternal or infant serum or plasma. In case of antibodies to extremely rare antigens, antigen-typed red cells may not be available, but antiglobulin phase cross-match must still be compatible.

  a. **Cross-matches are needed with each transfusion** until antibodies are no longer demonstrable in the neonate's serum or plasma.
  b. **The presence of multiple antibodies** increases the difficulty of identifying compatible donors and delays blood availability.

II. Routine blood donation

  A. Voluntary blood donations. These are from donors with both a negative history for and negative screening tests for transfusion-transmissible diseases. All blood donors are tested using serologic enzyme immunoassays (EIAs) and nucleic acid amplification tests (NATs) for viral risks that include HIV (1 and 2), hepatitis viruses B and C (HBV and HCV), human T-cell lymphotropic viruses (HTLV [I and II]), West Nile virus (WNV), and Zika virus. The only screening assay for parasites currently is an EIA for antibodies to *Trypanosoma cruzi* (cause of Chagas disease; once in donor's lifetime). In addition, EIA or microhemagglutination testing for *Treponema pallidum* (syphilis) is still required. Testing obviously is not performed for all blood-borne threats; testing for the following viruses is *not* routinely done: cytomegalovirus (CMV), parvovirus B19, hepatitis A virus (HAV), Epstein-Barr virus (EBV), and human herpes virus-8 (HHV-8 or Kaposi sarcoma–associated herpes virus [KSHV]).

  B. The residual risks of transfusion per unit transfused are estimated to be:
  1. **Human immunodeficiency virus types 1 and 2.** 1 per 1,467,000.
  2. **Hepatitis C virus.** 1 per 1,149,000.
  3. **Hepatitis B virus.** 1 per 280,000 to 1 per 843,000 depending on length of infectious period
  4. **Human T-cell lymphotropic virus types I and II.** 1 per 2,993,000 to 1 per 4,364,000 (2007–2008 estimate). An accurate risk estimate applicable to the United States is not currently possible.
  5. **West Nile virus.** Risk for WNV varies with location, date, and test method (mini pool NAT vs individual NAT) and has been decreasing in recent years, so a single risk estimate applicable to the Unites States is not possible. Similar considerations apply to **Zika virus**, except incidence has been increasing in recent years.
  6. **Risk for transfusion-transmitted** *T cruzi* **is unknown;** 20 cases have been reported as transfusion transmitted globally in nonendemic areas. Prevalence in blood donors is estimated as 1 per 38,500.
  7. **For perspective, selected comparative mortality odds ratios are: anesthesia**—1 per 7000 to 340,000; **flood**—1 per 455,000; and **lightning strike**—1 per 10,000,000.

III. Donor-directed blood products. Blood provided by a relative or friend of the family for a specified infant.

  A. This technique cannot be used in an emergency setting because it takes up to 48 hours to process the blood for use.
  B. There is no evidence that donor-directed transfusion is safer than blood provided by routine donation. In fact, donor-directed transfusions are positive for transmissible disease markers at the same rate as first-time donors (higher than the rate for repeat volunteer donors).
  C. Mothers are not ideal donors because maternal plasma frequently contains a variety of antibodies (against leukocyte and platelet antigens) that could interact with antigens expressed on neonatal cells. Similarly, transfusions from paternal donors present a risk because the neonate may have been passively immunized against paternal blood cellular antigens (by transplacental transfer of maternal antibodies against paternal antigens).

IV. Autologous blood donation. In adults, safety of transfusion is enhanced by the use of autologous blood collected preoperatively.

  A. The fetoplacental blood reservoir contains a blood volume of approximately 110 mL/kg, with 30% to 50% of this volume contained in the placenta. Thus, placental blood is autologous blood. Approximately 20 mL/kg can be harvested at birth and used for future transfusions.

1. **The potential for bacterial contamination** and the additional expense of collection have limited the widespread adoption of placental autologous blood transfusion.
2. **Placental autologous blood,** in selected cases, is collected and stored as umbilical cord blood and used as a source of hematopoietic progenitor cells for transplantation.

B. **As an alternative, delayed cord clamping** for 30 to 60 seconds after birth allows the transfer of a significant amount of blood from the placenta to the infant. The blood volume of a newborn subjected to delayed cord clamping is 15 to 30 mL/kg larger than that of neonates with early cord clamping. **Beneficial effects** from this procedure are a reduction in transfusions needed, decreased iron deficiency at a later age, decreased hospital mortality, and possibly decreased risk of intraventricular hemorrhage in preterm infants.

V. **Irradiated/filtered blood components**
   A. **The following adverse outcomes to blood transfusion** are caused by contaminant leukocytes (white blood cells [WBCs]), whose numbers are maximal when fresh blood is used.
      1. **Sensitization** to human leukocyte antigens (HLAs).
      2. **Febrile transfusion reactions.**
      3. **Immune modulation,** which may increase the risk of postoperative infection.
      4. **Transmission of cytomegalovirus** and other herpes and retroviral leukocyte passenger viruses.
      5. **Transfusion-associated graft-versus-host disease** (TA-GVHD) from engraftment of donor T lymphocytes.
   B. **Human leukocyte antigen sensitization and febrile transfusion reactions** are unusual in infants, whereas transfusion-transmitted CMV and TA-GVHD can be life threatening.
      1. **At greatest risk of severe cytomegalovirus infection** are preterm infants (<1200 g) born to CMV-seronegative mothers and infants with immunodeficiency. For these high-risk patients, transfused blood components must be processed to remove passenger WBCs.
         a. **Leukoreduction (removal of passenger white blood cells)**
            i. Such so-called **leukoreduction** is almost always performed by filtration of the blood component through proprietary hollow-fiber filters to which intact WBCs adhere. (Centrifugation-based techniques are outdated.) Leukocyte counts can be reduced from 10^9 to $4–6 \times 10^5$ per RBC unit (4-log unit reduction) with fourth-generation filters.
            ii. **Leukoreduction** is effective in reducing HLA alloimmunization and transmission of cell-associated viruses, especially herpes viruses (eg, CMV, HHV-8, and EBV), as well as preventing some febrile transfusion reactions.
      2. **Patients at risk** for TA-GVHD include recipients of donor-directed units from first- and second-degree blood relatives, HLA-matched platelets, intrauterine transfusions, and massive fresh blood transfusions or exchange transfusions, as well as patients with suspected or proven severe T-lymphocyte immunodeficiency states (eg, DiGeorge syndrome).
         a. **Gamma-irradiation** of cellular blood components delivers a dose of 25 Gy and prevents subsequent WBC mitoses, and thereby TA-GVHD.

VI. **Emergency transfusions.** For patients >4 months old, uncross-matched (or "emergency release") blood is rarely transfused, because most blood banks can complete an IAT cross-match within 1 hour. In cases of massive exsanguinating hemorrhage, "type-specific" blood (wherein ABO and Rh[D] match the patient's antigens) is given as either uncross-matched or "immediate spin" cross-match compatible (directly tested in saline without anti-human globulin) and is usually available in 10 minutes. If this delay is too long (as in severe fetomaternal hemorrhage), type O Rh(D)-negative RBCs should be used.

VII. Blood bank products
  A. Red blood cells
   1. Packed red blood cells (PRBCs)
     a. Indications. PRBC transfusions are given to maintain hemoglobin (Hgb)/ hematocrit (Hct) at levels judged "best" for the clinical condition of the baby. Dueling proponents are split between those favoring "restrictive" Hgb thresholds ("transfusion triggers") of 7 to 8 g/dL and those favoring "liberal" Hgb thresholds of 9 to 10 g/dL. In general, restrictive practice has been shown (in randomized controlled trials [RCTs]) not to be inferior to liberal practice (since it was not associated with higher rates of adverse outcomes) and to result in fewer total transfusions.
     b. In the multicenter Premature Infants in Need of Transfusion randomized controlled trial, 451 very low birthweight infants were assigned to transfusions using either restrictive or liberal criteria. Outcome rates for death, severe retinopathy, bronchopulmonary dysplasia, and brain injury supported the use of restrictive transfusion criteria. In addition, 11% of infants in the restrictive group avoided transfusion completely compared to 5% in the liberal group.
     c. In a single-center randomized controlled trial, Bell et al assigned 100 preterm infants to either restrictive or liberal transfusion practice. Again, a reduction in the number of transfusions in the restrictive group was seen but with more episodes of apnea and neurologic events than in the liberal group.
     d. More recent meta-analysis contrasting documented benefits of a restrictive transfusion practice (decreased number of transfusions and exposure to fewer RBC donors) to those of a liberal transfusion practice (decreased apnea and brain injury) called for additional clinical studies to clarify the impact of practice type on long-term neonatal outcomes.
     e. Currently, the selected posttransfusion hemoglobin/hematocrit target is quite *controversial* and may vary greatly among neonatal units. In general, an advocate of a liberal transfusion practice would list Hct goals as:
       i. >35% to 40% in the presence of severe cardiopulmonary disease. The severity of cardiopulmonary disease is assessed based on the level of respiratory support required (intermittent positive pressure ventilation [IPPV], continuous positive airway pressure [CPAP], FiO_2), symptoms of unexplained apnea and/or tachycardia, and/or poor growth.
       ii. 30% to 35% for moderate cardiopulmonary disease or major surgery.
       iii. 20% to 25% for infants with stable, so-called asymptomatic anemia (primarily due to iatrogenic blood loss for laboratory testing and/or inadequate hematopoiesis).
     f. Administration
       i. Type. PRBCs transfused throughout infancy should be screened in order to exclude donations from blood donors containing Hgb S.
       ii. Dosage. 10 to 20 mL/kg given over 1 to 3 hours (4 hours maximum). **Use the following formula as a guide:**

Volume PRBC to transfuse (mL) = 1.6 × weight (kg) × desired rise in Hct (%)

   2. "Adsol" packed red blood cells. The traditional use of relatively fresh RBCs (<7 days in storage) has been largely replaced by the practice of transfusing aliquots of RBCs from a dedicated unit of PRBCs stored for up to 42 days. This requires a sterile connecting device and is done to diminish the number of donor exposures among infants expected to require numerous transfusions during their stay in the neonatal intensive care unit (infants whose birthweight is <1500 g).
     a. Packed red blood cells are suspended in a citrate-anticoagulated storage solution at an Hct of 55% to 60% stored at 1°C to 6°C.

    b. These additive solutions (AS or Adsol-1, -3, or -5) contain various combinations of preservatives (dextrose, sodium chloride, phosphate, adenine, and mannitol) with citrate anticoagulant.

  3. Citrate phosphate dextrose packed red blood cells. Because of concern about potential hepatorenal toxicity of adenine and mannitol, units of RBCs without extended storage AS media are used for large-volume transfusions such as exchange transfusion and transfusions for major surgical procedures.

    a. Citrate phosphate dextrose with adenine (CPDA-1) PRBC units with only small amounts of adenine and devoid of mannitol have an Hct of 65% to 80% and a shelf life of 35 days.

    b. Citrate phosphate dextrose (CPD) PRBC units lacking both adenine and mannitol also have an Hct of 65% to 80% but a shelf life of only 21 days.

    c. Washed AS or Adsol PRBC units are an alternative if these other PRBC units are unavailable.

  4. Washed packed red blood cells. During storage, potassium is progressively released from RBCs so that, by the end of the storage period, extracellular (plasma) potassium levels approximate 50 and 80 mEq/L for Adsol and CPD units, respectively. This leakage is increased in irradiated blood. For small-volume transfusions, the amount of infused potassium is, in general, of little clinical significance (0.3–0.4 mEq/kg per 15 mL/kg RBC transfusion). But it may become hazardous for larger transfusion volumes such as in exchange transfusion. In such an event and in the absence of fresh whole blood (<2–3 days old), RBCs (typically O Rh[D] negative) washed free of their potentially hyperkalemic supernatant using normal saline and then resuspended to an Hct of 50% to 55% with fresh frozen plasma (typically AB, termed "reconstituted whole blood") can be used. Irradiated reconstituted whole blood should be used for total (or "double blood volume") exchange transfusions.

  5. Fresh PRBCs. RCTs demonstrating advantages of fresh PRBCs compared to standard-issue (within licensed time frame) PRBCs have not been replicated or dominated meta-analyses.

B. Plasma—fresh-frozen plasma, thawed plasma. Donated whole blood is centrifuged to separate the cells (RBCs, WBCs, and platelets) and the liquid (plasma). Plasma separated and frozen within 8 hours of the blood being donated is called fresh-frozen plasma (FFP); plasma separated and frozen within 24 hours is called plasma frozen 24 (PF24). Beyond 24 hours after thawing, FFP and PF24 are known as thawed plasma, which is usable for 5 days after donation. Plasma contains albumin, immune globulins, and clotting factors. Some clotting factors retain much of their activity after thawing (eg, von Willebrand factor [vWF]), but the activity of others is progressively reduced during refrigerated storage after thawing (factors V, VII, and VIII).

  1. Indications

    a. Correction of coagulopathy due to deficiencies of multiple clotting factors in vitamin K deficiency (hemorrhagic disease of the newborn) or disseminated intravascular coagulation (DIC).

    b. Prophylaxis for or treatment of bleeding for a known single coagulation factor deficiency for which no concentrate is available.

      i. When available, clotting factor concentrates are preferred to plasma in case of a single, inherited clotting factor deficiency.

      ii. There are no US Food and Drug Administration–approved single factor concentrates available in the United States for factors II, V, and XI.

      iii. Concentrate for treatment of acute angioedema or preoperative prophylaxis in hereditary C1-inhibitor deficiency may not be immediately available.

    c. Prothrombin complex concentrates (PCC) containing factors II, VII, IX, and X are used for factor II and X deficiencies and warfarin reversal in case of severe bleeding or pending surgical procedures. If PCC is unavailable, use FFP.

  d. **Prophylaxis for or treatment of dilutional coagulopathy** ("coagulopathic bleeding") that may ensue during massive RBC transfusion administered for replacement of blood loss in excess of half of the blood volume.

  e. **Preparation of reconstituted whole blood from washed PRBCs** for total exchange transfusion.

  f. **Although fresh-frozen plasma provides excellent colloid volume support,** it is not recommended for volume expansion, albumin supplementation, or antibody replacement because safer components (albumin, intravenous immunoglobulin) are available for these purposes.

  g. **Fresh-frozen plasma should not be given for abnormal coagulation screen results** in the absence of bleeding or for coagulopathies that can be corrected by adjusting warfarin dose and/or administration of vitamin K.

 2. **Administration**

  a. **Transfused plasma should be ABO compatible with the patient's blood group.** Incompatible antibodies in the donor plasma (eg, anti-A or -B antibodies in group O plasma) may rarely, if given in sufficient volume, result in an acute hemolytic reaction in the transfused patient.

  b. **Dosage:** 10 to 20 mL/kg over 1 to 2 hours (4 hours maximum).

  c. **Rapid transfusion may result in transient hypocalcemia due to the sodium citrate anticoagulant that is added to donated blood.** If rapid infusion of FFP is needed, a small bolus of calcium chloride (3–5 mg/kg) may be considered.

 C. **Cryoprecipitate.** This is prepared from FFP by thawing it at 1°C to 6°C. In this temperature range, a cryoprecipitate forms and is separated from so-called cryo-poor supernatant plasma by centrifugation at 1°C to 6°C. The pellet is then frozen as cryoprecipitate. Prior to use, it must again be thawed and dissolved off the interior surface of its plastic bag with sterile, normal saline (total volume of 10–15 mL). Cryoprecipitate is a concentrated source of the following blood clotting proteins: factor VIII, vWF, fibrinogen, and factor XIII (with some other proteins, eg, fibronectin).

 1. **Indications**

  a. **To restore fibrinogen levels** in patients with acquired hypofibrinogenemia (as occurs in DIC and massive transfusion)

  b. **Factor XIII in deficient patients,** if Food and Drug Administration–approved Corifact concentrate is unavailable.

 2. **Administration**

  a. **Unlike plasma, it does not need to be ABO compatible with the recipient's blood group.**

  b. **Dosage:** 10 mL/kg (0.1–0.2 U/kg raises fibrinogen by 60–100 mg/dL).

  c. **Infusion should be completed within 6 hours of thawing.**

 D. **Platelets.** This component is prepared from whole blood donations by centrifugation (termed *random donor*) or by automated apheresis (termed *single donor* or *platelets, pheresis*). Each random donor unit contains 5.5×10^{10} platelets in 50 to 70 mL of anticoagulated plasma. Each single-donor unit contains 3×10^{11} platelets, typically in 200 to 300 mL of anticoagulated plasma. Both are stored at room temperature (20–24°C) with agitation for a maximum of 5 days.

 1. **Indications.** There are no absolute guidelines regarding platelet counts that necessitate transfusion.

  a. **In general, prophylactic platelet transfusions are indicated** for platelet counts of <20,000/μL for stable neonates at term or <30,000/μL for stable premature neonates.

  b. **For high-risk neonates at an increased risk of intraventricular hemorrhage,** prophylactic platelet transfusions may be given at <30,000/μL at term or <50,000/μL if premature.

      i. Such high-risk neonates include those with extremely low birthweight, perinatal asphyxia, sepsis, ventilatory assistance with an FiO_2 >40%, or clinical instability.

    c. In the presence of clinically significant, active bleeding or prior to undergoing invasive or surgical procedures, this "transfusion trigger" may be raised to <50,000/μL.

    d. Infants on extracorporeal life support/extracorporeal membrane oxygenation are usually prophylactically transfused to maintain a platelet count of >80,000 to 100,000/μL.

    e. In septic patients, platelet increments after transfusion may only be transient.

    f. Because of room temperature storage, bacterial contamination of platelet units is actively sought, typically by culture or direct testing of each component.

    g. Increased mortality and morbidity have been described among preterm infants receiving multiple platelet transfusions; causality is unclear.

  2. Administration

    a. Infant and donor should be ABO identical if possible. When ABO-identical platelets are unavailable, group AB platelets are the most suitable substitute. However, the frequent unavailability of group AB platelets causes the use of group A platelets for group B recipients and vice versa. Group O platelets are the least suitable for non–group-O infants, because passively transfused anti-A or anti-B antibodies may lead to hemolysis.

    b. Rh(D)-negative platelets should be given whenever possible to Rh(D)-negative patients, especially female infants. If this is impossible, consider administration of Rh immune globulin.

      i. The Alloimmunization After D-Incompatible Platelet Transfusions study in nonneonates, which included Rh(D)-negative recipients with hematologic, oncologic, and various other conditions who received Rh(D)-positive apheresis platelets, found anti-D antibody in approximately 1.4% of recipients upon follow-up after a median of 77 days.

    c. For infants with alloimmune thrombocytopenia (AIT), platelets lacking human platelet antigens (HPAs) to which antibodies are directed are required. If such platelets are unavailable, then HPA-1a/5b–negative platelets may be given since these will be compatible in 95% of AIT cases among white patients. For Asian patients, HPA-4a–negative platelets would be chosen. If anti-HPA antibodies are not demonstrated, then anti-HLA antibodies may be present, requiring HLA-matched platelets.

    d. Dosage: 10 to 20 mL/kg intravenously should raise neonatal platelet counts by 60,000 to 100,000/μL.

VIII. Transfusion reactions

  A. Acute intravascular hemolysis. Occurs due to incompatibility of donor RBCs with antibodies in the patient plasma. The most common antibodies responsible for complement-mediated acute hemolysis are isohemagglutinins (anti-A, anti-B). Newborns do not all make isohemagglutinins in high titer until 4 to 6 months of age.

    1. However, transfusion of ABO-incompatible donor red blood cells (most commonly due to clerical error) may result in hemolysis if isoagglutinin titers are high enough. Accordingly, some neonatal units may transfuse all neonates with O Rh(D)-negative PRBCs (if the blood supplier can support this policy).

    2. Incompatible isohemagglutinins are more often found in the neonatal circulation due to transfusion of the ABO-incompatible plasma in platelet units.

    3. Transplacental passage of group O maternal isohemagglutinins to a non–group-O fetus may also cause hemolysis of the neonate's own RBCs in the absence of transfusion (often mild; hemolytic disease of the fetus and newborn). Note that passively acquired anti-A and anti-B, whether of blood donor or maternal origin, are not detected by antibody screens but do cause incompatible cross-matches. Accordingly, cross-matches using an IAT are always necessary when clinically significant RBC antibodies, including isohemagglutinins, are present in neonatal plasma.

4. **Red cell T-antigen is present on all human erythrocytes** but expressed only after exposure to neuraminidase produced by a variety of infectious organisms—in particular *Streptococcus*, *Clostridium*, and influenza viruses. Anti-T antibodies are present in almost all adults but are not present in the plasma of infants until 6 months of age. Anti-T may be associated with hemolysis in patients whose RBCs are "activated" (eg, infants with necrotizing enterocolitis [NEC] or sepsis). When intravascular hemolysis occurs and T activation of neonatal RBCs is identified through peanut lectin testing, donor RBCs and platelets should be washed prior to use.

5. **Possible symptoms of intravascular hemolysis include** hypotension, fever, tachycardia, hematuria, and hemoglobinuria. Diagnosis may be confirmed by an elevated free serum Hgb, absent haptoglobin (if it is not congenitally absent, as in about 10% of African-American infants), as well as the presence of schistocytes on a peripheral blood smear.

B. **Nonhemolytic febrile reactions.** Usually mild and due to transfusion of cytokines released from donor WBCs during storage or of fragmented donor WBCs.

C. **Allergic transfusion reactions.** Unusual in neonatal transfusion recipients. Due to antibodies in the patient's plasma reacting to epitopes on donor plasma proteins.

D. **Transfusion-associated acute lung injury.** Transfusion-related acute lung injury (TRALI) is typically due to antibodies in donor plasma that react with the patient's HLA antigens. More likely to occur with blood components containing a large volume of plasma such as FFP or platelets.

E. **Bacterial contamination.** There is a small but potentially fatal risk of bacterial infection on the order of 1 per million for PRBCs but of 1 per 100,000 for platelets (because of room temperature storage). Platelet components are bacterially contaminated at a rate of 1 per 1000 to 3000; false-negative results of platelet screening for bacterial contamination are unavoidable. (To address the risk, the AABB Standard 5.15.1 was first added on March 1, 2004 to "implement measures to limit bacterial contamination in all platelet components.") Transfusion-transmitted sepsis with culture confirmation occurs in at least 1 per 100,000 recipients, and 1 of every 5 cases has an immediate fatal outcome (1 in 500,000 recipients).

1. **For several consecutive years, bacterial contamination of platelets has been the top transfusion-transmitted infection in the United States and the second leading cause of blood transfusion-related death in the United States** (after TRALI). However, it is widely suspected that bacterial contamination of blood components is underreported.

2. *Escherichia coli, Pseudomonas, Serratia, Salmonella, Enterobacter,* **and** *Yersinia* are the most commonly implicated gram-negative bacteria causing severe or fatal infections. Gram-positive bacteria (eg, *Staphylococcus epidermidis*) are the most frequent contaminants of platelet units (from blood donor's skin).

3. **Immediate notification of public health authorities is required for:**

   a. **Bacterial category A agents of bioterrorism:** *Bacillus anthracis, Yersinia pestis, Francisella tularensis,* and *Clostridium botulinum.* Individual isolates of these organisms must be saved for confirmatory testing at public health laboratories.

   b. **Multiple other, selected bacteria are listed as nationally notifiable diseases;** consult the Centers for Disease Control and Prevention's National Notifiable Diseases Surveillance System for a complete list.

F. **Hypothermia.** Large-volume transfusions of either reconstituted whole blood (exchange transfusion) or PRBCs (major surgery, large fetomaternal hemorrhages), which are stored at 1°C to 6°C, will result in hypothermia unless a blood warmer is used.

G. Hyperkalemia. At risk are infants receiving a large transfusion of RBCs such as in exchange transfusion, major surgery, or extracorporeal life support (ECLS). Reconstituted whole blood (washed PRBCs [<14 days old] with Hct adjusted using FFP) is recommended. In some neonatal units, fresh whole blood (2–3 days old) may be available.

H. Necrotizing enterocolitis. In the past 15 years, several case reports and retrospective studies have reported that up to one third of all very low birthweight (VLBW) infants who develop NEC may have received 1 or more RBC transfusions in the 24 to 72 hours prior to onset of NEC. The causality of the "transfusion-associated" NEC has been hypothesized to share the same TRALI immunologic mechanisms, such as transfusion of biologic response mediators such as donor antibodies against the HLA, biologically active lipids, free Hgb, RBC membrane fragments, and inflammatory cytokines present in stored blood.

More recently, 2 published prospective studies failed to demonstrate this association between RBC transfusion and NEC, with 1 of the studies suggesting that it is the underlying anemia, not the transfusion, that may increase the risk of NEC.

20 Extracorporeal Life Support in the Neonate

I. **Introduction.** Extracorporeal life support (ECLS), also referred to as extracorporeal membrane oxygenation (ECMO), provides either direct cardiac/pulmonary support (venoarterial [VA] ECLS) or indirect cardiac/pulmonary support (venovenous [VV] ECLS) by providing oxygen (O_2) delivery and carbon dioxide (CO_2) removal in neonates with reversible life-threatening respiratory or cardiac disease. While on ECLS, blood is drained from the right atrium through a cannula with the aid of a pump and then propelled through an oxygenator where gas exchange occurs. From there, it is returned to the aorta (VA) or right atrium (VV) (Figure 20–1). Uniform guidelines have been established to describe essential equipment, procedures, personnel, and training required for ECLS and can be found in *Extracorporeal Life Support: The ELSO Red Book*, 5th Edition, and *Extracorporeal Membrane Oxygenation (ECLS) Specialist Training Manual* published by the Extracorporeal Life Support Organization (ELSO) and on the ELSO website.

II. **Indications.** ECLS is used in critically ill term and late preterm newborns with reversible respiratory and/or cardiac failure who have failed maximal medical management. Neonatal conditions supported with ECLS include meconium aspiration syndrome (MAS), congenital diaphragmatic hernia (CDH), persistent pulmonary hypertension of the newborn (PPHN), respiratory distress syndrome (RDS), sepsis, pneumonia, severe air leak, and airway anomalies awaiting surgical repair and postoperatively during recovery. VV-ECLS is preferred in most neonates with respiratory failure because it appears safer. VA-ECLS is used in patients with cardiac failure due to congenital heart disease, postcardiotomy heart failure, cardiomyopathy, cardiac failure due to sepsis, severe rhythm disturbances, situations of cardiac arrest, and as a bridge to cardiac transplantation. VA-ECLS is often favored in patients with CDH where vessel anatomy prevents cannulation with a double-lumen venous catheter. (However, comparison studies provide data supporting successful VV-ECLS use in the CDH population). VA-ECLS is also preferred in patients with septic shock in whom higher flow rates may be required to provide support.

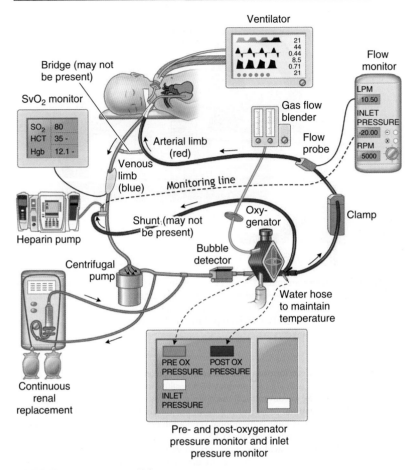

FIGURE 20–1. Extracorporeal life support circuit.

III. **Appropriate patients for extracorporeal life support**
  A. **Weight ≥1800 to 2000 g and/or gestational age ≥32 to 34 weeks.** The cannula size is determined by the infant's weight; the lower limit in weight is based on the limitation of cannula sizes available.
  B. **Cardiopulmonary criteria for extracorporeal life support**
    1. **Oxygenation index.** Most centers use a combination of persistently elevated oxygenation index (OI) calculations (OI of 30–40) and the inability to wean from 100% oxygen within a period of time as criteria for initiating ECLS support.

$$OI = \frac{FiO_2 \times MAP \times 100}{PaO_2}$$

(FiO$_2$, fraction of inspired O$_2$; MAP, mean airway pressure; PaO$_2$, partial pressure of oxygen, arterial)

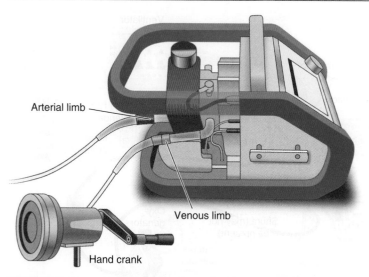

Arterial limb

Venous limb

Hand crank

FIGURE 20–2. Maquet Cardiohelp (Maquet Cardiopulmonary, Hirrlingen, Germany) incorporates the pump, gas exchanger, and heat exchanger into a single unit. Oxygenator (*red*) and centrifugal pump (*silver*) are in one unit. The arterial limb is above the venous limb (shown as tubes on the left). Hand crank is pictured to the lower left. (*Maquet Cardiopulmonary, Hirrlingen, Germany.*)

     2. **Acute deterioration with intractable hypoxemia.** Neonates who have a PaO_2 <30–40 mm Hg or a preductal SaO_2 <80% for greater than an hour with no response to conventional therapies should be considered for ECLS support.
     3. **Barotrauma.** Severe air leak from pneumothoraces that is not responsive to low tidal volume conventional ventilation or high-frequency ventilation may benefit from lung rest on ECLS.
     4. **Severe lactic acidosis.** Indicators of circulatory failure including hypotension and a rising lactate despite circulatory support strategies including volume expansion and inotropic/vasopressor support should prompt ECLS as well.
     5. **Cardiac arrest.** ECLS during cardiopulmonary resuscitation (ECPR) is available in many centers for patients with or without primary heart disease in situations where the cardiac arrest is witnessed.
  IV. **Relative contraindications to extracorporeal life support.** Decisions for determining contraindications to ECLS are institution based.
    A. **Gestational age <32 to 34 weeks and/or a birthweight <1800 to 2000 g** are relative contraindications to ECLS due to increased mortality and morbidity. ECLS may be accomplished in neonates <34 weeks if their vessels are large enough to accommodate the cannula/cannulae. A Doppler ultrasound of the internal jugular vessel and carotid artery may help determine if the vessel size is appropriate. Current ECLS circuit technology requires the use of systemic heparinization for anticoagulation, increasing the risk for developing an intraventricular hemorrhage or parenchymal hemorrhage, particularly during the first week of life. Preterm neonates older than a week of life appear to gain some cerebrovascular stability and are less likely to have an intracranial hemorrhage when on ECLS. Newer technologies, improved anticoagulation strategies, and smaller cannulae sizes are being developed that may allow ECLS support in younger and smaller patients.

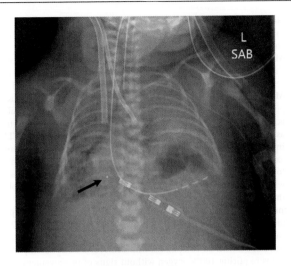

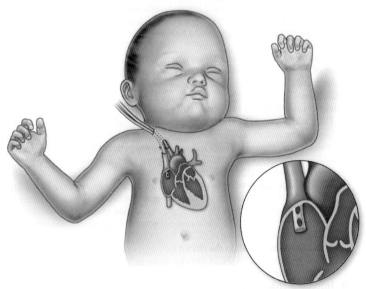

FIGURE 20–3. Venoarterial extracorporeal life support cannulae placement. The echogenic dot denoting the end of the venous cannula is shown near the arrow.

    B. **Intracranial hemorrhage grade >II due to a higher risk of extending the hemorrhage.** Neonates with grade III or IV intracranial hemorrhages and those with severe brain damage are likely to have significant neurologic sequelae and may extend the area of central nervous system (CNS) hemorrhage if placed on ECLS. Generally, ECLS support is weaned off under circumstances of a grade III or IV intracranial hemorrhage or extending parenchymal hemorrhage.

    C. **Severe congenital anomalies** incompatible with long-term survival.

    D. **Cardiac lesions** that cannot be corrected or palliated.

E. **Neonates with congenital diaphragmatic hernia** who have never had a preductal saturation >80% or $PaCO_2$ <80 mm Hg may be excluded from ECLS therapy in some centers.

F. **Marked perinatal asphyxia** with severe neurologic sequelae (ongoing stupor, flaccidity, dilated and fixed pupils, and absent primitive reflexes) persisting after respiratory and metabolic resuscitation will not benefit from ECLS.

G. **Multiple organ dysfunction** in neonates can develop with septic shock, hypoperfusion, or hypoxia. Such neonates often develop respiratory failure, metabolic acidosis, and coagulopathy that do not resolve with transfusion therapy, as well as cardiac, renal, and gastrointestinal dysfunction. Although ECLS can support infants in multiorgan failure and provide time for improvement, neonates in extremis with such significant multiple-organ derangements that are not likely to survive should not receive ECLS. Interdisciplinary discussions are important when making a decision about placing an infant on ECLS and, if placed on ECLS, throughout the ECLS course.

V. **Transfer of neonates possibly needing extracorporeal life support.** Neonates should be transferred early in their course, if possible. An OI of >25 suggests significant hypoxic respiratory failure and equates to a neonate on a mean airway pressure of 15 with an FiO_2 of 1.0 who achieves a PaO_2 of only 60 mm Hg. Any neonates requiring 100% oxygen without signs of improvement on conventional or high-frequency ventilation and inhaled nitric oxide within 4 to 6 hours or those who have persistent hypotension, respiratory acidosis, and/or lactic acidosis despite vasopressor/inotropic therapy should be considered candidates for transport to an ECLS center.

VI. **Parental consent.** Prior to ECLS initiation, parents or guardians should be made aware of the risks and benefits of ECLS. The physician should emphasize that ECLS provides supportive treatment rather than curative therapy and that neonates may not survive.

VII. **Potential complications to discuss with parents**

A. **Difficulties may arise during cannulation,** including the inability to achieve adequate venous drainage or infusion secondary to a venous web, valve, or vessel spasm. Perforation of the right atrium leading to pericardial tamponade can occur suddenly and be life threatening, requiring massive transfusion of blood products and immediate surgical evacuation.

B. **Hemorrhage may develop in any organ.** Blood accumulation in the pericardium, abdomen, retroperitoneum, or chest can result in decreased pulse pressure, low venous oxygen saturations (SvO_2), hypotension, and inability to maintain ECLS flows and may need to be evacuated. Significant intracranial hemorrhage may necessitate discontinuation of ECLS.

C. **Thrombosis or emboli in the circuit** may lead to an infarction in the brain. This is usually seen with VA-ECLS but can occur in VV-ECLS when an intracardiac shunt is present.

D. **Infectious risks** increase with prolonged ECLS and are more common in VA-ECLS patients. Coagulase-negative staphylococci and *Candida* are the most common organisms identified. However, routine prophylactic antibiotics while on ECLS are not warranted.

E. **Acute kidney injury** (AKI) can increase the length of time on ECLS and is independently associated with mortality. Continuous renal replacement therapy is used for AKI or for massive fluid overload.

F. **Development of chronic lung disease** may lead to future hospitalizations and have long-term effects on pulmonary function. Data suggest that allowing the lung to rest using minimal ventilator settings and by supporting with ECLS in the interim limits pulmonary complications. Evaluations at 1 year show slightly better lung function in those treated with ECLS than with conventional therapy.

G. **Extracorporeal life support survivors are at risk for neurologic sequelae** resulting from the underlying disease process and/or their treatments. See Section XXIII.

H. **Accidental decannulation, arrhythmias** (due to the venous catheter being positioned in the atrium), **and mechanical problems** (eg, oxygenator failure, fracture of the tubing or connector sites) are other possible ECLS complications.

VIII. **Pre-extracorporeal life support studies, preparation, and monitoring**

A. **Before initiating extracorporeal life support,** patients should be evaluated for structural heart disease and intracranial hemorrhage with an **echocardiogram and head ultrasound** if time allows. Ninety percent of intracranial hemorrhages occur in the first 5 days of ECLS therapy, so serial ultrasound studies should be done daily for 5 days followed by an every-other-day regimen at a minimum.

B. **Screening lab assessments** should include electrolytes, ionized calcium, blood urea nitrogen, creatinine, glucose, complete blood count, differential, coagulation studies including international normalized ratio (INR), total and direct bilirubin, arterial blood gas, lactate, heparin assay, antithrombin III antigen assay, blood culture, and a blood type and screen. Lab assessments should be followed daily to twice daily.

C. **A bladder catheter, enteral feeding tube or gastric sump tube, and a rectal temperature probe (if the patient is undergoing therapeutic hypothermia) should be inserted as needed.** It is extremely important to place these tubes prior to the initiation of anticoagulation for ECLS given the risks of bleeding when they are placed while on ECLS. Generally, gastric sump tubes are placed to gravity to avoid any risk of bleeding that low intermittent suction may cause.

D. **For venovenous extracorporeal life support, a percutaneously placed internal jugular central line** can serve as a guide for placement of the VV cannula. Other access for IV infusions or radial arterial, femoral venous, or umbilical catheters should be placed prior to the initiation of ECLS, if possible.

E. **Monitoring.** Because of the administration of sedatives, or muscle relaxants for severe illness, seizures may be difficult to detect in this population. Patients benefit from monitoring amplitude-integrated electroencephalogram or continuous electroencephalogram (especially after ECPR), near-infrared spectroscopy (NIRS), and oximetry prior to and during support on ECLS.

IX. **Pretreatment with glucocorticoids.** During ECLS, patient blood, exposed to plastic, silicone, polymethylpentene, and other circuit components, causes activation of the immune system, which releases inflammatory mediators (complement, leukotrienes, cytokines, and leukocytes). The coagulation cascade, complement, and fibrinolytic systems are also activated, and capillary leak ensues. Consumption of platelets by the oxygenator or filter used for continuous renal replacement can exacerbate the coagulopathy and inflammatory reaction. This process may be mitigated somewhat by pretreating neonates with glucocorticoids, but the evidence for this has not been well established. Some centers use **dexamethasone** (generally 0.1–0.5 mg/kg prior to the initiation of ECLS or with circuit changes). If patients are on hydrocortisone due to hypotension associated with adrenal insufficiency, dosing with hydrocortisone should be continued, but additional steroid therapy is unnecessary for the initiation of ECLS or circuit changes.

X. **Gas exchange devices (extracorporeal lungs): hollow-fiber oxygenators and membrane oxygenators.** The oxygen concentration from the wall source is adjusted via the gas flow blender and delivered to both types of oxygenators via the gas flow blender tubing (Figure 20–1). To increase the removal of CO_2, the **flow** to the oxygenator is increased, analogous to increasing alveolar ventilation in the native lung. This provides gas flow or "sweep gas" through the gas exchange unit and serves to wash out CO_2.

A. **Hollow-fiber oxygenators.** Gas exchange occurs in the hollow fibers. **Blood flows** around the fibers, in constant contact with the fiber surface. **Oxygen flow,** on the other hand, occurs through the hollow fibers. The microporous nature of the fibers allows gas exchange by diffusion across the fiber based on concentration gradients, allowing O_2 delivery and CO_2 removal. Most oxygen is carried by hemoglobin, with the dissolved fraction being a relatively minor component.

  B. Membrane oxygenators. Membrane oxygenators are designed to allow blood to flow on one side of the membrane while gas flows on the other side. Again, concentration gradients determine the driving force for diffusion of gases. Membrane oxygenators are more likely to have complications with plasma leaks, air emboli, water vapor condensation, and thrombus formation.

  C. Factors affecting oxygen delivery on extracorporeal life support
    1. **Oxygen content** of the blood after it passes through the **oxygenator.**
    2. **Oxygen content** of the blood after it passes through the **neonate's lung.**
    3. **Native cardiac output in combination with circuit flow on extracorporeal life support**
    4. **Patient hemoglobin**

  D. Factors affecting oxygenation through the circuit:
    1. **Driving concentration gradient:** the amount of O_2 in the gas phase.
    2. **Permeability:** the ease with which O_2 crosses the hollow fibers or membrane
    3. **Solubility:** the ability of O_2 to diffuse through the blood layer. Because there is more O_2 in the sweep gas than in the blood, there is always a large concentration gradient favoring oxygen diffusion into the blood. The sweep gas flow rate has little influence on oxygen exchange, again similar to native alveolar ventilation.
    4. **In hollow-fiber oxygenators,** gas exchange is rapid at all degrees of flow. However, in **membrane oxygenators,** where the surface area and blood path mixing determine the maximum oxygenation capacity, oxygenation may be influenced by the rate of blood flow. If the blood flows faster than the time it takes to achieve complete saturation of the hemoglobin with oxygen, blood will leave the **oxygenator** incompletely saturated. The **rated flow** is the pump blood flow rate at which maximal O_2 delivery is achieved (ie, where venous blood with a saturation of 75% and hemoglobin of 12 g/dL achieves a saturation of 95% when exiting the membrane oxygenator). Oxygenation decreases at flows that exceed the rated flow. In addition, the likelihood of hemolysis increases directly proportional to high flows. Oxygenators have a flow-rated graph on the manufacturers' websites.

  E. Factors affecting carbon dioxide exchange on extracorporeal life support
    1. **The concentration of carbon dioxide** is usually at least 45 to 50 mm Hg in the venous blood and 0 in the sweep gas of the oxygenator, allowing efficient transfer of CO_2.
    2. **The movement of gas through the oxygenator or sweep gas flow rate** constantly refreshes the concentration gradient, determining ventilation.
    3. **The surface area of the hollow fibers or membrane** allows for rapid gas exchange. Because the diffusion of CO_2 through blood and the hollow fibers or membrane occurs rapidly (6 times faster than O_2), it remains independent of blood flow rate through the oxygenator. Factors that decrease the functional surface area, however, will limit CO_2 transfer before affecting oxygenation.

XI. Comparison of venoarterial and venovenous extracorporeal life support
  A. Venoarterial extracorporeal life support provides cardiopulmonary bypass that runs in **parallel** to the native cardiac output. Access for VA-ECLS is usually through the **right internal jugular vein** and **right common carotid artery**, each using a single lumen cannula. (Central cannulation is generally used after cardiac surgery in neonates). Venous blood from the right atrium serves as the source for ECLS pump preload that is oxygenated and then infused into the systemic circulation via the brachiocephalic artery. The path of this blood flow augments the native cardiac output. In VA-ECLS, the majority of blood flows into the aorta,

but some blood continues to flow through the heart and lungs. Because there is less blood ejected from the left ventricle, the pulse contour decreases.

1. **Advantages of venoarterial extracorporeal life support**
   a. **Provides full cardiac and respiratory support for the nonfunctioning heart and/or lungs.** Oxygen delivery is enhanced because of the extracorporeal output.
   b. **Decreases the load on the heart, allowing for recovery.**
2. **Disadvantages of venoarterial extracorporeal life support**
   a. **Results in increased left ventricular afterload that can delay myocardial recovery.** With very poor left ventricular function, increased afterload may cause acute cardiac dilation, resulting in pulmonary hemorrhage and death.
   b. **Necessitates ligation of the carotid artery when cervical cannulation is used; reconstruction may or may not be possible.** VA-ECLS causes temporary interruption of isohemispheric cerebral blood flow patterns when carotid cannulation is used. To date, studies following NIRS during cannulation do not demonstrate long-standing asymmetric effect on cerebral oxygenation or hemodynamics.
   c. **Appears to cause a higher incidence of central nervous system injury** because any emboli entering the arterial circulation can potentially cause CNS infarction.
   d. **May compromise organ tolerance to hypoxia** (especially in the brain, myocardium, splanchnic bed, and kidneys) because of the lack of pulsatility in blood flow.
B. **Venovenous extracorporeal life support** provides respiratory support that runs in **series** with the native cardiac output. For VV-ECLS, the right internal jugular vein is cannulated with a dual lumen cannula. Venous blood from the drainage ports in the right atrium serves as the source for ECLS pump preload that is oxygenated, then infused back into the right atrium via the other side of the cannula, the reinfusion port; consequently, there is no net effect on the right atrial volume, intracardiac flow, or aortic blood flow. **Ideally, the output from the reinfusion port should be directed toward the tricuspid valve.** The native cardiac output propels oxygenated blood from the pump forward to the systemic arterial system and tissues. Saturations depend on the amount of ECLS flow, native venous flow, lung function, and cardiac output.

1. **Venovenous extracorporeal life support advantages**
   a. **Maintains function of the carotid artery** since it is not used for cannulation.
   b. **Delivers highly oxygenated blood to the pulmonary vascular bed** that can help attenuate high pulmonary pressures, improve hypoxic vasoconstriction, and decrease right ventricular afterload, potentially allowing faster recovery.
   c. **Increases the availability of oxygen to the coronary circulation,** which can improve myocardial function as blood is ejected from the left ventricle.
   d. **Preserves pulsatile flow,** which may better protect organ function and reverse organ failure.
   e. **Is protective of the systemic circulation from emboli because the lungs serve as filters** (unless intracardiac shunts are present).
2. **Venovenous extracorporeal life support disadvantages**
   a. **Provides only indirect circulatory support by improving myocardial oxygenation** but does not provide additional cardiac output. Patients may continue to require vasopressors.
   b. **May not provide full oxygen delivery.** The oxygen delivery is dependent on the mixing of extracorporeal oxygen content with the oxygen content of the body. Maintaining some degree of lung expansion helps keep the pulmonary vascular resistance lower and may allow some patient contribution

to gas exchange in circumstances where perfect cannula placement cannot be achieved and recirculation limits oxygenation. In this case, some native lung function may be necessary to sustain appropriate gas exchange, so the lung cannot fully be "rested."

c. **Is more prone to challenges with flow due to the risk of the cannula being malpositioned compared to venoarterial extracorporeal life support.** Blood flow can be limited by the resistance to flow in the venous side of the cannula, the suction produced by the pump, and the size of the cannulated vessel.

d. **Provides less support for gas exchange than venoarterial extracorporeal life support** due to **recirculation** caused by oxygenated blood coming from the circuit through the reinfusion port then streaming back into the drainage side of the double lumen cannula. In situations where there is a high degree of recirculation causing suboptimal oxygen delivery, the cannula should be adjusted. (See Section XIX.B.3.)

XII. **Cannulation guidelines and preparation**

A. **Circuit preparation.** Once a patient has been determined to be a candidate for ECLS, the circuit tubing is "primed," generally with leukoreduced, irradiated packed red blood cells, fresh-frozen plasma (FFP), sodium bicarbonate, calcium gluconate, and heparin. Albumin is used instead of FFP for ECLS initiated while a neonate is undergoing cardiopulmonary resuscitation (ECPR).

B. **Neonatal vascular access.** For **cervical cannulation**, neonates should be positioned with the head turned to the left and the neck extended using a small neck roll under the shoulders to achieve appropriate surgical access. In many centers, a pediatric cardiologist is present for the cannulation to verify correct placement of the catheter(s) with an echocardiogram due to difficulty confirming correct placement using x-ray alone. Other centers use fluoroscopy. **Because adverse events can occur during cannulation, such as perforation of the atrium by the guidewire in the cannula with accompanying cardiac tamponade, teams should be prepared to provide medications and volume for resuscitation during the cannulation.**

C. **Medications.** To provide analgesia/anesthesia and surgical preparedness, neonates should receive a narcotic and a neuromuscular blocking agent before the procedure and subsequent narcotic doses during the cannulation procedure. Sedatives and narcotics are usually provided throughout the ECLS course; however, most patients do not require ongoing therapy with neuromuscular blocking agents after cannulation. When neuromuscular blockade is used for cannulation or during the course with VV-ECLS, the ventilator settings should be adjusted and the end-tidal CO_2 followed closely.

D. **X-ray placement.** Some centers place an x-ray cassette under the patient before initiation of surgical placement of the cannula(e). Others may simply insert it in the warmer tray at the time the x-ray is taken.

E. **Heparin anticoagulation.** Neonates should be given a **heparin bolus between 50 and 100 U/kg immediately prior to the insertion of the cannula(e)** to prevent clot formation in the cannula(e). It is paramount to correct a coagulopathy prior to the initiation of ECLS if there is time. Nevertheless, even in situations where a coagulopathy is present, it is still important to give the loading dose of heparin prior to cannulation, but a dose adjustment may prove advisable. The initial bolus is followed by a continuous heparin infusion at 10 to 20 U/kg/h typically, and a steady-state infusion rate between 20 and 40 U/kg/h is common.

F. **Appropriate cannula positions/sizes** (see Figures 20–3 and 20–4).

1. **Venoarterial cannulation.** Generally, a wire-wound, kink-resistant 8- to 10-F Bio-Medicus arterial cannula with a single end hole and a 12- to 14-F Bio-Medicus venous cannula (Medtronic, Dublin, Ireland) with several side holes are used. The arterial cannula tip is advanced 2 to 3 cm in the

brachiocephalic artery, at or just above the junction of the aortic arch. Optimal positioning is achieved when the cannula tip is at T3–4 on x-ray (just above the carina) after the neck roll is removed. If the arterial cannula is positioned high in the right common carotid artery, streaming of blood can occur into the right subclavian artery, causing the right arm to appear more oxygenated than the rest of the body and invalidating any arterial blood gas sampling from the right radial artery. In this case, adjusting the catheter position may be necessary.

The tip of the venous cannula should be advanced 6 to 8 cm in the right atrium near the junction of the inferior vena cava (IVC). On x-ray, the opaque metal "dot" on the cannula should be located about 1 cm above the diaphragm.

2. **Venovenous cannulation.** The size of the venous cannula is critical because restricted flow due to high resistance may cause high shear forces resulting in hemolysis and may also limit flow to the oxygenator. Commonly used VV catheters include the 13- or 16-F OriGen dual lumen PEBAX wire reinforced atrial cannula (OriGen Biomedical, Austin, TX) and the 13-F Avalon Elite bi-caval dual lumen cannula (Maquet Cardiovascular, Wayne, NJ). The 13-F OriGen catheter is used in neonates weighing 2 to 5 kg and advanced to a maximum insertion length of 8.2 cm. The 16-F OriGen catheter is used in neonates weighing 5 to 8 kg and advanced to a length of 9.5 cm. The 13- or 16-F OriGen catheter cannula tip should be well into the right atrium at T7–8 or about 1 to 2 cm above the diaphragm. The 13-F Avalon catheter should be positioned slightly into the IVC using echocardiography or fluoroscopy (Figure 20–4).

Removal of the neck roll may advance the VV catheter as much as 1 cm. Proper cannula position helps maintain appropriate flows, a critical feature of VV-ECLS. Flows of 120 mL/kg/min should be achievable following intravascular volume expansion and removal of the neck roll.

It is imperative to assess the position of the cannula with echocardiography to assure directed flow toward the tricuspid valve. If the cannula is not ideally placed to achieve optimal drainage and appropriate directed flow, there can be significant recirculation.

Recirculation occurs when oxygenated blood being delivered to the patient loops back to the drainage ports of the cannula, lowering the oxygenation potential of the blood flow. It can be detected by decreased saturations in the patient and increased saturations in the venous catheter. When this occurs, venous saturations may be >85% to 90% and arterial saturations lower than their baseline levels. (See Section XIX.B.3.)

Problems with flow after VV cannulation can also occur if the cannula is butting up against the Eustachian valve, impeding venous drainage. Echocardiography should help identify this problem, prompting adjustment of the cannula position.

G. **Intravascular volume needs at the time of cannulation.** Before connecting the ECLS cannula(e) to the circuit, surgeons may allow backflow of the neonate's blood in the cannula(e) to assure that there is no air in the circuit. During these times, blood pressures may be low momentarily, and administration of intravascular volume may be necessary.

H. **Pericardial tamponade** can occur due to malposition of the cannula at the time of cannulation or subsequently on ECLS. If there is hemodynamic compromise with inability of the circuit to flow, an echocardiogram should be obtained immediately to diagnose the problem. Sometimes the circuit may be flowing and the only clue to pericardial tamponade may be decreased pulse pressures and diminished heart tones. An emergent pericardiocentesis or drainage with a pericardial tube and repair of the intracardiac injury via a median sternotomy may be necessary.

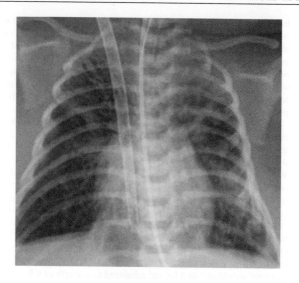

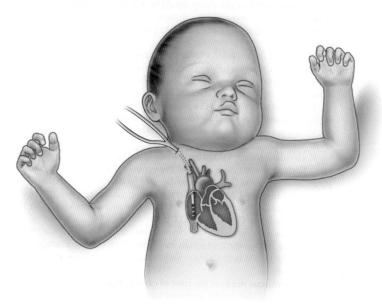

FIGURE 20–4. Venovenous extracorporeal life support cannulae placement showing the Origen catheter on x-ray and graphically. The Avalon catheter would extend farther into the inferior vena cava.

XIII. **Monitoring and ongoing management during extracorporeal life support**
    A. **Managing coagulation/anticoagulation on extracorporeal life support**
        1. **Role of unfractionated heparin administration for anticoagulation.** The artificial surfaces of the ECLS circuit activate coagulation factors, platelets,

complement, and leukocytes, leading to clot formation. Flow through the circuit creates turbulence and shearing of cells, causing platelet activation with clot formation as well, particularly in areas of low flow and stasis. To prevent excessive clot formation, unfractionated heparin (UNFH) is used. **UNFH is a** mixture of mucopolysaccharide chains ranging from 5000 to 30,000 Daltons that undergoes hepatic metabolism and renal excretion with a plasma half-life of 30 to 60 minutes. UNFH anticoagulates by binding to and accelerating the activity of the enzyme antithrombin. This complex then inactivates thrombin and other proteases, especially factor Xa, decreasing clot formation by preventing the conversion of fibrinogen to fibrin and formation of a cross-linked fibrin clot.

2. **Measures of coagulation/anticoagulation**
    a. **Activated clotting time.** Anticoagulation with heparin is a balance between the heparin activity mediated through binding to antithrombin and coagulation factor levels. An **activated clotting time (ACT)** is a whole blood clot assay that relies on contact activation by activating factor XII. Because the hematocrit, platelets, factors, and inhibitors can affect the clotting time in the ACT assay, it may track the actual heparin level directly and thus is not the best measure of heparin-dependent anticoagulation during ECLS.

    For centers using ACTs, the desired range depends on the type of monitoring equipment and institution-specific standards. Common ACT targets are **between 200 and 220 seconds.** When disseminated intravascular coagulation (DIC) or bleeding occurs, clinicians may target a lower ACT goal, typically between 180 and 200 seconds. A heparin bolus may be necessary if the ACT falls below 180 seconds.

    b. **Unfractionated heparin (antifactor Xa, anti-Xa) assay.** Several centers are using a more reliable measure of heparin effect to titrate heparin, the anti-Xa assay. This test is a chromogenic plasma assay that is sensitive to the level of both antithrombin and heparin. Anti-Xa activity is based on the ability of the heparin–antithrombin complexes to inhibit a predetermined amount of factor Xa in vitro. This test measures residual factor Xa activity that is inversely proportional to the heparin concentration in the sample. Use of the anti-Xa assay to monitor heparin effect has been shown to decrease blood product use, decrease hemorrhagic complications, and increase circuit life. Increased plasma free hemoglobin and hyperbilirubinemia can interfere with the anti-Xa assay and result in the underestimation of anti-Xa activity. (See Section XIII.F.)

    Anti-Xa activity goals are generally between **0.2 and 0.5 U/mL.** If the anti-Xa is at the lower end or below the target range, a bolus of heparin (5–10 U/kg) may be needed, or the drip may need to be increased by 10% to 20%. The reverse is true if the anti-Xa activity is above the range, allowing the heparin drip to be decreased by 10% to 20%. One approach to maintaining the anti-Xa activity in goal range is to treat the neonate with 25 U/kg of heparin prior to transfusing platelets.

    The anti-Xa activity can help to determine whether a prolonged ACT is due to overheparinization or coagulopathy and should be used in conjunction with the prothrombin time (PT) to assess coagulation factors (Table 20–1). If the PT is normal, the coagulation factor concentrations can be presumed to be normal and the heparin activity can be maintained with anti-Xa activity in the reference range. If the PT is prolonged, the neonate probably has low concentrations of coagulation factors, and treating with 10 mL/kg of FFP can correct this.

    Because the circuit flow rate also has an impact on thrombus formation, an attempt should be made to maintain ECLS flows >80 mL/kg/min whenever the anti-Xa activity or ACT is low.

Table 20–1. HEPARIN MONITORING DURING ECLS

Test	Treatment
Anti-Xa assay	Measures the activity of the heparin–AT complex. Base the heparin dose adjustments on heparin activity. Goal level is 0.2–0.5 U/mL.
PT normal (heparin independent)	Used to assess coagulation factor levels. If normal, coagulation factors are normal. Maintain heparin activity in the targeted range.
PT prolonged	Indicates that factors are low; consider treating with FFP. Use PTT to assess combined coagulation factors and heparin effect. Keep PTT <150 and keep heparin in the targeted range.
AT level <50	If the heparin is not increasing as expected with dose changes, check the AT antigen and consider an AT infusion.

AT, antithrombin; ECLS, extracorporeal life support; FFP, fresh-frozen plasma; PT, prothrombin time; PTT, partial thromboplastin time.

If ongoing bleeding and coagulopathy remain a concern or if the neonate has recently had surgery, heparin administration can be decreased and a balance between coagulation and anticoagulation achieved with infusions of FFP. For neonates requiring surgery on ECLS, aminocaproic acid, an antifibrinolytic agent, can be used. The loading dose of aminocaproic acid is 100 mg/kg IV to be given immediately prior to surgery with a maintenance dose of 30 to 33 mg/kg/h for 40 to 72 hours after surgery.

3. **Factor and blood replacement.** Aberrations in coagulation labs should be corrected. However, a balance needs to be maintained between overaggressive therapy to correct a coagulopathy or anemia and fluid overload.

   a. **Fibrinogen concentrations.** The normal goal while on ECLS is >150 mg/dL and is most often maintained using infusions of 1 unit of cryoprecipitate.

   b. **International normalized ratio levels.** The normal goal while on ECLS is ≤1.4; levels >1.5 to 2 are generally treated with 10 to 15 mL/kg of FFP and/or 1 unit of cryoprecipitate.

   c. **Platelet counts.** The normal goal while on ECLS is >80,000/μL or >100,000/μL if there is bleeding. A 10- to 15-mL/kg volume of platelets will increase the platelet count by 50,000 to 100,000/μL.

   d. **Hematocrit levels.** To avoid volume overload, values for neonates can be maintained at >30% to 35% for VA-ECLS and >35% to 40% for VV-ECLS (generally kept higher because oxygen delivery is not as efficient as in VA-ECLS). If a coagulopathy is observed in neonates, hematocrit values are generally kept toward the higher side due to concerns for possible hemorrhage.

   e. **Antithrombin levels.** Antithrombin, a serine protease inhibitor produced by the liver, is essential to endogenous anticoagulation by inhibiting the activity of thrombin and factor Xa. It also inactivates plasmin and factors IXa, XIa, and XIIa. Antithrombin is necessary for an adequate response to heparin. Heparin is a glycosaminoglycan produced by basophils and mast cells that works by binding to and upregulating the catalytic activity of antithrombin 1000-fold.

   Some centers strive to keep antithrombin antigen levels >60% of normal, especially with excessive clot buildup in the circuit, and/or a high heparin infusion rate (eg, >40 U/kg/h). The evidence for this remains inconclusive. Infants demonstrate physiologically low antithrombin levels until 6 to 9 months of age depending on their gestational age and other illnesses. Furthermore, low antithrombin levels may result from DIC, endothelial injury, ongoing protein losses from a chylothorax or nephrotic syndrome, dilutional effects of cardiac bypass, liver disease with synthetic failure, or rarely congenital deficiencies.

FFP has approximately 1 U of antithrombin/mL. Antithrombin concentrate, however, increases the serum level with a much smaller volume, so it may be appropriate to use if a goal antithrombin antigen level is targeted. Larger protein losses, with the loss of other coagulation factors, may be treated more efficiently with FFP.

B. Managing edema. Neonates on ECLS frequently develop edema because of diffusely increased permeability and reduced lymphatic function. Furosemide may be used to promote diuresis and improve fluid balance. Diuresis increases heparin clearance, often necessitating an increase in the heparin infusion rate. Likewise, a spontaneous increase in urine output, continuous renal replacement therapy, or platelet transfusions often require an increase in the heparin rate to maintain the target ACT or anti-Xa activity. Some centers use intermittent furosemide, whereas others use a continuous infusion. **If continuous furosemide is used, caution must be taken to avoid intravascular volume depletion that can affect circuit flow and increase inlet pressures, setting off alarms.** (See Section XIII.H.)

C. Monitoring centrifugal pump inlet pressures. Large negative pressure spikes at the inlet and outlet of the centrifugal pump can occur when there is an abrupt cessation of venous flow and can lead to intimal damage at the venous cannula site, especially in circumstances where excessive negative pressures collapse the vasculature around the drainage cannula. Prepump negative pressures in the drainage line can be monitored by the incorporation of a Better Bladder (Circulatory Technology, Oster Bay, NY), a safety device housing a flexible balloon within a rigid chamber with a noninvasive pressure transducer placed between the drainage line and pump inlet. The bladder serves as a reservoir or pressure buffer by providing compliance in the venous line, reduces large negative pressure inflections at the pump inlet, and protects from accidental air entrapment. This safety measure can prevent negative pressures from developing when the pump flow exceeds the return. Measurement of the inlet pressure allows time for the centrifugal pump to servo-regulate the flow, reducing the negative pressure.

D. Managing circuit thrombi and monitoring pre- and postoxygenator pressures. During the ECLS course, a balance between bleeding and clotting can be difficult to achieve. Clot formation in the circuit occurs commonly during the ECLS course. A thrombus in the oxygenator is suspected when there is an increase in the preoxygenator pressure and a fall in the postoxygenator pressure (see Figure 20–1). Trends in the change in pressures across the oxygenator (Δ pressure) should be followed. If the Δ pressure value doubles, one should investigate oxygenator performance. If it increases above acceptable parameters, the oxygenator or circuit should be changed.

Depending on the estimated length of time needed for ECLS therapy, the oxygenator or entire circuit may need to be changed. In addition, evidence for excessive consumption of clotting factors and platelets along with hematuria suggests the presence of thrombi in the circuit, so-called "circuit disseminated intravascular coagulation." This often requires a change of the entire circuit. Ideal flow through the circuit can be gauged by achieving the lowest Δ pressure with the lowest revolutions per minute of the centrifugal pump.

Clots in the cannula(e) can be challenging to manage because removal of these by flushing out the cannula(e) with normal saline requires temporary discontinuation of ECLS. The neonate may not be ready to efficiently exchange gases even with increased ventilator settings providing full support. Flushing the clots can result in dislodgement of small thrombi not removed by this process that may inadvertently be infused into the neonate when the cannula is reattached to the circuit.

Table 20–2. DECREASED SvO$_2$ LEVELS DURING ECLS

O$_2$	Causes	Etiologies
↓ O$_2$ delivery	↓ CO	Heart failure, cardiac depressants, arrhythmias, ↑ PEEP, ↓ preload
	↓ SaO$_2$	↓ Respiratory function, poor native lung function, and desaturated pulmonary venous return, oxygenator failure, insufficient ECLS flow, ↓ ECLS blender FiO$_2$
	↓ Hb	Anemia, methemoglobinemia (abnormal Hb)
↑ O$_2$ demand	↑ VO$_2$	Fever, shivering, agitation, pain, seizures, infection
	↑ CO	↑ Work of breathing

CO, cardiac output; ECLS, extracorporeal life support; Hb, hemoglobin concentration; PEEP, positive end-expiratory pressure; VO$_2$, oxygen consumption.

E. **Monitoring the mixed venous oxygen saturation. During ECLS, the mixed venous oxygen saturation (SvO$_2$) reflects the degree of O$_2$ extraction** and should normally be in the **65% to 70% range for VA- and VV-ECLS.** SvO$_2$ <60% indicates a marginal oxygen delivery and critical level of O$_2$ extraction, suggesting that the rate of tissue metabolism is approaching the rate of O$_2$ delivery. Once the balance between delivery and extraction reaches the critical level, cells begin to use anaerobic metabolism, producing lactic acid. The SvO$_2$ presents a useful parameter to follow in VA-ECLS. Due to recirculation in VV-ECLS, the SvO$_2$ may sometimes be more difficult to interpret but can provide a useful trend. (See Tables 20–2 and 20–3.)

F. **Monitoring blood pressures**
   1. **Hypertension.** Elevated blood pressures are common with VA-ECLS in neonates. Nicardipine is a common drug used under these circumstances. The initial dose is 0.5 mcg/kg/min by continuous infusion and titrated every 10 minutes to maintenance doses of 0.5 to 5 mcg/kg/min to achieve the desired blood pressure.
   2. **Hypotension.** Because VV-ECLS does not provide direct cardiovascular support, neonates can have lower blood pressures that may require vasopressor/inotropic support. Dopamine has traditionally been a first-line choice for many centers, starting at 5 mcg/kg/min and titrated upward 2 to 5 mcg/kg/min every few minutes to 20 mcg/kg/min. Epinephrine has also been used as a primary agent or added to dopamine. The starting dose is 0.1 mcg/kg/min and titrated upward 0.1 mcg/kg/min to 1 mcg/kg/min. In situations of distributive shock

Table 20–3. INCREASED SvO$_2$ LEVELS DURING ECLS

O$_2$	Causes	Etiologies
↑ O$_2$ delivery	↑ CO	Improved cardiac function
	↑ SaO$_2$	Improved lung function, excess ECLS flow, ↑ FiO$_2$
	↑ Hb	Blood transfusion
	↑ Flow	Recirculation with VV-ECLS
↓ O$_2$ demand	↓ VO$_2$	Hypothermia, anesthesia, muscle relaxation
	↓ Utilization	Sepsis, cyanide toxicity (from sodium nitroprusside), severe neurologic injury

CO, cardiac output; ECLS, extracorporeal life support; Hb, hemoglobin concentration; VO$_2$, oxygen consumption; VV, venovenous.

from sepsis associated with systemic vasodilation, normal saline volume and the initiation of norepinephrine at 0.1 mcg/kg/min titrating to 1 mcg/kg/min or vasopressin starting at 10 milliunits/kg/h and titrating to 50 milliunits/kg/h can be therapeutic. Many centers also start hydrocortisone in neonates with hypotension regardless of the etiology.

G. **Monitoring for hemolysis.** Plasma free hemoglobin (pfHb) measures hemoglobin that has leaked into the serum when red blood cells undergo hemolysis. A normal pfHg is <10 mg/dL. The ELSO registry defines **hemolysis** as pfHb concentrations >50 mg/dL. pfHb can increase dramatically due to increased ECLS pump flows causing extreme negative pressures, elevated temperature in the water bath, clots in the oxygenator, or kinks in the circuit leading to high shear stresses from turbulent flow. Differences in tubing sizes and connection points throughout the circuit add to the shear stress and turbulence, further damaging red blood cells and causing local thrombus formation. Hemolysis also occurs when using centrifugal pumps due to the shearing force on blood components created by the vortex in the pump head. Elevated pfHb can cause vasoconstriction in the pulmonary vascular bed, direct injury to the kidney by obstructing the renal tubules, and damage to other organs as well. Neonates are particularly prone to hemolysis because of the differences in flow and pressure dynamics as well as small cannula sizes. Studies suggest that neonates on centrifugal pumps have higher rates of hemolysis, hyperbilirubinemia, hypertension, and acute renal failure than those on roller pumps. Centrifugal pumps designed more recently have less stagnation in the pump head and decreased hemolysis. Measures to alleviate high pfHb levels should be undertaken, in particular avoiding high flow rates. Circuit changes may be necessary if the pfHb level is extremely high (>200 mg/dL), although lower levels are of concern as well.

H. **Monitoring for loss of pump flow, retrograde flow, air embolism, chattering, and cavitation.** Loss of pump flow is an emergency and can be due to malposition of the cannula, low volume status, air in the circuit, or cardiac tamponade. Measures to recover pump flow include lowering flow rates, repositioning the patient, and, if persistent, evaluating for the possibility of cardiac tamponade with an echocardiogram. Frequently fluid boluses are used to increase venous filling when pump flow is challenged. However, the benefit is short lived and can lead to fluid overload. Attempts should be made to adjust a malpositioned cannula, if this is the cause, rather than using excessive volume.

1. **Retrograde or reversed flow** can occur if the pump flow is too low or if a shunt is open. In this situation, the distal pressure exceeds the pressure generated by the pump. It can be detected by the flow alarm and alleviated by running the pump flow faster.

2. **Air embolism** can occur when air is introduced inadvertently into the circuit through loose connections on the circuit. Emergent ventilator settings providing full support need to be used while these problems are alleviated. The problem is corrected by tapping the circuit line to get the air bubbles to the pump head or connector site where the air can be extracted with a syringe. The oxygenator has an escape port for air as well.

3. **"Chattering" or surging of the drainage line** of the circuit can occur when the centrifugal pump flow rate is excessive, causing a high negative pressure that occludes the blood flow returning to the neonate. Chattering is caused by hypovolemia, changes in the cannula position, and changes in intrathoracic pressure induced by coughing or moving and results in a fall in blood flow. If blood flow is interrupted but the pump rotor continues to spin at a high speed, the pump head ejects blood, but no volume refills the voided space. A vacuum forms within the pump head, and cavitation occurs.

4. **"Cavitation" or "outgassing"** appears when dissolved gases, oxygen and carbon dioxide, come out of solution during times of excessive negative pressure

generated by the centrifugal pump. **Cavitation can create gaseous microemboli that cause hemolysis of the red blood cells.** When the pressure normalizes, the gas will go back into solution; however, free hemoglobin remains in circulation. Generally, flows are run so that inlet pressures do not become more negative than −40 mm Hg in neonates.

XIV. **Lung rest during extracorporeal life support.** Neonates who receive ECLS usually have substantial primary lung disease complicated by ventilator-associated lung inflammation and injury. An important benefit of ECLS is to provide cardiopulmonary support while on "resting" or decreased ventilator settings. Although rest ventilator settings vary, for **VA-ECLS,** widely accepted settings for neonates include a rate of 10 breaths/min (10–20), positive end-expiratory pressure (PEEP) of 8 to 14 cm H_2O, and peak inspiratory pressure (PIP) in the 12 to 20 cm H_2O range. With VA-ECLS, a ventilator FiO_2 of approximately 0.3 to 0.4 may improve oxygenation of coronary blood, which is dependent on the blood flow and saturations from the left ventricle.

Higher ventilator settings may be required in VV-ECLS compared to VA-ECLS. Blood in VV-ECLS flows from the circuit to the right heart and must either go through the pulmonary vascular bed or extrapulmonary shunt pathways. Some degree of lung inflation and tidal ventilation is probably necessary to enhance pulmonary blood flow. Additionally, since VV-ECLS may not add as much oxygen content to the blood due to suboptimal cannula position and/or recirculation (see Section XIX.B.3), the rest settings are frequently higher than on VA-ECLS (ie, conventional rate of 20–30 breaths/min, PIP 15–25 cm H_2O, PEEP 8–14 cm H_2O, and FiO_2 0.3–0.5). High-frequency ventilation can also provide more cardiopulmonary support to the patient yet maintain gentle ventilatory assistance. For the Life Pulse High-Frequency Ventilator (Bunnell Incorporated, Salt Lake City, UT), general settings would include a rate of 420 (360 if the neonate has CDH), PIP of 16–20 cm H_2O, I time of 0.02, and PEEP of 10 to 14 cm H_2O from the corollary conventional ventilator without a conventional rate. On high-frequency oscillatory ventilation (3100A Neonatal and Pediatric High-Frequency Ventilator; CareFusion, Yorba Linda, CA), routine settings would include a mean airway pressure of 10 to 14 cm H_2O with low amplitudes of 15 to 20 cm H_2O and frequency between 8 and 10 Hz.

Higher vent settings to achieve improved gas exchange should be discouraged and are inappropriate in situations where ventilator-induced injury or air leak has occurred. The goal of ECLS is to avoid exacerbating lung injury, so noxious stimuli to the lungs should be avoided as much as possible. Improving oxygen delivery from ECLS can be accomplished by administering sedatives and, on occasion, neuromuscular blockers or converting to VA-ECLS when poor gas exchange, hypotension, and elevated lactate levels occur, suggesting that VV-ECLS is not sufficient.

Inhaled nitric oxide is generally discontinued when patients are placed on ECLS. To date, no studies have shown a benefit of inhaled nitric oxide (iNO) in decreasing pulmonary hypertension when the lung volumes are small. However, once the inflammatory process wanes and lung inflation improves, theoretically iNO could help lower pulmonary pressures and expedite successful transition off ECLS.

XV. **Renal function during extracorporeal life support.** Because fluid overload commonly occurs with critical illness, ECLS patients frequently require pharmacologic diuresis once capillary leak subsides. Furthermore, when using VA-ECLS, the kidneys may be perfused with nonpulsatile flow, resulting in a decrease in renal function. For patients with preexisting or developing AKI and/or those with anasarca, hemofiltration may be added in parallel to the ECLS circuit via a small shunt. This system allows for removal of excess fluid and stabilizes electrolyte abnormalities. (See Figure 20–1.) Studies have reported increased mortality associated with AKI in the setting of ECLS.

XVI. **Medications and nutrition.** Antibiotics, sedatives, narcotics, proton pump inhibitors, and total parenteral nutrition should be delivered directly to the patient, and not via the ECLS circuit, if possible. However, in neonates with limited vascular access, these agents can be delivered into the ECLS circuit at venous access locations. Because the volume of distribution is higher with the added ECLS circuit volume, higher doses may be needed to achieve therapeutic concentrations, particularly for sedatives and narcotics, regardless of where the medications are delivered. Sedatives are particularly beneficial because of the risk that excessive movements may have on circuit flow and function and are useful in reducing oxygen consumption. Medications used most frequently include morphine, lorazepam, fentanyl, and dexmedetomidine. Due to the fact that fentanyl binds to the plastic in the circuit, many centers avoid using it. With AKI, dosing may need to be decreased with medications cleared by the kidney. Discussion with a pharmacist will help with correct dosing.

Because of hypotension, neonates are often treated with fluid resuscitation. However, caution should be taken not to fluid overload prior to the initiation of ECLS or during ECLS. Adequate nutrition can generally be provided with fluids running at 100 to 120 mL/kg/d with an increase in protein daily by 1 g/kg/d to a goal of 4 g/kg/d. Enteral nutrition is of vital importance and should be started once infants have stabilized.

XVII. **Myocardial dysfunction.** Initiation of VA-ECLS is associated with an increased after-load because the extracorporeal flow is delivered to the aortic arch. This can lead to decreased myocardial contractility and dysfunction.

Myocardial stun, an extreme form of cardiac dysfunction, is a transient phenomenon that can be recognized by a **dampening of the arterial waveform and patient PaO$_2$ that approximates the postoxygenator PO$_2$.** It is more likely to occur in neonates with myocardial dysfunction prior to being placed on ECLS from disorders such as myocarditis and intractable arrhythmias and after cardiac surgery or cardiopulmonary arrest. Patients usually recover in 3 to 7 days.

Myocardial stun is less likely to occur with the initiation of VV-ECLS because there is no increase in left ventricular (LV) afterload and there is higher oxygen content provided to the coronary arteries than with VA-ECLS. Echocardiography has shown similar function of the ventricles before and after the initiation of VV-ECLS. However, cardiac stun will lead to cardiovascular collapse or arrest if it occurs on VV-ECLS because, in contrast to VA-ECLS, there is no cardiovascular support. Under these circumstances, a neonate would need to be converted to VA-ECLS.

Myocardial stun may be confused with **poor cardiac output due to hypovolemia, pneumothorax, pneumopericardium, hemothorax, or hemopericardium**. An echocardiogram showing minimal LV wall motion can confirm the diagnosis.

Right ventricular (RV) dysfunction can occur, particularly in neonates with severe pulmonary hypertension before the initiation of ECLS. In some cases, even while on VV- ECLS, the RV becomes further dilated with poor function, causing it to bow into the LV and compromising LV filling and cardiac output. Assessment by echocardiography may diagnose poor RV function and the use of agents to reduce RV afterload, such as iNO, milrinone, and/or medications such as sildenafil (Revatio; Pfizer), treprostinil (Remodulin; United Therapeutics Corporation), or epoprostenol (Flolan; GlaxoSmithKline) may be warranted.

On occasion RV, LV, or biventricular dysfunction or the need for higher flows due to sepsis may necessitate conversion from VV-ECLS to VA-ECLS. If the neonate is too unstable to be off ECLS for more than a few seconds, the arterial cannula can be placed and then both lumens of the VV cannula used for drainage. Under these circumstances, the arterial lumen of the VV catheter is at risk for clotting. Alternatively, the VV arterial limb can continue to be used for patient inflow, but this may be limited by venous return. If lung function can support the infant for a few minutes, VA-ECLS can be accomplished by placing the arterial cannula and then replacing the venous cannula.

XVIII. **Circuit changes.** Circuit changes are undertaken if there is large thrombus formation or excessive need for blood products and/or hematuria suggesting circuit DIC or poor oxygenator function, indicated by a need to increase the sweep gas flow to achieve the appropriate goal CO$_2$ or noting a decrease in the postoxygenator PaO$_2$. During circuit changes, a large percentage of blood volume is exchanged, potentially causing electrolyte imbalances and arrhythmias. Drug doses may need to be adjusted. Narcotics, in particular, may need to be redosed or increased significantly.

XIX. **Practical considerations for extracorporeal life support management**
  A. **Venoarterial extracorporeal life support**
    1. **Venoarterial extracorporeal life support blood flows.** After cannulation, ECLS flow is increased gently over several minutes. After initiation of ECLS and particularly during cardiopulmonary arrest when ECPR is initiated, care should be taken to minimize hyperoxia and hypocarbia. Adjustments should be made in the FiO_2 and sweep gas flow to normalize gases and saturations.

       Typically VA-ECLS flow is maintained at approximately 100 to 150 mL/kg/min, and the pulse pressure is often approximately 10–20 mm Hg if the heart contracts effectively. As more blood is routed through the circuit with a high flow rate, the systemic arterial **pulse contour may become dampened** and then flatten if total bypass is achieved. In this situation, more blood drains into the circuit, decreasing both right and left heart preload and resulting in a decrease in the left ventricular stroke volume. Despite the lack of pulsatility, the mean blood pressure remains fairly constant and is the best gauge of blood pressure. Flow should be optimized to attain reasonable saturations and arterial pulse pressures as well as appropriate venous saturations, the best indicator of adequate oxygen delivery. As noted earlier, severe cardiac dysfunction may cause the arterial pulse contour to flatten.

    2. **Oxygen delivery/carbon dioxide removal.** In VA-ECLS, part of the blood from the right atrium also circulates through the neonate's lungs into the left heart and out through the aorta, returning again to the right heart. This blood will be exposed to variable ventilation depending on lung function and status of the disease process. With improvement in native lung function and cardiac output, the oxygen content of the blood returning to the right heart will increase.

       A major strategy to improve oxygen delivery includes maintaining a high hemoglobin concentration. Increasing the ECLS flow rate increases oxygen delivery as well. However, increasing the ECLS blender O_2 or ventilator FiO_2 will only minimally improve arterial saturations. A failing oxygenator with markedly reduced functional surface area may decrease oxygen content, but generally because of the large surface area in current oxygenators, this is rarely an issue.

       Increasing the sweep gas flow rate to the oxygenator lowers the arterial $PaCO_2$. An increasing $PaCO_2$ level may be the first sign that the oxygenator is malfunctioning.

    3. **Trialing off Venoarterial extracorporeal life support.** Patients should be ready to wean off VA-ECLS after the initial disease processes and inflammatory responses have subsided, appropriate fluid balance is achieved, and lungs have cleared. The surgical team should be notified of the estimated time of possible decannulation.
       a. **Starting 12 hours prior to the anticipated trial off, the extracorporeal life support blood flows are decreased slowly** and ventilator settings adjusted as needed to maintain gas exchange. Conventional ventilator settings may include a rate of 40 to 60 breaths/min, PEEP level of 8 to 10 cm H_2O, and PIP of 25 to 30 cm H_2O. Acceptable high-frequency oscillator settings generally include a mean airway pressure of 14 to 16 cm H_2O, amplitude of 30 to 35 cm H_2O, and frequency of 8 to 10 Hz. Life Pulse high-frequency ventilator settings are similar with a rate of 420 (360 in CDH patients), PEEP of 14 to 16 cm H_2O, PIP of 25 to 30 cm H_2O, and inspiratory time of 0.02 (which may vary depending on the disease process).

          In conducting the trial, all dextrose, antibiotic, and sedative or narcotic infusions should be moved from the ECLS circuit to the patient. Heparin may be split, so that half is infused to the patient and half to the circuit, or given all to the patient. Centers may also choose to give a single bolus dose to help prevent cannula thrombosis during this time or increase the rate of anticoagulation. The pump flow can be weaned hourly by 10 to 20 mL/min while gradually increasing ventilator support. ECLS blood flows can be weaned to a target "idling" flow of approximately 100 mL/kg/min. A bridge (connecting the venous and arterial sides of the circuit) is used to allow continued flow through the circuit but not to the patient. Continued flow through the circuit prevents clotting while the cannulae are clamped for the trial. The bridge can be part of the circuit or added at the time of the trial off. The venous and arterial cannulae are then clamped and the sweep gas line removed from the oxygenator.

To maintain the integrity of the cannulae and circuit while trialing off, the cannulae are flushed every 10 to 15 minutes per institutional guidelines to avoid stagnation. Patient blood gases are obtained every 10 to 15 minutes as well to assure adequate lung function throughout the trial. The low-flow state of the trial increases the possibility of thrombus formation in the circuit; the length of time for the trial may depend on cannulae and circuit integrity as well as patient response. If the neonate does well for 60 to 90 minutes and is not at the limits of acceptable ventilator support, he or she is ready to be separated from ECLS.

B. Venovenous extracorporeal life support

1. **Venovenous extracorporeal life support blood flows.** As with VA-ECLS, the initiation of VV-ECLS flow is gradually increased to 100 to 120 mL/kg/min. O_2 delivery can be augmented by increasing the O_2 content of the venous blood in the right atrium (increasing the FiO_2 to the oxygenator) or by maneuvers that decrease recirculation (eg, increasing native cardiac output, repositioning the cannula). Because oxygenated blood entering the right atrium mixes continuously with desaturated venous blood, the final O_2 content of the blood reaching the aorta and tissues is limited by the amount of blood that can be drained into the ECLS circuit, oxygenated, and returned to the venous system. The optimal pump flow rate is one that provides the highest effective pump flow at the lowest revolutions per minute of the pump, resulting in the highest O_2 delivery and causing the least degree of hemolysis.

2. **Oxygen delivery/carbon dioxide removal on venovenous extracorporeal life support.** Neonates usually have arterial saturations between 80% and 95% and PaO_2 of 40 to 80 mm Hg on VV-ECLS. During VV-ECLS, only indirect circulatory support is achieved, and lower PaO_2 and oxygen saturations often need to be tolerated as long as there are indications of adequate oxygen delivery. No evidence exists to show that this is detrimental. Major strategies to improve oxygen delivery include increasing the hemoglobin concentration, increasing ECLS flow, and augmenting native cardiac output. PaO_2s often rise as native pulmonary function improves. Increasing the sweep gas flow rate lowers the $PaCO_2$.

3. **Recirculation.** During VV-ECLS, recirculation occurs when oxygenated blood from the ECLS circuit delivered to the reinfusion lumen is siphoned back to the venous drainage side of the cannula instead of flowing across the tricuspid valve. When pump flow rises above optimal flow, recirculation increases and effective forward flow through the tricuspid valve decreases. **Clinically significant recirculation is recognized by decreased neonatal arterial saturations and a rise in SvO_2 with increasing pump flow.** Higher degrees of recirculation decrease the effective O_2 delivery from the circuit, possibly contributing to increased hemolysis as well. Factors that increase recirculation include the following:

     a. Decreased right atrial volume causes a higher percentage of returned oxygenated blood to be drained back to the pump.

     b. Inappropriate positioning of the outflow ports of the arterial side of the cannula may result in blood being directed away from the tricuspid valve, thus increasing the **recirculation fraction.** Catheters may migrate with changes in lung volume, changing edema of the neck, alterations in patient positioning, or movement, necessitating adjustment of the cannula to maintain adequate flows and minimize recirculation. Appropriate catheter position is critical in VV-ECLS and should be assessed by echocardiography.

     c. Poor cardiac output leads to greater recirculation because a smaller fraction of the oxygenated pump blood is propelled forward out of the right atrium.

     d. Pump flows need to be adjusted to achieve the least amount of recirculation. High flows can cause collapse of the right atrium, loss of pump flow, and hemolysis.

   4. Trialing off venovenous extracorporeal life support. Given the flow and physiology of VV-ECLS, weaning of circuit flow provides no benefit. Blood flow may remain constant (usually 100–120 mL/kg/min) followed by weaning the FiO_2 sweep gas flow rate and oxygen. During this time, the ventilator settings are increased to those expected to achieve suitable gas exchange. Then the sweep gas tubing is disconnected from the blender source (the oxygenator is "capped off"), which functionally removes the patient from ECLS. Blood gases and SvO_2 are followed, and once assured of success after 1 to 2 hours, the patient may be separated from ECLS and the heparin drip discontinued. Since the integrity of the cannula and circuit is maintained during the trial off because blood continues to flow through the entire circuit, longer trials are possible. If a percutaneous technique was used for VV cannula insertion, simply removing any sutures and then pulling the cannula and holding pressure at the insertion site for 15 to 20 minutes should achieve adequate hemostasis. In some cases, patients require a suture to close the skin over the entry site.

XX. Length of extracorporeal life support therapy. Typically, neonatal patients with MAS, PPHN, and sepsis require ECLS for 5 to 7 days. Patients with respiratory syncytial virus may require 2 to 4 weeks. Those with CDH usually require longer courses (10–14 days), but may need up to 21 days if the pulmonary pressures are slow to fall. If there is lack of improvement within 10 to 14 days in non-CDH neonates, a lung biopsy while on ECLS should be considered to rule out lethal anomalies such as alveolar capillary dysplasia or acinar dysplasia. If the suspicion for anomalies is high at birth, biopsies should be done sooner. Antifibrinolytics generally are not necessary for the biopsy. The heparin infusion can be decreased to a rate where the ACT or anti-Xa levels are in the low range of normal, or heparin can be discontinued for a period of time. Platelet counts are most frequently kept >100 to 150,000 and the fibrinogen >150 mg/dL. Air leaks are generally a rare complication.

XXI. Complications of extracorporeal life support

   A. Patient complications of ECLS per the Extracorporeal Life Support Organization (ELSO) International Summary data as of January 2019 for neonatal respiratory patients are as follows: acute renal failure (continuous renal replacement required, 31.1%); hypertension requiring vasodilators, 8.4%; hypotension requiring inotropes, 32.9%; CNS infarction, 3.2%; CNS hemorrhage 10.1%; culture-proven infection, 4.1%; surgical bleeding, 6.4%; pulmonary hemorrhage, 4.8%; pneumothorax requiring treatment, 5.2%; DIC, 4.6%; hemolysis, 15.3%; seizures by EEG, 3.7%; brain death, 0.3%.

   B. Mechanical problems include the following: circuit component clots, 36.8%; cannula problems, 12.8%; oxygenator failure, 4%; air in the circuit, 4%; pump malfunction, 0.9%.

XXII. Prognosis. As of January 2019, the Neonatal ECLS Registry lists 41,707 neonatal runs. From 2014 to current, the overall cumulative neonatal survival rate is 67% for pulmonary cases, 49% for cardiac, and 42% for ECPR. The cumulative drop in survival rates over the years reflects a larger proportion of patients treated with more severe disease. CDH accounts for the majority of respiratory mortality. Survival rates for specific diseases are: MAS, 92%; PPHN, 73%; RDS, 82%; sepsis, 50%; pneumonia, 53%; air leak syndrome 88%; CDH, 50%; congenital heart defect, 46%; cardiac arrest, 40%; cardiogenic shock, 55%; cardiomyopathy, 55%; and myocarditis, 52%. While 77% of neonates with pulmonary disease survived VV-ECLS, only 63% survived VA-ECLS. The diagnosis of CDH in neonates with lower birth weight treated for respiratory failure are factors associated with increased mortality and morbidity.

XXIII. Outcomes. Head ultrasounds should be obtained during the ECLS course and an MRI post ECLS to better define potential injury.

Bilateral sensorineural hearing loss (SNHL) can occur when pre-ECLS risk factors are present such as seizures, $PaCO_2$ <30 mmHg, pH >7.5, and is associated with the use of furosemide, aminoglycosides, or neuromuscular blocking agents. Early audiologic evaluations are necessary and should be continued throughout childhood because late presentation of SNHL can occur.

Despite neurophsychological development showing favorable trends, hyperactivity, or behavioral difficulties can occur at later ages so children need to be followed long term. Difficulties in visual-spatial and memory tasks can occur in those evaluated at age 5. Adolescents with a history of being treated with ECLS have been noted to have problems with short- and long-term verbal memory, visual-spatial memory, and working memory. This group also reported more withdrawn/depressed behavior, somatic complaints, and social problems. Problems with gross motor function may become more obvious as the child ages. Despite these stated complications, many children can have excellent morbidity-free outcomes.

21 Follow-Up of High-Risk Infants

Whenever an infant requires neonatal intensive care, concerns about survival are followed by concerns about the infant's quality of life. Neonatal intensive care follow-up clinics are a necessary adjunct to neonatal intensive care. They provide families with the support and advice they need following neonatal intensive care unit (NICU) discharge. They provide feedback regarding the child's ongoing health and development to families, pediatricians, neonatologists, and obstetricians. Most important, to optimize neurodevelopmental outcomes, serial developmental assessments facilitate early diagnosis and referral for specific early interventions when neuroplasticity may be at its peak.

I. **Goals of a neonatal follow-up clinic**
   A. **Early identification of neurodevelopmental disability.** High-risk NICU infants need comprehensive neurodevelopmental evaluations and appropriate intervention services. There is a growing body of evidence suggesting that early detection can take advantage of periods of the most active neuroplasticity after brain injury. **Neuroplasticity** refers to the ability of the central nervous system (CNS) to change both structurally and functionally in response to experience and to adapt following injury. In the postnatal brain, there is a very active period of proliferation and pruning of synapses through neurogenesis and apoptosis. This period of neuroplasticity is most active during the first 3 years. An additional mechanism of brain plasticity in the developing child is activity-dependent shaping of neuronal circuits by experience

or injury. There is growing evidence extracted from adult and animal literature that there is a finite period of injury-induced neuroplasticity where most recovery occurs. This will be missed without early identification and appropriate intervention services in high-risk infants.

B. **Assessment of a child's need for early interventions.** Although NICUs refer many infants directly to community early intervention programs, a child's needs change with neuromaturation, requiring periodic review of community service needs.

C. **Parent counseling.** Reassurance that their child is making good neurodevelopmental progress is always welcome, as the anxiety of uncertainty is a heavy burden for parents. Parents of children with developmental delay need realistic information about its significance and whether it will lead to impairment. A comprehensive neurodevelopmental evaluation can provide parents with essential information and recommendations for how to promote their child's neurodevelopment. Physical and occupational therapists provide valuable suggestions regarding positioning, handling, and feeding infants. Even if their infant does well, parents of high-risk infants should be warned about their child's risk for and early indicators of school or behavior problems.

D. **Identification and treatment of medical complications** that were not recognized or anticipated at the time of discharge from the NICU (eg, hypertension, sleep problems).

E. **Referral for comprehensive evaluations and services as indicated.**

F. **Feedback for neonatologists, pediatricians, obstetricians, pediatric surgeons, and others** regarding neurodevelopmental outcomes, ongoing medical problems, and unusual or unforeseen complications in these infants is essential.

II. **Staff of the neonatal follow-up clinic.** Pediatricians, neurodevelopmental pediatricians, and neonatologists make up the regular staff of the clinic, and many clinics include neuropsychologists and physical, occupational, and/or speech and language therapists. In addition, many need referrals to audiologists, social workers, ophthalmologists, neuropsychologists, pulmonologists, nutritionists, gastroenterologists, orthopedic surgeons, or other subspecialists.

III. **Risk factors for developmental disability.** It is virtually impossible to diagnose developmental disability with certainty in the neonatal period, but a number of perinatal risk factors have been identified for selecting high-risk infants for close follow-up.

A. **Preterm birth.** The risks of cerebral palsy, intellectual disability, and sensory deficits increase with decreasing gestational age and severity of brain injury. Risk of disability, especially cognitive impairments, is highest in survivors born at the limit of viability (at or before 25 weeks' gestation). Children born preterm have higher rates of language disorders, visual perception problems, minor neuromotor dysfunction, attention deficits, executive dysfunction, learning disabilities, social-communicative problems, and emotional difficulties than full-term controls. Although most do well, children born at 33 to 36 weeks' gestation have higher rates of cognitive impairments, cerebral palsy, and school problems than children born full term. Besides gestational age, predictors of neurodevelopmental disability include poor growth (especially head growth), asphyxia, sepsis (especially meningitis), chronic lung disease, necrotizing enterocolitis, and retinopathy of prematurity. Risk is highest in infants with signs of brain injury on neonatal neurodevelopmental examination and neuroimaging studies (see Chapter 18).

B. **Intrauterine growth restriction (IUGR).** Full-term infants who are small for gestational age (SGA) have a higher risk of motor or cognitive impairments, attention deficits, specific learning disability, and school and behavior problems than appropriate for gestational age (AGA) infants. The etiology and severity of their IUGR, timing of the insult, and subsequent perinatal complications (eg, asphyxia, hypoglycemia, feeding difficulties, polycythemia, brain injury) influence their degree of risk (see Chapter 104). After 30 weeks' gestation, compensatory mechanisms for adverse intrauterine circumstances include accelerated maturation to improve survival if born preterm. Adverse intrauterine circumstances, preterm birth, and accelerated neuromaturation can adversely influence neurodevelopmental (especially cognitive) outcomes in preterm SGA infants.

C. **Neonatal encephalopathy.** Neonatal encephalopathy (NE) is a clinical syndrome characterized by a constellation of findings, including seizures and abnormalities of consciousness, muscle tone, reflexes, respiratory control, and feeding. Etiologies include infection, inflammation, metabolic errors, drug exposures, brain malformations, stroke, hypoxia, ischemia, or any combination of these conditions. Etiology, severity of clinical symptoms, abnormal electroencephalogram (EEG) pattern (especially low voltage or burst-suppression patterns), and patterns of brain injury (eg, injury to the basal ganglia and thalamus) are much stronger predictors of neurodevelopmental disability than signs of fetal distress, cord pH, or Apgar scores. Infants with mild or moderate NE who do not develop major disability are at risk for more subtle disorders, including attention deficit, learning disability, and other school problems. Infants with severe NE have a high mortality rate; many of the survivors have severe multiple disabilities, including intellectual disability, spastic quadriplegia, microcephaly, seizures, and sensory impairment. Treatment of infants with moderate to severe NE with hypothermia improves neurodevelopmental outcomes.

D. **Respiratory failure.** Some late preterm and full-term infants develop respiratory failure that can be due to pulmonary hypoplasia, pneumonia, meconium aspiration, and/or persistent pulmonary hypertension. Outcome studies for randomized controlled trials of treatments for severe respiratory failure (eg, inhaled nitric oxide, ECLS) report cognitive impairment in up to one-quarter of survivors, cerebral palsy in up to 15%, and hearing impairment in up to 30%. When followed to school age, many have problems with attention deficit, specific learning disability, minor neuromotor dysfunction, and behavior problems. Health sequelae include poor growth, reactive airway disease, and increased frequency of respiratory infections. Some survivors have demonstrated progressive hearing loss, so these children need serial hearing assessments.

E. **Infection and/or inflammation.** Maternal, fetal, and neonatal infection or inflammation has been implicated as an etiology of preterm birth, brain injury (eg, white matter injury), cerebral palsy, and cognitive impairments.

F. **Other risk factors**
   1. **Congenital infections (TORCHZ—*t*oxoplasmosis, *o*ther, *r*ubella, *c*ytomegalovirus, *h*erpes simplex virus, and now *Z*ika virus).** Infants with congenital cytomegalovirus infection, toxoplasmosis, rubella, or Zika virus who are symptomatic at birth have a high incidence of neurodevelopmental disability. Asymptomatic infants are at risk for sensory impairment and learning disability.
   2. **In utero exposures.** Maternal drugs reported to influence fetal development include narcotics, cocaine, alcohol, phenytoin, trimethadione, valproate, warfarin, aminopterin, retinoic acid, and environmental toxicants.
   3. **Complex medical healthcare needs.** Children discharged home from NICUs with complex medical healthcare needs have a high risk of neurologic impairment and need close follow-up of their neurodevelopment.

IV. **Terminology.** Communicating about preterm outcomes entails consistent definitions.
   A. **Gestational age.** Time between mother's first day of the last menstrual cycle and birth.
   B. **Postmenstrual age (PMA).** Infant's gestational age (GA) plus chronological age (from birth).
   C. **Corrected age.** Calculated from the infant's due date, the infant's age corrected for degree of prematurity (ie, chronological age minus number of weeks born preterm).
   D. **Use PMA for preterm infants in a NICU and corrected age for preterm follow-up.**
V. **Parameters requiring follow-up**
   A. **Growth (height, weight, head circumference, weight for height).** Assess at each follow-up visit. Poor head growth is associated with lower cognitive scores. Most

preterm infants "catch up" in growth, but some infants with IUGR, extremely preterm birth, chronic lung disease, or short gut syndrome remain smaller than their peers. Too rapid weight gain and overweight raise concerns for increased risk for metabolic syndrome.

B. Vital signs with blood pressure. High blood pressure is a serious NICU sequela and occurs more frequently in infants who had umbilical catheters or renal problems.

C. Breathing disorders

1. **Apnea.** For infants discharged home on monitors, there is often uncertainty as to when to discontinue the monitor.

2. **Chronic lung disease.** Infants with chronic lung disease have higher rates of respiratory infections, reactive airway disease, rehospitalization, and neurodevelopmental disability. Those on supplemental oxygen, monitors, diuretics, and other medications need subspecialty follow-up.

3. **All infants need protection from secondhand smoke** and anticipatory guidance against ever smoking themselves.

D. Hearing. Hearing is essential for language acquisition, so it should be identified as early as possible. Before hospital discharge, all neonates should have their hearing screened (**eg, brainstem auditory evoked potentials, transient evoked otoacoustic emissions**) and referred for a comprehensive audiologic evaluation if there are concerns. Hearing aids, cochlear implants, and other treatment strategies have had a profound effect on language acquisition. Infants who had congenital or perinatal (eg, TORCHZ) infection, congenital malformations of the head or neck, persistent pulmonary hypertension, chronic otitis, a family history of hearing impairment, or a language delay warrant serial hearing assessments.

E. Vision. Retinopathy of prematurity (ROP) is a disease of the developing retina in preterm infants (see Chapter 118). Infants at risk for ROP need serial eye examinations until their retinas are fully vascularized. Ophthalmologic examinations are also indicated in infants with congenital infection, congenital anomalies, and NE. All high-risk infants should have their visual acuity assessed when 1 to 5 years old. Infants with injury to the visual cortex need to be assessed for signs of cortical visual impairment (CVI) because early intervention for CVI can improve their visual function.

F. Neuromaturation, the functional development of the central nervous system, is a dynamic process: what is typical at one age is often abnormal at another age. Extremely preterm infants are hypotonic at birth and typically develop flexor tone, first in the legs then in the arms (eg, in a caudocephalad direction) as they approach term. Typical preterm infants at term and full-term infants have strong flexor tone (ie, flexor hypertonia), as well as a number of primitive (eg, Moro) and pathologic (eg, Babinski) reflexes. In the months following term, emergence of higher cortical control suppresses flexor tone and pathologic and primitive reflexes. Examiners must know typical infant development and the significance of deviations from the norm.

G. Neurodevelopmental examination. Includes an assessment of posture, extremity and axial (neck and trunk) muscle tone, deep tendon reflexes, primitive reflexes, pathologic reflexes, postural reactions (eg, automatic movements that keep the body upright), and quality of motor function.

H. Neuromotor abnormalities. Abnormalities on neuromotor exam are common in high-risk infants during the first year, but they often resolve or become less prominent by age 1 to 2 years. They persist and are accompanied by motor delay in infants who develop cerebral palsy. These infants should have a comprehensive multidisciplinary evaluation because infants with cerebral palsy may have associated deficits that interfere with function. Infants with neuromotor abnormalities and mild or no motor delay have minor neuromotor dysfunction, which signifies increased risk of balance and coordination difficulties (developmental coordination disorder), learning disability, attention deficit, and behavior problems.

1. **Hypotonia (generalized or axial hypotonia) is common in preterm infants,** infants with chronic lung disease, and infants with genetic syndromes.

2. **Hypertonia is most common at the ankles and hips.** Persistent hypertonia (especially extensor) and hyperreflexia indicate spasticity. In preterm children, spastic diplegia (ie, of both lower extremities) is the most common type of cerebral palsy. Avoid standing activities until infants can pull themselves up to stand against furniture.

3. **Asymmetry of function, tone, posture, or reflexes.** Encourage parents to position infants in their crib so they will turn their head to each side, as a strong head preference can influence neuromuscular and motor milestone development. Some NICU infants develop such a strong head preference that they develop torticollis and plagiocephaly. Infants generally do not develop a hand preference until between 1 and 2 years. Spastic hemiplegia is spasticity of an arm and ipsilateral leg. Early handedness and significant persistent asymmetry are indications for referral for intensive physical therapy, including possible constraint-induced therapy.

4. **Neck, trunk, and lower extremity extensor hypertonia and shoulder retraction** (ie, excessive arching, shoulders back) can interfere with head control, hand use, rolling over, sitting, and getting in and out of a sitting position. Encourage families to hold and position infants with their head and shoulders in line with their body and to avoid standing activities until their children pull themselves up to stand.

5. **Fine motor dysfunction** is difficulty using the hands for manipulating objects. Fine motor milestones include reaching and grabbing for toys, transferring them from hand to hand, and developing a pincer grasp (using index finger and thumb).

6. **Feeding problems.** Tube-fed infants need oromotor stimulation programs to prevent oral aversion (eg, not tolerating anything in their mouth). Coughing, choking, and/or gagging with feedings are indications for referral for an oral motor evaluation.

I. **Cognitive development.** Language and visual attention are early signs of cognitive development. Refer infants with language delay for an audiologic evaluation to be sure there is no subtle hearing impairment. The primary way that infants and young children learn is by face-to-face interactions with family. Encourage families to talk and read to their infant, reinforce vocalizations, and by 9 to 10 months, identify objects by name. Avoid any screen time before 2 years. Accuracy of cognitive assessments improves with age.

J. **Developmental assessment.** A number of standardized tests are available for developmental screening or assessment. Many of them are easy to learn and administer.
1. **Infant developmental milestones.** History and observation of language, motor, and adaptive milestone attainment provide a quick overview of developmental progress.
2. **Standardized screening and assessment tests.** A number of standardized tests are available for use in infants and children at different ages.

VI. **Correction for degree of prematurity.** Most agree that one should correct for degree of prematurity in preterm infants, but correcting beyond 2 to 3 years is *controversial*. The older a child, the less important correction is: by 5 years, arithmetically a difference of 4 months (eg, 60 vs 56 months) matters little. Motor milestone attainment up to independent walking proceeds according to age corrected for degree of prematurity. Some data suggest correction influences cognitive scores in children born extremely preterm beyond age 2 to 3 years.

VII. **Comprehensive evaluations.** Recognizing delay or disability is an indication for comprehensive evaluation of all areas of function. Brain damage is seldom focal and often diffuse. A comprehensive multidisciplinary evaluation recognizes areas of a child's strength and challenges, helps develop strategies for intervention, provides realistic information for parent counseling, and provides recommendations for promoting the child's neurodevelopment during critical periods of infancy and early childhood.

22 Complementary and Integrative Medical Therapies in Neonatology

I. **Introduction.** The use of complementary and alternative therapies continues to grow in this country and abroad. **Integrative medicine** is a newer term that emphasizes integration of complementary therapies with conventional medicine. In integrative medicine, health professionals are expanding their view of Western medicine to a more holistic perspective. Integrative care has emerged in neonatal intensive care units (NICUs) throughout the globe as an attempt to create a more neuroprotective environment and provide a more nurturing, family-friendly environment.

Early exposure to the ex utero environment, long before development is capable of handling it, has a myriad of sequelae. We cannot escape the evolving realization of environmental and epigenetic influences on the development of the immature brain. These infants require developmental care equal to their acute and chronic medical care. Integrative therapies give us some options that might help ameliorate some of the routinely expected morbidities.

This chapter briefly describes some of the most popular and promising integrative therapies, explores how these options are used in the NICU, provides some evidence-based support of integrative therapies, and presents ideas on potential future integrative expansions. **Broad categories that integrative therapies address include the following:**

   A. **Lifestyle therapies (called "developmental care" in neonatology).** Examples include light and color therapies, music therapy, aromatherapy, kangaroo care, and attention to environmental influences, such as bright lights and loud noises.

   B. **Biomechanical therapies.** Example include massage, reflexology, and osteopathy/craniosacral therapy.

   C. **Bioenergetic therapies.** Examples include acupuncture/acupressure, therapeutic/healing touch, and reiki.

   D. **Biochemical therapies.** Examples include homeopathy and herbal medicine.

II. **Lifestyle therapies.** Lifestyle therapies are more commonly referred to in the NICU as developmental care intervention. Research shows that the environment of a newborn is an important influence on sensory, neural, and behavioral development.

   A. **Developmental care** includes many interventions, both on the macro- and microenvironmental level. Many neonatal units have made tremendous efforts to modify existing nurseries or have designed new units with environmental modifications that include particular attention to noise levels, light exposure, organization of care, and family-centered care.

      1. **Noise.** Adverse environmental auditory stimuli are a common concern. Many NICUs incorporate a system of noise assessment and regulation. Ex utero, the auditory system is not shielded by the maternal tissues, which significantly attenuate frequencies. Ambient noise in the NICU may cause distress, and attempts have been made to minimize the noise using ear plugs or using sound to negate other sounds, called sonic acoustic masking. Single-family rooms create a more home-like environment and have proved to be successful in terms of noise abatement. However, there is concern of lack of stimulation for infants who do not have regular visitation by family members.

      2. **Light.** Regulation of ambient light in the NICU is also an important concern. Constant exposure to light can result in disorganization of an infant's state. Unit lighting is now designed or modified to regulate light and to include developmentally supportive circadian dark/light cycling. Focused lighting for procedures and the use of eye covers or incubator drapes are all great adjuncts.

3. **Care organization.** Infant-specific care plans help better regulate the myriad intrusions of intensive care. Positioning, handling, and interactions should be coordinated when possible with cues of readiness from the infant. This is felt to help the infant minimize energy losses and allow for more optimal conditions for neurodevelopment maturation. Infants need more conscious developmental care when the situation allows.

4. **Family involvement.** Having an infant in intensive care not only causes acute stress but also can lead to posttraumatic stress disorder, which can continue or manifest months later. There is a current trend that allows parents to be present 24/7 and to participate in the daily rounds on their infant. Many professionals, who would not otherwise even consider some of the integrative therapies that follow, now look at these therapies as opportunities that allow more parental participation and connection, encourage parent–neonate interactions, and enhance bonding. Parents can create a loving environment, instill a sense of security, and foster a trusting responsiveness; however, when they are met with an authoritarian, "You can't touch your baby," they can feel pushed aside and confused.

Parents are integral team members who should be included in our expanded focus on the developmental aspects of care. What parents need is a context for their interactions; they need someone to teach them how to titrate interactions while becoming aware of their infant's cues. The **Newborn Individualized Developmental Care and Assessment Program (NIDCAP)** has been especially influential in encouraging awareness of the use of an infant's communications as a basis for individualized care delivery. These can be detected by reading the infant's sign language or state-related behaviors such as finger splaying, frequent fisting, trunk arching, gaze aversion, or more typical behaviors such as cooing, babbling, or fussing with a frowning face. Awareness of these states has changed our understanding from thinking of an infant as a passive organism to an active partner in a feedback system of rich human interactions.

Maternal administration of physical activity such as passive limb movements has been shown to enhance bone mineral acquisition in very low birthweight (VLBW) infants. This could be a great way for a father to also feel included in the care of his baby. These care practices can also provide an opportunity for infants to hear their parents' voices, as speech and language development are believed to be influenced by prenatal maternal speech.

5. **Kangaroo care (KC)** is usually used to promote bonding and attachment between the infant and the parent (the infant is usually wearing nothing more than a diaper while held on the parent's bare chest). KC was originally developed for a different purpose. Preterm infants in Bogota, Colombia, were dying of infection caused by cross-contamination from shared bedding space and equipment in the nursery. Colombian physicians decided to try having mothers stay in the hospital and incubate their infants next to their bodies until the babies were stable and discharged home.

KC has many cogent justifications. It supports the growing consumer interest in participation in the care of hospitalized infants while giving a significant feeling of autonomy to the parents. When a parent holds their infant against his or her skin, the infant's breathing, oxygen saturation, heart rate, and tone improve. It has also been shown that skin-to-skin care results in less episodes of apnea, less disorganized sleep states, and a doubling in the periods of quiet regular sleep. In addition, varying body positions seems to affect gastric emptying and reflux. Recent evidence confirms that KC promotes physiologic stability with very immature and ventilated infants.

6. **Aromatherapy.** Researchers have reported that newborns have an acute sense of smell. Odor forms part of the complex bonding process. The soothing effects of a mother's odor are in stark contrast to the noxious odors of alcohol, skin cleansers,

and adhesives normally found in a NICU. In some cultures, familiar odors are often left in a newborn's crib to calm an infant in the mother's absence. Through the use of aromas, neurotransmitters are released that calm, sedate, and decrease painful sensations or can be used for stimulation. **Lavender** has been the most studied; for example, when lavender is placed on pillows of adults, it is known to alleviate insomnia and stress. Aromatherapy could be helpful for NICU staff as well. A recent study showed that aromatherapy with lavender oil decreased stress levels in nurses who worked in the adult trauma intensive care setting. In a study from Japan, male college students who were exposed to lavender scent during work showed improved concentration. In another Japanese study, female students exposed to lemon fragrance had diminished fatigue.

Several recent articles address the role of olfaction as a tool in preterm infant care. A study published in 2016 showed that *Rosa damascena* **(rose) distillate** reduced the incidence of apnea, bradycardia, and decrease in oxygen saturation in preterm infants. Other studies have shown a decrease in apnea and apnea with bradycardia using **vanillin**. The explanation for the reduction in apnea and bradycardia is unclear but may be due to a direct or indirect effect on the respiratory centers and the ability of these compounds to be absorbed by the nasal mucosa, allowing a direct pathway to the brain centers. Another explanation is that the presence of a pleasant odor in the environment may help the infant to self-regulate. Aromatherapy with **lavender and mother's breast milk** has also been shown to reduce the pain with blood drawing in newborns.

7. **Music therapy.** Lullabies have been linked with infants throughout history; music therapy carries this tradition over into the NICU. Music therapy has also been shown to calm distress after painful stimuli, resulting in a faster return to a more organized state and improving the hypersensitivity that is associated with stimulation. A number of studies have documented improvements in feedings and weight gain, decreased salivary cortisol levels, and enhanced development and parental bonding. We know that by 16 to 18 weeks of gestation, the auditory capabilities of the fetus are present. In utero, the uterine blood flow provides a soothing musical waterfall, and the maternal heartbeat provides a continuous tick-tock.

In a recent study, Loewy et al reported that intentional, therapeutic use of live sounds, inclusive of breath, rhythm, and parent-preferred lullabies, applied by a certified music therapist can influence cardiac and respiratory function. Particularly when entrained with a premature infant's observed vital signs, sound and lullaby can enhance quiet alert and sleep states, sucking patterns, and oxygen saturation. Parent-preferred lullabies, sung live, and contextualized in a 6/8 meter, can enhance bonding and have the potential to significantly reduce parental stress. Music therapists can work with fathers as well and thereby increase their presence in the NICU, implementing a family-centered approach. Dr. Loewy is the founder of the Rhythm, Breath, and Lullaby (RBL) international training.

Music, both live and recorded, has been studied in a variety of conditions and contexts. Music may alleviate some of the distress infants sustain with suctioning and heel sticks. In the first meta-analysis of music therapy in the NICU, Standley reported heart and respiratory rates, oxygen saturations, weight gain, length of stay, and sucking and feeding ability as all being positively influenced. A recent meta-analysis replicated these findings and found that live music therapy and early music therapy showed the greatest benefit. The Pacifier-Activated Lullaby (PAL) is a medical device that has been used to reinforce sucking patterns, which may lead to enhanced sucking patterns. Studies involving the live use of music therapy as integrative in the treatment of neonatal abstinence syndrome are ongoing and compelling because they involve parents in the discipline, which ensures continuity of care at home, enhancing bonding potential for infants with parents.

Environmental music therapy involves the intentional use of music and sound to modulate the soundscape of a noisy hospital area such as the NICU.

A noxious sound environment is converted into a quieter treatment area, one that is more conducive to healing and well-being. Infants, families, and staff reap the benefits.

8. **Color and light therapy.** Healthcare workers tend to dismiss color and light therapy as something from the distant annals of medicine, but certainly neonatologists could expand awareness in this area due to the near omnipresent use of phototherapy in neonatal units. Research on phototherapy has shown the biologic significance of light exposure. Aside from the classically recognized effects of diminishing bilirubin and activation of vitamin D, numerous studies have shown other metabolic alterations with phototherapy, including thyroid stimulation, alterations in renal and vascular parameters, and increased gut transit times. Could it be that other wavelengths of light might have other physiologic effects? This has become the basis for the field of study for color and light therapy.

The current interest for light therapy in the NICU has less emphasis on the effect of different wavelengths (colors) on an infant's metabolic milieu; rather, it focuses on generalized lighting in the unit. Establishing circadian rhythmicity by varying light cycles in the infant's environment seems to minimize endocrine fluctuations, as well as the states of disorganization that come from constant light stimulation. One study used acrylic helmets to reduced infant exposure to light on a defined schedule. Infants in the intervention group had improved weight gain and earlier hospital discharge. Another study that used a special light filter placed over the incubator for a specified time each day found similar improvements in weight gain prior to 28 weeks; when not using incubator covers or eye patches, it has been suggested that overexposure to light may interfere with the development of the other senses.

III. **Biomechanical therapies**

A. **Massage therapy** has been used in the care of premature infants for many years, and a significant body of research has already shown its effectiveness. Tiffany Fields has conducted infant massage research since the 1970s, much of which has focused on the premature infant. Fields reported that massaged infants have improved weight gain and better organized sleep states; they become more responsive to social stimulation, have more organized motor development, and are commonly discharged 6 to 10 days earlier from the hospital. Fields's studies suggest that massage increases vagal activity, which in turn releases gastrin and insulin and also increases levels of insulin-like growth factor-1. These findings may explain the weight gain in massaged premature infants. Recent studies have shown that massaged infants are found to be calmer upon discharge with improved neurodevelopmental outcome at 2 years of corrected age.

The amount of massage or stimulation applied should be altered according to the infant's maturation, acuity, engagement cues, and response to touch. There are many types of massage and touch therapy, including gentle stroking, gentle touch without stroking, M-technique (structured touch), Yakson touch (a Korean therapeutic touch), containment, kinesthetic (bicycling) stimulation, or even confinement holds mimicking the womb. Being aware of the infant and his or her receptivity and alertness is important in determining the best time for a massage rather than relying on a predetermined time. Numerous studies have shown benefits of all types of massage, including improved weight gain, improved sleep, and decrease in stress hormone levels and reduced hospital stay. A Japanese study showed that touch modified changes of cerebral oxygenation in response to a sensory punctate stimulus using near-infrared spectroscopy.

A significant emphasis has been placed on fathers performing massage as a bonding tool, similar to what breast feeding would be for the mother. It can also be a great way to get other family members, such as grandparents, involved. Data suggest that the masseuse also benefits, with lower stress hormone levels and decreased postnatal depression and anxiety. KC is probably the most widely accepted and used form of touch therapy.

B. **Osteopathy/craniosacral therapy.** Osteopaths believe that many problems begin at birth. Labor is seen as quite traumatic, and an infant may be altered both physically and psychologically by the experience. A multicenter Italian trial of osteopathic manipulative treatment on preterm infants showed decreased length of stay. A study exploring the effectiveness of osteopathic treatment in reducing pain in a sample of preterm infants is ongoing.

Craniosacral therapists feel that misalignment of structure that is not corrected can lead to potential alterations in function. Problems such as sucking/swallowing difficulties, suboptimal breast feeding, and recurrent reflux after birth are so common that many mothers and doctors consider them to be normal; however, in osteopathy, they are believed to be based in craniosacral abnormalities. Recognition and treatment of these dysfunctions in the immediate postpartum period are considered an essential preventive measure. According to craniosacral theory, these can be easily rectified.

The occipital area is thought to sustain most of the trauma at delivery. A complex study by osteopath Viola Frymann explored the relationship between symptomatology in the newborn and anatomic disturbances. The study suggested that strains within the unfused fragments of the occipital bones produce problems in the nervous system, such as vomiting, reflux, hyperactive peristalsis, tremor, hypertonicity, and irritability. Frymann notes that compression at the point of the hypoglossal nerve egress can cause an infant to suck ineffectively. Symptoms left untreated may result in tongue thrust, deviant swallowing, speech problems, and, in later life, malocclusion. If the condylar parts of the occiput are decompressed, the vomiting stops. In temporal bone development, misalignment may cause recurrent otitis media. If the sphenoid sinuses are involved, the child may have headaches. When the vagus nerve is compressed, recurrent vomiting or reflux can occur.

Craniosacral therapy has been used successfully in the NICU to improve feeding. Since adequate feeding is an important criterion for safe discharge, this therapy may be a useful adjunct to care. Craniosacral therapy has also been shown to be beneficial for infants with colic, improving sleep and reducing crying.

IV. **Bioenergetic therapies**
   A. **Acupuncture** is part of the traditional system of Chinese medicine. The main concept behind this system is that of chi (body energy not currently measurable by current instrumentation), which underlies and supports all aspects of the physical body. This chi/energy circulates throughout the body along specific pathways called meridians. Obstructions in the flow of chi may cause disease. By gently placing thin, solid, disposable, metallic needles into the skin along the meridians where chi is blocked, acupuncturists rebalance the flow of energy.

   Acupuncture has shown promising results in use for anesthesia, postoperative pain, and addiction recovery. A study from Turkey concluded that acupuncture decreased pain scores in preterm infants and crying time during heel prick. However, noninvasive electrical stimulation of acupuncture points did not reduce pain from heel stick in another study. Auricular acupuncture has been used since the early 1970s for various forms of maternal addiction and withdrawal prenatally. It is also used to help reduce the effects of neonatal drug withdrawal. In a study conducted in Austria, laser acupuncture, using a **LABpen MED 10** (Behounek Medizintechnik GMBH, Graz, Austria) and a specific protocol on ear and body points, was found to be an effective in reducing the duration of morphine therapy in infants with neonatal abstinence syndrome.

   Currently in China, acupuncture is used to treat infants with jaundice (augmenting hepatic chi), skin problems, teething, ear infections, constipation, conjunctivitis, and peripheral nerve injury. It is also used in intraoperative and postoperative pain control. Auricular acupuncture is used in China for the treatment of hypogalactia in mothers.

B. **Acupressure,** similar to acupuncture but without the needles, is popular in pediatrics. Acupressure involves applying pressure along the 14 major energy meridians to promote the flow of chi. Noninsertive acupuncture can also be used as an adjunctive treatment for infants with neonatal abstinence syndrome. However, noninvasive electrical stimulation of acupuncture points did not reduce heel stick pain in a recent study. More research is needed.

C. **Healing touch (HT) and therapeutic touch (TT)** are energy-based therapies based on clearing, aligning, and balancing the human energy system through touch or near-body touch to promote health and healing. The treatments are based on the idea that a universal life force energy flows through all of us. HT was developed by Janet Mentgen and the American Holistic Nurses Association. One example of an HT technique that can empower parents to feel like they are actively participating in care of their infant is called **comfort infusion** and is used to relieve pain. Parents are taught to place their left palm over the infant, encouraging any pain the infant may be having to move up from the infant to the parent's palm and then through their body to drain out of their right hand. When parents no longer sense pain, the right hand is placed over the infant and the left one turned upward to infuse healing energy. When the parents are at a point of feeling totally helpless in their infant's plight, this can restore a feeling of energetic connection with no touch involved, so they can do this no matter how ill their infant may be.

   TT was developed by Dora Kunz, a healer, and Dolores Krieger, a professor of nursing. TT does not require physical contact. Through the compassion and intention of the practitioner, the flow of energy between the practitioner and the infant is modulated to promote the infant's natural energy flow and support the infant's own healing abilities. The steps in TT include centering, assessment, unruffling (clearing extraneous energy), balancing and rebalancing, and closure. Limited studies have shown that TT improves vital signs, decreases pain scores, and promotes relaxation.

D. **Reiki** is a form of noninvasive energy healing, similar to HT, in which energy is transferred from the hands of a reiki master to a patient using a sequence of hand positions above the body. Reiki relaxes and heals by clearing energy meridians and chakras (vortices of energy along the spine). Energy blockages are dissolved, allowing the vibration frequency of the body to increase, thus restoring balance. As a calming balance occurs, respirations slow, blood pressure normalizes, and pain is relieved—all of which are felt to accelerate the healing process. Reiki is beneficial to the practitioner as well, increasing relaxation and enhancing focus.

E. **Reflexology** is an ancient form of healing, somewhat similar to traditional acupuncture. In this modality, chi is restored by manipulation of reflex points in the hands and feet that have specific correlates to organs, glands, and body parts. Reflexology may benefit infants by increasing blood flow to specific organs such as increasing perfusion to the kidneys or increasing cardiac output.

V. **Biochemical interventions**

A. **Homeopathy.** The basic idea behind homeopathy is that the body's internal wisdom will defend and heal itself by choosing the most beneficial response. Homeopathy is based on the "like cures like" principle: a symptom in a patient is treated with a remedy that causes this same symptom, thus further stimulating the body's natural responses (similar in philosophy to a vaccine). Homeopathy can be considered a catalyst to jumpstart the body's healing process.

   Homeopaths prescribe medicine that is very patient specific, and they base these prescriptions on past health history, past medical treatments, genetic inheritance, and a constellation of physical, emotional, mental, and spiritual symptomatology. Apparently, titrating individualized medicine(s) for newborns is not always easy. Chubby infants require different constitutional remedies than small or low birthweight infants, as do infants who sleep through the night compared to those who do not. Although homeopathic preparations are used globally, there is concern regarding efficacy and safety.

Some examples of homeopathic therapies are for infants who endure traumatic labors with bruising or other injuries (eg, postnatal intravenous infiltrates). They are considered to benefit from a remedy called **arnica** and *Hypericum perforatum*, which are thought to optimize the body's attempts to heal wounds, both physical and psychological. In Europe, where homeopathic remedies are much more commonly used, **carbovege** is used for apnea and bradycardia. *Aethusa* is used for milk intolerance as well as for reflux. **Nux vomica** and **chamomilla** are used for colic. **Magnesium phosphorica** is used to relieve symptoms of gas, bloating, and burping. **Topical calendula** is used for diaper dermatitis. Topical emollient therapy (vegetable oil, sunflower oil, and coconut oil) has been studied in preterm infants and newborns and was associated with improved weight gain and linear growth (vegetable oil).

B. **Herbal medicine.** The World Health Organization (WHO) considers herbal medicine part of traditional medicine, which is "the knowledge, skills and practices based on the theories, beliefs and experiences indigenous to different cultures, used in the maintenance of health and in the prevention, diagnosis, improvement or treatment of physical and mental illness." The WHO estimates that approximately 80% of the world's population relies on botanical medicines; indeed, 30% of Americans also use botanical remedies. It behooves healthcare professionals to be familiar with the expanding field of herbal medicine. Many mothers use herbal remedies during pregnancy. They are especially popular among breast-feeding women. Knowing what, if any, herbal remedies nursing mothers use is essential because the substances can be passed through breast milk to children. **Galactagogue herbs** have gained a reputation for increasing breast milk, but must be used with caution and more selectively because recent studies have shown limited benefits and possibility of significant side effects. (See Section VI.C.) **St. John's wort** is commonly used for postpartum depression. **Caffeine** is probably the herbal medicine most used in neonatal care. Many consider the use of probiotics, a hot topic in neonatology, for prevention of necrotizing enterocolitis as originating from the field of herbal medicine. A recent study showed that **arnica echinacea powder** applied to the umbilical cord after birth was safe and effective in preventing infection after umbilical cord detachment. Many others are herbal folk remedies. **Aloe vera** is used as a skin protectant or for burns and skin irritations. Creams made from **comfrey, plantain,** or **marigolds** are used for treatment of rashes and cradle cap. **Thyme tea solution** was studied retrospectively for treatment of staphylococcal skin infection in preterm and term newborns and found to be effective. **Calendula** is used in Russia for conjunctivitis. **Tree tea oil** is used as an antifungal.

VI. **Supportive care**

A. **Palliative care and hospice care.** Neonatal palliative care has been evolving within the auspices of neonatal intensive care. Palliative care is focused on the prevention and relief of suffering and includes medical treatments intended to improve the baby's life. Increasingly, NICUs are developing palliative, comfort care programs to care for families whose infants have life-limiting conditions. Palliative care is multidisciplinary and interdisciplinary. Teams typically consist of medical and nursing personnel, spiritual advisors, social service personnel, and therapists, including child life and music. Advances in technology and genetics have made it easier to detect a fetus with a life-limiting abnormality. Other NICU populations who benefit from palliative care are infants born at the limits of viability, infants with overwhelming illness not responding to disease-directed intervention, and infants with chronic life-limiting conditions.

Integrative medicine therapies used in palliative care include family-centered care with attention to environmental light and noise, KC, infant massage, and music therapy. Palliative care and hospice care are often used synonymously. However, in general, hospice care falls under the umbrella of palliative care. Hospice care is a particular form of palliative care delivered in the United States by licensed hospice agencies. Palliative care is discussed in detail in Chapter 24.

B. Emotional care. Parents are at risk for acute stress as well as posttraumatic stress disorders and depression. Support groups can help parents cope. A study conducted by Shaw et al showed that trauma-focused therapy reduced symptoms of trauma and depression in mothers of preterm infants. Shaw also showed that fathers may manifest symptoms of posttraumatic stress disorder several months after the infant is discharged. Support groups may also be helpful to meet the often overlooked needs of siblings.

C. Galactagogues. Therapies in the management of inadequate breast milk supply are of special concern to neonatologists. Prescription galactagogues and increased fluid intake are traditional mainstays, but many mothers prefer more natural therapies when breast feeding. Herbal galactagogues include **fenugreek, goat's rue, milk thistle (*Silybum marianum*), oats, dandelion, millet, seaweed, anise, basil, blessed thistle, fennel seeds, marshmallow, and trobangun leaves** (thought to antagonize the dopamine receptors, thereby increasing prolactin release). **Milk thistle** and **fenugreek** have limited safety data, and the evidence for using other herbs has grown weaker. Eidelman sites a recent human study showing benefits of **ginger supplements** in the immediate postpartum period, and a study in animals using traditional Chinese herbal mixture was shown to increase breast milk production and aquaporins in the mammary tissue. (Aquaporins are a family of membrane proteins that facilitate water transport and may have a possible role in milk secretion). More studies are needed.

VII. Conclusion. As neuroprotective care in neonatology continues to evolve as neonatology's new frontier, integrative therapies challenge us to think of the many options for supporting and nurturing the complexities of health and healing in infants. Many of these provide the possibility of using structured stimuli to help reduce stress and other noxious environmental factors. Family-focused integrative therapies may also mitigate the toxic stress of the infant as well as the parent. As mainstream medicine is embracing integrative therapies, research will be needed to demonstrate the efficacy of these therapies as well as to assess the short- and long-term benefits and burdens.

23 Neonatal Bioethics

I. Introduction. Neonatology has evolved significantly in the past 30 years. Although care of premature infants and their specific disease processes has been studied for the past century, it was the development of the ventilator that truly birthed the field of neonatology. This occurred in the 1960s and was a time of rapid technologic development. These technologies were applied to this new field of neonatology rapidly. We were able to care for children who had previously had no hope of survival. Many of these new technologies had never been used before, and innovation was the hallmark of neonatal care. Although this was essential in saving the lives of literally millions of premature infants during this time period, it also made it difficult to predict outcome or effectiveness of treatment. Issues such as effectiveness of treatment, potential risk to the patient, or quality of life were difficult to determine. However, any treatment was considered better than the hopelessness that these children faced before this era. This "frontier" mentality spurred the application of technology, even in instances where we were unsure of the outcome. This sometimes caused conflict in choosing the best course of action. It was difficult to know when application of technology might be ineffective or might have unintended consequence on the patient's quality of life.

The present day of neonatology is quite a bit different. We now have a much better idea of quality of life and prognosis. Indeed, the neonatal intensive care unit (NICU) for the most part has become a field of fairly routine but technologically advanced care where the expectation is a minimum of complications and a quality of life and development that are indistinguishable from children who did not require this care. This has allowed us to look more closely at the effectiveness of care and quality of life. We are able to back away from the idea that any care is better than no care and look at our treatment of these patients in a more standard and less pressured framework. As in any field of medicine, this is not to say that there are not ethical dilemmas that occur. There are still significant issues related to the benefits of treatment versus risk and questions about long-term disability, cost of care, and harm to the patient who cannot speak for himself or herself. To answer some of these questions, we would need for framework to discuss the ethical issues involved as well as the medical decision making.

II. **Bioethical framework.** Ethical discussion in medicine has been highly influenced by the ideas of principlism, which have been eloquently described in the foundational textbook of bioethics, *Principles of Biomedical Ethics*, by Beauchamp and Childress. They describe 4 overriding principles that must be considered when making ethical decisions for patients. These principles are beneficence, nonmaleficence, respect for autonomy, and justice.

A. **Principles that must be considered when making ethical decisions for patients**

1. **Beneficence** means that the action or treatment provides some benefit to the patient. This idea encompasses the concept of effectiveness as well. Beneficial actions or treatment may be short term or long term.

2. **Nonmaleficence** means the action or treatment must not harm the patient. This certainly includes the concept that we should not intentionally harm patients but also that we should evaluate possible unintended outcomes or complications related to treatment.

3. **Respect for autonomy.** We should always respect patients' wishes to guide their own fate. If the patients are competent, their wishes and matters of treatment should never be abrogated. In neonatal care, this respect for autonomy is usually for the parents and their decisions for their young child.

4. **Justice.** Justice defines the social and legal obligations we have in applying action or treatment. This principal includes a broader idea of what is fair within society.

   In ethical decision making, these 4 principles are weighed against one another to discern which might be superior in resolving various aspects of conflict. This is proven to be very useful in focusing bioethical dialogue and decision making on the patient and avoiding bias and conflicting values that are not in the patient's best interest. However, this process is not without difficulties. In many instances, it is difficult to find complete resolution between the tensions of the 4 overriding principles. Indeed, there are times when these principles will be in direct conflict with one another, making the dilemma appear insolvent. Another issue with the principlism approach is that it does not account for the other participants in the healthcare process. How does the integrity or virtue of the healthcare provider influence the patient's welfare? Should we factor in the cost of care and impact to society in making decisions?

   Jonsen and colleagues have developed a practical case-based approach to ethical decision making that builds on the 4 principles. They proposed the idea that ethical decision making is much like clinical decision making and that information must be sorted and prioritized to make a practical decision. Their method is directed much more toward a practical solution for individual cases as opposed to the finding overarching answers for every case. The proposed 4 topics provide a way to collect, sort, and prioritize data to provide a practical solution and are reviewed here.

Table 23–1. CASE-BASED APPROACH TO ETHICAL DECISION MAKING (4-BOX PARADIGM)

Medical Indications	Patient Preferences

Principle: Beneficence and Nonmaleficence
Examples:
• What is the patient's medical problem? Acuity? Prognosis?
• What are the goals of treatment?
• Are there circumstances in which treatment is not indicated?
• How likely is it that medical treatment(s) will be successful?
• How can the patient be benefited by medical care? How can harm be avoided?
	Principle: Respect for Autonomy
	Examples:
	• Is the patient mentally capable and legally competent?
	  ○ Has the patient stated preferences?
	  ○ If incapacitated, did the patient previously state preferences?
	  ○ Who is the appropriate proxy (surrogate) to make decisions?
	  ○ Is the patient unwilling or unable to cooperate?
	• Has the patient been informed of benefits, risks, and possible complications, and does the patient understand the information and give consent?

Quality of Life	**Contextual Features**
Principle: Beneficence, Nonmaleficence, and Respect for Autonomy Examples: • What are the prospects of returning to a normal life? What deficits might the patient incur? • Can a surrogate make reasonable judgment about the patient's quality of life? • Are there biases or prejudice that might influence the healthcare provider? • Does improving quality of life create ethical issues? • Does quality-of-life assessment influence treatment plan? • What quality-of-life assessment would be grounds to forgo life-sustaining treatment?	*Principle: Justice and Fairness* Examples: • Are there conflicts of interest (professional, business, social)? • Are there other parties affected by the clinical decisions? • Are there financial factors? • Are there issues with allocation of scarce health resource? • Are there religious issues? • Are there legal issues? • Are there public health issues?

B. **Practical case-based approach to ethical decision making (Table 23–1)**
   1. **Medical indications.** Medical indications refer to the diagnostic and therapeutic interventions that are being used to evaluate and treat the medical problem in the case.
   2. **Patient preferences.** Patient preferences state the express choices of the patient about his or her treatment or the decisions of those who are authorized to speak for the patient when the patient is incapable of doing so.
   3. **Quality of life.** Quality of life describes the degree of satisfaction, pleasure, and well-being or the degree of distress and malfunction that people experience in their life prior to and following treatment.
   4. **Contextual features.** Contextual features identify the social, institutional, financial, and legal setting within which any particular case of patient care takes place, in so far as these influence medical decisions.

   The case-based approach to ethical decision-making method allows the clinician to gather information about the ethical issues involved with the case in a nonbiased manner and place them in a priority schema that will help provide a practical answer in the individualized case (Table 23–1). Once this has been performed, a final step is to reflect on the dilemma as well as a resolution with cases that have occurred in the past. These "paradigm cases" serve as a way to test the decision making and reasoning involved in the case resolution. The resolution does not necessarily have to agree with the paradigm case; however, it will be useful to make sure the participants have thought of all aspects of the case.

III. **Specific issues in Neonatology**

A. **Delivery room resuscitation.** Neonatal care in the delivery room requires rapid assessment and quick decision making. In infants with severe congenital anomalies or extreme prematurity, these first few moments of life are critical. In these instances, the pediatrician is called on to make critical decisions within seconds concerning viability, quality of life, and prognosis. Care during this period should be guided by the following general principles.

1. **Discuss as fully as possible with the parents their wishes and expectations before actual delivery of the child.** Coordination between the pediatricians and obstetricians can facilitate this dialogue (counseling parents before high-risk delivery is discussed in Chapter 55).

2. **Err on the side of life.** If the mother is unable to express her wishes, then emergency therapy must be performed. It is much better to err on the side of life-sustaining therapy than to withhold such therapy. If in the aftermath of this crisis, it is discovered that the parents wish no such therapy, then it is appropriate to withdraw therapy. This gives the parents the opportunity to form their own opinion and exercise their right in protecting the child's best interest.

3. **Noninitiation of resuscitation in the extremely immature infant or in cases of severe congenital anomaly is a challenging problem in neonatology.** According to guidelines from the American Heart Association and American Academy of Pediatrics, noninitiation of resuscitation appears appropriate in confirmed gestation of <23 weeks or birthweight <400 g, anencephaly, or confirmed trisomy 13 or 18. In these cases, all data suggest that resuscitation of these infants is highly unlikely to result in survival or survival without severe disability. In cases in which the antenatal information may be unreliable or with uncertain prognosis, options include a period of resuscitation with the option of discontinuation of the resuscitation if assessment of the infant after delivery does not support the continued efforts. Initial resuscitation and subsequent withdrawal of support may allow time to gather key clinical information and to counsel the family appropriately.

4. **Discontinuation of resuscitation may be appropriate if the infant fails to have return of spontaneous circulation within 15 minutes.** This is based on strong data suggesting that after a period of 10 minutes of asystole, survival or survival without severe disability is highly unlikely. The Guideline Committee of the American Academy of Pediatrics and American Heart Association recommends that each institution develop local discussions of these issues based on the availability of resources and outcome data.

B. **Withholding or withdrawing care**

1. **Withholding care.** There is sometimes a feeling among family members and/ or healthcare providers that, to provide optimal care, patients should be offered every technologic treatment or procedure possible. In many cases, however, the application of highly technical procedures is not in the best interest of the patient. Frequently, critically ill infants who are not responding to present therapy should have further therapy or have more advanced therapy withheld. The decision in these cases rests on whether further therapy will **have its intended effect, reverse the process, or restore the quality of life that is acceptable to the patient or the caregivers**.

   With these goals in mind, one can see that it is as important to obtain informed consent for withholding care as it is for the application of procedures. The physician should not withhold care without discussing this course of action with the parents. Likewise, the decision to withhold care should be discussed with the other physicians and nursing staff involved. The indications for and benefits of withholding care should be clearly defined.

2. **Withdrawing care.** In some cases, care can and should be withdrawn for a number of reasons.

   a. **The care or treatment rendered no longer accomplishes its intended purpose** (ie, futility of care).

   b. **Ongoing evaluations or tests reveal information changing the diagnosis or prognosis of the patient.** In these cases, reevaluation and discussion with the patient's parents are required to provide for the patient's best interest with this new information.

   c. **Care given in an emergency should be withdrawn if it is contrary to the parents' wishes when they are informed.** As noted, there are a few legal exceptions to this rule. Overall, the withdrawal of care hinges on the idea of futility. Does the patient benefit from such care? Can we expect the therapy to accomplish both short- and long-term goals? As an example, the use of vasopressor agents in a moribund infant may reach the point of futility. If the short-term goal (ie, raising the blood pressure) is not accomplished and neither is the long-term goal (ie, restoring health), then therapy is no longer useful and should be withdrawn. At every step, the patient's parents should be clearly informed of the decisions and possible outcomes.

3. **Nutrition and patient comfort.** Nutrition has been classified as a therapy, that is, as a medicine that could potentially be withdrawn or, in other instances, as one of the patient's basic rights for comfort. In any discussion of ethics and patient care, there is consensus that the patient should be provided some basic comforts despite what other circumstance may be in question. The comfort of nursing care, cleanliness, pain relief, and mere presence are factors considered to be basic to human life and not subject to diminution or withdrawal, secondary to end-of-life issues. In most cases, nutrition (ie, food and water) is classified as one of these basic comfort cares. This has been contested in the legal system in a variety of cases, with a broad spectrum of opinions. With this in mind, it is probably wise to assume nutrition and feeding to be basic rights for patient care and to challenge this position only in extreme circumstances. The parents' understanding of nutrition as therapy or as a basic right is important. Agreement among the parents, caregivers, administration, and legal authorities must be obtained if the withdrawal of nutrition is contemplated. The activation and opinion of the institution's bioethics committee may be very helpful in resolving these issues.

C. **Determining quality of life.** Although quality of life is often a focal point of ethical dilemmas in the NICU, it is very difficult to define this term. The word *quality* can be used in many different ways. It can describe the efficiency or usefulness of an object. Another use of the descriptor would be to describe how closely this subject of the description matches the ideal. ("The quality of the metal is like pure gold"). None of these definitions applies directly to a human life. **A broad definition in this instance could be as follows: the ability to lead an unencumbered life to its fullest potential.**

There have been several attempts to measure quality of life. These can be difficult due to the subjective nature of quality. Self-reporting of quality of life is problematic in the NICU because children are not able to give an account for themselves. Even in older patients, there is little correlation between disability and subjective evaluation of individual quality of life. This "disability paradox" makes it very difficult to use potential disability or loss of function as a measure of quality of life or personal sense of significance.

In many cases, health professions view quality as a biologic process. They are biased by their clinical thinking in this perspective. There are certainly cases in the NICU where we can easily predict a poor biologic quality. Examples would be high-grade interventricular hemorrhage or short gut syndrome. However, this biologic certainty does not necessarily correlate with the predicted quality of life both from the patient's perspective and the family's. Although it is important for us to define these issues clearly for the family, we must be careful not to transpose this perspective to the patient and parents.

Because the concept of quality of life is both conceptually difficult and subjective in nature, neonatologists and NICU nurses should be careful in how they frame their interpretation of these issues. Instead of stating that a patient may have a "poor quality of life," it would be more helpful to state the biologic difficulties the child might have and how that might impact the patient's ability to function normally. This leaves the subjective judgment concerning these issues to the parents and their thoughts on their child's life.

IV. **Ethics resources.** Conflict is any dispute or disagreement of opinion. This may occur between the physician and the patient or the patient's guardian. Alternatively, conflicts can arise between the physician and the nursing staff, healthcare workers, and administrative staff, or any combination of these. Most ethical issues arise as conflict between differing values or moral ideals. Therefore, the identification of conflict is a key or essential ingredient in bioethical decisions. Conflict is best identified by ongoing communication. Normally, we think of this as communication between physician and patient. However, this is just the first step. Continued communication among members of the healthcare team, parents, family members, and others involved in the case will uncover unvoiced concerns and opinions. These should be dealt with in an open and honest fashion to obtain consensus about ethical issues.

A. **Family conference.** When there is disagreement about the best course of action for a patient, the first step in resolution is to have an open and clear conversation about all of the issues that are involved. To accomplish this, it is often best to have all of the involved parties meet and discuss the issue itself as well as the patient's history and surrounding social issues. In many instances, there is an incomplete knowledge about treatment or prognosis by the parents or the healthcare team, which can be rectified in such a meeting. The goals of the meeting should be clearly stated, and all members should be reassured that there is not a pejorative nature to the discussion. At the conclusion of discussion, a clear action plan with each step detailed should be formulated. This helps to ensure continued open conversation and increases trust between the family and healthcare team in times of disagreement.

B. **Bioethics consultation.** Most institutions have standing bioethics committees or departments that can aid in resolving bioethical conflicts. Despite our best intentions, we are sometimes unable to resolve conflict with patients or cannot fully explain the necessity of action to patients, causing confusion. In these instances, an outside perspective may be of value. A consultation from the bioethics committee is simply an outside review of the facts and values associated with a particular crisis. This outside observer may be a physician, another healthcare worker, or a member of the clergy. The purpose of the consult is not to render a "more expert" opinion but to uncover differing moral values and miscommunication that lead to conflict. In many instances, this is all that is needed to resolve these problems. If consensus cannot be obtained in this manner, further interventions are warranted.

C. **Bioethics committee.** The bioethics committee is usually multidisciplinary in membership. Composed of administrators, lawyers, physicians, nursing staff, and clergy, the committee reviews ethical dilemmas put before it. Many bioethics committees also have a standing role in monitoring the ethical behavior of physicians and healthcare workers at their institution. Activation of the bioethics committee, as opposed to a consult, is a more involved process. The committee's purpose is to not only resolve conflict in particular instances, but also to provide policy and general guidelines for ethical behavior at that institution. Because of the potential legal ramifications, this group may routinely consult the judiciary system for further advice. It is the usual policy of most committees that physicians or other healthcare workers, family members, clergy, or other interested parties may query the group. These queries can be put forth without fear of retribution or chastisement from other staff members. The procedure for activating the bioethics committee should be posted in the residents' or physicians' handbook or nursing manual for that patient unit.

   D. **Legal intervention.** On occasion, conflict arises that cannot be resolved by the physician, bioethics consult, or committee opinion. In these instances, outside judiciary opinions should be sought. The bioethics committee can usually be helpful in obtaining this legal opinion. Not only does the committee have familiarity with accessing the judiciary system, but they should also be able to frame the question in such a way to provide the most concise legal response. Activation of the legal system in this way also protects the physician from direct consequence from legal action.

V. **Summary.** The field of neonatal bioethics, much like neonatology itself, has changed and evolved over the past 30 years. The NICU is now an environment where most patients have a fairly predictable outcome, and many of the dilemmas we faced in the pioneering days of neonatology have much less impact. However, we continue to care for very ill children who have a variety of potential medical complications that will impact them throughout their life. These issues require good communication concerning both objective biologic processes and prediction of outcome as well as subjective understanding of issues such as quality of life. When these dilemmas arise, employment of a practical clinical decision-making tool as described by the 4-box method (Table 23–1) can be very useful in identifying all of the issues involved and finding practical solutions. If the dilemma remains unresolved, outside reflection by a bioethics consultation or discussion via a bioethics committee can be helpful.

24 Neonatal Palliative Care

I. **General principles**
   A. **The World Health Organization's definition of palliative care (PC) is as follows:** "Palliative care is an approach that improves the quality of life of patients and their families facing the problem associated with life-threatening illness, through the prevention and relief of suffering by means of early identification and impeccable assessment and treatment of pain and other problems, physical, psychosocial and spiritual."
      1. **Provides relief from pain** and other distressing symptoms.
      2. **Affirms life and regards dying** as a normal process.
      3. **Intends neither to hasten** nor postpone death.
      4. **Integrates the psychological** and spiritual aspects of patient care.
      5. **Offers a support system** to help patients live as actively as possible until death [and] to help the family cope during the patient's illness and in their own bereavement.
      6. **Uses a team approach** to address the needs of patients and their families, including bereavement counseling, if indicated.
      7. **Will enhance quality of life,** and may also positively influence the course of illness.
      8. **Is applicable early in the course of illness,** in conjunction with other therapies that are intended to prolong life.
   B. **World Health Organization's definition of palliative care for children:**
      1. **The active total care of the child's body, mind, and spirit,** and also involves giving support to the family.
      2. **Begins when illness is diagnosed** and continues regardless of whether or not a child receives treatment directed at the disease. HCP must evaluate and alleviate

a child's physical, psychological and social distress. Requires a broad multidisciplinary approach that includes the family.

3. **Can be provided at home,** community health centers or in tertiary care facilities.

C. **American Academy of Pediatrics definition of pediatric palliative care:** "Pediatric palliative care addresses the needs of *infants*, children, and the needs of their families, providing treatments that aim to:

1. **Relieve suffering across multiple realms,** including the physical, psychological, social (isolation), practical (home-based services or financial stress), and existential/spiritual (why is this happening?).
2. **Improve the child's quality and enjoyment of life** while helping families adapt and function during the illness and through bereavement.
3. **Facilitate informed decision-making** by patients, families, and health care professionals.
4. **Assist with ongoing coordination** of care among clinicians and across various sites of care."

D. **Hospice**

1. **All hospice care is palliative care, but not all palliative care is hospice.**

   a. **Hospice care is palliative care.** For example, the family of a baby with trisomy 18 and complex congenital heart disease receiving nasogastric feedings may choose to care for their baby at home instead of in the neonatal intensive care unit (NICU) during the baby's expected shortened life span. With a skilled in-home hospice supportive program, the family's goal of having meaningful time with their child at home may be supported with intermittent nursing visits, multidisciplinary support, and bereavement support. Nasogastric feedings and attention to the baby's comfort level can be continued at home, and the family may or may not choose to pursue hospitalizations or surgical interventions if the baby's respiratory status deteriorates.

   b. **Not all palliative care is hospice care.** For example, a 23-week-old baby with bilateral grade 4 intraventricular hemorrhages with a predicted high mortality or poor neurodevelopmental outcome can benefit from a PC model of extra support. PC for this baby and family includes skilled supportive communication to establish unique goals of care, shared decision making surrounding all reasonable options in care (continuation of life-prolonging interventions, placing limits on care such as do not resuscitate/do not attempt resuscitation orders, or discontinuation of life-sustaining interventions), and intentionally making memories and creating opportunities for parenting experiences.

2. **Hospice is not a place; it is a model of care** that ideally is a comprehensive multidisciplinary team approach with a focus on quality of life. It can include physicians, nurses, clergy, social workers, genetic counselors, midwives, traditional hospice professionals, and others.

3. **Professionals skilled in pediatric hospice** may provide supportive in-home outpatient hospice care for neonates and families whose goal is to continue care outside of a hospital setting. Hospice resources vary for neonates, and it is important to be aware of local resources. Hospice care can begin to be integrated during an inpatient hospitalization; there is increasing overlap with inpatient hospice models and outpatient PC resources.

4. **Historically, a predicted life expectancy of <6 months** is a criterion to meet hospice eligibility.

E. **Patient criteria**

1. **Diagnoses.** Neonatal patients with a **life-limiting or life-threatening condition or uncertain prognosis benefit from a PC approach.**

   a. **Life-limiting diagnoses** such as trisomy 13 or 18, anencephaly, holoprosencephaly, hydranencephaly, renal agenesis, or multiple congenital anomalies with severe differences.

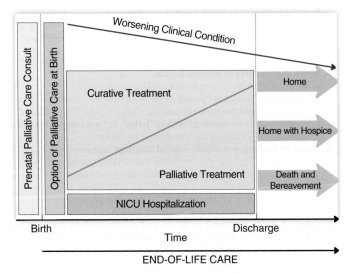

FIGURE 24–1. Schematic of palliative care planning. NICU, neonatal intensive care unit. (*Reproduced with permission from Bidegain M, Younge N: Comfort Care vs Palliative Care: Is There a Difference in Neonates? NeoReviews 2015 June;16(6):e333-339.*)

        b. Life-threatening diagnoses such as extreme prematurity, overwhelming sepsis, severe hypoxic ischemic/neonatal encephalopathy, overwhelming necrotizing enterocolitis totalis, or severe pulmonary hypoplasia.

        c. Patients not responding to aggressive medical interventions.

        d. Families with an established birth plan after a prenatal diagnosis.

    2. Timing. A PC approach is appropriate for both families that choose to pursue full aggressive medical interventions and families that choose limits on care—at any age and any stage of illness—and can be provided along with curative treatment (Figure 24–1).

II. Components of neonatal palliative care support

    A. Palliative care implementation. Interhospital variation exists regarding available **integrated** PC resources and practices versus **consultative** PC team structures.

        1. Determine local resources.

        2. Multidisciplinary palliative care teams may include physicians, neonatal nurse practitioners, nurses, social work, hospital chaplains, and others.

        3. Palliative care teams support both the primary medical team and patient and often work in collaboration to optimize quality of care, communication, and neonatal quality of life as defined by each individual family.

           a. Provide time to devote to intensive family meetings and patient/family counseling.

           b. Provide expertise in managing complex physical symptoms such as pain and symptoms around the end of life.

           c. Provide skilled communication and support for resolving patient/family/physician questions concerning goals of care.

    B. Skilled communication. The PC "procedure" is skilled communication to establish neonatal goals of care, offer support, and guide decision making.

        1. Use honest, compassionate, and clear communication in establishing a supportive relationship to enable shared decision making.

    a. Parents want to be heard. Explore understanding and invite questions. A helpful phrase is: "Can you share with me how others have explained . . . ?"

    b. Parents want to be validated that their baby's life has meaning.

        i. Use baby's first name in conversations.

        ii. Be aware of the baby's gender prior to conversations.

  2. Avoid euphemisms or medical jargon.

    a. Be mindful to avoid complicated medical terminology.

    b. Avoid phrases such as "passed away" or "moved on." Instead, use unambiguous terms or phrases such as "is dying," "has died," or "I'm worried will die."

    c. Parents report terminology such as "lethal" or "not compatible with life" as hurtful (life-limiting or life-threatening is preferred).

  3. Avoid misleading, potentially hurtful language such as:

    a. "We can't do anything else" or "We've done everything we can."

        i. Care can be redirected to focus on comfort and loving.

    b. "Withdraw support"

        i. Support is not withdrawn; medical interventions are.

    c. "You will have another baby" or "It will be okay."

  4. Spiritual. Respect cultural, religious, and spiritual beliefs and/or life philosophy. Parents often desire inquiry into how these beliefs contribute to medical decision making. Helpful phrases include:

    a. "From where do you obtain your strength in hard times?"

    b. "How do you make sense out of what is happening?"

    c. "What guides decision making for you and your family?"

    d. "What religious or spiritual beliefs are important for the medical team to be aware of to incorporate in your care?"

  5. Social. Identify important and helpful individualized family support and other stressors.

    a. Determine who the parents or decision makers request to be present for important conversations or family meetings.

    b. Identify other supportive resources such as friends/family, hospital chaplain and/or religious leader, hospital/local support groups, social work, or supportive literature/online resources.

C. Decision making (see also Chapter 23, "Neonatal Bioethics")

  1. Palliative care teams may offer assistance with shared decision making (between family and medical providers) and establishment of goals of care for a patient, weighing the risks and benefits of care/interventions.

  2. Avoid providing a menu of options or being directive in care. Recommend a path forward after assessing family values and goals.

  3. Recognize that parents (or surrogate decision maker) use the best interest standard in decision making.

D. Around the time of death

  1. Provide anticipatory guidance about what to expect: visual changes, next steps, necessary decisions to make, and so on.

  2. Identify a provider whose primary role is communication with the family.

  3. Parental presence is most often appropriate during an acute resuscitation.

  4. Restore control where possible. Helpful phrase: "We cannot control that your baby is dying, but we can control . . ." (eg, where, how, when, who).

  5. Consider pharmacologic and nonpharmacologic pain management. (See also Chapter 81, "Sedation and Analgesia.")

    a. Adequate pain control does not hasten death in limited studies.

    b. Rule of Double Effect states that given the intent is to do good, foreseeable yet undesirable consequences are acceptable.

E. Postmortem support

  1. Be aware of local guidelines regarding the timing of final decision making, postmortem care, and the potential use of cooling blankets. Allow desired time for parents and family to hold their deceased baby prior to transfer to the morgue or other location.

2. **Autopsy considerations** (see also Chapter 57, "Death of an Infant")
   a. **Review potential benefits and available options** (partial or directed vs full autopsy, radiology autopsy, molecular autopsy).
   b. **Discuss expectations for timing of results and plan follow-up.**

III. **Communication frameworks.** Skilled communication is essential to establish neonatal goals of care and guide decision making regarding options in care.
   A. **Helpful phrases**
      1. **"I'm sorry . . ." or "I wish . . ."** (empathizes with a family's hope/wish if their desire is not possible while acknowledging the reality of the situation).
      2. **"Tell me more about . . ."** (rather than make an assumption, explore any uncertainty).
      3. **"What are you hoping for?"**
      4. **"What is important to you as you face these hard times?"**
      5. **"What outcomes are you willing to accept/go through?"**
      6. **NURSE statements for articulating empathy:**
         a. **Naming:** "It sounds like you are very upset."
         b. **Understanding:** "This helps me understand what you are thinking," but do not say, "*I know* how hard this is."
         c. **Respecting:** "I can see you have really been trying to show your baby as much love as possible," or "I think you've been so thoughtful in your decisions."
         d. **Supporting:** "We will do our best to make sure you have what you need and to help you through this."
         e. **Exploring:** "Could you say more about what you mean when you say . . ." or "Tell me more about . . . ."
   B. **Sharing bad news**
      1. **Setting.** Find a quiet location that is private if possible, invite the important people to be present, have tissues available, have enough chairs, and turn off the ringer on your phone or pager.
      2. **Assess understanding about the upcoming news.** "What have the other doctors told you about why we obtained an ultrasound for your baby?"
      3. **Ask permission.** "Would it be okay for me to discuss the results of the tests with you now?" "Is there anybody else who needs to be present?"
      4. **Give a warning.** "I have something serious we need to discuss." "I was hoping I would have better news to share today."
      5. **Say "the news" simply and stop.**
      6. **Wait quietly for the family** to start speaking.
      7. **Follow the family's guidance** about what to discuss next and invite questions.
      8. **Describe next steps** and discuss a follow-up plan.
      9. **Ensure understanding.** "I want to be sure I communicated as well as possible about what I just told you. Can you please tell me what you heard me say?" Use the "Ask, Tell, Ask" framework.
   C. **Goals of care.** All possible medical interventions are thoughtfully considered, focusing on the likely benefits and burdens of each intervention and the family's interpretation of acceptable quality of life.
      1. **Determine short- and long-term goals** such as:
         a. **Resuscitation status** (do not resuscitate/do not attempt resuscitation, allow a natural death, full attempts at resuscitation and medical interventions, or consider a trial of interventions with frequent reassessment).
         b. **Any treatment limitations** (intubation/mechanical ventilation, continuation or limitation of intravenous hydration/nutrition or enteral nutrition, or options such as "do not escalate care").
         c. **Withdrawal of life-prolonging interventions** already initiated (compassionate extubation/removal of endotracheal tube or other life-sustaining interventions, discontinuation of vasopressors).

      d. Location of care or location of death (hospital NICU, home with or without hospice, or less acute inpatient setting).

      e. Pain management (oral or systemic analgesia).

      f. Memory-making experiences to accomplish (see Section IV).

  2. **Helpful phrases**

      a. "Given this news, it seems like a good time to talk about what to do now."

      b. "We're in a different place."

      c. "Tell me more about that. What are you worried about?" "Is it okay for us to talk about what this means?"

      d. "Given this situation, what's most important for your family?"

      e. "As I listen to you, it sounds like the most important things are . . . ."

IV. Memory-making opportunities should be considered during goal setting or during care for a baby using a PC approach. (see also Chapter 57, "Death of an Infant").

  A. Offer "normal" parenting experiences to encourage bonding and memory making, such as holding, bathing, dressing, changing the diaper, sleeping together in a "family bed" within the hospital, reading special books, listening to music/meaningful songs, tasting breast milk or other tastes, or going outside.

  B. Offer memorabilia to be obtained such as foot or hand prints (in special places such as a meaningful text/religious text), foot or hand impressions (molds), a lock of hair, or pictures. Considerations for pictures:

    1. With family/siblings (with twin or triplet, etc, if multiple gestation)

    2. With special stuffed animal (parent may hold while leaving the hospital)

  C. Ritualistic experiences to consider

    1. Religious ceremony such as baptism, blessing, naming ceremony, or prayer

    2. Meeting other family members or friends

V. Other relevant literature

  A. Cummings J. Antenatal counseling regarding resuscitation and intensive care before 25 weeks of gestation. *Pediatrics.* 2015;136(3):588-595.

  B. Nakagawa TA, Ashwal S, Mathur M, et al. Guidelines for the determination of brain death in infants and children: an update of the 1987 task force recommendations. *Ann Neurol.* 2012;71(4):573-585.

  C. Diekema DS, Botkin JR, Committee on Bioethics. Clinical report: forgoing medically provided nutrition and hydration in children. *Pediatrics.* 2009;124(2):813-822.

25 Principles of Neonatal Procedures

I. **Informed consent.** Upon admission to the neonatal intensive care unit (NICU), most facilities provide a parental blanket or general informed consent for routine procedures performed on newborns (eg, phlebotomy, intravenous placement) and emergency procedures for life-threatening situations. For nonemergent invasive bedside procedures that may carry significant risk, parental or guardian permission should be obtained. Risks, benefits, and alternative procedures, if appropriate, should be discussed. Major surgical procedures require informed consent. Refer to your local unit policy manual for detailed guidance.

II. **Standard precautions.** Standard precautions integrate and expand the elements of the previously adopted universal precautions and are designed to protect both healthcare workers and patients. Standard precautions apply to contact with all body fluids including blood, secretions, and excretions (except sweat), nonintact skin, and mucous membranes. Standard precautions must be used in the care of all patients, regardless of their infection status. In the case of a known transmissible infection, additional precautions known as expanded or transmission-based precautions are recommended. These are used to interrupt the spread of diseases that are transmitted by airborne, droplet, or contact transmission. Most bedside procedures incorporate principles of standard precautions. Refer to your local unit policy manual for detailed guidance.

  A. **Standard precautions key components**

  1. **Hand hygiene** before and after patient contact.

     a. **Hand washing** (40–60 seconds): Wet hands and apply soap; rub all surfaces; rinse hands and dry thoroughly with a single-use towel; use towel to turn off faucet.

     b. **Hand rubbing** (20–30 seconds): Apply enough product (alcohol-based products gels, rinses, foams) to cover all areas of the hands; rub hands until dry.

     c. **Wearing gloves without correct hand hygiene can contaminate the gloves.** Studies show that less direct patient care also occurs when clinicians wear gloves. A randomized trial found that wearing gloves after hand washing protects premies from infections. Infants <8 days old, <29 weeks, and <1000 g who were handled with nonsterile gloves after handwashing had less late-onset invasive infections, less necrotizing enterocolitis, less gram-positive infections, and less central line–associated bloodstream infections when compared to infants handled with hand washing only.

     d. **Clean versus sterile gloves.** The World Health Organization (WHO) recommends that **clean gloves** are to be worn prior to insertion of peripheral intravascular catheterization and that **sterile gloves** are to be worn for insertion of arterial, central, and midline catheters, when guidewire exchanges are performed. Wear either clean or sterile gloves when changing the dressing on intravascular catheters. **Nonlatex gloves** are recommended for contact with blood, body fluids, secretions, contaminated items, mucous membranes, and nonintact skin.

  2. **Personal protective equipment (masks, goggles, and/or face masks).** Assess the risk of exposure to body substances or contaminated surfaces **before** any healthcare activity when contact with blood and body fluids is likely. **For facial protection (eyes, nose, and mouth)**, wear a surgical or procedure mask and eye protection (eye visor, goggles) or a face shield to protect mucous membranes of the eyes, nose, and mouth during activities that are likely to generate splashes or sprays of blood, body fluids, secretions, and excretions.

    3. **Gowns.** Wear gowns for blood or body fluid contact and to prevent soiling of clothing. Remove soiled gown as soon as possible, and perform immediate hand hygiene.

    4. **Sharps precautions.** Avoid recapping used needles; avoid bending, breaking, or manipulating used needles by hand; and place used sharps in puncture-resistant containers. Use self-shielding safety needle devices whenever possible.

    5. **Respiratory hygiene and cough etiquette.** Persons with respiratory symptoms should apply source control measures: cover their nose and mouth when coughing/sneezing with tissue or mask, dispose of used tissues and masks, and perform hand hygiene after contact with respiratory secretions.

III. **Time out.** The Joint Commission has produced a universal protocol for the prevention of wrong site, wrong procedure, and wrong person surgery. The 3 principal components of the universal protocol include a preprocedure verification, site marking, and a time out. Originally developed for the operating room, many facilities use this before bedside invasive procedures. All activity ceases, a moment will be taken ("time out"), and the following will be verified verbally by each member of the team:

    A. **Correct patient identity**

    B. **Correct side and site**

    C. **Agreement on the procedure to be done**

    D. **Correct patient position**

    E. **Availability of correct equipment and/or special requirements**

IV. **Neonatal intensive care unit procedure considerations**

    A. **Latex allergy.** There is a growing concern over latex exposure in the hospital. Certain pediatric populations are at higher risk for latex allergies such as in spina bifida. Only latex-free equipment (including gloves) should be used in the NICU.

    B. **Hand hygiene.** Hand hygiene is the single most effective method of decreasing healthcare-related infections. The term *hand hygiene* includes both hand washing with either plain or antiseptic-containing soap and water and use of alcohol-based products (gels, rinses, foams) that do not require the use of water. In the absence of visible soiling of hands, approved alcohol-based products for hand disinfection are preferred over antimicrobial or plain soap and water because of their superior micro-biocidal activity, reduced drying of the skin, and convenience. WHO has instituted the "Clean Care Is Safer Care" campaign to improve compliance because studies still show it is unsatisfactory. Artificial fingernails should not be worn by healthcare providers with direct patient contact in neonatal intensive care since they have been associated with *Pseudomonas aeruginosa*, *Klebsiella pneumoniae*, and fungi. Always follow your hospital-based infection prevention protocols.

        1. **A 3- to 5-minute scrub (washing up to the elbows) is usually required before entering the neonatal intensive care unit.** This is also necessary before all major procedures (eg, lumbar puncture, chest tube, central line placement, or cut down).

        2. **A 2- to 3-minute scrub (up to elbows)** is recommended for a minor procedure (eg, bladder aspiration, blood drawing, intravenous placement).

        3. **A 30-second hand wash or shorter alcohol-based hand rub** is indicated before and after each patient contact.

    C. **Minimal sterile barrier precautions.** These precautions include sterile gloves and small drape.

    D. **Maximum sterile barrier precautions.** These precautions are defined as wearing a sterile gown, sterile gloves, cap, and full-body drape (entire patient is covered, with a small opening for the site of insertion). Using these precautions during a central venous catheter insertion resulted in fewer episodes of infection and colonization as compared to using a minimal sterile barrier.

    E. **Antiseptic solutions.** The use of topical antiseptic agents for skin disinfection is important in reducing and preventing healthcare-associated infections. The Centers for Disease Control and Prevention (CDC) has specific recommendations for cannulation and central venous catheter insertion in infants age 2 months or older, but no recommendations for infants <2 months. The stratum corneum, which is the epidermal barrier, is not developed until 32 to 34 weeks' gestation; therefore, preterm infants are prone to infection. There is a paucity of evidence in neonates to state which topical antiseptic agent is preferred prior to blood culture, venipuncture, or intravenous cannulation. General rules for procedure site preparation include the following:

1. **A 30-second cleansing was more effective than 5- to 10-second cleansing in decreasing bacterial colony counts from skin swabs.**
   a. **Always allow antiseptics to dry on the site** (at least 30 seconds is recommended). Read manufacturers' recommendations on time to dry.
   b. **Remove iodophor solutions off the wider area at the end of the procedure** except right at the procedure insertion site.
   c. **Verify that antiseptic is not collecting under the infant because it can cause skin damage.**
2. **Commonly used antiseptics.** The most commonly used agents in the NICU are alcohols, iodine preparations, and chlorhexidine solutions.
   a. **Alcohol** (70%–90% ethyl or isopropyl) is effective against gram-positive and gram-negative bacteria, methicillin-resistant *Staphylococcus aureus* (MRSA), vancomycin-resistant *Enterococcus* (VRE), mycobacteria, and fungi. It is commonly used for skin prep of minor procedures (eg, phlebotomy), not for mucous membranes. It can be used alone or in combination (with CHG). Apply 3 times in a circle starting at the center of the site and going outward. Alcohol is not used for major procedures and may cause burns in premature infants.
   b. **Iodine preparations** have broad-spectrum antimicrobial activity (bacteria, viruses, fungi, spores).
      i. **Topical iodine** (1%) is not recommended because it can cause skin hypersensitivity, iodine overload, and transient hypothyroidism. Topical iodine has been replaced by iodophors.
      ii. **Iodophor solutions** (iodine plus a solubilizing agent such as surfactant or povidone). One example is **povidone-iodine** (polyvinylpyrrolidone plus elemental iodine), which releases iodine slowly. It is not recommended for antisepsis in extreme premature newborns, but can be used in term newborns (small risk of transient hypothyroidism with large area of the body or >5 days of use). Typically, 10% solutions of povidone-iodine (Betadine, Wescodyne) are recommended for major procedures.
   c. **Chlorhexidine (also known as chlorhexidine gluconate, CHG) solutions are the most widely used antiseptic agent.** These solutions are effective against gram-positive bacteria, but less effective against gram-negative bacteria, MRSA, VRE, streptococci, and *Pseudomonas*. CHG 2% was more effective than 0.5%, and CHG 0.5% was superior to 0.05%. Studies show that alcohol-containing CHG is more effective than aqueous solution, but it has not been studied in neonates. Alcohol can cause chemical burns, and a recent review showed that alcohol and aqueous solutions are similar in effectiveness. CDC states that no recommendation can be made for the safety or efficacy of chlorhexidine in infants <2 months old.
      i. **Hibiclens** (CHG 4% solution) is good for hand washing and used in the following procedures in preparation or maintenance: central venous catheter insertion, umbilical venous catheter prep, and others. Use with care in premature infants or infants <2 months old. May cause irritation or chemical burns.
      ii. **ChloraPrep** (2% chlorhexidine gluconate in 70% isopropyl alcohol) is used on the skin prior to peripheral intravenous lines, peripherally inserted central catheters, umbilical line arterial puncture, and chest tube insertion. Do not use on nonintact skin, below neck, in infants <26 weeks, in infants <1000 g, for lumbar punctures, or for urethral catheter. Approved for infants >2 months of age.

    d. phisoHex (brand of hexachlorophene) is effective against gram-positive organisms (especially *Staphylococcus* strains) but is less effective against gram-negative organisms, fungi, and mycobacteria. Infants in the 1970s were bathed with hexachlorophene, and some developed vacuolar degeneration (nonlipid vacuoles form in the cytoplasm). Infants who have had 6% hexachlorophene powder applied have developed irritability, dermatitis, generalized clonic muscular contractions, decerebrate rigidity, and death. Indications per the US Food and Drug Administration (FDA) are as follows: "Bacteriostatic skin cleanser for surgical scrubbing or handwashing as part of patient care, for topical application to control an outbreak of gram positive infection where other infection control procedures have been unsuccessful. Use only as long as necessary for infection control." The FDA states that hexachlorophene is "not for routine prophylactic total body bathing, and not for use on burned or denuded skin or on mucous membranes." Some sources note that hexachlorophene should not be used in infants <2000 g or in infants with a high bilirubin. It should never be used on skin excoriations or burns or on any mucous membranes.

    e. Octenidine hydrochloride is effective against gram-positive and gram-negative organisms, MRSA, vancomycin-resistant *S aureus*, extended-spectrum β-lactamase–producing bacteria, and *Pseudomonas* and is mainly used in Europe.

V. Assist devices for procedures

    A. Transillumination. See Chapter 44. Transillumination is the use of a strong light source as a noninvasive tool to aid in procedures. It can help localize a vessel for cannulation or blood sampling, verify the presence of urine in the bladder, aid in oro/nasoduodenal feeding tube insertion and document the success of air removal in thoracentesis or pericardiocentesis.

    B. Point-of-care ultrasound. See Chapter 44. Point-of-care ultrasound (POCUS) is the use of a portable ultrasound at the bedside by a nonradiologist imager (eg, neonatologist) that can be used to help with a procedure. Two techniques are used in such procedures:

        1. Static technique involves the use of ultrasound prior to the procedure and can identify anatomy (eg, key landmarks for lumbar puncture), locate a vessel (eg, a peripheral artery for arterial line placement), locate the position of the endotracheal tube or catheter tip (eg, PICC, UVC, UAC), determine needle placement (eg, suprapubic aspiration), or determine if the procedure should be done (eg, POCUS of the bladder to identify urine volume amount).

        2. Dynamic technique involves the use of the ultrasound during the procedure : such as seeing the needle go into the bladder in suprapubic aspiration or helping guide the needle into the interspace while doing a lumbar puncture or direct visualization of the needle into the pericardial space.

    C. Near-infrared spectroscopy imaging. These devices (VascuLuminator, Vein Viewer Vision, AccuVein AV300) are all noninvasive methods used to locate an artery or vein for phlebotomy or cannulation. A near-infrared light source is used that transilluminates the puncture site, which is processed by a camera that projects the 2-dimensional image on the skin or on a display (VascuLuminator). The bulk of research using these devices has been inconclusive. In a randomized controlled trial, the vein viewer was found to improve successful placement, with the greatest benefit in infants of greater gestational age.

VI. Pain management in the neonate. The American Academy of Pediatrics (AAP) has recommended that every healthcare facility caring for neonates have an effective pain prevention program that includes strategies to reduce the number of painful procedures performed, and the use of pharmacologic and nonpharmacologic therapies to prevent pain with procedures. Procedures in this manual each discuss pain management. This information is based on the AAP recommendations plus a review of international guidelines (see Selected References). Chapters 15 and 81 provide additional details on neonatal pain management.

26 Arterial Access: Arterial Puncture

I. **Indications**
   A. **To obtain blood** for arterial blood gas measurements.
   B. **When blood is needed and venous or capillary blood samples cannot be obtained.** Not preferred.
   C. **To obtain ammonia levels.** Venous blood can be used if it is collected, transported appropriately, and done quickly, but because ammonia levels in peripheral venous blood can be affected by many variables, arterial blood is preferred.
   D. **To obtain lactate and pyruvate levels.** Free-flowing arterial blood; stasis of blood increases lactate.
   E. **To obtain a large quantity of blood that would be difficult to obtain from a peripheral vein.**

II. **Equipment.** Sterile gloves, a 23- (preferred for term infants) or 25-gauge (preferred for preterm infants) butterfly needle with extension tubing or venipuncture needle (safety-engineered self-shielding), 1- or 3-mL syringe, povidone-iodine and alcohol swabs, 4 × 4 gauze pad, preheparinized syringes (if not available, use a thin coat of 1:1000 IU/mL heparin in the syringe and plunger to prevent coagulation) or self-contained blood gas kit, high-intensity fiberoptic light for transillumination, Doppler ultrasound, a portable ultrasound (can be useful to locate the artery). Use a cap, mask, sterile gloves, and small sterile drape if obtaining a blood culture.

III. **Procedure**
   A. **For a blood gas, most hospitals have kits with 1-mL syringes coated with heparin.** If this is not available, draw a small amount of heparin (1:1000) into the blood gas syringe (coat the surfaces and discard excess heparin from the syringe). The small amount of heparin coating the syringe is sufficient to prevent coagulation. Excessive heparin may falsely lower pH and $PaCO_2$. If any other laboratory test is to be performed, use another syringe without heparin. **Available arteries to use:**
      1. **Low-risk preferred sites. Radial, posterior tibial, and dorsalis pedis arteries.**
         a. **Radial artery.** The radial artery is the **most frequently used site**, is the recommended site, and is described in detail here. The radial artery lies superficially at the underside of the forearm between the radial styloid process and lateral to the flexor carpi radialis tendon. **Advantages of the radial artery site include the following:** its superficial location is easily accessed, it is easy to palpate and puncture, there are no large veins nearby, there is good collateral circulation, and there are no nerves adjacent to the artery that could be injured.
         b. **Posterior tibial artery** (preferred second site). The posterior tibial artery lies posterior to the medial malleolus and is in the best position for puncture when the foot is in dorsiflexion. It has good collateral circulation, it is easy to puncture, and there are no large veins nearby.
         c. **Dorsalis pedis artery** (preferred third site). The dorsalis pedis artery is on the dorsal surface of the midfoot, draw an imaginary vertical line between the first and second toe. It has good collateral circulation, but because it is a small artery, it may be difficult to puncture. If using this artery, do an Allen test to assess collateral circulation of the posterior tibial artery.
      2. **High-risk not preferred sites. Femoral, brachial, temporal, and ulnar arteries.**
         a. **Femoral arteries** should be avoided in newborns and only used for emergency situations. There are serious complications that can occur; embolus, spasm, or significant thrombus could cause damage to the leg because there is no collateral circulation (loss of the extremity or infection at the hip joint).

      b. Brachial arteries should not be used (unless absolutely necessary) because there is minimal collateral circulation (only via 3 small arteries) and a risk of median nerve damage.

      c. Temporal arteries should not be used in newborns. There is a high risk of neurologic complications and the possibility of a thrombus or embolus stopping blood supply to that area of the brain.

      d. Ulnar arteries should not be used in newborns. It can result in impaired collateral circulation of the hand and damage to the median and ulnar nerves that lie close to the ulnar artery.

B. Check for collateral circulation and patency of the ulnar artery by means of the modified Allen's test. Elevate the infant's hand and simultaneously occlude the radial and ulnar arteries at the wrist; massage the palm toward the wrist to cause blanching. Release occlusion of the ulnar artery. If normal color returns in <10 seconds, adequate collateral circulation from the ulnar artery is present. If normal color does not return for >15 seconds, the collateral circulation is inadequate, and it is best not to use the radial artery in this arm. The radial and ulnar arteries in the other arm should then be tested for collateral circulation. Because of concern regarding the reliability of the modified Allen test in neonates, other methods such as the modified Allen test with Doppler ultrasound evaluation of collateral flow are being used.

C. Pain management

    1. Nonpharmacologic methods of pain control. Swaddling, facilitated tucking with positioning, nonnutritive sucking, breast feeding, or other methods can be used. A recent article found that a recording of the mother's voice played 10 minutes before, during, and 10 minutes after sampling reduces arterial blood sampling pain in term neonates.

    2. Topical local anesthetic agents. Use of topical local anesthetic agents (eutectic mixture of lidocaine and prilocaine [EMLA]) has been found to decrease measures of pain during a peripheral arterial puncture. There is concern for use of topical anesthetics in preterm infants.

    3. Sucrose. Sucrose can be used, but a recent Cochrane review (2016) found that the effectiveness of sucrose for reducing pain or stress from an arterial puncture was inconclusive.

    4. Subcutaneous local anesthesia. If time permits, consider infiltrating the skin subcutaneously with 0.1 to 0.2 mL of 0.5% to 1.0% buffered lidocaine (buffered lidocaine with sodium bicarbonate decreases the burning) using the smallest needle.

D. Perform appropriate hand hygiene and put on sterile gloves.

E. To obtain the sample. Take the patient's hand in your left hand (for a right-handed operator), and slightly extend the wrist beyond neutral position. Avoid hyperextension because it can occlude the vessel and will obscure the pulse. Techniques in locating the artery include: transillumination, palpation, Doppler auditory assistance, and point-of-care ultrasound. Mark the skin at the location of the artery with a fingernail imprint or sterile pen.

    1. Palpate the radial artery by feeling through the skin for the pulse (Figure 26–1). Difficulty in palpation can occur because the artery is small or a weak pulse if the infant is dehydrated or hemodynamically unstable.

    2. Transillumination with a high-intensity fiberoptic light to visualize the vessel. It will be a dark, linear line that is fixed (see Chapter 44).

    3. Doppler auditory assistance uses high frequency sound waves and notes a characteristic sound (area of maximum sound with a higher pitch) when the exact location of the artery is found.

    4. Point-of-care ultrasound using the static technique can be used to identify the artery location. Using the linear probe, scan the area in transverse and longitudinal planes where the artery should be. One can identify the artery because it will be pulsatile and will not collapse like the vein with compression. (See Chapter 44.)

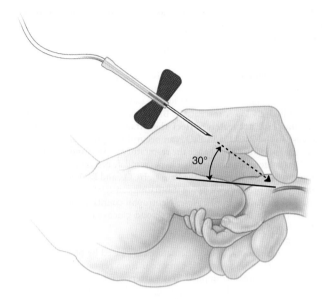

FIGURE 26–1. Technique of radial arterial puncture in the neonate.

  F. **Clean the puncture site.** Clean with antiseptic solution per hospital policy. If doing a blood culture, sterile technique is required.
  G. **Puncture the skin at about a 30-degree angle.** Then slowly advance the needle and penetrate the artery with the bevel up until blood appears in the tubing (see Figure 26–1). If the entire artery is perforated (anterior and posterior wall) and no blood is obtained, slowly withdraw the needle until blood is obtained. Because the artery can spasm, you may need to wait for blood return. **For a more superficial artery or in a premature or extremely low birthweight infant,** puncture the skin at approximately 15 degrees with the bevel down. With arterial blood samples, little aspiration is usually needed to fill the syringe. If there is no return of blood, withdraw the needle slowly because the artery may have been punctured through and through. Best to limit to 2 attempts.
  H. **Collect the least amount of blood needed.** The volume of blood taken at one time should not exceed 3% to 5% of the total blood volume (the total blood volume in a neonate is ~80 mL/kg).
  I. **Withdraw the needle and apply firm, but not occlusive, pressure to the site for a minimum of 3 minutes (≥5 minutes in very sick infants or those with a pro-longed clotting time) with a 4 × 4 gauze pad to ensure adequate hemostasis.** Shield and dispose of the needle in an appropriate container. Check fingers for adequate circulation.
  J. **If the hand starts to discolor or turn white during or after the procedure,** this occurs when the artery has a spasm. Wrap the opposite arm and hand with a warm, not hot, compresses. This will cause the blood vessels to dilate in the unaffected arm and hand and may cause the vessels in the affected hand to dilate (sympathetic response). Do not wrap the affected hand because this will increase the metabolic demand and blood flow in an area where there is already compromise.

K. **Before submitting an arterial blood gas sample, expel air bubbles from the sample and tightly cap the syringe.** Failure to do this can lead to errors in testing.

L. **Take the sample to the laboratory immediately or place it on ice if there is a delay.** Note the collection time and the patient's temperature and hemoglobin on the laboratory slip.

M. **Inaccurate blood gas results.** Excessive heparin in the syringe may result in a falsely low pH and $PaCO_2$. Remove excess heparin before obtaining the blood sample. Air bubbles caused by failure to cap the syringe may falsely elevate the PaO_2 and falsely lower the $PaCO_2$. **Blood gases by intermittent arterial punctures may not accurately reflect the infant's respiratory status.** A sudden decrease in the $PaCO_2$ and PaO_2 can occur during the puncture. Crying during an arterial puncture can change the respiratory pattern and significantly alter the blood gas values. Infants can either hyperventilate or stop ventilating. Hyperventilation can cause a decrease in the $PaCO_2$, HCO_3, and PaO_2 and oxygen saturation. Holding their breath or stopping ventilating can cause an increase in $PaCO_2$ and a decrease in PaO_2 and pH. *Note:* Neutrophil counts are lower in samples from arterial blood than venous samples. Blood glucose levels are 10% higher than venous blood levels.

IV. **Complications**

A. **Bleeding/hematoma.** A local hematoma is caused by bleeding from the vessel into the surrounding tissue. It can occur from repeated punctures or probing or not enough pressure applied to the artery after the procedure. To minimize hematoma risk, use the smallest gauge needle possible and hold pressure for 5 minutes immediately after withdrawing the needle. Hematomas usually resolve spontaneously.

B. **Vasospasm, thrombosis, and embolism.** These can cause distal ischemia and can be minimized by using the smallest gauge needle possible. With thrombosis, the vessel usually recanalizes over a period of time. Temporary arteriospasm can occur but usually resolves spontaneously (see Chapter 84).

C. **Infection.** Risk is rare and can be minimized by using strict sterile technique. Infection is commonly caused by gram-positive organisms such as *Staphylococcus epidermidis*, which should be treated with nafcillin or vancomycin and gentamicin (see Chapter 155). Drug sensitivities at the specific hospital should be checked. Osteomyelitis can occur if the bone is penetrated but is very rare.

D. **Arteriovenous fistula.** May occur after multiple arterial punctures and is treated surgically. Because the brachial artery and median cubital vein are anatomically very close, a single puncture can cause a fistula. Diagnosis is by Doppler flow of the brachial vessels.

E. **Nerve damage. Nerves usually run parallel to the arteries and may be damaged if punctured multiple times.** Median nerve damage has been reported after brachial artery puncture (high incidence of median nerve damage, ~13%). Posterior tibial and femoral nerve damage have also been reported. Nerve damage can also be caused by pressure from a hematoma.

F. **Rare complications. Forearm compartment syndrome** can occur with a brachial artery puncture. **Extensor tendon sheath injury** can occur from repeated radial artery punctures. **Pseudoaneurysm** formation is a rare complication of an arterial puncture. It can occur from trauma to the wall of the artery and may require surgical treatment (removal with primary end-to-end anastomosis).

27 Arterial Access: Percutaneous Arterial Catheterization

I. **Indications**
   A. **Frequent arterial blood sampling is required** and an umbilical arterial catheter cannot be placed or has been removed.
   B. **Intra-arterial blood pressure monitoring.**
   C. **Measure preductal PaO$_2$.** Requires right upper extremity catheterization.
   D. **Exchange transfusions (removal of blood only).** Used in peripheral vessel exchange transfusion (PVET) when drawing blood from a peripheral artery and infusing through a peripheral vein.

II. **Equipment.** Safety-engineered catheter over needle access device based on local practices (22 or 24 gauge; 24 gauge preferred for infants <1500 g), arm board (or 2 tongue blades taped together), adhesive tape, cap, mask, sterile fenestrated drape, povidone-iodine or skin disinfectant, sterile gloves, suture material (optional; needle holder, suture scissors, 4–0 or 5–0 silk sutures) or Steri-Strips or Tegaderm, 0.5% or 0.25% normal saline flush solution (0.25% preferred in premature infants to decrease hypernatremia risk) with heparin (0.5–2 units of heparin/mL saline), pressure bag (to prevent backflow and keep the line free of clots), connecting tubing, pressure transducer for continuous blood pressure monitoring, fiberoptic light for transillumination, a Doppler device or a portable ultrasound to locate the artery.

III. **Procedure. The radial, dorsalis pedis, and posterior tibial sites are the preferred sites.** Two methods are described here using the **radial artery**, which is the most common access site because of low complication rates. Methods can be adapted to other arteries. Another common site is the **posterior tibial artery**, as both the radial and posterior tibial arteries have good collateral circulation. The **dorsalis pedis** artery can be used as an alternative site but is often too small. The temporal, brachial, and femoral arteries are **not** recommended. Temporal artery catheterization may have adverse neurologic sequelae. The brachial artery is not recommended because it does not have good collateral flow and the median nerve can be damaged. The ulnar artery should also not be used because of poor collateral circulation or potential for damage to the ulnar nerve.
   A. **Locate the artery by palpation, transillumination, Doppler auditory assistance, or point-of-care ultrasound (POCUS).** Palpation of the artery can be done at the following sites: radial artery (lateral wrist), ulnar artery (medial wrist), posterior tibial artery (posterior to the medial malleolus), and dorsalis pedis artery (on top of the foot). For technique in transillumination see Chapter 44. Doppler device can identify the artery by a characteristic high sound. Using POCUS, one can find the artery which will be pulsatile and will not collapse like the vein when compressed.
   B. **Point-of-care ultrasound during cannulation.** The use of ultrasound during radial arterial cannulation is considered standard of care in adults and pediatrics. Use in neonates depends upon the clinician's training and experience and availability of equipment. It can help guide the catheter during the procedure, can lead to a shorter procedure time, a higher first and second attempt success rate, and a decrease in complications (hematoma or ischemia) as compared to palpation or Doppler auditory assistance as noted in a 2016 Cochrane review. The procedure involves using a linear probe transverse to the artery to first find the vessel. The artery will appear pulsatile and will not collapse with compression. Place the small linear probe over the vessel, insert the needle near the probe, and advance the needle until the vessel wall is punctured. The advantage is that one can directly visualize the needle passing into the vessel on the image.

C. **Verify adequate collateral circulation in the hand using the modified Allen test or Doppler evaluation.** (See Chapter 26.) Do this also on the foot for the dorsalis pedis and posterior tibial arteries, but it is not as reliable as in the hand. Raise the foot, occlude both the dorsalis pedis and posterior tibial artery, release them one at a time, and see if perfusion comes back within 10 seconds.

D. **Pain management.** Oral sucrose, breast milk, and/or pacifier are recommended with other nonpharmacologic pain prevention and relief techniques. Use of topical local anesthetic agents (eutectic mixture of lidocaine and prilocaine [EMLA]) or subcutaneous infiltration of lidocaine can also be considered. Consider a dose of opioids if intravenous access is available. (See Chapters 15 and 81.)

E. **Place the infant's wrist in a slightly hyperextended position.** Some choose to use a board with gauze under the wrist (Figure 27–1).

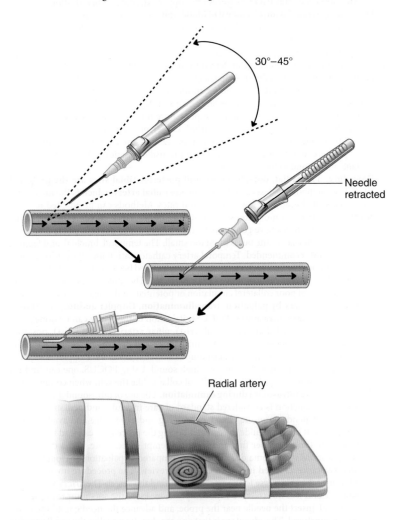

FIGURE 27–1. When placing an indwelling arterial catheter, the wrist should be secured as shown. The catheter assembly is introduced at a 30- to 45-degree angle.

F. **Perform hand hygiene and put on sterile gloves.** The Centers for Disease Control and Prevention recommend a minimum of cap, mask, sterile gloves, and a small sterile fenestrated (opening in the center) drape. During axillary or femoral insertion, maximum sterile precautions are recommended to include a gown and larger sterile field. **Cleanse the site** with antiseptic solution, and place sterile drapes around the puncture site.

G. **Methods of arterial catheter insertion**

1. **Standard method;** preferred for any newborn infant who is not premature.

   a. **Puncture (with bevel up) both the anterior and posterior walls of the artery** at a 30- to 45-degree angle and remove the stylet. There should be little or no backflow of blood.

   b. **Pull the catheter back slowly until blood is seen;** this signifies that the arterial lumen has been entered.

   c. **Advance the catheter** after attaching the syringe and flush the catheter. Never use hypertonic solutions to flush an arterial catheter.

   d. **Securely tape the catheter** with Steri-Strips and Tegaderm (preferred), or secure the catheter with 4–0 or 5–0 silk sutures in 2 places (may promote skin infection and is not recommended). Always allow for visualization of insertion site.

   e. **Connect the tubing with or without the transducer** from the heparinized saline pressure bag to the catheter.

   f. **Iodophor or other iodine-based ointments** on the area are no longer recommended because they can obscure the site and may promote infection.

2. **Premature infant method**

   a. **With the bevel down, at an angle of 10 to 15 degrees, puncture the anterior wall of the artery until blood return is seen.** At this point, the catheter should be in the lumen of the artery. Vasospasm is common, and the procedure should be performed slowly.

   b. **Advance the catheter into the artery while simultaneously withdrawing the needle.** The blood should be flowing freely from the catheter if the catheter is properly positioned.

   c. **Attach the syringe and flush the catheter.** Secure the line as in the standard method described earlier.

IV. **Additives**

A. **Heparin is recommended in the flushes and the pressure line.** Dosage range: 0.5 to 2 U/mL, per Pediatric Advanced Life Support for the American Heart Association. American College of Chest Physicians Evidence-Based Clinical Practice Guidelines recommend continuous heparin infusion at 0.5 U/mL at 1 mL/h for neonates with peripheral arterial catheters. Follow your institution's guidelines.

B. **Papaverine.** Added to the arterial line infusion (30 mg/250 mL), papaverine may prolong patency and reduce the risk of failure of peripheral arterial lines (***controversial***).

C. **Lidocaine.** Sometimes given intra-arterially to prevent vasospasm or treat vasospasm (***controversial***).

V. **Radial artery catheter removal**

A. **Remove the dressing** and sutures if present.

B. **Slowly remove the catheter.** Have sterile gauze available.

C. **Apply pressure to the site for 5 to 10** minutes and dress site.

VI. **Complications**

A. **Vasospasm/embolism/thrombosis.** Temporary arteriospasm can occur but usually resolves spontaneously (see Chapter 84).

   Vascular endothelium, injured from catheters, reacts by eliciting an inflammatory response with hemostasis and thrombus formation, resulting in tissue ischemia and release of potent vasoconstrictors. Use the smallest gauge catheter possible, minimize the infusion rate, and avoid large or rapid infusions and withdrawals. Avoid hypertonic solutions and blood products. Remove catheter at the earliest signs of ischemia. These events can cause a wide spectrum of complications:

1. **Temporary blanching of the extremity.**
2. **Skin ulcers** with sloughing of skin.
3. **Tissue ischemia, skin necrosis, gangrene, and partial loss of digits.** Transient ischemia of the forearm and hand has been reported with radial artery cannulation. Topical 2% nitroglycerin ointment on the site (dose 4 mm/kg) has been used to reverse tissue ischemia in infants who do not respond to noninvasive treatments (warming of the contralateral limb to promote reflex vasodilation). Intra-arterial administration of lidocaine and papaverine has also been used to reverse skin discoloration and tissue ischemia. See Chapter 84.
4. **Cerebral embolization** from a clot from a catheter in the radial or temporal artery and retrograde thrombosis of the posterior auricular artery have been reported from a temporal artery catheterization. Retrograde embolization of air or thrombus to the central nervous system can occur if the catheter is flushed too vigorously.
5. **Temporary occlusion.** Reversible total occlusion of the artery has been reported after a radial arterial catheterization.

B. **Air embolism.** Can be prevented by making certain that air is not introduced into the catheter and the catheter is flushed with heparinized saline.

C. **Hemorrhage/hematoma at puncture site.** If the catheter becomes dislodged, bleeding can occur. Tightly secure connections.

D. **Infection.** Low infection risk; rarely associated with bloodstream infection. Local infection, sepsis, cellulitis, and abscess have been reported. Prophylactic antibiotics are not recommended

E. **Extravasation/infiltration of solution.** See Chapter 42.

F. **Nerve damage.** Median, ulnar, posterior tibial, and peroneal nerve damage based on the catheter site.

G. **Hypernatremia.** Use 0.25% normal saline in low birthweight infants.

H. **Pseudoaneurysm.** Rare.

28 Arterial Access: Umbilical Artery Catheterization

I. **Indications**
   A. **Frequent or continuous measurements of arterial blood gases.**
   B. **Continuous arterial blood pressure monitoring.**
   C. **Access for exchange transfusion (to withdraw blood).**
   D. **Angiography.**
   E. **Infusion of maintenance solutions.**
   F. **Administration of emergency resuscitation medications and emergency infusion of volume expanders and fluids.** (*Note:* Umbilical vein preferred.)
   G. **Short-term infusions, parenteral nutrition, and/or medications (*controversial*).** Parenteral nutrition can be given through an umbilical artery catheter (UAC) and has been used in some centers, especially in very low birthweight (VLBW) infants; however, the umbilical artery is not preferred and should be used with caution. The maximum dextrose concentration that can be administered using this method is 15%. Antibiotics can be given via UAC, but this also is not preferred. Indomethacin,

vasopressor medications (epinephrine, dopamine, dobutamine), calcium boluses, and anticonvulsants **should not** be given via the UAC.

H. **Blood products (*controversial,* emergency only)** Blood products can be given via a UAC (less preferred, as this may enhance risk of thrombosis).

II. **Equipment**

A. **Basic.** Prepackaged UAC trays (usually include sterile drapes, tape measure, a needle holder, suture scissors, hemostat, forceps, scalpel, 3-way stopcock), umbilical tape, 2–0 to 4–0 silk suture, gauze pads, antiseptic solution, sterile gown, gloves, mask, hat, 10-mL syringe, 0.5% normal saline (NS) flush solution (0.25% NS for very small infants to reduce hypernatremia risk), and NS with heparin (0.25–1.0 U/mL) in continuous infusion calibrated pressure transducer for pressure monitoring; point-of-care ultrasound (if available) to guide catheter insertion and verify location of the catheter.

B. **Umbilical artery catheter (sizes 3.5 and 5F).** Size recommendations vary based on institutional guidelines. Some general guidelines:

   1. **UAC size:** infant <1.5 kg, use 3.5F; infant >1.5 kg, use 5F.
   2. **Perinatal Continuing Education Program recommendations:** <1000 g, use 3.5F; >1000 g, use 5F. Recommend use of single-lumen UAC.
   3. **End-hole catheters** are preferred and are associated with a decreased risk of aortic thrombosis when compared with side-hole catheters based on a Cochrane review.
   4. **Feeding tubes used as umbilical artery catheters** are associated with increased thrombosis risk and should be avoided.
   5. **Cochrane review notes that there is no benefit of using a heparin-bonded polyurethane catheter versus the standard polyvinyl chloride catheter.** A catheter made of Silastic (silicone) is more difficult to use because it is softer but may reduce aortic thrombosis compared with polyvinyl chloride (PVC) tubing. Teflon or polyurethane catheters have been associated with fewer infections and thrombogenicity than PVC or polyethylene catheters.

III. **Procedure**

A. **Umbilical artery catheterization practical tips**

   1. **The 2 umbilical arteries** (1 umbilical artery in ~1% of births) are muscular walled vessels (2–3 mm) that carry deoxygenated blood from the fetus to the placenta. The umbilical arteries are the direct continuation of the internal iliac arteries. The catheter enters the umbilical artery at the umbilicus; it courses downward into the internal iliac artery and then superiorly into the common iliac and then the aorta.
   2. **The umbilical arteries usually constrict within seconds after birth and close a few minutes later.** They can be dilated and used for the first 3 to 4 days (some sources 5–7 days) after birth and are easiest to place on the first day. After the first day, it helps to place a saline-soaked gauze on the umbilical stump for 45 to 60 minutes before attempting the procedure.
   3. **Unless it is an emergency (in which case you put the umbilical vein catheter (UVC) in first), put the umbilical artery catheter in first if putting in both an umbilical artery catheter and umbilical vein catheter.** The UAC is the more difficult one to insert, and often a second amputation of the umbilical stump needs to be done when inserting a UAC.
   4. **Blood cultures can be drawn** from the UAC for up to 6 hours after insertion (right after insertion preferred; venipuncture preferred overall).
   5. **Heparin use.** Cochrane reviews note the use of heparin (as low as 0.25 U/mL) is recommended to prolong the life of the catheter by decreasing the incidence of catheter occlusion or thrombosis. Heparinization with intermittent flushes alone is ineffective in preventing occlusion. Using heparinized fluid does not decrease the incidence of aortic thrombosis or affect the frequency of intraventricular hemorrhage.

The **American Academy of Pediatrics (AAP)** recommends low doses of heparin (0.25–1.0 U/L) through the UAC. The **American College of Chest Physicians Evidence-Based Clinical Practice Guidelines (2012)** recommend prophylaxis with a low-dose unfractionated heparin infusion via the UAC (heparin concentration of 0.25–1.0 U/mL; total heparin dose of 25–200 U/kg/d) to maintain patency. The Centers for Disease Control and Prevention (CDC) recommends low doses of heparin (0.25–1.0 U/mL) added to the fluid infused through the UAC.

6. **Prophylactic antibiotic use (*controversial*).** One review found that there was not enough evidence to support or refute the use of prophylactic antibiotics when UACs are inserted or to continue antibiotics once initial cultures rule out an infection.

7. **Point-of-care ultrasound in UAC placement. Ultrasound guided umbilical catheter insertion allows for direct visualization and localization of the vessel and can help guide catheter placement and accurately place the catheter in the optimal position.** It resulted in a faster method of placement (average saving 64 min in one study per Fleming et al) and required fewer x-rays and a decreased number of manipulations when compared to routine placement without ultrasound guidance. Technique in one study involved using a linear probe placed over the middle of the chest with scanning done in the sagittal plane. Malpositioned catheters could be seen and manipulations of the umbilical artery catheter could be done real time based on images seen. Injection of sterile saline helped locate the tip by seeing turbulence on the ultrasound. Use of POCUS is limited by many factors including lack of training in neonates, medicolegal issues, lack of availability, and high cost of equipment.

B. **High versus low umbilical artery catheter**

1. **High catheter/line.** UAC tip lies above the diaphragm at the level of T6–9. This position is above the celiac artery (T12), the renal arteries (L1), and the superior mesenteric artery (T12–L1).

2. **Low catheter/line.** UAC tip lies between the level of L3 and L4 (above the L4–5 aortic bifurcation).

3. **Catheter position was once determined by institutional guidelines.** High catheters were previously thought to be associated with a higher risk of vascular complications, but a recent analysis showed a decreased risk of vascular complications and no increased risk of hypertension, necrotizing enterocolitis (NEC), intraventricular hemorrhage, or hematuria. High catheters may be associated with glucose abnormalities. Low catheters are associated with an increased risk of lower extremity vasospasms. **Cochrane review states there is no evidence to support the use of low UACs.** They found that high catheters have fewer complications (decreased ischemic complications and decreased aortic thrombosis) and lesser need for replacement and reinsertion. The **American College of Chest Physicians Evidence-Based Clinical Practice Guidelines** (2012) suggest high UAC placement. A low position may only be needed if there is a problem placing a high catheter. See Figure 28–1 for vascular landmarks.

C. **Determining the length** of UAC can be obtained from multiple methods, with no universally accepted and no universal formula that applies to all infants. Remember to add the umbilical stump length. There are various methods (eg, birthweight, body measurements, surface anatomy) to determine the length of UAC placement. **Lean et al (2018) did a study of 11 published formulas to guide UAC placement and found that the formulas using body part measurements (not body weight) were the most accurate. Weight based formulas tend to overestimate the distance of insertion and do not do a good job at predicting catheter placement in smaller preterm infants.** Follow institutional guidelines.

1. **Dunn method (1966).** Uses the shoulder to umbilicus length and a nomogram to determine the insertion length. (Do not measure from the shoulder to the umbilicus on a diagonal.) It can be used for **high or low UAC** placement (Figure 28–2).

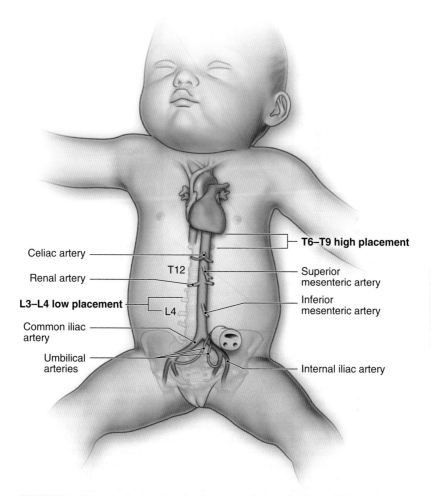

FIGURE 28–1. Important landmarks, related vessels, and the path of the umbilical artery. The internal iliac is also called the hypogastric artery.

2. **Shukla and Ferrara method(1986)** is more accurate for UAC than the Dunn method. It consistently overestimates the length in VLBW infants. Uses the birthweight and the following formula for a **high UAC:**

$$\text{UAC insertion length (cm)} = 3 \times \text{Birthweight (kg)} + 9$$

3. **Wright et al formula (2008)** for high UAC. The Wright formula in VLBW infants was found to be superior to the Shukla method. The correct insertion rate was higher in the Wright formula than the Dunn method for term newborns, low birthweight (LBW) newborns, VLBW newborns, and small for gestational age (SGA) newborns. The Wright formula in VLBW infants involves less repositioning than using the Shukla method. This formula results in more accurate placement and less overinsertion in VLBW newborns, especially in infants <1000 g. A study by

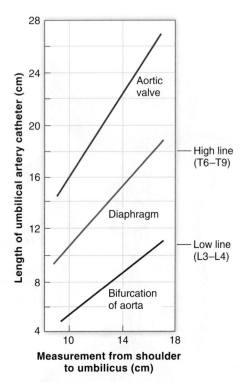

FIGURE 28–2. The umbilical artery catheter can be placed in 1 of 2 positions. The **low catheter** is placed below the level of L3 to avoid the renal and mesenteric vessels. The **high catheter** is placed between the thoracic vertebrae from T6 to T9. The graph is used as a guide to help determine the catheter length for each position. The **low line** corresponds to the aortic bifurcation in the graph, whereas a **high line** corresponds to the diaphragm. To determine catheter length, measure (in centimeters) a perpendicular line from the top of the shoulder to the umbilicus. This determines the shoulder-umbilical length. Plot this number on the graph to determine the proper catheter length for the umbilical artery catheter. Add the length of the umbilical stump to the catheter length. (*Modified with permission from Dunn PM: Localization of the umbilical catheter by post-mortem measurement,* Arch Dis Child. *1966 Feb;41(215):69-75.*)

Kumar and colleagues found there is no universal formula but that the Wright formula is the closest and can be applied to all neonates.

UAC length (cm) = (Birthweight in kg × 4) + 7 cm

D. **Surface anatomy measurements to determine high umbilical artery catheter insertion.** Gupta et al described a new method for estimation of insertion length that provided a better estimate in all birthweights than birthweight-based formulas.

(UN – 1 cm) + 2 × USp

UN is the distance from the umbilicus to the nipple, and USp is distance from the umbilicus to the symphysis pubis.

E. **Other measurements used**
   1. **Total body length (Weaver and Ahlgren formula, 1971):** One-third of total body length in centimeters.
   2. **Suprasternal notch to left superior iliac spine length (Sritipsukho and Sritip-sukho, 2007).** Measure suprasternal notch to superior iliac spine.
   3. **Shoulder to umbilicus length.** Shoulder to umbilicus + 2 cm.
F. **Pain management.** Because the umbilical cord is denervated, pain will be minimal. Avoid placement of the hemostat or any sutures on the skin around the umbilicus, as this will cause pain. Consider any nonpharmacologic methods of pain relief (see Chapter 15).
G. **Umbilical artery catheterization technique**
   1. **Place the patient supine.** Wrap a diaper around both legs and tape the diaper to the bed. This stabilizes the patient for the procedure and allows observation of the feet for vasospasm. Another option is to use commercial prefabricated restraints on all 4 extremities.
   2. **Put on sterile gloves, a mask, a hat, and a sterile gown.** Prepare a sterile field for the supplies.
   3. **Prepare the umbilical artery catheter.** Attach the stopcock to the catheter. Fill the 10-mL syringe with flush solution, and inject it through the stopcock and catheter.
   4. **Clean the umbilical cord area with antiseptic solution (povidone-iodine). Avoid tincture of iodine because of effect on the thyroid.** Place sterile drapes around the umbilicus, leaving the feet and head exposed.
   5. **Tie a piece of umbilical tape around the base of the umbilical cord tight enough to minimize blood loss** but loose enough so that the catheter can be passed easily through the vessel.
   6. **Cut off the excess umbilical cord with a scalpel,** leaving a 1-cm stump (Figure 28–3A). There are *usually* 2 umbilical arteries (1 and 7 o'clock positions). The vein usually has a large floppy thin wall at the 12 o'clock position (Figure 28–3B). If there is difficulty determining the vessels by observation, rub the flat side of the scalpel across the stump; the arteries can be felt with resistance, the vein cannot. Bloom et al and Gupta et al have described an alternative method: the umbilical stump is incised from the side and not the top.
   7. **If bleeding occurs,** tighten the umbilical tape or pinch base of the umbilicus tightly for a minimum of 5 minutes.
   8. **Using the curved hemostat, grasp the end of the umbilicus to hold it upright and steady.**
   9. **Use the iris forceps to open and dilate the umbilical artery.** Remember, the diameter is only 2 to 3 mm. First, place 1 arm of the forceps in the artery, and then use both arms to gently dilate the vessel (Figure 28–3, C and D).
      a. **An alternative technique** described by Wallenstein and Stevenson (2015) is useful for 1 practitioner performing the procedure. Pass a 4–0 or 5–0 silk suture needle directly into the arterial lumen and then drive the needle out of the sidewall 3 to 4 mm below the opening of the lumen. The needle is then brought back to the surface of the transected stump. When the suture is pulled upward, the lumen of the artery is opened and the catheter can be inserted.
   10. **Once the artery is sufficiently opened or dilated, insert the catheter caudally or toward the feet.** It is common to have some resistance at either the abdominal wall or at the level of the bladder. If resistance is met, apply gentle pressure for about 30 to 60 seconds. Avoid repeated probing. Approximately 5% to 10% will have difficulty passing the catheter. If there is spasm of the vessel, some centers recommend inserting the catheter 2 cm into the lumen and dripping 0.5 mL of 2% lidocaine hydrochloride solution without epinephrine into the vessel to dilate it. Topical nitroglycerin (NTG), used on peripheral veins to make them easier to cannulate, has been used to enhance UAC passage. Dose ranges from 0.12

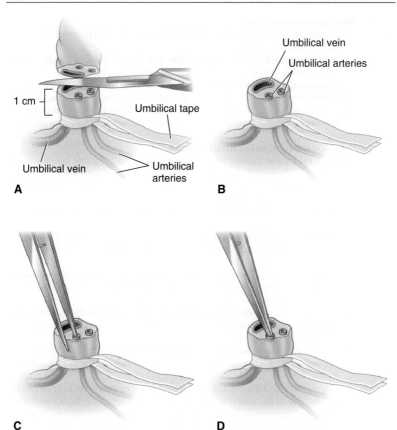

FIGURE 28–3. (**A**) The umbilical cord should be amputated, leaving a 1-cm stump. (**B**) Identification of the umbilical cord vessels. (**C–D**) A forcep is used to gently dilate the umbilical artery.

to 0.6 mg/kg, and application time is 5 to 10 minutes. One study suggests that topical application of NTG does not increase cannulation of umbilical arteries.

    a. The most common cause of failure to catheterize an umbilical artery is inadequate dilation of the artery.

    b. Use of the **"double catheter technique,"** as often used for UVC **is not recommended** due to greater risk of perforation.

    c. If in a false channel suggested by no blood return, remove and use other artery.

    d. Incorrect path. Rarely, the UAC will go from the umbilical artery to the femoral artery (by way of the internal, common, and external iliac arteries) or to the gluteal artery (by way of the internal iliac artery). Using too small a catheter in a large infant increases the risk of the gluteal artery entry. These incorrect path lines are not usable and should be removed.

 11. Once the catheter is in position, aspirate to verify blood return. Never advance the catheter once sterile technique is broken. It is better to have it too high and withdraw it. Connect to the tubing and transducer if appropriate.

12. **Secure the catheter.** It is very important that the umbilical artery catheter is securely placed because an unrecognized hemorrhage can lead to death if it accidently dislodges. Catheters that can move and become malpositioned can cause serious complications (myocardial perforation, liver injury, intestinal necrosis and thrombosis, cardiac arrhythmias, pleural or pericardial effusions). **There are 4 methods of securing an umbilical catheter, and the literature does not state that one method is better than another.** The goal is to keep the line secure while protecting the integrity of the abdominal skin. Choosing which method depends on the infant, the infant's health status, the healthcare provider inserting it, and what each institutional guideline recommends.

  a. **Method 1. Anchoring (with or without stitches).** The silk tape is folded over part way, the catheter is placed, and the remaining portion of the tape is folded over (Figure 28–4A). Suture the silk tape to the base of the umbilical cord (through the Wharton jelly, not the skin or vessels) using 3–0 silk sutures. No special dressing is needed. The umbilical stump with the catheter in place is left open to the air. Once the catheter is secure, loosen the umbilical tape.

  b. **Method 2. "Tape bridge" or "goal post" method (most popular method).** Secure the catheter with a tape bridge. (See Figure 28–4B, "goal post" method.) Make 2 tabs from tape and place on either side of the umbilicus. Then take another piece of tape and wrap it around the 2 tabs to make a T shape. This technique has 2 disadvantages: skin irritation and infection may occur, and sometimes the tape does not adhere to the skin well and does not last.

  c. **Method 3. DuoDERM technique.** This is the easiest and quickest method of securing an umbilical line. A DuoDERM (ConvaTec, Bridgewater, NJ) patch is cut and placed over the coiled up umbilical catheter. Skin irritation may sometimes occur. Image not shown.

  d. **Method 4. A commercially available umbilical line securement device** (eg, NeoBridge; Neotech, Valencia, CA) can also be used (Figure 28–5). It is an umbilical catheter holder that attaches to the skin with a hydrocolloid gel; 2 flaps come up from the base that hold 2 catheters. Advantages are that the flaps can be opened and closed repeatedly. This is the most expensive method of securing the line. Skin irritation and infection can occur.

13. **Do not use topical antibiotic ointment or creams on the umbilical catheter insertion site.** This can promote fungal infections and antimicrobial resistance.

14. **Obtain a radiograph of either abdomen (verify position of a low catheter) or chest (verify position of a high catheter).** Best position for low catheter: between L3–4, just above the aortic bifurcation and to avoid the renal and mesenteric arteries. Best position for high catheter: between T6–9, above the origin of the celiac axis. Radiographs showing positioning can be found in Chapter 12 (high UAC, see Figure 12–14; and low UAC, see Figure 12–15).

15. **Point-of-care ultrasound confirmation of UAC tip placement.** A bedside **ultrasound** can be used to assess catheter tip position and was found to more accurately confirm the position than a radiograph. Because catheters are often not placed at the correct position (Lean et al found that >25% UACs placed needed manipulation), some suggest that ultrasound should be the gold standard to confirm correct catheter placement. Evidence shows that ultrasound has good sensitivity, specificity, and positive and negative predictive value when comparing it to a radiograph. Place the linear transducer in the subxiphoid position aimed toward the left of the midline pointed toward the back to the aorta. The aorta is pulsatile and straight. The UAC tip will pass up the descending aorta and end near the diaphragm.

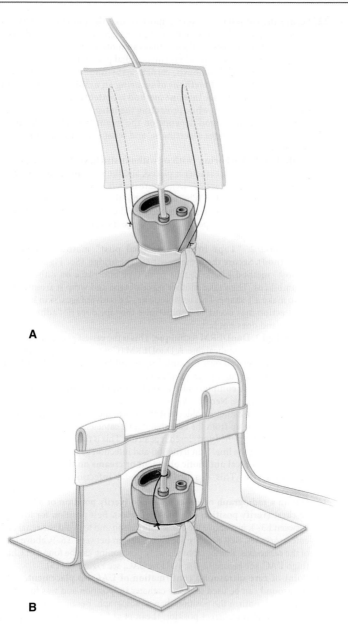

A

B

FIGURE 28–4. (**A**) The umbilical artery catheter is secured with silk tape, which is attached to the base of the cord (through the Wharton jelly, not the skin or vessels). (**B**) The umbilical catheter is secured with a tape bridge ("goal post" method). (*Reproduced with permission from Tshudy MM, Arcara KM: The Harriet Lane Handbook, 19th ed. Philadelphia, PA: Elsevier; 2012.*)

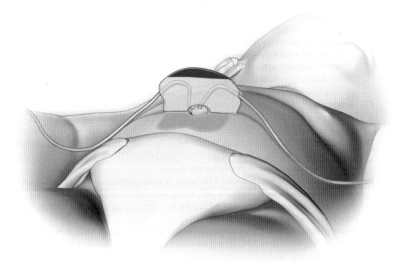

Figure 28–5. NeoBridge (inspiration-healthcare.com) is an umbilical catheter holder that attaches to the skin.

16. **The Centers for Disease Control and Prevention recommends that UACs stay in for no more than 5 days.** Other sources state 5 to 7 days. The duration of UACs is a risk factor for aortic thrombosis. CDC states that a malfunctioning umbilical catheter can be replaced if the total duration is not greater than 5 days and there is no other indication for catheter removal.

IV. **Umbilical artery catheter removal**

A. **Make sure the umbilical tie is lightly tied around the stump.** Cut any sutures or tape that holds the catheter.

B. **Withdraw the catheter slowly** until about 5 cm remains in the vessel.

C. **Tighten the umbilical tie.**

D. **Discontinue the infusion, and pull the catheter slowly (1 cm/min).**

E. **If bleeding, apply pressure to the base of the cord.**

V. **Complications of umbilical artery catheterization** have been reported in the range of 5% to 32%.

A. **Infection (septic emboli, cellulitis, omphalitis, sepsis).** The catheter disrupts the integrity of the skin, introducing bacteria or fungi and causing an infection; minimize by using strict sterile technique. **No attempt should be made to advance a catheter once it has been placed in position; instead, if needed, the catheter should be replaced.** AAP and CDC recommend the catheter to be removed and not replaced if there are any signs of central line–associated bloodstream infection. Prophylactic antibiotics are not recommended. VLBW infants who received antibiotics for >10 days were at increased risk for catheter-related bloodstream infections in one study.

B. **Vascular complications. Vasospasm, thrombosis, embolism, and infarction can occur.** Heparin use in UACs did not decrease the rate of aortic thrombi. Air embolism has also been reported. Doppler ultrasound is useful to examine the aorta and renal vessels. AAP and CDC recommend removing the UAC if thrombosis is present. See Chapter 84 for other treatment plans for vasospasm and thromboembolism.

1. **Arterial vasospasm** can cause blanching and cyanosis of the buttocks, legs, feet, and toes. It is increased in low-lying catheters. Loss of extremity is rare but can occur. If the leg blanches, warm the other leg to cause reflex vasodilatation.

    2. **Thrombosis.** This can cause dampening of the arterial tracing and is further classified as follows:

       a. **Femoral artery thrombosis.** Limb ischemia, gangrene.

       b. **Renal artery thrombosis.** Hematuria, hypertension, renal failure.

       c. **Mesenteric artery thrombosis.** Ischemia of the gut, NEC.

       d. **Aortic thrombosis.** Congestive heart failure, hematuria, paraplegia, renovascular hypertension, leg-growth discrepancy.

  C. **Hemorrhage.** This can be secondary to perforation of the vessel, umbilical cord site bleeding around the catheter, disconnection of the catheter at any point in the system, or accidental line dislodgment. The tubing stopcocks must be securely fastened.

  D. **Vessel perforation.** The catheter should never be forced into position. If the catheter cannot be easily advanced, use of the other vessel should be attempted. If perforation occurs, surgical intervention may be necessary.

  E. **Gastrointestinal complications.** UACs may lead to gastrointestinal ischemia, intestinal necrosis (embolization to the gut), or localized perforation. Data do not support that UACs alter the incidence of NEC whether they are high or low or regardless of enteral feeding status.

  F. **Improperly placed catheter** can cause perforation of a vessel, false aneurysm, perforation of the peritoneum, hematoma formation, sciatic nerve palsy, retrograde arterial bleeding, and refractory hypoglycemia (catheter tip opposite celiac axis).

  G. **Hematuria** can occur secondary to renal vein thrombosis or injury to the bladder.

  H. **Hypertension secondary to renal artery embolus** can occur as a long-term complication caused by stenosis of the renal artery as a result of improper catheter placement near the renal arteries.

  I. **Patent urachus.** If the urachal tract is not obliterated during embryonic development, a patent urachus can result. If urine is obtained from a UAC and not blood, there may be a patent urachus. Urology or pediatric surgery consult is required.

  J. **Other complications.** Urinary ascites, scrotal hypoperfusion (may be secondary to catheter-induced vasospasm of pudendal arteries), Wharton jelly or cotton fiber embolus, hypernatremia, peroneal nerve palsy, broken umbilical artery catheter fragment causing thrombosis, infection, distal embolization, factitious hypernatremia or hyperkalemia, and hypoglycemia.

29 Bladder Aspiration (Suprapubic Urine Collection)

I. **Indication.** To obtain urine for culture when a less invasive technique is not possible. It is the most invasive method of urine collection, but also the most accurate culture source for infants and children <2 years of age when compared with urethral catheterization and bag urine specimens. It is considered the **gold standard of urine specimen collections** because it has a relative rate of urine culture contamination of only 1%. Any bacteria or growth (unless clearly a contaminant) from a suprapubic culture is considered abnormal and may indicate an infection. The American Academy of Pediatrics (AAP) has made recommendations for infants age 2 to 24 months to obtain a catheterization or suprapubic aspiration for any urine specimen (urinalysis and urine culture) obtained in a febrile ill infant who has no apparent source for the fever and who is planning on receiving antibiotics.

II. Equipment. Safety-engineered needle: 23- or 25-gauge 5/8- or 1-inch needle or 21-, 22-, or 23-gauge 1.5-inch needle (larger infant) or 23-gauge butterfly (for preemie), 3- or 5-mL syringe, sterile gloves, antiseptic solution, 4 × 4 gauze pads, sterile urine culture container (per institutional guidelines), topical anesthetic cream, 1% lidocaine (with or without epinephrine), transillumination light source, or portable ultrasound (optional).

III. Procedure

A. **Contraindications.** Empty bladder, significant bleeding disorders, significant abdominal distension, massive organomegaly, cellulitis/infection at the puncture site, major genitourinary anomalies, or recent lower abdominal or urologic surgery.

B. **Verify that voiding has not occurred** within the previous hour so there will be enough urine in the bladder for the procedure by one of the following methods:

1. **Palpate or percuss the bladder.** Dullness to percussion 2 fingers above the pubic symphysis suggests urine in the bladder. The neonatal bladder extends above the pubic symphysis as it fills.

2. **Transillumination** can determine bladder height and verify the presence of urine. With the lights dim, the transillumination source is pointed at the bladder. The area will glow red if urine is present. (See Chapter 44.)

3. **Point-of-care ultrasound of the bladder can be used** to help determine the presence and volume of urine in the bladder before attempting the procedure, thus increasing the likelihood of a successful tap. Using a high frequency linear-array transducer probe, apply it in a transverse position in the midline of the lower abdomen to locate the bladder. The bladder will be a dark cavity (if filled with urine) just below the abdominal musculature, usually round, with bright margins. A minimum volume on ultrasound of 10 mL in children <2 years of age is associated with a 90% successful bladder aspiration. If the cephalocaudal diameter of the bladder (sagittal view) is >20 mm and the anteroposterior diameter is >15 to 20 mm, the success rate approaches 100%.

C. **Pain management.** The majority of studies found that pain scores were significantly higher with suprapubic aspiration when compared to transurethral catheterization.

1. **Nonpharmacologic pain reduction procedures** can be used such as sucrose on a pacifier.

2. **Topical local anesthesia.** EMLA (eutectic mixture of lidocaine and prilocaine) can be used. In one study, EMLA use 1 hour before the suprapubic aspiration was found to reduce pain scores more than without EMLA.

3. **Local injection of lidocaine** can be used, but it is often reserved for older infants with thicker abdominal walls.

4. **EMLA plus local injection of lidocaine.**

D. **Point-of-care ultrasound can also be used to assist one in performing the procedure.** It can identify the site of needle insertion in the bladder (static technique, mark location with a sterile pen) and guide the needle insertion and puncture of the bladder wall (dynamic technique). When used, fewer needle insertions are necessary. Using the linear probe, apply it in a transverse position in the lower midline of the abdomen. Locate the bladder and mark the site of insertion. Leave the probe on the abdomen, while imaging in the sagittal plane. The needle can be inserted just inferior to the probe site in the plane of the ultrasound beam. The needle tip can be seen on the ultrasound screen as it advances through the skin and then the bladder. Ultrasound-guided suprapubic bladder aspiration is more successful than a blind suprapubic bladder aspiration in infants <4 months old, especially if the anterior-posterior and transverse diameter of the bladder is >2 cm.

E. **An assistant should hold the infant** in a supine position with the legs in the frog-leg position. The arms and legs need to be held.

F. **Locate the site of bladder puncture,** which is approximately 1 to 2 cm above the pubic symphysis in the midline of the lower abdomen (look for the transverse lower abdominal skin crease just above the pubic symphysis). *Note:* The urinary bladder of the neonate and infant is more of an abdominal organ and easier to access since as it fills it rises above the level of the pubic symphysis. As the infant grows, the bladder assumes more of a pelvic position. The bladder lies posterior to the pubic symphysis and anterior to the female uterus. See Figure 29–1A.

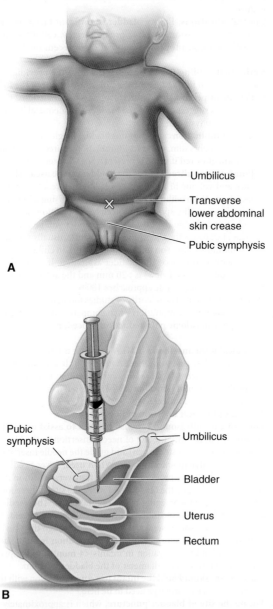

FIGURE 29–1. Technique of suprapubic bladder aspiration. (**A**) Landmarks and recommended site for suprapubic bladder aspiration. (**B**) Technique of suprapubic aspiration.

G. **To avoid the bladder from emptying** (reflex urination) when the needle is inserted, have an assistant apply gentle pressure at the base of the penis in a male infant, or in a female infant, apply anterior rectal pressure with a fingertip in the anus.

H. **Put on sterile gloves,** and clean the entire suprapubic area of skin (from pubic symphysis to the umbilicus) with antiseptic solution 3 times. Place sterile drapes around the insertion site.

I. **Palpate the pubic symphysis.** Insert the needle with syringe attached 1 to 2 cm above the pubic symphysis (at the transverse lower abdominal skin crease in the midline) at a 90-degree angle (Figure 29–1B). Some suggest angling the needle slightly caudad (10–20 degrees posteriorly).

J. **Advance the needle approximately 2 to 3 cm while aspirating.** Do not advance the needle once urine is seen in the syringe to reduce the risk of posterior wall bladder perforation. Use only gentle aspiration to prevent suctioning the posterior bladder wall.

K. **If no urine appears,** do not advance or redirect the needle. Withdraw the needle and reattempt the procedure in a minimum of 1 hour; consider ultrasound to more accurately evaluate bladder filling.

L. **Collect sample,** withdraw the needle, maintain pressure over the site of puncture, and apply a bandage (optional). Place a sterile cap on the syringe or transfer the specimen to a sterile urine cup, and submit the specimen to the laboratory.

IV. **Complications.** Serious complications are rare.

A. **Bleeding and hematomas.** Hematuria is the most common complication; it is usually microscopic, rarely causes concern, and usually resolves. Gross hemorrhage is more likely if there is a bleeding disorder; transient gross hematuria is reported in up to 3.4% of cases. Hematomas (abdominal wall, pelvic, and bladder wall), massive hemoperitoneum, and vaginal bleeding are rare.

B. **Infection.** Rare and not likely to occur if strict sterile technique is used. Sepsis, bacteremia, abdominal wall abscess, cellulitis of the abdominal wall, suprapubic abscess formation, and osteomyelitis of the pubic bone have all been reported.

C. **Perforation of the bowel.** With careful identification of the landmarks, preferably using ultrasound guidance, and not advancing the needle too far, this complication is rare. Bowel perforation can occur if a loop of the bowel is over the bladder. Usually the perforation is not clinically significant because the small puncture rarely causes peritonitis. If the bowel is perforated (aspiration of bowel contents), one can reattempt the procedure with a new sterile needle and syringe.

30 Bladder Catheterization

I. **Indications**

A. **To collect a urine specimen for culture when a suprapubic aspiration is contraindicated or cannot be performed and a clean-catch specimen is unsatisfactory.** Bladder catheterization is an alternative to suprapubic aspiration. It has a higher false-positive rate than suprapubic aspiration (relative rate of urine culture contamination of 6%–12%) and can also introduce bacteria and cause a urinary tract infection. The American Academy of Pediatrics (AAP) has made recommendations to obtain a catheterization or suprapubic aspiration for any urine specimen (urinalysis and urine culture) obtained in a febrile ill infant who is >2 months of age, who has no apparent source for the fever, and who is planning on getting antibiotics.

B. **To monitor urinary output, relieve urinary retention, or to instill contrast** to perform cystourethrography.

   C. **To determine a bladder residual urine volume.**
   D. **To place contrast for diagnostic cystography.**
II. **Equipment.** Sterile gloves, cotton balls, povidone-iodine solution, sterile drapes, lubri-cant gel, a sterile collection bottle (often packaged together as a commercial set), and choice of catheter (see below); point-of-care ultrasound, if available.
   A. **Urethral catheters. Use the smallest catheter possible.** (*Note:* balloon retention catheters [eg, Foley] are not used in newborns.) Recommendations on urethral cath-eter choice vary widely; follow your institution's guidelines if available.
      1. **Commercially available urethral catheter sizes:** 3.5, 5.0, 6.5, and 8F.
      2. **Urethral catheter size recommendations by weight**
         a. **3.5F for weight <1000 g.**
         b. **5F for weight 1000 to 1800 g.**
         c. **6.5F for weight 1800 to 4000 g.**
         d. **8F for weight >4000 g.**
      3. **National Association of Neonatal Nurses (NANN) recommendations:** 3.5F for weight <1000 g; 5F for weight 1000 to 1800 g; 8F for weight >1800 g.
      4. **Feeding tubes.** When used as an alternative, they may increase the risk of trauma or knotting (commercial urethral catheters are softer and not as long). A 5F feed-ing tube is sometimes used but not generally preferred.
      5. **Umbilical catheter.** May be used as an alternative: 3.5F for weight <1000 g; 5F for weight >1000 g.
III. **Procedure**
   A. **When performing catheterization to obtain a specimen,** it is best to wait until 1 to 2 hours after voiding.
   B. **POCUS of the bladder.** Ultrasound of the bladder can help determine if there is sufficient urine in the bladder. Use a high frequency linear array transducer probe and apply it in a transverse position in the midline of the lower abdomen to locate the bladder. The bladder will be a dark cavity with a thin wall that is echogenic. Mea-sure the **sonographic urinary bladder index measurement** (product of anteroposte-rior and transverse diameters, expressed in centimeters squared), which will identify whether there is sufficient urine in the bladder. A urinary bladder index <2.4 cm^2 means there is lack of urine volume and the catheterization may be unsuccessful. A urinary bladder index >2.4 cm^2 suggests an adequate urine volume. An ultrasound of the bladder at the bedside led to an increased success rate of urethral catheteriza-tion in children <2 months of age. **Ultrasound directed bladder catheterization** has been used in pediatrics for guiding the catheter in the bladder and is more successful than blind catheterization.
   C. **Pain management.** Nonpharmacologic pain-reducing methods are recom-mended (see examples in Chapter 15). Intraurethral lidocaine gel 1% can also be considered (*controversial*). A recent study showed that lidocaine gel did not reduce pain from urethral catheterization versus nonanesthetic gel in children <4 years of age.
   D. **Technique for male catheterization.** See Figure 30–1.
      1. **Place the infant supine, with the thighs abducted** (frog-leg position).
      2. **Wash hands thoroughly,** put on sterile gloves, and drape the area with sterile towels.
      3. **The newborn male infant has a physiologic phimosis, and the foreskin cannot be retracted fully.** Gently retract the foreskin just enough to expose the meatus with the nondominant hand (now considered contaminated); do not force retrac-tion of the foreskin. The meatus can usually be aligned with the opening in the prepuce.
      4. **Cleanse the penis with povidone-iodine solution using your free sterile hand.** Begin with the meatus and move in a proximal direction. Clean it 3 times in a circular fashion.
      5. **Place the tip of the catheter in sterile lubricant gel.**

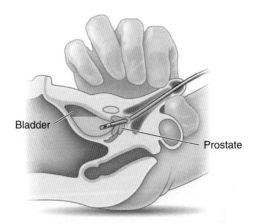

FIGURE 30–1. Bladder catheterization in the newborn male.

6. **Hold the penis approximately perpendicular to the body to straighten the penile urethra and help prevent false passage.** Use a small amount of pressure at the base of the penis to avoid reflex urination.

7. **Advance the catheter until urine appears. A newborn male urethra (preterm to term) measures 3.5 to 7 cm.** Length of catheter insertion in males is generally as follows: weight <750 g, <5 cm; weight >750 g, approximately 6 cm. A **slight resistance may be felt** as the catheter passes the external sphincter; therefore, hold the catheter in place with minimal pressure. Gentle continuous pressure enables the catheter to pass when the sphincter relaxes. Never force the catheter because urethral trauma or false passage can occur.

8. **Collect the urine specimen.** Discard the first few drops of urine to avoid any chance of contamination of the early stream of urine. If the catheter is to remain in place, connect it to a closed urinary collection system. It should be taped to the lower abdomen rather than to the leg in males to help decrease stricture formation caused by pressure on the posterior urethra. Contrast can be injected at this point if the catheter has been placed for a radiographic study.

E. **Female catheterization.** See Figure 30–2.
   1. **Supine position technique**
      a. **Place the infant supine, with the thighs abducted (frog-leg position).**
      b. **Wash hands thoroughly,** put on sterile gloves, and drape sterile towels around the labia.
      c. **Separate the labia with the nondominant hand (now considered contaminated),** and cleanse the area around the meatus with povidone-iodine solution 3 times. Use anterior-to-posterior strokes to prevent fecal contamination.
      d. **Keep the labia spread with the nondominant hand** with 2 fingers. See Figure 30–2 for landmarks. The meatus is found between the clitoris and vagina and may be difficult to see if the vaginal introitus is covering it. Lubricate the catheter, and advance it in the urethra until urine appears. A newborn female (preterm to term) urethra measures 1 to 2 cm. **General length of catheter insertion:** weight <750 g, generally <2.5 cm; weight >750 g, approximately 5 cm.
      e. **Collect the urine.** Discard the first few drops of urine to avoid any chance of contamination of the early stream of urine.
      f. **Tape the catheter to the leg** if it is to remain in position.
      g. **If urine does not appear in the catheter, the catheter may be in the vagina.** Check the catheter position and replace if necessary.

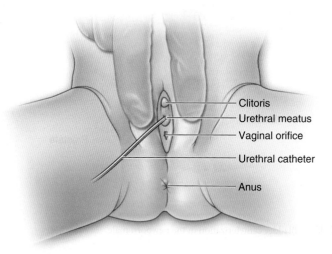

FIGURE 30–2. Landmarks used in catheterization of the bladder in newborn females in supine position.

> 2. **Prone position technique.** Used for a female infant who cannot be placed in the supine position (eg, infant with meningomyelocele).
>> a. **Place the infant prone on blankets,** so the upper body is elevated as compared with the lower body.
>> b. **Tape a gauze pad over the anus to avoid contamination.** Place sterile drapes.
>> c. **Then proceed from step b as for supine position (see Section III.E.1.b).**

IV. **Catheter removal.** Once urine has been obtained and flow has stopped, gently withdraw the catheter. Observe after the procedure for urine output.

V. **Complications**

> A. **Infection.** Sterile technique is necessary to prevent infection. There is a risk of introducing bacteria into the urinary tract and then the bloodstream. "In-and-out" catheterization carries a small (<5%) risk of urinary tract infection. The longer a catheter is left in place, the greater is the infection risk. Infections that can occur include sepsis, cystitis, pyelonephritis, urethritis, and epididymitis.
>
> B. **Trauma to the urethra or the bladder.** Urethral tear, urethral false passage, erosion, stricture, meatal stenosis, or bladder injury (perforation) is more common in males. Minimize by adequately lubricating the catheter and stretching the penis to straighten the male urethra. Never force the catheter if resistance is felt. Use the smallest catheter possible, and advance only until urine is obtained.
>
> C. **Hematuria** is usually transient but may require irrigation with normal saline solution. Gross hematuria on insertion may indicate a false passage.
>
> D. **Urethral stricture.** A longer term complication more common in males. It is usually caused by a catheter that is too large or by prolonged or traumatic catheterization. In males, taping the catheter to the anterior abdominal wall helps decrease the pressure on the posterior urethra.
>
> E. **Urinary retention.** Secondary to urethral edema.
>
> F. **Catheter knot.** Rare (0.2 per 100,000 catheterizations) but can happen if the catheter advances too far (too long of a flexible catheter may form a loop and knot on itself). More common if feeding tubes are used. Overdistension of the bladder and bladder

spasm are also a risk. This is also more common in males, neonates, and children rather than adults. Using appropriate lengths based on age and sex may help prevent this complication. Removal (traction under general anesthesia, unraveling the knot using a guidewire through the catheter under fluoroscopy, suprapubic cystotomy, and endoscopic retrieval) can cause significant morbidity involving general anesthesia, fluoroscopy, and transient hematuria. If this occurs, a urology consultation may be necessary.

   G. Malpositioned catheter. In males, the catheter may coil in the urethra before it reaches the bladder. The catheter can be accidently placed in the vagina in females. If this happens during cystography, the vagina can mimic the bladder. The clue to this is that fluid is in the peritoneal cavity (contrast material flowed through the uterus and fallopian tubes into the peritoneal cavity).

   H. Obstructive bilateral hydroureteronephrosis. Rare.

31 Chest Tube Placement

I. **Indications**
   A. **Evacuation of pneumothorax** compromising ventilation and causing increased work of breathing, hypoxia, and increased $PaCO_2$.
   B. **Relieve tension pneumothorax** causing respiratory compromise and decreased venous return to the heart, resulting in decreased cardiac output and hypotension. **This is an emergency that should be handled by immediate needle aspiration before chest tube placement.** (See Chapter 75.)
   C. **Drainage of significant pleural fluid** (pleural effusion, empyema, chylothorax, hemothorax, extravasation from a central venous line).
   D. **Postsurgical drainage** after repair of a tracheoesophageal fistula, bronchopleural fistula, esophageal atresia, or other thoracic procedure.

II. **Equipment.** Prepackaged chest tube tray (typically includes sterile towels, gauze pads, 3–0 silk suture, a needle holder, curved hemostats, a no. 15 scalpel, scissors, antiseptic solution, antibiotic ointment, 1% lidocaine, 3-mL syringe, 25-gauge needle), sterile gloves, mask, eye protection, hat, gown, suction-drainage system (eg, Pleur-Evac system). A high-intensity fiberoptic light for transillumination or point-of-care ultrasound is helpful (see Chapter 44). Chest tube types and sizes are as follows:
   A. **Standard (traditional) chest tube insertion.** Requires a skin incision with blunt chest wall dissection and sutures. Use polyvinyl chloride chest tubes with or without trocars (8, 10, or 12F). Recommended chest tube size for weight: <2000 g, 8 or 10F; >2000 g, 12F.
   B. **Percutaneous chest tube with pigtail catheter.** Does not require a skin incision. The pigtail catheter is inserted through a needle. This is an easier and less invasive technique requiring less anesthesia. Disadvantages are that the catheter may kink and become obstructed since they are softer. **Pigtail catheter sizes** range from 5 to 12F, with 8 or 10F most commonly used.

III. **Procedure**
   A. **The site of skin insertion** for the elective chest tube insertion is the same for both air and fluid, but the direction of the tube is determined by examining the anteroposterior (AP) and cross-table lateral or lateral decubitus chest films for air or fluid. Air collects in the uppermost areas of the chest, and fluid in the most dependent areas. **For air collections, place the tube anteriorly. For fluid collections, place the tube posteriorly and laterally.**

B. **Transillumination** of the chest may help detect a pneumothorax but not a small pneumothorax (see Chapter 44). It can also document the success of air removal. With the room lights turned down, a strong light source is placed on the anterior chest wall above the nipple and in the axilla. The affected side usually appears hyperlucent ("lights up") and radiates across the chest as compared with the unaffected side. Unless the infant's status is rapidly deteriorating, a chest radiograph (both AP and lateral decubitus or cross-table lateral) should be obtained to confirm pneumothorax before the chest tube is inserted. If air is suspected, the infant should be lying on his or her side with the suspect side up; if fluid is suspected, the infant should be placed with the suspect side down. See Figure 12–23 for a radiograph showing a left tension pneumothorax.

   1. **False-positive transillumination.** Can occur in infants with subcutaneous air, severe pulmonary interstitial emphysema, congenital lobar emphysema, pneumomediastinum, large air bubble in the stomach, and a weak light source.

   2. **False-negative transillumination.** Can occur in infants with a small pneumothorax, thick chest wall with increased subcutaneous fat or edema, thick skin folds, dark pigmented skin, and a weak light source and bright room lights.

C. **Use of point-of-care ultrasound for diagnosis.** Lung ultrasound is useful in identifying a **pneumothorax** in a newborn and is just as accurate a chest x-ray. Findings include lung sliding disappearance (100%), a pleural line and A line (100%), absence of B lines (100%), no area of lung consolidation in the area of the pneumothorax (100%), and lung point (75%). Ultrasound findings of a **pleural effusion** include: absent lung sliding, absent A lines, present anechoic zone, +/− jellyfish sign, sinusoid sign, or quad sign. These findings are described in detail in Chapters 44 and 75.

D. **Use of POCUS during the procedure.** POCUS (static and ultrasound guidance) in adult thoracentesis is recommended and a standard of care to increase the success rate and decrease complications. It is used in pediatrics and there are some reports in neonatology. POCUS static technique can be used to identify landmarks and the optimal location of the needle or chest tube insertion. Dynamic technique can be used to aid in doing the thoracentesis for air or fluid with direct visualization of the needle and increases the rate of success and decreases the rate of complications. See Chapter 44 for technique.

E. **Position the patient** so the site of insertion is accessible. Place the infant with the affected side at a 60-degree upright angle using a towel roll behind the infant's back to evacuate air. Use a 15- to 30-degree angle for fluid, chyle, blood, or pus evacuation. Make sure the arm is over the head because this position allows air to rise. Secure the infant's arm above his or her head.

F. **Select the appropriate site.** Make sure the team takes a "time out" to confirm the side that you plan to aspirate.

   1. **Emergency needle aspiration (tension pneumothorax).** Needle aspiration is done at the **second intercostal space** in **the midclavicular line** on the suspected side of the pneumothorax. The needle is inserted above the third rib. See Chapter 75 and Figure 75–1. The **fourth intercostal space at the anterior axillary line** can also be used (needle would be inserted above the fifth rib).

   2. **Emergency needle aspiration (pleural effusion)** (per American Heart Association Neonatal Resuscitation, seventh edition): Needle aspiration is done at the fifth and sixth intercostal space along the posterior axillary line. For needle aspiration, make sure the infant is supine to allow fluid to collect in the posterior position of the chest.

   3. **Chest tube placement (for air or fluid).** The chest tube should be at the **fourth or fifth intercostal space at the anterior axillary line in between the anterior axillary line and midaxillary line (modified Buelau position).** This site is safe for both thoracic sides, for both preterm and term infants, as only lung

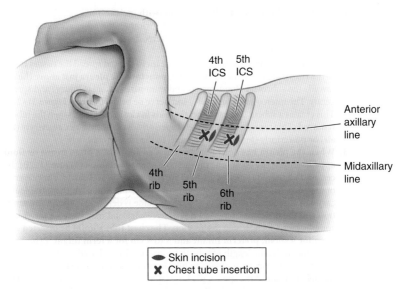

4th   5th
ICS   ICS

Anterior
axillary
line

Midaxillary
line

4th
rib   5th
         rib   6th
                  rib

◗━ Skin incision
✗ Chest tube insertion

FIGURE 31–1. Recommended site for skin incision and chest tube insertion in the neonate: fourth and fifth intercostal space between the anterior and midaxillary line. ICS, intercostal space.

parenchyma and no organ structures are found. See Figure 31–1. This lateral site avoids a scar on the anterior chest and nipple area.

    a. Air. Insert the tube anteriorly (upward) and toward the apex.

    b. Fluid. Insert the tube posteriorly (downward) and inferiorly.

  4. The nipple is a landmark for the fourth intercostal space. *Do not place the tube in the nipple area or surrounding breast tissue* (especially in females, as this can cause future asymmetrical breast tissue development.) Avoid the midclavicular approach in females.

G. Put on a sterile gown, mask, hat, and gloves. Cleanse the area of insertion with antiseptic solution, and drape appropriately.

H. Prophylactic antibiotics for newborn infants with chest tubes. Because chest tubes breach the skin barrier, there is a risk of infection. Some neonatologists use preventive antibiotics. Cochrane review states: "There is no data from randomized trials to either support or refute the use of antibiotic prophylaxis for intercostal catheter insertion in neonates."

I. Pain management. There are no prospective studies on pain management for chest tube insertion. The American Academy of Pediatrics (AAP) recommends routine pain management during chest tube insertion.

  1. The American Academy of Pediatrics recommends slow infiltration of the area with a local anesthetic before incision (unless life-threatening instability) and the use of systemic analgesia with a rapidly acting opiate (fentanyl). If there is not enough time to infiltrate before the chest tube is inserted, infiltration should be done after the chest tube is in (may decrease later pain responses).

    a. Local anesthetic. Slowly infiltrate the area superficially with 0.125 to 0.25 mL of 1% lidocaine and then down to the rib. Infiltrate into the intercostal muscles and along the parietal pleura. Do not use more than 0.5 mL of 1% lidocaine.

    b. Systemic analgesia with a rapidly acting opiate (fentanyl).

    c. General nonpharmacologic measures should also be used.

J. **Standard (traditional) chest tube insertion (with incision)**
1. **Make a small incision** (approximately the width of the tube, usually 3–4 mm) in the skin over the rib just below the intercostal space where the tube is to be inserted (see Figure 31–1).
2. **Insert a closed curved hemostat into the incision,** and spread the tissues down to the rib. Using the tip of the hemostat, **puncture the pleura just above the rib** (avoids the subcostal blood vessels and minimizes vascular injury) and spread gently. The intercostal vein, artery, and nerve lie below the ribs (Figure 31–2A). This creates a subcutaneous tunnel that aids in closing the tract when the tube is removed. This tunnel can be carried superiorly over the next rib, anteriorly (for air) or posteriorly (for effusion) parallel to the ribs, or obliquely.
3. **When the pleura has been penetrated, a rush of air is often heard or fluid appears.** Insert the chest tube through the opened hemostat (Figure 31–2B). Be certain that the side holes of the tube are within the pleural cavity. The presence of moisture in the tube usually confirms proper placement in the intrapleural cavity in a pneumothorax. Use of a trocar guide is dependent upon the institution and the operator. Some feel it is unnecessary and may increase the risk of complications such as lung perforation. **The chest tube should be inserted 2 to 3 cm for a small, preterm infant and 3 to 4 cm for a term infant.** (These are guidelines only; the length of tube to be inserted varies based on the size of the infant.) An alternative approach to tube insertion is to measure the length from the insertion site to the apex of the lung (approximately the mid clavicle) and tie a silk suture around the tube the same distance from the tip. Position the tube until the silk suture is just outside the skin.

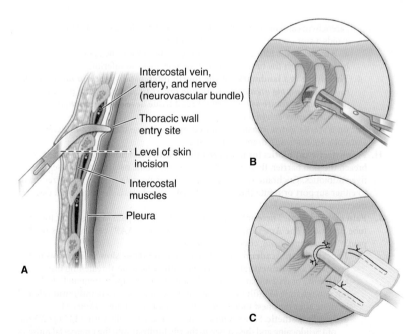

FIGURE 31–2. Standard chest tube insertion. (**A**) Level of skin incision and thoracic wall entry site in relation to the rib and the neurovascular bundle. (**B**) Opened hemostat, through which the chest tube is inserted. (**C**) The chest tube is then secured to the skin with silk sutures.

    4. **Hold the tube steady first,** and then allow an assistant to connect the tube to a water seal vacuum drainage system (eg, Pleur-Evac system). Five to 10 cm of suction is usually used. Start at the lower level of suction and increase as needed if the pneumothorax or effusion does not resolve. Some recommend starting at 10 cm and increasing 20 cm, if necessary. Excessive suction can draw tissue into the side holes of the tube. Systems such as the Pleur-Evac provide both continuous suction and a water seal. A water seal prevents air from being drawn back into the pleural space.

    5. **Secure the chest tube** with 3–0 silk sutures and silk tape (Figure 31–2C). Close the skin opening with sutures, if necessary. Use a purse-string suture around the tube or a single interrupted suture on either side of the tube.

    6. **Obtain an immediate chest radiograph (anteroposterior and lateral) to verify placement** and check for residual fluid or pneumothorax. One can also use transillumination to document success of air removal. Figure 31–3 shows a standard chest tube in position.

    7. **Place a sterile clear occlusive dressing at the site.**

K. Percutaneous chest tube placement (modified Seldinger technique using a pigtail [Fuhrman] catheter). Pigtail catheters are a safe and effective alternative to traditional chest tubes. Advantages include speed and ease of placement, safety (fewer complications), less discomfort, and easily learned. **This is the preferred chest tube placement in premature infants.** The catheter is a coiled, single-lumen polyurethane catheter (5–12F), with 8- or 10F being commonly used.

    1. **Follow the site and anesthetic selections as noted earlier.**

    2. **Insert an 18-gauge needle with the syringe attached** (or an 18-gauge intravenous [IV] catheter) into the skin over the top of the rib at the designated site into the pleural space. Pull back on the syringe while inserting the needle. Do not advance >2 cm in depth. Stop insertion when air or fluid is obtained.

    3. **Secure the needle and remove the syringe; keep the lumen occluded.** If an 18-gauge IV catheter is used, the IV catheter will act as the introducing needle.

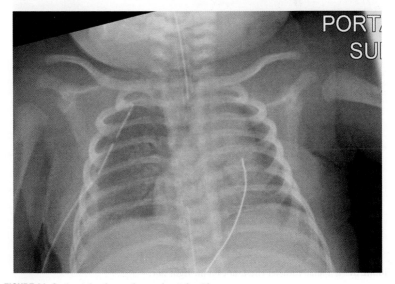

FIGURE 31–3. Straight chest tube on the right side.

4. **Straighten the J tip of the guidewire and insert into the hub of the needle or the intravenous catheter.** Advance the guide wire into the needle about 2 to 3 cm past the tip of the needle or until the colored line on the wire is at the level of the hub.

5. **Withdraw the needle or intravenous catheter while holding the guidewire.**

6. **Thread the dilator down over the guidewire.** Twist the dilator to dilate the skin, muscles, and pleura. The site has to be well dilated so the catheter will fit. Once dilated, remove the dilator while securing the guidewire.

7. **Straighten the pigtail catheter and insert over the guidewire.** Advance until all holes are inside the skin and pleural cavity and then 1 to 2 cm further.

8. **Slowly remove the guidewire while holding the tube in place.** The pigtail catheter will curl up inside the pleural cavity. Immediately connect the tube to the underwater sealed drainage (see Section III.J.4).

9. **Secure the tube using suture and tape and** place a sterile clear occlusive dressing at the site.

10. **Obtain an immediate chest radiograph (anteroposterior and lateral)** to verify placement and check for residual fluid or pneumothorax (see Section III.I.6). **One can also use transillumination to document success of air removal.** Figure 31–4 shows a pigtail catheter in position.

IV. **Chest tube removal**

A. **Pain management.** Removing a chest tube is known to be painful. **AAP recommends routine pain management during chest tube removal,** including general nonpharmacologic measures and a short-acting rapid-onset systemic analgesic.

B. **For pneumothorax.** If there is no more bubbling in the underwater seal or presence of air for 24 to 48 hours, discontinue the suction and leave to water seal for 4 to 12 hours (some units will leave it for 24 hours). Transilluminate, or preferably check an x-ray. If there is no air on x-ray or transillumination, it is okay to remove the chest tube. *Never* clamp a chest tube (tension pneumothorax risk).

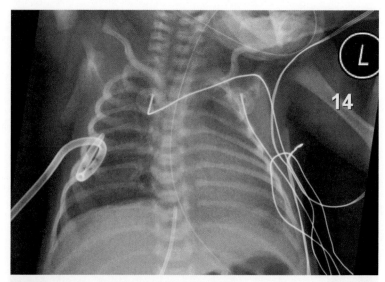

FIGURE 31–4. Pigtail catheter chest tube on the right side.

C. **Clean the skin area around the chest tube with an antiseptic solution.** Remove any tape or sutures but leave the wound suture. Cover entry site with gauze and your fingertips to prevent air from entering the chest as the tube is withdrawn, and then cover with petroleum gauze. Keep pressure on it. Cover with gauze and remove sutures when healed.

D. **Clinical signs and symptoms of respiratory distress** will identify almost all patients with significant pneumothoraces following chest tube removal. Monitor for tachypnea, dyspnea, increasing oxygen requirement, hypotension, or worsening arterial blood gas. Transillumination and chest x-ray may be necessary.

V. **Complications**

A. **Infection.** Strict sterile technique minimizes infections. Cellulitis is common. Intrapleural inoculation of *Candida* has been reported after chest tube placement. Many institutions recommend prophylactic antibiotics (eg, nafcillin) when a chest tube is placed (***controversial***). Empyema requires antibiotics and drainage.

B. **Bleeding.** May occur if a major vessel (intercostal, axillary, pulmonary, or internal mammary) or the myocardium is perforated or if the lung is damaged during the procedure. It can cause a hematoma or hemothorax. This complication can be avoided if landmarks are properly identified. Bleeding is less likely if a trocar is not used. Bleeding may stop during suctioning; however, if significant bleeding continues, immediate surgical consultation is necessary. Bleeding can be more significant with a coagulopathy.

C. **Nerve damage.** Passing the tube over the top of the rib helps avoid injury to the intercostal nerve running under the rib. Horner syndrome, diaphragmatic paralysis, or eventration from **phrenic nerve injury** has been reported. The medial end of the chest tube should be no less than 1 cm from the spine on frontal chest radiograph (phrenic nerve paralysis is related to the abnormal location of the medial end of the chest tube).

D. **Trauma.** The premature lung is at a greater risk of trauma because the chest wall is thin and the lung tissue is fragile. Lung trauma (perforation or laceration) can be minimized by never forcing the tube into position. Trauma can also occur to the breast tissue. Iatrogenic tracheobronchial perforation (tube through esophagus, carina, or right main bronchus) and tracheoesophageal fistula have been reported.

E. **Subcutaneous emphysema.** Secondary to a leak through the pleural opening.

F. **Chylothorax.** Results if the catheter causes trauma to the thoracic duct. It is best to avoid penetration into the posterior superior mediastinum.

G. **Cardiac tamponade.** See Chapter 41.

H. **Fluid and electrolyte imbalance/hypoproteinemia.** Secondary to significant pleural fluid output.

I. **Rare complications.** Myocardial perforation, severing the phrenic nerve, subclavian vessel tear with blood loss, thymic trauma with blood loss, trauma to the liver with hemoperitoneum, traumatic arteriovenous fistula, aortic obstruction, compression of the aorta, and displacement of the trachea can all occur.

J. **Complications from percutaneous thoracostomy (pigtail catheter).** Percutaneous thoracostomy with pigtail catheters has always been felt to be safer with less complications than straight chest tubes. Recent reviews from autopsy cases suggest that complications from pigtail catheters are more prevalent than previously believed. These complications may be from tubing that is too long. The pigtail catheters enter structures outside of the pleural cavity. These include lung perforation (usually upper), pleural effusion, and tube entering and wrapping around cardiac and mediastinal structures.

32 Defibrillation and Cardioversion

Defibrillation and cardioversion are procedures that involve giving a controlled electrical shock to the heart through the chest wall and are used for rapid termination of a tachyarrhythmia (a fast, abnormal rhythm originating either in the atrium or ventricle) that is unresponsive to baseline treatment or is causing the patient to have cardiovascular compromise (inadequate systemic perfusion). Baseline treatment consists of correcting metabolic problems, use of vagal maneuvers which work by stimulating the vagal tone that slows the heart rate (eg, diving reflex, bag filled with ice and cold water applied on the whole face for 15–30 seconds without obstructing the airway, rectal stimulation using a thermometer, bending legs and bringing the knees to the chest for 15–30 seconds), use of medications (adenosine, digoxin, propranolol, verapamil, amiodarone, procainamide, lidocaine, or magnesium sulfate), or transesophageal pacing. It is best to try these maneuvers or medical therapy if intravenous access is available. **Neonatal arrhythmias are rare, and the majority can be treated with these initial measures.**

Current defibrillators can deliver 2 modes of shock: synchronized and unsynchronized. **Synchronized shocks are lower dose and used for cardioversion. Unsynchronized shocks are higher dose and used for defibrillation. Pediatric cardiology consultation is recommended for all infants with a tachyarrhythmia.**

I. Indications
  A. **Cardioversion (synchronized delivery of energy [shock] during the QRS complex)**
    1. **Unstable patients** with tachyarrhythmias who have a perfusing rhythm but evidence of poor perfusion, heart failure, or hypotension (signs of cardiovascular compromise). Tachyarrhythmias appropriate for cardioversion include:
      a. **Supraventricular tachycardia or ventricular tachycardia** with a pulse and poor perfusion.
      b. **Supraventricular tachycardia with shock** and no vascular access.
      c. **Atrial flutter with shock.**
      d. **Atrial fibrillation with shock** (very rare in infants).
    2. **Elective cardioversion** in infants with **stable supraventricular tachycardia (SVT), ventricular tachycardia (VT), or atrial flutter** (good tissue perfusion and pulses) unresponsive to other treatments. This is always done under the close supervision of a pediatric cardiologist. Sedation and a 12-lead electrocardiogram are recommended before cardioversion.
  B. **Defibrillation (asynchronized, random delivery of energy [shock] during the cardiac cycle).** Used in pulseless arrest with a shockable rhythm (VT and ventricular fibrillation) and in between cardiopulmonary resuscitation (CPR) but **not in asystole or pulseless electrical activity (PEA).** The most common cause of a ventricular arrhythmia in a neonate is electrolyte imbalance. Defibrillation will not stop the arrhythmia in these patients. **Defibrillation is recommended and is the most effective treatment for documented ventricular fibrillation and pulseless ventricular tachycardia.**
II. Equipment
  A. **Manual external defibrillator, (where the operator preselects the energy to be used); two paddle electrodes of the correct sizes, and conductive gel pads.** For infants, use the smallest size of paddle (usually measuring 4.5 cm) or hands-free, multifunction, self-adhesive electrode pads (SAEP) can be used instead of paddles for cardioversion, defibrillation, and monitoring. It is important to be familiar with your institution's equipment because there are many different types and models. Pediatric-capable automated external defibrillators (AEDS) (adult automated external defibrillators with pediatric attenuated pads are recommended for children ages 1 to 8 years but may be used in infants <1 year of age if a manual external defibrillator (preferred) is not available.

B. **Other equipment.** Heart rate monitor, airway equipment, resuscitation medications, antiarrhythmic medications, and equipment used in basic and advanced life support.

III. **Procedure**

A. **Preoxygenation and continuous heart monitoring are essential.** Emergency airway equipment should be readily available.

B. **Adequate systemic sedation and pain management (may not be possible in emergency situations).** During an emergency cardiac event, pain relief is not a focus. Depending on the type of procedure, sedation may be considered.

1. **Planned cardioversion.** Use propofol (short acting; side effects are rare). Induction dosing: 2.5 to 3.5 mg/kg over 20 to 30 seconds, then 200 to 300 mcg/kg/min.

2. **Emergent cardioversion.** These patients are usually too unstable to wait for appropriate sedation. It is best to proceed with cardioversion without sedation.

3. **Defibrillation.** These patients are unconscious and thus do not require sedation.

C. **Wipe any cream or soap off the chest.**

D. **Place the electroconductive pads firmly on dry clean skin of the chest wall.** To prevent skin burns, be sure the conductive pad totally covers the paddle and that the skin is not in contact with any noninsulated part of the paddle. The pads must not touch each other, at least one inch is required between electrodes for safe use. If the pads are in contact with each other, this can cause the electric current to arch across the chest instead of toward the heart. Alternatively, self-adhesive electrode pads can be used in place of the paddles. If pediatric pads are too large for the neonate, hand-held paddles may need to be used as pediatric pads should not be folded, crushed, or bent. There are 2 different positions for pad placement.

1. **Anterolateral positioning (Figure 32–1).** The anterior pad is placed to the right of the upper sternum, and the posterior pad is placed below the left nipple toward the axilla.

2. **Antero-posterior positioning (Figure 32–2).** This may be preferred in atrial tachycardia. The anterior pad is placed on the midsternal border, and the posterior pad is placed between the scapulae. The paddles or pads should not be in contact with one another. **With dextrocardia, the pads need to be placed across the right chest.**

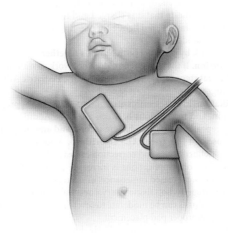

FIGURE 32–1. Location for anterolateral pad or paddle placement.

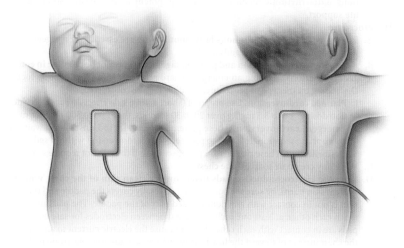

FIGURE 32–2. Anteroposterior pad or paddle placement.

    E. **Charge the defibrillator**
        1. **Cardioversion uses lower energy.** Charge the defibrillator to **0.5-1.0 J/kg** (initial charge) and synchronize. The SYNC button must be activated each time because the default setting on a defibrillator is on the asynchronized setting.
        2. **Defibrillation uses higher energy.** Charge the defibrillator to **2 J/kg** (initial charge).
        3. **Once charged, make sure everybody is clear of the patient, including the person holding the oxygen.** Ask if everyone is clear, and visually check while they answer. Use the accepted phrase, **"I'm clear, you're clear, oxygen clear."** Verify that oxygen is not flowing across the area. It is best to disconnect the bag and verify that no one is touching the endotracheal tube or any part of the ventilation circuit. The machine will indicate that it is charged and ready for discharge with an audible signal and/or a flashing red light either on the machine or the end of the paddle based on the model.
    F. **Deliver the shock by pressing both buttons together**
        1. **Cardioversion.** If the first attempt does not work, additional attempts should be made. **Repeat steps C to E using 2 J/kg per the Pediatric Advanced Life Support (PALS) algorithm.**
        2. **Defibrillation.** In pulseless infants, continue CPR with appropriate compressions, ventilation, and medications between attempts. Additional attempts should be made by repeating steps C to E. **The second and any subsequent shocks should have a dose of 4 J/kg (per PALS algorithm).** Acidosis and hypoxia decrease the success of defibrillation, and correction increases the likelihood of success.
IV. Complications. Risk of complications is increased when there is an increased energy dose, multiple shocks, increased impedance, or decreased interval between shocks.
    A. **Altered skin integrity.** Soft tissue injury, chest wall lesions, skin burns, bruising, and pain can occur. Burns can be moderate to severe in 20% to 25% of patients. They are usually due to improper pad placement.
    B. **Pulmonary edema** (rare). It is most likely due to left ventricular dysfunction, but true mechanism is unknown.

C. **Neurologic impairment.** This can occur from a stroke from a thromboembolic event after cardioversion, most often when cardioverting atrial flutter or atrial fibrillation. A preelective cardioversion echocardiogram to evaluate for atrial clots could aid in determining whether the patient is at risk for an embolic event.

D. **Cardiac arrhythmias.** Dysrhythmias due to enhanced automaticity, such as digitalis toxicity or catecholamine-induced arrhythmias, have an increased risk of VT or ventricular fibrillation with shock. Premature beats can occur. Ventricular fibrillation can also occur with poor synchronization of the shock administration.

E. **Myocardial necrosis.** When excessive energy is delivered, heart tissue can be damaged. This can cause necrosis with elevated ST segments seen on electrocardiogram. If myocardial damage is severe enough, this can cause shock.

F. **Cardiogenic shock.** Patients can develop transient decreased cardiac output with left ventricular diastolic dysfunction and damage of the myocardium after cardioversion or defibrillation.

G. **Fire (rare).** Fire has resulted from sparks with flammable material (eg, oxygen). Most reports involve the use of older paddles. If using older paddles, make sure there is good contact with the body surface and no other metallic surfaces are near the paddles. If the infant is on oxygen, place the oxygen source at least 1 meter away from the patient before defibrillation.

H. **Electrical shock to healthcare providers.** This can result in tingling, minor burns, or transient lethargy.

33 Endotracheal Intubation and Extubation

I. **Indications**
   A. **Provide mechanical respiratory support.**
   B. **Administration of surfactant.**
   C. **Management of apnea.**
   D. **Alleviate upper airway obstruction (subglottic stenosis).**
   E. **Assist in the management of congenital diaphragmatic hernia** to avoid bowel distention.
   F. **Administer medications** (see Section III.R.) in the emergency setting.
   G. **Obtain aspirates for culture.**
   H. **Assist in bronchopulmonary hygiene** ("pulmonary toilet").
   I. **Selective bronchial ventilation.**

II. **Equipment.** Correct endotracheal tube (ETT) (Table 33–1), a pediatric laryngoscope handle with a Miller blade ("No. 00" blade for extremely preterm infants, "No. 0" blade for preterm infants, "No. 1" blade for term infants), an ETT adapter, a suction apparatus, suction catheters, tape, scissors, tincture of benzoin, a malleable stylet (*optional*), personal protection equipment, a stethoscope, bag-and-mask apparatus, humidified oxygen/air source and blender, and pressure manometer should be available at the bedside. A colorimetric device or capnograph should be available to confirm the position of the tube. The mechanical ventilator set up should be ready. Cardiorespiratory monitoring is essential if not an emergent intubation.

III. **Procedure**
   A. **Orotracheal versus nasotracheal intubation**
      1. **Orotracheal intubation.** More commonly performed emergently and is described here. It is easier and quicker than nasotracheal intubation.

Table 33–1. GUIDELINES FOR ENDOTRACHEAL TUBE (ETT) SIZE AND SUCTION CATHETER SIZE BASED ON WEIGHT AND GESTATIONAL AGE

Weight (g)	Gestational Age (wks)	ETT Size, Inside Diameter (mm)	Suction Catheter Size (based on inner diameter of ETT)
<1000	<28	2.5	5–6F
1000–2000	28–34	3.0	6–8F
>2000	>34	3.5	8F

Data from American Academy of Pediatrics, American Heart Association, Weiner GM, et al: *Textbook of Neonatal Resuscitation*, 7th ed. Chicago, IL: American Heart Association and American Academy of Pediatrics Chicago; 2016.

2. **Nasotracheal intubation.** More commonly performed in the elective setting or if anatomy precludes the oral route. Nasotracheal intubation can be used in overly active infants or in those infants who have copious secretions. It offers tube stability but can be associated with an increase in postextubation atelectasis and a risk of nasal damage. In nasotracheal intubation, the procedure is similar except the lubricated nasotracheal tube is passed into the nostril and then pharynx and into cords following to the back of the throat. Small doses of intranasal 2% lidocaine gel can be used. Postextubation atelectasis maybe more frequent after nasal intubation, but one route of intubation does not seem to be preferable over the other.

B. **Video laryngoscopy.** A newer technique that uses a video laryngoscope (eg, GlideScope AVL Preterm/Small Child Video Laryngoscope; Verathon) to assist in the placement of the ETT. There is a high-resolution micro camera mounted on the blade that is connected to a small portable digital monitor. It is a form of indirect laryngoscopy that allows enhanced visualization of the glottis. It has also been used in teaching neonatal trainees with improvement in intubation success rates. A Cochrane review (2015) notes there was insufficient evidence to recommend or refute the use of video laryngoscopy for endotracheal intubation in neonates.

C. **Pain/premedication**

1. **Premedication is not necessary** for an emergency intubation in the delivery room or after an acute deterioration in a neonatal intensive care unit. It is also not necessary in some cases of infants with upper airway anomalies (such as Pierre Robin sequence) or in infants in whom the instrumentation of the airway is presumed to be extremely difficult.

2. **If intravenous access is not available,** the intramuscular route should be considered for premedications.

3. **Premedication can decrease pain and discomfort of a nonemergent intubation. Practical evidence suggests that it may also improve intubation success, decrease the time it takes to intubate, and prevent some of the complications.** Neonates who undergo "awake intubation" without premedication have the following physiologic responses: systemic hypertension, bradycardia, hypoxemia, and increased intracranial pressure. Premedication for nonemergency intubation in the neonate is safer and more effective than when awake, but the ideal combination of premedication has not been established. No validated scoring systems to assess the level of sedation prior to intubation exist in the literature. Preferred medications have rapid onset and short duration of action. One preferred sequence is as follows:

a. **Administer oxygen** to maximize levels.

b. **Vagolytic agents prevent reflex bradycardia during intubation.** Atropine is the American Academy of Pediatrics (AAP) preferred vagolytic agent.

  c. **Analgesia agents decrease pain and discomfort during intubation.** Fentanyl is the AAP preferred agent. Other acceptable medications are remifentanil and morphine but only if no other option is feasible.

  d. **Sedative/hypnotic agents depress the activity of the brain.** The AAP does not list any preferred agents and notes that propofol and thiopental are acceptable hypnotic agents for preterm and term infants and that midazolam is the only acceptable sedative for term infants along with an analgesic agent.

  e. **Neuromuscular blocking agents (ie, muscle relaxants) block the transmission of neurotransmitters between neurons resulting in paralysis.** The AAP states that no ideal muscle relaxant exists. The preferred agent is vecuronium or rocuronium with succinylcholine and pancuronium also acceptable agents.

 4. **Because optimal protocols and medications have not been established,** each unit should adopt its own pain and premedication protocols. See Table 33–2 for a listing of elective intubation medications reviewed by the AAP. The AAP recommends to either give an analgesic or hypnotic medication and to consider vagolytic agents and rapid-onset paralytics. They recommend to not give a sedative or paralytic agent by itself. The Canadian Pediatric Society recommends the combination of atropine, fentanyl, and succinylcholine for premedication of intubation. Key premedication points:

  a. **Do not use a muscle relaxant** without an analgesic agent.

  b. **Analgesic or anesthetic dose of a hypnotic drug** should be given.

  c. **Vagolytic and muscle relaxants (rapid onset)** should also be considered.

 5. **Rapid sequence intubation.** Involves premedication prior to intubation with atropine, an analgesic, and a neuromuscular blocker. It is commonly used in the emergency department for rapid intubation. When rapid sequence intubation (RSI) is used in neonates, there is better visualization of the airway and no movement from the infant, and intubation is quicker with fewer attempts. One recommendation is atropine intravenous (IV) push (0.01–0.03 mg/kg, minimum dose 0.1 mg), fentanyl (2–3 mcg/kg per dose), and lastly vecuronium (0.1 mg/kg per dose). Further research is needed before definite recommendations can be made on using RSI in the neonate.

D. **Confirm that the laryngoscope light source is working** before beginning the procedure. Check to make sure the integrity of the equipment is okay (no loose laryngoscope parts).

E. **Stylets. A stylet is a malleable metal wire that is inserted into the endotracheal tube. Malleable stylets** are optional but may aid intubation and help guide the tube into position more efficiently (***controversial***). A Cochrane review (2017) suggests that use of a stylet during neonatal orotracheal intubation does not significantly improve success rates of neonatal trainees. However, only 1 brand of stylet and ETT have been tested, and therefore, the results cannot be generalized. **If using a stylet, place it in the ETT and be sure the tip of the stylet does not protrude out of the end of the ETT.** The stylet should be 1 to 2 cm proximal to the distal end of the ETT.

F. **Place the infant in the "sniffing position"** (the neck slightly extended); a small roll behind the neck may help with positioning. Hyperextension of the neck in infants may cause the trachea to collapse. It displaces the cords anteriorly and makes it difficult to pass the ETT. The infant's head should be at the same level as the operator.

G. **Cautiously suction the oropharynx** as needed to make the landmarks clearly visible. Routine suctioning is not recommended as excessive secretions were found to be rare in elective and premedicated intubations in neonates.

H. **Preoxygenate the infant with a bag-and-mask device,** and monitor the heart rate, color, and oxygen saturations. **To decrease hypoxia, limit each intubation attempt to <20 seconds before reoxygenation. Infants frequently deteriorate during an intubation attempt.**

I. **Hold the laryngoscope with your left hand.** Insert the scope into the right side of the mouth, and sweep the tongue to the left side. Some practitioners move the tongue

Table 33–2. PREMEDICATIONS FOR NONEMERGENCY INTUBATION

Drug	Route/Dose	Onset of Action	Duration of Action	Common Adverse Effects	Comments[a]
Analgesic					
Fentanyl	IV or IM[b]: 1–4 mcg/kg	IV, almost immediate; IM, 7–15 minutes	IV, 30–60 minutes; IM, 1–2 hours	Apnea, hypotension, CNS depression, chest wall rigidity	Preferred analgesic Effects reversible with naloxone Give slowly (preferably over 3–5 minutes, at least over 1–2 minutes) to avoid chest wall rigidity Chest wall rigidity can be treated with naloxone and muscle relaxants
Remifentanil	IV: 1–3 mcg/kg; may repeat in 2–3 minutes if needed	IV, almost immediate	IV, 3–10 minutes	Apnea, hypotension, CNS depression, chest wall rigidity	Acceptable analgesic Short duration of action and limited experience in neonates Effects reversible with naloxone Give slowly over 1–2 minutes to avoid chest wall rigidity Chest wall rigidity can be treated with naloxone and muscle relaxants Rapid administration
Morphine	IV or IM: 0.05–0.1 mg/kg	IV, 5–15 minutes; IM, 10–30 minutes	IV, 3–5 hours; IM, 3–5 hours	Apnea, hypotension, CNS depression	Acceptable analgesic agent Use only if other opioids are not available; if selected, must wait at least 5 minutes for onset of action Effects reversible with naloxone
Hypnotic/sedative					
Midazolam	IV or IM: 0.05–0.1 mg/kg	IV, 1–5 minutes; IM, within 5–15 minutes	IV, 20–30 minutes; IM, 1–6 hours	Apnea, hypotension, CNS depression	Acceptable sedative for use in term infants in combination with analgesic agents Hypotension more likely when used in combination with fentanyl Not recommended in premature infants Effects reversible with flumazenil

	Dose	Onset	Duration	Adverse effects	Comments
Thiopental	IV: 3–4 mg/kg	IV, 30–60 seconds	IV, 5–30 minutes	Histamine release, apnea, hypotension, bronchospasm	Acceptable hypnotic agent Hypotension more likely when used in combination with fentanyl and/or midazolam
Propofol	IV: 2.5 mg/kg	Within 30 seconds	3–10 minutes	Histamine release, apnea, hypotension, bronchospasm, bradycardia; often causes pain at injection site	Acceptable hypnotic agent Limited experience in newborns Neonatal dosing has not been well established
Muscle relaxant					
Pancuronium	IV: 0.05–0.10 mg/kg	1–3 minutes	40–60 minutes	Mild histamine release, hypotension, tachycardia, bronchospasm, excessive salivation	Acceptable muscle relaxant Relatively longer duration of action Effects reversible with atropine and neostigmine
Vecuronium	IV: 0.1 mg/kg	2–3 minutes	30–40 minutes	Mild histamine release, hypertension/hypotension, tachycardia, arrhythmias, bronchospasm	Preferred muscle relaxant Effects reversible with atropine and neostigmine
Rocuronium	IV: 0.6–1.2 mg/kg	1–2 minutes	20–30 minutes	Mild histamine release, hypertension/hypotension, tachycardia, arrhythmias, bronchospasm	Preferred muscle relaxant Effects reversible with atropine and neostigmine
Succinylcholine	IV: 1–2 mg/kg; IM[b]: 2 mg/kg	IV, 30–60 seconds; IM, 2–3 minutes	IV, 4–6 minutes; IM, 10–30 minutes	Hypertension, hypotension, tachycardia, arrhythmias, bronchospasm, hyperkalemia, myoglobinemia, malignant hyperthermia	Acceptable muscle relaxant Contraindicated in presence of hyperkalemia and family history of malignant hyperthermia

(Continued)

Table 33–2. PREMEDICATIONS FOR NONEMERGENCY INTUBATION (CONTINUED)

Drug	Route/Dose	Onset of Action	Duration of Action	Common Adverse Effects	Comments[a]
Vagolytic					
Atropine	IV or IM: 0.02 mg/kg	1–2 minutes	0.5–2 hours	Tachycardia, dry hot skin	Preferred vagolytic agent
Glycopyrrolate	IV: 4–10 mcg/kg	1–10 minutes	~6 hours	Tachycardia, arrhythmias, bronchospasm	Acceptable vagolytic agent Limited experience in newborns Contains benzyl alcohol as preservative

Note: Most of these drugs have limited pharmacokinetics data from newborns and are not approved for use in the newborn, but they have been used in newborns. Rapid administration of remifentanil provided inadequate sedation and is associated with chest wall rigidity in preterm infants.

CNS, central nervous system; IM, intramuscularly; IV, intravenously.

[a]Preferred and acceptable designation of medications is based on consensus opinion after review of available evidence.

[b]Consider only if no intravenous access.

Reproduced with permission from Kumar P, Denson SE, Mancuso TJ, et al: Premedication for nonemergency endotracheal intubation in the neonate, *Pediatrics.* 2010 Mar;125(3):608-615.

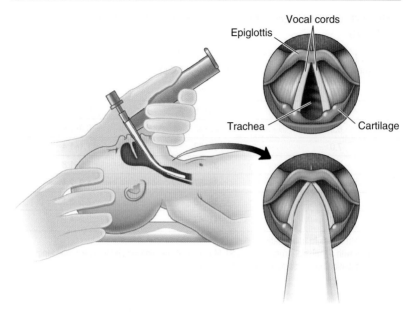

FIGURE 33–1. Endotracheal intubation in the neonate.

to the left by using the index finger of the right hand placed alongside the head. To perform this maneuver, stabilize the head and hold the mouth open. (**Do not use the laryngoscope blade to open the mouth**).

J. **Advance the blade a few millimeters,** passing it beneath the epiglottis.

K. **Lift the blade vertically to elevate the epiglottis** and visualize the glottis (Figure 33–1). *Note:* The purpose of the laryngoscope is to lift the epiglottis vertically, not to pry it open. To better visualize the vocal cords, an assistant may place gentle external pressure on the thyroid cartilage. If the cords are together, wait for them to open (never force a tube between closed cords). Do not touch the closed cords because this may cause spasm.

L. **Pass the endotracheal tube along the right side of the mouth** and down past the vocal cords during inspiration. Advance the tube *only* 2 to 2.5 cm into the trachea to avoid placement in the right mainstem bronchus (no more than 1–2 cm below the vocal cords). If a stylet was used, it should be removed gently while the tube is held in position.

M. **Multiple endotracheal tube depths of insertion methods have been described:**

1. **7-8-9 rule (Tochen rule)/(weight plus 6).** Most commonly used formula in one study. The depth of ETT insertion in centimeters ("tip to lip") is estimated as 6 plus the weight in kilograms. Tape the ETT at the lip when the tube has been advanced 7 cm in a 1-kg infant, 8 cm in a 2-kg infant, 9 cm in a 3-kg infant, or 10 cm in a 4-kg infant (**"1, 2, 3, 4 – 7, 8, 9, 10"**). Do not use this in infants <750 g (it overestimates the depth of insertion) or in infants with severe neck or orofacial deformities. Infants weighing <750 g may only require a 6-cm insertion (see Table 33–3). Interestingly Tochen's rule was not found to be suitable for neonates in Taiwan, as the final ideal ETT depth was shallower.

2. **Endotracheal tube length based on gestation-based guidelines.** (NRP recommended.) ETT length is more related to gestation in a linear manner than to birth-weight. Using gestation-based guidelines is associated with a decrease in uneven lung expansion and a decrease in the number of tubes that need to be repositioned.

Table 33–3. ENDOTRACHEAL TUBE (ETT) LENGTH BASED ON GESTATIONAL AGE–BASED GUIDELINES

ETT Length at Lips (cm; "tip to lip")	Gestational Age (wks)	Actual Weight[a] (kg)
5.5	23–24	0.5–0.6
6.0	25–26	0.7–0.8
6.5	27–29	0.9–1.0
7.0	30–32	1.1–1.4
7.5	33–34	1.5–1.8
8.0	35–37	1.9–2.4
8.5	38–40	2.5–3.1
9.0	41–43	3.2–4.2

[a]Actual weight is weight at intubation.
Reproduced with permission from Kempley ST, Moreiras JW, Petrone FL: Endotracheal tube length for neonatal intubation, *Resuscitation*. 2008 Jun;77(3):369-373.

Using gestational age or a weight-based chart outperformed the nasal tragus length (NTL) formula, described below, in a recent study. See Table 33–3.
3. **Nasal-tragus length and sternal length.** (NRP recommended.) One method that allows length assessment in approximately 10 seconds and does not require weight is the NTL (base of the nasal septum to the tragus of the ear); the other method is the sternal length (STL; suprasternal notch to the tip of the xiphoid process). The NTL method has been validated in both term and preterm infants.
   a. **Orotracheal route.** NTL or STL plus 1.
   b. **Nasotracheal route.** NTL or STL plus 2.
N. **Regardless of technique used, rapidly confirm the position of the tube immediately after insertion.** Detection of exhaled carbon dioxide plus clinical assessment (rapidly increasing heart rate) are considered the most primary initial methods of confirming the ETT is within the trachea. A Cochrane review (2014) states: "There is insufficient evidence to determine the most effective technique for the assessment of correct ETT placement either in the delivery room or the neonatal intensive care unit."
   1. **Auscultation.** The resuscitation bag or Neopuff Infant T-Piece Resuscitator (Fisher & Paykel Healthcare) is attached to the tube using the adapter, and an assistant provides mechanical breaths while the operator listens for equal breath sounds on both sides of the chest. Auscultate the stomach to be certain that the esophagus was not intubated. **Caution is necessary** because breath sounds heard over the anterior part of the chest can come from the stomach or esophagus. If correctly intubated, there should be an increase in heart rate and color. There should be vapor condensing on the inside of the tube during exhalation. Other clinical observations that the tube is in the trachea include no air entering over the stomach (no gastric distension), little or no air leak from the mouth, symmetrical and slight rise of chest movement with breathing, and equal bilateral breath sounds near both axillae.
   2. **External digital tracheal palpation of the suprasternal notch.** The suprasternal notch corresponds to the interclavicular midpoint on a chest x ray and midpoint of the trachea which approximates the correct ETT tube position. Suprasternal palpation is a simple and safe method of confirming ETT placement in neonates. During

ETT intubation, palpate the tip in the suprasternal notch with the index finger of the left hand while holding the tube with the right hand. One can adjust the tube so the edge is palpable in the notch. It was found to be as accurate as the 7-8-9 rule.

3. **Carbon dioxide detectors**

    a. **Colorimetric devices** change color in the presence of carbon dioxide (CO_2) and are the most commonly used devices. End-tidal CO_2 detectors connected to the ETT are commercially available that rapidly confirm proper endotracheal placement. One such device (Pedi-Cap CO_2 detector; Nellcor) displays violet in the absence of CO_2 and yellow in the presence of CO_2 (tube in trachea).

    b. **Capnographs** have a special electrode at the ETT connector, and a waveform shows oscillation with each breath if the tube is in the correct place. A flat wave usually means the ETT is in the esophagus but other clinical scenarios may also show this (ETT obstruction, prolonged cardiac arrest, technical malfunction of the monitor).

    c. **Limitations of endotracheal tube carbon dioxide detectors.** Recent studies have shown that end-tidal CO2 monitoring did not correctly identify ETT placement in up to 30% of cases in the delivery room. With some cyanotic congenital heart disease, they may underestimate the true arterial CO_2 level. If the cardiac output is low, the infant has a low heart rate, there is no heartbeat, the lungs are not adequately ventilated, the lungs are collapsed, there are secretions in the ETT or trachea that are causing an obstruction, or there are large bilateral pneumothoraces, the CO_2 monitor may not change color because not enough CO_2 is exhaled to detect. Any acidic substance (gastric acid, endotracheal epinephrine) can contaminate the colorimetric device and cause a false-positive result. If the detector is yellow in the package, it means it changed color in the package, is defective, and should not be used.

4. **Respiratory function monitor** (RFM) is a newer method used to detect the accurate position of ETT by measuring the airway pressure and gas flow in and out of the ETT. It can identify if the ETT is in the trachea by showing inspiratory as well as expiratory flow. Difficulties with this include operator experience in interpretation of flow signals and judging the depth of the ETT.

O. **Secure the endotracheal tube in place.** There are many ways to secure an ETT in a ventilated infant. Some of these include water-resistant tape, sutures, silk ties, ETT holders, head restraints, bonnets, umbilical cord clamps, or a combination of techniques. A Cochrane review (2014) indicates that "evidence is lacking to determine the most effective and safe method to stabilize the ETT in the ventilated neonate."

    1. **Paint the skin with tincture of benzoin, and tape the tube securely in place.**

    2. **Commercial devices** may be provided in your unit for securing an ETT without tape. Some examples include the NEO-fit tube grip (Cooper Surgical, Trumbull, CT), which eliminates the need for tape use and provides stabilization for ETT sizes 2.5 to 4.0 mm. The Neobar (Neotech, Valencia, CA) is another device.

P. **After the endotracheal tube is secured, obtain a chest radiograph with the infant's head in neutral position to confirm proper placement of the tube.** Figure 12–10 shows proper placement of a neonatal ETT. Some sources indicate that the ETT tip should be placed at the level of the body of the **first to second thoracic vertebra** and to not use the medial end of the clavicles (most common reference point) because their position may be variable. Others state that the ETT tip should be placed 2 cm above the carina. Thayyil et al found that infants who had a ETT tip lower than T1–T2 were more likely to have localized PIE, pneumothorax, and right upper lobe collapse. **Bedside ultrasound (POCUS) of the chest** (due to a cartilaginous sternum in newborns) allows one to directly visualize the ETT position in preterm and term infants and can be used to identify the ETT position. It can also be used for the rapid assessment of the ETT position (as quick as 17 seconds) using a US curvilinear probe. It is well tolerated but less studied in infants and children than in adults. It was found to be as accurate as capnography and a chest x ray. See Technique in Chapter 44.

Q. **Best position for newborns on assisted ventilation.** A Cochrane review (2016) states that the prone position is favored for slightly improved oxygenation in neonates undergoing mechanical ventilation.

R. **Certain emergency medications can be given through the endotracheal tube** if IV access is limited. These medications are *l*idocaine, *a*tropine, *n*aloxone, and *e*pinephrine. These can be remembered by the mnemonic **"LANE" or "NEAL."** **Epinephrine given by IV route is recommended as the most effective route, since absorption by the lungs is slow and unpredictable**; however, it can be given emergently by the ETT route while the vascular access is obtained. A higher dose of epinephrine (0.5–1 mL/kg of 1:10,000) is necessary even though studies have not validated the safety of this. There are no studies confirming that endotracheal naloxone is effective.

S. **Other drug therapy administered by endotracheal tube.** Efficacious inhaled drugs in infants include the following: **proven:** surfactant, nitric oxide; **unproven:** diuretics, bronchodilators, mucolytics; **more evidence needed:** inhaled corticosteroids, prostacyclin, budesonide with surfactant, colistin, heliox, pentoxifylline, superoxide dismutase, xenon.

IV. **Endotracheal extubation**

A. **The decision to remove an endotracheal tube is a complex clinical decision.** Issues surrounding ventilatory support are discussed in Chapter 9. When adequate ventilation is maintained with minimal settings, extubation should be attempted. Manage postextubation atelectasis intensively with chest physiotherapy.

B. **Use of medications prior to extubation**

1. **Dexamethasone use is *controversial*.**

a. **Stridor.** Some advocate systemic dexamethasone given before and after extubation to reduce the incidence of stridor. A Cochrane review (2009) states: "Using corticosteroids to prevent (or treat) stridor after extubation has not proven effective for neonates or children. However, given the consistent trends towards benefit, this intervention does merit further study, particularly for high risk children or neonates."

b. **Reintubation risk.** Dexamethasone IV given prior to extubation reduces the need for reintubation in high-risk neonates. A Cochrane review (2017) states that it is best to use in infants at risk (repeated and prolonged intubations) for airway edema and obstruction.

c. **Systemic corticosteroids.** Early corticosteroid therapy (first 2 weeks after birth) reduced the risk of bronchopulmonary dysplasia/chronic lung disease (BPD/CLD) and shortened the time to extubation. However, a Cochrane review (2017) notes that the benefits of early postnatal corticosteroid treatment (≤7 days), particularly dexamethasone, may not outweigh adverse effects associated with this treatment (gastrointestinal bleeding, intestinal perforation, hyperglycemia, hypertension, hypertrophic cardiomyopathy, and growth failure). Another Cochrane review (2017) states that late corticosteroids (after 7 days) for BPD/CLD reduced mortality without significantly increasing risk of adverse long-term neurodevelopmental outcomes, but there is still concern about the limitations of these studies. Therefore, late corticosteroid use should be reserved for infants who cannot be weaned from mechanical ventilation and to minimize the dose and duration of any course of treatment.

d. **Inhaled steroids.** In infants on invasive mechanical ventilation with birthweight ≤1500 g or gestational age ≤32 weeks, a Cochrane review (2017) suggests that there is no evidence that inhaled steroids compared to systemic steroids prevented the primary outcome of death or BPD. The number of days the baby needed mechanical ventilation support or additional oxygen were increased in infants who received inhaled steroids versus infants who received systemic steroids.

2. **Methylxanthines (caffeine)** used prophylactically increase the chance of successful extubation of preterm infants within 1 week of life. The caffeine group had lower rates of patent ductus arteriosus ligation, cerebral palsy, death, BPD/CLD, or major disability at 18 to 21 months. The majority of preterm infants are given caffeine before extubation and are maintained on this medication while on nasal continuous positive airway pressure (nCPAP) or nasal ventilation.

3. **Other medications.** A Cochrane review (2000) indicates: "The evidence does not support the routine use of doxapram to assist endotracheal extubation in preterm infants who are eligible for methylxanthine and/or CPAP [continuous positive airway pressure]." It also notes the following: "There is no evidence either supporting or refuting the use of inhaled nebulized racemic epinephrine in newborn infants."

C. **Extubation procedure**

1. **Perform chest physiotherapy and suction.**

2. **Remove tape and any devices** that are holding the ETT in place.

3. **Remove the tube.** It is best to use your own unit's recommendation on how and when to remove the tube. Recommendations vary:

   a. **Give positive-pressure inspiration** while slowly removing the tube.

   b. **Suction, give positive-pressure breaths,** and remove the ETT.

   c. **Using manual ventilation,** give the infant a sigh breath, and withdraw the tube during exhalation.

4. **Chest physiotherapy.** Some studies have found that fewer babies had to go back on ventilator support when chest physiotherapy was used after extubation, but these were older studies that did not use modern humidification systems. The use of physiotherapy in this setting is unclear.

D. **Other postextubation procedures.** Level of respiratory support varies and depends on the clinical status of the patient (see also Chapter 9). Possibilities include:

1. **Supplemental oxygen by hood or high-flow nasal cannula >3 to 6 L/min.** Limit flows in extremely low birthweight infants to <6 L/min (***controversial***). Cochrane review (2016) states that high-flow nasal cannula (HFNC) has similar rates of efficacy as other forms of noninvasive respiratory support in preterm infants for preventing treatment failure, death, and CLD. HFNC is also associated with less nasal trauma and potentially less pneumothorax compared with nCPAP. Further evaluation is needed for extremely preterm infants.

2. **Nasal continuous positive airway pressure.** A Cochrane review (2016) indicates that short binasal prongs are more effective than single prongs after weaning in reducing reintubation. nCPAP is used with a nasal interface such as nasal prongs (eg, Hudson type). Other forms of postextubation support are **bubble CPAP**, and **nasal biphasic positive airway pressure**.

3. **Nasal intermittent positive pressure is better than nasal continuous positive airway pressure** in preventing reintubation on extubated infants. Both nasal intermittent positive-pressure ventilation (NIPPV) and synchronized NIPPV (SNIPPV) seem to be equally effective.

E. **Observe for atelectasis.** If the infant has an increasing oxygen requirement and signs of respiratory distress, a chest radiograph should be obtained.

V. **Complications**

A. **Hypoxia, apnea, hypoventilation, and bradycardia can all occur during the intubation process.** This can be secondary to a prolonged attempt or vagal reflex.

B. **Hypopharyngeal or tracheal perforation/rupture and trauma.** Tracheal perforation is a rare complication requiring surgical intervention and is prevented by careful use of the laryngoscope and the ETT. Hemorrhage, edema of the larynx, and injury to the vocal cords can occur. Tracheal injury usually presents with rapid occurrence of subcutaneous emphysema, pneumomediastinum, and respiratory failure. Contusions of the gums, tongue, and airway can occur.

C. **Esophageal perforation.** Usually caused by traumatic intubation, and treatment depends on the degree of perforation. Most injuries can be managed conservatively by use of parenteral nutrition until the leak seals, use of broad-spectrum antibiotics, and observation for signs of infection. A barium swallow contrast study may be necessary after several weeks to evaluate healing and rule out stricture formation.

D. **Laryngeal edema.** Usually seen after extubation and may cause respiratory distress. A short course of steroids (eg, dexamethasone) can be given intravenously before and just after extubation.

E. **Improper tube positioning (esophageal intubation, right mainstem bronchus).** Signs of esophageal intubation include poor chest movement, no breath sounds heard, no condensation in the tube, continued cyanosis, gastric distension, and air heard over the stomach. Signs of right mainstem bronchus intubation include breath sounds heard over the right chest and none heard over the left and no improvement in color. ETT in right mainstem bronchus causes overventilation of the right lung and hypoventilation or atelectasis of the left lung. If the tube is in the right mainstem bronchus, it needs to be pulled back to the position where the breath sounds become equal on both sides of the chest.

F. **Tube obstruction or kinking.** Try suctioning or possibly reintubation.

G. **Infection.** Pneumonia and tracheobronchitis can occur.

H. **Palatal/alveolar grooves.** Palatal and alveolar grooves are usually seen in cases of long-term intubation and typically resolve with time.

I. **Subglottic stenosis.** Subglottic stenosis is most often associated with long-term (>3–4 weeks) endotracheal intubation. It is the most serious long-term complication and is secondary to posttraumatic fibrosis of the infant larynx. Surgical correction is usually necessary. With prolonged intubation, consideration may be given to surgical tracheostomy to help prevent stenosis (*timing is controversial*).

J. **Ingestion of the laryngoscope light bulb** (very rare complication reported during intubation).

K. **Other complications.** Aspiration, atelectasis, pneumothorax, increased intracranial pressure, and hypertension can all occur.

34 Exchange Transfusion

I. **Indications**

A. **Unconjugated hyperbilirubinemia.** Exchange transfusion (ET) is most commonly performed for infants with hyperbilirubinemia of any origin when the serum bilirubin level reaches or exceeds a level that puts the infant at risk for central nervous system toxicity (see Chapters 63 and 99). Double-volume ETs (DVETs) taking 50 to 70 minutes are usually recommended for removal and reduction of serum bilirubin. Efficiency of bilirubin removal is increased in slower paced exchanges to allow for time of extravascular and intravascular bilirubin equilibration. The American Academy of Pediatrics (AAP) has recommendations for indications of ET for unconjugated hyperbilirubinemia (see Figure 99–3).

B. **Hemolytic disease of the newborn** (HDN) results from destruction of fetal red blood cells (RBCs) by passively acquired maternal antibodies. ET aids in removing antibody-coated RBCs and replaces them with uncoated donor RBCs that lack sensitizing antigen, thereby prolonging intravascular RBC survival. It also reduces a potentially toxic bilirubin concentration, the result of the antibody destruction of RBCs. Intravenous immunoglobulin administration has been shown to decrease the need for ET in infants with hemolytic disease of the newborn caused by Rhesus (Rh) or ABO incompatibility and is recommended by the AAP if the total serum bilirubin level is rising with intensive phototherapy or within 2 to 3 mg/dL of the exchange level. Recent Cochrane review (2018) feels further studies are needed before recommending the use of IVIG for the treatment of alloimmune HDN.

C. **Severe anemia** (normovolemic or hypervolemic) causing congestive cardiac failure, as in hydrops fetalis, or chronic fetal–maternal or fetal–fetal posthemorrhagic anemia, which is best treated by partial ET (PET) using packed RBCs.

D. **Polycythemia/hyperviscosity syndrome** is best treated by PET using normal saline. Normal saline is preferred because it reduces both the polycythemia and the hyperviscosity of the infant's circulating blood volume. A Cochrane review (2010) states that "there are no proven clinically significant short or long term benefits of PET in polycythemic newborn infants who are clinically well or who have minor symptoms related to hyperviscosity. PET may increase the risk of NEC [necrotizing enterocolitis]. The true risks and benefits of PET are unclear."

E. **Other less common indications**
   1. **Metabolic disorders** causing severe acidosis or hyperammonemia (organic acidemia, hyperammonemia).
   2. **Extreme thrombocytosis**
   3. **Congenital leukemia.** ET is effective in improving hyperleukocytosis.
   4. **Neonatal sepsis.** Recent studies indicate that mortality rate was lower (36%) in infants with septic shock treated with ET than with standard of care treatment (51%). In infants <1000 g with severe sepsis, DVET was associated with a 21% decrease in mortality.
   5. **Malaria**
   6. **Neonatal hemochromatosis**
   7. **Severe fluid or electrolyte imbalance** (eg, hyperkalemia)
   8. **Renal failure**
   9. **Drug overdose/toxicity**
   10. **Removal of abnormal proteins or antibodies**

II. **Types of exchange transfusions**
   A. **Three types of ETs are commonly used: single-volume, double-volume, and partial exchange.**
      1. **Single-volume exchange blood transfusion** refers to replacing 1 times the estimated blood volume at 60% of infant's blood volume.
      2. **Double-volume exchange blood transfusion** refers to replacing 2 times the estimated blood volume at 85% of the infant's blood volume. Recommended for infants with severe hyperbilirubinemia and Rh hemolytic disease. Cochrane review states there is insufficient data to support or refute the use of single-volume exchange transfusion as opposed to double-volume exchange transfusion in jaundiced newborns.
      3. **Partial exchange transfusion** with normal saline is indicated in neonates with polycythemia to decrease the hematocrit and whole blood viscosity. A partial exchange with packed RBCs is used to treat severe anemia (usually associated with congestive cardiac failure.)
   B. **Two methods can be used for the exchange transfusion procedure:** isovolumetric method or push-pull method.
      1. **Isovolumetric double-volume exchange blood transfusion** is the simultaneous pulling of blood out of the umbilical artery or peripheral arterial line (usually radial arterial line) and pushing blood into the umbilical vein or peripheral intravenous (IV) catheter. It is indicated in sick and unstable neonates because of less fluctuation of blood pressure and cerebral hemodynamics and in cases where only peripheral vascular access is available. It is the **preferred method** and can be done automatically using infusion pumps.

2. **Push-pull method (classical "one-way" exchange transfusion).** This method uses the same vascular access (usually central access through the umbilical vein) to push in and pull out the volume of blood to be removed and transfused. Blood is withdrawn and then replaced with equal volume from the donor blood. If the infant is hypovolemic or has a low CVP, start with a transfusion of the donor blood; if the infant is hypervolemic or has a high CVP, start the exchange by withdrawing blood. This was the standard or traditional technique used and may cause fluctuations in blood volume and intravascular pressure.

III. **Equipment.** Radiant warming bed or hybrid incubator; infant restraints; equipment for cardiorespiratory monitoring, support, and resuscitation; immediate access to blood gas determinations; equipment for umbilical artery and umbilical vein catheterization (see Chapters 28 and 48) or equipment for peripheral venous and arterial access; nasogastric tube for evacuating the stomach before beginning the transfusion; preassembled disposable ET set or a nonassembled set with two 3-way stopcocks, 5- to 20-mL syringes, waste receptacle, IV connecting tubing, and appropriate blood product or fluid. A temperature-controlled device must be used for warming of the blood/fluid (37°C) before and during the transfusion. There must be an assistant whose role is to help maintain a sterile field, monitor and assess the infant, and record the procedure and exchanged volumes.

IV. **Choice of blood product for exchange transfusion**
   A. **Blood collection**
      1. **Homologous blood.** Blood donated by an anonymous donor with a compatible blood type is most commonly used. Donor-directed blood (blood donated by a selected blood type–compatible person) is another option.
      2. **Cytomegalovirus.** Seronegative donor blood is preferred. White blood cells harboring cytomegalovirus (CMV) can be removed using leukodepletion filters during blood preparation.
      3. **Hemoglobin S (sickle cell trait).** Precautions should be taken to avoid ET with donor blood from a carrier. If the donor blood with sickle trait becomes acidic, sickling can occur with expected complications to the patient.
      4. **Graft-versus-host disease.** Consideration should be given for using irradiated donor blood to avoid graft-versus-host disease in known immunocompromised infants and low birthweight infants. Preterm infants who have been transfused in utero or who have received >50 mL of transfused blood are candidates for irradiated blood.
   B. **Blood typing and cross-matching**
      1. **Infants with Rh incompatibility.** The blood must be type O, Rh-negative, low-titer anti-A, anti-B blood. It must be cross-matched with the mother's plasma and RBCs.
      2. **Infants with ABO incompatibility.** The blood must be type O, Rh-compatible (with the mother and the infant) or Rh-negative, low-titer anti-A, anti-B blood. It must be cross-matched with both the infant's and mother's blood.
      3. **Other blood group incompatibilities.** For other hemolytic diseases (eg, anti-Rhc, anti-Kell, anti-Duffy), blood must be cross-matched to the mother's blood to avoid offending antigens.
      4. **Hyperbilirubinemia, metabolic imbalance, or hemolysis not caused by isoimmune disorders.** The blood must be cross-matched against the infant's plasma and RBCs.
   C. **Freshness and preservation of blood.** Fresh blood (<24 hours old) is preferred, as older blood may have higher potassium values and lower pH. For newborn infants, it is preferable to use blood that has been collected in citrate phosphate dextrose (CPD). Use of irradiated blood is recommended to decrease graft-versus-host disease.
   D. **Hematocrit.** Most blood banks can reconstitute a unit of blood to a desired hematocrit (Hct) of 50% to 65%. The blood should be agitated periodically during the transfusion to maintain a constant Hct.

E. **Potassium levels in donor blood** should be determined if the infant is asphyxiated or in shock or renal impairment is suspected. If potassium levels are >7 mEq/L, consider using a unit of blood that has been collected more recently.

F. **Temperature of the blood.** Warming of blood (37°C) is especially important in low birthweight and sick newborn infants.

V. **Procedure**

A. **Double-volume exchange transfusion used for uncomplicated hyperbilirubinemia**

1. **The normal blood volume in a full-term newborn infant is 80 mL/kg.** In an infant weighing 2 kg, the volume would be 160 mL, and twice the volume of blood is exchanged in a 2-volume transfusion. Therefore, the amount of blood needed for a 2-kg infant would be 320 mL. Blood volume of low birthweight and extremely low birthweight newborns, which may be up to 95 mL/kg, should be taken into account when calculating exchange volumes.

2. **Allow adequate time for blood typing and cross-matching.** The infant's bilirubin level increases during this time, and this increase must be taken into account when ordering the blood.

3. **Perform the transfusion in an intensive care setting.** Place the infant in the supine position. Restraints must be snug but not tight. A nasogastric tube should be passed to evacuate the stomach and should be left in place to maintain gastric decompression and prevent regurgitation and aspiration of gastric juices. Feedings should be held for 2 to 3 hours prior to the procedure.

4. **Intensive phototherapy** should be continued as much as possible during the preparation and the ET procedure.

5. **Give albumin infusion (1 g/kg of 25% albumin) (*controversial*) 1 to 2 hours before the procedure.** Albumin causes a shift of extravascular bilirubin into the circulation so more bilirubin can be removed. Using albumin did not decrease the incidence of repeat ET. Studies are conflicting on whether this decreases phototherapy duration or bilirubin amount removed. A randomized controlled trial found that in healthy late preterm and term neonates with nonhemolytic hyperbilirubinemia, giving albumin did not reduce post-ET phototherapy duration or bilirubin amount removed.

6. **Scrub and put on a sterile gown and gloves.** Perform a procedure time-out.

7. **Perform umbilical vein catheterization** (see technique Chapter 48) and confirm the position by radiograph. If an isovolumetric exchange is to be performed, then an umbilical artery catheter (Chapter 28) must also be placed and confirmed by radiograph. Radiographs of catheter positions can be found in Chapter 12.

8. Alternatively, a peripheral IV can be used for infusion of blood and a peripheral arterial line for removal of blood.

9. **Have the unit of blood prepared.**

   a. **Check the blood types of the donor and the infant.**

   b. **Check the temperature of the blood and warming procedures.**

   c. **Check the hematocrit of the product.**

10. **Attach the bag of blood to the tubing and stopcocks according to the directions on the transfusion tray.** The orientation of the stopcocks for infusion and withdrawal must also be checked by the assistant as part of the procedure time-out.

11. **Establish the volume of each aliquot** (Table 34–1).

B. **Isovolumetric double-volume exchange transfusion.** Isovolumetric DVET is performed using a double setup, with infusion via the umbilical vein (or peripheral IV) and withdrawal via the umbilical artery (or peripheral arterial line). This method is preferred when volume shifts during simple exchange might cause or aggravate myocardial insufficiency (eg, hydrops fetalis). Two operators are needed; one to perform the infusion and the other to handle the withdrawal.

1. **Perform steps 1–6** as in a simple 2-volume ET. In addition, perform umbilical artery catheterization (Chapter 28) or peripheral arterial line insertion (Chapter 27). Confirm the blood product parameters (see step V.A.9 above).

Table 34–1. ALIQUOTS USUALLY USED IN NEONATAL EXCHANGE TRANSFUSION

Infant Weight	Aliquot (mL)
>3 kg	20
2–3 kg	15
1–2 kg	10
850 g–1 kg	5
<850 g	1–3

   2. **Attach the unit of blood to the tubing and stopcocks attached to the umbilical vein catheter or peripheral intravenous line.** The umbilical catheter may be left in place after the ET to monitor central venous pressure.
   3. **The tubing and the stopcocks of the second setup** are attached to the umbilical artery catheter and to a sterile plastic bag for discarding the exchanged blood.
   4. **If isovolumetric exchange is being performed because of cardiac failure,** the central venous pressure can be determined via the umbilical vein catheter placed in the inferior vena cava above the diaphragm.
  C. **Partial exchange transfusion** is performed in the same manner as DVET. If a partial exchange is for polycythemia (using normal saline) or for anemia (using packed RBCs), the following formulas can be used to determine the volume of the transfusion. (*Note:* Estimated blood volume is 80 mL/kg for term and 95 mL/kg for preterm.)
   1. **To calculate volume to exchange for polycythemia:**

$$\text{Volume of exchange (mL)} =$$

$$\frac{\text{Estimated blood volume (mL / kg)} \times \text{Weight (kg)} \times (\text{Observed Hct} - \text{Desired Hct})}{\text{Observed Hct}}$$

   2. **To calculate volume to exchange for anemia:**

$$\text{Volume of exchange (mL)} =$$

$$\frac{\text{Estimated blood volume (mL / kg)} \times \text{Weight (kg)} \times (\text{Desired Hct} - \text{Observed Hct})}{\text{Packed RBC Hct} - \text{Observed Hct}}$$

  D. **Isovolumetric partial exchange transfusion** with packed RBCs is the best procedure for severe hydrops fetalis.
  E. **Ancillary procedures**
   1. **Laboratory studies.** Blood should be obtained for laboratory studies before and after ET.
      a. **Blood chemistries:** Total calcium, sodium, potassium, chloride, pH, $PaCO_2$, acid-base status, bicarbonate, and serum glucose.
      b. **Hematologic studies:** Hct, platelet count, white blood cell count, and differential count. Blood for retyping and cross-matching after exchange is often requested by the blood bank to verify typing and re-cross-matching and for study of transfusion reaction, if needed.
   2. **Administration of calcium gluconate.** The CPD buffer in stored blood binds calcium and transiently lowers ionized calcium levels. Treatment of suspected hypocalcemia in patients receiving transfusions is **controversial.** Some physicians routinely administer 1 to 2 mL of 10% calcium gluconate by slow infusion

after 100 to 200 mL of exchange donor blood. Others maintain that this treatment has no therapeutic effect unless hypocalcemia is documented by electrocardiogram showing a change in the QT interval. Cochrane review states the following: "Due to very low quality of evidence available, it is difficult to support or reject the continual use of prophylactic intravenous calcium in newborn infants receiving exchange blood transfusion."

3. **Monitor serum bilirubin levels after transfusion at 2, 4, and 6 hours and then at 6-hour intervals.** A rebound of bilirubin level is expected 2 to 4 hours after the ET and is more common in hemolytic disease of the newborn as the breakdown of the remaining innate sensitized RBCs will continue.

4. **Re-medication.** Patients receiving antibiotics or anticonvulsants need to be re-medicated. Determination of drug levels after ET is advisable because the percentage of lost drug levels is variable.

5. **Antibiotic prophylaxis after the transfusion should be considered on an individual basis.** Infection is uncommon but is the most frequent complication.

6. **Delay feedings for at least 24 hours** after completion to observe the infant for the possibility of a post-ET ileus.

VI. **Complications. Mortality risk is approximately 0.5%.**

A. **Infection.** Bacteremia (usually caused by a *Staphylococcus* organism), hepatitis, CMV, malaria, and HIV have been reported.

B. **Vascular complications.** Clot or air embolism, vasospasm of the lower limbs, thrombosis, and infarction of major organs may occur. Portal vein thrombosis can occur.

C. **Cardiac arrhythmias,** arrest, and volume overload can occur.

D. **Coagulopathies** may result from thrombocytopenia or diminished coagulation factors. Platelets may decrease by >50% after a DVET. Disseminated intravascular coagulation and bleeding can occur.

E. **Electrolyte abnormalities.** Hyperkalemia, hypernatremia, hyperglycemia, hypercalcemia or hypocalcemia, and hypomagnesemia can occur. **Hypoglycemia** is especially likely in infants of diabetic mothers and in those with erythroblastosis fetalis because of islet cell hyperplasia and hyperinsulinism. Rebound hypoglycemia may result in these infants in response to the concentrated glucose (300 mg/dL) contained in CPD donor blood.

F. **Metabolic acidosis.** Metabolic acidosis from stored donor blood (secondary to the acid load) occurs less often in CPD blood.

G. **Metabolic alkalosis.** Metabolic alkalosis may occur as a result of delayed clearing of citrate preservative from the donated blood by the liver.

H. **Necrotizing enterocolitis.** An increased incidence of NEC after exchange transfusion has been reported. It is thought to occur from ischemic injury to the gastrointestinal tract possibly from larger aliquots of blood being used and how quickly the exchange of blood is. For this reason, the umbilical vein catheter should be removed after the procedure unless central venous pressure monitoring is required.

I. **Anemia or polycythemia can occur.**

J. **Feeding intolerance.**

K. **Mortality risk** is approximately 0.5%.

L. **Miscellaneous:** Hypothermia, hyperthermia, graft-versus-host disease, apnea and bradycardia, hypotension, hypertension.

35 Gastric and Postpyloric Tube Placement

Gastric tube placement involves placing a tube through the nose (nasogastric [NG]) or mouth (orogastric [OG]) into the stomach. In a **postpyloric (sometimes referred to as transpyloric) tube placement,** a tube is inserted through the nose or mouth through the pylorus into the small bowel (duodenum or jejunum).

GASTRIC TUBE PLACEMENT

I. **Indications**
   A. **To perform enteric feeding in the following situations:**
      1. **High respiratory rate.** Enteric feedings are used at some centers if the respiratory rate is >60 breaths/min to reduce the risk of aspiration pneumonia (*controversial*).
      2. **Nutritional support in premature infants** who may have immature sucking and swallow mechanisms that normally develop after 32 weeks.
      3. **Neurologic disease** that impairs the sucking reflex or the infant's ability to feed. An abnormal gag reflex is also an indication for a gastric tube.
      4. **Insufficient oral intake.**
   B. **Gastric decompression** in infants with necrotizing enterocolitis (NEC), bowel obstruction, congenital diaphragmatic hernia, intestinal malformations, or ileus.
   C. **Administration of medications.** Consult a pharmacist for medications that are administered into the stomach.
   D. **When a postpyloric tube is placed,** a gastric tube is needed to empty gastric contents and administer medications.
   E. **Analysis of gastric contents.**
II. **Equipment.** Infant feeding single-lumen tube (3.5 or 5F if <1000 g or 5–8F if ≥1000 g), dual-lumen vented Replogle tube for decompression (6, 8, or 10F; *Note:* tubes come with and without stylets; stylet use is **not recommended** in neonatal population), stethoscope, sterile water (to lubricate the tube), syringes (10–20 mL), 1/2-inch adhesive tape, benzoin, gloves, suctioning equipment, cardiac monitor, pulse oximeter, stethoscope, pH paper, and bag-and-mask ventilation with 100% oxygen (in case of emergency). Strongly recommended is a colorimetric device (eg, Kangaroo CO_2 Detector; Covidien, Mansfield, MA) or capnograph to help confirm the position of the tube by absence of carbon dioxide (CO_2) within the tube.
III. **Procedure**
   A. **Monitor heart rate and respiratory function throughout the procedure.** Place the infant in the supine position, with the head of the bed elevated. The infant can be swaddled to provide comfort.
   B. **There are several methods of estimating gastric tube insertion length:**
      1. **Orogastric tube insertion in very low birthweight infants.** Table 35–1 provides OG guidelines for infants <1500 g.
      2. **NEX method.** This method measures from the *n*ose to the *e*ar to the *x*iphoid (NEX) process. This method has been used for years but may misplace tubes, usually in the esophagus (up to 21%). This method is no longer recommended.
      3. **Age-related/height-based method.** In the age-related/height-based (ARHB) method, heights in age groups are used; this method requires multiple calculations that are time consuming and may lead to errors.
         a. **Less than 1 month of age: nasogastric only**
            i. **Nasogastric tube insertion length (cm)** = 1.950 cm + 0.372 × (infant's length in centimeters)

Table 35–1. GUIDELINES FOR MINIMUM OROGASTRIC TUBE INSERTION LENGTH TO PROVIDE ADEQUATE INTRAGASTRIC POSITIONING IN VERY LOW BIRTHWEIGHT INFANTS

Weight (g)	Insertion Length (cm)
<750	13
750–999	15
1000–1249	16
1250–1500	17

Data from Gallaher KJ, Cashwell S, Hall V, Lowe W, et al: Orogastric tube insertion length in very low birth weight infants, *J Perinatol*. 1993 Mar-Apr;13(2):128-131.

      b. Greater than 1 month of age (if >44.5 cm in length)
         i. Orogastric tube insertion distance = 13.3 cm + 0.19 × (infant's length in centimeters)
         ii. Nasogastric tube insertion distance = 14.8 cm + 0.19 × (infant's length in centimeters)
    4. Nose/ear/mid-umbilicus for nasogastric/orogastric tubes. In general, the nose/ear/mid-umbilicus (NEMU) method is considered to be the safest, most accurate, and most recommended method to use. Measure the distance from the tip of the nose (for nasogastric) or corner of the mouth (orogastric) to the bottom of the ear (earlobe) to the mid-umbilicus (distance halfway between the xiphoid process and umbilicus). This measurement, compared to measuring to the xiphoid process (NEX process) or umbilicus, has been shown to be the **most accurate.**
  C. Mark the length on the tube. Measure based on choice of the preceding calculations and lubricate the tube by moistening the end of the tube with sterile water. Note that smaller tubes (eg, 3.5F) clog easily.
  D. Pain management. Consider nonpharmacologic methods (see page 215).
  E. The tube can be placed in 1 of 2 insertion points, oral or nasal. There is controversy on whether the tubes should be placed orally or nasally. Nasal tubes are more secure and less prone to movement but may partially obstruct breathing. A Cochrane review (2013) states that there are insufficient data to support the use of one over the other in preterm or low birthweight infants.
    1. Many centers preferentially use nasogastric tubes because they do not limit breast or bottle feeds. Do not use nasal insertion with nasal trauma, recent esophageal surgery, choanal atresia, nasal prong continuous positive airway pressure, or significant respiratory distress. In these cases, the oral route is preferred.
    2. Nasal insertion. Avoid NG in very low birthweight infants because of increased incidence of respiratory compromise.
      a. Check nostrils for patency. Moisten end of tube with sterile water.
      b. Flex the neck, push the nose up, and insert the tube, directing it straight back (toward the occiput).
      c. Tilt head slightly forward. Advance the tube to the desired distance.
    3. Oral insertion is less traumatic and does not usually impact respiration. Push the tongue down with a tongue depressor and pass the tube into the oropharynx. Slowly advance the tube the desired distance. It is easier for the infant to dislodge and may limit breast and bottle feeding.
  F. Do not push against any resistance (perforation potential).
  G. Continue to observe the infant for respiratory distress and/or bradycardia. A brief period of coughing or gagging and a decrease in heart rate are considered normal. Stop procedure immediately until the patient appears unstable.

H. **Determine the location of the tube after placed and also before each use. Never instill materials into the tube until the position is verified.** The optimum position for a gastric tube is within the body of the stomach. Error rates for malposition are common and can range from 21% to 56%. If misplaced in the esophagus or lungs, the infant can have aspiration, apnea, bradycardia, and desaturations. If placed near the pyloric junction and duodenum, the infant can manifest diarrhea, poor weight gain, or malabsorption. See Figure 35–1 for algorithm for performing and verifying optimal placement of gastric enteral tubes.

1. **Radiologic verification** is considered the **gold standard** and is recommended at the time of initial tube placement or tube change. It should provide 100% accuracy in determining the location. *Note:* An abnormally positioned NG/OG feeding tube on a radiograph may suggest an underlying serious condition that needs to be ruled out.

2. **Point-of-care ultrasound for verification.** This method to confirm correct placement of the gastric tube has been used in adults. A small study in neonates showed it is not a reliable technique. Further studies are needed to confirm the efficacy of using POCUS in neonates to verify gastric tube positioning.

3. **Nonradiologic verification** can be done by the following methods. A recent study showed that for verification of tube placement, the most frequently used method was aspiration with inspection, followed by auscultation, assessment and verification of measurement marking, pH assessment, and, finally, radiographic study.

   a. **Measurement marking.** Because the tube is commonly marked at the nose (NG tube) or lip (OG tube), check to see if the marking has moved as a way of verifying the tube is in the correct place. Unfortunately, this method is prone to error because the tube can migrate or coil.

   b. **Auscultation** is not reliable as the only method to verify placement and should be used along with other assessment methods. While listening with the stethoscope over the stomach, inject 1 to 2 mL of air into the tube with a syringe and listen for a rush of air (swoosh sound) as the air enters the stomach (also known as the "whoosh test"). This may be unreliable because a rush of air can occur when the tip is in the distal esophagus and respiratory tract air can be heard by auscultation. It is difficult to distinguish from lung, esophageal, or abdominal sounds. This method is no longer recommended.

   c. **Visual inspection of the aspirate** has not been reliable when used alone because gastric contents can vary in color. It can be affected by the time of the last feeding. Respiratory and gastric aspirates may be similar in color; therefore, the result may be misinterpreted. If used with pH assessment, it may be more beneficial.

      i. **Normal gastric aspirate:** clear, tan, off white, pale yellow.
      ii. **Intestinal aspirate:** green, greenish brown, golden yellow, bile stained.
      iii. **Pleural space aspirate:** pale white or yellow
      iv. **Tracheal aspirate:** clear, tan, off white, straw colored.
      v. **Perforation of esophagus, stomach:** grossly bloody aspirate.

   d. **Capnography and capnometry.** Both use CO_2 detection technology to determine if the tube is in the respiratory tract or anywhere in the gastrointestinal (GI) tract (note that the exact location in GI tract not known).

      i. **Capnography** detects a CO_2 waveform that is emitted from the enteral tube. Absence of a CO_2 waveform suggests placement in the GI tract, and presence of a CO_2 waveform suggests placement in the trachea and distal airways.
      ii. **Capnometry** uses an end-tidal CO_2 detecting device that is attached to the end of the tube. If there is CO_2, a color change occurs, indicating the tube is placed incorrectly in the respiratory tract.

   e. **Gastric aspirate pH testing using pH paper or a pH meter** (pH paper is preferred and recommended (per National Patient Safety Agency) over litmus

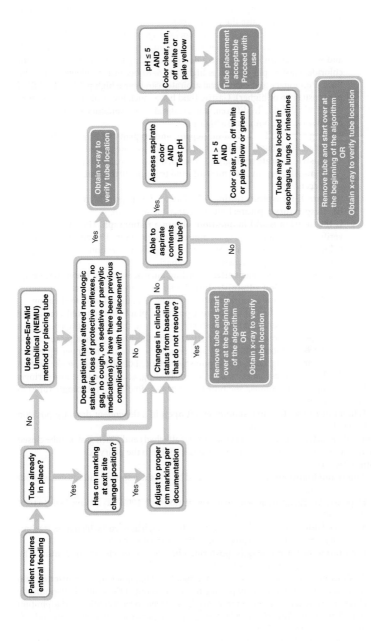

FIGURE 35–1. Algorithm for performing and verifying optimal placement of gastric enteral tubes. (*Adapted with permission from Clifford P, Heimall L, Brittingham L, et al: Following the Evidence Enteral Tube Placement and Verification in Neonates and Young Children, J Perinat Neonatal Nurs. 2015 Apr-Jun;29(2):149-161.*)

paper. Gastric fluid usually has a pH ≤5 to 5.55, and the intestine has a pH of ≥6. A pH aspirate <5 suggests gastric placement. If the pH is >6, then the placement of a gastric tube should be questioned. The mean values of pH may be affected by feeding status (pH of formula is 6.6 and pH of breast milk is 7–7.4), which may raise the pH, but studies found it was not statistically significant. Medications such as acid-blocking agents were not found to alter the pH aspirates. *Note:* Swallowed amniotic fluid may transiently raise gastric pH, and some preterm infants have a decreased ability to produce gastric hydrochloride. Gastric pH at birth is high (pH 6–8) because of alkaline amniotic fluid. Pulmonary and esophageal aspirates can have a high pH (tracheal fluid pH is usually 6 or higher). Gastric fluid has a much lower pH than respiratory or intestinal fluid. To differentiate intestinal and respiratory fluid, pH is less effective because both have a high pH.

  f. **Testing aspirate for bilirubin, pepsin, and trypsin** can help identify site of tube placement but is usually not practical for routine procedures.
     i. **Gastric aspirate testing:** bilirubin <5, high pepsin, low trypsin. A bilirubin <5 mg/dL, pepsin ≥100 mcg/mL, and trypsin ≤30 mcg/mL indicate gastric placement.
     ii. **Intestinal aspirate testing:** bilirubin >5, low pepsin, high trypsin.
     iii. **Respiratory aspirate:** little or no trypsin or pepsin.
  g. **If the location is still in question, obtain a radiograph.** However, this only verifies the location at the exact time of the radiograph. The tube tip should be below T12 for a gastric tube. See Figure 12–11, which demonstrates a nasogastric tube properly positioned in the stomach.
  4. **It is best to verify placement after insertion, once per shift, before each feeding, and with medication administration.** Some recommend radiography to verify placement if planning to initiate enteral feeding or administering medication.

  I. **Once the tube is verified in the correct position, place that marked area at the lip or nares.** Aspirate the gastric contents and secure the tube to the cheek with benzoin and 1/2-inch tape. Another effective method is to place a piece of tape on the upper lip ("moustache tape") and secure the tube on the upper lip with a small loop and taping again to the moustache tape. For NG tubes, make certain the tube does not press on the nasal ala. For feeding, attach the tube to a syringe. For decompression, connect the tube (preferably a dual-lumen **Replogle tube**) to low continuous suction.
  J. **When not in use, the tube should be left open** in a dependent drainage position below the level of the stomach.

IV. **Removal of gastric tube.** Disconnect suction (if attached) and pinch gastric tube closed when withdrawing the tube so contents will not spill into the pharynx.

V. **Complications**
   A. **Apnea and bradycardia.** Usually mediated by a vagal response and resolve without specific treatment.
   B. **Hypoxia.** Always have bag-and-mask ventilation with 100% oxygen available to treat this problem.
   C. **Misplaced tube.** Incorrect placement in trachea, esophagus, eustachian tube, trachea, or oropharynx. Twisting, coiling, or knotting of the tube can occur.
   D. **Perforation of the esophagus, posterior pharynx, stomach, or duodenum.** The tube should never be forced during insertion.
   E. **Aspiration.** If feeding has been initiated in a tube that is accidentally inserted into the lung or if the GI tract is not passing the feedings out of the stomach. Periodically check the residual volumes in the stomach to prevent overdistention and aspiration (see Chapter 59). Any NG or OG tube may increase gastroesophageal reflux and risk of aspiration pneumonia.
   F. **Nasopharyngeal complications.** Irritation, bleeding, infections. Grooved palate with prolonged OG placement.

POSTPYLORIC TUBE PLACEMENT

Postpyloric (transpyloric) tube placement requires a gastric tube for aspiration, drainage, and medication administration. A Cochrane review (2013) found that transpyloric tubes are not recommended in premature infants because there was no evidence of any benefit of transpyloric feeding in preterm infants, with increased adverse effects. Feedings with human milk via transpyloric tubes may reduce apnea and bradycardia in preterm infants with suspected gastroesophageal reflux.

I. **Indications**
   A. **Enteric feeding in the following conditions:**
      1. **Not tolerating gastric feeding** (eg, severe gastroesophageal reflux, persistent emesis).
      2. **Infants at risk for aspiration.**
      3. **Delayed gastric emptying and other motility disorders.**
      4. **Severe gastric distension.**
   B. **To test duodenal and jejunal contents**
   C. **Postoperative management of duodenal atresia**
II. **Equipment.** Weighted infant feeding tube (silastic tubes preferred with or without stylet; 6F <1500 g, 8F >1500 g), stethoscope, sterile water (to lubricate the tube), a syringe (20 mL), 1/2-inch adhesive tape, pH paper, continuous infusion pump and tubing, gloves, suctioning equipment, and bag-and-mask ventilation with 100% oxygen.
III. **Procedure**
   A. **Determine insertion length.** Measure using the ARHB or NEMU method noted for gastric intubation. Add the distance from the designated point to the right lateral costal margin. Mark the point on the tube with tape.
   B. **Follow initial steps for gastric intubation as noted on page 357.** Confirm the initial gastric position as previously described.
   C. **Metoclopramide has been previously recommended to assist placement of the postpyloric feeding tubes.** Based on reviews, it appears that metoclopramide enhances tube placement.
   D. **Place infant into a right lateral position.** With the patient on his or her right side, elevate the head of the bed 30 to 45 degrees. Distend the stomach by injecting 10 mL/kg of air into the gastric tube and close the tube.
   E. **Insert the tube (lubricated at the tip with sterile water) to the desired length.** Keep the infant in the right side down position for 1 to 2 hours to allow the weighted tube to migrate into the duodenum.
   F. **It is essential to place an orogastric/nasogastric tube,** as described earlier, for aspiration and medication delivery.
   G. **Check postpyloric tube placement and patency.**
      1. **The "snap test."** When air is aspirated, the plunger snaps right back to the tip of the syringe; if no air is aspirated, this means the tube is in the pylorus. Proper placement is characterized by high-pitched crackling sounds and the inability to withdraw air, but many providers consider this an unreliable test.
      2. **Checking the pH and color of the aspirate.** If pH >6 and the color of the aspirate is golden yellow, the tube is probably in the transpyloric position. To further confirm, **check bilirubin** level in the aspirate (a value >5 is seen if tube is in transpyloric position).
   H. **Confirm placement with a radiograph.** The tip of the tube should be just beyond the second portion of the duodenum. See Figure 12–12. **Aspirate contents** or initiate tube feeding. **Using bedside ultrasound** is a potential alternative to confirm placement of the transpyloric tube.
   I. **Flushing the tube with 3 mL of water after each use will limit tube obstruction.** Avoid flushing tubes with small-caliber syringes (1–5 mL) because they generate high pressure and may rupture tubing.
   J. **If long-term use is anticipated, consider changing the tube every 2 to 4 weeks or per manufacturer's recommendations.**

IV. **Removal of tube.** Discontinue the infusion, pinch off the tube, and withdraw slowly. Gastric tube can be left in place or removed as described earlier for gastric tubes.

V. **Complications.** These are similar to NG/OG tube placement, as noted earlier. Other complications may include:

A. **Inability to pass tube beyond pylorus.** Fluoroscopic guidance may be necessary.

B. **Aspiration.**

C. **Infection.** Local infection or sepsis can occur. Enterocolitis can occur secondary to *Staphylococcus* or NEC.

D. **Malabsorption.** Enteral feeds bypass the stomach, leading to fat malabsorption and increased frequency of bowel movements; in addition, some medications may not be absorbed.

E. **Rare complications.** Intussusception, pyloric stenosis, enterocutaneous fistula, methemoglobinemia in very premature infants from intestinal obstruction and inflammation induced by the transpyloric tube, pyloric stenosis, bronchopleural fistula, and pneumothorax.

36 Heelstick (Capillary Blood Sampling)

I. **Indications**

A. **Blood collection,** when only a small sample (1 drop to <1 mL) is needed or when there is difficulty obtaining samples by venipuncture of other sources.

1. **Common capillary blood studies:** Complete blood count (CBC), general chemistry labs, bedside glucose estimation, liver function tests, thyroid levels, bilirubin levels, toxicology/therapeutic drug levels, and newborn metabolic screening.

2. **The following laboratory tests are not recommended by capillary blood sampling:** Coagulation studies, chromosomal analyses, erythrocyte sedimentation rate, immunoglobulin titers, some other, more sophisticated tests, any tests that require a lot of blood.

B. **Capillary blood gas determination** gives satisfactory pH and PCO_2, but not PO_2.

C. **Blood cultures** when venous access or other access is not possible. Sterile technique is required, but heel stick is not the preferred method.

D. **Not recommended for blood sampling in term infants.** Most sources confirm that **venipuncture, not capillary blood sampling,** by a skilled operator is the method of choice for blood sampling in term neonates. Lower pain scores are seen with venipuncture in infants.

II. **Equipment.** Automated self-shielding lancets are preferred in neonates (full-term neonate: incision depth of 1 mm and length of 2.5 mm; preterm neonate: incision depth of 0.85 mm and length of 1.75 mm; see Table 36–1); sterile manual lancets are not recommended but may be used in some units (sizes: 2 mm for <1500 g and 4 mm for >1500 g); capillary collection tube (for rapid hematocrit and bilirubin tests) or appropriate microcollection tubes (if more blood is needed [eg, for chemistry determinations]), preheparinized capillary tubes for blood gas analysis, filter paper card for newborn screening (if appropriate), clay or caps to seal the capillary tube, a warm washcloth with a diaper or heel warming device (eg, a chemically activated packet), antiseptic solution/swabs (alcohol/chlorhexidine swabs); nonsterile or sterile gloves.

Table 36–1. SOME COMMONLY USED AUTOMATED SELF-SHIELDING LANCETS FOR SAMPLE COLLECTION IN NEWBORNS

Device	Infant	Characteristics
Tenderfoot MicroPreemie[a]	<1000 g	Blue: depth 0.65 mm, length 1.40 mm Incision type
Tenderfoot Preemie[a]	Low birthweight, 1000–2500 g	White: depth 0.85 mm, length 1.75 mm Incision type
Tenderfoot Newborn[a]	Birth to 3–6 months, >2500 g	Pink/blue: depth 1.0 mm, length 2.5 mm Incision type
BD Microtainer Quikheel Preemie Lancet[b]	Low birthweight (>1.0 kg and <1.5 kg) premature infants or full term for lower blood volume	Pink: depth 0.85 mm, length 1.75 mm Incision type
BD Microtainer Genie Lancet[b,c]	Infant heel sticks for glucose testing	Purple: 1.25 mm × 28 g Puncture type
BD Microtainer Quikheel Infant Lancet[b]	Infants who need high flow, full term with high blood volume needed	Teal: depth 1.0 mm, length 2.5 mm Incision type
babyLance Preemie: BLP[d]	Preemie	Green: depth 0.85 mm Incision type
babyLance Newborn[d]	Newborn	Blue: depth 1.0 mm Incision type
Gentleheel Micropreemie[e]	<1000 g	Yellow: depth 0.65 mm, length 1.4 mm Incision type
Gentleheel Preemie[e]	Low birthweight, 1000–2500 g	Pink: depth 0.85 mm, length 1.75 mm Incision type
Gentleheel Newborn[e]	>2500 g	Green: depth 1.0 mm, length 2.5 mm Incision type

Other devices include: Natus Medical NeatNick; Natus SugarPlum; Sarstedt Safety Heel; and Vitrex Steriheel Baby.

[a]Accriva Diagnostics, Bedford, MA.
[b]BD, Franklin Lakes, NJ.
[c]BD Microtainer Genie Lancets (pink/green/blue) are for finger sticks and not for heel sticks in infants.
[d]MediPurpose, Duluth, GA.
[e]Cardinal Health, Dublin, OH.

III. Procedure

    A. **Automated self-shielding lancets are preferred in neonates** because they are more effective and associated with fewer complications, decreased tissue damage, and in infants with respiratory distress, decreased pain and enhanced cerebral oxygenation. Automated devices cause less hemolysis and less lab value error and provide an exact width and depth of incision. **Manual unshielded lancets** are no longer recommended (unless automated lancets are not available) because they cause more pain, may penetrate too deeply, and are more likely to injure healthcare providers.

Consider vascular puncture if an automatic lancet is not available. There are 2 types of lancet devices: **puncture** and **incision.**

1. **Puncture devices. Automated lancets** (eg, BD Microtainer contact-activated lancet; Becton, Dickinson and Company, Franklin Lakes, NJ) activate only when positioned and pressed against the skin. These puncture the skin by inserting a blade or needle vertically into the tissue. Puncture-style devices typically deliver a single drop of blood and are better for repeated punctures (eg, for glucose testing). SugarPlum glucose lancet is used to draw just one drop of blood to measure glucose.

2. **Incision devices** (eg, BD Microtainer Quickheel Lancets, Tenderfoot, babyLance, gentleheel). These slice through the capillary beds. These are less painful and require fewer repeat incisions and shorter collection times and are recommended for infant heel sticks. Incision devices deliver a small flow of blood as opposed to a drop and are better to fill Microtainer tubes.

B. **Capillary blood sampling is considered the most common painful blood drawing methods but the least invasive and safest of those done on neonates.** Sampling is done by puncturing the dermis layer of the skin to access capillaries running through the subcutaneous layer. The sample is a mixture of arterial and venous blood (from arterioles, venules, and capillaries) plus interstitial and intracellular fluids. The proportion of arterial blood is greater than that of venous, due to increased pressure in the arterioles leading into the capillaries. Warming of the puncture site further arterializes the blood. The areas on the bottom surface of the heel contain the best capillary bed. Infant heels are appropriate for blood collection until approximately 6 months to 1 year of age.

C. **Heel stick contraindications.** Local infection, poor perfusion, significant edema, injury of the foot, or any congenital anomaly of the foot.

D. **Infant should be supine.** Some advocate for infant to be on stomach with the limb lower than the level of the heart to increase blood flow.

E. **Warm the heel to increase arterial inflow (arterialization of the puncture site)** *(controversial).* Apply a heel warmer (specially designed heel pack for single use that is temperature controlled and safer) or warm washcloth with a diaper wrapped around it, or submerge the heel in warm water (need to control the temperature). This prewarming may increase the local blood flow in the capillaries (hyperemia) and reduce the difference between the arterial and venous gas pressures. It is often done when collecting a sample for a blood gas or pH determination. *Note:* Some feel if the heel is well perfused this step is not necessary, and 2 studies note that warming the heel does not increase blood flow or facilitate blood collection (studies not blinded). In another study, topical nitroglycerine did not facilitate blood collection in a heel stick study.

F. **Pain management. Heel sticks are very painful.** Factors that contribute to pain responses are size of needle, gestational age, repeated exposure, squeezing of the heel, severity of illness, and behavioral state of the infant. Pain from a heel stick cannot be completely eliminated. It is best not to squeeze the heel because this is very painful.

1. **The American Academy of Pediatrics recommends nonpharmacologic pain prevention** such as oral sucrose/glucose, breast feeding, kangaroo care, swaddling, rocking, nonnutritive sucking, facilitated tucking, gentle human touch (but no analgesic effects on very premature infants), or other methods. A combination of these methods seems to be more effective in controlling pain. **Multiple sensorial stimuli** (3 Ts: taste, touch, and talk) have been proven to be more effective than just oral sweet solution.

2. **EMLA (eutectic mixture of lidocaine and prilocaine)** has not been found to be effective in heel stick pain reduction.

3. **Systemic analgesia (acetaminophen)**, therapeutic touch, music therapy, co-bedding, heel warming, and noninvasive electrical stimulation at acupuncture points are not effective in relieving pain in neonates during a heel stick.

4. **Automated devices, compared with conventional lancets,** reduce the duration of blood collection, thereby indirectly reducing the pain. Blade-shaped automatic lancets are recommended over needle-shaped lancets. It is preferable to have an automatic lancet with an arched cutting edge. Two studies assessed which automated lancet was the least painful (one study supported the Exxe Safe Blade and the other study found the Tenderfoot device to be superior).

G. **Choose the area of puncture** (Figure 36–1; red area is preferred). Always avoid the end (crown) of the heel (the posterior curvature where the calcaneus bone is close to the skin), as this area is associated with an increased incidence of osteomyelitis. Vary the sites to prevent bruising, tissue injury, and inflammation.

1. **Recommended site.** There are 2 sites that are recommended based on a study by Blumenfeld et al. One site is medial to the visual line from the middle of the big toe to the posterior of the heel; the other is lateral to a line drawn between the fourth and fifth toes that extends posterior to the heel. These areas avoid the medial and lateral plantar nerve and artery and the medial calcaneal nerves.

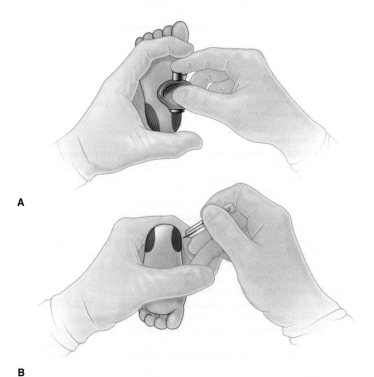

A

B

FIGURE 36–1. Preferred sites and technique for heel stick in an infant. Use the red shaded area when performing a heel stick. (**A**) Use of an automated self-retracting lancet (BD Quikheel) for heel stick illustrated. (**B**) Standard lancet technique is shown. The automated lancet is held at 90 degrees to the axis of the foot and activated. (*Reproduced with permission from Gomella LG, Haist SA: Clinician's Pocket Reference, 11th ed. New York, NY: McGraw-Hill Education; 2007.*)

2. **Alternative site.** Based on a study by Jain and Rutter, a heel stick can also be safely done on any part of the plantar surface of the heel except the posterior aspect of the heel (standard lancet punctures 2.4 mm; shortest depth of perichondrium is in the center of the heel at 3 to 8 mm). Some sources recommend an alternative site (between the sides of the heel in the plantar area) to be used if the other areas have been used extensively because repeated heel sticks can cause tissue injury and inflammation. *Note:* Be aware of the nerves and arteries in this location. Always avoid the end (crown) of the heel (the posterior curvature where the calcaneus bone is close to the skin), as this area is associated with an increased incidence of osteomyelitis. Vary the sites to prevent bruising, tissue injury, and inflammation.

3. **Fingertips and toes are not recommended in infants** and are only recommended in children >1 year old.

H. **Wash hands and wear gloves prior to procedure.** Wipe the proposed heel stick area with povidone-iodine, followed by a saline wipe, and let dry for approximately 30 seconds. Some sources advocate using only a 70% alcohol prep pad and letting it dry. Do not use cotton balls. (*Note:* Povidone-iodine can interfere with potassium, bilirubin, phosphorus, and uric acid. If the area is wet with alcohol, hemolysis may occur, altering the results.)

I. **As noted earlier, 2 general devices are available: automated and manual.** Automated devices (spring loaded) are recommended.

1. **Using an automated lancet (preferred method).** Prepare the unit and hold the device either perpendicularly to the skin or at 90 degrees to the long axis of the foot (see Figure 36–1A). Depress the trigger to activate the device and automatically make the puncture. Immediately discard the device.

2. **Using a standard (not automated) lancet.** Encircle the heel with the palm of your hand and index finger (see Figure 36–1B). Make a quick puncture. Never puncture >2.4 mm to avoid complications. Incision depths recommended:

a. **<1 kg:** 0.65-mm incision depth.

b. **>1 kg:** 0.85-mm incision depth.

c. **Term infants:** 1-mm incision depth.

J. **Wipe off the first drop of blood with gauze,** as it is often contaminated with interstitial and intracellular fluid and may have a high potassium level, causing specimen dilution, hemolysis, and clotting. Wiping off the first drop also permits the sample to flow better as platelets may otherwise aggregate at the site. Gently apply pressure to the heel ("tennis racket grip"), hold heel in a dependent position, and place the collection tube at the site of the puncture. Capillary tubes will automatically fill by capillary action; gently "pump" the heel to continue the blood flow to collect drops in a larger tube. Allow time for capillary refill of the heel, and apply pressure so the incision is opened with each pumping maneuver. Do not squeeze, milk, scoop, scrape, or massage the area, as these actions may affect the test results and because squeezing the heel causes much pain.

K. **Seal the end of the capillary tube with clay** (if necessary).

L. **Order of collection/draw. Example using BD Microtainer blood collection tubes. Note that this differs from a venipuncture collection sequence.**

1. **Collect the blood gas sample first.** The blood becomes more venous if its collection is delayed. Run the sample promptly, making sure there are no air bubbles.

2. **Hematology studies should be done next.** If the CBC is delayed, there is an increased chance of erroneous cell counts due to platelet clumping.

3. **Lastly, take chemistry/toxicology samples.** Use the following order of draw for the specific color of microtainer tubes (minimizes the effect of platelet clumping):

a. **Blood gas always first.**

b. **Lavender (purple-topped) tubes** (additive: ethylenediaminetetraacetic acid) (EDTA): For whole blood hematology (CBC with or without differential, erythrocyte sedimentation rate, reticulocyte count) and others.

    c. **Green-topped tubes** (additive: sodium or lithium heparin): For biochemistry tests that require a heparinized plasma sample such as ammonia, insulin, renin, or aldosterone.

    d. **Gold-topped tubes** (additive: clot activator and gel for serum separation): For serum determinations in chemistry, such as bilirubin, creatinine, urea, calcium, sodium, potassium, chloride, chemistry panels (eg, liver function tests).

    e. **Red-topped tube** (no additive): For chemistry testing, serology, blood bank tests, and therapeutic drug and antibiotic levels (eg, phenobarbital, theophylline).

M. For filter paper newborn screening. (See Chapter 16.) The paper can be directly applied to the heel, or the blood can be transferred from a capillary tube (without anticoagulants) to the filter paper.

N. Maintain pressure on the site with a dry sterile gauze pad until the bleeding stops and elevate the foot. Gauze can be wrapped around the heel and left on to provide hemostasis.

O. Inaccurate laboratory results. Relative to venous or arterial sampling, heel stick can alter results:

    1. **Elevated:** Glucose, potassium, lactate, ionized calcium, hematocrit, white blood cell count, red blood cell count, mean corpuscular volume, mean corpuscular hemoglobin, lactate dehydrogenase, and aspartate aminotransferase.

    2. **Decreased:** Platelet counts, total protein, calcium, and electrolytes.

    3. **Blood gas values:** Slightly lower pH, slightly higher PCO_2, and markedly lower PO_2.

IV. Complications

A. Infectious

    1. **Cellulitis.** Risk can be minimized with sterile technique. If present, a culture from the affected area should be obtained and the use of broad-spectrum antibiotics considered.

    2. **Osteomyelitis.** Usually occurs in the calcaneus bone. Avoid the posterior curvature of the heel, and do not puncture too deep. If osteomyelitis occurs, tissue should be obtained for culture, and broad-spectrum antibiotics should be started until a specific organism is identified. Infectious disease and orthopedic consultation is usually obtained.

    3. **Other infections.** Abscess and perichondritis have been reported.

B. Scarring of the heel. Occurs when there have been multiple punctures in the same area. If extensive scarring is present, consider another technique or site for blood collection.

C. Pain and hypoxemia. Heel stick related pain can cause declines in hemoglobin oxygen saturation as measured by pulse oximetry.

D. Calcified nodules. These can occur because of repetitive punctures but usually disappear by 30 months of age.

E. Other complications. Nerve damage, tibial artery laceration (medial aspect of heel), burning of the skin with too hot of water while warming the heel, bleeding, bruising, hematoma, and bone calcification.

37 Laryngeal Mask Airway

The laryngeal mask airway (LMA) is an alternative airway device that consists of a soft elliptical mask with an inflatable cuff that is attached to a flexible airway tube. The mask covers the glottis (laryngeal opening), and the inflatable cuff occludes the esophagus. Placement of the LMA is feasible in neonates. A study shows it was successfully placed in <35 seconds in most patients with only 1 attempt with minimal fluctuations in heart rate and oxygen saturation (SaO_2). It is intended for use in babies who weigh >2000 g. The seventh edition of the American Academy of Pediatrics/American Heart Association *Textbook of Neonatal Resuscitation* states: "When you 'can't ventilate and can't intubate,' a laryngeal mask may provide a successful rescue airway." The International Liaison Committee on Resuscitation and the European Resuscitation Council recommend that LMA can be used as an alternative to intubation with an ETT in late preterm, term, and infants >2000 g when face mask ventilation is unsuccessful or intubation is not possible. A recent Cochrane review (2018) states: The LMA can achieve effective ventilation during neonatal resuscitation in a time frame consistent with current guidelines. It is more effective than bag-mask ventilation in terms of shorter resuscitation and ventilation times, and less need for endotracheal intubation. Bansal et al in a critical review of the LMA in neonatal resuscitation suggests that the use of the LMA is a feasible and safe alternative to mask ventilation of late preterm and term infants in the DR, but state it is not recommended as initial respiratory support since evidence is still insufficient.

I. **Indications**

  A. **Ineffective face mask ventilation in neonates with:**

    1. **Abnormal facial anatomy** (eg, cleft lip, cleft palate)

    2. **Unstable cervical spine** (eg, osteogenesis imperfecta, arthrogryposis, and trisomy 21)

    3. **Upper airway obstruction** (eg, Pierre-Robin sequence, micrognathia, large tongue, redundant tissues, and oral, pharyngeal, or neck tumors)

  B. **Rescue procedure after failed intubation or intubation not feasible.**

  C. **Short-term mechanical ventilation for procedures in the neonatal intensive care unit.**

  D. **Resuscitation in delivery room.** Use of LMA was found to be a safe alternative to mask ventilation of late preterm and term infants in the delivery suite.

  E. **Administration of medications *(controversial).*** Medications may leak from the mask and not enter the lungs. The seventh edition American Academy of Pediatrics/American Heart Association *Textbook of Neonatal Resuscitation* states: "There is insufficient evidence to recommend using a laryngeal mask to administer intratracheal medications." Recent studies have shown that surfactant therapy through the LMA may be effective (results showed a decreased rate of intubation and mechanical ventilation in premature infants with RDS), but since there is not enough sufficient evidence it is not recommended for routine use.

  F. **Infants undergoing minor elective procedures.** LMA in infants undergoing minor elective procedures had clinically significantly fewer perioperative respiratory adverse events (PRAEs) and decreased incidence of major PRAEs than with endotracheal tubes.

II. **Equipment.** There are various LMA devices for use in newborns (eg, LMA Classic, LMA ProSeal, LMA Supreme [LMA North America Inc, San Diego, CA], i-gel supraglottic airway [Intersurgical, Liverpool, NY], Ambu® AuraOnce [Ambu A/S, Ballerup, Denmark], Air-Q disposable laryngeal mask airway [Mercury Medical, Clearwater FL], Shiley™ LMA [Medtronic, USA]). For a basic laryngeal airway design, see Figure 37–1. Appropriate-size LMA: all neonatal LMA are size 1 for infants <5 kg, except Air-Q disposable LMA available size 0.5 for infants with BW <4 kg. Other equipment: water-soluble lubricant, 5-mL syringe, carbon dioxide (CO_2) detector, gloves. Optional: orogastric tube (5 to 6F).

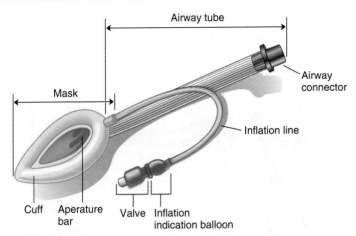

FIGURE 37-1. Basic laryngeal mask airway design.

III. **Procedure**

A. **Pain management/premedication.** Because this is usually an emergent procedure, premedication is not necessary in the delivery room or after an acute deterioration in the neonatal intensive care unit. In older children, propofol and midazolam have been used.

B. **Use size 1 laryngeal mask airway.** Designed for infants >2000 g, but can be used for smaller infants (>1500 g) if needed.

C. **Wash hands and put on gloves** following standard precautions.

D. **Inspect the entire laryngeal mask airway device (airway connector, airway tube, inflatable cuff, aperture bar, inflation line, and inflation indication balloon)** to ensure there are no tears, cuts, or kinks.

E. **Check cuff for leakage by inflating with 2 to 3 mL of air.** Be sure to fully deflate the cuff before insertion.

F. **If the infant has a distended stomach and you are using a laryngeal mask airway that does not have a gastric port:** Prior to inserting the LMA, place an orogastric tube in the infant and aspirate any air in the stomach.

G. **Lubricate the back of the mask with a water-soluble lubricant** if needed. Make sure the lubricant does not get near the openings on the inside of the mask.

H. **Stand as if you were intubating the infant. Position patient on back in sniffing position.** Hold the LMA in the right or left hand.

I. **With the aperture facing anteriorly, insert the laryngeal mask airway against hard palate and, using your index finger, guide the laryngeal mask airway.** The mask will follow the path of the mouth and palate, mimicking the swallowing of food. Insert until resistance is felt.

J. **Inflate the mask with 2 to 4 mL of air (do not exceed maximum recommended by manufacturers)** to provide adequate seal (Figure 37-2). The mask will move slightly upward when it is inflated. Remove the syringe.

K. **Attach a carbon dioxide detector** to airway tube

L. **Connect the end of tube to bag, T-piece, or ventilator.**

M. **Give 8 to 10 positive-pressure breaths.** Assess chest movement and breath sounds. One should notice an increase in heart rate, movement of the chest wall, increasing SpO_2, and equal breath sounds when listening to both sides of chest. Confirm the presence of CO_2 on the detector. All of these findings verify that the laryngeal mask is correctly placed.

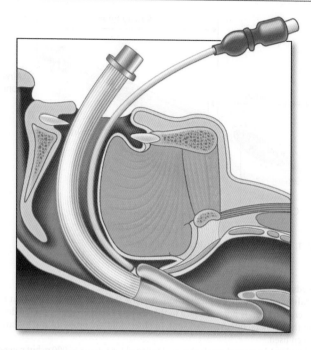

FIGURE 37-2. Demonstration of correct anatomic positioning of the laryngeal mask airway cuff around laryngeal inlet.

   N. Secure laryngeal mask airway similar to an endotracheal tube. Grunting and crying when the infant breathes spontaneously through the device is normal. A large leak of air or presence of a bulge in the neck could indicate that the LMA is not properly placed.
   O. Optional: If there is a gastric drain tube, a size 5- or 6-F lubricated gastric tube can be inserted and the air aspirated out of the stomach. The syringe can be disconnected and left to air.
IV. **Complications**
   A. **Air leak around LMA** may result in ineffective ventilation.
   B. **Gastric distention and aspiration.**
   C. **Malposition.**
   D. **Laryngospasm and bronchospasm.**
   E. **Soft tissue trauma of the uvula and epiglottis.**
   F. **LMA obstruction of the laryngeal inlet** by a supraglottic mucus plug in a premature infant with tracheoesophageal fistula. Vomiting and regurgitation can occur.
   G. **Partial airway obstruction secondary to an improperly placed LMA.**
V. **Removal of the laryngeal mask airway**
   A. **Indications:** Infant has effective spontaneous respirations, or an endotracheal tube can be safely placed.
   B. **Procedure:** Suction secretions around the mouth and throat, deflate the cuff, and remove the LMA.

38 Lumbar Puncture (Spinal Tap)

I. **Indications**
   A. **Obtain cerebrospinal fluid for the diagnosis of central nervous system disorders such as meningitis/encephalitis.**
      1. **Infections** that can be diagnosed are bacterial, viral, fungal, and TORCHZ (*t*oxoplasmosis, *o*ther [usually syphilis], *r*ubella, *c*ytomegalovirus, *h*erpes simplex virus, and *z*ika virus). Meningitis can be present in as many as 23% of cases of neonatal sepsis, and blood cultures can be negative in up to 38% of infants with meningitis.
      2. **Initial sepsis workup (*controversial*).** If central nervous system (CNS) involvement is suspected or blood cultures are positive, some sources recommend a lumbar puncture (LP). Because signs and symptoms of neonatal meningitis are vague and nonspecific, some clinicians advise that all infants with proven or suspected sepsis undergo LP. The American Academy of Pediatrics (AAP) recommends that an LP be performed in any infant with a positive blood culture, when clinical course or laboratory findings highly suggest sepsis, or in an infant with worsening clinical status on antibiotic therapy. Delay the LP in any infant who is critically ill who will not be able to tolerate the procedure. (Confirm that the antibiotic dosage will cover for meningitis.)
   B. **Diagnose an inborn error of metabolism.** Multiple cerebrospinal fluid (CSF) studies exist that can help delineate different inborn errors of metabolism, including but not limited to amino acid analysis for nonketotic hyperglycinemia and CSF lactate-to-pyruvate ratio for mitochondrial disorders.
   C. **Drainage of cerebrospinal fluid in communicating hydrocephalus associated with intraventricular hemorrhage.** (Serial LPs for this are *controversial*.) A Cochrane review (2017) found the following: "There was no evidence that repeated removal of CSF via LP, ventricular puncture or from a ventricular reservoir produces any benefit over conservative management in neonates with or at risk for developing post hemorrhagic hydrocephalus in terms of reduction of disability, death or need for placement of a permanent shunt."
   D. **Aid in the diagnosis of intracranial hemorrhage.** CSF studies are indicative but not diagnostic for intracranial hemorrhage. Signs include a large number of red blood cells (RBCs), xanthochromia, increased protein content, and hypoglycorrhachia (abnormally low CSF glucose).
   E. **Administration of intrathecal medications.** Chemotherapy, antibiotics, anesthetic agents, or contrast material.
   F. **Evaluation of antibiotic efficacy in CNS infections by examining CSF fluid.**
   G. **Diagnose CNS involvement with leukemia.**
II. **Equipment.** LP kit (usually contains 3–4 sterile specimen tubes; 4 are often necessary); sterile drapes; sterile gauze; 20-, 22-, or 24-guage, 1.5-inch spinal needle with stylet (**do not use a butterfly needle** as it may introduce skin into the subarachnoid space and form a dermoid cyst); 1% buffered lidocaine and/or topical anesthetic (EMLA [eutectic mixture of lidocaine and prilocaine]); 25- to 27-gauge needle, 1-mL syringe; sterile gloves; mask; gown; hat; and skin disinfectant (10% povidone-iodine solution or other unit-approved type), point-of-care ultrasound.
III. **Procedure**
   A. **Contraindications to lumbar puncture** include increased intracranial pressure (ICP) (risk of CNS herniation), uncorrected bleeding abnormality (thrombocytopenia or bleeding diathesis), overlying skin infection near puncture site, severe cardiorespiratory instability, and lumbosacral abnormalities that interfere with identification of key structures. If significant increased ICP is suspected, consider a magnetic resonance imaging (MRI) of the head. Herniation rarely occurs in the neonate with open cranial sutures but is reported.

B. Pain management

    1. The American Academy of Pediatrics recommends that topical anesthetics (EMLA) be applied 30 minutes before the procedure. Cochrane review (2017) found 2 individual studies with a statistically significant reduction in pain using EMLA during an LP. An AAP update notes that EMLA may decrease pain during an LP, especially if the infant is given oral sucrose or glucose at the same time. Nonpharmacologic pain management alone, if appropriate, can be used (ie, sucrose with pacifier).

    2. Lidocaine (buffered with bicarbonate) 0.5% to 1% can be injected subcutaneously. Warming the lidocaine, using a small-gauge needle, and injecting slowly will help.

    3. Systemic therapy. Other recommendations include sedation with a slow intravenous opiate bolus if the infant is intubated; if not intubated, a bolus of midazolam in a term infant can be considered (see Chapter 81).

C. Use of POCUS for lumbar puncture. Typically done as a blind stick, with the added difficulty of the small interspinous spaces in neonates, use of bedside ultrasound is recommended since it can be used to identify key landmarks (spinous processes, interspinous spaces, and the terminal end of the conus medullaris). A static technique is used prior to the procedure to help determine the best location for needle insertion and maximum safe depth. Using dynamic guidance, one can see the passage of the needle into the skin. Of the few studies done in young infants, two-thirds showed an improved success rate using ultrasound. See Chapter 44 for technique.

D. An assistant should restrain the infant in either a lateral decubitus position (Figure 38–1) with the knees and hip flexed toward the chest or in a sitting

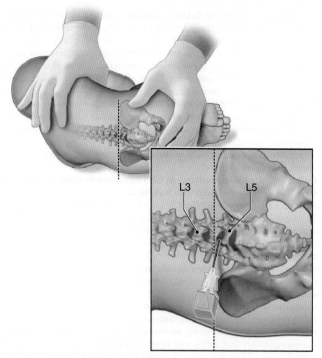

FIGURE 38–1. Positioning and landmarks used for lumbar puncture. The iliac crest (*dashed line*) marks the approximate level of L4.

position with the legs straightened depending on personal preference. The spine should be flexed to open the interlaminar spaces. The neck should not be flexed because of an increased incidence of airway compromise. An intubated infant must be placed in the lateral decubitus position. Some advocate that if CSF cannot be obtained in the lateral decubitus position, the sitting position should be used. Supplemental oxygen can help prevent hypoxemia. Monitor vital signs and pulse oximetry during the procedure. A recent study found that there was no difference in LP success between the lateral and sitting positions.

E. **Once the infant is in position, check landmarks** (see Figure 38–1). Palpate the top of iliac crest. The intercristal line/Tuffier's line is the line across the top of the superior aspect of the iliac crests and is used to estimate the L4 vertebra. Just below the line is usually the L4–5 interspace. Slide your finger down to the L4 vertebral body. The L4–5 interspace is the preferred site of LP to avoid cord penetration because a neonate's cord terminates lower than that of older patients. **Use of point-of-care ultrasound** is recommended if the health care provider is properly trained and the equipment is available.

F. **Prepare materials.** Determine the amount of CSF needed based on the tests desired. Put sterile gloves on, open sterile containers, and have antiseptic solution poured into the plastic well located in the LP kit.

G. **With sterile gloves on, clean the lumbar area with antiseptic solution, starting at the interspace selected.** Prep in a widening circle, up and over the iliac crest.

H. **Drape the area with 1 towel under the infant and 1 towel covering everything but the selected interspace.** Keep the infant's face exposed. Palpate again to find the selected intervertebral space. Keep a finger on the vertebral process above the selected space.

I. **Insert the needle in the midline with steady pressure,** aiming toward the umbilicus.
   1. **Guidelines for spinal needle depth:** 1 to 1.5 cm in term infant and <1 cm in a preterm; or calculate depth of needle insertion: $0.03 \times$ body length (in centimeters). Advance the needle slowly and then remove the stylet to check for appearance of fluid. The fluid should be clear but may be slightly xanthochromic (common).
   2. **Remove the stylet frequently to keep from going too far and getting a bloody specimen.** Some studies suggest that early stylet removal—including not replacing the stylet after initial dermal penetration—can improve the success rate. Compared with older patients, a "pop" as the ligamentum flavum and dura are penetrated is not usually found. Rotate the needle if no fluid is seen, and **never aspirate with a syringe.**

J. **Collect 0.5 to 1 mL of cerebrospinal fluid** in each of the necessary sterile specimen tubes by allowing the fluid to drip into the tubes. **CSF white blood cell (WBC) and glucose values can decrease over time after collection**; therefore, send these immediately. For routine CSF examination, send 3 to 4 tubes of CSF in the following recommended order:
   1. **Tube 1.** Gram stain, bacterial culture, and sensitivity testing.
   2. **Tube 2.** Glucose and protein levels. Other metabolic testing if desired.
   3. **Tube 3.** Cell count and differential.
   4. **Tube 4.** Optional/other studies. Rapid antigen tests for specific pathogens (eg, group B *Streptococcus*) or polymerase chain reaction (PCR) or reverse transcriptase PCR (eg, herpes, enterovirus), viral cultures, CSF metabolic studies.

K. **If treating communicating hydrocephalus with intraventricular hemorrhage,** remove 10 to 15 mL/kg of CSF.

L. **If a bloody specimen is obtained in the first tube:**
   1. **Observe for clearing in subsequent tubes.** An RBC count on the first and last tubes helps determine if the tap was traumatic (usually puncture of the epidural venous plexus on the posterior surface of the vertebral body) by comparing the difference in the number of RBCs/mm³. *Note:* Adjustment of WBC counts in a traumatic LP does not aid in the diagnosis of meningitis. A recent study found that for every 1000 CSF RBCs/mm³, the CSF protein increased by 1.1 mg/dL.

Table 38-1. NORMAL CEREBROSPINAL FLUID VALUES IN NEONATOLOGY

	WBC (mm³)	Protein (mg/dL)	Glucose (mg/dL)
Term	0–32 (mean 61% PMN)	20–170	34–119
Preterm (970–2500 g)	0–29 (mean 57% PMN)	65–170	24–63
VLBW (550–1500 g)	0–44 (range 0%–66% PMN)	45–370	29–217

PMN, polymorphonuclear neutrophils; VLBW, very low birthweight.
Data from Rodriguez AF, Kaplan SL, Mason EO Jr. Cerebrospinal fluid values in the very low birth weight infant. *J Pediatr.* 1990;116(6):971-974; Sarff LD, Platt LH, McCracken GH Jr. Cerebrospinal fluid evaluation in neonates: comparison of high-risk infants with and without meningitis. *J Pediatr.* 1976;88(3):473-477; and Martín-Ancel A, García-Alix A, Salas S, et al. Cerebrospinal fluid leucocyte counts in healthy neonates. *Arch Dis Child Fetal Neonatal Ed.* 2006;91(5):F357-F358.

2. **If blood does not clear, but forms clots,** a blood vessel was probably punctured.
3. **If blood does not clear and does not clot and there are equal numbers of red blood cells in the first and last tubes,** there could be intracranial bleeding.
M. **Replace the stylet before removing the needle** to prevent trapping the spinal nerve roots. Withdraw the needle. Maintain temporary pressure, and then clean and bandage the site.
N. **A repeat tap in 24 to 48 hours may be recommended** if the first tap is not diagnostic and the clinical picture is concerning.
IV. **Interpretation of cerebrospinal fluid findings.** Normal CSF values are listed in Table 38-1. Note that neonatal meningitis can occur with normal CSF values and no single value can exclude meningitis. Specific neonatal values that indicate meningitis are *controversial*. Use caution when interpreting results in the premature infant, because data suggest that results cannot be reliably used to exclude meningitis in this population.
A. **Bloody cerebrospinal fluid.** See Section III.L.
B. **Cerebrospinal fluid protein and white blood cell count.** Decreases with increasing postnatal age.
C. **Elevated cerebrospinal fluid protein without increased cerebrospinal fluid white blood cell counts.** Seen in congenital infections, intracranial hemorrhage, and parameningeal infections (eg, brain abscess).
D. **Cerebrospinal fluid white blood cell count.** Higher in gram-negative than gram-positive meningitis.
E. **Number of bands in cerebrospinal fluid.** Does not predict meningitis.
F. **Cerebrospinal fluid glucose.** A normal CSF value would be 80% of a term infant's blood glucose; 75% if preterm. **A low CSF glucose** has the greatest specificity for meningitis.
G. **Generally, cerebrospinal fluid protein is higher in term infants with meningitis** when compared to preterm infants. CSF glucose values are lower in term infants with meningitis when compared to preterm infants.
H. **Other values suggestive of meningitis**
1. **Cerebrospinal fluid white blood cell count** >20 to 30 cells with predominance of polymorphonuclear leukocytes (for infants >34 weeks with bacterial meningitis, the median WBC is 477/mm³; for infants <34 weeks, median WBC is 110/mm³).
2. **Cerebrospinal fluid protein** >150 mg/dL in preterm infants, >100 mg/dL in term (96% of infants with meningitis have a CSF protein >90 mg/dL).

   3. **Cerebrospinal fluid glucose** <20 mg/dL in preterm infants, <30 mg/dL in term infants.
   4. **Meningitis can be present** with normal CSF values.
 I. **Values suggesting meningitis is not present**
   1. **Cerebrospinal fluid white blood cell count (in any infant)** <10 cells/mm³.
   2. **Cerebrospinal fluid protein in term infants** <100 mg/dL. With preterm infants, it varies with gestational age.
   3. **Age-specific normal mean protein values:** 0–14 days: 79 mg/dL; 15–28 days: 69 mg/dL; 29–42 days: 58 mg/dL.
 V. **Complications.** There is no evidence that LP-related headache occurs in infants.
   A. **Contamination of cerebrospinal fluid specimen with blood.** (See Section III.L.)
   B. **Infection.** Sterile technique reduces risk. Bacteremia may result if a blood vessel is punctured after passage through contaminated CSF. Meningitis can occur if LP is performed during bacteremia. Abscesses (spinal and epidural) and vertebral osteomyelitis are rare.
   C. **Intraspinal epidermoid tumor.** Results from performing an LP with a needle without a stylet, causing the displacement of a "plug" of epithelial tissue into the dura. The incidence of traumatic LP is not reduced by the use of a needle without a stylet. Early stylet removal, however, can be recommended (see Section III.I.2).
   D. **Herniation of cerebral tissue through the foramen magnum.** Uncommon in neonates because of the open fontanelle.
   E. **Spinal cord and nerve damage.** To avoid this complication, use the L4–5 interspace. Between 25 and 40 weeks' gestation, the spinal cord terminates between the second and fourth lumbar vertebrae. After 2 months postterm, the cord is in the normal adult position (T12–L3).
   F. **Intramedullary hemorrhage/intratumoral hemorrhage resulting in paraplegia.** It is important to consider the location of the conus medullaris in a preterm infant. An infant developed paraplegia following an LP because of an **intratumoral hemorrhage** from a congenital neuroblastoma.
   G. **Bleeding/hematoma.** Spinal epidural hematoma, intracranial or spinal subdural hematoma, and intracranial or spinal subarachnoid hematoma have all been reported.
   H. **Cerebrospinal fluid leakage into epidural space.**
   I. **Apnea and bradycardia.** Can occur from respiratory compromise caused by the infant being held too tightly during the procedure.
   J. **Hypoxemia.** Commonly seen; increasing oxygen before or during the procedure may help.
   K. **Cardiopulmonary arrest** (rare).

39 Ostomy Care

 I. **Indications.** A variety of surgical procedures may require an **ostomy, a temporary or permanent artificial opening in the intestine (enterostomy) or urinary tract (urostomy).** An ostomy is performed for gastrointestinal or urinary diversion. Ostomies in the neonatal intensive care unit are most commonly intestinal for the management of necrotizing enterocolitis (NEC), anorectal malformations, meconium ileus, Hirschsprung disease, volvulus, and intestinal atresias, and these disease entities are discussed elsewhere in this book. **A gastrostomy (surgical opening in the stomach)** may be necessary for feeding or decompression in a variety of conditions, such as the inability to swallow (neurologic or congenital anomalies), esophageal abnormalities, and prolonged poor oral feeding. Urinary diversions are sometimes performed. This chapter will only discuss ostomy care in gastrointestinal diversions since they are the more common in neonates.

II. **Ostomy classification**

    A. Ileostomy. Stoma opening from the ileum used for NEC, intestinal malrotation or volvulus, and small bowel atresia or stenosis.

    B. Colostomy. Stoma opening from the colon used for NEC, Hirschsprung disease, malrotation or volvulus, imperforate anus, and colonic atresia.

    C. Mucous fistula. Distal nonfunctioning limb of intestine secured flush to skin with a mucocutaneous anastomosis.

    D. Hartman pouch. Distal intestine is left in the abdominal cavity rather than removed or secured as mucous fistula, allowing reconnection to stoma at later date.

    E. Double-barrel stoma. Loop of bowel is completely divided and 2 ends brought out as stomas to abdominal surface. Skin and fascia are closed between ends to provide separation of stomas.

    F. End ostomy. Intestine is completely divided. The functioning proximal end is everted, elevated above skin, and secured circumferentially.

    G. Loop ostomy. The intestine is incompletely divided with an opening at the antimesenteric side, while leaving the mesenteric side intact. This is used when temporary diversion or minimal surgical procedure is needed and not performed as often as end ostomy.

    H. Gastrostomy. Surgical opening into the stomach, where a gastrostomy tube is inserted into the opening for nutritional support, medications, or gastrointestinal decompression. It can also be placed by interventional radiology in a less invasive way.

    I. Urostomy. Opening made to divert urine from the urinary tract to the outside of the body through an intestinal stoma. Rare in the neonate.

    J. Vesicostomy. Surgical opening from the bladder to the skin for urinary diversion. More common in neonate (posterior urethral valves, neurogenic bladder).

III. **Equipment**

    A. Ostomy. Ostomy bag or pouch (1-piece or 2-piece system), skin barrier wafer, skin preparation agents, sterile water, gauze pads, petroleum gauze, and gloves. Products that improve security of pouch include plasticizing or liquid skin sealants (use on intact or damaged skin), skin barrier paste (protect exposed skin), adhesive agents (improve adherence), and skin barrier powder (dusted onto denuded skin to form protective crust).

    B. Gastrostomy tube. 12- to 14-F balloon or mushroom gastrostomy tube. Silicone is preferred over latex skin barrier.

IV. **Procedures**

    A. Ileostomy and colostomy

        1. Postoperative ileostomy and colostomy care

            a. No bag is applied for first 24 to 48 hours postoperative due to minimal stool production.

            b. Apply petrolatum gauze to stoma to maintain moisture until first stool output appears. (When attaching pouch, remove residual petroleum because it will interfere with adherence.)

            c. Measure effluent output. Volume >2 mL/kg/h should be replaced with 1/2 normal saline. Some institutions add 10 to 20 mEq of potassium chloride per liter.

        2. Changing ostomy bags. Not a sterile procedure, but regular hand washing and clean gloves are important. Goals are containment of stool/odor and protection of the peristomal skin. Minimize skin sealants, adhesives, and adhesive removers in premature infants due to more permeable skin.

            a. Empty bag and carefully remove from skin.

    b. Clean skin and stoma with warm water and dry thoroughly. Inspect stoma and peristomal skin. Mild bleeding of the stoma is common with cleaning. Soap is not recommended.

    c. Measure stoma at base using stoma-measuring guide or template. Cut appropriate-size hole (usually 2–3 mm larger than stoma) in soft silicone-bordered dressing or wafer for bag; do not constrict stoma, but ensure that the skin is covered by the appliance.

    d. Prepare skin for wafer application. If there is no skin compromise, apply skin sealant to surface area. Apply stoma adhesive paste around stoma for better adherence. Apply skin barrier powder to denuded skin to form protective crust.

    e. Position wafer on skin around stoma and mold to contour of skin.

    f. Adhere closed-ended ostomy bag or pouch to wafer.

    g. Position bag in lateral position to allow for easy drainage.

    h. Empty bag regularly when one-third to one-half full. Change bag with any evidence of leaking.

B. Gastrostomy tubes

  1. Types of gastrostomy tubes

    a. Balloon tip. Initial placement requires abdominal surgery. Tube has a retention balloon on distal end, similar to indwelling urinary catheter.

    b. Mushroom tip portion creates resistance to tube displacement.

    c. Percutaneous endoscopic gastrostomy tube. Placed by endoscopy. Tube has internal bumper secured against abdominal mucosa and external bumper to stabilize the tube.

    d. Low-profile gastrostomy ("button"). Replaces original gastrostomy tube once the stoma tract has matured 6 to 8 weeks. Access device is flush to the skin.

  2. Care of all gastrostomy tubes

    a. Flush tubing every 4 hours during continuous feedings or before and after intermittent feedings with at least 3 mL of warm water.

    b. Give only 1 medication at a time and flush between medications.

    c. Assess site daily for breakdown, warmth, redness, edema, purulent drainage, leakage, foul odor, or pain.

    d. Clean gastrostomy tube site with warm water and mild soap to remove drainage or crusting. Dry skin thoroughly. Site should be kept clean and dry.

    e. Do not use hydrogen peroxide to clean site.

V. Complications

  A. Ileostomy and colostomy. Consider consultation with an ostomy nurse specialist for persistent dermatitis or ostomy issues.

  1. Peristomal skin breakdown. Common problem as small bowel effluent contains a high concentration of digestive enzymes.

    a. Careful cleansing of the stoma and surrounding skin requires gentle technique to avoid abrasions.

    b. To minimize contact dermatitis from digestive fluids, fecal materials, or adhesives, select a correctly sized bagging system to minimize skin exposure.

    c. Use protective skin products (see earlier) to further prevent contact between skin and ostomy output.

  2. Excessive output may cause dehydration and/or electrolyte imbalance. Daily liquid output is normally 10 to 15 mL/kg; ileostomy output is usually greater than colostomy.

    a. Replace excessive output with appropriate fluids (1/2 normal saline). Some institutions add 10 to 20 mEq of potassium chloride per liter to the replacement fluids or supplement potassium in the daily fluids.

    b. Malabsorption. A risk with surgical loss of overall small intestine length.

    c. **Diarrhea** secondary to infectious agents or osmotic enteral loads is a constant threat. Replace fluid losses intravenously and evaluate electrolyte balance.

    d. **Management.** May involve changes in enteral feeds such as continuous feeds or elemental formulas to improve absorption or tolerance. Probiotics (controversial) may improve gut flora. Cholestyramine may reduce diarrhea related to short gut and excessive bile acids.

3. **If dermatitis is suspected (contact, fungal, or otherwise), change bag and barrier every 24 to 48 hours to reassess for further treatment.** Fungal skin infections may appear in the form of pustules or papules. Apply antifungal (eg, nystatin) powder to area before applying skin barrier wafer and bag.

4. **Bleeding.** A small amount of blood from the stoma tissue itself after cleaning is normal. Notify pediatric surgeon about excessive bleeding or blood coming from lumen of the stoma.

5. **Peristomal hernia.** A defect in abdominal fascia that allows intestine to bulge into peristomal area. Surgical intervention will be necessary if hernia is incarcerated.

6. **Stomal stenosis.** An impairment of drainage due to narrowing or contraction of stoma tissue at the skin or subcutaneous fascial level; may require revision.

7. **Retraction of a stoma.** Stoma tissue being pulled below skin level. Surgical reevaluation is suggested. Adequate bag adherence can be challenging if the stoma cannot be revised.

8. **Necrosis of stoma tissue can occur from impaired blood flow.** Stomas are usually moist and pink-red in color. Color changes can occur when infant cries, but should return to normal when infant is calm. A dark maroon or black stoma may indicate necrosis.

9. **Prolapse is a telescoping of intestine through the stoma beyond skin level.** This requires surgical assessment for perfusion, length, and stoma function. If ischemia or obstruction is suspected, then surgical intervention will be required.

B. **Gastrostomy**

1. **Leaking around tube.** This can result from tube displacement, improper balloon inflation, inadequate tube stabilization, or increased abdominal pressure.

2. **Skin irritation.** Possible causes include leakage, sutures, and infection. Topical treatments include antifungal powder or ointment, zinc oxide, and skin barrier wafer. Cover site with dry gauze or foam dressing under stabilizer to pull drainage off skin.

3. **Infection.** Most likely occurs within first 2 weeks after tube placement. Risk factors include skin breakdown, immunosuppressed patient, chronic corticosteroids, and excessive handling/manipulation of tube.

4. **Granulation tissue formation.** A proliferation of capillaries that present as red, raw, beefy, painful, or bleeding tissue protruding from stoma. Possible causes include moisture, infection, tube not stabilized, and use of hydrogen peroxide. Treatment may include cauterization with silver nitrate. Surgery may also recommend steroid cream until resolved.

5. **Tube occlusion.** May be caused by inadequate tube flushing, kink in tube, or formula or medication precipitation in tube.

6. **Accidental removal.** Site can close within 1 to 4 hours. Immediately place appropriate-sized Foley catheter in stoma if tube is removed to maintain patency while the correct tube can be replaced.

40 Paracentesis (Abdominal)

I. Indications

A. To obtain peritoneal fluid for diagnostic tests to determine the cause of ascites. **Ascites is an excessive amount of fluid in the peritoneal cavity,** and in the neonate, it is usually urinary, biliary, or chylous. Other causes can occur but are less common.

1. **Urinary ascites.** Due to perforation of the ureter, renal pelvis, or bladder (often caused by a distal urinary tract obstruction and proximal buildup of pressure). The most common neonatal cause is posterior urethral valves. Rare causes: ureterocele, ureteral or urethral stenosis, persistent cloaca, neurogenic bladder, urogenital sinus, congenital nephrotic syndrome, bladder neck obstruction, and renal vein thrombosis.

2. **Biliary ascites.** Due to perforation in the extrahepatic biliary tree (most common site is junction of common bile duct with cystic duct), injury to the bile ducts, or a choledochal cyst.

3. **Chylous ascites.** Usually idiopathic. Causes include: congenital chylous ascites (most commonly caused by a malformation of the lymphatic duct causing an obstruction or inadequate drainage of the intraabdominal lymphatic system), "leaky lymphatics," lymphangiectasia, external compression (malrotation, intussusception, mesenteric cyst, incarcerated hernia), complication following neonatal surgery and others.

4. **Hepatocellular ascites.** Can be caused by neonatal hepatitis, viral hepatitis, α_1-antitrypsin deficiency, congenital hepatic fibrosis, storage disorders, Budd-Chiari syndrome, or hepatic/portal vein thrombosis.

5. **Pancreatic ascites.** Usually caused by trauma, infection, anatomical lesions, congenital pancreatic pseudocyst.

6. **Gastrointestinal tract causes of ascites.** Any perforation of the gastrointestinal tract: necrotizing enterocolitis (NEC) with perforation/peritonitis, meconium peritonitis, perforation of the Meckel diverticulum, atresia, malrotation, volvulus, gastroschisis, omphalocele, post abdominal surgery, or intussusception. **Peritonitis** in neonates is most commonly associated with gastrointestinal perforations.

7. **Infections.** Most commonly congenital (cytomegalovirus [CMV], toxoplasmosis, syphilis, and others) but can also be from fungal (most common *Candida albicans*), viral (parvovirus, enterovirus), or bacterial infections (tuberculosis, salmonella).

8. **Inborn errors of metabolism.** Glycogen storage disorders, lysosomal storage disorders, and galactosemia can all cause ascites. Examples include infantile free sialic acid storage disorder (ISSD), Salla disease, GM1 gangliosidosis, Gaucher disease, and α_1-antitrypsin deficiency.

9. **Cardiac abnormalities.** Congestive heart failure, arrhythmias, and right-sided heart obstruction.

10. **Chromosomal causes.** Turner syndrome and trisomy 21.

11. **Iatrogenic.** Can occur from fluid from central venous catheters or intraperitoneal extravasation of fluids from an umbilical vein catheterization–related perforation, gastric perforation from gastric tubes.

12. **Hemoperitoneum (bloody ascites).** Uncommon but can be nontraumatic (hepatoblastoma), secondary to birth trauma (hepatic, splenic, or adrenal), or secondary to a ruptured internal organ. Splenic trauma can be associated with consumptive coagulopathy.

    B. As a therapeutic procedure to relieve pressure and aid in ventilation in a patient with cardiorespiratory compromise. **Examples include removal of peritoneal fluid from massive ascites or air from a pneumoperitoneum.**

 II. Equipment. Sterile drapes, sterile gloves, topical disinfectant (eg, povidone-iodine solution), sterile gauze pads, tuberculin syringe, 1% lidocaine (see pain management options later in this chapter [Section III.G]), appropriate sterile collection tubes for fluid, a 5- to 20-mL syringe on a 3-way stopcock, 22- or 24-gauge catheter-over-needle assembly (24 gauge for <2000 g, 22–24 gauge for >2000 g); self-shielding device preferred. Consider the use of bedside ultrasound to guide needle placement.

III. Procedure

    A. Contraindications and precautions. Paracentesis can be done with thrombocytopenia or coagulopathy if corrected before the procedure. Decompress bowel and empty bladder to minimize puncture of organs. Avoid surgical scar sites.

    B. Diagnosis of ascites is usually done by clinical examination and ultrasound. Ascites is usually obvious on examination (abdominal distention, increasing abdominal girth, increased weight gain, bulging flanks, dullness to percussion, and dilated superficial veins). Most infants are also very edematous. Ascites obvious by clinical examination in a neonate usually indicates a fluid volume of ≥200 mL. Ascites not obvious on examination usually means the volume is <100 mL. Point-of-care ultrasound can be used for rapid diagnosis of ascites as it can identify small amounts of free fluid in the abdominal cavity.

    C. Position the infant supine with both legs restrained, such as with a diaper wrapped around the legs. Slightly elevate the flank side you are not using, so the intestines float up to that side and the fluid becomes more dependent.

    D. Choose the site for paracentesis. The area between the umbilicus and the pubic bone is not generally used because of the risk of bladder or intestinal perforation. The sites most frequently used are the right and left flanks. A good rule is to draw a line from the umbilicus to the anterior superior iliac spine and plan to use the area two-thirds of the way from the umbilicus to the anterior superior iliac spine (Figure 40–1).

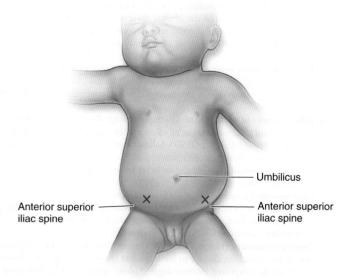

FIGURE 40–1. Recommended sites for abdominal paracentesis noted by the Xs.

E. **Point-of-care ultrasound.** Static technique can be used to localize the intraabdominal fluid and to identify landmarks to determine the optimal location of the needle. Dynamic technique uses real time imaging to show the direct trajectory of the needle to assist with fluid sampling. Use of POCUS in adults has not only helped with the decision for the need of procedure, but it also improves the success rate and lessens the adverse events. Studies evaluating POCUS for paracentesis in pediatrics are lacking (see Chapter 44).

F. **Prepare the area with povidone-iodine in a circular fashion,** starting at the puncture site. Put on sterile gloves, and drape the area. Perform a "time-out" per unit protocol.

G. **Pain management.** Topical anesthetic (eutectic mixture of lidocaine and prilocaine [EMLA]) can be used if the procedure is not emergent, or the area can be infiltrated with a tuberculin needle (skin to peritoneum) with lidocaine 0.5% to 1%. Use nonpharmacologic pain prevention (eg, oral sucrose or breastmilk) if possible.

H. **Connect the 10- to 20-mL syringe to the catheter and needle assembly.** If using an Angiocath with an auto-retractable needle, the syringe is connected to the catheter after the needle is retracted.

I. **Insert the needle at the selected site** (Section III.D). To minimize persistent fluid leak, aim the needle toward the back at a 45-degree angle and use a **Z-track technique.** Displace the cutaneous tissue 0.5 to 1 cm caudad from its original placement over the deeper tissues. Then insert the needle perpendicular to the skin; when the catheter is withdrawn at the end of the procedure, the cutaneous and peritoneal insertion sites will not align.

J. **Advance the needle, gently aspirating until fluid appears in the barrel of the syringe or until a flash is seen in the Angiocath.** Hold the assembly steady and remove the needle. Aspirate the contents slowly with the syringe and stopcock connected to the catheter. It may be necessary to reposition the catheter to obtain an adequate amount of fluid. Once the necessary amount of fluid is taken (usually 5–10 mL for tests and at least 10–15 mL if aiding ventilation), remove the catheter. **If too much fluid is removed, or it is removed too rapidly, hypotension may result.** If there is no fluid, the catheter could be attached to the intestine or in the retroperitoneum; reposition, withdraw, or remove the catheter and retry. If air is aspirated and there was no pneumoperitoneum, it usually means you have entered a hollow viscus and you need to withdraw the needle. If bright red blood is aspirated, it may mean an artery was punctured.

K. **Cover the site with a sterile gauze pad until leakage has stopped.**

L. **Distribute the fluid in containers as needed for testing.** Examples include complete blood count and differential, Gram stain and culture, protein, albumin, triglycerides, cholesterol, bilirubin, glucose, electrolytes, creatinine, inclusion bodies and treponemes, sialic acid, and amylase.

M. **Ascitic fluid analysis and appearance**
1. **Gross appearance of the fluid.**
   a. **Translucent or straw colored sterile fluid:** Normal fluid.
   b. **Brown with debris:** Fecal matter, bacteria, and white blood cells suggests intestinal perforation. Dark brown fluid may indicate biliary ascites.
   c. **Bloody (hemorrhagic) fluid:** Organ trauma, a ruptured internal organ, or from a traumatic tap.
   d. **Milky appearance (if the infant is being orally fed); otherwise, it is usually straw colored or cloudy:** Suggests chylous ascites.
   e. **Cloudy, turbid color:** Suggests infection.
2. **Analysis of fluid:**
   a. **Gram stain positive for bacteria:** Suggests perforation or peritonitis.
   b. **Elevated creatinine level (ascites creatinine > serum creatinine):** Urinary ascites.
   c. **Elevated bilirubin:** Biliary or intestinal leak.

    d. Elevated triglycerides and lymphocyte predominance (>75%): Suggests chylous ascites. Triglyceride levels may be low if the infant has never been fed.

    e. Elevated amylase and lipase: Suggests pancreatic ascites.

    f. Elevated serum-to-ascites albumin gradient >1.1 g/dL: Suggests hepatocellular disease (hepatitis, α_1-antitrypsin deficiency).

    g. Values consistent with infusate (check for glucose): Iatrogenic fluid or total parenteral nutrition ascites.

    h. Inclusion bodies: Congenital infections (CMV, tuberculosis, toxoplasmosis).

    i. Treponemes: Syphilis.

    j. Sialic acid: Infantile free sialic acid storage disease.

IV. Complications

    A. Cardiovascular effects. Hypotension, tachycardia, and decreased cardiac output can occur. Hypotension can be caused by removing too much fluid or removing fluid too rapidly.

    B. Infection. The risk of peritonitis is minimized by using strict sterile technique.

    C. Perforation of a viscus. To help prevent perforation, use the shortest needle possible and take careful note of landmarks (see Section III.D). If perforation occurs, broad-spectrum antibiotics may be indicated with close observation for signs of infection. Usually the puncture site heals spontaneously. **Perforation of the bladder** is normally self-limited and requires no specific treatment.

    D. Persistent peritoneal fluid leak. The Z-track technique (see Section III.I) helps prevent the persistent leakage of fluid. Leaks may have to be bagged to quantify the volume. Apply pressure over the site or apply a pressure dressing, and monitor the site.

    E. Pneumoperitoneum. Observation is usually required (see Figure 12–25 for a radiograph of a pneumoperitoneum).

    F. Bleeding. Severe bleeding from the liver or intra-abdominal vessels may require emergency surgery consultation. An **abdominal wall hematoma** can occur but is usually self-limiting. Correct abnormal clotting factors if necessary.

    G. Scrotal swelling. Occurs in males with extravasation of ascitic fluid between body wall layers and is usually self-limiting.

41 Pericardiocentesis

I. Indications

    A. Emergency evacuation of air or fluid from the pericardial space in the **treatment of cardiac tamponade** (inability of the heart to expand with decreased stroke volume and cardiac output) and hemodynamic instability caused by **pericardial effusion** (accumulation of excess fluid in the pericardial space) or **pneumopericardium** (accumulation of air in pericardial space). Early recognition and intervention are paramount and can be lifesaving because mortality can be high (up to 67%).

        1. Cardiac tamponade secondary to a pericardial effusion. A rare but life-threatening complication of central venous catheters, including PICC and UVC. Incidence is 1% to 3%. Etiology is unclear, but proposed causes include a direct puncture of a vessel or myocardium (areas of weakness and incomplete muscularization may occur in neonates) by the catheter tip during insertion or delayed perforation secondary to erosion of the cardiac or vascular wall. **Keep a high index of clinical suspicion in a neonate who has a central line and suddenly has**

cardiovascular collapse that does not respond to resuscitation or has resistance to external cardiac compressions and has no air leak by thoracic transillumination. Possible signs include hypotension, tachycardia, decreased/diminished heart signs, poor perfusion, decreasing arterial saturation, decreased heart sounds, increased jugular venous pressure (very difficult to assess in an infant), pulseless electrical activity with a central line, and pulsus paradoxus (a drop in systolic blood pressure >10 mm Hg during inspiration seen on blood pressure waveform and on echocardiography). The **Beck triad** (hypotension, increased jugular venous pressure, and distant heart sounds) is described in cardiac tamponade. Pericardial effusion is more common with lines in the right atrium; the median time to occurrence is 3 days after catheter insertion (range, 0–37 days). A chest radiograph may not be diagnostic; an echocardiogram is, but may delay treatment. *Note:* Pericardial effusion and cardiac tamponade can occur with a central venous catheter in the correct position. It is felt that total parenteral nutrition (especially intralipid) permeates into the interstitium and into the pericardial sac.

2. **Cardiac tamponade secondary to a pneumopericardium.** Rare but very dangerous, and usually occurs with other air leak syndromes, severe lung pathology, a history of vigorous resuscitation, and/or a history of assisted ventilation. **Early recognition (see signs above) and intervention are important. A chest radiograph can be diagnostic with lucency around the cardiac border.** (See Figure 12–21)

B. **To obtain pericardial fluid for diagnostic studies** in cases of **pericardial effusion.** Pericardial effusion is rare in neonates and most commonly occurs in a hydropic or septic infant. Other causes include thyroid dysfunction, cardiac and pericardial tumors (intrapericardial mixed germ cell tumor and intrapericardial teratoma have been reported in infants), congenital anomalies (diaphragmatic hernia/eventration, ruptured ventricular diverticulum), postoperative, and idiopathic.

II. **Equipment.** Antiseptic solution (eg, povidone-iodine solution, chlorhexidine); sterile gloves; gown; sterile drapes; a safety-engineered, 22- or 24-gauge, 1-inch catheter-over-needle assembly; 21- or 23-gauge butterfly needles; extension tubing (if catheter to be left indwelling); 10-mL syringe; 3-way stopcock; lidocaine; underwater seal if the catheter is to be left indwelling; telemetry; fiberoptic light for transillumination (pneumopericardium); portable ultrasound device.

III. **Procedure.** *Note:* **If a central venous catheter is in place and a pericardial effusion is suspected, stop infusion of fluids into the catheter immediately.**

A. **Contraindications.** There are no absolute contraindications for this procedure in the case of a cardiac tamponade. For a diagnostic pericardiocentesis, a coagulopathy may be a contraindication.

B. **This is a 2- or 3-person procedure.** Three people are preferred, but 2 are able to do it. One will insert the needle, 1 will operate the stopcock, and 1 will monitor telemetry for any changes in the cardiac rhythm during the procedure.

IV. **Point-of-care ultrasound of the heart. (See Chapter 44.)** Ideally, pericardiocentesis is performed with the help of ultrasound because it can determine the site and angle of entry, allow an estimation of necessary needle depth, and can be used in real time imaging to aid in the procedure to reduce complications. Use of ultrasound for pericardiocentesis is supported by adult literature but use of POCUS for pericardiocentesis in pediatric literature is extremely limited and based on case reports. With a pneumopericardium, **thoracic transillumination** may be helpful to diagnose and monitor air evacuation while the procedure is done. **With sudden cardiovascular collapse, time does not allow these tests, and an immediate lifesaving aspiration is necessary.** In these cases, a quick betadine prep followed by a "blind" needle insertion with aspiration is necessary.

A. **Monitor electrocardiogram and vital signs.**

B. **Prep the area (xiphoid and precordium) with antiseptic solution.** Wash hands, put on sterile gloves and gown, and drape the area, leaving the xiphoid and a 2-cm circular area around it exposed.

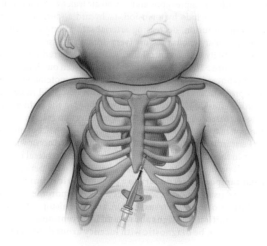

FIGURE 41–1. Recommended site for pericardiocentesis.

C. **Pain management.** If time permits, local anesthesia can be administered (0.25–1 mL of 1% lidocaine subcutaneously). A narcotic/analgesic drug can also be given.

D. **Prepare the needle assembly. There are 2 methods:**
   1. **Attach the catheter-over-needle** to a short piece of extension tubing that is attached to a 3-way stopcock. Attach a syringe to the stopcock. More common method used.
   2. **Use a 22- to 24-gauge needle or butterfly attached directly to a syringe** (no cannula is placed; when fluid or air can no longer be aspirated, the needle is removed). Used in extreme emergencies when time does not permit other set up.

E. **Identify the site where the needle is to be inserted.** Most commonly, approximately 0.5 cm to the left of and just below the infant's xiphoid (left sternocostal margin) (Figure 41–1).

F. **Insert the needle at about a 30- to 45-degree angle (smaller degree angle for lower gestational age), aiming toward the midclavicular line on the left.** The 3-way stopcock is closed to the syringe and needle during the initial insertion. After insertion, the assistant should then open the 3-way stopcock to the needle and syringe. The needle should then be advanced toward the left shoulder while the assistant applies constant suction on the syringe until fluid or air is obtained.

G. **Monitor the infant with telemetry** to check for any changes in the cardiac rhythm while advancing the needle and during aspiration. If any ectopic beats occur, stop advancing or withdrawing air and retract the needle slightly. If ectopy continues, stop the procedure and remove the needle.

H. **Stop advancing once air or fluid is obtained (depending on which is to be evacuated).** Advance the cannula over the needle, remove the needle from the catheter, and reconnect the cannula to the extension tubing. If using a butterfly needle, connect the cannula to the extension tubing.

I. **Withdraw as much air or fluid as possible.** The goal is to relieve the symptoms or obtain sufficient fluid for laboratory studies. Once there is no more fluid or air that can be aspirated, the needle can be removed or an indwelling catheter can be left in place.

J. **If an indwelling catheter is to be left in place (depends on the likelihood of reaccumulation)**, secure it with tape and attach the tubing to continuous suction (10–15 cm H_2O).

K. **Obtain a chest radiograph or echocardiogram/ultrasound.** Confirm the position of the catheter and/or the effectiveness of drainage. Transillumination can also be done.

V. **Complications**

A. **Cardiac puncture/perforation.** Grossly bloody fluid may indicate that the needle punctured the heart, which can be avoided by advancing the needle only far enough to obtain fluid or air. **Ultrasound guidance** is recommended if time permits. **Another technique to avoid puncturing the heart (if ultrasound is not available)** is to attach the electrocardiogram (ECG) anterior chest lead to the needle with an alligator clip. If changes are seen on the ECG (eg, ectopic beats, changes in the ST segment (elevation), increase in the QRS voltage), the needle has contacted the myocardium and should be withdrawn. Most needle perforations heal spontaneously. If cardiac perforation occurs, emergency intervention and cardiac surgeon consultation are needed.

B. **Pneumothorax or hemothorax.** Higher risk if landmarks are not used and "blind" punctures are done. If this complication occurs, a chest tube on the affected side is usually needed.

C. **Infection.** Strict sterile technique minimizes the risk of infection.

D. **Arrhythmias.** Usually transient. Repositioning the needle is usually effective, but with persistent arrhythmia, treatment may be necessary.

E. **Hemorrhage.** Bleeding is usually superficial and controlled with pressure. Hepatic puncture can occur.

F. **Hypotension.** May occur if a significant amount of fluid is drained. A fluid bolus may be necessary.

G. **Pneumomediastinum.** Only observation is required.

H. **Pneumopericardium.** Treat as above.

42 Peripheral Intravenous Extravasation and Infiltration: Initial Management

I. **Indication.** To manage and minimize the initial injury resulting from infiltration of intravenous (IV) fluids or medications into tissue. Infiltration rates are high among neonates (up to 70%), with extravasation occurring in up to 23%. Risk factors associated with a higher risk of complications within 48 hours after puncture were: endotracheal intubation, total parenteral nutrition, blood transfusion, other medications, presence of infection, body weight at the day of insertion, and type of infusion (intermittent vs continuous).

A. **Infiltration** refers to the leakage of **nonvesicant** (nonirritating) fluid from a catheter into the surrounding tissues. Infiltrates are usually benign unless a large amount of fluid causes compression of nerves or compartment syndrome. Typically involves routine IV solutions.

B. **Extravasation** refers to the inadvertent leakage of **vesicants** (highly caustic fluid or medication that is capable of causing tissue necrosis) from a catheter into the surrounding tissues; this can occur from displacement of the catheter or increased vascular permeability. Common vesicants include total parenteral nutrition (TPN), potassium, bicarbonate, and high-dextrose concentrates. Extravasation can cause a mild skin reaction, severe tissue necrosis, or an injury so severe it leads to surgical intervention, including amputation.

II. **Procedures**

A. **Prevention of extravasation and infiltration should be the goal.** This strategy includes frequent monitoring of puncture sites, appropriate infusion rates for the size of the catheter, and prompt evaluation if concerns of infiltration exist. Implementation of an IV infiltration management program or evidence-based guideline and checklist for IV infiltrate injuries was found to be effective in decreasing the IV infiltration rate and increasing the rate of early detection of infiltration. Cochrane review found insufficient evidence to recommend a single dressing or securement method over another for peripheral IVs and percutaneously inserted central catheters to prevent complications. Another consideration for prevention is to minimize vesicant administration through peripheral catheters as opposed to central lines.

B. **Initial treatment is determined by the stage of the infiltration/extravasation, the type of solution, and the availability of specific antidotes.** There is a lack of conclusive evidence regarding optimal care after IV extravasation in the newborn. Available literature is primarily anecdotal or descriptive case reports. A staging system has been proposed that provides guidance concerning the appropriate initial treatment options (Table 42–1). This chapter refers only to initial management and not to the management of long-term complications (scarring, tissue loss, vascular compromise).

Table 42–1. STAGING OF IV INFILTRATES[a]

Stage	Description	Treatment Options[a]
I	Painful IV site No redness or swelling Catheter flushes with difficulty	1. Remove intravenous (IV) cannula. 2. Elevate extremity.
II	Painful IV site Redness and light swelling (0%–20%)	1. Remove IV cannula. 2. Elevate extremity.
III	Painful IV site Moderate swelling (30%–50%) Blanching Skin cool to touch, but with good pulse and brisk capillary refill below infiltration site	1. Leave IV cannula in place. Using 1-mL syringe, aspirate as much fluid as possible. 2. Remove cannula unless it is needed for administration of an antidote. 3. Elevate extremity. 4. Consider antidote (eg, hyaluronidase, phentolamine).
IV	Painful IV site Severe swelling (>50%) Blanching Skin cool to touch Decreased or absent pulse Delayed capillary refill >4 seconds Skin breakdown, blistering, or necrosis	1. Leave cannula in place. Using 1-mL syringe, aspirate as much fluid as possible. 2. Remove cannula unless needed for administration of antidote. 3. Elevate extremity. 4. Consider antidote. 5. If site is tense with swelling and skin is blanched, use multiple needle puncture technique (see Section II.D).

[a]Data from Millam D. Managing complications of IV therapy. *Nursing.* 1988;18:34-43; and Thigpen JL. Peripheral intravenous extravasation: nursing procedure for initial treatment. *Neonatal Netw.* 2007;26(6):379-384.

C. **Specific antidotes**
1. **Hyaluronidase.** Indicated for high osmotic solutions and drugs such as high-dextrose solutions, TPN, blood, calcium, penicillin, nafcillin, methicillin, potassium chloride, and vancomycin.
   a. **Appropriate for stage III extravasation of IV fluids** except vasoconstrictors.
   b. **Administer within 1 hour** after insult if possible, and no later than 3 hours.
   c. **Clean area with antimicrobial agent** and maintain aseptic conditions.
   d. **Inject 1 mL (150 U) as 5 separate 0.2-mL subcutaneous injections** around the periphery of the extravasation site. Change the needle after each injection.
   e. **Cover with hydrogel dressing** (IntraSite; Smith and Nephew, Andover MA) and elevate for 48 hours.
2. **Saline irrigation is suggested to help prevent further damage in stage III or IV extravasation,** although no randomized control data exist on the intervention. When saline injection is performed, it can be done alone or following the injection of hyaluronidase. A Cochrane review (2017) states the following: "Saline irrigation is frequently reported in the literature as an intervention. No randomized controlled trials have examined the effects of saline irrigation with or without prior hyaluronidase infiltration for management of extravasation injury in neonates."
   a. **If done in conjunction with hyaluronidase injection,** perform saline irrigation soon after hyaluronidase.
   b. **Make 4 to 5 small stab incisions around the periphery;** if hyaluronidase was injected, these sites can serve as the stab incision sites.
   c. **Infiltrate the subcutaneous tissue where extravasation occurred** with aliquots of up to 50 mL of normal saline. This allows saline and diluted extravasate to exit the stab incisions and flush out the area.
   d. **Promote further fluid removal by massaging area,** followed by elevation for 24 to 48 hours.
3. **Phentolamine (Regitine)**
   a. **The drug of choice for extravasation of dopamine and other vasoconstrictors** (eg, norepinephrine, epinephrine, dobutamine). It is an α-adrenergic blocking agent that decreases local vasoconstriction and ischemia (US Food and Drug Administration label for use as an antihypertensive).
   b. **Clean area with antimicrobial agent** and maintain aseptic technique.
   c. **Inject a 0.5-mg/mL solution subcutaneously into the affected area.** Usual amount needed is 1 to 5 mL, depending on size of infiltrate. May repeat if necessary.
4. **Topical nitroglycerin.** This agent promotes local vasodilation, which improves perfusion to the area.
   a. **Effective treatment for extravasation of dopamine.**
   b. **Clean area with antimicrobial agent** and maintain aseptic technique.
   c. **Apply 2% nitroglycerine ointment** (4 mm/kg) to area. May repeat every 8 hours if necessary.
D. **Multiple needle puncture technique**
1. **May be used to create an avenue for fluid to escape** and help to minimize tissue damage.
2. **Clean with antimicrobial agent** and maintain aseptic technique.
3. **Using a 20-gauge needle, puncture the skin subcutaneously** multiple times in the affected area. Change the needle after each puncture.
4. **Cover with saline-soaked gauze** to absorb the fluid, and elevate the extremity.
5. **Evaluate** every 1 to 2 hours for 48 hours.

III. **Complications.** Initial management may cause the following:
A. **Infection.** Use strict aseptic technique during injections.
B. **Trauma to site.** Handle skin gently; remove skin disinfectant with sterile saline pad.
C. **Hypotension.** Could potentially occur with a large dose of phentolamine or with absorption of topical nitroglycerin.

43 Therapeutic Hypothermia

Therapeutic hypothermia (TH) is now the gold standard treatment for infants with moderate to severe hypoxic ischemic encephalopathy, whereby the infant's core body temperature is decreased within 6 hours after birth followed by slow rewarming for neuroprotection. This treatment slows the metabolic rate so cells can recover and prevent further damage. Neonatal encephalopathy can be due to different causes; care providers should take careful assessment of possible etiologies because this could lead to specific therapy that may improve prognosis. When a clear diagnosis of hypoxia-ischemia is known to be the reason for moderate to severe encephalopathy, TH is implemented if the infant meets the criteria. It has been shown to improve survival and outcome and reduce the risk of death or major neurodevelopmental disability at 18 months of age with data suggesting that the long term benefits resulted in improved neurocognitive outcomes persisting into middle childhood. The benefits of cooling outweigh the short-term risks related to hypothermia. Published hypothermia protocols have consistently used gestational age of at least ≥36 weeks at birth to qualify for TH and starting treatment within the first 6 hours after birth with systemic temperatures between 33°C and 35°C and continuing treatment for a total of 72 hours. Deviating from this protocol is not recommended as it may result in an increase in adverse outcomes; longer or deeper hypothermia showed an increase in mortality. **Cooling infants who are <36 weeks' gestation is not recommended because of insufficient evidence to evaluate risks and benefit in this patient population.** The best benefit of TH is when it is started before 6 hours of life, but there may be a small benefit and low risk for infants with moderate HIE who have it started between 6 and 24 hours of life. A Cochrane review provided evidence from 11 randomized controlled trials (n = 1505 infants) that TH is beneficial in term and late preterm newborns with moderate to severe HIE.

There are 2 types of cooling, **selective head cooling (SHC)** and **whole-body cooling (WBC), which is more common. Selective head cooling** is done by using a cooling cap that circulates cold water that is placed on the infant's head to lower the core temperature. **Whole body cooling** is done by using a cooling blanket or different types of wraps or mattresses that circulate cold water that is placed under the baby to lower the total body temperature. Both methods have been shown to be effective, and several recent studies showed no significant differences in adverse effects, neuromotor development at 12 months, or mortality rate between SHC and WBC when treating HIE. Further trials to determine the appropriate cooling technique are necessary to better understand the advantage of WBC versus SHC. Some neonatal intensive care units (NICUs) prefer using WBC because it is easier to administer and allows one to perform electroencephalogram monitoring on the infant. It is recommended that application of TH should only be done by following published guidelines. **The protocol discussed in this chapter is based on WBC published by Shankaran et al** (*New England Journal of Medicine,* 2005).

I. **Indication.** Treatment of newborn infants who fulfill the criteria for diagnosis of moderate to severe HIE (see Chapter 110).

II. **Eligibility for therapeutic hypothermia.** Newborn infants ≥36 weeks' gestation admitted to NICU for perinatal depression should be sequentially evaluated for eligibility for TH by clinical and physiologic criteria followed by complete neurologic examination.

A. **Clinical and physiologic criteria**

1. **Blood gas pH of ≤7.0 or base deficit of ≥16 mmol/L** in a sample of umbilical cord blood or any blood during the first hour after birth; proceed to step B.

2. **Blood pH of 7.0 to 7.15 or base deficit of 10 to 15.9 mmol/L** *plus* **history of an acute perinatal event*** *and* **Apgar score of <5 at 10 minutes** *or* **continued need for assisted ventilation for at least 10 minutes; proceed to step B.** (*Examples of acute perinatal event include abruption placenta, cord prolapse, severe fetal heart rate abnormality, variable or late decelerations, maternal trauma, hemorrhage, or cardiorespiratory arrest.)

Table 43-1. SIGNS OF MODERATE OR SEVERE ENCEPHALOPATHY

Category	Moderate Encephalopathy	Severe Encephalopathy
Level of consciousness	Lethargic	Stupor/coma
Spontaneous activity	Decreased activity	No activity
Posture	Distal flexion, full extension	Decerebrate
Tone	Hypotonia (focal, general)	Flaccid
Primitive reflexes		
Suck	Weak	Absent
Moro	Incomplete	Absent
Autonomic system		
Pupils	Constricted	Skew deviation/dilated/nonreactive
Heart rate	Bradycardia	Variable heart rate
Respirations	Periodic breathing	Apnea

    B. **Complete neurologic examination.** Once infant meets clinical and physiologic criteria, **a complete standardized neurologic examination is to be performed.** Moderate to severe encephalopathy is defined as seizures or presence of 1 or more signs in 3 of the 6 categories in staging of HIE. The number of moderate or severe signs will determine the extent of encephalopathy; if signs were equally distributed, the designation is based on the level of consciousness.

      1. **If seizure is documented or reported, infant is automatically eligible for cooling.**

      2. **If no seizure is documented or reported,** infant has to have at least 3 of 6 signs of moderate or severe encephalopathy to be eligible for cooling (Table 43-1).

III. **Equipment (Whole-Body Cooling)**

    A. **Hyper-hypothermia machine** used to raise or lower a patient's temperature to a target level through conductive heat transfer. Use 2 to 3 gallons of distilled water for initial setup.

    B. **Infant-size hyper-hypothermia blanket.** A single-patient use blanket to provide both heating and cooling to maintain patient's target temperature. (**Note:** Low cost alternatives such as ice packs, frozen gel packs, and phase changing materials can be used in resource limited settings and is beneficial, but require careful monitoring to avoid temperatures outside the therapeutic range.)

    C. **Infant esophageal probe and cable.** Allows continuous monitoring of patient's core temperature while on the hyper-hypothermia machine. (Some centers use rectal temperature probes.)

    D. **Drainage hose.** Use to drain water from the hyper-hypothermia machine.

    E. **Available open infant radiant warmer bed with warming capability** at the conclusion of the TH period.

IV. **Procedure**

    A. **Confirm eligibility** for hypothermia therapy, per Section II.

    B. **Pain management.** There is no specific recommendation for sedation and pain control during cooling; however, based on the author's experience, low-dose morphine or fentanyl drip has been effective in keeping the infant comfortable during the cooling process. Close monitoring for evidence of respiratory depression in patients who are not intubated is recommended.

    C. **Gather equipment.** Follow preparation instructions of the hyper-hypothermia machine per operation manual.

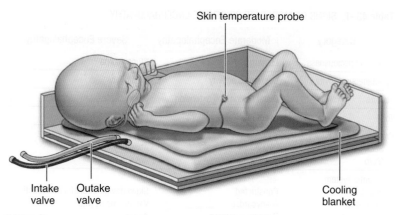

Skin temperature probe

Intake valve   Outake valve   Cooling blanket

FIGURE 43–1. Whole-body cooling hypothermia patient setup.

D. **Precool the blanket to 5°C for whole-body cooling to maintain an esophageal temperature of 33.5°C ± 5°C.** Lay infant supine on the precooled blanket with occiput resting on the blanket. A single-layer thin blanket may be placed between the infant and the cooling blanket to prevent soiling of equipment (Figure 43–1).

E. **Insert the esophageal temperature probe into an external naris.** Probe may be softened by placing in warm water for a few minutes. The probe should be positioned in the lower third of the esophagus (desired length = distance from nares to ear to the mid-sternum minus 2 cm). Secure the probe by taping with adhesive to the side of the infant's nose. Connect the probe to the cooling unit. Confirm probe placement with a radiograph. However, do not wait for a radiograph; connect the probe to the cooling unit and begin temperature monitoring straight away. Some recommend a **rectal temperature sensor.** Measure and mark the sensor, lubricate the tip, insert the rectal probe 5 to 6 cm into the rectum, and secure to the buttocks with tape.

F. **Use an open radiant warmer bed for optimal monitoring.** Skin temperature will be monitored by skin temperature probe on the lower abdomen attached to the radiant warmer. The radiant warmer is set to "manual mode" with the heat turned off (allows for continuous skin temperature monitoring without any heat output from the warmer). Do not use any other source of exogenous heat.

G. **Operate the cooling unit in automatic mode** with a core temperature goal of 33.5°C ± 0.5°C (follow your NICU-specific cooling unit instruction manual).

H. **The infant's esophageal temperature will begin to decrease soon after the initiation of the cooling therapy.** The cooling blanket system adjusts automatically to achieve 33.5°C by approximately 90 to 120 minutes. Once stable at 33.5°C, some esophageal temperature fluctuation around the setpoint is to be expected, but should not be greater than ± 0.5°C. Monitor and record esophageal, skin, and water temperatures, as well as all vital signs at 15-minute intervals during cooling (or follow unit-specific policy). **Total period of cooling is 72 hours.**

I. **Gradual rewarming is done over 6 hours after completion of 72-hour cooling period.** The automatic cooling unit setpoint temperature is increased by 0.5°C every hour to maximum setpoint of 36.5°C. The goal is to slowly increase the temperature by 0.5°C per hour to reach normothermia by the end of 6 hours. Smaller or sicker infants may require a longer period to reach normothermia. Monitor vital signs (especially temperature) throughout the rewarming period. **Hyperthermia must be avoided.** New-onset or rebound seizures have been reported during and after rewarming.

J. **When normothermia is achieved, turn off hyper-hypothermia unit and remove cooling blanket and esophageal probe.** Return to temperature maintenance per local NICU protocol.

K. **During the cooling and rewarming process,** infant should receive routine clinical care appropriate for the level of acuity, including laboratory blood studies for surveillance of respiratory, cardiovascular, hematologic, and renal dysfunction. Blood gas measurements must be corrected for body temperature during hypothermia.

L. **Adjuvant therapies.** The incidence of death and disability with therapeutic hypothermia is approximately 40%. Promising adjunctive therapies to augment therapeutic hypothermia include erythropoietin, melatonin, xenon, 2-iminobiotin, stem cells, and antiepileptic medications. Erythropoietin has shown promise in preliminary studies.

V. **Complications.** The following is a list of potential complications of systemic hypothermia; note that all complications may not be included.

A. **Cardiovascular and respiratory**

1. **Arrhythmia.** Hypothermia can decrease depolarization of cardiac pacemaker cells, causing bradycardia (most common cardiovascular complication). Maintain infant's temperature within the target range of 33.5°C ± 0.5°C to prevent more severe arrhythmias.

2. **Hypotension.** Decreases in stroke volume and heart rate may contribute to the decrease in cardiac output, leading to hypotension.

3. **Pulmonary hypertension.** Increased pulmonary vascular resistance has been reported in hypothermic infants; however, the number of hypoxic-ischemic infants with persistent pulmonary hypertension in large clinical trials was similar between cooled and noncooled infants.

4. **Blood gases.** Hypothermia decreases oxygen consumption and carbon dioxide production; therefore, ventilator settings need to be monitored and adjusted to avoid hyperventilation that can cause cerebral vasoconstriction. **Blood gas values are temperature dependent,** and if blood samples are warmed to 37°C before analysis (as is common in most laboratories), PO_2 and PCO_2 will be overestimated and pH underestimated in hypothermic patients. For accurate blood gas interpretation, blood samples should be analyzed at the patient's real temperature. If this is not possible, the blood gas values assayed at 37°C can be estimated in the following way, as described by Polderman (2009):

   a. **Subtract 5 mm Hg PO_2 per 1°C** that the patient's temperature is <37°C.

   b. **Subtract 2 mm Hg PCO_2 per 1°C** that the patient's temperature is <37°C.

   c. **Add 0.012 pH units per 1°C** that the patient's temperature is <37°C.

B. **Dermatologic**

1. **Skin breakdown.** Vasoconstriction during extreme cold can lead to decreased blood flow and localized damage to skin and other tissues. Regular inspection of the infant's skin is part of routine care during cooling.

2. **Subcutaneous fat necrosis.** The cause of subcutaneous fat necrosis is unknown. It has been associated with perinatal asphyxia. Hypothermia causes vasocontriction that worsens skin perfusion that has already been compromised by asphyxia, thereby leading to fat necrosis. Most of the reported cases occurred after completion of cooling. Serum calcium levels have to be monitored in affected infants due to risk of hypercalcemia.

C. **Hematologic.** Serial follow-up of hematologic parameters is an important part of surveillance during hypothermia therapy.

1. **Hypothermia-induced thrombocytopenia** is due to **increased platelet destruction** (platelet sequestration in the liver and spleen) and **disseminated intravascular coagulopathy** resulting in early thrombocytopenia and bone marrow suppression.

2. **Coagulopathy induced by mild hypothermia** with the risk of severe bleeding associated with TH is small.

D. Metabolic
   1. Metabolic acidosis. Decreased cardiac output leading to reduced clearance of lactic acid.
   2. Altered glucose metabolism. Hypothermia decreases insulin sensitivity and secretion, leading to hyperglycemia; higher doses of insulin maybe needed. During rewarming, infants treated with insulin for hyperglycemia may be at risk for hypoglycemia as sensitivity to insulin is restored.
   3. Drug metabolism and excretion of drugs and metabolites might be modified by cooling, as well as the presence of hepatocellular and renal impaiment complicating HIE. Metabolism of drugs such as phenobarbital, morphine, and vecuronium is slowed by effects of the temperature-dependent hepatic cytochrome P450 enzyme system. **Potentially toxic levels of drugs can accumulate in the system if metabolism and excretion are impaired.** Check antibiotic levels if being used.
E. Infections. Cooling has immunosuppressive and anti-inflammatory effects. Meta-analysis of large trials did not show any increase in incidence of infection in cooled infants.

44 Transillumination and Point-of-Care Ultrasound

Transillumination and point-of-care ultrasound (POCUS) are techniques that can be used as an aid in performing procedures, to diagnose specific conditions, and to help in clinical decision making. Both **transillumination and POCUS** can be performed at the bedside, require no sedation, and have no significant complications. Although transillumination has been around since 1831 (Richard Bright's first description using a candlelight to shine through the head of a macrocephalic adult and diagnose hydrocephalus), it has only been used in neonatology since the 1970s. The first ultrasound studies can be traced back to 1794, but diagnostic ultrasound did not enter medicine until the 1950s. The first portable ultrasound unit was initially developed in 1988 to help identify and diagnose serious injuries in troops in the field. POCUS was used in the late 1990s by emergency room physicians as a trauma screening tool and is now gaining popularity in other medical disciplines.

I. Transillumination
   A. Indications. Transillumination is the use of a strong light source as a noninvasive tool for bedside diagnosis and to aid in procedures. By shining a bright light through an area of the body or an organ, abnormal air, fluid, or a nonsolid mass can be potentially diagnosed. One of the best uses of transillumination in the neonatal care unit is that it can provide a rapid diagnosis in an unstable infant with a tension pneumothorax, pneumopericardium, or abdominal perforation and allow for immediate intervention if necessary. Individuals with deutan color vision (red-green blindness) may have difficulty with transillumination techniques.
     1. Procedures
       a. Localize an artery or vein for vessel cannulation or blood sampling.
       b. Bladder aspiration. Verify the presence of urine in the bladder and show the size and location of the bladder.
       c. Cannulation of umbilical vessels. Identify the path of vessels and identify a false passage of an umbilical catheter.

    d. Aid in oro-/nasoduodenal feeding tube insertion by gauging distension of stomach with air.

    e. Thoracentesis, chest tube thoracostomy, or pericardiocentesis. Document the success of air removal in a pneumothorax or in a pneumopericardium.

  2. **Diagnosis.** Air, fluid, or nonsolid masses light up brightly when transilluminated, whereas solid masses appear dark. Normally there is a 2-cm area of lucency around the probe. If there is >2 cm lucency, it is considered abnormal, and further testing may have to be done.

    a. Chest abnormalities. Air leaks (eg, pneumothorax, pneumomediastinum, and pneumopericardium) can be suspected and some diagnosed with transillumination. The thin wall of the infant's chest makes it easy to transilluminate, and as little as 10 mL of free air can be detected. Obtain a baseline on any infant at high risk for an air leak.

    b. Abnormalities in the head such as hydrocephalus, intracranial hemorrhage, subdural effusion or hematoma, skull fractures, hydranencephaly, anencephaly, porencephaly, encephalocele, and large cerebral cysts. Transillumination of the skull is known as **skull diaphanoscopy.**

    c. Differentiate cystic from solid masses such as cystic hygroma, a congenital macrocystic lymphatic malformation commonly found in the left base of the neck.

    d. Abdominal abnormalities such as ascites, distended bowel, pneumoperitoneum, cysts, and perforated bowel in male infants with a patent processus vaginalis.

    e. Genitourinary abnormalities such as distended bladder, hydrocele, hydronephrosis, and cystic kidneys.

    f. Differentiate between a meningocele and meningomyelocele.

B. Equipment. Light source such as mini–light-emitting diode light, high-intensity fiberoptic light source, commercially available transilluminators (eg, Veinlite, TransLite LLC, Sugarland, TX; Pediascan, Sylvan Fiberoptics, Irwin, PA), or otoscope with light; disposable plastic cover or sterile glove to cover light source for aseptic technique; alcohol swab.

C. Procedure. Clinical examination is always necessary with transillumination; transilluminate the contralateral side of the body for comparison.

  1. **Clean end of light source with an alcohol swab** and cover with either a disposable plastic cover or sterile glove. Ensure that it is not hot.

  2. **Turn the lights in the room down to darken the room as much as possible.** Turn on the fiberoptic light at low intensity and increase as needed. Remember to place the tip of the light as firmly as possible.

  3. **Head exam.** Place light on the anterior fontanel; if the light spreads beyond >2 to 2.5 cm in the frontal or parietal area and beyond 1 to 2 cm in the occipital region or asymmetry is noted, this may be abnormal, and further studies are needed. It can imply there is increased fluid or a decrease in brain tissue. There is always a false glow across the suture lines, fontanels, and areas of craniotabes. Transillumination may not be reliable if there is scalp edema, thick black hair, or a bony cortex >2 cm. The light source should be moved around all over the skull.

    a. Increased transillumination

      i. Subdural effusion: Increased supratentorial transillumination.

      ii. Hydrocephalus: Increased supratentorial lucency.

      iii. Hydranencephaly: Entire skull will be transilluminant, or with increased lucency superior to the posterior fossa, entire skull may be transilluminant.

      iv. Porencephalic or leptomeningeal cyst: Focal swelling with increased transillumination.

      v. Caput succedaneum: Diffuse scalp swelling with increased transillumination.

   b. **Decreased transillumination**
       i. **Subgaleal hematoma:** Diffuse scalp swelling with decreased transillumination.
      ii. **Cephalohematoma:** Parietal swelling and decreased transillumination.
     iii. **Subdural hematoma:** Overall decreased transillumination.
   4. **Vessel localization.** Place light source opposite the puncture site (eg, the palm for hand cannulation) so the light goes through to show the vessel. Vessels are dark lines against an illuminated background; arteries are fixed, whereas veins move with the skin.
   5. **Genitourinary system/abdomen**
       a. **Scrotum.** Place the light underneath the scrotum. If the entire scrotum lights up, a collection of fluid (hydrocele or patent processus vaginalis) is likely. The testicles will appear as marble-sized shadows. Particulate matter or gas bubbles in the scrotum suggest intestinal perforation.
       b. **Kidneys/ureter/bladder**
           i. **Kidney.** Place infant on his or her side, and place transilluminator anteriorly over the kidney area with the kidney manipulated against the abdominal wall. Normal kidneys do not transilluminate.
          ii. **Bladder.** Point the transilluminator at the bladder area above the pubic symphysis. The area will glow red if urine is present. The size of the bladder on transillumination correlates with the size on excretory urography.
       c. **Abdomen.** Place the transilluminator in the left paramedian position and direct the probe toward the midline. If the peritoneal cavity glows brightly, suspect a pneumoperitoneum. The falciform ligament can usually be seen as a dark band. In differentiating air from fluid, place the infant in a lateral decubitus position; ascites will light up inferiorly, and free air will light up superiorly.
   6. **Chest**
       a. **Pneumothorax.** Place transilluminator on the anterior chest wall above the nipple, in the axilla, or along the posterior axillary line on the side where air is suspected. Normally, there is approximately a 1-cm ring around the light. In a pneumothorax, the area of lucency is usually >2 cm (sometimes the entire side of the chest). The chest lights up like a "jack-o'-lantern." Compare to the other side of the chest and look for a difference in the amount of transillumination. Note that a small pneumothorax may not be seen. Once a chest tube or pigtail catheter has been inserted, transilluminate the area to verify the air is gone.
       b. **Pneumopericardium.** Place the transilluminator over the third or fourth intercostal space on the left midclavicular line and angle toward the xiphoid process. The pericardium will light up. It will appear as a crown in the lower left chest.
       c. **Pneumomediastinum.** Differentiating between a pneumomediastinum and a pneumothorax is difficult. Cardiac pulsations within the lucent area suggest air in the mediastinum.
       d. **Hydrothorax and chylothorax.** Abnormal accumulations of fluid in the pleural space will light up.
   7. **Spine.** Place the transilluminator on the swelling/sac on the back in the lumbosacral area. In a meningocele, one will not see any nerves, only fluid. When transilluminating the myelomeningocele, nerve roots will be seen floating in the sac.
D. **Complications**
   1. **Burns and thermal blisters from the light source.** Limit light source contact time; burns can also occur from a faulty transillumination device. Contamination from an unclean transilluminator device can cause superficial infections.

    2. **False-positive and false-negative results for pneumothorax.** Limit these by using a sufficiently bright light source and dimming the room lights.

      a. **False positive.** Pneumothorax example: subcutaneous air or edema, pulmonary interstitial emphysema, pneumomediastinum, large stomach air bubble. Very premature infants with thin skin can appear to have a pneumothorax when it is not present (ie, the chest lights up).

      b. **False negative.** Pneumothorax example: small air leak, increased skin thickness, thick/edematous chest wall, darkly pigmented skin, light not bright enough, room not dark enough.

II. **Point-of-care ultrasound (POCUS)** is also called **bedside ultrasound imaging (BUSI), clinical ultrasound (CUS),** or **focused ultrasound**. POCUS in the neonatal intensive care unit (NICU) or newborn nursery is done with a portable ultrasound device to perform a focused ultrasound exam at the bedside to help with a procedure or answer a specific clinical question by a nonradiologist imager (eg, neonatologist). The Society of Point of Care Ultrasound considers it complementary (not adjunctive) to the physical examination because it adds anatomic, functional, and physiologic information. Historically ultrasound use in the NICU has only been done by cardiologists or radiologists. An increasing number of NICUs and providers are becoming familiar with the benefits of POCUS but it still remains underused. Some clinicians have even recommended that it become part of the routine physical examination, with the handheld ultrasound acting as a "visual stethoscope." The American Academy of Pediatrics has already published a policy statement for POCUS for pediatric emergency physicians.

    Premature infants are perfect POCUS candidates because they have less subcutaneous fat and muscle. Providers in certain countries (eg, Canada, United Kingdom, Australia, New Zealand) are already using POCUS in their NICUs. A recent survey validated that neonatal perinatal fellowship programs agree that POCUS is beneficial and neonatology fellows should receive necessary training.

    Advantages of POCUS include timely and accurate diagnosis at the bedside, aid in procedures, acceleration of clinical decisions, and no ionizing radiation exposure; in addition, it is ideal for the nonmobile patient who cannot be transported, can be performed and repeated any time, may decrease unnecessary testing, and also decreases costs compared to other diagnostic modalities.

    Disadvantages of POCUS include lack of training, length of training involved (targeted neonatal echocardiography recommendation is a minimum of 4–6 months), lack of knowledge of ultrasound anatomy, limited penetration through air and bones so deeper structures cannot be seen well, loss of control by radiology, lack of access to ultrasound equipment, paucity of positive impact studies, and medicolegal implications. The potential utility of POCUS in the NICU or newborn nursery includes use in certain procedures and clinical applications. **The majority of these applications and techniques have been based on experience with pediatric emergency POCUS and use in adults, some with very limited studies.** Integration of POCUS into neonatology practice will ultimately depend on multiple factors, including sufficient training and experience and access to ultrasound equipment.

A. **Point-of-care ultrasound indications: Procedure Applications**

    1. **Central and peripheral catheters.** The majority of catheters placed in the NICU are done "blindly." POCUS allows for direct visualization and localization of the vessel and can help guide catheter placement. It can also more accurately confirm the position of the catheter and its tip when compared to radiography. It can result in faster placement, fewer manipulations, decreased complications, and fewer radiographs ordered.

      a. **Umbilical venous catheter.** Umbilical venous catheter (UVC) tip placement is not precise in a typical radiograph. With ultrasound, the UVC can be placed in a perfect position (UVC beyond the inferior vena cava [IVC]–right atrium [RA] junction). Look at subxiphoid long axis below and above the diaphragm and identify location of the hepatic segment of the IVC, hepatic vein, and ductus venosus. Hepatic veins and IVC should not be obstructed.

b. **Peripherally inserted central catheters.** Imaging and assessment are similar to UVC. Upper peripherally inserted central catheter (PICC) line position should be 1 cm before SVC-RA junction; lower PICC position should be at 1 to 2 cm below IVC-RA junction.

c. **Umbilical artery catheter.** Look for umbilical artery catheter (UAC) in the subxiphoid view (best view is subxiphoid long axis view below and above the diaphragm). Identify the tip. Best position is behind the heart in T7–8 position. Doppler ultrasound can be beneficial to examine the aortal and renal vessels.

d. **Peripheral arterial line.** POCUS allows one to locate the artery, and Doppler ultrasound allows one to identify the flow and perform a modified Allen test for collateral flow.

e. **Peripheral venous access.** Ultrasound-guided peripheral intravenous catheter placement is associated with a decreased use of central venous catheter use. It has been referred to as "one stick vascular access." **Static technique:** allows optimal location for needle insertion (mark the skin). **Dynamic technique:** allows direct observation of the needle passing into the vessel.

f. **Intraosseous placement.** POCUS using color Doppler can assess placement of intraosseous needles. After infusion of crystalloid, visualization of color flow in the bone confirms the correct placement of the line.

2. **Endotracheal tube.** POCUS can be used to visualize the anatomic position of the endotracheal tube (ETT) in term and preterm infants through the chest since their sternum is cartilaginous. It compares to radiography.

3. **Bladder/suprapubic aspiration.** Ultrasound of the bladder can be used to determine the size and location of the bladder and the volume of urine in the bladder. A minimum volume of 10 mL of urine on ultrasound is associated with a 90% successful bladder aspiration in children <2 years of age. POCUS can also be used to help guide needle insertion and puncture of the bladder wall and is more successful than a blind suprapubic bladder aspiration in infants <4 months of age. In infants <2 years of age, the urinary bladder index of >2.4 cm^2 correlated with a bladder volume of 2 mL and a successful catheterization. Urinary bladder index is expressed in cm^2 and is determined using the following equation: Anteroposterior diameter of the bladder × Transverse diameter of the bladder.

4. **Bladder catheterization.** Pediatric application of guiding the catheter in bladder catheterization has been used. In infants <2 years of age, ultrasound-directed bladder catheterization is more successful than blind catheterization.

5. **Lumbar puncture.** Typically done as a blind stick, POCUS can be used to identify key landmarks (spinous processes, interspinous spaces, level of conus medullaris) and can help guide needle placement via static or dynamic imaging. It has also been used to identify reasons for a failed lumbar puncture. Studies have found that ultrasound was better when the infant was in a seated position with flexed hip (interspinous space is maximized) versus the lateral decubitus position. Use of an ultrasound may increase the chances of a successful spinal tap because it may identify the best position for the spinal tap, the terminal end of the conus medullaris, the maximum safe depth of the needle, and the appropriate intervertebral space. In fact, one study did an ultrasound evaluation of lumbar spine anatomy and came up with optimal conditions for performing a lumbar puncture (infant sitting with hips flexed, needle entry angle of 65–70 degrees, and a needle insertion depth calculated by the following equation = 2.5 × weight in kg + 6).

6. **Paracentesis.** Identify small amounts of free fluid in the abdominal cavity for ascites. It cannot differentiate different types of fluid. **Static:** identify anatomic landmarks and amount of peritoneal fluid, determine optimal location of needle. **Dynamic:** directly observe needle trajectory into fluid.

7. **Thoracentesis.** POCUS can detect air or fluid in the pleural space and may help with removal (ultrasound-guided thoracentesis). There has been a case report of an ultrasound used to assist with needle aspiration of a spontaneous pneumothorax in a preemie.

8. **Pericardiocentesis.** POCUS can detect the presence of pericardial fluid, assess its significance, and help guide pericardiocentesis. **Static:** identify the location of the effusion and mark area of needle insertion. **Dynamic:** direct visualization of the needle into the pericardial space.

9. **Extracorporeal life support.** Evaluate cannula position and function with ultrasound methods more accurate than chest radiograph. Assess cardiac function, ductal shunting, and presence of atrial communication.

B. **Point-of-care ultrasound indications: Clinical Applications.** To aid in diagnosis and clinical decision making. POCUS should always be combined with a detailed clinical examination.

1. **Head/neck.** Emergency assessment of an intracranial hemorrhage (infant deteriorates and hemorrhage suspected), hydrocephalus, ventriculomegaly, asymmetry of the ventricles, calcifications, early ischemia, periventricular leukomalacia, Doppler assessment of cerebral arteries, determination of change in resistive index in intracranial pressure in infants with hydrocephalus and posthemorrhagic hydrocephalus, and laryngeal ultrasound to assess vocal cord palsy and paralysis.

2. **Heart. Focused cardiac ultrasound (FOCUS)/point-of-care echocardiography is the greatest indication for ultrasound in the NICU. Functional echocardiography** describes the use in the clinical assessment of the hemodynamic status in neonates. **Targeted neonatal echocardiography** is the term used for focused studies. These studies enable monitoring of cardiac function, evaluating murmurs, and obtaining cardiac and hemodynamic information. The following can be evaluated: left ventricular systolic and diastolic function, right ventricular systolic pressure and pulmonary artery pressure, atrial-level shunt, presence of physiologically significant patent ductus arteriosus (hemodynamic significance and effect of treatment), need for and response to inotropic agents, systemic and pulmonary blood flow, organ perfusion, pericardial fluid, left ventricular preload/volume depletion for oliguria, pulmonary hypertension, and coarctation of the aorta. (See consensus statement Targeted Neonatal Echocardiography in the Neonatal Intensive Care Unit: Practice Guidelines and Recommendations for Training in Selected References).

3. **Persistent pulmonary hypertension of the newborn.** Targeted neonatal echocardiography allows assessment of effect of treatment on right ventricular function, pulmonary artery pressures, and shunt directions at atrial and ductal level.

4. **Hypotension not related to structural heart disease.** May help determine the cause and direct management. Evaluate IVC to estimate intravascular volume status; gauge response to fluid boluses and inotropic support.

5. **Abdomen.** Bowel viability assessment: Ultrasound is limited in GI pathology because gas-filled bowel reflects the ultrasound beam.

   a. **Necrotizing enterocolitis.** US can detect a small amount of intramural gas or changes in bowel wall thickness or peristalsis. Able to better detect pneumatosis intestinalis (see small echogenic dots within the bowel wall) and portal venous gas than with x-ray. Can also see intestinal ischemia, bowel wall thickening, abnormal bowel wall perfusion, and reduced peristalsis. US may also aid in diagnosis of perforation and abscess formation (see loculated right lower quadrant mass and intra-abdominal fluid containing debris). Color Doppler can estimate bowel wall perfusion and show loss of blood flow with nonviable bowel.

b. **Intussusception and volvulus.** Ultrasound is the first-choice test for intussusception. In ileocolic intussusception (most common type), one sees a peripheral hypoechoic ring with a central echogenicity (pseudokidney sign). In volvulus, ultrasound can visualize the twisting of the mesenteric vessels.

c. **Hypertrophic pyloric stenosis.** Ultrasound is the gold standard for diagnosis. Diagnosis is based on elongation of pyloric channel >17 mm, anteroposterior diameter of pylorus >12 mm, and wall thickness >2 mm.

d. **Kidney/ureter/bladder.** Evaluate hydronephrosis, calyceal dilatation, renal abnormalities, distended bladder from outlet obstruction, and ascites.

6. **Lung ultrasound** can be used to differentiate normal lung from lung diseases and disorders. Studies suggest lung ultrasound has better sensitivity and specificity than chest x-ray in diagnosing a pneumothorax. It has also been used as a predictor of the need for intubation by seeing a persistence of a white lung in 1 small study. Lung ultrasound is based on the presence or absence of lung sliding, A lines, B lines, lung consolidation, shred sign, B profile lung point, dynamic air/fluid bronchograms, anechoic zone, jellyfish sign, sinusoid sign, or quad sign (see descriptions of these findings in Section II.D.4). **A recent article has published algorithms for lung ultrasound for immediate postnatal respiratory distress and for late-onset neonatal respiratory distress (Kurepa et al, 2018).** Some lung ultrasound examples include the following:

a. **Normal lung findings:** Well-defined A lines, regular pleural line and presence of lung sliding, rare or absent B lines.

b. **Transient tachypnea of the newborn:** Regular pleural line and presence of lung sliding, absent A lines, present B profile with double lung point.

c. **Meconium aspiration syndrome:** Present lung sliding, absent A lines, absent B profile with double lung point.

d. **Pneumothorax (confirmed):** Absent lung sliding, present A lines, present lung point (specific sign of pneumothorax).

e. **Pneumothorax (possible):** Absent lung sliding, present A lines, absent lung point, presence of **stratosphere sign** (barcode sign). Presence of B lines has almost 100% negative predictive value for pneumothorax.

f. **Respiratory distress syndrome:** Absent lung sliding, absent A lines, absent anechoic zone with or without jellyfish sign, sinusoid sign, quad sign, present bilateral/uniform consolidation.

g. **Pneumonia:** Absent lung sliding (25% have this), absent A lines, absent anechoic zone with or without jellyfish sign, sinusoid sign, quad sign, absent bilateral/uniform consolidation, present shred sign and/or dynamic air/fluid bronchograms.

h. **Atelectasis:** Absent lung sliding, absent A lines, absent anechoic zone with or without jellyfish sign, sinusoid sign, quad sign, absent bilateral/uniform consolidation, absent shred sign and/or dynamic air/fluid bronchograms.

i. **Lung edema:** Present lung sliding, absent A lines, present bilateral uniform B profile.

j. **Pleural effusion:** Absent lung sliding, absent A lines, present anechoic zone with or without jellyfish sign, sinusoid sign, quad sign.

k. **Pulmonary hemorrhage:** Lung consolidation with air bronchograms, shred sign, pleural effusion, disappearing A lines.

l. **Bronchopulmonary dysplasia:** Present lung sliding, thick pleural line with scattered small consolidations, possible white lung to coalescent B lines, absent A lines, absent bilateral/uniform B profile.

m. **Amniotic fluid aspiration:** Homogenous pattern of B lines and variable subpleural consolidation alternating with spared areas.

7. **Use in neonatal peripheral intravenous extravasation injuries.** POCUS can provide direct visualization of the skin tissue and therefore may provide a better objective staging of peripheral intravenous extravasation injuries.

8. **Use of cardiopulmonary point-of-care ultrasound in neonatal transport.** Use of cardiopulmonary POCUS before transport helped improve diagnostic accuracy in determining cardiac or respiratory failure in 1 study of critically ill neonates.

C. **Equipment.** Portable ultrasound equipment (SonoSite [FUJIFILM SonoSite, Bothell, WA], Mindray [Mindray North America, Mahwah, NJ], others), ultrasound gel, transducers (also known as probes) or specific neonatal transducers available for specific body areas (eg, neonatal abdominal, neonatal head), high-frequency probes (8–12 MHz; should be available for use in neonates). For imaging neonatal hearts, use an ultrasound system that is two dimensional with M-mode and full Doppler with electrocardiogram tracing.

1. **Ultrasound terms: Echogenicity** is the ability of a tissue to reflect or transmit an ultrasound wave. **Anechoic** (absence of echoes) appears black on screen. **Hypoechoic** (less echogenicity) appears gray on the screen. **Hyperechoic** (more echogenic) appears white on the screen.

2. **Types of transducers/probes:** High-frequency probes penetrate less and produce high-resolution images. Low-frequency probes penetrate more and produce lower resolution images.

   a. **Linear transducers** use high frequency (5–15 MHz) to produce a high-resolution image and are the most commonly used transducers in neonates; they are also used for blood vessel visualization.

   b. **Convex/curved/curvilinear transducers** use low to midrange frequency (2–5 MHz) to visualize deep structures such as transabdominal imaging.

   c. **Phased array transducers** use a low frequency (1–5 MHz) and can be used for cardiac/brain imaging. Phased arrays and 3-dimensional transducers are used for cardiac imaging.

3. **Scanning modes:** Imaging modes commonly used in ultrasound include:

   a. **B or brightness mode(now known as 2D mode):** Most commonly used ultrasound mode; a transducer scans a plane through the body that can be viewed as a two dimensional image on the screen.

   b. **M or motion mode:** A rapid sequence of B mode scans that are in sequence, allowing one to see and measure range of motion. Used for cardiac scanning and lung sliding.

   c. **Doppler mode**

      i. **Color Doppler:** Most common Doppler type; measures mean velocity and direction of flow (most often blood flow) on B-mode image.

      ii. **Power Doppler:** Displays intensity of the Doppler signal by a variation in color; averages flow over multiple frames.

      iii. **Spectral Doppler:** Distinguishes arterial versus venous waveforms.

4. **Knobs on point-of-care ultrasound**

   a. **Gain knob:** Increases or decreases the brightness of returning echoes on the screen. It changes the amount of black, white, or gray on the screen.

   b. **Depth knob:** Adjusts the field of view. Higher depth will get a bigger picture; use lower depth for a more focused picture.

D. **Procedure.** Perform in incubator or radiant warmer. Consider warming the gel. Apply gel to the probe. **Static technique is the use of ultrasound prior to a procedure** to identify anatomy, locate vessels, determine needle placement, determine catheter tips, and help decide if a procedure should be done, but the procedure is performed without the use of ultrasound. **Dynamic technique is the use of ultrasound during the procedure,** where the ultrasound provides direct visualization of the procedure (eg, observe the passage of needle from skin into spinal canal). Most of these procedure techniques have been based on pediatric and adult literature.

1. **Cranial ultrasound.** Look at coronal (front to back), sagittal (left to right), and axial views (posterior fossa). Place a linear transducer over the anterior fontanelle, and visualize the brain in a coronal (sweep beam from anterior to posterior

aspect of head) and sagittal plane (sweep beam from left to right direction). Look at 2 ventricles, and evaluate for hemorrhage, calcifications, or early ischemia. Look at the superior sagittal sinus above the interhemispheric fissure and examine for signs of extra-axial fluid; rule out a subdural hematoma here. For color Doppler: evaluate flow velocities in cerebral arteries and veins.

2. **Cardiac ultrasound.** FOCUS includes evaluation of the heart and IVC. Standard assessment includes views in parasternal short axis, apical 4-chamber windows, subxiphoid, and parasternal short and long axis. Assess the IVC in subxiphoid longitudinal plane. **Dynamic:** use M-mode and measure vessel diameter during inspiration and expiration, view aorta in subxiphoid location, and measure size of aorta during systole.

3. **Abdominal ultrasound.** Use linear probe of 8 to 15 MHz. Look for bowel wall thickening >2.6 mm, portal venous air, pneumatosis intestinalis, free air, intra-abdominal fluid, and an increase in bowel wall echogenicity. Color Doppler can estimate bowel wall perfusion.

4. **Lung ultrasound.** Use high-frequency (≥10 MHz) linear transducer set to lung preset. Orient transducer in a sagittal plane. Examine in supine, lateral, or prone position and examine anterior, lateral, and posterior areas. Scan each lung in the longitudinal and transverse orientation. Scan from clavicles to the diaphragm; use M-mode to confirm the presence or absence of lung sliding. Note that all signs of lung ultrasound arise from the pleural line.

   a. **Normal lung findings.** Air completely scatters the ultrasound waves, and parietal and visceral pleura slide against each other with every respiration. Presence of A lines and lung sliding indicates normal lung with no lung pathology.

      i. **Pleural line** is a curvilinear smooth echogenic line that comes from the reflection of the pleural surface.

      ii. **Lung sliding** is the movement of the parietal against the visceral pleura during respiration. It creates a "**seashore sign,**" indicating a healthy lung.

      iii. **A lines** are horizontal hyperechogenic lines distal to the pleural line that are a demonstration of air below the pleura. They are present in normal lungs and also in a pneumothorax.

      iv. **Bat sign** appears when there are 2 adjacent ribs with shadowing (looks like wings of bat) on top of the pleural line (looks like body of bat).

   b. **Abnormal lung ultrasound findings**

      i. **B lines/B line artifacts** are either unilateral or bilateral vertical lines that are hyperechoic and extend from the pleura to the edge of the screen and do not fade. They erase A lines. They indicate lung fluid. May be normal in infants during the first 48 hours of life, or longer in premature infants, until fluid reabsorbs. The appearance of compact B lines indicates white lung.

      ii. **Lung point** represents the zone between normal (lung sliding) and abnormal (no lung sliding) lung.

      iii. **Double lung point:** The difference in lung echogenicity between the upper lung fields that are improved and the lower lung fields that are still wet.

      iv. **Barcode or stratosphere sign:** The absence of lung sliding in a pneumothorax. There is free air that separates the lung from the pleura that looks like a barcode.

      v. **Lung consolidation:** Appears as a tissue-like density like the liver. It erases both A lines and pleural line. The **shred sign,** an irregular shredded image, is specific for lung consolidation.

      vi. **Air bronchograms** appear as tiny hyperechoic lines.

      vii. **Jellyfish sign:** Seen with pleural effusion when the lung is partially collapsed from fluid; the lung tip flaps freely in the effusion.

      viii. **Sinusoid sign** occurs when the lung moves toward and away from the pleural line with inspiration and expiration and is seen in pleural effusion.

      ix. **Curtain sign** occurs in a pleural effusion during inspiration when the image appears to vanish when the lung expands and is interposed between the probe and the effusion.

      x. **Quad sign** occurs with a pleural effusion; 4 boundaries are as follows: pleural line forms the upper border, lung surface line forms the lower border, and the side borders are shadowing of the ribs.

5. **Vascular access ultrasound:** For peripheral intravenous access, peripheral arterial access, central venous access, umbilical artery and vein placement, and intraosseous placement. Using the linear high-frequency transducer, scan in longitudinal and transverse planes to identify structures, anatomic anomalies, and optimal site of cannulation. Vessels can be cannulated in the short (out of plane; image is perpendicular to the course of vessel) or long (in the plane; image is parallel to the course of the vessel) axis. Differentiates nerves from arteries from veins. Both arteries and veins have an echoic (black) lumen, but arteries have thicker walls that are brighter than veins. Veins are collapsible with compression; arteries are not. Nerves will show internal echoes when the scanning plane is perpendicular to the nerve, and arteries will show arterial pulsations. **Doppler color flow** can also distinguish arteries from veins. **For UAC placement,** flow in aorta should be unobstructed and the antegrade systolic peak pulse wave of velocity should be <1 per second on pulsed Doppler. **For UVC placement,** the UVC is seen passing down the umbilicus recess (echolucent large vessel) and through the ductus venosus. If the UVC is not in the ductus venosus, it is not in the correct position. **For intraosseous placement,** scan distal to the insertion site of the intraosseous needle, and angle it slightly cephalad to intercept the plane of the intraosseous needle.

6. **Bladder ultrasound:** For suprapubic aspiration or urethral catheterization. Use a high-frequency linear-array transducer and apply it in the transverse position in the midline of the abdomen. Image the bladder in the sagittal plane. Note that the bladder is an anechoic structure when filled with urine with the wall appearing as a thin echogenic line. To visualize the entire needle length, introduce the needle into the plane of the ultrasound beam.

    a. **Calculate the urinary bladder index** by measuring the transverse and anteroposterior measurements of the bladder in the transverse plane. Note that the bladder is anechoic, fluid filled, and extends above the pubic symphysis when full.

    b. **Measure the cephalocaudal and anteroposterior diameter of the bladder.** If the cephalocaudal diameter is >20 mm and the anteroposterior diameter is >15 mm, bladder aspiration success rate is near 100%.

7. **Thoracentesis.** Perform static and dynamic technique. Use a linear probe and apply it parallel to the spine on the affected hemithorax. Start at the lower ribs and move the probe toward the head, while looking for the pleural effusion. The pleural effusion will appear dark, whereas the lung tissue will be bright. Verify the pleural effusion by moving the probe parallel inside the intercostal space. Mark the site for needle/chest tube insertion. Site should be on the posterior axillary line. Alternatively, one can scan the hemithorax from the inferior border of the scapula to the upper lumbar region. Evaluate the costophrenic sulcus from the paravertebral region posteriorly to the parasternal region anteriorly. Identify pertinent structures prior to the procedure.

8. **Lumbar puncture.** Estimate landmarks by palpation first. Use a 7- to 15-MHz hockey stick (linear array transducer). Use either the transverse or longitudinal approach. Move the probe up and down the spine. Perform static technique to identify the spinous processes (most superficial bony prominence that is

visualized on ultrasound), interspinous spaces, epidural space, subarachnoid space, and level of conus medullaris. The cerebrospinal fluid is anechoic, the strands of the cauda equine are hyperechoic, and the conus is a hypoechoic tapering structure. Dynamic technique is not well studied in neonates but can help guide the needle into the interspace.

9. **Paracentesis.** Use an 8- to 15-MHz linear probe. Do static and dynamic technique. Examine bilateral upper and lower quadrants, splenorenal and hepatorenal spaces, and pelvis. Note that the pockets of fluid are anechoic or hyperechoic and the peritoneal lining is hyperechoic. Identify largest pocket of fluid and intra-abdominal structures (urinary bladder, bowel, and inferior epigastric vessels) to avoid. Set color Doppler threshold low and identify the inferior epigastric vessels.

10. **Pericardiocentesis.** Do static and dynamic technique. Obtain images in the parasternal long, apical, or subxiphoid view. Note the pericardial effusion will be an anechoic (black) space surrounding the bright echogenic pericardium. Measure from the epicardial surface of the heart to its maximum dimension on 2-dimensional imaging at end diastole. Identify right and left ventricle, liver, pericardium, and pericardial space. Identify the internal mammary artery (note that it is 3–5 cm lateral to the lower sternal border) and neurovascular bundles so these may be avoided. Note that the pericardial effusion will be an anechoic space surrounding the bright echogenic pericardium. A pneumopericardium will show bright spots/echogenic bubbles moving along the pericardial layer during diastole. A tamponade will show poor filling and/or diastolic collapse of the right side of the heart (right atria or right ventricle).

11. **Urinary tract ultrasound.** Scan each kidney in the longitudinal and transverse orientation. Evaluate kidneys, collecting system, and bladder. Normal bladder: see earlier in chapter (Section II.A.3).

12. **Endotracheal tube ultrasound.** Using high parasternal view or suprasternal approach, ultrasound exam can be done to confirm the ETT tip. Studies used either a 13-MHz linear transducer or a probe with a 5- to 8-MHz frequency. Correct ETT placement was 0.5 to 1.0 cm from the upper border of arch of aorta, between the thoracic inlet and the carina. The distance of the tip of the ETT from the carina can be measured. Tip of the probe is seen as a white or hyperechoic line that can help identify the tip of the ETT.

E. **Complications.** Although the safety profile of ultrasound is excellent, POCUS should only be performed by those healthcare workers who are fully trained. Knowledge of equipment settings and potential thermal and other bioeffects is essential.

1. **Maintain body temperature.** Monitor the infant's temperature and keep the infant warm during the scan. Warm the gel and open the incubators as few times as possible.

2. **Attention to immature skin and prevention of infection.** Minimize skin trauma and use infection prevention protocols per specific NICU.

3. **Cardiorespiratory monitoring.** Minimize the duration of the scan, and monitor cardiorespiratory status during the procedure.

4. **Prolonged duration of scanning may cause small risk of cell damage.** Use of the "as low as reasonably achievable" principle is recommended. Examination times should be as short as possible. Output levels should be as low as possible.

5. **Incorrect interpretation ("misreadings").** Following is a partial listing of errors that can be made on POCUS interpretation:

a. **Confusing vein for artery or nerve.**

b. **Misinterpreting pericardial fat for pericardial effusion.**

c. **Mistaking inferior vena cava for aorta.**

d. **Reversing right and left heart chamber.**

e. **Mistaking other fluid-filled structures for the bladder.**

f. **Combination of spleen and air in stomach can look like pneumonia.**

45 Venous Access: Intraosseous Infusion

I. **Indications.** Intraosseous (IO) infusion is the infusion of fluids or medications into the bone marrow cavity of a large bone. It is used for emergency vascular access (fluids and medications) when other access methods have been attempted and cannot be quickly established or have failed. In neonates during resuscitation, it is difficult to give medications through a peripheral vein because of insufficient perfusion. The bone medullary cavity does not collapse during circulatory failure or hypovolemia. Some recommend IO access if venous access is not established within 3 attempts or within 90 seconds. The **umbilical vein is the preferred route in the delivery room in a hospital setting,** but IO access can be considered if rapid intravenous (IV) access is essential and the operator is not experienced in umbilical vein catheter placement. IO access is an acceptable alternative in prehospital settings and emergency rooms. IO infusion of medications and fluids has the same hemodynamic effect as medications and fluids infused by the IV route.

II. **Equipment.** Antiseptic solution, 4 × 4 sterile gauze pads, sterile towels, gloves, IO device (devices approved for newborns are available; Table 45-1), syringe with saline flush, IV fluid, and infusion setup (Luer lock catheter with a 3-way stopcock).

III. **Procedure**

   A. **Contraindications** include prior unsuccessful attempt in the same bone, bone diseases (eg, osteogenesis imperfecta, osteopetrosis, osteomyelitis), infection of the overlying skin, presence of a fracture, hemophilia or other coagulopathies, and thermal injury to the overlying skin. There are limited data, but IO seems safe in preterm infants.

Table 45–1. COMPARISON OF SOME INTRAOSSEOUS (IO) DEVICES USED IN NEONATOLOGY

IO Device	Features
Butterfly needles or short hypodermic needles	18–20 gauge (*Note:* needles without stylet usually not recommended but have been used in preterm infants; absence of stylet may increase incidence of obstruction of needle by bony spicules)
Spinal/lumbar puncture needle[a]	Straight needle with stylet, 18–20 gauge
Bone marrow biopsy needle[a]	Hollow needle with handle and stylet, 18 gauge
IO infusion needle (eg, Sussmane-Raszynski IO infusion needle; Jamshidi Illinois IO infusion needle)	Specialized handles and stylets with short needle shafts, 15.5 and 18 gauge
EZ-IO Pediatric (Teleflex, Morrisville, NC)	Reusable lithium-powered drill that drills the IO needle into the IO space; 15-gauge needle; length 15 mm for infants 3–39 kg
Bone Injection Gun, Pediatric (B.I.G., WaisMed, Houston, TX)	Automatic impact driven (spring-loaded) device; uses the "position and press" mechanism; 18 gauge <12 years; dial in age for needle depth

[a]Best for emergency use where specifically designed IO device is not available.
Data from Tobias JD, Ross AK: Intraosseous infusions: a review for the anesthesiologist with a focus on pediatric use, *Anesth Analg.* 2010 Feb 1;110(2):391-401.

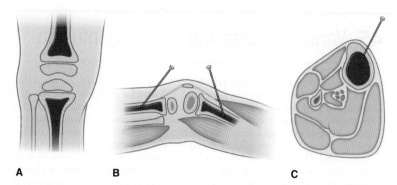

A   **B**   **C**

FIGURE 45–1. Technique of intraosseous infusion. (**A**) Anterior view of sites on the tibia and the fibula. (**B**) Sagittal view. (**C**) Cross-section through the tibia. (*Reproduced with permission from Hodge D: Intraosseous infusions: a review,* Pediatr Emerg Care. *1985 Dec;1(4):215-218.*)

B. **The proximal tibia (anteromedial surface) is the preferred site in the infant** (vs the sternum in adults) and is described here (Figure 45–1). Benefits include a flat wide surface, less amount of soft tissue to obscure the bony landmark, and that it does not interfere with airway management or chest compressions, if needed. The intramedullary vessel in the tibial marrow empties into the popliteal vein and into the femoral vein. The preferred second site in the infant is the **distal femur.** Both sites avoid the epiphyseal plates of the bone. In some references the distal tibia is mentioned as an alternative site for infants but in other references it is recommended only for children >1 year. A theoretical alternative intraosseous infusion site that has been suggested is the greater tubercle of the humerus 9.5 to 11.1 mm from the acromion.

C. **Select the area in the midline on the flat surface of the anterior tibia, approximately 2 cm below and 1 to 2 cm medial to the tibial tuberosity (bony bulge below knee cap).** This area avoids the epiphyseal growth plate injury, and the thinner cortex here ensures an easier insertion. The mean medullary diameter of the proximal tibia at the site that is recommended is only 7 mm in the neonate and 10 mm in a 1- to 12-month-old infant.

D. **Restrain the patient's lower leg,** and place a small sandbag/rolled towel or IV bag behind the knee for support.

E. **Wash hands and put on gloves.** Clean the area with antiseptic solution. Sterile drapes can be placed around the area.

F. **Pain management.** Lidocaine (0.5%–1%) can be injected into the skin, soft tissue, and periosteum, but this is optional because this is usually an emergency procedure.

G. **Intraosseous needle insertion.** (See specific devices in Table 45–1.) Insertion site should be at least 10 mm distal to tibial tuberosity to avoid epiphyseal growth plate. Preference depends upon the study, some health care providers recommend manual needles or power driven devices over impact driven devices in infants. One study compared different devices and techniques and found that intraosseous access for premature and neonatal infants was best achieved by using a manually twisted butterfly needle.

1. **Manual technique (butterfly or short hypodermic needle, spinal, bone marrow biopsy, or intraosseous needles).** Stabilize the limb above and lateral to the insertion site with the nondominant hand. Insert the needle perpendicular to the skin to avoid the growth plate. Advance the needle firmly, using hand-delivered steady force with a twisting and rotating, not rocking, motion until a

lack of resistance is felt, a "pop", usually no more than 1 cm is necessary, at which point entry into the marrow space should have occurred. The needle will stand up without support, and it will feel firm in the bone, although it may not be as firm in a neonate with a thin cortex. **Note** that it is best not to place the other hand under the tibia for stabilization, as excessive force may cause the needle to pass through the bone and exit on the other side.

2. **Impact driven or spring loaded device technique (eg, B.I.G. Pediatric device** [Bone Injection Gun; WaisMed Medical, Houston, TX]). Dial the age to get the appropriate needle depth. Position device at 90 degrees to the skin and hold firmly with one hand while the other hand pulls out the safety latch. It uses a "position and press" mechanism with a spring-loaded device that penetrates the cortex when the button is pushed. No additional force is needed other than holding the device firmly against the skin. Manufacturer-recommended site for infants is 0.5 inches medial and distal to the tibial tuberosity.

3. **Drill assisted technique (eg, EZ-IO Pediatric** [Teleflex, Morrisville, NC]; only recommended for infants >3 kg). Device operates like a power drill. It has a tip that rotates into the IO space at a preset depth. Once the needle enters the space, the stylet is withdrawn, and a metal catheter remains with a Luer lock attachment. Manufacturer recommends removal within 24 hours.

H. **Once the catheter is in place, remove the stylet and tape needle in place.**

I. **Confirm appropriate IO needle placement.** Some healthcare providers will aspirate blood or bone marrow, but the recommendations from the American Heart Association *Textbook of Neonatal Resuscitation* state that this is not a reliable indicator of correct needle placement. They feel if the needle is in the correct place it will stand and feel firm in the bone and not wiggle because it is supported by bony cortex. One recommendation to make sure the IO needle is in the correct place is to slowly infuse 2 to 3 mL of a saline flush solution. There should be no extravasation or swelling with correct placement. **POCUS using color Doppler** can assess correct and incorrect placement (extravasation of fluid) of an intraosseous needle, but there is limited experience in pediatrics. Usually a plain radiograph is obtained to confirm position and rule out a fracture.

J. **Bone marrow aspiration for laboratory studies** can be done, if needed. Bone marrow aspirates can be sent for bedside glucose testing, electrolyte concentrations, pH, PCO_2, hemoglobin, culture and sensitivity, blood type and crossmatch, and drug levels. CBC is not recommended because of immature cells found in the bone marrow. Even if marrow cannot be aspirated, the IO needle can be used if it flushes without extravasation. If appropriate, secure the needle to the skin with tape to prevent it from dislodging.

K. **Attach the needle to the intravenous infusion set (Luer lock with 3-way stopcock) and infuse at the same rate used for intravenous route.** Hypertonic and alkaline solutions may be diluted 1:2 with normal saline. Administer at the same rate as that for an IV infusion. Any fluid or medication that can be used via an umbilical venous catheter can be used via the IO route (Table 45–2).

L. **Secure the needle and catheter with tape and an arm board,** allowing one to be able to visualize the area. Secure IV tubing with tape to the leg.

M. **Intraosseous vascular access should optimally be used for <2 hours** to minimize the risk of infectious complications, with some devices approved by the US Food and Drug Administration for longer use. When completed, withdraw the needle, apply pressure, and dress the site. Use for >24 hours is not recommended.

N. **With unsuccessful intraosseous placement,** do not repeat attempts at the same site or use the same site for 1 to 2 days.

O. **Monitor the site frequently for redness, bruising, inflammation, swelling, or any fluid extravasation.** Monitor limb circulation. Measuring the leg circumference hourly is recommended.

P. **It is important to note that the needle should be removed as soon as the infant has stabilized** or an alternative access has been successful.

Table 45–2. FLUIDS AND MEDICATIONS THAT HAVE BEEN ADMINISTERED BY THE INTRAOSSEOUS ROUTE

Intravenous Fluids

Blood and blood products (eg, fresh frozen plasma, whole blood)	Crystalloids (lactated Ringer's, sodium chloride solutions [0.9% and hypertonic])	Dextrose solutions (D50 should be diluted)	Colloids

Medications

Adenosine	Digoxin	Lorazepam	Prostaglandin
Amikacin	Dobutamine	Magnesium sulfate	Rocuronium
Aminophylline	Dopamine	Methylene blue	Sodium bicarbonate
Amiodarone	Ephedrine	Methylprednisolone	(diluted)
Ampicillin	Epinephrine	Midazolam	Succinylcholine
Atracurium	Fentanyl	Morphine	Sulfadiazine
Atropine	Furosemide	Naloxone	Thiamine
Calcium chloride and gluconate	Gentamicin	Pancuronium	Thiopental
	Heparin	Pentothal	Vancomycin
Cefotaxime	Isoproterenol	Phenobarbital	Vasopressin
Ceftriaxone	Insulin	Phenytoin	Vecuronium
Clindamycin	Ketamine	Potassium chloride	Vitamins
Contrast media (dilute if possible)	Labetalol	Propofol	
	Levarterenol	Propranolol	
Dexamethasone	Lidocaine		
Dextrose (D50; dilute)			
Diazepam			
Diazoxide			

Data Dubick MA, Holcomb JB. A review of intraosseous vascular access: current status and military application, *Mil Med.* 2000 Jul;165(7):552-559 and MacDonald M, Ramasethu J, Rais-Bahrami K: *Atlas of Procedures in Neonatology*, 5th ed. Philadelphia, PA: Wolters Kluwer; 2012.

IV. **Removal**
   A. **Remove any dressing or tape.** Stabilize the extremity.
   B. **Use aseptic technique.** Gently rotate the needle while withdrawing it.
   C. **Apply pressure to the site for a minimum of 5 minutes** and cover with sterile dressing.
   D. **Continue to observe the limb for 24 hours.**
V. **Complications**
   A. **Extravasation.** (Most common complication.) If giving caustic/vasoactive medications, such as dopamine, and extravasation occurs, tissue damage is possible. Subperiosteal infiltration of fluid can also occur.
   B. **Infections.** Introduction of pathogens during needle insertion can occur and lead to an infection. Localized cellulitis, subcutaneous abscess, periostitis, and sepsis have all been reported. Osteomyelitis is rare (<0.6%). To prevent osteomyelitis, hypertonic and alkaline solutions and all medications should be diluted. Sterile technique is important, and if compromised, consider antibiotic coverage.
   C. **Clotting of bone marrow.** Results in loss of vascular access.
   D. **Iatrogenic bone fracture.** Fractures can occur in infants secondary to the increased force required to penetrate the bone and also are increased in infants with osteopenia. Radiograph confirmation of the needle should be done to confirm position and rule out fracture (tibial fracture is most common).

E. **Compartment syndrome.** Due to prolonged infusion and extravasation. The leaking fluid collects in the spaces between the muscles of the leg.

F. **Blasts in the peripheral blood.** These have been noted after IO infusions.

G. **Fat embolism.** Much less likely in infants than adults. Before the age of 5 years, the intramedullary space consists mainly of red marrow, which is more vascular and has a lower fat component. No adverse outcomes have been related to embolic events.

H. **Bone growth concerns have been ruled out.** Studies have shown there is no long-term effect on tibial growth after IO infusion with a properly placed IO needle trocar. At the tibia, IO blood transfusions may result in transient radiologic changes but do not impact actual bone growth. If the catheter is placed in the growth plate, an injury may occur, but has not been reported in pediatric literature.

I. **Needle dislodgement.**

J. **Amputation of the leg.** Rare case reports (one that was treated with therapeutic hypothermia).

46 Venous Access: Peripherally Inserted Central Catheter

I. **Indications. Peripherally inserted central catheter (PICC) or percutaneous central venous catheterization (PCVC)** involves inserting a long small-gauge catheter into a peripheral vein and threading it into a central venous location. The catheter can be placed in large vessels such as the temporal vein in the scalp, cephalic and basilic veins in the arm, or the saphenous vein in the leg.

A. **When intravenous access is anticipated for an extended period.** The Centers for Disease Control and Prevention (CDC) recommends placing PICC access if therapy is needed for >6 days.

B. **High-risk patient populations (surgical).**

C. **In low birthweight infants when it is anticipated that full enteral feedings will not be achieved within a short period.** Cochrane review found in one small study that the use of percutaneous central venous catheters increases nutrient output. Three trials suggested that the use of percutaneous central venous catheters decreased the number of catheters needed to deliver nutrition.

D. **Fluid delivery, nutritional solutions, and medications when other venous access is not acceptable or able to be obtained** (eg, hypertonic intravenous [IV] solutions).

II. **Equipment**

A. **Basic supplies.** Cap, mask, sterile gloves, sterile gown, transparent dressing, sterile tape strips, a sterile tray, locally approved bactericidal skin prep, a sterile tourniquet, sterile transilluminator cover (optional), saline flush solution, sterile saline wipes, sterile gauge, and a T-connector.

B. **Percutaneous catheter device.** Silicone catheters and polyurethane catheters (typically with guidewire) are available. Some infants may benefit from dual lumen catheters due to multiple infusions or medication incompatibility. Ensure careful consideration when using dual lumen catheters due to increased associated risks, including catheter thrombosis and infection. According to the National Association of Neonatal Nurses (NANN) guidelines, the most commonly used PICC catheters are 1.1 to 2F (28- to 23-gauge) catheter. Use the smallest catheter possible to accommodate the vein. Choose proper-sized catheters because a catheter too large for a vessel may cause the vessel to spasm.

1. **Specialty antibiotic-coated catheters.** Cochrane review (2015) found that although data from one trial did indicate that antimicrobial-impregnated central venous catheters might prevent catheter-related bloodstream infection in newborns, the available evidence is insufficient to guide clinical practice.

2. **Specialty heparin-bonded catheters.** Cochrane review (2014) found 2 studies on heparin-bonded catheters that revealed no decrease in catheter-related thrombosis; 1 study did report a decrease in catheter-related bloodstream infections and colonization with the use of heparin-bonded catheters.

III. **Procedure.** If a guidewire is present, it needs to be removed before blood is withdrawn or the catheter is flushed. Providers placing lines need to be trained with competency check off, to maintain skills with a designated minimum number of insertions per year, and to be comfortable with manufacturer guidelines specific to catheter devices. A review of the NANN Guideline for Peripherally Inserted Central Catheters (see Selected References) is suggested.

A. **Obtain informed consent and perform a time-out.** Gather the equipment and assemble the tray with the catheter using sterile technique.

B. **Consider utilization of available technology including transillumination or ultrasound-guided insertion techniques.** These techniques have been shown to improve success rates. **Ultrasound-guided PICC line placement** is very effective in very low and extremely low birthweight infants. The inserter should be proficient with associated technology. See Chapter 44.

C. **Select a suitable large vessel. The right saphenous vein is an ideal site associated with lower complication rates** (Figure 47–1). Position the infant with the selected vessel accessible. An assistant is helpful to maintain sterility and provide nonpharmacologic pain management (see Section III.G).

D. **Determine the length of the catheter.** Measure the distance between the insertion site and the desired catheter tip location.

1. **Upper extremity position:** Measure to the level of the superior vena cava (SVC).

2. **Lower extremity position:** Measure to the inferior vena cava (IVC).

E. **Put on the cap and mask, wash your hands, and then put on the sterile gown and gloves (provider placing line).** Anyone within about 3 feet of the bedside should have a cap and mask on and observe maximal sterile barrier precautions.

F. **Prepare the area of insertion** using a unit-approved bactericidal agent and allow the solution to dry. Avoid alcohol because it can cause degradation of some catheters. Tourniquet proximal to the insertion site.

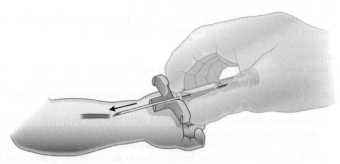

FIGURE 46–1. Technique for insertion of the introducer needle into the vein.

G. **Pain.** The American Academy of Pediatrics policy statement indicates that the goal for pediatricians is to prevent or minimize pain in the neonate.

   1. **Guidelines should be written by the local unit** to address pharmacologic and nonpharmacologic pain management strategies for PICC insertion.

   2. **Pharmacologic pain management** may include topical anesthesia (EMLA [eutectic mixture of lidocaine and prilocaine]) or systemic opiate-based anesthesia. Sucrose pacifier may provide sufficient analgesia.

H. **Place sterile drapes over the patient.** Use maximal sterile barrier precautions with a large sterile field around the area of insertion that covers most of the infant.

I. **Remove the plastic protector from the introducer needle.**

J. **Insert the introducer and needle into the vein.** Confirm entry into the vein by observing for a flashback of blood in the needle. Do not advance the introducer and needle once the flashback has been noted due to risk for puncturing through the opposite side of the vessel (see Figure 46–1).

K. **Release the tourniquet.**

L. **Hold the introducer and needle to maintain the position in the vein and withdraw the needle.** Slowly advance the catheter through the introducer with a pair of smooth forceps or fingers into the vein. **Ridged forceps may damage the catheter** (Figure 46–2).

M. **Once the catheter has been advanced to the premeasured location, stabilize the catheter by placing a finger 1 to 2 cm above the tip of the introducer.** Carefully withdraw the introducer completely out of the skin. Hold sterile gauze to the area until hemostasis is achieved (Figure 46–3).

N. **Separate the introducer from the catheter.** Grasp the opposite halves of the introducer, and carefully peel each half apart until the needle splits completely (Figure 46–4).

O. **During removal of the introducer needle, the catheter may partially withdraw.** Readvance to the desired location.

P. **If a guidewire is present, remove the wire slowly and steadily from the catheter.** Do not attempt to reintroduce the wire once it has been removed from the catheter.

Q. **As the introducer wire is withdrawn, blood return may or may not be observed in the catheter.** Smaller catheters are less likely to have blood return. Using a 3-mL syringe, aspirate blood through the catheter until blood reaches the hub. (Slightly more

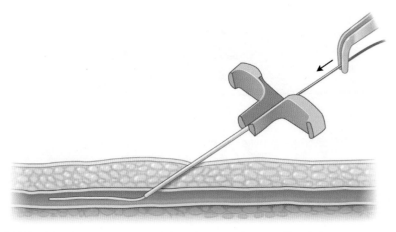

FIGURE 46–2. The catheter is inserted through the introducer needle with forceps.

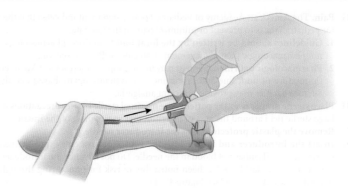

FIGURE 46–3. The catheter is stabilized while withdrawing the needle.

pressure is necessary to withdraw blood through the very small diameter of the catheter. If you achieve blood return, the catheter is patent and in the intravascular system.) Once blood has been aspirated back to the catheter hub, place a T-connector and flush the catheter with normal saline. Avoid excessive pressure when flushing the catheter as it can result in catheter rupture or fragmentation with possible embolization.

R. **Secure the catheter to the extremity by placing a sterile tape strip over the disc to anchor the catheter** (damage may occur if placed directly on the catheter). Coil the external catheter, making sure there are no kinks, and cover with a sterile transparent dressing. **Do not suture the catheter in place.**

S. **Connect the intravenous fluid.** New fresh sterile IV fluids should be connected to the new catheter. The necessary use of heparin for patency is *controversial*. The lowest PICC maintenance infusion rate has been widely reported as 1 mL/h. Cochrane review (2014) recommends prophylactic use of **heparin** in PICC lines because it allows a higher number of infants to complete their therapy and reduces the risk of catheter occlusion. The American College of Chest Physicians Evidence-Based Clinical Guidelines (2012) recommends continuous infusion of unfractionated heparin 0.5 U/kg/h to maintain patency in neonates with central venous access devices.

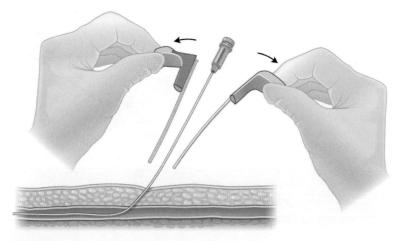

FIGURE 46–4. Technique for removing the needle wing assembly of most catheters.

T. **Obtain a radiograph to verify the central catheter tip location.** Most catheters are radiopaque. Occasionally, they are too small to visualize the catheter tip location. In some instances, 0.3 to 1 mL of contrast is used prior to radiograph to assess tip location. The position of the catheter tip should be in a central location such as the SVC or IVC because these locations are associated with a lower risk of complications. If unable to advance to a central location, the line may be used as a midline catheter with the tip in the proximal portion of the extremity (avoid placing the tip in a flexed position). Hypertonic solutions should not be infused through a midline catheter. Midline catheters are typically used for a shorter duration (<1 week). **Sonography** has been used in a pilot study to localize the position of the catheter.

U. **Lower extremity peripherally inserted central catheter.** A cross-table lateral x-ray should be done to assess the proper placement of the catheter in the IVC (risk for spinal vein insertion).

V. **Chart the size and the length of catheter that has been inserted** and the position of the catheter on radiograph.

W. **Precautions**
1. **Avoid blood pressure measurements on the extremity containing the catheter.**
2. **Only trim catheters prior to placement if directed by manufacturer.** A rough-cut end may increase thrombus formation.
3. **During insertion through the introducer needle, avoid pulling the catheter back through the introducer needle.** Risk for the catheter to sever.
4. **Do not suture the catheter.**
5. **Blood product administration is controversial.** In general, try to avoid due to the risk of catheter occlusion.
6. **Avoid excessive pressure when flushing the line due to risk of rupture** (do not use syringe <3 mL).

X. **Maintenance of the catheter**
1. **Prevention of central line–associated bloodstream infection.** Line insertion bundles, care guidelines, and specially trained insertion teams have been associated with decreased incidence of infection.
2. **The transparent dressing should remain in place over the catheter.** Routine dressing changes are not recommended. The dressing should be changed using sterile technique if the current dressing is soiled or is no longer occlusive.
3. **Examine the site for inflammation or tenderness.**
4. **Fluids and medications** running through the catheter should be prepared using sterile conditions and heparinized according to hospital or unit protocol.
5. **Limit the number of times the catheter is accessed to decrease infection.** Research suggests that the hub is a common site of contamination and subsequent infection. Clean hubs with antiseptic each time the line is entered.
6. **Use the exchange technique for occluded or malpositioned catheters in limited circumstances** because it has been associated with a higher risk of central line–associated bloodstream infection (CLABSI).

Y. **Removal of the catheter.** The catheter can remain in place for several weeks. Several studies have shown an increase in the infection rate after 2 weeks.
1. **The use of antibiotic administration prior to removal is controversial** and has been studied on a limited scale. A small trial suggests that antibiotics given 12 hours prior to removal, whether for treatment or prophylaxis, has been associated with a decreased incidence of late-onset sepsis after catheter removal. The theory is that this reduces the risk of bacterial showering with line removal. Prophylactic antibiotic administration has not yet been introduced widely into practice and needs to be studied on a larger scale.
2. **Gently remove the occlusive dressing** from the extremity and the catheter.
3. **Grasp the catheter tubing near the insertion site** and gently pull the catheter in a continuous movement. If resistance is met, do not apply force and do not stretch the catheter. Doing so could cause the catheter to rupture.

4. **Apply a moist, warm compress to the area above the catheter tract for several minutes, and then reattempt removal of the catheter.** If the catheter is still resistant, it may take several hours to days to remove some catheters.

5. **Once the catheter is removed, inspect and measure it to make sure the entire catheter was removed from the vein.** Compare this to the initial insertion note.

6. **Cover the site with petroleum-based gauze and occlusive dressing for 24 to 48 hours.** This technique reduces the risk of air embolism. A Cochrane review found the following: "Chlorhexidine dressing/alcohol skin cleansing reduced catheter colonization, but had a risk of contact dermatitis in preterm infants and did not affect major outcomes like sepsis and CLABSI compared to polyurethane dressing/povidone iodine cleansing. Silver alginate patch appears safe but cannot be recommended because of insufficient evidence."

IV. **Complications.** Common complications are listed.

A. **Infiltration.** Assess for swelling at the insertion site up to the catheter tip location.

B. **Catheter occlusion.** PICCs are at risk for occlusion due to the size, fragility of the catheter, and the potential for neonatal flexion of extremities. Take care to avoid kinking the catheter during securement because it could lead to catheter occlusion. If resistance is met when flushing the catheter, do not attempt to flush it any further because it could result in catheter rupture and ultimately possible embolization. Tissue plasminogen activator/alteplase therapy may be indicated in certain clinical situations (refer to your local unit protocol).

C. **Infection or sepsis. A catheter-associated bloodstream infection is the most common healthcare-associated infection in the neonatal intensive care unit.** Each unit should develop a strategy to track CLABSI and develop strategies for prevention. Refer to NANN guidelines (see Selected References) and CDC guidelines for risk reduction strategies. Infants requiring a PICC are at an increased risk for nosocomial infections (poor skin integrity, immature immune system, multiple invasive procedures, exposure to multiple pieces of equipment). Coagulase-negative staphylococci account for >50% of infections. Other pathogens include gram-negative organisms (20%), *Staphylococcus aureus* (4%–9%), *Enterococcus* (3%–5%), and *Candida* (10%). Paired samples should be drawn (catheter and a peripheral vein) from neonates with suspected sepsis to isolate a potentially infected catheter. Neonates with suspected CLABSI should be treated with broad-spectrum antibiotics to cover both gram-positive and gram-negative organisms. Line stewardship focuses on daily review of the need for central access.

D. **Air embolism.** Special precautions should be taken to avoid air in the line.

E. **Catheter embolus.** Risk for catheter shearing if the catheter is pulled back through the introducer needle.

F. **Catheter migration/malposition.** Catheters can move after initial placement. Assess the catheter position with an x-ray the first 2 to 3 days after insertion and at minimum weekly.

G. **Pericardial effusions are a rare but life-threatening complication of percutaneous central venous catheters.** Keep a high index of clinical suspicion in a neonate who has a central line and suddenly has cardiovascular collapse that does not respond to resuscitation, resistance to external cardiac compressions, and no transilluminated air leak. It is more common with lines in the right atrium, and the median time to occurrence is 3 days after percutaneous central catheter insertion. Chest radiograph may not be diagnostic; echocardiography is diagnostic but may delay treatment, and mortality is high.

47 Venous Access: Peripheral Intravenous Catheterization

I. **Indications.** Peripheral intravenous (IV) catheterization involves inserting an IV catheter into a peripheral vein.
   A. **Vascular access in nonemergent and emergent situations** for the administration of IV fluids and medications.
   B. **Administration of parenteral nutrition.**
   C. **Administration of blood and blood products.**
   D. **Blood sampling only if associated with initial intravenous placement.**
II. **Equipment**
   A. **Basic.** Armboard, adhesive tape, tourniquet, alcohol swabs, normal saline for flush (0.5% normal saline if hypernatremia is a concern), povidone-iodine solution/swabs, transparent dressing material, appropriate IV fluid, and connecting tubing. For difficult venous access, transillumination, near-infrared light, or ultrasound can be used, and these are considered optional. In-line filters are sometimes used; however, a Cochrane review (2015) found that there was insufficient evidence to recommend the use of IV in-line filters to prevent morbidity and mortality in neonates.
   B. **Intravenous catheter.** Safety-engineered/self-shielding devices preferred: 23- to 25-gauge scalp vein ("butterfly") needle or a 22- to 24-gauge catheter-over-needle. Use at least 24 gauge for blood transfusion.
III. **Procedure**
   A. **Catheter-over-needle assembly**
      1. **Select the vein.** Common neonatal IV insertion sites are shown in Figure 47–1. Several techniques have been described based on personal preference.
         a. **The vessel can be entered directly after puncture of the skin on the top of the vein.**
         b. **Enter the vein at the "crotch" or "Y region," the location where 2 veins join together** (Figure 47–2A).
         c. **Insert alongside the vein and advance approximately 0.5 cm before entry into the side of the vessel** (Figure 47–2B).
      2. **To help identify the vein, use visualization, palpation, near infrared spectroscopy imaging, transillumination, or point-of-care ultrasound using static technique (see Chapters 25 and 44).** The dorsum of the hand is the best choice to preserve the sites for potential central venous catheters (cephalic, brachial, greater saphenous veins) if needed. Avoid areas of flexion.
         a. **Scalp.** Supratrochlear (frontal), superficial temporal, or posterior auricular vein (last resort).
         b. **Back of the hand.** Preferred site using the dorsal venous network.
         c. **Forearm.** At the wrist area is the cephalic and basilic vein. Median antebrachial vein and accessory cephalic vein are higher up on the forearm.
         d. **Foot.** Dorsal venous arch.
         e. **Antecubital fossa.** Basilic or cubital veins.
         f. **Ankle.** Greater and small saphenous veins.
      3. **Use of point-of-care ultrasound for peripheral intravenous catheterization.** One can use real time imaging to help guide the peripheral IV placement. Benefits include less time for placement, better success, decreased attempts and needle redirections, and less complications. See Chapter 44 for technique.
      4. **Shave the area if a scalp vein is to be used.** Try to place needle behind the hair line in the event of cosmetic scarring.

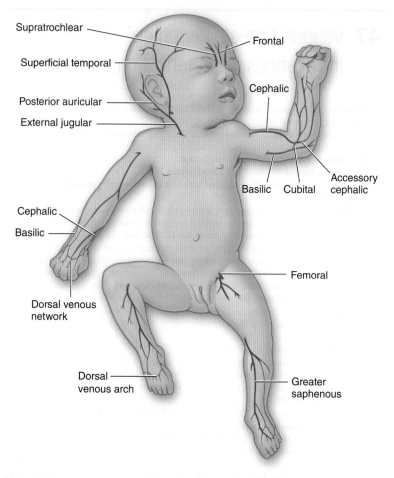

FIGURE 47–1. Frequently used sites for venous access in the neonate.

5. **Restrain the extremity on an armboard** or have an assistant help hold the extremity or the head.
6. **Pain management.** Oral sucrose/glucose, pacifier, swaddling, and other non-pharmacologic methods can be used for pain reduction. The American Academy of Pediatrics recommends eutectic mixture of lidocaine and prilocaine (EMLA) applied 30 minutes before the procedure.
7. **Apply a tourniquet proximal to the puncture site.** If a scalp vein is to be used, a rubber band can be placed around the head, just above the eyebrows.
8. **Wash hands and put on nonsterile gloves.** Glove use after hand hygiene prior to patient and line contact is associated with a decreased incidence of gram-positive infections in preterm infants.
9. **Clean the area with antiseptic solution.** Allow to dry and wipe off with sterile water or saline.

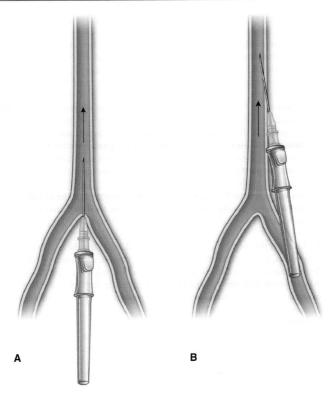

A   **B**

FIGURE 47–2. Two commonly used techniques for entering the vein for intravenous access in the neonate (see text). (**A**) Enter vein at the "crotch" or "Y region" where 2 veins come together. (**B**) Side entry technique where the needle is inserted into the skin and then advanced 0.5 cm before puncturing the vein on the side. Some providers will enter the vein from the top as well.

10. **Fill the needle and the hub with flush via syringe (if possible),** and then remove the syringe.
11. **Pull the skin taut** to stabilize the vein.
12. **Puncture the skin** and then enter the side of the vein in a separate motion. Alternately, the skin and the vein can be entered in one motion.
13. **Carefully advance the needle** until a flash of blood appears in the hub.
14. **Activate the shield** to safely sheathe the needle and advance the catheter. Injecting a small amount of flush solution into the vein before advancing the catheter may help.
15. **Remove the tourniquet** and gently inject some normal saline into the catheter to verify patency and position.
16. **Connect the intravenous tubing and fluid** and tape securely in place using transparent dressing.
17. **Heparin for peripheral intravenous lines** *(controversial).* Heparin is usually not recommended for peripheral IV lines. A 2013 review found that low-dose heparin in peripheral IV catheters prolonged the catheter life with a decrease in infusion failure rates when a continuous infusion was used. Cochrane review states that there are insufficient data concerning the effect of heparin for prolonging IV use in neonates and that recommendations cannot be made.

One study found that heparinized saline flushes increased the functional duration of peripheral IV catheters.

B. **Scalp vein or butterfly needle.** Used for short-term therapy, for small scalp veins, or for smaller veins in which a catheter-over-needle assembly cannot be used. Scalp veins provide an option for IV access in infants because of limited subcutaneous fat and less movement. The needles are often easier to insert but do not have much durability.

1. **Follow steps 1 to 9 for catheter-over-needle procedure (see Section III.A).**
2. **Foot.** Dorsal arch veins are very small but are very good to use. A vein that runs behind the malleolus on the lateral aspect of the foot is easy to access.
3. **Antecubital fossa.** The median antecubital, cephalic, and basilic veins are excellent veins but need to be splinted well for them to maintain the site.
4. **Grasp the plastic wings.** Using your free index finger, **pull the skin taut** to help stabilize the vein.
5. **Insert the needle through the skin in the direction of the blood flow.**
6. **Advance the needle when blood appears in the flash chamber or tubing.** Gently inject some of the flush to ensure patency and proper positioning of the needle.
7. **Connect the intravenous tubing and fluid, and tape the needle into position.**

IV. **Complications.** In one study, the incidence of IV complications was up to 63%.

A. **Hematoma** at the site can often be managed effectively by gentle pressure.
B. **Phlebitis (inflammation of the vein) risk** increases the longer a catheter is left in place, especially if >72 to 96 hours. Sites are rotated at 72- to 96-hour intervals to decrease phlebitis and infection.
C. **Occlusion/obstruction** is a common complication.
D. **Vasospasm** rarely occurs when veins are accessed and usually resolves spontaneously.
E. **Infection risk** can be minimized by using sterile technique, including antiseptic preparation. The risk of infection increases after 72 hours. Peripheral IV catheterization is rarely associated with bloodstream infection. Presence of blood in the hub is universal and may facilitate infection.
F. **Embolus (air or clot).** Never allow the end of the catheter to be open to the air, and make sure that the IV catheter is flushed free of air bubbles before it is connected. Do not use excessive force when flushing.
G. **Infiltration/extravasation injury** results from the leakage of fluid from a vein into the surrounding tissue, usually due to improper catheter placement or damage to the vessel. See Chapter 42 for details on management of infiltration and extravasation.

1. **Infiltration of nonvesicant fluid** does not cause tissue loss, but a large volume can cause compression of the neurovascular structures, leading to compartment syndrome.
2. **Extravasation can cause a mild injury or severe necrosis** (blisters, tissue injury, and necrosis) and may result in the need for skin grafting. To limit this, confirm intravascular placement of the catheter with the flush solution before the catheter is connected to the IV tubing. Infiltration often means that the catheter needs to be removed. Avoid hyperosmolar solutions for peripheral infusion, and use caution with dopamine, which can cause constriction. Vialon catheter material was found to reduce the risk of infiltration (35% in infants <1500 g) as compared to Teflon in one study.

H. **Calcification of subcutaneous tissue** secondary to infusion of a calcium-containing solution.
I. **Fluid overload,** electrolyte problems (hypernatremia).

48 Venous Access: Umbilical Vein Catheterization

I. **Indications**

 A. **Immediate, postnatal access** for intravenous (IV) fluids or emergency medications.

 B. **Long-term central venous access** in low birthweight (BW) infants or sick infants for administration of IV fluids, total parenteral nutrition, other hypertonic or hyperosmotic solutions, and medications.

 C. **Exchange or partial exchange transfusion.**

 D. **Delivery of blood and blood products.**

 E. **Central venous pressure monitoring** (if umbilical venous catheter [UVC] passes through the ductus venosus).

 F. **Secondary aid** in the diagnosis of cardiovascular or other anomalies by an unusual course of the UVC or the blood gas values are suspicious.

  1. **Congenital diaphragmatic hernia.** UVC is left of the midline because of the anomalous positioning of the liver in the chest.

  2. **Persistent left superior vena cava.** UVC extends beyond the lung (it enters the persistent left superior vena cava and then the left jugular vein).

  3. **Congenital absence of the ductus venosus.** This can cause an abnormal path of UVC (caudal loop is seen on radiograph).

  4. **Infracardiac total anomalous pulmonary venous return.** Diagnosed by high partial pressure of oxygen in an infradiaphragmatic UVC.

II. **Equipment**

 A. **Basic.** Identical to umbilical artery catheterization (see Chapter 28).

 B. **Umbilical venous catheters**

  1. **Types. Single lumen:** 2.5, 3.5, or 5F; **dual lumen:** 3.5 or 5F; **triple lumen:** 5 or 8F.

  2. **Size guideline.** Preterm: 3.5 or 5F; term and late preterm: 5F. Other guidelines: 3.5 or 5F catheter <3.5 kg, 5 or 8F >3.5 kg. An 8F catheter is recommended for exchange transfusion or large-volume replacement. **American Academy of Pediatrics (AAP) Perinatal Continuing Education Program recommendations:** 5F for all infants for emergency medications, 8F for exchange transfusions for large infants. **Dual (double-lumen) catheters** are sometimes recommended in infants <28 weeks and <1000 g, in infants who need several different medications, in infants who need inotropes or insulin, and in critically ill infants such as those with severe cases of persistent pulmonary hypertension or meconium aspiration syndrome.

III. **Procedure**

 A. **Important umbilical vein catheter tips**

  1. **There is only 1 umbilical vein, and it remains a viable option for cannulation up to 1 week after birth.** The umbilical vein carries oxygenated blood from the placenta to the fetus. The UVC passes into the umbilical vein through the umbilicus and follows this path: junction of the right and left portal vein in the liver, across the ductus venosus, across the level of the right and left hepatic vein, and into the inferior vena cava (IVC) to the junction of the IVC and right atrium.

  2. **In an emergency postnatal situation (eg, delivery room),** a UVC can be rapidly inserted until blood return is obtained (usually 2–4 cm in a term infant; some sources insert 5 cm plus cord length with less distance in preterm) as emergency venous access. Resuscitation medications, volume, and blood can be given.

3. **Single- versus multiple-lumen catheters. Cochrane review** (2005) makes no recommendation on using single- versus multiple-lumen catheters. Double-lumen catheters decreased the number of additional venous lines during the first week of life, but they broke, leaked, and clogged more (smaller diameter). No differences in UVC placement difficulty, misplacement, catheter-related infections or blood clots, or rate of infant mortality were noted. Consider using the least number of lumens required.

4. **Suspect cardiac tamponade in a neonate with an umbilical vein catheter (even if properly placed) who develops a sudden unexplained clinical deterioration in cardiopulmonary status.** Urgent echocardiography or pericardiocentesis should be considered. Routine radiography/ultrasound to verify placement is recommended by some to check for tip migration. Positional changes in the upper extremity may cause migration of the catheter tip. When obtaining a chest radiograph, note arm position. Minimize infant mobilization while the catheter is in place to prevent the catheter from migrating to the right atrium.

5. **Catheter duration recommendations** from the Centers for Disease Control and Prevention (CDC), 14 days; other sources, 7 days, up to 28 days if absolutely necessary. The AAP notes catheters can be used up to 14 days if used aseptically. A Cochrane review (2017) analyzed whether early planned removal of UVCs would decrease the chance of an infection in newborn infants but found the following: "There was only one RCT [randomized controlled trial] and it did not show that early planned removal could reduce the chance of developing a bloodstream infection."

6. **Heparin use in umbilical vein catheters is *controversial*.** Literature is conflicting; there are recommendations for and against its use. The majority of neonatal intensive care units use heparin in UVCs. A common practice is as follows: heparin (typical range, 0.5–1 U/mL) in all fluids via the UVC. Use of heparin flushes alone is not effective in maintaining patency. The American College of Chest Physicians Evidence-Based Clinical Practice Guidelines recommend heparin in central venous access devices at a continuous infusion at 0.5 U/kg/h; the AAP recommends a starting dose of 0.12 U/kg/h.

7. **Blood cultures** can be obtained from a UVC right after placement; otherwise, venipuncture is preferred.

8. **Point-of-care ultrasound (POCUS) during placement of UVC.** Ultrasound guidance can help guide the catheter and allow for faster placement and results in fewer manipulations and x-rays compared with conventional placement. See Chapter 44.

B. **Estimate the depth of insertion for umbilical vein catheter.** Multiple methods have been reported; refer to institutional guidelines if possible. It is important to standardize the calculation method, since this improves the accuracy of placement. Some recommendations are to insert it 2 cm longer than the recommended length, since it is easier to withdraw the catheter than to insert it deeper. Remember to add the umbilical stump length to the calculation.

1. **Dunn method (early method).** Measures the shoulder-umbilicus length and uses a nomogram to determine the insertion length. Do not measure the shoulder diagonally to the umbilicus (it needs to be a straight line from the shoulder to the level of the umbilicus). This method was more accurate than the Shukla-Ferrara method (see below) in 1 study. **The catheter tip should be placed between the level of the diaphragm and the left atrium on the graph (see Figure 48–1).**

2. **Shukla-Ferrara method.** Based on BW, may lead to overinsertion in very low BW infants.

$$(3 \times BW \text{ in kg} + 9)/2 + 1 \text{ cm}$$

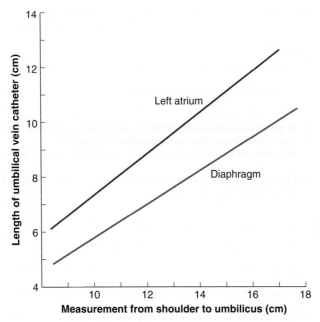

FIGURE 48–1. The umbilical venous catheter is placed above the level of the diaphragm and below the left atrium. Determine the shoulder-umbilical length as for the umbilical artery catheter. Use this number and determine the catheter length using the graph. Add the length of the umbilical stump to the length of the catheter. The catheter length should be between the diaphragm and left atrium on the graph. (*Data from Dunn PM. Localization of the umbilical catheter by post-mortem measurement.* Arch Dis Child. *1966;41:69.*)

If the umbilical artery length has been previously calculated (page 315), use the following formula:

UVC length: ½ × umbilical artery line calculation + 1

a. Modified (revised) Shukla (birthweight) equation. May reduce the rate of overinsertion.

$$(3 \times BW \text{ in kg} + 9)/2 \text{ cm}$$

3. Another method relies on external anatomic landmarks to determine the appropriate insertion length. It can be used in infants with all BWs. The measurement "UN" was found to be more accurate in infants with all BWs than any BW-based formula in one study.

UN (distance in cm from the umbilicus to the nipple) – 1 cm
= distance to place the UVC

4. Other measurements used:
   a. Xiphoid to umbilicus length: Measure from the xiphoid to the umbilicus and add 0.5 to 1 cm.
   b. Shoulder to umbilicus length: Measure the shoulder (end of clavicle) to umbilicus length and then multiply by 0.66.

C. **Pain management.** Since the umbilical cord is denervated, pain may be minimal. No formal anesthesia is usually needed if you avoid traumatizing the skin. Use non-pharmacologic pain prevention and relief techniques if possible.

D. **Technique**

1. **Place the infant supine with a diaper wrapped around both legs for stabilization.**

2. **Prepare the tray as you would for the umbilical artery catheterization.** (See Chapter 28.) Fill the lumen with infusion solution so it is air free. Don a gown, mask, and sterile gloves.

3. **Prepare the area around the umbilicus with antiseptic solution per local policy.**

4. **Place sterile drapes, leaving the umbilical area exposed.**

5. **Tie a piece of umbilical tape** or a purse string suture around the base of the umbilicus.

6. **Cleanly cut the excess umbilical cord with a knife blade (scalpel), leaving a stump of about 0.5 cm.** Scissors are not recommended because they can crush the vessels. If bleeding occurs, tighten the umbilical tape, or press downward just above the umbilicus on the infant's abdomen (since the umbilical vein travels toward the head). Identify the umbilical vein; it is thin walled, larger than the arteries, and close to the periphery of the stump (see Figure 28-3B). Normally one can determine the vessels by visual observation. If not, rub the flat side of the instrument across the stump; the arteries can be felt with resistance, but the vein will not.

7. **Grasp the end of the umbilicus with the curved hemostat to hold it upright and steady** (Figure 48-2A).

8. **Open and dilate the umbilical vein with the forceps.** If any clots are visible in the lumen, remove them with forceps. **Insert the flushed catheter** (Figure 48-2B) the desired length. Direct the UVC toward the head/cephalad with a hand providing liver immobilization (this improves the rate of insertion into the IVC). Some units use **ultrasound to help guide the catheter,** and this has been found to reduce complications during UVC insertion.

9. **Occasionally, a catheter enters the portal vein** (Figure 48-3). Suspect portal vein entry if you meet resistance and cannot advance the catheter the desired

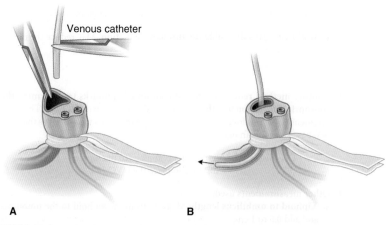

Venous catheter

A   B

FIGURE 48–2. Umbilical vein catheterization. (**A**) The umbilical stump is held upright before the catheter is inserted. (**B**) The catheter is passed into the umbilical vein.

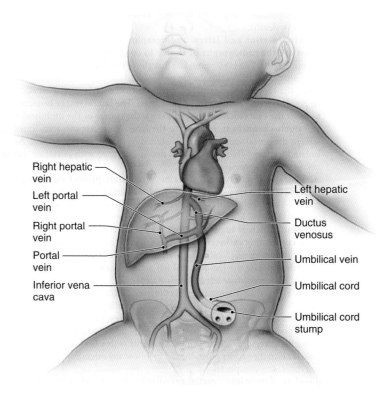

Right hepatic vein

Left portal vein

Right portal vein

Portal vein

Inferior vena cava

Left hepatic vein

Ductus venosus

Umbilical vein

Umbilical cord

Umbilical cord stump

FIGURE 48–3. Anatomic relationships used in the placement of an umbilical venous catheter.

distance or if you detect a "bobbing" motion of the catheter. Several options are available to correct this:

    a. **Withdraw the catheter 2 to 3 cm,** rotate it, and try to reinsert it.

    b. **Try injecting flush as you advance the catheter.** Sometimes this makes it easier to pass the catheter through the ductus venosus.

    c. **Double-catheter technique** is based on the concept that if the first catheter occupies the wrong vessel (portal system), the second catheter will enter the correct vessel (and pass through the ductus venosus) because the wrong one is blocked. Leave the misplaced catheter in place and pass another catheter through the vein; the misplaced one can then be removed (reported 50% success rate). This technique increases the risk of perforation.

10. **Connect the catheter to the fluid and tubing.**

11. **Secure the catheter similar to an umbilical artery catheter** (see Figures 28–4 and 28–5). Never advance a catheter once it is secured in place.

12. **Minimize infant mobilization while the catheter is in place to prevent the catheter from migrating to the right atrium.**

13. **Confirm placement.** Incorrect placement is associated with higher complication rates. The UVC should be at the junction of the inferior vena cava and the right atrium (in the inferior vena cava, below the level of the right atrium and above the level of the ductus venosus). Incorrect placement is associated with higher complication rates (pericardial or peritoneal effusion,

cardiac tamponade, arrhythmia, thrombosis, liver tissue necrosis, intracardiac thrombosis, death).

  a. Anteroposterior and lateral radiographs that include abdomen and chest are the radiographs of choice to confirm catheter position (see Figure 12–13). The UVC should be just **above the diaphragm** but below the right atrium. The UVC tip should be 0.5 to 1.0 cm (reported range, 0–2 cm) above the right diaphragm (UVC tip at thoracic vertebrae 8–9 usually corresponding to the right cavoatrial junction). **The lateral image is necessary to show the exact location and will show the course of the umbilical vein and ductus venosus in relation to the liver.** *Note:* Air can sometimes be seen in the portal venous branches immediately after UVC insertion. As an isolated transient finding, it should not be confused with portal air due to necrotizing enterocolitis.

    i. Thoracic level on x-ray does not accurately predict catheter position. UVCs were found to be located at a wide range of vertebral bodies (T6–11) by echocardiogram. Recommendations vary on what thoracic level the UVC line should be at (T8–9, T9, or T9–10).

    ii. Some clinicians suggest radiography is unreliable and very imprecise in confirming catheter tip position. Lateral radiographs do not always accurately predict catheter placement. Anteroposterior radiographs underestimate the incidence of left atrial placement, and lateral radiographs overestimate left atrial placement.

  b. POCUS. Present evidence supports the use of ultrasound for localization of the UVC. It has been suggested as the best modality since it more accurately confirms the position of the catheter tip and resulted in decreased radiation exposure than x-ray. Some also recommend the routine use of POCUS screening at regular intervals in all newborns with a UVC to make sure the catheter is in the proper position, and to follow any migration of the catheter and detect any complications.

  c. Blood gas determining partial pressure of oxygen and saturation can be obtained to confirm venous sampling (sensitivity 45% and specificity 95%).

  d. Gold standard is considered echocardiography with saline contrast injection to document distal catheter location.

  e. If bright red (arterial) blood is obtained, the UVC has either crossed the foramen ovale and needs to be pulled back, or the catheter is in an artery.

  f. If the catheter needs to be repositioned, you can withdraw (whether the sterile field is intact or not) if necessary. If you need to insert it further, you can only do this if the sterile field was kept intact. If the sterile field is not intact, you will have to remove and repeat with a clean setup.

  14. There is insufficient evidence to support or refute the routine use of prophylactic antibiotics with umbilical vein catheterization (Cochrane review, 2005). Do not use topical antibiotic ointments or creams at umbilical insertion sites because these will promote fungal infections and antimicrobial resistance.

IV. Umbilical vein catheter removal. UVC removal should be done as soon as possible because of the higher risk of colonization and infection with longer indwelling times.

  A. Make sure the umbilical tie is loose and cut and remove any sutures or tape that would hinder removal.

  B. Withdraw the catheter slowly 1 to 2 cm at a time over a few minutes until about 2 to 5 cm remain.

  C. Tighten the umbilical tie and stop any infusions.

  D. Pull the rest of the catheter out slowly (rate of 1 cm/min).

  E. Apply gentle pressure above the umbilicus until bleeding has stopped; loosen the umbilical tie.

  F. Send tip for culture if infection is suspected. Observe for excessive oozing or hemorrhage.

V. Complications. Risk of complication is high (10%–50%). Keep the catheter tip in the IVC and not at the foramen ovale, portal vein, or hepatic vein. Remember, complications can occur even with appropriately placed UVCs.

   A. Infection. Most commonly reported adverse effect. Minimize the risk by strict sterile technique, never advancing a secured catheter, and limiting indwelling time. Sepsis is most common, but cellulitis, omphalitis, endocarditis, septic emboli, liver abscess, and lung abscess can also occur. The AAP and CDC recommend to remove and not replace the line if any signs of a central line–associated bloodstream infection are present.

   B. Cardiac complications. Pericardial effusion is the second most common complication. It can be asymptomatic; suspect in infants with a UVC and progressive cardiomegaly. Right atrial arrhythmias can be caused by a UVC inserted too far that irritates the heart. Cardiac tamponade, cardiac perforation, pneumopericardium, and thrombotic endocarditis have also been reported.

   C. Thrombotic or embolic phenomenon. Largest risk factor is placement of central catheters. Make sure to flush catheters prior to insertion and never allow air to enter the end of the catheter. Nonfunctioning catheters should be removed. Never try to flush clots from the end of the catheter. Emboli can be in the lungs, liver, or anywhere in systemic circulation. Careful monitoring is indicated in very low BW infants who have a hematocrit >55% because they have an increase in UVC-associated thrombosis. The AAP and CDC recommend removing the line if thrombosis is present.

   D. Blood loss/hemorrhage can occur if tubing becomes disconnected.

   E. Retroperitoneal fluid extravasation (genital, buttocks, thigh, abdominal), ascites, hemoperitoneum.

   F. Necrotizing enterocolitis is thought to be a complication of UVCs, especially if in place for >24 hours. Studies suggest a higher cumulative risk in premature infants, especially if the UVC migrates to the portal vein or ductus venosus.

   G. Fungal infections of the right atrium. Reported complication rate of 13%.

   H. Pulmonary edema, hemorrhage, infarction, and hydrothorax can occur from a catheter that has lodged in or has perforated a pulmonary vein.

   I. Portal vein hypertension. Caused by a catheter positioned in the portal system.

   J. Hepatic complications include necrosis, calcification, laceration, abscess, biliary venous fistula formation, hematoma, infusate ascites, and portal venous air/hematoma/erosion. Do not allow a catheter to remain in the portal system. In case of emergency placement, the catheter should be advanced only 2 to 5 cm (just until blood returns) to avoid hepatic infusion.

   K. Other rare complications reported. Creation of a false luminal tract, vessel perforation, hepatic cyst, digital ischemia, perforation of the peritoneum, hemorrhagic infarction of the lungs, colon perforation, perforation of a Meckel diverticulum, persistent neonatal hypoglycemia, Wharton jelly embolism, and gangrene of an extremity.

49 Venous Access: Venipuncture (Phlebotomy)

I. Indications. Cochrane review states that **venipuncture**, by a skilled operator, is the **method of choice for blood sampling** in term infants. It was found to be less painful than heel stick sampling and a more effective sampling method.

   A. Blood sampling for routine analysis or blood culture. Venipuncture typically allows a larger volume of blood (recommended if ≥1 mL is needed) to be collected and is the method of choice for obtaining **blood cultures**. It is preferred over capillary blood sampling for certain tests (drug levels, hemoglobin/hematocrit, karyotype, coagulation studies, and cross-matching blood). Arterial blood sampling is preferred for lactate, pyruvate, and ammonia.

B. **Central hematocrit.** Venipuncture hematocrit is more reliable than heel stick hematocrit.

C. **Venous blood gas.** This can be used in some diseases (neonatal sepsis/respiratory distress syndrome) to diagnose acid-base imbalance if an arterial blood gas cannot be obtained. Venous samples show good validity in terms of pH, PCO_2, and HCO_3.

D. **Administration of medications** (infrequent application of venipuncture).

II. **Equipment.** Whenever possible, use safety needles that are self-shielding; 23- or 25-gauge syringe-mounted needles or 23- to 25-gauge winged infusion needles (butterfly needles; 23 gauge preferred to reduce risk of hemolysis or clotting), gloves (sterile for blood culture), 1- to 5-mL syringe, alcohol swabs, 3 povidone-iodine swabs (for blood culture), appropriate specimen containers (eg, red-topped tube, blood culture bottle[s]), a tourniquet or rubber band (for the scalp), 4 × 4 sterile gauze pads, optional localization devices if available (transilluminator, near-infrared visualization unit; eg, AccuVein, Palatine, IL, ultrasound).

III. **Procedure**

A. **Use distal venous sites first to preserve venous access.** Decide which vein to use. Use Figure 47–1 as a guide. Veins to use commonly include basilic, cephalic, or cubital veins in the antecubital fossa, veins on the dorsum of the hand (dorsal venous network) or foot (dorsal venous arch), wrist, greater saphenous vein at the ankle, scalp vein. Blood sampling proximal to intravenous sites should not be done.

B. **In cases of difficult vein localization.** Transillumination (see Chapter 44), near-infrared spectroscopy vein imaging (eg, AccuVein AV300; see Chapter 25), or possible bedside ultrasound (more commonly used for peripheral intravenous IV access) can be used (see Chapter 44).

C. **Restrain the infant as appropriate.**

D. **Pain management.** The American Academy of Pediatrics (AAP) recommends topical anesthesia (eg, eutectic mixture of lidocaine and prilocaine [EMLA], applied 30 minutes prior to procedure), oral sucrose or glucose, and nonpharmacologic pain prevention and relief techniques, with a combination of sucrose or glucose and nonpharmacologic techniques considered more effective.

1. **Topical local anesthetics.** AAP reports that topical anesthesia did decrease measures of pain during venipuncture. Cochrane review found there was not enough quality evidence to determine whether topical local anesthetics applied to the skin help relieve pain during needle-related procedures in newborn infants.

2. **Sucrose/glucose.** Sucrose is more commonly used, but glucose can be used as an alternative. Cochrane review states the following: "Sucrose is effective for reducing procedural pain from single events such as venipuncture. Optimal dose could not be identified and use in extremely preterm, unstable or ventilated neonates and needs to be addressed." AAP recommends an oral dose of 0.1 to 1 mL of 24% sucrose (or 0.2–0.5 mL/kg) 2 minutes before a painful procedure.

3. **Nonpharmacologic pain prevention during venipuncture**

a. **Breast feeding.** Cochrane review found that breast feeding during venipuncture was associated with lower pain responses in term infants compared with other nonpharmacologic interventions. The effect of breast feeding was similar to oral sucrose or glucose. Giving human milk via a pacifier or syringe seems to be as effective as giving sucrose or glucose for pain in term infants.

b. **Massage.** A recent review found that, when comparing massage to breast feeding during venipuncture, massage caused the lowest pain score followed by breast feeding. Another study found that upper limb massage may be effective in decreasing the infants' venipuncture pain perceptions.

c. **Maternal milk odor** (through a diffuser) was found to have an analgesic effect and to decrease the variability of the infant's heart rate and blood oxygen saturation in preterm infants during a venipuncture.

d. **Maternal voice** is effective in decreasing physiologic parameters during and after the painful procedure of venipuncture.

e. **Swaddling and skin-to-skin care.** There was no difference between swaddling and skin-to-skin kangaroo care on physiologic pain and other indices in neonatal premature infants during venipuncture.

f. **Sensorial stimulation** was found to be effective at decreasing pain during minor procedures, and 1 review found it to be more effective than sucrose.

4. **Combination of methods.** When using a combination of oral sucrose with nonpharmacologic measures, there is added analgesic effect.

E. **"Tourniquet" the extremity to occlude the vein.** Use a rubber band (for the head), a tourniquet, or an assistant's hand to encircle the area proximal to the vein. Removing and reapplying may optimize the distension of the vein.

F. **Prepare the site with antiseptic solution.** For blood cultures, wipe at least 3 times in concentric circles starting at the puncture site.

G. **Attach syringe (1–5 mL) to needle.**

H. **Puncture the skin with the bevel up** (for optimal blood flow and less chance of occlusion by vein wall). Direct the needle into the vein at a 15- to 30-degree angle. Use the vessel bifurcation if possible.

I. **Once blood enters the tubing,** collect the blood slowly with gentle suction to avoid hemolysis or vein wall occlusion (or administer the medication).

J. **Remove the tourniquet.** Remove and press the button to shield the needle. Apply gentle pressure on the area until hemostasis has occurred (usually 2–3 minutes). Distribute blood samples to the appropriate containers and invert or store as indicated.

IV. **Complications**

A. **Infection is a rare complication,** minimized by sterile technique. Septic arthritis of the hip has been reported from femoral venipuncture.

B. **Venous thrombosis/embolus** is often unavoidable, especially when multiple punctures are performed on the same vein and the vein is large.

C. **Hematoma or hemorrhage** is avoided by applying pressure to the site after the needle is removed to ensure hemostasis. If a coagulation defect is present, hemorrhage can occur.

D. **Scarring of the dorsum of the hand** from multiple venipunctures can occur in very low birthweight neonates.

E. **Cervical dural puncture can occur** from internal jugular venipuncture in an infant secondary to insertion of the needle at excessive depth.

F. **Laceration of artery** near the vein.

50 Abdominal Distension

I. **Problem.** <u>The nurse calls you to the bedside to assess a newborn infant with abdominal distention.</u> How is abdominal distension defined? There is no statistical definition of abdominal distension. Some reported definitions include: actual increase in abdominal size, measurable change in abdominal circumference, or "when the abdominal wall is on a higher plane than the xiphisternum in an infant lying on their back on a flat surface." Abdominal distension will frequently be evaluated as increased girth in comparison to the neonate's baseline. This can be associated with other concerning symptoms or be an isolated finding.

II. **Immediate questions**

A. **Are there additional gastrointestinal symptoms?** Bilious emesis is an emergent condition that suggests intestinal malrotation with volvulus until proven otherwise. Perform a physical exam to determine whether the abdomen is firm or soft and whether bowel sounds are present. A distended abdomen that is soft with normal bowel sounds is usually benign. In contrast, a firm abdomen with no bowel sounds and taut and discolored skin is significantly more concerning and will likely require immediate intervention. Presence of bilious or nonbilious emesis, increased gastric residuals, and bloody stools will also help guide acuity and the differential.

B. **Are there concerning systemic symptoms?** If the distention is associated with tachycardia, tachypnea, apnea, temperature instability, and irritability, the etiology of the distention becomes more concerning for infection, and the evaluation should include a sepsis workup in addition to further evaluation of the gastrointestinal (GI) system. The neonate's state (comfortable vs distressed) will also guide the differential diagnosis.

C. **Was the baby feeding and how?** Neonates can present with abdominal distention during a feed advance or a change in type of feed. Neonates may be receiving large quantities of feeds or feeds via a nasogastric (NG) or orogastric (OG) tube faster than they can digest them.

D. **Has the neonate stooled recently?** If the baby has not stooled in >12 to 24 hours, consider constipation. If the neonate is only a few days old and has never stooled, consider an intestinal obstruction. If there has been a recent stool, quality of stool and presence of blood should be assessed. See also Chapter 72.

E. **Is the neonate on continuous positive airway pressure?** If the neonate is receiving continuous positive airway pressure (CPAP) or other noninvasive ventilation, the abdomen can become distended because positive pressure will push air through the esophagus and subsequently the stomach and intestines.

F. **Is the stomach being vented?** If the neonate is receiving CPAP, it is important that the stomach be vented to relieve the abdomen of increased air pressure. If there is concern for abdominal distention, an OG or NG tube should be passed for decompression. If it cannot be passed or loops within the esophagus, this is concerning for esophageal atresia with a distal tracheoesophageal fistula. Continuing with CPAP in this situation will fill the stomach and intestines with air without an outlet. In this case, CPAP should be minimized and discontinued if possible.

G. **Does the neonate look edematous?** Abdominal distention could be secondary to third spacing from ascites or other fluid. Palpation of the abdomen and other signs of edema elsewhere in the body should help identify whether the distention is secondary to air or fluid.

III. **Differential diagnosis.** (See Figure 50–1.) The differential includes acute emergent concerns and benign causes. It is important to rule out the etiologies that need immediate intervention first because abdominal distention can be the first presenting sign of conditions that will have significant adverse outcomes if not treated immediately.

    A. **Obstruction.** A small bowel obstruction with intestinal malrotation/volvulus typically occurs with bilious emesis. Large bowel obstructions typically present with no stooling and distension.

        1. **Small bowel obstruction**

            a. **Malrotation with volvulus.** This is an emergent concern for which a surgical consultation is required. One-third of infants with malrotation present with volvulus before 1 month of age.

            b. **Intestinal atresias.** Occur in the ileum > duodenum > jejunum > colon. May have bilious or nonbilious emesis with a failure to pass stool.

            c. **Meconium ileus.** Meconium obstructs the terminal ileum, leading to distension. Approximately 90% of patients with meconium ileus have cystic fibrosis.

        2. **Large bowel obstruction**

            a. **Hirschsprung disease.** Aganglionosis of distal colon/rectum leading to delayed passage of stool. Approximately 75% of infants with Hirschsprung disease fail to pass meconium in the first 48 hours after birth. More common in males.

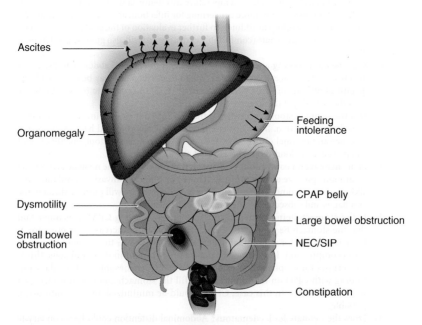

FIGURE 50–1. Causes of abdominal distention in a neonate. CPAP, continuous positive airway pressure; NEC, necrotizing enterocolitis; SIP, spontaneous intestinal perforation. *(Used with permission from Namrita Odackal, DO.)*

    b. Small left colon. Typically seen in term infants born to mothers with a history of diabetes. Fail to pass stool in the first 48 hours. Transient disease that usually resolves spontaneously.

    c. Anorectal malformation. May be imperforate anus with or without a fistula or simply anal stenosis. Anal atresia is highly associated with other anomalies including VATER/VACTERL (vertebral anomalies, anal atresia, tracheoesophageal fistula, and radial or renal dysplasia/vertebral defects, anal atresia, cardiac defects, tracheoesophageal fistula, renal and radial abnormalities, and limb abnormalities).

    d. Meconium plug. Meconium obstructs the rectum and/or lower colon. Increased incidence of Hirschsprung disease. More commonly seen in infants of diabetic mothers.

B. Perforation. Perforation of the bowel (pneumoperitoneum) can occur from congenital defects or secondary to acquired intestinal diseases. Plain radiographs will indicate free air lying over the liver. (See Figure 12–25.) Surgical evaluation is required.

    1. Congenital. More likely to occur secondary to bowel obstructions or atresias. Bowel perforation in utero may lead to meconium peritonitis and secondary abdominal distension.

    2. Acquired

      a. Necrotizing enterocolitis. Perforation occurs in approximately 30% of necrotizing enterocolitis (NEC) cases. Terminal ileum and ascending colon are the most common locations.

      b. Spontaneous intestinal perforation. Isolated perforation, typically in the ileum, that occurs most commonly in extremely low birthweight infants with an incidence of 5%. Risk factors include concomitant use of steroids and indomethacin and extreme prematurity. Presents in the first 2 weeks, often with a bluish discoloration of the abdomen and abdominal distension.

    3. Other. Traumatic perforations of the stomach may occur from NG/OG tube misplacement or excessive positive-pressure ventilation.

C. Necrotizing enterocolitis. NEC can present with isolated GI symptoms, including abdominal distention and bloody stools, and also with systemic symptoms of sepsis, such as apnea and temperature instability. Concern for NEC is greater with a history of prematurity, hypoxemia, and formula feeds. NEC occurs in approximately 6% of infants <1500 g. Red blood cell transfusion (controversial) or significant anemia in the prior 48 hours may also be a risk factor. Overall mortality is between 10% and 15%, with an increase to 30% if intestinal perforation occurs. Pneumatosis intestinalis is the classic sign on abdominal radiograph (See Figure 12–26), and thrombocytopenia is also classically seen.

D. Sepsis. Abdominal distention and other signs of feeding intolerance can be clinical signs of sepsis, particularly in premature patients who may not mount a fever. This should be considered with or without NEC based on the entire clinical picture. Sepsis occurs in approximately one-third of very low birthweight infants, and incidence is indirectly related to gestational age.

E. Anatomic abnormality or organomegaly. If the baby is 1 to 2 days old, has been in the well-baby nursery where close monitoring is less likely, or has received late prenatal care, consider an undiagnosed anatomic abnormality that is presenting with abdominal distention (eg, a tracheoesophageal fistula, abdominal mass, or hepatosplenomegaly associated with an inborn error of metabolism).

F. Dysmotility/gastroparesis. It may take several days for premature neonates to have normal gut motility, and they may present with abdominal distention if feeds are relatively larger or faster than they can handle. Alternatively, the neonate could have pathologic dysmotility secondary to Hirschsprung disease, cystic fibrosis, or other genetic disorders.

G. Constipation. If the neonate has yet to stool or is stooling infrequently, abdominal distention may present secondary to backup of GI contents.

H. **Ascites.** If the patient is septic or has leaky capillaries secondary to extracorporeal membrane oxygenation or some other systemic or local source of inflammation, a loss of protein or other liver function, hydrops, impaired right ventricular function, or high-output cardiac failure, the neonate could have fluid collecting into the abdominal interstitial space, causing abdominal distention.

I. **Continuous positive airway pressure belly.** When receiving positive pressure through a noninvasive route (ie, no endotracheal tube), the air cannot differentiate between passing through the esophagus or trachea. This can cause inflation within the GI tract, leading to abdominal distention. This is more likely if the stomach is not being intermittently vented. This occurs in >75% of infants <1000 g and less frequently in larger infants.

J. **Feeding intolerance.** Some neonates will not tolerate specific types of formula or may have a milk protein allergy. This can present with malabsorption, bloating, and abdominal distention, with or without bloody stools.

IV. **Database**

A. **Physical examination.** Examination of the abdomen should include auscultation and palpation of the abdomen. Examine for discoloration of the abdominal skin. Look for systemic signs of distress such as increased work of breathing from increased abdominal girth; edema in the face, hands, or feet; and hypotonia. Some neonatal intensive care units measure abdominal girth, although this is *controversial* because it is can be affected by many variables such as time since last feed/stool and amount of body fat/edema. If performed, measurements should be taken 1 cm above the umbilicus in a supine position. A change of up to 1.5 cm suggests normal variability.

1. **If the examination is abnormal beyond abdominal distension,** place the infant on nothing by mouth (NPO) while continuing the evaluation. Abdominal radiographs and gastric decompression are indicated, and consider a sepsis evaluation and surgical consultation.

2. **If the examination is normal beyond abdominal distension** and the infant is tolerating feeds, continue close examination and consider a baseline radiograph.

B. **Laboratory studies**

1. **Complete blood count and/or C-reactive protein.** Thrombocytopenia and other complete blood count abnormalities may indicate sepsis. Some institutions use C-reactive protein to help guide sepsis evaluations.

2. **Blood and urine cultures.** If concerned for sepsis, a blood and urine culture should be obtained to assess for both aerobic and anaerobic bacteria.

3. **Liver function tests.** Liver function tests can help evaluate when concerned for hepatomegaly or ascites secondary to liver pathology. If abnormal, coagulation studies may be indicated.

C. **Imaging and other studies**

1. **Abdominal radiograph.** The abdominal radiograph is a good screening study that may reveal ileus, distended loops of intestine, pneumoperitoneum (Figure 12–26), or pneumatosis intestinalis (Figure 12–27). This can be followed by serial imaging depending on severity and level of concern. If free air is suspected, a lateral decubitus film should be done in addition. Alternatively, an abdominal x-ray can confirm that there is air passing through to the rectum, indicating less concern for obstruction.

2. **Abdominal ultrasound.** Ultrasound can be used for diagnosing masses, ascites, or debris indicating perforation. May also be used to assess for pneumatosis intestinalis (NEC).

3. **Fluoroscopy.** If obstruction is suspected, a fluoroscopic upper GI study should be conducted emergently. Immediate evaluation to look for flow of contrast from the esophagus, through the stomach, and through the duodenum and remainder of the intestinal tract is indicated.

V. **Plan**
  A. **Rule out emergent conditions.** Intestinal obstruction and infection (either systemic or NEC) are the most serious pathologies associated with abdominal distention.
  B. **Decide whether to stop or continue feeds.** Enteric feeds may or may not be a contributing factor to abdominal distention. If the etiology is considered to be benign, continuing feeds is reasonable. If imaging is concerning for ileus or slow motility through the GI tract, slowing feeds or holding a feed advance at the current volume of feeds may be appropriate. If there is concern for significant illness, NEC, spontaneous intestinal perforation, or sepsis, stopping feeds is appropriate to avoid ischemia to the GI tract, which would potentially cause further damage. The duration of holding feeds depends on clinical improvement. Intravenous fluid hydration or nutrition should be started if feeds are held.
  C. **Treat the symptoms.** Acutely, venting the abdomen via an NG or OG tube and helping the baby stool with glycerin suppositories can relieve abdominal pressure, which may be affecting respiratory status. If there is ascites causing distention, diuresis or a peritoneal tap may be indicated. If treating the neonate for pain, careful thought should be given to treating with opiates as this will further delay gut motility.
  D. **Treat the underlying cause.** Once the etiology has been established, ultimately symptoms will resolve when the underlying cause is treated. In severe cases, treatment may require surgical intervention, antibiotics, and long-term parenteral nutrition.
  E. **Monitor for worsening abdominal distention.** Routine measuring of abdominal girth once a shift (center dependent) or with serial x-rays (to continue to monitor for ileus, ascites, or free air) may be indicated to monitor for worsening abdominal distention.

51 Abnormal Blood Gas

  I. **Problem.** An abnormal blood gas value for a neonate is reported by the laboratory. A blood gas measures pH, PCO_2, and oxygen (O_2), and all the other components (base excess, bicarbonate concentration, and oxygen saturation) are calculated based on the 3 levels measured. Accepted normal values for an arterial blood gas on room air are pH 7.35 to 7.45 (pH varies with age; a pH >7.30 is generally acceptable), $PaCO_2$ 35 to 45 mm Hg (slightly higher accepted if the blood pH remains normal), and PaO_2 50 to 95 mm Hg (based on gestational age). (See Table 9–1, page 98, for normal range of arterial blood gas values for term and preterm infants.)
  II. **Immediate questions**
    A. **What component of the blood gas is abnormal?**
      1. **What is the pH?** The pH determines the presence of acidemia or alkalemia. Is it acidic (pH <7.35) or alkalotic (pH >7.45)?
        a. **pH is proportional to HCO_3 (base excess)**
           i. **Metabolic acidosis.** Abnormal ↓ in HCO_3 ↓ pH.
           ii. **Metabolic alkalosis.** Abnormal ↑ HCO_3 ↑ pH.
        b. **pH is inversely proportional to PCO_2**
           i. **Respiratory acidosis.** Abnormal ↑ PCO_2 ↓ pH.
           ii. **Respiratory alkalosis.** Abnormal ↓ PCO_2 ↑ pH.
      2. **What is the PCO_2?** Is it increased or decreased? PCO_2 reflects alveolar ventilation and is mediated by the respiratory system, and the only way to remove it is through the lungs. If it is abnormal, it suggests a respiratory disorder.

3. **What is the PaO$_2$? Is it increased or decreased?** Hypoxia (inadequate oxygenation) or hyperoxia (excess supply of oxygen) can occur.
4. **What is the HCO$_3$? Is it increased or decreased?** Bicarbonate is a weak base that is mediated by the renal system as part of the acid-base homeostasis. It is retained or excreted by the kidney to regulate acid-base balance. If bicarbonate is abnormal, it is a metabolic disorder.

B. **Is this blood gas value very different from the patient's previous blood gas determination?** If the patient has had metabolic acidosis on the last 5 blood gas measurements and now has metabolic alkalosis, it might be best to repeat the blood gas measurements before initiating treatment. **Do not treat the infant based on 1 abnormal gas value,** especially if the infant's clinical status has not changed.

C. **How was the sample collected?** Blood gas measurements can be reported on **arterial, venous, or capillary (heel stick)** blood samples.
1. **Arterial blood samples. Best indicator of pH, PaCO$_2$, and PaO$_2$.** The **gold standard** of obtaining a blood gas is to obtain one from an indwelling arterial catheter (peripheral or umbilical). Blood gases by **intermittent arterial punctures** may not accurately reflect the infant's respiratory status. A sudden decrease in the PaCO$_2$ and PaO$_2$ can occur during the puncture. Crying can decrease the PaCO$_2$, HCO$_3$, and oxygen saturation. Arterial blood gas reference values per the Perinatal Continuing Education Program (PCEP) are as follows: pH, 7.30 to 7.40; PaCO$_2$, 40 to 50 mm Hg; and PaO$_2$, 45 to 65 mm Hg.
2. **Venous blood samples.** Gives a lower pH value, a significantly lower PO$_2$, and a higher PCO$_2$ than arterial samples. It is good for HCO$_3$ estimation. Venous blood gas reference values per PCEP are as follows: pH, 7.25 to 7.35; PCO$_2$, 45 to 55 mm Hg; and PO$_2$, unreliable.
3. **Capillary (heel stick) samples.** Gives a satisfactory assessment of the infant's pH and PCO$_2$ but does not give an accurate PaO$_2$. Capillary blood gases (CBG) give a similar or lower pH value (not as low as venous pH), similar or slightly higher PCO$_2$, and lower PO$_2$ than arterial samples; capillary blood gas measurements are not reliable in an infant who is cold or has decreased perfusion (hypotensive or in shock). CBG reference values with proper technique per PCEP are as follows: pH, 7.25 to 7.35; PCO$_2$, 45 to 55 mm Hg; and PO$_2$, unreliable.

D. **Is the infant on ventilatory support?** Management of abnormal blood gas levels is approached differently in an intubated infant than in a patient breathing room air.

E. **Is there a sudden change in the blood gas or a gradual change over several blood gases? A sudden change in a blood gas accompanied by a sudden deterioration in the infant's clinical status is an emergency situation and is more urgent than a gradual change in a blood gas.** The differential of the 2 conditions is also different.
1. A sudden change in the blood gas (a sudden decrease in PaO$_2$ and an increase in PaCO$_2$) with **a sudden clinical deterioration in the infant** can be a result of a blocked or displaced endotracheal tube, a pneumothorax (tension or unilateral), the endotracheal tube in the mainstem bronchus, or a malfunctioning ventilator.
2. **A gradual change in the blood gas with a gradual deterioration in the infant.** Gradual changes can reflect that there is increasing respiratory failure or inadequate ventilation requiring that the settings be changed. Examples include:
   a. **Gradual decrease in PaO$_2$, gradual increase in PaCO$_2$:** Inappropriate ventilator settings, atelectasis that is causing increased intrapulmonary shunting.
   b. **Gradual increase in PaCO$_2$, no changes in PaO$_2$:** Inadequate alveolar ventilation or an increased dead space (from tubing or airway issues).

F. **Is there a nonrespiratory cause of the change in blood gas in an infant on a ventilator?** Nonrespiratory causes can result in changes in blood gases. These include intraventricular hemorrhage, seizures, hypoglycemia, overwhelming sepsis, pneumopericardium, patent ductus arteriosus (PDA), and hypotension. **Note that any severe illness can cause a metabolic acidosis.**

III. **Differential diagnosis**
   A. **Metabolic acidosis (pH <7.30–7.35 with a normal to low carbon dioxide).** After birth, it is normal for an infant to have a mild metabolic acidosis. Metabolic acidosis is very common in the neonatal intensive care unit (NICU), especially in the very sick neonate. The **3 main causes of metabolic acidosis** are **loss of base (mainly bicarbonate) from renal or gastrointestinal causes, decreased renal excretion of acid,** or **an increased production of acid.** Metabolic acidosis is classified as increased anion gap, normal or nonanion gap, or low anion gap acidosis. **Determining the anion gap will help decide the cause of the acidosis.**
      1. **Anion gap.** Difference in measured cations and anions in serum or plasma. Calculated by:

      $$\text{Anion gap (mEq/L)} = \text{sodium (mEq/L)} - [\text{chloride (mEq/L)} + \text{bicarbonate (mEq/L)}]$$

      a. **Normal range.** 8 to 16 mEq/L (up to 18 mEq/L in premature infants <1000 g).
      b. **Increased.** >16 mEq/L in infants (>18 mEq/L in premature infants <1000 g).
      2. **Common causes of metabolic acidosis in the newborn**
      a. **Increased anion gap metabolic acidosis (normal chloride)** implies presence of other acids.
         i. **Lactic acidosis associated with clinical evidence of decreased tissue perfusion is common in the neonate.** A serum anion gap >16 mEq/L is highly predictive of lactic acidosis (<8 mEq/L lactic acidosis is highly unlikely). Some infants may not have an increased anion gap with lactic acidosis. **Causes:** asphyxia, hypoxia, respiratory distress syndrome (RDS), sepsis, compromised cardiac output (cardiogenic, septic, and hypovolemic shock), circulatory or respiratory failure, massive hemorrhage/severe anemia, periventricular hemorrhage (PVH)/intraventricular hemorrhage (IVH), hypothermia/cold stress, hypotension, PDA, necrotizing enterocolitis (NEC) or any intestinal ischemia, excessive ventilator pressures with decreased cardiac output, seizures, and ascites/third spacing of fluids.
         ii. **Inborn errors of metabolism.** Inborn errors have lactic acidosis not associated with clinical evidence of poor tissue perfusion. An anion gap of >16 is seen in many inborn errors of metabolism secondary to accumulation of fixed acids. Examples include: **organic acidemias** (most common), galactosemia, hereditary fructose intolerance, maple syrup disease, congenital/primary lactic acidosis, type I glycogen storage disease and pyruvate dehydrogenase/carboxylase deficiency, mitochondrial respiratory chain defects, multiple carboxylase deficiency, and fatty acid oxidation defects. In an infant with persistent metabolic acidosis with increased anion gap, negative urine ketones, whose mother had HELLP (hemolysis, elevated liver enzymes, and low platelet count) syndrome, think fatty acid oxidation defects.
         iii. **Acute kidney injury and chronic kidney disease.** Results in failure of excretion of hydrogen ions and other unmeasured acid anions.
         iv. **Late metabolic acidosis of prematurity (first to third week of life)** occurs in healthy premature infants who have a mild to moderate metabolic acidosis and decreased growth. It is caused by an excessive acid load from high-protein formula (casein-based formulas), amino acid intake, or intravenous (IV) alimentation on the premature kidney with decreased renal clearance.
         v. **Toxins and medications.** Maternal use of salicylates and maternal acidosis. Benzyl alcohol in doxapram. Others: alcohols and glycols, acetaminophen, α-adrenergic agents, cocaine, nitroprusside, ibuprofen, iron, isoniazid, paraldehyde, sulfasalazine, valproic acid.

    b. Normal or non–anion gap metabolic acidosis (normal anion gap, elevated serum chloride, hyperchloremic acidosis). A low serum potassium indicates loss of base; a high serum potassium suggests renal tubular acidosis (RTA). Most common causes are RTA and diarrhea.

        i. Renal loss of bicarbonate

            (a) Immature kidneys. Bicarbonate wasting.

            (b) Renal tubular acidosis. Defect in either the reabsorption of bicarbonate or the secretion of the hydrogen ion. (Most common cause in preterm infants is proximal RTA.) Check urine pH; <7 suggests proximal RTA, whereas >5.5 suggests distal RTA.

            (c) Acute kidney injury.

            (d) Renal dysplasia.

            (e) Medications. Carbonic anhydrase inhibitors can cause reduced uptake of bicarbonate ions (acetazolamide, dorzolamide, methazolamide, hydroxyurea). Aldosterone inhibitors: spironolactone and eplerenone.

            (f) Hypoaldosteronism. Low Na^+, elevated K^+.

            (g) Hyperparathyroidism.

        ii. Gastrointestinal loss of bicarbonate

            (a) Diarrhea (usually secretory).

            (b) Urologic and gastrointestinal procedures. Surgery for NEC, ileostomy, enterocutaneous or bowel fistula, small bowel or pancreatic drainage, any bowel diversion in contact with urine.

            (c) Medications. Ion exchange resins, cholestyramine, calcium chloride, magnesium sulfate.

        iii. Dilutional acidosis. Rapid volume expansion with lactated Ringer's solution, saline, or dextrose with dilution of bicarbonate.

        iv. Factitious acidosis. Due to excessive heparin in the syringe. Air contamination can give a large base deficit.

        v. Excessive chloride in intravenous fluids.

        vi. Hyperalimentation acidosis caused by the acid load.

        vii. Potassium-sparing diuretics and hyperkalemia.

    c. Low anion gap metabolic acidosis. (Low or negative anion gap.) Rare; usually caused by laboratory error or hypoalbuminemia.

B. Metabolic alkalosis (pH >7.45 with base excess of >5). First clue is often an elevated bicarbonate. It is usually iatrogenic and uncommon in the neonatal period and due to an excess of base (HCO_3) or loss of acid H^+. In the neonatal period, the most common causes of an excess of base is chronic administration of alkali administration. In the neonate, the most common cause of loss of acid is continuous nasogastric suction, diuretic treatment, and persistent vomiting. There are 2 types: chloride resistant (high urinary chloride) and chloride responsive (low urinary chloride). **Obtain a spot urinary chloride** to help determine the etiology.

    1. High urinary chloride >20 mEq/L (chloride-resistant metabolic alkalosis; increased extracellular fluid volume). Excess alkali administration (acetate, citrate, bicarbonate, lactate); early diuretic therapy (especially furosemide); hypokalemia; large blood product transfusion; Bartter syndrome (mineralocorticoid administration); exogenous steroid therapy; Cushing, Conn, or Liddle syndrome; primary aldosteronism, congenital adrenal hyperplasia variant (deoxycorticosterone excess syndrome); milk-alkali syndrome; neonatal pseudo-Bartter syndrome (secondary to maternal eating disorder).

    2. Low urinary chloride <10 mEq/L (chloride-responsive metabolic alkalosis; low serum chloride and decreased extracellular fluid volume). Loss of gastric secretions (persistent vomiting, continuous nasogastric/orogastric suction), secretory diarrhea (congenital chloride-wasting diarrhea), acute correction of chronically compensated respiratory acidosis, late diuretic therapy, post hypercapnia syndrome.

3. **Common causes of metabolic alkalosis in the newborn**
   a. **Prolonged nasogastric/orogastric suction.**
   b. **Diuretic therapy** (especially furosemide in patients with bronchopulmonary dysplasia/chronic lung disease [BPD/CLD]).
   c. **Excess alkali administration** (eg, sodium bicarbonate, citrate, acetate, or lactate infusion) as in parenteral nutrition or increased alkali load from feedings.
   d. **Potassium depletion.**
   e. **Compensation for respiratory acidosis** (eg, infant with BPD/CLD/chronic ventilation).
4. **Less common causes.** Pyloric stenosis (persistent vomiting), Bartter syndrome (rare), pseudo-Bartter syndrome due to maternal eating disorder, primary hyperaldosteronism, congenital chloride-wasting diarrhea, congenital adrenal hyperplasia (certain types).

C. **Respiratory alkalosis (a decrease in carbon dioxide with an increase in pH).** Alkalosis can be associated with decreased cerebral blood flow and a decrease in tissue oxygen delivery. Hypocarbia is associated with periventricular leukomalacia and deafness.
   1. **Overventilation by the ventilator.** Most common cause in NICU.
   2. **Air bubble in the blood gas collection syringe.** This can falsely lower the PaO_2 and $PaCO_2$.
   3. **Heparin can falsely lower the $PaCO_2$.** Make sure minimal heparin remains in the syringe.
   4. **Hyperventilation therapy.** Used to be a treatment of persistent pulmonary hypertension but is no longer recommended.
   5. **Central hyperventilation.** Central nervous system (CNS) stimulation of the respiratory drive caused by a CNS disorder or transient hyperammonemia (ammonia stimulates the respiratory center, resulting in hyperventilation).
   6. **Hypoxemia can cause a low carbon dioxide.** Respiratory centers are stimulated through chemoreceptors.
   7. **Hyperventilation.** Seen in a spontaneously breathing infant secondary to sepsis, fever, aspiration pneumonia, or retained fluid.
   8. **Compensation for a primary metabolic acidosis.**

D. **Respiratory acidosis (increase in $PaCO_2$ with decrease in pH).** A gradual increase in PCO_2 is usually secondary to insufficient alveolar ventilation.
   1. **Obstructed endotracheal tube (eg, mucus plug).** Tube blockage can occur after a few days of ventilation because of increased secretions.
   2. **Improper endotracheal tube position.** An endotracheal tube positioned in the oropharynx, down the right mainstem bronchus, or at the carina.
   3. **Ventilator malfunction or insufficient respiratory support.** Disconnect the ventilator and manually inflate the infant's lungs; if the condition improves, then the problem is with the ventilator. There can be a mechanical failure, tubing can be disconnected, leak may be present, or there can be electrical failure.
   4. **Ventilator strategy that allows permissive hypercapnia (controlled mechanical hypoventilation) is *controversial*.** Use caution with permissive hypercapnia until further studies are done. Severe hypercapnia or hypocapnia should be avoided. In infants with BPD/CLD, higher carbon dioxide (CO_2) is sometimes tolerated to wean them from mechanical ventilation.
   5. **Increasing respiratory failure.** Lung diseases such as RDS, pneumonia, transient tachypnea, BPD/CLD, pleural effusion, pulmonary hypoplasia, atelectasis.
   6. **Pneumothorax.**
   7. **Hypoventilation or poor respiratory effort** from maternal anesthesia, medications, neuromuscular disorders, congenital central hypoventilation syndrome, sepsis, intracranial hemorrhage, or hypoglycemia.

8. **Patent ductus arteriosus with pulmonary edema.** Suspect a PDA if the infant has a systolic murmur, active precordium, bounding pulses, and increased pulse pressure. Other clinical signs and symptoms may include congestive heart failure, deteriorating blood gases with an increase in the ventilator settings, and cardiomegaly with increased pulmonary vascularity on chest radiograph.

9. **Others.** Congenital diaphragmatic hernia, phrenic nerve paralysis, and other causes.

E. **Low oxygen (hypoxia)**
   1. **Agitation**
   2. **Improper endotracheal tube position**
   3. **Inadequate ventilatory support**
   4. **Congenital heart disease (cyanotic);** see Chapter 56
   5. **Respiratory diseases**
      a. **Primary lung disease.** Respiratory distress syndrome, transient tachypnea of the newborn, BPD/CLD, and others.
      b. **Airway obstruction.** Mucus plug, choanal atresia, other congenital malformations (eg, macroglossia, cystic hygroma).
      c. **External compression of the lungs.** Air leak syndrome (eg, pneumothorax) or congenital defects (eg, congenital diaphragmatic hernia).
   6. **Apnea of prematurity**
   7. **Persistent pulmonary hypertension**
   8. **Central nervous system/neuromuscular disorders**
   9. **Metabolic abnormalities**
   10. **Hematologic disorders**
   11. **Sepsis /hypotension**

F. **High oxygen (hyperoxia).** Hyperoxia can cause severe retinopathy of prematurity, CLD, and brain injury in preterm infants. Overventilation (high FiO_2, high positive end-expiratory pressure (PEEP), high peak inspiratory pressure (PIP) or tidal volume, high inspiratory time, high flow, high rate) can cause a high PaO_2. Nitrogen washout therapy using 100% oxygen to rapidly resolve a pneumothorax can cause hyperoxia but is no longer recommended. Decrease the oxygenation first before reducing any of the other ventilator parameters.

IV. **Database**
   A. **Physical examination.** Evaluate for signs of sepsis (eg, hypotension or poor perfusion). Check for equal breath sounds; asymmetric breath sounds suggest pneumothorax or incorrect endotracheal tube (ETT) placement. Observe for chest wall movement. Listen for breath sounds over the chest versus the epigastric region, which may help determine whether the ETT is malpositioned. Listen to the heart for any murmur, and palpate for cardiac displacement.

   B. **Laboratory studies**
      1. **Repeat blood gas measurement if the result is unexpected.** Do not make a major clinical decision based on a venous or capillary blood gas values or on just 1 arterial blood gas result.
      2. **Serum electrolytes.** To include blood urea nitrogen, creatinine, glucose, and potassium (severe metabolic alkalosis can cause hypokalemia). Serum Na^+, K^+, Cl^-, and bicarbonate (from arterial blood gas) to determine anion gap.
      3. **Urine chloride.** To evaluate metabolic alkalosis. May not be valid in the setting of diuretic use.
      4. **Urinary ketones.** If absent or small, consider lactic acidosis; if moderate or large, suspect organic acidemias (maple syrup urine disease, glycogen storage disease, disorders of pyruvate metabolism, others).
      5. **Plasma ammonia level.** If normal, may be RTA; may be increased in urea cycle defects and in some organic acidemias (acidosis and hyperammonemia).
      6. **Serum potassium level.** Severe metabolic alkalosis can cause hypokalemia.

7. **Measure the anion gap.** Correct for hypoalbuminemia by adding 2.5 mEq/L to the anion gap for every gram per deciliter that the concentration of serum albumin is reduced below the normal value of 3.5 g/dL.

8. **Plasma lactate is increased in lactic acidosis.** Measure lactate in infants who have a normal anion gap but in whom lactic acidosis is suspected. Normal and elevated lactate can be seen in organic acidemias; lactate is elevated in sepsis (predictor of mortality) and hypoperfusion.

9. **Complete blood count with differential.** If sepsis is being considered.

10. **Further sepsis workup if indicated.** Blood culture, urinalysis and culture, and lumbar puncture if indicated.

11. **Metabolic screen if indicated.** Urine and plasma for amino acids and organic acids.

C. **Imaging and other studies**

1. **Pulmonary mechanics.** Check the tidal volume (VT) delivered on the ventilator. The normal VT is 5 to 6 mL/kg. If the VT is low, it could mean that not enough pressure is given or there is an obstruction in the ETT.

2. **Transillumination of the chest.** If pneumothorax is suspected (see Chapter 44).

3. **Chest radiograph.** Should be performed if an abnormal blood gas value is reported, unless there is an obvious cause. An anteroposterior view should be obtained to check ETT placement (see Figure 12–10), rule out air leak (eg, pneumothorax; see Figure 12–23), check heart size and pulmonary vascularity (increased or decreased), and determine whether the infant is being hypoventilated or hyperventilated.

4. **Abdominal radiograph.** If NEC is suspected in a patient with **severe metabolic acidosis.** See Figure 12–26.

5. **Ultrasonography of the head.** To diagnose IVH. See Figures 12–1 through 12–4 for examples of IVH.

6. **Echocardiography.** May detect PDA or other cardiac abnormality and can be used to diagnose low cardiac output.

7. **Ultrasonography of the abdomen with color Doppler studies.** To evaluate for NEC and bowel necrosis.

V. **Plan**

A. **Overall plan.** Verify the blood gas result, determine the cause of the problem, and provide specific treatment. First, examine the infant. If the infant's clinical status has not changed, repeat a blood gas to verify the report. If the clinical status has changed, the abnormal report is probably correct; repeat the blood gas and begin further evaluation of the infant.

B. **Specific management of blood gas abnormalities**

1. **Metabolic acidosis**

a. **Understand and treat** the underlying cause of the acidosis.

b. **Correct any treatable causes** such as hypoxia, hypovolemia, sepsis, hemorrhage, low cardiac output, or severe anemia.

c. **Do not treat metabolic acidosis** with hyperventilation.

d. **Volume expansion should not be used to treat acidosis** unless there are signs of hypovolemia. Severe acidosis causes a decrease in myocardial contractility. **Cochrane review** states that there is insufficient evidence to state that a fluid bolus reduces morbidity and mortality in preterm infants with metabolic acidosis.

e. **Watch for hypokalemia** as metabolic acidosis is corrected.

f. **If metabolic acidosis is persistent and the infant does not respond to treatment,** consider an inborn error of metabolism.

g. **Controversy over sodium bicarbonate use in metabolic acidosis.** Treatment with sodium bicarbonate is no longer routinely recommended as supportive therapy in metabolic acidosis. It has been quoted as being "basically useless therapy" and is associated with adverse sequelae, such as hypernatremia, intracranial hemorrhage (increases IVH), transient fluctuations in the cerebral blood flow and cardiovascular hemodynamics in extremely premature infants, decreased oxygen delivery to tissues, aggravated myocardial injury and cardiac function deterioration, worsening intracellular acidosis, and increased risk of death. **It is no longer recommended in the following situations:**

  i. **Sodium bicarbonate in the delivery room.** The American Academy of Pediatrics (AAP) and American Heart Association (AHA) guidelines do not recommend the use of sodium bicarbonate in the delivery room.

  ii. **Sodium bicarbonate in postresuscitation care.** AAP and AHA do not recommend giving sodium bicarbonate to an infant with metabolic acidosis after resuscitation. They state it might be helpful early on and might actually improve the acid pH, but if the infant's lungs cannot exhale the CO_2 that is formed, the acidosis will worsen.

  iii. **Sodium bicarbonate in a newborn** with perinatal asphyxia, ischemia (NEC), or prolonged hypoxia (persistent pulmonary hypertension) is not recommended.

  iv. **Sodium bicarbonate in preterm or extremely premature infants.** No evidence of benefit. Cochrane review states there is insufficient evidence to state that use of sodium bicarbonate in preterm infants with metabolic acidosis reduces mortality and morbidity.

  v. **Sodium bicarbonate in a cardiac arrest.** Sodium bicarbonate infusion during a cardiac arrest is not recommended in neonatal patients. May cause harm as noted earlier.

  vi. **Sodium bicarbonate in sepsis.** Sodium bicarbonate in sepsis is accepted in adults with a pH <7.15. Limited data in neonates.

h. **Some other less controversial recommendations** concerning sodium bicarbonate use in metabolic acidosis.

  i. **Sodium bicarbonate is part of the European and United Kingdom neonatal resuscitation guidelines** because there is some evidence that using alkali to reverse intracardiac acidosis may sometimes restore the heart rate when all else fails.

  ii. **Sodium bicarbonate use in an infant with severe metabolic acidosis (pH <7.15)** with certain life-threatening conditions (eg, cardiac dysfunction, ventricular tachycardia requiring cardioversion, severe hyperkalemia with electrocardiogram changes, certain inborn errors of metabolism with acute metabolic decompensation). Use of sodium bicarbonate in each individual patient must be evaluated and the potential risks and benefits considered.

  iii. **Sodium bicarbonate use in replacement of base for ongoing gastrointestinal and renal losses.** Not proven but is often accepted as reasonable therapy. Bicarbonate therapy has been used for conditions such as diarrhea and proximal RTA type 2.

  iv. **Sodium bicarbonate use in inborn errors of metabolism.** Sodium bicarbonate has been used to correct metabolic acidosis in some inborn errors of metabolism (eg, organic acidemia) and is used if the infant has an acute metabolic decompensation with metabolic acidosis (pH 7.0–7.2).

  v. **Sodium bicarbonate use in hyperkalemia.** Sodium bicarbonate decreases the serum potassium level by moving potassium into the cells. It accepted in the emergent treatment of hyperkalemia. See Chapter 65.

i. **Medications for metabolic acidosis**

  i. **Sodium bicarbonate administration.** As reviewed earlier, administration of sodium bicarbonate has very limited use. However, if there are specific indications for its use, it should be a diluted formulation and a slow correction. Verify there is adequate ventilation and circulation to prevent an increase in CO_2 retention. Give in a large vein because it is hypertonic and can be caustic. Initial dose is 1 to 2 mEq/kg/dose IV administered slowly over 30 minutes. Use a 0.5-mEq/mL solution or dilute the 1-mEq/mL solution 1:1 with sterile water for injection; maximum rate in neonates and infants is 10 mEq/min. (See also Chapter 155.)

ii. **Tromethamine (tromethamine acetate) is no longer available in the United States.** It has been used in infants who have metabolic acidosis with significant hypercarbia (high PCO_2 of >65 mm Hg) or significant hypernatremia (serum sodium >150 mEq/L) despite aggressive assisted ventilation.

iii. **Sodium or potassium acetate (intravenous preparations)** can be used to treat metabolic acidosis through the conversion of acetate to bicarbonate at a 1:1 ratio. It is used in hyperalimentation or IV fluids for bicarbonate replacement as part of urinary losses in preterm infants and treatment of chronic metabolic acidosis. The dosing for sodium or potassium acetate is similar to sodium bicarbonate. See dosing in Chapter 155.

iv. **Citrate and citric acid solutions (oral medications).** Used in the treatment of chronic metabolic acidosis, as in RTA or chronic kidney disease, because sodium and potassium citrate salts have the ability to buffer gastric acidity and are metabolized to bicarbonate. See Chapter 155 for dosing information.

j. **Conditions with metabolic acidosis and their specific treatments**

i. **Sepsis.** Initiate a septic workup and consider broad-spectrum antibiotics. (See Chapter 146.)

ii. **Necrotizing enterocolitis.** See Chapter 109.

iii. **Hypothermia or cold stress.** See Chapter 8.

iv. **Periventricular/intraventricular hemorrhage.** Weekly ultrasonographic examinations of the head and daily head circumferences are indicated. Monitor the infant for signs of increased intracranial pressure (convulsions, vomiting, and/or hypotension). (See Chapter 103.)

v. **Patent ductus arteriosus.** If hemodynamically significant, PDA should be treated. (See Chapter 114.)

vi. **Shock/low cardiac output.** Give volume expansion if hypovolemic or vasoactive medications based on cardiac function. (See Chapter 70.)

vii. **Renal tubular acidosis.** Treat with alkaline therapy such as sodium bicarbonate or citrate or citric acid solution.

viii. **Inborn errors of metabolism.** Rare cause (see Chapter 100).

ix. **Maternal use of salicylates.** Acidosis usually resolves without treatment.

x. **Acute kidney injury.** See Chapter 86.

xi. **Congenital lactic acidosis.** Supportive care, correction of the metabolic acidosis with sodium bicarbonate.

xii. **Parenteral hyperalimentation.** Preterm infants usually need acetate supplementation in hyperalimentation to correct for ongoing bicarbonate losses. It should be given to infants with a base deficit >-5. The use of acetate in total parenteral nutrition reduces the severity of the acidosis and the incidence of hyperchloremia.

xiii. **Late metabolic acidosis of prematurity.** Use a low casein formula; this may alleviate the acidosis. In some cases, giving a base such as sodium acetate may be necessary.

2. **Metabolic alkalosis.** Mild or moderate alkalosis may not require correction. Severe metabolic alkalosis is associated with increased mortality, and chronic metabolic acidosis may increase the risk of sensorineural hearing loss. **First**

treat any underlying cause. Volume replacement can be used in cases of volume contraction and chloride depletion. If hypokalemia is present, that should be treated. Chloride replacement as potassium chloride (KCl) can be used, but infusion rate may have to be limited. Dilute hydrochloride acid or ammonium hydrochloride can be considered in severe persistent cases but must be given carefully and can be associated with serious complications. **Acetazolamide** may be effective in decreasing serum bicarbonate and has been used in pediatric cardiac patients with congenital heart disease with chloride-resistant metabolic alkalosis and in some carefully selected infants with chronic metabolic alkalosis with chronic respiratory insufficiency.

a. **Reduce excess administered alkali.** Adjust or discontinue the dose of sodium bicarbonate or potassium citrate and citric acid solutions; reduce acetate in hyperalimentation.

b. **Hypokalemia.** This can cause a shift of hydrogen ions into cells as potassium is lost. The infant's potassium level should be corrected (see Chapter 68).

c. **Prolonged nasogastric suction.** Treated with IV fluid replacement, usually with 1/2 normal saline with 10 to 20 mEq KCl/L, replaced mL/mL each shift.

d. **Vomiting and loss of chloride from diarrhea.** Give IV fluids and replace deficits, as described earlier.

e. **Compensation for respiratory acidosis.** Correct ventilation.

f. **Diuretics.** These can cause mild alkalosis; no specific treatment is usually necessary. Stop the dose temporarily, decrease the diuretic dose if necessary, or add a potassium-sparing diuretic such as spironolactone.

g. **Bartter syndrome.** Correct dehydration and electrolyte imbalance (replace electrolyte losses). Treatment includes potassium supplements, and after 6 to 12 weeks, indomethacin is given.

h. **Primary hyperaldosteronism.** Treatment depends on the cause. Acute therapies include diuretics, angiotensin-converting enzyme inhibitors, and steroids.

3. **Other causes of abnormal blood gases**

a. **Endotracheal tube problems.** Determine whether there are any changes in the pulmonary function test measurements on the ventilator that may indicate a problem with the ETT. **Colorimetric CO_2 detectors** can be used to determine airway patency, with a color change from purple to yellow if there is exhaled CO_2 gas. If there is no color change, there is airway obstruction and a possible ETT problem. Mark position on the ETT when it is correctly placed to note whether the tube is out of position.

   i. **Mucus plug.** With decreased bilateral breath sounds and retractions, a plugged ETT is possible. Pulmonary function measurements on specific ventilators may also define this if the VT is low. The infant can be suctioned, and if clinically stable, repeat blood gas measurements can be obtained. If the infant is in extreme distress, replace the tube.

   ii. **Endotracheal tube placement problems.** An infant with a tube placed down the **right mainstem bronchus** has breath sounds on the right only and decreased breath sounds on the left. Withdraw the tube 0.5 to 1 cm. Listen for equal breath sounds and check an x-ray. An infant with a **tube that has dislodged or is in the nasopharynx** has decreased or no breath sounds on chest auscultation. Listen from breath sounds over the stomach or see if air is escaping from the mouth. Need to replace the tube.

b. **Ventilator issues.** Changes in blood gas levels based on changes in routine ventilator settings can be found in Table 51–1. Advanced ventilator management for high-frequency devices can be found in Chapter 9.

   i. **Overventilation.** If the blood gas levels reveal overventilation, the ventilation parameters need to be adjusted. Deciding which parameter to adjust depends on the patient's lung disease and the disease course.

Table 51–1. CHANGES IN BLOOD GAS LEVELS CAUSED BY CHANGES IN VENTILATOR SETTINGS

Variable	Rate	PIP	PEEP	IT	FiO$_2$
To increase PaCO$_2$	↓	↓	NA	NA	NA
To decrease PaCO$_2$	↑	↑	NA[a]	NA[b]	NA
To increase PaO$_2$	↑	↑	↑	↑	↑
To decrease PaO$_2$	NA	↓	↓	NA	↓

FiO$_2$, fraction of inspired oxygen; IT, inspiratory time; NA, not applicable; PEEP, positive end-expiratory pressure; PIP, peak inspiratory pressure.
[a]In severe pulmonary edema and pulmonary hemorrhage, increased PEEP can decrease PaCO$_2$.
[b]Not applicable unless the inspiratory-to-expiratory ratio is excessive.

(a) **If the oxygen level is high.** Easiest solution is to decrease the FiO$_2$. Other options include decreasing the PEEP, PIP, VT, inspiratory time, rate, and flow.

(b) **If the carbon dioxide level is low.** Decrease the rate. Other options include decreasing the PIP or VT, expiratory time, or flow.

ii. **Insufficient respiratory support.** If the infant's chest is not moving, the PIP is not high enough; an adjustment of the ventilator setting is needed. Also check the VT; if it is low, it could mean not enough pressure is given.

(a) **If the oxygen is low, with increase in PaCO$_2$ and gradual deterioration in the infant.** One or more of the following can be increased: FiO$_2$, PIP, PEEP, inspiratory time, or VT. Increase FiO$_2$ by 5% to 10%, and increase PIP and PEEP by increments of 1 to 2 cm H$_2$O. Increase inspiratory time (preterm infants not >0.4 seconds; term infants not >0.5 seconds). Increase the VT by 1 to 2 mL/kg (volume ventilator).

(b) **If the CO$_2$ is high and no changes in PaO$_2$.** One or more of the following can be increased: ventilator rate by increments of 5 to 10 breaths/min, PIP by 2 to 5 cm H$_2$O (pressure ventilator), VT by 1 to 2 mL/kg (volume ventilator), flow rate, or expiratory time. Decreasing PEEP will increase VT and decrease CO$_2$. **Increased dead space from tubing can cause this;** cut the endotracheal tube to make it shorter.

iii. **Ventilator malfunction. This can cause an acute change in the blood gas.** To check to see if there is ventilator malfunction, disconnect the ventilator from the infant and manually inflate the infant's lung. If the infant improves, then it is the ventilator. Ventilator problems include the following: the concentration of O$_2$ going to the ventilator may be wrong, there may be a leak, the tubing may be disconnected, or there may be electrical or mechanical failure. Notify respiratory therapy to check the ventilator and replace it if necessary.

iv. **Agitation.** May cause oxygenation to drop in the infant; sedation may be needed (***controversial***) or ventilator settings may need to be adjusted.

(a) *Note:* **Agitation can be a sign of hypoxia, so a blood gas level should be obtained before ordering sedation.** If there is documented hypoxia, attempt to increase oxygenation.

(b) **Sit by the bedside and try different ventilator rates** to see whether the infant fights less.

(c) **Routine sedation.** Usually not recommended because in very low birthweight infants and premature infants, it is associated with an increase in severe IVH, delay in diuresis, and ileus. **If sedation is used,** use the preferred agent at your institution (see Chapter 81 for agents used: diazepam, lorazepam, midazolam, fentanyl, chloral hydrate, morphine).

c. **Acute change in clinical pulmonary status**
  i. **Pneumothorax.** See Chapter 75.
  ii. **Endotracheal tube problems, ventilator malfunction.** See Sections V.B.3.a.i and ii, and V.B.3.b.iii.
  iii. **Atelectasis.** Treatment consists of percussion and postural drainage and possibly increased PIP or PEEP. Avoid percussion in small preterm infants; a study showed a strong link between IVH and porencephaly with chest physiotherapy in extremely premature infants.
  iv. **Pulmonary edema.** Diuretics (eg, furosemide) are the primary treatment with mechanical ventilation as indicated.
  v. **Persistent pulmonary hypertension.** See Chapter 115.

52 Apnea and Bradycardia (A's and B's): On Call

I. **Problem.** An infant has just had an apneic episode with bradycardia (often referred to as "A's and B's"). American Academy of Pediatrics (AAP) has defined apnea as follows: "**Apnea** is the absence of breathing for 20 seconds or longer or a shorter pause associated with **bradycardia** (<100 beats per minute), cyanosis, or pallor." Shorter apnea <10 seconds without hypoxemia or bradycardia is usually due to immaturity and is not clinically important. (See also Chapter 89.)

A. **The 3 types of apnea** with approximate incidence are:
  1. **Central apnea.** Complete absence of the brainstem stimulus to breathe, resulting in no respiratory effort (10%–25%). Preterm infants can have central apnea due to their immature brains. Other causes include: inborn errors of metabolism, metabolic issues (hypoglycemia, hypocalcemia, acidosis), congenital anomalies, CNS infections, birth asphyxia, head trauma, toxin exposure.
  2. **Obstructive apnea.** Infant breathes but no airflow is present because of an obstruction usually at the pharyngeal level by mucus or airway collapse (10%–20%). Preterm infants have an increase in obstructive apnea due to difficulty maintaining their airway as a result of positioning.
  3. **Mixed apnea.** Elements of both central and obstructive apnea. Mixed apnea involves a period of central apnea usually followed by airway obstruction or vice versa. This is the **most common type found in most premature infants** (50%–75%). Other causes include gastroesophageal reflux, pertussis, and bronchiolitis.

B. **Definitions**
  1. **Apnea of infancy.** The AAP definition of apnea of infancy (AOI) is as follows: "an unexplained episode of cessation of breathing for 20 seconds or longer or a shorter respiratory pause associated with bradycardia, cyanosis, pallor, and/or marked hypotonia" in an infant >37 weeks' gestational age at the onset of the apnea. It

occurs in 1 per 1000 infants. **AOI** and **apnea in term infants** are interchangeable terms. **Apnea in a term infant** is not common and is usually pathologic and secondary to a long list of causes (eg, infection, seizure disorder, severe birth asphyxia, stroke, drug depression, intracranial hemorrhage, cerebral infarction, polycythemia, micrognathia).

2. **Apnea of prematurity.** AAP defines apnea of prematurity (AOP) as follows: "Sudden cessation of breathing that lasts for at least 20 seconds or is associated with bradycardia or oxygen desaturation (cyanosis) in an infant <37 weeks' gestational age." It may start as obstructive or central but involves elements of both and is most commonly mixed apnea. AOP is a developmental disorder usually of **physiologic immaturity of respiratory control**, but other diseases may contribute. Factors found in the pathogenesis of AOP include central mechanisms and peripheral reflex pathways. **Central mechanisms** include decreased central chemosensitivity, hypoxic ventilatory depression, upregulated inhibitory neurotransmitters, and delayed central nervous system development. **Peripheral reflex pathways** include decreased or increased carotid body activity, laryngeal chemoreflex, and excessive bradycardic response. The incidence of AOP is inversely correlated with gestational age and birthweight. It affects almost all infants born ≤28 weeks of gestation or with a birthweight <1000 g. AOP may be hereditary. AOP usually presents on days 2 to 7. It usually resolves by 36 to 37 weeks of postmenstrual age (PMA) in 92% of infants born at ≥28 weeks' gestation and by 40 weeks of PMA in >98% of infants. Infants born at <28 weeks' gestation can have apnea to or beyond term gestation. **If apnea presents in the first 24 hours of life or after day 7, it is very unlikely to be AOP. Note: AOP is a diagnosis of exclusion.**

3. **Persistent apnea.** Apnea that persists in a neonate ≥37 weeks of PMA. It usually occurs in infants born at <28 weeks' gestation.

4. **Extreme apnea event.** AAP defines this as apnea >30 seconds and/or heart rate <60 beats/min for >10 seconds.

5. **Periodic breathing.** Periodic breathing is a normal variation of breathing found in premature and full-term infants. There are pauses of breathing for no more than 5 to 10 seconds at a time (may have minor oxygen desaturation and bradycardia) followed by a series of rapid breathing episodes and then a return to normal breathing without stimulation. It occurs mainly during quiet sleep. It is absent the first few days of life, is more frequent at 2 to 4 weeks of age, and is usually gone by 6 months.

6. **Brief resolved unexplained event** (BRUE), formerly known as apparent life threatening event (ALTE), is not synonymous with apnea and has specific defining criteria. It applies to a well-appearing infant (no underlying health problems) <1 year old who has a brief, <1-minute (usually <20–30 seconds) event that resolves, is unexplained after a history and physical examination, and includes 1 or more of the following: cyanosis or pallor; decreased, absent, or irregular breathing; altered level of responsiveness; or marked change in tone (hypertonia or hypotonia).

C. **Secondary causes of apnea (apnea with identified causes).** Apnea that results from an underlying disorder (eg, sepsis, anemia, asphyxia, temperature instability, pneumonia, others). Some will classify this as **pathologic apnea** (apnea from pathologic causes such as sepsis or pneumonia). Note that **immaturity** can worsen any apnea that is associated with a specific cause.

II. **Immediate questions**

A. **Did you observe the apnea? What was going on when the apnea occurred? Do you know what type of apnea it is?** Try to distinguish the type; **obstructive apnea** is the easiest to detect visually, whereas central and mixed are more difficult. A thorough history of the event may help differentiate the type of apnea. **If it occurred during feeding with a nasogastric/orogastric tube, is the tube in proper position?** (Stimulation of laryngeal receptors causes **central apnea**.) **Did it occur with insertion of a nasogastric/orogastric tube?** Consider a vagal response (vagal nerve stimulation resulting in **central apnea**.) If the infant has no respiratory effort on the monitor or on physical examination (absent breath sounds, chest wall not moving), think **central apnea. What position was the infant in when it occurred?** Neck flexion can obstruct the airway and cause **obstructive apnea. Was the infant just suctioned when the apnea occurred?** Aggressive pharyngeal suctioning can cause **central apnea. Does the infant have excessive secretions?** If so, this suggests **obstructive apnea**.

B. **What is the gestational age of the infant? The incidence of apnea is inversely related to gestational age.** A's and B's are common in **premature infants** (all infants <28 weeks' gestation have apnea; 80% of infants at 30 weeks and 20% of infants at 34 weeks have apnea) and uncommon in **term infants.** In **term infants,** the incidence is 0.8 to 1.0 per 1000 term births. Apnea in term infants is usually associated with a serious disorder or related to a maternal condition (magnesium treatment or maternal exposure to narcotics). **Apnea in a term infant is usually never physiologic; it requires a full workup to determine the cause.**

C. **What is the birthweight of the infant?** Apnea increases as birthweight decreases. All babies <1000 g will have at least 1 apneic spell. Thirty percent of all babies weighing <1800 g will have at least 1 apneic spell.

D. **Was significant stimulation needed to return the heart rate to normal?** An infant requiring significant stimulation (eg, oxygen by bag-and-mask ventilation) usually needs an immediate evaluation. An infant who has had 1 episode of apnea and bradycardia not requiring oxygen supplementation may not need a full evaluation unless the infant is term.

E. **If the patient is already receiving medication (eg, methylxanthine) for apnea and bradycardia, is the dosage adequate?** Determine the serum drug level.

F. **Did the episode occur during or after feeding?**
   1. **Feeding hypoxemia** is more common in premature infants and can be seen in term infants. When infants start oral feedings, they can experience hypoxemia, cyanosis, and bradycardia. Apnea occurs more commonly during feeding due to the following reasons: obvious increased work of breathing, diaphragmatic fatigue, abdominal distension causing a decrease in lung volume, and immaturity of coordination of sucking, swallowing, and breathing such that ventilation is impaired during sucking and swallowing. Feeding hypoxemia resolves with maturation.
   2. **Gastroesophageal reflux.** It has been stated that **gastroesophageal reflux (GER) causes apnea and bradycardia** because it was observed when regurgitation of formula into the pharynx occurred after feeding. This has been a source of much debate, with recent studies showing no relationship between the 2 conditions. Evidence now shows that apnea is rarely temporally related to GER episodes and GER does not make apnea worse.
   3. **Insertion of a nasogastric tube** may cause a **vagal reflex,** resulting in apnea and bradycardia.

G. **How old is the infant? Apnea in the first 24 hours is usually pathologic.** The peak incidence of AOP occurs between 5 and 7 days of postnatal age.

H. **Is there a change in the frequency or an increase in severity of episodes? Is this the first episode, or has the pattern changed?** If the pattern changes or the amount and severity of each episode increase, then something new may be going on and a workup should be done.

I. **What is the temperature of the infant and the environment?** Hyperthermia and hypothermia can cause apnea. Overwarming an infant can cause apnea, and cold-stressed infants being warmed can have apnea.

III. **Differential diagnosis.** Causes of A's and B's can be classified according to diseases and disorders of various organ systems, gestational age, or postnatal age. **AOP is a diagnosis of exclusion; therefore, it is important to diagnose and treat any secondary cause.**

A. **Diseases and disorders of various organ systems**
   1. **Head and central nervous system**
      a. **Perinatal asphyxia**

    b. Intraventricular/intracranial or subarachnoid hemorrhage
    c. Meningitis
    d. Hydrocephalus with increased intracranial pressure
    e. Cerebral infarct with seizures
    f. **Seizures (apnea is an uncommon presentation of a subtle seizure).** Consider a seizure if apnea occurs without bradycardia; tachycardia can be seen before or during the apneic attack.
    g. Birth trauma
    h. Congenital myopathies or neuropathies
    i. Congenital malformations
    j. Congenital central hypoventilation syndrome
    k. Encephalopathy
2. **Respiratory system**
    a. Hypoxia, hypercarbia
    b. **Upper airway obstruction/malformation** (eg, Pierre Robin sequence), nasal obstruction
    c. **Lung disease/pneumonia/respiratory distress syndrome/aspiration/bronchopulmonary dysplasia**
    d. **Hypercarbia, inadequate ventilatory support, or performing extubation too early**
    e. Surfactant deficiency
    f. Pulmonary hemorrhage
    g. Pneumothorax
    h. Reparatory syncytial virus
    i. Vocal cord paralysis
3. **Cardiovascular system**
    a. Congestive heart failure
    b. Patent ductus arteriosus
    c. **Cardiac disorders** such as cyanotic congenital heart disease, congenital heart block, hypoplastic left heart syndrome, and transposition of the great vessels.
    d. **Severe hypovolemia/hypotension/hypertension**
    e. **Increased vagal tone.** There is increased vagal tone in newborns, especially in the postdelivery period. Vagal hyperreactivity has been described in sudden infant death syndrome (SIDS).
4. **Gastrointestinal tract**
    a. **Necrotizing enterocolitis.** Apnea is associated with the onset of necrotizing enterocolitis (NEC).
    b. **Gastroesophageal reflux disease.** All preterm infants and many term infants have GER. GER disease (GERD) is when GER occurs with many of the symptoms or complications associated with it. Some of the signs attributed to GERD in infants include apnea, desaturation, and bradycardia. Studies have shown that in premature infants the timing of reflux episodes to apnea is rarely related. In full-term infants, GER is an infrequent cause of apnea.
    c. **Feeding intolerance**
    d. **Oral feeding.** Introduction of oral feeding in premature infants can cause changes in color and heart rate due to ineffective feeding (sucking, swallowing, and breathing).
    e. **Abdominal distension** (decreases lung volume and increases vagal stimulation).
    f. **Bowel movement**
    g. **Nonrotavirus infection; esophageal hematoma.** Both rare.
5. **Hematologic system**
    a. **Severe anemia** has been implicated in the pathophysiology of AOP. There is no specific hematocrit at which apnea and bradycardia occur, and they

can be seen in infants with anemia of prematurity. Although it makes sense that giving blood transfusions would increase the respiratory drive and decrease AOP, studies on this are conflicting. One study showed decreased apnea 3 days after blood transfusions were given in preterm infants when compared to 3 days before, but there are no data on long-term reduction in apnea after a blood transfusion. It has been shown that liberal blood transfusion may reduce apnea compared with more restrictive blood transfusion.

    b. Polycythemia. More common in term infants.

6. Other diseases and disorders

    a. Temperature instability. Most often hyperthermia, but also hypothermia, can cause apnea and bradycardia. Note the incubator temperature; the infant may have a normal body temperature but may have a rise in incubator temperature (the infant is hypothermic) or may require a lower incubator temperature (the infant is hyperthermic). Any rapid fluctuation of temperature can cause apnea. Cold stress can occur after birth or during transport or a procedure, and it may produce apnea.

    b. Infection (sepsis). Check for bacterial, fungal, and viral infections. Respiratory syncytial virus, *Ureaplasma urealyticum*, and botulism can all cause apnea in preterm infants. Human *Parechovirus* type 3 causes apnea in premature infants.

    c. Metabolic/electrolyte imbalance and inborn errors of metabolism. Hypoglycemia, hypo-/hypernatremia, hypermagnesemia (during parenteral nutrition), hyperkalemia, hyperammonemia, and hypo-/hypercalcemia can cause apnea and bradycardia. Hypothyroidism and inborn errors of metabolism can also cause apnea and bradycardia. Magnesium given to the mother for preeclampsia has been associated with apnea and hypoventilation in the newborn.

    d. Vagal reflex secondary to nasogastric tube insertion, feeding, and suctioning.

    e. Acute/chronic pain.

    f. Head/body position (neck flexion). Improper neck positioning (especially hyperextension and hyperflexion of the neck) can cause tracheal occlusion and obstructive apnea.

    g. Drugs/drug withdrawal. Oversedation from **maternal drugs** such as magnesium sulfate, opiates, and general anesthesia can cause apnea in the newborn. Apnea can be seen in drug withdrawal of infants born to drug-addicted mothers. In the infant, high levels of phenobarbital or other narcotics or sedatives, such as diazepam and chloral hydrate, may cause apnea and bradycardia. Topical eye drops for routine eye examinations can sometimes cause changes in apnea pattern. Prostaglandin E_1, γ-aminobutyric acid (GABA), and adenosine therapy can cause apnea.

    h. Immunization. Apnea (with or without bradycardia) is reported in extremely low birthweight (ELBW) infants (<1000 g) after the use of DTwP (diphtheria and tetanus toxoids with the whole-cell pertussis vaccine), but more recent reports did not support this in ELBW with DTaP (diphtheria and tetanus toxoids with acellular pertussis). Apnea and bradycardia with oxygen desaturation are increased in very low birthweight infants when they are given the combination DTaP, inactivated poliovirus, hepatitis B, and *Haemophilus influenzae* b (Hib) conjugate vaccines. Postimmunization apnea has been seen in the following circumstances: infants with apnea within 24 hours prior to immunization, younger age, or weight <2000 g at the time of immunization and a 12-hour Score for Neonatal Acute Physiology II (SNAP II) (illness severity score) <10. If these infants at risk are still in the hospital when they get an immunization, some feel they should be monitored for 48 hours after immunization. One strategy for infants at risk is to vaccinate in the hospital so they can be observed. These postimmunization events do not appear to have a detrimental effect on the clinical course of immunized infants.

i. **Kangaroo care.** Studies are conflicting as to whether kangaroo care (KC) increases or decreases apnea. Recently it was found that the effect of KC on apnea rates was the same as that seen with prone positioning. Infants in the neonatal intensive care unit (NICU) should have continuous cardiovascular monitoring. Make sure there is correct head positioning for patency of the airway, and make sure the endotracheal tube, arterial and venous lines, and any other equipment are not compromised. Cochrane review found that KC is an effective and safe alternative to conventional neonatal care for low birthweight infants in resource-limited countries but did not specifically evaluate the effects of KC on apnea and bradycardia.

j. **Surgery.** This can cause postoperative apnea in premature infants.

k. **Ophthalmologic examinations.** Retinopathy of prematurity (ROP) examination has been reported as a cause of apnea and bradycardia. From 19% to 25% of infants (usually younger gestational age and lower birthweight) experienced an increase in cardiorespiratory events in the 24 hours after eye exams.

l. **Jaundice (unconjugated hyperbilirubinemia)** is associated with central apnea in premature infants.

m. **Genetic basis of apnea of prematurity.** Recent studies have suggested a genetic basis to AOP because it has a higher incidence in first-degree relatives. A study showed a higher rate of AOP among monozygotic twins compared to dizygotic twins of the same sex. Single nucleotide polymorphisms of genes encoding for adenosine receptors A1 and A2A are linked to the highest risk of having apnea. Certain gene polymorphisms of A2A and A2B receptors are associated with a lower incidence of apnea. Central infantile apnea may be familial.

B. **Gestational age.** See Table 52–1.

1. **Full-term infants.** Term infants rarely have apnea; the incidence is low, and it is usually not due to physiologic causes as in premature infants. The cause is usually serious and pathologic, and the disease or disorder must be identified. The onset of apnea in a term infant at any time is a **critical event** that requires immediate investigation. The causes of apnea in a term infant can be quite different depending on the age when the infant presents.

Table 52–1. **SOME COMMON CAUSES OF APNEA AND BRADYCARDIA ACCORDING TO GESTATIONAL AGE**

Premature Infant	Full-Term Infant	All Ages
Apnea of prematurity	Seizure disorder	Sepsis
Patent ductus arteriosus	Infection	Necrotizing enterocolitis
Respiratory distress syndrome	Severe birth asphyxia	Meningitis
Periventricular-intraventricular hemorrhage	Intracranial hemorrhage	Aspiration
Anemia of prematurity	Stroke	Gastroesophageal reflux
Posthemorrhagic hydrocephalus	Drug depression	Pneumonia
	Cerebral infarction	Cardiac disorder
	Polycythemia	Postextubation atelectasis
		Seizures
		Cold stress
		Asphyxia

    a. **Apnea in a term infant <3 days old**

       i. **Apnea in the delivery room:** Intrapartum maternal drugs (narcotics, anesthetic agents, magnesium sulfate), brain injury secondary to hypoxia and ischemia (with hypotension, hypoxemia, and metabolic acidosis), general anesthesia, early onset sepsis.

      ii. **Other conditions presenting with central apnea early on:** Infections (early-onset sepsis, pneumonia, meningitis), congenital central nervous system malformations (Dandy-Walker syndrome, Arnold-Chiari malformation), seizures (stroke or infarction), metabolic causes (abnormal glucose, calcium, electrolytes), traumatic brain injury, spinal cord transection, intracranial hemorrhage, temporal lobe lesions, feeding-related hypoventilation/apnea (infants suck vigorously up to 30–60 times per minute; since there is a protective upper airway closure with each swallow, infants can have apnea), upper airway obstruction (anomalies, craniofacial abnormalities, choanal atresia, Pierre Robin sequence, Treacher Collins syndrome, Goldenhar syndrome, Crouzon disease, Down syndrome, airway mass lesions, tracheal web/stenosis, vocal cord paralysis, and others), positional (asphyxiating position after delivery during KC), congenital central hypoventilation syndrome (healthy newborn with apnea and cyanosis), phrenic nerve palsy, and unexplained causes.

    b. **Apnea in a term infant >3 days old.** The focus is on GER, respiratory syncytial virus, seizures, central nervous system disorder, cardiac disease (arrhythmias, structural, cardiomyopathies, conduction defects), metabolic/inborn errors of metabolism (mitochondrial disease, Pompe disease, Leigh syndrome, mucopolysaccharidoses), anaphylaxis, bacterial infections (eg, urinary tract infection), anemia, upper airway obstruction, and bilirubin encephalopathy. Beyond the neonatal period, the presumed apnea may be a **brief resolved unexplained event (BRUE)** (see page 443).

    c. **Apnea of immaturity in a term infant.** There are some term infants in whom the **workup is negative** and no cause can be found. Some term infants may not have a fully mature respiratory control network and may have changes in the brain and peripheral chemoreceptor systems that could put them at risk for apnea. This apnea is considered secondary to physiologic immaturity in a term infant.

  2. **Preterm infants.** The most common cause is AOP, usually presenting between days 2 and 7 of life (usually <34 weeks' gestation, <1800 g, and no other identifiable cause). It is a diagnosis of exclusion **and other causes need to be considered and ruled out before this diagnosis can be made.** AOP is related to immaturity of the central and autonomic nervous and neurotransmitter systems.

C. **Postnatal age can be a clue to the cause of apnea with common causes noted:**

  1. **Apnea onset within hours after birth.** Oversedation from maternal drugs, birth asphyxia, seizures, hypermagnesemia.

  2. **Apnea on day 1.** Usually pathologic; consider sepsis or respiratory failure.

  3. **Apnea on day 1 or 2.** Sepsis, hypoglycemia, respiratory failure, polycythemia.

  4. **Apnea onset <1 week.** Patent ductus arteriosus, periventricular-intraventricular hemorrhage, sepsis, respiratory failure, AOP.

  5. **Apnea onset >1 week of age.** Posthemorrhagic hydrocephalus with increased intracranial pressure or seizures, postextubation atelectasis, outgrown dose of caffeine or theophylline.

  6. **Apnea onset after 2 weeks in a previously well premature infant.** This requires immediate evaluation because it is usually indicative of a serious illness such as sepsis, meningitis, or other condition.

  7. **Apnea onset at 4 to 6 weeks.** Respiratory syncytial virus infection.

  8. **Variable onset of apnea.** Sepsis, NEC, meningitis, aspiration, GER, cardiac disorder, pneumonia, cold stress, fluctuations in temperature.

IV. Database. Complete history and review of maternal, prenatal, intrapartum, resuscitation, and postpartum history. Determine any prenatal risk of sepsis. A thorough history of any feeding problems is important. A history of feeding intolerance increases the suspicion of NEC. Was the mother on magnesium or opioids? Did the infant receive opioids? Was there any perinatal asphyxia? Is the infant jittery or lethargic? Is there any evidence of temperature instability?

A. Complete physical examination. Overall, does the infant appear sick or well? Pay particular attention to the following signs:

1. **Head.** Signs of increased intracranial pressure, central nervous system depression, or irritability.

2. **Nares.** Pass a small-diameter feeding tube through the nares to rule out choanal atresia.

3. **Heart.** Listen for a murmur or gallop.

4. **Lungs.** Check for adequate movement of the chest if mechanical ventilation is being used; otherwise, note signs of respiratory distress.

5. **Abdomen.** Check for abdominal distention (early sign of NEC). Other signs of NEC are decreased bowel sounds and visible bowel loops. Note any bloody stools.

6. **Skin.** An infant with polycythemia has a ruddy appearance; pallor is associated with anemia.

7. **Neurologic examination.** Do a complete neurologic examination and observe for seizure activity. Is there hypotonia?

B. Laboratory studies

1. **Immediate studies**

    a. **Arterial blood gas.** To rule out hypoxia and acidosis.

    b. **Complete blood count with differential.** May suggest infection, anemia, or polycythemia.

    c. **Cultures of the blood, urine, and cerebrospinal fluid.** If infection is suspected and these specific tests are indicated. **C-reactive protein** at 36 to 48 hours after birth may be useful as an infection screen. Polymerase chain reaction analyses and viral cultures are appropriate if a viral infection is suspected. **Lumbar puncture and cerebrospinal fluid (CSF) analysis** are appropriate if meningitis is suspected or if increased intracranial pressure from hydrocephalus is causing apnea and bradycardia.

    d. **Serum electrolyte, calcium, magnesium, and glucose levels.** To rule out metabolic abnormality.

    e. **Serum phenobarbital and methylxanthine levels.** To check levels if indicated.

2. **Additional studies**

    a. **If an inborn error of metabolism is suspected.** Test for organic acid levels, amino acid profiles, ammonia, pyruvate, and lactate. Ketones in the urine may indicate an organic acidemia.

    b. **Stool analysis.** To rule out infectious organisms.

C. Imaging and other studies may be needed depending on the differential

1. **Immediate studies**

    a. **Chest radiograph.** Should be performed immediately if there is any suspicion of heart or lung disease.

    b. **Electrocardiogram.** If cardiac disease is suspected. Electrocardiogram changes in the R-wave amplitude and QRS duration appear at the onset and termination of apnea and bradycardia episodes. Also rules out prolonged QT syndrome.

    c. **Abdominal radiograph.** Should be performed immediately if indicated. It may detect signs of NEC (see Figure 12–26).

    d. **Ultrasonography of the head.** To rule out periventricular-intraventricular hemorrhage, hydrocephalus, or any congenital abnormalities. To screen for any abnormal findings.

2. **Additional studies**

    a. **Echocardiography.** To rule out congenital heart disease.

b. **Electroencephalography.** Apnea and bradycardia may be manifestations of seizure activity.

c. **Computed tomography of the head.** To detect cerebral infarction and subarachnoid hemorrhage. Use adjusted scanning protocol to limit radiation exposure. The **AAP recommends early noncontrast computed tomography (CT)** in term encephalopathic infants to rule out hemorrhage.

d. **Magnetic resonance imaging (MRI)** may be used because of the concern for radiation exposure. Term infants may require an MRI for a more extensive workup; sedation may be necessary for the study.

e. **If concerned about gastroesophageal reflux:** Upper gastrointestinal (GI) series is no longer recommended.

   i. **Contrast fluoroscopy** can show episodes of reflux but cannot determine if it is significant GER or if it correlates with symptoms.

   ii. **Gastroesophageal reflux scintigraphy (termed *milk scan* if used with milk or formula)** is used to document GER. It is comparable to the pH probe and superior to the barium swallow. Technetium-99m–sulfur colloid is put in a water-based solution or milk (milk scan) and is instilled in the stomach. The patient is scanned in the supine position for 1 to 2 hours with the gamma camera. Positive scintigraphy has no correlation with clinical signs.

   iii. **Esophageal pH probe monitoring.** A small-caliber tube with a pH electrode is passed into the distal esophagus. Continuous monitoring can be carried out over 4 to 24 hours. This can determine the number of reflux episodes, the duration of the longest episode, and the reflux index (RI; percentage of total recording time of esophageal pH <4). RI >7% is abnormal, RI <3% is normal, and RI of 3% to 7% is indeterminate. If abnormal, it still does not verify that reflux is causing the symptoms. Most reflux in infants is not acidic. pH monitoring is of limited use in preemies because their gastric pH is >4 approximately 90% of the time.

   iv. **Multichannel intraluminal impedance.** Most accurate method of detecting GER. It is often combined with pH measurement to determine acidity. It detects the bolus movement of liquid and air in the esophagus via a catheter with electrodes and can determine if there is reflux in the esophagus and the height of the reflux.

f. **Lateral neck radiography, head and neck tomography (3-dimensional), and otolaryngology evaluation** to evaluate the upper airway in obstructive apnea.

g. **Polygraphic recording.** Can be done but may not be useful in infants near discharge. Usually multichannel, which can include many physiologic parameters such as heart rate, nasal thermistor detection of airflow, and impedance pneumography. Continuous recordings for up to 24 hours may help in the differential diagnosis of apnea. There are many different types of devices used.

   i. **Polysomnography.** This is the collective process of monitoring and recording physiologic data during sleep. It includes respiration, perioral electromyography, oxygen saturation, heart rate, electroencephalography, electrocardiography, and electrooculography.

   ii. **Thermistor pneumocardiogram.** This incorporates a thermistor, which detects changes in nasal and mouth airflow. It incorporates a pH probe to study the acidity in the esophagus.

   iii. **Impedance pneumography.** This measures chest wall movements, oronasal flow, heart rate, and oxygen saturation by a multichannel recorder to help identify different types of apnea.

V. **Plan.** See also Chapter 89.

A. **Prophylactic therapy and recommended monitoring**

1. **At-risk infants.** In the Caffeine for Apnea of Prematurity (**CAP**) study where the inclusion criterion was documented apnea, to facilitate extubation or prophylaxis

(only 20%), the infants who did the best (survival without neurodevelopmental disability at 18–21 months) were the very low birthweight infants (<1250 g) who were treated early with caffeine (<3 days compared to >3 days). Rates of bronchopulmonary dysplasia (BPD) were also decreased. In a Canadian study on infants <31 weeks' gestation, prophylactic caffeine was associated with decreased rates of death, BPD, and patent ductus arteriosus (PDA). Even though the use of prophylactic caffeine in the CAP trial was only 20% and there are limited data stating that prophylactic caffeine is beneficial, **the majority of NICUs routinely give prophylactic caffeine to infants <1000 g (or some <1250 g) soon after birth to avoid intubation and mechanical ventilation.** Some recommend caffeine for infants ≤28 weeks' gestation. It is also given prophylactically in preterm infants on mechanical ventilation getting ready to be extubated to enhance extubation. The AAP states that further trials are needed to study the safety and benefits of prophylactic caffeine in regard to potential neurobehavioral benefits and in infants who require mechanical ventilation. A recent follow-up of infants in the CAP trial found no adverse effects of caffeine on attention, executive function, intelligence, and behavior when compared to controls. At 11 years of age, the caffeine group performed better on certain tests (visual perception, fine motor coordination, and others). Cochrane review does not support the use of prophylactic caffeine for preterm infants at risk of apnea. It is best to follow your institution's protocol.

2. **Prophylactic use of kinesthetic stimulation (oscillating mattresses) to prevent apnea in preterm infants** is not recommended, and a Cochrane review found it to be ineffective.

3. **Postoperative apnea/bradycardia.** Caffeine can be used to prevent postoperative apnea/bradycardia and oxygen desaturation in preterm infants. Infants <46 weeks' postconceptional age should be monitored for a minimum of 12 hours postoperatively. Cochrane review indicates the following: "After general anesthesia, caffeine can be used to prevent postoperative apnea/bradycardia and episodes of oxygen desaturation in growing preterm infants if this is deemed clinically necessary."

4. **Postimmunization of preemies.** Infants who had apnea after their first immunization should receive cardiorespiratory monitoring for a minimum of 24 hours after immunization.

5. **Postretinopathy of prematurity exams.** As noted, ROP exams may increase the risk of a cardiorespiratory event for 24 hours after the exam (similar to the incidence after immunization). Monitor these infants for 24 hours after the exam.

6. **Co-bedding of preterm twins.** Cochrane review found no difference between the co-bedded group and the group receiving care separately in terms of apnea, bradycardia, or desaturation episodes.

B. **General plan**

1. **Assess the infant first.**

   a. **Is the infant blue?** Use tactile stimulation (gently stroking or rubbing baby's back or extremities; sometimes, more vigorous rubbing is necessary to resume breathing). If the infant does not respond, do not continue the tactile stimulation.

      i. **Bag-and-mask ventilation** until heart rate and respirations normalize.

      ii. **Supplemental oxygen** if cyanosis persists.

      iii. **Intubation** may be necessary if the infant is not responding.

      iv. **Send stat labs, and obtain a chest x-ray and possible abdominal radiograph.**

      v. **Rule out simple causes:** Is temperature okay in isolette? Is the nasogastric or endotracheal tube in the correct position? Is the position of the infant okay?

   b. **Is the infant pink and breathing, and is the heart rate acceptable?** The infant may have had a true apneic spell with spontaneous remission of breathing by the infant. Malfunction of the monitor could also have been the cause.

    c. **Apnea in the delivery room.** Apnea is an indication for positive-pressure ventilation in the delivery room per the *Textbook of Neonatal Resuscitation,* seventh edition.

2. **Determine the cause of apnea and bradycardia and treat if possible.** Sepsis is a cause that cannot be overlooked because antibiotics need to be started. Rule out sepsis/infection and other treatable causes (eg, intraventricular hemorrhage [IVH], seizures, PDA, anemia, NEC) before diagnosing and treating the infant with AOP.

3. **Apnea in a term infant** is approached differently because it is more likely to be pathologic and is usually secondary to an underlying known cause. Term infants require a detailed evaluation (thorough maternal, prenatal, intrapartum, resuscitation, postpartum, and feeding history and physical examination) to identify the cause (a long differential) and treat it accordingly. These infants should be admitted and observed with cardiorespiratory and pulse oximetry monitoring. A full workup depending on the specific history is necessary. Minimal laboratory studies to be ordered include complete blood count, electrolytes, calcium blood glucose, and arterial blood gas. Other studies (CT scan, radiographs, electroencephalogram, otorhinolaryngology consult, genetics consult, MRI, pneumogram, polysomnogram) may be necessary depending on the history and findings on the physical examination. Management and guidelines are lacking for this group. Caffeine is not recommended in this group of infants. It is best to identify the cause and target treatment based on that. If no cause can be found, a pneumogram or polysomnogram may be helpful. If a BRUE event is being considered, review BRUE clinical guidelines.

4. **Apnea of prematurity**
    a. **Nonpharmacologic treatments**
        i. **Environmental temperature.** Because overheating may play a role in apnea, keep the environmental thermostat neutral or at the lower end of the range; a specific environmental temperature cannot be recommended. Some recommend humidification of warm gas. Body temperature between 36.5°C and 37°C seems to be effective in decreasing apnea episodes.
        ii. **Infant body positioning.** Often used as a first-line intervention in infants with AOP. Studies are conflicting on whether different body positions decrease apnea in the premature infant. Several studies have shown that certain positions can decrease AOP; decrease episodes of oxygen desaturation; or improve apnea, bradycardia, and desaturation. A recent Cochrane review (2017) found insufficient evidence to determine effects of body positioning on apnea, bradycardia, and oxygen saturation in preterm infants and do not recommend the use of one position over another for premature infants with apnea. **It is important to avoid extreme flexion or extension, which decreases the patency of the airway** and may cause obstruction and apnea. Three positions (prone position, head elevated tilt position [HETP], and 3-stair position [TSP]) are used in the NICU.
          (a) **Prone position (body lying face down).** Avoid neck flexion or extension, which can decrease the patency of the airway. Several studies show that the prone position stabilizes the chest wall and decreases AOP. It also increases ventilation, and reduces GER and energy expenditure in respiration. Only recommended for infants with apnea with NICU monitoring.
          (b) **Head elevated tilt position.** The bed is tilted in an inclined position of 15 degrees so the head and neck are elevated 15 degrees from the prone position; this position reduces episodes of oxygen desaturation. It does not improve AOP in an infant receiving aminophylline treatment.

      (c) **Three-stair position.** The head and abdomen are maintained at horizontal position. The head is on 3 blankets, the thorax is on 2 blankets, and the pelvis is on 1 blanket. Airway obstruction and neck inclination do not occur. This position was shown to improve apnea, bradycardia, and desaturation. It does not improve AOP in an infant receiving aminophylline treatment.

  iii. **Stimulation**

      (a) **Tactile stimulation** provides excitatory activity in the brainstem to stimulate respiratory activity and represents the most common intervention. Tactile stimulation includes rubbing the skin, stroking the back, patting the infant, and tapping or tickling the feet.

      (b) **Olfactory stimulation.** Introducing a pleasant odor (vanillin) into the incubator (15 drops of saturated vanillin solution to the infant's pillow at the periphery) decreased the frequency of apnea by 45% in one 24-hour study in infants who were unresponsive to caffeine or doxapram (see Chapter 22).

      (c) **Kangaroo care for the treatment of AOP** is controversial, with conflicting studies on whether it increased or decreased apnea and bradycardia events. It was found to have the same effect as prone positioning. Cochrane review states that evidence supports KC in low birthweight infants as an alternative to conventional neonatal care, especially in resource-limited settings.

      (d) **Kinesthetic stimulation (oscillating mattress).** Not effective in clinically significant apnea. Use of stochastic mechanosensory stimulation (mattress with embedded actuators that delivers subarousal vibration to infants) stabilized breathing during sleep and helped to decrease the incidence of AOP, oxygen desaturation, and some aspects of bradycardia.

  iv. **Maintain nasal patency.** Because nasogastric tubes increase nasal airway resistance and an increase in upper airway resistance may increase AOP, **orogastric tubes** have been preferred in premature infants with apnea. Cochrane review indicates that there is insufficient evidence that the route of feeding tube placement affects the incidence or frequency of apnea or bradycardia. Tube placement should be based on clinician preference.

  v. **Feeding.** One observational study found that transpyloric feeding (especially with human milk) may decrease the frequency or degree of apnea and bradycardia in preemies with GER. A Cochrane review of transpyloric versus gastric feeding for preterm infants found no trials that addressed the issue of whether transpyloric versus gastric feeding affected the incidence of GER-related apnea or bradycardia. They found that transpyloric feedings do not have benefits for preterm infants and there is a higher risk of adverse effects (GI disturbance and mortality).

C. **Specific management.** Deciding on which infants to treat usually depends on how many episodes of apnea are occurring, the severity of each episode, and the required intervention to stop the episode of apnea. If there are multiple or severe apneic episodes, medical treatment may be necessary. Different institutions have varying guidelines on when to start medical treatment. **Some recommendations** include the following: >6 apneic episodes every 12 hours requiring only minimal stimulation; >2 apneic episodes per hour requiring minimal stimulation over a couple of hours; >1 to 2 apneic episodes in 24 hours requiring vigorous stimulation; any episode during which the infant does not respond to tactile stimulation; or when the infant requires bag-and-mask ventilation with oxygen. These infants are usually managed with noninvasive respiratory support, with medications added as needed. It is best to follow your institution's guidelines. **Combination therapy** (nasal continuous positive airway pressure [nCPAP] in conjunction with xanthine therapy) is very effective.

1. **Respiratory support.** Maintain adequate oxygen saturation with supplemental oxygen (indicated if there is desaturation or bradycardia). Avoid vigorous suctioning.
   a. **Low-flow oxygen** may decrease the rate of intermittent hypoxia and apnea. Avoid hyperoxia.
   b. **Nasal cannula oxygen.** This is a small, tapered cannula that is used to deliver oxygen or blended oxygen. It can cause nasal irritation, causing arousal, and may help to prevent apnea.
      i. **Low-flow nasal cannula** (<1 L/min) can be used as an adjunct for apnea. Low-flow oxygen decreases the rate of intermittent hypoxia and apnea.
      ii. **High-flow nasal cannula** can provide high concentrations of oxygen and also deliver a positive end-expiratory pressure and can be used as an alternative to nCPAP. The rates are 1 to 6 L/min. One study showed that nasal cannula oxygen was just as effective as nCPAP. Heated humidified high-flow nasal cannula is preferred over high-flow nasal cannula.
   c. **Nasal continuous positive airway pressure.** Continuous positive airway pressure (CPAP) via nasal prongs reduces the frequency and severity of apneic spells. It decreases the risk of obstructive apnea. (**Note:** Different sources cite different CPAP parameters. Variable-flow CPAP may be better than ventilator or bubble CPAP. Ranges reported: 2–4, 3–6, 4–6, and 5–8 cm H_2O.) **A range of 4 to 6 cm H_2O seems to be cited frequently and is considered safe.** Use the settings recommended by your institution. It can be used in conjunction with medication (after a therapeutic level has been obtained). Side effects of CPAP include bowel distension, nasal trauma, barotrauma, and pneumothorax.
   d. **Noninvasive ventilation.** Noninvasive ventilation is a method of ventilation without tracheal intubation that uses constant or variable pressure to provide ventilatory support. It is often used with CPAP. **Nasal intermittent positive-pressure ventilation (NIPPV)** is a type of noninvasive ventilation that combines nCPAP with superimposed positive-pressure breaths. Cochrane review states that NIPPV reduced the frequency of apneas more effectively than nCPAP. NIPPV via nasal prongs is more effective than nCPAP alone in AOP. NIPPV also reduces the incidence of extubation failure more effectively when compared with nCPAP.
   e. **Mechanical ventilation.** Should only be used if apnea and bradycardia cannot be controlled by other less invasive interventions (drug therapy, nCPAP, or NIPPV). Low pressures (minimal peak inspiratory pressure) are used at the rate necessary to prevent apnea.
2. **Pharmacotherapy.** See detailed dosing information in Chapter 155.
   a. **Caffeine is the drug of choice for apnea.** Theophylline and caffeine seem to have equal efficacy (both reduce apnea and the use of mechanical ventilation within 2–7 days of beginning treatment), but **caffeine** offers multiple benefits over theophylline (ie, longer half-life, fewer side effects, lower toxicity, once-daily dosing, increased CSF penetration, better longer term outcomes, and no drug level monitoring required). Some authors have called caffeine the "silver bullet" or "magic bullet" in neonatology. **Long-term dose is 20 mg/kg loading dose and 5 to 10 mg/kg/d for maintenance.** Caffeine therapy reduces the rate of severe retinopathy, BPD, and neurodevelopmental disability at 18 months. Long-term follow-up at 11 years showed benefit of a reduced risk of motor impairment in children who were very low birthweight. It is associated with improved neurodevelopmental outcome at 18 months, improved survival at 18 to 21 months in infants 500 to 1250 g, a reduction in death, decreased incidence of BPD, less time on mechanical ventilation, and a decreased incidence of cerebral palsy, cognitive delay, and severe ROP. A recent follow-up study of infants in the CAP trial found no adverse effects of caffeine on attention, executive function, or behavior and found that the

caffeine group performed better on tests for visual perception, visuospatial organization, and visuomotor integration at the age of 11 years.
  i. **When to start caffeine therapy?** The optimal time to start therapy is not known. Early caffeine therapy (<3 days) is associated with a decreased incidence of BPD and a shorter course of mechanical ventilation. The AAP states that it would be reasonable to start caffeine therapy in infants >28 weeks' gestation who are not on positive-pressure support once they have their first apnea episode.
  ii. **When to discontinue caffeine therapy?** The optimal time to stop therapy is not known, and no trials have addressed this. The AAP suggests considering a trial off caffeine when the infant is no longer on positive-pressure ventilation and the infant has either been free of apnea for 5 to 7 days or is 33 to 34 weeks of PMA.
  b. **If apnea persists, begin doxapram hydrochloride.** (*Controversial*, not recommended as routine therapy.) The package insert notes it should not be used in neonates due to the benzyl alcohol component. Doxapram appears to be efficacious when theophylline, caffeine, and CPAP have failed; it can reduce apnea within 48 hours after other methods have failed. A recent article stated that both oral and intravenous (IV) doxapram treated most cases of apnea in preterm infants, avoiding the need for endotracheal intubation and invasive ventilation. There are concerns regarding side effects: risk of reduced cerebral blood flow with mental delay later; increased QTc interval, second-degree heart block, severe hypokalemia, and lower mental developmental index at 18 months; irritability, gastric retention, electroencephalogram changes in preterm infants, hypertension, seizures, and GI disturbance; and metabolic acidosis (has benzyl alcohol preservative). If acidosis occurs, consider stopping doxapram. A recent review concluded that the routine use of doxapram could not be recommended because there were no conclusions on safety and efficacy as a result of the limited studies and low level of evidence. Cochrane review states the following: "IV doxapram might reduce apnea within the first 48 hours of treatment; further studies are needed to determine the role of it in clinical practice."
D. **Cause-specific treatment of apnea and bradycardia**
  1. **Anemia**
    a. **Transfusion is not routinely recommended** because data are conflicting and evidence is insufficient. The rationale is that if you give red blood cells to an infant, you increase the total content of oxygen in the blood, increase tissue oxygenation, and increase oxygen-carrying capacity, thereby increasing the respiratory drive and decreasing the episodes of apnea. Most institutions do not treat anemia if the infant is asymptomatic, the infant is feeding and growing, and the reticulocyte count is >5% to 6%. If the hematocrit (Hct) is very low (<25% based on institutional guidelines), transfusion may be indicated. If the infant is symptomatic (significant apnea and bradycardia, defined as >9 episodes in 12 hours or >2 episodes in 24 hours requiring bag-and-mask ventilation), on therapeutic doses of methylxanthines, not feeding well, or on oxygen or respiratory support and the reticulocyte count is not appropriate for the low hematocrit (ie, reticulocyte count <2%–3%), transfusion may be indicated to an Hct level of ≥30% (*controversial*). Note that **transfusion-associated NEC** (ie, NEC that appears 48 hours after a blood transfusion) is a concern and has been associated with approximately 25% to 35% of NEC cases. One survey showed that the majority of neonatologists support the following guidelines for transfusion:
      i. Without symptoms but Hct is 20% to 25%.
      ii. Symptomatic (ie, FiO_2 >40% per nasal cannula) with Hct of 25% to 30%.
      iii. Require ventilator assistance with FiO_2 >40% and have an Hct of 30% to 35%.

   b. **Erythropoiesis-stimulating agents such as recombinant human erythro-poietin and darbepoetin.** The use of recombinant human erythropoietin (EPO) with iron for anemia of prematurity, decreasing the need for transfusions, is ***controversial***, with early studies showing an increase in the risk of development and progression of ROP, although later studies showed no difference in stage 3 or greater ROP in EPO versus placebo groups. **Early and late recombinant human EPO treatment is not recommended.** There may be benefit in infants <1000 g, in whom a significant reduction in transfusions was found at 1 month.

2. **Gastroesophageal reflux.** There is normal physiologic GER (no signs other than spitting up) and pathologic GER or GERD (acidic reflux that causes injury to the lower esophageal mucosa and complications such as respiratory problems and poor growth). Signs of pathologic GER/GERD include frequent regurgitation, apnea, bradycardia, desaturation, poor weight gain, feeding aversion, irritability, and discomfort. The majority of signs of pathologic GER/GERD do not correlate with multichannel intraluminal impedance or pH measurements (see page 450). Physiologic GER is considered a normal developmental process that will resolve with maturation. In the majority of infants with apnea, GER is not the cause. Furthermore, research has not shown a relationship between GER and AOP. Nonpharmacologic therapy does not seem to decrease signs of GER in preterm infants, and medications are not recommended in this group. **This guideline is only included here for the uncommon circumstance where there is a definitive relationship between symptoms and GER or in a term infant with apnea with severe GER.**
   a. **Feeding modifications**
      i. **Breast-fed infants.** Modify maternal diet if breast fed. Restrict maternal cow's milk and eggs for 2 to 4 weeks for any infant with GERD who is breast feeding (to rule out milk protein allergy in the infant, which can mimic GERD).
      ii. **Formula-fed infants.** Milk protein sensitivity may cause vomiting and crying in infants. Infants with recurrent vomiting may benefit from a 2- to 4-week trial of an extensively hydrolyzed protein formula. Hydrolyzed protein formulas decrease reflux and symptoms of GER in term infants but only decrease reflux episodes in preterm infants, not symptoms. Hydrolyzed protein formula can be tried in term infants and in preterm infants with severe reflux.
      iii. **Small-volume feeds or hourly feeding.** No randomized trials have been done studying different feedings (bolus intragastric tube vs transpyloric vs continuous intragastric) on symptoms and severity of GER. Overfeeding can aggravate reflux, so decreasing the volume of feeds while increasing the frequency is recommended. Hourly feedings decreased the total GER episodes but increased the acidic reflux episodes in premature infants. Another study found that longer feeding duration and slower milk flow rates were associated with decreased GER events.
      iv. **Thickened feedings.** Thickening feeds decreases GER in term infants but does not decrease the acidic GER. North American Society for Pediatric Gastroenterology, Hepatology, and Nutrition (NASPGHAN) states that thickening feeds decreases visible regurgitation but does not cause a measurable decrease in the frequency of episodes. For **term infants** with GER and GERD, add 1 Tbsp of dry rice cereal per 1 oz of formula. For **preterm** infants, the US Food and Drug Administration and AAP issued a warning about thickened feedings and NEC in premature infants. **The following should not be used in infants <37 weeks:** pectin-based thickeners, carob bean gum–based products, SimplyThick, and xanthan gum–based products. Commercial anti-regurgitant formulas decrease overt regurgitation and frequency of

vomiting compared with formula with rice or unthickened formula. Cochrane review found with moderate certainty evidence that feed thickeners should be considered if regurgitation symptoms persist in term bottle-fed infants. The reduction of 2 episodes of regurgitation per day is likely to be of clinical significance.

v. **Continuous or transpyloric feedings.** Transpyloric feedings (especially with human milk) may reduce apnea and bradycardia in preterm infants with GER. Cochrane review on transpyloric versus gastric feeding in preterm infants showed that transpyloric enteral feeding did not improve feeding tolerance, had an increased risk of stopping feeds, and increased mortality. There is no evidence to support the use of continuous feedings or transpyloric feeding for the treatment of GER.

b. **Position. Head up angle is ineffective in decreasing acid reflux in older infants; this position has not been studied in preterm infants.** Left lateral and prone positioning after feeding may decrease reflux episodes but showed no decrease in behavioral manifestations of reflux in one small study. Right lateral positioning may increase reflux episodes but was also found to enhance gastric emptying. Therefore, it is uncertain whether positioning techniques actually decrease signs of GER in infants with reflux. One group recommended to place infants in the right lateral position right after feeding for 1 hour and then place them in the left lateral position. The North American Society for Pediatric Gastroenterology, Hepatology, and Nutrition states that prone positioning is acceptable if the infant is awake and being observed, especially right after feeding. Because of the increased risk of SIDS with the lateral and prone positioning, the AAP and NASPGHAN have stated the following: "All infants with GER should be placed for sleep in the supine position with the exception of the rare infants for whom the risk of death from GER is greater that the risk of SIDS." An example of an exception is infants with upper airway disorders with an impaired airway protective mechanism such as type 3 or 4 laryngeal clefts who have not had surgery yet.

3. **Medications.** The **Choosing Wisely campaign** states to avoid routine use of acid blockers and motility agents for physiologic GER that is effortless, painless, and not affecting growth. If GER is associated with poor growth or significant respiratory symptoms, the infant needs further evaluation. Avoid routine use of antireflux medications for treatment of symptomatic GERD or for the treatment of apnea and desaturation in preterm infants because there is no evidence that pharmacologic treatment of GER with medications that either decrease acidity or increase motility decrease the risk of apnea and bradycardia in preterm infants. These medications should be used sparingly or not at all in preterm infants (see Chapter 155 for details).

a. **Prokinetic, promotility agents (metoclopramide, domperidone, and erythromycin).** These agents increase the muscle tone of the digestive tract and should decrease the volume of the refluxate. In older infants, these agents improve gastric emptying, decrease regurgitation, and enhance lower esophageal sphincter tone. These medications have not been shown to decrease GER symptoms in preterm infants. These medications all have significant side effects and are not recommended in preterm infants if the only indication is GER. Side effects include increased risk of infantile pyloric stenosis and increased risk of cardiac arrhythmia (erythromycin) and neurologic side effects (domperidone, metoclopramide). Metoclopramide now has a black box warning for tardive dyskinesia.

b. **Antacids (Maalox and Mylanta).** Antacids neutralize and buffer the gastric acid, raise the pH of the gastric refluxate, and may improve the symptoms and signs of GER. Their use increases the risk of infection and feeding intolerance in infants receiving gavage feedings, and there is a risk of concretion formation. Side effects include diarrhea or constipation. If used, the dosage is 0.5 to 1 mL/kg by mouth every 4 hours by nasogastric tube.

c. **Sodium alginate with sodium bicarbonate (Gaviscon).** These medications work by protecting the esophagus from acidification. They may decrease the signs of GER in older infants. In preterm infants, these medications decreased the frequency of regurgitation, decreased the number of acidic GER episodes, and decreased the total esophageal acid exposure. The long-term safety has not been evaluated in preterm infants. Side effects have included bezoar formation and adverse effects from the aluminum content. (**Note:** Gaviscon is now aluminum free.) None of these agents are recommended as the only treatment. Further studies need to be done.

d. **Histamine (H_2) receptor blockers (ranitidine, famotidine)** inhibit histamine-stimulated acid secretion by the gastric parietal cells, decrease hydrochloric acid secretion, and increase intragastric pH. Of the 4 H_2 blockers available, **ranitidine and famotidine are most commonly used in infants** and are preferred because of fewer side effects. No studies of these medications have been done in preterm infants. Use of these medications in preterm infants is associated with an increased incidence of NEC, late-onset infections (*Candida* and gram-negative sepsis), possibly IVH, and death in some studies.

e. **Proton pump inhibitors (omeprazole, lansoprazole)** block the proton pump in the gastric parietal cell, which is the last step in the acid secretory pathway, and decrease both basal and stimulated parietal cell acid secretion. Proton pump inhibitors in preterm infants will maintain the stomach pH >4 but do not relieve the clinical signs of GER in clinical trials. Like the H_2 blockers, they also increase the risk of *Candida* infections. There is also increased risk of gram-negative sepsis. Lansoprazole was associated with a higher rate of adverse events.

E. **Persistent apnea.** AOP usually resolves by 37 weeks. Persistent apnea is apnea that persists ≥37 weeks of PMA. It usually occurs in infants born at ≤28 weeks' (24–26 weeks) gestation. These infants can have apnea that persists to term gestation or after. These infants are usually ready to go home except they continue to have apnea. These infants can be at risk for serious episodes of apnea, bradycardia, and cyanosis for several months. How to manage these infants at home is not well studied, and recommendations are lacking. Sometimes a comprehensive polygraphic recording (pneumogram) is done prior to discharge to give a more detailed explanation of the apnea and help in the decision process, but studies have shown it is not useful. The **Choosing Wisely campaign** states the following "Avoid routine use of pneumograms for predischarge assessment of ongoing or prolonged apnea of prematurity." A pneumogram does not predict the risk of SIDS or recurrence of a significant event, a severe cardiopulmonary event, or the need for readmission. Medication is usually continued in these infants after discharge. There is no evidence that AOP increases the risk of SIDS. Cardiorespiratory monitoring at home with an event recorder can be recommended. Parents should be told that home monitoring does not prevent SIDS. Parents need to be instructed in the use of the monitor and be trained in cardiopulmonary resuscitation. **AAP recommendations for home monitoring** may be justified in some premature infants with an unusually prolonged course of recurrent extreme apnea. It can be discontinued at 44 weeks of PMA unless there is a significant medical condition that necessitates that it be continued. Use is limited after episodes stop or at approximately 43 weeks of PMA. It is not recommended in preterm infants with resolved AOP. After 43 weeks, extreme apnea events (apnea >30 seconds and or heart rate <60 beats/min for >10 seconds) are very rare.

F. **Discharge considerations for apnea of prematurity**

1. Discontinue caffeine therapy (see page 455).

2. Observe the infant for apnea and bradycardia for a few days after caffeine has been stopped since the half-life of caffeine is 50 to 100 hours. Most physicians

agree that the infant needs to be apnea free for a period of time before discharge. The period of time that most neonatologists recommend before discharge is 5 to 7 days of being apnea free after caffeine therapy has been discontinued. Based on studies, this period of time should be customized for the individual newborn (shorter duration for older gestational ages and longer duration for younger gestational ages, especially <26 weeks).

3. **Bradycardic episodes that are brief and isolated** and resolve on their own or are feeding related that resolve with stopping feeding do not need to delay discharge.

G. **Close monitoring with readmission may be indicated in certain situations** (general anesthesia, viral illnesses, immunizations) in preterm infants until 44 weeks of PMA. Preterm infants who have had immunizations or ROP exam may need to be observed and monitored for 24 hours because there have been reports of apnea in these situations.

53 Arrhythmia

I. **Problem.** <u>An infant has an abnormal tracing on the heart rate monitor.</u> Arrhythmias in neonates can be classified as benign or pathologic. They can be found in 1% to 5% of all neonates.

II. **Immediate questions**

A. **What is the heart rate?** The heart rate in newborns varies from 70 to 190 beats/min (normally 120–140 beats/min; may decrease to 70–90 beats/min during sleep and increase to 170–190 beats/min with increased activity such as crying). See Table 53–1 for normal heart rate values.

B. **Is the abnormality continuous or transient?** Transient episodes of sinus bradycardia, tachycardia, or arrhythmias (usually lasting <15 seconds) are benign and do not require further workup. Episodes lasting >15 seconds usually require full electrocardiogram (ECG) assessment.

C. **Is the infant symptomatic?** A symptomatic infant may need immediate treatment. Signs of some pathologic arrhythmias include tachypnea, poor skin perfusion, lethargy, hepatomegaly, and rales on pulmonary examination. All of these signs and symptoms may signify congestive heart failure (CHF), which may accompany arrhythmias. If an infant shows clinical signs of heart failure that are believed to be have been caused by an arrhythmia, then this suggests the infant was in an abnormal rhythm for a significant period of time (hours to days). CHF resulting from rapid cardiac rhythms is unusual with heart rates <240 beats/min.

III. **Differential diagnosis**

A. **Heart rate abnormalities.** Heart rates in the normal newborn vary dramatically. Some evidence, using computer programs to assess heart rate variability in the neonatal period, suggests that the lower heart rates early on are due to the inability of the infant's sympathetic system to inhibit the parasympathetic (or vagal) response.

1. **Tachycardia.** Heart rate >2 standard deviations (SDs) above the mean for age (see Table 53–1).

a. **Benign causes.** Postdelivery, heat or cold stress, painful stimuli, medications (eg, atropine, caffeine, epinephrine, intravenous glucagon, pancuronium bromide, tolazoline, and isoproterenol).

Table 53–1. HEART RATES IN NEWBORNS

	Term Infants		Preterm Infants	
Age	Mean HR	Range HR	Mean HR	Range HR
1 minute	80	20–140	100	50–145
2 minutes	140	80–200	120	80–160
3 minutes	150	100–200	140	105–175
4 minutes	160	120–195	155	120–183
5 minutes	160	120–190	160	120–180
10 minutes	160	110–185	160	129–195
Normal Newborns				
Up to 24 hours	119	84–145		
1–7 days	133	100–175		
8–30 days	163	115–190		

HR, heart rate.
Data from Hastreiter AR, et al. The electrocardiogram in the newborn period: I. The normal infant, *J Pediatr* 1971 Jan;78(1):146-156; Dawson JA, et al. Changes in heart rate in the first minutes after birth. *Arch Dis Child Fetal Neonat Ed.* 2010;95:F177-F181; Brady JP, et al. Heart rate changes in the fetus and newborn infant during labor, delivery and immediate neonatal period. *Am J Obstet Gynecol.* 1962;84:1-12; Davidson S, et al. Spectral analysis of heart rate fluctuations and optimal thermal management for low birth weight infants. *Med Biol Eng Comput.* 1997;35:619-625.

b. Pathologic causes

i. Common. Fever, shock, hypoxia, anemia, sepsis, patent ductus arteriosus, and CHF.

ii. Uncommon. Hyperthyroidism, metabolic disorders, cardiac arrhythmias, and hyperammonemia.

2. **Bradycardia.** Bradycardia is a heart rate >2 SDs below the mean for age (see Table 53–1). Transient bradycardia is fairly common in newborns (particularly premature infants); rates range from 60 to 70 beats/min.

a. Benign causes. During defecation, vomiting or micturition, gavage feedings, suctioning, medications (eg, propranolol, digitalis, atropine, and infusion of calcium; maternal long-acting β-blockers to treat hypertension given within 24 hours of delivery).

b. Pathologic causes

i. Common. Hypoxia, apnea, convulsions, airway obstruction, air leak (eg, pneumothorax), CHF, intracranial bleeding, severe acidosis, and severe hypothermia.

ii. Uncommon. Hyperkalemia, cardiac arrhythmias, pulmonary hemorrhage, diaphragmatic hernia, hypothyroidism, and hydrocephalus.

B. Arrhythmias

1. **Benign arrhythmias.** Includes any transient episode (<15 seconds) of sinus bradycardia and tachycardia and any of the benign causes of sinus tachycardia and bradycardia noted in Section III.A.1 and III.A.2. Sinus arrhythmia, a phasic variation in the heart rate often associated with respiration, is also benign.

a. **Premature atrial beats.** These can occur in the newborn and are usually benign. The QRS is narrow, and the T waves are often discordant. (See the example in Figure 53–1A.) They tend to decrease in number or resolve entirely in the first few months of life. If the premature atrial contraction (PACs), premature beats that occur in the upper chambers of the heart, are frequent or occur at a particular time in the cardiac cycle (during ventricular repolarization, when the lower chambers are refractory), they can cause paradoxical bradycardia from "blocked" PACs. A workup is usually not indicated unless the infant has the premature atrial beats in association with structural cardiac disease or if there is significant bradycardia. The most common cause of PACs in the neonatal intensive care unit setting is usually a deep central line in the right atrium.

b. **Unifocal premature ventricular beats.** Fairly frequent in the newborn. The QRS is wide, and the T wave is discordant with the sinus T wave. (See Figure 53–1B.) If seen in a newborn, obtain a 12-lead ECG. Do not treat unless the infant is symptomatic. Sometimes premature ventricular contractions (PVCs), premature beats that occur in the lower chambers of the heart, become less frequent when the sinus rate increases. PVCs tend to decrease in number or go away entirely in the first few months of life. If the PVC burden is frequent (usually assessed by review of telemetry), the mother's perinatal history should be pursued to rule out the possibility of myocarditis from a perinatal infection. If myocarditis is suspected, an echocardiogram with a pediatric cardiology consult should be part of the diagnostic evaluation.

c. **Sinus bradycardia.** Usually benign but is a diagnosis of exclusion after review of telemetry, a 12-lead ECG, echocardiogram, and evaluation of any clinical symptoms that may be related to the bradycardia. It is important to correlate clinical symptoms with heart rate and rhythm. Consider a head ultrasound to ensure no neurologic injury, because increased intracranial pressure can be missed and is a common etiology of low heart rates.

2. **Pathologic arrhythmias**

a. **Reentry supraventricular tachycardia.** Most common type of cardiac arrhythmia seen in the neonate (Figure 53–1D). Supraventricular tachycardia (SVT) is usually due to an accessory connection between the atria and ventricles and creates the substrate for paroxysms of tachycardia; it requires vagal maneuvers and other measures to terminate (adenosine, antiarrhythmics, direct current cardioversion).

b. **Atrial flutter.** Difficult to distinguish from other SVTs, unless the block is >2:1. Administration of adenosine may increase the block to 3:1 or 4:1, allowing the flutter waves to become more visible on the ECG tracing. The typical finding is "saw-tooth" P waves in the inferior leads; usually the P waves do not return to baseline (no isoelectric segment, Figure 53–1E).

c. **Atrial fibrillation.** Less common than SVT or atrial flutter. Defined by an irregular ventricular rate with no discernible P waves.

d. **Wolff-Parkinson-White pattern/ventricular preexcitation.** A short PR interval and delta wave and slow upstroke of the QRS complex with a wider than normal QRS. Difficult to identify when the rate is fast (Figure 53–1C) or if in SVT.

e. **Ectopic beats.** These are beats that start from anywhere outside the sinus node. Figure 53–1A shows an ectopic atrial beat (the P wave of the fourth beat is different in morphology than the preceding beats) and Figure 53–1B shows a premature ventricular complex/beat. The term "premature" is used when the ectopic beat comes in earlier than when one would expect the sinus node to initiate a beat.

f. **Ventricular tachycardia.** Usually a wide QRS complex rhythm (with more QRS complexes than P waves) in an infant who may or may not be hemodynamically stable. Treatment depends on the etiology and workup (Figure 53–1F).

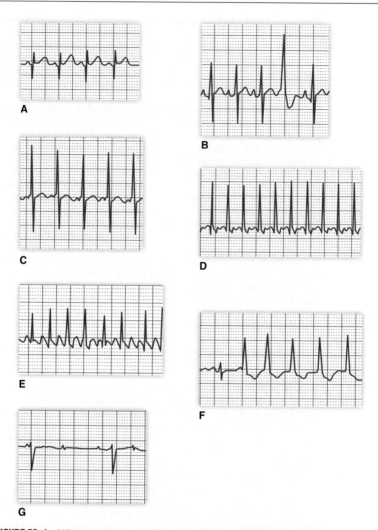

FIGURE 53–1. (**A**) A **premature atrial beat** that is blocked (blocked premature atrial contraction). Note the deformation of the T wave in the last beat; this is the ectopic P wave, and if early enough, it will block and there will be a pause afterward until the sinus node conducts. (**B**) A **premature ventricular beat.** The QRS is wide, and the T wave is discordant with the sinus T wave. (**C**) **Sinus rhythm with ventricular preexcitation** (Wolf-Parkinson-White pattern); note the short PR and delta wave with no appreciable flat PR segment between the P wave and onset of delta wave. (**D**) **Supraventricular tachycardia,** a narrow-complex QRS tachycardia with a rate of almost 300 beats/min. The P waves are retrograde following the QRS before the T wave, likely atrioventricular reentrant tachycardia. (**E**) **Atrial flutter,** a narrow QRS tachycardia with flutter waves in between; there is variable conduction to the ventricles. (**F**) **Ventricular tachycardia,** a wide QRS tachycardia (rate 160–185 beats/min) that starts with a wide QRS complex; there is no relationship between the P waves and QRS. (**G**) **Complete heart block** with more P waves than QRS complexes and no relationship between top and bottom chambers; ventricular rate is 52 beats/min, and atrial rate is 125 beats/min.

g. **Atrioventricular block with symptoms.** Occurs in newborns with complete block and ventricular rates <55 beats/min (Figure 53–1G). Premature infants may even require a higher rate. Because cardiac output in premature and young term babies can increase only by rate increase (their stroke volume is fixed by the small size of the ventricles), fevers, sepsis, and other stressors are tolerated poorly by babies with complete heart block.

3. **Arrhythmias secondary to extracardiac disease**

a. **Sepsis (usually tachycardia).**

b. **Diseases of the central nervous system (usually bradycardia).**

c. **Hypoglycemia.**

d. **Drug toxicity.** Digoxin dysrhythmias, such as PACs or PVCs and atrioventricular (AV) blocks (potentiated by hypokalemia, alkalosis, hypercalcemia, and hypomagnesemia); theophylline (less frequently used in neonatal intensive care units).

e. **Electrolyte abnormalities** such as potassium, sodium, magnesium, or calcium abnormalities.

f. **Other.** Metabolic acidosis or alkalosis, adrenal insufficiency.

IV. **Database**

A. **History and physical examination.** Assess whether the mother was ill during the pregnancy because neonatal myocarditis can occur from certain maternal viral illnesses. Also assess whether the mother had taken medications during the pregnancy or has connective tissue disease or hyperthyroidism. Check for signs of CHF (ie, tachypnea, rales on pulmonary examination, enlarged liver, and cardiomegaly). Vomiting and lethargy may be seen in patients with digoxin toxicity. Hypokalemia can cause ileus.

B. **Laboratory studies**

1. **Electrolyte, calcium, and magnesium levels**

2. **Blood gas may reveal acidosis or hypoxia**

3. **Drug levels to evaluate for toxicity**

a. **Digoxin.** Normal 0.5 to 2.0 mcg/mL (some assays up to 4 mcg/mL). Elevated levels of digoxin alone are not diagnostic of toxicity; clinical and ECG findings consistent with toxicity are also needed, and many neonates have naturally occurring substances that interfere with the radioimmunoassay test for digoxin.

b. **Caffeine.** Toxicity is manifested by tachycardia and feeding intolerance. Reduce dose or skip dose.

C. **Imaging and other studies**

1. **Electrocardiogram.** Should be performed in all infants who have an abnormal rhythm that lasts >15 seconds or is not related to a benign condition. Diagnostic features of the common arrhythmias are listed next. Although PR interval varies with heart rate, a **PR interval of >160 milliseconds** is abnormal in any newborn.

a. **Supraventricular tachycardia** (see Figure 53–1D)

i. Ventricular rate of 180 to 300 beats/min

ii. No change in heart rate with activity or crying

iii. An abnormal P wave (maybe retrograde) or PR interval

iv. A fixed R-R interval

b. **Atrial flutter**

i. Atrial rate is 220 to 400 beats/min.

ii. A saw-tooth configuration seen best in leads V_1 to V_3 or the inferior leads (II, III, and aVF) but often difficult to identify when a 2:1 block or rapid ventricular rate is present (see Figure 53–1E).

iii. The QRS complex is usually normal.

c. **Atrial fibrillation**

i. Irregular atrial waves that vary in size and shape from beat to beat.

ii. The atrial rate is 350 to 600 beats/min.

iii. The QRS complex is normal, but ventricular response is irregular.

    d. **Wolff-Parkinson-White pattern/ventricular preexcitation** (see Figure 53–1C)
        i. A short PR interval
        ii. A widened QRS complex
        iii. Presence of a delta wave
    e. **Ventricular tachycardia**
        i. Ventricular beats at a rate of 120 to 200 beats/min and a widened QRS complex (see Figure 53–1F). Can be difficult to differentiate from SVT with aberrancy and should mandate involvement by pediatric cardiology.
    f. **Ectopic beats (supraventricular or ventricular)**
        i. Abnormal P wave and may have a widened QRS if conducts to ventricles due to aberrant conduction
        ii. Wide QRS without a preceding P wave
    g. **Atrioventricular block**
        i. **First-degree AV block** (Figure 53–2A)
            (a) A prolonged PR interval (normal range, 0.08–0.12 seconds)
            (b) Normal sinus rhythm
            (c) A normal QRS complex
        ii. **Second-degree AV block**
            (a) Mobitz type I (Figure 53–2B)
                (i) A progressively prolonged PR interval until a ventricular beat is dropped (Wenckebach)
                (ii) A normal QRS complex
            (b) Mobitz type II (Figure 53–2C). A constant PR interval with dropped ventricular beats or nonconducted P waves.
        iii. **Third-degree AV block** (Figure 53–2D$_1$ and D$_2$)
            (a) Regular atrial beat.
            (b) Slower ventricular rate.
            (c) Independent atrial and ventricular beats.
            (d) Atrial rate increases with crying and level of activity. The ventricular rate usually stays the same.
    h. **Hyperkalemia**
        i. Tall, tented T waves
        ii. A widened QRS complex
        iii. A flat and wide P wave
        iv. Ventricular fibrillation and late asystole
    i. **Hypokalemia**
        i. Prolonged QT and PR intervals
        ii. Depressed ST segment
        iii. Flat T wave
    j. **Hypocalcemia.** A prolonged corrected QT interval. QTc interval prolongation may also be due to myocardial stress at the time of delivery and may resolve. Persistent prolongation of the QTc interval with normocalcemia mandates questions about family history of arrhythmia or sudden death. An ECG on the parents may be indicated.
    k. **Hypercalcemia.** Shortened corrected QT interval.
    l. **Hypomagnesemia.** Same as for hyperkalemia.
    m.**Hyponatremia.** Increased duration of the QRS complex.
    n. **Hypernatremia.** Decreased duration of the QRS complex.
    o. **Metabolic acidosis**
        i. Prolonged PR and QRS intervals
        ii. Increased amplitude of the P wave
        iii. Tall, peaked T waves
    p. **Metabolic alkalosis.** Inverted T wave.
    q. **Digoxin**

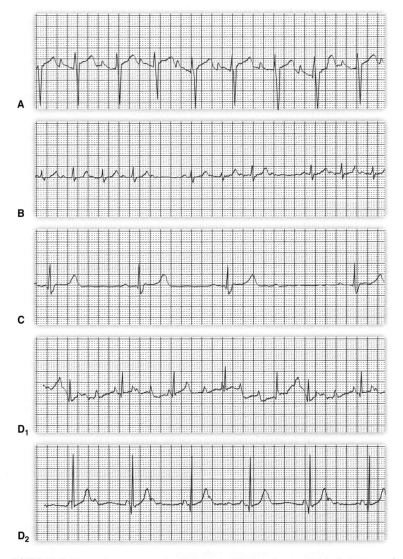

FIGURE 53–2. Types of atrioventricular (AV) block. (**A**) **First-degree AV block:** PR interval is long. (**B**) **Mobitz type I second-degree AV block** (Wenckebach): progressive lengthening of PR interval until ventricular beat is blocked. (**C**) **Mobitz type II second-degree AV block:** PR interval is constant; ventricular beat is blocked. (**D$_1$**) **Infant with complete or third-degree AV block:** atrial rate is 175 beats/min, ventricular rate is 62 beats/min; no relationship between P waves and QRS complexes. (**D$_2$**) **Same infant at 2 months of age:** atrial rate is 119 beats/min, ventricular rate is 54 beats/min; still no relationship between P waves and QRS complexes.

   i. **Therapeutic levels.** Prolonged PR interval and a short QT interval.
   ii. **Toxic levels.** Most common are sinoatrial block, second-degree AV block, and multiple ectopic beats; also seen are AV block and bradycardia.
  r. **Caffeine**
   i. **Therapeutic levels.** Desired effect is decreased frequency and duration of apneic spells; no significant changes on ECG.
   ii. **Toxic levels.** Tachycardia with feeding intolerance.
2. **Chest radiograph.** Perform in all infants with suspected heart failure or air leak. Ensure proper central line placement and position.
3. **Echocardiogram**
  a. **Certain deficits in atrioventricular conduction** (higher grade heart block or complete heart block) can be a manifestation of certain forms of congenital heart disease or cardiomyopathy.
  b. **Supraventricular tachycardia or ventricular tachycardia** almost always requires an echocardiogram to evaluate ventricular function and to ensure no coincident congenital heart disease.

V. **Plan**
  A. **General management.** Decide whether the arrhythmia is benign or pathologic, as noted. If it is pathologic, full ECG evaluation must be performed. Any acid-base disorder, hypoxia, or electrolyte abnormality needs to be corrected.
  B. **Specific management**
   1. **Heart rate abnormalities**
    a. **Sinus tachycardia**
     i. **Benign.** No treatment is necessary because the tachycardia is usually secondary to a self-limited event.
     ii. **Medications.** With certain medications, such as caffeine, observe infant for other signs of toxicity and decrease or skip the next dose.
     iii. **Pathologic conditions.** The underlying disease should be treated.
    b. **Sinus bradycardia.** Confirm it is sinus bradycardia and not complete heart block.
     i. **Benign.** No treatment is usually necessary.
     ii. **Drug related.** Check the serum drug level if possible and then consider lowering the dosage or discontinuing the drug unless it is necessary.
     iii. **Pathologic.** Treat the underlying disease.
      (a) **In severe hypotension or cardiac arrest,** check the airway and initiate breathing and cardiac compressions.
      (b) **Administer atropine, epinephrine, or isoproterenol** to restore normal rhythm. (See Chapter 155 for detailed dosing.)
   2. **Arrhythmias.** For dosages and other pharmacologic information, see Chapter 155; for details on cardioversion, see Chapter 32.
    a. **Benign.** Observation.
    b. **Pathologic.** Treat any underlying acid-base disorders, hypoxia, or electrolyte abnormalities. Note position of umbilical lines, which might be triggering arrhythmias if deep in the right atrium.
     i. **Supraventricular tachycardia**
      (a) **If the infant's condition is critical.** Electrical cardioversion is indicated, with an antiarrhythmic medication started for maintenance therapy. Digoxin is contraindicated if the patient has Wolff-Parkinson-White (WPW)/preexcitation.
      (b) **If the infant's condition is stable.** Vagal stimulation (ice or an ice-cold washcloth applied to the infant's face for a few seconds) can be tried. Adenosine, 100 mcg/kg intravenous push into a central vein, converts SVT to sinus rhythm. It may be necessary to double the dose to 200 mcg/kg (300 mcg/kg maximum). **Never use verapamil in infants.** An antiarrhythmic is started for maintenance therapy

(usually digoxin or propranolol, depending on the presence of WPW). SVT refractory to digoxin and propranolol may be treated with other antiarrhythmic medications (flecainide, sotalol, or amiodarone).

  ii. **Atrial flutter**
      (a) **If the infant's condition is critical (severe congestive heart failure or unstable hemodynamic state).** Perform synchronized electrical cardioversion.
      (b) **If the infant is stable.** Start digoxin, which slows the ventricular rate. A combination of digoxin and propranolol may be used instead of digoxin alone. If the infant spontaneously converts, medication maybe discontinued. This plan should be made in concert with a pediatric cardiologist.
      (c) **If rate is rapid and 2:1 block is present.** Atrial flutter may be hard to identify on ECG. May give adenosine (see earlier) to increase block to 3 or 4:1.
  iii. **Recurrent atrial flutter management.** Same as that for atrial flutter.
  iv. **Atrial fibrillation (unusual in infants).** Management is the same as for atrial flutter.
  v. **Wolff-Parkinson-White pattern/ventricular preexcitation.** Often accompanied by SVT. β-Blockers are preferred because digoxin may promote 1:1 conduction during rapidly conducted atrial fibrillation and demise.
  vi. **Ventricular tachycardia.** Perform electrical cardioversion (except in digitalis toxicity) if unstable. Drugs that maybe used include lidocaine, esmolol, procainamide, phenytoin, or amiodarone. The choice is usually determined by the cause of the ventricular tachycardia and the hemodynamic status of the patient.

3. **Ectopic beats**
   a. **Asymptomatic.** No treatment is necessary.
   b. **Symptomatic.** With underlying heart disease, in the unlikely event that ectopic beats compromise cardiac output, suppress with phenytoin, propranolol, or amiodarone.

4. **Atrioventricular block**
   a. **First degree.** No specific treatment necessary.
   b. **Second degree.** Treat the underlying cause. Consider congenital long QT syndrome because neonates with this syndrome can present with 2:1 heart block in the neonatal period.
   c. **Third degree (complete heart block)**
      i. **Rate >70 beats/min.** If the infant is asymptomatic, observe and evaluate for congenital/structural heart disease or autoimmune causes (see later in chapter). Generally at this rate, no problems develop.
      ii. **Rate <55 beats/min.** The patient usually needs emergency pacing if hemodynamically unstable, with the need for subsequent permanent pacing. The decision for permanent pacing also depends on the presence of coincident congenital heart disease, ventricular function, and the type of escape rhythm.
      iii. **Rate between 55 and 70 beats/min.** Gray zone. Monitor urine output as an index of end-organ perfusion and measure serum lactate. Check the mother for SAA or SSA antinuclear antibodies (associated with complete heart block and cardiomyopathy). Infants with nonimmune complete heart block generally fare better than those whose heart block is caused by maternal antibodies. Mothers who have given birth to an infant with complete heart block because of autoimmune-related SSA or SAA antibodies have a 50% to 69% chance of subsequent infants having complete heart block. Standard of care for these mothers' subsequent pregnancies

includes maternal treatment with hydroxychloroquine (Plaquenil) and following PR interval of the fetus weekly starting at 12 weeks. In an effort to increase fetal heart rate, maternal terbutaline is sometimes used if the infant's heart rate is slow enough to worry about fetal demise.

5. **Arrhythmias secondary to an extracardiac cause**
   a. **Pathologic conditions.** Treat the underlying disease.
   b. **Digoxin toxicity.** Check the PR interval before each dose, obtain a stat serum digoxin level, and hold the dose. Consider digoxin immune Fab (Digibind).
   c. **Theophylline toxicity.** Reduce the dosage or discontinue medication.

6. **Electrolyte abnormalities**
   a. **Check serum electrolyte levels with repeat determinations.**
   b. **Treat electrolyte abnormalities accordingly.**

VI. **Technique of defibrillation/cardioversion** is discussed in Chapter 32. Defibrillation and cardioversion are used for rapid termination of a tachyarrhythmia from the atrium or ventricle that is unresponsive to basic treatment or is causing the patient to have cardiovascular compromise.

VII. **Fetal considerations.** A multidisciplinary approach in any fetus with any arrhythmia serious enough to cause fetal hydrops is mandatory. Perinatologists, neonatologists, and cardiologists must be prepared to exert efforts in concert if such infants are to survive. Usually there is at least some warning that such an infant is being delivered, but in the event that specialists are not all in attendance, the physician assuming responsibility for care must be ready to intubate, perform pleural and pericardial taps and a paracentesis if necessary, and treat the arrhythmia responsible for fetal CHF.

54 Bloody Stool

I. **Problem.** <u>A newborn infant has passed a bloody stool.</u> A bloody stool in a neonate can represent a spectrum of conditions from benign (eg, anal fissure, swallowed maternal blood, cows' milk protein sensitivity) to life threatening (eg, necrotizing enterocolitis [NEC], malrotation with volvulus). It is critical to detect the cases that have significant underlying pathology, especially those that require emergent operative care.

II. **Immediate questions**

A. **Is the stool grossly bloody? Hematochezia** is passage of fresh blood through the anus. It can be pure blood, bright red or maroon colored, or blood mixed with stool. A grossly bloody stool usually signifies **lower gastrointestinal (GI) bleeding** (typically below the ligament of Treitz, the anatomic landmark of the duodenojejunal junction), which includes the jejunum, ileum, cecum, colon, rectum, and anus. Hematochezia can occur rarely with massive upper GI tract bleeding with a rapid transit time. **Necrotizing enterocolitis (NEC)** is the most common cause of bloody stool in premature infants and is critical to identify.

B. **Is the stool otherwise normal in color but with streaks of blood?** This is more characteristic of a lesion in the anal canal, such as an anal fissure. **Anal fissure** is the **most common cause of rectal bleeding** in the first 2 years of life and is the most common cause in well-appearing infants.

C. **What is the consistency of the stool?** A hard stool usually signifies constipation, which can cause a fissure, whereas a loose or diarrheal stool usually signifies colitis.

D. **Is the stool black and tarry looking? Melena** is the passage of black or tarry stools through the anus. Melena usually suggests the blood is from the upper GI tract (proximal to the ligament of Treitz which includes the esophagus, stomach, or duodenum).

Melena can also be from bleeding from the small bowel or proximal ascending colon if transit time is slow enough to allow bacteria to denature the hemoglobin. Nasogastric trauma and swallowed maternal blood are common causes.

E. **Is the stool occult blood (fecal occult blood testing) positive only?** Microscopic blood as an isolated finding is usually not significant in the neonate. Tests for occult blood are very sensitive and can be positive with conditions such as repeated rectal temperature measurements or perianal dermatitis.

F. **How old is the infant?** The age of the infant is important as it can give clues to the diagnosis. **For the first week of life consider:** swallowed maternal blood syndrome, vitamin K deficiency bleeding (early or classic onset), Hirshsprung disease, malrotation with midgut volvulus, term infant with NEC. **For infants less than 1 month of age, consider:** anal fissure, malrotation with midgut volvulus, NEC, colitis, and milk allergy. **For infants usually 1 month or older consider:** lymphonodular/nodular lymphoid hyperplasia, milk protein allergy, late onset VKDB, intussusception.

G. **Was the infant given vitamin K at birth? What were the maternal medications during her pregnancy?** This should be asked of all parents especially if the infant is breast fed (breast milk has less vitamin K than cow's milk formula) or was born out of the hospital (did not receive vitamin K). An infant with **vitamin K deficiency bleeding (VKDB)** may present with hematemesis, melena, or blood flecks/streaks in the stool. If the mother was on certain medications that can cross the placenta and interfere with vitamin K metabolism (eg, phenobarbital, phenytoin, carbamazepine, primidone, warfarin, aspirin, cephalosporins, rifampin, isoniazid, anticoagulants), these may cause early-onset VKDB.

H. **What medications is the infant on?** Certain medications can cause bleeding in the newborn. If the infant has been given nonsteroidal anti-inflammatory drugs, heparin, indomethacin, or dexamethasone, these are all associated with bleeding.

I. **Does the infant appear well, or is the infant ill and toxic appearing? Are there other significant clinical findings?** Infants with NEC, Hirschsprung enterocolitis, bleeding disorders, intussusception, or malrotation with volvulus are typically ill appearing. Infants with an anal fissure, swallowed maternal blood, milk protein allergy, or nodular lymphoid hyperplasia usually appear well. Remember that a **bloody stool with other significant clinical findings is worrisome**.

J. **Was there any recent surgery?** Circumcision can cause blood staining, and any GI surgery may cause bloody stools as a routine consequence or potential complication.

III. **Differential diagnosis.** The most common reasons are swallowed maternal blood from delivery and anal fissures. Significant hemorrhages are often caused by a duodenal or gastric ulcer. Etiology can often be based on the color or type of stool. The common causes are listed in Table 54–1. Verify non-GI causes before starting an entire GI evaluation (see Section III.F).

A. **Melena (black tarry stools).** Usually from the upper GI tract but can be from the small bowel or proximal colon, as noted previously. The appearance of the black tarry stool is because of the oxidation by intestinal bacteria that convert hemoglobin to hematin. **Emergent considerations** include coagulopathies, hemorrhagic gastritis, stress ulcer with massive bleed, and congenital GI tract malformations.

1. **Maternal blood.** Swallowing of maternal blood during delivery, called **melena neonatorum**, accounts for 30% of infant "GI bleeding." In infants with normal meconium, swallowed blood usually appears in the stool on the second or third day of life (or second or third stool has blood). **Swallowing of blood during breast feeding** (secondary to cracked and bleeding nipples, case reports of fibrocystic breast disease) can also be a cause. **Swallowing of bloody amniotic fluid** from antepartum hemorrhage associated with bleeding into the amniotic fluid for several hours before birth is rare. This usually presents in the first stool.

2. **Trauma** from nasogastric tube, suctioning, or intubation.

3. **Coagulopathies.** VKDB occurs from a deficiency in vitamin K–dependent coagulation factors and can be prevented if vitamin K is administered at birth.

Table 54–1. CAUSES OF BLOODY STOOL IN A NEONATE

Exogenous (External Source)
Swallowed maternal blood syndrome
Swallowed blood during breast feeding (cracked/
 bleeding nipples), fibrocystic disease
Swallowed bloody amniotic fluid

Trauma
Nasogastric tube
Suctioning
Intubation
Rectal (temperature probes, rectal thermometer)

Hematologic Disorders
Vitamin K deficiency bleeding
Thrombocytopenia
Disseminated intravascular coagulation
Liver failure
Inherited coagulation disorder

Maternal Medications
Thiazides
Phenobarbital
Oral anticoagulants
Anticonvulsants

Infant Medications
Nonsteroidal anti-inflammatory drugs
Heparin
Indomethacin
Dexamethasone

Gastrointestinal
Anal fissure
Stress gastritis/erosions
Ulcer (gastric/duodenal ulcer)
Necrotizing enterocolitis
Malrotation with volvulus
Meckel diverticulum
Hirschsprung disease with enterocolitis
Intussusception
Atrioventricular malformation
Hemangioma
Gastrointestinal duplication cyst
Incarcerated hernia
Rectal prolapse
Lymphonodular hyperplasia
Prolapsed rectal polyp
Vascular malformations

Infectious
Sepsis (bacterial): group B *Streptococcus*,
 Escherichia coli, Listeria
Sepsis (viral): Cytomegalovirus (CMV), herpes
Infectious enterocolitis:
 Salmonella, Shigella, E coli
 CMV, rotavirus

Allergy
Milk protein allergy
Eosinophilic gastrointestinal disorders
Food protein–induced enterocolitis syndrome
Allergic proctocolitis
Perianal dermatitis

It is categorized based on timing of symptoms: early onset (within 24 hours), classic onset (2–7 days), or late onset (rare; 2 weeks to 6 months). Infants can have hematemesis, melena, petechiae, oozing from the umbilicus, and retinal hemorrhages. Severe hemorrhage occurs in about 0.25% to 0.50% of neonates. **Other coagulopathies to consider** include the following: thrombocytopenia, disseminated intravascular coagulation (DIC), inherited clotting factor deficiency, liver failure found in some metabolic disorders (iron storage disorder), ischemic injuries, and infections (sepsis).

4. **Formula intolerance/dietary protein intolerance.** Milk protein sensitivity is secondary to cow's milk or soybean formula, and symptoms of blood in the stool usually occur in the second or third week of life. Infants usually have a mucoid bloody diarrhea and rarely melena.

5. **Eosinophilic gastrointestinal disorders (eosinophilic esophagitis, gastroen-teritis, and colitis)** can present with melena.

6. **Other gastrointestinal causes**
   a. **Gastritis/stress ulcer/esophagitis/erosions.** Occurs in up to 20% of infants in the neonatal intensive care unit (NICU). Prematurity, stress, and mechanical ventilation are associated with stress gastritis. **Hemorrhagic gastritis** can occur from NSAIDS, steroids, and theophylline therapy. Indomethacin is

associated with gastric mucosal injury. **Stress ulcer** is a common cause and can occur in the stomach or duodenum and is associated with prolonged severe illness or steroid therapy. Stress-induced gastric ulcers should be suspected in any infant presenting with massive GI bleeding after birth asphyxia and difficult delivery. Maternal stress in the third trimester may increase maternal gastrin secretion and contribute to a peptic ulcer in the newborn. **Esophagitis** can occur from trauma from pharyngeal, esophageal, or gastric suction at birth. A gastric and esophageal lesion together is unique to neonates. **Erosions** of the esophageal, duodenal, and gastric mucosa are a common cause of bloody stool. **Mallory-Weiss syndrome** is a tear in the distal esophagus and proximal stomach that is an unusual cause of upper GI bleeding in an infant.

- **b. Congenital gastrointestinal tract malformations**
    - **i. Anatomic.** Intestinal malrotation, duplication cysts, anatomic duplications, Meckel diverticulum, Hirschsprung disease. Meckel diverticulum is the most common congenital abnormality of the small intestine.
    - **ii. Vascular.** GI infantile hemangiomas can present with GI bleeding (melena and hematochezia), often with profound anemia. AV malformations or venous malformations are rare causes. **Associated syndromes with vascular malformations** of the GI tract are Down syndrome, Klippel-Trenaunay syndrome, Osler-Weber-Rendu disease, and blue rubber bleb nevus syndrome.
- **7. Isolated rectal bleeding in preterm and term infants.** Many cases of bloody stool in an infant with no other clinical signs of illness have no identifiable cause. Fortunately most resolve in several days. Controversial whether to stop feedings or give antibiotics. Breast feeding should be encouraged.
- **8. Rare causes.** Gastric teratoma, gastric Dieulafoy lesion, GI tract telangiectasia, heterotopic pancreatic tissue in the stomach, pyloroduodenal intestinal duplication, and dengue shock syndrome.

B. Grossly bloody stool (hematochezia). Usually from lower GI tract (jejunum, ileum, colon) but can be from the upper GI tract with rapid transit time (rare). **Emergent considerations** include NEC, coagulopathies, malrotation with volvulus, Hirschsprung disease, infectious colitis, and incarcerated hernia.

- **1. Swallowing of maternal blood** with rapid transit time.
- **2. Necrotizing enterocolitis.** NEC is usually seen in premature infants but can be seen in term infants. Term infants usually present within the first week of life and account for less than 10% of all NEC cases, preterm infants present later. It should be ruled out in any infant who presents with a grossly bloody stool.
- **3. Coagulopathies.** DIC is usually associated with bleeding from other sites and may be secondary to an infection.
- **4. Bleeding diathesis** (eg, platelet abnormalities and clotting factor deficiencies) can cause bloody stools. Hemophilia can present as GI hemorrhage. **Severe liver disease** can cause coagulopathy.
- **5. Surgical diseases**
    - **a. Malrotation with midgut volvulus.** Obstruction after birth can cause bleeding with ischemic damage or other causes of volvulus. Classically presents with bilious emesis and abdominal distension.
    - **b. Meckel diverticulum** is the vestigial remnant of the vitelline duct, which contains mainly gastric mucosa that can secrete acid and cause ulceration of tissue, which in turn causes **rectal bleeding.** (Meckel diverticulum rule of 2s: 2% of population, length 2 inches, within 2 ft of ileocecal valve, 2 times as common in males, diagnosed in the first 2 years of life, 2 types of tissue present).
    - **c. Hirschsprung enterocolitis.** Ten to 30% of patients present with GI bleeding and abdominal distension; failure to pass meconium and feeding intolerance are typical.

d. Intussusception. Rare in the neonatal period; incidence is greatest in infants 3 months to 1 year of age. Most present with typical symptoms: bloody stool ("currant jelly" stool), abdominal mass, vomiting, and intermittent screaming. Intrauterine intussusception presents with a complete ileus.

e. Gastrointestinal tract duplications (duplication cysts). Rare, abnormal extra portions of the intestine that are congenital anomalies of unknown etiology. They are called duplication cysts because they are attached to the normal intestine and share its blood supply. **Colonic and tubular** are least common but do occur; presents with intestinal obstruction, abdominal mass, and bleeding. Bleeding occurs due to presence of ectopic gastric mucosa or stasis.

f. Hernias. An incarcerated inguinal hernia typically presents with a very irritable infant who refuses to eat and, on physical examination, has a tender firm mass in the inguinal region. An infant with an **internal hernia** caused by a congenital defect in the mesentery can present with bilious vomiting, grossly bloody stool, and abdominal distension. An internal hernia secondary to a congenital defect in the mesentery can mimic NEC but requires emergency operative care.

g. Rare causes. Rectal polyp (more common in toddlers but can occur in newborns); acute appendicitis

6. Colitis can be secondary to the following:

a. Intestinal infections (bacterial enteritis). Rare in the neonatal period and more common in older children and adults. Pathogens that can cause lower GI bleeding include **bacterial**: *Salmonella, Shigella, Campylobacter, Clostridium difficile, Escherichia coli, Yersinia enterocolitica*; **viral**: cytomegalovirus, herpes simplex; or **parasitic**: *Entamoeba histolytica*. **Dysbiosis (low numbers of normal flora)** may play a role in grossly blood stools in preterm infants. Microbiota composition differs in infants who have a bloody stool and those who do not.

b. Food allergy is a common cause of GI bleeding due to colitis in newborns and is less common in preterm infants or those who are breast fed. Food allergy is a clinical diagnosis. The mechanism is a hypersensitivity reaction of the bowel mucosa to digested antigens with resulting enterocolitis. It can occur in breast-fed infants exposed to cow's milk proteins in human breast milk. Dietary formula–related intolerance factors include allergic and dietary protein–induced colitis. The top ingested allergens are cow's milk products (most common, 76%) and soy protein. The most common clinical sign of cow's milk protein allergy is a bloody stool in a well-appearing infant. **There are multiple types of food-related GI disorders:**

i. Allergic enterocolitis can present with massive bloody stool, and routine lab data show no eosinophilia. However, rectal mucosal biopsy shows eosinophilic infiltration.

ii. Eosinophilic gastrointestinal disorders (mixed immunoglobulin E [IgE] and non-IgE cell mediated) are noted by the overproduction of eosinophils. The primary eosinophil inflammation can be anywhere in the GI tract (esophagitis, gastroenteritis, colitis). A new disease that is part of eosinophilic gastrointestinal disorders is called **neonatal transient eosinophilic colitis (NTEC)** and occurs in infants with lower GI bleeding with no known allergic component involved (no prior feeding had occurred). It may start in the fetal stage.

iii. Food protein–induced enterocolitis syndrome/dietary protein–induced enterocolitis syndrome is non-IgE cell mediated. The entire GI tract is affected, and the symptoms can be severe (vomiting, diarrhea, lethargy, metabolic acidosis, shock). Acute food protein–induced enterocolitis syndrome (FPIES) can have frank or occult blood in the stool.

Cow's milk and soy protein in formula are the most common triggers; therefore, it is rare in breast-fed infants.

iv. **Hematochezia in exclusively breast-fed infants** presents at an average age of 7.4 weeks. Diarrhea is the most common symptom (other symptoms include mild anemia, red and white blood cells in stool, negative culture, or colitis on colonoscopy) and may represent sensitivity to protein eaten by the mother. The hematochezia disappears after the mother is on a protein-free diet.

C. **Streaks of bright red blood coating a normal or hard formed stool.** Most commonly associated with a perianal disorder.

1. **Anal fissure** can be secondary to constipation and straining. This is the **most common cause of bleeding in infants**: spots of blood in the diaper or a strip of blood on the outside of one side of the stool. Etiology is a tear of the anal canal at the mucocutaneous line from a hard stool. Deeper rectal fissures can also occur.

2. **Rectal trauma** may be secondary to temperature probes or thermometer.

3. **Perianal irritation and excoriations** can cause small amounts of blood. This can be from a diaper rash.

4. **Rare causes.** Rectal prolapse is reported with chronic constipation, cow's milk allergy, *Shigella* diarrhea, rectal ulcer, β-hemolytic streptococcal cryptitis, ulcerative proctitis, rectal parasite infections, Hirschsprung disease, high anorectal malformations, and cystic fibrosis. **Perianal abscess/fistula in ano** is common in infants <1 year of age. It can originate from anal cryptitis, which then forms a perianal abscess.

D. **Bright red blood with moderately loose/frothy/mucus-laden stools**

1. **Food protein–induced (allergic) proctocolitis** (non-IgE cell mediated) presents with bright red rectal bleeding with mucus in a healthy infant. (See page 472.)

2. **Lymphonodular/nodular lymphoid hyperplasia (of the rectosigmoid area).** Usually presents in infants age 1 month or older. Characterized by multiple masses of lymphoid nodules that are usually present in the terminal ileum or colon. It disrupts the normal mucosa and leads to thinning of the mucosa and bleeding. Etiology is unknown. It can occur from cow's milk allergy or an immunologic response.

E. **Occult gastrointestinal blood by fecal occult blood testing/Hemoccult test.** Occult blood in the stool is very common, with up to 60% of neonates <1800 g having at least 1 occult blood–positive stool in the first 6 weeks of life. Stools may be heme positive after indomethacin for patent ductus arteriosus. It is transient and not clinically significant.

1. **Positive fecal occult blood test/Hemoccult test.** As an isolated finding, it is usually not significant. Tests for occult blood are very sensitive and can be positive with **repeated rectal temperatures or any perianal dermatitis.**

2. **A positive fecal occult blood test can be a finding in exclusively breast-fed infants (secondary to cow milk soy protein induced allergic colitis) and an early finding** with more significant diseases such as NEC, esophagitis, gastritis, Meckel diverticulum, acid peptic disease, polyposis, vascular malformations, eosinophilic gastroenteritis, polyps, vascular malformation, eosinophilic colitis, and others such as food protein–induced allergic proctocolitis (FPIES).

3. **Necrotizing enterocolitis.** Presence of occult blood does not directly correlate with the development of NEC.

F. **Blood spots in a diaper (nongastrointestinal causes).** This can be from other **etiologies besides the GI tract:** hematuria, severe diaper rash with excoriation, blood from a circumcision, or vaginal bleeding in a female infant (also called **pseudomenses;** withdrawal of maternal hormones). Reddish-orange spots ("brick stain") in the diaper are from uric acid crystals in the urine and are usually benign but may

indicate concentrated urine. A red-stained diaper can also be from bile pigments or porphyrins.
IV. **Database.** The age of the infant is important. If the infant is <7 days old, swallowed maternal blood is a likely cause; in older infants, this is unlikely. Cow's milk protein allergy usually presents in the first few months of life. NEC is unlikely in the first few days of life. Lymphonodular/nodular lymphoid hyperplasia presents in infants age 1 month or older. Ask the mother about medications taken during pregnancy. Is the infant breast feeding? Get a detailed description of the stool because type of stool and color of blood can help to differentiate the bleeding source (see Section III). Some advocate using a grading system (grade 1, 1 to 3 specks of blood; grade 2, 4 to 20 specks; grade 3, distinct blotch of blood staining the diaper; grade 4, gross blood with occasional blood clumps; and grade 5, all gross blood, no stool) to assess the severity of visible blood in the stool.
A. **Physical examination**
  1. **Evaluate the infant's peripheral perfusion.** An infant with NEC can be poorly perfused and may appear to be in early or impending shock. Bruising may suggest a coagulopathy.
  2. **Examine naso-/oropharyngeal area** for a source of bleeding.
  3. **Abdominal examination.** Check for bowel sounds and tenderness. Hyperactive bowel sounds are more common in upper GI bleeding. If the abdomen is soft and nontender and there is no erythema, a major intra-abdominal process is unlikely. If the abdomen is distended, rigid, or tender, an intra-abdominal pathologic process is likely. Abdominal distention is the most common sign of NEC. Abdominal distention may also suggest intussusception or midgut volvulus. If there are red streaks and erythema on the abdominal wall, suspect NEC with peritonitis. Malrotation with ischemic bowel can also present with peritonitis. If there is an abdominal mass, consider duplication. Consider Hirschsprung disease or malrotation if there is obstruction. Hepatomegaly, splenomegaly, or jaundice may indicate liver disease.
  4. **Genitourinary/anal examination.** Does the infant have a rash? If the infant's condition is stable, perform a visual examination of the anus to check for anal fissure or tear. Look for polyps, masses, or fistulas. Gentle digital rectal examination with a lubricated fifth digit may reveal fissures or polyps. Bedside "anoscopy" can be done by placing a well-lubricated blood collection tube into the anus.
B. **Laboratory studies**
  1. **Initial studies**
    a. **Fecal occult blood testing.** Hemoccult or other test should be obtained to confirm the presence of blood in the stool.
    b. **Apt test.** To differentiate maternal from fetal blood if swallowed maternal blood is suspected. A positive Apt test indicates that the blood is due to either GI or pulmonary bleeding from the neonate. A negative test would indicate that the blood is of maternal origin suggesting that the infant swallowed or aspirated maternal blood.
    c. **Complete blood count with differential.** If a large amount of blood is lost acutely, it takes time for it to be evident on hemoglobin results; therefore, initial hemoglobin values may be unreliable. An increased white blood cell count suggests infection or thrombocytopenia (can be associated with NEC or sepsis). Eosinophilia can be present in the serum with allergic enterocolitis, but it is not a uniform finding.
    d. **Chemistry panel.** High blood urea nitrogen can be seen in upper GI bleeding due to resorption of blood in GI tract.
    e. **Coagulation studies** rule out DIC or a bleeding diathesis. The usual studies are partial thromboplastin time (PTT), prothrombin time (PT), fibrinogen level, and platelet count. Thrombocytopenia can also be seen with cow's

milk–protein allergy. An elevated PT can indicate a coagulopathy, and a prolonged PTT may indicate hemophilia.

   f. **Suspected NEC.** If NEC is suspected, the following studies should be performed:

      i. **Complete blood count with differential.** To establish an inflammatory response and to check for thrombocytopenia and anemia.

      ii. **Serum potassium levels.** Hyperkalemia secondary to hemolysis may occur.

      iii. **Serum sodium levels.** Hyponatremia can be seen secondary to third spacing of fluids.

      iv. **Blood gas levels.** To rule out metabolic acidosis, often associated with sepsis or NEC.

2. **Further studies**

   a. **Stool studies.** Certain pathogens cause bloody stools, but they are rare in the neonatal nursery. Obtain **stool cultures** for common pathogens, ova, and parasites. **Stool smear** for white blood cells (elevated with colitis) and eosinophils (suggests allergic type of colitis).

   b. **Rectal biopsy.** A rectal mucosal biopsy can show eosinophilic infiltration suggestive of an allergic origin.

   c. **Serum radioallergosorbent test for cow's milk protein** with a specific IgE for whole cow's milk.

C. **Imaging and other studies**

1. **Immediate study**

   a. **Abdominal radiograph.** A plain radiograph of the abdomen is useful if NEC or a surgical abdomen is suspected. Look for an abnormal gas pattern, a thickened bowel wall, pneumatosis intestinalis, or perforation. Pneumatosis can appear as a "soap bubble" area (see Figure 12–26). If a suspicious area appears on the abdominal radiograph in the right upper quadrant, it is usually not stool. A left lateral decubitus view of the abdomen may show free air if perforation has occurred and it cannot be seen on a routine anteroposterior film. Surgical conditions usually show signs of intestinal obstruction. Most common sign in intussusception in premature infants is dilated bowel loops.

   b. **Ultrasound** can detect most of the common abdominal masses. It is the diagnostic modality of choice for suspected ileocolic intussusception. The "pseudokidney of intussusception" which is the longitudinal appearance of the intussuscepted segment of bowel which looks like a kidney is seen. Ultrasound can also be used to aid in the diagnosis of necrotizing enterocolitis.

   c. **Contrast studies** can be done for diagnosis of obstruction. An upper GI study can diagnose malrotation; the "bird beak" sign (contrast in the dilated proximal duodenum) can be seen.

   d. **Endoscopy of upper gastrointestinal tract** allows visualization of the esophagus, stomach, and duodenum and helps to identify the site of bleeding in the upper tract.

   e. **Meckel scan** (technetium-99m pertechnetate nuclear scan) can help diagnose Meckel diverticulum.

   f. **Radioactive tagged red blood cell scan** can localize the site of lower GI bleeding if the source is unknown.

   g. **Colonoscopy/flexible sigmoidoscopy** can be done to rule out colitis, polyps, or other masses. It can reveal nodular lymphoid hyperplasia. Can be done on infants who do not respond to elimination of formula for food protein–induced proctocolitis.

   h. **Rectal mucosal biopsy** can show eosinophilia in the lamina propria in cases of allergic enterocolitis.

      i. **Computed tomography scan** to evaluate for obstruction or see GI hemangiomas. Considered a suboptimal image quality with risks of ionizing radiation.

      j. **Magnetic resonance imaging** can be used for more complex cases. The magnetic resonance imaging (MRI)-compatible incubator is a promising method for safer imaging of smaller and less stable infants. MRI provides excellent anatomic details and aids in identification of congenital anomalies.

V. Plan. Based on the clinical status of the infant: Is the infant critically ill? Is the infant in shock? Is the infant who presents with blood in the stool well?

  A. Critically ill infant. Follow basic airway, breathing, and circulation measures, and pass nasogastric/orogastric tube. Begin aggressive volume replacement if hypotension/hypovolemia is present. Consider broad-spectrum antibiotics. Correct acidosis and fluid disturbances if appropriate. Do immediate laboratory and radiograph studies. Consider surgical consultation and initiation of peripheral nutritional support.

    1. **Place the infant NPO.**

    2. **Start the workup.** Initial laboratory tests and abdominal radiograph.

    3. **Antibiotics.** Some institutions will start the infant on antibiotics while the workup is done depending on the clinical status of the infant.

  B. Non–critically ill infant. Rule out non-GI causes of blood, especially if there was just blood on a diaper (see Section III.F above). Rule out swallowed maternal blood, blood from breast feeding, and anal fissure.

  C. Individual plans as follows:

    1. **Swallowed maternal blood.** Observation only.

    2. **Anal fissure and rectal trauma.** Observation is indicated. Petroleum jelly applied to the anus may promote healing. Constipation is treated with glycerin suppositories.

    3. **Necrotizing enterocolitis.** See Chapter 109.

    4. **Nasogastric trauma.** In most cases of bloody stool involving nasogastric tubes, trauma is mild and requires only observation. If the tube is too large, replacing it with a smaller one may resolve the problem. If there has been significant bleeding, **gastric lavages** are helpful; it is *controversial* whether tepid water or normal saline is best. Then, if possible, removal of the nasogastric tube is recommended.

    5. **Formula intolerance.** Difficult to document acutely and is usually diagnosed if the patient has remission of symptoms when the formula is eliminated. In breast-fed infants with rectal bleeding, the use of *Lactobacillus* was not supported by the literature. Cow's milk allergy should be treated with a cow's milk–free diet, and then those who become symptom free should be rechallenged to reduce the number of false-positive diagnoses.

    6. **Gastritis or ulcers.** Treatment usually consists of ranitidine (preferred because of fewer side effects) or famotidine. Use of antacids in neonates is *controversial*; some clinicians believe that concretions may result from the use of antacids. Use of antacids increases the risk of infection and feeding intolerance in infants receiving gavage feedings. (See Chapter 60.)

    7. **Unknown cause.** If no cause is found, the infant is usually closely monitored. In the majority of the cases, the bleeding subsides.

    8. **Nodular lymphoid hyperplasia.** Change the infant's formula to a hypoallergenic type.

    9. **Intestinal infections.** Antibiotic treatment and isolation are standard treatment.

    10. **Vitamin K deficiency bleeding** is usually adequately treated with vitamin K (see Chapter 92). Fresh-frozen plasma and red blood cell transfusions are sometimes needed.

    11. **Surgical conditions** (eg, NEC, perforation, volvulus). All require immediate surgical evaluation. Intussusception can be reduced with an enema in most cases.

55 Counseling Parents Before High-Risk Delivery

I. **Problem.** <u>The nurse calls to notify you of a pending high-risk delivery.</u> You are on delivery room duty, and you are asked to counsel the parents before their infant is delivered.

II. **Immediate questions**

  A. **Are both parents and other important family members available? What language do they speak? Is an interpreter needed?** Discuss the situation with the obstetric staff, and call for an interpreter if needed. Avoid using family members to translate because they need to be listening, may not have the expertise to provide appropriate translation of medical details, and may at times dominate questioning during the counseling session.

  B. **Is the mother too sick or uncomfortable to be able to adequately participate in the discussion?** In this situation, time is critical; be sure to include other family members.

  C. **How well do the parents understand their current situation?** Discuss the circumstances with the obstetric staff, and ask the parents what they understand. Some practitioners ask parents to repeat what they have heard at the end of the session.

  D. **What do they know about neonatal intensive care units (NICUs), pregnancy and neonatal complications, chronic health problems, and neurodevelopmental disability?** This helps you in beginning and planning the discussion.

III. **Differential diagnosis.** Neonatologists are called to counsel expectant parents in a wide variety of circumstances. These generally include:

  A. **Preterm birth**

  B. **Fetal growth restriction (FGR) (also known as intrauterine growth restriction [IUGR])**

  C. **Maternal substance use disorders (SUDS)**

  D. **Signs of fetal distress**

  E. **Congenital anomalies**

IV. **Database**

  A. **Maternal/paternal data.** Obtain information regarding the age of both parents; mother's obstetric, past medical, and social history; history of the pregnancy, medications, and pertinent laboratory data; and family history.

  B. **Fetal data.** Review fetal information with the obstetric staff, including accuracy of pregnancy dating, findings on prenatal ultrasounds, and signs of fetal distress.

V. **Plan**

  A. **General approach to parent counseling.** Although circumstances are often less than ideal, it is important to communicate as effectively and empathetically as possible. Sit down, communicate at eye level, take time to introduce yourself and your role, and talk in a clear and unhurried manner. Explain all medical terms, avoid using abbreviations, keep in mind that most people cannot think in percentages, acknowledge uncertainties, and try to give the parents an idea of what to expect. Ask if they understand, and summarize the most important points. Ask if they have any questions and offer to follow-up with them if they have more questions.

  B. **Goal of counseling session.** Because a complete discussion is often unrealistic, your goal is to help parents anticipate and to provide a framework for understanding what happens during delivery and in the neonatal intensive care unit (NICU).

  C. **Content of discussion.** As appropriate, discuss the infant's chances of survival, possible complications, and the range of long-term outcomes. (In preparation for counseling the parents, review appropriate references, other chapters in this book, and other textbooks for more information.) Describe anticipated activity during delivery and transition to the NICU. Giving the parents the opportunity to tour the NICU allows them to see the monitoring and life support equipment, so that they can better see their own baby attached to it all.

D. **Bedside manner.** For many, the shock and anxiety of facing difficult circumstances challenge their ability to process information, especially when a lot of medical and technical terms are used. Avoid overloading the family with information. Your communication is most effective if conveyed in a caring, empathetic, and unhurried manner. *Understand that hope helps people get through the most dire situations.*

VI. **Specific counseling issues.** Although medical terms are used in this section, use simple language when counseling parents. Stress influences the ability to process information in even the most medically sophisticated parents.

A. **Preterm delivery.** The more immature the infant, the greater are the risks of death, complications, health sequelae, and neurodevelopmental disability (see Table 55–1 for **estimate only** of survival by gestational age and birthweight [Mednax, 2018], and Table 55–2 for **estimates** of morbidity based on gestational age). Gestational age serves as a proxy for maturity when counseling parents before delivery.

1. **Immediate questions.** Why is the mother delivering preterm? What is the gestational age of the fetus? Are there concerns about fetal growth, fetal distress, infection, or anomalies that may influence fetal outcome?

2. **Specific issues to address with the parents**

a. **Mortality.** Even with aggressive intervention, the lower limit of viability is 23 to 24 weeks' gestation, with occasional survival reported at 22 weeks' gestation.

b. **Complications of prematurity.** Complications of prematurity include respiratory distress syndrome (RDS); electrolyte and metabolic problems; infection; necrotizing enterocolitis (NEC); patent ductus arteriosus (PDA); apnea and bradycardia; anemia; and intraventricular hemorrhage (IVH) and other signs of brain injury. Chronic complications include bronchopulmonary dysplasia/ chronic lung disease (BPD/CLD); retinopathy of prematurity (ROP) with subsequent visual problems, hearing impairment, and neurodevelopmental impairment. Complication rates increase with decreasing gestational age.

c. **Long-term neurodevelopmental outcome.** Rates of neurodevelopmental disabilities increase with decreasing gestational age at birth, with the highest rates in those born before 25 weeks' gestation (see Table 55–2). Even late preterm children (born at 34–36 weeks' gestation) have higher rates of cerebral palsy and school problems than do infants born full term. Learning disability, language delays, visual perceptual deficits, minor neuromotor dysfunction, executive dysfunction, attention deficits, and behavior problems are more frequent in school-age children born preterm than in controls born full term. Nonetheless, the majority of preterm survivors have normal intelligence, graduate from high school, and become functioning adults in their communities.

B. **Fetal growth restriction.** See also Chapter 104.

1. **Immediate questions.** What is the cause of the FGR and when was it detected? Does the fetus have anomalies? Are there signs of fetal decompensation?

2. **Specific issues to address with parents**

a. **Prediction of outcome.** The most important determinant of FGR outcome is its cause. Infants with chromosomal disorders and congenital infections (eg, toxoplasmosis, cytomegalovirus) experience early FGR, often do not tolerate labor and delivery well, and commonly have a disability. When there is fetal deprivation of uterine supply, the fetus initially compensates by reducing weight and length before head growth and, after 30 weeks' gestation, may accelerate fetal maturation. Although accelerated maturation improves fetal survival if delivered preterm, there is a cost in terms of cognitive development. Adverse intrauterine circumstances that overwhelm compensatory mechanisms lead to progressive damage to fetal organs (eg, liver, gut, brain) and may result in fetal death.

Table 55-1 SURVIVAL BY ESTIMATED GESTATIONAL AGE AND BIRTH WEIGHT[a]

Weight Group (gm)	Estimated Gestational Age (wks)										Overall
	22	23	24	25	26	27	28	29	30	31	
250 to 500	15.6%	28.1%	40.4%	46.3%	50.0%						37.5%
501 to 750	28.8%	46.8%	65.6%	77.2%	87.1%	85.1%	92.6%	87.1%			69.8%
751 to 1000			77.1%	84.6%	90.5%	95.8%	98.0%	97.2%	97.9%	93.4%	92.3%
1001 to 1250				91.3%	90.6%	95.9%	97.5%	98.5%	98.7%	99.7%	97.7%
1251 to 1500						95.9%	96.4%	98.8%	98.9%	99.9%	99.0%
1501 to 1750							97.3%	99.5%	99.5%	99.4%	99.7%
1751 to 2000								95.5%	99.0%	99.6%	99.8%
2001 to 2250									93.3%	98.3%	99.9%
Overall for EGA	22.9%	43.3%	65.1%	78.8%	88.7%	94.0%	97.2%	98.2%	98.9%	99.4%	
Total Patient Count	131	467	814	904	1195	1442	1797	2089	2893	3752	

[a]The outcomes of 119,139 non-anomalous neonates born at, cared for in, and discharged from 272 hospitals in 34 states from 2016 to 2017. Estimated gestational age range was 22 to 42 weeks. Birth weight range was 0.3 to 6.0 kg. For calculations the minimum cell sample size was 20 patients. Data on outcome of infants more than 31 weeks is not presented as their percent survival and percent survival without morbidity approached 100%. **These numbers represent an estimate.** The likelihood of a good outcome is influenced by many variables, only two of which are estimated gestational age and birth weight. Source: Pediatrix Clinical Data Warehouse.

Table 55–2. ESTIMATES OF MORBIDITY USEFUL IN COUNSELING PARENTS

Risk Factor	Cerebral Palsy (%)	Intellectual Disability (%)	Sensory Impairment (%)
None	0.1	1–2	0.1–0.2
Prematurity			
GA 33–36 weeks	0.3–0.7	1–2	0.1–0.2
GA 29–32 weeks	2–5	2–3	0.4–2
GA ≤28 weeks	6–15	3–8	2–4
GA ≤25 weeks	7–25	27–35	3–5

GA, completed weeks of gestation at birth (birthweight data are difficult to accurately determine for prenatal counseling).

   b. **Complications of fetal growth restriction.** IUGR infants are vulnerable to postnatal complications, including perinatal asphyxia, cold stress, polycythemia, hypoglycemia, and feeding problems.
   c. **Long-term outcome.** Full-term FGR infants with fetal deprivation of supply have an increased risk of motor and cognitive impairments (eg, cerebral palsy, minor neuromotor dysfunction, learning disability, attention deficits, behavior problems) and, as adults, cardiovascular disease, obesity, and diabetes. Preterm FGR infants are vulnerable to the complications of both preterm delivery and FGR.
C. **Maternal substance use disorder**
   1. **Immediate questions.** Which drugs did the mother use? When and how much?
   2. **Specific issues to address with parents**
      a. **Fetal growth restriction.** Infants with intrauterine exposure to opiates, cocaine, alcohol, cigarettes, and some prescription drugs may have FGR (see preceding Section VI.B).
      b. **Specific syndromes and risks.** Fetal alcohol and fetal hydantoin syndromes are well defined but often difficult to diagnose in the neonatal period. Both carry an increased risk of intellectual disability. (See Chapter 93.)
      c. **Neonatal abstinence syndrome (NAS).** Infants with intrauterine exposure to opiates, cocaine, alcohol, or some prescription medications may demonstrate signs of neonatal withdrawal (see Chapter 102). These infants require close observation after delivery and may require medications to help them through the withdrawal period. Later, these infants have an increased incidence of school and behavior problems.
      d. **Maternal cocaine use** is associated with increased rates of miscarriage, stillbirth, abruption, preterm labor, and FGR. Infants with central nervous system infarctions resulting from intrauterine cocaine exposure are at high risk for cerebral palsy, especially hemiplegia, as well as cognitive and sensory impairments.
D. **Signs of fetal distress**
   1. **Immediate questions.** Which signs of fetal distress are evident and for how long?
   2. **Specific issues to address.** Fetal distress is a risk factor for respiratory distress at birth requiring resuscitation, persistent pulmonary hypertension, neonatal encephalopathy, and metabolic problems (eg, hypoglycemia). The type of fetal distress and perinatal and postnatal complications, especially neonatal encephalopathy and brain injury on neuroimaging, electroencephalogram, and neurodevelopmental examination (see Chapter 18), are prognostic indicators. Nonetheless,

the majority of infants with fetal distress who recover quickly after birth have a good prognosis.

E. **Congenital anomalies**

1. **Immediate questions.** What anomalies have been detected, and how were they noted? Is the anomaly life threatening? What workup and/or fetal therapy has been done? Have any other anomalies been detected?

2. **Specific issues to address with the parents.** See also Chapter 93.

   a. **Diagnosis.** The type of congenital anomaly, its severity, and whether further evaluation has identified other anomalies or etiology determine how you should counsel the parents. Identification of an anomaly should trigger a search for other anomalies.

   b. **Prognosis.** Clinical courses and outcomes have been well described for most chromosomal disorders (eg, trisomy 21, 22q11 deletion), many multiple congenital anomaly syndromes (eg, VATER/VACTERL [*v*ertebral defects, *a*nal atresia, *t*racheo*e*sophageal fistula, and *r*adial or *r*enal dysplasia/*v*ertebral defects, *a*nal atresia, *c*ardiac malformations, *t*racheo*e*sophageal fistula, *r*enal dysplasia, and *l*imb abnormalities] association, arthrogryposis), and some specific single anomalies (eg, meningomyelocele, congenital heart disease). The presence of a congenital anomaly increases an infant's risks of FGR, preterm birth, and neurodevelopmental disability.

   c. **Counseling parents.** A study of mothers who were counseled after prenatal diagnosis of a congenital anomaly who were interviewed a week after delivery found that the consultation helped to prepare them. They authors concluded that "parents want realistic medical information, specific to their situation, provided in an empathetic manner and want to be allowed to hope for the best possible outcome."

56 Cyanosis

I. **Problem.** During a physical examination, an infant appears blue. **Cyanosis** is a physical sign indicating a bluish/purplish discoloration of the skin and/or mucous membranes. There are many different types of cyanosis, and it is important to differentiate physiologic versus pathologic cyanosis. **This chapter will focus mainly on central cyanosis because it is a potentially serious condition that requires an immediate evaluation.** The differential diagnosis of central cyanosis includes disorders involving an increase in deoxygenated hemoglobin (respiratory, cardiovascular, neurologic, or other) or hematologic disorders involving abnormal hemoglobin (methemoglobinemia/sulfhemoglobinemia). **Early diagnosis and treatment for any cyanotic infant is essential.**

II. **Immediate questions**

A. **What type of cyanosis does the infant have?** Some types of cyanosis are not considered pathologic and require no workup; others such as central cyanosis can be associated with a life-threatening disease. Differentiate the type of cyanosis to help guide the workup and treatment.

1. **Central cyanosis: bluish skin, including the tongue, mucosal membranes, and lips.** This is caused by lack of oxygen in the blood (low PaO_2 and low SaO_2). While this can occur immediately after birth, persistent central cyanosis is never normal and needs to be evaluated to rule out major cardiac, lung, central nervous system (CNS), metabolic, or hematologic diseases.

2. **Peripheral cyanosis: bluish skin with pink lips, mucous membranes, and tongue.** Associated with normal PaO_2 and normal (or falsely low if sensor wrapped around a cold blue finger or toe) arterial oxygen saturation. It is caused by decreased/sluggish local circulation leading to an increase in deoxygenated blood on the venous side. This is a consequence of increased oxygen extraction by the tissues and may be a physiologic response. Peripheral cyanosis can be a normal finding; can be associated with causes of central cyanosis; or can be caused by vasomotor instability, venous obstruction (venous thrombosis), polycythemia, low cardiac output (cardiomyopathies, hypocalcemia), shock, sepsis, hypothermia, hypoadrenalism, hypoglycemia, vasoconstriction secondary to cold exposure, and elevated venous pressure. Peripheral cyanosis is common in Down syndrome (vasomotor instability).
3. **Acrocyanosis (bluish hands and feet only).** There is normal oxygen saturation in the blood. A type of peripheral cyanosis, it is cyanosis of the extremities and around the mouth and may be considered a normal finding immediately after birth, within the first 1 to 2 days, or with cold stress. Spasm of smaller arterioles is the cause. In a normothermic older infant, consider hypovolemia as the main cause.
4. **Perioral/cirumoral cyanosis (bluish color around the lips and philtrum [nose to upper lip]).** There is normal oxygen saturation in the blood. It is common after birth and is due to the close proximity of the blood vessels to the skin. Infants have a prominent superficial perioral venous plexus that can engorge with feeding, and this is not a sign of peripheral or central cyanosis and usually resolves after 48 hours.
5. **Traumatic cyanosis.** There is normal oxygen saturation in the blood. This is cyanosis of the head and face usually found with petechiae. This is a result of venous congestion during delivery caused by a face presentation or nuchal cord.
6. **Pseudo-cyanosis.** Bluish color of the skin without hypoxemia, hemoglobin abnormality, or peripheral vasoconstriction. The mucous membranes of the mouth are pink, and with pressure on the skin, the color does not blanch. This can mimic peripheral cyanosis. Most commonly caused by fluorescent lighting in neonatal units, but can also be caused by drug exposure.
7. **Cyanosis caused by methemoglobinemia** causes a diffuse persistent **slate gray bluish appearance** of the infant. Drugs such as lidocaine, benzocaine, and nitrates may result in acquired methemoglobinemia.
8. **Differential cyanosis.** See Section II.I below.

B. **Does the infant have respiratory distress?** If the infant has increased respiratory effort with increased rate, retractions, and nasal flaring, **respiratory disease** should be high on the list of differential diagnoses. **Cyanotic heart disease** usually presents without respiratory symptoms ("happy blue baby") but can have effortless tachypnea (rapid respiratory rate without retractions). **Methemoglobinemia syndromes** usually present without respiratory symptoms, but **polycythemia** can present with or without respiratory symptoms. **CNS disease** can present with respiratory symptoms (ie, respiratory muscle weakness, hypoventilation with a decreased respiratory drive).
C. **Does the infant have a murmur?** A murmur usually implies heart disease, but in infants with congenital heart malformations, <50% have a murmur in the newborn period. Transposition of the great vessels can present without a murmur (~60%). **Muffled heart sounds** can indicate pericardial effusions or pneumopericardium.
D. **Was the infant cyanotic at birth?** Infants just born can have central cyanosis for a brief period after birth. Once their oxygen saturation normalizes, they are no longer cyanotic. They can also have differential cyanosis soon after birth while transitioning. If cyanotic at birth and cyanosis persists, consider that transposition of the great vessels (transposition of the great arteries [TGA]) and tricuspid atresia can present immediately at birth. Infants with TGA with ventricular septal defect (VSD), left ventricular outflow obstruction (LVOTO), and restricted pulmonary blood flow (PBF) present with intense cyanosis at birth. In the perinatal period, infants with

truncus arteriosus, total anomalous pulmonary venous return, and tetralogy of Fallot can present with persistent cyanosis. Most infants with airway abnormalities or congenital diaphragmatic hernia will usually present shortly after birth and will have persistent cyanosis. Infants with hereditary methemoglobinemia usually have cyanosis present at birth.

E. **Is the cyanosis continuous, intermittent, cyclical, sudden in onset, or occurring only with feeding or crying?**

1. **Continuous cyanosis** is more commonly associated with intrinsic lung disease or heart disease.
2. **Recurrent episodes of cyanosis.** Consider phrenic nerve paralysis.
3. **Intermittent cyanosis** is more common with neurologic disorders; these infants may have apneic spells alternating with periods of normal breathing.
4. **Cyclical cyanosis** can occur with nasal obstruction.
5. **Sudden onset of cyanosis** may occur with an air leak, such as pneumothorax.
6. **Cyanosis with feeding** can occur with esophageal atresia, tracheoesophageal atresia, and severe gastroesophageal reflux. **Feeding hypoxia** occurs more commonly with bottle feeding than breast feeding.
7. **Cyanosis in supine position that decreases when the infant is placed in prone position.** Micrognathia, retrognathia, Pierre Robin sequence.
8. **Cyanosis only with crying** can occur in infants with tetralogy of Fallot.
9. **Cyanosis that disappears with crying** may mean bilateral choanal atresia. These infants are cyanotic when quiet and at rest and pink when crying with their mouth open.
10. **Cyanosis that gets worse with crying, feeding, respiratory infections, and supine position.** Severe laryngomalacia and tracheomalacia.
11. **Crying may improve cyanosis in respiratory disease** and worsen it in cardiac disease.
12. **Cyanosis after crying.** Some term infants have a prolonged apnea after crying that results in a marked decrease in oxygen saturation and **central cyanosis** (central apnea immediately after crying with a decrease in SpO_2 to 60%).

F. **Is the pulse oximeter reading low in an infant who is cyanotic with a normal PaO_2 on arterial blood gases?** Consider methemoglobinemia, hemoglobin variants, or some cases of peripheral cyanosis. The pulse oximeter estimates oxygen saturation by using light absorbance measurements at 2 wavelengths to determine the percentage of hemoglobin that is saturated with oxygen. It is inaccurate when more than 2 types of hemoglobin are present, as in methemoglobinemia. In infants with a high concentration of methemoglobin, the pulse oximeter will show a falsely low reading (regardless of the real hemoglobin oxygen saturation. **It falsely indicates arterial hypoxemia in infants with peripheral cyanosis or with abnormal hemoglobin.** Laboratory blood gas analysis can differentiate deoxyhemoglobin from abnormal hemoglobin; therefore, it only indicates hypoxia in infants with central cyanosis. Some newer pulse oximeters can measure methemoglobin and oxygen saturation (eg, Masimo Rainbow SET Radical-7 pulse oximeter; Masimo, Irvine, CA). **In some infants with peripheral cyanosis** with poor perfusion in the extremities, deeply pigmented skin, or jaundice, the pulse oximeter can be inaccurate and can indicate arterial hypoxemia in patients with normal arterial oxygenation.

G. **What is the hemoglobin concentration?** The degree of visible cyanosis on physical examination depends on both oxygen saturation and hemoglobin concentration. The appearance of cyanosis depends upon the absolute amount of reduced hemoglobin. Normally cyanosis is perceptible at 85% saturation when the hemoglobin concentration is 15 g/dL and the reduced hemoglobin is >3 g/dL. In a polycythemic infant one will detect cyanosis at a higher level of oxygen saturation (Hbg 20 g/dL detects cyanosis at 87% saturation) and in anemic infant cyanosis may not be apparent since one will only detect cyanosis at a lower level of oxygen saturation (Hgb of 6 g/dL detects cyanosis at 62.5% saturation).

H. **Has the baby had the pulse oximetry screening test for critical congenital heart disease (CCHD)?** This increases the detection rate of CCHD by 28% as physical examination can miss up to 50% of cyanotic congenital heart disease. This is a required test now in all newborns (see Chapter 7) as a useful method for screening for cyanotic CCHD. It can identify the following 7 core heart conditions that present with hypoxemia before cyanosis develops: hypoplastic left heart syndrome, pulmonary atresia with an intact septum, tetralogy of Fallot, total anomalous pulmonary venous connection, TGA, tricuspid atresia, and truncus arteriosus.

I. **Is there differential cyanosis?** Differential cyanosis (DC) is when there is cyanosis of the upper or lower part of the body only, and it usually signifies serious heart disease. **The prerequisite for this is the presence of a right-to-left shunt through the patent ductus arteriosus (PDA).** To diagnose this, oxygen saturation should be measured preductal (right hand is preferred since it accurately reflects preductal value) and postductal (foot). There are 2 different types of DC.

1. **Pink upper half of the body, cyanosis lower part of body (more common).** Oxygen saturation is greater in the right hand than in the foot. It usually occurs with severe coarctation of the aorta with PDA, interrupted aortic arch with a PDA, mitral stenosis with a PDA, persistent pulmonary hypertension with a PDA, and Eisenmenger syndrome (PDA with severe pulmonary hypertension.

2. **Cyanosis in the upper half of the body, pink lower part of the body.** This type is very rare (reversed differential cyanosis [RDC]) and occurs when oxygen saturation is lower in the right hand than in the foot. This is usually seen in TGA and a PDA associated with severe coarctation of the aorta, interrupted aortic arch, or pulmonary hypertension. It can also be seen in an infant with supracardiac total anomalous pulmonary venous connection (TAPVC) to the superior vena cava with a shunt through the PDA.

J. **What is the prenatal and delivery history?** Did the mother have a prenatal sonogram? It may show a cardiac anomaly. Certain perinatal conditions increase the incidence of congenital heart disease. The delivery history may provide clues for the diagnosis of cyanosis.

1. **An infant of a diabetic mother** has an increased risk of hypoglycemia, transient tachypnea of the newborn (TTN), polycythemia, respiratory distress syndrome, and congenital heart disease (TGA, VSD, hypertrophic cardiomyopathy).

2. **Mother with connective tissue disorder:** causes heart block (anti-Ro/SSA and anti-La/SSB antibodies).

3. **Risk of infection** (eg, premature rupture of membranes, maternal fever, chorioamniotis) can all increase the risk of infection in the neonate which can be associated with cyanosis. Coxsackie B viral infection in the mom can cause myocarditis in newborn infants. Congenital intrauterine infections (eg, cytomegalovirus, herpesvirus, rubella) can cause cardiac abnormalities and cyanosis.

4. **Amniotic fluid abnormalities,** such as oligohydramnios (associated with pulmonary hypoplasia and renal defects) or polyhydramnios (associated with esophageal atresia or neurologic or airway conditions), may suggest a cause for the cyanosis.

5. **Cesarean section** is associated with increased respiratory distress, TTN, and persistent pulmonary hypertension of the newborn (PPHN). If sedatives or general anesthesia were used, suspect apnea or respiratory depression.

6. **Hypertension early in pregnancy increases the risk of a congenital heart defect.** Pregnancy-induced hypertension can be associated with intrauterine growth restriction, polycythemia, and hypoglycemia.

7. **Advanced maternal age** can be associated with birth defects such as Down syndrome and Turner syndrome, which include heart defects.

8. **Meconium at delivery** can be associated with meconium aspiration syndrome and PPHN.

9. **Preterm delivery.** Consider respiratory distress syndrome.
10. **Medications used by the mother can cause an increase in congenital heart disease.** Anticonvulsants, lithium, indomethacin, nonsteroidal anti-inflammatory drugs (NSAIDs), ibuprofen, sulfasalazine, thalidomide, trimethoprim, sulfonamide, high-dose vitamin A, antihypertensive medications, selective serotonin reuptake inhibitors (SSRIs), marijuana, alcohol, cigarette smoking, cocaine, and exposure to organic solvents. Maternal lithium treatment increases the risk of Ebstein anomaly.
11. **Maternal illnesses that increase the risk of congenital heart disease.** Untreated phenylketonuria, maternal pregestational diabetes, febrile illness during the first trimester, influenza, maternal rubella (increased risk pulmonary artery stenosis and PDA), epilepsy, and maternal lupus/connective tissue disease.
12. **Maternal congenital heart disease and/or congenital heart disease in a first-degree relative.** Increased incidence of heart disease in the infant.

III. **Differential diagnosis.** Cyanosis becomes visible when there is >3 g/dL of deoxygenated hemoglobin in arterial blood. Cyanosis is caused by either a disorder involving deoxygenated hemoglobin or disorders involving abnormal hemoglobin. The causes of cyanosis can be classified as arising from respiratory, infectious, cardiac, CNS, hematologic, or other disorders. **Central cyanosis** in the neonate is secondary to hypoxia by one or more of the following reasons: **hypoventilation** (eg, CNS depression, neuromuscular disorders, obstruction of the airway, metabolic causes), **impairment of alveolar arterial diffusion** (eg, congestive heart failure/pulmonary edema), **right to left shunting** (eg, PPHN, cyanotic congenital heart disease), or **ventilation perfusion mismatch** (eg, RDS, pulmonary hemorrhage, pneumonia, pleural effusion, pneumothorax, atelectasis, pulmonary hypoplasia, TTN). **The most common etiology of cyanosis in a newborn infant is respiratory, and this should be excluded first.**

A. **Respiratory diseases.** These include: primary pulmonary diseases, airway obstruction, extrinsic compression of the lungs, congenital defects, hypoventilation, and pulmonary edema. The majority of airway abnormalities usually present right after birth. Newborns with lung disease will usually present with respiratory distress.
   1. **Primary pulmonary diseases.** Respiratory distress syndrome, TTN (rarely associated with visible cyanosis), aspiration (meconium, blood, amniotic fluid) syndromes, pneumonia, bronchopulmonary dysplasia/chronic lung disease, pulmonary hemorrhage, atelectasis, pulmonary edema.
   2. **Airway obstruction.** Choanal atresia/stenosis, micrognathia, retrognathia (Pierre Robin sequence), laryngomalacia and tracheomalacia, bilateral vocal cord paralysis (severe respiratory distress and cyanosis), tracheal stenosis, macroglossia, subglottic stenosis, atelectasis, mucus plug, and others. Vascular rings cause compression of the trachea and cyanosis.
   3. **External compression of the lungs.** Any air leak syndrome (eg, pneumothorax, pulmonary interstitial emphysema), pleural effusion, chylo-/hemothorax, thoracic dystrophy, and others.
   4. **Congenital defects.** Congenital diaphragmatic hernia, pulmonary hypoplasia, cystic pulmonary airway malformation, tracheoesophageal fistula/esophageal atresia, congenital lobar emphysema (rarely presents at birth), subglottic stenosis, pulmonary artery sling, asphyxiating thoracic dystrophy/dysplasia (Jeune syndrome), congenital laryngomalacia, arteriovenous fistulas, Pierre Robin sequence, and others.
   5. **Hypoventilation.** Sedation, sepsis, neuromuscular diseases, CNS depression or lesions.
B. **Infections. Sepsis is the second most common cause of cyanosis in infants.** Sepsis causes increased oxygen utilization, capillary leak, and pulmonary edema, which results in cyanosis.
C. **Cardiac diseases.** The majority of congenital heart diseases that present in the first couple of weeks of life are ductal-dependent cardiac lesions.

1. **More common cyanotic heart diseases include the 5 Ts.** Central cyanosis results from right-to-left shunting.
   a. **Transposition of the great arteries.** This is the most common cause of cardiac cyanosis in newborns.
   b. **Total anomalous pulmonary venous return/connection.**
   c. **Tricuspid valve abnormalities (tricuspid atresia).**
   d. **Tetralogy of Fallot is the most common cyanotic congenital heart disease in older children.**
   e. **Truncus arteriosus.**
   f. **Often a 6th and 7th T are added to the mnemonic of the 5 Ts:**
      i. **Tiny heart (hypoplastic left heart syndrome)**
      ii. **Seventh T ("tons of others"/"terrible Ts")** includes all the others: critical pulmonary stenosis, double outlet right ventricle, pulmonary atresia with intact ventricular septum or with VSD, variations on single ventricle, Ebstein anomaly of the tricuspid valve, total anomalous pulmonary venous connection with and without obstruction, single-ventricle complexes, and absent pulmonary valve syndrome.
2. **Severe congestive heart failure.** This can occur from cardiomyopathies (infant of diabetic mother [IDM], inborn errors of metabolism, genetic or neuromuscular disease), myocarditis (bacterial or viral), congenital cardiac disease, sepsis, perinatal asphyxia, and sustained tachyarrhythmias. **Cyanosis and heart failure can be seen in left-sided obstructive lesions** (hypoplastic left heart syndrome [HLHS], severe coarctation of the aorta, interrupted aortic arch, and critical valvar aortic stenosis). These lesions are ductal dependent for systemic flow, and when it closes, these patients become cyanotic and experience shock and hypotension, pulmonary edema, and metabolic acidosis.
3. **Pneumopericardium or pericardial effusion.**
4. **Other congenital anomalies** such as those associated with cardiac malformations: Turner syndrome, Noonan syndrome, and others. **Pulmonary arteriovenous malformation** is a rare cause of cyanosis in the newborn. See Table 94–1 for congenital anomalies associated with heart defects.
5. **Primary intracardiac tumors** with obstructive symptoms (eg, cardiac rhabdomyoma presenting with cyanosis in a 3-day-old infant).

D. **Persistent pulmonary hypertension of the newborn causes right-to-left shunting with resultant cyanosis.** In PPHN, infants do not transition from fetal to newborn circulation. Pulmonary hypertension causes **right-to-left shunting of blood,** a decrease in PBF, and cyanosis.

E. **Central nervous system disorders** can cause apnea, seizures, and decreased respiratory drive (hypoventilation and cyanosis).
   1. **Infectious.** Bacterial or viral CNS infection (meningitis, encephalitis).
   2. **Seizures.** Infection, metabolic, CNS injury, genetic syndrome, congenital disorder, primary seizure disorder.
   3. **Neonatal encephalopathy/hypoxic ischemic encephalopathy.**
   4. **Hemorrhage.** Periventricular/intraventricular hemorrhage, subdural hemorrhage, subarachnoid hemorrhage, intracerebellar hemorrhage, infarction.
   5. **Congenital disorders.** Congenital hydrocephalus, spinal muscle atrophy, congenital central hypoventilation syndrome.
   6. **Drug toxicity (eg, opioid toxicity).**

F. **Neuromuscular disorders cause hypoventilation.** Werdnig-Hoffmann disease, Pompe disease, Barth syndrome, Duchenne or Becker muscular dystrophy, limb girdle muscular dystrophy, congenital myopathy, neonatal myasthenia gravis, phrenic nerve injury, and congenital myotonic dystrophy.

G. **Hematologic disorders.** A hemoglobin disorder can interfere with the transport of oxygen and cause cyanosis. Suspect methemoglobinemia when administration of oxygen does not resolve the cyanosis. The typical infant with methemoglobinemia is cyanotic, has no respiratory distress, and has a low oxygen saturation and normal PaO_2.

1. **Methemoglobinemia (normal arterial oxygen)** is characterized when red blood cells contain a high level of methemoglobin. Methemoglobin is caused by iron being oxidized from the normal ferrous state to the abnormal ferric form within the heme moiety of hemoglobin, and it is incapable of transporting oxygen or carbon dioxide. Because the arterial blood is brown in color, it gives off a bluish hue in the skin of white people ("chocolate cyanosis"). It can be congenital (genetic) or acquired.

    a. **Congenital methemoglobinemia** is typically caused by autosomal recessive inheritance of the deficient *cv5R* gene.

    b. **Acquired methemoglobinemia** can be caused by exposure to certain medications (eg, eutectic mixture of lidocaine and prilocaine [EMLA], metoclopramide, nitrites, sulfonamides, benzocaine, dapsone, lidocaine, amyl nitrate, nitric oxide, nitroglycerin, nitroprusside, phenazopyridine, prilocaine, quinones, sulfonamides) or toxin oxidizing chemicals (eg, nitrates, nitrous gases, chlorobenzene, isobutyl nitrate, aniline dye derivatives, naphthalene), environmental substances, or dietary etiologies. Transient neonatal methemoglobinemia can be caused by maternal pudendal anesthesia with prilocaine.

2. **Congenital familial sulfhemoglobinemia** is an extremely rare disease caused by excess sulfhemoglobin in the blood and can cause cyanosis. It is caused by sulfur-containing drugs or intestinal microbiota (eg, *Morganella morganii*).

3. **Other rare variants of hemoglobin.** Fetal HB and fetal M hemoglobin variants are rare causes of cyanosis. Clinical clues are a positive family history in an infant with a decreased hemoglobin oxygen saturation with a normal PaO_2. Six identified mutations can cause cyanosis at birth, with the cyanosis resolving as the adult β-globin chain replaces the fetal γ-globin chain.

4. **Polycythemia/hyperviscosity syndrome (normal arterial oxygen)** presents with peripheral cyanosis, tachypnea, congestive heart failure (CHF), and cardiomegaly. Infants can appear cyanotic because of an elevated hemoglobin even though their oxygen saturations are normal. Cyanosis is detectable at a higher value of SaO_2 (eg, in polycythemic infants [polycythemia can cause persistent pulmonary hypertension and cyanosis]). Mild hypoxia can cause cyanosis in polycythemia.

5. **Severe anemia** from hemorrhage or bleeding disorders. Patients who have anemia do not develop cyanosis until the oxygen saturation falls below normal hemoglobin levels.

H. **Metabolic abnormalities can present with cyanosis secondary to hypoventilation from lethargy, apnea, and seizures.**

1. **Drug withdrawal.**

2. **Severe hypoglycemia, hypermagnesemia, severe metabolic acidosis.**

3. **Inborn errors of metabolism.**

4. **Rarely abnormalities of calcium, potassium, and phosphorus** can cause hypoxia and cyanosis. Calcium and potassium abnormalities can cause cardiac arrhythmias.

I. **Other disorders**

1. **Apnea and bradycardia/apnea of prematurity.**

2. **Hypothermia.**

3. **Hypoadrenalism/hypopituitarism.**

4. **Hypotension and shock.** This can be secondary to sepsis or cardiogenic, neurogenic, or hypovolemic, and all can present with cyanosis. (See Chapter 70.)

5. **Abdominal distension** with elevation of the diaphragm.

6. **Respiratory depression** secondary to maternal medications (eg, magnesium sulfate and narcotics) or maternal sedation.

7. **BRUE (brief resolved unexplained events) replaces ALTE (apparent life threatening event).** A BRUE applies to a well-appearing infant (no underlying

health problems) age <1 year who has a brief, <1 minute (usually <20–30 seconds) sudden event that resolves, is unexplained after a history and physical examination, and includes 1 or more of the following: **cyanosis** or pallor; decreased, absent, or irregular breathing; altered level of responsiveness; or marked change in tone (hypertonia or hypotonia).

J. **Pseudo-cyanosis.** Caused by fluorescent lighting.

IV. **Database.** Obtain a prenatal and delivery history (see Section II.J). Measure oxygen saturation by a pulse oximeter to confirm central cyanosis.

A. **Physical examination**

1. **Assess the infant for central, peripheral, acrocyanosis, perioral/circumoral, or differential cyanosis.** See Section II.A.

   a. **Central cyanosis.** Skin, lips, and tongue appear blue. It may be difficult to assess cyanosis in infants with darker skin pigmentation. Focus on nailbeds, tongue, and mucous membranes.

   b. **Peripheral cyanosis.** Skin is bluish, but the oral mucous membranes are pink.

   c. **Acrocyanosis.** Hands and feet are blue but nothing else.

   d. **Perioral/circumoral cyanosis.** Blue appearance around the mouth.

   e. **Poor peripheral perfusion with cyanosis.** These infants "don't look good," "look mottled," or "look washed out or have poor perfusion." (See Chapter 77.)

   f. **Differential cyanosis.** Cyanosis of the upper or lower part of the body only (see Section II.I).

2. **Assess the heart.** Check for any murmurs and the heart rate and blood pressure. Blood pressure ≥10 mm Hg higher in the arms than the legs is suggestive of coarctation of the aorta or other aortic arch obstruction. Increased second heart sound can be seen in pulmonary hypertension. Single second heart sound can be seen with transposition of the great vessels, teratology of Fallot, hypoplastic left heart syndrome, severe pulmonary stenosis, tricuspid atresia, aortic atresia, truncus arteriosus, pulmonary atresia with intact ventricular septum, and conditions with pulmonary hypertension. A split S_2 can be seen with total anomalous pulmonary venous connection and Ebstein anomaly. Remember that not all infants with congenital heart disease have a murmur (eg, transposition of the great vessels can have no detectable murmur). Muffled heart sounds can signify pneumopericardium or pericardial effusion. A displaced cardiac impulse may mean dextrocardia or dextroposition.

3. **Assess the respiratory system.** Are there retractions, nasal flaring, or grunting? Retractions are usually minimal in heart disease. Check the nasal passage for choanal atresia. Try to pass a suction catheter through each nostril into the oropharynx; if it will not pass, then the infant has choanal atresia. Infants with pulmonary disease will have tachypnea and distressed breathing, whereas infants with cardiac disease do not.

4. **Assess the abdomen.** Check for an enlarged liver. The liver can be enlarged in CHF and hyperexpansion of the lungs. A scaphoid abdomen may suggest a diaphragmatic hernia. Hepatomegaly can indicate high venous pressure.

5. **Check the pulses.** In coarctation of the aorta or other aortic arch obstruction, the pulses in the lower extremities are decreased or absent, whereas the pulses are strong in the upper extremities. In PDA, the pulses are bounding.

6. **Consider neurologic problems.** Check for apnea and periodic breathing, which may be associated with immaturity of the nervous system. Observe the infant for seizures, which can cause cyanosis if the infant is not breathing during seizures.

7. **Assess for multiple malformations on the examination.** These may suggest underlying heart or pulmonary defects (CHARGE [coloboma, CNS abnormalities, heart defects, atresia of the choanae, restricted growth and/or development, genital abnormalities, and ear anomalies] or VATER/VACTERL [vertebral anomalies, anal atresia, tracheoesophageal fistula, and radial or renal

dysplasia/vertebral defects, anal atresia, cardiac defects, tracheoesophageal fistula, renal and radial abnormalities, and limb abnormalities] anomalies).

B. **Laboratory studies**

1. **Arterial blood gas measurements on room air.** If the patient is not hypoxic, it suggests methemoglobinemia, polycythemia, or CNS disease. If the patient is hypoxic, perform the hyperoxia test, described later. Pulse oximetry can be used to check arterial saturation but is not a good indicator of central cyanosis. An **increased PaCO$_2$** can indicate pulmonary disorders, PPHN, heart failure, or CNS disorders. **Metabolic acidosis** can indicate sepsis, severe hypoxemia, or shock from poor perfusion. A **low or normal carbon dioxide** can indicate cardiac disease. **Methemoglobinemia** will have decreased SaO$_2$, normal PaO$_2$, and "chocolate brown" blood.

2. **Complete blood count with differential.** This may reveal an infectious process (with a low white blood cell count more common). A central hematocrit of >65% confirms polycythemia.

3. **Sepsis workup.** Blood culture and C-reactive protein, urine culture, and lumbar puncture if indicated.

4. **Serum glucose level.** To detect hypoglycemia.

5. **Methemoglobin level.** If the infant has methemoglobinemia, the blood will not turn red when exposed to air and have a chocolate hue ("chocolate cyanosis"). Examine a drop of blood on white filter paper, and allow the paper to dry; after exposure to room air, it will remain dark brown. To confirm the diagnosis, the laboratory should perform a hemoglobin electrophoresis.

6. **Next-generation sequencing.** Next-generation sequencing (NGS)-based diagnostic approaches can be used to diagnose rare cases of fetal methemoglobinemia. Genetic testing for mutations is important if other laboratory tests are nonconclusive. DNA analysis of the globin gene should be done to diagnose the mutation if a γ-globin gene mutation is suspected.

C. **Imaging and other studies**

1. **Transillumination of the chest** should be done on an emergent basis if pneumothorax is suspected (see Chapter 44).

2. **Chest radiograph.** If normal, it suggests a CNS disease or other cause for the cyanosis (see Section III). It can verify lung disease, air leak, or diaphragmatic hernia. (See radiographic pearls on page 184). It can also help diagnose heart disease by evaluating the heart size and pulmonary vascularity. Is there detrocardia or situs inversus (suggests cardiac disease)? The **heart size** may be normal or enlarged in hypoglycemia, polycythemia, shock, and sepsis. In cardiac lesions with cyanosis and increased PBF, there will be **cardiomegaly. Decreased pulmonary vascular markings** represent decreased blood flow through the pulmonary circulation and can be seen in tetralogy of Fallot, pulmonary atresia/stenosis, tricuspid atresia, Ebstein anomaly, and idiopathic pulmonary hypertension of the newborn. **Increased pulmonary arterial markings** can be seen in truncus arteriosus, single ventricle, total anomalous pulmonary venous connection without obstruction, and TGA. **Increased venous markings (venous congestion)** can be seen in hypoplastic left heart syndrome and total anomalous pulmonary venous return. The **shape of the heart** can be informative:

   a. **Boot-shaped heart.** Tetralogy of Fallot, tricuspid atresia.

   b. **Egg-shaped heart ("egg on a string").** TGA.

   c. **Large globular heart/massive cardiomegaly.** Ebstein anomaly

   d. **Dextrocardia/mesocardia.** Congenital heart disease

   e. **"Snowman" or "figure 8."** Total anomalous pulmonary venous return.

3. **Hyperoxia test** is used to differentiate cyanotic congenital heart disease (with right-to-left shunting) from pulmonary and other causes of cyanosis. Because of intracardiac right-to-left shunting, the infant with cyanotic congenital heart disease, in contrast to the infant with pulmonary disease, is unable to increase the

arterial saturation. Some institutions do not use this test because of the concern of using 100% oxygen in preterm infants and instead rely on echocardiography.

a. Measure PaO_2 in the right radial artery (preductal) on room air.
b. Then place the infant on 100% oxygen for 10 minutes and repeat the arterial oxygen (**note:** best not to use pulse oximetry).
c. If the oxygen saturation and PaO_2 do not increase, cardiac causes of cyanosis should be considered. **Note:** A value of >150 mm Hg does not always rule out cyanotic heart disease. Diagnosis of cardiac disease can be delayed due to a misleading hyperoxia test, and this has been reported (severe cases of pulmonary disease with intrapulmonary shunts or PPHN, pulmonary disease with cardiac disease, infracardiac total anomalous pulmonary venous connection with PaO_2 >250 mm Hg). Echocardiogram should be done if unsure.
d. **Hyperoxia test interpretation**
   i. PaO_2 >300 mm Hg: Normal result.
   ii. PaO_2 >150 but <300 mm Hg: Pulmonary disorders, CNS disorders, methemoglobinemia. In an infant with severe pulmonary disease, the arterial oxygen saturation may not increase significantly.
   iii. PaO_2 >100 but <150 mm Hg: PPHN, truncus arteriosus, hypoplastic left heart syndrome, total anomalous pulmonary venous return without obstruction.
   iv. PaO_2 <100 mm Hg: Dextro-TGA, tricuspid atresia, pulmonary atresia or stenosis, tetralogy of Fallot.
   v. **Neurologic disease.** PaO_2 >150 but <300 mm Hg.
   vi. **Methemoglobinemia.** PaO_2 >150 but <300 mm Hg but pulse oximetry remains low.
4. **Right-to-left shunt test.** Done to rule out PPHN; the best way to do this is with pulse oximetry. Place 2 pulse oximeters on the infant (1 preductal on the right hand and 1 postductal on either foot). If the simultaneous difference is >5% to 10% between preductal and postductal oxygen saturations, it is indicative of a right-to-left shunt. Alternatively, draw a simultaneous sample of blood from the right radial artery (preductal) and the descending aorta or the left radial artery (postductal). If there is a difference of >10 to 20 mm Hg (preductal more than postductal), the shunt is significant.
5. **Hyperventilation test.** Hyperventilating the infant for 10 minutes (lowering $PaCO_2$ and increasing the pH) will result in a marked improvement in oxygenation (>30 mm Hg increase in PaO_2) in PPHN. This may help differentiate the infant with PPHN from the infant with cyanotic congenital heart disease (little or no response in congenital heart disease).
6. **Electrocardiography.** Usually normal in patients with methemoglobinemia or hypoglycemia. With polycythemia, pulmonary hypertension, or primary lung disease, the electrocardiogram (ECG) is usually normal but may show right ventricular hypertrophy. The **ECG is usually nondiagnostic in CCHD** because it is normal for a newborn to have right axis deviation (up to 180 degrees) and right ventricular dominance in the right chest leads, which is seen in the majority of CCHD ECGs. Tall P waves have been seen in approximately 40% of infants with hypoplastic left heart syndrome. **The ECG is helpful in identifying patients with 2 congenital heart diseases: tricuspid atresia and atrioventricular septal defect.** Both show a left superior axis deviation because of the inferior and posterior displacement of the atrioventricular node. The only difference is that tricuspid atresia has diminished right ventricular forces and atrioventricular septal defect show right ventricular hypertrophy.
   a. **Tricuspid atresia:** Left superior axis deviation and diminished right ventricular forces.
   b. **Atrioventricular septal defect:** Left superior axis deviation and right ventricular hypertrophy.

7. **Echocardiography.** Should be performed immediately if cardiac disease is suspected or if the cause of cyanosis is unclear. It is the **gold standard** and definitive diagnostic test for congenital heart disease. It can confirm pulmonary hypertension. See Table 94–1.

8. **Computed tomography and computed tomography angiography.** May help identify anomalies of the pulmonary venous return and identify choanal atresia.

9. **Ultrasonography of the head** to rule out periventricular/intraventricular hemorrhage, subependymal cyst (increased echogenicity or cyst in ganglionic eminence), or respiratory inhibition after crying in term infants.

10. **Polysomnographic recording** to diagnose apnea and its type.

11. **Electroencephalogram.** If seizure disorder is suspected.

12. **Bronchoscopy.** Direct bronchoscopic visualization confirms the diagnosis of tracheal stenosis.

V. **Pan**

A. **General management.**

1. **Act quickly and accomplish many of the diagnostic tasks at once.** Perform resuscitation (airway, breathing, and circulation), if necessary. Perform rapid physical examination. Is the infant breathing normally? Is the infant having episodes of apnea? Is there upper airway obstruction? What are the vital signs?

   a. **Provide respiratory support,** if needed (establish an airway if necessary, provide oxygenation, and make sure there is adequate ventilation). **Give oxygen first, prior to full evaluation.** Assisted ventilation may be necessary in infants with severe cyanosis. Prone position and oral airway may be required. If pneumothorax suspected, transilluminate the chest. If a tension pneumothorax is present, rapid needle decompression may be needed.

   b. **Establish vascular access for blood sampling** (intraarterial and intravenous) and administering volume and medications. Give volume resuscitation if necessary, especially in infants with hypotension and poor perfusion. Inotropic support may be required for hypotension and correcting metabolic acidosis are essential.

2. **Order immediate laboratory studies and a radiograph.** For example, stat blood gas level, complete blood count, blood glucose, blood culture, electrolytes, and chest radiograph.

3. **Give antibiotics as indicated** for sepsis or pneumonia (usually started unless obvious reason for cyanosis) after doing a sepsis work up.

4. **Symptomatic hypoglycemia and hypocalcemia** should be corrected.

5. **Prostaglandin E_1 (PGE$_1$) is indicated in infants** with or who have a clinical suspicion for a ductal-dependent congenital heart defect and should be given until a definitive diagnosis or treatment is established. See below.

6. **Perform the hyperoxia test to differentiate pulmonary from cardiac from other causes,** or perform an echocardiogram. See Section IV.C.3.

7. **Suspect methemoglobinemia** when the cyanosis does not improve with oxygen.

8. **Obtain a pediatric cardiology consult if cardiac disease is suspected.**

B. **Specific management.**

1. **Lung disease.** (See the appropriate disease chapter.) Respiratory depression caused by narcotics at birth should be treated with respiratory support with positive-pressure ventilation and possible laryngeal mask airway placement or endotracheal tube placement if apnea is prolonged.

2. **Air leak (pneumothorax).** See Chapter 75. Depending on the severity of the pneumothorax, urgent needle aspiration or chest tube placement may be necessary.

3. **Congenital defects (eg, upper respiratory).** Surgery may be indicated.

4. **Cardiac disease.** Correction of metabolic acidosis if present, supplemental oxygen, and maintain adequate respiratory support. Prostaglandin E_1 (PGE$_1$) is indicated in infants with or who have a clinical suspicion for a ductal-dependent congenital heart defect and should be given until a definitive diagnosis or

treatment is established. PGE_1 is indicated for any clinical condition in which blood flow must be maintained through the ductus arteriosus to sustain pulmonary or systemic circulation until surgery can be performed. Dose is 0.01 mcg/kg/min initial intravenous infusion.

a. **Give prostaglandin E_1 to increase pulmonary blood flow** for pulmonary atresia/stenosis, TGA, tetralogy of Fallot, and tricuspid atresia (if PBF restricted). Other ways of improving PBF are with supplemental oxygen, maintaining a respiratory alkalosis, sildenafil, and inhaled nitric oxide.

b. **Give prostaglandin E_1 to increase systemic blood flow** for hypoplastic left heart syndrome, coarctation of the aorta, critical aortic stenosis, and aortic arch interruption.

c. **Give prostaglandin E_1 to improve mixing in transposition of the great arteries.**

d. **Prostaglandin E_1 is not recommended** in respiratory distress syndrome, PPHN, total anomalous venous return with obstruction (PGE_1 may minimize obstruction but does not help clinically), and dominant left-to-right shunt (PDA, truncus arteriosus, or VSD).

e. **If the diagnosis is uncertain,** a trial of PGE_1 can be given over 30 minutes in an effort to improve blood gas values.

f. **Other management**

  i. **Dextro-transposition of the great arteries with severe cyanosis and restrictive atrial communication.** Urgent Rashkind atrial septostomy under echocardiogram in the nursery will maintain oxygenation until surgery is performed (arterial switch operation). Total anomalous pulmonary venous return, TGA with VSD, and truncus arteriosus require further cardiac evaluation and possible surgery.

  ii. **Tetralogy of Fallot.** If there is cyanosis in the first 2 weeks, give PGE_1 until surgery can be done. For **tetralogy spells** (usually not seen in the neonatal intensive care unit but can be if the infant has a prolonged stay), treatment includes blow-by oxygen, comforting and feeding, and holding the infant in knee-chest position (decreases right-to-left shunting and increases systemic vascular resistance). If the infant remains cyanotic, give propranolol (0.05 mg/kg) to decrease the heart rate and myocardial contractility. Other treatments include intravenous phenylephrine, ketamine, intubation, and sedation (last resort). A Blalock-Taussig shunt can be done if surgery cannot be done. Surgery consists of closure of VSD, resecting the hypertrophied muscle bundles, and pulmonary valvuloplasty.

  iii. **Hypoplastic left heart syndrome.** Give PGE_1 infusion, correct metabolic acidosis, avoid oxygen if possible (worsens pulmonary congestion), and avoid excess fluids or inotropic agents. If atrial communication is severe, an urgent Rashkind atrial septostomy can be done. Surgery involves the Norwood procedure in 3 stages.

  iv. **Tricuspid atresia.** Treatment depends on PBF. If restricted: PGE_1 infusion, Rashkind atrial septostomy, Blalock-Taussig shunt. If increased: pulmonary arterial banding. If normal: observation for cyanosis. Surgery involves 3 procedures: aortopulmonary shunt or pulmonary artery banding procedure, bidirectional Glenn procedure, and then modified Fontan procedure.

  v. **Truncus arteriosus.** Manage medically in the neonatal unit with diuretics and angiotensin-converting enzyme (ACE) inhibitors. Surgery is required in the first few months once heart failure symptoms worsen.

  vi. **Total anomalous pulmonary venous connection.** If veins are obstructed: surgical emergency. If veins are not obstructed: avoid PGE_1. Use diuretics and ACE inhibitors. Surgery is needed in all cases, once the infant is stable.

5. **Persistent pulmonary hypertension of the newborn.** See Chapter 115.
6. **Central nervous system disorders.** Treat the underlying disease.
7. **Methemoglobinemia.** Treat the infant with methylene blue only if the methemoglobin level is markedly increased and the infant is in cardiopulmonary distress (tachypnea and tachycardia). Administer intravenously 1 mg/kg of a 1% solution of **methylene blue** in normal saline. The cyanosis should clear within 1 to 2 hours. Methylene blue is not recommended in infants with glucose-6-phosphate dehydrogenase deficiency. Ascorbic acid can be added if needed. If the combination does not work, consider exchange transfusion or hyperbaric oxygen. Recall that methylene blue can cause a low SpO_2.
8. **Shock.** See Chapter 70.
9. **Polycythemia.** See Chapters 76 and 116.
10. **Choanal atresia requires an evaluation by otorhinolaryngology.** Place an oral airway, which should immediately improve the infant's condition until surgery can be performed (see Chapter 125).
11. **Micrognathia, retrognathia, Pierre Robin sequence.** Treatment includes, placing an infant prone, possibly using an oral airway, possible surgical mandibular surgery, possible tracheostomy until the mandible grows.
12. **Tracheal stenosis** requires extensive surgical repair.
13. **Hypothermia.** Rewarming is necessary, as described in Chapter 8.
14. **Hypoglycemia.** See Chapter 67.

57 Death of an Infant

I. **Problem.** <u>A newborn infant is dying or has just died.</u> Even though the overall infant mortality rate in the United States has improved, >23,000 infants die each year, with >15,000 dying in the neonatal intensive care unit (NICU). The mortality rate in the United States for newborns is 5.82 per 1000 live births. The leading causes of infant death are shown in Table 57–1, with the top 5 being birth defects/congenital malformations, preterm birth and low birthweight, sudden infant death syndrome (SIDS), maternal pregnancy complications, and infant accidents (unintentional injuries).

Some researchers found that parents experience more intense grief reactions for an infant who died in the NICU than earlier pregnancy losses, possibly because of the longer time for a stronger attachment. Studies show that bereaved parents who experience an infant death or stillbirth have an increased mortality for up to 25 years compared to

Table 57–1. TOP 10 LEADING CAUSES OF NEONATAL DEATH IN THE UNITED STATES

1. Birth defects/congenital anomalies/malformations
2. Preterm birth and low birthweight
3. Sudden infant death syndrome (SIDS)
4. Maternal pregnancy complications
5. Infant accidents (unintentional injuries)
6. Umbilical cord and placental complications
7. Bacterial sepsis
8. Respiratory distress syndrome
9. Circulatory system diseases
10. Neonatal hemorrhage

parents who did not experience an infant death or stillbirth. Infants in the NICU are usually very ill, and parents may experience prolonged grief. Many bereaved families lack the necessary support at critical times. Recent studies have focused on the importance of bereavement support and the profound effect healthcare providers can have on parents who have lost an infant. A healthcare provider's insensitivity to a parent can contribute to difficulties in coping and may increase the risk of a complicated grief reaction. Nurses, who are more likely than physicians to have received bereavement training, are more likely to have a positive attitude in these difficult situations. Hospitals should be encouraged to establish formal training and defined protocols for an infant death to improve everyone's experience. Good-quality bereavement care decreases the negative psychological, emotional, and social effects for parents. Every bereaved parent is entitled to the best possible care.

II. **Immediate questions**
   A. **Has the family been prepared for the death, or was it unexpected?** It is important to prepare the family in advance, if possible, for the death of an infant. Be ready and available to answer questions after the event.
   B. **Was this an early or late neonatal death?** Early neonatal death describes the death of a live-born infant at <7 days of age. Late neonatal death is the death of a live-born infant at 7 to 27 days of age. A postnatal death is a live birth that results in death at 28 to 364 days. Late neonatal deaths result in more protracted grief reactions than early neonatal deaths.
   C. **Which family members are present?** Usually, several immediate family members in addition to the parents are present at the hospital, which is usually beneficial for emotional support. Each of the family members may adopt a special role. The family should be allowed to go through the immediate process of grieving the way they feel most comfortable (eg, on their own, with the chaplain, with their favorite nurse, or with the physician they trust) and in the location they feel most comfortable (eg, the NICU or family conference room). Attention should focus on both parents if appropriate.
   D. **If the family members are not present, is a telephone contact available?** It is standard practice to ensure there is a contact telephone number available for any sick infant. If the family members are not present, telephone contact must be made as soon as possible to alert the family that their infant is dying or has already passed away. In either case, urge the family to come in and be with their infant.
   E. **Are there any religious needs expressed by the family?** The religious needs must be respected and the necessary support provided (eg, priest, rabbi, appropriate clergy, chaplain, or pastoral care). Every hospital has pastoral services, and it is useful to inform the chaplain in advance because some parents may request that their child be baptized before death. It is essential to be sensitive to the family's culture or religion as this may influence the family's decision on how to handle the death, autopsy, and funeral.

III. **Differential diagnosis.** Although there is not a differential diagnosis for this situation, when a death occurs, it is important to accurately report and define the perinatal death. The American Academy of Pediatrics Committee on Fetus and Newborn established standard terminology for fetal, infant, and perinatal deaths based on standards set by the World Health Organization and the National Center for Health Statistics of the Centers for Disease Control and Prevention (2016). The following definitions are recommended:
   A. **Live birth.** "Extraction or complete expulsion from the mother of a product of human conception, irrespective of the duration of pregnancy, which after such expulsion or extraction, breathes or shows any other evidence of life, such as beating of the heart, pulsation of the umbilical cord, or definite movement of voluntary muscles, regardless of whether the umbilical cord has been cut or the placenta is attached." It is important to distinguish heartbeats from transient cardiac contractions and respirations from fleeting respiratory efforts or gasps.

B. **Fetal death.** "Death before the complete expulsion/extraction from the mother of a product of human conception, irrespective of the duration of the pregnancy, that is not an induced pregnancy termination. After expulsion, the fetus does not show any evidence of life (breathing, beating of the heart, pulsation of the umbilical cord, or movement of voluntary muscles).
   1. **Early fetal death:** 20 to 27 weeks' gestation.
   2. **Late fetal death:** >28 weeks' gestation.
C. **Infant death.** A live birth that results in death within the first year (<365 days).
   1. **Early neonatal death:** A live birth that results in death at <7 days of age.
   2. **Late neonatal death:** A live birth that results in death at 7 to 27 days of age.
   3. **Postnatal death:** A live birth that results in death at 28 to 364 days of age.
D. **Perinatal death.** This is a combination of fetal deaths and live births with only a brief survival. Perinatal death is not reportable but is used for statistical purposes. Three definitions are used:
   1. **Infant deaths** that occur at <7 days of age and fetal deaths with a period of gestation of ≥28 weeks.
   2. **Infant deaths** that occur at <28 days of age and fetal deaths with a period of gestation of ≥20 weeks.
   3. **Infant deaths** that occur at <7 days of age and fetal deaths with a period of gestation of ≥20 weeks.
IV. **Database.** It is essential to recall that the dying infant may continue with a gasp reflex for some time even without spontaneous respiration and movement. The heart beat may be very faint; therefore, auscultation for 2 to 5 minutes is advisable. Legal definitions of "death" vary by state or other jurisdiction. Providers must be familiar with the local legal requirements for declaring death.
V. **Plan**
A. **Preparations.** A review has reported on the provider behaviors viewed most favorably by parents after their infant has died; these are outlined in Table 57–2.
   1. **The neonatal intensive care unit environment.** The noise level should be kept to a minimum. The staff should be sensitive to the emotions of the parents and the family. In one study, sensitivity, kindness of staff, and time spent with the baby were ranked as very important. The infant and family members should be provided privacy (but should not be abandoned) in an isolated quiet room or a screened-off area in the NICU. Examination of the infant by the physician to confirm the death may be done in that same private area, with the family.
   2. **The infant.** The equipment (eg, intravenous [IV] lines and endotracheal tubes) may be removed from the infant unless an autopsy is anticipated. In that case, it is best to leave in place central catheters and possibly the endotracheal tube. The parents should be allowed to hold the infant for as long as they desire. This type of visual and physical contact is important to begin the grieving process in a healthy manner and try to relieve any future guilt. Careless treatment of the infant by staff members is not tolerated well by parents. The practice reported in the literature of placing the deceased infant on an uncovered metal table or into a bucket after delivery is unacceptable. Parents are acutely aware of how staff cares for the deceased infant. Bathing and dressing the infant in a caring manner and treating the deceased infant with respect are appreciated by the family. Families may also appreciate if nurses take special photos of the infant and provide the family with special mementos so they can have some memories.
B. **Discussion of death with the family**
   1. **Location.** Parents and immediate family members should be in a quiet, private consultation room, and the physician should calmly explain the cause and inevitability of death.
   2. **News of the death.** Studies show that parents value clear communication. The physician needs to offer condolences to the family concerning their loss. News

Table 57–2. BEHAVIORS VIEWED MOST FAVORABLY BY PARENTS AFTER PERINATAL DEATH

Offering emotional support
Stay with the family and spend extra time with them as much as practical.
Talk about the baby by name.
Allow parents to grieve or cry.
Be sensitive to comments that could be perceived as trite or minimizing of grief.
Return to see family on multiple occasions, if possible.

Attending to physical needs of parents and baby
Continue routine postpartum nursing and medical care for mother.
Treat infant's body respectfully.
Consider dressing, bathing, or wrapping infant as for a live baby.
Be flexible about hospital policies that may not be appropriate for bereaved families.
Help parents create tangible memories of their infants.

Educating parents
Communicate loss to all staff to help avoid inappropriate comments or actions.
Help parents anticipate what normal grieving will be like.
Provide straightforward information about cause of death if known. Use lay language.
Take time to sit down with parents when discussing information.

Reproduced with permission from Gold KJ: Navigating care after a baby dies: a systematic review of parent experiences with health providers, *J Perinatol.* 2007 Apr;27(4):230-237.

of the infant's death can be very difficult for the physician to convey and the family to accept. The physician must be sensitive to the emotional reactions of the family. **Nurses, in one review, were perceived as the healthcare providers who were most likely to provide key emotional support.** The nurse's ability to partner with the family is very important in helping the family take steps in their ability to grieve. It is important that nurses participate in this process because they can provide more ongoing support through this difficult time. They can also guide new mothers and fathers of caring tasks that they can perform for their baby and create memories that will provide them a sense of comfort later on. **Communicate the news of the death to all staff members who will be taking care of the mother if she is still hospitalized at the time of the infant death. This includes dietary staff and housekeepers so they know the appropriate way to act.**

3. **Areas of dissatisfaction noted by parents.** Reviews have emphasized that parents are upset by lack of communication between staff members. Staff who did not know the infant had died and made comments, staff who avoided or were silent with the family, and staff who showed insensitivity or lack of emotional support all created great stress in the families of the deceased. Treating the mother and deceased infant with respect is important.

C. **Effects on the family**

1. **Emotional (grieving).** A brief outline of the normal grieving process may be discussed with the family members. The stages **Kübler-Ross identified** are **denial** ("This isn't happening to me!"); **anger** ("Why is this happening to me?"); **bargaining** ("I promise I'll be a better person if . . ."); **depression** ("I don't care anymore"); and **acceptance** ("I'm ready for whatever comes"). **Temes has described 3 particular types of behavior** exhibited by those suffering from grief and loss: **numbness** (mechanical functioning and social insulation), **disorganization**

(intensely painful feelings of loss), and **reorganization** (reentry into a more "normal" social life). Physicians who offered specifics to the family regarding what to expect in the grieving process were rated as the most competent physicians. In one study, 3% of mothers experienced prolonged periods of grief and 18% had posttraumatic stress.

2. **Physical.** Loss of appetite and disruption of sleep patterns can occur.
3. **Siblings.** It is important to discuss the impact of the death on a sibling. A study was done to assess the developmental impact of surviving a sibling who died in the NICU; it showed that siblings born both before and after a death of an infant are at emotional risk and are in need of psychological support. Photos and family rituals are important for parents and siblings. Clinicians should allow siblings to be active participants in the infant's life and death.
4. **Surviving twin or multiple.** Staff must be aware of the added stress on the parents looking in on a surviving twin or multiple birth.

D. **Practical aspects**

1. **Perinatal bereavement programs.** Because the neonatal staff plays a major role in helping families cope with the loss of their infant, it is important for each unit to set up a comprehensive program to help families deal with their grief. Some units have set up a bereavement support service that includes a bereavement suite, bereavement coordinators, and bereavement support (funerals and blessings, 24-hour communication, financial advice and benefits, provision of mementos and keepsakes, sibling involvement and counseling, and follow-up). It is important to not only focus on the neonate's physical needs, but also to address the family's spiritual, religious, and existential needs. Recent studies show that intergenerational services should be offered and provide benefit for the entire family.
2. **Hospice care teams** are becoming more involved in the prenatal arena, such as for mothers with infants with known lethal anomalies, and give support while the infant is in utero and also in the NICU to address the process of dying and stages of grief for parents. See also Chapter 24 on palliative care.
3. **Multiple organizations are offering practice guidelines or direct help.** Some of these include: Pregnancy Loss and Infant Death Alliance, M.E.N.D. (Mommies Enduring Neonatal Death; www.mend.org), HAND (Helping After Neonatal Death), MISS Foundation (www.missfoundation.org), Now I Lay Me Down to Sleep (www.nowilaymedowntosleep.org), and others including at the local medical center level. The ATTEND model (attunement, trust, touch, egalitarianism, nuance, and death education) is an interdisciplinary paradigm for providers that is a mindfulness-based bereavement care model (Figure 57–1).
4. **Parental education.** Recent reviews have reported that parents appreciated education from the healthcare providers. Parents want to have information regarding why the infant died and also specific information on the grieving process. Parents have indicated that staff members who kept them informed and provided honest answers with consistent information were valued the most. *When Hello Means Goodbye* by Paul Kirk and Pat Schwiebert (www.griefwatch.com) is an often-recommended lay book that can help the family cope with the loss of an infant.
5. **Additional support.** Family members should be asked whether they need any support for transport or funeral arrangements and whether they need a note to the employer regarding time off from work and so on. Social workers or case workers are usually available to assist in these practical matters in the hospital setting. Questions regarding maternity leave benefits and returning to work can be answered. Some units offer a 24-hour dedicated telephone line for bereaved families.

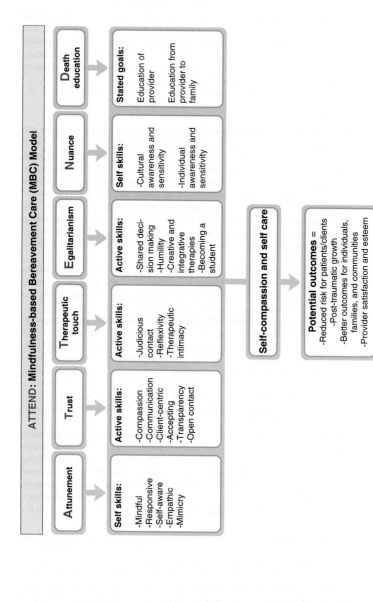

FIGURE 57–1. The ATTEND bereavement care model is useful in the setting of neonatal death. (*Data from Cacciatore J, Flint M: ATTEND: toward a mindfulness-based bereavement care model, Death Stud. 2012 Jan;36(1):61-82.*)

6. **Bereavement photography (also called "memento mori photography").** Photographs were positively regarded by most parents after perinatal death. This includes pictures of the infant either alone or with family members done by staff, a professional photographer, or other organizations that help to ease the grief of NICU parents by taking professional photographs. These images can serve as a link to memories and feelings and help parents grieve and heal. Parents may wish to dress their baby in clothes or include mementos in the pictures. It is most important to respect the parents' wishes. It is considered essential to obtain parental consent for any bereavement photograph.

7. **Rituals.** Rituals provide an ordered way to say goodbye to a loved one. They can be beneficial to individuals and families who have experienced the death of a child. These can include funerals, memory boxes (with name bands, cord clamp, lock of baby's hair, etc.), naming the baby, religious practices, and specific cultural traditions.

8. **Written permission.** Should be obtained for the following: bereavement photography, obtaining mementos, autopsy, or biopsy of the deceased for any further inquiry.

9. **Organ donation.** Occasionally, parents and immediate family members may have discussed organ donation before the death of the infant. If not, it can be brought up gently with the family, who will be given adequate time to reflect on it, taking into consideration the requirements for organ donation. Sometimes the parents may want to donate an organ, but this may not be possible because of the presence of infection or inadequate function of the organ before death. This should be explained carefully to the parents. Follow your institution's defined procedure for discussing requests for organ procurement with the family.

10. **Autopsy.** Autopsy can be a vital part of determining the cause of death and may be important in counseling the parents for future pregnancies. It is always a very sensitive issue to discuss with the parents, especially after the loss of their loved one. Parents should always be allowed adequate time to discuss this themselves and with the family if they have not already made up their minds. A recent study on bereaved parents' perception on autopsy revealed that it is important to openly discuss the benefits of an autopsy; 90% of parents valued autopsy as a way to find out why their child died, and 77% knew it contributed to medical knowledge. Forty-two percent felt that the autopsy examination added to their grief, 30% found it a comfort, and 41% said it helped them with their loss.

11. **Documentation (Figure 57-2).** Refer to local hospital guidelines for proper reporting of live births, infant deaths, fetal deaths, and induced terminations of pregnancy.
    a. **Neonatal death summary note.** The physician may include a brief synopsis of the infant's history or a problem list. The events leading up to the infant's death that day, whether it was sudden or gradual, and the treatment or interventions performed must be noted. It is also important to note conversations with family members while the infant was dying, if not written earlier in separate notes.
    b. **Death certificate.** The physician declaring the infant dead initiates the death certificate; it is important to obtain accurate information on state/country law to file the fetal death certificate according to the state/country requirements.

E. **Follow-up arrangements**
    1. **Family contact.** A telephone call from a medical team member should be arranged within the first week of death. A letter of sympathy is strongly encouraged based on local policy. Another contact can be made at the end of the first month to comfort the family, share any further information, and answer questions. Some NICU teams may choose to make contact again at the 1-year anniversary.

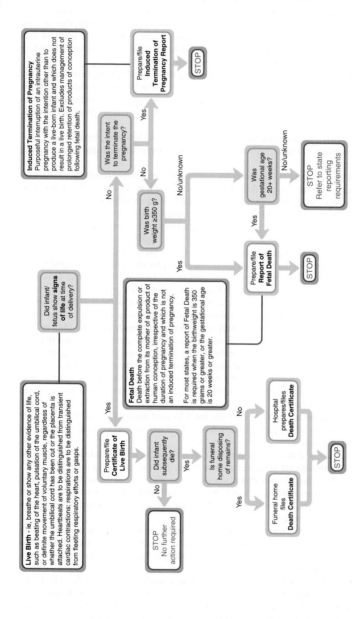

FIGURE 57–2. Hospital guidelines for reporting live births, infant deaths, fetal deaths, and induced terminations of pregnancy. (*Reproduced with permission from Barfield WD; Committee on Fetus and Newborn: Standard Terminology for Fetal, Infant, and Perinatal Deaths, Pediatrics. 2016 May;137(5). pii: e20160551.*)

2. **Counseling.** It is extremely important to discuss the arrangements for future counseling and refer the parents to high-risk obstetrics if appropriate. Genetic counseling may also be appropriate based on the specific case. Parents should be allowed to grieve for the death of their child and should be given the opportunity to contact the physician at a later date when they are more receptive emotionally. Siblings are at risk and may require psychological support. Recent study shows that having another child after infant loss may promote resilience, so parents should not be discouraged or asked to wait a certain amount of time if they choose to have another child.

3. **Autopsy follow-up.** If consent for autopsy has been obtained, an autopsy follow-up conference at approximately 6 to 8 weeks is essential. The presence of a geneticist at this follow-up may be appropriate. This autopsy conference not only provides the parents with concrete information but also assists in the process of grieving.

4. **The obstetrician, pediatrician, and family physician** involved with the care of the mother or family should be notified of the death.

5. **The needs of the caregivers also should be considered.** Dealing with grief, loss, and bereavement is one of the major stressors to the staff in the NICU setting. Several units have developed specific programs in this area, and resources should be made available to the staff as well. Some units have a palliative care team that receives specific training. They offer debriefing sessions for anyone in the NICU to attend.

58 Eye Discharge and Conjunctivitis

I. **Problem.** <u>A purulent eye discharge is noted in a 3-day-old infant.</u> Eye discharge in a neonate is usually caused by neonatal conjunctivitis (also known as **ophthalmia neonatorum**) or **congenital nasolacrimal duct obstruction** (CNLDO or congenital dacryostenosis). **Neonatal conjunctivitis** (conjunctivitis occurring within the first 4 weeks of life) is an inflammation of the surface or covering of the eye that presents with eye discharge and hyperemia. It is the most common ocular disease in neonates. Etiology is chemical, bacterial, or viral. Most infections are acquired during vaginal delivery, but ascending infection can occur. In the United States, the incidence of infectious conjunctivitis is 1% to 2%, and in the world, it is 0.9% to 21%. Neonates with conjunctivitis require a thorough clinical and appropriate laboratory evaluation so appropriate treatment can be started as soon as possible if necessary. **CNLDO** is a membranous obstruction at the valve of Hasner, which is at the distal end of the nasolacrimal duct. Incidence is 6% to 20% in infants (studies show higher incidence in preterm infants when compared to full-term infants). The symptoms are persistent tearing and a mucoid discharge in the inner corner of the eye.

II. **Immediate questions**

A. **How old is the infant?** Age may be helpful in determining the cause of eye discharge, noting that bacterial infections can occur anytime.

1. **First day of life.** Conjunctivitis is most often due to ocular prophylaxis secondary to medications such as silver nitrate drops, tetracycline, erythromycin, gentamicin, povidone iodine solution, and chloramphenicol.

2. **2 to 5 days old.** Conjunctivitis is most often due to *Neisseria gonorrhoeae* (but can present earlier with premature rupture of membranes).

3. **5 to 12 days old.** Conjunctivitis is most often due to *Chlamydia trachomatis*. It is usually seen during this time and can present as late as the second or third week.

4. **5 to 14 days old.** Conjunctivitis is often due to other bacterial microbes. This includes pathogens from the skin, respiratory, gastrointestinal, or vaginal tract. See Table 58-3.

5. **5 to 28 days old.** *Pseudomonas aeruginosa* infections are typical during this time.

6. **6 to 14 days old.** Conjunctivitis can be due to herpes simplex virus (HSV).

7. **2 weeks old.** CNLDO usually manifests at 2 weeks of age but can sometimes be seen in the first few days to the first few weeks after birth.

B. **Is the discharge unilateral or bilateral?** Typical symptoms are persistent tearing and a mucoid discharge in the inner corner of the eye.

1. **Unilateral conjunctivitis** is most often seen with *Staphylococcus aureus*, *P aeruginosa*, HSV, and adenovirus.

2. **Bilateral conjunctivitis** is seen with infection caused by *N gonorrhoeae* or by the use of ocular prophylaxis.

3. **Unilateral, then bilateral.** Chlamydia usually develops in 1 eye but affects the other after 2 to 7 days. Lacrimal duct obstruction usually causes unilateral discharge, but up to 20% of infants have bilateral obstruction.

C. **What are the characteristics of the discharge (eg, purulent, serous, greenish)?**

1. **Purulent discharge:** More common with bacterial infection. Gonorrhea has a classic profuse purulent discharge.

2. **Serous discharge:** More common with a viral infection.

3. **Greenish discharge:** More characteristic of *P aeruginosa*.

4. **Serosanguinous (light/pale red) discharge:** Watery with a mixture of serum and blood can be seen with herpes conjunctivitis. Nonpurulent discharge can also be seen with herpes.

5. **Watery early, purulent later** (may be blood stained): Chlamydial infection.

6. **Watery tears or mucus or yellow discharge in eye:** CLNLDO can cause watery tears in the corner of the eye or tears draining from the eyelid down the cheek. It can also cause mucus or yellowish discharge in the eye.

D. **Did the infant receive eye prophylaxis, and was it properly given?** Ocular prophylaxis against gonococcal ophthalmia neonatorum is used to prevent gonorrheal infection (prevent blindness), and certain prophylactic agents (silver nitrate, povidone-iodine, and erythromycin) prevent **nongonococcal and nonchlamydial conjunctivitis** during the first 2 weeks of life. The majority of medical groups recommend prophylactic ocular topical medication for all newborns for the prevention of gonococcal ophthalmia neonatorum (Table 58-1). Various conjunctivitis prophylactic regimens are presented in Table 58-2. Infants can still get gonococcal conjunctivitis with prophylaxis, but the risk drops from 50% to 2%. **Gonorrheal ophthalmia neonatorum prophylaxis is mandatory in the United States** but may not be in other countries (eg, Denmark, Norway, Sweden, Great Britian, Belgium, Australia, The Netherlands). A reevaluation of the mandatory prophylaxis is being considered by the American Academy of Pediatrics (AAP) because of improved prenatal screening, testing at the time of delivery, and maternal treatment to prevent exposure to the neonate, especially in areas where the maternal infection is low. There is concern that some strains of gonorrhea have shown resistance to erythromycin.

1. **Proper ocular administration technique is as follows:** Give shortly after birth or within 1 hour of birth (to facilitate parent–infant bonding), whether cesarean or vaginal delivery.

a. **For the term infant,** wipe each eyelid with sterile cotton or gauze; instill the prophylactic agent (single-dose tubes or ampules preferred, 1-cm ribbon of ointment or 2 drops of solution) in each of the lower conjunctival sacs. Massage the eyelids gently to spread the agent. Wipe away any excess ointment after 1 minute. Do not irrigate or flush the eyes.

Table 58–1. SOCIETY AND ORGANIZATION RECOMMENDATIONS FOR OPHTHALMIC NEONATORUM PROPHYLAXIS

AAP	Universal prophylaxis of all newborns shortly after birth with 0.5% ophthalmic erythromycin ointment. Erythromycin is the only antibiotic ointment recommended. If not available, see AAP alternative recommendations.
USPSTF	All newborns within 24 hours after birth: 0.5% erythromycin ophthalmic ointment, 1% silver nitrate solution, 1% tetracycline ointment. All equally effective but latter 2 not available in the United States.
CDC	All newborns as soon as possible after birth. Erythromycin 0.5% ophthalmic ointment in each eye single application. If not available, in infants at risk for *Neisseria gonorrhoeae*, give ceftriaxone 25–50 mg/kg intravenously or intramuscularly (125-mg maximum single dose).
CPS	Erythromycin ocular prophylaxis may no longer be useful and should not be routinely recommended. The CPS recommends maternal screening over eye prophylaxis. If prophylaxis must be given (based on territorial regulations), use erythromycin ophthalmic ointment 0.5%.
WHO	For all infants, topical application to both eyes immediately after birth. WHO suggests 1 of the following: erythromycin 0.5% eye ointment, tetracycline hydrochloride 1% eye ointment, silver nitrate 1% solution, povidone-iodine 2.5% solution (water based); do not use alcohol-based povidone-iodine solution or chloramphenicol 1% eye ointment.

AAP, American Academy of Pediatrics (https://redbook.solutions.aap.org/chapter.aspx?sectionid=88187322&bookid=1484); CDC, Centers for Disease Control and Prevention (https://www.cdc.gov/std/tg2015/gonorrhea.htm#op-neo); CPS, Canadian Pediatric Society (https://www.cps.ca/en/documents/position/ophthalmia-neonatorum); USPSTF, US Preventive Services Task Force (https://www.uspreventiveservicestaskforce.org/Page/Document/UpdateSummaryFinal/ocular-prophylaxis-for-gonococcal-ophthalmia-neonatorum-preventive-medication); WHO, World Health Organization (http://apps.who.int/medicinedocs/en/d/Jh2942e/4.1.3.html).

     b. For the very premature infant with fused eyes, apply the prophylactic agent without separating the eyelids.
    2. **Agents used for prophylaxis:** 0.5% erythromycin ophthalmic ointment, 2.5% povidone-iodine solution, 1% silver nitrate solution, and 1% tetracycline ophthalmic ointment.
       a. **0.5% erythromycin ophthalmic ointment.** A 1-cm ribbon is given in each eye. AAP, Centers for Disease Control and Prevention (CDC), and US Preventive Services Task Force (USPSTF) recommend only erythromycin ophthalmic ointment for prophylaxis, and it is the only approved agent in the United States. It causes less chemical conjunctivitis than other agents such as silver nitrate. There is some concern for *N gonorrhoeae* strains being resistant to erythromycin.
       b. **1% silver nitrate solution.** This is recommended over erythromycin if the patient population has a high number of penicillinase-producing *N gonorrhoeae*. It is highly irritating and frequently causes a chemical conjunctivitis (see later in chapter). It is not available in the United States but is used elsewhere. The World Health Organization (WHO) recommends 2 drops in each eye.
       c. **1% tetracycline ophthalmic ointment** is as effective as silver nitrate but is not available in the United States.
       d. **2.5% povidone-iodine ophthalmic solution (water based; do not use alcohol-based solution)** is widely available, low cost, and effective. It is used in

Table 58–2. AGENTS FOR CONJUNCTIVITIS PROPHYLAXIS

Medication	Form	Concentration	Frequency	Class	Indication	Side Effects	Availability	Organizations That Recommend Agent
Erythromycin	Ophthalmic ointment	0.50%	1 time	Macrolide antibiotic	Prophylaxis of gonococcal ophthalmia neonatorum	Contact dermatitis[a]	Global	AAP, CDC, USPSTF, WHO
Silver nitrate	Ophthalmic solution	1%	1 time	Astringent	Prophylaxis of gonococcal ophthalmia neonatorum	Contact dermatitis	Not in United States	USPSTF, WHO
Tetracycline	Ophthalmic ointment	1%	1 time	Tetracycline antibiotic	Prophylaxis of gonococcal ophthalmia neonatorum	Contact dermatitis	Not in United States	USPSTF, WHO
Povidone-iodine	Ophthalmic solution	1.25%, 2.5%	1 time	Antiseptic	Prophylaxis of gonococcal ophthalmia neonatorum	Contact dermatitis	Global	WHO
Chloramphenicol	Ophthalmic solution	0.50%	1 time	Synthetic antibiotic	Prophylaxis of gonococcal ophthalmia neonatorum	Contact dermatitis	Not in United States	WHO

AAP, American Academy of Pediatrics; CDC, Centers for Disease and Prevention; USPSTF, US Preventive Services Task Force; WHO, World Health Organization.
Note. Routine prophylaxis with topical antibiotics carries the risk of resistance, especially in patients with ophthalmia neonatorum due to gonococcal infection. Povidone-iodine as a topical anti-infective appears to be an effective and cheap alternative. Further epidemiologic research and monitoring on the incidence of ophthalmia neonatorum and the prevalence of the various agents in different parts of the world are needed, so that prevention and treatment can be adjusted accordingly and experience with new options can be analyzed for wide use. See https://www.ncbi.nlm.nih.gov/pmc/articles/PMC2566367.
[a]Contact dermatitis side effects include blurred vision, eye irritation, eyelid erythema and edema, conjunctival hyperemia, and punctate keratitis.

developing countries and is not available in the United States. Some data suggest that povidone-iodine is more effective against *C trachomatis* than silver nitrate or erythromycin. There are 3 doses available (5%, 2.5%, and 1.25%); 5% is used for preoperative use. The 2.5% solution is most commonly used. **Note:** Use the ophthalmic solution and not the detergent version of povidone-iodine, which can damage the cornea.

    e. Other topical agents that have been used when erythromycin is not available. Recommended backup agents per the AAP *Red Book* include the following:

        i. Use first: Azithromycin ophthalmic solution 1%; 1 to 2 drops are placed in each conjunctival sac. Note this is not an ointment but a solution, so care must be used when placing these drops. CDC recommendations for this medication: 2 people are required to administer this medication. One person holds the lids open, while the other instills the drops.

        ii. Use second: Either gentamicin ophthalmic ointment 0.3% or tobramycin ophthalmic ointment 3%.

        iii. Use last: Ciprofloxacin ophthalmic ointment 0.3% is generally not recommended because of high gonococcal resistance.

    f. Fatty acid–based formulas (monocaprin and myristoleic acid), which are bactericidal against virulent bacteria and effective against *S aureus*, are being studied for prevention of ophthalmia neonatorum.

  3. Society and organization recommendations for ophthalmic neonatorum prophylaxis can be found in Table 58–1.

E. Does the mother have a history of sexually transmitted infections? Infants who pass through the birth canal of an infected mother with gonorrhea or chlamydia have an increased conjunctivitis risk. Neonatal conjunctivitis is frequently diagnosed in infants born to human immunodeficiency virus (HIV)-infected mothers.

F. Is the infant at high risk?

  1. Conjunctivitis. Neonates are at increased risk for conjunctivitis and more serious cases of conjunctivitis because of decreased tear production, lack of immunoglobulin A (IgA) in tears, decreased immune function, absence of lymphoid tissue of the conjunctiva, and decreased lysozyme activity. Risk factors may include mode of delivery, exposure of the infant to infectious organisms, no or inadequate prophylaxis after birth, ocular trauma/local eye injury during delivery, poor hygienic conditions, premature rupture of membranes, prolonged delivery, prematurity, mechanical ventilation, increased birthweight, history of midwife interference, HIV-infected mother, poor prenatal care, documented or suspected sexually transmitted infection, infection after delivery from direct contact from health care worker, or aerosolization. **Performing red reflex examinations** increases the rate of neonatal conjunctivitis.

  2. Congenital nasolacrimal duct obstruction. Neonates are at **an increased risk for CNLDO** if they have Down syndrome, Goldenhar sequence, clefting syndromes, any midline facial anomaly, hemifacial microsomia, or craniosynostosis.

G. Is the infant low birthweight and low gestational age? An infant with conjunctivitis who has a low birthweight and low gestational age has a higher risk of having a conjunctivitis caused by a **gram-negative organism** (*Klebsiella* spp., *Escherichia coli, Serratia marcescens, P aeruginosa,* and *Enterobacter* spp.). Premature infants have an increased risk of CNLDO.

III. Differential diagnosis. As noted, eye discharge in the neonate most commonly is caused by **conjunctivitis** (chemical/inflammatory, bacterial, or viral) or is due to an **obstruction** (CNLDO). **Other less common diagnoses that may cause an eye discharge in an infant** are foreign body, orbital or preseptal cellulitis, entropion, trichiasis, eye trauma (corneal abrasion following delivery), dacryocystitis, infectious keratitis, subconjunctival hemorrhage (breakage of vessels during delivery), vitreous hemorrhage (associated with

Table 58–3. COMMON CAUSES OF INFECTIOUS AND NONINFECTIOUS CONJUNCTIVITIS IN THE NEONATE

Chemical	Viral	Bacterial Gram Negative	Bacterial Gram Positive
Silver nitrate (most common) Povidone-iodine solution Tetracycline Gentamicin Erythromycin Chloramphenicol	Herpes simplex virus Adenovirus Enterovirus Parechovirus Zika virus (perinatal transmission) Chikungunya (perinatal transmission)	Chlamydia trachomatis Neisseria gonorrhoeae Pseudomonas aeruginosa Klebsiella pneumoniae Escherichia coli Serratia marcescens Enterobacter spp. Haemophilus influenzae Neisseria mucosa Proteus spp. Neisseria cinerea Eikenella corrodens Acinetobacter baumannii Moraxella catarrhalis Neisseria meningitides Stenotrophomonas maltophilia	Staphylococcus aureus Staphylococcus epidermidis Streptococcus pneumoniae Streptococcus viridans Methicillin-resistant S aureus (MRSA) Streptococcus haemolyticus Streptococcus mitis Streptococcus marcescens Group A and B Streptococcus Corynebacterium spp.

thrombocytopenia and polycythemia), congenital anomalies of the nasolacrimal system, corneal epithelial disease, neonatal abstinence syndrome (lacrimation), and congenital glaucoma. Common causes of infectious and noninfectious conjunctivitis can be found in Table 58–3.

A. **Chemical/inflammatory conjunctivitis.** Usually secondary to silver nitrate ocular drops (causes a transient chemical conjunctivitis in 50%–90% of infants) and is the most common cause of conjunctivitis in underdeveloped countries. **The incidence of chemical/inflammatory conjunctivitis has decreased in the United States since silver nitrate drops are no longer being used.** Chemical conjunctivitis can occur from all the other prophylactic ocular antibiotics but less often. It is a nonpurulent inflammation of the eye with a watery discharge, conjunctival injection, and swelling within several hours of instilling the medication. The conjunctivitis shows a maximum inflammatory response around 48 hours and usually clears by the third or fourth day.

B. **Infectious conjunctivitis.** (See Table 58–3.) Infectious conjunctivitis in the newborn is caused by either a bacteria or virus. Causes and their incidence include C trachomatis (2%–40%), N gonorrhoeae (<1%), P aeruginosa (<1%), HSV (<1%), and other bacterial microbes (30%–50%). Common gram-negative organisms are Klebsiella spp. (23%), E coli (17%), S marcescens (17%), P aeruginosa (3%), Enterobacter spp. (2%), and Haemophilus influenzae. Gram-negative isolates cause 38% of conjunctivitis in the neonatal intensive care unit (NICU). Look for a gram-negative etiology in a very low birthweight infant with low gestational age in the NICU. The most common viral cause is herpes, with others including adenovirus, Enterovirus, and Parechovirus.

   1. **Mechanisms of infection**
      a. **Infections acquired through an infected maternal genital tract during birth** are typically N gonorrhoeae, C trachomatis, group B streptococci, or HSV. They tend to reflect sexually transmitted infections in the community. Any bacteria that are normally present in the vagina (not sexually transmitted) can also cause neonatal conjunctivitis.

b. **Cesarean section can be associated with ascending infections through ruptured or intact amniotic membranes (transplacental or transmembrane transmission).** Risk factors include amniotic fluid leak, vaginal examinations, and use of internal monitors.

c. **Postnatally acquired infections from organisms that are present in the environment** (normal skin flora or nasopharyngeal flora). Infection can occur through direct contact, by contamination of parent's or caregiver's hands or mouth, or respiratory tract spread. Examples are *S aureus* (coagulase negative most common in one study), *Staphylococcus epidermidis*, *Streptococcus* spp., *Pseudomonas* spp., *Serratia* spp., *Klebsiella* spp., and *Enterococcus* spp. *Pseudomonas* infections are more typical in hospitalized preemies beyond 5 days of birth.

2. **Chlamydial (inclusion) conjunctivitis. Most common cause of ophthalmia neonatorum** transmitted from the mother and develops in 20% to 50% of infants delivered vaginally to infected untreated mothers. **Topical prophylaxis with erythromycin does not prevent the incidence of chlamydial ophthalmia neonatorum.** Prophylaxis does not eradicate nasopharyngeal colonization or pneumonia. Infected eyes have a mucopurulent discharge, ocular congestion, and eyelid swelling; membranes form on the palpebral conjunctiva, and there is no follicular response. Infection can be unilateral or bilateral and usually starts out as a watery discharge that becomes purulent and copious later. Corneal opacification, chemosis (thickened conjunctivae), and pseudomembranes may be present. Pneumonia is present in 10% to 20% of infants with chlamydial conjunctivitis. Otitis, pharyngeal, and rectal colonization can occur. Repeated and chronic infections of *C trachomatis* can cause **trachoma** (rare in the United States), which is a **chronic follicular keratoconjunctivitis** that causes scarring and neovascularization of the cornea that can result in blindness.

3. **Gonococcal conjunctivitis. Second most commonly reported communicable disease and is the most feared cause of neonatal conjunctivitis.** Approximately 28% of infants born to women with gonorrheal disease in the United States will develop gonococcal ophthalmia neonatorum. It accounts for <1% of neonatal ophthalmia in the United States and is most commonly transmitted from the mother during vaginal birth. The transmission rate from an infected mother to her newborn is up to 50%. Ocular manifestations tend to occur 3 to 5 days after birth with abrupt onset. Usually bilateral, the eyes are very red (hyperacute conjunctivitis) with a thick, purulent drainage and swelling. The lid has chemosis (edema), and a conjunctival membrane may be present. **This is an emergency because, left untreated, it can cause a corneal ulcer and perforation within hours.** The incidence is low because of prophylactic ocular treatment immediately after birth. Infants can manifest systemic manifestations, including sepsis, meningitis, arthritis, vaginitis, and urethritis.

4. *Pseudomonas* **conjunctivitis.** A nosocomial infection that used to be rare but is becoming more common in nurseries. It presents with a purulent discharge, eyelid edema and erythema, and pannus formation. It can lead to a devastating and rapid corneal ulceration and perforation, blindness, endophthalmitis, and death. The organism thrives in moisture-filled environments such as respiratory equipment, and infection occurs most often in hospitalized premature infants or those with depressed immunity. It can be responsible for an epidemic conjunctivitis in premature infants. Infants with *Pseudomonas* conjunctivitis can have systemic complications (sepsis/meningitis).

5. **Herpes simplex keratoconjunctivitis.** There are 3 different types of presentation of herpes in the neonate. The one that will be discussed here is disease localized to the skin, eyes, or mouth (SEM disease). HSV type 2 (HSV-2) can cause unilateral or bilateral conjunctivitis (especially keratoconjunctivitis), optic

neuritis, chorioretinitis, cataracts encephalitis, and permanent vision impairment and is the most frequent viral cause of conjunctivitis. The conjunctivitis can be superficial or may involve the deeper layers of the cornea; vesicles may appear on the nearby skin (80% of infants with SEM have skin vesicles). The infants can have lid edema, conjunctival injection, and a watery nonpurulent discharge. A conjunctival membrane may be present. Most of these infections are secondary to HSV-2 sexually transmitted infection (maternal genital tract ascending infection, through the birth canal, or by transplacental mechanisms); 15% to 20% are caused by HSV-1. Suspect herpes if the conjunctivitis is not responding to antibiotic therapy. Most neonatal HSV-1 infections are related to contact with someone with an active infection (fever blister or cold sore) in the perinatal period.

6. **Viral causes (other than herpes).** Infection usually occurs through direct contact, through contamination of the hands, or via respiratory tract spread. These are usually associated with other symptoms of respiratory tract disease due to adenovirus (most common), *Enterovirus*, or *Parechovirus*. There is usually redness, and it is more commonly unilateral. Infants with adenovirus can have petechial hemorrhages. The discharge is usually mild and watery and is rarely purulent. Lymphadenopathy and preauricular adenopathy can be seen in approximately 50% of cases. Epidemic keratoconjunctivitis from adenovirus can occur by direct contact or from equipment during an eye examination. The CDC site states that Zika virus can cause a conjunctivitis when an infant acquires the infection perinatally (from women who become infected within 2 weeks of delivery). Perinatal transmission of chikungunya virus can also cause conjunctivitis.

7. **Other bacterial infections (nongonococcal, nonchlamydial).** (See Table 58–3.) Conjunctivitis can be caused by other microbial agents (not listed earlier), and these usually present **as a milder form of conjunctivitis.** There may be conjunctival injection, chemosis, and a discharge. Infections caused by *Haemophilus* spp. and *Streptococcus pneumoniae* are associated with **dacryocystitis** (inflammation of the nasolacrimal sac). Staphylococcal conjunctivitis is usually a nosocomial infection. It is the most frequent isolate but may not be a cause of conjunctivitis in infants who are colonized and can cause mild conjunctival hyperemia. Methicillin-resistant *S aureus* conjunctivitis can also occur and has been associated with nurseries and NICUs.

C. **Congenital nasolacrimal duct obstruction (dacryostenosis) occurs in approximately 5% to 20% of infants.** The nasolacrimal duct may fail to canalize completely at birth, and the obstruction is usually at the nasal end of the duct (distal nasolacrimal duct). It is usually unilateral. The symptoms are persistent tearing and a mucoid discharge in the inner corner of the eye. One in 5 infants may have transient discharge (watery and sticky, particularly after sleep) due to a delay in the normal development and opening of the tear duct that resolves spontaneously. CNLDO is the most common of the lacrimal duct anomalies in congenital rubella syndrome. **Dacryocystitis** is a secondary infection in the lacrimal sac.

IV. **Database**

A. **Physical examination**

1. **Ophthalmic examination.** Examine both eyes/eyelids for swelling and edema, and check the conjunctiva for injection (congestion of blood vessels) and chemosis (conjunctival swelling). A purulent discharge, edema, and erythema of the lids and injection of the conjunctiva are suggestive of bacterial conjunctivitis. Check for ulcerations and the presence of a red reflex.

2. **Perform a complete physical examination** to rule out signs of respiratory or systemic infection. Evaluate for any adenopathy.

B. **Laboratory studies**

1. **Gram-stained smear of the exudate discharge** to check for white blood cells (WBCs) (a sign of infection) and bacteria (to identify the organism). **A sample**

of the discharge should also be submitted for culture and sensitivity testing (chocolate agar and/or Thayer-Martin agar for *N gonorrhoeae* and blood agar for other bacteria). Typical findings on Gram stain:

a. ***N gonorrhoeae* conjunctivitis.** Gram-negative intracellular diplococci (kidney bean shaped) and increased WBCs (neutrophils). *Note:* A presumptive diagnosis can be made based on the Gram stain, but remember that other nonpathogenic *Neisseria* species and *Moraxella catarrhalis* can look like *N gonorrhoeae* on Gram stain, so it is best to support the diagnosis with a culture.

b. ***S aureus* conjunctivitis.** Gram-positive cocci in clusters and WBCs.

c. ***P aeruginosa* conjunctivitis.** Gram-negative bacilli and WBCs.

d. **Conjunctivitis caused by *Haemophilus* spp.** Gram-negative coccoid rods.

e. **Streptococcal or enterococci.** Streptococci are gram-positive spherical cocci, and enterococci are gram-positive lancet-shaped encapsulated diplococci.

f. **Other gram-positive organisms.** *S pneumoniae, Streptococcus viridans, S epidermidis,* group A and B streptococci, and *Corynebacterium* species.

g. **Other gram-negative organisms.** *E coli, Klebsiella pneumoniae, S marcescens, Proteus, Enterobacter, H influenzae, Acinetobacter, P aeruginosa, Neisseria cinerea, M catarrhalis, Eikenella corrodens,* and *Stenotrophomonas* maltophilia.

h. **Herpes simplex.** See lymphocytes, plasma cells, and multinucleated giant cells.

i. ***C trachomatis.*** Difficult to stain but classified as gram negative, typically coccoid or rod shaped bacteria. Neutrophils, lymphocytes, and plasma cells.

j. **Chemical conjunctivitis.** Neutrophils and lymphocytes (occasionally).

k. **CNLDO.** The Gram stain is negative, or there is normal conjunctival flora unless there is a secondary infection.

2. **If a chlamydial infection is suspected, methods to diagnose chlamydia ophthalmia** include:

a. **Culture identification of the organism (gold standard)** by a conjunctival swab specimen with 100% specificity and sensitivity. A result can be obtained after 48 to 72 hours.

b. **Nonculture testing**

i. **Antigen detection methods** include direct fluorescent antibody (DFA) and enzyme immunoassay (EIA) tests. DFA is the only US Food and Drug Administration (FDA)-approved nonculture test for chlamydia conjunctivitis in the neonate. An example of one such platform is the commercially available Pathfinder Chlamydia DFA (Bio-Rad Laboratories, Hercules, CA).

ii. **Nucleic acid amplification tests, which use a method of amplifying *C trachomatis* DNA or RNA sequences.** Nucleic acid amplification tests (NAATs) are not FDA approved for use in conjunctivitis in infants but can be used if available through a Clinical Laboratory Improvement Amendments–certified laboratory. Some believe that NAAT has higher sensitivity and specificity than the DFA assays and may actually outperform culture results.

c. **To obtain the swab specimen,** use a Dacron-tipped swab or swab from the manufacturer (do not use calcium alginate or wood shafted swabs) and evert the eyelid; then swab the everted eyelid to obtain conjunctival cells. The exudate is not adequate for the test.

3. **If herpes is suspected.** Historically a histologic exam of lesions for multinucleated giant cells and eosinophilic intranuclear inclusions was performed (Tzanck smear), but is no longer recommended due to low sensitivity. Recommended test is the cell culture of swab specimens (surface and other), skin vesicles, and cerebrospinal fluid (CSF). HSV polymerase chain reaction (PCR) assay can be done on all the specimens including whole blood sample (a positive result does not mean disseminated disease) but has not been studied in neonates. Rapid

diagnostic techniques such as DFA and EIA are available but less sensitive than cultures. A rapid culture test, ELVIS ID HSV test system (Quidel Corporation, San Diego, CA), is available.

4. **In gonococcal infection, cell culture is the most widely used test for nongenital sites.** NAATs are not FDA approved for *N gonorrhoeae* testing on nongenital sites.

5. *Pseudomonas* **infection.** Suspect based on Gram stain and send culture of the exudate.

C. **Imaging and other studies.** Imaging tests usually do not have a role in the workup of conjunctivitis but neuroimaging may be done in herpes conjunctivitis.

1. **Blot test for nasolacrimal duct obstruction.** Apply gentle digital pressure over the lacrimal sac. If there is moisture, it indicates an obstruction. If there is a mucopurulent reflux (positive blot test) from the punctum, this suggests a complete obstruction.

2. **Fluorescein dye disappearance test.** Best test to rule out CNLDO. Instill 1 drop of 0.5% proparacaine followed by 1 drop of 2% fluorescein/moistened fluorescein strip into the lower conjunctiva of each eye. Wipe away any excess dye. After 5 to 10 minutes, evaluate if any dye is still present. If there is significant dye present in the eye and failure of the dye to appear in the nose after 10 to 15 minutes, then an obstruction may exist. If the dye disappears, then there is no obstruction. Alternatively, dim the room and use a cobalt blue light or Burton lamp to see if the dye is still present.

3. **Slit lamp examination with fluorescein staining by an ophthalmologist.** Can help differentiate viral versus bacterial conjunctivitis. With viral one can see conjunctival follicles, with bacterial one can see papillae. One will see dendritic keratitis with HSV keratitis.

4. **Tests for viral conjunctivitis.** Viral cell culture with immunofluorescence assay and PCR. Rapid antigen testing (Adeno Plus, Rapid Pathogen Screening, Inc.) is available for adenovirus.

V. **Plan.** Complications (perforation of the cornea, blindness, *Chlamydia* pneumonia, sepsis, meningitis) can be severe, so it is important to treat as soon as possible. **Do not wait for the culture results to treat the infant.** Send the culture, and based on the Gram stain, start empirical treatment,

A. **Important facts in the management of conjunctivitis**

1. **Infection can spread easily from one eye to another** or to other people by touching the eye or drainage. Proper and frequent hand washing and wearing gloves are essential. **Isolation is recommended for gonococcal, herpes, and** *Pseudomonas* **conjunctivitis.** See Appendix F for specific isolation guidelines.

2. **Drainage is contagious for 24 to 48 hours** after beginning treatment.

3. **Irrigate eye with sterile isotonic saline** to remove accumulated purulent drainage.

4. **Systemic treatment is required for gonococcal,** *Chlamydia, Pseudomonas,* **and herpetic conjunctivitis.** Some recommend systemic treatment for *H influenzae* conjunctivitis since it is often associated with otitis media or other severe infections such as sepsis and meningitis. **Topical and systemic treatment** is recommended for *Pseudomonas* and herpes infection.

5. **Avoid eye patching.**

6. **Consultation with a pediatric ophthalmologist or pediatric infectious disease specialist should be considered.**

7. **Evaluate for signs of systemic disease.** Infants with conjunctivitis are at risk for secondary infections such as sepsis, meningitis, and pneumonia.

8. **Follow daily for signs of improvement** or worsening.

9. **Breast milk/colostrum to treat conjunctivitis.** Colostrum and breast milk contain antimicrobial and anti-inflammatory properties and have been used to treat conjunctivitis or mucopurulent discharge from nasolacrimal duct obstruction.

Colostrum is more effective than mature breast milk because it contains leuko-cytes and has higher concentrations of antibodies, especially IgA. Studies suggest that the use of breast milk or colostrum is safe, has no side effects, and may help as a treatment for blocked tear ducts and that the use of colostrum may be effec-tive against certain type of infections. However, because evidence is limited and studies are conflicting, this treatment is not recommended. Preventive effects of colostrum (2 drops in each eye) against neonatal conjunctivitis have been documented when compared to no prophylaxis.

B. **Chemical conjunctivitis.** Observation only is needed because this usually resolves within 2 to 4 days. Lubrication with artificial tears (4 times a day) may be helpful.

C. **Gonococcal conjunctivitis.** This is considered an emergency, as it can result in per-foration of the globe, corneal scarring, and blindness. Because of the high prevalence of penicillin-resistant *N gonorrhoeae*, the treatment is not penicillin but a third-gen-eration cephalosporin (eg, ceftriaxone). *Note:* Gonococcal conjunctivitis can occur even with appropriate eye prophylaxis in infants delivered to mothers with positive maternal gonococcal infection.

1. **Infants with evidence of gonococcal conjunctivitis, scalp abscess, or dissemi-nated infection** need to be hospitalized.

2. **Isolate the infant during the first 24 hours** of parenteral antibiotic therapy. Both **mother and partner need full medical examinations and treatment** for *N gonorrhoeae*. Mother cannot visit the baby, breast feed, or room-in until she receives 24 hours of antibiotics.

3. **Evaluate for disseminated disease if the infant has gonococcal ophthal-mia** (arthritis, meningitis, sepsis, scalp abscess caused by scalp electrodes from fetal monitoring). Cultures should include blood, eye discharge, CSF, joint aspi-rate, and any other sites, as noted earlier. Conjunctival exudates need to be cul-tured for *N gonorrhoeae* and tested for antibiotic susceptibility.

4. **Tests for concomitant infection** with *C trachomatis*, congenital syphilis, and HIV. The mother and her sexual partner should also be evaluated and presump-tively treated for gonorrhea. Check maternal hepatitis B surface antigen results. Do not treat empirically for chlamydia unless the test comes back positive.

5. **Parenteral antibiotics.** Ceftriaxone is the preferred antibiotic treatment because of the high frequency of penicillin-resistant *N gonorrhoeae*. **Ceftri-axone is not recommended** in a neonate with hyperbilirubinemia or in a neonate receiving or planning on receiving calcium-containing intravenous (IV) fluids. Ceftriaxone can displace bilirubin from binding to serum albu-min, possibly causing bilirubin encephalopathy. **Cefotaxime is recommended in any infant** with hyperbilirubinemia and in infants on calcium-containing IV fluids.

6. **For uncomplicated gonococcal conjunctivitis (without dissemination),** administer a single dose of ceftriaxone 25 to 50 mg/kg IV or intramuscularly (IM) (up to a maximum of 125 mg). **WHO recommends** 1 of the following: ceftriaxone (50 mg/kg IM single dose [maximum 150 mg]), kanamycin (25 mg/kg IM single dose [maximum 756 mg]), or spectinomycin (25 mg/kg IM single dose [maximum 75 mg]).

7. **For gonococcal conjunctivitis with dissemination (arthritis, septicemia) and scalp abscess,** ceftriaxone 25 to 50 mg/kg IV or IM may be given once every day for 7 days. An alternative therapy is cefotaxime (recommended for hyperbiliru-binemic infants or infants receiving calcium-containing IV fluids) at 25 mg/kg every 12 hours, given IV or IM for 7 days. If **meningitis is present,** treatment should be given for a total of 10 to 14 days.

8. **Healthy infants (no conjunctivitis) born to mothers with untreated or inad-equately treated gonococcal infection.** These infants are treated with systemic antibiotics because gonococcal ophthalmia or disseminated infection can occur. A single dose of ceftriaxone (25–50 mg/kg IV or IM; not to exceed 125 mg) is

given. Topical antimicrobial therapy is not necessary if systemic therapy has been given.

9. **Irrigate the eyes with sterile isotonic saline (normal saline) solution** immediately and at frequent intervals (every 1–2 hours) to remove mucopurulent discharge until clear. **Topical antibiotics are not necessary** when systemic antibiotics are used and are only recommended when a corneal ulcer is present. Use topical atropine if there is corneal involvement.

10. **Pediatric ophthalmologic consultation** is usually requested because gonococcal ophthalmia can lead to corneal perforation and blindness. **Infectious disease consultation** is usually requested also to help manage the infant.

D. **Chlamydial conjunctivitis.** Evaluate for systemic disease (pneumonia, otitis, pharyngeal and rectal colonization). Pneumonia has been reported in 20% of infants with chlamydial conjunctivitis.

1. **Recommended neonatal prophylaxis** does not prevent neonatal chlamydial conjunctivitis, extraocular infection, or nasopharyngeal colonization.

2. **Topical treatment with antibiotics is ineffective and unnecessary** when systemic therapy is given, but some institutions use erythromycin drops (4 times a day).

3. **Oral erythromycin base or ethylsuccinate,** 50 mg/kg/d, in 4 divided doses for 14 days by mouth, is recommended. Azithromycin suspension (20 mg/kg/d for 3 days) is an alternative regimen. A second course of erythromycin is sometimes required because approximately 20% of cases recur after therapy because erythromycin is only about 80% effective. **Infantile hypertrophic pyloric stenosis (IHPS) has been seen in infants <6 weeks old (especially <2 weeks) treated with erythromycin. It has been seen with azithromycin, but the risk is unknown.** These infants should be followed and parents should be counseled about the risk and signs of IHPS. The AAP still recommends erythromycin because other treatments have not been well studied. **WHO recommends** azithromycin (20 mg/kg/d orally; 1 dose daily for 3 days) over erythromycin.

4. **Infants born to mothers with untreated chlamydia are at high risk for infection.** Prophylactic antibiotic treatment is not indicated. Monitor for infection. If adequate follow-up is not possible, treatment should be considered.

5. **Treat the mother and sexual partner** if the infant has *C trachomatis* infection.

E. *Pseudomonas* **conjunctivitis**

1. **Isolate the patient and implement standard precautions** unless infection is resistant, in which case contact precautions are indicated.

2. **Evaluate for systemic disease because superficial infection can progress rapidly to serious systemic infection (sepsis, meningitis).** Infants with low birthweight and lower gestational age have an increased risk for systemic disease. *Pseudomonas* infection can lead to devastating consequences: corneal ulceration and perforation, endophthalmitis, blindness, serious systemic infection, and subsequent death.

3. **Parenteral therapy is recommended** because *Pseudomonas* is a virulent organism. Use an aminoglycoside for a minimum of 10 to 14 days. Systemic therapy with an antipseudomonal β-lactam may also be indicated.

4. **Topical therapy is required** because systemic antibiotics have poor penetration in the eye. Treat with topical therapy for 2 weeks with an aminoglycoside, such as gentamicin ophthalmic ointment or tobramycin ophthalmic ointment/ solution. Some will treat with ciprofloxacin ophthalmic ointment/solution because gentamicin and tobramycin can cause a chemical conjunctivitis. See doses in Table 58–4.

5. **Ophthalmology consultation is critical** because the infection may be devastating. **Infectious disease consult** may also be helpful, especially with *Pseudomonas* meningitis. For *Pseudomonas* meningitis, careful follow-up is recommended (check for hearing loss, developmental delay, and neurologic abnormalities).

Table 58–4. COMMON TOPICAL AGENTS TO TREAT CONJUNCTIVITIS

Medication	Form	Concentration	Frequency	Class	Indication	Side Effects
Acyclovir	Ophthalmic ointment	3%	3–6 times daily	Antiviral	Not currently commercially available	Contact dermatitis[a]
Bacitracin	Ophthalmic ointment	500 U/g	3–6 times daily	Polypeptide antibiotic	Gram-positive organisms such as staphylo-cocci (including some penicillin-resistant staphylococci), streptococci, anaerobic cocci, corynebacteria, and clostridia	Contact dermatitis
Chloramphenicol	Ophthalmic solution	0.50%	3–6 times daily	Synthetic antibiotic	Aerobic gram-positive bacteria and many gram-negative aerobic bacteria	Contact dermatitis
Ciprofloxacin	Ophthalmic ointment or solution	0.30%	3–6 times daily	Fluoroquinolone antibiotic	Most gram-negative aerobic bacteria and many gram-positive aerobic bacteria including Pseudomonas and *methicillin-resistant Staphylococcus*	Contact dermatitis
Erythromycin	Ophthalmic ointment	0.50%	3–6 times daily	Macrolide antibiotic	Gram-positive cocci (staphylococci and streptococci) and gram-positive bacilli. Erythromycin also effective against some gram-negative cocci (Neisseria spp.) and some gram-negative bacilli including some H. influenzae and Moraxella lacunata. Erythromycin also active against Chla-mydia and *Treponema.*	Contact dermatitis
Ganciclovir	Ophthalmic gel	0.15%	5 times daily	Antiviral	Herpetic keratitis caused by herpes simplex virus (HSV) type I or 2 (HSV-1 or HSV-2)	Contact dermatitis
Gentamicin	Ophthalmic ointment	0.30%	3–6 times daily	Aminoglycoside antibiotic	Aerobic gram-negative bacteria and some aerobic gram-positive bacteria	Contact dermatitis

(Continued)

513

Table 58–4. COMMON TOPICAL AGENTS TO TREAT CONJUNCTIVITIS (*CONTINUED*)

Medication	Form	Concentration	Frequency	Class	Indication	Side Effects
Iododeoxyuridine	Ophthalmic solution	0.1%	4–6 times daily	Antiviral	Herpetic keratitis caused by herpes simplex virus (HSV) type 1 or 2 (HSV-1 or HSV-2)	Conjunctival scarring
Moxifloxacin	Ophthalmic solution	0.50%	3–6 times daily	Fluoroquinolone antibiotic	Aerobic gram-positive bacteria, some aerobic gram-negative bacteria	Contact dermatitis
Neomycin	Ophthalmic ointment	0.35%	3–6 times daily	Aminoglycoside antibiotic	Aerobic gram-negative bacteria and some aerobic gram-positive bacteria	Contact dermatitis
Polymyxin B	Ophthalmic ointment	10,000 U/g	3–6 times daily	Polymyxin antibiotic	Aerobic and anaerobic gram-negative organisms	Contact dermatitis
Povidone-iodine	Ophthalmic solution	1.25%, 2.5%, 5%	1–6 times daily	Antiseptic	Wide range of bacteria, viruses, fungi, protozoa, and spores	Contact dermatitis
Sulfacetamide	Ophthalmic ointment or solution	10%	3–6 times daily	Sulfonamide antibiotic	Aerobic and anaerobic gram-negative organisms	Contact dermatitis
Tetracycline	Ophthalmic ointment	1%	3–6 times daily	Tetracycline antibiotic	Aerobic and anaerobic gram-negative and gram-positive bacteria	Contact dermatitis
Tobramycin	Ophthalmic ointment or solution	0.3% or 15 mg/mL	3–6 times daily	Aminoglycoside antibiotic	Aerobic gram-negative bacteria and some aerobic gram-positive bacteria	Contact dermatitis
Trifluridine	Ophthalmic ointment	1%	6 times daily	Antiviral	Herpetic keratitis caused by herpes simplex virus (HSV) type 1 or 2 (HSV-1 or HSV-2)	Contact dermatitis
Vancomycin	Ophthalmic solution	25 mg/mL	3–6 times daily	Tricyclic gly-copeptide antibiotic	Aerobic and anaerobic gram-positive bacteria	Contact dermatitis
Vidarabine	Ophthalmic ointment	3%	3–6 times daily	Antiviral	Not currently commercially available	Contact dermatitis

aBlurred vision, eye irritation, eyelid erythema and edema, conjunctival hyperemia, punctate keratitis.

F. **Herpes simplex conjunctivitis**
 1. **Isolate the patient and implement contact precautions.** Infant can room-in if low risk of infection, and mother can visit and breast feed if there are no vesicular herpetic lesions in the breast area and all lesions are covered.
 2. **Obtain a complete set of viral cultures** (PCR assays on skin and mucus have not been studied in neonates; do this in addition to the gold standard cultures). A positive culture obtained from any of the surface sites >12 to 24 hours after birth is considered positive and not intrapartum exposure contamination.
   a. **Obtain a surface culture from the mouth, nasopharynx, conjunctivae, and anus for HSV surface culture and HSV PCR assay (if desired).** Any positive culture from any surface area >12 to 24 hours after birth indicates viral replication and is suggestive of an infection in the infant and not contamination by intrapartum exposure.
   b. **Skin vesicle (if present) culture** for HSV and PCR assay.
   c. **Cerebrospinal fluid and whole blood culture for HSV and PCR assay,** as clinical findings may be absent in CSF disease early on.
   d. **Whole blood sample for serum alanine aminotransferase.** Can be elevated in HSV hepatitis.
   e. **Direct fluorescent antibody staining of vesicle scrapings** or EIA detection of HSV antigens. These methods are specific but less sensitive than a culture.
 3. **Administer a topical therapy with ocular herpes simplex virus:** 1% trifluridine solution/drops or 0.15% ganciclovir gel (both are proven to be effective) 5 times per day for 10 days (every 2 hours).
 4. **Parenteral acyclovir for all neonates with herpes simplex virus disease (including conjunctivitis):** 60 mg/kg/d IV divided 3 times a day for a minimum of 14 days for SEM disease. If central nervous system (CNS) disease or disseminated disease is present, treat for a minimum of 21 days. (For dosage, see Chapter 155.)
 5. **Ophthalmologic evaluation and follow up** are required for all infants with neonatal HSV disease because chorioretinitis, cataracts, and retinopathy may develop. **Infectious disease consultation** is also recommended.
 6. **Neuroimaging** should be done for a baseline brain anatomy (magnetic resonance imaging is the most sensitive, but computed tomography or ultrasound is also acceptable). Neurologic follow-up is important.
 7. **With cerebrospinal fluid involvement,** a repeat lumbar puncture (LP) needs to be done near the end of the therapy to document that CSF is negative for HSV DNA on PCR assay; if positive, another week of therapy needs to be given and another repeat LP needs to be done. Parenteral treatment should not be stopped until CSF PCR is negative.
 8. **Suppression therapy with oral acyclovir** (300 mg/m^2/dose) 3 times a day for 6 months is recommended following acute neonatal HSV disease. Adjust dose for growth. This prevents skin recurrences and improves neurodevelopmental outcomes in infants with CNS disease. Check absolute neutrophil counts at 2 and 4 weeks after starting therapy and then monthly.
G. **Other bacterial infections once gonococcal, chlamydial, and *Pseudomonas* infections have been ruled out.**
 1. **Local saline irrigation.**
 2. **Topical antibiotics** only are usually required. (See Table 58–4.) For gram-positive organisms: bacitracin or erythromycin. For gram-negative organisms: gentamicin, tobramycin, or ciprofloxacin ointment or solution. Ointments are preferred over eye drops for neonates because they have reduced washout effect.
   a. **Ophthalmic ointment:** 0.5- to 1-cm ribbon in each eye every 6 hours for 7 to 14 days.
   b. **Ophthalmic solution:** 1 to 2 drops into each eye every 4 hours for 7 to 14 days.

3. **H influenzae infection** may require further evaluation of the infant (rule out sepsis, meningitis, and other infections if indicated), and systemic antibiotics may be necessary. Topical conjunctivitis can be treated with any fluoroquinolone topical antibiotic.

4. **Methicillin-resistant S aureus conjunctivitis.** Treatment depends on the clinical situation; some do not need to be treated. Topical chloramphenicol eye drops and fortified vancomycin drops can be compounded under the direction of an ophthalmologist. See Chapter 141.

5. **For gram-negative conjunctivitis in premature low birthweight infants** and increasing antibiotic resistance (especially noted among the β-lactam antibiotics), third- and fourth-generation antibiotics are recommended.

6. **Viral infections other than herpes simplex conjunctivitis.** Treatment of viral conjunctivitis is mainly supportive (artificial tears, cool compresses). It usually resolves without specific treatment. One study found that conjunctival irrigation with 2.5% povidone-iodine was effective for the treatment of adenoviral conjunctivitis ("pink eye") in infants and reduced the spread of infection.

H. **Congenital nasolacrimal duct obstruction** is the most common cause of persistent tearing and discharge in infants. Treatment can involve nonsurgical or surgical methods. Nonsurgical treatment consists of observation or digital massage (**Crigler massage**). Surgical treatment consists of probing the nasolacrimal duct to open the membranous obstruction, nasolacrimal duct stent insertion, balloon catheter dilation, or dacryocystorhinostomy.

1. **Observation.** Most cases clear spontaneously without treatment. Studies show varying results (66% to 88% to 96% resolution in 6 to 10 months to 1 year). Some physicians will treat with topical antibiotic eye drops to treat the discharge or mattering around the eye.

2. **Digital (Crigler) massage.** Massaging the inside corner of the eye over the lacrimal sac, in a downward motion with expression toward the nose, can exert hydrostatic pressure on the lower end of the lacrimal duct and may help to open any obstruction and establish patency. The massage method involves 5 to 10 strokes 4 times a day.

3. **Nasolacrimal probing.** If the problem does not resolve and symptoms persist (usually after 6 months), the infant should be evaluated by an ophthalmologist. Probing of the duct is usually indicated. It can be done as an office procedure or under general anesthesia. Probing will not work if the duct is swollen due to infection or if the obstruction is caused by a bony protrusion of the inferior turbinate. Probing is not without risk of complications, which can include creation of a false passage, injury to the nasolacrimal duct, bleeding, aspiration, and laryngospasm. There is controversy as to when this should be done (early or later). A Cochrane group performed a review to see if immediate probing versus delayed probing resulted in more treatment success. Results noted that the effects of immediate versus deferred probing are uncertain but found that children who had unilateral CNLDO and immediate office probing had a higher success of treatment compared to deferred probing.

4. **Nasolacrimal duct stent insertion, balloon catheter tear duct dilation, and dacryocystorhinostomy** are reserved for those cases that have failed other procedures.

I. **Dacryocystitis.** This is an infection of the lacrimal (tear) sac. It is almost always related to nasolacrimal duct obstruction. It can cause redness, swelling, and pain near the nose just below the lower lid.

1. **Congenital dacryocystitis** is a serious disease that can cause orbital cellulitis, brain abscess, meningitis, sepsis, and death if not treated immediately and aggressively with systemic antibiotics. Urgent ophthalmology consult is necessary.

2. **Acquired dacryocystitis can be acute or chronic.**

a. **Acute dacryocystitis.** Sudden onset of redness and edema over the lacrimal sac and may have injection of the conjunctiva and preseptal cellulitis. Orbital cellulitis can also occur, and urgent ophthalmology consultation is recommended. Treatment includes heat, systemic antibiotics, and percutaneous drainage of the abscess.
b. **Chronic dacryocystitis.** Infant presents with tearing and mattering. Inside the lacrimal sac is a chronic low-grade bacterial infection. Treatment includes dacryocystorhinostomy.

59 Gastric Residuals

I. **Problem.** The nurse alerts you that a bloody gastric residual has been obtained in an infant. Gastric residuals (also known as a gastric aspirates) can be abnormal in appearance or abnormal in volume. **Gastric aspiration** is a procedure by which the stomach is aspirated with an oral or nasogastric tube. The procedure is typically performed before each feeding or at a predetermined interval during continuous feeding to verify correct orogastric/nasogastric tube placement, to assess if feedings are being tolerated and digested (feeding intolerance), and to prevent aspiration of contents of the stomach (prevent ventilator-associated pneumonia). The color is noted. The amount of residual is measured and recorded as the **gastric residual.** Once a standard procedure in the neonatal unit, performing routine gastric residuals is now *controversial* because of the lack of consensus and supporting evidence. Because there is lack of evidence and recommendations, each neonatal intensive care unit (NICU) should develop a standardized protocol to determine the role of gastric residuals in their unit. Recent reviews have found the following:

A. **There is no formal consensus on the definition of an abnormal gastric residual.** Definitions include a percentage of previous feedings (range 20%–50%), a preset volume of the previous feeding (range 2–5 mL), or a preset volume based on body weight (>2 mL/kg to >5 mL/kg). **The most common definition used of an abnormal gastric residual is >50% of the previous feeding.**
B. **It is not a reliable indicator of the placement of the feeding tube.** Straw-colored gastric aspirates can be seen from a nasogastric tube abnormally placed in the respiratory system.
C. **It does not give an accurate estimate of gastric contents.** The volume of the gastric contents is influenced by body position, size of feeding tube, technique, temperature of feed, and viscosity. Abdominal ultrasound has been recommended as an alternative method of measurement of gastric contents.
D. **There is lack of evidence that increased residuals indicate feeding intolerance.** Some neonatologists will equate gastric residuals with feeding intolerance. The amount or characteristic of the gastric residual is not predictive of feeding intolerance.
E. **The use of gastric residuals prolongs the time to reach full feeds.** The response to a gastric residual can cause interruption of enteral feeding, delay in achieving full enteral feedings, prolonged use of TPN, and decreased growth. A recent review found omitting the evaluation of prefeed gastric residuals in extremely premature infants increased the delivery of enteral nutrition and improved weight gain.
F. **It is not an indication of necrotizing enterocolitis.** Studies show there is a possible increased volume of gastric residuals prior to necrotizing enterocolitis (NEC), but there is no definition of the exact volume to guide decisions. Recent survey of 173

physicians from 26 countries showed that neonatologists do rely on increased gastric residuals and abdominal distension to help diagnose NEC.

G. **Although refeeding is supported in adults** (ie, returning the tube feed residual), there is no evidence in neonates.

H. **An isolated gastric residual in very low birthweight infants** can reflect delayed gut maturation and decreased intestinal motility and may not signify a gastrointestinal (GI) problem.

I. **Bilious and bloody residuals were once considered a red flag,** and feedings were stopped and complete workups were initiated. Bilious or bloody residuals in the absence of other clinical signs may not indicate serious disease and are not predictive of NEC or feeding intolerance. Bilious residuals can be secondary to immaturity, and bloody residuals maybe secondary to irritations from trauma. Consider the gestational age of the infant and the infant's clinical status before withholding feeds.

II. **Immediate questions**

A. **Is the gastric residual volume abnormal?** The stomach is a secretory organ, and basal gastric secretions average 2.8 mL over 4 hours in preterm infants; therefore, a gastric residual could contain normal basal gastric secretions plus enteral feeding. There is great variation in definitions of abnormal gastric residuals (see definitions provided earlier). The most common definition of an abnormal gastric residual appears to be >50% of the previous feeding. The volume of the gastric residual can be influenced by:

   1. **Body position of the infant.** Larger residuals if the infant was in the left lateral position or supine compared to prone and right lateral positions.

   2. **Size of the feeding tube.** Bigger feeding tube residual volumes are greater than those of smaller feeding tubes.

   3. **Feeding viscosity and temperature of the milk.** Cool and or room temperature milk produced greater gastric residuals than body temperature milk. Expressed breast milk emptied faster from the stomach than formula. Fortification of breast milk delayed gastric emptying.

   4. **Position of the feeding tube and the aspiration technique** can also affect the amount of gastric contents.

   5. **Infusion rate of the feeding.** Slow rate of infusion caused greater gastric emptying when compared to the fast rate of infusion.

B. **Color of the residual used to define a clinically or nonclinically significant gastric residual** (eg, bloody, bilious, nonbilious nonyellow, or yellow) and is important in the differential diagnosis (see Section III.A–D). Some NICUs are introducing color charts to help identify bilious residuals because there is lack of consensus when trying to identify a bilious gastric residual.

C. **Is the abdomen soft, with good bowel sounds, or distended, with visible bowel loops? Is there abdominal distension? Has the abdominal girth increased?** Absence of bowel sounds, distention, tenderness, and erythema are all abnormal signs and may indicate a pathologic process. Absence of bowel sounds suggests an ileus. For abdominal distension, a change of up to 1.5 cm suggests normal variability, but studies showed an increase of 3.5 cm was seen with 1 feeding in normal premature infants.

D. **When was the last stool passed?** Constipation resulting in abdominal distention may cause feeding intolerance and increased gastric residuals.

E. **What medications is the infant receiving?** Theophylline delays gastric emptying in very low birthweight infants. Doxapram can cause gastric residuals.

F. **Is the infant premature? Delayed gastric emptying and feeding intolerance** are common in premature infants. There is an inverse relationship between gestational age and rate of gastric emptying. **Premature infants** have delayed gut maturation, decreased duodenal motor activity, GI dysmotility, and slower intestinal transit time.

G. **Is the infant ill appearing?** Gastric emptying is delayed in acutely ill infants, especially in those infants with respiratory distress.

III. **Differential diagnosis.** The characteristics of the residual can provide important clinical clues to the cause of the problem and are outlined next.

   A. **Bilious residual.** A bilious residual is a residual that is light to dark green but can be yellow in the initial phases. It is important to be able to correctly identify a bilious residual because overidentification of bilious residuals can lead to infants being placed nothing by mouth (NPO) and getting unnecessary evaluations. Yellow and light green gastric residuals, especially with a normal exam, were not found to correlate with feeding intolerance or the need to delay feedings. **Dark green (color of collard greens)** may indicate an obstruction or ileus. It is important to remember that a bilious aspirate in a term infant should be approached differently than a bilious aspirate in a preterm infant.

   1. **Term infant.** In the term infant, especially if the residual is persistent and dark green and there are other clinical signs, it can mean an **intestinal obstruction** distal to the ampulla of Vater, usually in the proximal small bowel. GI pathology needs to be investigated, and immediate surgical consultation should be obtained.

   2. **Preterm infant.** In the **premature infant**, bilious residuals, especially isolated green or light green residuals, can occur without serious bowel pathology and may indicate **immaturity of the bowel** (duodenogastric reflux from immaturity of the duodenal motor activity and pyloric sphincter tone).

   3. **Causes of bilious residual**

      a. **Malpositioned nasogastric tube.** Passage of the feeding tube into the duodenum or the jejunum instead of the stomach can cause a bilious residual.

      b. **Overaggressive/zealous aspiration** can cause a bilious residual by sucking back duodenal contents.

      c. **Bowel obstruction.** Bilious gastric aspirates or emesis may indicate bowel obstruction. Studies show that 30% to 38% of infants with bilious vomiting in the first 72 hours of life had obstruction, of whom 20% required surgery. **Bowel perforation with pneumoperitoneum** can present with increased bilious gastric residuals.

         i. **Malrotation with midgut volvulus.** Most common obstruction and was present in 22% of infants with bilious vomiting. Presents at 3 to 7 days of age. Bilious gastric residual may be the only early sign of small bowel volvulus.

         ii. **Duodenal atresia.** If atresia is distal to ampulla of Vater (seen in 80% of cases), one can see bilious emesis without abdominal distension. If atresia is proximal to the ampulla, one can see nonbilious vomiting. Duodenal obstruction is seen with associated anomalies (Down syndrome, VATER/VACTERL [vertebral anomalies, anal atresia, tracheoesophageal fistula, and radial or renal dysplasia/vertebral defects, anal atresia, cardiac defects, tracheoesophageal fistula, renal and radial abnormalities, and limb abnormalities], and others).

         iii. **Jejunoileal atresia.** Small bowel atresia, including distal duodenum and jejunal and ileal atresia, can cause bilious residuals.

         iv. **Meconium ileus/plug.** Presents soon after birth with abdominal distention and bilious residuals/vomiting.

         v. **Hirschsprung disease.** Usually presents with abdominal distension and no stool but can have bilious or yellow residual or vomiting.

      d. **Ileus** can cause bilious residuals and can be associated with sepsis, prematurity, hypokalemia, effects of maternal drugs (especially magnesium sulfate), pneumonia, hypothyroidism, and other etiologies.

      e. **Prematurity and bilious residuals.** Some premature infants will have bilious residuals from gastric dysmotility and immaturity. These infants do not have a bowel obstruction or pathologic process.

      f. **Gastroesophageal and duodenogastric reflux** can cause bilious residuals/vomiting.

      g. Necrotizing enterocolitis. Bilious residuals can be seen with NEC, **but bloody residuals are more common**
      h. Idiopathic. No cause is found.

B. **Nonbilious, nonyellow residual (white, clear, straw colored, cloudy, undigested or digested formula)**
   1. **Problems with the feeding regimen.** Undigested or digested formula may be seen in the residual if the feeding regimen is too aggressive and is more likely in small premature infants who are given a small amount of formula initially and then are given larger volumes too rapidly, or after adding fortifier to breast milk.
      a. Residual containing undigested formula. May be seen if the interval between feedings is too short or if too much formula is being given.
      b. Residual containing digested formula. May be a sign of delayed gastric emptying or overfeeding. Also, if the osmolarity of the formula is increased by the addition of vitamins, retained digested formula may be seen.
   2. **Other causes**
      a. Formula intolerance. An uncommon cause of residual but should be considered. Some infants do not tolerate the carbohydrate source in some formulas. If the infant is receiving a lactose-containing formula (eg, Similac or Enfamil), perform a stool pH to rule out lactose intolerance. If the stool pH is acidic (>5.0), lactose intolerance may be present. Diarrhea is more common than gastric residuals with lactose intolerance.
      b. Constipation. This is a factor especially if the abdomen is full but soft and no stool has passed in 48 to 72 hours.
      c. Pyloric stenosis. Pyloric stenosis typically presents at 3 to 4 weeks with nonbilious projectile vomiting.
      d. Infections can cause gastric residuals.
      e. Hypermagnesemia. This can present with increased gastric residuals and delayed passage of meconium.
      f. Retinopathy of prematurity examination. Gastric residuals are associated with retinopathy of prematurity (ROP) eye examination. Feeding is recommended 1 hour before ROP examination.
      g. Rare causes. Incarcerated hernia, bowel obstruction, inborn errors of metabolism, and congenital adrenal hyperplasia can present with nonbilious residuals.

C. **Bloody residual.** Includes any color of red or coffee ground color. (See also Chapter 60.) Upper GI bleeding is blood loss proximal to the ligament of Treitz (from the esophagus, stomach, or duodenum).
   1. **Swallowed maternal blood.** Must be ruled out to verify true neonatal bleeding.
   2. **Trauma from nasogastric intubation** is a common cause. Upper airway suctioning can also cause blood-tinged residuals.
   3. **Coagulopathies.** Vitamin K deficiency bleeding, disseminated intravascular coagulation due to infection, coagulopathy from liver failure, and any congenital coagulation factor deficiency.
   4. **Stress-related mucosal lesions.** Gastritis; esophagitis; erosions of the esophageal, gastric, or duodenal mucosa; and gastroduodenal ulcers can all have a bloody residual. Absence of bloody residual does not exclude stress-related mucosal lesions.
   5. **Necrotizing enterocolitis.** Hemorrhagic residuals can be seen in NEC, are hypothesized to be a result of disruption in the bowel integrity, and are considered a marker for NEC.
   6. **Allergic colitis.** Causes include milk or soy enterocolitis, milk protein intolerance, and cow milk intolerance. Lower GI bleeding is the more common presentation.
   7. **Severe fetal asphyxia.**
   8. **Medications.** Theophylline, indomethacin, heparin, nonsteroidal anti-inflammatory drugs, and corticosteroids. Maternal use of aspirin, cephalothin, and phenobarbital can cause coagulation abnormalities in infants.

9. **Rare causes.** GI perforations, gastric volvulus or duplication, intestinal duplications, duplication cyst, and vascular anomalies including hemangiomas, telangiectasias, arteriovenous malformations, Hirschsprung enterocolitis, and Meckel diverticulitis.

D. **Yellow residuals.** Non–bile-stained yellow residuals can be associated with intestinal obstruction (early on) and should not be ignored if the infant has other abnormal clinical findings. Clinical evaluation may be warranted in this situation, and further workup may be required depending on the evaluation. Colostrum may also be yellow in color. **Isolated yellow gastric residuals** may be unimportant in very low birthweight infants or in infants with a normal examination.

IV. **Database**

A. **Physical examination.** Check for any temperature instability or any new subtle signs that could indicate a pathologic process. How is the infant's perfusion? Is there any apnea? Is there anything else going on besides gastric residuals? Are the stools normal? Pay particular attention to the **abdominal examination.** Check for bowel sounds (absent bowel sounds may indicate ileus), abdominal distention, tenderness to palpation and erythema of the abdomen (may signify peritonitis), or visible bowel loops.

B. **Laboratory studies.** Testing depends on the physical examination of the infant and the infant's clinical status.

1. **Initial studies**

a. **Complete blood count with differential and platelets.** To evaluate for sepsis or NEC, if suspected. The hematocrit and platelet count may be checked if bleeding has occurred. Acute NEC is commonly associated with thrombocytopenia.

b. **Blood culture.** If sepsis or NEC is suspected and before antibiotics are started.

c. **Serum potassium level if ileus is present.** To rule out hypokalemia.

d. **Arterial blood gas.** If metabolic acidosis is seen, this is a red flag in this setting, and a further workup should be done.

e. **Serum electrolytes.** Hyponatremia can be seen with third spacing of fluid.

f. **C-reactive protein for necrotizing enterocolitis.**

2. **Additional studies**

a. **Stool pH.** (See Section III.B.2.a.) If there is a family history of milk intolerance, a stool pH can rule out lactose intolerance (stool pH is usually >5.0).

b. **Coagulation profile.** (Prothrombin time, partial thromboplastin time, fibrinogen, and platelets.) A bloody residual may signify the presence of a coagulopathy.

C. **Imaging and other studies**

1. **Immediate studies**

a. **Plain radiograph (flat plate) of the abdomen** should be obtained if the residual is persistently bilious or very dark green (especially in a term infant), if there is any abnormality on physical examination, or if residuals continue. The radiograph will show whether the nasogastric tube is in the correct position and will define the bowel gas pattern. Look for an unusual gas pattern, pneumatosis intestinalis, ileus, or evidence of bowel obstruction. Dilated bowel loops and air fluid levels suggest a surgical abdomen. Duodenal atresia has a double bubble sign. (See Chapter 12 for radiographic examples of tube placements and intra-abdominal diseases.)

b. **A left lateral abdominal decubitus film** is useful because a perforation can be easily missed on the anteroposterior film. A gasless abdomen can be seen with midgut volvulus.

2. **Additional studies**

a. **Gastroesophageal reflux scintigraphy ("milk scan").** See page 450.

b. **Endoscopy** should be considered for ulcer evaluation.

c. **Abdominal ultrasound and contrast studies of the gastrointestinal tract** if indicated. Point-of-care ultrasound can be used to diagnose NEC (small intramural gas or changes in bowel wall thickness or peristalsis).

V. **Plan.** The approach to management of the neonate with an abnormal gastric residual is initially based on the nature of the residual and most important if the physical examination is abnormal. **It is so important to not just react to the gastric aspirate. Evaluate the entire clinical picture. Current treatment modalities include:** refeeding or discarding the residual, continuing or stopping feedings, placing the infant NPO, checking an abdominal x-ray, and doing laboratory work to evaluate for sepsis and other conditions.

A. **General recommendations when called to the bedside of an infant with an abnormal gastric aspirate** (>50% of the feeding volume)

1. **Are there any other concerning characteristics of the aspirate?** For example, is it increasing with each feed, bloody, bilious in a term infant, or persistently bilious in a preterm infant? These may signify a more serious condition.

2. **Evaluate the infant.**

   a. **If infant has a normal physical examination, normal abdominal examination** (eg, no distension, tenderness, discoloration, palpable loop), **and no other clinical signs that would be concerning** (eg, increasing apnea and bradycardia, temperature instability, frequent emesis, bloody stool, no stool, decreased stooling), keep feeding with close observation. Gastric residuals are usually discarded or refed. Refeed gastric aspirate if it is undigested formula and discard if it is bilious, contains excess mucus, or is very bloody. If the infant is term, consider a baseline abdominal radiograph.

   b. **If infant has an abnormal physical examination and/or worrisome clinical signs,** do an abdominal radiograph.

      i. **If abnormal radiograph** (free air, NEC, pneumatosis, gasless, fixed dilated loops, ileus), place NPO, start intravenous (IV) fluids, do laboratory testing, place a nasogastric tube for gastric decompression, and consult pediatric surgery.

      ii. **If questionable radiograph,** consider making the infant NPO and reevaluate and repeat radiograph in the next 6 to 8 hours. If improvement is noted and radiograph normal, reinitiate feeding. If no improvement and radiograph still the same or worse, hold feeds and initiate formal workup.

      iii. **If normal radiograph but concerning physical examination and or other clinical signs with no obvious reason for abdominal distension (eg, CPAP belly).** Place NPO and reevaluate over the next 6 to 8 hours.

B. **Treatment of specific types of residuals**

1. **Bilious residual**

   a. **Malpositioned nasogastric tube. Rule this out first.** An abdominal radiograph will confirm the position of the nasogastric tube distally in the duodenum. Replace or reposition the tube in the stomach.

   b. **Gastrointestinal pathology.** The majority are initially managed by making the infant NPO and placing a nasogastric tube to rest and decompress the gut while doing a workup. Start an IV and give fluids. Obtain laboratory studies, consider antibiotics if indicated, and consult pediatric surgery if indicated.

      i. **Necrotizing enterocolitis.** See Chapter 109.

      ii. **Ileus.** May be secondary to sepsis, hypokalemia, effects of maternal drugs (especially magnesium sulfate), pneumonia, and hypothyroidism. Place the infant NPO and insert a nasogastric tube for decompression. Diagnose and treat the underlying cause.

      iii. **Other surgical problems** (eg, bowel obstruction, malrotation, volvulus, meconium plug). Pediatric surgery consultation should be obtained immediately. Specific radiologic studies may be indicated (other radiologic films, ultrasound, or contrast studies) based on the infant. Surgery may be indicated.

    c. **Prematurity and bilious residuals.** If the infant has a normal examination and it is an isolated bilious residual, it is acceptable to feed with close observation. If the bilious residuals persist or anything changes on the vitals or clinical examination, then the infant needs to be reevaluated, a baseline radiograph should be obtained, and a bowel obstruction needs to be ruled out.

    d. **Gastroesophageal and duodenogastric reflux.** See Chapter 52.

2. **Nonbilious, nonyellow residual.** Usually means residual involves undigested or digested formula.

    a. **Residual containing undigested formula.** If the volume of undigested formula in the residual does not exceed 50% of the previous feeding and the physical examination and vital signs are normal, the gastric residual can be replaced. There is no evidence that refeeding is supported in neonates, only in adults. Gastric residuals do contain important essential acids and enzymes that aid in digestion, including hydrochloric acid (necessary for limiting intestinal overgrowth of bacteria) and pepsin (enzyme used in digestion in the stomach). Discarding gastric residuals can cause loss of hydrochloric acid (which can increase the bacteria in the intestine and intestinal inflammation and may increase risk of NEC and late-onset sepsis) and loss of pepsin. If gastric residuals continue and the examination of the infant is normal, the following can be tried:

        i. **The time interval between feedings may not be long enough for digestion to take place.** If the infant is being fed every 2 hours and residuals continue, the feeding interval may be increased to 3 hours.

        ii. **Decreasing the volume of the feeds.**

        iii. **Continuous gavage feedings.** The patient may also have to be fed IV to allow the gut to rest.

        iv. **If elevated residuals still continue or if the residual exceeds >50% of the previous feeding,** the patient must be reevaluated. If the infant has physical findings, work up the infant and withhold feeds. An abdominal radiograph should be obtained.

    b. **Residual containing digested formula.** The residual is usually discarded, especially if it contains a large amount of mucus. If the physical examination and vital signs are normal, continue feedings. If elevated residuals continue, the patient must be reassessed. If the examination is normal, consider **decreasing the amount of feeds.** The number of calories should be calculated to make certain that overfeeding (usually >130 kcal/kg/d) is not occurring. If the examination is not normal, further workup must be done.

    c. **Other**

        i. **Formula intolerance.** A trial of lactose-free formula (eg, ProSobee or Isomil) can be instituted if lactose intolerance is verified. (See formula components in Chapter 11.)

        ii. **Necrotizing enterocolitis or post–necrotizing enterocolitis stricture.** See Chapter 109.

        iii. **Pyloric stenosis.**

        iv. **Constipation.** Anal stimulation can be attempted. If this fails, a glycerin suppository can be given. (See Chapter 72.)

        v. **Infections.** If sepsis is likely, broad-spectrum antibiotics are started after a laboratory workup is performed. A penicillin (usually ampicillin) and an aminoglycoside (usually gentamicin) are given initially until culture results are available. The patient is usually not fed orally if this diagnosis is entertained; an infant with sepsis usually does not tolerate oral feedings.

        vi. **Inborn errors of metabolism.** See Chapter 100.

        vii. **Congenital adrenal hyperplasia.** Hormone/steroid replacement, fluid and electrolyte management, and possible surgery are indicated.

        viii. **Hypermagnesemia.** See Chapter 105.

3. **Bloody residual.** See also Chapter 60.
   a. **Swallowed maternal blood.** Observation only.
   b. **Nasogastric trauma.** Nasogastric trauma may occur if the nasogastric tube is too large or insertion is traumatic. Use the smallest nasogastric tube possible. Observation is indicated. Because the bleeds are usually minimal, active management is not necessary.
   c. **Coagulopathies.** GI hemorrhage from disseminated intravascular coagulation, vitamin K deficiency bleeding, and others are discussed in detail in Chapter 87.
   d. **Stress-related mucosal lesions.** See Chapter 60.
   e. **Necrotizing enterocolitis.** See Chapter 109.
   f. **Allergic colitis.** Change formula.
4. **Non–bile-stained yellow residual.** If isolated, it is probably unimportant. If it continues or increases in volume, then a full clinical examination and possible abdominal radiograph are warranted. If anything abnormal is found, further studies are needed to rule out any intestinal obstruction. These infants need to be followed closely.

C. **Medications for feeding intolerance with gastric residuals** *(controversial).* Infants can have GI motility immaturity that causes feeding intolerance. Some institutions have used prokinetic agents such as metoclopramide and erythromycin to improve feeding intolerance (to stimulate and improve gastric emptying [promote motility], improve lower esophageal sphincter tone, decrease gastric residual volume, and decrease time to full enteral feeding). These medications have been shown to improve gastric emptying, decrease regurgitation, and enhance lower esophageal sphincter tone in older infants. They have not been shown to decrease gastroesophageal reflux symptoms in preterm infants. These medications are associated with a lack of data for efficacy and safety and have major side effects (some can cause significant harm) and are not recommended in preterm infants.

60 Gastrointestinal Bleeding from the Upper Tract

I. **Problem.** Vomiting of bright red blood or active bleeding from the nasogastric (NG) tube is seen in a newborn. **Upper gastrointestinal (GI) bleeding** is bleeding that occurs proximal to the ligament of Treitz (duodenojejunal flexure) which arises from the esophagus, stomach, or duodenum. It usually presents with hematemesis (vomiting of blood) most commonly bright red or less commonly the color of coffee grounds, or it can present with melena (black tarry stools). Rarely, a brisk upper GI (UGI) bleed has such a short intestinal transit time that it presents with hematochezia (fresh blood through the anus). Coffee ground emesis means the blood has been altered by gastric contents, which indicates slow bleeding from the esophagus and duodenum. Diagnosis is made most commonly by blood-stained aspirates in the NG or orogastric (OG) tube, by hematemesis, or by endoscopy (gastric mucosa shows bleeding). UGI bleeding is more common in sick newborns in the NICU, than in term neonates. The majority of UGI bleeds in neonates are benign, self-limiting, and require minimal workup and treatment, but some can be severe, especially those associated with other underlying conditions.

II. **Immediate questions**
   A. **What are the vital signs?** If the blood pressure is dropping and there is active bleeding, urgent crystalloid volume replacement is necessary.

B. **Is the infant ill or well appearing?** Is the bleeding mild or severe? **If the infant looks well,** consider swallowed maternal blood first, mild trauma from nasopharyngeal bleeding, esophagitis, or gastritis (most cases are asymptomatic), clinically relevant mucosal lesions of the upper GI tract (seen in healthy term infants), or milk protein intolerance. **If the infant is severely ill** (hypovolemia, shock, near death) with significant upper GI bleeding, most of these cases are related to other problems such as hypoxemia, infection, perinatal stress, respiratory failure, congenital heart disease, increased intracranial pressure. **Milder bleeding:** gastritis, esophagitis, milk protein intolerance. **More severe bleeding:** coagulopathies (VKDB), NEC, Stress ulcer.

C. **What is the hematocrit?** A hematocrit should be done as soon as possible. The result is used as a baseline value and to determine whether blood replacement is needed. **With any acute bleeding, the hematocrit may not reflect the blood loss for several hours.**

D. **Is blood available in the blood bank should transfusion be necessary?** Verify that the infant has been typed and cross-matched so that blood will be quickly available if necessary.

E. **Is there bleeding from other sites?** Bleeding from other sites suggests disseminated intravascular coagulation (DIC), vitamin K deficiency bleeding, or other coagulopathy. If bleeding is only from the NG tube, disorders such as stress-related mucosal lesions, NG trauma, and swallowing of maternal blood are likely causes to consider.

F. **How old is the infant?** During the first day of life, vomiting of bright red blood or the presence of bright red blood in the NG tube is frequently secondary to swallowing of maternal blood during delivery. Infants with this problem are clinically stable with normal vital signs. Vitamin K deficiency bleeding can occur at different times depending on the type (see Chapter 92). Age of the infant can help narrow down the differential diagnosis, but there can be overlap between ages.
   1. **Newborns (<1 month old). Common:** stress gastritis, stress-induced ulcer, vitamin K deficiency, sepsis, trauma from NG tube, cow's milk protein allergy medications (nonsteroidal anti-inflammatory drugs [NSAIDS]), idiopathic. **Less common:** vascular anomalies, GI duplications, congenital coagulation factor deficiency, ulcer, esophagitis.
   2. **Infants (≥1 month old).** Stress esophagitis, peptic ulcer bleeding, vascular anomalies, GI duplications, duodenal or gastric webs, bowel obstruction, varices, medication induced (NSAIDs), Mallory-Weiss syndrome, gastric and duodenal ulcers.

G. **What medications are being given?** Certain medications are associated with an increased incidence of GI bleeding.
   1. **Maternal medications.** Some maternal medications can cross the placenta (aspirin, cephalothin, and phenobarbital) and cause coagulation disorders in the infant. Thiazides in pregnancy can be associated with neonatal thrombocytopenia.
   2. **Infant medications.** The most common are indomethacin, NSAIDs, theophylline (rare), heparin, and corticosteroids.

H. **Was vitamin K given at birth?** Failure to give vitamin K at birth may result in a vitamin K deficiency bleeding, which can present at different times. See Section III.B.4a.

I. **Is there a history of melena?** Melena signifies significant UGI bleeding or possibly swallowed maternal blood with rapid transit time.

J. **Does the infant have a syndrome or condition that is associated with gastrointestinal bleeding?** These are rare causes of UGI bleeding in a neonate.
   1. **Down syndrome:** Meckel diverticulum, Hirschsprung disease, pyloric stenosis.
   2. **Turner syndrome:** Venous ectasia, inflammatory bowel disease.
   3. **Klippel-Trenaunay syndrome and blue rubber bleb nevus syndrome:** Vascular malformations.

4. **Osler-Weber-Rendu syndrome (hereditary hemorrhagic telangiectasia):** Epistaxis and vascular malformations, acute and chronic digestive tract bleeding.

5. **Epidermolysis bullosa:** Anal fissures, esophageal lesions, and strictures of the colon.

6. **Ehlers-Danlos syndrome and pseudoxanthoma elasticum:** Fragile blood vessel wall structure.

7. **Hermansky-Pudlak syndrome:** Platelet dysfunction, inflammatory bowel disease.

8. **Glycogen storage disease type 1b:** Inflammatory bowel disease.

9. **Zellweger cerebrohepatorenal syndrome:** GI bleeding.

10. **Curry-Jones syndrome:** UGI bleeding.

III. **Differential diagnosis**

A. **Conditions that are not a true gastrointestinal bleed**

1. **Swallowing of maternal blood accounts for approximately 10% of cases.** Typically, blood is swallowed during cesarean delivery, but can be swallowed during a vaginal birth as well. Swallowed blood irritates the stomach and can cause vomiting. Infants with this problem are usually only a few hours old, are not sick, and usually have a positive Apt test result. Infants with swallowed maternal blood can present with hematemesis or melena.

2. **Swallowing of blood from a cracked nipple or fissure** during breast feeding can also cause it.

3. **Swallowing of amniotic fluid** with an antepartum hemorrhage bleeding into the amniotic fluid normally presents with melena stools but can present with UGI bleeding.

4. **Trauma from nasopharyngeal bleeding or endotracheal intubation.**

5. **Medications** that can alter the color of the stool or emesis are rifampin, bismuth, and iron.

B. **True gastrointestinal bleed.** UGI bleeding in newborns is usually associated with clinically relevant mucosal lesions of the UGI tract, with gastric ulcers more common than duodenal ulcers. Based on 1 study, 20% of infants admitted to the neonatal intensive care unit and 53% of mechanically ventilated infants have signs of GI bleeding. The most common causes of UGI bleeding are idiopathic, trauma from NG tube, stress-induced gastritis/ulcers, vitamin K deficiency disease, sepsis, and cow's milk protein allergy.

1. **Idiopathic.** A large percentage of cases have no clear diagnosis and usually resolve within several days.

2. **Trauma**

a. **Nasogastric trauma.** Forceful insertion or too large a tube can cause trauma. Frequent aspiration to identify gastric residuals can cause trauma. The bleeding from this is usually minimal.

b. **Vigorous/continuous suctioning or lavage.**

c. **Traumatic esophagitis.** This has been reported in newborns possibly from pharyngeal, esophageal, or gastric suction at birth.

3. **Stress-related mucosal lesions occur in the esophagus, stomach, or duodenum (up to 75% of preterm infants).** These can be caused by an increase in gastric acid secretion and laxity of gastric sphincters in infants. Prematurity, neonatal distress, and mechanical ventilation are associated with stress gastritis. Stress-induced ulceration in the stomach is secondary to birth asphyxia, prolonged labor, RDS, sepsis, caesarean deliveries. Maternal stress in the third trimester with increased maternal gastrin may also play a part. UGI bleeding in healthy full-term infants is often associated with clinically relevant mucosal lesions of the UGI tract. Absence of bloody aspirate does not exclude stress-related mucosal lesions. Many infants with these lesions on endoscopy do not have UGI bleeding.

     a. Esophagus. Esophagitis (hemorrhage or ulcerative), Mallory-Weiss tear (associated with vomiting).

     b. Gastric. Stress gastritis from illness, trauma, increased ICP, stress induced ulcer (occur more frequent in stomach than duodenum in neonates), gastritis due to viral infections including cytomegalovirus.

     c. Duodenum. Duodenitis, duodenal mucosal lesions, vascular malformation single stress ulcers.

     d. Gastroesophageal lesions. Infants tend to have gastric and esophageal lesions together.

4. **Coagulopathy.** Vitamin K deficiency bleeding and DIC account for 20% of the cases of UGI bleeding in newborns.

     a. Vitamin K deficiency disease. There are 3 forms:

        i. Early form (first day of life) is related to maternal medications affecting production of vitamin K by the neonate (barbiturates, oral anticoagulant, anticonvulsants, phenytoin, rifampin, isoniazid, warfarin).

        ii. Classic form (between days 2 and 7) of life is more commonly seen in infants with inadequate intake of breast milk and when an infant has not received vitamin K at birth (eg, home delivery).

        iii. Late form (between 2 weeks and 6 months of age) is secondary to inadequate vitamin K intake (breast-fed infants) or hepatobiliary disease.

     b. Disseminated intravascular coagulation. This can occur after infection, shock, liver failure, and severe fetal asphyxia.

     c. Congenital coagulopathies. Most commonly factor VIII deficiency (hemophilia A) and factor IX deficiency (hemophilia B).

5. **Allergic colitis** is caused by allergy to cow's milk (milk protein intolerance) or soy protein after it has been introduced. Can present with esophagitis but lower GI bleeding is more common.

6. **Medications (drug-induced bleeding).** Indomethacin, corticosteroids, heparin, NSAIDs, sulindac, theophylline (rare), and other drugs may cause UGI tract bleeding. High-dose dexamethasone is associated with stress and perforated ulcers and hemorrhage in the newborn. **Maternal use** of aspirin, cephalothin, and phenobarbital can cause coagulation disorders in the infant. Thiazides in pregnancy can be associated with neonatal thrombocytopenia.

7. **Congenital gastrointestinal defects** such as intestinal duplications (most common) (eg, esophageal duplication). Less common: gastric volvulus, duodenal web, antral web, heterotopic pancreatic tissue in the stomach, malrotation with volvulus, Hirschsprung disease with enterocolitis, intussusception, duplication cyst, and Meckel diverticulitis. Bowel obstruction can cause UGI bleeding.

8. **Congenital vascular anomalies** such as arteriovenous malformations, hemangiomas (isolated cavernous hemangioma of the stomach), extensive telangiectasias, and GI hemangiomas with or without a related syndrome can present with GI hemorrhage. Arteriovenous malformations associated with Osler-Weber-Rendu syndrome or blue rubber bleb nevus syndrome can cause bleeding.

9. **Liver disease/failure in the newborn.** Usually presents in older infants. Severe bleeding can occur from the following:

     a. Esophageal varices from portal hypertension from intrinsic liver disease caused by cirrhosis from biliary atresia, parenteral nutrition–induced liver disease, hemochromatosis, or extrahepatic causes (portal vein thrombosis due to umbilical vein catheterization or sepsis).

     b. Metabolic disorders that cause liver failure have associated coagulopathies that can present with GI bleeds.

     c. Ischemic injury to the liver.

10. **Necrotizing enterocolitis** is a rare cause of UGI tract bleeding.

11. **Pyloric stenosis** presents at the third to fourth weeks of life with nonbilious projectile vomiting (occasionally bloody). Hypertrophic pyloric stenosis has presented with hematemesis in the newborn.

12. **Rare causes:** Gastric teratoma/gastric tumors, Dieulafoy lesion, infection with *Serratia marcescens*, complication from intrapulmonary percussive ventilation therapy, telangiectasia involving the entire GI tract, pyloroduodenal intestinal duplication, heterotopic pancreatic tissue in the stomach, and focal foveolar hyperplasia of the gastric mucosa.

IV. **Database**

  A. **Physical examination** should focus attention on other potential bleeding sites. Carefully examine the nares and oropharynx to rule out respiratory causes of bleeding. Bruising or petechiae suggest a bleeding disorder. Note bowel sounds, abdominal distension, splenomegaly, and if there is any abdominal wall erythema. Is there evidence of portal hypertension (splenomegaly, prominent abdominal vessels)?

  B. **Laboratory studies**

   1. **Initial tests**

      a. **Testing for blood.** The Hemoccult ICT (HemoCue), an immunochemical test that gives fewer false-positive results, can be used to test the emesis or stool. Gastroccult (HemoCue) is used to test gastric fluid for blood.

      b. **Apt-Downey test** is performed to determine if swallowed maternal blood is a possible cause. This test differentiates maternal from fetal blood; fetal/newborn hemoglobin F is not hydrolyzed by a strong base, whereas maternal hemoglobin A hydrolyzes to a yellow brown. A negative test does not completely rule out swallowed maternal blood.

      c. **Hematocrit.** Should be checked as a baseline and serially to gauge the extent of blood loss. It is not a reliable index of the severity of the acute GI bleed.

      d. **Complete blood count with differential.** A change in the white blood cell count may indicate infection. Thrombocytopenia is associated with necrotizing enterocolitis (NEC) and sepsis. A low mean corpuscular volume of red cells suggests a chronic bleed.

      e. **Coagulation studies** (platelet count, prothrombin time [PT], partial thromboplastin time [PTT], fibrinogen, thrombin time, and international normalized ratio). See Table 60–1. All neonates with UGI bleeding should be screened for coagulopathy. An elevated PT and prolonged PTT suggest a coagulopathy.

      f. **Chemistry panel.** An elevated blood urea nitrogen can be seen in a massive UGI bleed.

      g. **Type and cross match** blood in case of transfusion is necessary.

Table 60–1. **COAGULATION TESTING IN VARIOUS DISEASE STATES**

Test	Vitamin K Deficiency	DIC	Liver Disease	Hemophilia Bleeding
Platelets	Normal	Reduced	Normal	Normal
PT	Prolonged	Prolonged	Prolonged	Normal
PTT	Prolonged	Prolonged	Prolonged	Prolonged
TT	Normal	Prolonged	Prolonged	Normal
Fibrinogen	Normal	Reduced	Reduced	Normal

DIC, disseminated intravascular coagulation; PT, prothrombin time; PTT, partial thromboplastin time; TT, thrombin time.

2. **Additional tests**
   a. **Liver function tests.** If cholestasis is a concern, total and direct bilirubin and liver function tests should be done. Elevated liver enzymes may indicate liver disease.
   b. **Serum pepsinogen level.** Elevated levels can indicate severe atrophic gastritis and gastric atrophy; levels can be elevated in infants with gastric and duodenal lesions.

C. **Nasogastric lavage.** Used to confirm the diagnosis and determine whether the bleeding is ongoing. Place NG tube for gastric lavage.
   1. **Nasogastric lavage is negative (no blood is seen):** No active UGI bleeding or the bleeding has stopped.
   2. **Nasogastric lavage is positive (fresh blood in stomach):** Diagnostic of UGI bleeding, including duodenal hemorrhages.
   3. **Repeated nasogastric lavage**
      a. **Clearing of the fluid:** Bleeding has stopped.
      b. **Persistent red or pink fluid:** Ongoing bleed.

D. **Imaging and other studies**
   1. **Immediate tests**
      a. **Abdominal radiograph.** Assess the bowel gas pattern and rule out NEC. The film also shows the position of the NG tube and indicates a possible surgical problem. It can help identify a bowel obstruction, pneumoperitoneum, small bowel dilatation, and pneumatosis intestinalis.
   2. **Additional tests**
      a. **Upper gastrointestinal series.** A barium contrast study can be done for nonemergent bleeding. It can evaluate for UGI bleed or midgut volvulus. Not recommended when acute bleeding is occurring.
      b. **Endoscopy.** Fiberoptic/flexible UGI endoscopy (esophagogastroduodenoscopy) is the test of choice to evaluate for hematemesis. It is used for both diagnosis and therapy. It reveals the source of bleeding in 90% of patients with UGI bleeding. It is safe (smaller endoscopes) and should be considered in bleeding that is persistent or recurrent or in cases of severe hemorrhage requiring blood transfusion. Gastric lavage and intravenous (IV) erythromycin (*controversial*) can be used prior to the test to clean the area and improve visualization of the gastric mucosa. In 1 study, the most common lesion identified by endoscopy was gastroesophagitis (unique to neonates). Erythema, erosions, diffuse bleeding, or ulcerations can also be seen.
      c. **Ultrasound.** Ultrasound can show portal hypertension. If pyloric stenosis is suspected, ultrasound of the abdomen should be done.
      d. **Hepatobiliary scan.** To rule out biliary atresia and neonatal hepatitis.

V. **Plan**
   A. **Prophylactic treatment of high-risk neonates** at risk for stress-induced gastric UGI bleeding. Cochrane review (July, 2019) found that use of an H_2 receptor antagonist decreases the risk of GI bleeding in newborns at high risk of GI bleeding.
   B. **Consider giving parenteral vitamin K** to infants if vitamin K deficiency bleeding is suspected, even before the coagulation results are done.
   C. **General measures.** Evaluate the infant, verify if the bleed is a true GI bleed (eg, rule out swallowed maternal blood, trauma from ETT, nasopharyngeal trauma), assess if bleeding is minimal or significant, if the bleeding is ongoing, if there is any hemodynamic compromise (check heart rate, blood pressure, capillary refill).
   D. **If the infant appears well and bleeding is minimal and there is no evidence of hemodynamic compromise**, rule out more benign causes (mild esophagitis or gastritis, milk protein allergy, and other causes). Do the Apt test if swallowed maternal blood is suspected as the cause. Treatment depends upon the cause: observation, possible antisecretory medications can be used (if indicated), possible formula change.

E. **If the infant is actively bleeding, and the bleeding is significant/severe:** Do a quick airway, breathing, and circulation assessment. Order stat laboratory tests including a type and cross to ensure blood is available if needed. These infants may show signs of hemodynamic instability with decreased vascular volume, hypotension, and impending shock. The most important goal is to stabilize the infant and stop the active bleeding. Pediatric gastroenterologist/pediatric surgery consultation is recommended for a significant UGI bleeding.

1. **Airway/breathing.** Assess the airway and breathing and make sure the infant does not require intubation and mechanical ventilation. Supplemental oxygen should be started.

2. **Circulation.** Verify vascular access. Assess if volume replacement is necessary. Check blood pressure, heart rate, and capillary refill. If the blood pressure is low or dropping, crystalloid (usually normal saline) can be given immediately. **Blood replacement** may be indicated, depending on the amount of blood loss and the result of hematocrit values obtained from the laboratory. Fresh-frozen plasma and platelet transfusions may be necessary.

3. **Stop the acute episode of gastrointestinal bleeding**

   a. **Gastric lavage** (with room temperature or tepid water, 1/2 normal saline [NS], or NS 5 mL/kg) by NG tube until the bleeding has subsided. This should not be done beyond 10 minutes if the NG fluid does not clear. (*Note:* There is *controversy* about which fluid to use. Hyponatremia may occur if water is used and hypernatremia if NS is used. Follow your institution's guidelines.) **Never use ice or cold water lavages** as it lowers the infant's core temperature. Gastric lavage is *controversial*, and there is no definitive evidence to support that it controls hemorrhage.

   b. **Epinephrine lavage** (*controversial*). Use 0.1 mL (1:10,000 solution) diluted in 10 mL of sterile water. Considered if tepid water lavages do not stop the bleeding.

   c. **Therapeutic endoscopy.** This has been recommended in patients with active bleeding that cannot be controlled to avoid surgery. Gastric lavage and IV erythromycin (*controversial*) can be used prior to the test to clean the area and improve visualization of the gastric mucosa. **Endoscopic hemostatic techniques may be necessary in massive bleeds** and include cautery (electrocoagulation, laser photocoagulation, heater probe thermocoagulation), injection therapy (sclerosing agents, dilute epinephrine), and mechanical therapy (hemoclips and endoscopic band ligation).

   d. **Intravenous acid suppression therapy** has been used in adults and has reduced the rate of rebleeding. Cochrane review (July, 2019) found that there is low-quality evidence that the use of an H_2 receptor antagonist or proton pump inhibitor decreases the duration of UGI bleeding. Many physicians will treat infants with GI bleeding with acid suppression medications. **Use of ranitidine (H_2 blocker) has been shown to control mild-to-moderate bleeding in 24 to 48 hours.**

   e. **Somatostatin and a long-acting synthetic peptide analog octreotide.** These are typically used to decreased bleeding in some cases of variceal bleeding. These medications decrease blood flow to the portal system, thereby decreasing variceal bleeding. These medications have been associated with a decreased risk of continued bleeding in some patients. Their use in acute bleeding ulcer disease is *controversial* because they also decrease splanchnic blood flow and prevent gastric acid secretion.

F. **Disease-specific measures**

1. **Swallowing of maternal blood.** Observation only.

2. **Trauma** is usually self-limiting, requiring observation only.

3. **Stress-related mucosal lesions.** Commonly diagnosed after an episode of GI bleeding by endoscopy. This disorder is difficult to confirm using radiologic

studies. Remission usually occurs, and recurrence is rare. Acid suppression agents are used even though evidence-based recommendations are not available. The following medications have been used: antacids, acid suppression medications (proton pump inhibitors [PPIs], H_2 receptor antagonists), and mucosal protective agents (sucralfate and bismuth salts).

    a. **Antacids neutralize gastric acid in the lumen of the esophagus or stomach and inhibit pepsin activity** such as aluminum/magnesium hydroxide (eg, Maalox) 0.5 to 1 mL/kg or 0.25 mL/kg, 6 times per day, placed in the NG tube until bleeding has subsided. This is *controversial* because it may cause concretions in the GI tract and may increase the risk of infection and feeding intolerance in infants receiving gavage feedings. Calcium- and aluminum-containing antacids cause diarrhea, and magnesium-containing antacids can cause constipation. Possible side effects include hypermagnesemia, hypophosphatemia, and intestinal obstruction. Chronic use of antacids can be associated with aluminum toxicity and milk-alkali syndrome.

    b. **Acid suppression medications** are recommended for erosive esophagitis and gastric and duodenal ulcers and are only beneficial if the infants have acid-related problems. The majority of these medications are not approved for infants <1 month of age. A few are approved for infants >1 month of age.

        i. **Proton pump inhibitors** block gastric acid production and decrease pepsin secretion. They are superior to H_2 blockers in the treatment of peptic ulcers after endoscopy. Studies show they have faster healing times than H_2 blockers. These include esomeprazole (Nexium), omeprazole (Prilosec), lansoprazole (Prevacid), rabeprazole (AcipHex), and pantoprazole (Protonix). Studies with these agents are promising, but they are not all approved in neonates. Esomeprazole is currently recommended only as treatment for erosive esophagitis. Esomeprazole and omeprazole are approved in infants >1 month of age for erosive esophagitis. There is an increased risk of pneumonia and diarrhea. See doses in Chapter 155.

        ii. **H_2 receptor antagonists** suppress gastric acid production by binding to H_2 receptors, which inhibits the effects of histamine. They have a faster onset of action but shorter duration of action than PPIs. These are less effective than PPIs in decreasing gastric acidity. **Ranitidine and famotidine are preferred** because they have fewer side effects. See Chapter 155 for dosing information. Follow your institution's guidelines. Cimetidine is rarely used because of adverse effects and clinically significant drug interactions. H_2-blocker therapy is associated with higher rates of NEC in very low birthweight infants and infections.

        iii. **Mucosal protective agents (sucralfate or bismuth salts)** are medications that provide physical protection of the gastric mucosa and promote mucosal healing. These may play a role in prophylaxis of UGI bleeding in neonates.

4. **Coagulation disorders.** See also Chapter 92.

    a. **Vitamin K deficiency bleeding.** When vitamin K deficiency is suspected, vitamin K should be administered IV or subcutaneously. Intramuscular injection can result in severe hematoma. One milligram of vitamin K IV stops the hemorrhage within 2 hours.

    b. **Disseminated intravascular coagulation.** Associated with bleeding from other sites. Coagulation studies are abnormal (increased PT and PTT with decreased fibrinogen levels; see Table 60–1). Treat the underlying condition and support blood pressure with multiple transfusions of colloid as needed. Platelets may be required. The cause of DIC (eg, hypoxia, acidosis, bacterial or viral disease, toxoplasmosis, NEC, shock, or erythroblastosis fetalis) must be investigated. Several obstetric disorders, including abruptio placentae, chorioangioma, eclampsia, and fetal death associated with twin gestation, may give rise to DIC.

    c. **Congenital coagulopathies.** The most common that present with bleeding are secondary to factor VIII deficiency (hemophilia A) and factor IX deficiency (hemophilia B). Specific laboratory testing and appropriate consultation with a pediatric hematologist are appropriate.

5. **Allergic colitis.** Eliminate the formula and change to a hypoallergenic formula.

6. **Drug-induced bleeding.** The drug responsible for the bleeding should be stopped, if possible.

7. **Congenital defects** such as gastric volvulus, malrotation with volvulus, Hirschsprung disease with enterocolitis, and gastric duplication require urgent surgical consultation.

8. **Gastrointestinal bleeding due to liver disease.** Usually due to variceal bleeding. The following medications decrease blood flow to the portal system, thereby decreasing variceal bleeding.

    a. **Octreotide (Sandostatin) is an analog of somatostatin.** Dosage recommended (safety and dosing not firmly established) is 1 mcg/kg IV bolus, followed by 1 mcg/kg/h IV infusion. If no bleeding occurs in 12 hours, decrease the dose by 50%. Then stop the medication when the dose is 25% of the initial dose.

    b. **Vasopressin (Pitressin).** Used in neonates but has many adverse effects, so it is not recommended.

    c. **Terlipressin** is a long-acting analog of vasopressin with a good safety profile, but hyponatremia and seizures have been reported in the pediatric population.

9. **Necrotizing enterocolitis.** See Chapter 109.

10. **Pyloric stenosis.** Hydration and surgical pyloromyotomy are necessary.

61 Hematuria

I. **Problem.** A nurse reports that an infant has a red-stained diaper and states the infant may have hematuria. **Hematuria is the presence of gross or microscopic blood in the urine.** It is more common in premature infants in the neonatal intensive care unit than in healthy newborns. Studies on incidence are lacking, but one older retrospective study reporting gross hematuria in 0.21 per 1000 admitted infants <1 month old. The differential diagnosis in neonates is different than in older children. Gross hematuria requires an immediate evaluation, whereas microscopic hematuria is usually transient and benign in the neonate.

II. **Immediate questions**

  A. **Does the infant really have hematuria?** A red-stained diaper usually signifies hematuria but may be due to **pseudohematuria** (red-colored urine in the absence of red cells or hemoglobin) or **blood from a nonurinary source** that is mistaken for gross hematuria in the diaper or **myoglobinuria or hemoglobinuria**. First it needs to be decided whether the urine dipstick is positive or negative for blood. If urine is negative for blood then it is pseudohematuria. If it positive for blood microscopic urinalysis needs to be done to confirm RBCs are from the urine.

    1. **Negative dipstick for blood**

      a. **Urate crystals** can present as pinkish to reddish brown discoloration in the diaper. It is more commonly seen in volume depletion, especially in breast-fed neonates. This is a benign condition, and treatment is increased fluid intake.

   b. **Congenital erythropoietic porphyria** (Gunther disease) is a rare autosomal recessive disease due to deficiency of the uroporphyrinogen III cosynthetase enzyme, which results in an accumulation of type I porphyrins. It can present as pink to brown staining of the diaper because of porphyrin pigment in the urine. Red fluorescence of urine on a diaper under a Wood's light (ultraviolet) indicates porphyria (normal urine shows greenish blue/yellow).

   c. **Medications that cause urine to look red or pink** include rifampin, phenytoin, methyldopa, chloroquine, nitrofurantoin, senna, heparin, salicylates, ibuprofen, phenothiazines, phenylbutazone, daunorubicin, and doxorubicin.

2. **Positive dipstick for blood**

   a. **Nonurinary sources of bleeding that can be mistaken for gross hematuria in the diaper.**

      i. **Vaginal bleeding (pseudomenses)** from maternal hormonal withdrawal.

      ii. **Rectal or other gastrointestinal bleeding**

      iii. **Postcircumcision bleeding**

      iv. **Severe diaper rash with excoriation**

   b. **Myoglobinuria and hemoglobinuria.** In myoglobinuria (seen in severe perinatal asphyxia) or hemoglobinuria (seen with ABO incompatibility with intravascular hemolysis), the urine looks red and the dipstick is positive for blood, but there are no red blood cells on microscopic examination.

   c. **Urinary source of bleeding.** See causes below.

B. **What is the degree of hematuria?** Hematuria is classified as **gross hematuria** (urine that is visibly discolored (seen by naked eye) by blood that can be red or brown colored or frank blood) or **microscopic hematuria** (defined as ≥5 red blood cells per high-power field on a spun urine sample). Gross hematuria requires immediate evaluation. Microscopic hematuria is more common in premature infants and increases with a lower birth weight and gestation. If present in a neonate with no renal or urologic abnormalities, it is usually transient and requires no treatment, but if prolonged a work up should be done.

C. **What is the urine output?** Low urine output should raise concern for obstruction of the urinary tract. Beyond the first 24 hours of life, urine output should be 1 to 2 mL/kg/h. Spontaneous voiding may not occur until after 24 hours of life. If the newborn is not symptomatic and does not have a distended bladder, continuing observation for the wet diaper is appropriate.

D. **Were prenatal ultrasounds normal?** Abnormalities including obstructive uropathies, hydronephrosisrenal/abdominal masses, tumors, and renal cystic changes may cause hematuria. Most cases of autosomal recessive polycystic kidney disease and some cases of autosomal dominant polycystic kidney disease are diagnosed by prenatal ultrasound.

E. **Has there been any instrumentation of the urinary tract?** Traumatic catheterization, bladder aspiration, or other instrumentation of the urinary tract may lead to hematuria that is usually transient.

F. **Was there a maternal history of diabetes?** Maternal diabetes should raise suspicion of renal vein thrombosis.

G. **Has vitamin K been given? Was the mother on any medications that would affect vitamin K in the newborn?** Consider vitamin K deficiency bleeding. Babies of mothers on certain medications that decrease vitamin K storage and function in the infant are at increased risk of having bleeding in the first 24 hours from vitamin K deficiency. These medications include anticonvulsants, antituberculosis drugs, some antibiotics (cephalosporins), and vitamin K antagonists (warfarin).

H. **Is there an umbilical artery catheter?** Presence of a catheter with hematuria should raise suspicion for possible aortic or renal artery thrombosis.

III. **Differential diagnosis.** Hematuria is not common in newborns, and most normal newborns do not have hematuria. However, hematuria is still one of the most common reasons for referral to a pediatric urologist or pediatric nephrologist. Transient hematuria is common in critically ill infants. The most common cause of gross hematuria is renal vein thrombosis.

A. Verify it is true hematuria. Rule out causes that are not hematuria first. See Section II.A above.

B. Causes of hematuria

1. **Trauma.** Gross hematuria can be seen after a traumatic birth (rare) or after a suprapubic bladder aspiration (more common up to 3.4%), urethral catheterization (especially if urethra narrow or obstructed), cystoscopy, or placement of percutaneous nephrostomy tubes. Trauma to the urethral mucosa usually causes microscopic hematuria. Bladder hematomas or a lacerated vessel on the anterior bladder wall can occur from a suprapubic bladder aspiration and cause hematuria. It is important to note that mild birth trauma can cause bleeding in a kidney with hydronephrosis.

2. **Vascular thrombosis of an artery or vein can cause hematuria.** Neonates are at an increased risk for thrombosis because of their small-caliber vasculature, their kidney has a lower perfusion pressure, imbalance of coagulation factors, and decreased level of clotting inhibitors. Multiple maternal factors (diabetes, chorioamnionitis, thrombotic states) and infant factors (sepsis, hypotension, hypoxia, dehydration, polycythemia, umbilical artery catheterization) also increase their risk.

   a. **Renal vein thrombosis.** Renal vein thrombosis (RVT) is the most common thrombosis in newborns not associated with an intravascular catheter. It is most common in males and on the left side and is more commonly unilateral. It usually presents within 24 hours or on the second day of life. The classic triad (only present in up to 22% of patients) is gross hematuria, flank mass, and thrombocytopenia. Consider RVT in an infant of a diabetic mother or an infant with cyanotic congenital heart disease, birth asphyxia or in utero fetal distress, dehydration, coagulation abnormalities (activated protein C-resistance, factor V Leiden mutation), polycythemia, infection, prematurity, conjoined twin, or an umbilical venous catheter.

   b. **Renal artery thrombosis.** Less common than RVT, renal artery thrombosis (RAT) is associated with aortic thrombus (often) and an umbilical artery catheter (almost always). Infants present with gross or microscopic hematuria, thrombocytopenia, and hypertension.

3. **Renal diseases**

   a. **Renal cortical necrosis** can be secondary to a kidney insult (cortical ischemia secondary to sepsis, blood loss, NEC, dehydration, severe hypoxic ischemic injury, placental abruption, twin–twin transfusion, or nephrotoxic medications). It can cause microscopic or gross hematuria and oliguria, hypertension, abnormal electrolytes, and an increased creatinine.

   b. **Acute tubular necrosis** rarely causes gross hematuria.

   c. **Glomerulonephritis** (rare in neonates) causes microscopic or gross hematuria, proteinuria, hypertension, and edema. Neonatal lupus, syphilis, and neonatal hemolytic-uremic syndrome are potential causes.

4. **Structural abnormalities/malformations in the urinary tract.** Any cause of obstruction or anatomic anomaly can cause hematuria.

   a. **Posterior urethral valves.** Most common cause of lower urinary tract obstruction (males). Most are diagnosed prenatally with hydronephrosis. A small percent of neonates can have gross hematuria within the first month of life.

   b. **Congenital ureteropelvic junction obstruction (rare).** Presents with hydronephrosis and gross hematuria.

   c. **Cystic kidney disease.** Autosomal recessive polycystic kidney disease and autosomal dominant polycystic kidney disease can present with gross or microscopic hematuria and proteinuria. Infants with ARPKD can have a flank mass and respiratory symptoms.

    d. Medullary sponge kidney and ureterocele (rare causes of hematuria in newborn).

  5. Urolithiasis

    a. Nephrocalcinosis (calcium salts within the renal tissue) or nephrolithiasis (formation of stones in the kidney). Nephrocalcinosis caused by calcium oxalate (most common) or calcium phosphate is more common in preterm infants (up to 40%) because of renal immaturity and use of medications. Both nephrocalcinosis and nephrolithiasis can cause hematuria, but it is more common in nephroliathisis. Term infants with distal renal tubular acidosis, Dent disease, or hyperparathyroidism can have nephrocalcinosis associated with hypercalciuria. Certain medications can cause nephrocalcinosis (dexamethasone, glucocorticoids, methylxanthines).

    b. Urolithiasis (formation of stones anywhere in the urinary track) can be seen after chronic furosemide administration.

  6. Tumors. Renal tumors are very rare in neonates, with the majority identified by prenatal ultrasound. Clinically, they present with an abdominal mass (more common) and hematuria. The most common renal tumor in neonates is congenital mesoblastic nephroma, followed by Wilms tumor. Renal tumors are associated with several syndromes (Beckwith-Wiedemann, Denys-Drash, and WAGR [Wilms tumor, aniridia, genitourinary anomalies, and intellectual disability] syndrome). Other tumors include rhabdomyosarcoma, nephroblastoma, angiomas, ossifying renal tumor of infancy, and bladder hemangioma (rare).

  7. Infection. Infections can cause hematuria specifically: sepsis, UTI, viral infections, infectious endocarditis. Infants with a UTI can have hematuria, but it is not common. Neonates with urosepsis not caused by *Escherichia coli* have an increased risk of structural abnormalities. Viral infections (adenovirus and BK virus) can cause hematuria in immunocompromised children. Infectious endocarditis (rare) is more common in neonates who have congenital heart disease or sepsis and can present with a new or changed heart murmur and hematuria.

  8. Hematologic disorders

    a. Vitamin K deficiency bleeding, previously called hemorrhagic disease of the newborn, can manifest with gross or microscopic hematuria. However, infants more commonly present with bleeding elsewhere (eg, umbilical stump, gastrointestinal tract, skin). It is seen in infants who did not receive vitamin K prophylaxis and exclusively breast-fed infants, and the risk is increased in infants of mothers on certain medications (anticonvulsants, rifampin, isoniazid, and warfarin).

    b. Thrombocytopenia. Severe thrombocytopenia (platelets <60,000 μL) can cause microscopic hematuria and is more common in premature infants.

    c. Disseminated intravascular coagulation. Seen in asphyxia, sepsis, and respiratory distress syndrome.

    d. Polycythemia can cause hematuria.

  9. Medications. Most common are nonsteroidal anti-inflammatory drugs, especially indomethacin, which can cause interstitial nephritis and microscopic hematuria.

IV. Database

  A. History

    1. Include timing of onset of hematuria, persistent or intermittent, correlation with illnesses or trauma, and association with other symptoms (eg, fever). History can guide the full evaluation.

    2. Prenatal history. Was there a maternal prenatal ultrasound? Was it abnormal? (Any masses or kidney abnormalities? Was amniotic fluid volume within normal limits?)

    3. Maternal history. Does the mother have kidney disease (genetic, kidney stones, glomerulonephritis, autoimmune disorders)? Any diabetes or bleeding disorders?

What medications was the mother on? Are there any bleeding disorders in the mother? Previous pregnancies?

4. **Family history** should focus on genetic kidney disease, stone disease, or bleeding disorders.
5. **Birth history** should focus on prematurity or if any resuscitation was required. Was vitamin K given at birth? When did the infant first urinate?
6. **Postnatal history.** Urine output? Weight gain or loss? Breast fed or bottle? Is the infant on a high calcium formula or on TPN (increased risk of nephrocalcinosis)? Any evidence of syndromes (hemihypertrophy and Beckwith-Wiedemann syndrome associated with medullary sponge kidney)? Beckwith-Wiedemann and Denys-Drash and WAGR are associated with renal tumors.

B. **Physical examination.** Note temperature (infection?), blood pressure (hypertension suggests kidney involvement or ARPKD, hypotension suggests infection or cardiac dysfunction), bruising, petechiae (suggest bleeding disorder), or edema (glomerulonephritis). Abdominal mass (obstruction, neoplasm, ARPKD [flank mass], renal vein thrombosis) may be noted. Is there subcutaneous fat necrosis (hypercalcemia)? Remove the diaper to examine the genitalia and rectum. Note the presence of urinary or umbilical artery catheters.

C. **Laboratory studies**
   1. **Urinalysis**
      a. **Urine dipstick evaluation. A positive urine dipstick confirms the presence of red blood cells or free myoglobin or hemoglobin.** Protein, leukocytes, and nitrates should be evaluated as well. Association with proteinuria is concerning and indicates significant abnormality in the kidney (eg, glomerulonephritis). White blood cells (WBCs) and nitrates suggest infection.
      b. **Microscopic examination of urine** is done on any positive dipstick of the urine and helps to identify the origin of the hematuria. Normal red blood cells (RBCs) suggest lower tract origin, whereas dysmorphic RBCs suggest upper tract disease. RBC casts are seen in glomerulonephritis, and WBCs with bacteria on a properly collected specimen suggest infection. There are no RBCs in the microscopic examination of urine in hemoglobinuria or myoglobinuria.
   2. **Urine culture.** Collection of urine by catheterization or suprapubic bladder aspiration to rule out UTI.
   3. **Complete blood count and differential and platelet count.** This may help diagnose an infection, thrombocytopenia, or polycythemia.
   4. **Serum blood urea nitrogen and creatinine levels.** Abnormal levels may indicate renal insufficiency; they may also reflect maternal renal function during the first week of life.
   5. **Coagulation studies.** Thrombocytopenia may indicate renal vein thrombosis. Abnormal prothrombin time and partial thromboplastin time may indicate disseminated intravascular coagulation or hemorrhagic diseases of the newborn.
   6. **Electrolytes, calcium, phosphorus, and spot urine calcium/creatinine (if term infant)** and parathyroid hormone level for nephrocalcinosis.

D. **Imaging and other studies**
   1. **Renal and bladder ultrasonography is usually the first test** to show upper urinary tract dilation, congenital anomalies of the urinary tract or neoplasms, or renal calcification. In renal cortical necrosis, atrophy of the kidney can be seen with increased echogenicity and loss of cortical medullary differentiation. Ultrasound findings of RVT vary depending on when the scan is done (early: enlarged kidney with increased echogenicity; later: decreased kidney size, calcification of thrombus).
   2. **Renal Doppler ultrasonography** evaluates renal blood flow. In renal cortical necrosis there is decreased perfusion with patent renal vessels. In RVT there is decreased flow in the main renal vein or abnormal flow in the renal vein branches.
   3. **Voiding cystourethrogram** to rule out bladder outlet obstruction.

4. **Computed tomography/magnetic resonance imaging** may be used for evaluation of neoplasms and renal vein thrombosis.
5. **Radioisotope renography** is rarely required but may be used to assess for functional renal parenchyma. In cortical necrosis, it will show no perfusion of the kidney.
6. **Cystoscopy is rarely required.** For evaluation of recurrent gross hematuria or for urethral and bladder pathology or if ultrasound shows something suspicious in the bladder.
7. **Echocardiogram to rule out cardiac vegetations** if infectious endocarditis is suspected.

V. **Plan.** Most cases of microhematuria are transient and resolve without any specific therapy. Some authors recommend that 2 of 3 urinalyses show microhematuria before an evaluation is undertaken. Persistent hematuria or gross hematuria requires urologic or nephrology consultation. **It is important to note that gross hematuria may cause obstructive ureteropelvic junction clots that may cause hydronephrosis.** Some clinicians recommend serial ultrasounds during the time of the gross hematuria.

A. **Trauma.** Expectant management for minor birth trauma or instrumentation of the urinary tract. The hematuria is typically self-limited and resolves quickly. Intervention is rarely required.
B. **Vascular.** RVT and RAT: supportive care, removal of arterial catheter for RAT, thrombolytic agents, heparin (see Chapter 92).
C. **Infections.** Treat with appropriate antibiotics.
D. **Obstruction.** Indwelling urethral catheter for bladder outlet obstruction; may require acute or nonurgent operative intervention for congenital anomalies of the urinary tract based on urology consultation.
E. **Nephrocalcinosis.** Treat with increased fluids and thiazide diuretic. Long-term follow-up is recommended.
F. **Tumors.** Operative intervention may be needed, and consultation with pediatric urologist and oncologist is suggested. For congenital mesoblastic nephroma and Wilms tumor, the treatment is based on stage and may involve radical nephrectomy or a combination of surgery and chemotherapy (see Chapter 127).
G. **Hematologic.** Correct coagulopathies if present (see Chapter 92). For vitamin K deficiency bleeding, give vitamin K; for severe bleeding, fresh-frozen plasma may be necessary. For microscopic hematuria and thrombocytopenia no treatment is necessary. For gross hematuria and thrombocytopenia consider platelet transfusion.
H. **Renal.** Supportive measures and treatment of the specific cause. Restrict fluid intake and replace insensible losses. May require renal replacement therapy (dialysis or transplantation). (See Chapter 86.) With renal cortical necrosis, acute dialysis may be needed with risk of kidney failure.

62 Hyperbilirubinemia: Conjugated, On Call

I. **Problem.** An infant's direct (conjugated) serum bilirubin level is elevated at 3 mg/dL. Conjugated bilirubin is the fraction of bilirubin that is conjugated with glucuronic acid in the liver to form bilirubin diglucuronide. It is a biochemical marker of cholestasis. Neonatal cholestasis is **conjugated hyperbilirubinemia** in the newborn period and is an accumulation of bile substances in the liver. It is secondary to decreased bile secretion from the liver to the duodenum and usually signifies an underlying hepatobiliary or metabolic dysfunction. Cholestasis can be **extrahepatic/obstructive** (most commonly biliary atresia, other causes include choledochal/biliary cyst, inspissated bile syndrome, obstructive tumors, gallstones) or **intrahepatic/nonobstructive** (idiopathic, infectious, metabolic/genetic, autoimmune, or toxic). This chapter incorporates recommendations from the North American Society for Pediatric Gastroenterology, Hepatology, and Nutrition (NASPGHAN), the European Society for Pediatric Gastroenterology, Hepatology, and Nutrition (ESPGHAN), and the American Academy of Pediatrics (AAP) on the management of conjugated hyperbilirubinemia in the newborn infant 35 or more weeks of gestation. **NASPGHAN defines an abnormal direct bilirubin** as >1 mg/dL. The **AAP defines an abnormal direct bilirubin** as >1 mg/dL if the total serum bilirubin (TSB) level is ≤5 mg/dL. If the TSB level is >5 mg/dL, a direct bilirubin >20% of the TSB is abnormal. The majority of prolonged physiologic jaundice is secondary to breast milk jaundice, but it is important not to misdiagnose cholestasis as physiologic jaundice because this will delay the early diagnosis that is essential for treatment. **Conjugated hyperbilirubinemia is never normal or physiologic and indicates hepatobiliary dysfunction.** It occurs in 1 in every 2500 term infants, and common causes in the newborn infant are biliary atresia (25%–40%), monogenic disorders (25%), and multifactorial or unknown etiologies. The more common causes in premature infants are prolonged parenteral nutrition and sepsis. Timely diagnosis is critical for successful treatment and optimal prognosis, in particular for biliary atresia. Kasai hepatic portoenterostomy should be done as soon as possible to establish bile flow and is best performed within the first 60 days of life (approximately 70% with bile flow vs <25% with bile flow at >90 days). See also Chapter 98 for additional discussion on conjugated hyperbilirubinemia management.

II. **Immediate questions**
  A. **What is the stool and urine color?**
    1. **Dark urine.** The presence of dark urine is a nonspecific indicator of increased conjugated bilirubin.
    2. **Stool color.** A stool examination is vital to the workup of every infant with cholestasis. A persistent pale or clay-colored stool suggests an extrahepatic obstruction/biliary obstruction. When bile flow decreases, the stool starts to lose its normal pigmentation. One or 2 pale stools usually do not indicate disease, and infants with biliary atresia can have normal stools.
      a. **Pale/clay/depigmented stool** with increased serum bilirubin can be associated with biliary atresia, choledochal/biliary cyst, biliary sludge (inspissated bile syndrome), Alagille syndrome, neonatal sclerosing cholangitis, cystic fibrosis, and α_1-antitrypsin deficiency.
      b. **Normal stool with increased serum bilirubin:** Consider infection, hypothyroidism, panhypopituitarism, cystic fibrosis, α_1-antitrypsin, progressive familial intrahepatic cholestasis (PFIC), and metabolic and storage disorders.
  B. **Does the infant appear sick?** Infants with intrahepatic cholestasis often appear ill, whereas those with extrahepatic cholestasis usually do not. **Infants with cholestasis who are ill appearing warrant an immediate evaluation for bacterial sepsis** because an infection can cause hepatocellular damage and increase bilirubin levels. Other disorders that can present with cholestasis and an ill-appearing infant include urinary tract infection, galactosemia, tyrosinemia, hypopituitarism, fructosemia, gestational alloimmune liver disease (fetal demise with acute liver failure), any metabolic disorder, an acute common duct obstruction, or hemolysis. These disorders also require a rapid diagnosis and treatment.
  C. **Is the infant receiving total parenteral nutrition? Parenteral nutrition–associated liver disease (PNALD)** does not occur until the infant has been on total parenteral nutrition (TPN) for >2 weeks. It is more common in premature infants. Resumption of enteral foods improves cholestasis.
  D. **Have any risk factors been identified?** The **most important risk factors** are prematurity, prolonged exposure to parenteral nutrition, lack of enteral feeding, and infection. Other risk factors include small for gestational age, congenital infections, hemolytic process (Rh or ABO incompatibility), and trisomy 21.

E. **At what age did the direct hyperbilirubinemia occur?** Age at which the direct hyperbilirubinemia occurs may provide a clue to the diagnosis.

   1. **Early-onset conjugated hyperbilirubinemia** (≤14 days). More likely due to nonhepatic causes and more infants were likely to be sick. Causes include: multifactorial liver injury (eg, antibiotics, TPN, sedatives, mechanical ventilation, surgery), sepsis, inborn error of metabolism, idiopathic, biliary atresia, choledochal cyst.

   2. **Late-onset conjugated hyperbilirubinemia** (15–28 days). Idiopathic, multifactorial liver injury (eg, antibiotics, TPN, sedatives, mechanical ventilation, surgery, inotropic support), biliary atresia, sepsis, cytomegalovirus (CMV) infection/choledochal cyst, inborn errors of metabolism.

   3. **Presence of direct hyperbilirubinemia immediately after birth** (within hours or few days) may be secondary to congenital infection, hemolysis (with biliary sludging), gestational alloimmune liver disease, genetic disorders, or inborn errors of metabolism.

   4. **Presence of direct hyperbilirubinemia after feedings** are established suggests that a metabolic disorder such as galactosemia may be present.

   5. **Onset of jaundice in an asymptomatic infant after the first week of life** may be secondary to an underlying infection such as urinary tract infection.

F. **Is there evidence of liver dysfunction or failure?** If presentation is accompanied by evidence of liver dysfunction or failure, the following should be highly considered in the differential diagnosis: gestational alloimmune liver disease (formerly known as neonatal hemochromatosis), infection (congenital herpes simplex virus [HSV], CMV, viral hepatitis), α_1-antitrypsin deficiency, inborn error of metabolism (tyrosinemia, galactosemia), congenital leukemia, neuroblastoma, hypoxic-ischemic event, biliary atresia, and hemoglobinopathy.

III. **Differential diagnosis.** There is a significant listing for the differential diagnosis of conjugated hyperbilirubinemia in the neonate. Clues in the history and physical examination may help to narrow the diagnosis. **Remember that any condition that alters the systemic circulation** can causes an acute ischemic injury to the liver that can cause a temporary increase in direct bilirubin 24 to 48 hours after the insult. These conditions include: shock, hypoxia, severe metabolic acidosis, birth asphyxia, and cardiopulmonary arrest. Based on 1 extensive study, causes in order of frequency included: idiopathic neonatal hepatitis, extrahepatic biliary atresia, infection (CMV most common), TPN, metabolic disease (galactosemia most common), α_1-antitrypsin deficiency, and perinatal hypoxia-ischemia. Another study reported biliary atresia, idiopathic neonatal hepatitis, metabolic and endocrine causes, PFIC, preterm birth, infectious diseases, mitochondriopathies, and biliary sludge as the most common causes. The **single most common cause in the neonatal intensive care unit is parenteral nutrition related,** especially in premature infants. See Table 98–1 for selected causes of conjugated hyperbilirubinemia.

A. **Common causes**

   1. **Biliary atresia.** This is a progressive obliterative process involving the bile ducts and is fatal if untreated. It may present as part of a syndrome with associated malformations (30% of cases) such as polysplenia, situs inversus, cardiac anomalies, and/or vascular malformations (absent inferior vena cava). It is the most common cause of end-stage liver disease resulting in liver transplantation in children. Clinical findings that should raise index of suspicion include unexplained cholestasis associated with acholic/clay-colored stools and dark urine. These infants typically appear well except for presence of jaundice and associated clinical findings. High γ-glutamyl transferase (GGT) and a small or absent gallbladder on ultrasound are suggestive of biliary atresia. **Mimickers of biliary atresia include α_1-antitrypsin deficiency, Alagille syndrome, PNALD, and cystic fibrosis.**

   2. **Idiopathic neonatal hepatitis/neonatal giant cell hepatitis.** Idiopathic neonatal hepatitis is the term given to any hepatitis that is diagnosed from birth up to

the fourth month of life with no known cause, after all other causes have been excluded by clinical and laboratory evaluation. No known infectious or metabolic cause can be found. Most occur sporadically, but some (up to 20%) run in families. Idiopathic neonatal hepatitis can occur in premature infants due to an immature biliary tree and can manifest as feeding difficulties and hypoglycemia.

3. **Genetic intrahepatic cholestasis.** Includes many proposed subtypes of intrahepatic cholestasis. Each of these diseases is rare, but collectively as a group, they may be a common cause of conjugated hyperbilirubinemia. These are chronic diseases, and many progress and require liver transplantation.

   a. **Progressive familial intrahepatic cholestasis** is a group of autosomal recessive disorders characterized by defective bile export leading to subsequent cholestasis (includes PFIC1 [formerly Byler disease], PFIC2, and PFIC3).

   b. **Alagille syndrome** is a genetic disorder with multisystem involvement characterized by paucity of the intrahepatic bile ducts (cholestasis), cardiovascular anomalies (peripheral pulmonic stenosis), skeletal abnormalities (butterfly vertebrae), ophthalmologic findings (posterior embryotoxon), and "typical facies" (triangular face, low-set ears, hypertelorism). It is inherited in an autosomal dominant fashion but may occur sporadically due to de novo mutation. Most individuals carry a mutation in *JAG1* gene located in chromosome 30; however, some have mutations in *NOTCH2*.

4. **Hyperalimentation/parenteral nutrition–associated liver disease (PNALD). The most common drug-induced liver injury is caused by parenteral nutrition. Incidence is 20% in infants receiving parenteral nutrition for >2 weeks.** The etiology of PNALD is multifactorial. Several theories have been proposed as to the role of soybean-based intralipid in its pathophysiology, including modulation of oxidative stress and inflammation and phytosterols causing inhibition of bile acid–induced bile salt export pump expression. The most important cause of parenteral nutrition–related pathology appears to be the disruption of normal enterohepatic circulation due to lack of feedings, as evidenced by improvement of cholestasis with resumption of enteral feeds. Risk factors identified that contribute to development of PNALD include prematurity, low birthweight, infection, and overall prolonged exposure to TPN. It is rare that cholestasis will develop if exposure is <2 weeks.

5. **Infections.** Bacterial, viral, and protozoal infections have been reported to cause cholestasis. Sepsis and UTI can both cause direct hyperbilirubinemia. Jaundice may be the only presenting sign of urinary tract infection (*Escherichia coli* being the most common organism). Congenital infections such as CMV, toxoplasmosis, rubella, herpes, syphilis, and human immunodeficiency virus may present with early-onset cholestasis (jaundice in the first 24 hours), coagulopathy, and growth restriction. CMV is the most common congenital infectious cause of cholestasis. Adenovirus, enterovirus, echovirus, and parvovirus B19 are less common causes. Viral hepatitis A, B, and C typically do not cause neonatal cholestasis, but case reports exist.

6. **Inspissated bile syndrome.** This condition was first described in infants with blood group incompatibility, in particular Rh disease, complicated by severe hemolysis that can lead to excessive unconjugated hyperbilirubinemia, biliary sludging, and subsequent development of cholestasis. Most cholestasis due to sludge is mild and transient; however, some report a more severe and protracted course of cholestatic liver disease attributed to iron overload in neonates who received multiple intrauterine transfusions. Other reported causes include vitamin K deficiency bleeding, parenteral nutrition, sepsis, ABO incompatibility, medication (ceftriaxone pseudolithiasis, diuretics), and extracorporeal life support.

7. **Choledochal cysts (biliary cysts).** Extrahepatic bile duct cysts have been reclassified to include intrahepatic cysts (now called biliary cysts), and there are 6

different types of cysts. The most common is cystic dilatation of the common bile duct (type 1). They typically present with jaundice at 1 to 3 weeks of life; some may have obvious hepatomegaly, palpable mass in right upper quadrant, and rarely vomiting or fever. It is critical that biliary atresia is ruled out. Diagnosis can be made by performing a fasting abdominal ultrasound.

8. **α₁-Antitrypsin deficiency. Most common genetic cause of cholestasis, inherited as an autosomal disorder.** These infants can present with intrauterine growth restriction and hepatomegaly, usually with acholic stools.

9. **Galactosemia.** Autosomal recessive disorder and the **most well-known metabolic disorder** that presents with prolonged jaundice. It can be caused by deficiencies in 1 of 3 enzymes involved in the metabolism of galactose: galactose-1-phosphate uridyltransferase (GALT), galactokinase (GALK), and uridine diphosphate galactose-4-epimerase (GALE). Deficiency of the enzyme GALT is most common and most severe. *E coli* sepsis with liver cell dysfunction is characteristic of galactosemia.

10. **Perinatal hypoxia-ischemia.** This has been identified as an important causal factor in transient neonatal cholestasis. Shock can cause hepatic insult. Acute circulatory failure from congenital heart disease, myocarditis, and severe asphyxia can cause fulminant liver failure and conjugated hyperbilirubinemia.

B. **Less common causes of direct hyperbilirubinemia**
1. **Cholelithiasis (gallstones), biliary sludge.**
2. **Paucity of intrahepatic bile ducts.**
3. **Cholecystitis (acute and chronic).**
4. **Bile duct stenosis/spontaneous perforation of the bile duct.**
5. **Neonatal sclerosing cholangitis.** Etiology is unknown; presents in early infancy and then resolves.
6. **Select inborn errors of metabolism.** Wolman disease, Niemann-Pick diseases A and C, glycogen storage disease type IV, Gaucher disease, Zellweger syndrome (cerebrohepatorenal syndrome), neonatal hemochromatosis, tyrosinemia, fructosemia, mevalonic aciduria, and citrin deficiency. Cystic fibrosis can rarely present with cholestatic jaundice. Look for early signs of intestinal obstruction and low serum cholesterol. Bile acid synthetic defects, disorders of fatty acid oxidation, and citrin deficiency can all cause cholestasis. Mitochondrial respiratory chain defects can cause liver failure and usually present with a metabolic crisis.
7. **Endocrine disorders.** Congenital hypothyroidism, panhypopituitarism (infant with increased total and direct bilirubin, normal GGT, possible hypoglycemia, and shock).
8. **Congenital disorders.** Rotor syndrome and Dubin-Johnson syndrome are rare disorders of bilirubin metabolism that are noncholestatic; they have high direct and indirect hyperbilirubinemia but normal excretion of bile acid. Caroli disease is a congenital disease that has saccular dilatations of the intrahepatic bile ducts and is associated with polycystic kidney disease. Other rare diseases include: arthrogryposis-renal dysfunction–cholestasis, Aagenaes syndrome, Budd-Chiari syndrome, North American Indian familial cirrhosis, and hair-like bile duct syndrome.
9. **Chromosomal syndromes.** Trisomies 21, 18, and 13; monosomy X; partial trisomy 11; cat eye syndrome.
10. **Immunologic disorder. Neonatal hemochromatosis** is severe liver disease with extrahepatic siderosis in the neonate. It is mainly caused by **gestational alloimmune liver disease (GALD),** now referred to as **GALD-NH.** Suspect this if there is if severe coagulopathy not responsive to parenteral vitamin K and liver failure. Neonatal lupus erythematosus can also cause cholestatic jaundice.
11. **Bile acid synthesis disorders.** Rare disorders of synthesis of bile acids; some present with cholestasis. Patients often have normal or low GGTP and low serum bile acids.

12. **Neoplasms (rare)** include mesenchymal hamartoma, rhabdomyosarcoma of the biliary tree, neuroblastoma, hepatoblastoma, histiocyosis X, and neonatal leukemia.

13. **Medications.** There are case reports of maternal use of carbamazepine and methamphetamine causing neonatal cholestasis. Postnatal infant drugs include prolonged use of chloral hydrate, anticonvulsants, cephalosporins (ceftriaxone), erythromycin, ethanol, isoniazid, sulfa-containing products, rifampin, methotrexate, tetracycline, trimethoprim-sulfamethoxazole, fluconazole, and micafungin.

IV. **Database.** The physical examination alone cannot distinguish jaundice caused by cholestasis from jaundice caused by physiologic unconjugated hyperbilirubinemia. Physiologic unconjugated hyperbilirubinemia and cholestasis can coexist. That is why it is important to have screening recommendations regarding who to screen for cholestasis. Note that these are only recommendations because any infant in whom you suspect cholestatic disease should be tested. When screening, always measure fractionated bilirubin into unconjugated and conjugated.

A. **Who to screen for cholestasis**

1. **Testing recommendations from the North American Society for Pediatric Gastroenterology, Hepatology, and Nutrition:** any formula-fed infant noted to be jaundiced after 2 weeks of age. For exclusively breast-fed infants, this can be delayed by another week (until the third week of life) as long as they have a normal history and physical examination and no history of acholic stools or dark urine. If the first follow-up is at 4 weeks of age, any jaundiced infant should be tested. Other indications to test is any infant with a red flag (eg, ill infant, poor growth, dysmorphic features, acholic stools, and others).

2. **Testing recommendations from American Academy of Pediatrics guidelines for jaundiced infants ≥35 weeks' gestation:** Any infant receiving phototherapy or if TSB is rising rapidly and unexplained by history and physical examination; also, any sick infant or if jaundice is present at or beyond 3 weeks of age.

B. **History should include family, prenatal, and infant history.** Asking the appropriate questions in order to reveal signs and symptoms that may have been overlooked is critical to getting a good picture of what is going on with the patient.

1. **Family history**

a. **Any family members have neonatal cholestasis?** Consider genetic disease: cystic fibrosis, Alagille syndrome, α_1-antitrypsin deficiency, PFIC.

b. **History of consanguinity?** Consider autosomal recessive inheritance.

c. **History of fetal loss or early neonatal death?** Rule out gestational alloimmune liver disease.

d. **History of hemolytic disease or spherocytosis?** These can worsen conjugated hyperbilirubinemia.

2. **Prenatal history**

a. **Did the mother have a prenatal ultrasound?** Rule out biliary cyst, bowel abnormalities, possible syndromes, and cholelithiasis.

b. **Was the mother ill during pregnancy?** Rule out intrauterine infections (toxoplasmosis, rubella, CMV, HSV, other)

c. **Did the mother have cholestasis of pregnancy?** Rule out mitochondrial disorder or PFIC gene mutations.

d. **Did the mother have acute fatty liver of pregnancy?** Rule out neonatal long-chain L-3-hydroxyacyl-CoA dehydrogenase deficiency.

3. **Infant history**

a. **Is the infant premature?** Increased risk of neonatal hepatitis.

b. **Is the infant small for gestation age?** Risk factor for developing neonatal cholestasis and increased risk of congenital infections and neonatal cholestasis.

      c. **Is there a history of acholic or pale stools or dark urine?** Suggestive of biliary atresia. Acholic stools are difficult to assess; they are identified in only 63% of cases by health care providers. Stool color cards are being used in some countries (eg, Taiwan) to help parents identify the correct color of stool and increase awareness of acholic stools.

      d. **What is the infant being fed? Is it breast milk, formula, or parenteral nutrition?** Consider galactosemia, fructose intolerance, TPN-associated cholestasis.

      e. **When did the infant present with cholestasis relative to feeding?** A clue to galactosemia.

      f. **Did the infant have delayed passage of meconium?** Consider cystic fibrosis, panhypopituitarism.

      g. **Does the infant have vomiting?** Bowel obstruction, pyloric stenosis, metabolic disease.

      h. **Is the infant lethargic or irritable?** Lethargy suggests hypothyroidism or panhypopituitarism. Irritability can mean sepsis, metabolic disease.

      i. **Any signs of failure to thrive?** Metabolic or genetic disorder.

      j. **Any excessive bleeding?** Vitamin K deficiency bleeding or a coagulopathy. Did the infant receive vitamin K?

C. **Physical examination.** NASPGHAN states: "A thorough physical examination is crucial to the proper evaluation of the jaundiced infant. Attention to hepatomegaly and splenomegaly (which are classic hallmarks of the disease) and ill appearance warrants special consideration. Direct visualization of the stool pigment is a key aspect of the complete evaluation of the jaundiced infant."

   1. **Ill-appearing infant.** Consider infectious process first and rule that out. Other causes in an ill appearing infant see Section II.B. Infants with biliary atresia usually appear well.

   2. **Presence of characteristic physical features or accompanying congenital anomalies?** Consider syndromic etiologies (syndromic biliary atresia). The characteristic facial features of Alagille syndrome are rare in the newborn and appear approximately at 6 months.

      a. **Hearing issues.** Consider congenital infections, PFIC1, mitochondrial disease.

      b. **Eye examination.** May suggest congenital infection, storage disease, septo-optic dysplasia.

      c. **Cardiac.** Murmur, signs of heart failure: peripheral pulmonic stenosis or teratology of Fallot in Alagille syndrome, septal defects in biliary atresia.

      d. **Abdominal exam:**

         i. **Palpable mass in the right side of the abdomen.** Choledochal/biliary cyst.

         ii. **Prominent left or middle lobe of liver (hepatomegaly).** Biliary atresia.

         iii. **Splenomegaly.** More common in neonatal hepatitis but can be seen at 2 to 4 weeks in storage or hematologic disorders and as a late sign in biliary atresia.

      e. **Hypoplastic male genitalia.** Consider panhypopituitarism.

      f. **Jaundice skin color.** Jaundice has a greenish hue compared with unconjugated jaundice, which is more yellow. "Bronze baby syndrome" (a bronze discoloration of the skin as a result of dermal accumulation of coproporphyrins) occurs in infants with direct hyperbilirubinemia who are exposed to phototherapy.

D. **Laboratory and imaging studies**

   1. **Newborn screening.** The routine newborn screen will pick up congenital hypothyroidism, tyrosinemia, classical galactosemia, cystic fibrosis, and other inborn errors of metabolism. Verify these results because these conditions require urgent treatment to prevent serious sequelae. In case of galactosemia,

elimination of galactose in the diet pending confirmatory testing is a must. For congenital hypothyroidism, an immediate confirmatory test with serum thyroid-stimulating hormone (TSH) and thyroid hormone levels should be done.

2. **American Academy of Pediatrics guidelines for infants with hyperbilirubinemia at >35 weeks with elevated direct bilirubin.** Obtain urinalysis and urine culture, and perform a sepsis evaluation if indicated by history and physical examination. Check the results of the newborn thyroid and galactosemia screen, and evaluate the infant for hypothyroidism. Additional evaluation for the causes of cholestasis is recommended. **If the direct bilirubin is ≥50% of the total bilirubin,** consultation with an expert in the field is recommended.

3. **Testing guidelines from NASPGHAN and ESPGHAN.** The NASPGHAN and ESPGHAN has recently published guidelines for laboratory evaluation of conjugated hyperbilirubinemia in neonates. They jointly recommend that any infant with an **elevated serum direct bilirubin level of >1 mg** warrants timely evaluation and referral to a gastroenterologist or hepatologist to reduce the time to diagnosis of pediatric liver disease. This includes Tier 1 testing for infants when cholestasis is suspected and Tier 2 testing for confirmed cholestasis to be done in concert with the pediatric gastroenterologist/hepatologist. This enables a focused and targeted workup. (See Figure 98–1.)

   a. **Tier 1 testing**

      i. **Serum:** Complete blood count/differential, international normalized ratio (rule out coagulation disorders), aspartate aminotransferase (AST) and alanine aminotransferase (ALT) (liver inflammation), alkaline phosphatase/GGT (marker for biliary obstruction/inflammation), total bilirubin/direct bilirubin/albumin (rule out liver failure), and glucose (rule out hypoglycemia). Check α_1-antitrypsin phenotype and level. If newborn screening results not available, check thyroxine (T_4) and TSH. Some important facts: GGT is usually elevated in cholestasis, especially disorders such as biliary atresia, α_1-antitrypsin deficiency, Alagille syndrome, and idiopathic neonatal hepatitis. GGT is normal or low in PFIC1 and PFIC2, some cases of hypopituitarism, and some inborn errors of bile acid metabolism. With increased AST and a normal to mildly increased ALT, total bilirubin, or direct bilirubin, suspect a hematologic or muscle process. With severe coagulopathy, suspect GALT, metabolic disease, and sepsis.

      ii. **Urine:** Urinalysis and urine culture to rule out urinary tract infection (UTI); check reducing substances (rule out galactosemia).

      iii. **Consider sepsis workup** if infant is critically ill: blood, urine, cerebrospinal fluid, and other fluid cultures if appropriate.

      iv. **Obtain a fasting abdominal ultrasound.** Rule out biliary cyst and gallstone disease; look for advanced liver disease and splenic/vascular abnormalities. **Signs of biliary atresia:** a small/undetectable gallbladder, triangular cord sign, abnormal morphology of gallbladder, common bile duct not visualized, diameter of hepatic artery, subcapsular blood flow. Biliary atresia splenic malformation syndrome: polysplenia/asplenia, midline liver, abdominal heterotaxy, preduodenal portal vein, interrupted inferior vena cava.

   b. **Tier 2 testing.** Confirmed cholestasis with further targeted evaluation with a pediatric gastroenterologist/hepatologist.

      i. **General:** TSH and T_4 values, serum cortisol, serum bile acids.

      ii. **Metabolic:** Serum ammonia, lactate, cholesterol, red blood cell GALT. Urine for organic acids, succinylacetone, and bile salt species profiling.

      iii. **Infectious disease:** Polymerase chain reaction for CMV, HSV, *Listeria*.

      iv. **Genetics:** Discuss with pediatric gastroenterologist/hepatologist about gene panels or exome sequencing.

     v. Sweat chloride analysis: Serum immunoreactive trypsinogen level or *CFTR* genetic testing.

     vi. Chest x-ray: Rule out heart or lung disease.

     vii. Spine: Detect spine abnormalities (butterfly vertebrae).

     viii. Echocardiogram: Evaluate for cardiac anomalies (24% of infants with Alagille syndrome have structural heart disease, as do some infants with biliary atresia).

     ix. Intraoperative cholangiogram and histologic exam of the duct remnant: Gold standard to diagnose biliary atresia.

     x. Liver biopsy: Most supportive test for diagnosis. Approach and timing vary.

     xi. Other consultations may be necessary: Ophthalmology, metabolic/genetic, cardiology/ECHO (if murmur, hypoxic, poor cardiac function), pediatric surgery, nutrition/dietician.

     xii. Other diagnostic imaging may be necessary: Hepatobiliary scintigraphy, endoscopic retrograde cholangiopancreatography, and magnetic resonance cholangiopancreatography have all been used to diagnose biliary atresia but have limited specificity and availability.

V. Plan. The list of causes of cholestasis can be extensive, and diagnosis can be difficult. Early treatment is essential (eg, improved outcome in biliary atresia; prevent bacteremia/sepsis in UTI; prevent severe hypoglycemia in hypopituitarism). It is important to identify the life-threatening and treatable causes of cholestasis. Even with causes that have no specific treatment available, early medical management and dietary modifications are beneficial. It is best to follow a stepwise approach.

   A. Focus on any ill infants who have conditions that can be treated:

     1. **Bacterial sepsis.** If signs of sepsis are present, appropriate cultures should be performed and empirical antibiotic therapy initiated.

     2. **Viral/intrauterine infections.** Appropriate antiviral agents.

     3. **Urinary tract infection.** Appropriate antibiotic therapy.

     4. **Galactosemia.** Galactose-free diet.

     5. **Tyrosinemia.** Low-tyrosine diet, phenylalanine diet, 2-2-nitro-4 trifluoromethylbenzoyl-1,3-cyclohexanedione (NTBC).

     6. **Hereditary fructosemia.** Fructose/sucrose-free diet.

     7. **Gestational alloimmune liver disease.** Any infant with a suspicion of GALD-NH should be given 1 dose of intravenous immunoglobulin (IVIG) while a workup is being done (eg, biopsy of oral mucosa for iron staining and magnetic resonance imaging, possible liver biopsy). Supportive care and treatment with double volume exchange transfusion and IVIG. Liver transplantation may be necessary.

     8. **Hypothyroidism.** Treatment is L-thyroxine. See Chapter 129.

     9. **Hemolytic disease/hemolysis.** Treatment depends on etiology (eg, vitamin K).

     10. **Panhypopituitarism.** Hormone replacement (thyroid hormone, growth hormone, and cortisol replacement), fluid and electrolyte therapy.

     11. **Acute obstructive gallstones.** Surgery is indicated.

   B. Focus on infants who will benefit from early surgery to restore bile flow

     1. **Biliary atresia.** Early intervention is critical for successful treatment and optimal prognosis. Kasai hepatoportoenterostomy should be done as soon as possible to establish bile flow and is best performed with the first 60 days of life. Liver transplantation if end-stage liver disease.

     2. **Choledochal/biliary cyst.** Resection of the cyst to create bile flow from the liver to the small intestine (eg, type 1 cysts: total cyst excision with Roux-en-Y hepaticojejunostomy).

     3. **Inspissated bile duct syndrome.** Treatment includes removal of the precipitating factor, biliary tract irrigation, or surgery/endoscopic procedures for refractory cases.

     4. **Spontaneous perforation of the common bile duct.** Surgical drainage.

C. **Other causes and treatment plans**
1. **Parenteral nutrition–associated liver disease.** First confirm the diagnosis and verify the infant does not have biliary atresia or other diagnosis; cases of biliary atresia have been mistaken for PNALD. Treatment involves starting enteral feeding as soon as possible as this stimulates bile flow and prevents biliary stasis. Small oral feedings are recommended. Lipid restriction (1 g/kg/d or less) reduces exposure to parenteral soybean oil, which contributes to hepatotoxicity. Lipid modification replaces parenteral soybean oil with parenteral fish oil.
2. **α_1-Antitrypsin deficiency.** Treatment is mostly supportive or liver transplantation if cirrhosis is progressive.
3. **Cystic fibrosis.** Pancreatic enzymes, ursodeoxycholic acid.
4. **Bile acid synthetic defects.** Treatment with primary bile acids (cholic acid or chenodeoxycholic acid).
5. **Alagille syndrome.** Check an α-fetoprotein and ultrasound every 6 months as part of hepatocellular carcinoma screening. No specific treatment and may require liver transplantation.
D. **Supportive measures.** Medical management and optimal nutritional support are beneficial even when there is no curative treatment. These include nutrition, vitamin supplementation, and medications.
1. **Nutrition.** Many of these infants suffer from growth failure because of an increase in metabolic demand, a decreased absorption of fats, and impaired protein and carbohydrate metabolism. Most of these infants require high caloric diets (125% of recommended dietary allowance based on ideal body weight). Protein intake should be 2 to 3 g/kg/d. Special formulas (eg, Pregestimil, Enfaport, Portagen) may be necessary that include medium-chain triglycerides (MCTs) that can be absorbed without the action of bile salts. Oral feeding is preferred for formula, but sometimes nasogastric feedings are required at night to make sure the caloric need is met. Supplemental MCTs can be given to breast-fed infants. Special formulas are recommended for galactosemia, fructosemia, and tyrosinemia. Some infants may require other dietary restrictions.
2. **Vitamins.** Supplemental fat-soluble vitamins (A, D, E, K) are needed in many of these infants since intestinal absorption of these vitamins is impaired. Blood levels should be routinely monitored. See doses of vitamins in Chapter 155.
3. **Medications** are used to promote bile flow and decrease the pruritus (especially in Alagille syndrome and PFIC). Ursodeoxycholic acid, phenobarbital, and cholestyramine are used often and are discussed in detail in Chapters 98 and 155. Rifampin has been used for pruritus but has limited experience in neonates.

63 Hyperbilirubinemia: Unconjugated, On Call

I. **Problem.** An infant's indirect (unconjugated) serum bilirubin level is elevated at 10 mg/dL. Unconjugated (indirect) bilirubin is the fraction of serum bilirubin that has not been conjugated with glucuronic acid in the liver. The exact definition of a physiologic range and management of indirect hyperbilirubinemia are complex and based on many factors, including gestational age (GA), postnatal age, birthweight, disease state, risk factors, ethnicity, and hydration and nutritional status. **Total serum bilirubin (TSB)** is the sum of direct (conjugated) and indirect (unconjugated) bilirubin. The **indirect** bilirubin is calculated by subtracting the direct bilirubin from the total bilirubin. **Transcutaneous bilirubin (TcB)** is a measurement of TSB from an instrument that uses reflectance measurements on the skin and correlates well with the laboratory TSB value. **Unconjugated hyperbilirubinemia** is usually transient and physiologic in the newborn period, but it is important to note that kernicterus (chronic bilirubin encephalopathy) is still occurring in the developed world.

II. **Immediate questions**

A. **How old is the infant? What is the gestational age? High indirect serum bilirubin levels during the first 24 hours of life are never physiologic.** Hemolytic disease (Rh isoimmunization or ABO incompatibility), infection, occult hemorrhage, and polycythemia are common causes of early-onset jaundice. GA and age in hours of the infant determine the bilirubin level at which phototherapy should be initiated. The risk of unconjugated hyperbilirubinemia is inversely proportional with GA. In premature infants, hyperbilirubinemia is usually more severe and lasts longer.

B. **Is the infant being breast fed? Breast-feeding jaundice (early onset)** occurs within the first week of life and is secondary to decreased intake of breast milk resulting in dehydration and caloric deprivation. **Breast milk jaundice (late onset)** occurs after the first week of life and can last up to the third or fourth week. Current literature supports a genetic predisposition. High levels of the enzyme β-glucuronidase can also be a contributing factor leading to increased enterohepatic circulation.

C. **What is the family ethnicity?** The incidence of neonatal jaundice is increased in infants of Native American Indian, Inuit, Mediterranean (Greece, Turkey, Sardinia), Sephardic Jewish, Nigerian, and Eastern Asian descent. Native Greeks have a higher incidence than Greeks in the United States. The incidence is lower in African Americans. Glucose-6-phosphate dehydrogenase (G6PD) deficiency, which is a cause of unconjugated hyperbilirubinemia, is more common in many of these groups and may be partially responsible. Immigration and intermarriage have increased the incidence of G6PD in the United States.

D. **Is the infant dehydrated?** If **evidence of dehydration exists** (eg, weight loss of >12% from birthweight, increased sodium, decreased urine out), fluid administration may help to lower serum bilirubin level. Supplemental formula feedings or expressed breast milk should be considered if breast-feeding failure is the reason for hyperbilirubinemia; otherwise, intravenous (IV) fluids should be given. Adequate hydration is essential, but excess hydration by causing dilutional effects of IV fluids and enhancing peristalsis to decrease enterohepatic circulation by oral fluid supplements will not clear bilirubin any faster. **Cochrane review found that there is no evidence that IV fluid supplementation affects major clinical outcomes associated with excessive bilirubin in healthy full term infants.**

E. **What are the important risk factors for severe hyperbilirubinemia in infants ≥35 weeks' gestation?** Lower gestational age, predischarge total serum, or transcutaneous bilirubin measurement in the high-risk or high-intermediate risk zone, exclusive breastfeeding, especially if nursing is not going well and weight loss is exclusive, jaundice observed in the first 24 hours, isoimmune or other hemolytic disease (G6PD deficiency), previous sibling with jaundice, cephalhematoma or significant bruising, east Asian race.

F. **Are there any factors increasing risk for bilirubin-induced neurologic dysfunction (BIND)?** BIND occurs when bilirubin crosses the blood–brain barrier and targets brain tissue producing clinical signs associated with bilirubin toxicity. Bilirubin-induced neurotoxicity risk factors include isoimmune hemolytic disease, G6PD deficiency, asphyxia, sepsis, acidosis, and albumin <3.0 mg/dL. Infants with lower GA, significant lethargy, and temperature instability are at much higher risk of developing bilirubin toxicity. In this context of increased risk factors, the bilirubin threshold for starting phototherapy and exchange transfusion is at a much lower level.

III. Differential diagnosis. Indirect (unconjugated) bilirubin is derived mainly from hemoglobin metabolism. Hemoglobin by-products must be conjugated by the liver before they can be excreted in the bile, stool, or urine. Unconjugated bilirubin cannot be directly measured in the blood and is never present in urine. Newborn jaundice can be caused by an increase in enterohepatic circulation, decrease in the clearance of bilirubin, decrease in conjugation and hepatic uptake, impaired bile flow, and increase in production. In premature infants, bilirubin can reach a higher level and lasts longer than in term infants, some up to 6 weeks of age. See also Chapter 99 for further discussion on unconjugated hyperbilirubinemia.

A. Common causes of indirect hyperbilirubinemia. The majority of infants have hyperbilirubinemia in the first week of life. It is important to differentiate **physiologic from nonphysiologic hyperbilirubinemia.** The timing of onset and duration aid in diagnosis. The following are more likely associated with **nonphysiologic indirect hyperbilirubinemia**: onset of jaundice before 24 hours of life, jaundice lasting >2 weeks in full-term infants, higher level requiring treatment, or jaundice present in a clinically ill infant.

1. **Physiologic hyperbilirubinemia** is a transient and common process that almost all newborns will experience. It is secondary to 2 factors: (1) the shorter life span of red blood cells (RBCs), which causes mildly elevated bilirubin levels due to increased turnover of heme, and (2) the relative deficiency of uridine 5′-diphospho-glucuronosyltransferase leading to decreased conjugation, which causes a decrease in bilirubin clearance. It commonly appears after the second day, peaks between the third and fifth days, and resolves within 1 week of life. **Exaggerated or severe physiologic jaundice** can occur when higher bilirubin levels require therapy and hyperbilirubinemia lasts longer than 2 weeks.

2. **Nonphysiologic hyperbilirubinemia**
   a. **Breast-feeding failure or breast milk jaundice.** Breast-feeding failure jaundice is due to dehydration and decreased caloric intake. **Breast milk jaundice** has a genetic etiology and once was considered an extension of physiologic jaundice, but serious complications can occur, such as kernicterus.
   b. **Infection.** Jaundice as the only sign of sepsis is rare. Jaundice secondary to congenital viral infection may be associated with conjugated hyperbilirubinemia.
   c. **Hemolysis.** Major and minor blood group incompatibilities may cause exaggerated hyperbilirubinemia. Signs of hemolytic disease of the newborn include a positive direct Coombs test, elevated cord bilirubin, and hemolytic anemia.
   d. **Increased bilirubin load from a breakdown of red blood cells.** Subdural hematoma, intraventricular hemorrhage in premature infants, cephalohematoma, excessive bruising, pulmonary hemorrhage, and polycythemia/hyperviscosity can contribute.
   e. **Infant of a diabetic mother.** Polycythemia seems to be the most important factor associated with hyperbilirubinemia. Other factors related to hyperbilirubinemia in an infant of a diabetic mother include prematurity, macrosomia, and poor maternal glycemic control.

B. Other causes of indirect hyperbilirubinemia
1. **Glucose-6-phosphate dehydrogenase deficiency.**
2. **Pyruvate kinase deficiency.**
3. **Red blood cell membrane defects:** Hereditary spherocytosis, hereditary elliptocytosis, pyknocytosis.
4. **Disorders of bilirubin clearance:** Lucey-Driscoll syndrome (familial neonatal jaundice), Crigler-Najjar syndrome (CNS) (type I and type II), and Gilbert syndrome.
5. **Hypothyroidism/hypopituitarism.**
6. **Hemoglobinopathies:** α- and γ-Thalassemia.

7. **Metabolic disorders:** Early galactosemia or fructose intolerance.
8. **Medications:** Penicillin, oxytocin, sulfonamides, vitamin K, nitrofurantoin, novobiocin (not available in United States). Maternal use of naproxen, atazanavir, or methyldopa can cause a positive direct antiglobulin test and jaundice in the newborn. Maternal oxytocin and valium are risk factors.

IV. **Database**

A. **History.** What is the infant's feeding regimen and frequency of voiding (hydration status)? Ask about jaundice in previous siblings and family ethnicity. Is there a familial history of significant hemolytic disease? Is there a history of light-colored stools or dark urine? Any maternal medication use? History of lethargy?

B. **Physical examination.** The accumulation of bilirubin in body tissues produces jaundice (yellow skin) and scleral icterus. Jaundice is first seen in the face (forehead) and progresses caudally to the trunk and extremities. Pressure on the skin often reveals jaundice. The TSB can be roughly estimated (not 100% reliable, note that visual estimation can lead to errors especially in darkly pigmented infants or difficult to assess in polycythemic infants) by examining the skin of different areas of the body for jaundice (face, ~5 mg/dL; upper chest, ~10 mg/dL; abdomen, ~12 mg/dL; palms and soles, usually >15 mg/dL). Note signs of bruising, cephalohematoma, or intracranial bleeding. Check for hepatosplenomegaly. A complete neurologic examination should be performed because bilirubin encephalopathy can occur. Look for signs such as poor feeding, lethargy, hypotonia, or seizures.

C. **Laboratory studies.** In normal and healthy term infants whose jaundice appears within physiologic time line, few tests are necessary. It is useful to save cord blood for future testing if necessary.

1. **Jaundiced infant of ≥35 weeks' gestational age.** These recommendations are based on the American Academy of Pediatrics (AAP) Subcommittee on Hyperbilirubinemia. All bilirubin levels should be interpreted based on infant's age in hours. See also the algorithm in Figure 63–1 for when to perform laboratory studies and on the management of jaundice in the newborn nursery.

a. **Infant jaundiced in the first 24 hours.** Measure TSB and TcB. TcB is determined by a portable transcutaneous instrument that measures the amount of yellow color in the skin, which correlates with the laboratory measurement of TSB. Repeat TSB or TcB depends on initial result, age of the infant, and evolution of the hyperbilirubinemia.

b. **Jaundice seems excessive for the infant's age or there is uncertainty regarding the degree of jaundice.** Obtain TcB and TSB.

c. **Infant is receiving phototherapy or total serum bilirubin is rising rapidly and unexplained by history and physical examination.** Obtain:

   i. **Direct (conjugated) bilirubin.**

   ii. **Blood type and Coombs test.** If not obtained on the cord blood.

   iii. **Complete blood count with differential and smear.** Observe RBC morphology.

   iv. **Reticulocyte count (optional).**

   v. **Glucose-6-phosphate dehydrogenase level (optional).**

   vi. **End-tidal carbon monoxide (concentration) if available (optional).** End-tidal carbon monoxide corrected for ambient carbon monoxide (ETCOc) is a measurement of the rate of heme catabolism and rate of bilirubin production. It is used to confirm hemolysis and can help identify infants at risk for developing high bilirubin levels.

   vii. **Repeat total serum bilirubin in 4 to 24 hours,** depending on infant's age and TSB level.

d. **TSB is approaching exchange levels (see Figure 99–3) or is not responding to phototherapy:**

   i. **Reticulocyte count.**

   ii. **Glucose-6-phosphate dehydrogenase level.**

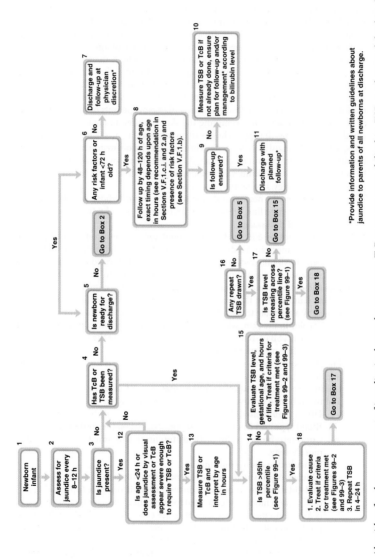

FIGURE 63–1. Algorithm for the management of jaundice in the newborn nursery. TcB, transcutaneous bilirubin; TSB, total serum bilirubin. (*Reproduced with permission from American Academy of Pediatrics Subcommittee on Hyperbilirubinemia: Management of hyperbilirubinemia in the newborn infant 35 or more weeks of gestation, Pediatrics. 2004 Jul;114(1):297-316.*)

      iii. **Albumin.** An albumin of <3.0 g/dL is a risk factor for lowering the threshold for phototherapy. Obtaining a serum albumin will allow you to calculate the bilirubin-to-albumin (B/A) ratio, which can help determine the need for exchange transfusion (see Figure 99–3).

      iv. **End-tidal carbon monoxide (concentration).** See Section IV.C.1.c.vi.

  2. **Jaundiced infant <35 weeks' gestational age (*controversial*).** There are no formal guidelines for laboratory values for jaundiced infants age <35 weeks. Follow institutional guidelines. (See also tests for infant >35 weeks, discussed earlier.)

V. Plan

  A. **Phototherapy**

    1. **Principles of phototherapy.** Bilirubin absorption of visible light in the blue region of the spectrum transforms unconjugated bilirubin (bound to albumin) into bilirubin "photoproducts," mostly isomers of bilirubin. Practice considerations for devices and the optimal administration of phototherapy in infants >35 weeks' gestation per AAP Committee on Fetus and Newborn are as follows:

      a. **Ensure maximum exposure of patient's body surface area under phototherapy.**

      b. **Irradiance level of ≥30 μW/cm^{-2}/nm^{-1} over waveband of 460 to 490 nm (blue-green region).**

      c. **Phototherapy should be implemented in a timely/urgent fashion.**

      d. **Briefly interrupt for feeding and other care.**

      e. **Measure bilirubin load reduction and discontinue when desired level reached.** Beware of rebound increase in bilirubin.

    2. **Phototherapy for the hospitalized infant ≥35 weeks' gestation (per AAP guidelines, 2004).** (See Figure 99–2.) Phototherapy is started when the TSB exceeds the line (or an option is to start 2–3 levels below the line) indicated for each category. The risk factors were selected because these conditions have a negative effect on the albumin binding of bilirubin, the blood–brain barrier, and the susceptibility of the brain cells to damage by bilirubin. When using this figure, follow the following guidelines:

      a. **Use total serum bilirubin.** Do not subtract direct bilirubin from the total.

      b. **Measure serum albumin.** If <3 g/dL, it is considered a risk factor. Lower the phototherapy threshold.

      c. **Risk factors.** Isoimmune hemolytic disease, G6PD deficiency, asphyxia, significant lethargy, temperature instability, sepsis, acidosis, or albumin <3.0 g/dL.

      d. **Infants at low risk.** Infants who are ≥38 weeks and well.

      e. **Infants at medium risk.** Infants who are ≥38 weeks and have risk factors (see earlier). Other infants at medium risk include those infants who are 35 to 37 6/7 weeks and well. It is optional to intervene at a lower TSB level for those infants who are closer to 35 weeks and at a higher level for those infants who are closer to 37 6/7 weeks.

      f. **Infants at high risk.** Infants who are 35 to 37 6/7 weeks with risk factors listed earlier.

    3. **Preterm infants <35 weeks' gestation.** There are no good evidence-based bilirubin level guidelines for initiation of phototherapy or exchange transfusion in preterm infants. Maisels and colleagues published their recommendations on bilirubin threshold for initiation of treatment in this patient population (Table 63–1).

      a. **Use the lower range number if the infant is at a greater risk for bilirubin toxicity.** Risk includes lower GA, serum albumin <2.5 g/dL, rapidly rising TSB (suggesting hemolytic disease), and those who are clinically unstable (see later).

      b. **When a decision is being made about the initiation of phototherapy or exchange transfusion,** infants are considered to be clinically unstable if they have 1 or more of the following conditions:

Table 63–1. SUGGESTED USE OF PHOTOTHERAPY AND EXCHANGE TRANSFUSION IN
PRETERM INFANTS <35 WEEKS' GESTATIONAL AGE

Gestational Age (weeks)	Initiate Phototherapy Total Serum Bilirubin (mg/dL)	Exchange Transfusion Total Serum Bilirubin (mg/dL)
<28 0/7	5–6	11–14
28 0/7 to 29 6/7	6–8	12–14
30 0/7 to 31 6/7	8–10	13–16
32 0/7 to 33 6/7	10–12	15–18
34 0/7 to 34 6/7	12–14	17–19

This table reflects the authors' recommendations for operational or therapeutic total serum bilirubin
threshold levels at or above which treatment is likely to do more good than harm.
Reproduced with permission from Maisels MJ, Watchko JF, Bhutani VK, et al: An approach to the management of hyperbilirubinemia in the preterm infant less than 35 weeks of gestation, *J Perinatol.* 2012
Sep;32(9):660-664.

      i. Blood pH <7.15.
     ii. Blood culture–positive sepsis in the prior 24 hours.
   iii. Apnea and bradycardia requiring cardiorespiratory resuscitation
        (bagging and/or intubation) during the previous 24 hours.
    iv. Hypotension requiring pressor treatment during the previous 24 hours.
     v. Mechanical ventilation at the time of blood sampling.
  c. **Prophylactic phototherapy.** Some institutions use prophylactic phototherapy
(at birth) for ELBW infants. Maisels et al state that it is an option to use PT
prophylactically soon after birth in infants <26 weeks of age. Cochrane review
found that "prophylactic phototherapy helps to maintain a lower serum bilirubin concentration and may have an effect on the rate of exchange transfusion
and the risk of neurodevelopmental impairment, but further studies are needed
to determine the efficacy and safety on long term outcomes." Studies have
shown that prophylactic phototherapy does not decrease the total bilirubin
or the duration of phototherapy. Aggressive phototherapy (started earlier and
continued at lower bilirubin levels) in one trial was found to increase mortality in the smallest and sickest infants while decreasing their impairment and
profound impairment.
  d. **For infants <1000 g, start phototherapy at lower irradiance levels.** If TSB
continues to rise, additional phototherapy should be provided by increasing
the surface area exposed (consider adding bili-blanket); if TSB continues to rise
despite increased surface area exposed, increase irradiance level by switching
to higher intensity settings.
  e. **For infants < 35 weeks. Special blue fluorescent lamps or light-emitting
diode (LED) systems** that will deliver irradiance predominately in the 430- to
490-nm band are recommended. Fluorescent and LED light sources can be
brought closer to the infant than halogen or tungsten lamps (burn risk).
  f. **Discontinue phototherapy when total serum bilirubin is 1 to 2 mg/dL** below
the initiation level for the infant's postmenstrual age.
  g. **Attempt regular feedings if possible, and feed frequently.** Feeding inhibits
the enterohepatic form of bilirubin and helps lower the serum bilirubin level.
Studies indicate that increasing the frequency of breast feeding will not have a
significant effect on the serum bilirubin level in the first 3 days of life.
  4. **There is no universal standard for discontinuing phototherapy.** Phototherapy may be discontinued once serum bilirubin levels have fallen 1 to 2 mg/dL

below the level at which phototherapy was initiated. Factors to consider when stopping phototherapy are the cause and the age at which it was initiated. A repeat TSB measurement is recommended in all infants within 24 hours of stopping phototherapy.

5. **If total serum bilirubin continues to rise or does not decrease on phototherapy,** hemolysis may be present.

6. **If infant has an elevated direct bilirubin level and is receiving phototherapy,** the infant may develop **bronze baby syndrome.** This is not a contraindication to phototherapy.

7. **Contraindications to phototherapy.** Congenital porphyria and use of medications that are photosensitizers.

B. **Exchange transfusion.** (See Chapter 34.) Exchange transfusions should be performed only by trained personnel in a neonatal intensive care unit. There is considerable *controversy* concerning the exact level at which to initiate exchange transfusion.

1. **Exchange transfusion for infants ≥35 weeks' gestation.** See Figure 99–3. This figure is based on guidelines from the AAP and displays the suggested levels for exchange transfusion (see lines) in jaundiced infants >35 weeks' GA despite phototherapy. When using this figure, follow these guidelines:

   a. **Use total serum bilirubin.** Do not subtract direct bilirubin.

   b. **Risk factors.** G6PD deficiency, asphyxia, sepsis, temperature instability, acidosis, isoimmune hemolytic disease, and lethargy that is significant.

   c. **The first 24 hours.** (See dashed lines on Figure 99–3.) Represents uncertainty secondary to the wide range of clinical circumstances and a range of responses to phototherapy.

   d. **Immediate exchange transfusion.** Indicated if the infant shows signs of bilirubin encephalopathy (hypertonia, arching, retrocollis, opisthotonos, fever, or high-pitched cry) even if the TSB is falling or if the TSB is 5 mg/dL above these lines in Figure 99–3.

   e. **Measure serum albumin and calculate bilirubin-to-albumin ratio at which exchange transfusion should be considered.** If an exchange transfusion is being considered, the serum albumin should be measured so the B/A ratio can be calculated and used with the TSB levels to help decide whether an exchange transfusion needs to be done. The ratio of B/A correlates with measured unbound bilirubin in newborns, which if elevated can be associated with kernicterus in sick preterm newborns and transient abnormalities in audiometric brainstem response in infants.

2. **Exchange transfusion for infants <35 weeks.** See consensus guidelines in Table 63–1. Recommendations for exchange transfusion are only for those infants whose TSB levels are rising who are on intensive phototherapy to the maximal surface area. Exchange transfusion is recommended for any infant who shows signs of **acute bilirubin encephalopathy** (hypertonia, arching, retrocollis, opisthotonos, high-pitched cry), although these signs rarely occur in very low birthweight infants. Exchange transfusion is recommended at lower levels in infants with hemolytic disease and at high risk, as discussed earlier.

C. **Drug therapy.** Medications can be used to inhibit hemolysis, increase conjugation/elimination, and inhibit formation of bilirubin. These agents include phenobarbital, metalloporphyrins, albumin, and IV immunoglobulin. See Chapter 99 for detailed discussion.

1. **Phenobarbital** increases the concentration of ligandin in liver cells, which induces production of uridine diphosphate glucuronyl transferase (UDPGT) and enhances bilirubin excretion. It is used for treatment of CNS type II and Gilbert syndrome and can also be used as an adjunct therapy for treatment of exaggerated unconjugated hyperbilirubinemia in the newborn period. It is not helpful in acute management since it takes 3 to 7 days to be effective.

2. **Metalloporphyrins** reduce bilirubin production by competitive inhibition of heme oxygenase, the rate-limiting enzyme in the catabolism of heme. A recent (2016) clinical trial showed that prophylactic predischarge administration of a single intramuscular injection of 4.5 mg/kg of Sn-mesoporphyrin (SnMP) decreased the duration of phototherapy, reversed total bilirubin trajectory, and reduced the severity of subsequent hyperbilirubinemia. Long-term safety of SnMP remains to be studied. It remains an unlicensed drug and is available on an investigational or "compassionate use" basis.

3. **Albumin** increases bilirubin binding capacity and results in a decreased free bilirubin. Albumin infusion may be considered when albumin level is <3.0 mg/dL, when TSB/albumin ratio is >6, and prior to double-volume exchange transfusion.

4. **Intravenous immunoglobulin** works by competing with sensitized neonatal RBCs at the Fc receptors in the reticuloendothelial system, thus preventing further hemolysis. It is recommended in patients with isoimmune hemolysis when TSB is rising despite intensive phototherapy. Dose is 1 g/kg given over 2 to 4 hours; it can be repeated if needed in 12 to 24 hours (2 doses).

D. **Breast-fed infants.** The AAP does not recommend interruption of breast feeding in healthy term newborns with hyperbilirubinemia and encourages continued and frequent breast feeding. Infants who require phototherapy should continue breast feeding. The AAP recommends that mothers nurse their infants at least 8 to 12 times per day the first several days. The AAP does not recommend routine supplementation of non-dehydrated breast-fed infants with water or sugar water. **Supplementing with water or dextrose water does not lower the bilirubin level.** Different options are available, and the decision regarding which treatment option to use depends on the specific infant, whether phototherapy is indicated, the physician's judgment, and the family circumstances.

1. **If phototherapy is not recommended:**
   a. Observation and close follow-up of serial total serum bilirubin levels.
   b. **Continue breast feeding but supplement with formula,** while following serial TSB levels.
   c. **Interrupt breast feeding and substitute formula,** while following serial TSB levels.

2. **If phototherapy is recommended:**
   a. **Continue breast feeding, and administer phototherapy (American Academy of Pediatrics recommendation). Supplementation with expressed breast milk** is indicated if the infant's intake is inadequate, weight loss is excessive, or there is a question of dehydration. Although phototherapy does not reduce the serum bilirubin concentration in breast-fed infants as quickly as it does in formula-fed infants, it is still effective.
   b. **Continue breast feeding, and administer phototherapy (American Academy of Pediatrics recommendation). Supplementation with formula** is indicated if the infant's intake is inadequate, weight loss is excessive, or there is a question of dehydration.
   c. **Interrupt breast feeding temporarily and substitute formula and administer phototherapy (American Academy of Pediatrics optional recommendation).** This reduces bilirubin levels and improves the efficacy of phototherapy.

E. **Breast-fed infants with persistent jaundice after 2 weeks.** Approximately 30% of healthy term infants have persistent jaundice after 2 weeks of age. Treat as follows:

1. **Observe.** If the physical examination is normal and pale stools and dark yellow urine are not present.

2. **Screen for congenital hypothyroidism.** A rare cause of direct hyperbilirubinemia.

3. **If jaundice is still present at 3 weeks, total and direct serum bilirubin should be obtained to evaluate for cholestasis.** If elevated direct bilirubin level, proceed with cholestasis workup (see Chapter 62).

F. **Early follow-up should be provided for all neonates (especially those discharged at <72 hours of age) to monitor for bilirubin-related problems.**

   1. **Perform a risk assessment of all infants before discharge.** The AAP recommends 2 clinical options used individually or in combination: the predischarge TSB or TcB and/or a thorough evaluation of clinical risk factors. Recent studies state that combining these 2 options offers the best estimate for predicting the risk of later hyperbilirubinemia. Appropriate follow-up is always recommended, because even with a low predischarge level, the risk of subsequent hyperbilirubinemia is never zero.

     a. **Predischarge measurement of total serum bilirubin or transcutaneous bilirubin level can then be plotted on the nomogram on Figure 99–1.** This predicts subsequent significant hyperbilirubinemia. This table is for risk in well newborns at 36 weeks' GA with birthweight ≥2000 g or 35 weeks' GA with birthweight >2500 g.

       i. **Total serum bilirubin at discharge in the low-risk zone.** 0% risk of developing a TSB level >95th percentile.

       ii. **Total serum bilirubin at discharge in the low-intermediate–risk zone.** 12% risk of developing a TSB level >95th percentile.

       iii. **Total serum bilirubin at discharge in the high-intermediate–risk zone.** 46% risk of developing a TSB level >95%.

       iv. **Total serum bilirubin at discharge in the high-risk zone.** 68% risk of developing a TSB level >95%.

     b. **Risk factors based on American Academy of Pediatrics recommendations in order of importance.** The greater the number of risk factors present, the greater is the risk of significant hyperbilirubinemia. Certain risk factors before discharge were noted to be more frequently associated with hyperbilirubinemia: breast feeding, significant jaundice in a previous sibling, GA <38 weeks, and jaundice noted before discharge. Factors that are most predictive of hyperbilirubinemia when combined with the risk zone are lower GA and exclusive breast feeding.

       i. **Decreased risk.** TSB or TcB in low-risk zone, GA ≥41 weeks, exclusive bottle feeding, black race, discharge after 72 hours.

       ii. **Minor risk factors.** Predischarge TSB or TcB in the high-intermediate–risk zone, GA 37–38 weeks, jaundice observed before discharge, previous sibling with jaundice, macrosomic infant of a diabetic mother, maternal age ≥25 years, and male gender.

       iii. **Major risk factors.** Predischarge TSB or TcB in the high-risk zone, jaundice observed in the first 24 hours, blood group incompatibility with positive direct antiglobulin test (other known hemolytic disease, elevated ETCOc), GA 35–36 weeks, previous sibling who received phototherapy, cephalohematoma or significant bruising, exclusive breast feeding (especially if nursing is not going well, with excessive weight loss), and East Asian race.

     c. **Key points**

       i. **Clinical judgment is necessary in determining follow up.** For some neonates sent home before 48 hours, 2 follow up visits may be necessary (first between 24 and 72 hours, second between 72 and 100 hours).

       ii. **Infant with risk factors for severe hyperbilirubinemia.** Earlier and more frequent follow-ups are recommended.

       iii. **If follow up cannot be guaranteed, consider delaying discharge for infants with increased risk for severe hyperbilirubinemia.**

2. **Follow-up schedules.**
   a. **AAP recommendations for follow up:**
      i. Infant discharged before 24 hours of age: see by 72 hours.
      ii. Infant discharged between 24 and 47.9 hours of age: see by 96 hours.
      iii. Infant discharged between 48 and 72 hours of age: see by 120 hours.
   b. **Combining the risk zone (as per bilirubin nomogram) and clinical risk factors** can be used to predict subsequent risk for hyperbilirubinemia and to formulate plans for management and follow-up (Maisels et al). See Figures 63–2A through C for management and follow-up according to predischarge bilirubin measurements, gestation, and risk factors.
3. **Follow-up assessment.** Should include weight, intake, voiding and stooling pattern, and presence of jaundice. Use clinical judgment in deciding whether a TSB should be obtained.

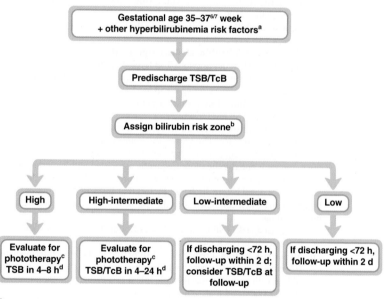

FIGURE 63–2. Algorithm providing recommendations for management and follow-up according to predischarge bilirubin measurements, gestation (≥35 weeks), and risk factors for subsequent hyperbilirubinemia. Provide lactation evaluation and support for all breast feeding mothers. Recommendation for timing of repeat TSB or TcB measurement depends on infants' age at measurement and how far the level is above the 95th percentile (see Figure 99–1); higher and earlier initial levels require an earlier repeat measurement. Perform standard clinical evaluation at all follow up visits. For evaluation of jaundice see the 2004 American Academy of Pediatrics guideline.TcB, transcutaneous bilirubin; TSB, total serum bilirubin. (*Reproduced with permission from Maisels MJ, Bhutani VK, Bogen D, et al: Hyperbilirubinemia in the newborn infant > or = 35 weeks' gestation: an update with clarifications,* Pediatrics. *2009 Oct;124(4):1193-1198.*)

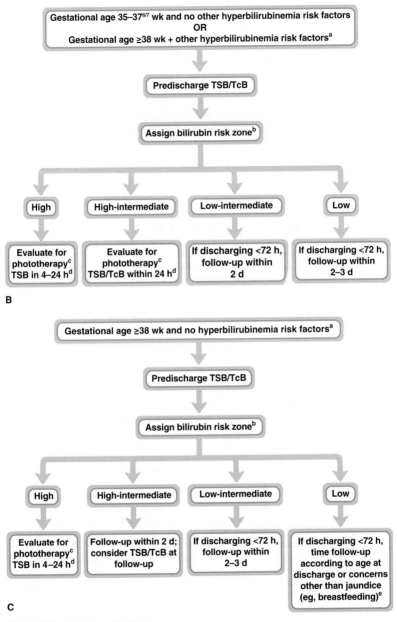

Gestational age 35–37⁶ᐟ⁷ wk and no other hyperbilirubinemia risk factors
OR
Gestational age ≥38 wk + other hyperbilirubinemia risk factors[a]

Predischarge TSB/TcB

Assign bilirubin risk zone[b]

| High | High-intermediate | Low-intermediate | Low |

| Evaluate for phototherapy[c] TSB in 4–24 h[d] | Evaluate for phototherapy[c] TSB/TcB within 24 h[d] | If discharging <72 h, follow-up within 2 d | If discharging <72 h, follow-up within 2–3 d |

B

Gestational age ≥38 wk and no hyperbilirubinemia risk factors[a]

Predischarge TSB/TcB

Assign bilirubin risk zone[b]

| High | High-intermediate | Low-intermediate | Low |

| Evaluate for phototherapy[c] TSB in 4–24 h[d] | Follow-up within 2 d; consider TSB/TcB at follow-up | If discharging <72 h, follow-up within 2–3 d | If discharging <72 h, time follow-up according to age at discharge or concerns other than jaundice (eg, breastfeeding)[e] |

C

[a]Other risk factors for hyperbilirubinemia.
[b]Figure 99–1.
[c]Figure 99–2.
[d]In hospital or as outpatient.
[e]Follow up recommendations can be modified according to level of risk for hyperbilirubinemia: depending on the circumstances in infants at low risk, later follow-up can be considered.

FIGURE 63–2.

64 Hyperglycemia

I. **Problem.** <u>The nurse reports an infant has a high blood glucose level of 240 mg/dL.</u> Hyperglycemia is very common in premature low birthweight and extremely low birthweight infants and in extremely sick or stressed newborn infants. There is no universally accepted set definition of hyperglycemia in the newborn. An operational definition, a blood glucose level that triggers an osmotic diuresis, has yet to be defined by sufficient evidence. The treatment of hyperglycemia is also ***controversial.*** Following are some of the definitions used in the literature:

   A. **Whole blood glucose >120 to 125 mg/dL or a plasma glucose >145 to 150 mg/dL regardless of gestational or postnatal age or weight.**

   B. **Whole blood glucose >125 mg/dL in term and >150 mg/dL in preterm infant.**

   C. **Whole blood glucose >215 mg/dL (operational definition), proposed by Dr. Edmund Hey.**

   A major concern with hyperglycemia is that it can cause hyperosmolality, osmotic diuresis, and subsequent dehydration. For every 18 mg/dL increase in plasma glucose, the plasma osmolality increases by 1 mOsm/L. In hyperglycemia, the high filtered load of glucose exceeds the amount the kidney tubules can reabsorb, and the excess glucose ends up in the urine. Because glucose is a solute, it draws water into the urine by osmosis (**osmotic diuresis**). Therefore, a high volume of glucose-containing urine is produced, which can lead to dehydration. It is difficult to know the exact level of blood glucose that triggers an osmotic diuresis in neonates. Significant osmolar changes have been reported to occur at a serum glucose >360 mg/dL.

   The other concern is that preterm infants with hyperglycemia are at an increased risk of mortality, infection, intracranial hemorrhage, neurodevelopmental impairment (prolonged or symptomatic hyperglycemia), white matter reduction on magnetic resonance imaging, retinopathy of prematurity, and developmental delay. Hyperglycemia is an independent risk factor for the prediction of death (57% likelihood of death when present in critically ill neonates). In the first 12 hours in asphyxiated term infants, it is associated with poor gross motor outcome, and if it occurs on the first day in infants undergoing therapeutic hypothermia for hypoxic ischemic encephalopathy, it is associated with a poor outcome. Hyperglycemia is common in infants with NEC and is associated with a poor outcome (increase in late mortality and longer NICU stay).

II. **Immediate questions**

   A. **Are there any signs of hyperglycemia?** Hyperglycemia is most common during the first week of birth, and most infants are asymptomatic or can have signs of an underlying disorder (eg, sepsis). Signs that are specific but unreliable in hyperglycemia include weight loss, fever, failure to thrive, glycosuria, metabolic acidosis, and dehydration secondary to an osmotic diuresis. Signs that are common in transient or permanent neonatal diabetes are glycosuria, ketosis, and metabolic acidosis.

   B. **What is the serum glucose value on plasma laboratory testing?** Plasma glucose measurement by a laboratory performed method is the gold standard for measuring blood glucose levels. Point-of-care bedside glucose testing using reagent strips and glucose reflectance meters are widely used for screening but are not always accurate or reliable. Contamination of the blood sample with alcohol has been shown to increase the blood glucose level in reagent strips. The reagent strips measure glucose concentration in whole blood, which is 10% to 15% lower than laboratory plasma glucose levels. Confirm a serum glucose level from the laboratory before initiating treatment.

C. **Is glucose being spilled in the urine (glucosuria)?** The amount of glucose in the urine, which is an indication of the renal threshold for glucose, has been used to evaluate hyperglycemia and whether too much glucose is being administered. In neonates, glycosuria can be an unreliable marker for both hyperglycemia and the evaluation of the glucose infusion rate. Glycosuria can occur with normal blood levels, and hyperglycemia can be associated with mild or no glycosuria. It is important to remember the renal threshold is lower in premature infants, because nephrogenesis is not complete until 36 weeks' gestation. Normal renal threshold for glucose is 160 to 180 mg/dL; urinary glucose will start to be detected above this level. General findings on reagent strip testing of the urine are as follows:

1. **Trace glucose:** Urine contains 100mg/dL glucose.
2. **+1 glucose:** Serum glucose >180 mg/dL; urine contains 250 mg/dL of glucose.
3. **+2 glucose:** Serum glucose >200 mg/dL; urine contains >500 mg/dL of glucose.
4. **+3 glucose:** Serum glucose >300 mg/dL; urine contains >1000 mg/dL glucose.
5. **+4 glucose:** Serum glucose >400 mg/dL; urine contains >2000 mg/dL glucose.

A trace amount of glucose in the urine is accepted as normal. If the **urinary glucose level is +1, +2, or greater, the renal threshold has been reached with an increased chance of osmotic diuresis.** Significant glycosuria is uncommon, and some sources indicate that osmotic diuresis is not a concern until the urine contains greater than +2 to +3 glucose. Some institutions accept a urinary glucose level of +1 without treating the patient (*controversial*), whereas some authors suggest that greater than +1 glucosuria indicates early osmolar changes and should be treated.

D. **How much glucose is the patient receiving?** High glucose intake is a common cause of hyperglycemia in a preterm infant. Dextrose (D-glucose) infusions >10 to 12 mg/kg/min may result in hyperglycemia, and hyperglycemia may occur at lower levels if the infant is stressed. Normal initial maintenance dextrose therapy in infants not being fed orally is 6 to 7 mg/kg/min on days 1 to 8 or 9 mg/kg/min on days 2 to 7. ELBW infants should be started at 4 to 6 mg/kg/min (see Chapter 13).

E. **Are there signs of stress?** Stressful situations such as surgery may cause hyperglycemia by inducing a catecholamine-mediated stress response. When an infant who has had normal glucose levels develops hyperglycemia and there is no change in intravenous (IV) fluids, or if an infant who is being fed only enterally suddenly develops hyperglycemia, suspect either sepsis or necrotizing enterocolitis (NEC).

F. **What is the birthweight of the infant? Is the infant preterm?** Low birthweight and lower gestational age are significant risk factors for hyperglycemia. The incidence is ≤5% in full-term infants, 68% in infants weighing 1000 to 1500 g, 72% in infants weighing <1000 g, and 80% in infants weighing <750 g.

G. **Does the infant have any of the high-risk factors for hyperglycemia?** Risk factors include gestational age <37 weeks, postnatal age <72 hours, weight <2500 g (lower birthweight), hypoxia, infection, use of inotropes, lipid infusions, high glucose infusion rate, respiratory distress syndrome, and sepsis. These infants should have frequent monitoring of their blood sugars. Low phosphate can be associated with hyperglycemia in ELBW neonates.

H. **What are the current medications?** Steroids (most common), methylxanthines, and vasoactive drugs can cause hyperglycemia. Caffeine rarely has an effect on blood glucose levels, but an overdose can cause hyperglycemia.

III. **Differential diagnosis.** Hyperglycemia in preterm or low birthweight infants used to be attributed only to excess IV glucose infusion, but other mechanisms may be responsible. These infants have limited reserve since glycogen storage does not occur until the third trimester. There is also immaturity or defective glucoregulatory hormone control, poor insulin response to elevated blood glucose levels, insulin resistance in peripheral tissues, a lack of negative feedback on hepatic glucose production during dextrose infusion, inability to suppress glucose production, and glucose intolerance. **Neonatal** hyperglycemia is usually related to a clinical condition and not a specific abnormality in glucose metabolism.

A. **Factitious hyperglycemia**
  1. **Blood drawn from an intravenous line** containing glucose or shortly after a bolus of glucose was given.
  2. **False bedside hyperglycemia from a glucose meter.** Some glucose meters will overestimate the serum glucose in an infant with **galactosemia** because of the lack of specificity of the enzyme used by the assay. Always confirm with a serum sample if glucose meter is high.

B. **True hyperglycemia**
  1. **Glucose infusion** can play a major role in hyperglycemia. Giving infants more glucose than they can handle needs to be evaluated first. Incorrect calculation of glucose levels or errors in the formulation of IV fluids may cause hyperglycemia. Infants often need their glucose infusion rates frequently adjusted because their needs have changed or other factors are causing hyperglycemia (sepsis, prematurity, stress).
     a. **Extremely low birthweight infants (<1000 g).** These infants have greater fluid requirements because of their immature renal function and increased insensible water loss. This often leads to a high volume of fluid and administering too much glucose. They also may have insulin resistance or an immature insulin response and thus may be unable to stop gluconeogenesis when IV glucose is given.
     b. **Preterm infants/small for gestational age infants.** Preterm infants receiving a glucose challenge show variable increases in insulin levels consistent with **insulin resistance.** This resistance may be related to immaturity or down-regulation of peripheral receptors or inadequate development of the insulin dependent GLUT-4–mediated glucose transport system. Transient hyperglycemia can also be seen in small for gestational age (SGA) infants from impaired glucose homeostasis.
  2. **Sepsis.** Suspect sepsis-related hyperglycemia in a neonate who had normal glucose levels with no change in the rate or amount of IV glucose. The etiologies can include the stress response, a reduction in the peripheral utilization of glucose, or a decrease in release of insulin. Hyperglycemia is more frequent in **fungal** than bacterial sepsis in the neonate. Hyperglycemia may be the first sign in neonatal sepsis; in *Candida* sepsis, it can appear 2 to 3 days before other signs.
  3. **Hypoxia** can cause increased glucose production and hyperglycemia.
  4. **Hyperosmolar formula.** Ask how the formula was made. An inappropriate dilution can lead to a hyperosmolar formula, which in turn can cause transient hyperglycemia. Signs can look the same as those of transient neonatal diabetes (hyperglycemia, glycosuria, dehydration).
  5. **Lipid infusion.** Lipids and lipid components (especially free fatty acids) can cause hyperglycemia. Infants who receive lipid infusion even with low rates of glucose administration may develop hyperglycemia. Lipids are emulsified in a dextran solution, a glucose polymer which can increases blood glucose levels. The lipid component may also cause a glycemic response and a decrease in peripheral glucose utilization and may inhibit insulin's effect. One study found that giving lipid infusion increased plasma glucose concentrations by 24% over baseline values. If the lipid infusion is given rapidly at a rate >0.25 g/kg/h, it can cause hyperglycemia.
  6. **Stress/surgical procedures/therapeutic hypothermia.** Pain, painful procedures (venipuncture, vascular cutdowns, and others), surgical procedures (during surgery and postoperative), mechanical ventilation, NEC, acute intracerebral bleeding, hypoxia, catecholamine infusions, and respiratory distress can all cause hyperglycemia secondary to increased stress hormones. During surgical procedures and postoperatively, infants are often given too much glucose-containing

IV fluids, which can lead to hyperglycemia. Increased cortisol secretion during surgery and increased catecholamine release after induction of anesthesia also play a role. Infants undergoing therapeutic hyperthermia can become hyperglycemic and often require insulin therapy. Hypothermia can decrease insulin sensitivity and the amount of insulin secretion by the pancreas, which leads to hyperglycemia.

7. **Medications**
   a. **Maternal use of diazoxide** can cause hyperglycemia in the infant.
   b. **Medications used in infants** that have been associated with hyperglycemia include steroids (most common, especially in ELBW infants), theophylline, caffeine, inotropic agents, diazoxide, and phenytoin. Inhaled fluticasone propionate can cause hyperglycemia.

8. **Chromosome 13 deletion (46,xxDq–)** has been associated with hyperglycemia in an SGA neonate.

9. **Neonatal diabetes mellitus is a rare form (1 in 500,000 live births) of diabetes and usually has a monogenic etiology.** It is defined as persistent hyperglycemia that lasts >2 weeks and requires insulin therapy. Neonatal diabetes mellitus (NDM) occurs in infants <6 months old; it is not an autoimmune disease and is most commonly caused by genetic defects. Molecular analysis of chromosome 6 anomalies and the *KCNJ11* and *ABCC8* genes can provide a way of differentiating transient from permanent neonatal diabetes. Infants with NDM can have hyperglycemia, metabolic acidosis, ketosis, weight loss, polyuria, volume depletion, and glycosuria. **There are 2 types of NDM, and it is clinically difficult to differentiate whether an infant has transient NDM (TNDM) or permanent NDM (PNDM):**
   a. **Transient neonatal diabetes mellitus (40%–60% of cases)** is a developmental disorder of the production of insulin that usually resolves. It is primarily a genetic disorder, and the gene responsible can be ascertained in 90% of the cases (mutation of imprinting gene *ZAC/PLAGL1* on chromosome 6q24 a major cause; mutation of the *ABCC8* gene, which encodes SUR1, can cause transient and permanent diabetes mellitus). Most infants are SGA or have intrauterine growth restriction (IUGR); they present from 2 days to 6 weeks of age with hyperglycemia and require insulin therapy. TNDM persists for >2 weeks and usually resolves by 18 months. It lasts a median of 12 weeks. Common findings are hyperglycemia, dehydration, glycosuria, polyuria, progressive wasting, hypoinsulinism, ketosis, metabolic acidosis, absent ketonuria, and normal or transiently low C-peptide levels in urine and serum. There is a positive family history in approximately 33% of cases. About half of these patients relapse later in life (in adolescence or adulthood) and require medication.
   b. **Permanent neonatal diabetes mellitus.** PNDM is less common than TNDM. It develops in the neonatal period, does not go into remission, and requires lifelong medical treatment. It is genetically heterogeneous with mutations in >20 different genes (most common are the *KCNJ11* gene encoding Kir6.2; mutation of the *ABCC8* gene, which encodes SUR1; and mutations in *INS* gene). These infants are usually SGA, and some may have DEND syndrome (developmental delay, epilepsy, neonatal diabetes). **Preterm infants can have neonatal diabetes mellitus** secondary to a monogenic etiology (*GATA6* mutations and chromosome 6q24 imprinting abnormalities are more common).

10. **Idiopathic hyperglycemia.** No identifiable cause is found; a diagnosis of exclusion.

11. **Rare causes.** Pancreatic lesions (pancreatic aplasia, pancreatic hypoplasia, congenital absence of insulin-secreting B cells) are extremely rare in neonates and they rarely survive. The prevalence of cystic fibrosis–related diabetes mellitus

(CFRD) in infants <10 years is 2%. The majority of infants with inborn errors of metabolism have hypoglycemia, but organic acidemias (isovaleric, methanolic, and propionic acidemias) can present with hyperglycemia.

IV. **Database**

   A. **Physical examination and history.** Is the infant premature or SGA, or does the infant have IUGR? Determine whether there is a family history of diabetes and ask about maternal and infant medications. Infants with hyperglycemia usually have no obvious signs. Look for dehydration, weight loss, and fever. Evaluate for subtle signs of sepsis (eg, temperature instability, changes in peripheral perfusion) or changes in gastric aspirates if the infant is feeding. Look for signs of NEC.

   B. **Laboratory studies**

   1. **Initial studies**

      a. **Serum glucose level.** Confirm any rapid bedside paper-strip test result with a serum glucose level. It is advisable to repeat serum blood glucose before treating.

      b. **Urine dipstick testing for glucose.** Because of the immaturity of the proximal tubule in premature infants, glucosuria is not the most accurate marker of hyperglycemia. Glucosuria can occur at normal blood glucose levels. High levels may indicate osmotic diuresis.

      c. **Complete blood count with differential** as a screening test for sepsis.

      d. **Blood, urine, and spinal cultures.** For sepsis workup if indicated.

      e. **Serum electrolytes.** Hyperglycemia may cause osmotic diuresis, which may lead to electrolyte losses and dehydration. Monitor serum electrolyte levels in significantly hyperglycemic patients.

      f. **Arterial blood gas.** If concerned about hypoxia; metabolic acidosis can be seen in sepsis and neonatal diabetes.

      g. **Phosphate levels.** Hypophosphatemia can be associated with hyperglycemia in ELBW neonates.

      h. **Liver transaminases** can be elevated secondary to steatosis and impairment in secretion of hepatic triglycerides.

   2. **Further studies**

      a. **Serum ketones** can be positive in NDM. **Ketonuria** can be absent or mild.

      b. **Serum insulin level** is low to normal in TNDM and normal to high in sepsis.

      c. **Serum or urine C-peptide levels** are low in TNDM.

      d. **Genetic evaluation and testing (molecular diagnosis) for neonatal diabetes are recommended** for all patients diagnosed with diabetes in the first 6 months of life. It is important because the results may change the treatment plan, predict prognosis, and improve glycemic control. Testing identifies which types of PNDM will respond to oral sulfonylurea therapy and which will require insulin. Molecular analysis of chromosome 6q24 anomalies and the *KCNJ11* and *ABCC8* genes will help to differentiate TNDM from PNDM.

   C. **Imaging and other studies.** None are usually required; however, a **chest radiograph** may be useful in the evaluation of respiratory distress and sepsis, and an **abdominal film** may be useful for NEC. **Head ultrasound** is recommended in premature infants to rule out a bleed.

V. **Plan.** The standard treatments of hyperglycemia are observation, glucose restriction, insulin therapy, or a combination of glucose restriction and insulin therapy. A Cochrane review of trials of interventions (decreasing amount of glucose or giving insulin) for treatment of neonatal hyperglycemia in very low birthweight (VLBW) infants found "evidence from randomized trials was insufficient to determine the effects of treatment on death or major morbidities and it remains uncertain whether the hyperglycemia per se is a cause of adverse clinical outcomes or how the hyperglycemia is treated." Recommended treatment is conservative since most cases of hyperglycemia are transient. Treatment values and method of treatment vary; follow institution's guidelines.

A. **Early insulin therapy and low versus high glucose infusion rates to prevent hyperglycemia.** Routine early continuous insulin infusion is not recommended in VLBW infants. A multicenter trial of early insulin therapy in VLBW infants addressed whether early insulin therapy reduced hyperglycemia. It showed that the infants who received early insulin therapy had lower glucose levels, were less likely to be hyperglycemic, had less weight loss, and received more calories because of the increased amount of glucose infusion. It did not improve growth and increased the episodes of hypoglycemia and death before 28 days. A Cochrane review states there is insufficient evidence comparing lower or higher glucose rates **to prevent hyperglycemia in VLBW infants.** They also found that the evidence does not support the routine use of insulin infusions to prevent hyperglycemia in VLBW neonates.

B. **Permissive hyperglycemia in extremely low birthweight infants.** Permissive hyperglycemia (allowing a higher than normal serum glucose to give additional calories to promote growth) is practiced in some neonatal intensive care units. A study was done in ELBW infants that showed that permissive hyperglycemia up to <300 mg/dL without insulin in the first 14 days of life was associated with faster weight gain and was not associated with osmotic diuresis or increased mortality or morbidity. **Permissive hyperglycemia allows increased caloric intake** to support nutrition and prevents the frequent episodes of hypoglycemia and increase in mortality associated with early insulin treatment.

C. **Initial management**
   1. **Rule out factitious hyperglycemia.** Check to see how the blood glucose was drawn, make sure to get a serum blood glucose, and recheck another one before treatment to confirm.
   2. **Recalculate how much glucose the infant is receiving** and make sure the infant is not getting too much glucose (see Chapter 13). ELBW infants, especially <1000 g, cannot tolerate high glucose loads, and giving >4 mg/kg/min may cause hyperglycemia. Some infants may need less glucose because of stress or sepsis or some other clinical situation.
   3. **Treat any underlying causes of hyperglycemia,** such as sepsis, hypoxia, pain, respiratory distress, or postsurgery; stop medications that may cause hyperglycemia; check formula dilution; and institute other measures to address underlying cause. **Monitor blood glucose levels and glycosuria frequently,** especially in preterm, low birthweight, ELBW, stressed, or septic infants and infants with symptoms suggestive of hyperglycemia or whose glucose levels have not been stable. Monitor all infants on parenteral glucose therapy and insulin therapy. It is important to monitor blood glucose levels during observation and treatment since hypoglycemia can occur.
   4. **Enteral feeding.** Feed as early as possible since early feeding promotes pancreatic function and secretion of insulin and can be beneficial for maintaining euglycemia. Even minimal enteral feeds induce insulin secretion. If the clinical situation is severe, feeding may not be possible.
   5. **Parenteral nutrition and lipids.** Early introduction of parenteral infusion is associated with a decreased incidence of hyperglycemia. It provides a substrate for gluconeogenesis and helps stimulate insulin release in infants receiving glucose. If the infant is on lipids, some institutions decrease the lipid infusion rate to help decrease the hyperglycemia. Infants with persistent hyperglycemia on parenteral nutrition may warrant treatment with insulin. **Clinical guidelines from the American Society for Parenteral and Enteral Nutrition for infants on parenteral nutrition and hyperglycemia include the following:**
      a. **Check blood glucose by laboratory serum glucose** or glucose electrode measurements. Keep serum glucose concentration <150 mg/dL.
      b. **Avoid excess dextrose and add fat emulsion.** Lower the dose of fat emulsion if hyperglycemia occurs.
      c. **Do not use early insulin therapy.**

    d. Persistent hyperglycemia in the neonate receiving parenteral nutrition may require treatment with insulin. First try other methods to decrease glucose: decrease amount of glucose infusion rate, remove medications that cause hyperglycemia, and correct any underlying causes of hyperglycemia.

D. Treatment of hyperglycemia

  1. Observation only. If the glucose is not too high (usually <180 mg/dL) and the urinary glucose is negative or trace, observation with close monitoring of blood glucose levels is usually all that is needed. Some providers accept +1 glucose in the urine and will not treat. Monitor with bedside glucose testing every 4 to 6 hours, and check for glucose in the urine with each void.

  2. Decrease the amount of glucose administered. This can be done by decreasing the concentration of glucose or the rate of infusion until a normal serum glucose level is present. If the glucose is >180 to 200 mg/dL or if the infant is spilling greater than +2 glucose in the urine, treatment is usually necessary. The presence of glucose in the urine may indicate osmolar changes, which could indicate hyperosmolarity, osmotic diuresis, and dehydration. Monitor with bedside glucose testing every 4 to 6 hours, and check for glucose in the urine with each void.

    a. Decrease the concentration of glucose. Typically, the concentration can be reduced from 10% to 5%. Do not use a solution that has a dextrose concentration of <5%. Such a solution is hypo-osmolar and could cause hemolysis, with resulting hyperkalemia.

    b. Decrease the rate of glucose infusion. The rate can be safely decreased by 1 to 2 mg/kg/min every 2 to 4 hours. Typically, the rate can be decreased to 4 to 6 mg/kg/min, with some sources reporting 3 to 4 mg/kg/min.

  3. Insulin therapy. Although routine early insulin is not recommended, persistent hyperglycemia may warrant treatment with insulin. Indications for insulin therapy are controversial. Most physicians treat infants with persistent hyperglycemia that occurs after the amount of glucose is decreased, infants with osmotic diuresis, or infants on a decreased glucose infusion rate who need more calories because they are not gaining weight (failure to thrive). Levels vary widely on recommendations, but many will treat the infant with insulin for persistent blood glucose levels >200 to 250 mg/dL (some sources use 300 mg/dL). Guidelines are institutional dependent and ***controversial*. Use regular insulin (100 U/mL)** diluted in normal saline to a concentration of 0.5 U/mL or 0.1 U/mL. Several regimens are available for insulin dosing.

    a. Bolus infusion

      i. Insulin 0.05 to 0.1 U/kg/dose over 15 minutes every 4 to 6 hours as needed.

      ii. Monitor glucose every 30 to 60 minutes after dose.

      iii. Consider continuous infusion if the bolus does not work after 2 to 3 doses (blood glucose >200 mg/dL).

    b. Continuous insulin infusion (most common and preferred method)

      i. Insulin infusion rate: 0.01 to 0.2 U/kg/h.

      ii. Usual starting dose is between 0.01 and 0.05 U/kg/h.

      iii. Adjust in small increments (0.01 U/kg/h) as needed.

      iv. Flush the tubing with >25 mL of the insulin-containing solution for at least 20 minutes so that all sites in the tubing will be saturated satisfactorily before beginning the infusion. This is done because insulin binds to the tubing, preventing the entire dose of insulin getting to the infant. Adding albumin to the bag to prevent insulin from adhering to the plastic tubing is now considered unnecessary.

      v. Potassium should be added to the solution to limit hypokalemia; monitor potassium levels.

      vi. Bedside glucose testing must be performed within 30 minutes of starting the infusion and after every change made. Check every hour until the blood glucose is stable.

       vii. **When to stop.** Once the serum glucose improves (serum glucose <150 mg/dL), infusion rates can be decreased in increments between 0.01 and 0.05 U/kg/h. Once the achieved glucose level is obtained and remains stable, the infusion can be discontinued. Monitor the glucose levels closely after that for a minimum of 24 hours.

    c. **Subcutaneous insulin.** Subcutaneous route is typically only used in neonatal diabetes. TNDM is typically treated with subcutaneous insulin, but it is difficult for some caregivers to use it. **Dose varies, but some providers use** 0.1 to 0.2 U/kg/dose every 6 to 12 hours. Bedside glucose testing must be performed every 60 minutes until the glucose level is stable. **Insulin glargine and insulin lispro** have both been used in neonates.

    d. **Potassium and glucose levels need to be monitored when giving insulin therapy.** Insulin can cause hypokalemia and hypoglycemia. Several studies found the risk of hypoglycemia to be small in ELBW infants receiving insulin infusion.

  E. **Transient or permanent neonatal diabetes mellitus**

    1. **Give intravenous or oral fluids** and monitor the urine output, blood pH, and serum electrolyte levels.

    2. **Give insulin** either by **constant infusion** or **subcutaneously** (see Section V.D.3). Monitor glucose levels with bedside testing every 4 to 6 hours.

    3. **Continuous subcutaneous insulin infusion** is administered with an insulin pump and has been used in neonates with diabetes with less variability in glucose. **Continuous subcutaneous insulin infusion (CSII) is felt to be safe, more accurate, more physiologic, and easier to manage insulin. CSII has been used with continuous glucose monitoring system** successfully in 4 young infants.

    4. **Oral sulfonylurea therapy** is recommended for infants with activating mutations in the *KCNJ11* and *ABCC8* genes. It has been successfully used in >300 patients who have been able to stop insulin completely and have better control with less hypoglycemia. Infants are transitioned from insulin to an oral sulfonylurea. The majority of infants unable to transfer to oral therapy had profound developmental delay and epilepsy before 6 months of age. There are many different sulfonylureas (glyburide, glipizide, glimepiride).

    5. **Repeat serum insulin values** to rule out PNDM. Early genetic testing should be considered.

    6. **Consult a pediatric endocrinologist and pediatric geneticist.**

  F. **Medications**

    1. **If the infant is receiving theophylline,** the serum theophylline level should be checked to detect possible toxicity, with resulting hyperglycemia. Other signs of theophylline toxicity include tachycardia, jitteriness, feeding intolerance, and seizures. If the level is high, the dosage must be decreased or the drug discontinued.

    2. **With maternal use of diazoxide,** the infant may have tachycardia and hypotension as well as hyperglycemia. Toxicity in the infant is usually self-limited, and only observation is usually necessary.

    3. **Caffeine and phenytoin** should be adjusted or discontinued if possible.

    4. **Steroids.** Prolonged courses and pharmacologic dosing of corticosteroids are being used in some infants with chronic lung disease. When steroid use is deemed necessary, reducing the dose or frequency may limit the hyperglycemic effects.

  G. **Hyperosmolar formula–induced hyperglycemia.** Rehydration is necessary. Stop the formula and give detailed instructions on how to make formula using powder or concentrated formula.

  H. **Pain control for stress following surgery or invasive procedures.** Pain recommendations are listed with each procedure in this book. Fentanyl has been used during and after surgery and has decreased the incidence of hyperglycemia.

65 Hyperkalemia

I. **Problem.** The serum potassium level is 7.0 mEq/L in an extremely low birthweight (ELBW) infant. Normal potassium levels are generally between 3.5 and 5.5 mEq/L, with a potassium >5.5 mEq/L indicating hyperkalemia. The exact definition varies and can be based on maturity or severity. Some reported definitions of hyperkalemia include the following:

   A. **Serum potassium >6 mEq/L in full-term neonates.**
   B. **Serum potassium >6.5 mEq/L in premature infants.**
   C. **Moderate hyperkalemia: Serum potassium 6 to 7 mEq/L**
   D. **Severe hyperkalemia: Serum potassium >7 mEq/L**

   Hyperkalemia is common in preterm and ELBW infants because of an immature tubular function and a decreased potassium excretion caused by a lower glomerular filtration rate. Plasma potassium concentration also increases in ELBW infants in the first few days after birth from the shift of potassium from the intracellular to the extracellular compartment. **This is the most serious of electrolyte abnormalities because it can cause fatal arrhythmias.** If electrocardiogram (ECG) changes relating to hyperkalemia are present, this is an emergency situation. Plasma potassium should be monitored in all premature infants <30 weeks postmenstrual age during the first 3 days of life because they can develop nonoliguric hyperkalemia (NOHK) and have serious complications (cardiac arrhythmias, periventricular leukomalacia, brain hemorrhage, and sudden death).

II. **Immediate questions**

   A. **How was the specimen collected? What is the central serum potassium level? Is it a true level or factitious level?** Blood obtained from a heel stick or drawn through a small-bore intravenous (IV) line or tiny needle may yield falsely elevated potassium levels secondary to hemolysis. Clot formation can also cause a falsely elevated potassium. The blood should not be obtained from a heparin-coated umbilical catheter (release of benzalkonium from a heparin-coated umbilical catheter can elevate the potassium reading). *Note:* Serum potassium level is 0.4 mEq/L higher than the plasma level. Always do a serum potassium level from a venous sample (free flowing) before treatment.

   B. **Does the electrocardiogram show cardiac changes characteristic of hyperkalemia?** This may be the first indication of hyperkalemia. In neonates, serum potassium >6.7 mEq/L is associated with ECG changes. Early cardiac changes include tall, peaked, "tented" T waves, followed by loss of or flattened P wave, widening QRS, ST-segment depression, bradycardia, sine wave QRS-T, first-degree atrioventricular block, ventricular tachyarrhythmias, and finally cardiac arrest if the potassium levels continue to increase. Classic ECG changes include the following:

      1. **Serum potassium of 5.5 to 6.5 mEq/L.** Tall peaked T waves with a narrow base, shortening of PR interval, normal or decreased QT.
      2. **Serum potassium of 6.5 to 8 mEq/L.** Tall peaked T waves, prolonged PR interval, loss or decreased P wave, amplified R wave, widening of QRS.
      3. **Serum potassium >8 mEq/L.** Absent P wave, wide bizarre diphasic QRS, progressive QRS widening merging with the T wave, bundle branch blocks, ventricular fibrillation or asystole.

   C. **How much potassium is the infant receiving?** Normal amounts of potassium given for maintenance are 1 to 3 mEq/kg/d.

   D. **What are the blood urea nitrogen and creatinine levels? What are the urine output and body weight?** Elevated blood urea nitrogen (BUN) and creatinine levels suggest renal insufficiency. Another indication of renal failure is decreasing or inadequate urine output with weight gain.

E. **Is there associated hyponatremia, hypoglycemia, and hypotension?** With low sodium and glucose, high potassium, and hypotension, consider adrenal insufficiency.

F. **Does the infant have any of the common characteristics of premature newborns prone to hyperkalemia?** These include small for gestational age, female sex, severe respiratory distress syndrome, very low birthweight, requirement of exogenous surfactant, need for inotropic medications, and delayed feeding. Mildly elevated potassium (>5.6 mEq/L) and phosphate levels (>2 mEq/L) within 6 hours of birth may predict the development of hyperkalemia. NOHK risk factors in ELBW infants are younger gestational age and infants whose mothers did not use antenatal steroids. Electrolyte imbalance (hypernatremia, hypocalcemia, and hyperphosphatemia) occurs more often in infants with NOHK.

III. **Differential diagnosis.** True hyperkalemia can be caused by an increase in potassium intake (usually not a problem if kidneys able to excrete potassium), an increase in potassium release, a decrease in potassium excretion or inability to excrete potassium by the kidneys, medications, a shift of potassium into the extracellular space, or impaired aldosterone activity causing decreased renal excretion.

A. **Pseudohyperkalemia is a falsely elevated potassium level (plasma potassium is normal).** It can be due to hemolysis (trauma causes destruction of red blood cells [RBCs] with leakage of potassium into serum samples) during **phlebotomy or heel stick** or by drawing the sample proximal to an IV site infusing potassium. If an unspun sample is allowed to sit or if there is a delay in processing (after 2 hours), potassium release from the cells and causes pseudohyperkalemia. Laboratory error (multiple processing variables) can also be a reason. **Thrombocytosis (increase in platelets) and leukocytosis (increase in WBCs)** can lead to a false elevation of **serum potassium levels** because potassium leaks out of an increased number of white blood cells and platelets during clotting. The serum potassium increases by 0.15 mEq/L for every 100,000/mL elevation of the platelet count. Two rare genetic syndromes that can cause pseudohyperkalemia are **familial pseudohyperkalemia** and **hereditary spherocytosis.**

B. **True hyperkalemia**

1. **Common causes of hyperkalemia**

   a. **Increased potassium administration or intake.** Excessive amount in IV fluids, excessive oral supplementation (excess potassium chloride supplementation in an infant with bronchopulmonary dysplasia/chronic lung disease), or potassium-containing medications. Potassium supplements usually are not necessary on the first day of life and often are not necessary until day 3, with the typical requirement of 1 to 3 mEq/kg/d. This is a rare cause because the kidneys usually excrete any excess potassium.

   b. **Pathologic hemolysis of red blood cells.** May be secondary to intraventricular hemorrhage, use of a hypotonic glucose solution (<4.7% dextrose), sepsis (most commonly *Pseudomonas*), intravascular hemolysis, cephalohematoma, bleeding, asphyxia, or Rh incompatibility.

   c. **Tissue necrosis and breakdown.** In certain disease states, such as necrotizing enterocolitis (NEC) or bowel infarction, tissue necrosis can occur and hyperkalemia may result. Trauma and severe hypothermia can cause rhabdomyolysis.

   d. **Renal failure/insufficiency.** Impaired kidney function can lead to hyperkalemia. Oliguria can cause decreased potassium clearance and hyperkalemia. **Acute kidney injury or chronic kidney disease** can impair potassium excretion in the urine.

   e. **Nonoliguric hyperkalemia (NOKH). NOKH is hyperkalemia in the absence of oliguria and potassium intake.** There are multiple definitions of NOHK, one that is frequently used is serum potassium ≥7 mmol/L in the presence of urine output of ≥1 mL/kg/h during the first 72 hours of life. Incidence varies between 11% and 52%. It occurs more commonly in ELBW infants than term infants, with 80% of NOHK cases in ELBW infants <28 weeks' gestation. These infants usually did not have exposure to antenatal steroids, which seems to protect some infants. Pathophysiology is unknown but current evidence states that NOHK results from a shift of potassium from the intracellular to extracellular space due to the immature function of Na/K-ATPase activity in premature neonates.It can cause life-threatening cardiac arrhythmias.

f. **Metabolic acidosis.** Causes potassium to move out of cells, resulting in hyperkalemia. For every 0.1-unit decrease in pH, the serum potassium increases approximately 0.3 to 1.3 mEq/L. Respiratory acidosis rarely causes significant hyperkalemia.

g. **Dehydration.** Volume depletion and congestive heart failure can cause renal hypoperfusion and therefore hyperkalemia.

h. **Medications. Medication error is one of the most common causes of hyperkalemia in the neonatal intensive care unit. Penicillin G potassium** contains potassium salts and can cause hyperkalemia. **Digoxin therapy** can lead to hyperkalemia secondary to redistribution of potassium. **Potassium-sparing diuretics** cause decreased potassium losses. Both **propranolol** and **phenylephrine** are associated with hyperkalemia. **High glucose load** can lead to hyperkalemia secondary to increases in plasma osmolality. **Heparin** can cause hyperkalemia by blocking aldosterone biosynthesis in the adrenal gland. **Other medications**, including tromethamine, enalapril, indomethacin, angiotensin-converting enzyme inhibitors, α-blockers, trimethoprim, captopril, amiloride, and nonsteroidal anti-inflammatory drugs, have been associated with hyperkalemia. **Medications that cause decreased potassium output include** potassium-sparing diuretics (spironolactone, triamterene, amiloride), cyclosporine, angiotensin-converting enzyme inhibitors, nonsteroidal anti-inflammatory drugs, heparin, tacrolimus, pentamidine, and trimethoprim.

i. **Adrenal insufficiency seen in congenital adrenal hyperplasia and bilateral adrenal hemorrhage.** In salt-losing congenital adrenal hyperplasia, infants have low serum sodium, chloride, and glucose and elevated levels of potassium and hypotension. In bilateral adrenal hemorrhage, anemia, thrombocytopenia, and jaundice are seen, and bilateral adrenal masses are often palpable. Renal tubular hyperkalemia/hyperkalemic distal renal tubular acidosis type IV occurs secondary to hypoaldosteronism. Infants present with metabolic acidosis and hyperkalemia. Hyperkalemia is seen in adrenal disorders (hypoaldosteronism, congenital adrenal hyperplasia), obstructive uropathy, reduced renal mass, renal reflux, urinary tract infection, and pseudohypoaldosteronism.

j. **Decreased insulin levels** can cause hyperkalemia as insulin drives potassium into cells.

k. **Transfusion-induced hyperkalemia.** Transfusions that require a large amount of blood transfused (eg, exchange transfusion and major surgery) can contribute to hyperkalemia. Smaller volume transfusions do not cause hyperkalemia. Irradiation of RBCs accelerates the leakage of potassium out of stored RBCs, which can increase the risk of transfusion-induced arrhythmias from hyperkalemia. Washing of irradiated RBCs reduces potassium and lactate loads. It is best to use fresh blood when possible.

l. **Hyperosmolality.** Caused by inappropriately diluted formula, hyperosmolar amino acid solution, or glucose infusions.

2. **Less common causes**

a. **Neonatal Bartter syndrome (a variant of this with *ROMK* mutation presents with early hyperkalemia).** This is a group of renal tubular disorders usually characterized by hypokalemic metabolic alkalosis.

b. **Hereditary hyperkalemic disorders.** Hereditary pseudohyperkalemia, hereditary hyperkalemic periodic paralysis, various types of hypoaldosteronism, and hereditary tubular defects that cause hyperkalemia.

     c. Disorders that cause decreased renal excretion of potassium. Renal failure, Addison disease, mineralocorticoid deficiency, primary hypoaldosteronism, aldosterone synthase deficiency, and pseudohypoaldosteronism.

IV. Database

  A. Physical examination. Typical clinical manifestations of symptomatic hyperkalemia include muscular or respiratory paralysis, bradycardia, ventricular arrhythmias (ventricular fibrillation/tachycardia), shock, and cardiac arrest. It is difficult to state an exact potassium level when clinical signs will appear, but most agree that when the serum potassium increases to >7 mEq/L, signs can be identified. Signs include polyuria and abdominal distension; lethargy with muscle weakness occurs if potassium level is >8 mEq/L but is hard to evaluate in a newborn. Tendon reflexes can be decreased. Pay special attention to the abdomen for signs of NEC (abdominal distention, decreased bowel sounds, and visible bowel loops). Evaluate for signs of other underlying diseases.

  B. Laboratory studies

    1. Immediate tests

      a. Serum potassium level measured by a properly collected venous sample. A repeat serum potassium level is usually recommended before treatment.

      b. Serum and urine electrolytes.

      c. Complete blood count and differential. To rule out sepsis and hemolysis.

      d. Serum ionized and total calcium levels. Hypocalcemia may potentiate the effects of hyperkalemia. Maintain normal serum calcium concentrations.

      e. Serum pH and bicarbonate. To rule out acidosis, which may potentiate hyperkalemia.

      f. Blood urea nitrogen and serum creatinine levels. May reveal renal insufficiency.

      g. Urine dipstick and specific gravity. To assess renal status and blood and hemoglobin for tissue breakdown secondary to hemolysis. Examine for casts or sediment.

    2. Further testing

      a. 17-hydroxyprogesterone (17-OHP) by tandem mass spectrometry for classic congenital adrenal hyperplasia. Other tests include serum cortisol, 11-deoxycortisol, 17-hydroxypregnenolone, androstenendione, and dehydroepiandrosterone.

      b. Serum renin, angiotensin, and aldosterone for hypoaldosteronism and pseudohypoaldosteronism.

  C. Imaging and other studies

    1. Abdominal radiograph if NEC is suspected.

    2. Electrocardiogram may reveal the cardiac changes characteristic of hyperkalemia and provides a baseline study (see Section II.B).

V. Plan. First, rule out pseudohyperkalemia and confirm true hyperkalemia with a repeat stat serum potassium level (make sure it is free flowing venous sample). Obtain an ECG and place the infant on a cardiac monitor. **Document any ECG changes, and if present, this is a medical emergency and needs to be treated immediately.** Treatment is also recommended when the serum potassium reaches a certain level (>6.0–6.5 mEq/L) but level recommendations vary depending upon the source.

  A. General management for hyperkalemia (see Table 65–1)

    1. Stop all exogenous potassium intake. Check the calculation of potassium in the IV fluids/TPN to verify that excess potassium was not given. Consider stopping any potassium containing medications, oral potassium supplements or medications known to induce hyperkalemia.

    2. If hypocalcemia is also present, treat it by infusing 100 to 200 mg/kg of calcium gluconate (diluted in appropriate fluid given over 10–30 minutes). This will lower the cell membrane threshold and be cardioprotective. Use caution

Table 65–1. HYPERKALEMIA MANAGEMENT IN NEONATES

Drug	Dosing Regimen	Onset	Comments and Side Effects
MOA: Cardiac membrane stabilization			
Calcium gluconate 10%	60 mg/kg IV over 5–10 minutes	Immediate	Vesicant—undiluted drug must be given via CENTRAL line only. Dilute with equal volume of D5W or NS to yield final concentration of 50 mg/mL to be given via peripheral IV. Do not administer in the same line with sodium bicarbonate due to possible precipitation
Calcium chloride 10%	20 mg/kg IV over 3–5 minutes	Immediate	Vesicant—must be given via CENTRAL line only
MOA: Intracellular shifting of potassium			
Insulin regular and dextrose (bolus)	0.1 unit/kg mix in 5 mL/kg D10W OR 2 mL/kg D25W IV over 15–30 minutes	10–20 minutes	Insulin: **Regular** only for intravenous administration. Prime and flush IV tubing with insulin continuous infusion solution prior to administration to minimize insulin adsorption to plastic
(Continuous infusion)	0.05–0.1 units/kg/h co-infuse with D10W at 2–4 mL/kg/h		
Albuterol inhalation	1.25–2.5 mg/dose every 2–6 hours	20–30 minutes	Do not use as sole agent for treating severe hyperkalemia
Premature neonates use only:	0.4 mg in 2 mL NS, may repeat after 2 hours if needed		
Sodium bicarbonate 4.2%	1 mEq/kg IV over 10–15 minutes; may repeat after 10–15 minutes if needed	15 minutes	Do not use as sole agent for treating severe hyperkalemia. Do not administer in the same line with calcium product due to possible precipitation
MOA: Potassium removal			
Sodium polystyrene sulfonate (without sorbitol)	1 g/kg PO or PR; may repeat after 4-6 hours if needed	1–2 hours	1 g resin binds 1 mEq of potassium. Use is contraindicated in preterm neonates or term neonates with bowel obstruction or ileus, intestinal hypomotility, or at risk for necrotizing enterocolitis. Avoid sorbitol containing product due to concern for intestinal necrosis. Consider lactulose use to prevent colonic impaction

(Continued)

Table 65–1. HYPERKALEMIA MANAGEMENT IN NEONATES (*CONTINUED*)

Drug	Dosing Regimen	Onset	Comments and Side Effects
Furosemide	1 mg/kg IV; repeat after 6 hours	1–2 hours	Monitor fluid losses and replace as needed
Renal replacement therapy: hemodialysis/ peritoneal dialysis			Hemodialysis is more effective in removing potassium, but peritoneal dialysis is generally used since it is easier to perform

MOA, mechanism of action.
Data from Lexi-Comp OnlineTM, Pediatric & Neonatal Lexi-Drugs OnlineTM, Hudson, Ohio: Lexi-Comp, Inc.; 2018; April 19, 2018; Michael J. Somers MD. Management of hyperkalemia in children. Post TW, ed. UpToDate. Waltham, MA: UpToDate Inc. http://www.uptodate.com (accessed April 19, 2018).

in giving calcium to infants on digitalis because it may increase the risk of arrhythmias.
3. **Rule out and treat any specific cause/disease** that may be contributing to the hyperkalemia.
    a. **Renal failure** can be treated with fluid restriction.
    b. **Congenital adrenal hyperplasia.** Cortisol therapy.
    c. **Hypovolemia.** Give isotonic fluids to promote tubular secretion of potassium.
    d. **Metabolic acidosis.** Correct metabolic acidosis with sodium bicarbonate. The most rapid method is hyperventilation but it is not recommended as decreases reported in serum potassium has only been 0.1 to 0.3 mE/L for every 0.1 increase in serum pH and there is a risk of decreased cerebral perfusion.
4. **Monitor electrocardiogram changes, serial potassium and calcium levels** during therapy.
5. **Remember the role of each medication and its use.**
    a. **Calcium** prevents cardiac arrhythmias by stabilizing the cell membrane of the myocardium; it does nothing to the serum potassium.
    b. **Insulin and glucose, albuterol, and sodium bicarbonate** decrease the serum potassium level by moving potassium into cells, which reduces the risk of immediate complications but does not remove potassium from the body.
    c. **Furosemide, sodium polystyrene (Kayexalate), and dialysis (exchange transfusion, peritoneal dialysis)** remove potassium from the body by renal excretion, gastrointestinal loss, or removal by dialysis.
6. **If the renal status is abnormal.** Consider the following to treat hyperkalemia: albuterol, furosemide (if oliguric), sodium polystyrene (Kayexalate), and dialysis (exchange transfusion, peritoneal dialysis).
7. **Preterm infants.** The combination of insulin and glucose as a treatment has more immediate results and is preferred over the treatment with Kayexalate (sodium polystyrene).
B. **Hyperkalemia with ECG changes.** Arrhythmias from hyperkalemia are difficult to treat. The usual steps of defibrillation, epinephrine, and antiarrhythmic drugs will not work without lowering the potassium level.
1. **First, give calcium to protect the heart from the toxic effects of potassium with calcium.** It stabilizes the myocardium and lowers the threshold potential to protect against arrhythmias. **For ECG changes or arrhythmia:** dose is calcium gluconate 10% solution (60–100 mg/kg/dose) IV diluted in appropriate fluid (NS or D5W to yield a concentration of 50 mg/mL or less) and given over 5 to 10 minutes. It can be repeated every 10 minutes as needed. Administer slow IV

infusion over 10 minutes, optimally through a central line, not a scalp IV. Observe the ECG while infusing the medication; improvement in the ECG should occur within 1 to 5 minutes. Once the arrhythmia or ECG changes disappear, the bolus can be stopped. It is necessary to give a medication immediately that will begin to decrease potassium. If the infant is on digoxin therapy, remember that calcium therapy can worsen digoxin toxicity and a slower infusion may be necessary. **For cardiac arrest, calcium chloride can be used** since it results in a more rapid increase in serum calcium. Dose is 20 mg/kg IV given over 10 minutes. Repeat dose may be needed if ECG changes persist. If effective, consider IV infusion 20 to 50 mg/kg/h.

2. **Second, start a medication (glucose and insulin or β-adrenergic agonists or sodium bicarbonate)** that causes cellular intake of potassium which will reduce serum potassium levels but does not reduce total body stores. Sodium bicarbonate has a more immediate onset; glucose, insulin, and albuterol take a minimum of 15 minutes to work. If there is no IV access, one can start a β-adrenergic agonist while starting an IV. Deciding which one to use depends on your unit's preference.

   a. **Insulin and glucose.** Insulin drives potassium into the cells. The usual dose is 0.1 to 0.2 U/kg/h insulin in combination with a continuous infusion of 0.5 g/kg/h of dextrose. If the infant is hyperglycemic, only insulin is recommended. Adjust infusion rates based on serum glucose and potassium concentrations. Time to onset is 10 to 20 minutes. Monitor the glucose levels.

   b. **Sodium bicarbonate** is considered most effective if the infant is acidotic but can be used even when blood pH is normal (***controversial***). Sodium bicarbonate use is no longer recommended in the management of the majority of cases of metabolic acidosis in a neonate (see Chapter 51); in addition, it is not recommended as monotherapy and is to be used with caution in premature infants. Some suggest using it only in life-threatening hyperkalemia or not at all. For every 0.1 increase in serum pH, serum potassium will decrease by approximately 0.6 mEq/L. Dose, **give sodium bicarbonate 1 to 2 mEq/kg over 10 to 15 minutes IV (some recommend over 30–60 minutes; works in 5–15 minutes).** Inducing alkalosis drives potassium ions into the cells. In very tiny infants, sodium bicarbonate may have associated risks. Avoid rapid infusion of sodium bicarbonate to decrease the risk of intraventricular hemorrhage. Use with caution in infants with renal failure or heart failure because the extra sodium could cause fluid retention. Use is not recommended in infants with respiratory failure.

   c. **β-Adrenergic agonists (albuterol and others).** Most studies have been in infants with hyperkalemia with chronic renal failure. Some infants do not respond to the effect of albuterol, so this should not be used as first line treatment for urgent hyperkalemia. Onset of action is approximately 20 to 30 minutes. (Case studies report a decrease of potassium 1–1.5 mEq/L within an hour of giving the medication.) The most commonly used medication is albuterol, nebulized 1.25 to 2.5 mg/dose every 2 to 6 hours as needed. Dosage for premature infants: 0.4 mg in 2 mL of saline. If no IV access is available this can be used while obtaining access.

3. **Third, give medications to cause potassium excretion** and lower total body stores, such as furosemide, sodium polystyrene (Kayexalate).

   a. **Diuretics (furosemide [Lasix]).** Enhances potassium excretion in the urine and can be given if **renal function is adequate**; the usual dose is 1 mg/kg IV every 6 hours (***controversial***). It takes 5 to 10 minutes to work. Value is limited in renal failure, with higher doses required. Remember that the amount of potassium excretion is variable and does not always correlate with the furosemide dose. Useful in hyperkalemia associated with congestive heart failure and hypoaldosteronism.

   b. **Sodium polystyrene sulfonate (Kayexalate), a potassium-exchange resin, can be given.** It removes potassium from the gut (1 g of resin removes ~1 mEq of potassium) in exchange for sodium. (Sorbitol free is recommended in neonates as sorbitol can cause bowel necrosis and sodium retention.) The usual dose is 1 g/kg/dose orally every 6 hours or rectally every 2 to 6 hours. **Rectal route is preferred** as it has a faster onset of 1 to 2 hours. Administered orally, it lowers the potassium level slowly and therefore is of limited value acutely. Cochrane review states that oral and rectal ion exchange resins should be avoided. **This therapy should not be used in ELBW infants because of risk of irritation, concretions, hemorrhagic colitis, gastrointestinal hemorrhage, colonic necrosis, sodium overload, and NEC.** This treatment can cause an increase in sodium and calcium. Repetitive rectal use can cause local bleeding. Do not use with obstructive bowel disease and infants with decreased gut motility (risk of intestinal necrosis). Complications include hypernatremia and NEC. **Use in refractory cases only.**

C. **Hyperkalemia without electrocardiogram changes.** Treatment is recommended when serum potassium is >6 to 6.5 mEq/L (*controversial*). Deciding which medication to use to decrease potassium and to cause excretion of potassium depends on your institution.

   1. **Follow recommendations in general management above.**
   2. **Start a medication (glucose and insulin or β-adrenergic agonists or sodium bicarbonate)** that causes cellular intake of potassium which will reduce serum potassium levels. See doses above.
   3. **Third, give medications to cause potassium excretion** and lower total body stores, such as furosemide, sodium polystyrene (Kayexalate). See doses above.

D. **Persistent hyperkalemia.** Continuous infusion of insulin with glucose is recommended. Infants with chronic kidney disease and renal insufficiency may require dialysis.

E. **Refractory hyperkalemia.** If all of these measures fail to lower the potassium level, other measures, such as renal replacement therapy must be considered. The methods used include hemodialysis, peritoneal dialysis, and continuous renal replacement therapy. Deciding on which one depends upon the clinical status of the infant and the availability of the different therapies. Hemodialysis is more effective than peritoneal dialysis and is preferred when hyperkalemia is secondary to cell breakdown. See Chapter 73.

F. **Nonoliguric hyperkalemia**
   1. **Prophylactic treatments**
      a. **Antenatal steroid use in the mother** results in maturation of the kidneys (Na/K-ATP enzyme maturation) and decreases the risk and possibly prevents NOHK in ELBW infants.
      b. **Early aggressive nutrition and high-dose calcium supplementation** significantly reduced the incidence of NOHK after 24 hours of life in one study.
   2. **Treatment guidelines vary and most are adapted from hyperkalemia from renal failure.** Follow guidelines for treatment as stated above or based on your recommendations from your institution. Cochrane review has no firm recommendations for treatment of hyperkalemia in NOHK in the preterm infant, except that the combination of insulin and glucose is preferred over treatment with a rectal cation resin. IV calcium use is recommended with ECG changes. Some recommend using insulin and glucose when the serum potassium is >6.5 mmol/L.
      a. **Potassium should not be administered in the first days of life** until good urinary output is established and serum potassium is normal and not rising. Potassium levels should be monitored every 6 hours in the first few days of life. Remember potassium can rise rapidly and lead to cardiac disturbances in these infants.
      b. **Because of increased electrolyte imbalances** (eg, hypocalcemia, hypernatremia, hyperphosphatemia, increased BUN), monitor these labs.
      c. **Early administration of amino acids (first day of life)** may stimulate endogenous insulin secretions and prevent the need for insulin infusion.

66 Hypertension

I. **Problem.** A premature infant has a systolic blood pressure (BP) of >95 mm Hg. **Normal BP values depend on the infant's gestational age, postnatal age, and birthweight.** There is no set definition of hypertension in newborns. American Academy of Pediatrics (AAP) clinical practice guidelines for children and adolescents state that normal BP is <90th percentile, but no guidelines have been established for infants. Hypertension has been defined as follows:

A. **Blood pressure >2 standard deviations above the mean.**

B. **Blood pressure >95th percentile for postmenstrual age.**

C. **The Task Force on Blood Pressure Control in Children defines hypertension as a blood pressure reading ≥95th percentile on 3 separate occasions.**

Hypertension occurs in 1% to 2% of all neonates in the neonatal intensive care unit (NICU); it is less common in term infants (0.2%), and more common in premature infants (75% of hypertensive infants in NICU). It typically occurs either early on (within the first couple of weeks of life) or later on (infant who is a couple of months old with a chronic condition). Persistent hypertension should be treated because it can cause hypertensive cardiomyopathy, nephropathy, encephalopathy, and retinopathy. For a rapid reference of BP ranges for premature and term infants, see Table 70–1. For estimated BP levels at the 95th and 99th percentiles in infants after 2 weeks of age, see Table 66–1. For other detailed BP values, see Appendix C.

II. **Immediate questions**

A. **How was the blood pressure measured?** BP can be measured either by invasive or noninvasive methods. Invasive methods include an indwelling intra-arterial catheter. Noninvasive methods include palpation, auscultation, Doppler ultrasound, and use of an oscillometric device. The most common methods used in the NICU are the indwelling intra-arterial catheter and the oscillometric device.

1. **Invasive method. BP reading from an indwelling intra-arterial catheter** is the most accurate (**gold standard**) of all methods and is the preferred method. It is most commonly placed in the umbilical artery or the radial artery, but can also be in the posterior tibial artery. This system uses a pressure transducer where the pressure waveform of the arterial pulse is transmitted by a column of

Table 66–1. ESTIMATED BLOOD PRESSURE LEVELS AT THE 95TH AND 99TH PERCENTILES IN INFANTS AFTER 2 WEEKS OF AGE

	Postconceptional Age in Weeks									
	26	28	30	32	34	36	38	40	42	44
95th percentile (systolic/diastolic)	72/50	75/50	80/55	83/55	85/55	87/65	92/65	95/65	98/65	105/68
99th percentile (systolic/diastolic)	77/56	80/54	85/60	88/60	90/60	92/70	97/70	100/70	102/70	110/73

Data from Dionne JM, Abitbol CL, Flynn JT: Hypertension in infancy: diagnosis, management and outcome, *Pediatr Nephrol.* 2012 Jan;27(1):17-32. Based on studies using Doppler and oscillometric blood pressure measurements.

fluid to an electrical signal. If measurements are taken by means of an umbilical artery catheter (UAC), be certain that the catheter is free of bubbles or clots and the transducer is calibrated; otherwise, erroneous results will occur. It provides continuous readings.

2. **Noninvasive methods**
   a. **Blood pressure measurement by palpation.** This is not used because it only measures the systolic BP.
   b. **Blood pressure measurement by auscultation.** The systolic pressure determination is the appearance of Korotkoff sounds, and the diastolic pressure is the disappearance or muffling of the Korotkoff sounds. This is not recommended because the arterial sounds are either unobtainable or are not reliable in newborns.
   c. **Doppler ultrasound method** is time consuming and labor intensive and underestimates the systolic BP.
   d. **Automated oscillometric devices** (electronic pressure sensor) are the **most common noninvasive method** used in the NICU. This device uses a BP cuff to detect oscillations in the artery to measure the mean arterial pressure. An algorithm is then used to give the systolic and diastolic BP. Oscillometric devices compare to intra-arterial measurements in well infants. Intra-arterial measurements may be preferred in ill infants. There are conflicting studies because one study showed that the oscillometric method overestimated the systolic and diastolic BP in ill preterm and term neonates, and another study showed that oscillometric measurements underestimated systolic and diastolic BP in small for gestational age infants. Dionne and colleagues state that oscillometric measurements are generally 3 to 8 mm Hg higher than intra-arterial measures for mean arterial pressure.
      i. **Choosing the appropriate site.** The site most often used is the upper extremity, most often the right upper extremity. Do not place the cuff on the extremity where an intravenous (IV) or intra-arterial line is placed or where there is injured skin.
      ii. **Blood pressure cuff size is important in noninvasive methods.** Often providers will choose a cuff that is too small, which can lead to high BP readings. The BP cuff should encircle two-thirds of the length of the upper extremity. Some cuffs have index lines to ensure the correct size of cuff is used. If the cuff is too narrow, the BP will be falsely elevated. **The AAP recommendations for BP cuff bladder width are as follows:** newborn—4 cm; infant—6 cm. **For length:** newborn—8 cm; infant—12 cm. **Maximum arm circumference:** newborn—10 cm; infant—15 cm. The **American Heart Association** recommends a 4 × 8 cm cuff size for newborns and infants.
      iii. **Choose the correct placement of the cuff.** The majority of cuffs have an artery mark indicator, so one can palpate the brachial artery and align it with the artery mark on the cuff.
      iv. **Make sure all the air is out of the cuff** and that it is snug around the arm; it should not impede venous return by being too tight.
      v. **Blood pressure protocols have been established to standardize blood pressure measurement in infants.** This was done to minimize incorrect readings since multiple factors can influence BP. Because the first reading is usually the highest, it is best to take at least 3 confirmatory measurements. BP rises when the infant is feeding (by 20 mm Hg), is crying, has pain, is agitated, is sucking on a pacifier, or has the head in an upright position. BP is 5 mm Hg lower in sleeping infants than in infants who are awake. Most BP data are from measurements taken from the right arm. One standardized method using an oscillometric device suggested by Nwankwo and colleagues is as follows:

(a) **Measure blood pressure 1.5 hours after feeding** or a medical intervention.

(b) **Make sure the infant is asleep or in a quiet state,** lying prone or supine.

(c) **Place an appropriate-sized cuff** on the right upper arm, and let the infant rest undisturbed after cuff placement for 15 minutes.

(d) **Measure by oscillometric device,** and do 3 successive BP readings at 2-minute intervals.

vi. **The American Academy of Pediatrics** does not recommend universal screening in term healthy newborns but states it is important to screen BP in infants in whom coarctation of the aorta or renal disease is suspected.

B. **Is an umbilical artery catheter in place, or has one been in place in the past?** Incidence of hypertension is approximately 9% with a UAC. UACs are associated with an increased incidence of renovascular hypertension. The hypertension is probably related to endothelial disruption and thrombus formation at the time of line placement. The longer the UAC is in, the higher is the risk of thrombus formation. Thrombi have been demonstrated to be present on 25% to 81% of catheters studied. The following conditions are risk factors for thrombus formation in the aorta: bronchopulmonary dysplasia/chronic lung disease (BPD/CLD), patent ductus arteriosus (PDA), hypervolemia, and certain central nervous system (CNS) disorders. Improved catheter design and the use of heparin have helped decrease the incidence of thrombus formation. A Cochrane review found that hypertension appears with equal frequency in infants with high versus low catheters.

C. **Are signs of hypertension present?** The presentation of hypertension varies and can range from no signs to massive heart failure and cardiogenic shock. Infants with high blood pressure usually show no signs, and the hypertension is noted incidentally on routine continuous monitoring. Alternatively, it can manifest the following signs: irritability, tachypnea, cyanosis, seizures, lethargy, increased tone, apnea, abdominal distention, failure to thrive, irritability, feeding difficulty, respiratory distress, fever, and mottling. Infants with severe hypertension can have congestive heart failure (CHF), cardiogenic shock/hypotension masking hypertension, seizures, renal dysfunction, and/or hypertensive retinopathy. Specific causes can cause specific presentations: hypertension causing CHF with respiratory distress, tachypnea, and hypoxia; kidney-related hypertension with oliguria/polyuria; or neurologic symptoms mimicking intraventricular hemorrhage (IVH) with apnea, seizures, lethargy, and tremors.

D. **What is the blood pressure in the extremities?** The BP in a healthy infant should be higher in the legs than in the arms. If the pressure is lower in the legs, **coarctation of the aorta** may be the cause of the hypertension. **Coarctation of the aorta** is the most common heart malformation that causes hypertension in a neonate.

E. **What is the birthweight, gestational age, postmenstrual age, and postnatal age of the infant?** Gestational age, birthweight, and postmenstrual age have the strongest influence on determining BP. **Normal BP values increase with increasing birthweight (data on birthweight are conflicting in term infants), gestational age, and postconceptual age.** Values rise approximately 1 to 2 mm Hg per day during the first week of life and then approximately 1 to 2 mm Hg per week over the next 6 weeks. Postmenstrual age is a primary determinant of BP in preterm infants after day 1, and there is a progressive increase in BP over 2 weeks in infants <31 weeks. Normal term infants experience a significant rise only from day 1 to day 2. In infants <27 weeks' gestation, the BP decreases over the first 3 hours of life, with the lowest point at 4 to 5 hours of life, and then it increases.

F. **Is the infant in pain or agitated?** Pain from an invasive procedure, crying, agitation, or suctioning can cause a transient rise in BP. The systolic pressure can be 5 mm Hg lower in sleeping infants.

G. **Does the infant have bronchopulmonary dysplasia/chronic lung disease or an intraventricular hemorrhage?** Infants with BPD/CLD have a significant problem with hypertension (6% up to 40%). It often occurs after discharge from the nursery. Infants with an IVH (3% incidence) also have an increased risk of hypertension.

H. **Does the infant have any risk factors that would be associated with the development of hypertension?** Risk factors from 2 different studies include the following: lower birthweight, renal failure, acute kidney injury (AKI), renal disease/chronic renal failure, necrotizing enterocolitis, seizure, asphyxia, UAC catheterization, neonatal abstinence syndrome, extracorporeal membrane oxygenation/extracorporeal life support treatment, IVH, maternal hypertension, antenatal steroids, BPD/CLD, PDA, and indomethacin treatment. Other reported risk factors include congenital anomalies of the kidney and urinary tract (CAKUT), prematurity, low birthweight, coarctation of the aorta, perinatal hypoxia, increasing severity of illness, hemolytic uremic syndrome, and cytochrome P450 (CYP2D6) CC genotype in preterm infants.

I. **Were recent boluses of fluids or blood products given?** Fluid overload is a common iatrogenic cause of hypertension, especially in infants with decreased urine output.

J. **Was there maternal drug use (cocaine or heroin)?** Maternal drug use of cocaine and heroin has been associated with hypertension in newborn infants because of drug withdrawal or the direct effects on the developing kidney.

K. **Are there any maternal factors that would contribute to the hypertension?** Maternal factors include maternal body mass index >30, maternal diabetes, hypertension, certain maternal medications, maternal anesthesia, mode of delivery, preeclampsia, and abnormal uteroplacental perfusion. Antenatal steroid treatment resulted in an increased BP in the neonate in the first 24 to 48 hours of life with a decreased need for BP support. There is scant and conflicting evidence about whether maternal age, maternal anesthesia, mode of delivery, and maternal medications (eg, magnesium sulfate, β-blockers, α_2-adrenergic agonists, calcium antagonists, and direct vasodilators) affect neonatal BP. Maternal hypertension and diabetes may increase the risk of neonatal hypertension in the first month of life.

L. **Did the mother have a prenatal ultrasound?** Congenital abnormalities of the genitourinary tract are the most common malformations identified on ultrasound (15%–20% of all prenatal diagnosed congenital anomalies). Polyhydramnios and oligohydramnios are strong risk factors for CAKUT.

III. **Differential diagnosis.** Hypertension is rare in the healthy term newborn infant. The incidence ranges from 0.2% (healthy newborn) up to 43% (in infants with BPD/CLD). Hypertension in the neonate is most commonly secondary hypertension, which means that it is caused by an underlying identifiable condition or cause. Hypertension in newborns is most commonly renal in origin (renal vascular and renal parenchymal diseases). BPD/CLD is the most common nonrenal cause. One study reported the 3 most common causes are UAC-associated thrombosis, BPD/CLD, and coarctation of the aorta. Common causes are listed here. See Table 66–2 for a comprehensive list.

A. **Renal and vascular causes**

1. **Umbilical artery catheter–associated thrombosis.** Thromboembolic occlusion of the renal artery occurring after umbilical artery catheterization is the most common cause of hypertension in neonates. The thrombi embolize to the renal vessels, causing occlusion and infarction and increased release of renin and hypertension.

2. **Renal artery stenosis.** The infant is hypertensive from birth and has symptoms of CHF, cardiomegaly on chest x-ray, and left ventricular hypertrophy on electrocardiogram. This accounts for 20% of cases of hypertension in infants. It can be secondary to fibromuscular dysplasia. Congenital rubella infection can cause arterial calcification and renal artery stenosis.

3. **Renal vein thrombosis.** Seen in hypovolemic or asphyxiated infants, infants of diabetic mothers, and infants with coagulopathies. Only 13% of neonates present with the classical triad of hypertension, gross hematuria, and an abdominal mass.

Table 66–2. CAUSES OF HYPERTENSION IN NEWBORNS

Cardiac	Coarctation of the aorta, aortic arch interruption, hypoplastic aorta, patent ductus arteriosus
Drugs: infant	Glucocorticoids (dexamethasone), theophylline, caffeine, vitamin D intoxication, pancuronium (prolonged use), high dose of adrenergic agents, phenylephrine eye drops, doxapram, opiate withdrawal
Drugs: maternal	Cocaine (may harm neonatal kidney and cause withdrawal) and heroin (causes withdrawal), antenatal steroid administration (*controversial*)
Endocrine	Adrenal hemorrhage/hematoma/tumors, adrenogenital syndrome, congenital adrenal hyperplasia (secondary to 11β- and 17α-hydroxylase deficiencies), Cushing syndrome, primary hyperaldosteronism, hyperthyroidism, pseudohyperaldosteronism type II, familial hyperaldosteronism type II, Gordon syndrome, pheochromocytoma
Metabolic	Hypercalcemia
Neurologic	Elevated intracranial pressure secondary to intracranial hemorrhage, hydrocephalus, meningitis or subdural hemorrhage/hematoma, seizures, subdural hematoma, familial dysautonomia, drug withdrawal (opiate), neural crest tumor, cerebral angioma
Pain/agitation	Usually causes episodic hypertension
Pulmonary	Bronchopulmonary dysplasia/chronic lung disease, pneumothorax (rare)
Renal parenchymal diseases (acquired)	Acute tubular necrosis, cortical and medullary necrosis, interstitial nephritis, hemolytic uremic syndrome, nephrolithiasis/nephrocalcinosis, obstructive uropathy (eg, tumor or stones), pyelonephritis, glomerulonephritis, perirenal hematoma or urinoma, renal failure/renal insufficiency, renal infection
Renal parenchymal diseases (congenital)	Polycystic kidney disease (autosomal recessive or autosomal dominant), multicystic dysplastic kidney disease, hypoplastic/dysplastic kidney, congenital nephrotic syndrome, unilateral renal hypoplasia, tuberous sclerosis, renal tubular dysgenesis, obstructive uropathy (posterior urethral valves, ureteropelvic junction obstruction), congenital mesoblastic nephroma
Renovascular/vascular	Renal artery thrombosis, renal artery stenosis, renal vein thrombosis, midaortic syndrome (abdominal coarctation), congenital rubella syndrome (causes arterial calcification), idiopathic arterial calcification, renal artery compression, hypoplastic aorta, abdominal aorta aneurysm, aortic thrombosis, thrombosis of the ductus arteriosus, intimal hyperplasia, mechanical compression of 1 or both arteries (abdominal mass or tumor)
Syndromes/malformation syndromes	Noonan, Williams, Turner, Liddle (glucocorticoid remediable aldosteronism), and Cockayne syndromes; neurofibromatosis; tuberous sclerosis complex
Tumors (compression of renal vessels or production of vasoactive substances)	Wilms tumor, mesoblastic nephroma, neuroblastoma, nephroblastoma, pheochromocytoma

(Continued)

Table 66–2. CAUSES OF HYPERTENSION IN NEWBORNS (*CONTINUED*)

Miscellaneous	Birth asphyxia, closure of abdominal wall defects (eg, omphalocele or gastroschisis), abdominal surgery, ECLS, essential hypertension, iatrogenic (volume overload secondary to excess administration of sodium or intravenous fluids), idiopathic, long-term total parenteral nutrition related, infantile polyarteritis nodosa, maternal hypertension, environmental cold or noise stress, cytochrome P450 (CYP2D6) genotype in preterm infants (elevated systolic blood pressure after discharge from neonatal intensive care unit), idiopathic (5%–57%)

4. **Acute kidney injury.** Postnatal AKI is associated with hypertension. Acute tubular necrosis (ATN) is the most common cause of AKI. ATN can be secondary to perinatal asphyxia or sepsis.
5. **Persistent nephrocalcinosis in infants** can cause hypertension.
6. **Congenital anomalies of the kidney and urinary tract** cause hypertension more often than acquired kidney abnormalities. Autosomal dominant or autosomal recessive polycystic kidney disease can present in the neonate with hypertension and enlarged kidneys. Multicystic dysplastic kidney rarely causes hypertension. Ureteropelvic junction obstruction can activate the renin-angiotensin system and cause hypertension.
B. **Bronchopulmonary dysplasia/chronic lung disease is the most common cause of nonrenal hypertension in the neonate.** The origin is unclear but is probably multifactorial (increased renin activity and catecholamine secretion and chronic hypoxemia may be associated with CLD). The majority of these infants develop hypertension after being discharged from the hospital at 4 to 5 months of age and present with irritability and failure to thrive.
C. **Coarctation of the aorta.** A common cause of hypertension in newborns. Occurs with an increased incidence in Turner syndrome.
D. **Neurologic.** Increased intracranial pressure and seizures can cause episodic hypertension. IVH can cause increased intracranial pressure.
E. **Medications.** Such as corticosteroids (antenatal and postnatal), theophylline, caffeine, adrenergic agents, pancuronium, and topical mydriatic agents (phenylephrine eye drops). Maternal use of cocaine can cause damage to the kidneys of the fetus and resultant hypertension. Drug withdrawal from heroin can cause hypertension.
F. **Fluid/electrolyte overload.** Chronic total parenteral nutrition can cause chronic solute and water overload.
G. **Pain or agitation.** This usually causes episodic hypertension.
H. **Other.** ECLS (up to 50% of infants), abdominal surgery (closure of an abdominal wall defect), pneumothorax, PDA, and indomethacin treatment.
I. **Endocrine disorders.** Hyperthyroidism, congenital adrenal hyperplasia, hyperaldosteronism, and pheochromocytoma.
J. **Idiopathic/essential hypertension.** In 5% to 57% of neonates (depending on the study), there is no identifiable cause.
IV. **Database.** In a hypertensive crisis, data gathering is not the first priority. In some cases, treatment will need to be the priority before investigation of the cause.
A. **History.** Evaluate maternal factors: Was cocaine or heroin used during pregnancy, or were antenatal steroids used? Did the mom have diabetes or preeclampsia? Was a prenatal ultrasound done? Was there prenatal oligohydramnios/polyhydramnios (these are strong risk factors for CAKUT, and oligohydramnios is a good indicator of renal dysfunction)? Does the infant have a predisposing illness that would account for the

hypertension (eg, BPD/CLD, CNS disorder, PDA)? Evaluate the current medication list. Does or did the infant have a UAC?

B. **Physical examination.** In most infants, hypertension is discovered on vital signs with no other overt signs. Focus on the cardiovascular and abdominal (to include genito-urinary) examination. What is the volume status of the infant (is there weight gain)? **Life-threatening presentations** can include CHF with cardiogenic shock or seizures. Some infants present with apnea, feeding difficulties, failure to thrive, irritability, lethargy, unexplained tachypnea, and mottling of the skin. Check for tachycardia and flushing for hyperthyroidism.

1. **Perform a complete cardiac examination to rule out CHF.** Is there a heart murmur (coarctation of the aorta)? Is there cyanosis? Is there tachycardia? Are there mottling and signs of vasomotor instability? Are there absent or decreased femoral pulses? Check the femoral pulses in both legs, which are absent or decreased in coarctation of the aorta. Is there a difference in the BP in the upper and lower extremities? Check BP in all 4 extremities (BP discrepancies between the upper and lower extremities, arterial hypertension in the upper extremities with normal to low BP in the lower extremities, which is a hallmark of coarctation of the aorta).

2. **Are there any dysmorphic features** that would indicate a genetic abnormality or a syndrome that would explain the hypertension? Are there widely spaced nipples and webbed neck to suggest Turner syndrome? Is there elfin facies? Consider Williams syndrome.

3. **Respiratory.** Is there tachypnea or cyanosis?

4. **Examine the abdomen** for masses and to determine the size of the kidneys. Is there abdominal distension? An enlarged kidney or flank mass may indicate tumor, polycystic kidneys, obstruction, or renal vein thrombosis. An epigastric/flank bruit can indicate renal artery stenosis. Palpable kidneys can indicate hydronephrosis, polycystic kidney disease, or multicystic dysplastic kidney.

5. **Examine the genitalia (is it ambiguous/is there virilization?)** to look for signs of congenital adrenal hyperplasia.

6. **Neurologic signs** may include apnea, lethargy, tremors, seizures, asymmetric reflexes, and hypertonicity.

C. **Laboratory studies.** Few tests are usually needed and should be dictated by history and physical examination. **Common tests should include:** complete blood count and platelet count, serum electrolytes (sodium, potassium, chloride, bicarbonate), blood urea nitrogen and creatinine, urinalysis, renal ultrasound with Doppler, and echocardiography. **More detailed tests include:** serum calcium, serum cortisol, thyroid studies, plasma renin activity, aldosterone, head ultrasound, angiography, and renal scintigraphy. Assessment of renal function is important and is as follows:

1. **Assess renal function** with the following:
   a. **Serum creatinine and blood urea nitrogen.** Elevation suggests renal insufficiency, which may be associated with hypertension.
   b. **Urinalysis.** May show gross or microscopic hematuria or proteinuria. Red blood cells in the urine suggest obstruction, infection, or renal vein thrombosis.
   c. **Urine culture.** To evaluate for urinary tract infection.
   d. **Serum electrolytes and carbon dioxide.** A low serum potassium level and a high carbon dioxide level suggest primary hyperaldosteronism. Hypokalemia suggests congenital adrenal hypoplasia.
   e. **Urine protein/creatinine ratio, urine albumin/creatinine ratio.** To evaluate significant proteinuria and renal parenchymal disease.

2. **Other useful tests in selected infants**
   a. **Plasma renin levels (plasma renin activity)** may be elevated in patients with renovascular disease. Levels will be low in primary hyperaldosteronism. Rarely elevated in normal infants, plasma renin activity can be falsely elevated because of medications such as aminophylline. Direct renin assay has been used, but normal neonatal values are not readily available.

      b. Thyroid studies (thyroid-stimulating hormone, free thyroxine) to rule out hyperthyroidism.

      c. Serum cortisol.

      d. Serum aldosterone.

      e. Urine vanillylmandelic acid/homovanillic acid. Twenty-four–hour urinary catecholamines to evaluate for pheochromocytoma or neuroblastoma.

      f. Urinary 17-hydroxysteroid and 17-ketosteroid levels to evaluate for Cushing syndrome and congenital adrenal hyperplasia.

      g. Urine toxicology screen.

      h. Coagulation panel.

D. Imaging and other studies

  1. **Ultrasound.** Renal ultrasound with Doppler evaluation is the preferred screening test in neonates and should be done in all hypertensive infants. It will identify congenital anomalies of the urinary tract, renal masses, tumors, and renal cystic disease; assess adrenals; and check for renal vein thrombosis as well as kidney obstruction. Color Doppler flow ultrasonography can be used to screen for arterial or venous problems (thrombosis), renal and aortic thrombi, renal venous thrombosis, and renal artery stenosis. Infants who had a UAC should have their aorta and renal arteries studied for thrombi.

  2. **Chest radiograph.** Evaluate heart size. May help in infants with CHF and infants with a murmur. Cardiomegaly can be seen.

  3. **Echocardiography.** To assess structural lesions (if coarctation of the aorta is suspected) or to evaluate end-organ damage and dysfunction caused by hypertension (eg, left ventricular hypertrophy/dysfunction or decreased contractility). Severe hypertension can cause hypertensive cardiomyopathy.

  4. **Cranial imaging with ultrasound.** To rule out IVH.

  5. **Further studies.** The following procedures and studies are sometimes necessary to further evaluate the infant with hypertension:

    a. Angiography to evaluate renovascular disease or venacavography to evaluate renal vein thrombosis. This is most commonly done through the UAC. Renal angiography or scan helps quantitate the function of each kidney. Magnetic resonance angiography is the gold standard for renal vascular hypertension and is recommended in infants >3 kg.

    b. Abdominal computed tomography scan if needed to obtain more specific anatomic information on an abdominal mass (pheochromocytoma). A computed tomography angiogram can evaluate the aorta and renal arteries.

    c. Voiding cystourethrography if urinary tract pathology is possible.

    d. Nuclear medicine studies. Radionuclide imaging (nuclear scan) of the kidneys (renal scintigraphy/renal scans) can show renal perfusion abnormalities and increased isotope concentration in an obstructed kidney. A **dimercaptosuccinic acid (DMSA) renal scan** can rule out arterial infarctions. **Percutaneous femoral renal arteriography** with bilateral renal vein renin measurement is usually needed to rule out renovascular hypertension. **Captopril-enhanced renal scintigraphy** can detect significant renovascular disease.

V. Plan

A. General. First confirm the BP measurement. Treat any obvious or correctable causes of hypertension. Some infants may require antihypertensive medications while corrective therapy is being done. Consultations with pediatric cardiology and nephrology to help manage hypertension are recommended. Other consults may be required such as endocrinology, urology, or surgery depending on the underlying cause of hypertension. **The following are treatable causes of hypertension:**

  1. **Fluid overload.** Restrict sodium and fluids. Consider diuretics.

  2. **Pain.** Administer pain medications. See Chapter 15.

  3. **Stop any medications,** if possible, that can cause hypertension (adjust inotropic medications, steroids, caffeine).

4. **Hyperthyroidism.** Medications include methimazole, iodine preparations, and propranolol for tachycardia. See Chapter 129.
5. **Congenital adrenal hyperplasia.** Steroid therapy. See Chapter 95.
6. **Hypercalcemia.** See Chapter 91.
7. **Aortic or renal thromboembolic events** should be treated with close monitoring and supportive care unless severe enough that they need anticoagulation or fibrinolytic therapy. Remove UAC if possible. See Chapter 92.
8. **Surgical intervention. This is an option in <10% of infants.** Used for relief of obstructive uropathy, repair of coarctation of the aorta, nephrectomy for unilateral renovascular disease, and angioplasty for renal artery stenosis. Others that may require surgery include Wilms tumor and neuroblastoma, arterial or venous renal thrombosis (usually medically treated first), rare cases of autosomal recessive polycystic kidney disease, and multicystic dysplastic kidney.

B. **Drug therapy.** (See Chapter 155.) To guide drug therapy, determine whether the hypertension is **mild, moderate, or malignant/life threatening. Note that treatment thresholds are unclear, and many of the recommendations are** *controversial.* One important consideration is end-organ damage (damage to organs affected by hypertension). The most prominent evidence of end-organ damage is thickening of the left ventricle (left ventricular hypertrophy), which is a sign of hypertensive cardiomyopathy. Other examples are hypertensive retinopathy, hypertensive encephalopathy, and hypertensive nephropathy. Some experts believe that **any asymptomatic infant with hypertension with no end-organ involvement should only be observed.** Most believe that hypertension should be treated if there is evidence of target organ dysfunction, if BP is >95th percentile with end-organ involvement, if BP is consistently >99th percentile, if there is underlying renal disease, or if the infant is symptomatic. **Which medication and route should be used?** This depends on the severity of the hypertension, whether the infant can tolerate an oral medication, the gestational age of the infant, if the infant's kidneys can handle the medication, and if the infant has CLD.

1. **Important points when using antihypertensive medications in the neonate:**
   a. **Avoid the use of β-blockers** (propranolol, esmolol) or **α-/β-blockers** (labetalol, carvedilol) **in infants with BPD/CLD** because of a potential risk of bronchoconstriction. **β-Blockers** should not be used in emergency hypertension or as long-term therapy.
   b. **Do not use angiotensin-converting enzyme inhibitors (captopril, enalapril, or lisinopril) until the end of 44 weeks of postmenstrual age** or in infants with bilateral renovascular disease or disease in a solitary kidney, infants with acute renal failure, or infants with hyperkalemia. These drugs cause a profound decrease in BP. These medications, if given before 36 weeks of age, have the following effects on postnatal kidney development: atrophy of the renal papilla, tubular alterations (fibrosis and atrophy), urinary concentration impairment, and reduction in the nephron number. These medications are contraindicated in bilateral renovascular disease or renovascular disease in a solitary kidney because they can cause acute renal failure. Captopril in premature infants has been associated with severe drops in BP that do not respond to fluids or inotropes. Up to 20% of infants on enalapril have experienced hyperkalemia, hypotension, or death.
   c. **Do not use furosemide for chronic treatment in neonates** because it may result in hypokalemia, hypercalciuria, nephrocalcinosis, and nephrolithiasis. Furosemide may also have an effect on renal development as it has been shown to reduce nephron formation in organ culture. Furosemide should be used in neonates with oliguric renal insufficiency and edema.
   d. **Spironolactone, a potassium-sparing diuretic,** is recommended for hypertension with hypokalemic metabolic acidosis (hyperaldosteronism).
   e. **Esmolol** is a good choice in infants who cannot tolerate β-blockers.

f. **Isradipine and amlodipine are good choices** for long-term antihypertensive therapy.

g. **Vasodilators are the most common class of antihypertensive medications used in NICUs,** with hydralazine being the most common.

h. **Many infants will require >1 medication (up to 51%).** Start with 1 medication and increase the dose if necessary. If at the maximum dose and there is still hypertension, a second drug can be added. Term infants usually require more medications than preterm infants.

i. **Continuous intravenous medications to consider for severe hypertensive crisis:** Nicardipine, labetalol, esmolol, sodium nitroprusside, and fenoldopam mesylate.

j. **Intermittent intravenous medication to consider for mild to moderate hypertension or if oral therapy is not tolerated:** Furosemide, hydralazine, propranolol, labetalol, and enalapril.

k. **Oral medications for hypertension (mild to moderate hypertension, infants being converted to oral long-term therapy):** Furosemide, captopril, clonidine, enalapril, hydralazine, isradipine, amlodipine, minoxidil, propranolol, labetalol, spironolactone, furosemide, hydrochlorothiazide, and chlorothiazide.

2. **Recommendations for treatment depending on the type of hypertension.** See Table 66–3 for agents and doses.

a. **Life-threatening hypertension or hypertensive crisis.** If BP is well above the 99th percentile or >30% above mean value for age with signs of end-organ dysfunction (left ventricular hypertrophy, CHF, neonatal encephalopathy, cardiogenic shock, seizures) or without signs of end-organ dysfunction but with the potential to cause end-organ damage, parenteral treatment for hypertension is recommended. **Avoid too rapid of a decrease in the BP**, as this may cause cerebral ischemia and hemorrhage, especially in the premature infant. Monitor the BP every 5 to 15 minutes. One recommendation is to decrease the BP by 33% in the first 6 hours, by another 33 % over the next 24 to 36 hours, and by the last 33% over the next 48 to 72 hours. AAP target BP goal has not been established for infants, but for children, it is <90th percentile. The medications chosen depend on your institutional guidelines. **With life-threatening hypertension, short-acting continuous IV infusions should be used** and are preferred because these can be titrated, and the BP should begin to fall within 15 minutes to an hour. It is best to monitor BP continuously through an intra-arterial catheter in these infants. The following medications can be used for hypertensive crisis:

i. **Nicardipine.** A calcium channel blocker, nicardipine is considered the **drug of choice** because of its advantages and few side effects (reflex tachycardia and edema). **If the infant does not respond or the BP remains elevated,** one can add or substitute 1 of the following medications based on institutional guidelines: labetalol, esmolol, sodium nitroprusside, or fenoldopam mesylate. **See Table 66–3** for doses, concerns, and side effects.

ii. **If intravenous infusion medication is not available,** short-acting IV or oral antihypertensives can be used. Examples include short-acting IV medications (hydralazine or labetalol) or short-acting oral antihypertensives (isradipine [used successfully in neonates with severe acute hypertension] or clonidine).

b. **Moderate hypertension.** There are no data on choice of medication and no clinical trials comparing the specific medications. Which medication to use depends on your institution. Medications that can be used include diuretics, calcium channel blockers, β-blockers (avoid in CLD), and angiotensinogen-converting enzyme (ACE) inhibitors (if infant is >44 weeks of postconceptional age). Oral medications can be used depending on the infant's condition and the ability to tolerate oral medications. Follow your institution's guidelines.

Table 66–3 MEDICATIONS FOR NEONATAL HYPERTENSION: EMERGENCY AND ROUTINE

Drug Dosing Regimen	Drug Class	Comments and Side Effects
Hypertensive Crisis Medications		
Nicardipine: 0.5–4 mcg/kg/**min** as continuous infusion	Calcium channel blocker[a]	Infusion via central line is advised Caution use in perinatal asphyxia May cause reflex tachycardia
Labetalol: 0.25–3 mg/kg/**h** as continuous infusion OR **Labetalol:** 0.2–1 mg/kg/**dose** as **IV bolus** undiluted over 2 minutes; do not exceed 10 mg/min OR **Labetalol:** 1 mg/kg/**dose** PO every 8–12 hours scheduled; do not exceed 12 mg/kg/**d**	α- and β-Blocker[b]	Caution use in chronic lung disease, heart block, unstable heart failure, and neurological injury
Esmolol: 50–500 mcg/kg/**min** as continuous infusion; may titrate to a maximum of 1000 mcg/kg/**min**	β-Blocker[b]	Caution in chronic lung disease, heart block, and unstable heart failure
Fenoldopam: 0.2 mcg/kg/**min** as continuous infusion; may titrate every 20–30 minutes up to a maximum of 0.8 mcg/kg/**min**	Dopamine agonist[c]	Dose-related tachycardia can occur; tachycardia has been shown to persist for at least 4 hours with infusion rate >0.8 mcg/kg/min in pediatric patients. Monitor blood pressure closely; hypotension can occur.
Nitroprusside: 0.25–8 mcg/kg/min as continuous infusion; may titrate up to a maximum of 10 mcg/kg/min	Vasodilator[d]	Caution in elevated intracranial pressure, renal and hepatic failure Monitor for thiocyanate and cyanide toxicity, especially when used in high infusion rates (≥2 mcg/kg/min) or for prolonged period (>72 hours). May consider co-administering nitroprusside with sodium thiosulfate at a 1:10 ratio when infusion rate is ≥4 mcg/kg/min.
Other Antihypertensive Medications		
Amlodipine: 0.1–0.3 mg/kg/**dose** PO every 12 hours; do not exceed 0.6 mg/kg/**d** or 20 mg/**d**	Calcium channel blocker[a]	Caution in hepatic failure requiring lower starting dose
Captopril: • Premature and term neonates, PNA ≤7 days: 0.01 mg/kg/**dose** PO every 8 to 12 hours • Term neonates, PNA >7 days: 0.05–0.5 mg/kg/**dose** PO every 6 to 24 hours	ACE inhibitor[e]	Caution in renal failure, hyponatremia, hypovolemia, severe CHF, and concurrent diuretics use May cause hyperkalemia, cholestatic jaundice, cough, and angioedema

(Continued)

Table 66–3 MEDICATIONS FOR NEONATAL HYPERTENSION: EMERGENCY AND ROUTINE (*CONTINUED*)

Drug Dosing Regimen	Drug Class	Comments and Side Effects
Chlorothiazide: 2.5–10 mg/kg/dose IV every 12 hours OR Chlorothiazide: 5–20 mg/kg/dose PO every 12 hours	Diuretic	May cause hypokalemia, hyponatremia, hypochloremic alkalosis, and hypercalcemia; IV not generally recommended in infants
Clonidine: 2–5 mcg/kg/dose PO every 6–8 hours PRN	Central α-agonist[f]	May cause somnolence, xerostomia, and rebound hypertension with abrupt discontinuation
Enalapril: 0.04–0.3 mg/kg/dose PO every 12 to 24 hours scheduled	ACE inhibitor[e]	Caution in renal failure, hyponatremia, hypovolemia, severe CHF, and concurrent diuretic use May cause hyperkalemia, cholestatic jaundice, cough, and angioedema
Furosemide: 1–2 mg/kg/dose IV every 6 to 24 hours OR Furosemide: 1–6 mg/kg/dose PO every 6–24 hours	Diuretic, loop	May cause hypokalemia, hyponatremia, ototoxicity, and nephrocalcinosis
Hydralazine: 0.1–0.6 mg/kg/dose every 4–6 hours PRN as IV bolus undiluted over 1–2 minutes; do not exceed 5 mg/min OR Hydralazine: 0.25–1 mg/kg/dose PO every 6–8 hours; do not exceed 7.5 mg/kg/d	Vasodilator[d]	Caution in renal failure requiring lower starting dose May cause blood dyscrasias, tachycardia
Hydrochlorothiazide: 1–3 mg/kg/d PO every 24 hours or divided every 12 hours	Diuretic	May cause hypokalemia, hyponatremia, hypochloremic alkalosis, and hypercalcemia
Isradipine: 0.05–0.15 mg/kg/dose PO every 6–8 hours PRN; do not exceed 0.8 mg/kg/d or 20 mg/d	Calcium channel blocker[a]	Caution in hepatic failure and QTc prolongation
Minoxidil: 0.1–0.2 mg/kg/dose PO every 8–12 hours	Vasodilator[d]	Most potent oral vasodilator and **not** a first-choice agent Caution in renal failure, ischemic heart disease, pericardial effusion May cause fluid retention and tachycardia. Concurrent use with a diuretic and a β-blocker is recommended.
Propranolol: 0.25–0.5 mg/kg/dose PO every 8 hours; do not exceed 5 mg/kg/d	β-Blocker	May cause bradycardia and not a first-choice agent Caution in chronic lung disease and unstable heart failure

(*Continued*)

Table 66–3 MEDICATIONS FOR NEONATAL HYPERTENSION: EMERGENCY AND ROUTINE (*CONTINUED*)

Drug Dosing Regimen	Drug Class	Comments and Side Effects
Spironolactone: 1–3 mg/kg/d PO every 24 hours or divided every 12 hours	Diuretic, potassium sparing	May cause hyperkalemia Caution in renal failure

ACE, angiotensin-converting enzyme; CHF, congestive heart failure; IV, intravenous; PNA, postnatal age; PO, oral; PRN, as needed.

Neonate indicates birth to 28 days PNA.

Mechanisms of action are as follows:

[a]**Calcium channel blockers:** prevent calcium from entering vascular smooth muscle and myocardium cells, which leads to relaxation of the vascular smooth muscle, resulting in coronary vasodilation and reduction in blood pressure.

[b]**α- and β-blockers:** block norepinephrine and epinephrine, which causes the blood vessel to dilate, thereby lowering the **blood pressure.**

[c]**Dopamine agonists:** bind to dopamine receptors on vascular smooth muscle cells and within the sympathetic nervous system, which causes a decrease in peripheral vascular resistance and inhibition of sympathetic nervous system activity, which results in lower blood pressure.

[d]**Vasodilators:** cause relaxation of smooth muscle cells within the vessel walls, which causes the vessels to dilate, thereby lowering blood pressure.

[e]**ACE inhibitors:** decrease angiotensin II, which allows blood vessels to relax and widen, and decrease amount of water the body retains, which lowers the blood pressure.

[f]**Central α-agonists:** stimulate α_2-adrenoceptors in the brainstem, thus activating an inhibitory neuron and leading to a reduction in sympathetic outflow, which ultimately decreases peripheral resistance and blood pressure.

Data from Nickavar A, Assadi F. Managing hypertension in the newborn infants. *Int J Prev Med.* 2014;5(Suppl 1):S39-S43; Flynn JT, Kaelber DC, Baker-Smith CM, et al. Clinical practice guideline for screening and management of high blood pressure in children and adolescents. *Pediatrics.* 2017; 140(3):e20171904; Lexi-Comp Online. *Pediatric & Neonatal Lexi-Drugs Online.* Hudson, OH: Lexi-Comp, Inc.; 2017; November 5, 2017.

    Begin diuretics first, such as furosemide, hydrochlorothiazide, or chlorothiazide. Thiazide diuretics (chlorothiazide and hydrochlorothiazide) are preferred to loop diuretics (furosemide) due to less side effects. Add a second-line drug if necessary.

   c. Mild hypertension. Usually managed by observation (recommended) or oral medications (usually diuretics).

      i. Simple observation is best for asymptomatic patients with no readily identifiable cause and no evidence of end-organ involvement and is supported in recent reviews. Observe closely with BP measurements every 6 to 8 hours.

      ii. Consider treatment (medication) if there is proven underlying renal disease, if the BP elevation continues or increases, or if there is evidence of end-organ involvement (eg, left ventricular hypertrophy or decreased contractility on echocardiography). If medication is needed, **thiazide diuretics** are considered **first-line treatment** and are preferred over furosemide because of fewer electrolyte disturbances. They work well in cases of volume overload but may cause hypotension when used with other agents.

   d. Infants with mild to moderate hypertension who cannot tolerate oral therapy because of gastrointestinal problems. These infants are good candidates for IV bolus or intermittently administered IV agents:

   i. **Diuretics.** Furosemide can be used short term. Monitor electrolytes.
  ii. **Hydralazine.** Side effects include tachycardia.
 iii. **Labetalol.** Side effects include heart failure. Avoid in BPD/CLD patients.
   e. **Long-term oral antihypertensive medications.** These are typically used in infants with moderate to severe hypertension who are ready to go on long-term oral therapy. Medication choice depends on your institution's preference. The most common classes recommended are ACE inhibitors, α- and β-blockers, calcium channel blockers, vasodilators, and diuretics. See doses in Table 66–3.
   i. **Angiotensin-converting enzyme inhibitors.** Do not use if renal vascular disease is suspected.
      (a) **Captopril.** A commonly used oral drug, but because of the concern of renal development problems, especially in premature infants, it is preferred in infants at least 38 to 40 weeks (some state 44 weeks). Contraindicated in hyperkalemia and unilateral renal disease. Avoid use in preterm infants. Do not use in neonates with glomerular filtration rate <30 mL/min/1.73 m^2.
      (b) **Enalapril.** Close monitoring is recommended. Monitor serum sodium, potassium, and creatinine. Up to 21% of infants exposed to enalapril for hypertension and CHF in the first 120 days of life suffered an adverse event, most commonly hyperkalemia (13%).
      (c) **Lisinopril.** Not approved in infancy.
   ii. **β-Blockers, α-/β-blockers.** Do not use in infants with BPD/CLD.
      (a) **Propranolol (β-blocker).** This is the most commonly used β-blocker.
      (b) **Labetalol (α-/β-blocker).**
      (c) **Carvedilol (α-/β-blocker).** May be good to use in heart failure.
  iii. **Vasodilators**
      (a) **Hydralazine.** May cause increase in heart rate, flushing, and edema.
      (b) **Minoxidil.** Most useful for refractory hypertension.
  iv. **Calcium channel blockers**
      (a) **Amlodipine.** Due to its slow onset, it is useful in chronic hypertension.
      (b) **Isradipine.** Optimal dosing is difficult for smaller preemies due to small volumes needed for doses from the drug's stable suspension.
   v. **Central α-agonists** Clonidine can be used.
  vi. **Diuretics.** Diuretics are good for hypertension with BPD/CLD. Monitor electrolytes. Hydrochlorothiazide and chlorothiazide are preferred over furosemide. Spironolactone can be used for hypertension with hyperaldosteronism.

67 Hypoglycemia

I. **Problem.** <u>An infant has a low blood glucose level on bedside glucose testing.</u> **Hypoglycemia is the most common metabolic problem in neonates in the newborn nursery and neonatal intensive care unit (NICU).** Neonatal hypoglycemia occurs most often (47%–52%) in at-risk infants who are small for gestational age (SGA) or large for gestational age (LGA), late preterm infants, or infants of diabetic mothers (IDM). It can occur in up to 10% of healthy term newborns. There is controversy surrounding neonatal hypoglycemia, including **no absolute definition of hypoglycemia.** Low glucose values may or may not result in clinical signs; the low value and duration of hypoglycemia that result in neurologic injury are unknown, and there are differing viewpoints from the **American Academy of Pediatrics (AAP) and Pediatric Endocrine Society (PES)** on hypoglycemia screening and guidelines. There is agreement that there are 2 forms of hypoglycemia in neonates: **transitional hypoglycemia**, which usually resolves within 48 hours after birth, and **persistent hypoglycemia**, which continues and can be pathologic. The AAP Committee on Fetus and Newborn states that the "absolute definition of hypoglycemia as a specific value or range cannot be given, as no evidence-based studies can define what clinically relevant neonatal hypoglycemia is." **Hypoglycemia definitions are based on treatment recommendation target threshold values:**

A. **American Academy of Pediatrics:** In late preterm (34–36 6/7 weeks), term SGA infants, IDM, and LGA infants, hypoglycemia is defined as:
   1. **Symptomatic infants at any age and asymptomatic infants from birth to 4 hours of age:** <40 mg/dL.
   2. **Asymptomatic infants (4–24 hours):** <45 mg/dL.
B. **Pediatric Endocrine Society.** Defines hypoglycemia as "a plasma glucose concentration low enough to cause symptoms and signs of impaired brain function."
   1. **Infants:** <60 mg/dL (normal threshold for neurogenic responses)
   2. **Neonates with persistent hypoglycemia disorder:**
      a. **High-risk infants without a suspected congenital hypoglycemia disorder:** <48 hours, <50 mg/dL; >48 hours, <60 mg/dL.
      b. **Neonates with a suspected congenital hypoglycemia disorder:** <70 mg/dL.

This underscores the challenge in addressing the treatment for hypoglycemia. Because hypoglycemia can present as a neonatal emergency (seizures, loss of consciousness) and it is known to cause neurologic impairment (dose-dependent increased risk of poor executive function and visual motor function) per the Children with Hypoglycemia and Their Later Development (CHYLD) study, it is critical to recognize hypoglycemia and initiate treatment to avoid long-term neurologic impairment.

II. **Immediate questions**
   A. **Was a serum sample sent to the laboratory stat?** The blood glucose level should be repeated at the bedside, and a serum glucose should be sent to the laboratory stat. There are multiple ways to test for glucose (point-of-care blood glucose reagent test strips/point-of-care glucose meters, subcutaneous continuous glucose monitoring system [CGMS], and formal laboratory test). At present, there is no point-of-care method that is reliable and accurate enough to be used as the sole method for hypoglycemia screening.
      1. **Point-of-care bedside reagent test strips/point-of-care glucose meter.** Blood is obtained (heel stick or other method), and a drop of blood is placed on the strip. It is read by visual color change or by a glucose meter at the bedside. It is quick, inexpensive, and practical but not highly accurate, especially at the low levels of glucose (<40–50 mg/dL). The reading is based on whole blood, which can be 15 mg lower than the plasma blood level. The readings are affected by high hematocrit value, presence of bilirubin, and high viscosity, which can all falsely lower the level of glucose. Commercially available glucose meters will overestimate serum glucose level in the setting of galactosemia. Capillary blood is considered more accurate than venous. US Food and Drug Administration (FDA) guidelines state that 95% of glucose results have to fall within 15 mg/dL at glucose concentrations <75mg/dL. (Therefore, an infant with a glucose of 40 mg/dL can range from 25 to 55 mg/dL.) If the bedside value is very low or the infant is showing signs of hypoglycemia, draw a stat serum blood glucose for the lab, and empirically treat the infant.
      2. **Subcutaneous continuous glucose monitoring system** is a method that aims to improve glucose control and decrease the frequency of blood samples needed. A small flexible glucose oxidase sensor is inserted under the skin usually in the abdomen or arm. A water-resistant transmitter sits on the skin and sends glucose readings wirelessly to a receiver. The CGMS sensors measure glucose values every

5 minutes and require calibration twice a day. CGMS was studied in variety of infants at risk for hypoglycemia and was found to be accurate with a reduced exposure to procedural pain. It can also detect trends in glucose levels. Three CGMSs have been approved as of this writing by the FDA for use in newborns: DexCom Seven (DexCom Inc.), Guardian RT (Medtronic Diabetes, Inc.), and Navigator 40 (Abbott Diabetes). CGMSs are not yet used routinely in clinical practice.

3. **Laboratory diagnosis of blood glucose.** This is the **gold standard** and uses an enzymatic-based laboratory analyzer. PES guidelines indicate to only use plasma glucose concentrations determined by a clinical laboratory method. It measures plasma/serum glucose using 1 of 3 reactions (glucose oxidase, dehydrogenase, or hexokinase). It is not affected by the hematocrit. The only disadvantages include the time it takes, need for blood draw, and risk of pain and infection. It should always be ordered stat. Considerations specific to this method include the following:

   a. **Plasma glucose** can be lower by 6 mg/dL per hour if it is not processed soon in the laboratory (erythrocytes in the sample metabolize the glucose).

   b. **Whole blood glucose** values are approximately 15% lower than plasma blood glucose values.

   c. **An arterial sample has a higher glucose concentration** compared to a venous or capillary sample.

B. **How old is the infant?** If the infant was just born or is <48 hours of age, consider transitional hypoglycemia. If the infant is >48 hours, suspect persistent hypoglycemia.

C. **Has the infant been normoglycemic and then suddenly become hypoglycemic, consider the following:**

   1. **Intravenous line issues** such as abrupt cessation of high-glucose infusion in a neonate or infiltration of intravenous (IV) line containing a high-glucose infusion.

   2. **Insulin dosing issues** if the infant is on insulin.

   3. **Malpositioned umbilical artery catheter** near vessels supplying the pancreas (celiac and superior mesenteric arteries) at T11–12: stimulates insulin release.

   4. **Postexchange blood transfusion** with fluids containing high glucose concentration.

   5. **Other underlying disorders** such as infection should also be considered.

D. **Was there a delayed onset of feeding after birth?** Infants need to be fed soon after birth (breast/bottle feed usually right after birth or within the first hour of life) or they can become hypoglycemic. AAP recommends that healthy full-term infants "be placed and remain in direct skin-to-skin contact with their mothers immediately after delivery until the first feeding is accomplished."

E. **What is the caloric intake?** Inadequate caloric intake can lead to decreased glycogen stores and cause hypoglycemia.

F. **Does the infant have any physical signs of low blood sugar?** Infants can have documented hypoglycemia and show no outward signs. There is no pathognomonic sign of hypoglycemia; most signs are nonspecific and are commonly seen in sick neonates with other disorders. If these signs disappear with treatment for hypoglycemia and there is normalization of the glucose level, then they can most likely be attributed to hypoglycemia and not another disorder.

   1. **Absence of physical signs that are seen with a low blood glucose.** The majority of infants are diagnosed with hypoglycemia during a routine screening.

   2. **Clinical signs/symptoms from American Academy of Pediatrics:** Jitteriness, irritability, cyanosis, seizures, apnea, tachypnea, weak or high-pitched cry, floppiness, lethargy, exaggerated Moro reflex, poor feeding, and eye rolling. Coma and seizures can occur with severe and prolonged hypoglycemia and repetitive hypoglycemia.

   3. **Clinical signs/symptoms from Pediatric Endocrine Society:** Symptoms/signs can be neurogenic or neuroglycopenic.

   a. **Neurogenic (autonomic activation of the sympathetic nervous system)**
   signs appear earlier: Pallor, jitteriness, tremors, tachypnea, sweating, irritability, tremulousness, vomiting, temperature instability, tachycardia.
   b. **Neuroglycopenic (central nervous system deprivation of glucose supply):**
   Weak or high-pitched cry, apnea, hypotonia, seizures, lethargy, coma.
G. **Is the infant receiving glucose, and if so, how much?** Glucose requirement depends on the gestational age, weight, and how many days old the infant is. The normal initial glucose requirement in term infants during the first 24 hours of life is 5 to 8 mg/kg/min. If the glucose order was not calculated based on body weight, the infant may not be getting the right amount of glucose. (For glucose calculations, see Chapter 10.)
H. **Does the mother have any risk factors that would increase her infant's risk of hypoglycemia, such as pregestational/gestational or insulin-dependent diabetes? Is she on any medications that would cause the infant to be hypoglycemic?** Approximately 40% of IDMs have hypoglycemia. Throughout pregnancy, diabetic mothers can have episodes of hyperglycemia, resulting in fetal hyperglycemia. This fetal hyperglycemia induces pancreatic β-cell hyperplasia, which results in hyperinsulinism. After delivery, hyperinsulinism persists, and hypoglycemia results. An infant of a mother with high body mass index (BMI) but without glucose intolerance can also increase the risk of hypoglycemia in the infant. Infants born to mothers who had preeclampsia, have hypertension, or received IV glucose infusion during delivery can have an infant with hypoglycemia. **Maternal medication history** is very important because certain medications can cause hypoglycemia in the infant. These medications include insulin, oral antidiabetic medications (sulfonylureas, others), β-blockers (propranolol, labetalol), β-sympathomimetic drugs (terbutaline, ritodrine, fenoterol, salbutamol, isoxsuprine), chlorothiazide, and chlorpropamide.
I. **Is the infant at risk for hypoglycemia, and does the infant require glucose screening?**
   1. **American Academy of Pediatrics screening recommendations:** Late preterm infants (34–36 6/7 weeks), term SGA infants, IDM infants, and LGA infants.
   2. **Pediatric Endocrine Society screening recommendations:** Symptoms of hypoglycemia, LGA (even without maternal diabetes), perinatal stress (birth asphyxia/ischemia, cesarean delivery for fetal distress, maternal preeclampsia/eclampsia or hypertension), intrauterine growth restriction (IUGR; SGA), meconium aspiration syndrome, erythroblastosis fetalis, polycythemia, hypothermia, premature or postmature infants, IDM, family history of a genetic form of hypoglycemia, congenital syndromes (Beckwith-Wiedemann), or any abnormal physical features (microphallus, midline facial malformations).
III. **Differential diagnosis.** Hypoglycemia is classified as **transitional hypoglycemia** or **persistent** mainly based on the duration of the hypoglycemia. It is often difficult to distinguish between the 2 types, especially in the first 48 hours of life. The majority of hypoglycemia in the newborn period is transient/nonpathologic and lasts only a few days.
A. **Rule out other disorders that may mimic hypoglycemia and cause the same symptoms of hypoglycemia.** There are no pathognomonic signs of hypoglycemia, and many of these signs can be seen in other disorders such as sepsis, central nervous system disease, toxic exposure, encephalopathy secondary to perinatal asphyxia, congenital heart disease/heart failure, severe respiratory distress syndrome, renal and liver failure, adrenal insufficiency, opioid withdrawal, inborn errors of metabolism, and metabolic abnormalities (hypocalcemia, hypo-/hypernatremia, hypomagnesemia/pyridoxine deficiency). **If the signs of hypoglycemia disappear with treatment for hypoglycemia and there is normalization of the glucose level, then they are most likely attributed to hypoglycemia.** If the signs do not disappear with treatment for hypoglycemia and there is normalization of the glucose level, then one needs to rule out those disorders that can present with the same signs as hypoglycemia.

B. **Transitional hypoglycemia only lasts a few days after birth (usually 24 hours but can last up to 72 hours) and is nonpathologic (usually self-limiting and not caused by a disease).** It is often related to events occurring during birth and can occur in healthy or sick infants. In utero, the fetus has a constant supply of glucose from his or her mother. At delivery, with the cutting of the umbilical cord, this stops, and the neonate must be able to regulate insulin and maintain his or her glucose level. Blood glucose normally drops after birth and can be as low as 30 mg/dL. Some infants are able to regulate their blood glucose, and thus the level goes up in 2 to 3 hours, but some are not able to (usually at-risk infants, but some infants have no risk factors). Many of these infants are asymptomatic. Infants normally compensate for this drop, and blood glucose levels rise within 48 to 72 hours to values similar to adults. Transitional hypoglycemia probably represents an adaptation to early life because it is seen in other mammals. One concept is that infants with **transitional hypoglycemia** have lower levels of free fatty acids (FFAs; alternate fuel source), have inadequate muscle stores as a source of amino acids, are not efficient at producing ketones, are hyperinsulinemic due to immaturity in B-cell gene expression and regulation, and have inadequate/deficient hepatic glycogen stores. Recent studies suggest that transitional hypoglycemia is a regulated process in normal newborns; it is a hypoketotic form of hypoglycemia felt to be secondary to a lower glucose threshold for suppression of insulin secretion that is normal for infants. **Some cases of transitional hypoglycemia may last longer** than several days (a few weeks up to 6 months). Kallem et al (2017) define transitional hypoglycemia as lasting <7 days and has further divided transient hypoglycemia into **early transitional adaptive hypoglycemia** (due to adaption: IDM, infants with hypothermia, asphyxiated infants), **secondary associated hypoglycemia** (due to illnesses: sepsis, perinatal asphyxia, intracranial hemorrhage), and **classic transient neonatal hypoglycemia** (SGA). **Common causes of transitional hypoglycemia include the following:**

1. **Maternal:** Maternal diabetes mellitus/gestational diabetes, IV dextrose during delivery, hypoglycemic agents during pregnancy (eg, chlorpropamide), maternal use of ritodrine, tocolytic therapy with β-sympathomimetic agents (terbutaline, isoxsuprine, salbutamol), high BMI, preeclampsia/eclampsia/hypertension, other maternal conditions.

2. **Infant:** Delayed adaptation, prematurity, postmaturity SGA, LGA (even without diabetes), IDM, late preterm, hypothermia, asphyxia, IUGR, sepsis, erythroblastosis fetalis, polycythemia, transient hyperinsulinemia, stress-induced hyperinsulinemia, *HNF4A/HNF1A* mutation

3. **Syndromes that can cause transient (and persistent) hypoglycemia:** Beckwith-Wiedemann, Sotos, Kabuki, and Costello syndromes; mosaic Turner syndrome; and congenital disorders of glycosylation (CDG).

C. **Persistent hypoglycemia.** Usually defined as hypoglycemia that persists longer than 48 to 72 hours after birth and has been referred to as pathologic hypoglycemia. Infants who require higher amounts of glucose (>10–12 mg/kg/min) to maintain a normal glucose, especially over 72 hours, may have persistent hypoglycemia (lasting >7 days). Because some types of transitional hypoglycemia can persist past 6 months, persistent hypoglycemia is typically used to describe the more severe and prolonged hypoglycemia that is caused by rarer disorders such as congenital hyperinsulinemia (CHI), endocrine disorders, or inborn errors of metabolism. Persistent hypoglycemia is also more likely associated with possible neurologic sequelae. Causes of persistent hypoglycemia include the following:

1. **Congenital hyperinsulinism.** (Older terms include nesidioblastosis, idiopathic hypoglycemia of infancy, persistent hyperinsulinemic hypoglycemia of infancy, and hyperinsulinemic hypoglycemia of infancy.) CHI is an inappropriate or excessive amount of insulin secreted by the pancreatic islet β-cells caused by a group of genetic disorders. It is the **most common cause of persistent hypoglycemia.** Mutations in 9 different key genes have been identified in CHI.

Mutations in the *ABCC8/KCNJ11* genes, which cause diffuse forms of CHI and account for 60% to 75% of the cases, are the most common cause. Focal CHI is due to paternally inherited *ABCC8/KCNJ11* mutation. Incidence is from 1 per 2500 to 1 per 50,000.

2. **Insulin-producing tumors.** Includes nesidioblastosis, B-cell adenoma or islet adenomatosis, islet cell dysmaturity, B-cell hyperplasia/dysplasia including adenoma spectrum, sulfonylurea receptor defect. Insulinoma is rare in children.

3. **Syndromes associated with hyperinsulinemia (syndromic hyperinsulinemia).** Most common is Beckwith-Wiedemann syndrome (hypoglycemia, macroglossia, visceromegaly, omphalocele, ear creases/pits, renal abnormalities, macrosomia). Others include hyperinsulinism/hyperammonemia syndrome and Perlman, Kabuki, Ondine, Usher type IC, Simpson-Golabi-Behmel, and Sotos syndromes. Hypoglycemia associated with growth hormone (GH) and cortisol deficiency is Costello syndrome, and hypoglycemia associated with GH deficiency is Turner mosaicism.

4. **Congenital defects of glycosylation (CDG).** Inherited defects of protein glycosylation. Certain types of CDG can cause hypoglycemia.

5. **Insulin resistance syndromes.** These can cause hyperinsulinemic fasting hypoglycemia and can be genetic or autoimmune.

6. **Endocrine disorders.** Hormone deficiency disorders (rare) caused by deficiencies in cortisol, epinephrine, glucagon, and GH. Some of these disorders may have coexisting hyperinsulinemia.

   a. **Growth hormone deficiency (isolated).**

   b. **Adrenal insufficiency (cortisol deficiency).** Congenital adrenal hyperplasia, X-linked adrenal hypoplasia, adrenal hemorrhage, adrenogenital syndrome.

   c. **Congenital hypopituitarism.** Due to hypoplasia or aplasia of the anterior pituitary gland. Causes GH and cortisol deficiency.

   d. **Congenital adrenocorticotropic hormone deficiency or familial glucocorticoid deficiency.**

   e. **Other rare disorders.** Midline central nervous malformations such as congenital optic nerve hypoplasia, congenital hypothyroidism, glucagon deficiency, and epinephrine deficiency.

7. **Inborn errors of metabolism.** Hypoglycemia is more commonly seen in disorders of carbohydrate metabolism or fatty acid oxidation but may be seen in disorders of amino acid metabolism, organic acidurias, and respiratory chain defects.

   a. **Disorders of carbohydrate metabolism.** These include galactosemia, hereditary fructose intolerance, and glycogen storage diseases.

   b. **Fatty acid oxidation defects.** Present with isolated nonketotic hypoglycemia or may also have hyperammonemia, metabolic acidosis, and elevated transaminases. The most common is medium-chain acyl-CoA dehydrogenase deficiency. Others include short-chain acyl-CoA dehydrogenase deficiency, long-chain 3-hydroxyacyl-CoA and very-long-chain acyl-CoA dehydrogenase deficiency, and carnitine deficiency disorders (carnitine palmitoyl transferase deficiency types I and II).

   c. **Disorders of amino acid metabolism.** Maple syrup urine disease and hereditary tyrosinemia are disorders of amino acid metabolism that can present with hypoglycemia.

   d. **Disorders of organic acidurias that may present with hypoglycemia.** Methylmalonic acidemia, propionic acidemia glutaric acidemia type II, 3-hydroxy-3-methylglutaric aciduria.

   e. **Respiratory chain defects (oxidative phosphorylation deficiency).** May present only with hypoglycemia.

      f. **Glucose transporter deficiency syndrome.** **Neurohypoglycemia** is a rare condition in which the infant lacks the transport protein glucose transporter 1 (GLUT-1) that causes glucose to be transported across the blood–brain barrier.

      g. **Drugs/toxins.** The following drugs are associated with hypoglycemia: insulin, alcohol, sulfonylureas, β-blockers, and salicylates.

      h. **Rare.** Primary lactic acidosis, phosphoenolpyruvate carboxykinase deficiency.

IV. Database

  A. History

    1. **Family history.** Is there a history of diabetes in the family? If there are siblings, did they have a problem with hypoglycemia? Did they have any infantile seizures? Parental consanguinity suggests autosomal recessive disorders.

    2. **Pregnancy history.** Perform a detailed history of the pregnancy (Was there gestational diabetes during the pregnancy, any hypertension, or insulin use? What medications did the mother receive? Was the mother on IV glucose during delivery?).

    3. **Delivery history.** Cesarean section, vaginal delivery, Apgar (appearance, pulse, grimace, activity, respirations) score, any asphyxia, any resuscitation, any meconium, or hypothermia.

    4. **Gestational age (term, preterm) and weight of the infant.** Note low/high birthweight, SGA, LGA.

    5. **Infant history.** When did the episode of hypoglycemia occur? What was the timing of the episode to feeding history? What was the method of determining the blood sugar?

  B. Physical examination. Evaluate the infant for signs of hypoglycemia (see Section II.F). **Many of the findings below are suggestive of disorders causing persistent hypoglycemia and are more pertinent to that workup.**

    1. **Suggestive findings.** Are there signs of sepsis or shock? Is there dysmorphism that may suggest a syndrome? Is the infant plethoric (polycythemia)? Does the infant have atypical genitalia (congenital adrenal hyperplasia)? Is there a midline defect and a micropenis (panhypopituitarism)? Are cataracts present (galactosemia and intrauterine infections)? Does the urine smell like maple syrup (inborn error of metabolism)? Is the growth abnormal (IUGR/SGA and LGA)? Is there a large liver and/or tongue (Beckwith-Wiedemann syndrome, galactosemia, fructosemia)? Is the infant macrosomic (maternal diabetes, Beckwith-Wiedemann syndrome)? Does the infant have hairy pinna (suggests IDM)? Infantile spasms (rare) can be seen in hyperinsulinemic hypoglycemia. Infants with congenital forms of hyperinsulinism may have facial dysmorphism (high forehead, small nasal tip and short columella, and square face).

    2. **Specific exam findings for syndromic hyperinsulinemia.** **Beckwith-Wiedemann syndrome:** LGA, large protruding tongue (macroglossia), large prominent eyes, creases in earlobes, low-set ears, abdominal wall defect/omphalocele, undescended testicles, diastasis recti. **Perlman syndrome:** fetal gigantism, heart defect/malformation, risk of Wilms tumor, deep-set eyes, depressed nasal bridge, agenesis of the corpus callosum. **Costello syndrome:** heart defect/malformation, cutis laxa (loose folds of skin), large mouth. **Usher syndrome type IC:** intestinal malformation, deafness, retinitis pigmentosa. **Sotos syndrome:** LGA, macrocephaly, skeletal malformation, heart defect/malformation. **Timothy syndrome:** syndactyly, heart defect/malformation, long QT syndrome. **Kabuki syndrome:** skeletal malformation, urinary tract anomalies, heart defect/malformation, intestinal malformation. **Simpson-Golabi-Behmel syndrome:** widely spaced eyes, macrostomia, LGA, skeletal malformation, heart defect/malformation, intestinal malformation, tumor risk, corpus callosum agenesis, cerebellar atrophy/hypoplasia, deafness.

  C. Laboratory studies. (Who to screen?) Screening depends on risk factors and/or signs of hypoglycemia. AAP and PES guidelines differ on not only who to screen but also the target glucose to maintain. It is best to follow your institutional guidelines. **Some providers recommend AAP guidelines for infants <48 hours old and then use PES guidelines for those infants >48 hours old.**

1. **American Academy of Pediatrics guidelines for hypoglycemia screening.** Neonatal hypoglycemia occurs most commonly in infants who are SGA, IDM/ LGA, and late preterm infants. Screen and monitor glucose only in infants who are late preterm and term SGA or IDM/LGA infants unless an infant is symptomatic. AAP does not recommend routine screening in a healthy term newborn after a normal pregnancy and delivery. **AAP recommendations on who to screen:**

   a. **Any infant who manifests clinical signs that suggest hypoglycemia** needs a **stat blood glucose** immediately (within minutes) should be screened and monitored.

   b. **Any asymptomatic late preterm (34–36 6/7 weeks) and term SGA infants or IDM/LGA infants.** At-risk infants should be screened based on risk factors. IDM can be hypoglycemic as early as 1 hour after birth, SGA or LGA infants can be hypoglycemic by 3 hours of age but can be hypoglycemic for 10 days after birth.

   c. **Screening the asymptomatic at-risk infant.** Should include blood glucose within the first few hours of birth and continued through multiple feeding cycles. Gavage feeding can be considered if infant is not feeding well. The target glucose before each feed is 45 mg/dL.

      i. **Birth to 4 hours of age.** Infants should be fed by 1 hour of age and screened 30 minutes after the first feeding.

      ii. **4 to 24 hours of age.** Screen glucose before each feed. Continue feeds every 2 to 3 hours. Continue this screening for 12 hours for IDM and LGA infants. Continue this screening for 24 hours for late preterm and term SGA infants.

      iii. **After 24 hours of age.** If glucose is still <45 mg/dL, continue screening before each feeding.

2. **Pediatric Endocrine Society guidelines for hypoglycemia screening.** PES states there is not a definite glucose level to define hypoglycemia, and their definition of clinical hypoglycemia is a plasma glucose concentration low enough to cause symptoms and/or signs of impaired brain function. The guideline recommends to stabilize glucose levels in the first 24 to 48 hours, and after 48 hours, it is important to focus on the etiology of the hypoglycemia. It is important to identify infants with persistent hypoglycemia syndromes (after 48 hours) so serious neurologic sequelae can be prevented. The Pediatric Endocrine Society discusses screening **in terms of evaluating, recognizing, and managing infants.**

   a. **Neonates at risk for hypoglycemia and in whom screening is recommended:** Neonates who have symptoms of hypoglycemia, LGA (even without maternal diabetes), perinatal stress (birth asphyxia/ischemia, cesarean section for fetal distress, maternal preeclampsia/eclampsia or hypertension, IUGR, SGA, meconium aspiration syndrome, erythroblastosis fetalis, polycythemia, hypothermia), premature or postmature infants, IDM, family history of a genetic form of hypoglycemia, congenital syndromes (Beckwith-Wiedemann), or any abnormal physical features (microphallus, midline facial malformations).

   b. **Neonates who need to have persistent hypoglycemia ruled out before discharge:** Family history of genetic form of hypoglycemia, severe hypoglycemia (symptomatic hypoglycemia or need IV glucose), inability to maintain a preprandial glucose concentration >50 mg/dL up to 48 hours and >60 mg/dL after 48 hours, congenital syndrome (Beckwith-Wiedemann), or any abnormal physical features (microphallus, midline facial malformations).

    c. **High-risk neonates (without a suspected congenital hypoglycemia disorder) on normal feedings:**

        i. **<48 hours of age:** Evaluate infants whose blood glucose is <50 mg/dL. Any infant who is unable to maintain a glucose level >50 mg/dL in the first 48 hours is at risk for persistent hypoglycemia. If IV glucose is required, then these infants probably have more severe and prolonged hypoglycemia and should maintain a target blood glucose of >60 mg/dL. Once the blood glucose level is stabilized, normal feedings can be resumed.

        ii. **>48 hours of age:** Evaluate infants whose blood glucose is <60 mg/dL.

    d. **Neonates with a suspected congenital hypoglycemia disorder** (infants with increased risk for a persistent hypoglycemia disorder in whom it needs to be excluded before discharge).

        i. **Maintain a blood glucose >70 mg/dL.**

        ii. **Evaluate when the infant is >48 hours of age,** so that the transitional period has passed.

        iii. **Thorough history and physical examination.**

    e. **High-risk neonates in whom persistent hypoglycemia needs to be ruled out (before discharge):** Any infant with severe hypoglycemia (defined as episode of symptomatic hypoglycemia or need for IV dextrose), any infant not able to maintain a preprandial plasma glucose >50 mg/dL up to 48 hours of age or >60 mg/dL after 48 hours of age, any infant with a family history of a genetic form of hypoglycemia, or any infant with a congenital syndrome or any abnormal physical features.

3. **PES guidelines for laboratory screening of persistent hypoglycemia.** If possible, draw a critical sample at the time of hypoglycemia and before treatment. It is best to draw plasma glucose, bicarbonate, β-hydroxybutyrate (BOHB), and lactate. At the same time, draw an extra tube of blood to hold for other testing (plasma insulin, FFA, C-peptide for hyperinsulinemia; plasma total and free carnitine and acylcarnitine profile for fatty acid oxidation).

    a. **Metabolic clues based on bicarbonate, β-hydroxybutyrate, lactate, and free fatty acid lab testing:**

        i. **If acidemia is present based on bicarbonate result:**

           (a) **If β-hydroxybutyrate level is increased:** Suspect ketotic hypoglycemia, glycogenosis, GH deficiency, cortisol deficiency.

           (b) **If lactate is increased:** Suspect gluconeogenesis defects.

        ii. **If no acidemia is present based on bicarbonate result:**

           (a) **β-Hydroxybutyrate decreased, free fatty acids increased:** Suspect fatty acid oxidation defects.

           (b) **β-Hydroxybutyrate decreased, free fatty acids decreased:** Suspect genetic hyperinsulinism, hypopituitarism, transitional neonatal hypoglycemia, perinatal stress hyperinsulinism.

    b. **If critical sample at the time of hypoglycemia is not possible, "a provocative fasting test" can be done.** A plasma glucose of 50 mg/dL is low enough to perform the tests. Monitor vital signs, plasma glucose, and BOHB concentrations during the test. Draw necessary labs and stop the fast. Stop the fast if there are symptoms of distress or plasma BOHB is >2.5 mmol/L. Once the fast has been stopped, do the glucagon test. (See below.)

        i. **Suspected hyperinsulinism:** Give the glucagon test (1 mg IV, intramuscularly [IM], or subcutaneously) when the plasma glucose is <50 mg/dL to measure the glycemic response (>30 mg/dL nearly pathognomonic of hyperinsulinemia). Plasma BOHB and FFA are both low in hyperinsulinemia.

        ii. **Additional tests to consider:** GH, cortisol, total and free carnitine, acylcarnitine profile, C-peptide, proinsulin, and drug screening. Consider genetic mutation analysis.

      iii. Suspected adrenal insufficiency: Obtain plasma adrenocorticotropic hormone and cortisol.

      iv. Suspected drug/toxin: Obtain drug/toxicology screen. For exogenous insulin administration: see high plasma insulin level with low C-peptide level during hypoglycemia.

4. Other screening recommendations (not American Academy of Pediatrics/ Pediatric Endocrine Society)

   a. Laboratory recommendations for infants <34 weeks. There are no formal guidelines for these infants. Many of these infants will be admitted to a transitional care or special care nursery based on their weight and gestational age, so they will already be getting frequent glucose monitoring.

   b. Studies for persistent hypoglycemia in all infants. Draw any necessary labs at the time of hypoglycemia (plasma glucose <50 mg/dL). There are multiple tests that can be performed, but the primary goal is to determine whether the infant has hyperinsulinemia.

      i. Initial studies.

        (a) Serum glucose and insulin (insulin-to-glucose level). Serum insulin will be high at the time of hypoglycemia with hyperinsulinemia. Some clinicians obtain serum glucose and insulin to determine the ratio of insulin to glucose (I/G). Normal I/G is <0.30. A level >0.30 suggests hyperinsulinemia.

        (b) Serum ketones. Low to absent in the presence of hyperinsulinemia and high in GH and cortisol deficiency.

        (c) Hydroxybutyrate and free fatty acids. Decreased levels can indicate excessive insulin.

        (d) Serum lactate. This can be elevated in metabolic defects.

        (e) Serum ammonia. To rule out hyperinsulinism/hyperammonemia syndrome.

        (f) C-peptide levels. Elevated in hyperinsulinemia and insulinoma.

        (g) Insulin-like growth factor binding protein 1. Decreased in hyperinsulinemia.

        (h) Increased serum insulin, C-peptide, and proinsulin level and decreased glucose, FFAs, ketones, and insulin-like growth factor binding protein 1, and an exaggerated glycemic response after glucagon challenge can diagnose CHI.

      ii. Critical labs to diagnose hyperinsulinism

        (a) Plasma insulin >2 U/mL.

        (b) Plasma free fatty acids <1.0 to 1.5 mmol/L (<28–42 mg/dL).

        (c) Plasma <1.5 mmol/L (<15 mg/dL).

        (d) Glucagon challenge 1 mg IV, IM, or subcutaneously results in >30 mg/dL rise in blood sugar.

   c. Other tests. Serum pH (metabolic disorders), cortisol and adrenocorticotropic hormone stimulation test (adrenal insufficiency), GH levels (GH deficiency), blood ammonia (galactosemia, hyperinsulinism/hyperammonemia), thyroxine (T_4) and thyroid-stimulating hormone (TSH) (hypothyroidism), blood lactate levels (glycogen storage disorders), urine ketones and reducing substances or amino acids and organic acids (inborn error of metabolism), FFA levels (fatty acid oxidation defect), plasma acylcarnitines (3-hydroxyacyl-CoA dehydrogenase [HADH] deficiency).

      i. Genetic testing. To diagnose inherited syndromes or certain disorders of inborn errors of metabolism.

      ii. To differentiate a metabolic defect from hypopituitarism and hyperinsulinism. Obtain a set of laboratory tests before and 15 minutes after the administration of glucagon (1 mg/dose IV, IM, or subcutaneously). These tests include serum glucose, ketones, FFAs, lactate, alanine, uric

Table 67–1. DIAGNOSIS OF PERSISTENT HYPOGLYCEMIA BEFORE AND AFTER
PARENTERAL GLUCAGON ADMINISTRATION

Variable	Hyperinsulinism		Hypopituitarism		Metabolic Defect	
	Before	After	Before	After	Before	After
Glucose	↓	↑↑↑	↓	↑/N	↓	↓/N
Ketones	↓	↓	N/↓	N	↑	↑
Free fatty acids	↓	↑	N/↓	N	↑	↑
Lactate	N	N	N	N	↑	↑↑
Alanine	N	?	N	N	↑	↑↑
Uric acid	N	N	N	N	↑	↑↑
Insulin	↑↑	↑↑↑	N/↑	↑	N	↑
Growth hormone	↑	↓	↓	↓	↑	↑
Cortisol	↑	↓	↓[a]	↓[a]	↑	↑
TSH and T$_4$	N	N	↓[a]	↓[a]	N	N

N, normal or no change; ↑, elevated; ↓, lowered; ?, unknown; T$_4$, thyroxine; TSH, thyroid-stimulating
hormone.
[a]Response may vary depending on the degree of hypopituitarism.

acid, insulin, GH, cortisol, glucagon, T$_4$, and TSH. The results are
interpreted as shown in Table 67–1, courtesy of the late Dr. Marvin
Cornblath.
  D. **Imaging and other studies**
    1. **Ultrasound/computed tomography of the pancreas** to look for adenoma.
    2. **Echocardiogram** may show hypertrophic cardiomyopathy in IDM with transient
       hyperinsulinism.
    3. **Electrospray ionization tandem mass spectrometry** can identify inborn errors
       of metabolism more rapidly (see Chapter 100).
    4. **^{18}F-dihydroxyphenylalanine positron emission tomography/computed
       tomography** allows preoperative differentiation of focal from diffuse CHI.
    5. **Contrast-enhanced computed tomography** technique permits precise preopera-
       tive localization of the lesion.
    6. **Head magnetic resonance imaging** to rule out pituitary or hypothalamic neo-
       plasms or congenital abnormalities.
V. **Plan**
  A. **Transitional hypoglycemia.** There are many different recommendations on treat-
     ments for **transitional hypoglycemia**. The majority of cases of transitional hypo-
     glycemia respond well to treatment and are associated with an excellent prognosis.
     **Treatments include early feeding (bottle/breast/gavage), dextrose gel or IV fluids
     (mini-bolus and/or IV), or a combination of any of these.** There are many guide-
     lines, and they differ in their recommendations (AAP, PES, Sugar Babies dextrose
     gel trial). It is best to follow the guidelines of your institution. **Some advocate that
     it is best to follow the AAP guidelines for the first 48 hours.** The overall goal is to
     maintain normoglycemia. Infants at risk for hypoglycemia and those with established
     hypoglycemia should have glucose screening every 1 to 2 hours until glucose levels
     are stable and then every 3 hours. Once the glucose level is stable, the next step is

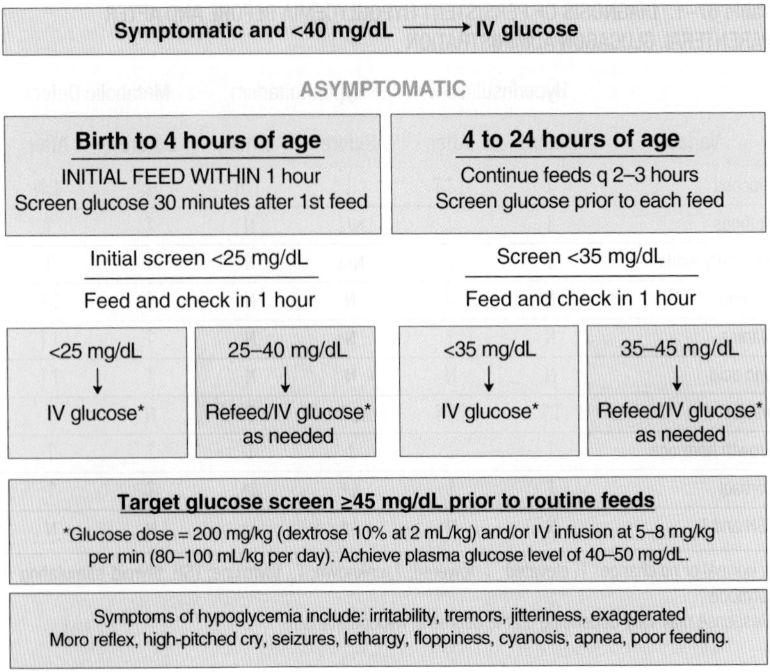

Symptomatic and <40 mg/dL ——→ IV glucose

ASYMPTOMATIC

Birth to 4 hours of age	**4 to 24 hours of age**
INITIAL FEED WITHIN 1 hour	Continue feeds q 2–3 hours
Screen glucose 30 minutes after 1st feed	Screen glucose prior to each feed

Initial screen <25 mg/dL	Screen <35 mg/dL
Feed and check in 1 hour	Feed and check in 1 hour

<25 mg/dL	25–40 mg/dL	<35 mg/dL	35–45 mg/dL
↓	↓	↓	↓
IV glucose*	Refeed/IV glucose* as needed	IV glucose*	Refeed/IV glucose* as needed

Target glucose screen ≥45 mg/dL prior to routine feeds
*Glucose dose = 200 mg/kg (dextrose 10% at 2 mL/kg) and/or IV infusion at 5–8 mg/kg per min (80–100 mL/kg per day). Achieve plasma glucose level of 40–50 mg/dL.

Symptoms of hypoglycemia include: irritability, tremors, jitteriness, exaggerated Moro reflex, high-pitched cry, seizures, lethargy, floppiness, cyanosis, apnea, poor feeding.

FIGURE 67–1. Screening for and management of postnatal glucose homeostasis in late-preterm (LPT 34–36 6/7 weeks), term small for gestational age (SGA) infants, and infants who were born to mothers with diabetes (IDM)/large for gestational age (LGA) infants. For LPT and SGA, screen at 0 to 24 hours; for IDM and LGA ≥34 weeks, screen at 0 to 12 hours. IV, intravenous. (*Modified with permission from Committee on Fetus and Newborn, Adamkin DH: Postnatal glucose homeostasis in late-preterm and term infants, Pediatrics. 2011 Mar;127(3):575-579.*)

to determine why the patient is hypoglycemic. Sometimes the cause is obvious, as in the case of an IDM or an infant with IUGR. If the cause is not obvious, further workup is necessary.

1. **The following American Academy of Pediatrics recommendations focus mainly on transitional hypoglycemia:**
   a. **At-risk late preterm (34–36 6/7 weeks) and term small for gestational age infants and infants of diabetic mothers/large for gestational age infants (American Academy of Pediatrics). (See Figure 67–1.)**
      i. **The following are key management concepts:**
         (a) **Signs of hypoglycemia** can be irritability, jitteriness, tremors, exaggerated Moro reflex, high-pitched cry, seizures, lethargy, floppiness, cyanosis, apnea, and poor feeding.
         (b) **Target blood glucose screen** ≥45 mg/dL prior to feeds.
         (c) **Gavage feedings can be considered** if the infant is not feeding well.
      ii. **Symptomatic infants:** If blood glucose is <40 mg/dL, treat with IV glucose. Give a 2 mL/kg dextrose 10% in water (D10W) mini-bolus at a rate of 1 mL/min and/or a continuous infusion of D10W at a rate of 5 to 8 mg/kg/ min glucose intake (80–100 mL/kg/d D10W infusion) to achieve a plasma glucose of 40 to 50 mg/dL.

    iii. **Asymptomatic infants from birth to 4 hours of age:**
- (a) Feed within 1 hour of birth.
- (b) Obtain serum glucose 30 minutes after first feed.
  - (i) **Serum glucose <25 mg/dL:** Refeed and check in 1 hour.
  - (ii) **If serum glucose <25 mg/dL:** Use IV glucose. Give a 2 mL/kg D10W mini-bolus at a rate of 1 mL/min and/or continuous infusion of D10W at a rate of 5 to 8 mg/kg/min glucose intake (80–100 mL/kg/d D10W infusion). Achieve blood glucose level of 40 to 50 mg/dL.
  - (iii) **If serum glucose is 25 to 40 mg/dL:** Refeed/IV glucose as needed.

    iv. **Asymptomatic infants 4 to 24 hours of age**
- (a) **Continue feeds** every 2 to 3 hours.
- (b) **Obtain serum glucose** prior to each feed.
- (c) **Serum glucose <35 mg/dL:** Refeed and check in 1 hour.
- (d) **If serum glucose <35 mg/dL:** IV glucose (see earlier).
- (e) **If serum glucose is 35 to 45 mg/dL:** Refeed/IV glucose as needed.

Note for American Academy of Pediatrics recommendations: Correction of hypoglycemia is recommended by infusion of glucose by mini-bolus and/or continuous infusion. Some authors have found that rapid correction of hypoglycemia in asymptomatic newborns >35 weeks of gestational age and at risk for hypoglycemia (maternal diabetes, LGA, fetal growth restriction, and prematurity [gestational age <37 weeks]) had a worse neurodevelopmental outcome at 2 years of age. Because of this finding, **some physicians are advocating bypassing the mini-bolus and just starting a continuous glucose infusion of 4 to 6 mg/kg/min.**

2. **Pediatric Endocrine Society recommendations for high-risk neonate without a suspected congenital hypoglycemia disorder**
   - a. **High-risk neonates without a suspected congenital hypoglycemia disorder <48 hours of age:** Maintain a blood glucose >50 mg/dL. Evaluate infants whose blood glucose is <50 mg/dL. Any infant who is unable to maintain a glucose level >50 mg/dL in the first 48 hours is at risk for persistent hypoglycemia. **If IV glucose is required,** then these infants probably have more severe and prolonged hypoglycemia, and a target blood glucose of >60 mg/dL should be maintained. Once the blood glucose level is stabilized, normal feedings can be resumed.
   - b. **High-risk neonates without a suspected congenital hypoglycemia disorder >48 hours of age:** Maintain a glucose level >60 mg/dL.

3. **Dextrose oral gel (40%)**
   - a. **Dextrose gel as prophylaxis.** A Cochrane review (2017) found insufficient evidence, so this practice cannot be recommended.
   - b. **Treatment of neonatal hypoglycemia.** The Sugar Babies Study in 2013 reported that buccal treatment with 40% dextrose gel (200 mg/kg; Table 67–2) was more effective than feeding alone for reversing neonatal hypoglycemia in at-risk term and late preterm infants (35–42 weeks' gestation) in the first 48 hours after birth. This method decreased the number of episodes and recurrence rate of hypoglycemia, decreased the need for admission to the NICU, increased exclusive breast-feeding rates at discharge, did not exhibit rebound hypoglycemia, and supported family bonding. Authors recommend it for first-line management of the late preterm and term hypoglycemic neonate up to 48 hours after birth. Developmental follow-up study at 2 years showed that treatment with dextrose gel did not decrease or increase the rate of neurosensory impairment or processing difficulties compared with placebo. **Cochrane review (2016)** concluded that treatment with 40% dextrose gel decreases the incidence of mother–infant separation for treatment and increases the likelihood of full breast feeding after discharge. There are no adverse effects at 2 years of corrected age. They state it should be considered **a first-line**

Table 67–2 DOSING OF ORAL GLUCOSE (40%) GEL

Neonate Birthweight, kg	Dose of 40% Glucose Gel, g	Amount, mL
2.0	0.4	1.00
2.5	0.5	1.25
3.0	0.6	1.50
3.5	0.7	1.75
4.0	0.8	2.00
4.5	0.9	2.25
5.0	1.0	2.50

Data from Harris DL, Weston PJ, Signal M, et al: Dextrose gel for neonatal hypoglycaemia (the Sugar Babies Study): a randomised, double-blind, placebo-controlled trial, *Lancet.* 2013 Dec 21;382(9910):2077–2083.

treatment for infants with hypoglycemia. Some institutions recommend buccal dextrose gel only for managing asymptomatic infants with hypoglycemia, not for managing symptomatic infants. Many different protocols exist, and it is best to follow your own institutional guidelines.

c. **One example of a protocol implementing glucose gel for treating neonatal hypoglycemia** is based on a study by Bennett and colleagues (*Nursing for Women's Health*, Volume 20, Issue 1, February–March 2016). This protocol resulted in a 73% decrease in NICU admissions for neonatal hypoglycemia diagnosis. Use Table 67–2 for dosing of oral glucose gel.

   i. **Any infant with symptomatic hypoglycemia. Check bedside glucose; if <40 mg/dL,** apply dose of dextrose gel by syringe to the neonate's buccal cavity, place skin-to-skin to breast feed, and obtain a serum glucose. Observe neonate closely. Recheck bedside glucose in 30 minutes after the glucose gel is given and check serum glucose.

   ii. **Any infant at risk for hypoglycemia** (SGA, LGA, late preterm, IDM, Apgar score <7 at 5 minutes of age)
      (a) **Breast feed infant within first hour of birth.**
      (b) **Check blood glucose level** 30 minutes after feeding is complete.
      (c) **If blood glucose <35 mg/dL,** give a weight-based dose of 40% glucose gel by syringe to the infant's buccal cavity. Place infant back with mother to feed.
      (d) **Repeat blood glucose level in 1 hour** after gel is given.
      (e) **If the blood glucose is >35 mg/dL:** Check levels before feedings until 2 consecutive readings are >45 mg/dL.
      (f) **If the blood glucose is <35 mg/dL,** give a second dose of glucose gel. Place infant back with mother to feed. Obtain a blood glucose 1 hour after the dextrose was given. If low, contact physician.

B. **Persistent hypoglycemia.** The management of these infants can be complicated, because they can have fluid overload and cardiac failure. Many require a central line to deliver high levels of glucose. Some will require a gastrostomy for frequent feedings. **Endocrinology and possible surgical consultation** should be obtained. Long-term therapy depends on the specific disorder with consultation with specialists in the area.

1. **Pediatric Endocrine Society recommendations for neonates with a suspected congenital hypoglycemia disorder**
    a. **Maintain a blood glucose >70 mg/dL.**
    b. **Any episode of severe symptomatic hypoglycemia should be rapidly corrected with intravenous dextrose infusion.** The initial dose is 200 mg/kg, followed by continuous infusion of 10% dextrose at maintenance rate.
    c. **Glucagon can support to normalize hypoglycemia** caused by hyperinsulinism. Glucagon dose is 0.5 to 1.0 mg IV, IM, or subcutaneously.
    d. **Long-term therapy** should be based on the etiology of the disorder. Medications, surgery, and nutritional therapy are some of the treatments used.
    e. **Testing should be done on neonates with ketotic hypoglycemia** who have recurrent episodes for glycogen synthase deficiency (GSD types 0, VI, IX) and *MCT1* gene deficiency.
    f. **Hyperinsulinemia:** Aim is to prevent recurrent hypoglycemia.
    g. **Defects in glycogen metabolism and gluconeogenesis:** Aim is to maintain plasma glucose level to prevent metabolic acidosis and growth failure.
2. **General recommendations. Continue IV glucose and increase the rate of IV glucose to 16 to 20 mg/kg/min.** Rates >20 mg/kg/min are usually not helpful. If it is evident at this point that the infant still has problems with hypoglycemia, medications to treat the hypoglycemia should be started.
    a. **Glucocorticoids (dexamethasone and hydrocortisone).** Formerly used in the nonspecific treatment of persistent hypoglycemia. Some units may still be using corticosteroids as first-line therapy. It **is no longer recommended** because of side effects and is now only used if there is evidence of adrenal insufficiency. (See dosage in Chapter 155.)
    b. **The following medications can be tried.** It is not necessary to stop the previous agent when trying a new medication. Choice of treatment can be variable and depends on the institution. **Knowledge of the genetic subtype can guide treatment.** Infants with *GLUD1, HNF4A, HADH, GCK,* and *UCP2* mutations respond better to diazoxide than those with *ABCC8* and *KCNJ11* mutations. The type caused by paternal *ABCC8* or *KCNJ11* mutations may be focal and may respond to surgery (lesionectomy). The homozygous/compound heterozygous *ABCC8/KCNJ11* mutations may need near-total pancreatectomy if medical treatment does not work. *Note:* **Infants with transitional hyperinsulinemia from perinatal stress and syndromic hyperinsulinemia also respond to diazoxide.** See Chapter 155 for dosages.
        i. **Diazoxide. First treatment of choice for persistent/pathologic hypoglycemia.** Initial dose is 10 mg/kg/d orally in divided doses every 8 hours. Range is 5 to 15 mg/kg/d divided every 8 hours. **Chlorothiazide** is often used with diazoxide for its synergistic effect and to decrease retention of fluid. Diazoxide is started for a trial of 5 days. Responsiveness is based on absence of hypoglycemia on normal feedings and during a 4-hour fast. If nonresponsive, octreotide is tried next.
        ii. **Octreotide.** A long-acting analog of somatostatin; preferred over somatostatin because the latter has a very short half-life. It can be used if the infant with persistent/pathologic hypoglycemia is nonresponsive to diazoxide. The starting dose is 2 to 10 mcg/kg/d subcutaneously divided every 6–12 hours or by continuous IV infusion. Doses up to 40 mcg/kg/d divided every 6 to 8 hours can be used. It has been used long term in combination with feeding.
        iii. **Glucagon.** Used if the infant has good glycogen stores. It converts stores of glycogen to glucose. Usually it is only given in temporary situations (eg, waiting for IV/central line access, waiting for surgery, used with octreotide in short-term stabilization of infants with hyperinsulinemia). Lower dose of 0.02 to 0.30 mg/kg/dose IV may work. PES recommends using a 0.5- to 1.0-mg dose (independent of weight) IV, IM, or subcutaneously.

iv. **Nifedipine reduces glucose tolerance and insulin secretion.** It has been used in some infants, but because of severe hypotension and lack of long-term experience, it is not used often.

v. **Sirolimus** has been used in a few infants unresponsive to high doses of diazoxide and octreotide with promising results.

vi. **Medications for endocrine deficiency disorders.** GH should be used if there is a GH deficiency. Epinephrine can be used in epinephrine deficiency. Zinc protamine glucagon is indicated for infants with glucagon deficiency.

3. **Other management strategies for persistent hypoglycemia**

   a. **Pancreatic surgery.** Considered if medical treatment does not work for neonatal hyperinsulinism. It is also recommended for infants with focal lesions (partial pancreatectomy) and some infants with diffuse lesions such as I-cell hyperplasia (subtotal pancreatectomy). Pancreatectomy (removes at least 95% of the organ) is often necessary. Partial pancreatectomy can be done when hypersecretion is shown to be confined to a small area of the pancreas. Studies have shown that some cases of CHI have been managed effectively with diazoxide and octreotide for decades.

   b. **Congenital hypopituitarism.** Usually responds to administration of cortisone and IV glucose. Administration of human GH may be necessary. (For dosages, see Chapter 155.)

   c. **Metabolic defects**

      i. **Type I glycogen storage disease.** Frequent small feedings and avoiding fructose or galactose may be beneficial.

      ii. **Hereditary fructose intolerance.** Begin a fructose-free diet.

      iii. **Galactosemia.** Begin a galactose-free diet immediately on suspicion of the diagnosis.

      iv. **Glucose transporter deficiency syndrome** is treated with a ketogenic diet.

C. **Discharge recommendations by AAP and PES**

   1. **American Academy of Pediatrics: If inadequate postnatal glucose homeostasis is documented:** Make sure the infant can maintain normal plasma glucose concentrations on a routine diet for at least 3 feed fast periods before discharge.

   2. **Pediatric Endocrine Society**

      a. **Any high-risk neonates without a suspected congenital hypoglycemia disorder on normal feedings:** Consider a safety fast of 6 to 8 hours before discharge to see if the glucose level is maintained >60 mg/dL. If not, additional investigation may be necessary.

      b. **Any infant with a known genetic or persistent form of hypoglycemia:** Obtain a consultation with a specialist before discharge. Before discharge, do a safety fasting test to make sure the infant can maintain a plasma glucose >70 mg/dL after a feeding is missed (minimum 6–8 hours).

68 Hypokalemia

I. **Problem.** The nurse reports a serum potassium of 2.8 mEq/L in a normal newborn. Normal serum potassium values vary with technique used by the laboratory but are usually between **3.5 and 5.5 mEq/L. Hypokalemia is defined as a serum potassium <3.5 mEq/L.** Most sources use the following designations:

A. **Mild hypokalemia** is 3.0 to <3.5 mEq/L,

B. **Moderate hypokalemia** is 2.5 to 3.0 mEq/L,

C. **Severe hypokalemia** is <2.5 mEq/L.

Hypokalemia causes membrane hyperpolarization and impairs muscle contraction; therefore, the clinical manifestations involve changes to muscle and cardiovascular function. Severe hypokalemia can cause cardiac arrhythmias (can be fatal), respiratory depression, skeletal muscle impairment and weakness, ileus, lethargy, and in extreme cases, rhabdomyolysis. Since 98% of potassium is intracellular and 2% is extracellular, serum potassium levels do not correlate with intracellular potassium levels; therefore, hypokalemia does not reflect total body potassium stores. The body must maintain a normal extracellular potassium in order to avoid any cardiac or neurologic signs or symptoms.

II. **Immediate questions**
   A. **What is the central serum potassium?** If a low value is obtained by heel stick, central values should be obtained because they may actually be lower than values obtained by heel stick (potassium release from hemolysis of red blood cells). Was the sample sent immediately to the lab? If a sample sat for hours in a warm area, "pseudohypokalemia" can occur.
   B. **Is the infant on diuretics? Are potassium-wasting medications or digitalis being given?** Hypokalemia in a neonate usually occurs from chronic diuretic use. Hypokalemia may cause significant arrhythmias if digitalis is being administered.
   C. **How much potassium is the infant receiving?** Normal maintenance doses are 1 to 2 mEq/kg/d.
   D. **Are there any gastrointestinal losses from diarrhea, a nasogastric/orogastric tube, or ileostomy?** Loss of large amounts of gastrointestinal (GI) fluids can cause hypokalemia. Severe vomiting can also cause hypokalemia such as in infantile hypertrophic pyloric stenosis.
   E. **What is the infant's magnesium level?** Hypomagnesemia can cause hypokalemia. Consider this diagnosis if the hypokalemia does not correct despite potassium supplementation.
   F. **Does the infant have hypertension?** Consider mineralocorticoid excess: primary aldosteronism, congenital adrenal hyperplasia, or Cushing syndrome.

III. **Differential diagnosis.** Hypokalemia can be caused by a prolonged inadequate intake of potassium, increased GI losses, increased renal losses, transcellular shifts of potassium from extracellular to intracellular spaces, and medications. **Medications (diuretics, specifically loop or thiazide diuretics) are the most common cause in the neonatal intensive care unit, followed by increased GI losses from the nasogastric (NG) tube.**
   A. **Pseudohypokalemia** can occur if the blood sample has a very high WBC count kept at room temperature for a long time, whereby uptake of extracellular potassium by the WBC occurs. If the blood sample sits at an increased temperature too long ("summertime pseudohypokalemia"), this increases Na+/K+-ATPase activity, which shifts potassium into cells. A blood specimen collected after insulin administration that sits too long can cause pseudohypokalemia. Avoid this by either storing the blood at 4°C or rapidly separating the plasma or serum from the cells.
   B. **True hypokalemia (total body deficit)**
      1. **Inadequate intake (rare)** of maintenance infusion, inadequate oral intake of potassium, or insufficient support in total parenteral nutrition. Extremely preterm small for gestational age infants on recommended early parenteral nutrition are at high risk of hypokalemia. For further discussion, see Chapter 10.
      2. **Gastrointestinal losses**
         a. **Loss of fluid via nasogastric tube, ostomies, or gastrointestinal fistulas.** Unreplaced electrolyte loss from NG tube (most common) or intestinal drainage (ostomies, GI fistulas). Infants with necrotizing enterocolitis or intestinal anomalies requiring surgery are at risk.
         b. **Diarrhea.** Congenital chloride diarrhea, any GI fistula, short bowel syndrome.
         c. **Vomiting.** May cause hypokalemia such as infantile hypertrophic pyloric stenosis with vomiting. In hypertrophic pyloric stenosis in infants, an enlarged pylorus, or **"pyloric olive,"** may be felt in 23% of cases (best felt during or at the end of a feeding).

    d. Medications. Kayexalate causes fecal potassium loss.
3. **Renal losses**
   a. Medications
     i. Diuretic use, especially long-term therapy with any **thiazide or loop diuretic,** is the most common medication-related cause.
     ii. Steroids and steroid-like medications.
     iii. Antibiotics. High-dose penicillin, ampicillin, carbenicillin, vancomycin, aminoglycosides. Combined treatment of aminoglycosides and vancomycin can cause tubular disturbances in extremely low birthweight infants with renal tubular wasting of potassium. Intravenous colistin use was significantly associated with hypokalemia.
     iv. Magnesium-depleting medications, such as amphotericin B, cisplatin, or carboplatin, cause renal magnesium wasting. Amphotericin B can cause direct renal tubular damage with potassium loss.
   b. Any cause of polyuria
   c. Renal tubular losses
     i. Renal tubular acidosis types 1 and 2 can both cause hypokalemia.
     ii. Hypomagnesemia. Exacerbates potassium loss by increasing distal potassium secretion.
     iii. Bartter syndrome (antenatal or neonatal). Antenatal Bartter syndrome is a rare autosomal recessive renal tubular disorder caused by mutations in the transporters in the thick ascending limb of the loop of Henle (defective gene *NKCC2*, type I Bartter syndrome; defective gene *ROMK*, type II Bartter syndrome). The infant presents at birth with hypokalemia, hypochloremia, and metabolic alkalosis and also has failure to thrive and recurrent episodes of dehydration. The hypokalemia is a form of potassium wasting, secondary to chloride channel abnormality. **Neonatal Bartter syndrome with sensorineural deafness (type IV)** can be caused by mutations in the *BSND* gene or *CLCNKB* and *CLCNKA* genes (type IVb). **Pseudo-Bartter syndrome** presents with the same clinical and biologic characteristics as Bartter syndrome but without the primary renal tubule abnormalities. It occurs most commonly from administration of diuretic agents or prostaglandin E, from prolonged vomiting and diarrhea, or from a maternal eating disorder. **Congenital hypokalemia with hypercalciuria** resembles Bartter syndrome.
     iv. Other syndromes. Liddle, Gitelman, and Fanconi syndromes.
4. **Transcellular shifts of potassium from serum to cells**
   a. Alkalosis (metabolic or respiratory) drives potassium into cells, causing hypokalemia. An increase in blood pH by 0.1 unit causes a decrease in the serum potassium by 0.6 mEq/L. The decrease is less in respiratory than in metabolic alkalosis.
   b. Insulin therapy causes intracellular uptake of potassium.
   c. Medications that cause an increase in intracellular uptake of potassium include β-adrenergic agonists (eg, epinephrine, decongestants, bronchodilators, tocolytic drugs) and **xanthine derivatives** (eg, theophylline, caffeine). Overdose related: insulin, verapamil, and epinephrine.
   d. Hypothermia can drive potassium into cells and lower the plasma potassium concentration.
   e. Endocrinopathies causing potassium loss (less common)
     i. Congenital adrenal hyperplasia. 11β-Hydroxylase deficiency accounts for approximately 5% to 10% of cases and causes hypertension, hypokalemic alkalosis, and salt retention.
     ii. Primary hyperaldosteronism/Conn syndrome. Hypertension, hypokalemia, and suppressed renin activity are the 3 laboratory hallmarks of

this disease. **Secondary hyperaldosteronism** can occur from renal artery stenosis, renin-secreting tumors, and coarctation of the aorta.

iii. **Cushing syndrome.** The most common cause of Cushing syndrome in infants is an adrenal tumor (bilateral hyperplasia, adenoma, or carcinoma).

iv. **Syndrome of apparent mineralocorticoid excess.** This can be congenital and causes hypokalemia.

v. **Hyperthyroidism (thyrotoxicosis).**

IV. **Database**

A. **Physical examination.** Signs of hypokalemia (muscle weakness, lethargy, myalgia, paresthesia, muscle cramps) are very difficult to assess in the neonate.

1. **Mild hypokalemia** may not cause any signs or symptoms. There may be slight muscle weakness.

2. **Moderate hypokalemia** can cause musculoskeletal symptoms (weakness, decreased tendon reflexes, myalgia, muscle cramps, paresthesias, paralysis), GI symptoms (nausea, vomiting, diarrhea, constipation, ileus), and central nervous system signs (lethargy). These are very difficult to evaluate in an infant.

3. **Severe hypokalemia** can cause lethargy, severe muscle weakness, paralysis, ileus (abdominal distension and hypoactive bowel sounds), cardiac arrhythmias (rare unless <2.5 mEq/L), respiratory depression (flaccid or diaphragmatic paralysis), respiratory arrest, or bradycardia with cardiovascular collapse. Rhabdomyolysis (skeletal muscle destruction) and myoglobinuria (leakage of muscle protein myoglobin in the urine) can occur. Muscle fasciculation and tetany can occur.

B. **Laboratory studies**

1. **Repeat the serum potassium level** to confirm the potassium level.

2. **Spot check urinary electrolytes.** Perform periodic spot checks of urinary potassium levels to determine whether urinary losses are high. This is not accurate with recent diuretic use.

a. **Urine potassium is <20 mmol/L:** Suspect nonrenal losses.

b. **Urine potassium is >20 mmol/L:** Suspect renal losses and Bartter syndrome.

c. **Urinary chloride level is low (<10 mEq/L):** Consider GI losses (vomiting, drainage, fistulas, ileostomy, diarrhea).

d. **Urine chloride** is normal in Bartter syndrome and diuretic therapy.

e. **A low urine sodium level with a high urine potassium level** is associated with secondary hyperaldosteronism.

f. **If urine magnesium is high,** consider renal magnesium loss.

3. **Urinary dipstick for blood.** Severe hypokalemia can induce rhabdomyolysis. A red or dark brown urine may indicate myoglobin (breakdown of muscle cells). If the urine is dark brown and positive for blood, then send the serum and urine for myoglobin.

4. **Serum electrolytes and creatinine.** To evaluate renal status and other electrolyte abnormalities.

a. **A low serum sodium** suggests GI loss or thiazide diuretic use.

b. **Urinary potassium-to-creatinine ratio.** If the ratio is <1.5, consider low potassium intake, GI losses, or thyrotoxicosis. If the ratio is ≥1.5, consider aldosteronism, Cushing syndrome, congenital adrenal hyperplasia, renal tubular acidosis (RTA), diuretic use, Bartter/Gitelman syndrome, or vomiting.

5. **Blood gas levels.** An alkalosis may cause or aggravate hypokalemia (ie, as hydrogen ions leave the cells, potassium ions enter the cells, causing decreased serum potassium levels). **Treatment of acidosis may worsen hypokalemia.** Acidosis is seen with RTA. Alkalosis is seen with Bartter syndrome, diuretic use, emesis, and NG losses. A high serum bicarbonate can be seen with hyperaldosteronism or Bartter syndrome. A low serum bicarbonate can be seen with RTA, diarrhea, or carbonic anhydrase inhibitors.

6. **Serum magnesium.** To rule out hypomagnesemia.
7. **Drug screen.** If the infant is on any medication that can cause hypokalemia, check the levels if available (methylxanthines such as theophylline, aminophylline, caffeine). Check digoxin level if the patient is on a digitalis preparation because hypokalemia can potentiate digitalis-induced arrhythmias.
8. **Serum adrenocorticotropic hormone, cortisol, renin activity, and aldosterone levels.** To evaluate for Cushing and Conn syndromes or adrenal hyperplasia. Low renin and low aldosterone suggest adrenal hyperplasia; low renin and high aldosterone suggest hyperaldosteronism.
9. **Serum insulin and C-peptide tests.** To evaluate for hyperinsulinism.
10. **Rhabdomyolysis.** Send aspartate aminotransferase, alanine aminotransferase, creatinine kinase, and creatinine kinase isoenzyme MB.
11. **Genetic testing in Bartter syndrome** can be performed.

C. **Imaging and other studies**
   1. **Abdominal radiograph.** If ileus is suspected.
   2. **Abdominal ultrasound.** In infants in whom pyloric stenosis is suspected, ultrasound is the diagnostic procedure of choice. Can also check for adrenal tumor or hyperplasia.
   3. **Electrocardiography.** The electrocardiogram (ECG) may appear normal in hypokalemia or may show conduction defects. The ECG changes do not always correlate with a specific potassium level as they do in hyperkalemia. ECG changes that are seen with hypokalemia include ST-segment depression, presence of or prominent U wave, flattening or inversion of or biphasic T wave, increase in P wave amplitude, prolonged PR interval, and decreased T-wave amplitude. Ventricular and atrial arrhythmias may also develop. The U-wave appearance may mimic atrial flutter. Note that these ECG findings are also seen in hypomagnesemia. There is a risk of significant cardiac arrhythmias if the infant has hypokalemia and is receiving digoxin. Digoxin toxicity is worsened in hypokalemia because digoxin binds to the ATPase pump on the same site as potassium. If potassium levels are low, it enables digoxin to bind more to the ATPase pump and increases digoxin toxicity.
   4. **Magnetic resonance image of the head** to rule out pituitary tumor if indicated.

V. **Plan**
   A. **General measures.** The following are generally accepted approaches to hypokalemia. Follow local institutional protocols if available. Treatment depends on whether the infant has ECG changes, whether the infant has any signs of hypokalemia, the severity of the signs, and the degree of hypokalemia present. Hypokalemia is increasing in neonatal intensive care units because of the widespread use of diuretics.
      1. **Prevent life-threatening cardiac and muscular complications first,** and then replenish total potassium stores so that normal blood levels are maintained.
      2. **Rapid correction of hypokalemia is not recommended** because of hyperkalemia risk with potential cardiac complications (arrhythmias and cardiac arrest).
      3. **Bolus intravenous potassium administration is not recommended** as it may cause damage to the veins and occasionally hyperkalemia, because potassium does not rapidly equilibrate.
      4. **Oral replacement is always preferred.**
      5. **If an infant is unable to tolerate oral replacement** (ileus, emesis) IV potassium is recommended.
      6. **Formula for slow correction (over 24 hours) of potassium replacement is:**

$$\text{Potassium deficit (mEq/L)} = (\text{Normal potassium} - \text{Observed potassium}) \times \text{Body weight in kg} \times 0.3$$

7. **The maximum recommended intravenous concentration is 40 mEq/100 mL (400 mEq/L) of potassium chloride** in patients with a central line. Peripheral intravenous (IV) line should be limited to 20 mEq/L.

8. **Serum potassium levels should be monitored every 4 to 6 hours** until correction is achieved. Once levels reach high normal, decrease the amount of potassium given.

9. **If alkalosis is present,** treatment is potassium chloride to replenish chloride.

10. **If the infant is acidotic,** preferred treatment is potassium acetate (IV) or potassium bicarbonate (oral). **Rapid correction of acidosis may worsen hypokalemia.**

11. **Correct low magnesium before treating with potassium** (see Chapter 105). It is ineffective to treat hypokalemia without treating the hypomagnesemia. If the low serum magnesium is not treated, the hypokalemia may get worse and become refractory to treatment. Dosage of magnesium sulfate is 25 to 50 mg/kg/dose IV every 8 to 12 hours for 2 to 3 doses.

12. **Do not dilute potassium salts in a dextrose-containing solution** because it causes secretion of insulin and cellular potassium uptake, which can further lower the potassium. It should be diluted in normal saline.

13. **Remember that excessive correction of hypokalemia** may result in hyperkalemia.

14. **Oral potassium supplements** are available as chloride, bicarbonate, citrate, gluconate, and phosphate salts. Recommendations for treatment with oral potassium supplements are as follows:

    a. **Potassium bicarbonate:** Used in infants with hypokalemia with metabolic acidosis (eg, RTA or diarrhea).

    b. **Potassium phosphate:** Used only in infants with hypokalemia and hypophosphatemia (eg, proximal RTA with Fanconi syndrome or phosphate wasting).

    c. **Potassium chloride:** Used in infants with hypokalemia, hypochloremia, and metabolic alkalosis (eg, diuretic therapy–induced hypokalemia, vomiting). Used in infants with hypovolemia.

B. **Emergency treatment.** Limited to infants with life-threatening symptoms of hypokalemia (cardiac arrhythmias, severe respiratory depression/distress, extreme muscle weakness/paralysis) or for a serum potassium level <2.0 to 2.5 mEq/L (*controversial* as to what critical level to treat regardless of clinical signs; varies from 1.5 to 2.5 mEq/L). Aggressive treatment with IV potassium requires ECG monitoring. Never give a bolus of potassium; give potassium chloride 0.5 to 1 mEq/kg/dose over 1 hour (some sources suggest 2 hours) with continuous ECG monitoring (maximum infusion rate: 1 mEq/kg/h).

C. **Moderate symptomatic hypokalemia.** Use IV potassium with ECG monitoring.

    1. **Abnormal electrocardiogram: ST-segment depression, T-wave depression, U-wave elevation:** Treat with potassium chloride 0.5 to 1 mEq/kg IV over 3 to 4 hours with ECG monitoring.

    2. **Normal electrocardiogram:** Add 20 mEq of potassium chloride per liter to peripheral vein IV fluids. If higher concentrations are needed a central line is necessary. Otherwise increase the amount in the IV fluids (preferred) or a slow correction over 24 hours (see formula Section V.A.6).

D. **Mild asymptomatic hypokalemia.** May resolve without treatment. The majority of cases can be corrected by increasing the daily potassium intake by 1 to 2 mEq/kg. If the infant is not on potassium supplements and is on oral feeding, oral supplementation with potassium chloride may be given, usually 2 to 3 mEq/kg/d in 3 to 4 divided doses (diluted with feedings), adjusted depending on serum potassium levels.

E. **Hypokalemia with hypovolemia/polyuria.** IV fluid with potassium chloride is indicated.

F. **Specific measures.** Any specific defects (eg, renal defects, adrenal disorders, and certain metabolic problems) require specific evaluation and therapy.

1. **Inadequate maintenance infusion of potassium.** Calculate the normal maintenance infusion of potassium that should be given and increase the amount accordingly (normal maintenance infusion is 1–2 mEq/kg/d, usually only necessary after the first day of life). Make sure potassium intake in early parenteral nutrition is adequate.

2. **Abnormal potassium losses**

   a. **Medications.** If the infant is receiving potassium-wasting medications, increase the maintenance dose of potassium (eg, patients with bronchopulmonary dysplasia on long-term furosemide therapy). Oral supplementation with potassium chloride may be given, 1 to 2 mEq/kg/d in 3 to 4 divided doses (with feedings), adjusted depending on serum potassium levels. It was once thought that a potassium-sparing diuretic decreased the amount of potassium supplementation; however, a randomized study showed that the serum electrolytes sodium and potassium were not affected by the addition of spironolactone.

   b. **Gastrointestinal losses**

      i. **Severe diarrhea correction.** Withhold oral feedings to allow the gut to rest and give IV fluids to correct dehydration. Add potassium to the IV fluids (initial dose of potassium chloride: 1–2 mEq/kg/d). Serum potassium levels are monitored, and the IV dose is adjusted.

      ii. **Nasogastric drainage/severe vomiting.** This amount should be measured each shift and replaced milliliter per milliliter with 1/2 normal saline with 10 to 20 mEq of potassium chloride per liter.

      iii. **Pyloric stenosis.** Correct dehydration or electrolyte issues if present. Surgery (pyloromyotomy) is indicated.

G. **Renal loss of potassium.** Other than induced by medications.

   1. **Bartter syndrome.** Correction of fluid and electrolyte imbalance. Potassium supplementation is given orally with a starting dosage of 2 to 3 mEq/kg/d, which is increased as necessary to maintain a normal serum potassium level. Treatment consists of using indomethacin, a prostaglandin synthetase inhibitor that corrects the biochemical abnormalities and decreases the urine volume.

   2. **Hyperaldosteronism.** Surgery and dexamethasone therapy may be indicated.

   3. **Cushing syndrome.** Surgical resection and postoperative glucocorticoid replacement are necessary.

   4. **Renal tubular acidosis types 1 and 2.** Alkaline therapy and potassium supplementation if needed.

H. **Redistribution of potassium**

   1. **Alkalosis.** Determine the cause of metabolic or respiratory alkalosis and treat the underlying disorder. Treat the alkalosis before increasing potassium intake.

   2. **Medications.** Should be discontinued if possible, or alternatives should be used that do not affect potassium (see Section III.B.3.a).

69 Hyponatremia

I. **Problem.** An infant has a serum sodium of 127 mEq/L, below the normal accepted value of 135 mEq/L. **Hyponatremia, defined as a low sodium, is the most common electrolyte disorder in neonates.** It occurs in approximately 33% of very low birthweight infants and is seen in up to 65% of very sick neonates. It is controversial as to what level of sodium constitutes hyponatremia in neonates. In adults, a level <135 mEq/L is considered hyponatremia; in neonates, various levels have been quoted (from <130 mEq/L to <136 mEq/L). **Most sources agree that hyponatremia in neonates is defined as a serum sodium <135 mEq/L.**

Hyponatremia is not benign and is frequently associated with significant morbidity (poor neurologic outcome [at 2 and 10–13 years of age], intracranial hemorrhage, sensorineural hearing loss, cerebral palsy, and poor growth [at 10–13 years of age]). Infants with late-onset hyponatremia have an increased risk of bronchopulmonary dysplasia (BPD) and retinopathy of prematurity (ROP) requiring surgery and longer hospital stays. If the infant has hyponatremia for >7 days, the infant has an increased risk of moderate to severe BPD, periventricular leukomalacia, and extrauterine growth retardation.

II. **Immediate questions**

A. **Is there any seizure activity?** Seizure activity can be seen in patients with extremely low serum sodium levels (usually <120 mEq/L). Most often, seizures are generalized tonic clonic but they can also be focal. **This is a medical emergency,** and urgent correction of intravenous (IV) sodium is needed.

B. **How much sodium and free water is the patient receiving? Is weight gain or loss occurring?** Be certain that an adequate amount of sodium is being given and that free water intake is not excessive. The normal amount of sodium intake is 2 to 4 mEq/kg/d. Weight gain with low serum sodium levels is most likely a result of volume overload, especially in the first day or 2 of life, when weight loss is expected.

C. **What is the urine output?** With syndrome of inappropriate secretion of antidiuretic hormone (SIADH), urine output is decreased. If the urine output is increased (>4 mL/kg/h), perform a spot check of urine sodium to determine whether urinary sodium losses are high.

D. **What medications is the infant receiving? Are renal salt-wasting medications being given?** Diuretics such as furosemide may cause hypovolemic hyponatremia. Other medications that cause hyponatremia include indomethacin, amphotericin B, theophylline, carbamazepine, chlorpromazine, indapamide, amiodarone, and selective serotonin reuptake inhibitors. Most of these cause SIADH (euvolemic hyponatremia). Morphine and barbiturates can also cause hyponatremia. Aminoglycosides and diuretics have natriuretic effects (cause excessive sodium loss in the urine). Caffeine and corticosteroids may also play a role because they increase sodium excretion in adults.

E. **Did the mother receive hypotonic intravenous fluids or an excessive amount of oxytocin? Was the mother hyponatremic in the intrapartum period?** If so, the infant can have hyponatremia at birth. Infants of mothers with hyponatremia (eg, diet deficient of sodium) can have low levels of sodium after delivery and are at a risk for early-onset hyponatremia. Increased maternal intake of water (psychogenic drinking during labor) can cause maternal hyponatremia, resulting in hyponatremia after birth. Fetal sodium levels mimic maternal levels. Fetal hyponatremia can cause tachypnea, jaundice, and seizures in the fetus and occurs when the fetal sodium equilibrates with the maternal sodium during pregnancy.

F. **What medications was the mother getting during pregnancy?** Maternal medication use during pregnancy (eg, diuretics, infusion of oxytocin and glucose, nebivolol) can cause hyponatremia in the infant. Tocolytic therapy with nonsteroidal antiinflammatory drugs (NSAIDs) can cause hyponatremia after birth.

G. **Is the infant premature and <1 week old (early-onset hyponatremia), or is the infant 2 weeks of age or older after achieving full feeding (late-onset hyponatremia)?**

1. **Early-onset hyponatremia** is usually due to free total water excess with a normal total body sodium from either increased maternal free water in labor or perinatal nonosmotic release of vasopressin (antidiuretic hormone [ADH]) (occurs in perinatal asphyxia, respiratory distress syndrome, bilateral pneumothoraces, intraventricular hemorrhage [IVH], and with certain medications). It can also occur from too much free water being given or not enough sodium intake in fluids.

2. **Late-onset hyponatremia** is usually from a negative sodium balance. It is usually caused by inadequate or low sodium intake or excessive salt losses (most common in preterm infant due to immature renal or intestinal function). Common causes are low sodium intake, diuretic therapy, and mineralocorticoid deficiency (congenital adrenal hyperplasia most commonly caused by 21-hydroxylase deficiency). Late-onset hyponatremia can also be from excessive ADH release, renal failure in infants, or edema causing retention of free water, but these causes are less common. Preterm infants >28 weeks have a high fractional excretion of sodium. Risk factors for late-onset hyponatremia include lower gestational age, respiratory distress syndrome, shorter duration of parenteral nutrition, use of furosemide, and breast feeding. Infants with late-onset hyponatremia have an increased risk of BPD and ROP requiring surgery and longer hospital stays. If an infant has late-onset hyponatremia for >7 days, the infant is at increased risk of moderate to severe BPD, periventricular leukomalacia, and extrauterine growth retardation.

III. **Differential diagnosis. Hyponatremia can be categorized based on the osmolality of the serum** (hypotonic hyponatremia <280 mOsm/L, hypertonic hyponatremia >295 mOms/L, or isotonic hyponatremia 285–295 mOsm/L). When considering the differential, first rule out pseudohyponatremia (isotonic hyponatremia) and use of osmotic agents or high glucose (hypertonic hyponatremia). Once those are ruled out, **true hyponatremia is likely present, which is hypotonic.** True hyponatremia can be further divided into 3 categories based on the volume status (hypovolemia, euvolemia, and hypervolemia). **The most common cause of hyponatremia in the neonate is hypervolemia hyponatremia (dilutional) caused by excessive fluid administration or retention of free water.** Causes of hyponatremia in a newborn include the following:

A. **Pseudohyponatremia** (other names: isotonic hyponatremia, factitious hyponatremia). This occurs in infants with a normal osmolality. Both hyperlipidemia and hyperproteinemia can cause pseudohyponatremia. **Hyperlipidemia** (an increase in lipid levels in the plasma level) or **hyperproteinemia** (an increase in proteins in the plasma level) can cause a decreased sodium because there is less plasma water due to the increase in lipids or proteins. This used to occur with **older lab testing techniques** (flame emission spectrophotometry and indirect potentiometry). Today, because most labs use direct ion-specific electrode potentiometry, this is uncommon (verify local lab technique if isotonic hyponatremia is detected in a patient).

B. **Hypertonic hyponatremia** (other names: translocation or redistributive hyponatremia). This occurs in infants with a high serum osmolality. Mannitol, hyperglycemia, glycerol, sucrose, maltose, dextran, and IV radiocontrast substances can all cause a hypertonic hyponatremia, whereby an increase in serum osmolality causes water and potassium to be pushed out of cells with an increase in extracellular fluid (ECF) volume, resulting in hyponatremia. In the neonate, it is occasionally seen with **hyperglycemia;** an accumulation of extracellular glucose causes a shift of free water from the intracellular space to the extracellular space. **For every 100 mg/dL increase in glucose, the sodium falls by about 1.6 mEq/L.** Once the hyperglycemia is corrected, the sodium will correct.

C. **Spurious result.** Can occur from a diluted sample drawn from an indwelling catheter with a low-sodium fluid.

D. **True hyponatremia is hypo-osmolar** because of its low serum osmolality. It has also been called hypotonic hyponatremia. **There are 3 categories of hyponatremia based on the ECF volume: hyponatremia with hypervolemia, hyponatremia with normo-/euvolemia, and hyponatremia with hypovolemia.** Etiologies are based on whether urine sodium and fractional excretion of sodium are high or low.

1. **Hyponatremia with hypervolemia.** This occurs with excess of ECF. There is a positive water balance. The total body sodium and total body water are increased. ECF is very increased, resulting in edema and weight gain. One can also see increasing blood urea nitrogen (BUN) and increasing urine specific gravity. Causes include the following:

   a. Urine sodium <20 mEq/L and low fractional excretion of sodium: Edematous states, congestive heart failure, liver failure/cirrhosis, nephrotic syndrome, neuromuscular blockage/paralysis, indomethacin therapy (causes water retention), sepsis with decreasing cardiac output, hypoalbuminemia.

   b. Urine sodium >20 mEq/L and high fractional excretion of sodium: Acute kidney injury (AKI) and chronic kidney failure. Hyponatremia was the most common electrolyte disturbance in AKI.

2. **Hyponatremia with hypovolemia.** This occurs with a deficit of ECF and can be caused by either renal or extrarenal losses. The total body sodium and total body water and ECF are all decreased. Signs include weight loss, poor skin turgor, increasing BUN, metabolic acidosis, and tachycardia.

   a. Urine sodium >20 mEq/L and high fractional excretion of sodium (renal solute loss)

     i. Diuretics (most common cause of urinary sodium loss in the neonate).

     ii. Renal immaturity. Neonates can have immature kidneys. Preterm infants are prone to hyponatremia because of a lower glomerular filtration rate, lower proximal tubular reabsorption of sodium, and an increase arginine vasopressin level when sick. Often very low birthweight infants show increased renal tubular sodium and water loss causing hyponatremia.

     iii. Salt-losing nephropathies.

     iv. Metabolic alkalosis.

     v. Osmotic diuresis.

     vi. Renal tubular acidosis.

     vii. Obstructive uropathy correction can cause high urinary losses of sodium.

     viii. Bartter and Fanconi syndromes. Bartter syndrome is associated with polyhydramnios and hypokalemic alkalosis.

     ix. Hypertension-hyponatremia syndrome in neonates caused by renovascular pathology. Renal ischemia from renal microthrombi can be the cause. Suspect if umbilical artery catheter has been placed and unilateral renal arterial stenosis is present.

     x. Mineralocorticoid deficiency (adrenal salt-wasting disorders): Addison disease, hypoaldosteronism, congenital adrenal hyperplasia, hypopituitarism, pseudohypoaldosteronism types 1 and 2, bilateral adrenal hemorrhage.

     xi. Cerebral salt-wasting syndrome. Occurs when there is loss of sodium in the urine and is secondary to acute or chronic damage to the central nervous system (hemorrhage, increased intracranial pressure). Extracellular volume is decreased, and BUN, albumin, and hematocrit are increased.

   b. Urinary sodium <20 mEq/L and low fractional excretion of sodium (extrarenal losses). Gastrointestinal losses such as vomiting, diarrhea, nasogastric tubes, ostomies, and fistulas. Infants with intestinal surgical diversions (stomas) are at risk for sodium deficiency; **third spacing of fluids** such as ascites, pleural effusion, ileus, sepsis, early necrotizing enterocolitis, or sloughing of skin; chest tube fluid loss; cerebrospinal fluid drainage; radiant warmer skin loss.

3. **Hyponatremia with euvolemia/normovolemia (normal extracellular fluid).** Total body water is increased, total sodium is normal or slightly decreased, and ECF is minimally increased but there is no edema.

   a. Urine sodium >20 mEq/L and high fractional excretion of sodium

     i. Syndrome of inappropriate secretion of antidiuretic hormone. ADH is normally secreted when blood volume is decreased. SIADH occurs when there is an inappropriate secretion of ADH despite normovolemia.

It occurs when there is normal renal, hepatic, cardiac, adrenal, and thyroid function. It causes plasma hyponatremia and hypo-osmolality and hyperosmolality of the urine usually with a high urine sodium concentration (>20 mEq/L) unless sodium intake is low. On physical examination, there are no signs of volume depletion or edema. It occurs commonly in central nervous system disorders (eg, IVH, encephalitis, perinatal asphyxia, meningitis) and also with lung disease (eg, respiratory distress, pneumonia, pneumothorax). SIADH is often seen in critically ill premature and term neonates and is seen in association with pain, stress, and general anesthesia. Medications associated with SIADH include opiates, carbamazepine, barbiturates, indomethacin, theophylline, NSAIDs, thiazides, and maternal oxytocin. **Reset osmostat**, a subtype of SIADH, has a subnormal threshold for ADH secretion and is a rare cause of hyponatremia.

    ii. **Nephrogenic syndrome of inappropriate antidiuresis** is very rare, is hereditary, and is caused by a gain-of-function mutation in *AVPR2*, which causes prolonged euvolemic hyponatremia. **Nephrogenic syndrome of inappropriate antidiuresis has a low vasopressin level, whereas SIADH has a high vasopressin level.**

    iii. **Endocrine related.** Severe hypothyroidism or glucocorticoid deficiency. With unexplained hyponatremia, consider hypothyroidism.

  b. **Urine sodium <20 mEq/L and low fractional excretion of sodium**

    i. **Excessive intravenous fluids, free water, or using diluted (hypotonic) formulas.** Maternal fluid overload (with glucose-only sodium-free solutions) or maternal water intoxication can cause dilutional hyponatremia. This is associated with a low urine specific gravity, low urine sodium, low fractional excretion of sodium (FE_{Na}), and high urine output.

    ii. **Inadequate sodium intake, sodium restriction.** Preterm infants have increased sodium intake requirements, and it should be provided to maintain serum sodium values and to promote adequate growth. Maintenance sodium is usually 2 to 4 mEq/kg/d. For recommended sodium intake for gestational age and postnatal age, see Table 69–1.

E. **Drug-induced hyponatremia.** Diuretics (used frequently with BPD/chronic lung disease [CLD]) can lead to sodium losses. Indomethacin causes water retention (dilutional hyponatremia). SIADH can be due to medications, as noted previously. Infusion of mannitol or hypertonic glucose can cause hyperosmolality with salt wasting. Amphotericin B can lead to sodium and potassium imbalances. Maternal medication use during pregnancy (diuretics, infusion of oxytocin and glucose, nebivolol) can cause hyponatremia in the infant.

Table 69–1. RECOMMENDED SODIUM INTAKE (mEq/KG/D) ACCORDING TO GESTATIONAL AND POSTNATAL AGES

Gestational Age	Postnatal Age in Days				
	1–2	3	7	14	30
<28 weeks	3	6–12	4–8	3–6	2–4
29–31 weeks	2	4–7	2–4	2–4	1–2
32–36 weeks	1	3–5	2–3	1–2	1–2

Reproduced with permission from Bischoff AR, Tomlinson C, Belik J: Sodium Intake Requirements for Preterm Neonates: Review and Recommendations, *J Pediatr Gastroenterol Nutr.* 2016 Dec;63(6):e123-e129.

IV. Database
  A. Review the bedside data.
    1. Check for weight loss or gain. Weight gain is more likely to be associated with dilutional hyponatremia. Weight loss is seen with hyponatremia with decreased ECF.
    2. Check fluid intake and output over a 24-hour period. Normally, infants retain two-thirds of the fluid administered, and the rest is lost in the urine or by insensible loss. If the input is much greater than the output, the patient may be retaining fluid, and dilutional hyponatremia should be considered.
    3. Assess the urine output and specific gravity. A low urine output with a high specific gravity is more commonly seen with SIADH. In excessive fluid, one sees a low urine specific gravity and a high urine output.
  B. History and physical examination. Are there maternal factors present (hypotonic IV fluids or an excessive amount of oxytocin), or was there maternal hyponatremia in the intrapartum period? The neurologic status is very important because it might guide treatment. Note any signs of seizure activity (abnormal eye movements, jerking of the extremities, and tongue thrusting). Is there a bulging fontanel or any lethargy? Check for edema, a sign of volume overload (renal failure, congestive heart failure). Decreased skin turgor and dry mucous membranes are seen in dehydration. Is the infant in shock? Does the infant have genital hyperpigmentation (congenital adrenal hyperplasia)? Is there virilization or ambiguous genitalia in a female infant or hypospadias in a male (3-β-hydroxysteroid dehydrogenase deficiency)? Specific signs and symptoms of hypovolemic hyponatremia include decreased blood pressure, depressed fontanelle, reduced capillary refill time, decreased urine output, and decreased skin turgor. Specific signs and symptoms of hypervolemic hyponatremia include edema, ascites, and pulmonary edema.
  C. Laboratory studies. See Table 69–2 for laboratory findings in specific diagnoses.
    1. Specific tests

Table 69–2. HYPONATREMIA AND LABORATORY FINDINGS IN SPECIFIC DIAGNOSES

	Urine Output	Urine Sodium/FE_{Na}	Urine Osmolality	Urine Specific Gravity
Excess fluid intake	Increased	Decreased	Decreased	Decreased
SIADH	Decreased	Increased	Increased	Increased
GI/skin/third spacing	Decreased	Decreased	Increased	Increased
Renal losses	Increased	Increased	Increased	Increased
Insufficient Na supply	Normal	Decreased	Normal	Normal
AKI prerenal	Decreased	Decreased	Increased	Increased
AKI intrinsic	Increased	Increased	Isoosmolar	Isosthenuric
Dehydration	Decreased	Decreased	Increased	Increased
CHF, hepatic failure	Decreased unless on diuretics	Decreased unless on diuretics	Increased	Increased
Hypoalbuminemia	Decreased	Decreased	Decreased	Decreased

AKI, acute kidney injury; CHF, congestive heart failure; FENa, fractional excretion of sodium; GI, gastrointestinal; IV, intravenous; NA, sodium; SIADH, syndrome of inappropriate secretion of antidiuretic hormone.

a. **Serum sodium and osmolality** to verify true hyponatremia and rule out pseudohyponatremia and hypertonic hyponatremia.

b. **Urine sodium, osmolality, and specific gravity.** A urinary sodium content is accepted by many as reflecting total body sodium deficiency, but it can be misleading since the concentration of sodium in the urine is dependent on the free water amount in the urine. There is also no consensus on normal and abnormal urinary sodium values in newborns. Urinary sodium concentrations vary from <10 to 30 mEq/L or >20 to 40 mEq/L.

   i. **Low urine sodium:** Extrarenal losses (eg, vomiting, diarrhea, ostomies, nasogastric suction, drainage tubes, ileus, necrotizing enterocolitis, pleural effusions, ascites) and edematous states (congestive heart failure, nephrotic syndrome, liver failure/cirrhosis, indomethacin therapy, water intoxication, vomiting, diarrhea, ostomies, nasogastric suction, polydipsia).

   ii. **High urine sodium:** Diuretic use, renal tubular disorders, SIADH, mineralocorticoid or glucocorticoid deficiency, AKI, chronic renal failure, hypothyroidism, Fanconi/Bartter syndrome, obstructive uropathy and metabolic alkalosis, osmotic diuresis.

   iii. **Urine osmolality,** a measure of urine concentration, and urine specific gravity, a measure of solutes in the urine, can both help in the differential of hyponatremia.

c. **Urine creatinine and plasma creatinine to calculate fractional excretion of sodium.** FE_{Na} is the percentage of sodium filtered by the kidney that is excreted in the urine and is calculated by obtaining the urine and plasma sodium and the urine and plasma creatinine. It is considered more accurate than the urinary sodium since urinary sodium concentrations can vary with water reabsorption. FE_{Na} varies inversely with gestational age and postnatal age. Higher values are used in preterm infants. Normal values vary with reference. Some commonly used values are: FE_{Na} >5% is increased or high and FE_{Na} <3% is decreased or low.

$$FE_{Na} = \frac{\text{Urinary sodium} \times \text{Plasma creatinine}}{\text{Plasma sodium} \times \text{Urinary creatinine}} \times 100$$

d. **Serum electrolytes, blood urea nitrogen, creatinine, and total protein** to assess renal function. Serum glucose to rule out hypertonic hyponatremia.

e. **Syndrome of inappropriate secretion of antidiuretic hormone.** The diagnosis is made by documenting the following on simultaneous laboratory studies: low urine output, urine osmolality greater than serum osmolality, low serum sodium level and low serum osmolality, and high urinary sodium level and high specific gravity. A plasma ADH concentration and a plasma concentration of atrial natriuretic peptide can be obtained. If they show a high ADH concentration in the presence of low serum osmolality and elevated urinary osmolality, the diagnosis is confirmed.

D. **Imaging and other studies**

1. **Ultrasound of the head or brain magnetic resonance imaging** may reveal IVH as a cause of hyponatremia secondary to SIADH.

2. **Electroencephalogram** if seizure activity is present and cannot differentiate various electrolyte disturbances. The most prominent feature is slowing of the normal background activity with hyponatremia.

3. **Electrocardiogram** if there is suspected cardiac arrhythmia. Hyponatremia causes elevated T wave with wide QRS complex.

4. **Abdominal ultrasound** if obstructive uropathy is suspected; voiding cystourethrogram may also be helpful.

V. **Plan.** Treatment is essential, and an effort should be made to keep sodium in the normal range, especially in the preterm infant, because hyponatremia can cause future problems.
   A. **Preventive therapy**
      1. **Use of isotonic fluid is recommended in children** but is controversial in newborns. This is due to the risk of hypernatremia since the immature kidneys may not handle the sodium load.
      2. **Monitor serum electrolytes in any infant** after initiation of IV fluids.
      3. **Monitor high-risk infants at risk for hyponatremia,** including the risk of SIADH, especially in very premature infants.
      4. **Make sure sodium supplementation is adequate for gestational and postnatal age.** Sodium supplementation of enteral feedings in very premature infants prevents hyponatremia and enhances weight gain. Serum sodium values should be maintained between 135 and 145 mEq/L to promote adequate growth. See Table 69–1 for recommended sodium intake according to gestational age and postnatal age (in infants who are stable, euvolemic, and not receiving sodium-altering medications).
   B. **Treatment of hyponatremia.** If infant is symptomatic and hyponatremia is severe, immediate treatment is indicated. If not symptomatic, hyponatremia should be corrected slowly over 24 to 48 hours.
      1. **Emergency treatment.** For symptomatic infants with seizures or infants with repeated apnea requiring intubation, severe neurologic symptoms (**early symptoms:** weakness, irritability, vomiting; **later symptoms:** apnea, coma, arrhythmias, hypothermia) or refractory status epilepticus as a result of low sodium (usually <120 mEq/dL), immediate hypertonic saline solution (3% sodium chloride) should be given. **Rapid corrections** (especially in chronic hyponatremia or a >8–10 mEq/L increase in serum sodium over 24 hours) can cause brain damage (**central pontine myelinolysis**). Suspect this in a neonate who, in the course of the correction, develops cranial nerve dysfunction and quadriparesis. Magnetic resonance imaging shows a round lesion in the central pontine area. **Once symptoms resolve** and the serum sodium is >120 mEq/dL, a slow correction can be given over 24 to 48 hours There is *controversy* regarding the rate and how it should be given. Follow institutional guidelines.
         a. **Intravenous bolus over 10 to 15 minutes (1–2 mL/kg of 3% sodium chloride [513 mEq sodium/L]).** This method should be reserved for only those patients with severe hyponatremia with severe symptoms such as seizures, repeated apnea episodes requiring intubation, signs of brainstem herniation, or refractory status epilepticus (*controversial*). This method (2 mL/kg bolus of 3% sodium chloride over 10 minutes) is recommended for hyponatremic encephalopathy in children. Many NICUS will calculate the deficit to a level of 125 mEq/dL and use hypertonic saline for a correction over 4 to 8 hours.
         b. **Twenty-four-hour correction.** The total body deficit can be calculated (see Section V.D.2.c), and half of that is given over 12 to 24 hours. Recommendations include not to give >8 to 10 mEq/L over the first 24 hours for acute hyponatremia and not to give >6 to 8 mEq/L over 24 hours for chronic hyponatremia.
         c. **Anticonvulsant therapy.** Use of routine anticonvulsants for hyponatremic seizures may not be effective and can be associated with severe apnea.
   C. **General management.** Always treat the underlying disorder.
      1. **Hyponatremia with hypervolemia.** Sodium and water restriction while maintaining an effective circulating volume.
      2. **Hyponatremia with hypovolemia.** Volume expansion with sodium and water to replace losses.
      3. **Hyponatremia with euvolemia.** Water restriction.
   D. **Specific management**
      1. **Volume overload (dilutional hyponatremia).** Treat with fluid restriction. The total maintenance fluids can be decreased by 20 mL/kg/d, and serum sodium

levels should be monitored every 6 to 8 hours. The underlying cause must be investigated and treated.

2. **Inadequate sodium intake.** See Table 69–1 for recommended sodium intake.
   a. **The maintenance sodium requirement for term infants is 2 to 4 mEq/kg/d and higher in premature infants.** Calculate the amount of sodium the patient is receiving using the equations in Chapter 10. Readjust the IV sodium intake if it is the cause of hyponatremia.
   b. **If the infant is receiving oral formula only, check the formula being used.** Low-sodium formulas such as Similac PM 60/40 or breast milk (which is low in sodium) may contribute to hyponatremia. Use of supplemental sodium chloride or a formula with higher sodium content may be necessary.
   c. **Calculate the total sodium deficit using the following equation.** The result will be the amount of sodium needed to correct the hyponatremia. Usually, **only half of this amount** is given over 12 to 24 hours.

$$\text{Total sodium deficit} = (\text{Desired sodium } [135 \text{ mEq/L}] - \text{Infant's sodium value}) \times (\text{Weight } [\text{kg}] \times 0.6)$$

3. **Increased sodium losses.** Treat the underlying cause and increase the sodium administered to replace the losses.
4. **Drug-induced hyponatremia.** If a renal salt-wasting medication such as **furosemide** is being given, serum sodium levels will be low even though an adequate amount of sodium is being given in the diet. An increase in sodium intake may be required, as is often the case in infants with BPD/CLD who are receiving diuretics. Most are also receiving oral feedings, so an oral sodium chloride supplement can be used. Start with 1 mEq 3 times per day with feedings and adjust as needed. Some infants may require 12 to 15 mEq/d. Sodium levels should be kept in the low 130s because higher levels may result in fluid retention when diuretics are used. **Indomethacin-induced hyponatremia** is treated with fluid restriction.
5. **Syndrome of inappropriate secretion of antidiuretic hormone. Prevention is the best management** by monitoring infants at risk for SIADH. If diagnosed, the goal is to **identify and treat the underlying cause of SIADH.** The cause of SIADH is usually obvious; if it is not, further investigation is needed (eg, ultrasonography of the head or chest radiograph to rule out lung disease). The treatment is to gradually increase the sodium level by promoting free water excretion by fluid restriction. During treatment, monitor the serum sodium, osmolality, and urine output to determine whether the patient is responding.
   a. **Seizures present or serum sodium is <120 mEq/L**
      i. **Hypertonic saline solution (3% sodium chloride) is the treatment of choice.** See Section V.B.1.a. and b.
      ii. **Fluid restriction.** Usually 40 to 60 mL/kg/d free water. There are no clear recommendations on fluid restriction. Some recommend decreasing free water by 20%.
      iii. **Furosemide (Lasix).** Administer 1 mg/kg IV every 6 hours. Loop diuretics inhibit free water absorption.
      iv. **Anticonvulsant therapy if seizing (*controversial*).** Treatment of hyponatremic seizures with anticonvulsants may be ineffective and associated with apnea.
      v. **Urea administration** increases water excretion and is associated with a decrease in urinary sodium excretion.
      vi. **Vaptans** inhibit vasopressin receptor and increase free water excretion. Tolvaptan (oral vasopressin receptor antagonist) has been used successfully in limited reports. Dose is 0.1 to 0.6 mg/kg/d; crush the tablets and mix with water.

b. **Serum sodium is >120 mEq/L without seizures.** Treat underlying cause.
   i. **Fluid restriction.** Usually 40 to 60 mL/kg/d; some recommend decreasing free water by 20%. This regimen does not allow for fluid loss that accompanies the use of a radiant warmer or phototherapy.
   ii. **Other therapies include:** Furosemide, sodium supplementation, increase solute load (fortified breast milk/formula, oral urea powder [0.1–2 g/kg/d], urea treatment for chronic SIADH).

70 Hypotension and Shock

I. **Problem.** The nurse reports that an infant is hypotensive and may be showing signs of shock. **Hypotension is defined as a decreased blood pressure.** There is no consensus on the exact definition of a normal blood pressure range or a clear accepted definition of hypotension in the term or preterm neonate. Hypotension can occur in a neonate with normal tissue perfusion or poor perfusion and overwhelming shock. Hypotension is very common in premature infants; however, the blood pressure that indicates end-organ damage in the very low birthweight (VLBW) infant is unknown.

A. **Hypotension.** Data are conflicting on the exact blood pressure that requires treatment based on gestational age, postnatal age, and infant weight. There are many definitions of hypotension:
   1. **Mean blood pressure <5th to 10th percentile of normative blood pressure** values from a reference population for the infant's gestational age, birth weight, or postnatal age (term).
   2. **Mean blood pressure that is less than the gestational age of the infant in weeks** (preterm infants during the first 3–5 days of life). For example, in a 28-week-old neonate, hypotension would be a mean blood pressure <28 mm Hg.
   3. **Mean blood pressure <30 mm Hg.**
   4. **For a rapid reference of premature and term infant blood pressure ranges, see Table 70–1 and Figure 70–1,** and for more detailed blood pressure values, see Appendix C.

B. **Shock is a clinical syndrome** of inadequate tissue perfusion that frequently accompanies hypotension. The types of shock are: **hypovolemic, cardiogenic, obstructive, distributive, and dissociative.** Some clinical scenarios may constitute many types of shock such as sepsis (distributive, hypovolemic, and cardiogenic), necrotizing enterocolitis (NEC) (hypovolemic and distributive), or pulmonary hypertension (obstructive and cardiogenic).

II. **Immediate questions**
A. **What is the method of measurement?** Blood pressure can be measured by invasive and noninvasive techniques. The invasive technique is considered the gold standard and is performed by transducing an indwelling arterial or umbilical artery catheter. A dampened waveform suggests air in the system or inappropriate position of the transducer and may result in inaccurate measurements. Because small bubbles in the system can affect the systolic and diastolic values, **the mean blood pressure is considered the most accurate measurement of systemic perfusion pressure.** The noninvasive technique most commonly performed is the oscillometric method using a blood pressure cuff on an extremity. Ensure that the cuff size is appropriate and that the cuff is applied properly to the extremity. Other noninvasive techniques include auscultation, Doppler ultrasound, and palpation, all of which are less accurate in infants.

Table 70–1. RAPID REFERENCE BLOOD PRESSURE RANGES IN PREMATURE INFANTS ACCORDING TO BODY WEIGHT AND TERM INFANTS BASED ON DAY OF LIFE (DETAILED BLOOD PRESSURE VALUES ARE FOUND IN APPENDIX C)

Birthweight (g)	Mean (mm Hg)	Systolic (mm Hg)	Diastolic (mm Hg)
Premature infants[a]			
501–750	38–49	50–62	26–36
751–1000	35.5–47.5	48–59	23–36
1001–1250	37.5–48	49–61	26–35
1251–1500	34.5–44.5	46–56	23–33
1501–1750	34.5–45.5	46–58	23–33
1751–2000	36–48	48–61	24–35
Term infants[b]			
Day 1	31–63	46–94	42–57
Day 2	37–68	46–91	27–58
Day 3	36–70	51–93	26–61
Day 4	41–65	60–88	34–57

[a]Reproduced with permission from Hegyi T, Carbone MT, Anwar M, et al: Blood pressure ranges in premature infants. I. The first hours of life, J Pediatr. 1994 Apr;124(4):627-633.
[b]Data from Kent AL, Kecskes Z, Shadbolt B, et al: Normative blood pressure data in the early neonatal period, *Pediatr Nephrol.* 2007 Sep;22(9):1335-1341.

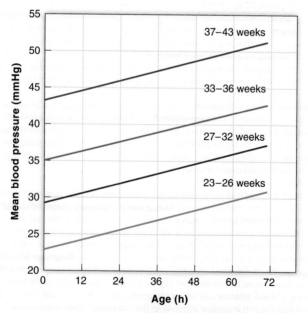

FIGURE 70–1. Currently suggested lower and upper limits for normal blood pressure in neonates. (*Reproduced with permission from Nuntnarumit P, Yang W, Bada-Ellzey HS: Blood pressure measurements in the newborn,* Clin Perinatol. *1999 Dec;26(4):981-996.*)

B. **Are signs of shock present?** Signs of shock include lethargy, poor tone, respiratory distress, tachypnea, apnea and bradycardia, tachycardia, narrow pulse pressure, weak pulses, prolonged capillary refill time (>3–4 seconds), pallor, and cold extremities (with a normal core temperature). Hypothermia is typically seen in infants with shock since they have an impaired autonomic nervous system. **Systolic hypotension** is a marker for decreased cardiac output secondary to impaired preload, contractility, and/or afterload. **Diastolic hypotension** is a marker for decreased systemic vascular resistance (SVR).

C. **Is the urine output acceptable?** Normal urine output is >1 to 2 mL/kg/h and is decreased in shock due to decreased renal perfusion. If the blood pressure is low but the urine output is adequate, aggressive treatment may not be necessary as renal perfusion is adequate (indirect measure of end-organ function). An exception would be the infant with septic shock and hyperglycemia resulting in osmotic diuresis and increased urine output.

III. **Differential diagnosis**

A. **Hypotension.** Low blood pressure can occur in term or preterm infants. It is very common in premature infants and managed differently from term infants. It can also be drug induced.

1. **Drug-induced hypotension** may cause vasodilation resulting in low blood pressure. Common types of medications include vasodilators, opiates, sedatives, and maternal antihypertensive agents. Some examples are, tubocurarine, nitroprusside, magnesium sulfate, digitalis, and barbiturates. Others include exogenous surfactant, topical timolol for infantile hemangioma, and intravitreal bevacizumab for the treatment of retinopathy of prematurity in premature infants.

2. **Extreme prematurity.** Hypotension is very common in extremely low birth-weight (ELBW) infants (60%–100% at 24–26 weeks' gestation) and VLBW infants (40% at 27–29 weeks' gestation) and is associated with an increased incidence of mortality and morbidity (specifically bronchopulmonary dysplasia, intraventricular hemorrhage [IVH]/periventricular leukomalacia, and neurodevelopmental delay). Etiology of hypotension in the immediate postnatal period is multifactorial and usually transient with improvement during the first few days of life. During this transitional period, hypotension in this group of infants is rarely secondary to hypovolemia and more likely due to due to the maladaptive transition to extrauterine circulation, immature preterm myocardium, delayed closure of the patent ductus arteriosus (PDA), adrenocortical insufficiency, poor vascular tone, immature catecholamine responses, and transient left ventricular (LV) dysfunction. After the immediate postnatal period, hypotension is usually secondary to an identifiable cause such as NEC, PDA, sepsis, or surgery.

B. **Shock**

1. **Hypovolemic shock.** Decreased intravascular volume causes decreased venous return, stroke volume, cardiac output, and tissue perfusion. It can be secondary to hemorrhagic shock (antepartum or postpartum blood loss) or nonhemorrhagic shock (fluid and electrolyte losses). The most common cause of hypovolemia in the neonate is hemorrhage. The majority of VLBW infants who are hypotensive are not hypovolemic.

a. **Antepartum/intrapartum blood loss** is often associated with asphyxia.

i. **Abruptio placentae**

ii. **Placenta previa**

iii. **Twin-twin transfusion**

iv. **Fetomaternal hemorrhage**

v. **Umbilical cord tear/prolapse/rupture**

vi. **Birth injury** (rupture of spleen or liver, adrenal hemorrhage, subgaleal hemorrhage, subdural hematoma)

    b. Postpartum blood loss
       i. Coagulation disorders (disseminated intravascular coagulation [DIC], coagulopathies)
      ii. Vitamin K deficiency bleeding
     iii. Iatrogenic (accidental dislodgement of vascular catheter)
     iv. Pulmonary hemorrhage
      v. Intracranial hemorrhage
     vi. Surgical blood loss (eg, circumcision-associated frenular artery bleed)
    vii. Tumor-associated hemorrhage (sacrococcygeal teratoma)
   viii. Massive internal bleeding (any major organ such as gastrointestinal [GI] tract)
    c. Fluid and electrolyte losses
       i. Insensible water loss
      ii. Diuretic use
     iii. Heat stress
     iv. Gastrointestinal abnormalities (vomiting, diarrhea)
      v. Polyuria (diabetes insipidus, osmotic diuresis)
     vi. Capillary leak syndrome (third space losses)

2. **Cardiogenic shock.** Myocardial dysfunction causes a decrease in cardiac output, resulting in inadequate tissue perfusion.

    a. Severe intrapartum or birth asphyxia, chronic fetal hypoxemia.

    b. Congenital heart disease with left-sided lesions (systemic outflow obstruction) is the most common condition to present with shock after the PDA closes. Examples include hypoplastic left heart syndrome, congenital aortic stenosis, coarctation of the aorta, and interruption of the aortic arch. Other congenital heart diseases can present with shock but are not as common.

    c. Congenital cardiomyopathy is rare and may present with hydrops fetalis. Other associations include inborn errors of metabolism (see Chapter 100) and infant of a diabetic mother.

    d. Patent ductus arteriosus can cause cardiac failure and hypotension due to a steal of systemic blood flow, which may cause decreased perfusion to postductal organs (intestine, kidneys). Increased left atrial pressure, pulmonary venous hypertension, and pulmonary edema/hemorrhage may occur.

    e. Cardiac dysrhythmias can cause poor cardiac output. Examples include supraventricular tachycardia, ventricular tachycardia, ventricular fibrillation, complete atrioventricular block, and atrial flutter. Complete congenital heart block can be due to Sjögren type A and B antigens in maternal Lupus and Sjögren syndrome.

    f. Myocarditis can cause cardiac failure in addition to septic shock and is usually secondary to a viral infection, most commonly coxsackievirus, in a neonate.

    g. Large arteriovenous malformation can cause shunting of blood.

    h. Congenital hypothyroidism can present with refractory cardiogenic shock (rare).

3. **Obstructive shock.** Obstruction of the great vessels of the heart can lead to decreased cardiac output and can be associated with cardiogenic shock. Causes include tension pneumothorax, cardiac tamponade, pulmonary embolism (air or thrombus), severe pulmonary hypertension, and pneumopericardium.

4. **Distributive shock.** Abnormalities within the vascular beds cause blood volume to be distributed inadequately to organs and tissues. There is no definitive volume loss, but rather inappropriate vasodilatation, dysfunction of the endothelium with capillary leak, loss of vascular tone, or a combination of these. Because the intravascular fluid volume is maldistributed, signs of shock appear.

   a. **Septic shock** is the most common cause of distributive shock and results from endotoxins released by various organisms. This can be complicated by DIC and the normal transition from fetal to neonatal circulation. With increased pulmonary vascular resistance (PVR) and the presence of a PDA, persistent pulmonary hypertension of the newborn (PPHN) results with increased right ventricular work. The incidence of hypotension in infants (any gestation) with sepsis is 38% to 69%. Neonatal herpes simplex virus infection can cause a rapid deterioration and should be considered in the setting of abnormal liver function tests and severe coagulopathy.
   b. **Neurogenic shock** is secondary to decreased sympathetic activity and lack of vascular tone, leading to vasodilation with decreased tissue perfusion. Although rare in neonates, it may occur with birth asphyxia or intracranial hemorrhage.
   c. **Anaphylactic shock** is caused by a hypersensitivity response with vasodilation, increased capillary permeability, and fluid shifts resulting in severe hypotension and circulatory collapse. Infants can become sensitized by antigens transferred through breast milk (peanuts, egg, cow's milk). Additional triggers include medications (β-lactam antibiotics, antipyretics), intravenous immune globulin, vaccinations, and natural rubber latex (bottle nipples, pacifiers).
   d. **Adrenal shock** is caused by adrenal insufficiency. The most common cause is congenital adrenal hyperplasia, whereby 21-hydroxylase deficiency accounts for the majority of cases (95%). Other causes include the nonclassical form of congenital adrenal hyperplasia, adrenal hemorrhage/infarction, and X-linked adrenal hypoplasia congenita (usually males). Clinical signs are hyponatremia, hypoglycemia, hyperkalemia, and masculinization of the external genitalia in females. Those with bilateral adrenal hemorrhage/infarction may not respond to volume resuscitation or inotropic medications.
   e. **Neonatal toxic shock syndrome** and neonatal toxic shock syndrome–like exanthematous disease are commonly caused by methicillin-resistant *Staphylococcus aureus*.
5. **Dissociative shock.** Cardiac function is preserved with intact and responsive blood vessels and adequate blood volume. However, poor perfusion results from inadequate ability to carry or release oxygen to tissues, such as in **severe anemia** (see Chapter 88) or **methemoglobinemia** (see Chapter 56).
6. **Mimics of shock in the neonate.** Some **inborn errors of metabolism** resulting in hypoglycemia or hyperammonemia can **mimic the presentation of shock** by an unexplained neonatal collapse (galactosemia, urea cycle defects, and others; see Chapter 100). Signs and symptoms of a possible inborn error of metabolism include hypoglycemia, vomiting, jaundice, seizures, hepatosplenomegaly, and cardiomyopathy. Appropriate laboratory tests should be obtained to rule out these conditions.
IV. **Database**
   A. **History**
      1. **What is the gestational age?** VLBW and ELBW infants have low cardiac output due to poor myocardial contractility and relative adrenal insufficiency.
      2. **What is the birth history?** Birth asphyxia may be associated with myocardial dysfunction and cardiogenic shock. Maternal bleeding or birth trauma may result in fetal hemorrhage and significant hypovolemia. Maternal intraamniotic infection can increase the risk for neonatal sepsis.
      3. **Is there known congenital heart disease?** Structural abnormalities or dysrhythmias can result in cardiogenic shock.
      4. **What medications are administered to the infant?** A common side effect of many drugs is hypotension.

B. **Physical examination**
   1. **Significant weight loss, sunken eyes, poor skin turgor, dry/cracked skin, immature skin, use of phototherapy or radiant warmer:** Consider insensible fluid losses (see Chapter 10).
   2. **Peripheral edema, heart murmur, hepatomegaly:** Consider cardiogenic shock
   3. **Tachycardia, poor urine output, cool extremities, skin mottling:** Consider sepsis.
   4. **Warm shock (early stage, warm extremities).** Loss of vascular tone resulting in peripheral vasodilation, capillary leak, tachycardia, increased cardiac output, bounding peripheral pulses, and hypotension (usually low diastolic blood pressure).
   5. **Cold shock (late stage, cool extremities).** Increase in vascular tone resulting in peripheral vasoconstriction, prolonged capillary refill time (>3 seconds), decreased peripheral pulses, depressed cardiac output, and hypotension (usually low systolic blood pressure or combined hypotension).
   6. **Compensated shock** maintains blood flow to vital organs.
   7. **Uncompensated shock** compromises blood flow to vital organs, resulting in tissue damage and multisystem organ failure.
   8. **Irreversible shock** results in death with irreversible damage to vital organs.
C. **Laboratory studies**
   1. **Complete blood count with differential** can assess for anemia and sepsis.
   2. **Coagulation studies (prothrombin time/partial thromboplastin time) and platelet count** if DIC is suspected.
   3. **Serum glucose, electrolytes, and calcium levels** may reveal a metabolic disorder.
   4. **Cultures** (blood, cerebrospinal fluid, urine if indicated) can assess for sepsis.
   5. **Kleihauer-Betke test** may reveal a suspected fetomaternal transfusion. The test detects the presence of fetal erythrocytes in the mother's blood by a slide elution technique. It causes adult hemoglobin to be eluted from erythrocytes, but fetal hemoglobin resists elution. After the slide is stained, fetal hemoglobin cells appear dark, whereas maternal erythrocytes appear clear. Ask the obstetrician to order this test on the mother.
   6. **Arterial blood gases** can assess for hypoxia and acidosis.
   7. **Serum lactate,** if increased, may signify anaerobic metabolism, sepsis, and poor tissue perfusion.
   8. **Serum histamine or tryptase levels** can be elevated with anaphylactic shock.
   9. **Baseline cortisol level** if considering hydrocortisone therapy.
   10. **Serum ammonia level** to rule out hyperammonemia in inborn errors of metabolism.
D. **Imaging and other studies**
   1. **Chest radiograph** can assess for a mechanical cause of shock (pneumothorax; transillumination may also be helpful), volume status (small cardiac silhouette suggests volume depletion), or cardiac disease (cardiomegaly may suggest a congenital heart defect).
   2. **Ultrasonography of the head** can identify intracranial hemorrhage.
   3. **Electrocardiogram** can assess for cardiac dysrhythmias.
   4. **Echocardiogram** can assess cardiac anatomy, cardiac output, right ventricular and LV function, and systemic and pulmonary blood flow. Decreased LV output or left ventricle underfilling may suggest hypovolemia. **Targeted neonatal echocardiography** is a shorter, more focused echocardiogram done at the bedside to assess a specific clinical problem and monitor the response to treatment.
   5. **Central venous pressure** is measured in the central veins near the heart and can be obtained via umbilical venous catheter placed at the junction of the inferior vena cava and right atrium. It approximates right atrial pressure and is an estimate of right ventricular preload. Normal values are 4 to 6 mm Hg (VLBW) and 5 to 8 mm Hg (newborn), with some sources reporting wider ranges of 2.8 to 13.9 mm Hg in VLBW infants. **Low values suggest hypovolemia, and high values suggest cardiogenic shock.**

6. **American College of Critical Care Medicine hemodynamic parameters for pediatric and neonatal septic shock**
   a. **Central venous oxygen saturation** is measured by a special catheter in the superior vena cava with goal levels >70%. **Less than 70%** is abnormal and indicative of shock.
   b. **Superior vena cava flow** can be obtained by Doppler echocardiography. **Less than 40 mL/kg/min** is abnormal and indicative of shock.
   c. **Cardiac index** measures the heart performance based on LV cardiac output in relation to body surface area. **Less than 3.3 L/min/m^2** is abnormal and indicative of shock.
7. **Near-infrared spectroscopy** provides a noninvasive measurement of venous oxygen saturation in the skin tissues to assess oxygen delivery to the brain, renal, and mesenteric regions (see Chapter 25).

V. **Plan**
A. **Follow the ABCDs** (airway, breathing, circulation, drugs). Immediately stabilize the infant's airway and respiratory status. Provide **adequate respiratory support** based on clinical exam, chest radiograph, and/or blood gas using noninvasive or invasive measures depending on the severity of respiratory failure. **Establish vascular access** and consider central venous and arterial access for invasive blood pressure monitoring and frequent blood draws. **Initiate fluid resuscitation** and **begin antibiotics** after obtaining cultures.
B. **Is treatment of hypotension necessary?** If the infant is hypotensive without clinical signs of shock and poor end-organ perfusion, aggressive treatment is usually not necessary, regardless of the blood pressure (consider permissive hypotension, especially in ELBW infants). Close observation and frequent reevaluation are important because the clinical picture may change quickly. Some clinicians recommend only treating hypotension if it is prolonged or associated with hypoxia, hypocapnia, hypercapnia, metabolic acidosis, or any condition associated with impaired cerebral autoregulation. If the infant is hypotensive with clinical signs of shock, early aggressive treatment should be considered.
C. **Immediate treatment based on etiology.** Remember to start prostaglandin infusion in the setting of shock with hepatomegaly, murmur, cyanosis, or upper/lower extremity blood pressure differential until an echocardiogram is performed to rule out ductal-dependent congenital heart disease.
   1. **Tension pneumothorax.** Use needle decompression and/or chest tube placement (see Chapter 75).
   2. **Pericardial effusion.** Manage with pericardiocentesis (see Chapter 41).
   3. **Anaphylaxis.** Remove source if possible and administer epinephrine.
   4. **Hemorrhage/anemia.** Give blood transfusion, see below.
   5. **Congenital heart disease.** Prostaglandin E$_1$ for ductal-dependent lesions.
   6. **Tachyarrhythmia.** Adenosine for supraventricular tachycardia.
   7. **Bradyarrhythmia.** Pacemaker for congenital heart block.
   8. **Critically large patent ductus arteriosus** should be considered for PDA closure.
   9. **Hypovolemia** is initially managed by fluid administration.
   10. **Sepsis** should be managed by empiric antibiotics within 1 hour.
   11. **Adrenal crisis/hypoadrenalism** treated by fluids, glucocorticoids, and mineralocorticoids.
   12. **Hypothyroidism.** Thyroid hormone replacement.
D. **Unknown etiology.** Consider empiric volume expansion with 10 mL/kg crystalloid (normal saline) given intravenously over 10 to 30 minutes.
   1. **If there is a response,** continue volume expansion to increase preload and improve cardiac output.
   2. **If there is no response or hypotension worsens,** consider cardiogenic shock and treatment with inotropic agents.

   3. **If there is no response to volume or inotropic agents,** consider treatment with glucocorticoids.
   4. **Preterm infants are known to have transient hypotension** secondary to relative adrenal insufficiency. Without a history of blood loss or evidence of hypovolemia, fluid administration is not recommended. Excess or unwarranted fluid in these infants is associated with increased mortality and morbidity (PDA, IVH, NEC, and abnormal neurodevelopment), and there is no evidence of benefit.
E. **Supportive therapy**
   1. **Correct hypothermia.**
   2. **Correct metabolic acidosis, electrolyte abnormalities** (hypoglycemia, hypocalcemia), and hormonal deficiencies (thyroid).
   3. **Correct coagulopathy and thrombocytopenia.**
   4. **Consider hydrocortisone at stress doses** if requiring >10 mcg/kg/min of vasopressors. It has been shown to hasten the weaning of vasopressors in VLBW infants.
F. **Blood replacement**
   1. **Consider transfusion** for hematocrit <35% to 40% with severe cardiopulmonary disease or hematocrit <30% with moderate cardiopulmonary disease.
   2. **Administer packed red blood cells** cautiously based on volume status of infant (5–10 mL/kg aliquots).
   3. **Consider fresh-frozen plasma, cryoprecipitate, and fibrinogen replacement** for DIC.
   4. **The following formula can be used to calculate the volume of packed red blood cells** required to achieve a desired hematocrit assuming the total blood volume is 80 mL/kg and the packed red blood cell (PRBC) hematocrit (Hct) is 70%.

$$\text{PRBC volume} = \frac{(\text{Weight [kg]} \times \text{Total blood volume}) \times (\text{Desired Hct} - \text{Patient Hct})}{\text{PRBC Hct}}$$

G. **Medications**
   1. **Commonly used medications for hypotension and shock** are listed in Table 70–2. Choose agent based on etiology and preferred effect.
VI. **Management of specific conditions**
   A. **Extreme prematurity (very low birthweight).** National Association of Neonatal Nurse Practitioners guidelines (American Academy of Pediatrics endorsed; Figure 70–2) recommend the following for hypotension in VLBW infants in the first 3 days of life:
      1. **Treat based on etiology.**
      2. **Use of volume expansion is not recommended** unless there is evidence of placenta previa, abruption, umbilical cord blood loss, fetal anemia, or fetal maternal transfusion. Treat with normal saline, lactated Ringer's, or O-/Rh-negative blood at 10 mL/kg over 5 to 10 minutes and repeat if necessary.
      3. **Dopamine alone should be used prior to dobutamine when the cause of hypotension is unknown.** In a VLBW infant with hypotension and low systemic blood flow during the first postnatal day, use dobutamine since it promotes systemic vasodilation, improves low systemic blood flow, and may increase cardiac output.
      4. **If the VLBW infant has hypotension and an infection, use dopamine** as first-line treatment and then epinephrine if it is not effective.
      5. **For VLBW infants with refractory hypotension, use hydrocortisone.** Obtain a baseline serum cortisol level. The use of hydrocortisone with indomethacin is associated with a high risk of GI perforation, and early postnatal use of dexamethasone is associated with cerebral palsy.

Table 70–2. COMMONLY USED MEDICATIONS FOR HYPOTENSION AND SHOCK

Vasopressor (Drug Class)	Dose	Receptors and Location	Effect	Clinical Use
Dopamine (adrenergic agonist)	Low: 1–5 mcg/kg/min	Dopamine (renal, mesenteric, coronary arteries)	Vasodilation in kidneys, intestines, coronary arteries ↑renal perfusion, urine output	First line for most clinical scenarios - PPHN without cardiac dysfunction - VLBW infant
	Intermediate: 5–15 mcg/kg/min	Beta (heart)	Positive inotropy Positive chronotropy ↑HR, ↑BP, renal perfusion, cardiac output	- Septic shock - Neurogenic shock - Perinatal hypoxic ischemia - **Infusion via central line is strongly advised (vesicant)**
	High: 15–20 mcg/kg/min	Alpha (vascular smooth muscle, heart) Beta (heart)	Vasoconstriction, Positive inotropy and chronotropy ↑HR, ↑BP, ↑SVR	
Dobutamine (adrenergic agonist)	2–20 mcg/kg/min	Beta (heart)	Positive inotropy Positive chronotropy Peripheral vasodilation ↑HR, ↑BP, ↑myocardial oxygen demand	- Hemodynamically significant PDA - Post-PDA ligation syndrome - Second/third line in cardiogenic shock - **Infusion via large vein**
Epinephrine (adrenergic agonist)	Low <0.3 mcg/kg/min	Beta (heart)	Positive inotropy Positive chronotropy Peripheral vasodilation ↑HR, ↑BP, ↑myocardial oxygen demand	- Anaphylactic shock - PPHN with cardiac dysfunction - Second line in septic shock - Third line in VLBW infants - **Infusion via central line is strongly advised (vesicant)**
	High >0.3 mcg/kg/min	Alpha (vascular smooth muscle, heart)	Vasoconstriction Positive inotropy ↑BP, ↑SVR, ↑PVR	

(Continued)

Table 70–2. COMMONLY USED MEDICATIONS FOR HYPOTENSION AND SHOCK (*CONTINUED*)

Vasopressor (Drug Class)	Dose	Receptors and Location	Effect	Clinical Use
Norepinephrine (adrenergic agonist)	0.02–2 mcg/kg/min	Alpha (vascular smooth muscle, heart)	Vasoconstriction Positive inotropy ↑BP, ↑SVR, ↑PVR	- Second or third line in cardiogenic shock - **Infusion via central line is strongly advised (vesicant)**
Vasopressin (antidiuretic hormone analog)	0.0001–0.0004 units/kg/min 0.17–10 milliunits/kg/min **Caution:** units of measure vary by indication and age	V1 (vascular smooth muscle) V2 (renal collecting duct system)	Vasoconstriction ↑BP, ↑SVR, ↑urine output	- PPHN without cardiac dysfunction - Hypertrophic obstructive cardiomyopathy - Rescue therapy if failed catecholamines and steroids - **Infusion via central line is strongly advised (vesicant)**
Milrinone	0.25–0.75 mcg/kg/min +/– loading dose	Phosphodiesterase 3 inhibitor (vascular smooth muscle, heart)	Positive inotropy Vasodilation Improved diastolic dysfunction ↓SVR, ↓PVR	- Post-PDA ligation syndrome - Omitting loading dose may decrease risk of hypotension
Hydrocortisone (glucocorticoid)	25 mg/m²/d divided every 6–8 hours **OR** 1 mg/kg/dose IV every 8 hours (physiologic dose) **OR** 50–100 mg/m²/d divided every 6–8 hours (stress dose)	Upregulates adrenergic receptors Treats adrenal insufficiency	↑BP, ↑urine output	- Adrenal shock - Second line in VLBW infants - Suspected or confirmed adrenal insufficiency (peak cortisol after ACTH stimulation: <18 mcg/dL or basal cortisol <4 mcg/dL or basal cortisol <18 mcg/dL with inotropic support)

ACTH, adrenocorticotropic hormone; BP, blood pressure; HR, heart rate; IV, intravenous; PPHN, persistent pulmonary hypertension of the newborn; PDA, patent ductus arteriosus; PVR, pulmonary vascular resistance; SVR, systemic vascular resistance; VLBW, very low birthweight.

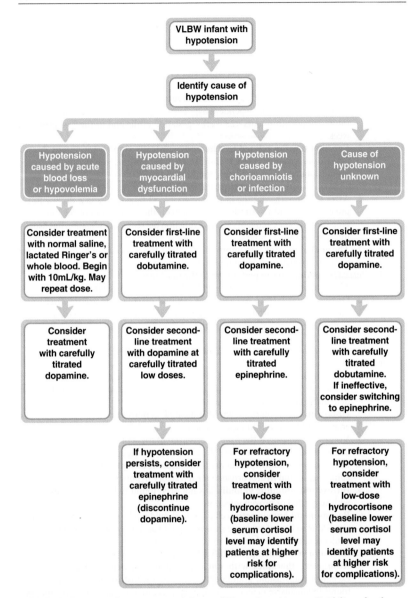

FIGURE 70–2. National Association of Neonatal Nurse Practitioners Guidelines for the treatment of transitional hypotension in very low birthweight infants (VLBW). (*Data from Vargo L, Seri I: New NANN Practice Guideline: the management of hypotension in the very-low-birth-weight infant,* Adv Neonatal Care. *2011 Aug;11(4):272-278.*)

6. **Use of milrinone in VLBW infants is not recommended** because it is not supported by evidence.

B. **Patent ductus arteriosus**

1. **Hypotension is common** due to systemic steal of blood flow to the pulmonary circulation, low diastolic pressure, and eventual systemic hypoperfusion and end-organ dysfunction.

2. **Prophylactic indomethacin (first 24 hours of birth)** to facilitate PDA closure decreases vasopressor-dependent hypotension and the need for escalating respiratory support in infants <28 weeks' gestation at the end of the first postnatal week.

3. **For hypotension related to a hemodynamically significant patent ductus arteriosus,** consider modest fluid restriction, optimal ventilation, inotropic agent (dobutamine is first line), and PDA closure.

C. **Post–patent ductus arteriosus ligation syndrome**

1. **After ligation,** the decline in pulmonary blood flow results in a decline in LV preload. SVR and LV afterload increase with the elimination of the low-resistance pulmonary circuit. Myocardial function decreases after ligation but usually improves within 24 hours.

2. **The goal of therapy** is to improve LV systolic function and reduce LV afterload with agents such as dobutamine and milrinone.

D. **Persistent pulmonary hypertension of the newborn**

1. **The goal of therapy** is to reduce PVR and improve left atrial filling.

2. **Optimal ventilation, oxygen, and inhaled nitric oxide** are the first treatments of choice, with inotropic agents, sedation, and muscle relaxation used as needed. Consider sildenafil, inhaled iloprost, and milrinone as additional therapies.

3. **ECLS** has been used in term infants with refractory PPHN.

E. **Sepsis** (see also Chapter 146)

1. **Hypotension is primarily caused by a decrease in SVR,** which increases heart rate and stroke volume. Acidosis, hypoperfusion, and high myocardial oxygen demand impair myocardial contractility.

2. **Obtain cultures (blood, urine if indicated, cerebrospinal fluid)** and initiate empiric antibiotics within the first hour.

3. **Volume expansion is the first-line treatment for septic shock** to optimize cardiac preload. If fluid-refractory shock persists, consider inotropic agents.

4. **Most common inotropic agents for treatment of septic shock** are dopamine, epinephrine, and hydrocortisone for refractory hypotension.

5. **Intravenous immune globulin** has not been found to be beneficial in infants with suspected or proven infection.

6. **Recombinant human activated protein** should not be used for severe neonatal sepsis due to lack of evidence showing benefit and increased risk of bleeding in adults resulting in withdrawal from the market.

7. **ECLS is a viable therapy for refractory septic shock** with 80% survival.

8. **Adjunctive therapies with unclear evidence of benefit.** Double-volume exchange transfusion, granulocyte/neutrophil transfusion (Cochrane review found inconclusive evidence to support or refute the use in neutropenic septic neonates), granulocyte colony-stimulating factor, pentoxifylline (Cochrane review found low-quality evidence to suggest it may decrease mortality in VLBW infants as an adjunct to antibiotics), continuous renal replacement therapy, and therapeutic plasma exchange.

9. **Term newborn septic shock algorithm.** Based on American College of Critical Care Medicine 2017 Clinical Practice Guidelines (Figure 70–3).

a. **Time-sensitive, goal-directed stepwise management of hemodynamic support** in newborns with septic shock.

b. **Proceed to next step** if shock persists.

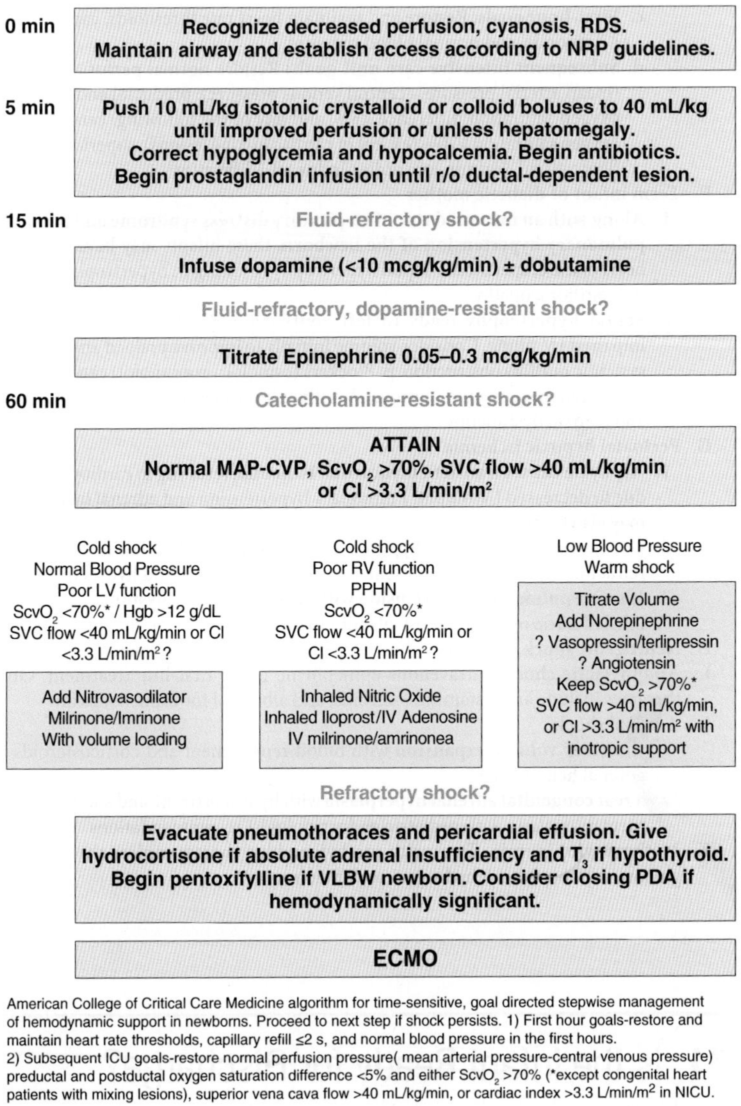

0 min — Recognize decreased perfusion, cyanosis, RDS.
Maintain airway and establish access according to NRP guidelines.

5 min — Push 10 mL/kg isotonic crystalloid or colloid boluses to 40 mL/kg until improved perfusion or unless hepatomegaly.
Correct hypoglycemia and hypocalcemia. Begin antibiotics.
Begin prostaglandin infusion until r/o ductal-dependent lesion.

15 min — Fluid-refractory shock?

Infuse dopamine (<10 mcg/kg/min) ± dobutamine

Fluid-refractory, dopamine-resistant shock?

Titrate Epinephrine 0.05–0.3 mcg/kg/min

60 min — Catecholamine-resistant shock?

ATTAIN
Normal MAP-CVP, ScvO$_2$ >70%, SVC flow >40 mL/kg/min
or CI >3.3 L/min/m^2

Cold shock	Cold shock	Low Blood Pressure
Normal Blood Pressure	Poor RV function	Warm shock
Poor LV function	PPHN	
ScvO$_2$ <70%* / Hgb >12 g/dL	ScvO$_2$ <70%*	Titrate Volume
SVC flow <40 mL/kg/min or CI <3.3 L/min/m^2?	SVC flow <40 mL/kg/min or CI <3.3 L/min/m^2?	Add Norepinephrine
		? Vasopressin/terlipressin
		? Angiotensin
Add Nitrovasodilator	Inhaled Nitric Oxide	Keep ScvO$_2$ >70%*
Milrinone/Imrinone	Inhaled Iloprost/IV Adenosine	SVC flow >40 mL/kg/min,
With volume loading	IV milrinone/amrinonea	or CI >3.3 L/min/m^2 with
		inotropic support

Refractory shock?

Evacuate pneumothoraces and pericardial effusion. Give
hydrocortisone if absolute adrenal insufficiency and T$_3$ if hypothyroid.
Begin pentoxifylline if VLBW newborn. Consider closing PDA if
hemodynamically significant.

ECMO

American College of Critical Care Medicine algorithm for time-sensitive, goal directed stepwise management of hemodynamic support in newborns. Proceed to next step if shock persists. 1) First hour goals-restore and maintain heart rate thresholds, capillary refill ≤2 s, and normal blood pressure in the first hours.
2) Subsequent ICU goals-restore normal perfusion pressure(mean arterial pressure-central venous pressure) preductal and postductal oxygen saturation difference <5% and either ScvO$_2$ >70% (*except congenital heart patients with mixing lesions), superior vena cava flow >40 mL/kg/min, or cardiac index >3.3 L/min/m^2 in NICU.

FIGURE 70–3. Term newborn septic shock algorithm based on the American College of Critical Care Medicine 2017 Clinical Practice Guidelines. CI, cardiac index; CVP, central venous pressure; ECMO, extracorporeal membrane oxygenation; IV, intravenous; LV, left ventricular; MAP, mean arterial pressure; NRP, Neonatal Resuscitation Program; PDA, patent ductus arteriosus; PPHN, persistent pulmonary hypertension of the newborn; RDS, respiratory distress syndrome; RV, right ventricular; ScvO$_2$, central venous oxygen saturation; SVC, superior vena cava; T3, triiodothyronine; VLBW, very low birthweight. (*Reproduced with permission from Davis AL, Carcillo JA, Aneja RK, et al: American College of Critical Care Medicine Clinical Practice Parameters for Hemodynamic Support of Pediatric and Neonatal Septic Shock, Crit Care Med. 2017 Jun;45(6):1061-1093.*)

    c. **First-hour goals:** Restore and maintain heart rate thresholds, capillary refill ≤2 seconds, and normal blood pressure

    d. **Subsequent intensive care unit goals:** Restore normal perfusion pressure (mean arterial pressure – central venous pressure), preductal and postductal oxygen saturation difference <5%, and any of the following: central venous oxygen saturation >70% (except in cardiac mixing lesions), superior vena cava flow >40 mL/kg/min, or cardiac index >3.3 L/min/m^2.

F. **Term infant of diabetic mother**
1. **Along with an increased risk of respiratory distress syndrome and persistent pulmonary hypertension of the newborn,** these infants may have congenital heart disease, specifically septal hypertrophy resulting in hypertrophic obstructive cardiomyopathy.
2. **Septal hypertrophy leads to left ventricular diastolic dysfunction** and impaired LV filling. Consider volume initially to improve preload and overcome systemic outflow obstruction. β-Blockers (esmolol, propranolol) can be used for chronic management to improve LV filling. Inotropes may worsen hypotension and cardiac dysfunction.

G. **Perinatal hypoxic ischemia**
1. **Asphyxia causes transient myocardial ischemia,** resulting in cardiogenic shock due to decreased LV output. Pulmonary hypertension and adrenal insufficiency may also occur.
2. **Use inotropic agents for hypotension.** First-line medication is dopamine. If refractory hypotension is present, consider epinephrine and hydrocortisone.
3. **If severe pulmonary hypertension with right ventricular dysfunction,** consider inhaled nitric oxide and prostaglandin to offload pressure on the right ventricle.

H. **Neurogenic shock.** Consider volume expansion and inotropic agents.

I. **Anaphylactic shock.** Intravenous epinephrine is the first-line treatment. Other therapies include antihistamines, steroids, and albuterol for bronchospasm.

J. **Adrenal shock**
1. **Consider volume expansion** with blood replacement and corticosteroids for adrenal hemorrhage.
2. **Treat congenital adrenal hyperplasia** with hydrocortisone and sodium supplementation along with pediatric endocrinologist recommendations.

K. **Methemoglobinemia.** Treat with methylene blue therapy unless the infant has glucose-6-phosphate dehydrogenase deficiency.

71 Is the Infant Ready for Discharge?

I. **Problem.** An infant in the newborn nursery or the neonatal intensive care unit (NICU) is ready to be discharged home. How can we ensure that discharge from the hospital is smooth, safe, and complete? **The American Academy of Pediatrics (AAP) has developed specific guidelines for discharge for the following infant types: high risk, late preterm, and healthy term.** The following section reviews the evaluation of infants prior to discharge.

II. **Immediate questions**

A. **What is the gestational age of the infant? Does the infant fit in a high-risk category?** It is important to accurately determine the gestational age of an infant to use the correct AAP guidelines. The guidelines for the late preterm infant differ from those for the healthy term infant. High-risk category guidelines are very specific for

4 subcategories: preterm infant, infant with special care needs or who is dependent on technology, infant at risk because of family issues, or infant with anticipated early death.

B. **Does the infant meet discharge criteria (infant readiness)?** The decision to discharge any infant is often a very complex decision. Careful preparation for discharge by ensuring infant readiness and other factors may decrease the incidence of readmission and reduce the risks of morbidity and mortality. These guidelines are only a framework for guiding decisions, as the final decision should be **individualized for each infant**. Historically, preterm infants were only discharged when they achieved a specific weight; now preterm infants are discharged based on physiologic criteria and not weight. In fact, the first, most important factor in deciding on discharge is infant readiness. Other considerations include family, community, and healthcare provider readiness; risk factors of the mother and infant; and safety concerns, among others.

1. **Are the vital signs stable?** Most discharge criteria require vital signs be documented within normal reference ranges for the infant for 12 hours preceding discharge. For late preterm and term infants, this includes a respiratory rate <60 breaths/min, a heart rate of 100 to 160 beats/min, and an axillary temperature of 36.5°C to 37.4°C in an open crib. For high-risk neonates, criteria include physiologic mature and stable cardiorespiratory function and adequate maintenance of normal body temperature in an open bed with normal ambient temperature. Most preterm infants are able to maintain normal body temperature at home between 36 and 37 weeks of postmenstrual age (PMA) but lag in achieving maturation of respiratory control, sometimes until up to 44 weeks of PMA.

2. **Have there been any recent episodes of apnea and bradycardia?** Episodes of apnea of prematurity along with associated bradycardia and desaturation typically resolve at approximately postconception age of 34 to 36 weeks, although infants born less than 28 weeks gestation may have prolonged apnea beyond term. If such episodes persist at 36 weeks of age, the infants may not yet be safe for discharge. Many NICUs will wait for an event-free period of time (typically 5–7 days) before considering these infants ready for discharge home. If events persist beyond term (42–44 weeks), some institutions will send infants home on varying combinations of cardiopulmonary event monitoring, respiratory stimulants (eg, theophylline or caffeine), and supplemental oxygen. In this situation, infant cardiopulmonary resuscitation training and monitor and oxygen use training are arranged for the parents. Complete caregiver understanding of the prescribed outpatient therapies must be verified before discharge. **It is important to note that the use of a home monitor** does not negate the fact that the infant still needs to show maturity of respiratory control prior to discharge. Home monitors do not prevent sudden infant death syndrome and should not be used to justify discharge of an infant with apnea or at risk of apnea.

3. **Is the infant feeding satisfactorily?** The ability of the infant to breast or bottle feed satisfactorily without cardiorespiratory compromise (ie, to be able to coordinate sucking and swallowing and breathing while taking in an adequate number of calories [120 kcal/kg/d] in reasonable frequency [every 3–4 hours], with each feed not taking >30–40 minutes) is of major importance. By 36 to 37 weeks of PMA, most preterm infants are able to feed satisfactorily. Gavage feeding and gastrostomy tube are alternative feeding practices that are used in infants who are not able to feed by breast or bottle. In addition, many premature infants require fortification of their milk to provide adequate nutrition even after discharge from the NICU. When preparing for the transition home, consideration must be given to the type and caloric content of the fortification that will continue after discharge.

4. **Is the infant showing consistent and sufficient weight gain (especially for the preterm, late preterm, and high-risk infants)?** At discharge, the infant should

be gaining weight steadily on breast or bottle feeds. Most healthy preterm or term infants with no ongoing problems show an average weight gain of 15 to 30 g/d. Sustained weight gain is more important than specific weight criteria for discharge.

5. **Has the late preterm and term infant passed 1 stool spontaneously and urinated regularly?** Delayed stooling and urination can indicate a serious medical problem (see Chapters 72 and 73).

6. **Is there any active bleeding from the circumcision site?** Make sure there has been no active bleeding for a minimum of 2 hours prior to discharge.

C. **Is the family ready for the infant's discharge?** The housing environment, caregiver comfort level, and access to community resources all play an important part in the successful transition to home.

1. **Has the family received discharge training?** Before discharge home, at least 2 family caregivers for the high-risk neonate and the mother and any other caregivers for the preterm and term infant should have received training in feeding, basic infant care (eg, bathing, skin cord and genital care, proper temperature measurement, comforting), and techniques to identify signs and symptoms of an acute illness; review of infant safety guidelines (eg, sleep safety, smoke-free environment, car seat use) is also needed.

2. **Are there medications that need to be continued after discharge?** Infants discharged on medications usually have the first prescription filled before discharge. Before the infant leaves the hospital, the caregivers should be trained in safely administering the medications. Caregivers are briefed on the duration of administration, importance of the medication, and probable duration of treatment, as well as side effects and risks of discontinuing too soon.

3. **Are any special feeding techniques necessary?** If clinical grounds indicate the need for a prolonged tube feeding or gastrostomy tube feeding, caregivers must be trained to carry out the feedings at home. Training on the specific method of feeding with the actual equipment the caregivers will be using at home is essential for safe discharge.

4. **Will the infant be discharged with technologic support?** If infants have bronchopulmonary dysplasia/chronic lung disease (BPD/CLD), a history of bradycardia, or other complications associated with prematurity, they may be sent home with a monitoring device, home oxygen, or both. Caregivers must have completed training on the specific devices they will be using in the home, and proper use of the devices should be verified before discharge. Rarely, infants will be discharged with more complex technologic support (eg, ventilators). The home environment must be safe for and supportive of all levels of support. If necessary, a home environmental assessment can be done to ensure appropriateness before discharge.

5. **Have the caregivers received training in cardiopulmonary resuscitation?** All caregivers should be aware of the procedures for emergency intervention. Parents of high-risk infants being discharged from the NICU should have infant cardiopulmonary resuscitation reviewed with them before discharge.

6. **Are there any risk factors in the family that require social services or child protective services to be involved?** These include mental illness in a parent at home, history of child abuse, neglect, untreated parenteral substance abuse or positive urine drug testing in the mother or infant, lack of social support for the mother, history of domestic violence, adolescent mother, mother who lives in a shelter or on the street, or person with a communicable disease living in the home. Discharge should be delayed until risk factors are resolved or a plan is in place for the infant to be safe.

D. **Is the community ready for the infant's discharge?** Identification of key local providers and support systems for both the infant and family is necessary before discharge of any infant but especially for the high-risk neonate.

1. **Has a primary care provider been identified and contacted?** Information on the name, location, and appointment time for the follow-up physician should be available at the time of discharge. In any given case, the specialty physician should personally contact the primary care physician by telephone to discuss the patient or to make arrangements for a preliminary discharge summary to be faxed to the primary physician. Most infants should be seen within 48 hours of discharge from the NICU.

2. **Will specialists be involved in outpatient care?** Caregivers should be made aware of all the clinical conditions that require outpatient follow-up as well as be given specific names and contact information for making follow-up appointments. In many cases, the inpatient team may be more successful at arranging follow-up than the caregivers, and every attempt should be made to solidify appointments before discharge. It is imperative that caregivers understand the importance of follow-up with subspecialists (eg, ophthalmologists, pediatric surgeons, pediatric cardiologists).

3. **Is the infant at high risk for neurodevelopmental disability?** High-risk NICU infants need comprehensive neurodevelopmental evaluations and appropriate intervention services. The initial examination and evaluation for developmental assessment are done in the NICU before discharge to assess the need for early interventional services. Early intervention is extremely important to beneficial long-term outcome in infants at highest risk for disability. There is a growing body of evidence suggesting that early detection can take advantage of periods of the most active neuroplasticity after brain injury. Many states have early intervention programs that are available to NICU graduates at high risk. These resources should be accessed before discharge in preparation for outpatient follow-up. Appointments at a neonatal follow-up clinic for monitoring growth and development, with input from a dietitian, social worker, physiotherapist, occupational therapist, and developmentalist, are mandatory for very-high-risk infants.

4. **Is the infant a candidate for in-home health visits?** At the request of the physician, follow-up house visits by a home health nurse to check clinical status, to repeat tests, and to ensure weight gain should be arranged for finite periods, depending on the needs of the individual infant and family. If the infant has an **anticipated early death**, has hospice care been notified and bereavement support been given?

5. **Have all screening tests, laboratory evaluations, radiologic evaluations, and appropriate immunizations been completed?**
   a. **Is the audiology screening complete?** An initial newborn hearing screen (either otoacoustic emissions [OAE] assessment, measuring the sound waves in the inner ear, or auditory brainstem response [ABR] assessment, measuring how the brain responds to sound) is recommended for all infants before discharge and no later than 1 month of age. Note that if OAE testing is done, it does not pick up neural dysfunction (eighth nerve or auditory brainstem pathway). All infants who do not pass the screen and subsequent rescreening need to have a medical evaluation including an audiologic evaluation no later than 3 months of age. The birth hospital and the state early hearing detection and intervention coordinator are responsible to convey the hearing screening results to the parents and medical home. Results are recorded in the patient's record and the discharge summary and are also mailed to each state's Newborn Hearing Screening Program. **ABR assessment** is essential in other clinical conditions in which there is an increased risk for hearing loss and for which progressive losses are possible. **Risk factors for hearing loss** include family history of permanent childhood hearing loss, in utero TORCHZ (toxoplasmosis, other infections, rubella virus, cytomegalovirus [CMV], herpes simplex virus, and Zika virus infection), ear

and craniofacial anomalies, hyperbilirubinemia requiring exchange transfusion, persistent pulmonary hypertension with mechanical ventilation, NICU stay >5 days, extracorporeal membrane oxygenation (ECMO), birthweight <1500 g, bacterial meningitis, low Apgar score of 0 to 3 at 5 minutes or 0 to 6 at 10 minutes, respiratory distress (meconium aspiration), assisted ventilation, exposure to ototoxic medication (gentamycin and tobramycin) or loop diuretics (furosemide), and physical features of a syndrome that includes hearing loss. Separate protocols exist for NICU and well infants.

   i. **Screening in the well infant nursery** includes 1 hearing screening using either OAE or ABR; if the infant does not pass, a repeat screening is done prior to discharge. If an infant passes the ABR, then no follow-up screen is required, but the pediatrician should follow-up with ongoing care which includes identifying and referring infants with risk indicators for late-onset hearing loss. If the infant fails the OAE screening but passes the ABR testing, the infant is considered a "screening pass." Infants who fail the ABR testing should not be rescreened using the OAE but need to be reevaluated within 1 month of discharge. Infants who did not receive screening in the hospital should have an outpatient screening no later than 1 month of age.

  ii. **Screening in the neonatal intensive care unit.** All infants need to be screened in the NICU, but infants admitted for >5 days require an ABR (not OAE) for screening to make sure neural hearing loss is not missed. If the infant does not pass, an audiologist needs to do the rescreening and, if indicated, a comprehensive evaluation with diagnostic ABR. The timing and number of hearing evaluations for infants with risk factors should be customized.

 iii. **Infant with risk factor indicators for hearing loss.** If the infant passes the hearing screen but is at high risk for hearing loss (1 or more of the high-risk indicators listed earlier), rescreening should be done by 3 months of age, and the infant should have at least 1 diagnostic audiology assessment by 24 to 30 months of age. **Perform early and more frequent assessment** in infants with CMV, infants who have a family history of permanent hearing loss or neurodegenerative disorders or trauma, infants who have received ECMO or chemotherapy, any infant with a syndrome associated with progressive hearing loss, and infants whose caregiver is concerned about the hearing. If an infant passes the ABR, then no follow-up screen is required, but the pediatrician should follow-up per standard practice. However, if the infant passes the hearing screen but is at high risk for hearing loss, rescreening should be done within 3 months. If the infant fails the ABR, rescreening should occur within 2 weeks.

b. **Is the newborn metabolic screen completed? If so, is it valid, or is a repeat test needed?** (See Chapter 16.) The content of the newborn metabolic screen varies among states. All initial newborn screens should be done per state protocol but essentially at 48 hours after birth and preferably after 24 hours of protein feeding. **Many screening tests are affected by** timing of the sample, diet, and whether the infant is preterm, had a transfusion, or is on total parenteral nutrition. Proper follow-up is essential for abnormal results. **Maple syrup urine disease, congenital adrenal hyperplasia, and galactosemia are 3 disorders that need to be treated since they can be fatal.** Any borderline values or abnormal initial metabolic screen results are repeated with more definitive diagnostic tests. It is important to remember that normal results do not totally rule out the presence of these diseases, because there can be false-positive results and some of these conditions have variants that present later on.

   c. **Has the mandatory pulse oximetry screening for critical congenital heart disease been done?** Routine screening is now recommended for all newborns after 24 hours of age but before discharge from the hospital to screen for low blood oxygen to detect critical cyanotic heart disease. Even though most infants will have had pulse oximetry as part of their management while in the NICU, routine care does not typically involve simultaneous measurement of both pre- and postductal saturations. For infants who have not had echocardiograms that rule out cyanotic heart lesions, critical congenital heart defect screening should be performed once they have been weaned from supplemental oxygen. If on oxygen, an echocardiogram is recommended. Some states mandate all infants have screening whether or not an echocardiogram has been performed. An infant passes the screening test if the oxygen saturation is ≥95% in the right hand and foot and the difference is ≤3 percentage points between the right hand and foot. See pulse oximetry screening recommendations in Chapter 7.

   d. **Have the infant's hips been screened for developmental dysplasia?** The AAP, Pediatric Orthopaedic Society of North America, American Academy of Orthopaedic Surgeons, and Canadian Developmental Dysplasia of the Hip (DDH) Task Force recommend the following: "All newborns should have a physical examination and periodic surveillance physical examination screening for DDH." This should include looking for limb length discrepancy and asymmetric thigh or buttock (gluteal) creases, performing the Ortolani test for stability, and testing for limited/asymmetric abduction. Routine ultrasound is usually not recommended but may be recommended for certain infants (those age 6 weeks to 6 months and at high risk [breech presentation at third trimester, positive family history, parenteral concern, history of previous clinical instability, history of improper swaddling, suspicious/inconclusive physical examination] with normal positive physical findings). Surveillance and periodic physical examinations by the primary care physician on subsequent visits are recommended until walking age. See Chapters 7 and 112 for further discussion on hip testing.

   e. **Does the infant require a car seat tolerance screening evaluation?** Preterm infants are at risk of adverse cardiorespiratory effects (oxygen desaturation, apnea, and bradycardia) when placed in a semi-upright position as when using a semi-reclined car safety seat. Specific recommendations per the AAP for transport of preterm and low birthweight infants at risk of apnea and bradycardia or oxygen desaturation are as follows:

      i. **Perform a car seat tolerance screening** (car seat test/infant car seat challenge) in all preterm infants (born <37 weeks of gestational age) to decide if physiologic maturity and stable cardiorespiratory function are present. This entails that the infant be placed in the infant's own personal car seat for a period of observation by trained hospital staff for 90 to 120 minutes or the duration of the car ride home, whichever is longer. Specific failure criteria were not provided by the AAP but include apnea (>20 seconds), bradycardia (heart rate < 80 beats/min), and oxygen desaturation (any desaturation <80% or ≥2 episodes of oxygen desaturation <88% for >10 seconds). If the infant fails or the events documented are significant, the following are recommended: use of car bed, supplemental oxygen, further medical assessment, or continued hospitalization. Travel in a Federal Motor Vehicle Safety Standard 213–approved car bed with the infant supine or prone is recommended for infants with documented oxygen desaturation, apnea, or bradycardia. **Other infants commonly tested using car seat tolerance screening** (AAP has no specific recommendations) include infants <2500 g, infants with hypotonia (Down syndrome/congenital neuromuscular disorders) or micrognathia (Pierre Robin sequence), or infants with congenital heart disease or who have undergone congenital heart surgery. **Low birthweight term infants** have a similar incidence of failure as preterm infants, with an association between maternal opiate use and increased risk of failure. It is ultimately up to each institution to decide which infants should be screened besides the AAP-recommended group.

(a) **Teach the family how to position the infant properly** in the car safety seat and to minimize the time in the seat. Only use the car safety seat for travel.

(b) **The American Academy of Pediatrics recommends that all infants ride rear facing until they are at least 2 years old** or have outgrown the height or weight allowed by the manufacturer of the car seat, at which point they need to continue to ride rear facing in a convertible or 3-in-1 seat. Infants in rear-facing seats are safer because these seats support the head, neck, and spine much better due to better distribution of the force of the collision.

(c) **Use infant-only car safety seats with 3- or 5-point harness systems** or convertible car safety seats with 5-point harness systems. Do not use a shield, abdominal pad, or arm rest for a small infant.

(d) **Choose a car safety seat with the shortest distance from the crotch strap to the seat back,** with a small cloth between the crotch strap and infant and blanket rolls on both sides of the infant. The car safety seat should be reclined approximately 45 degrees and always be placed in the back seat.

(e) **If the infant needs a home cardiac and apnea monitor,** this needs to be used during travel and should be carefully wedged on the floor or under a seat. It is advantageous to have an adult sit in the back with the infant.

(f) **Parents need to bring the car seat before discharge** for training on seating the infant, proper positioning, and support.

f. **Have all the required laboratory studies been completed and documented, if indicated?**

   i. **Hematocrit and reticulocyte count (preterm and high-risk neonates).** Anemia of prematurity and the physiologic nadir of the red cell line may combine to cause the hematocrit to be low at the time of discharge. Other diagnoses that can lead to poor red blood cell production must also be noted and potentially treated prior to consideration for discharge. A recent complete blood count and reticulocyte count should be documented prior to discharge. Each institution should have a guideline as to what is considered safe for discharge home.

   ii. **Serum calcium, phosphorus, and alkaline phosphatase.** Extremely premature infants and low birthweight infants are at risk for osteopenia of prematurity and must have these parameters checked during inpatient stay and prior to discharge. The AAP recommends that all breast-fed, mixed-fed, and formula-fed infants who consume <1000 mL of formula should be supplemented with oral vitamin D (minimum of 400 IU of vitamin D per day).

   iii. **Drug levels.** Infants being discharged home on medications such as phenobarbital or theophylline should have levels tested before discharge, and the results should be recorded with dose adjustment as necessary.

g. **Have all the required radiologic studies been completed and documented if indicated?**

    i. **Chest radiograph.** A copy of the most recent radiograph should be sent with the parents to the primary physician for follow-up care of chronic lung disease (eg, BPD/CLD).

    ii. **Head ultrasound scan.** Routine screening head ultrasound is recommended for all infants born <32 weeks' gestation. It is recommended to obtain an ultrasound at 2 weeks of life (diagnose hemorrhagic lesions) and at 6 weeks of life (detect cystic lesions/ventriculomegaly). Very low birthweight infants with multiple complications may require a diagnostic cranial ultrasound by the third day of life. Infants who have hemorrhagic lesions, cystic lesions, or any white matter lesions need close follow-up after NICU discharge. Clearly record the findings of the scans in chronologic order, with emphasis on hemorrhage, ventricular size, and areas of echogenicity suggestive of periventricular leukomalacia and porencephalic cysts.

    iii. **Computed tomography or magnetic resonance imaging.** If performed to evaluate any area in the infant's body, comment on the findings and interpretation.

  h. **Are any immunizations due before discharge?** Immunization recommendations are listed in Appendix E. Preterm infants should be immunized at the normal chronologic age with the same vaccine doses as term infants. (*Note:* Birthweight does not matter.) Infants still hospitalized when due for vaccinations should receive them during their stay if they are clinically stable and per individual NICU policy. **Any medically stable preterm infant who is still in the hospital at 2 months of age** should receive all the inactivated vaccines appropriate for the age. There are 2 immunizations that need to be either given or considered prior to discharge:

    i. **Hepatitis B.** All newborns should be vaccinated against hepatitis B before discharge from the hospital.

      (a) **Mother is hepatitis B surface antigen negative:** If infant is ≥2000 g, give 1 dose of hepatitis B vaccine to medically stable infants within 24 hours of birth. If infant is <2000 g, give one dose of hepatitis B vaccine at 1 month of age or at discharge.

      (b) **Mother is hepatitis B surface antigen positive:** Give hepatitis B vaccine and 0.5 mL of hepatitis B immune globulin (HBIG) (2 separate sites) within 12 hours of birth to the infant of any weight.

      (c) **Mother's hepatitis B surface antigen status is unknown:** If infant is ≥2000 g, give hepatitis B vaccine within 12 hours of birth to the infant. Determine mother's hepatitis B surface antigen status as soon as possible. **If positive,** give 0.5 mL of HBIG within 7 days of birth, or **if unknown,** give HBIG by 7 days of life or at hospital discharge. In infants <2000 g, give hepatitis B vaccine and 0.5 mL of HBIG within 12 hours of birth.

    ii. **Preterm or term infants at risk for respiratory syncytial virus** (RSV) should have palivizumab administered before discharge and monthly during RSV season. If the infant meets criteria for monthly palivizumab prophylaxis vaccine during the first or second year of life, then this information must be communicated with the primary care physician. Eligibility requirements include the following:

      (a) **Preterm infants with chronic lung disease of prematurity** (definition: gestational age <32 weeks 0 days; requirement of oxygen >21% for at least the first 28 days after birth).

      (b) **Infants with congenital heart disease and acyanotic heart disease** who are on medication to control congestive heart failure or who require cardiac surgical procedures and infants with moderate to severe pulmonary hypertension.

   (c) **Infants with cyanotic heart disease in the first year of life.** Consultation with pediatric cardiologist is recommended.

   (d) **Preterm infants without chronic lung disease or congenital heart disease.** Consider prophylaxis if born <29 weeks 0 days' gestation and <12 months of age. If >29 weeks 0 days' gestation, infants do not need prophylaxis unless they have congenital heart disease, CLD, or another condition.

   (e) **Infants with neuromuscular disease/congenital anomaly** who are at risk of a lower respiratory tract infection or prolonged hospitalization because of the inability to clear secretions from the upper airway. Consider prophylaxis during the first year of life.

  i. **Are there other studies that need to be completed or documented?**

   i. **Electroencephalogram.** Record the results, if done more than once, in chronologic order, indicating assessment of cerebral function in infants with seizures.

   ii. **Electrocardiogram.** Documentation is useful in cases of congenital heart defect, supraventricular tachycardia, or metabolic problems.

   iii. **Echocardiogram.** Useful to note results in case of persistent murmurs or the need for follow-up.

   iv. **Other tests.** Record the findings and recommendations of any other tests.

6. Discharge plan special considerations

 a. **Ophthalmologic examination.** An eye examination for evaluation of retinopathy of prematurity (ROP) is recommended for all infants of gestational age <30 weeks or ≤1500 g and selected infants with a birthweight between 1500 and 2000 g or gestational age >30 weeks with an unstable clinical course (requiring cardiorespiratory support with high risk of ROP); these infants should have dilated eye examinations starting at 4 to 6 weeks of age or 31 to 33 weeks of PMA. Examinations should continue every 2 to 3 weeks until retinal vascular maturity is reached and no disease is present. Infants with ROP or very immature vessels should be examined every 1 to 2 weeks until vessels are mature or the risk of disease is passed. Infants with the greatest risk should be examined every week. Parents need to be told the importance of follow-up examinations and the possible consequences of serious ROP. The examination schedule is initially determined by the neonatologist based on the AAP policy statement from the Section on Ophthalmology, and then follow-up examinations are usually scheduled by the examining ophthalmologist based on retinal findings. Follow-up recommendations are:

1-week or less follow-up:
Zone 1: immature vascularization, no ROP
Zone 1: stage 1 or stage 2 ROP;
Immature retina extending into posterior zone II, near the boundary of zone I-zone II;
Suspected presence of AP-ROP;
Stage 3 ROP, zone I requires treatment, not observation.

1- to 2-week follow-up:
Posterior zone II: immature vascularization
Zone II: stage 2 ROP
Zone I: unequivocally regressing ROP

2-week follow-up:
Zone II: stage 1 ROP
Zone II: no ROP, immature vascularization
Zone II: unequivocally regressing ROP

2- to 3-week follow-up:
Zone III: stage 1 or 2 ROP
Zone III: regressing ROP

    b. **Bilirubin assessment in infants >35 weeks' gestation**
      i. **Before discharge, every infant should be assessed for the risk of developing severe hyperbilirubinemia.** The AAP recommends doing a predischarge bilirubin using total serum bilirubin (TSB) or transcutaneous bilirubin and/or a clinical assessment of risk factors. New studies suggest that combining a predischarge measurement with clinical risk factors may improve the prediction of which infants will develop hyperbilirubinemia. Use the predischarge TSB and plot the results on the nomogram (see Figure 63–2) to assess the risk of subsequent hyperbilirubinemia. Once you have the predischarge bilirubin and assigned bilirubin risk zone, use the figure to help guide when the follow-up visit should be and when a repeat bilirubin needs to be done.

    c. **Male circumcision.** The AAP states that "the health benefits of newborn male circumcision outweigh the risks, but not enough to recommend universal newborn circumcision." The decision is up to the parents and can be performed at parental request and with their written consent before discharge. The procedure is elective, requires analgesia, and should not be done on any unstable infants or infants with serious medical conditions (ongoing apnea and bradycardia, infants with BPD/CLD on oxygen). Any infant with any penile edema or anomalies of the penis (eg, hypospadias with foreskin abnormalities, micropenis, torsion of the penis, webbed penis, chordee of the penis, any disorder of sexual development where reconstruction may be needed at a later date) should not be circumcised and be referred to a specialist. Premature infants should not have circumcision until they are healthy and being discharged. Older infants require formal anesthesia and analgesia.

III. **Discharge summary information**
  A. **Discharge diagnoses.** A concise list of all the diagnoses for a patient, listed in chronologic order of occurrence, including procedures, should be generated.
  B. **Database.** Review the initial history, NICU or newborn nursery hospital course, and physical examination at discharge. Compose an organized discharge summary by systems or by problems.
    1. **History.** Inclusive of maternal–fetal conditions (including prenatal diagnostic tests and medications), labor and delivery information, birth history (Apgar scores, head circumference, length, and weight), and neonatal history in the NICU or newborn nursery.
    2. **Physical examination.** List any significant abnormal findings noted at birth. Perform a complete physical examination, paying careful attention to note any significant changes or findings. See Chapter 7 for details on the newborn physical examination. List infant's condition at discharge with the discharge diagnoses listed.
    3. **Other important information.** Written feeding plan with specific breast-feeding or formula instructions, any medications at discharge, any medical equipment, follow-up appointments (eg, ophthalmology, orthopedics, audiology), car seat tolerance screening results, pulse oximetry results, newborn metabolic screening tests and dates when done, immunizations given, any pertinent lab results (hematocrit, bilirubin), any follow-up instructions for the first visit to healthcare provider.

IV. **Plan.** (Specific AAP guidelines for discharge of high-risk, late-preterm, and healthy term infants.)
  A. **American Academy of Pediatrics guidelines for high-risk infant discharge.** (Committee on Fetus and Newborn. Hospital discharge of the high-risk neonate. *Pediatrics.* 2008; 122[5]:1119-1126.) The decision to discharge a high-risk infant is dependent upon many factors: infant readiness, family and home readiness, and community and healthcare system. The AAP has also classified high-risk infants into 4 specific groups (the preterm infant, the infant with special healthcare needs or dependence on technology, the infant at risk because of family issues, and the infant with an

anticipated early death), and each group has additional minimal discharge guidelines that need to be followed.

1. **Infant readiness**
   a. **Demonstrate a pattern of weight gain** over a sufficient duration of time.
   b. **Make sure the infant can maintain normal body temperature** fully clothed in an open bed with normal ambient temperature (20–25°C).
   c. **Make sure the infant can feed by bottle or breast** without cardiorespiratory compromise.
   d. **Document for a sufficient duration a physiologically mature and stable cardiorespiratory function.**
   e. **Give appropriate immunizations.**
   f. **Perform metabolic screening.**
   g. **Assess hematologic status and give any appropriate therapy.**
   h. **Assess nutritional risks and institute any dietary changes.**
   i. **Perform hearing evaluation.**
   j. **Perform funduscopic examinations.**
   k. **Assess and demonstrate neurodevelopmental and neurobehavioral status.**
   l. **Perform car seat evaluation.**
   m. **Review hospital course,** identify any medical problems, and plan follow-up.
   n. **Plan an individualized home care plan,** with all necessary specialties.

2. **Family and home environmental readiness**
   a. **Identify at a minimum 2 caregivers** and assess their ability, commitment, and availability.
   b. **Do a psychosocial assessment of parenting strengths and risks.**
   c. **Do a home environmental assessment,** with on-site evaluation possibly included.
   d. **Review available financial resources.**
   e. **Document 24-hour telephone access, electricity, safe in-house water, and adequate heating in the home.**
   f. **Document parents'/caregivers' capability for feeding** including formula preparation.
   g. **Document basic infant care,** including comforting, bathing, skin and genital care, measuring temperature of the infant, and dressing.
   h. **Understand early signs and symptoms of illness** or any signs and symptoms that are specific to the condition of the infant.
   i. **Understand any specific precautions** for the artificial airway, feeding tube, intestinal stoma, infusion pump, or other devices needed, if indicated.
   j. **Understand giving medications,** including storing, dosage, timing, how to give medications, and recognition of signs of toxicity
   k. **Understand, if indicated, the operation, maintenance, and problem solving for any support equipment** the infant needs.
   l. **Go over the appropriate technique for any special care that the infant requires,** including maintenance of an artificial airway, physical therapy needs, oropharyngeal/tracheal suctioning, special dressing care for intestinal stoma, healing wounds, or infusion entry site.

3. **Community and healthcare readiness**
   a. **Identify and notify emergency medical service providers if indicated.** Make sure that an emergency intervention and transportation plan is in place.
   b. **Identify a primary care physician** who will take responsibility for the care of the infant.
   c. **Identify any surgical and/or pediatric medical specialties for follow-up care,** and make sure appointments have been made.
   d. **Identify neurodevelopmental referrals for follow-up,** and make sure appointments have been made.

e. **Arrange home nursing visits,** and verify home care plan with the home health agency.

f. **Give breast-feeding mothers information on breast-feeding support,** and give a list of lactation counselors who are available for questions.

4. **Special situations (eg, preterm infant or infant with special care needs or health dependent on technology, risk of family issues, or anticipated early death)** require certain considerations beyond the normal high-risk infant discharge factors.

a. **Preterm infants should be discharged based on physiologic criteria,** not body weight.

i. **Physiologic stability (most achieved at 36–37 weeks of postmenstrual age).** Oral feedings sufficient to support appropriate growth, ability to maintain body temperature at home, and sufficient mature respiratory control (may take up to 44 weeks of PMA). A home monitor should not be used to discharge infants who are at risk of apnea and should not stop the evaluation of mature respiratory control. Supine sleeping is recommended.

ii. **Arrange for healthcare after discharge with a healthcare provider experienced in high-risk infant care.**

iii. **Develop an active program of parental involvement, preparation for care of infant at home, and an organized program to track, and monitor growth and development.**

b. **Infant with special care needs or whose health is dependent on technology** (most commonly nutritional or respiratory needs)

i. **Nutritional support.** Gavage feeding, gastrostomy tube, parenteral nutrition.

ii. **Respiratory support.** Home oxygen therapy, cardiorespiratory monitor/pulse oximetry, tracheostomy care, home ventilator.

c. **Infant at risk because of family issues.** Risk factors for subsequent child abuse and dysfunction in the family include preterm birth, prolonged hospitalization, disabling conditions, and birth defects. Maternal factors include lower education level, unstable marriage, fewer prenatal care visits, lack of social support, fewer family visits, and parenteral substance abuse/drug-seeking behaviors of parents.

i. **Take a multidisciplinary team approach.**

ii. **Identify infants who require extra support or whose home environment is at risk.**

iii. **Plan follow-up monitoring and home visits.**

d. **Infant with anticipated early death (incurable terminal disorders).** Many of these infants will spend their last weeks of life at home cared for by the family with support of hospice care. Withdrawal of assisted ventilation can occur at home in some rare instances. The goal should be to enhance the remaining quality of life for the infant and the family. These additional aspects need to be addressed before discharge for home hospice care:

i. **Medical follow-up arrangements**

ii. **Home nursing visits**

iii. **Pain management and management of any distressing symptoms**

iv. **Arrangement of home oxygen and other equipment/supplies**

v. **Bereavement support information for the family/siblings/other**

vi. **Resources for respite care to caregivers**

vii. **Financial assistance**

viii. **If appropriate, a letter should be given to the family stating that the infant should not be resuscitated.**

B. **American Academy of Pediatrics clinical guidelines for late preterm infant discharge.** (Engle WA, Tomashek KM, Wallman C, et al. "Late-preterm" infants: a population at risk. *Pediatrics.* 2007; 120[6]:1390-1401.) Note that late preterm infants are more physiologically immature and are at a greater risk of morbidity and mortality than term infants. They are more likely to be readmitted for feeding difficulties, jaundice, dehydration, and sepsis. Recent studies show that mothers of **late preterm and early term infants** are more likely to smoke, less likely to start and continue breast feeding, and less likely to put infants in the supine position for sleep; therefore, it is important that this group of parents have more attention and special guidance in providing appropriate home care after discharge. **Discharge criteria for the late preterm infant include criteria from both the high-risk and normal term infant.** The following are **minimum criteria for late preterm infants on discharge:**

1. **Accurately determine the gestational age.**
2. **The timing of the discharge date is individualized** and based on ability to feed, ability to maintain body temperature, health status and absence of any medical illness, and absence of social risk factors. Do not expect a late preterm infant to meet these requirements before 48 hours of age.
3. **Choose a physician for continuing care,** and make sure a follow-up appointment has been made for 24 to 48 hours after discharge. Plan additional visits until a pattern of weight gain has been established and maintained.
4. **Vital signs need to be stable and within normal reference ranges for 12 hours prior to discharge,** and these should be recorded. Record stable vital signs for 12 hours prior to discharge; respiratory rate needs to be <60 breaths/min, heart rate should be 100 to 160 beats/min, and axillary temperature should be 36.5°C to 37°C (97.7–99.3°F) in an open crib with appropriate clothing.
5. **The infant should have passed 1 stool spontaneously.**
6. **Successful feeding for 24 hours** (breast or bottle; ability to coordinate sucking, swallowing, and breathing while feeding). Assess for dehydration if weight loss >2% to 3% of birthweight per day or a maximum of 7% of birthweight during hospitalization.
7. **A formal evaluation of breastfeeding should be done.** Observation of position, latch, and milk transfer should be documented in the chart by a trained caregiver for a minimum of 2 times a day after birth. The family needs to understand the feeding plan prior to discharge.
8. **Assess the infant for risk of hyperbilirubinemia prior to discharge** using the gestational age and hours of age nomogram, assign a bilirubin risk zone, and check Figure 63–2 to see when follow-up is recommended.
9. **Do a complete physical examination,** and make sure there are no abnormalities that require further hospitalization.
10. **Make sure the circumcision site** has no active bleeding for a minimum of 2 hours.
11. **Go over maternal and infant tests,** including maternal syphilis and hepatitis B surface antigen status, cord/infant blood type, and direct Coombs result if indicated and results of stat mandated screenings including human immunodeficiency virus (HIV) testing.
12. **Perform metabolic and genetic screenings** per your state's requirements. Assess the need for a repeat newborn screening if it was done before 24 hours of milk feeding.
13. **Give the initial hepatitis B vaccine at discharge.** See page 637 for recommendations. Stress the importance of immunizations to parents.
14. **Perform a car seat safety study by a trained professional.** Make sure the seated infant was observed for apnea, bradycardia, or oxygen desaturation and passed.
15. **Perform a hearing assessment, and go over results with the family.** Document results in the medical chart, and plan follow-up if needed.
16. **Assess family, environmental, and social risk factors.** Delay discharge if a risk factor has been identified. Examples of risk factors include history of child abuse or neglect, mental illness in parent in the home, untreated substance abuse in the parent, positive toxicology test results in mom or baby, homelessness (this

pregnancy), ongoing risk of domestic violence, and adolescent mother, especially if she has other risk factors.

17. **Train mother/caregivers and ensure competency in the following:**
    a. **Current condition of the baby and hospital course.**
    b. **Normal pattern of urine and stool frequency** for breast-fed or formula-fed infant. Best to give written and verbal instruction.
    c. **How to care for the umbilical cord, skin, and genital area** of a newborn.
    d. **Proper hand hygiene.** Discuss that this decreases the risk of infection.
    e. **How to use an axillary thermometer** in an infant.
    f. **Appropriate layers of clothing.**
    g. **How to identify jaundice for hyperbilirubinemia** and common signs and symptoms of sepsis and dehydration.
    h. **How to ensure there is a safe sleeping environment.** Instruct in the practice of "back to sleep."
    i. **Safety issues.** Car seat, smoke/fire alarms, hazards of secondhand smoke and any environmental pollutants, and what to do in an emergency.
    j. **Appropriate use of care by siblings and sibling's interactions.**

C. **American Academy of Pediatrics guidelines for healthy term infant discharge.** (Benitz WE; Committee on Fetus and Newborn, American Academy of Pediatrics. Hospital stay for healthy term newborn infants. *Pediatrics.* 2015; 135(5):948-953.) The decision to discharge a healthy term infant depends on many factors: the health and well-being of the mother and infant, the ability of the mother to care for the infant, the presence of an adequate support system at home, the access to follow-up, and the input from the mother, obstetrician, and nursing staff. Efforts should be made to discharge the mother and infant together. The following are **minimal discharge criteria for the healthy term infant** after an uncomplicated pregnancy, labor, and delivery with normal clinical course and normal physical examination:

1. **Document normal vital signs for 12 hours prior to discharge** (respiratory rate <60 breaths/min; no signs of respiratory distress; awake heart rate of 100–190 beats/min [heart rate <70 beats/min] if asleep okay if no signs of circulatory compromise], axillary temperature of 36.5–37.4°C (97.7–99.3°F) in open crib with appropriate clothing).
2. **Infant has urinated regularly and passed 1 stool.**
3. **Infant has fed twice successfully.** Document knowledge and success of breast feeding with a caregiver observing (latching on, swallowing, infant satiety) in the medical record. If bottle feeding, document that the infant can suck, swallow, and breathe successfully while feeding.
4. **Check circumcision site,** and make sure there is no significant bleeding for at least 2 hours.
5. **Assess the clinical risk of hyperbilirubinemia,** and make sure the AAP guidelines have been followed. See Chapters 63 and 99.
6. **Make sure the infant has been adequately evaluated for sepsis** based on maternal risk factors and current guidelines for infants with suspected or proven early-onset sepsis. See Chapter 146.
7. **Go over maternal blood test and screening results** (syphilis, hepatitis B antigen status, HIV test).
8. **Review infant blood tests** (eg, cord/infant blood type and direct Coombs test if indicated).
9. **Give initial hepatitis B vaccine** at discharge according to current immunization schedule and infant's risk status. (See Appendix E)
10. **Complete newborn metabolic screening, pulse oximetry screening, and hearing screenings** per hospital protocol and state regulations. Make sure a repeat metabolic screen is done on a follow-up visit if the infant has not been fed milk for 24 hours before the test.

11. **Verify that the mother is able to:**
    a. **State the importance of breast feeding benefits** for mother and child.
    b. **State what is the appropriate frequency of urinating and stooling of the infant.**
    c. **Understand umbilical cord, skin, newborn genital, and circumcision care.** Go over how to take a temperature and normal temperature assessment.
    d. **State the signs of illness and jaundice** and has the ability to recognize them.
    e. **Understand infant safety issues.** Car seat safety, supine positioning for sleeping, smoke-free environment, room sharing but not bed sharing.
    f. **Recognize the importance of hand hygiene.**
12. **Car safety seat is available and appropriate for the infant,** and mother has demonstrated appropriate car seat use with infant positioning.
13. **Make sure the mother has support people** who feel comfortable with newborn care and have a working knowledge of jaundice, dehydration, and lactation and who are available for the infant and her after discharge.
14. **Identify a medical home for continuing care for the mother and infant.** Provide instructions if there is an emergency and a number for the medical home; the first follow-up visit should be scheduled at discharge.
15. **Safe home environment counseling** (if risk factors are present, delay discharge until they are resolved, and consider discussing with social services/child protective services)
    a. **Untreated parental drug abuse** or positive urine toxicology screen in mother or infant
    b. **Child abuse/neglect history**
    c. **Mental illness** in parent at home
    d. **Lack of social support** (first-time mom)
    e. **No fixed home**
    f. **Domestic violence history,** especially during this pregnancy
    g. **Adolescent mother**
    h. **Barriers to adequate follow-up** (lack of transportation to medical visits and lack of telephone access, non–English-speaking parents)
16. **Discharge <48 hours after delivery.** Follow-up appointment needs to be made, and the infant needs to be seen by a licensed healthcare professional within 48 hours of discharge. If this cannot be done, the discharge should be delayed. Follow-up visit can be done anywhere as long as the healthcare professional is competent in newborn care and the visit is reported to the infant's physician. Follow-up visit purpose:
    a. **Establish a relationship with the medical home.**
    b. **Weigh the infant; check general health, hydration, jaundice, and feeding patterns;** obtain adequate stooling and urination patterns. Are there any new problems? If breast feeding is not going well, make a referral for lactation support.
    c. **Infant behavior? Mother–infant bonding/attachment?** Parental well-being? Any postpartum depression? Screen for postpartum depression.
    d. **Reinforce infant care and feeding** and safety issues such as back to sleep, no cosleeping, and child safety seats (only for travel; not for use in home) for the mom and family or support system.
    e. **Review any outstanding laboratory tests** performed at discharge (newborn metabolic screens).
    f. **Perform any necessary tests** such as any that are clinically indicated (eg, bilirubin) or any newborn screening tests mandated by the state.
    g. **Healthcare maintenance issues.** Verify the plan for healthcare maintenance, preventive care, emergency services, immunizations, periodic physical examinations, and necessary screenings.

72 No Stool in 48 Hours

I. **Problem.** The nurse reports that no stool has been passed in an infant for 48 hours. The first stool, meconium, is usually passed by 98.5% of term infants, 100% of postterm infants, and 76% of premature infants (majority are >32 weeks) in the first 24 hours of life. The majority of premature infants have delayed passage (37% in 24 hours, 32% beyond 48 hours, and 99% by 9 days in 1 study) (Table 72–1). Delayed passage of meconium was found to be in 81% of very low birthweight (VLBW) infants. Males were found to pass stool later than females. Delayed passage of meconium can be a predisposing factor for bowel perforation. The triad of failure to pass meconium, vomiting, and abdominal distention, is a sign that the infant may have intestinal obstruction.

II. **Immediate questions**

A. **What is the stooling history?** This history can give a clue to the diagnosis. An infant with a complete obstruction can pass meconium because the meconium was formed in utero distal to obstruction or a mucous stool (intestinal secretions can occur distal to the obstruction).

1. **Has the infant passed his or her first stool?** Meconium is composed of materials ingested while the infant is in the uterus and consists of **succus entericus** (intestinal epithelial cells, lanugo, mucus, amniotic fluid, bile salts, bile acids, and debris from the intestinal mucosa). It is not sterile because it contains enteric bacteria. The time when the first meconium stool passes has been used as a **marker for normal gastrointestinal functioning** and a delay can occur because of gestational immaturity, a severe illness, a bowel obstruction or other causes.

2. **If meconium has been passed and normal stooling has occurred,** but not in the past couple of days, consider simple constipation.

3. **If delayed passage of meconium occurs,** consider prematurity, distal intestinal obstruction, or Hirschsprung disease (observed in 90% of infants).

4. **If meconium has never been passed,** consider imperforate anus or some degree of distal bowel obstruction.

5. **If meconium has been passed and stooling has occurred and then slowed down or stopped completely,** consider small bowel obstruction.

Table 72–1. TIME OF FIRST STOOL BASED ON A STUDY OF 500 TERM AND PRETERM INFANTS

Hours	Preterm Infants (%) (Majority >32 wks)[a]	Full-Term Infants (%)	Postterm Infants (%)
Delivery room (0)	5.0	16.7	32
1–8	32.5	59.5	68
9–16	63.8	91.1	88
17–24	76.3	98.5	100
24–48	98.8	100.0	—
>48	100.0	—	—

Percentages are cumulative.
[a]Preterm: only 3 infants <32 weeks in the study.
Data from Clark DA: Times of first void and first stool in 500 newborns, *Pediatrics.* 1977 Oct;60(4):457-459.

B. **Is there abdominal distension?** Abdominal distension can be a sign of intestinal obstruction and may be present right after birth or at 24 to 48 hours, when it usually peaks. It is more common in lower obstructions, and the more distal the obstruction, the more severe is the abdominal distension. Proximal obstructions will have minimal to no abdominal distension.

If the abdominal distension is present at birth, consider antenatal intestinal obstruction/perforation from volvulus, intestinal atresia, or meconium ileus/peritonitis. Abdominal distension usually appears 24 hours or later after birth in infants with more distal or functional obstructions.

C. **Is there vomiting?** Secretions proximal to the obstruction build up and result in vomiting, which can be bilious or nonbilious. Bilious emesis is more common in proximal obstructions and suggests that the obstruction is located **distal to the ampulla of Vater** (where the fusion of the common bile duct and pancreatic duct enter the C-shaped curve of the duodenum). **Bilious vomiting** is seen with duodenal atresia, malrotation with midgut volvulus, jejunal ileal atresia, meconium ileus, small left colon syndrome, colorectal atresia, and Hirschsprung disease. **Nonbilious vomiting** occurs if the obstruction is proximal to the ampulla of Vater. **Sporadic bilious/nonbilious vomiting** may be seen in infants with a partial obstruction.

D. **How many hours or days old is the infant?** Infants with proximal intestinal obstructions usually present within 24 to 48 hours of birth. Infants with distal intestinal obstructions usually present a few days after birth. Infants with a functional obstruction (Hirschsprung disease) can present a few weeks after birth or later.

E. **What is the gestational age and birthweight of the infant?** An inverse relationship between gestational age, birthweight, and meconium passage exists. Studies show the older the gestational age, the shorter is the time to the first stool. Premature and VLBW infants commonly have a delayed passage of stool because of immaturity of interstitial cells of the colon, increased viscosity of meconium, and lack of triggering effect of enteral feeds on gut hormones when the patient is maintained nothing by mouth. **Failure of a full-term or postterm infant to pass meconium may signify a bowel obstruction, but in preterm infants, it may not.**

F. **Were maternal drugs used that could cause a paralytic ileus with delayed passage of stool?** Magnesium sulfate, which is used to slow the premature onset of labor, may cause a paralytic ileus. Some studies show it is associated with delayed stool passage. Narcotics for pain control or use of heroin or ganglionic blocking agents by the mother may also cause delayed passage of stool in the infant. Maternal ingestion of psychotropic drugs is associated with small left colon syndrome and delayed passage of stools.

G. **Are there any other congenital abnormalities, associated syndromes, or other diseases?** Many cases of bowel obstruction are associated with congenital anomalies, syndromes, or other diseases. **Cystic fibrosis (CF) should be considered in any infant with delayed meconium passage.**
   1. **Meconium plug syndrome:** Hirschsprung disease, neonatal hypothyroidism.
   2. **Hirschsprung disease:** Trisomy 21, neurofibromatosis, Waardenburg syndrome, multiple endocrine neoplasia type 2, central hypoventilation syndrome, and cardiac septal defects.
   3. **Anorectal malformation:** Genitourinary abnormalities most common; cardiovascular, spinal cord tethering, gastrointestinal (GI) complications, and VACTERL (vertebral defects, anal atresia, cardiac defects, tracheoesophageal fistula, renal and radial abnormalities, and limb abnormalities) association. **Eighty percent of cases of imperforate anus have associated abnormalities:** small intestine, esophagus, genitourinary system, cardiovascular system, and sacral area.
   4. **Small left colon syndrome:** Hypothyroidism, hypermagnesemia.
   5. **Colonic atresia:** Gastroschisis, omphalocele, Hirschsprung disease, ophthalmic and skeletal anomalies, bladder exstrophy, exomphalos, vesicointestinal fistula, choledochal cyst. Cases of colonic atresia have been reported with congenital varicella syndrome.

6. **Meconium ileus.** Approximately 90% to 95% of babies with meconium ileus have CF; 15% of CF patients will have meconium ileus as neonates.

7. **Duodenal atresia:** Trisomy 21 (most common in 30%), VACTERL association. Twenty to thirty percent have congenital heart disease.

8. **Jejunal and ileal atresia.** GI anomalies occur in up to 45% of cases (malrotation, meconium peritonitis, microcolon, duplication cysts, esophageal atresia, and volvulus).

9. **Meconium peritonitis.** CF is present in 8% to 40% of cases. Rare associations include biliary atresia, familial progressive intrahepatic cholestasis, and hemochromatosis.

10. **Malrotation and midgut volvulus:** Gastroschisis, omphalocele, diaphragmatic hernia, bowel atresia/stenosis (duodenal or jejunal atresia), and heterotaxy.

III. **Differential diagnosis.** The differential diagnosis of failure to pass a stool includes constipation, secondary to prematurity, and bowel obstruction, among many other causes. The main concern is being able to recognize a bowel obstruction.

A. **Constipation.** This occurs in infants who have already passed a stool and then fail to pass one. Infants have a mean of 4 stools per day during the first week of life; this gradually decreases to a mean average of 1.7 stools per day at age 2 years. Some breast-fed infants have only 1 stool a day during the first few days of life, but as the mothers' milk comes in, the frequency increases, and they tend to have more frequent stools in the first 3 months of life than standard formula-fed infants.

B. **Prematurity/very low birthweight infants.** Delayed passage of meconium is common in premature and VLBW infants. Immaturity of the colon, increased viscosity of meconium, and delayed first feeding are all associated with delayed passage in these infants. These infants also have a higher risk of respiratory distress syndrome, mechanical ventilation, patent ductus arteriosus, and uteroplacental insufficiency, which also contribute to delayed passage. These infants usually do not have abdominal distension or bilious nasogastric aspirates. Delayed meconium passage in VLBW infants can be a predisposing factor for **bowel perforation** (mortality rate of 50%). Prophylactic administration of glycerin laxatives in VLBW infants resulted in improved stool passage over the first 48 hours of life but did not shorten the time to full feeding or decrease time to discharge (Cochrane review, September 2015).

C. **Bowel obstruction** has an incidence of 1 in 2000 live births.

1. **Large bowel obstruction** usually presents with **abdominal distension and no stools.** This can be secondary to a meconium plug, Hirschsprung disease, anorectal malformations, small left colon syndrome, and colonic atresia.

a. **Meconium plug syndrome** has an incidence of 1 in 500 to 1000 births and is also known as functional immaturity of the colon, colonic immaturity, or functional colonic obstruction. This is the most common form of functional bowel obstruction in the neonate. It manifests as an obstruction in the lower left colon and rectum caused by abnormal meconium consistency creating a meconium plug. (**Note:** Consider rectal biopsy in all these patients due to the increased incidence of Hirschsprung disease.) Meconium plug syndrome is more common in infants of diabetic mothers, premature infants, and neonatal hypothyroidism.

b. **Hirschsprung disease (congenital aganglionic megacolon).** Accounts for approximately 15% of infants, usually male, who have delayed passage of stool. It occurs in 1 in 4000 live births. A functional obstruction is caused by congenital absence of ganglion cells in the rectum and distal colon (aganglionosis of cells in Meissner and Auerbach plexus in the rectum and variable amounts of the distal colon). The affected segment of colon and rectum fails to relax and is aperistaltic; therefore, no stool is passed. Typically, the infant is full term with delayed passage of meconium (usually after 48 hours of life) and symptoms in the first week of life (bilious vomiting, abdominal distension). It has a sex-dependent penetrance (4 males to 1 female), and 8% of patients have Down syndrome. It is more common in white males.

c. **Anorectal malformations** (1 in 4000–8000 infants) include imperforate anus, anal stenosis, and fistula. **The passage of meconium alone is not a sign of a correctly positioned anus.**

   i. **Imperforate anus or anal atresia** (absent anus) can be high or low type with a fistula or anal stenosis. An infant with an imperforate anus may pass meconium if a fistula exists (meconium per urethra with rectourethral fistula in male or per vagina with rectovaginal fistula in female). There are a high percentage of associated anomalies with anal atresia (70%), such as VATER (vertebral anomalies, anal atresia, tracheoesophageal fistula, and radial or renal dysplasia)/VACTERL association.

   ii. **Anal stenosis is a narrowing of the anal canal and accounts for 20% of anorectal malformations.** They present with a small, tight anus, sometimes with a dot of meconium present.

d. **Small left colon syndrome.** This syndrome involves a reduced caliber of the colon starting at the splenic flexure causing an intestinal obstruction that is not caused by aganglionosis or meconium. It is usually seen in large but immature infants. Approximately 50% have a history of maternal gestational diabetes, and most do not pass meconium in the first 24 hours of life. The others have sepsis, hypoglycemia, hypothyroidism, or increased magnesium. **Microcolon of prematurity** is the preterm equivalent of small left colon syndrome. The colon has an abnormally small caliber. It seems to be caused by a functional obstruction with failure of the small bowel contents to pass into the colon in utero and by ganglion cell dysfunction and depressive effects of magnesium sulfate. The majority of mothers had toxemia or received magnesium sulfate. The infants present with marked distension, failure to pass meconium, and no bilious vomiting.

e. **Colonic atresia is a congenital defect that causes complete obstruction of the lumen of the colon.** It is felt to be secondary to a vascular or mechanical event (intestinal volvulus). It may occur with Hirschsprung disease. The infant will usually present within the first 2 to 3 days after birth with severe abdominal distension, failure to pass meconium, and bilious vomiting.

2. **Small bowel obstruction** usually presents with **bilious vomiting with or without abdominal distension,** and meconium can be passed, but it usually progresses to **decreased or no stools.** This can be secondary to meconium ileus, meconium obstruction of prematurity, small bowel atresias, meconium peritonitis secondary to perforation, or malrotation and midgut volvulus.

a. **Meconium ileus.** The meconium is abnormal in consistency and obstructs the distal ileum. It presents with abdominal distension and a failure to pass meconium. It occurs in 10% to 20% of newborns with CF; 80% to 90% of patients with meconium ileum have CF and thus should be tested for it. It is the most common presentation of CF in the neonatal period. Median age of infants presenting with meconium ileus is 2 weeks.

b. **Meconium obstruction of prematurity** is a distinct clinical entity that occurs in VLBW premature infants. Maternal history of pregnancy-induced hypertension or chronic hypertension commonly exists in these infants. Meconium is most commonly found in the distal ileum with a predisposition of intestinal perforation. These infants usually pass some meconium and then develop obstructive symptoms a few days later. Feeding intolerance is common. None of these infants have CF.

c. **Small bowel atresias.** Atresias are congenital defects that cause complete obstruction of the lumen of the intestine. They are thought to be secondary to a vascular/mechanical event. Atresias most commonly occur in the ileum, followed by the duodenum and then jejunum. Bilious emesis, abdominal distension, and failure to pass meconium are seen; jaundice is possible.

    i. **Duodenal atresia** (1 in 10,000–40,000 births). Accounts for up to 60% of intestinal atresia. Infants have gastric distension and vomiting and may pass meconium.

    ii. **Jejunal and ileal atresia.** Abdominal distension and bilious vomiting within the first 2 days after birth. May pass meconium because it may remain in the distal bowel beyond the obstruction.

  d. **Meconium peritonitis** (1 in 30,000 births). Rare condition where the small bowel perforates proximal to the site of obstruction in utero and meconium leaks into the abdominal cavity and causes peritonitis from an inflammatory response. Most commonly caused by perforation in the small intestine (ileum most common). The obstruction can be caused by an atresia, stenosis, imperforate anus, volvulus, Meckel diverticulum, meconium ileus, intussusception, or peritoneal bands. In the majority of cases, the perforation has closed by the time of birth. Incidence of CF is 8% to 40%.

  e. **Malrotation and midgut volvulus.** Malrotation is a congenital anomaly in which there is a failure of normal rotation and fixation of the bowel. Because the intestine is not fixed in the normal position, it is prone to **volvulus,** which is a twisting of the small intestine that can cut off blood supply to the intestine. It usually presents with **bilious emesis;** meconium is passed, but then infants progress to decreased or no stools.

3. **Adhesions**

  a. **Necrotizing enterocolitis.** Postoperatively, such as after surgery for necrotizing enterocolitis (NEC), there is a 30% chance of having adhesions. It usually occurs in the segment of the intestine distal to the established enterostomy, most commonly the colon.

  b. **Non–necrotizing enterocolitis patients.** Acquired intestinal atresia in non-NEC patients is very rare. It can occur from an adhesive band that can entrap a jejunal or ileal segment with its mesentery.

4. **Infrequent causes**

  a. **Meckel diverticulum** is a congenital diverticulum in the small intestine and is a vestigial remnant of the vitelline duct. Rarely, it can present with obstruction with bilious vomiting, perforation, and pneumoperitoneum.

  b. **Hypoganglionosis** is a reduced number of ganglion cells; it presents with symptoms similar to Hirschsprung disease and can occur with Hirschsprung disease.

  c. **Neuronal intestinal dysplasia type A** is hypoplasia or aplasia of the sympathetic innervation of the myenteric plexus and mucosa, with inflammation of the mucosa; it presents with symptoms similar to Hirschsprung disease.

  d. **Neuronal intestinal dysplasia type B** is subtle malformation of the enteric nervous system of the submucosal plexus of the colon. It can manifest as meconium plug syndrome or small left colon syndrome.

  e. **Megacystis-microcolon intestinal hypoperistalsis syndrome (Berdon syndrome)** presents with urinary retention, dilated small bowel, microcolon, megacystis (giant bladder), and hydronephrosis. Pathology reveals that ganglion cells are present.

D. **Other medical conditions/causes/associations that can cause a delay in meconium passage.** Some of these conditions (eg, infection [sepsis], respiratory distress syndrome, electrolyte abnormalities) cause a functional ileus that can cause a delay in passage of stool.

1. **Infection.** Sepsis is the most common infection causing delayed passage of stool. Sepsis can cause a dynamic ileus and can be a mimicker of intestinal obstruction. Other infections that can result in intestinal dysfunction include pneumonia, enterovirus infection, omphalitis, and peritonitis.

2. **Respiratory distress syndrome** can cause delayed gastric emptying, which can cause dysmotility of the intestine.

3. **Electrolyte abnormalities.** Hypokalemia, hyponatremia, hypercalcemia, hypermagnesemia, and fetal hypoglycemia can also impair neonatal intestinal motility.

4. **Maternal medications.** Magnesium sulfate, narcotics, ganglionic blocking agents or illicit drugs (opiates, heroin), neuroleptics, antidepressants.

5. **Infant medications.** Theophylline, opiates, narcotic analgesics.

6. **Hypothyroidism (most common).** Other endocrinopathies—adrenal insufficiency, hyperparathyroidism, adrenal bleeding.

7. **Cystic fibrosis should be considered in any infant** with delayed meconium passage or in cholestatic infants with meconium ileus.

8. **Other less common causes.** Congestive heart failure, hyperbilirubinemia, renal vein thrombosis, hypovolemia, patent ductus arteriosus, embolism/thrombosis, uteroplacental insufficiency, mechanical ventilation.

9. **Idiopathic.** No identifiable cause.

IV. **Database**

A. **Prenatal history may reveal abnormalities on the fetal ultrasound.** One of the causes of polyhydramnios is proximal GI obstruction due to secretions proximal to the obstruction, and this can occur in intestinal atresia. Fetal bowel dilatation on ultrasound (fluid-filled intestinal loops at least 15 mm in length and 7 mm in diameter) is an indirect sign of a bowel obstruction. Obstruction in a newborn on a prenatal ultrasound is usually made in the late second or third trimester. The classic "double bubble" of duodenal atresia can be seen. Moderately dilated anechoic loops showing hyperperistalsis are seen in ileal atresia. Peritoneal wall calcifications, fetal ascites, and dilated thick-walled echogenic bowel with intra-abdominal cysts are seen in meconium ileus. Prenatal ultrasound findings of meconium peritonitis, bowel dilatation, and absent gallbladder warrant screening in the parents for prenatal CF carrier.

B. **Physical examination.** First, inspect the anus (eg, fifth digit exam, rectal thermometer, or soft feeding tube). Is the anus in the correct position? A normal anus location in a male is halfway between the base of the scrotum and the coccyx; in a female, it is halfway between the coccyx and vestibule (vaginal opening). A rectal exam will also determine if muscle tone is adequate, and it may reveal hardened stool in the rectum. If patency is in question, consult with surgery on the best way to further evaluate. **Special attention is paid to the abdomen.** Check for abdominal distention or rigidity, bowel sounds, and evidence of a mass. Erythema and tenderness are usually not seen with an obstruction unless there is perforation. Infants with Hirschsprung disease typically have a distended abdomen (63%–91% of neonates) and a tight anal canal with an empty rectum. Infants with Hirschsprung disease can also have the "squirt/blast sign" (explosive expulsion of stool after digital examination). Infants with hypothyroidism can have prolonged jaundice, lethargy, hypothermia, hoarse cry, macroglossia, umbilical hernia, large fontanels, hypotonia, and dry skin.

C. **Laboratory findings**

1. **Complete blood count with differential and blood culture to rule out sepsis.** A sterile urine culture should also be obtained.

2. **Urinary drug screening** on both mother and infant to detect maternal use of narcotics.

3. **Check newborn screening program for cystic fibrosis** because 63% of CF cases are diagnosed based on delayed stool passage issues. If screening returns positive results, newborns should have sweat chloride testing at 2 weeks of age and when the infant weighs >2 kg.

   a. **Genetic testing and sweat tests** are recommended to rule out or in CF in every intraoperative diagnosis of meconium ileus. CF is caused by mutations in the CFTR protein. Genetic testing should be done to rule out mutations in both alleles of the *CFTR* (CF transmembrane conductance regulator) gene.

CFTR-related metabolic syndrome describes infants with an equivocal diagnosis and is found in 3% to 4% of infants with a positive screen.
D. **Imaging and other studies**
   1. **Plain film abdominal radiographs.** A flat plate and lateral decubitus film of the abdomen should be obtained to look for ileus or bowel obstruction in any infant who has not passed a stool within 48 hours of birth. A neonate with GI obstruction will have abnormal air patterns, dilated loops of bowel, and multiple air fluid levels (fluid and gas collect in the intestine with an obstruction) at different areas depending on the obstruction. Do not order the film too early because you can miss an obstruction. Remember that at birth the GI tract is gasless and fluid filled. Air fills the stomach immediately after the first cry after birth, and within 5 minutes of life, you will see gas in the stomach; it reaches the small bowel by 3 to 4 hours, the colon by 6 to 8 hours, and the rectum by 12 hours. Important facts to remember when looking at the plain film include the following:
      a. **Small and large bowel cannot be differentiated on plain film** because of the nondevelopment of haustra; differentiation requires a barium enema.
      b. **The loop of bowel that is proximal to an obstruction is usually very dilated.** The loop of bowel that is distal to the obstruction will have paucity of gas in the bowel.
      c. **Dilated intestinal loops are defined if the diameter of the loop** is more than the transverse diameter of the vertebrae or as big as the surgeon's thumb ("thumb sign").
      d. **Intra-abdominal calcifications** can indicate antenatal perforation and can be seen in meconium ileus and meconium peritonitis.
      e. **Perforation can occur without free air** on the radiograph.
      f. **Absent colonic or rectal gas** may indicate a complete bowel obstruction.
      g. **With high intestinal obstruction,** <3 dilated bowel loops are seen. In low/distal intestinal obstruction, >3 dilated bowel loops are seen.
      h. **Neuhauser sign (air mixed with meconium)** is typically seen with meconium ileus but can be seen with Hirschsprung disease, ileal atresia, and NEC.
      i. **Other specific radiograph findings are as follows:**
         i. **Meconium plug:** Distal obstruction with multiple dilated/distended loops of bowel with absence of rectal gas.
         ii. **Hirschsprung disease:** Initial radiograph shows marked gaseous distension of colon with multiple dilated bowel loops with no gas in the rectum. Air fluid levels in the colon can be seen.
         iii. **Anorectal malformation** may show multiple dilated bowel loops with no rectal gas.
         iv. **Functional immaturity of the colon or small left colon syndrome:** Multiple dilated bowel loops with air-fluid levels.
         v. **Colonic atresia:** Distal obstruction with frothy appearance of air mixed with meconium in right lower quadrant.
         vi. **Meconium ileus:** Nonspecific; may show distended bowel loops proximal to the impaction. Can see Neuhauser sign (air mixed with meconium). Paucity of air-fluid levels. Calcifications, free air, and very large air fluid levels suggest complications/perforation.
         vii. **Meconium peritonitis:** Calcifications (linear and punctate) throughout the abdomen.
         viii. **Duodenal atresia:** Has classic "double bubble" sign: gas bubble in the stomach and the proximal duodenum and the absence of distal gas.
         ix. **Jejunal ileal atresia:** Air fluid levels often of different size, with largest being just proximal to the site of obstruction.
         x. **Malrotation and midgut volvulus:** Usually normal film, or gasless abdomen; intestinal dilatation suggesting small bowel obstruction or duodenal obstruction or normal. Sigmoid volvulus has a "coffee bean" sign.

2. **Ultrasound.** Targeted ultrasound of the GI tract is being used more often in the neonatal intensive care unit (NICU); it has no radiation, and infants do not need to be sedated. It can be used in infants with suspected intestinal obstructions to diagnose intestinal obstructions. Ultrasound should be done in infants with imperforate anus to also evaluate for urologic anomalies.

3. **Contrast enema.** Abdominal radiographs with contrast enema should be obtained in the majority of cases of delayed passage of stool if the patient is symptomatic. These will help define the disease process and may be therapeutic. It is contraindicated if a bowel perforation is suspected (calcifications on plain film may indicate perforation). Care must be taken because of risk of perforation in some cases (colonic atresia). Microcolon is a radiologic finding of an abnormally small caliber of colon and usually indicates distal ileal obstruction: ileal atresia, colonic atresia, colon aganglionosis, volvulus, or duplication. In some instances, such as duodenal atresia or jejunal ileal atresia, a contrast study is not necessary because the abdominal radiograph is diagnostic. Findings may include the following:

   a. **Meconium plug syndrome.** The contrast enema is a diagnostic test for meconium plug syndrome because it shows the outline of meconium and meconium plugs. Meconium plugs are seen in a small microcolon, with distal ileum obstruction. Can see distal ileum impacted with meconium.

   b. **Hirschsprung disease.** Contrast enema usually shows a distal, narrowed, aganglionic segment leading to a dilated proximal segment. A gradual transition zone may be seen with marked dilatation and presence of barium after 24 hours. Normal caliber left colon.

   c. **Small left colon syndrome.** A small left colon with a change in the splenic flexure. Narrow descending and rectosigmoid colon with an abrupt transition to a huge distended colon at the splenic flexure.

   d. **Colonic atresia.** In type 1 colonic atresia, "windsock sign" can be seen as contrast pushes against the membrane. In type 11, one can see a "hook sign" on the microcolon side of the colonic atresia.

   e. **Meconium ileus.** Contrast enema may reveal microcolon with proximal inspissated meconium proximally. Impacted meconium pellets may be seen in the right colon or distal ileum.

   f. **Malrotation and midgut volvulus.** The proximal duodenum is dilated and tapered to a beak shape, the distal duodenum may be spiral shaped (corkscrew appearance), and the duodenum is in a Z shape.

   g. **Meconium obstruction of prematurity.** Meconium plugs are seen in a small microcolon, with distal ileum obstruction. The distal ileum may be impacted with meconium.

4. **Upper gastrointestinal series is indicated in evaluating high obstructions.** It can differentiate between obstruction of the duodenum and malrotation with volvulus.

5. **Anorectal manometry** should be done in all newborns with symptoms suggesting lower bowel obstruction. It records changes in anal pressure during and after rectal distension by balloon dilation. A normal rectosphincteric reflex is seen with rectal distention, and there is a drop in anal pressure. In Hirschsprung disease, there is an absent rectosphincteric reflex, which means there is no drop in anal pressure. This test is difficult to perform, but serial manometry may prevent the need for rectal biopsy. If the rectosphincteric reflex is absent, a rectal suction biopsy is needed. High-resolution anorectal manometry (HR-ARM) is an effective, safe, and minimally invasive technique that has fewer limitations than ARM.

6. **Rectosigmoid ratio/index.** The rectosigmoid ratio is the measurement of the diameter of the rectum divided by the diameter of the sigmoid colon, which is done during a contrast enema. A value <0.9 or 1, depending on the reference, is suggestive of Hirschsprung disease.

7. **Rectal biopsy.** Biopsy either by suction anal biopsy or transanal wedge resection is the gold standard for diagnosis of Hirschsprung disease. Histology demonstrates the absence of ganglion cells and presence of acetyl cholinesterase–positive hypertrophic nerve fibers.

8. **Specific testing for Hirschsprung disease.** Three specific protein markers have been identified for Hirschsprung disease that allow for early screening and diagnosis, but they are not in widespread use. A 5-serum miRNA profile was identified and was found to be more accurate than contrast enema.

V. **Plan**

A. **Rule out simple constipation and rule out or treat any underlying etiologies** such as infection (sepsis), respiratory distress syndrome, electrolyte abnormalities, hypothyroidism, or maternal/infant medications.

B. **Premature infants.** Need to rule out pathologic cause versus normal delayed passage of stool before full workup is done. Because meconium passage can be normally delayed in infants who are premature and have a low birthweight, delayed passage of stool does not always predict GI disease. It is best to only do a diagnostic workup for intestinal obstruction in premature infants with other signs of GI disease (eg, progressive abdominal distension and vomiting).

C. **Term infants with delayed passage need to be evaluated earlier** because failure to pass meconium in a term infant is highly suspicious for intestinal obstruction.

D. **All infants with suspected intestinal obstruction.** Presentation can vary from asymptomatic to severe respiratory distress and cardiovascular collapse. Follow ABCs (airway, breathing, circulation) if infant is unstable and not doing well.

1. **Oxygen and ventilation** may be necessary in infants with severe abdominal distension and respiratory distress.

2. **Place nothing by mouth and start intravenous fluids.** If there are signs of **shock,** the infant may need fluid resuscitation.

3. **Nasogastric decompression.** A no. 8 nasogastric or no. 10 orogastric tube should be placed.

4. **Consider antibiotic therapy** if clinically indicated.

5. **Start with plain and lateral decubitus radiographs of the abdomen first.** Do a supine, upright (if possible), or lateral decubitus film to see the bowel gas pattern and to see if there are any air fluid levels. Look for dilated loops of bowel. Are there intraperitoneal calcifications?

6. **Perform contrast enema** if bowel gas is consistent with distal obstruction to identify lower bowel obstructions. It is the most useful test to distinguish the types of distal intestinal obstruction. A contrast enema can also be therapeutic in some cases. Consultation with pediatric radiology for the best contrast agent is recommended.

7. **Perform an upper gastrointestinal series** if bowel gas is consistent with proximal obstruction. Upper GI may be necessary to distinguish between malrotation and volvulus and duodenal atresia.

8. **Consider anorectal manometry and rectal biopsy** if indicated.

9. **Pediatric surgical consultation** is recommended.

E. **Specific treatment plans**

1. **Constipation**
   a. **Digital rectal stimulation is the first step.**
   b. **Glycerin suppositories** can be used if digital rectal stimulation is unsuccessful. Saline irrigation is used in some NICUs. **Enemas are not recommended. Mineral oil or stimulant laxatives are also not recommended.**

2. **Bowel obstruction**
   a. **Meconium plug**
      i. **The water soluble contrast enema to diagnose the meconium plug can also be therapeutic by clearing the meconium plug.**
      ii. **If the obstruction is not relieved, many agents have been used** (saline enemas, glycerin suppositories, *N*-acetylcysteine, or osmotic contrast

agents such as gastrograffin). Repeated water soluble enemas are usually recommended and given every 4 to 6 hours. Rectal stimulation and enemas usually relieve the obstruction.

   iii. **If normal stooling occurs,** monitor closely.

   iv. **If an abnormal pattern of stooling recurs.** Further workup (eg, rectal biopsy) to rule out Hirschsprung disease or blood work for hypothyroidism.

b. **Small left colon syndrome.** Treat with contrast enema as discussed earlier. If there is an intestinal perforation or if the obstruction is not relieved with medical management (contrast enema), surgery is indicated. Rule out Hirschsprung disease and CF.

c. **Hirschsprung disease**

   i. **Fluid resuscitation,** rectal irrigation, and antibiotics are important to initially treat the enterocolitis and decrease the risk of mortality.

   ii. **Surgical repair is always needed** and can be done laparoscopically, open, or transanally. Colostomy may be indicated if early surgery is contraindicated and the colon cannot be decompressed with rectal irrigation.

d. **Anorectal abnormality (imperforate anus)**

   i. **Obtain immediate pediatric surgical consultation.**

   ii. **Evaluate for other congenital anomalies.** Genitourinary tract abnormalities (approximately 50%) are frequently seen with imperforate anus.

   iii. **Corrective surgery is required.** Colostomy for high anomalies and perineal anoplasty or fistula dilation for low lesions.

e. **Functional immaturity of the colon or small left colon syndrome.** Contrast enema is usually diagnostic and therapeutic. Surgery is indicated if the obstruction is recurrent or if there is a perforation (rare).

f. **Colonic atresia.** Treatment is individualized for each patient based on the infant's clinical status. Some infants require a proximal colostomy with establishment of intestinal continuity done later or resection and primary anastomosis.

g. **Meconium ileus**

   i. **Obstruction can be treated with a water-soluble enema.** (See page 168.) Many agents have been used (saline enemas, glycerin suppositories, *N*-acetylcysteine, or osmotic contrast agents such as gastrograffin). Low osmolality water soluble contrast agents are preferred to decrease possible fluid shifts. Adequate fluid and electrolyte replacement must be given.

   ii. **Instillation of oral contrast agents in nasogastric tube** have been reported to decrease stool viscosity, but there is a potential for side effects and a lack of studies.

   iii. **Operative management** may be necessary in complicated meconium ileus (obstruction is not relieved by the enema or there are calcifications in the abdominal cavity).

h. **Duodenal atresia.** Decompression with nasogastric suction and surgery.

i. **Jejunal ileal atresia.** Surgery with resection and tapering of dilated proximal bowel with enteroenterostomy.

j. **Malrotation and midgut volvulus.** Treat immediately with emergent laparotomy and surgery. Fluid and antibiotics are necessary.

k. **Meconium obstruction of prematurity.** Water-soluble contrast enemas are diagnostic and therapeutic. Surgery (diversion) may be necessary for perforation or worsening symptoms of obstruction (increasing abdominal distention).

l. **Adhesions.** Surgery is usually necessary to lyse the adhesions if a trial of nasogastric decompression fails.

m. **Microcolon of prematurity.** Contrast enema examination and close observation of infants with possibility of surgical intervention if there are complications.

n. **Ileus caused by sepsis**

    i. **Broad-spectrum antibiotics are initiated** after a sepsis workup is performed (see Chapter 146). Intravenous ampicillin and gentamicin are usually recommended empirically. Vancomycin may be substituted for ampicillin if staphylococcal infection is suspected (for dosages, see Chapter 155).

    ii. **A nasogastric tube should be placed to decompress the bowel.** The infant should not be fed enterally.

o. **Ileus caused by necrotizing enterocolitis.** See Chapter 109.

p. **Ileus caused by hypokalemia**

    i. **Treat underlying metabolic abnormalities.** Correct potassium levels if low (see Chapter 68).

    ii. **Place a nasogastric tube to rest the bowel.**

3. **Prematurity and delayed passage of stool.** Conservative treatment is usually recommended in infants who are not vomiting but have progressive abdominal distention, even if microcolon is seen. Treatment consists of a low-osmolality, water-soluble contrast enema for passage of the stool. Consult a pediatric radiologist for appropriate contrast enema to be used. **Glycerin suppositories** are sometimes used in the NICU in infants for documented constipation and for premature infants who have not passed meconium in hope to improve feeding intolerance. They should not be used in infants who are sick or infants with congenital GI anomalies. The American Academy of Pediatrics states that the evidence for the use of glycerin suppositories or enemas in premature infants is inconclusive.

4. **Hypothyroidism.** If the serum thyroxine and thyroids-stimulating hormone levels confirm the presence of hypothyroidism, thyroid replacement therapy is indicated. Consult with an endocrinologist before starting therapy (see Chapter 129).

73 No Urine Output in 24 Hours

I. **Problem.** <u>The nurse alerts you that the infant has had decreased urine output for the past 24 hours.</u> In a newborn, passage of the first urine is usually a sign of well-being, and if no urine output is seen by 24 hours of life, the infant should be evaluated. The following are common definitions relating to urine output:

A. **Normal urine output:** ≥ 2 mL/kg/h after the first 24 to 48 hours (<1 mL/kg/h the first 12–18 hours of life).

B. **Oliguria** is defined as urine output <0.5 to 1.0 mL/kg/h for 24 hours.

C. **Anuria** is defined as absence of urine output usually by 48 hours of age.

    Decreased urine output can be from undocumented voiding, stressful or prolonged delivery, oliguria typically seen in the first 24 hours of life or in a premature infant, mild dehydration, syndrome of inappropriate antidiuretic hormone (SIADH), acute kidney injury (AKI), or chronic kidney disease.

II. **Immediate questions**

A. **Was the infant born in the past 24 hours?** At birth, a normal infant has approximately 6 to 44 mL of urine in the bladder. In 1977, Clark reported that 100% of healthy premature, full-term, and postterm infants void by 24 hours of age. Mataj

Table 73–1. TIME OF FIRST VOID BASED ON A STUDY OF 500
TERM AND PRETERM INFANTS

Hours	Full-Term Infants (%)[a]	Preterm Infants (%)[a]
Delivery room (0)	12.9	21.2
1–8	51.1	83.7
9–16	91.1	98.7
17–24	100.0	100.0

[a]Percentages are cumulative.
Data from Clark DA: Times of first void and first stool in 500 newborns,
Pediatrics. 1977 Oct;60(4):457-459.

and colleagues (2003) reported that 17% of infants void at birth, 92% by 24 hours,
and 99% by 48 hours.

B. **Is the bladder palpable?** If a distended bladder is present in an infant, it is usually
palpable. A palpable bladder suggests there is urine in the bladder. **Credé maneuver** (manual compression of the bladder) may initiate voiding, especially in infants
receiving medications causing muscle paralysis.

C. **Has bladder catheterization been performed?** Catheterization determines whether
urine is present in the bladder. It is commonly done in more mature infants.

D. **Is the infant term or premature?** Term infants are more likely to have delayed voiding than preterm infants (Table 73–1). Premature infants <32 weeks are at increased
risk of AKI because of their immature kidneys and increased risk of hypovolemia.

E. **What is the blood pressure? Hypotension** can cause decreased renal perfusion and
urine output. **Hypertension** may indicate renal/renovascular disease (if severe, suspect renal artery or venous thrombosis).

F. **Was the delivery prolonged or stressful?** Delayed voiding can be related to a
prolonged and stressful birth. A study showed that infants with delayed voiding
(>24 hours) were more likely to have primiparous mothers; in addition, the duration
of labor was longer (first and second stage) in these infants, and they had abnormal
electronic fetal monitoring. Stress increases ADH (arginine vasopressin) and aldosterone levels, which decreases urine output. Both ADH and aldosterone levels were
increased in these infants with delayed voiding and stressful birth.

G. **Has the infant ever voided? Did the infant void, and was it not recorded on the
bedside chart?** Table 73–1 shows the time after birth at which the first voiding
occurs. **Remember:** Voiding can be missed (occurred in the delivery room or with
the parents and was not recorded). Approximately 13% to 21% of infants void in the
delivery room.

H. **Did the mother have oligohydramnios?** One of the etiologies of oligohydramnios
(decrease in amniotic fluid) can be a decrease in fetal urine production. This can be
caused by renal problems such as decreased renal perfusion, obstructive uropathy,
and congenital absence of renal tissue (renal agenesis, cystic dysplasia, and ureteral
atresia).

I. **Is there gross hematuria?** Gross hematuria suggests intrinsic renal disease. See
Chapter 61.

J. **What medications was the mother on during her pregnancy?** Certain medications
(eg, angiotensin-converting enzyme [ACE] inhibitors, nonsteroidal anti-inflammatory
drugs [NSAIDs]) and high steroid level exposure if given to the mother during her
pregnancy may interfere with fetal nephrogenesis, which can result in fetal renal

injury and lead to AKI and decreased urine output in the newborn. ACE inhibitors during pregnancy can cause renal tubular dysgenesis in the infant. Maternal use of indomethacin as a tocolytic agent can cause AKI in the infant. Maternal use of valsartan is associated with the development of AKI.

K. **Does the infant have a congenital renal disease? Did the prenatal ultrasound suggest kidney disease?** Prenatal ultrasound can detect congenital anomalies of the kidney and urinary tract (CAKUT). **Fetal anomaly ultrasound scan at 18 to 20 weeks** of gestation will reveal absence of amniotic fluid, bladder, and kidneys in bilateral renal agenesis. Renal agenesis, renal dysplasia, polycystic kidney disease, congenital nephrotic syndrome, and any obstruction from congenital malformations can all cause decreased urine output in the newborn.

L. **Did the mother have diabetes?** Infants of diabetic mothers have an increased risk of renal anomalies (renal agenesis, hydronephrosis, and ureteral duplication).

M. **Are there any risk factors for acute kidney injury or predisposing factors that are associated with acute kidney injury?**
1. **High risk for acute kidney injury:** Infants on ECLS especially with a congenital diaphragmatic hernia (71%), infants post cardiac surgery (62%), infants who experienced perinatal asphyxia (38%), infants with sepsis (26%), sick near-term or term infants with low Apgar scores (18%), preterm very low birthweight (VLBW) infants (18%), and preterm extremely low birthweight (ELBW) infants (12.5%).
2. **Pregnancy- and delivery-related risk factors:** Pregnancy-induced hypertension, preterm premature rupture of membranes, antenatal corticosteroids, maternal NSAID use during pregnancy, low Apgar scores and lower 5-minute Apgar scores, lower cord pH, intubation at birth, and asystole at birth.
3. **Other risk factors:** CAKUT, clinical seizures before cooling, persistent pulmonary hypertension, transfusions, serum sodium variation, catecholamine treatment, nosocomial infections, bronchopulmonary disease, cerebral lesions, neonatal surgery, lower gestational age, patent ductus arteriosus (PDA), phototherapy, male sex, elevated gentamicin or vancomycin levels, umbilical artery catheterization, umbilical vein catheterization, mechanical ventilation (high mean airway pressures), pressor support, disseminated intravascular coagulation, shock, heart failure, left-sided congenital diaphragmatic hernia, respiratory distress syndrome, posterior urethral valves, ischemic events, renal venous thrombosis, and exposure to ampicillin, ceftazidime, ibuprofen, and catecholamine were all associated with AKI.

N. **What medications is the infant receiving?** Medications in the infant can cause prerenal, renal, and postrenal drug-induced kidney injuries. **Contrast media** during radiology procedures can cause contrast-induced nephropathy.
1. **Prerenal:** NSAIDs, angiotensin receptor blockers, ACE inhibitors (eg, captopril, enalapril), calcineurin inhibitors, tolazoline, and mydriatic eye drops (phenylephrine).
2. **Renal: Acute tubular necrosis:** aminoglycosides, amphotericin B; **papillary necrosis:** acetaminophen, NSAIDs; **glomerulonephritis:** ampicillin, rifampin, NSAIDS, foscarnet, lithium; **acute interstitial nephritis:** NSAIDS, vancomycin, β-lactam antibiotics, calcineurin inhibitors; **nephrocalcinosis:** loop diuretics; **intrinsic renal failure:** captopril, enalapril, contrast media.
3. **Postrenal:** Certain medications can precipitate within the tubules and cause obstruction: acyclovir (crystal-induced nephropathy), methotrexate, sulfadiazine, ciprofloxacin.

III. **Differential diagnosis.** A delay in first urination (more common in boys) can be due to failure to document or observe voiding, a prolonged or stressful delivery, physiologic oliguria seen in the first 24 hours of life or in a premature infant, or mild dehydration, SIADH, AKI, or CKD. At birth, the initial presentations of AKI and CKD are similar, and differentiating between the 2 conditions depends on the duration of the renal dysfunction. For a complete discussion of AKI, see Chapter 86. Urine output is often difficult to accurately access in the newborn because indwelling urinary catheters are not commonly used. Note that the presence of urine does not rule out AKI because some infants with AKI will have a normal urine output.

A. **Undocumented urine void in the delivery room** is the most common cause of a "lack of urine" in the first 24 hours of life. Remember that approximately 13% to 21% of infants void in the delivery room.

B. **Prolonged or stressful delivery.** See Section II.F.

C. **Oliguria in a newborn in the first 24 hours of life.** Oliguria may occur in the first day of life because of a high circulating ADH. A study showed extremely high concentrations of ADH present in the cord blood and infant at birth. Infants who were born with a difficult delivery and stressed infants also had higher plasma levels of ADH.

D. **Oliguria in a premature infant.** Oliguria can occur in a premature infant because infants have immature kidneys because nephrogenesis is not completed until 34 to 36 weeks. An infant's kidneys at birth also experience a decrease in cardiac output as compared to the adult kidney (at birth, 2.5%–4%; at 24 hours, 6%; at 1 week, 10%; at 6 weeks, 15%–18%).

E. **Mild dehydration.** An infant may have decreased urine output the first few days of life, especially if the infant is breast feeding (normal is considered a minimum of 2 wet diapers on day 2 and a minimum 3–5 wet diapers on days 3–5). Inadequate breast milk production can cause dehydration. Low volume of maternal milk intake causes dehydration. Laboratory findings are usually normal or may show a minimal change. Overclothing/overheating of infants can also contribute to dehydration.

F. **Syndrome of inappropriate antidiuretic hormone can cause oliguria.** SIADH is caused by too much ADH, which causes the infant to retain water. It consists of hyponatremia, serum hypo-osmolality, increased urine sodium, and increased urine osmolality. SIADH occurs more commonly in central nervous system disorders such as intraventricular hemorrhage, hydrocephalus, birth asphyxia, and meningitis, but may also be seen with lung disease (pneumothorax and positive-pressure ventilation). SIADH is often seen in critically ill premature and term neonates. It can also be seen in association with pain and with medications such as opiates, carbamazepine, barbiturates, theophylline, and thiazides.

G. **Acute kidney injury.** AKI is an acute renal dysfunction and occurs when there is a decrease in glomerular filtration rate (GFR) and an increase in creatinine and nitrogenous waste products with the loss of ability to regulate fluid and electrolytes. Definitions vary and can be based on serum creatinine (SCr) (see Section IV.F and Table 86–1). AKI is defined as an increase in SCr levels associated with or without a reduction in urine output. It can range from mild injury to complete kidney failure. It has an abrupt onset and is potentially reversible. Incidence of neonatal AKI is approximately 8% to 40% with a high mortality rate (up to 60%). The most prevalent causes were sepsis and asphyxia, with infants undergoing peritoneal dialysis having a higher mortality rate.

AKI can be caused by **prenatal, renal, and postrenal** causes. Etiology of AKI is different in term versus preterm infants. **In term infants,** the cause is most commonly CAKUT, obstructive uropathy, birth asphyxia, complications from surgery, or hypothermia. **Preterm infants** develop AKI from sepsis, necrotizing enterocolitis (NEC), PDA, hypotension, and medications that are nephrotoxic. AKI can present with normal urine output. Prognosis of AKI in infants is worse than in adults, and AKI can lead to chronic kidney damage and damage of nonrenal organs; therefore, it is important to identify risk factors in neonates to prevent AKI, and in infants with the disease, early treatment is essential. **AKI is prenatal in origin until proven otherwise.**

1. **Prerenal acute kidney injury (most common cause of acute kidney injury in the newborn, 85%).** Normal kidneys with **inadequate or decreased** renal blood flow (perfusion). This leads to decreased renal function. Prerenal failure

can be caused by **systemic hypovolemia** (a **true volume depletion**) or **renal hypoperfusion** (a disease process that results in decreased perfusion to the kidney). **Common causes in the NICU** are: perinatal asphyxia, hemorrhage (perinatal or postnatal), dehydration/hypovolemia, sepsis, NEC, polycythemia, hypoxemia, RDS, shock and hypotension, GI losses, third space losses, cardiac etiologies (CHF, PDA, congenital heart disease/cardiac surgery, pericarditis, cardiac tamponade), infants requiring ECLS (64% of infants on ECLS and 71% of neonates with congenital diaphragmatic hernia on ECLS have decreased renal blood flow), hypoalbuminemia, and any medication that can decrease renal blood flow (NSAIDs [indomethacin, ibuprofen {less toxic}], ACE inhibitors [captopril, enalapril], and adrenergic drugs [phenylephrine eye drops, tolazoline, angiotensin receptor blockers, calcineurin inhibitors]; aminoglycosides, amphotericin, and radiocontrast agents also cause prerenal AKI).

2. **Intrinsic/renal acute kidney injury (11%).** This occurs due to structural renal damage to the tubules, glomeruli, or interstitium. Most often, it is renal tubular dysfunction caused by an acute insult. Acute tubular necrosis (ischemic or drug or toxin induced), glomerular lesions (rare), and vascular lesions make up most of intrinsic renal failure cases. Sepsis can also cause direct tubular injury.

   a. **Acute tubular necrosis.** Most common cause of intrinsic renal disease and can be secondary to shock, dehydration, toxins, sepsis, perinatal asphyxia, cardiac surgery, ischemic or hypoxic insults, drugs, or intravenous (IV) contrast media. **Perinatal asphyxia is the most common cause of acute tubular necrosis.** A large percentage of infants with severe perinatal asphyxia have renal failure (25% of cases are oliguric and 15% are anuric). Prolonged prerenal failure that is not treated will progress to acute tubular necrosis.

   b. **Interstitial nephritis.** Either drug induced or idiopathic.

   c. **Congenital renal anomalies.** Renal tubular dysgenesis, renal agenesis (Potter syndrome), renal cysts, congenital nephrotic syndrome, or hypoplastic or dysplastic kidneys. **Bilateral renal agenesis** presents with no urine since birth and is rare (1 in 4000 livebirths), autosomal dominant, probably multifactorial genetic disorder in which there is absence of both kidneys, bladder, and urine in the baby. It is more common in male infants. There is oligohydramnios in the mother and pulmonary hypoplasia in the infant. **Potter sequence** is a term used to describe the atypical physical appearance of decreased amniotic fluid secondary to multiple reasons, one being bilateral renal agenesis (pulmonary hypoplasia, low-set ears, deformity in 1 or both feet).

   d. **Infections.** Acute pyelonephritis, sepsis, gram-negative infections, candidiasis, and intrauterine infections (toxoplasmosis, cytomegalovirus, syphilis).

   e. **Renal vascular events.** Bilateral renal vascular thrombosis, severe renal arterial thrombosis, and bilateral renal vein thrombosis can all cause intrinsic renal failure. Ischemic or hypoxic insults (twin-to-twin transfusion, abruptio placentae, or perinatal asphyxia) can cause renal cortical necrosis. Disseminated intravascular coagulation can also cause intrinsic AKI.

   f. **Nephrotoxic medications.** Nephrotoxic medications are commonly used in the NICU, with 1 study stating that 87% of VLBW neonates were exposed to a minimum of 1 nephrotoxic medication for an average of 14 days. Aminoglycosides, amphotericin, and radiocontrast agents cause intrinsic renal failure.

   g. **Endogenous toxins (rare).** Uric acid (uric acid nephropathy), myoglobin, free hemoglobin.

3. **Postrenal acute kidney injury (~3%; obstructive, where urine is formed but not passed).** More common in newborn infants than in older infants and caused by a mechanical or functional obstruction to the flow of urine. The obstruction causes AKI if the urinary flow is blocked in both kidneys. The obstruction can be

in the upper tract, such as bilateral ureteropelvic junction obstruction, or lower tract, such as posterior urethral valves.

   a. **Neurogenic bladder from myelomeningocele or medications** such as pancuronium or heavy sedation.

   b. **Obstruction for any reason in a solitary kidney.**

   c. **Meatal stenosis (usually males).**

   d. **Congenital malformations:** Urethral stricture, posterior urethral valves (males only; may be complicated by bladder rupture), primary vesicoureteral reflux, imperforate prepuce, urethral diverticulum, ureteropelvic junction obstruction, uterovesical obstruction, megacystic megaureter, Eagle-Barrett syndrome (vesicoureteral reflux).

   e. **Extrinsic compression/tumors** (eg, sacrococcygeal teratoma), neonatal hematocolpos (imperforate hymen).

   f. **Drugs.** Certain medications (eg, acyclovir, ciprofloxacin, methotrexate, sulfonamides) can precipitate within the tubules and cause obstruction. Morphine can cause functional bladder outlet obstruction.

   g. **Intrinsic obstruction:** Renal calculi, systemic candidiasis with bilateral ureteropelvic fungal bezoar formation (fungal balls causing obstruction).

   h. **Spontaneous or delivery-associated rupture of the bladder** with anuric renal insufficiency.

H. Chronic kidney disease. Chronic kidney disease is the gradual loss of kidney function (decreased renal function); it can initially present as AKI and progress to permanent renal failure. Neonatal CKD has an incidence of 1 in 10,000 live births. Causes include polycystic kidney disease (autosomal recessive and autosomal dominant), obstructive uropathy (eg, posterior urethral valves), hypoplastic or dysplastic kidney, glomerular disease, cortical necrosis, renal vascular thrombosis, genetic disorders, and unknown etiology. See Section IV.G.

IV. Database

  A. Family history. Any history of diabetes? Any history of urinary tract disease in other family members? History of polycystic kidney disease/congenital nephrotic syndrome may indicate chronic kidney failure rather than AKI.

  B. Detailed clinical history (prenatal, maternal, delivery, postnatal). Review for oligohydramnios, genetic renal disorders, and list of maternal/postnatal nephrotoxic medications. Was there any risk of infection? Did bleeding occur during the delivery? Did perinatal asphyxia occur? Was there maternal hypovolemia? Was there a prenatal ultrasound? Was it abnormal? Was the fetal heart rate monitoring normal? Is the infant premature? Did the infant require resuscitation? What were the Apgar scores?

  C. Physical examination. Gestational age assessment should be done. First, determine the state of hydration. It is important to evaluate the volume status to distinguish hypovolemia from hypervolemia. Tachycardia and low blood pressure may indicate hypovolemia. What is the body weight? (Weight loss indicates negative fluid balance, whereas weight gain indicates retained fluid.) Is the infant dehydrated? Is there depressed/sunken fontanelle? Is there evidence of congestive heart failure? Is the infant edematous? Does the infant have hypertension (renal disease) or hypotension (decreased renal perfusion)? Examination of the abdomen may reveal bladder distention (bladder outlet obstruction), abdominal masses, or ascites (ruptured obstructed urinary tract). Signs of renal disorders (eg, Potter facies [low-set ears, inner canthal crease]) should be noted. **Dysmorphic features suggestive of renal disease** include single umbilical artery, hypospadias, anorectal abnormalities, vertebral anomalies, abnormal ears, and esophageal atresia. Urinary ascites may be seen with posterior urethral valves. Oligohydramnios suggests possible renal problems. Does the infant have wide-set eyes; parrot beak nose; receding chin; excess dehydrated skin; large, low-set, floppy ears lacking cartilage; or deformities of the hands and feet (bilateral renal agenesis)?

1. **Prerenal acute kidney injury.** Signs of volume depletion (tachycardia and hypotension).
2. **Intrinsic acute kidney injury.** Edema, signs of congestive heart failure, hypertension. Palpable kidneys may mean polycystic kidney, hydronephrosis, or tumors.
3. **Postrenal acute kidney injury.** Poor urinary stream, enlarged bladder, and dribbling of urine; urinary ascites with rupture.

D. **Laboratory studies.** The following laboratory tests can help establish the diagnosis in cases of low urine output.
1. **Serum creatinine.** This is the most widely used test for AKI and to monitor renal function. Remember, creatinine at birth and the first 3 days of life reflects maternal creatinine, and it takes a couple of days to reach equilibrium. The use of creatinine in the first 48 to 72 hours to assess renal function (specifically for AKI diagnosis or GFR alteration) is not reliable. In addition, the SCr may not increase until after 25% to 50% of kidney function is lost. SCr is a marker of kidney function, not kidney damage, so it takes some time for the SCr to increase after the insult (48–72 hours). The National Kidney Disease Education Program recently created a creatinine standardization program to reduce error variation (Table 73–2).
2. **Serum electrolytes, serum osmolality, and blood urea nitrogen also help to evaluate renal function and volume status.** Hyponatremia can be seen because of decreased excretion of water and SIADH. An increased blood urea nitrogen (BUN) and BUN-to-creatinine ratio >30 are seen in prerenal oliguria. A BUN-to-creatinine ratio of <20 can be seen in intrinsic renal damage. Electrolytes can be abnormal, especially potassium (hyperkalemia), with renal failure. Hypokalemia can be seen in the recovering stage of AKI. Dilutional hyponatremia is commonly seen in AKI. In SIADH one will see hyponatremia and hypoosmolality.
3. **Calcium and phosphate levels.** Hypocalcemia and hyperphosphatemia can be seen.
4. **Complete blood count and platelet count.** An abnormal complete blood count can be seen in sepsis. Thrombocytopenia or polycythemia can be seen in bilateral renal vein thrombosis.
5. **Urinalysis and urine microscopy.** Most likely normal in prerenal disease (may see few hyaline casts) and postrenal disease. Microscopic hematuria and trace glucosuria may be normal. Protein in the urine can be normal, especially in a premature infant. The amount of protein increases in the urine with decreasing gestational age.
   a. **White blood cells** suggest urinary tract infection
   b. **Red blood cells, tubular cells, granular casts, renal tubular epithelial cells, and proteinuria** suggest intrinsic renal disease.

Table 73–2. **PLASMA CREATININE VALUES AT BIRTH**

Gestational Age (weeks)	Creatinine
23–26	0.77–1.05 mg/dL (73.1–92.8 μmol/L)
27–29	0.76–1.02 mg/dL (67.2–90.2 μmol/L)
30–32	0.70–0.80 mg/dL (61.9–70.7 μmol/L)
33–45	0.77–0.90 mg/dL (73.1–79.6 μmol/L)

Reproduced with permission from Singer SA: Acute Renal Failure in the Neonate, *NeoReviews.* 2010 May;11(5):e243-e251.

    c. **Protein in the urine** may indicate glomerular disease.

    d. **Renal tubular epithelia cells and granular (muddy brown), cellular, and tubular casts** can be seen in acute tubular necrosis.

    e. **Red blood cell casts** can be seen in glomerulonephritis.

    f. **Free or form casts** can be seen with ischemia or a nephrotoxic insult.

  6. **Arterial blood pH.** A metabolic acidosis can be seen in anything that causes hypovolemia, hypoperfusion, or hypotension, such as sepsis.

  7. **Urinary indices.** See Table 86–2. BUN-to-creatinine ratio, fractional excretion of sodium (FE_{Na}), urinary sodium, urine specific gravity, urine-to-plasma creatinine ratio, urine osmolality, fractional excretion of urea, and renal failure index can help in determining whether the renal failure is **prenatal or renal (intrinsic) disease. FE_{Na} varies inversely with gestational and postnatal age** and is difficult to interpret in premature infants. In term infants, a value <2% is seen in prerenal AKI and a value >2.5% is seen in intrinsic AKI. In preterm infants, the following have been used: <2% for prerenal AKI; for intrinsic AKI, FE_{Na} >3% in infants >31 weeks' gestation and FE_{Na} >6% in infants 29 to 30 weeks' gestation. Urine sodium and osmolality can be helpful in ruling out SIADH.

  8. **Diagnostic indices related to acute kidney injury.** Besides the urinary indices discussed earlier, response to fluid challenge (increase in urine output suggests prerenal cause; no change suggests intrinsic renal disease or postrenal obstruction) and renal/abdominal ultrasonography may be helpful (normal in prerenal AKI and may be abnormal in AKI).

  9. **Biomarkers of early detection of acute kidney injury in neonates.** Biomarkers are usually abnormally expressed proteins in renal structural or tissue injury. They allow for earlier identification of neonates with AKI, before the 48 hours it takes SCr to rise. The 2 most often studied urinary biomarkers in neonates are neutrophil gelatinase–associated lipocalin and cystatin C, both which show higher sensitivity than creatinine. Many other biomarkers are under study. Some of the serum and urine levels of biomarkers are early predictive biomarkers for AKI (serum and urine neutrophil gelatinase–associated lipocalin and cystatin C, urinary interleukin-18, serum cystatin C, kidney injury molecule-1). These markers in the urine and/or serum are higher in AKI and may be predictive for AKI. Some of the biomarkers correlate with drug-induced AKI. The use of "omics" (genomics, proteomics, metabolomics) in neonatal nephrology is increasing.

E. **Imaging and other studies**

  1. **Renal ultrasonography with Doppler flow studies of the bladder, kidneys, and ureters** should be done on any newborn with oliguria or anuria. It is normal in prerenal AKI and may be abnormal in renal AKI and postrenal AKI. It will rule out urinary tract obstruction and help evaluate for other CAKUTs, renal vascular abnormalities, and bladder outlet obstruction. It can help one differentiate AKI from CKD (autosomal polycystic kidney disease, renal hypodysplasia). **Doppler examination** of renal blood flow can diagnose renal vascular thrombosis.

  2. **Abdominal radiograph studies** may reveal ascites or masses. Spina bifida or an absent sacrum suggests neurogenic bladder.

  3. **Voiding cystourethrography** can help diagnose lesions of the lower tract that cause obstruction if bladder outlet obstruction is suspected. It can also rule out vesicoureteral reflux.

  4. **Radionuclide renal scanning** may be helpful in obstruction.

  5. **Cardiac echocardiogram** looking at left ventricular output may be necessary to help access intravascular fluid status.

F. **Acute kidney injury definition and staging.** There has been no standard definition of AKI in neonates. Originally, AKI was defined as a SCr ≥1.5 mg/dL. There have been multiple definitions including the Acute Kidney Injury Network criteria;

the Risk, Injury, Failure, Loss, and End-Stage Kidney Disease criteria; and the Kidney Disease: Improving Global Outcomes (KDIGO) criteria. **Much work has been done to standardize the definition and criteria.** The National Institute of Diabetes and Digestive and Kidney Diseases workshop in 2013 recommended that the neonatal KDIGO criteria be used for clinical care (see Table 86–1). Further studies are needed to address gaps in this evolving definition (use of biomarkers, use of urine output change, use of accurate SCr).

G. **Kidney Disease: Improving Global Outcomes classification of chronic kidney disease in infants <2 years old.** The GFR, which is low in neonatal life, increases after birth and reaches approximately 20 mL/min/1.73 m² at 1 month of age. Calculated GFR is based on SCr and is compared to age-appropriate values to determine renal impairment in CKD. A normal GFR is one that is ≤1 standard deviation (SD) below the mean. Infants with a moderately reduced GFR have a GFR >1 SD to ≤2 SDs below the mean. Infants with severely reduced GFR have a GFR >2 SDs below the mean. The KDIGO guidelines recommend that an infant with a GFR >1 SD below the mean is a red flag and the infant should be monitored.

V. **Plan.** If sufficient time has passed and it has been determined the bladder is not palpable, the following approaches are recommended.

A. **Fluid challenge for diagnosis and initial management.** A fluid challenge can be given without evidence of heart failure or fluid overload; 10 to 20 mL/kg of crystalloid (normal saline preferred) IV over 30 to 120 minutes. Colloid is only recommended if there is an indication such as bleeding or hypoalbuminemia. If there is no response, this can be repeated once. An increase in urine output of ≥1 to 2 mL/kg/h indicates a **prenal cause of AKI due to hypovolemia.** No increase in urine output suggests **intrinsic renal disease or postrenal obstruction.** If the infant **shows signs of fluid overload** after the fluid challenge, consider cardiac disease or third spacing (eg, sepsis, hypoalbuminemia, hydrops fetalis, or hepatic failure nephrotic syndrome).

B. **Mild dehydration.** For mild dehydration with decreased urine output (but no evidence of renal failure based on laboratory findings or clinical examination), only an increase in fluids (IV) or feedings may be necessary. For an infant only on breast feeding who is dehydrated, supplementation with formula may be considered.

C. **SIADH.** It is important to identify and treat the underlying cause of SIADH. The treatment is to gradually increase the sodium level by promoting free water excretion by fluid restriction. Treatment ultimately depends on the level of the sodium and whether seizures are present. See Chapter 69 on hyponatremia for treatment details.

D. **Initial evaluation if acute kidney injury is suspected**
   1. **Bladder catheterization** to determine if urine is being made and to rule out lower urinary tract obstruction. It will not help in renal dysfunction or upper urinary tract obstruction. It may be helpful to keep an **indwelling catheter** in the short term for accurate and strict intake and output, even though indwelling catheters are seldom used in neonates.
   2. **Evaluation of laboratory and ultrasound results.** (See also Table 86–2.) Based on the laboratory results and ultrasound, identify whether the infant has prenal, renal, or postrenal failure.

E. **Initial acute kidney injury management.** Nephrology consultation is recommended.
   1. **Identify high-risk infants** (any newborn with asphyxia, on ECMO, with sepsis, or requiring cardiac surgery; any sick near-term or term infant; any preterm ELBW or VLBW infant; or any infant with CAKUT) and monitor them very closely.
   2. **Be aware of the prophylaxis for asphyxiated infants at risk for acute kidney injury per Kidney Disease: Improving Global Outcomes guidelines.** Adenosine receptor antagonists (theophylline) inhibit adenosine-induced vasoconstriction

and may help prevent AKI. Give a single dose of theophylline (5–8 mg/kg) early after birth since it is associated with better kidney function.

3. **Caffeine in preterm neonates** is associated with a decreased incidence and severity of AKI. Further studies to focus on timing and dosage are needed.

4. **Identify and mitigate any risk factors**
   a. **Evaluate the infant's medications.** Be aware of any nephrotoxic medications. The most common medications used in the NICU that are nephrotoxic are ibuprofen, indomethacin, vancomycin, aminoglycosides, amphotericin B, and acyclovir. Adjust doses and discontinue if possible. Pharmacist support in adjusting levels can be useful.
   b. **Be aware of and treat any reversible conditions early on** that may result in hypotension and poor renal perfusion. These may include **sepsis** (antibiotics, fluid correction, and vasopressors), **PDA** (medical or surgical closure), **NEC** (IV fluids, vasopressors), **hypovolemia** (fluid replacement), **hemorrhage** (IV fluids, packed red blood cell transfusion), and **congenital heart disease** (depends on the cause) (refer to disease- and condition-specific chapters).

5. **Fluid management.** Try to maintain fluid and electrolyte balance until renal function returns.
   a. **Record strict intake and output.** Weigh the infant every 12 hours. Urine output can also be measured by weighing diapers every 3 hours. Remember that the measurement may be inaccurate because of evaporation by radiant warmers. Infants lose much of their body weight the first week of life. Weight gain can indicate fluid overload, whereas weight loss can indicate a need for more fluids. **Tachycardia and low blood pressure** indicate hypovolemia.
   b. **Replace insensible fluid losses (note that these may be increased with radiant warmer):**
      i. **Term infants:** 40 to 50 mL/kg/d.
      ii. **Preterm infants <750 g:** 100 to 150mL/kg/d.
      iii. **Preterm infants 750 to 1000 g:** 60 to 70 mL/kg/d.
      iv. **Preterm infants 1000 to 1250 g:** 35 to 65 mL/kg/d.
   c. **Avoid excessive fluid administration or dehydration.** Fluid overload with oliguria carries a poor prognosis. The majority of cases of oliguria are secondary to inadequate fluid or an increase in the loss of fluid. Diuretics, gastroschisis, and meningomyelocele (excessive insensible water loss), fluid restriction due to PDA, and pulmonary edema can all lead to fluid loss that needs to be addressed in these infants.

6. **Give a trial of diuretics (eg, furosemide) in oliguric neonates with acute kidney injury.** Loop diuretics are preferred over osmotic diuretics. It is an acceptable treatment despite lack of evidence in neonates. Diuretics are often used to maintain urine output. If the infant is unresponsive to diuretics, consideration of renal replacement therapy early on is recommended. With use, observe for electrolyte imbalances (hyponatremia, hypokalemia, and hypocalcemia) and a decrease in intravascular volume. Ototoxicity can occur with use of furosemide (especially with aminoglycosides). Furosemide can also be used if the infant has hypertension due to fluid overload.

7. **Management of hypotension.** (See also Chapter 70.) Blood pressure should be monitored closely. If hypotension is due to hypovolemia, fluid administration needs to be given. Dopamine can be used as a first-line vasopressor for treating hypotension. At lower doses, it improves renal perfusion and transiently improves SCr and urinary output. Dobutamine can be used in cases that do not respond to dopamine.

8. **Avoid any electrolyte and metabolic acidosis abnormalities.** Follow electrolytes closely for early changes and treat appropriately: dilutional hyponatremia, hyperglycemia, hyperkalemia, hyperphosphatemia, hypomagnesemia, hypocalcemia,

acidosis, and uremia. Restrict potassium unless there is hypokalemia. For metabolic acidosis, treatment with bicarbonate (*controversial*) or chronic oral replacement with acetate may be necessary.

9. **Nutritional management.** Because of an increasing BUN in AKI, protein was historically restricted to try to decrease the BUN. Fluid restriction also can contribute to lack of nutrition in these infants. It is best for the infant to receive protein early on to prevent growth failure and other poor neurodevelopmental outcomes. Maintain a minimum protein intake (1–2 g/kg/d). Human milk and formulas such as Similac PM 60/40 (low phosphate and renal solute load) are preferred for enteral nutrition. Parenteral nutrition may be necessary in critically ill infants.

F. **Specific management of prerenal, intrinsic, and postrenal failure**

1. **Prerenal failure.** The goal is to restore and maintain adequate renal perfusion. Because the kidneys are normal, prerenal failure is reversible once renal perfusion is restored. However, if not corrected, intrinsic renal tubular damage can occur.

   a. **Treat the specific cause** (eg, sepsis, NEC).

   b. **Provide volume resuscitation to restore renal perfusion.** Depending on how much fluid was given during the fluid challenge, another fluid challenge may be necessary to achieve euvolemia. Usual dose is 10 to 20 mL/kg of isotonic saline solution over 1 to 2 hours.

   c. **Maintain adequate volume maintenance** and replacement for any losses.

   d. **Dopamine.** Use of inotropic agents may be indicated in prerenal failure caused by hypoxia, acidosis, or indomethacin or in infants who develop hypotension. Renal dose of dopamine (1–3 mcg/kg/min) to improve renal perfusion is advocated by some, but no studies show that it improves survival. It increases urine output but does not prevent renal dysfunction or death. Cochrane review states that there is not enough evidence to give dopamine to prevent renal dysfunction specifically in indomethacin-treated preterm infants.

   e. **Furosemide.** May be indicated if there is oliguria and volume overload. Diuretics can help in fluid management but do not change the course of AKI. Furosemide (1–2 mg/kg/dose) can increase urine flow, but limit doses due to ototoxicity, especially if there is no response noted.

2. **Intrinsic renal disease.** Supportive measures, treatment of the specific cause, and recovery and prognosis depend on the etiology.

   a. **Discontinue any nephrotoxic medications.**

   b. **Restrict fluid intake, and only replace insensible losses plus urine output.** Consider potassium intake restriction.

   c. **Follow serum sodium, potassium, calcium, and phosphate, and acid-base balance.** Infants with AKI can have hyponatremia (usually dilutional), hyperkalemia, hypocalcemia, hyperphosphatemia, and metabolic acidosis.

   d. **Consider low-dose dopamine to increase renal blood flow (*controversial*).** See Section V.F.1.d.

   e. **Consider diuretics (eg, furosemide) if fluid overload.** Limit doses due to ototoxicity. See Section V.F.1.e.

   f. **Follow blood pressure.** Mild hypertension can occur.

   g. **For bilateral renal artery thrombosis:** Thrombolysis/thrombectomy is indicated in refractory hypertension.

3. **Postrenal acute kidney injury.** If an obstruction has been identified by renal ultrasound, it should immediately be treated to relieve it. The AKI can usually be reversed by relieving the obstruction.

   a. **Pediatric urologic consultation** should be obtained.

   b. **If obstruction is distal to the bladder.** Perform initial bladder catheterization. Surgical vesicostomy may be indicated.

    c. **If obstruction is proximal to the bladder.** Urologic surgical intervention should be considered (eg, nephrostomy tubes or cutaneous ureterostomy).

    d. **Neurogenic bladder.** Initially managed with catheterization.

    e. **Assessment of fluid balance** should be done.

    f. **Medications.** Medications that cause urinary retention should be discontinued.

    g. **Consider urinary tract infection prophylaxis** with antibiotics.

4. **Renal replacement therapy** replaces the normal blood-filtering function of kidneys. It is technically more difficult in the newborn, especially the VLBW infant, and is not routinely done. It also has a high rate of complications. There are **3 modes of therapy**: peritoneal dialysis, intermittent hemodialysis, and continuous renal replacement therapy. The most common modes of therapy in the neonate include peritoneal dialysis and continuous renal replacement therapy (CRRT). It is the **therapy of choice for severe cases of AKI.**

    a. **Indications are not absolute but include:** Refractory acidosis, uremia, electrolyte abnormalities (hyperkalemia not responding to usual medical management, high BUN and creatinine), fluid overload, metabolic disorders (hyperammonemia), congenital anomalies that result in end-stage renal disease (eg, polycystic/multicystic kidneys, oxalosis, CAKUT, inborn errors of metabolism, angiotensin receptor blockade fetopathy), and inability to provide adequate nutrition.

    b. **Modes of renal replacement therapy**

        i. **Peritoneal dialysis** is the **preferred method for neonates**, even in VLBW neonates. It is less difficult to do than CRRT. If peritoneal dialysis cannot be done (due to abdominal wall defect, previous abdominal surgery, hyperammonemia [ammonia best removed by ECMO or hemofiltration], anasarca, significant ascites, skin infections, or other causes), **venovenous CRRT** (hemofiltration-based dialysis modality) can be used.

        ii. **Continuous renal replacement therapy** is challenging in neonates. Current CRRT machines approved only for patients >20 kg are being used in patients <5 kg "off label." CRRT machines are needed with lower extracorporeal volume to provide safe renal support to small infants. There are neonatal CRRT machines (CARPEDIEM and Nidus), but they are only used outside of the United States. CRRT in neonates is still used only after medical management has failed, even though in pediatrics it is being used earlier in managing infants with AKI because it helps to maintain electrolyte homeostasis, decreases hypervolemia, and helps to provide adequate nutrition.

G. **Acute kidney injury follow-up.** Infants with oliguric AKI have a higher mortality rate (up to 89%) than infants with nonoliguric AKI. Any infant who had AKI is at increased risk (almost 50%) for CKD. The risk factors that carry a poor prognosis in AKI are low gestational age, low birthweight, oliguria, anuria, and multiorgan involvement. Studies show that evidence of renal dysfunction can be seen in childhood in neonates who were born VLBW. In fact, renal dysfunction can occur 3 to 5 years after the episode of AKI. These infants should be followed closely after discharge, with blood pressure closely monitored. Recommendations from KDIGO practice guidelines state that all infants who had AKI should be evaluated **after 3 months** for CKD.

H. **Chronic kidney disease.** Any infant who has a GFR value >1 SD below the mean needs to be monitored closely for CKD. Management focuses on replacing renal functions: 1, 25-hydroxylation of vitamin D, erythropoietin, fluid and electrolyte management, growth and nutrition, and renal replacement therapy for end-stage renal disease.

74 Pneumoperitoneum

I. **Problem.** <u>A pneumoperitoneum is seen on an abdominal radiograph.</u> A pneumoperitoneum is an abnormal collection of free air in the peritoneal cavity. The air can be secondary to perforation of the gastrointestinal (GI) tract (most common, approximately 90% of cases) or from the respiratory tract, or it can be idiopathic with no known cause. **Necrotizing enterocolitis (NEC) with perforation** is the most common cause of a pneumoperitoneum in the neonate, and it carries a high mortality rate. Approximately 78.5% of pneumoperitoneums were secondary to NEC; therefore, a neonate with a pneumoperitoneum requires immediate evaluation and treatment because early recognition is important in successful management. **It is important to note that a diagnosis of a pneumoperitoneum does not always imply a GI perforation.** Careful assessment of each case can limit unnecessary laparotomies and their surgical complications.

II. **Immediate questions**

   A. **Is a tension pneumoperitoneum present?** An emergency situation, this occurs when there is a large amount of air that impairs diaphragmatic excursion. A tension pneumoperitoneum can cause significant lung compression, severe respiratory distress, compression of the vena cava, and impaired venous return with cardiovascular compromise. If present, an emergency therapeutic paracentesis should be done (see Chapter 40).

   B. **Are signs of a pneumoperitoneum present?** These findings can include abdominal distension (most common sign), respiratory distress, deteriorating blood gas levels, and a decrease in blood pressure.

   C. **Were signs of necrotizing enterocolitis present before?** If so, the pneumoperitoneum is most likely to be associated with GI tract perforation. Bowel perforation typically occurs at a median interval of 1 day after clinical presentation of NEC. Risk factors for NEC are gestational age <32 weeks, birth weight <1500 g, and enteral feeding.

   D. **Does the infant have any dysmorphic features or congenital anomalies?** An infant with any dysmorphic features or congenital anomalies increases the likelihood that the perforation is GI in origin.

   E. **Are any signs of air leak present?** If a pneumomediastinum, pulmonary interstitial emphysema, or pneumothorax is present, the peritoneal air collection may be of respiratory tract origin.

   F. **Is mechanical ventilation being used?** High peak inspiratory pressures greater than a mean of 34 cm H_2O can be associated with a pneumoperitoneum.

   G. **Were antenatal nonsteroidal anti-inflammatory medications used? Is the infant presently on steroids or indomethacin?** These have all been associated with GI perforation.

   H. **Was an antenatal ultrasound done? Were any gastrointestinal anomalies detected?** If an antenatal ultrasound showed any GI anomalies, then the pneumoperitoneum is more likely to be from a GI perforation.

   I. **Did the infant recently undergo abdominal surgery or an invasive procedure such as paracentesis?** Intra-abdominal air is normal in the immediate postoperative period following abdominal surgery and usually resolves without treatment. Paracentesis can perforate a hollow organ.

III. **Differential diagnosis.** A pneumoperitoneum most commonly develops **secondary to perforation of the GI tract** (spontaneous, secondary from underlying GI disease, or traumatic). It can also be secondary **from the chest** (respiratory causes: air leak with or without mechanical ventilation) **or idiopathic, from no known cause** (no respiratory or GI cause found), or it can be a **normal immediate postoperative finding**. In a neonate, unless the infant is on high ventilator settings and has an air leak, **the cause is GI perforation until proven otherwise**. Some classify pneumoperitoneum into **medical (nonsurgical)** versus **surgical,** based on the need for surgical intervention. Some classify all pneumoperitoneums that are not surgical with various terms such as nonsurgical, asymptomatic, benign, misleading, or idiopathic. Some authors have suggested these terms should be changed to **benign,** indicating that their management is not surgery.

A. **Pneumoperitoneum associated with gastrointestinal perforation**

1. **Spontaneous intestinal perforation.** There is no demonstrable cause (no obvious GI disease, no evidence of trauma or obstruction that causes the perforation). **Proposed etiologies** include local ischemia in the perinatal period (from asphyxia or shock) or from noncommunication of the right and left gastroepiploic arteries, trauma during pregnancy or delivery, sepsis, prematurity, excessive gastric acidity, lack of intestinal Cajal cells (gastric perforation), maternal use of steroids or cocaine, or congenital defects in the muscular wall of the stomach. Spontaneous perforation occurs most commonly in the terminal ileum in premature infants (spontaneous intestinal perforation [SIP]) or in the stomach (preterm and term infants); it rarely occurs elsewhere in the GI tract.

   a. **Spontaneous gastric perforation.** Occurs most commonly between the second and seventh days of life in both full-term and preterm infants. It is more common in males and African American babies. Infants present with sudden abdominal distension, respiratory distress, vomiting, lethargy, and a massive pneumoperitoneum. Perinatal stress, prematurity, and postnatal steroid use are risk factors. Many of these infants have sepsis.

   b. **Spontaneous intestinal perforation.** Second most common presentation of neonatal intestinal perforation. **The single intestinal perforation** occurs primarily in the terminal ileum (rarely in the jejunum and transverse and descending colon) in infants <28 weeks' gestational age, with low birthweight <1500 g (2%–3%) or <1000 g (5%). Presentation is within the first week (hypotension and abdominal distension), it is more common in males, and is independent of feeding. There is no pneumatosis intestinalis and mortality rate is lower than with NEC. Prematurity is a major risk factor. Early exposure to postnatal steroids and postnatal exposure of indomethacin combined with steroids increases the risk of SIP. Conflicting evidence exists on whether indomethacin alone increases the risk of SIP. SIP is frequently associated with systemic candidiasis or coagulase-negative *Staphylococcus.*

   c. **Spontaneous colonic perforations.** These can occur but are very rare. They are more common in preterm infants and very difficult to diagnose. Signs include significant abdominal and scrotal distension, vomiting, cyanosis, respiratory distress, and tachypnea. Most infants have a massive pneumoperitoneum.

   d. **Other gastrointestinal perforations.** Isolated perforations can occur elsewhere in the intestine, including the appendix, cecum, and Meckel diverticulum.

   e. **Medications associated with spontaneous perforation** include indomethacin and steroids. A meta-analysis of the effect of early treatment (<96 hours) with high doses of steroids for chronic lung disease showed an increased risk of spontaneous GI perforation. **Gastroduodenal perforation** has been associated with steroid therapy. Combined therapy (early postnatal indomethacin and glucocorticoids) increases the risk of **SIP**.

   f. **Other causes.** Following exchange transfusion, perforation of the small and large intestine can occur. **Embolic phenomenon secondary to an umbilical artery catheter** can also contribute to perforation.

2. **Secondary perforations.** These are caused by an underlying disease: secondary to a GI disease process or an obstruction in the GI tract.

   a. **Necrotizing enterocolitis.** NEC is the most common cause of gastrointestinal perforation in neonates and is the most common cause of secondary perforation. It typically presents later in premature infants (second to third week) and after initiation of formula feeding. It carries a high mortality (up to 76% in premature infants). The perforation occurs because of local inflammation and intestinal necrosis leading to destruction of the bowel wall. The most commonly affected areas of perforation are the terminal ileum (MC ileocecal region) and proximal ascending colon, although any part of the GI tract may be involved. There is conflicting data on whether indomethacin increases the risk of NEC with intestinal perforation. **Perforation in NEC** can also be caused by a rupture of gas-filled cysts within the bowel wall (pneumatosis intestinalis). This diagnosis is a radiologic diagnosis (one sees linear or circular radiolucencies) because there are no clinical signs. It is most common in the colon but can also occur in the small bowel or stomach. It is important to note that pneumatosis intestinalis is a hallmark of NEC, but can also be seen in intestinal obstruction, vascular compromise, and milk intolerance.

b. **Gastrointestinal obstruction.** GI obstruction causes increasing intraluminal pressure, which can cause a perforation proximal to the obstruction. This can occur anywhere in the GI tract. Causes in the neonate include any GI atresia (esophageal atresia with tracheoesophageal fistula, duodenal/pylorus atresia, small/large intestine or anal atresia, and others), meconium ileus/plug, duplication cyst, small left colon syndrome, obstructive bands, Hirschsprung disease, and anorectal malformations (imperforate anus, incarcerated hernia, and others). Bowel perforation occurs in approximately 3% to 4% of infants with Hirschsprung disease.

c. **Gastritis or peptic ulcer disease.** Perforation can be the initial presentation of ulcer disease. Perforations of the stomach (most common), duodenum, pylorus, or esophagus can occur.

d. **Other rare causes.** Malrotation with midgut volvulus, omphalocele, ruptured appendix, gastroschisis, mesenteric thrombosis, perforated Meckel diverticulum, or idiopathic gastric necrosis.

3. **Traumatic perforations.** An iatrogenic pneumoperitoneum can be caused by an intervention. Most gastric perforations are secondary to nasogastric (NG) or orogastric (OG) tube placement or vigorous bag-and-mask or positive-pressure ventilation.

a. **Normal transient finding following laparotomy or laparoscopy.**

b. **Nasogastric tube trauma.** Most gastric perforations are along the greater curvature due to trauma by vigorous NG/OG tube placement. Use of a soft silastic feeding tube may reduce this risk. An NG tube in an unusual position on x-ray (eg, right upper quadrant) indicates a possible perforation.

c. **Intubation trauma.** During an intubation, the endotracheal tube (ETT) can be inadvertently placed in the esophagus and then through the posterior wall of the stomach. If the ETT on chest x-ray is seen more distally than expected, consider intubation trauma.

d. **Bag-and-mask/positive-pressure ventilation.** Traumatic **gastric perforation** can occur from vigorous bag-and-mask ventilation or be due to positive-pressure ventilation. Resuscitation with oxygen under pressure in patients with distal pyloric or duodenal obstruction can result in a perforation.

e. **Neonatal rectal perforations of the sigmoid colon or rectum** can be caused by a rectal thermometer or rectal tubes. Because of the shape of the neonatal rectum, when a rectal thermometer is placed to a depth of 2 cm, it impinges on the anterior wall. Therefore, insert a rectal thermometer <2 cm. An attempt to push it any further may result in perforation. **Enema-induced (colonic lavage) perforations** occur in the anterior wall of the rectum or rectosigmoid. A common factor in these colonic lavages in one study was inexperienced staff performing these procedures.

f. **Improperly performed suprapubic bladder aspiration or paracentesis** can perforate a hollow organ.

      g. Umbilical vein catheterization can cause perforation of Meckel diverticulum.

      h. Aerophagia (swallowing air) secondary to prolonged crying may cause gastric perforation. (There is a case report on an infant who had a circumcision with prolonged crying that may have caused a gastric rupture.)

  B. Pneumoperitoneum associated with a respiratory disorder (eg, pulmonary interstitial emphysema, pneumomediastinum, or pneumothorax). A pulmonary air leak, with or without mechanical ventilation or continuous positive airway pressure, can result in a pneumoperitoneum. It can be secondary to barotrauma in ventilated neonates with severe respiratory disease. A thoracic leak can dissect transdiaphragmatically or through the mediastinum along perivascular connective tissue to the abdominal cavity. Other pathways between the chest and abdomen include pleuroperitoneal fistula, retrograde path through pulmonary lymphatics, periaortic space, periesophageal space, or a congenital defect. *Note:* An infant can have a pneumoperitoneum from thoracic air dissection without evidence of a pulmonary air leak (pneumothorax or pneumomediastinum). In this case, an undetectable pulmonary rupture can occur with dissection into the peritoneal cavity. If there is a posterior pneumomediastinum, an air leak is probably the cause of the pneumoperitoneum.

  C. Idiopathic pneumoperitoneum. This is a pneumoperitoneum that has no identifiable cause, and there is no evidence of GI or respiratory pathology. It may be respiratory because a pulmonary rupture with a thoracic leak may not be apparent, or it may be GI because there could be a subclinical microperforation in a hollow viscus with no leakage of bowel contents.

  D. Pseudopneumoperitoneum occurs when there is a lucency with no free intraperitoneal air in the abdominal cavity. The lucency that mimics free air can be from a subphrenic fat pad, linear atelectasis, abnormal subphrenic anatomy, liver abscess, serosal enchancement after cardiac catheterization, transplacental transfer of nonionic contrast, gas-forming bacterial peritonitis (*Escherichia coli* [most common] *Pseudomonas, Clostridium, Staphylococcus, Streptococcus, Klebsiella, Candida*), subphrenic abscess, or Chilaiditi syndrome. **Chilaiditi syndrome,** a rare condition, is the interposition of the large intestine (usually gas filled transverse colon) between the liver and right hemidiaphragm; it can present with respiratory distress and can be misinterpreted as a true pneumoperitoneum.

IV. Database

  A. Physical examination. Although the clinical evaluation may not differentiate between respiratory or GI tract origin of the pneumoperitoneum, the examination should still focus on the pulmonary and abdominal aspects. **Abdominal distention (most common physical sign) and elevation of the diaphragm with increasing respiratory difficulty are hallmarks of a pneumoperitoneum.** Other signs and symptoms include vomiting (bilious), tachypnea, rectal bleeding, and failure or delay to pass meconium. **Is there respiratory compromise or unexplained tachypnea?** Large amounts of air in the abdominal cavity can impair diaphragmatic excursion and lung compression. Cardiovascular compromise can occur secondary to compression of the vena cava and impaired venous return. Feeding intolerance and poor activity can also be present. Is there a bluish-black discoloration of the abdominal wall (seen with SIP but not NEC)? **Scrotal swelling** may indicate gastric perforation (ie, **pneumoscrotum**) and can occur without significant abdominal distension. A pneumoscrotum can be secondary to a gastric perforation, perforation of Meckel diverticulum, or perforation of ileum secondary to atresia, or after aggressive resuscitation or mechanical ventilation.

  B. Laboratory studies

    1. Complete blood count and serum electrolytes. Elevation of the white blood cell count or a left shift may signify a GI tract perforation. Hyponatremia can be seen with NEC secondary to third spacing of fluid. Persistent or worsening thrombocytopenia can be indicative of bowel perforation.

2. **Arterial blood gas levels.** May reveal hypoxemia and increasing PCO_2 levels. Metabolic acidosis can be seen with peritonitis.
3. **Blood culture.** Should be obtained if bowel perforation or sepsis is suspected. Infants with bowel perforation can have a positive blood culture. In one study, 18 of 30 infants had a positive blood culture (*E coli* was the most common organism).
4. **C-reactive protein.** Correlates with the inflammatory response and may be increased in NEC.

C. **Imaging and other studies**
1. **Transillumination of the abdomen** with a cold fiberoptic light source can be done and acts as a useful tool for diagnosis, especially if radiographs are not readily available. Place the transilluminator in the left paramedian position and direct the probe toward the midline. If the peritoneal cavity lights up, the infant probably has a pneumoperitoneum (see Chapter 44).
2. **Radiographs.** Small amounts of air can be missed on a routine film; some infants have air, but it cannot be seen on x-ray. One study found a pneumoperitoneum in 63% of infants with GI perforation. Repeat radiographs frequently if air is suspected. Simple observation of free air is often sufficient, particularly if the air leak is large (see Figure 12–25). Supine films (some infants are too sick for an upright) are usually done. A **massive pneumoperitoneum** is suggestive of gastric or colonic perforation. Absence of pneumoperitoneum does not exclude perforation and may indicate gas reabsorption or nasogastric decompression.
   a. **Supine anteroposterior radiograph of the chest and abdomen.** The chest may show signs of air leak syndrome (pneumomediastinum or pneumothorax) if it is suspected that the intraperitoneal air is from the respiratory tract. The abdomen may show signs of NEC (pneumatosis intestinalis or portal venous gas; see Figures 12–26 and 12–27) or ileus. Air-fluid levels in the peritoneal cavity usually indicate ileus. SIP will have a pneumoperitoneum without pneumatosis intestinalis or portal venous gas. **Classically described x-ray findings pathognomonic of a pneumoperitoneum include the following:**
      i. **Right upper quadrant sign.** The most common finding is the presence of right upper quadrant subdiaphragmatic free air (collection of gas in the right upper quadrant adjacent to the liver, gas in the anterior subhepatic space).
      ii. **Doge's cap sign.** Air between the right kidney and liver. It is often the first sign and appears as an oval or triangular gas shadow.
      iii. **Cupola sign.** An inverted cup-shaped lucency (dome) of air accumulation that appears over the lower thoracic spine near the posterior part of the heart.
      iv. **Rigler sign (double wall sign).** Gas is seen on both sides of the bowel wall (the outer and inner walls of the bowel are seen). Normally only the inner wall of the bowel is seen. If the mean wall thickness of the bowel is >1 mm, it is a positive sign. If the thickness is ≤1 mm, it may be a false positive.
      v. **Falciform ligament sign.** Gas outlining the falciform ligament.
      vi. **Football sign.** A large oval radiolucency (gas outlining the peritoneal cavity) in the shape of an American football. It can also include when the falciform ligament is seen in the center as a vertical strip surrounded by gas (the radiographic appearance of pneumoperitoneum outlining the falciform ligament was renamed falciform ligament sign; see previous text). It appears as a white streak, which is surrounded by the oval lucency of a pneumoperitoneum. The football sign is most frequently seen in infants with spontaneous or iatrogenic gastric perforation.
      vii. **Inverted V sign.** Gas outlines the medial umbilical folds (umbilical arteries) on the supine radiograph.

      viii. **Saddle bag sign.** Spleen and liver are displaced downward toward the midline.

      ix. **Arcade sign.** Air is seen between bowel loops and creates triangular-shaped areas of gas.

      x. **A gasless abdomen.** May represent a perforation if there is no bowel gas to go into the peritoneal cavity (it is walled off).

      xi. **Persistent fixed dilated bowel loops with abnormal gas shadows (localized pseudocysts) on multiple films** on an abdominal x-ray may signify intestinal perforation.

   b. **Left lateral decubitus radiographic study of the abdomen.** With the right side up, the **left lateral decubitus study** is the best examination for the detection of free abdominal air; air (seen as a homogeneous lucency or streak-like lucencies) is seen over the liver if a perforation has occurred. This is also done to show smaller leaks not appreciated on the anteroposterior abdominal film. A lateral decubitus radiograph should be serially taken when NEC is suspected. **Lateral decubitus studies** have been shown to be more sensitive in detecting a pneumoperitoneum than upright view studies.

   c. **Upright view of the chest abdomen.** This will show air below the diaphragm but is rarely done because of the difficulty in positioning a sick infant.

3. **Ultrasound or color Doppler ultrasonography of the abdomen** can be used to detect free air, and some studies suggest it is more sensitive in the diagnosis of a pneumoperitoneum as compared to abdominal radiography. It can also diagnose free abdominal fluid, debris, and inflammatory masses. It may suggest NEC by visualizing pneumatosis intestinalis and portal venous air and can be obtained to assess ascites. The presence of intraperitoneal particulate matter strongly suggests perforation. **Complex ascites (ascites with debris) verifies bowel perforation.** Extraluminal calcifications usually indicate intrauterine intestinal perforation with intraperitoneal extravasation of meconium. It can also be used to diagnose NEC. (Central echogenic focus with hypoechoic rim can indicate necrotic bowel or presence of intermittent gas bubbles in the portal venous system and liver.) **Color Doppler studies** can detect bowel necrosis through altered blood flow.

4. **Computed tomography scan.** This may be necessary to better identify tiny free air in the intestinal wall such as to help better diagnose pneumatosis cystoides intestinalis.

5. **Paracentesis or diagnostic tap.** This can also help decide whether an infant needs to be surgically explored (eg, bilious or feculent fluid obtained). See Chapter 40.

   a. **Air.** Air obtained by paracentesis may be tested for its oxygen level. If the baby is receiving oxygen supplementation and the oxygen level is high (greater than room air, $FiO_2 = 0.21$), the air is probably from a respiratory tract leak. If the oxygen if similar to room air or lower, the air is probably from the GI tract.

   b. **Fluid (peritoneal lavage).** Fluid may be obtained by paracentesis if the diagnosis is still undetermined. If bilious or feculent (brownish) fluid is obtained, especially if bacteria are present on the Gram stain, the air is probably of GI tract origin. A positive microscopic smear of the fluid for white blood cells suggests peritonitis.

6. **Differentiate gastrointestinal perforation from nongastrointestinal perforation to guide treatment.** If the cause of the pneumoperitoneum is in doubt, attempts to distinguish between pneumoperitoneum from GI perforation and that of idiopathic etiology can be done using the following:

   a. **A table based on common criteria** to distinguish between a benign pneumoperitoneum (any pneumoperitoneum that is not caused by a GI perforation that requires only conservative management) and a pneumoperitoneum from a GI perforation (exploratory laparotomy) has been developed. See Table 74–1.

Table 74–1. CRITERIA TO DIFFERENTIATE BENIGN PNEUMOPERITONEUM FROM
PNEUMOPERITONEUM DUE TO GASTROINTESTINAL PERFORATION IN THE NEONATES

	Benign Pneumoperitoneum	GI Perforation
Birthweight	>1500 g	<1500 g
Gestational age	>32 weeks	<32 weeks
Feed	NPO	Fed
Age at diagnosis	Early, <5 days	Late, >5 days
Antenatal ultrasound	No GI anomalies detected	GI anomalies suspected/no antenatal care
Antenatal NSAID	None	Given
Postnatal steroids	None	Given
Postnatal indomethacin	None	Given
Family history	No history of GI anomalies/ Hirschsprung disease	History of GI anomalies/ Hirschsprung disease
General exam	No dysmorphic features No other congenital anomalies	Dysmorphic features Congenital anomalies present
Peritonitis signs	Absent	Present
Clinical status	Infant's status did not deteriorate by the time pneumoperitoneum was detected	Clinical status deteriorated
Pre–x-ray diagnosis	Line placement Part of chest x-ray Mild to moderate abdominal distension	Suspected NEC
X-ray findings	Absence of pneumatosis intestinalis No evidence of intestinal obstruction Free air in the abdomen Thoracic air leak	Pneumatosis intestinalis Intestinal obstruction Free air in the abdomen

GI, gastrointestinal; NEC, necrotizing enterocolitis; NPO, nothing by mouth; NSAID, nonsteroidal
anti-inflammatory drug.
Reproduced with permission from Al-Lawama M, Al-Momani HM, AboKwaik WM, et al: Benign pneumoperitoneum in newborns: which abdomen to open and which one to observe? *Clin Case Rep.* 2016
May 4;4(6):561-563.

      b. **Measurement of partial pressure of oxygen in peritoneal air.** See Section
        IV.C.5.a.
      c. **Presence of air leak in the chest.** Increases the chance the pneumoperitoneum
        is from an air leak.
    7. **Contrast studies.** A low or iso-osmolar, water-soluble contrast medium can be
      given through an NG tube. If there is a pneumoperitoneum secondary to a GI
      perforation, contrast material will pass into the peritoneal cavity and confirm
      the diagnosis. Hyperosmolar contrasts should never be used because they can
      cause further damage. **Barium should never be used** because of the morbidity
      of barium peritonitis.

V. **Plan.** Treatment approaches depend on the cause of the pneumoperitoneum and clinical status of the infant and includes observation only, paracentesis, (one time needle aspiration or repeated), placement of a peritoneal drain (primary peritoneal drainage), or surgical exploration. **Prompt surgical consultation is recommended for any neonate with a pneumoperitoneum, especially of GI origin.**

A. **Emergency measures. Rule out tension pneumoperitoneum.** A tension pneumoperitoneum is the abdominal equivalent of a tension pneumothorax. Infants can present with a tense, distended abdomen with respiratory failure and cardiovascular collapse. An emergency therapeutic paracentesis must be done to reduce the pressure and allow the diaphragm to mobilize (see Chapter 40).

B. **General measures/supportive care**

1. **Make the patient nothing by mouth.** Provide bowel rest, and stop all enteral foods and medications.

2. **Gastric decompression** with intermittent suction. One option is to place a double-lumen tube (Replogle) on low suction. This allows 1 lumen for drainage of fluid and 1 lumen as an air vent.

3. **Abdominal circumference is measured** and followed frequently to observe for accumulation of air. See Chapter 50.

4. **Fluid management.** Correct electrolyte abnormalities and any third space losses.

5. **Blood pressure support, if needed.**

6. **Correct any coagulopathy.**

7. **Parenteral nutrition, if indicated.**

8. **Sepsis evaluation and prompt antibiotic therapy** may be indicated. Infants with bowel perforation are put on empiric antibiotics that cover both aerobic and anaerobic organisms.

9. **Serial abdominal x-rays** should be done every 6 hours until stable.

C. **Surgical intervention, which typically is an exploratory laparotomy with bowel resection,** is usually indicated for perforated or necrotic intestine, peritonitis, pain, cardiovascular instability, clinical deterioration refractory to medical management, leukocytosis, positive paracentesis (evidence of leakage from the GI tract: bilious or feculent fluid), gas in the portal vein, erythema and cellulitis of the abdominal wall, fixed dilated intestinal segment on x-ray (sentinel loop), intraperitoneal fluid increasing in amount, rapid reaccumulation of air requiring >2 peritoneal taps a day, and conservative treatment failure.

D. **Nonsurgical intervention.** Conservative management, specifically meaning avoiding an exploratory laparotomy, is considered in some selective infants as initial management with a pneumoperitoneum secondary to GI perforation who do not have peritonitis, have a normal abdominal examination, and do not have any of the surgical indications listed earlier. A Cochrane review notes that evidence from 2 randomized trials suggests no significant benefits or harms of peritoneal drainage over laparotomy as initial surgical treatment for perforated NEC or SIP in preterm low birthweight infants. Survival rates were not statistically different between peritoneal drainage and laparotomy groups. No definitive recommendations could be made due to the very small sample size. Approximately 50% of infants who had a PPD avoided the need for laparotomy. Options include peritoneal tap or primary peritoneal drainage.

1. **Peritoneal tap/paracentesis** (see Chapter 40). Besides being diagnostic, peritoneal tapping provides peritoneal decompression and is less invasive than primary peritoneal drainage (PPD). It can aid in ventilation and also allow the bowel to heal. It is done until the abdomen is flat or the aspiration is negative. One time needle aspiration can also be effective for infants with a spontaneous intestinal pneumoperitoneum, which resulted in definitive treatment in 60% of cases. Tapping is repeated if there is reaccumulation of air as evident by an increase in abdominal circumference.

2. **Primary peritoneal drainage.** PPD is more invasive because it involves opening the peritoneal cavity and placing a drain at the bedside. Irrigation is sometimes

done. It can be done as a stabilizing or definitive treatment. It may be the preferred surgical procedure in ELBW infants who cannot be transported to the operating room.

E. **Specific measures**

1. **Pneumoperitoneum of gastrointestinal tract origin.** Stop all feedings, insert NG/OG tube to decompress the abdomen, provide supportive care (respiratory and circulatory support: correct hypoxia and acidosis, correct dehydration, correct any electrolyte disturbance), correct any coagulopathy, administer intravenous (IV) antibiotics, and call for an **immediate surgical consult**. The majority of cases require an exploratory laparotomy based on indications of surgical intervention above. Other alternative options include peritoneal tapping or PPD. It is best to discuss **options with the surgeon** and make the decision based on each individual patient. **If it is decided that surgery should be performed:**

   a. **Surgical management with exploratory laparotomy.** If surgery is decided upon, exploratory laparotomy is often the treatment of choice. Preoperative management includes the following:

      i. **Preoperative laboratory values** should be available.

      ii. **The infant should be stabilized** as much as possible before being taken to the operating room.

      iii. **Intravenous antibiotics** should be started. Choice depends on the institution but should include broad-spectrum antibiotics with anaerobic coverage.

      iv. **The surgical team may request a study** with a water-soluble contrast medium given through the NG tube to try to localize the perforation.

      v. **Laparotomy** with primary repair or laparoscopy. **Mini-laparotomy** is a newer bedside option in infants who cannot be transferred to the operating room.

   b. **Primary peritoneal drainage. This is considered conservative management, is used selectively, and is considered *controversial*.** Some suggest this approach for infants with the following: perforation without peritonitis, a normal abdominal examination or mild abdominal distension, normal blood gases and platelets, minimal free air, and no air-fluid levels on x-ray. **Others suggest this for isolated perforations or for infants who may be too sick for anesthesia and surgery.** Conservative management with PPD includes the following:

      i. **Place NPO, give fluids and antibiotics.** Make infant NPO, start IV fluids, total parenteral nutrition, blood transfusion if indicated, and IV antibiotics.

      ii. **Primary peritoneal drainage (closed abdominal drainage)** is done at the bedside. This procedure involves making a transverse incision midway between the umbilicus and anterior superior iliac crest in the right lower quadrant. A penrose drain is placed and secured after cultures are taken. The drain is removed once the drainage resolves.

      iii. **Close observation and frequent physical examinations,** serial radiographs, and follow-up laboratory evaluations are required.

      iv. **Delayed laparotomy** may be required in some of these infants if they fail to improve clinically (increasing need for respiratory support, ongoing sepsis, increasing inotrope requirement, increasing abdominal distension,) or have reaccumulation of free air after the drain is removed, or have persistent intestinal obstruction. Continued acidosis or free air that persists may also signify the need for laparotomy. Reviews have found that 38% to 74% infants required a delayed laparotomy.

2. **Pneumoperitoneum of respiratory tract origin.** The pulmonary air leak should be treated first if this is the cause of the pneumoperitoneum. Treatment depends upon if the infant is asymptomatic or symptomatic.

   a. **Asymptomatic patients.** Observation with close monitoring is often the treatment of choice, with frequent abdominal girth measurements and follow-up radiographic studies usually performed every 8 to 12 hours but more frequently if the patient's clinical course changes.

   b. **Symptomatic patients.** Emergency paracentesis may be necessary in some infants with compromised ventilation and can be performed with treatment of coexisting pneumothorax if present. Review the ventilator settings to avoid high pressures that will contribute to the problems. Conservative treatment can be done.

   3. **Traumatic pneumoperitoneum.** A pneumoperitoneum caused by rectal thermometers, NG/OG placement, suprapubic bladder aspiration, umbilical venous lines, enemas, attempted intubation, or paracentesis can usually be treated conservatively. Postlaparotomy or postlaparoscopy pneumoperitoneum associated with an uncomplicated surgical procedure will resolve spontaneously over several days.

F. **Benign neonatal pneumoperitoneum with no known cause.** Depending on the infant and his or her clinical examination, observation with conservative management is usually done. Peritoneal tapping/lavage may be necessary in some cases.

75 Pneumothorax

I. **Problem.** An infant with respiratory distress may have a pneumothorax. A pneumothorax is the abnormal accumulation of air in the pleural space, between the visceral and parietal pleura. It can develop spontaneously (idiopathic or from underlying lung disease) or be secondary to trauma. Pathophysiology involves an increased intra-alveolar pressure, which causes alveolar rupture and results in interstitial air; this air then dissects along the perivascular spaces and ruptures into the pleural space. A pneumothorax occurs more commonly in the neonatal period than any other time in life. Incidence is approximately 1% to 2% in term newborns and approximately 6% in premature infants. A pneumothorax is generally characterized as spontaneous, traumatic, tension, or persistent.

A. **Spontaneous pneumothorax**
   1. **Primary spontaneous pneumothorax.** Occurs when there is **no obvious precipitating factor and no clear cause;** it is **idiopathic,** without lung disease. **Familial spontaneous pneumothorax** (pneumothorax occurring in more than 1 neonate in the same family) is extremely rare but has been described in neonates.
   2. **Secondary spontaneous pneumothorax.** Occurs from a complication of **underlying lung disease** (respiratory distress syndrome [RDS], meconium aspiration syndrome [MAS]), pulmonary hypoplasia (can be bilateral), transient tachypnea of the newborn, pneumonia, or congenital pulmonary cystic malformations, among other causes.

B. **Traumatic pneumothorax**
   1. **Iatrogenic** occurs from an unintended insult during a procedure, such as central line placement, bronchoscopy, or thoracentesis.
   2. **Positive-pressure ventilation (mechanical or noninvasive ventilation)** can cause barotrauma and a subsequent pneumothorax. A Cochrane review (2015) found that in preterm infants with RDS, using continuous distending pressure (eg, continuous positive airway pressure or continuous negative pressure) is associated with an increased rate of pneumothorax.
   3. **Chest trauma** can occur when blunt or penetrating trauma occurs to the chest (rare in neonates).

    C. **Tension pneumothorax. A life-threatening condition that occurs when air is trapped in the pleural cavity under positive pressure.** Air enters the pleural cavity during inspiration, but no air is allowed to escape during expiration. It acts as a 1-way valve. Because air is trapped, intrathoracic positive pressure rises, lung volume decreases, and pressure compresses the mediastinum and causes a shift, with increased pulmonary vascular resistance. This results in an increase in central venous pressure, a decrease in venous return to the heart, and a decrease in cardiac output. In the latest stages, this causes displacement of mediastinal structures and cardiopulmonary compromise.

    D. **Persistent pneumothorax (persistent air leak).** A pneumothorax that persists >5 to 7 days in the absence of mechanical ventilatory problems. In 1 study, the major determinants of persistent pneumothorax and mortality were underlying lung pathology, need for mechanical ventilation, and bilateral pneumothorax.

II. **Immediate questions**

    A. **Are you sure it is a pneumothorax?** See Section IV.C.2 for classic findings of a pneumothorax on chest x-ray (CXR). Rule out artifacts and mimickers of a pneumothorax such as:

       1. **Skin folds** are the most common artifact projected over the thoracic cavity. They occur as a broad curvilinear line that travels across or the chest or diaphragm into the abdomen. If the line extends beyond the lung or if there are lung markings peripheral to the line then you know it is an artifact.

       2. **Neonatal incubator access port projection,** which produces lower density round images that can look like cystic lesions or a small pneumatocele.

       3. **Scapulae margins, clothing, or inserted and overlying lines or tubes** may cause a curvilinear shadow over the lung and be misinterpreted as a pneumothorax. Look for lung markings, which will be visible in the periphery, to rule out a pneumothorax.

       4. **Companion shadows along the inferior margins of the ribs** are smooth radiopaque shadows running parallel along the bones that can mimic a pneumothorax.

       5. **Bullae or lung cysts** can mimic a pneumothorax. Bullae have a concave surface facing the chest wall. A pneumothorax typically has a convex surface facing the chest wall.

       6. **Free air in the abdomen** can extend into the mediastinum and pleural space.

       7. **Gastric dilatation or a severely distended intrathoracic stomach** can simulate a pneumothorax.

    B. **Is the infant symptomatic?** Symptoms of a pneumothorax vary depending on the size and whether the pneumothorax is under tension. Respiratory distress signs are tachypnea, chest retractions, grunting, and nasal flaring.

       1. **A small pneumothorax** can be asymptomatic or can cause mild respiratory distress.

       2. **A large pneumothorax** can cause more symptoms: increasing respiratory distress, cyanosis, decreased breath sounds on the affected side, chest bulge with enlargement of the affected side, point of maximal cardiac impulse shifted away from the affected side, and an increase in heart rate and blood pressure.

       3. **A tension pneumothorax presents as a medical emergency, and the patient's status can suddenly deteriorate to a complete cardiovascular collapse.** The following signs may be seen with tension pneumothorax: severe respiratory distress, cyanosis, hypoxia, tachypnea, a sudden decrease in heart rate with bradycardia that persists, a sudden increase in systolic blood pressure followed by narrowing of pulse pressure and hypotension, an asymmetric chest (bulging on the affected side), distention of the abdomen (secondary to downward displacement of the diaphragm), decreased breath sounds on the affected side, and shift of the cardiac apical impulse (most consistent finding) away from the affected side. A cyanotic upper half of the body with a pale lower half can be seen.

C. **Is the infant asymptomatic?** An asymptomatic pneumothorax is present in approximately 1% of neonates. It occurs more frequently in males and term and postterm infants. It is usually unilateral, with most of these discovered on CXR at admission. Up to 15% of these infants can be meconium stained at birth with a pneumothorax.

D. **Is mechanical ventilation being used?** The incidence of pneumothorax in patients receiving positive-pressure ventilation is 15% to 30%. A life-threatening tension pneumothorax may result from mechanical ventilation.

E. **Are there risk factors for a pneumothorax?** Neonates delivered between 30 and 36 weeks, moderately preterm, or term by cesarean section have a higher incidence of pneumothorax. The following factors are associated with an increased risk: male infant, low birthweight, prematurity, meconium-stained amniotic fluid, vacuum extraction, a low 1-minute Apgar score, ventilator treatment, perinatal asphyxia, cardiopulmonary resuscitation, transient tachypnea of the newborn, RDS, MAS (10%–30%), pneumonia, pulmonary hypoplasia (often bilateral pneumothorax), urinary tract anomalies, need for resuscitation at birth, continuous positive airway pressure, and positive-pressure ventilation. α_1-Antitrypsin deficiency may play a role in some cases of spontaneous pneumothorax of the newborn.

III. **Differential diagnosis**

A. **Clinical differential diagnosis.** Clinically, a pneumothorax can present as any process that causes respiratory distress, diminished breath sounds, or a sudden deterioration in a neonate. All of these can signify a pneumothorax or another diagnosis. It is important to recognize the differential and exclude the other causes.

1. **Other causes of respiratory distress in a neonate:** RDS, endotracheal tube obstruction/displacement, aspiration, congenital heart disease, asphyxia, congenital diaphragmatic hernia (CDH), congenital cystic pulmonary malformation, or pleural effusions.

2. **Other causes of diminished breath sounds:** Inadequate ventilation, malpositioned endotracheal tube, tracheal obstruction, enlarged heart, pulmonary hypoplasia, pleural effusion, CDH, or positive-pressure ventilation equipment failure.

3. **Other causes of a sudden deterioration in a neonate:** Tension pneumothorax, pneumopericardium, massive pericardial effusion/cardiac tamponade (umbilical venous catheter, systemic air embolism), or other diseases (eg, septic shock).

B. **Radiographic differential diagnosis** can include pneumomediastinum, congenital lobar emphysema, atelectasis with compensatory hyperinflation, CDH, congenital cystic pulmonary malformation, a large pulmonary cyst, and the artifacts noted earlier.

C. **Pneumothorax**

1. **Symptomatic pneumothorax (includes tension vs nontension pneumothorax)**

a. **Nontension pneumothorax symptoms:** Irritability, pallor, cyanosis, restlessness, apnea, mild tachypnea, respiratory distress (flaring, grunting, tachypnea, retractions).

b. **Tension pneumothorax symptoms** are noted in Section II.B.3.

2. **Asymptomatic pneumothorax**

3. **Persistent pneumothorax**

D. **Pneumomediastinum. Air is in the mediastinal space.** Heart sounds are distant on physical examination. **Extrapleural air seen over the lung space or air in the mediastinal space may be misdiagnosed as a true pneumothorax.** On the radiograph, mediastinal air can elevate the lobes of the thymus (called "angel wing" or "spinnaker sail" sign), and the air can also track within the extrapleural space and outline the inferior aspect of the heart ("continuous diaphragm" sign). See Figure 12–22. Apical extrapleural air due to a pneumomediastinum is almost always seen bilaterally; in a pneumothorax, it is seen unilaterally.

E. **Congenital lobar emphysema.** A rare anomaly of lung development that presents with respiratory distress and pulmonary lobar hyperinflation. Overdistention of 1 lobe secondary to air trapping occurs most commonly (47%–50%) in the left upper lobe. Other lobe involvement includes right upper lobe (20%), right middle lobe (28%), and lower lobes (rare). The causes of congenital lobar emphysema are multifactorial.

F. **Atelectasis with compensatory hyperinflation.** Compensatory hyperinflation may appear as a pneumothorax on a CXR.

G. **Pneumopericardium. A pneumopericardium is air in the pericardial space.** In neonates, pneumopericardium and tension pneumothorax can both present as sudden and rapid clinical deterioration. In pneumopericardium, the blood pressure drops, heart sounds are distant or absent, and pulses are muffled or absent. Massive abdominal distention can also be seen. In tension pneumothorax, the blood pressure may initially increase, but then hypotension follows. The CXR easily differentiates the 2 conditions. A pneumopericardium has a halo of air around the heart (see Figure 12–21). Air never extends into the neck or along other mediastinal structures seen on a CXR of a pneumopericardium. The air seen on the film does not change with different positions of the infant. **The more common event is a tension pneumothorax.** If one is unsure and time does not permit radiographic verification, quick transillumination can be done. If not available or unsure of results, it is better to insert a needle in the chest on the suspected side. If no response, then a needle should be inserted on the other side. If there is still no response, then the diagnosis of pneumopericardium should be considered.

H. **Congenital diaphragmatic hernia.** A developmental defect in the diaphragm allows the abdominal viscera to protrude into the chest, which causes pulmonary hypoplasia and decreased pulmonary vasculature and dysfunction of the surfactant system. Ninety percent of cases are on the left side. **CDH is often mistaken as a left tension pneumothorax.** CDH presents with respiratory distress, cyanosis, and circulatory insufficiency. It can be hard to differentiate a left-sided pneumothorax from a typically left-sided CDH. With CDH, the abdomen is scaphoid, and the spleen cannot be palpated. There can be a mediastinal shift on radiograph. If chest tubes are placed, there is a risk of perforating the herniated viscus. This is the most common condition associated with a gastrothorax (a distended stomach herniates through a ruptured diaphragm) and may simulate a pneumothorax.

I. **Congenital pulmonary airway malformation (formerly known as congenital cystic adenomatoid malformation).** This rare congenital abnormality of the lung results from abnormal embryogenesis and reduced alveolar growth. Infants present with respiratory distress. Tachypnea and cyanosis can be presenting signs that are similar to a pneumothorax. Many of these are detected on ultrasound prenatally. A CXR usually identifies the mass containing air-filled cysts (see Chapter 125).

IV. **Clinical findings**

A. **Physical examination.** Signs of respiratory distress classically include tachypnea, retractions, grunting, and flaring. Other signs include decreased breath sounds on the affected side, chest bulge with enlargement of the affected side, point of maximal cardiac impulse shifted away from the affected side, and increase in heart rate and blood pressure. As air increases, hypotension and decreased blood pressure can occur.

B. **Laboratory studies.** Blood gas levels may show a decreased PaO_2, increased PCO_2, and decrease in blood pH with resultant respiratory acidosis. Metabolic acidosis due to a low cardiac output can be seen as a result of a tension pneumothorax. Both CRP and procalcitonin concentrations increase in response to a pneumothorax.

C. **Imaging and other studies**

1. **Chest transillumination** is a **rapid bedside method** to identify a pneumothorax. **Always verify the diagnosis of pneumothorax by a CXR if time permits.** (See Chapter 44 for details on transillumination techniques.) The room lights are lowered, and a fiberoptic transilluminator is placed firmly and flat against the baby's chest wall along the midaxillary area between the fourth and sixth interspaces on the side on which pneumothorax is suspected. If a pneumothorax is present, the chest "lights up" on that side. The transilluminator may be moved up and down

along the midaxillary line and may also be placed above the nipple. Transilluminate both sides of the chest and then compare the results. Premature infants
will normally transilluminate more than full-term infants. Large/obese or term
infants with thick chest walls do not transilluminate well. A recent study showed
chest transillumination to be the **least accurate** method in the diagnosis of pneumothorax when compared to CXR and ultrasound. *Note:* Pulmonary interstitial
emphysema (PIE) and pneumothorax can look the same on transillumination
because they both light up.

    a. **Normal (negative transillumination results):** No pneumothorax. The only
area that lights up will be a symmetric ring around the tip of the fiberoptic
light and will not extend over 1 cm. Both sides will have equal translucency.

    b. **Abnormal (positive transillumination results):** The translucency will be
larger on the 1 side, and it will have an irregular pattern. If severe subcutaneous
edema is present, transillumination may be falsely positive. Premature infants
with PIE may also have a false-positive transillumination because diffuse PIE
can give the same appearance as a large pneumothorax on transillumination.

    c. **Suspicious:** Difficult to assess if the area of translucency is larger than the
other side.

2. **Chest radiographs** are the **method of choice** for diagnosing pneumothorax. The
classic radiographic findings include displacement of the thin white line of the
visceral pleura lining the lung parenchyma from the chest wall. Lung markings
are absent peripherally beyond this white line. This is not a definite sign because
it can be seen in lung cysts or bullae. Early or small pneumothoraces are difficult
to diagnose. Early on, there is separation of lung from the chest wall with no
lung markings in that space. In infants, there is a tendency of pleural air to cloak
diaphragmatic and mediastinal surfaces. A pleural line is often not seen, but a
well-defined costophrenic sulcus (deep sulcus sign) can be observed. Of note, a
study showed that using a personal smart phone to view a CXR image of a neonatal
pneumothorax was just as accurate as viewing the image on a computer screen.

    a. **Subtle radiographic signs of a pneumothorax**

        i. **Deep sulcus sign.** A unilateral, abnormally deepened costophrenic angle
that is lower than normal. It looks like a sharp black shadow in the costophrenic angle that goes below the ribs.

        ii. **Black stripe sign.** Medially located air in the pleural space that extends
along the cardiac and mediastinal margins. It appears sharp and clear and
is unilateral.

        iii. **Black and white stripe sign.** With the black strip sign, a white stripe is
seen lateral to the black stripe.

        iv. **Inverted diaphragm sign.** The hemidiaphragm is flattened, depressed, or
inverted; this sign is seen in a tension pneumothorax or basal loculated
pneumothorax.

    b. **The following radiographs can aid the diagnosis:**

        i. **Anteroposterior view of the chest** (see Figure 12–23) will show the following:

            (a) **A shift of the mediastinum** away from the side of pneumothorax (this
is seen with tension pneumothorax).

            (b) **Depression of the diaphragm** on the side of the pneumothorax (with
tension pneumothorax).

            (c) **Displacement of the lung** on the affected side away from the chest
wall by a radiolucent band of air.

        ii. **Cross-table lateral view** will show a rim of air around the lung ("pancaking").
It will *not* help to identify the affected side. **You must have an
anteroposterior (AP) film to identify the side of the pneumothorax.**
This film must be considered together with the AP view to identify the
involved side. Pleural air tends to collect anteriorly and may require
computed tomography or the lateral decubitus view.

   iii. **Lateral decubitus view (shot through the anteroposterior position)** will detect even a **small pneumothorax** not seen on a routine CXR. A lateral view will show an anteriorly located pneumothorax or loculated pneumothorax in the major fissure that could be missed on the AP view. It can also differentiate a large dilated intrathoracic stomach from a pneumothorax. The infant should be positioned so the side of the suspected pneumothorax is up (eg, if pneumothorax is suspected on the left side, the film is taken with the left side up).

  3. **Ultrasound examination of the lungs. (See Chapter 44.) A point-of-care ultrasound is a useful tool** that may be quicker in obtaining a diagnosis of a pneumothorax than waiting for an x-ray. Studies suggest that lung ultrasound is just as accurate as a CXR in the diagnosis of a pneumothorax, outperforms the clinical evaluation, and reduces the time to the imaging diagnosis and treatment. **There are 4 sonographic signs of a pneumothorax:** (1) lung point sign (junction between the sliding lung and the absent sliding); (2) absence of lung sliding (grainy appearance, pleura and ribs move together); (3) absence of B lines (arise from normal pleura reflecting sound waves, narrow base, and form a ray spreading from transducer); and (4) absence of lung pulse (transmission of cardiac systoles on the pleural line). The lung point sign may be able to differentiate between a large and small pneumothorax.

  4. **Transcutaneous carbon dioxide reference percentiles with changes over time** can indicate a pneumothorax or a blocked or misplaced endotracheal tube.

  5. **Cardiac tracing on monitor.** Sudden decrease of voltage of the QRS complex is an early sign of pneumothorax.

  6. **Echocardiography and renal ultrasound** may be indicated in spontaneous pneumothorax in term infants, because some of these infants can have renal and cardiac anomalies.

V. Plan. Specific treatment guidelines for treating a pneumothorax in neonates are lacking. The treatment varies and is dependent on age and the degree of symptoms of the infant, the size of the pneumothorax, whether or not it is a continuous leak or a tension pneumothorax, if the infant has underlying lung disease, and whether the infant is on a ventilator or not. It is best to follow the guidelines of your institution.

  A. **Basic recommendations**

    1. **Maintain the infant's oxygenation.** Use supplemental oxygen for only those infants who are hypoxic, and use only enough oxygen to maintain a normal pulse oximeter (range of 92% to 95%) in the infant (targeted pulse oximetry).

    2. **Consider conservative treatment** (close observation, oxygenation to provide adequate saturation) in those pneumothoraces that are small and asymptomatic, those infants that have no underlying lung disease, that are not on a ventilator, or whose air leak is not ongoing.

    3. **Perform a needle aspiration and/or place a thoracostomy tube** if the pneumothorax is causing symptoms. Any approach should include a follow-up evaluation to determine resolution of the pneumothorax. **A Cochrane review (2019)** notes there is insufficient evidence to decide between needle aspiration versus intercostal tube drainage in terms of efficacy and safety in managing neonatal pneumothorax (based only on 2 small trials). Randomized controlled trials are needed comparing the 2 techniques. They did state that needle aspiration might reduce the need for intercostal tube drainage placement.

  B. **Specific recommendations.** The following are recommendations for different scenarios of a pneumothorax:

    1. **Symptomatic pneumothorax**

      a. **Tension pneumothorax. A tension pneumothorax is an emergency!** A 1- to 2-minute delay could be fatal. If a tension pneumothorax is suspected, act immediately. It is better to treat in this setting, even if it turns out that there is no pneumothorax. There is no time for x-ray confirmation. If the patient's status is deteriorating rapidly, a needle or catheter-over-needle can be placed for aspiration, followed by formal chest tube placement. There is no specific sign that distinguishes a tension from a nontension pneumothorax. The previously discussed signs of a tension pneumothorax can also occur in a nontension pneumothorax, except the signs and symptoms are more severe in a tension pneumothorax.

i. **Needle aspiration (see Figure 75–1) can be done as an emergency or as part of planned elective aspiration.** Often this is all that is necessary if the infant is not on a ventilator. If on a ventilator, a chest tube placement may need to be followed by needle aspiration. Confirm the side that you plan to aspirate with a procedural "time-out."

   The site of puncture should be at the second intercostal space along the midclavicular line on the suspected side of pneumothorax. Cleanse this area with antibacterial solution and prepare with sterile towels. The **fourth intercostal space at the anterior axillary line** can also be used (needle would be inserted above the fifth rib). Position the infant on his or her back with the affected side on a small blanket roll so that side is elevated. This allows the air to rise to the upper part of the chest. Appropriate

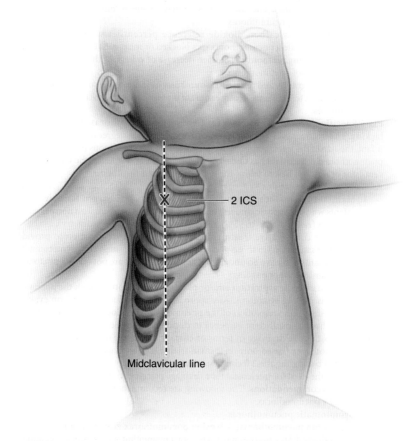

FIGURE 75–1. Site of emergency needle aspiration for tension pneumothorax is puncture at the second intercostal space (ICS) along the midclavicular line.

anesthetic for pain management should be used, but in the case of a tension pneumothorax, urgency of treatment may not allow it.

    ii. **Use a 18–20-gauge percutaneous catheter over needle (recommended by *Textbook of Resuscitation*)** or 19–21-gauge percutaneous catheter over needle (per Perinatal Continuing Education Program Neonatal Care), or connect a 21- or 23-gauge butterfly needle to a 10- to 20-mL syringe with a stopcock attached.

    iii. **Palpate the third rib at the midclavicular line. Avoid insertion at or near the nipple area.** Insert needle (perpendicular to the chest surface) over the top of the third rib (to avoid the blood vessels and the nerve that run below the rib) at the second intercostal space, and **advance the catheter upward** until air is withdrawn from the syringe. Stop inserting the needle once you get air into the syringe. Have an assistant hold the syringe to withdraw the air. **If using a catheter-over-needle (Angiocath-shielded IV catheter)**, the needle can be removed once the pleural space is entered (a "pop" is typically felt); a large syringe (20–60 mL) is then attached to the catheter with a 3-way stopcock. Open the stopcock between the syringe and catheter to evacuate air. When it is full, close the stopcock to the chest and empty the syringe. Continue to aspirate air until the infant improves. The needle may be removed before the chest tube is placed if the infant is relatively stable, or it may be left in place for continuous aspiration while the chest tube is being placed. Check a chest x-ray to make sure there is no residual pneumothorax.

  b. Chest tube/pigtail catheter placement. This may be necessary in most infants on mechanical ventilation with a tension pneumothorax, if the air leak is continuous, or if the pneumothorax does not clear after needle aspiration. See Chapter 31 for chest tube details.

  c. If the infant does not improve with a properly functioning chest tube, suspect extrapleural air leaks such as a pneumoretroperitoneum, pneumomediastinum, or pulmonary cyst.

  d. If the pneumothorax is persistent after chest tube drainage, consider the following trouble-shooting measures:

    i. **Check to see if there is an air leak in the tubing or if it is in the lung:** Remember, bubbling in the water seal chamber is normal and indicates air is entering the system. Persistent bubbling means there is an air leak or bronchopleural fistula.

    ii. **Check all tubing connections.** A nonfunctioning chest tube can result from disconnection of the tube from the suction mechanism, mechanical obstruction (blood clot or pleural fluid), kinked tube, or a malfunctioning suction apparatus.

    iii. **Clamp the chest tube near the entrance of the chest *cautiously*.** If there is **continuous bubbling,** it means there is an air leak in the tubing. If there is **no bubbling,** it means the chest tube is outside of the chest or there is an active leak.

    iv. **A malpositioned/incorrect tube placement** (most common cause) is a tube in the subcutaneous tissue or posterior pleural space.

    v. **Check for possibility of a new air leak.**

    vi. **Check for perforation of lung (most commonly injured organ) or diaphragm.**

  2. **Nontension pneumothorax.** Depending on the infant's symptoms, observation with room air only or oxygen supplementation if needed, needle aspiration, and chest tube placement are all options based on the clinical situation. In 1 study, only 7.5% of symptomatic term infants with a spontaneous pneumothorax required needle aspiration or chest tube placement.

    a. Mild symptoms. Typically, observation only with serial imaging.

      b. Symptomatic pneumothorax (not on ventilator). Close observation, supplemental oxygen to maintain saturation and needle aspiration. In 1 study, the majority of infants could be managed with supplemental oxygen or close observation.

      c. Symptomatic pneumothorax (on the ventilator). Needle aspiration and/or chest tube placement are typical options. If possible decrease the mean airway pressure (decrease PIP, PEEP, and inspiratory duration).

C. Asymptomatic pneumothorax

  1. If positive-pressure mechanical ventilation is being used:

      a. Needle aspiration/chest tube. A chest tube will probably need to be inserted because the ventilator pressure will prevent resolution of the pneumothorax, and a tension pneumothorax may develop. Sometimes **needle aspiration is all that is needed.** If a pneumothorax develops in a patient who is ready to be extubated, clinical judgment must be used in deciding whether a chest tube should be placed.

      b. Expectant management. Recent studies are showing that some select infants on a ventilator can be managed without a chest tube. These select infants are usually more mature, on lower ventilator settings, and have better gases at the time of the pneumothorax compared to infants who require a chest tube.

  2. If positive-pressure mechanical ventilation is not being administered and there is no underlying lung pathology, these approaches may be considered.

      a. Close observation with follow-up chest radiographs every 8 to 12 hours or sooner if the infant becomes symptomatic. The pneumothorax will likely resolve within 24 to 48 hours.

      b. Nitrogen washout therapy. (*This method is controversial and not used widely anymore*). Older studies showed that this therapy allowed a more rapid resolution of the asymptomatic pneumothorax, but it is infrequently used due to the toxicity of 100% oxygen. The infant receives 100% oxygen for 8 to 12 hours. The theory behind this therapy is that high oxygen therapy reduces the partial pressure of nitrogen in the alveolus when compared to the pleural space. This diffusion gradient causes the nitrogen to diffuse from the pleural space into the alveoli, which results in resorption of air from the pleural space into the alveoli, resulting in faster resolution of the pneumothorax. If used, this method should be reserved for only full-term infants in whom retinopathy of prematurity will not be a problem. Some neonatal intensive care units give only enough oxygen to maintain adequate saturation and have found resolution to be similar to the hyperoxic group. **More recent studies** indicate that nitrogen washout therapy (100% oxygen) is not associated with a faster resolution of spontaneous pneumothorax in term infants compared to room air. It resulted in infants being exposed to unnecessary oxygen, longer IV therapy, and delay in reaching full feeds. **If this technique is used, it is best to use oxygen saturation targeted therapy (use only enough oxygen to maintain a normal pulse oximeter and not any more).**

D. Persistent air leak pneumothorax is generally defined as a pneumothorax that persists >5 to 7 days in the absence of mechanical problems. Sometimes infants who have chest tubes still have air leaks that persist for more than a week. These infants tend to have episodes of instability when air reaccumulates; some require a new or replacement chest tube and an increase in their ventilator settings. These persistent leaks are treated to decrease the complications associated with air leaks (eg, air embolus, hypotension, intracranial hemorrhage). Techniques that have been used with variable success in adults for persistent air leaks in anecdotal reports include fibrin sealants, ethanol injection, metal coils, and Watanabe spigots, and in larger studies, chemical pleurodesis, autologous blood patch pleurodesis, and endoscopically placed endobronchial valves have been used. The following treatments have been reported:

  1. Observation. The American College of Chest Physicians states that the majority of persistent pneumothoraxes, in the absence of a bronchopleural fistula, will likely resolve spontaneously and recommends observation for spontaneous closure for 4 days.

2. **Placing the chest tube to water seal** has been successful in some cases of post-operatively persistent air leaks.

3. **Low lung volume strategy.** Reduce the inspiratory time, positive end-expiratory pressure, and peak inspiratory pressure if on conventional positive-pressure ventilation.

4. **Consider high-frequency oscillatory ventilation or high-frequency jet ventilation,** which can be used due to lower mean airway pressures.

5. **Unilateral lung intubation** has been reported as an efficient and relatively safe therapy for pneumothorax. Selective intubation of the contralateral bronchus causes the affected lung to collapse to enable the ruptured alveoli to heal. This is a very difficult procedure, especially if the left mainstem bronchus has to be intubated, with many complications. Duration of therapy should be a minimum of 48 hours.

6. **Pleurodesis with fibrin glue or povidone-iodine.** Agents are introduced into the pleural space through the chest drain that cause irritation between the parietal and visceral layers of the pleura, which closes the space between them, thus treating the pneumothorax and preventing any further air from accumulating. Fibrin glue and povidone-iodine have been used in neonates with persistent pneumothoraces.

   a. **Fibrin glue,** such as CryoSeal C (ThermoGenesis Corp, Rancho Cordova, CA), has been injected in the chest tube with a marked reduction in the air leak. It has been used in newborns (single case reports and 1 study with 8 patients) and is an effective treatment for an intractable persistent pneumothorax but has significant risks (hypercalcemia, localized tissue necrosis, bradycardia requiring manual ventilation, diaphragmatic paralysis, and pneumothorax on the contralateral side).

   b. **Povidone-iodine** has been used in case reports.

E. **Pneumomediastinum.** Most do not need any treatment and usually resolve spontaneously. **Close observation is required** because it may progress to a pneumothorax or pneumopericardium. If there is a **tension pneumomediastinum,** ultrasound-guided percutaneous drainage should be urgently performed.

F. **Congenital lobar emphysema.** If asymptomatic, conservative management with observation is recommended. If symptomatic or respiratory failure is occurring, the treatment is usually surgical excision of the affected lobe.

G. **Atelectasis with compensatory hyperinflation**

1. **Chest physiotherapy and postural drainage should be initiated.** Chest physiotherapy should be used with caution in premature infants. A study showed an association with intraventricular hemorrhage and porencephaly in extreme premature infants.

2. **Treatment with bronchodilators** is indicated.

3. **Positioning the infant with the affected (hyperinflated) side down** may speed resolution.

4. **Bronchoscopy.** May be necessary with a mucus plug.

H. **Pneumopericardium.** If symptomatic, the infant should be treated (urgently if experiencing cardiac tamponade) by a therapeutic pericardiocentesis (see Chapter 41). Sometimes a pericardial tube needs to be left in for continuous decompression. If asymptomatic, intervention may not be necessary, but the infant needs to be closely followed for any changes in physical examination or on CXR. Ventilator settings should be decreased if possible.

I. **Cystic pulmonary airway malformations (formerly known as congenital cystic adenomatoid malformation).** Surgery is the treatment of choice.

J. **Pulmonary interstitial emphysema.** Management is supportive with the goal of decreasing the mean airway pressure. For unilateral PIE, position the infant with the affected side down and decrease the inspiratory time and ventilator pressure (see Chapter 87).

76 Polycythemia: On Call

I. **Problem.** <u>The hematocrit (Hct) is 68% in a newborn.</u> **Polycythemia** is an increase in total erythrocyte mass empirically defined as a venous Hct >2 standard deviations above the normal value for postnatal and gestational age. **An infant who has a peripheral venous Hct >65% or a hemoglobin >22 g/dL is considered polycythemic.** Polycythemia occurs in 1% to 5% of healthy newborns (1%–2% at sea level and 5% at high altitude) and is rare in premature infants <34 weeks' gestation. The venous Hct level of 65% was chosen to define polycythemia based on an exponential increase in viscosity above this level. **Hyperviscosity** and the resultant impairment of blood flow are important in polycythemia because they cause most of the symptoms and complications. Increased blood viscosity impairs circulation of red blood cells through vessels and organs and interferes with delivery of oxygen, glucose, and amino acids to the tissues. Poor oxygen and nutrient delivery causes neurologic, gastrointestinal, metabolic, and cardiopulmonary problems. The Hct is the main determinant of blood viscosity (thickness); however, plasma proteins (especially fibrinogen), low plasma volume, and decreased erythrocyte deformability also affect blood viscosity. Blood is unable to flow freely due to increased viscosity of blood because of the increased number of erythrocytes that occurs in polycythemia. **Hyperviscosity** is defined as >14.6 centipoise (shear rate of 11.5 seconds) and is also defined as 2 standard deviations greater than the norm. Viscosity rises linearly until the Hct reaches 60% but increases exponentially when it reaches 70%.

    Polycythemia hyperviscosity syndrome (PHS) is the symptom complex that involves hyperviscosity resulting from polycythemia and the symptoms that accompany it. Not all polycythemic infants will have hyperviscosity: roughly 47% of polycythemic infants will have hyperviscosity, and 24% of infants with hyperviscosity have polycythemia.

II. **Immediate questions**

  A. **What is the central hematocrit?** If the Hct was obtained by a heel stick, it can be falsely elevated by up to 15% as compared to venous samples. Warming the heel prior to the heel stick will give a result that better correlates with the central Hct. However, treatment should **never** be initiated based on heel stick Hct values alone; **a central (peripheral venous phlebotomy) Hct is needed.** The Hct is highest in capillary samples and lowest in umbilical venous samples.

  B. **What method was used to determine the hematocrit?** There are two methods of determining the **Hct: automated hematology analyzer (cell counter),** which calculates the Hct from a measurement of the mean cell volume and hemoglobin, and the **microcentrifuge** (blood is centrifuged, plasma and packed cell volume separates, and the Hct is measured). A microcentrifuge Hct can be 2% higher than Hct by a hematology analyzer.

  C. **How old is the infant?** A newborn's Hct peaks at 2 hours of age, plateaus between 2 and 4 hours of age, and then decreases back to values close to cord blood values between 12 and 24 hours of age. A value up to 71% may be normal at 2 hours of age.

  D. **Does the infant have symptoms of polycythemia?** Most infants with polycythemia are **asymptomatic** (up to 90%). Symptoms of hypoperfusion correlate more with viscosity than the Hct. One study found that gastrointestinal symptoms (**poor feeding and vomiting**) were the most common symptoms. There are many signs of polycythemia, most of them nonspecific, and they include the following:

    1. **Central nervous system signs** are common in infants with polycythemia and can include lethargy, hypotonia, irritability, jitteriness, weak sucking reflex, vomiting, seizures, apnea, sleepiness, exaggerated startle, tremors, and cerebrovascular accidents.

   2. **Cardiovascular.** Murmurs, congestive heart failure, cyanosis, plethora, tachycardia, cardiomegaly, and prominent vascular markings on chest radiograph. Cyanosis and tachycardia are uncommon.
   3. **Respiratory.** Respiratory distress, tachypnea, and cyanosis.
   4. **Gastrointestinal.** Poor feeding, poor sucking, vomiting, abdominal distension, and necrotizing enterocolitis (NEC).
   5. **Renal.** Proteinuria, oliguria, hematuria, renal vein thrombosis, decreased glomerular filtration rate, and transient hypertension.
   6. **Hematologic.** Thrombocytopenia, hepatosplenomegaly, thrombosis, disseminated intravascular coagulation (rare), and elevated reticulocyte count.
   7. **Metabolic.** Hypoglycemia (most common; 12%–40%), hypocalcemia (1%–11%), and increased bilirubin (33%).
   8. **Skin.** Plethora or ruddiness, jaundiced.
   9. **Genitourinary.** Testicular infarcts or priapism (majority are idiopathic).
   10. **Eyes.** Vitreous hemorrhage seen in an infant with thrombocytopenia and polycythemia.

E. **Is the mother diabetic?** Poorly controlled maternal diabetes during pregnancy leads to chronic fetal hypoxia, which may result in increased fetal erythropoiesis. Infants of diabetic mothers (IDM) have a 13% to >40% incidence of polycythemia. Good maternal glycemic control will help prevent fetal hypoxia and polycythemia.

F. **Is the infant dehydrated?** Dehydration may cause hemoconcentration, resulting in a high Hct. It usually occurs in infants >48 hours old.

G. **Does the mother live at a high altitude?** Infants born to mothers at high altitudes have a higher incidence of polycythemia.

H. **Is the infant at high risk for polycythemia?** Infants who are small for gestational age, postterm, or intrauterine growth restricted; IDMs; large for gestational age infants; infants with twin-to-twin transfusion; and infants with chromosomal abnormalities (trisomy 21, 13, or 18) have an increased risk for polycythemia.

I. **Was there delayed clamping of the umbilical cord? Were the guidelines followed? Was the cord milked ?** Delayed cord clamping (DCC) is now recommended by the American College of Obstetricians and Gynecologists (ACOG), the World Health Organization (WHO), and the American Academy of Pediatrics (AAP) Neonatal Resuscitation Program for vigorous term and preterm infants. Randomized controlled trials of DCC in term and preterm infants have shown increased Hct, without increased incidence of polycythemia when following the guidelines. Umbilical cord milking (UCM), where the cord is held and blood is squeezed down the cord into the baby, is another way that newborns can receive extra blood volume at birth; however, it is not universally recommended or practiced.

III. **Differential diagnosis.** See also Chapter 116.

A. **Falsely elevated hematocrit.** Most often occurs when blood is obtained by a heel stick.

B. **Diseases that cause the same clinical signs as polycythemia that should be ruled out.**
   1. **Hypoglycemia:** Intrauterine growth restriction, IDM, inborn error of metabolism, Beckwith-Wiedemann syndrome, infection, nesidioblastosis, cortisol, or insulin production abnormalities.
   2. **Respiratory disorders:** Respiratory distress syndrome, transient tachypnea of the newborn, pneumonia.
   3. **Cardiovascular abnormalities:** Persistent pulmonary hypertension of the newborn, congenital heart disease.
   4. **Neurologic abnormalities:** Intracranial hemorrhage, intracranial abnormalities, hypoglycemia, hypocalcemia, perinatal hypoxia, genetic/metabolic syndromes, venous thrombosis, infant with a high magnesium level, peripheral neuromuscular disease.

5. **Renal failure:** Acute tubular necrosis, dehydration, renal dysplasia, obstruction of the urinary tract.
6. **Feeding intolerance.** NEC, bowel obstruction, formula intolerance, central nervous system or peripheral neuromuscular disease, genetic syndrome, IDM.
7. **Endocrine abnormalities:** Hypothyroidism or congenital adrenal hyperplasia.
8. **Neonatal sepsis.**

C. **Dehydration.** Also called "relative polycythemia," this condition is associated with weight loss and decreased urine output (sensitive indicators of dehydration). Hemoconcentration secondary to dehydration is suspected if >7% of the birthweight has been lost in the first 5 days of life. It usually occurs on the second or third day of life.

D. **Primary polycythemia (very rare in newborns).** Occurs when there is a problem with the production of red blood cells (excess production) in the bone marrow and occurs from inherited and acquired mutations. Polycythemia vera, idiopathic erythrocytosis, and primary familial and congenital polycythemia are examples.

E. **Secondary polycythemia.** Caused by an increase in the production of erythrocytes secondary to either **excess erythrocyte transfusion to the fetus or newborn** (which is considered passive) or **increased intrauterine fetal erythropoiesis** (which is considered active).

1. **Excess erythrocyte transfusion to the fetus or newborn**

   a. **Delayed cord clamping causes placental fetal transfusion** and results in an increase in red cell mass in the neonate, but does not cause polycythemia when the ACOG/AAP guidelines are followed. Polycythemia can occur from an unattended delivery, holding the infant below the mother after birth for too long before clamping the cord, aggressive cord milking, or clamping the cord way past the recommended time. There is no set definition of the time set for DCC because it varies depending on the study. Immediate cord clamping is right after delivery (usually before 30 seconds), whereas DCC is usually >30 seconds, >1 minute, or >3 minutes after delivery depending upon the reference. The term fetus has an approximate blood volume of 70 mL/kg with immediate cord clamping and an approximate blood volume of 90 mL/kg after DCC at 3 minutes. In preterm infants, a delay in cord clamping by 30 to 45 seconds results in an 8% to 24% increase in blood volume. **AAP and ACOG recommend DCC in vigorous term and preterm neonates for 30 to 60 seconds.** WHO recommends delaying umbilical cord clamping in term infants for 1 to 3 minutes. Studies show that polycythemia does not occur with the recommended time per ACOG for delayed cord clamping.

   b. **Type of delivery.** In a **vaginal birth**, because of contractions, there is an increased transfer of placental blood to the infant versus a caesarean delivery with absent contractions. Uterine contractions, especially strong ones, increase the blood volume in the fetus, and uterine contractions during the third stage of labor may cause most of the placental transfusion. **Use of oxytocin** in the mother can also increase contractions. An uncontrolled or precipitous delivery can lead to passive transfusion.

   c. **Position of the infant and effect of gravity on volume of placental transfusion.** If the cord is not clamped immediately at birth, blood will flow between the placenta and the infant. If the infant is held high above the placenta, there is a decrease in placental transfusion. If the infant is held a significant distance below the placenta, transfusion of blood can occur from the placenta to the infant. Holding the infant at the level of the abdomen, chest, or the introitus will prevent the effect of gravity.

   d. **Umbilical cord milking** is the practice of holding the infant in a neutral position while squeezing blood from the cord (either connected to the placenta or after it is cut) to the baby. **Recommendations are to milk the cord 4 times for a preterm infant and to milk the cord 5 times for a term infant.** This may lead to a higher Hct in infants, and the main advantage of UCM over DCC is a quicker improvement in the pulmonary blood flow at birth, which will help with lung expansion at the onset of respirations. UCM is shown to have a greater placental transfusion, higher blood pressure, higher systemic blood flow, and higher urine output in infants delivered by cesarean section than infants who had DCC. UCM may be an alternative to DCC for premature infants because it is completed much faster than DCC.

  e. **Twin-to-twin transfusion** can result in increased blood in 1 twin (10%–15% of monochorionic twins). Twin-to-twin transfusion occurs with discordant amniotic fluid volumes. **Twin anemia polycythemia sequence** is an atypical form of twin-to-twin transfusion in monochorionic twin pregnancies that does not have discordant amniotic fluid volumes.

  f. **Maternal-to-fetal transfusion (rare).**

  g. **Iatrogenic polycythemia** is uncommon and caused by overtransfusion of red blood cells during a transfusion.

  h. **Acute fetal hypoxia** will result in a transfer of blood from the placenta to the fetus to maintain fetal oxygenation and cardiac output.

2. **Increased intrauterine fetal erythropoiesis.** This can occur from chronic intrauterine hypoxia or insufficiency of the placenta. In an attempt to correct the chronic intrauterine fetal hypoxia, the production of erythropoietin increases, which leads to increased red blood cell production and an increased Hct. Intrapartum asphyxia can also cause blood volume to shift from the placenta to the fetus and cause polycythemia.

  a. **Infant.** Intrauterine hypoxia may be seen in small for gestational age infants, postmature/postterm infants, intrauterine growth restricted infants, and infants with perinatal asphyxia.

  b. **Mother.** Maternal smoking, heavy maternal alcohol use, chronic or recurrent abruptio placentae, maternal chronic hypertension, mothers with preeclampsia, and severe maternal cardiac, pulmonary, or primary renovascular disease may also cause intrauterine hypoxia. Severe maternal diabetes can cause reduced placental blood flow, and pregnancy at high altitudes can cause intrauterine hypoxia.

3. **Other causes/factors usually associated with increased erythropoiesis**

  a. **Infant of a diabetic mother.** The incidence of polycythemia is 22% to 29%. This occurs with gestational diabetes as well as with insulin-dependent diabetes and is due to increased erythropoiesis.

  b. **Chromosomal abnormalities:** Down syndrome (trisomy 21; 15%–33%), trisomy 13 (8%), trisomy 18 (17%), fumarate hydratase deficiency.

  c. **Endocrine abnormalities:** Hyperthyroidism, congenital hypothyroidism, congenital adrenal hyperplasia.

  d. **Large for gestational age infants.**

  e. **Beckwith-Wiedemann syndrome.**

  f. **Maternal use of β-blockers** (such as propranolol or nebivolol).

4. **Idiopathic.** No specific cause found.

IV. **Database**

  A. **Physical examination.** Evaluate for dehydration; weight loss will be present and the mucous membranes will be dry, but increased skin turgor is usually not seen. True polycythemia is often associated with visible skin changes. Ruddiness or plethora is most often seen, but one can also see poor perfusion, or "pink-on-blue" or "blue-on-pink" coloration. In males, priapism may be seen secondary to sludging of red blood cells causing venous congestion. Hypothermia is also a sign of polycythemia. Assess for macrosomia. Does the infant have large fontanels (congenital hypothyroidism)? Genitourinary exam should evaluate for disorders of sex development (congenital adrenal hypoplasia). Clinical signs are listed in Section II.D.

B. **Laboratory studies.** The AAP does not recommend universal screening for polycythemia, but it states that selective testing should be done in high-risk infants. **Hypoglycemia, thrombocytopenia, and hyperbilirubinemia** are commonly associated with polycythemia and need to be closely followed in these infants.

   1. **Hematocrit in cord blood** >56% may predict polycythemia at 2 hours of age (controversial).
   2. **Central hematocrit (venous or arterial) is essential.** Typically recommended at 2, 12, and 24 hours of age.
   3. **Serum glucose.** Hypoglycemia is commonly seen with polycythemia. Coexisting hypoglycemia may worsen long-term outcome.
   4. **Complete blood count with differential** to evaluate for sepsis.
   5. **Platelet count.** Thrombocytopenia occurs in 51% of infants with polycythemia. Disseminated intravascular coagulation is rare.
   6. **Serum bilirubin.** Infants with polycythemia have been shown to be at increased risk of hyperbilirubinemia thought to be related to an increased turnover of red blood cells.
   7. **Metabolic panel.** Serum electrolyte, blood urea nitrogen, and creatine levels. If dehydration is being considered, these labs are important. They are usually high, or higher than baseline values, if dehydration is present. These labs are also necessary to assess renal dysfunction.
   8. **Urine specific gravity** >1.015 is usually seen with dehydration.
   9. **Arterial blood gas.** Rule out inadequate oxygenation.
   10. **Calcium.** Hypocalcemia can also be seen but is uncommon.

C. **Imaging and other studies.** These studies are usually not needed acutely.
   1. **Chest radiograph.** Cardiomegaly, increased pulmonary vascular markings, and pleural effusions may be seen on chest radiography.
   2. **Abdominal x-ray if NEC is suspected.**
   3. **Electrocardiogram and electroencephalogram.** Electrocardiogram (ECG) and electroencephalogram may be abnormal, but these tests are not routinely indicated. An ECG can show right ventricular hypertrophy and right and left atrial hypertrophy.
   4. **Echocardiogram.** Echocardiogram may show increased pulmonary resistance and decreased cardiac output.

V. **Plan.** Exclude dehydration first. Rule out other diseases that cause the same symptoms as polycythemia. The suggested treatment strategies are based on low-quality evidence and therefore should be considered weak recommendations. Routine use of partial exchange transfusion (PET) is not recommended.

A. **Polycythemia preventive measures**
   1. **American Academy of Pediatrics and American College of Obstetricians and Gynecologists recommend** DCC in vigorous term and preterm neonates for at least 30 to 60 seconds. **WHO recommends** delaying umbilical cord clamping in all infants for 1 to 3 minutes, while initiating early neonatal care. Early cord clamping <30 seconds is not recommended unless the infant is asphyxiated or the infant needs positive-pressure ventilation.
   2. **Do not milk or strip the umbilical cord** until further studies are done since research is still insufficient on this practice.
   3. **Do not hold the infant significantly below the placenta** with an intact cord at delivery, since this may cause passive transfusion of placental blood to the infant. Holding the infant on the mother's abdomen, chest, or introitus does not affect the volume of placental transfusion.
   4. **Routine screening.** Screening is usually not recommended but may warranted in selective infants who are symptomatic or at high risk: small for gestational age, large for gestational age, or postterm infants; infants with intrauterine growth restriction; IDMs; monochorionic twins; and infants with chromosomal abnormalities (eg, Down syndrome, trisomy 13 or 18). It is best to screen with a

capillary Hct. Some institutions do not screen healthy high-risk asymptomatic infants since asymptomatic infants with polycythemia do not benefit from treatment. Screening recommendations vary, but screening can be done at 2, 6, 12, 24, 48, and 72 hours of age.

B. **Falsely elevated hematocrit (>65%).** If the confirmatory central Hct is normal, no further evaluation is needed. If the central Hct is high, either dehydration or polycythemia is present.

C. **Hemoconcentration secondary to dehydration.** Check weight loss. If the infant is dehydrated (usually the infant is >48 hours of age and has lost >7%–10% of body weight) but does not have symptoms of polycythemia, a trial of rehydration over 6 to 8 hours can be attempted. Usually, a minimum of 100 mL/kg/d up to 130 to 150 mL/kg/d is given. The Hct is checked every 4 to 6 hours and usually decreases with adequate rehydration.

D. **True polycythemia.** Treatment includes observation with or without intravenous (IV) hydration and/or PET. Treatment is usually based on whether the infant is symptomatic. Some clinicians will narrow it down further on whether the infant has **severe symptoms** (persistent hypoglycemia, severe GI symptoms, worsening apnea, worsening cyanosis) or **nonsevere symptoms**. Treatment is controversial and widely varies depending on the source of recommendations. Supportive care for hypoglycemia, thrombocytopenia, and hyperbilirubinemia should also be provided. It is best to follow your own institutional guidelines:

1. **Asymptomatic infants** should be observed with or without IV hydration no matter what the Hct is according to some sources. A recent study did not show any evidence of clinical benefit of giving supplemental IV fluids versus routine fluids in late preterm and term neonates with asymptomatic polycythemia with an Hct of 65% to 75%. The following is a recommendation, but it is best to follow your institutional guidelines.

   a. **Central hematocrit of 65% to 69%:** Close observation with or without IV hydration with monitoring of symptoms and follow-up Hct. The peripheral venous Hct should be reassessed every 4 to 6 hours for 12 to 24 hours. If the Hct remains stable and asymptomatic, the infant can be followed for 48 hours.

   b. **Central hematocrit of 70% to 75%:** Consider IV hydration. Many of these patients will respond to increased fluid therapy (controversial); consider increasing fluids by 20 to 40 mL/kg/d. Some advocate feedings be withheld until Hct is <70%. Note that liberal IV fluid therapy can be associated with problems in preterm infants. Rarely, clinicians will recommend a PET for an infant with an Hct >70%.

   c. **Central hematocrit >75%:** PET should be considered if a repeated Hct remains >75%.

2. **Symptomatic infants with a hematocrit >65%.** Some clinicians recommend that any infant with polycythemia and symptoms be treated. The 2 options are as follows:

   a. **Treat with observation and intravenous hydration.** IV hydration and close observation with follow-up Hct; if the infant gets worse (increasing symptoms, Hct is rising), treat with PET.

   b. **Treat with a partial exchange transfusion.** (See also Chapter 34.) If a PET is to be done, it should be done as soon as possible because the Hct and blood viscosity peak between 2 and 4 hours. In a PET, a calculated amount of blood volume is slowly removed and replaced with fluids (normal saline) to dilute the red blood cell concentration, which decreases the Hct. The goal of PET is to decrease blood viscosity and improve end-organ perfusion. PET may be administered via an umbilical venous catheter (UVC). **Care must be taken not to place the catheter in the liver** (see Chapter 48). A high umbilical artery catheter (UAC) or a peripheral IV catheter can also be used. **Normal saline is preferred as the replacement fluid of choice** as crystalloids are as effective as colloids in PET. Crystalloids do not carry the risk of infection or anaphylaxis and are cheaper and more readily available. Colloid products (plasmanate, 5% albumin, and FFP) have been used but are not currently recommended because of an association with NEC seen with their use. Serial Hct levels should be obtained after transfusion.

   i. **Exchange formula:** Desired Hct is 55%, and blood volume is 80 mL/kg.

$$\text{Volume exchanged (mL)} = \frac{[(\text{Weight (kg)} \times \text{Blood volume (mL/kg)}) \times (\text{Actual Hct} - \text{Desired Hct})]}{(\text{Actual Hct})}$$

   ii. **Use these guidelines when performing partial exchange transfusion:**
      (a) **Aliquots should not exceed 5 mL/kg** and should be removed or delivered over 2 to 3 minutes.
      (b) **Removal of blood can be from any arterial or venous line.** Arterial lines are not recommended for infusion.
      (c) **If there is both an umbilical artery catheter and an umbilical venous catheter,** withdraw blood from the UAC while giving the replacement fluid through the UVC.
      (d) **If only an umbilical venous catheter is in place,** use the push-pull method: pull out the blood, and then push in the replacement fluid. **Never remove >5 mL/kg.** Isovolumetric method through 2 vessels is preferred.
      (e) **If you have an umbilical venous catheter, umbilical artery catheter, and peripheral venous catheter in,** you can use either the UAC or UVC for blood withdrawal and then use the peripheral line for replacement fluid. Removal from the UVC and infusion in the peripheral venous catheter did not result in NEC in 1 study.

3. **Symptomatic infant with a central hematocrit of 60% to 65%.** If all other disease entities are ruled out, these infants may indeed be polycythemic and hyperviscous. Management is **controversial.** Use clinical judgment and institutional guidelines to decide if these infants should have a PET. Some would closely observe with IV hydration.

4. **Restrictive management protocol of neonatal polycythemia follows a more conservative approach.** Hct of 65% to 69%: no treatment. Hct of 70% to 75%: give IV fluids and no feedings until Hct is <70%. Hct ≥76% or in any symptomatic neonates: use PET. A review demonstrated that the groups did not differ in morbidities or hospital stay, nor was there an increase in risk of short-term complications.

E. **Observe for complications of polycythemia** and disorders that are more common in polycythemic infants.
   1. **Apnea.**
   2. **Hypoglycemia (most common).**
   3. **Hypocalcemia.**
   4. **Thrombocytopenia.**
   5. **Hyperbilirubinemia.**
   6. **Neurologic.** Seizures, stroke, cerebral vein thrombosis.
   7. **Vascular/thromboses.** Vasospasms, peripheral gangrene. Large-vessel thrombosis and stroke.
   8. **Cardiopulmonary complications.** Cardiomegaly, tachycardia, tachypnea, arrhythmia, congestive heart failure.
   9. **Gastrointestinal complications.**
      a. **Necrotizing enterocolitis risk** is increased in term or near-term neonates with polycythemia and hyperviscosity. Etiologies include gut mucosal injury secondary to altered splanchnic perfusion and infants who received a PET via a UVC with colloid (FFP, albumin, or Plasmanate). The development of NEC in these infants who had a partial exchange via a UVC with colloid may be related to PET with colloid, not the polycythemia.

  b. Ileus, spontaneous intestinal perforations, intestinal atresia.

  c. **Treated infants had more gastrointestinal complications** (bloody stools, emesis, and abdominal distension) in 1 study, but this may have been related to PET technique.

 10. **Genitourinary complications.** Decreased glomerular filtration rate, oliguria, hematuria, proteinuria, renal vein thrombosis, testicular infarcts, and priapism.

 11. **Air embolism.**

F. **Follow-up data.** PET has some benefit short term (decreases the Hct, decreases the viscosity, and reverses some physiologic abnormalities) but has not been show to improve long-term outcome. Further research is needed to assess the impact on newborns, because there is conflicting information in the literature.

 1. **Partial exchange transfusion benefits**

  a. **It lowers the hematocrit and decreases the viscosity.**

  b. **It may improve symptoms earlier on,** but this may be transient. It does not eliminate them.

  c. **It improves microcirculation in polycythemic neonates.** Near-infrared spectroscopy showed increased cerebral oxygenation and decreased fractional tissue oxygen extraction.

  d. **It has been shown to improve cerebral blood flow velocity and decrease pulmonary vascular resistance,** and may normalize cerebral hemodynamics (normal cerebral blood flow). Oxygen transport and systemic blood flow improve as well.

 2. **Controversial data on long-term outcome**

  a. **Partial exchange transfusion does not appear to significantly improve long-term neurologic outcomes.** Newborns with hyperviscosity had significantly more neonatal problems and motor delays at 2 and 7 years of age, and they have lower IQs and achievement test results and decreased gross motor skills compared with children with a normal Hct. At 7 years of age, children who had neonatal hyperviscosity had lower IQs and decreased visual motor and neurologic function. There was no difference between those who had and had not received a PET. Children with hyperviscosity who received either PET or symptomatic care both had lower spelling and arithmetic achievement test results and gross motor skill scores. Reading, visual motor integration, and neurologic scores did not differ from normal controls. However, decreased IQ scores and lower achievement were reported in infants with hyperviscosity syndrome who were not treated with PET.

  b. **There is no evidence of improvement** in long-term outcomes (neurologic outcome or early neurobehavioral assessment scores) following PET in symptomatic or asymptomatic infants.

 3. **Polycythemic infants are at risk** for speech abnormalities and for fine/gross motor delays.

 4. **Long-term outcome may be related** to other perinatal or clinical factors and not polycythemia or PET. Given that infants who are at higher risk for polycythemia and hyperviscosity include those undergoing chronic hypoxia in utero, the association with worse developmental outcomes may be related to the underlying cause of the polycythemia, instead of the polycythemia itself.

 5. **Partial exchange transfusion may lead to an increase in the risk of necrotizing enterocolitis** and gastrointestinal symptoms. **Partial exchange transfusion via umbilical vein with colloid** has been shown to increase the risk of NEC.

 6. **Intrauterine fetal hypoxia is related to polycythemia** and impaired long-term outcome.

 7. **Coexisting hypoglycemia** may worsen the long-term outcome.

 8. **Cochrane review** states there are no proven short- or long-term benefits to PET in infants with polycythemia who are well or who have minor symptoms. PET may increase the risk of NEC. The review notes that the risks and benefits of PET are not clear.

77 Poor Perfusion

I. **Problem.** You receive a report that an infant "doesn't look good" or looks "mottled." Other descriptors may include "poor perfusion" or "washed-out appearance." This can include pallor, which can be seen in poor perfusion or may be an early sign of hypoxia or anemia. **Most of these terms refer to poor perfusion and imply there is inadequate blood flow to the tissues of the skin.** Assessing peripheral tissue perfusion is important in the clinical examination of a neonate since it can help determine who may have low systemic blood flow or cardiovascular failure. Recent studies have shown correlations between poor outcomes and peripheral hypoperfusion in preterm infants.

II. **Immediate questions**

   A. **What is the age of the infant?** Hypoplastic left heart syndrome (HLHS) may cause poor perfusion and a mottled appearance. It may be seen at days 1 to 21 of life (more commonly at day 2 or 3). In an infant <3 days old (some definitions say <7 days) **early-onset sepsis** may be a cause. Associated risk factors for sepsis are premature rupture of membranes, maternal infection, and fever. **Late-onset sepsis** can occur at >3 days or after 7 days, depending upon which definition is used.

   B. **What are the vital signs?** If the temperature is lower than normal, cold stress or hypothermia associated with sepsis may be present. Hypotension may cause poor perfusion (see normal blood pressure values in Table 70–1 and Appendix C). Decreased urine output (<2 mL/kg/h) may indicate depleted intravascular volume or shock.

   C. **Is the liver enlarged? Are metabolic acidosis, poor peripheral pulse rate, and a gallop present?** These problems are signs of failure of the left side of the heart (eg, HLHS). Poor perfusion occurs because of reduced blood flow to the skin.

   D. **If mechanical ventilation is being used, are chest movements adequate and are blood gas levels improving?** Inadequate ventilation can result in poor perfusion.

   E. **Is the poor perfusion localized to only 1 area of the body?** Aortic thrombosis can present with weak femoral pulses, coldness, and **poor perfusion of the limbs.**

   F. **Are congenital anomalies present?** Persistent cutis marmorata (see Section III.A.15) may be seen in Cornelia de Lange syndrome, cutis marmorata telangiectatica congenita (CMTC), Edward syndrome (trisomy 18), and Down syndrome (trisomy 21). **Chromosome 22q11 deletion syndrome** can present with abnormal vascular tone with hypotension. **Cornelia de Lange syndrome** consists of multiple congenital anomalies: a distinctive facial appearance, pre- and postnatal growth deficiency, feeding problems, psychomotor delay, behavioral problems, and malformations that mainly involve the upper extremities.

III. **Differential diagnosis**

   A. **Common causes**

   1. **Sepsis.** Poor peripheral perfusion is seen as an early sign of sepsis.
   2. **Cold stress/hypothermia.** In general, associated with a skin temperature <36.5°C (97.7°F).
   3. **Hypotension** usually with shock.
   4. **Hypoventilation** can cause poor perfusion.
   5. **Respiratory distress syndrome.** Infants with respiratory distress syndrome have poor perfusion and lower perfusion index.
   6. **Apnea/apnea of prematurity** can cause a decrease in peripheral perfusion.
   7. **Pneumothorax.** A large pneumothorax or tension pneumothorax can cause poor perfusion.
   8. **Hypoglycemia** can mimic hypoxemia, and poor perfusion can be seen.
   9. **Polycythemia with hyperviscosity.** Infants have sluggish capillary refill and poor peripheral perfusion.

10. **Acute hemorrhagic anemia** due to acute blood loss can present with symptoms of hypovolemia including poor perfusion, hypotension, tachycardia, and pallor. A decrease in peripheral perfusion occurs with a 10% loss of blood volume.
11. **Necrotizing enterocolitis.** Systemic signs are nonspecific but can include decreased peripheral perfusion.
12. **Patent ductus arteriosus.** A hemodynamically significant patent ductus arteriosus in the first week of life can cause poor perfusion in infants <1000 g.
13. **Left-sided obstructive heart disease.** Newborns with critical left-sided obstructive lesions (ductal-dependent systemic circulation) generally appear normal at birth, and when the ductus arteriosus begins to close, they have cardiac failure with systemic hypoperfusion (poor perfusion with cold, clammy, mottled skin), poor peripheral pulses, increasing metabolic acidosis, and shock. Cyanosis may not be seen until later. One study showed that the majority of infants presented with shock, approximately one-third presented with heart failure, and a small percentage presented with profound cyanosis. These diseases include HLHS, critical aortic stenosis (AS), coarctation of the aorta (COA) (with or without septal defect), and interrupted aortic arch (IAA). When the ductus closes, infants with COA and IAA have hypoperfusion of the lower half of the body, and infants with AS and HLHS have hypoperfusion of the entire systemic circulation.
14. **Infant of substance-abusing mother.** Mottling can be a sign of neonatal abstinence.
15. **Cutis marmorata** is a common vascular disorder that affects newborns and a normal physiologic response of newborns to cold. When newborns are exposed to cold, a marbling, red/blue, lacy, reticulated mottling pattern appears on the skin (usually trunk and extremities) that disappears with warming of the skin. It is due to an immature neurologic and vascular system or an exaggerated physiologic vasomotor response. It can also indicate **poor perfusion** in septic infants or in infants with shock.
    a. **Persistent cutis marmorata** can occur in hypothyroidism, central nervous system dysfunction, cardiovascular hypertension, neonatal lupus erythematosus, Menke disease, familial dysautonomia, homocystinuria, Divry-Van Bogaert syndrome, and some congenital syndromes (Cornelia de Lange, Edward [trisomy 18], and Down [trisomy 21] syndromes).
    b. **Cutis marmorata telangiectatica congenita (CMTC), also known as Van Lohuizen syndrome. Cutis marmorata** needs to be distinguished from **CMTC,** which is a permanent rare congenial cutaneous vascular anomaly that presents as persistent cutis marmorata, telangiectasia, and phlebectasia (see Chapter 7). Vascular anomalies (Sturge-Weber syndrome and Klippel-Trenaunay-Weber syndrome) have been associated with CMTC. See Figure 7-2. CMTC does not disappear with warming of the skin.
B. **Less common causes**
    1. **Enteroviral/viral or fungal infection.** Presents with poor perfusion and overwhelming sepsis.
    2. **Periventricular hemorrhage/intraventricular hemorrhage.** Presentation varies but can present with extreme signs, including sudden onset of poor perfusion, pallor, and hypotonia.
    3. **Subgaleal hemorrhage (rare).** Most commonly associated with a vacuum evacuation or forceps delivery. It progresses after birth and can have a massive amount of blood.
    4. **Inborn errors of metabolism.** Present with a history of deterioration with poor perfusion. Organic acidemia, urea cycle defects, and certain disorders of amino acid metabolism can present with poor perfusion, lethargy, and other symptoms.
    5. **Seizures.**
    6. **Hematologic.** Bleeding disorders.

7. **Adrenal problems.** Congenital adrenal hyperplasia, Addison disease, adrenal hemorrhage.
8. **Renovascular hypertension.** Presents with apnea, irritability, and mottling of the skin.
9. **Gastrointestinal problems.** Necrotizing enterocolitis (NEC), perforation, and volvulus.
10. **Systemic air embolism.** Symptoms are sudden and include mottling of the skin with pallor.
11. **Aortic thrombosis** can present with weak femoral pulses, coldness, and poor perfusion of the limbs.
12. **Chronic pain.** Infants experiencing chronic pain can exhibit decreased and poor perfusion with cool extremities.

IV. **Database**
   A. **Peripheral parameters of poor perfusion.** Peripheral parameters have been used to assess peripheral circulation and cardiac output. They have not been very good indicators of low systemic blood flow; therefore, they are not great in predicting poor perfusion. Peripheral parameters include temperature, skin color, capillary refill time, acid-base balance, and urine output.
      1. **Temperature (central vs peripheral temperature gradient/difference).** A central temperature (usually axillary) and a peripheral temperature (usually sole of foot) are monitored with a thermal probe. If an infant is peripherally hypoperfused, the central temperature is higher than the peripheral temperature. A gradient increase of >2°C may be an early indication of cold stress and is noted in infants with sepsis.
      2. **Skin color.** Color change can be seen with poor perfusion (washed out, pallor, mottled appearance, acrocyanosis).
      3. **Capillary refill time** is the time required for the normal skin color to return after a blanching pressure has been applied. It is measured by pressing on the chest, midpoint of the sternum (better intraobserver repeatability), or forehead for 5 seconds with a finger and noting the time needed for the color to return. Upper limit of normal for capillary refill is <3 seconds. **Delayed capillary refill (>3–4 seconds)** is a sign of tissue hypoperfusion and had a sensitivity of 55% and a specificity of 81% for predicting low superior vena cava flow in 1 study. One study found that low birthweight infants have lower capillary refilling time when compared with infants >2500 g.
      4. **Acid-base balance.** Metabolic acidosis and base deficit are seen with poor perfusion.
      5. **Urine output.** Oliguria (decreased urine output) can be seen with poor perfusion and can indicate reduced kidney perfusion.
      6. **Other markers of poor perfusion**
         a. **Decreased pulses** can be seen with poor perfusion.
         b. **Warmth of extremities.** Cold extremities can indicate poor peripheral perfusion, and warm extremities can indicate normal peripheral perfusion. Warmth of extremities is not that reliable in neonatal intensive care unit infants since they are usually under the radiant warmer or in the incubator.
         c. **Blood pressure** is used as a marker of systemic organ perfusion, but there is a poor correlation between blood pressure and cardiac output, and it may not reflect blood flow in the end organs.
         d. **Left ventricular output** is a measurement of systemic blood flow in adults but not in infants since it not a true measure of systemic blood flow but a measure of systemic blood flow with shunt flow (through the patent ductus or foramen ovale).
   B. **Physical examination.** Check vital signs (heart rate, core temperature, blood pressure). Examine for weak pulses and look for signs of sepsis. The cardiovascular and pulmonary examinations are important because they may suggest cardiac problems

or pneumothorax. Does the infant have an S_3 gallop with or without a cardiac murmur (left-sided, obstructive, ductal-dependent heart lesion)? Signs of trisomy 18 include micrognathia and overlapping digits. Signs of trisomy 21 include a single palmar transverse crease and epicanthal folds. Look for scalp swelling to rule out subgaleal hemorrhage. Abdominal distension can be seen with gastrointestinal problems.

C. **Laboratory studies**

1. **Complete blood count to evaluate for sepsis or decreased/increased hematocrit** (eg, polycythemia or blood loss).

2. **Blood gas. Metabolic acidosis and base deficit** are markers of poor perfusion. The blood gas can reveal inadequate ventilation or the presence of acidosis (seen in sepsis, shock, NEC, and other disorders). Persistent metabolic acidosis can be seen in subgaleal hemorrhage.

3. **Serum lactate level** is a marker of poor perfusion. A level >3.0 mmol/L can predict low blood flow, and a level >6.0 mmol/L is associated with increased morbidity and mortality.

4. **Serum creatinine** is a marker and gauge for kidney function. It is a late marker because at least 50% loss of function has to occur before the serum creatinine increases.

5. **Blood glucose levels.** To rule out hypoglycemia.

6. **Cultures.** If sepsis is suspected, a complete workup should be considered, especially if antibiotics are to be started. This workup includes cultures of blood, urine, and spinal fluid (if indicated). If enteroviral infection is suspected, send for viral cultures.

7. **Polymerase chain reaction.** Studies of stool and cerebrospinal fluid and nasopharyngeal or throat swab for *Enterovirus* and other viruses.

8. **Inborn errors of metabolism.** See Chapter 100 for appropriate tests.

D. **Methods of measuring peripheral perfusion**

1. **Peripheral perfusion index.** The perfusion index is an indication of the blood flow to the peripheral tissue and can correlate with the capillary refill time. **This can be derived from the pulse oximeter.** As an example, the light-emitting diode–based infrared Masimo™ pulse oximeters such as Rad-5 and Rad-5v (Masimo, Irvine, CA) display perfusion index as the pulse amplitude index, where the height of the bar represents the pulse strength (info-america@masimo.com). It continuously measures the ratio of the pulsatile blood flow (arterial) to the nonpulsatile blood (static blood in peripheral tissue). It correlates with superior vena cava flow and is useful in monitoring changes in peripheral perfusion. A low value indicates low peripheral perfusion and is associated with low superior vena cava blood flow. **Normal median perfusion index values for stable preterm infants:** on day 1 is 0.9, day 3 is 1.2, and day 7 is 1.3.

2. **Near-infrared spectroscopy** is a noninvasive continuous measure of tissue oxygenation in a specific tissue bed. A spectrophotometer is used, and a cerebral probe is placed on the left or right side of the forehead or a somatic region (renal area, abdomen, upper or lower extremities) such as the INVOS™ Cerebral/Somatic Oximeter (Covidien, Boulder, CO). It is used to measure **regional hemoglobin oxygen saturation (rSO_2)** and can measure oxygenation in the brain, renal area, abdomen (liver), skeletal muscle, and upper and lower extremities. It can be used at the bedside to identify complications of low cardiac output, renal failure, shock, seizures, and neurologic damage. A downward trend in rSO_2 may be an early sign of low cardiac output. Somatic desaturations are an early sign of shock. Cerebral desaturations are a late sign of shock. It is used in left-sided obstructive lesions to monitor for low cardiac output.

3. **Orthogonal polarization spectral imaging and sidestream darkfield imaging** are other noninvasive, noncontinuous transdermal methods to measure capillary density and visualize microcirculation. They allow measurement or assessment of peripheral tissue perfusion in term and preterm infants. They also give an indirect measure of oxygen delivery.

4. **Laser Doppler flowmetry** has been used in evaluating peripheral perfusion in newborns. A laser beam penetrates an area of the skin and hits the red blood cells in the capillaries, venules, and arterioles; this is converted into scattered light, and a probe recognizes it and calculates a relative value of blood flow. One study found not only that blood flow in the skin correlated with systemic blood flow, but also that low skin blood flow of the feet by laser Doppler flowmetry at 18 and 24 hours after birth predicted intraventricular hemorrhage in very low birthweight infants.

5. **Targeted Doppler echocardiography measuring superior vena cava flow.** Superior vena cava flow is a marker for systemic blood flow but is difficult to measure. Studies show that a superior vena cava flow <40 mL/kg/min in preterm infants correlates with poor neurodevelopmental outcome and late-onset intraventricular hemorrhage.

6. **Cardiac magnetic resonance imaging measurements** of systemic blood flow are being investigated, but it is difficult to perform this procedure in infants who are extremely premature and ill.

7. **Markers of perfusion.** The various clinical measurements over time associated with progressive poor perfusion are illustrated in Figure 77–1. The daily baseline rSO_2 numbers in preterm infants (29–34 weeks' gestation) decrease over the first few weeks of life (cerebral baseline 66%–83% rSO_2; renal 64%–87% rSO_2; abdominal 32%–66% rSO_2).

E. **Imaging and other studies**

1. **Transillumination of the chest** (see Chapters 31 and 44) can be performed emergently to help determine whether or not a pneumothorax is present.

2. **Chest radiograph** if pneumonia, pneumothorax, congenital heart lesion, or hypoventilation is suspected. In left-sided heart lesions, the radiograph shows cardiomegaly with pulmonary venous congestion (except in HLHS, in which the size of the heart may be normal). If a view taken during lung expansion shows that the lungs are down only to the sixth rib or less, hypoventilation should be considered. With hyperventilation, lung expansion is down to the ninth or tenth rib. See Figure 12–18 for a radiograph of pneumonia. See Figure 12–23 for radiograph showing a pneumothorax.

3. **Abdominal radiograph** if NEC is suspected. See Figure 12–26 for a radiograph demonstrating pneumatosis intestinalis seen in NEC. Air can be seen with a perforation. Obstruction can be seen with malrotation with volvulus.

4. **Echocardiography** should be performed if a congenital heart lesion is suspected. In HLHS, a large right ventricle and a small left ventricle are seen on the echocardiogram, and there is failure to visualize the mitral or aortic valve. In AS, the echocardiogram reveals a deformed aortic valve. In COA, it reveals decreased aortic diameter. In venous air embolism, one can see acute obstruction of the right ventricle outflow tract.

5. **Head ultrasound** to rule out intraventricular bleed. Optimal imaging for subgaleal hemorrhage is by computed tomography or magnetic resonance imaging.

6. **Computed tomography of the head** to look for intracranial air bubbles if systemic air embolism suspected. CT is also used to rule out subgaleal hemorrhage.

7. **Karyotyping or molecular genetic testing** if trisomy 18 or 21 or a deletion is suspected. Cornelia de Lange syndrome has mutations in the *NIPBL* and *SMC3* genes.

V. **Plan**

A. **Immediate plan.** Infants with a low blood pressure and clinical signs of poor perfusion may be in shock and need to be urgently treated with fluids or pressors. An initial quick workup should be performed. While checking vital signs and quickly examining the patient, order a stat blood gas and a chest radiograph. Initiate oxygen supplementation and transilluminate the chest if a pneumothorax is suspected. Send a stat complete blood count and differential and blood culture.

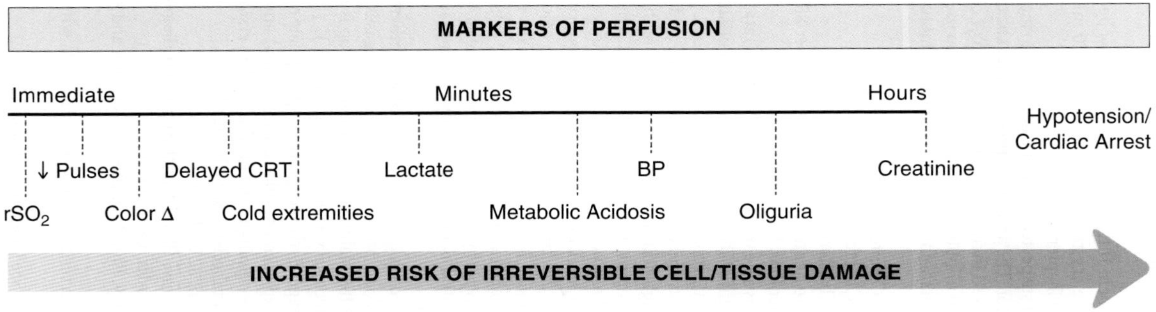

FIGURE 77–1. Time line illustrating progressive alterations in key markers of perfusion. BP, blood pressure; CRT, capillary refill time; rSO₂, regional hemoglobin oxygen saturation. (*Used with permission from William I. Douglas, M.D.*)

B. **Specific plans**
   1. **Sepsis.** Full cultures and empirical antibiotic therapy may be started at the discretion of the physician.
   2. **Cold stress.** Gradual rewarming is necessary, usually at a rate of ≤1°C/h. It can be accomplished by means of a radiant warmer, incubator, or heating pad. (See Chapter 8.)
   3. **Hypotension or shock.** If the blood pressure is low because of depleted intravascular volume, give crystalloid (normal saline) 10 mL/kg intravenously for 5 to 10 minutes. (See Chapter 70.)
   4. **Hypoventilation.** If suspected, it may be necessary to increase the pressure being given by the ventilator. The amount of pressure must be decided on an individual basis. One method is to increase the pressure by 2 to 4 cm H_2O and then obtain blood gas levels in 20 minutes. Another method is to use bag-and-mask ventilation, observing the manometer to determine the amount of pressure needed to move the chest.
   5. **Pneumothorax.** See Chapter 75.
   6. **Hypoglycemia.** See Chapter 67.
   7. **Polycythemia.** See Chapters 76 and 116.
   8. **Anemia secondary to acute blood loss.** See Chapter 88.
   9. **Necrotizing enterocolitis.** See Chapter 109.
   10. **Left-sided obstructive heart lesions.** Initial stabilization with respiratory support (endotracheal intubation and mechanical ventilation if poor respiratory effort and hypoxemia), volume resuscitation, inotropic support with dopamine for low cardiac output, and correction of metabolic acidosis. Immediate cardiac consultation. Prostaglandin E_1 is considered before diagnosis is confirmed if ductal-dependent systemic blood flow is suspected. The infant should be stabilized and transferred to a pediatric cardiac center. Surgery is usually indicated in all these patients. For a full discussion of cardiac abnormalities, see Chapter 94.
   11. **Cutis marmorata.** If this condition is secondary to cold stress, treat the patient as described in Section V.B.2. Cutis marmorata usually resolves within weeks to months, and no formal treatment is necessary. If the condition persists, consider thyroid testing for hypothyroidism or formal genetic testing for various syndromes noted. If central nervous system dysfunction is suspected, this should be evaluated further.
   12. **Periventricular hemorrhage/intraventricular hemorrhage.** Initial supportive care (eg, maintain blood pressure, stabilize blood gases, transfuse if necessary, treat for seizures). After stabilization, close follow-up is required. Serial lumbar punctures may be necessary. (See also Chapter 103.)
   13. **Subgaleal hemorrhage.** Early recognition, appropriate resuscitation, supportive care as in volume replacement, blood transfusion, and coagulation factors if necessary. Pressure wrapping of the head is *controversial*.
   14. **Inborn errors of metabolism.** See Chapter 100.
   15. **Seizures.** See Chapters 82 and 120.
   16. **Hematologic problems.** Blood transfusions and diagnosing and treating the specific bleeding disorder are necessary.
   17. **Adrenal insufficiency.** Blood volume replacement and steroid therapy are usually necessary.
   18. **Renovascular hypertension.** Usually treated with aggressive medical management.
   19. **Intestinal problems.** See Chapters 109 and 121.
   20. **Enteroviral infections.** Supportive management. See Chapter 134.
   21. **Systemic air embolism.** Supportive cardiac and respiratory care. One hundred percent oxygen therapy, hyperbaric oxygen.
   22. **Chronic pain.** See Chapter 15.

78 Postdelivery Antibiotics

I. **Problem.** <u>Two infants were born within the past hour. One infant's mother had premature rupture of membranes (PROM) but no antibiotics. The other infant's mother was pretreated with antibiotics for a positive group B *Streptococcus* (GBS) culture taken at 36 weeks. Who should be evaluated, and who should receive empiric antibiotics?</u> It is necessary to review some of the basic concepts of early-onset sepsis (EOS), such as definition, pathogenesis, incidence morbidity, and mortality, before treatment plans are discussed. Major organizations have varying recommendations on EOS. **This on-call problem focuses on postdelivery antibiotics for suspected EOS.** Late-onset sepsis is discussed in Chapter 146, and infections of premature infants with prolonged hospital stays may require a different workup and antibiotic choice.

A. **Definition of early-onset sepsis.** There are multiple definitions:

1. **The National Institute of Child Health and Human Development and Vermont Oxford Network:** The onset of sepsis at ≤72 hours of life. In term infants, it can be extended to <7 days of life.

2. **The Centers for Disease Control and Prevention:** Blood culture– and/or cerebrospinal fluid (CSF) culture–proven infection occurring in the newborn at <7 days.

3. **The American Academy of Pediatrics (2018):** Blood or CSF culture obtained within 72 hours after birth that is growing a pathogenic bacterial species.

4. **AAP definition of GBS EOS (2019).** Isolation of group B *Streptococcus* organisms from the blood, cerebrospinal fluid, or another normally sterile site from birth through 6 days of age.

B. **Pathogenesis of early-onset sepsis** differs in the term/late preterm infant and the preterm infant.

1. **Early-onset sepsis in the term/late term infants occurs most commonly during labor.**

a. **Vertically transmitted (ascending infection).** Ascending colonization with amniotic membrane rupture/leak before or during labor resulting in infection of the uterine compartment (amniotic fluid, placenta, umbilical cord, or fetus) with maternal gastrointestinal/genitourinary flora. The fetus can become infected by being colonized on the skin/mucous membranes (sepsis develops hours or days after birth), or the fetus aspirates or swallows infected amniotic fluid (sepsis begins in utero). GBS can also enter amniotic fluid through an occult tear. This is the most common cause of GBS early-onset disease (GBS EOD).

b. **Direct contact in the birth canal.** The neonate can acquire the pathogen as it passes through the colonized birth canal during delivery.

c. **Transplacentally by hematogenous spread.** Rarely, EOS develops before the onset of labor (eg, *Listeria monocytogenes* is typically transmitted from the mother to the fetus by hematogenous spread across the placenta).

2. **Early-onset sepsis in the preterm infant occurs most commonly before the onset of labor.**

a. **Intra-amniotic infection** from either microbial induced maternal inflammation (vaginal organisms) or the transplacental pathway (maternal oral flora or *Listeria monocytogenes*).

b. **Inflammation secondary to immune-mediated rejection** of the fetus or placenta from a maternal extrauterine infection or reproductive/nonreproductive microbiota.

C. **Incidence of early-onset sepsis** is highest among preterm and very low birthweight (VLBW) infants, and cases are inversely proportional to gestational age. EOS incidence is also higher among late preterm infants than term infants. The incidence of culture-proven EOS is approximately 0.8 cases per 1000 live births, 0.5 cases per 1000 live births at >37 weeks' gestation, 1 case per 1000 live births at 34 to 36 weeks' gestation, 6 cases per 1000 live births at <34 weeks' gestation, 20 cases per 1000 live births at <29 weeks' gestation, and 32 cases per 1000 live births at 22 to 24 weeks' gestation. Since the institution of the Centers for Disease Control and Prevention (CDC) guidelines (endorsed by the American Academy of Pediatrics [AAP]) for GBS prophylaxis, the incidence of early-onset GBS has decreased from an incidence of 1.8 cases per 1000 live births in 1990 to 0.23 cases per 1000 live births in 2015. Recent studies have shown that the incidence among VLBW infants (9–11 per 1000 live births in infants <1000 g) has also decreased.

D. **Organisms that cause early-onset sepsis.** Overall, GBS is most common, followed by *Escherichia coli*.

   1. **Term/late preterm infants:** GBS in 40% to 45% of cases and *E coli* in 10% to 15% of cases, with the remainder secondary to other gram-positive organisms (viridans and enterococci) and other gram-negative organisms (5%). Rare causes include *Staphylococcus aureus* (3%–4%) and *L monocytogenes* (1%–2%).

   2. **Preterm infants:** *E coli* in 50% of cases, GBS in 25%, 10% other gram-positive organisms (viridans and enterococci), and 20% other gram negatives. Rare causes include fungal (<1%), *S aureus* (1%–2%), and *L monocytogenes* (1%). Anaerobic bacteria are present in approximately 15% of EOS cases (*Bacteroides fragilis* most common).

E. **Morbidity and mortality in early-onset sepsis.** Mortality is 2% to 3% in term infants, with 75% of deaths attributable to EOS in VLBW infants. Mortality estimates based on gestational age are as follows: 1.6% at ≥37 weeks, 2% to 3% at ≥35 weeks, 30% at 25 to 28 weeks, and 50% at 22 to 24 weeks. Mortality by birthweight is as follows: 3.5% if born weighing >1500 g and 35% if weighing <1500 g. Up to 60% of term infants and 95% of preterm infants require neonatal intensive care unit (NICU) care for respiratory distress and/or blood pressure support. Up to 50% of term infants with GBS can suffer serious morbidity (seizures, blindness, deafness, and cognitive delays). GBS EOD is also associated with stillbirth.

F. **Multiple protocols exist. Which one should be used?** There are multiple protocols for evaluation and treatment of EOS. The AAP and ACOG have published new guidelines specifically for management of GBS EOD in 2019 that officially replace prior recommendations from the CDC (last updated in 2010). AAP also recently published separate guidelines on the management of early-onset sepsis in both term/late preterm infants, and preterm infants (2018). **The AAP describes 3 primary approaches to risk assessment for term/late preterm infants that can be used, and recommend that the clinical approach for infants at risk for GBS EOD should be the same as that used for all bacterial causes of early-onset sepsis.** The AAP also states that the best approach to GBS EOD management for preterm infants involves the circumstances of preterm birth and recommends strategies based on that. In addition, a National Institute of Child Health and Human Development (NICHD) workshop (2016) published recommendations for management, and there are also various septic scoring systems available (that are referenced in the AAP guidelines). In a review of 97 nurseries located throughout the United States, 51 reported using the AAP/CDC guidelines to evaluate infants, while 11 used published sepsis risk calculators (discussed later), and 2 used clinical observation alone.

II. **Immediate questions**

A. **Are there any risk factors in the infant?** Risk factors vary depending upon which protocol or scoring system is used.

1. **American Academy of Pediatrics EOS Guidelines (2018) risk factors in term/ late preterm or preterm infants**
   a. **Term/late preterm infants:** Gestational age, maternal intra-amniotic infection (formerly chorioamnionitis), duration of rupture of membranes (ROM), maternal GBS colonization, appropriate intrapartum antibiotics given, and infant's clinical condition. Other risk factors that are not independent predictors include African American race, twin gestation, fetal tachycardia, and meconium-stained amniotic fluid (MSAF).
   b. **Preterm infants:** The only risk factor that has been easy to quantify is gestational age. **Gestational age is the strongest predictor of EOS.** Infants who are born preterm because of the following are considered high risk for EOS: preterm labor, cervical incompetence, PROM, intra-amniotic infection (previously chorioamnionits), and unexplained onset of nonreassuring fetal status.
2. **AAP GBS EOD (2019) risk factors:** Lower gestational age, increased ROM, maternal intrapartum fever, African American race, maternal age <20 years, delivery of a previous infant with GBS, obstetric practices that may promote ascending bacterial infection (observational studies only) such as invasive fetal monitoring, membrane sweeping, frequent intrapartum vaginal examinations.
3. **NICHD.** Based on whether there was an isolated maternal fever (maternal oral temperature $\geq 39°C$ on any one occasion is documented fever), or suspected triple I, defined as fever without a clear source plus any of the following: fetal tachycardia (>160 bpm for 10 minutes or longer), maternal WBC >15,000 (in the absence of corticosteroids), purulent fluid from the cervical os. Confirmed triple I requires all of the above plus amniocentesis proven infection (positive gram stain), low glucose or positive amniotic fluid culture, or placental pathology revealing diagnostic features of infection.
4. **Kaiser Permanente septic score risk factors.** Local incidence of EOS, gestational age in weeks and days, highest maternal antepartum temperature, hours of ROM, maternal GBS status, and type and timing of intrapartum antibiotics. A risk for EOS is calculated at birth based on this information. An EOS risk after clinical exam is also calculated. (See Section V.D.2 below.)

B. **Are signs of sepsis present in the infant? In all guidelines for clinical management, distinguishing between asymptomatic infants and infants with signs of illness is critical when determining the next steps.** Signs of sepsis are nonspecific (80%–100% of infected infants exhibit signs within the first 48 hours after birth) and can include apnea and bradycardia, temperature instability (more frequently hypothermia), feeding intolerance, tachypnea, jaundice, cyanosis, poor peripheral perfusion, hypoglycemia, lethargy, poor sucking reflex, increased gastric aspirates, and irritability. Other signs include tachycardia, shock, vomiting, seizures, abnormal rash, abdominal distention, and hepatomegaly. Neonatal sepsis is associated with systolic and diastolic myocardial dysfunction. Bacteremia can also occur without clinical signs. Preterm infants who are septic may have bradycardia, cyanosis, and apnea. Newborn infants with GBS EOD present clinically at or shortly after birth. Most infants become symptomatic by 12 to 24 hours of age. They can present with the following: tachypnea, tachycardia, lethargy, severe cardiorespiratory failure, persistent pulmonary hypertension, and perinatal encephalopathy.

C. **Was the mother tested for group B** *Streptococcus*, **and did she receive adequate intrapartum antibiotic prophylaxis if she tested positive?** The AAP and ACOG have recently published guidelines for the prevention and management of GBS EOD in newborns (2019), which replace the prior guidelines published by the CDC (and endorsed by the AAP). All pregnant women should undergo antepartum screening for GBS at 36 0/7 to 37 6/7 weeks of gestation, and receive appropriate intrapartum antibiotic prophylaxis unless a cesarean section is performed prior to labor and with intact membranes. For the purposes of assessing risk of GBS disease in the infant, only penicillin, ampicillin, and cefazolin administered >4 hours prior to delivery are considered adequate intrapartum prophylaxis.

D. Did the mother have a fever? The incidence of intrapartum fever (≥38.0°C [≥100.4°F]) is estimated to be present in approximately 6% to 9% of deliveries ≥36 weeks' gestation. In a study of >6000 deliveries, 412 mothers had intrapartum fever and only 1 developed EOS, with no significant difference in the rate of EOS among those deliveries with intrapartum fever and those without. In VLBW infants, only approximately 23% of culture-proven sepsis was associated with a maternal fever.

E. Did the mother have signs of suspected intra-amniotic infection? Isolated maternal fever is not synonymous with an intra-amniotic infection (formerly chorioamnionitis; see later discussion regarding terminology changes). A confirmed diagnosis of intra-amniotic infection is difficult to make prior to delivery. Maternal signs concerning for suspected intra-amniotic infection include maternal intrapartum fever (single maternal temperature ≥39.0°C [102.2°F] or a persistent temperature of 38.0–38.9°C [100.4–102°F]) with 1 or more of the following: maternal leukocytosis, purulent cervical drainage, or fetal tachycardia.

　　1. **Recent recommended terminology updates.** In January 2015, the NICHD proposed replacing the term *CAM* (*chorioamnionitis*) with *intrauterine inflammation or infection or both* (*triple I*). Triple I is defined as maternal fever (>39°C [102.2°F] once or 38°C [100.4°F] twice) plus 1 of more of the following: fetal tachycardia (>160 beats/min for >10 minutes); maternal WBC >15,000/mm^3 in the absence of corticosteroids; purulent fluid from the cervical os; or biochemical or microbiologic amniotic fluid results consistent with microbial invasion. The NICHD further suggested categorizing cases as isolated maternal fever (when additional criteria are not met), suspected triple I (in the absence of objective evidence of infection in amniotic fluid), or confirmed triple I (when criteria are accompanied by objective evidence of amniotic fluid infection, which may ultimately be retrospective based on pathology). In 2017, the American College of Obstetricians and Gynecologists (ACOG) endorsed this change in terminology, suggesting that chorioamnionitis be replaced with intra-amniotic infection and adopting the distinction between confirmed and suspected cases. The AAP 2018 guidelines on EOS also reflect this change.

　　2. **Risk factors for intra-amniotic infection** include spontaneous labor, low parity, multiple digital vaginal examinations, MSAF, presence of genital tract microorganisms, prolonged active labor, prolonged ROM, and internal fetal or uterine monitoring. Studies of MSAF in isolation have not shown it to be an independent risk factor for early-onset neonatal sepsis. A recent Cochrane review identified 4 randomized controlled trials evaluating efficacy of antibiotics in preventing sepsis in infants born through MSAF and found no difference in the rate of confirmed sepsis.

III. Differential diagnosis. Helps to guide further workup and treatment.

　A. Culture-proven sepsis. Positive cultures (eg, blood or CSF) confirm sepsis diagnosis.

　B. Suspected sepsis. An infant has nonspecific signs of sepsis, or there is a high likelihood that the infant has sepsis based on clinical signs. Sepsis needs to be ruled out in the infant. From 18% to 33% of infants with negative blood cultures have sepsis confirmed at autopsy. Noninfectious syndromes (respiratory distress syndrome [RDS]) can mimic sepsis.

　C. Increased risk for sepsis. The infant has risk factors based on AAP or CDC guidelines or NICHD workshop.

D. **Infant at low risk for sepsis.** Newborns without the risk factors noted previously are at low risk of sepsis.

IV. **Database**

A. **Complete maternal, perinatal, and birth history** should be obtained and reviewed to identify risk factors, as noted previously. **Maternal history is just as important as the birth history.** It is important to discuss the possibility of intra-amniotic infection with the obstetrician and carefully consider whether the mother has a suspected or confirmed infection.

B. **Physical examination.** Most infants with EOS exhibit abnormal signs in the first 24 hours of life. Observe for signs of sepsis (see Section II.B). Clinical observation is important, such as affect, peripheral perfusion, and respiratory status were key predictors in sepsis compared with feeding patterns, level of activity, and level of alertness in 1 study. The maternal clinical examination should be reviewed with the obstetrics and gynecology service. **Key point: EOS does occur in infants who appear healthy at birth.**

C. **Laboratory studies**

1. **Definitive laboratory studies for early-onset sepsis:** Blood culture, LP.

   a. **Peripheral blood cultures are the gold standard for diagnosis of sepsis and should be obtained prior to starting antibiotics.** Small specimen volumes decrease the sensitivity (a minimum of 1 mL per single bottle is recommended for optimal recovery of organisms). Using 2 separate culture bottles is advantageous to allow comparison (contamination vs true infection). Using aerobic and anaerobic systems will allow one to rule out rare strict anaerobic species. Most neonatal pathogens (GBS, *E coli,* and *S aureus*) also grow on aerobic cultures. Contemporary blood cultures can reliably detect bacteremia at 1 to 10 colony-forming units/mL. Collection systems also contain antimicrobial neutralization elements. Optimum ways to obtain blood culture in a neonate include the following (fresh vein is preferred to reduce contamination): peripheral vein, arterial puncture, newly placed intravenous (IV) catheter, and umbilical artery catheter immediately after placement. Risk of contamination is greater with umbilical vein blood culture. Umbilical venous catheter at delivery is also acceptable if the cord is adequately prepared (double clamped and adequately prepared segment of the cord).

   b. **Lumbar puncture.** The use of an LP for CSF examination in EOS involves many factors. Is the infant stable enough for the procedure? Will obtaining the procedure delay starting antibiotics? **AAP guidelines for both term/ late preterm and preterm infants recommend that an LP be considered in infants who are "at the highest risk of infection, especially those with critical illness."**

      i. **Term and late preterm infants:** Infants with clinical signs of illness are considered to be at the highest risk for sepsis, and in those patients it is recommended that an LP is performed prior to initiating antibiotics, **if feasible, and ensuring it does not delay the initiation of antibiotics.** If the LP cannot be done prior to antibiotic initiation, it can be reserved for cases in which the blood culture is positive. If blood cultures are negative, the incidence of culture confirmed meningitis is low (1–2 cases/100,000 live births). Culture confirmed meningitis in term infants is rare (0.01–0.02 cases/1000 live births).

      ii. **Preterm infants:** The incidence of meningitis is higher among premature infants (0.7 cases per 1000 births) than among overall births. LP is recommended, as discussed earlier for term infants, prior to the start of antibiotics. If this is not possible, the physician needs to make the decision on whether to do an LP in a critically ill infant based on the clinical status of the infant, the risk of EOS, and the risk of prolonged antibiotic therapy.

iii. **The lumbar puncture also helps to rule out viral etiologies** such as enteroviral infection, herpes virus infection, *Parechovirus* meningitis, and meningoencephalitis.

iv. **Cerebrospinal fluid values in neonatal meningitis are controversial,** and meningitis can occur with normal CSF values. A study evaluating >9000 infants >34 weeks used a CSF WBC cutoff of 20 cells/mm^3, which resulted in missed diagnoses in 13% of infants with confirmed meningitis. While culture remains the gold standard for evaluation of the CSF, emerging technologies such as real-time polymerase chain reaction (PCR) have an overall higher detection rate, particularly in infants who have already received antibiotics. Examples from a study on meningitis CSF lab results include the following:

(a) **Uninfected preterm/term infants:** Mean WBC <10 cells/mm^3.

(b) **Infants >34 weeks' gestation with bacterial meningitis:** Median WBC >477 mm^3.

(c) **Infants <34 weeks' gestation with meningitis:** Median WBC 110/mm^3.

v. **Helpful facts when deciding on meningitis lab results:**

(a) **Infants with gram-negative meningitis** have a higher CSF WBC count than infants with gram-positive pathogens.

(b) **Number of bands** in the CSF does not predict meningitis.

(c) **If there is a >2-hour delay at the lab,** WBC and glucose decrease.

(d) **Cerebrospinal fluid protein concentrations in healthy term infants** are <100 mg/dL, and in preterm infants, they vary inversely with gestational age.

(e) **Low cerebrospinal fluid glucose** has the best specificity to diagnose meningitis.

(f) **In meningitis, protein concentrations are higher** and glucose concentrations are lower in term infants than preterm infants.

2. **Additional laboratory testing to be considered.** The most recent guidelines by the AAP (as well as NICHD and the Kaiser Sepsis Calculator) no longer explicitly recommend evaluating infants with additional laboratory testing other than blood culture (and lumbar puncture, if clinically indicated). There are no recommendations regarding early cessation of antibiotics based on additional laboratory testing, or continuing empiric antibiotics in the presence of a negative blood culture due to abnormal secondary laboratory testing. **Blood culture is the gold standard for identifying early onset sepsis.** The following tests can be considered in individualized cases when clinically appropriate:

a. **Complete blood count with differential.** AAP states that using complete blood counts (CBC) alone to determine the risk of GBS EOD is not justified since it has a poor test performance in predicting disease. Immature/total neutrophil ratio (I/T) and absolute neutrophil count (ANC) are the most commonly used WBC count parameters. Many factors affect the WBC count some of which are gestational age, sex, mode of delivery, maternal preeclampsia, and placental insufficiency as well as PROM can cause bone marrow depression in the fetus and an abnormal WBC without an infection. Studies have found that the CBC lacked sensitivity for predicting EOS. A single CBC is not helpful when compared to serial tests. Timing of the CBC is important; an early CBC is not recommended, a CBC at 6 to 12 hours is optimal, after the inflammatory response has occurred. In general, **a CBC has a better negative predictive value (ability to rule out infection) than a positive** predictive value (ability to rule in infection), especially when using serial measurements. Extreme values were associated with a higher likelihood of infection: WBC <1000 cells/uL, ANC <1000, I/T neutrophil >0.25 was associated with an infection in infants <34 weeks' gestation.

i. **Total white blood cell count.** Abnormally low or high WBC count is worrisome. Values <6000 cells/mm^3 or >30,000 cells/mm^3 in the first 24 hours of life are abnormal. Only half of infants with WBC <5000 cells/mm^3 or WBC >20,000 cells/mm^3 have positive blood cultures. As many as 50% of infants with culture-proven sepsis have normal WBC counts. Septic infants with a WBC count <5000 cells/mm^3 are more likely to have bacterial meningitis.

ii. **Total neutrophil count.** Includes segmented (fully mature) neutrophils and bands (almost mature neutrophils). Total neutrophil count is more sensitive than the total leukocyte count but is too often normal in cases of infection. It peaks in 12 hours, and it has a poor sensitivity and poor predictive accuracy for EOS. See Table 78–1 for total neutrophil counts for variable gestational ages, Table 78–2 for neutrophil values in late preterm and term infants, and Table 78–3 for neutrophil values in VLBW infants.

iii. **Immature neutrophil count (bands).** If >20%, it is considered abnormal. The total immature neutrophil count has poor sensitivity but better positive predictive value. See Table 78–2.

iv. **Ratio of immature to total neutrophils.** The greatest value relies in its negative predictive value; the likelihood of infection is minimal if the I: T ratio is normal. Reference ranges for late preterm and term infants are shown in Table 78–2. In most healthy preterm infants at <32 weeks (96%), the I: T ratio is <0.22. A study of serial neutrophil values demonstrated that a combination of 3 separate neutrophil values (total neutrophils, immature neutrophils, and I: T ratio), obtained serially over the first 24 hours of life, had the greatest negative predictive value for EOS among WBC markers.

v. **Neutropenia** is a decrease in the number of neutrophils and a good marker for sepsis because of its relatively small differential. It generally occurs only in sepsis, asphyxia, inborn errors of metabolism, hemolytic disease, and pregnancy-induced maternal hypertension. Neutropenia is more common in small for gestational age and low birthweight neonates. Early-onset neutropenia in small for gestational age infants, usually secondary to decreased production of neutrophils due to intrauterine hypoxia, can last up to 1 week, is associated with

Table 78–1. NEONATAL TOTAL NEUTROPHIL COUNT[a] REFERENCE RANGES (× 10^3/MM^3) (5%–95%)

Variable	Birth	12 Hours	24 Hours	48 Hours	72 Hours	>72 Hours
Term infants (>36 weeks)	3.5–18	7.5–27.5	7.0–22.5	4.2–15.8	2.8–12.9	2.7–13
28–36 weeks	1–10	3.5–25	2.8–19.2	1.7–15.8	0.5–12.5	1.0–12.5
<28 weeks	0.5–8	1.2–34	1.2–40	0.5–26	0.5–23	1.3–153

[a]Total count includes mature and immature forms.
Data from Schmutz N, Henry E, Jopling J, et al: Expected ranges for blood neutrophil concentrations of neonates: the Manroe and Mouzinho charts revisited, *J Perinatol.* 2008 Apr;28(4):275-281.

Table 78–2. NEONATAL NEUTROPHIL INDICES REFERENCE RANGES FOR LATE PRETERM AND TERM INFANTS (PER MM³)

Variable	Birth	12 Hours	24 Hours	48 Hours	72 Hours	>120 Hours
Absolute total neutrophil count[a]	1800–5400	7800–14,400	7200–12,600	4200–9000	1800–7000	1800–5400
Total immature neutrophil count[b]	≤1120	≤1440	≤1280	<800	<500	<500
I:T ratio[c]	<0.16	<0.16	<0.13	<0.13	<0.13	<0.12

[a]Total count includes mature and immature forms. Derived from the white blood cells and the percentage of neutrophils.
[b]Includes all neutrophils except segmented ones.
[c]Ratio of immature to total neutrophils (total immature neutrophil count divided by absolute total neutrophil count).
Data from Manroe BL, Weinberg AG, Rosenfeld CR, et al: The neonatal blood count in health and disease. I. Reference values for neutrophilic cells, *J Pediatr.* 1979 Jul;95(1):89-98.

Table 78–3. **REFERENCE RANGES FOR NEUTROPHIL COUNTS IN VERY LOW BIRTHWEIGHT INFANTS (<1500 G)**

Age	Absolute Total Neutrophil Count (mm^3) (range)
Birth	500–6000
18 hours	2200–14,000
60 hours	1100–8800
120 hours	1100–5600

Data from Mouzinho A, Rosenfeld CR, Sánchez PJ, et al: Revised reference ranges for circulating neutrophils in very-low-birth-weight neonates, *Pediatrics.* 1994 Jul;94(1):76-82.

thrombocytopenia, and has an increased risk of necrotizing enterocolitis (NEC). The neutropenia ranges depend on gestational age (WBC count increases with gestational age), type of delivery (vaginal births have higher WBC counts than cesarean section without labor), type of sample (arterial samples give lower WBC counts than venous samples), and altitude (WBC counts are higher at higher altitudes). Tables 78–2 and 78–3 show historical results for late preterm/term infants and low birthweight infants, respectively.

    b. **Acute phase reactants (C-reactive protein and procalcitonin)** have been studied to help identify infants with sepsis. Both CRP and procalcitonin concentrations can be increased in response to infections or noninfectious conditions such as asphyxia, pneumothorax, ischemic tissue injuries, hemolysis, and meconium aspiration syndrome. The AAP states that using CRP alone to determine the risk of GBS EOD is not justified since it has a poor test performance in predicting disease.

      i. **C-reactive protein** is the acute phase reactant that has been the best studied in sepsis. An increasing CRP is worrisome and is elevated in 50% to 90% of infants with sepsis. CRP increases at 6 to 8 hours and peaks at 24 hours. If CRPs remain normal, sepsis is less likely. Early CRP should not be used to rule out sepsis because it is unreliable at the initial time of a sepsis evaluation. In a study of almost 1000 infants with culture-proven sepsis, CRP was <1 mg/dL (normal) at the onset of clinical sepsis in 25% of cases. The main interest in CRP is its negative predictive value if repeated over 1 to 3 days when the value remains normal. One study showed that 2 normal CRPs (1 acquired 8–24 hours after birth and 1 acquired 24 hours later) have a negative predictive accuracy of 99.7% and a negative likelihood ratio of 0.15 for neonatal sepsis. No recommendations exist on using an elevated CRP to help determine duration of antibiotic therapy. An estimate of normal CRP values is as follows (ranges in parentheses):

        (a) **C-reactive protein (term). Birth:** 0.1 mg/dL (0.01–0.65 mg/dL); **21 hours:** 1.5 mg/dL (0.2–10.0 mg/dL); **56 to 70 hours:** 1.9 mg/dL (0.3–13 mg/dL); **96 hours:** 1.4 mg/dL (0.2–9 mg/dL).

        (b) **C-reactive protein (preterm). Birth:** 0.1 mg/dL (0.01–0.64 mg/dL); **27 to 36 hours:** 1.7 mg/dL (0.3–11 mg/dL); **90 hours:** 0.7 mg/dL (0.1–4.7 mg/dL).

      ii. **Serum procalcitonin.** A prohormone of calcitonin, procalcitonin (PCT) levels are elevated in sepsis and have been used as a marker for sepsis. A single value is not helpful, whereas serial negative values are associated with absence of EOS. PCT has better sensitivity and specificity than CRP. However, it can be increased due to asphyxia, pneumothorax, neonatal resuscitation, mothers with intra-amniotic infection (in the absence of neonatal infection), GBS colonization, and prolonged ROM (in the absence of neonatal infection). Serum PCT also increases normally in the first 24 to 36 hours of life. Normal levels over the first 48 hours are associated with no evidence of EOS. AAP does not recommend extending antibiotic therapy based on abnormal values. These factors currently limit its usefulness as a marker, and more high-quality studies are needed before it is incorporated into routine practice. Estimates of normal PCT levels are as follows (ranges in parentheses):

   (a) **Procalcitonin (term). Birth:** 0.08 mcg/L (0.01–0.55 mcg/L); **24 hours:** 2.9 mcg/L (0.4–18.7 mcg/L); **80 hours:** 0.3 (0.04–1.8 mcg/L).

   (b) **Procalcitonin (preterm). Birth:** 0.07 mcg/L (0.01–0.56 mcg/L); **21 to 22 hours:** 6.5 mcg/L (0.9–48.4 mcg/L); **5 days:** 0.10 mcg/L (0.01–0.8 mcg/L).

c. **Baseline serum glucose.** Hypoglycemia can be an early marker for sepsis, but there is no evidence that hypoglycemia occurring in isolation in an otherwise well appearing infant is a risk factor for GBS EOD or EOS. Studies have suggested that it can be an additional sign of severe sepsis and can be used in a model to predict failure of conventional antibiotic therapy. In addition, serum glucose can be helpful when interpreting CSF glucose, as they have a linear relationship. One study suggested that for every increase in serum glucose of 1.0 mg/dL, the CSF glucose increases by 0.56 mg/dL.

d. **Arterial blood gas.** To rule out metabolic acidosis if clinically indicated.

e. **Platelet count/coagulation studies.** These are used to rule out thrombocytopenia and disseminated intravascular coagulation. A low platelet count is a nonspecific and insensitive test for sepsis. A decreased platelet count is usually a late sign of sepsis.

f. **Molecular assays** include conventional and real-time PCR, PCR followed by post-PCR processing, multiplex PCR, staphylococcal PCR, and fungal PCR. They are newer methods of detecting infection based on detecting DNA from bacteria. Advantages of these tests are that they produce rapid results. Cochrane review states they may perform well as "add-on" tests. Compared to blood culture, they are more rapid, require less blood, can be more sensitive, and can be useful after the initiation of antibiotics when standard blood cultures may become sterile. They are limited in their ability to inform antibiotic choices. Blood culture remains the gold standard for antimicrobial drug susceptibility. The following is not an exhaustive list of these assays, but highlights a few that have been studied in neonates:

   i. **16S rRNA polymerase chain reaction** uses universal primers conserved among bacterial species to detect the presence of bacteria quicker than traditional blood cultures. It has been studied in neonates and is more sensitive than blood culture in EOS. **PCR restriction fragment length polymorphism,** a related assay, can be used to identify the specific bacterial species.

   ii. **Syndrome Evaluation System (SES).** Multiplex PCR-based diagnostic tool that has been studied in a randomized controlled trial of neonates. Detection of bacteria was 4-fold higher compared to traditional blood cultures, with 100% concordance.

   iii. **PCR coupled with electrospray ionization mass spectrometry (PCR/ESI-MS).** Analysis of blood samples of neonates with suspected sepsis using **PCR/ESI-MS** had a 98% negative predictive value when compared to blood cultures. It has been proposed as a tool to allow for earlier reassessment of antibiotic administration.

3. **Laboratory testing that is not routinely recommended in the evaluation of early onset sepsis:**
    a. **Urine culture** is no longer recommended in infants <72 hours of age in an EOS workup. It is more appropriate for late-onset sepsis workup.
    b. **Gastric aspirate analysis** is not recommended since it cannot be used to diagnose EOS. WBCs in the gastric aspirate at birth represent maternal response and do not correlate with sepsis in the neonate.
    c. **Newborn surface cultures** (usually obtained from the axilla, external ear canal, groin, etc) are not recommended since they cannot be used to diagnose EOS.
    d. **Tracheal aspirate** may be of benefit for Gram stain and culture if performed immediately after endotracheal tube placement. Some advocate this only if pneumonia is suspected or the volume of secretions increases or there is overwhelming newborn EOS. In a sample of 139 tracheal aspirate cultures taken within 12 hours of birth, 6.5% grew a pathogenic specimen. Tracheal aspirate cultures done after several days of intubation are of no value.
    e. **Erythrocyte sedimentation rate (ESR)** is increased with infection but has limited value in diagnosing or monitoring infection. A low value does not exclude the diagnosis of sepsis.
4. **Laboratory tests in development.** The following tests are all under investigation, and the list is not exhaustive. In general, there is a lack of confirmatory studies and a wide variation in results, cost, and turnaround time, which limit their use. There are no guidelines that recommend their use at this time.
    a. **Serum amyloid A.** An apolipoprotein synthesized by the liver secreted in response to injury or infection. Serum amyloid A levels have been shown to have high sensitivity in 2 high-quality studies. Limited in use due to the cost and turnaround time.
    b. **Cytokines.** Interleukin (IL)-6, IL-1B, soluble IL-2 receptor, IL-8, and tumor necrosis factor-α (TNF-α) all increase in response to a bacterial infection. Cytokines are also found in umbilical cord blood and can predict the risk of infection in the first few hours after birth and can predict late-onset sepsis. They are early biomarkers (2–12 hours) in sepsis and generally have very short half-lives, which creates a narrow window for detection.
    c. **Surface antigens** found on a variety of WBCs and endothelial cells include CD11b, CD64, sCD14, and E-selectin. They require sophisticated equipment, are very expensive, and have a long turnaround time.
    d. **Cord blood markers.** The most promising markers are IL-6, serum amyloid A, and PCT, but large studies are required.
    e. **Other markers** being studied include lipopolysaccharide binding protein, urinary neutrophil gelatinase–associated lipocalin, calprotectin, inter-α inhibitor proteins, and other protein biomarkers (eg, fibronectin, lactoferrin).
D. **Imaging and other studies**
    1. **Chest x-ray.** Pneumonia is a common presentation of EOS, and GBS pneumonia can mimic RDS. With signs of respiratory infection, obtain a chest radiograph to rule out pneumonia.
    2. **Echocardiography and Doppler imaging.** Can be used to assess myocardial function in infants with sepsis, which can cause systolic and diastolic myocardial dysfunction.
    3. **Head ultrasound or magnetic resonance imaging.** Neonatal central nervous system (CNS) infections are typically diagnosed based on clinical and laboratory findings. Imaging modalities can be useful in diagnosing complications of CNS infections, with magnetic resonance imaging (MRI) generally offering greater sensitivity and specificity. MRI can also be used to inform treatment duration.

V. **Plan**

A. **General comments.** For many cases, a decision about whether an infant requires a sepsis workup and antibiotic treatment can be straightforward. Infants who are clinically sick or have a positive history of known increased risk factors for sepsis with clinical signs should be evaluated. However, if an infant does not have a clear-cut history and clinical presentation, the decision is more difficult. Consideration must be made regarding the risks of missing early-onset sepsis in infants who are of low risk, and a need to be stewards of antibiotic use and limit overtreatment. Once the decision is made to treat the infant, treatment usually involves at least 36 to 48 hours of antibiotics after obtaining cultures. **For risk assessment and treatment it is important to remember that separate consideration of infants must be given to those born at ≥35 0/7 weeks' gestation and to those born ≤34 6/7 weeks' gestation.**

B. **Historical context.** The CDC guidelines for the prevention of GBS were initially published in 1996, and endorsed by AAP in 2002. The CDC published updated guidelines in 2010 which were endorsed by the AAP. While written for the evaluation and management of GBS disease in neonates, these guidelines have historically served as treatment algorithm for evaluating infants at risk for early-onset sepsis more generally. In 2017, a consensus between the CDC, AAP, ACOG, and other stakeholders determined that the AAP would revise and update neonatal care recommendations moving forward (while ACOG would update guidelines involving obstetric care). The AAP subsequently published guidelines on the management of newborns at risk for early onset sepsis in 2018, and the management of infants at risk for GBS specifically in 2019 (which officially replaces the 2010 CDC guidelines). **In the AAP GBS guidelines, they stress that "the clinical approach to risk of GBS EOD should be the same as that for all bacterial causes of early-onset sepsis", and therefore present the same options for clinical evaluation in both guidelines.** The NICHD workshop on the management of chorioamnionitis published recommendations regarding the care of neonates born to mothers with "suspected Triple I," based on their new terminology (2016). While the change in terminology has been endorsed by both ACOG and AAP, the management recommendations differ from the most recent AAP guidelines published in 2018. In these guidelines, we will primarily discuss the guidelines recommended by the AAP, but will make note of where the NICHD recommendations differ.

C. **Prevention.** Appropriate maternal intrapartum antibiotic prophylaxis is the only proven preventive measurement for EOS and should be given based on the newly updated AAP/ACOG Guidelines, published in 2019 and officially replacing the previous CDC guidelines. In brief, recommendations for maternal intrapartum antibiotic prophylaxis (IAP) are:

1. **Universal antepartum screening for GBS at 36 0/7 to 37 6/7 weeks of gestation** using vaginal-rectal cultures. Testing is also recommended for women who present in preterm labor and/or with PROM before 37 0/7 weeks' gestation. Women with GBS bacteriuria during pregnancy, or who had a prior child with GBS disease do not need to undergo routine screening (because IAP is already indicated).

2. **IAP is recommended in the following scenarios:**
   a. All women who screen positive unless a cesarean birth is planned and performed prior to the onset of labor, in the setting of intact membranes.
   b. Women with GBS bacteriuria identified during pregnancy.
   c. Women with a history of a previous infant with GBS disease.
   d. Women who present in preterm labor and/or with PROM at <37 0/7 weeks' gestation.
   e. Women who present in labor at ≥37 0/7 weeks' gestation with unknown GBS status if risk factors develop during labor (maternal temperature ≥100.4°F,

ROM ≥18 hours), or if point-of-care nucleic acid amplication testing (NAAT) is positive for GBS.

3. **IAP can be considered in women with GBS colonization** in a prior pregnancy whose current status is not yet known.

D. **Treatment plans for term and late preterm infants (≥35 weeks' gestation) can be based on three approaches (see page 1180, Figure 146–1):** Categorical risk factor assessment, multivariate risk assessment, or risk assessment based on clinical condition. All these approaches are considered acceptable and each has advantages and limitations. The AAP recommend that decisions are made at the institutional level regarding which approach to use, as resources need to be allocated accordingly.

   1. **Categorical risk factor assessment (see Figure 146–1A).** Classical approaches to evaluation for early onset sepsis have used categorical risk factor assessment, such as the prior CDC guidelines on management of neonates at risk for GBS. It is important to note that maternal intrapartum temperature ≥38°C (100.4°F) is used as a surrogate for intra-amniotic infection. If categorical risk factor assessment is the chosen approach, the AAP guidelines recommend the following:

      a. **If signs of clinical illness** (abnormal vital signs such as tachycardia, tachypnea, temperature instability, supplemental oxygen requirement; requiring CPAP or mechanical ventilation or blood pressure support): Blood cultures and empiric antibiotics should be initiated. Lumbar puncture should also be considered and CSF culture before initiation of empiric antibiotics for infants who are at the highest risk of infection, especially those with critical illness. A lumbar puncture should not be performed if the infants clinical condition would be compromised. Note that antibiotics should be given promptly and not deferred because of a delay in the procedure.

      b. **If no signs of clinical illness, but maternal intrapartum temperature ≥38°C (100.4°F).** Blood cultures and empiric antibiotics should be initiated. LP should also be considered and CSF culture before initiation of empiric antibiotics for infants who are at the highest risk of infection, especially those with critical illness. It should not be performed if the infants' clinical condition would be compromised and antibiotics should be given promptly and not deferred because of a delay in the procedure.

      c. **If neither of the above are true, is GBS IAP indicated for the mother?** (See Section V.C.)

         i. **If not indicated:** Routine newborn care
         ii. **If indicated, and adequate GBS IAP given** (adequate GBS IAP is defined as the administration of penicillin G, ampicillin or cefazolin ≥4 hours before delivery): Routine newborn care
         iii. **If indicated, and adequate GBS IAP not given:** Clinical observation for 36 to 48 hours after birth.
            (a) This includes women who receive other antibiotics (such as clindamycin or vancomycin) , or received antibiotics <4 hours prior to delivery.

      d. **Limitations.** While this is the traditional approach to management, categorical risk factor assessment means that many individual patients will have a relatively low risk of sepsis and still receive empiric treatment. This approach will therefore result in empirical treatment of many low-risk neonates.

   2. **Multivariate risk assessment (Sepsis calculator).** See Figure 146–1B. The best-studied scoring system is a multivariate prediction model developed by Kaiser Permanente (https://kp.org/eoscalc), which they have studied in a population of >50,000 infants born at 35 weeks or later. This estimates an individual infants' risk of EOS, including GBS EOD. The scoring system led

to a reduction in the use of antibiotics and blood cultures, while maintaining the same incidence of EOS and with no change in other adverse outcomes. The tool integrates an individual infant's combination of risk factors and clinical condition to estimate an individual infant's risk of EOS. This septic scoring system is based on incidence of early onset sepsis in your unit (or using the baseline national rate of 0.5/1000 live births), gestational age in weeks and days, highest maternal antepartum temperature, hours of ROM, maternal GBS status, and type and timing of intrapartum antibiotics (only penicillin, ampicillin, or cefazolin are considered GBS specific antibiotics; if clindamycin or vancomycin are given alone one should enter no antibiotics), where all this information is put in a interactor calculator tool and the EOS risk at birth per 1000 births is calculated as a percentage. An EOS risk after the clinical exam is also calculated with a clinical and vital sign recommendation based on that risk. Clinical recommendations depending upon the percentage of risk include: no blood culture recommended, obtain a blood culture, no antibiotics recommended, empiric antibiotics recommended, or strongly consider starting antibiotics. Vital sign recommendations depending upon the percentage of risk include: routine vital signs, vital signs every 4 hours for 24 hours, or vital signs per NICU.

  a. The classification of the infant's clinical presentation is:
    i. **Well appearing:** no persistent physiologic abnormalities.
    ii. **Equivocal:** persistent physiologic abnormality ≥4 hours or 2 or more physiologic abnormalities lasting for ≥2 hours: tachycardia or HR ≥160, tachypnea ≥60, temperature instability ≥100.4°C or <97.5°C, respiratory distress not requiring supplemental oxygen.
    iii. **Clinical illness:** persistent need for NCPAP/HFNC/mechanical ventilation outside of the delivery room, hemodynamic instability requiring vasoactive drugs, neonatal encephalopathy/perinatal depression (seizure or APGAR Score at 5 minutes <5), need for supplemental O_2 ≥2 hours to maintain oxygen saturations >90% outside the delivery room.
  b. **For the purposes of the calculator, "GBS-specific antibiotics" refers only to penicillin, ampicillin, or cefazolin.**
  c. **Limitations.** Ideally individual institutions should use local data to validate the use of the calculator at their own institution. Centers that adopt this approach need to plan ahead and provide the resources required for close clinical observation in infants who would otherwise receive empiric antibiotic prophylaxis. While expected to be rare, prompt recognition of a change in clinical condition is critical to properly reassessing those infants who receive monitoring only despite a higher than normal risk of sepsis.
3. **Risk assessment based on newborn clinical condition (enhanced observation).** See Figure 146–1C. Good clinical condition at birth is associated with a decreased risk of EOS by 60% to 70%. This approach leads to a decrease in the rate of antibiotic use. It requires significant changes to newborn care as it requires multiple physical examinations for the first 36 to 48 hours of life. Infants who appear ill at birth or those that develop signs of illness over the first 48 hours after birth are treated with antibiotics.
  a. **Who and when to examine?**
    i. **Conduct serial examinations on all newborn infants without regard to risk of EOS.** Physical examinations to detect the presence of clinical signs of illness would be performed serially (eg, every 4–6 hours) for the first 48 hours of life. This scenario would identify those low risk infants that develop EOS (1/10,000 live birth of term/late preterm infants).
    ii. **Decide a categorical or multivariate approach for those infants at risk.** Conduct serial physical examinations to detect the presence of

clinical signs of illness for the first 48 hours of life in those infants at risk. Physical examinations and vital signs ideally would be performed every 4 to 6 hours for the first 36 to 48 hours of life.

  iii. **Infants whose mothers had an intrapartum temperature ≥38°C (100.4°F) or inadequate indicated GBS IAP.** Serial physical examinations and vital signs for 36 to 48 hours.

  b. **Who to treat?**

  i. **Any infant who has signs of clinical illness at birth, or normal at birth but develops signs of clinical illness in the first 48 hours after birth.**

  (a) **Treat empirically with antibiotic agents.**

  (b) **Further evaluate with laboratory screening** (blood culture and consider LP and CSF culture prior to initiation of empiric antibiotics for infants; LP should not be performed if the infant's clinical condition would be compromised and antibiotics should not be deferred because of a delay in the procedure).

  c. **Who not to treat?** An infant with no signs of clinical illness, whose maternal intrapartum temperature was <38°C (100.4°F), or adequate indicated GBS IAP does not need treatment and should receive routine newborn care.

  d. **Limitations.** This approach places the largest proportion of infants into the category of "close observation," which requires formal processes to ensure that serial, well-documented physical examinations occur. Individual centers would also need clear criteria based on physical evaluation and empiric antibiotic administration.

4. **NICHD proposed algorithm.** The NICHD Workshop (2015) recommended a categorical approach which separates isolated maternal fever from suspected intra-amniotic infection (fever plus fetal tachycardia >160 bpm for 10 minutes or longer, maternal leukocytosis >15,000 per mm^3, or purulent fluid from the cervical os), while all three approaches described and endorsed by the AAP above use maternal fever as a surrogate for intra-amniotic infection (Kaiser sepsis calculator factors highest maternal temperature). In infants ≥34 weeks who are well appearing with either isolated maternal fever or suspected intra-amniotic infection, the NICHD risk assessment recommends clinical observation only with "frequent close observations" (but not specific recommendations regarding serial examination). They also endorse the use of the Kaiser Sepsis Calculator for patients who fall in the "suspected intra-amniotic infection" category.

E. **Treatment approach for infants ≤34 6/7 weeks' gestational age.** These infants are at the highest risk for early onset infection from all causes. **Preterm infants can be categorized by level of risk for EOS based on their circumstances of birth** (see page 1183 or Figure 146–2). Clear communication and documentation between OB and neonatology are critical in these cases to insure an accurate risk assessment. Clinicians can adopt one of the following strategies:

1. **Preterm infants at highest risk for EOS.** Any infant born preterm because of cervical insufficiency, preterm labor, PROM, intra-amniotic infection (consider when a pregnant woman presents with unexplained decreased fetal movement and/or there is sudden and unexplained poor fetal testing), and/or acute and otherwise unexplained onset of nonreassuring fetal status are at the highest risk of EOS and GBS EOD.

  a. **Obtain a blood culture and start empirical antibiotic treatment.**

  b. **Consider an LP for culture and analysis of CSF** in clinically ill infants with a high risk of infection, unless the procedure will compromise the infant's clinical condition.

  c. **Give antibiotics promptly,** do not defer because of a delay in a procedure.

2. **Preterm infants at lowest risk for EOS.** Are born under circumstances that include **all of these criteria:** maternal and/or fetal indications for preterm

birth (eg, maternal eclampsia or other noninfectious medical illness, placental insufficiency, fetal growth restriction), birth by cesarean delivery, absence of labor, attempts to induce labor, or any ROM before delivery. AAP guidelines state that acceptable initial approaches to management for these patients include:

    a. **No laboratory evaluation and no empiric antibiotic therapy.**

    b. **Blood culture and clinical monitoring.**

    c. **Infants who do not improve after initial stabilization** and or those infants who have severe systemic instability, giving empirical antibiotics may be reasonable but is not mandatory.

3. **Preterm infants at unclear risk for EOS.** Infants delivered for maternal and/or fetal indications but who are born by vaginal or cesarean section after attempted induction of labor and/or with ROM before delivery. These infants are at a potentially higher risk of GBS EOD.

    a. **If the mother has an indication for GBS IAP and adequate IAP (penicillin, ampicillin, or cefazolin ≥4 hours before delivery) is not given or if there is concern for intra-amniotic infection** (consider when a pregnant woman presents with unexplained decreased fetal movement and/or there is sudden and unexplained poor fetal testing), **or the infant has respiratory or cardiovascular instability.**

        i. **Obtain a blood culture and start empirical antibiotic treatment.**

        ii. **Consider an LP for culture and analysis of CSF** in clinically ill infants with a high suspicion for GBS EOD, unless the procedure will compromise the infant's clinical condition.

    b. **Infants that are well at birth:** close observation.

    c. **Infants with respiratory and/or cardiovascular instability after birth:** obtain a blood culture and initiate antibiotic therapy.

4. **NICHD proposed algorithm.** For infants ≤34 weeks' gestation, the NICHD proposed algorithm is in line with the AAP guidelines. They recommend blood culture and empiric antibiotics in the setting of suspected/confirmed Triple I, or isolated maternal fever. The algorithm does not address other risk factors for EOS aside from intra-amniotic infection.

F. **Antibiotic therapy.** Consider the risk/benefit balance before starting antibiotic therapy for the risk of EOS as well as continuing antibiotics if there is no documented infection. **If the decision is to treat** (empirical treatment based on risk factors, positive cultures, term infants who are critically ill with negative cultures):

1. **Obtain blood cultures prior to initiating antibiotic therapy,** and consider CSF analysis if clinically indicated at the initiation of therapy (infant is unwell but stable enough to undergo the procedure). LP is also indicated after initiating empiric antibiotic therapy if there is a positive blood culture, the infant develops clinical signs or lab values highly suspicious for sepsis or meningitis, or the infant does not respond to treatment. Any other cultures that seem appropriate should be sent to the laboratory (eg, if there is eye discharge, send a Gram stain and culture).

2. **Ampicillin and gentamicin, in combination are the first choice** for antibiotics as empirical initial therapy in newborn EOS. It will cover GBS, most other streptococcal and enterococcal species, and *L monocytogenes*. The majority of gram-negative isolates that cause EOS are sensitive to gentamicin. Once a pathogen is identified, narrow therapy if possible unless synergism is necessary. If GBS is identified in the culture, penicillin G is the drug of choice, with ampicillin as an acceptable alternative.

    a. **Antibiotic resistance:** Extended-spectrum β-lactamase producers are bacteria that contain enzymes that confer resistance to β-lactam antibiotics, as well as aminoglycosides. Between 1% and 2% of all cases of EOS are resistant to both ampicillin and gentamicin. Based on available data at this time, the organisms responsible for EOS in neonates remain generally susceptible to gentamicin, an aminoglycoside. The routine use of broader spectrum antibiotic agents is therefore not justified and may be harmful. This may change in the future, and it is important to keep up to date with local resistance patterns, which may necessitate changing empiric antibiotics to better cover resistance patterns.

    i. **Term infants who are critically ill.** Consider broader spectrum therapy until culture results are available.

    ii. **Preterm infants who are severely ill and at highest risk of gram-negative early-onset sepsis.** Consider broader spectrum antibiotic therapy until culture results are available.

3. **Third-generation cephalosporins** (eg, cefotaxime) are an alternative to gentamicin, but recent studies have shown cephalosporin-resistant strains with routine use for EOS and increased risk for candidiasis. Cefotaxime should be added to the treatment regimen for infants who have symptoms or laboratory testing concerning for meningitis to cover gram-negative bacterial meningitis. Cefotaxime and an aminoglycoside should be used in infants with gram-negative meningitis until susceptibility testing is back.

4. **If the cultures are positive, treat accordingly per expert references** (eg, AAP Red Book). Bacteremia without source: treat for 10 days. Uncomplicated GBS meningitis: treat for 14 days. Gram-negative meningitis: treat for 21 days or 14 days after obtaining a negative culture. Some recommend doing a second LP for CSF culture 24 to 48 hours after starting antibiotics.

G. **Antibiotic stewardship.** The AAP guidelines recognize the clinical challenges in this area. The concern of overtreatment is validated by recent data showing that prolonged antibiotic treatment in preterm infants is not safe at all and resulted in poorer outcomes (a higher incidence of NEC, late-onset sepsis, bronchopulmonary disease, and mortality). Even intrapartum antibiotics alone have been shown to alter the gut microbiota in infants. Term infants who receive empiric antibiotics have also been found to have delayed initiation of breast feeding and higher rates of formula use. Retrospective studies have shown that term infants who have early exposure to antibiotics in infancy have increased risks of wheezing, asthma, food allergy, obesity, and inflammatory bowel disease. Proper antibiotic stewardship involves considering 3 key aspects of treatment:

1. **Whether initiation of antibiotics is warranted.** Adherence to evidence-based guidelines can help ensure that only infants who meet high-risk criteria receive empiric antibiotic therapy. The use of the Kaiser Sepsis Calculator, or a risk assessment based on clinical condition, is aimed at reducing the number of infants who receive antibiotics in the first place.

2. **Duration of therapy and when antibiotics can be safely discontinued**

    a. **Empiric antibiotic treatment.** There are no strict guidelines for length of empiric antibiotic treatment. Using blood culture as the gold standard for diagnosis, when blood cultures are sterile, the standard course of treatment is for 36 to 48 hours in preterm and term infants, unless there is clear evidence of a site-specific infection.

    b. **Using laboratory tests to decide.** There are some studies and centers that suggest using normal laboratory measurements as indicators to stop antibiotics earlier (serial CRP or WBC measurements); however, there are no guidelines that recommend that practice at this point. The AAP position is that that laboratory test abnormalities alone do not justify prolonged antibiotic treatment, especially in preterm infants at low risk or well-appearing term infants.

    c. **Persistent cardiorespiratory instability. Should antibiotics be continued?**
       i. **Preterm and very low birthweight infants.** Continuing antibiotics for persistent cardiorespiratory instability, which can be common in these infants, does not justify prolonged antibiotic treatment.
      ii. **Term infants.** Continuing antibiotics for unexplained critical cardio-respiratory illness may be justified even without a culture-confirmed infection.
    d. **Duration of therapy.** Duration of therapy for a confirmed EOS by blood culture or LP should be guided by expert references (AAP Red Book) and by infectious disease specialists for complicated cases.
  3. **When antibiotic coverage can be narrowed appropriately.** Proper antibiotic stewardship also includes a consideration of antimicrobial resistance patterns. Although GBS continues to be generally susceptible to penicillin, ampicillin, and first-generation cephalosporins, there have been isolates identified with increasing resistance patterns. If an organism is identified, it is important to properly narrow antibiotic coverage as quickly as is feasible to avoid overexposure to critical broad-spectrum antibiotics.
H. **Treatment of early-onset sepsis beyond antibiotic therapy**
  1. **Immunoglobulin therapy is not recommended.** The 2015 Cochrane review states that "Routine administration of IVIG [intravenous immunoglobulin] or IgM [immunoglobulin M] enriched IVIG to prevent mortality in infants with suspected or proven neonatal infection is not recommended" and recommends no further trials on this intervention.
  2. **Fresh-frozen plasma** is only indicated in disseminated intravascular coagulation, and no benefit has been shown in septic infants.
  3. **Granulocyte or neutrophil transfusion** benefits have been documented. However, there are potential serious side effects. A Cochrane systematic review indicates there is not enough evidence to either support or refute the use in sepsis.
  4. **Cytokines.** Granulocyte-macrophage colony-stimulating factor (GM-CSF) and granulocyte colony-stimulating factor (G-CSF) are naturally occurring cytokines that stimulate bone marrow neutrophils. A Cochrane systematic review states that there is not enough evidence to support the use of GM-CSF or G-CSF as treatment to reduce mortality in a systemic infection or as prophylaxis to prevent a systemic infection. The review suggests limited data that treatment may decrease mortality in severe neutropenia with a systemic infection.
  5. **Double-volume exchange transfusion** with fresh whole blood is beneficial in severe or gram-negative neonatal sepsis, and it may be used as a last resort. Because of significant risks and because evidence from a few prospective studies is not strong on the subject, many institutions have not advocated its use.
  6. **Extracorporeal life support** (ECLS) is a viable therapy for refractory septic shock in neonates. Various extracorporeal therapies such as ECLS, continuous renal replacement therapy, and blood purification (hemofiltration, hemoperfusion, and therapeutic plasma exchange) have been reported with various successes in the management of pediatric sepsis and septic shock. ECLS is a viable therapy for refractory septic shock in neonates and children. Neonates have comparably good outcomes (≥80% survival) whether the indication for ECLS is refractory respiratory failure or refractory shock from sepsis.
  7. **Pentoxifylline** is a methylxanthine derivative and a phosphodiesterase inhibitor. It reduces the inflammatory response in septic neonates. Current evidence shows that pentoxifylline as an adjunct to antibiotics reduces mortality in neonatal sepsis without any adverse effects and decreases the

duration of hospitalization. The studies have been small, and larger trials are needed.

8. **Selenium/melatonin supplementation.** Melatonin has been studied as an adjuvant therapy in the treatment of neonatal sepsis in a few small studies and showed improvement in clinical and laboratory parameters. Selenium supplementation has been shown to reduce the incidence of sepsis in very preterm infants, but the studies were small and in countries with low selenium concentrations. More studies are needed.

9. **Zinc** is a cofactor for many enzymes and is needed for the immune system to work properly. There are limited data available on its use in sepsis. Two randomized controlled trials done in India compared antibiotic treatment with zinc as adjuvant to antibiotic treatment alone. One study showed a reduction in mortality and improved developmental scores at 12 months. The other study showed no improvement in mortality but improvement in neurologic outcome at 1 month.

10. **Lactoferrin** is a normal component of human colostrum and milk thought to enhance the host immune system. The most recent Cochrane systematic review found 6 randomized controlled trials evaluating its use. They found that lactoferrin added to enteral feeds decreased the incidence of late-onset sepsis and NEC stage 2 or 3, but the evidence was low quality. Ongoing trials will hopefully enhance the quality of evidence.

11. **Recombinant human activated protein.** There were no trials identified in the most recent Cochrane systematic review on its use. There are significant side effects noted in adult studies. It is not recommended for use in neonates at this time.

79 Pulmonary Hemorrhage

I. **Problem.** <u>A nurse informs you that an infant has bloody secretions from the endotracheal tube (ETT).</u> **Pulmonary hemorrhage is bleeding into the lungs.** It is typically an acute, catastrophic, often life-threatening event **that causes a sudden deterioration in the infant's clinical condition** and is characterized by fresh continuous bloody fluid from the ETT or lower respiratory tract. **Histologically,** it is defined as fresh hemorrhage in the alveolar spaces or interstitium of the lung. The incidence of pulmonary hemorrhage varies from 1 to 12 per 1000 live births. It can be as high as 50 per 1000 live births if high risk (eg, premature, intrauterine growth restriction [IUGR]). The mortality rate can be up to 50% in premature infants. Survivors of pulmonary hemorrhage require longer ventilator support, and many will develop bronchopulmonary dysplasia/chronic lung disease (60% of premature infants). Studies show an increased risk of death and survival with neurosensory impairment, increased incidence of cerebral palsy and cognitive delay, and an increased risk of seizures and periventricular leukomalacia at 18 months of age.

II. **Immediate questions**

A. **Are any other signs abnormal?** Typically, an infant with a pulmonary hemorrhage is a ventilated low birthweight infant, often from a multiple birth, and 2 to 4 days old (usually in the first week of life). Late-gestation infants with pulmonary hemorrhage usually have low 1- and 5-minute Apgar scores. The infant with a pulmonary hemorrhage can have a sudden deterioration: hypoxic, severe retractions, associated pallor, shock, apnea, bradycardia, and cyanosis.

B. **Is the infant hypoxic? Has a blood transfusion recently been given?** Hypoxia or hypervolemia (usually caused by overtransfusion) may cause an acute rise in the pulmonary capillary pressure and lead to pulmonary hemorrhage.

C. **Is there bleeding from other sites?** If so, coagulopathy may be present, and coagulation studies should be obtained. Volume replacement with colloid or blood products may be needed.

D. **What is the hematocrit of the endotracheal blood?** If the hematocrit (Hct) is close to the venous Hct, it represents a true hemorrhage, and the blood is usually from trauma or a bleeding diathesis. Aspiration of maternal blood will result in an Hct close to the venous Hct. If the Hct is 15 to 20 percentage points lower than the venous Hct, the bleeding is likely hemorrhagic edema fluid. This is seen with the majority of cases of pulmonary hemorrhage (such as those secondary to PDA, surfactant therapy, and left-sided heart failure; others discussed later).

E. **Has there been a recent procedure, or has suctioning just taken place? Was surfactant recently given?** Vigorous suctioning, traumatic intubation, or chest tube insertion may be a cause. Surfactant can also be associated.

F. **Did the mother or infant have any risk factors for pulmonary hemorrhage?** Major risk factors include IUGR, surfactant therapy, PDA, sepsis, and coagulopathy.

   1. **Maternal risk factors.** Breech delivery, maternal cocaine use, maternal hypertension during pregnancy, abruptio placentae, maternal antibiotic therapy, preeclampsia, possible previous pregnancy losses. **Note that antenatal steroids may be protective.**

   2. **Infant risk factors. Prematurity is the most common risk factor.** Others include IUGR, respiratory problems (hypoxia, asphyxia, RDS, meconium aspiration, pneumothorax, surfactant treatment, or any need for ventilator support), mechanical ventilation, PDA with left-to-right shunting, disseminated intravascular coagulation (DIC), cold injury, oxygen toxicity, urea cycle defects, multiple births, male sex, overwhelming sepsis, infections/sepsis, coagulopathy, hypothermia, polycythemia, IUGR, erythroblastosis fetalis, extracorporeal membrane oxygenation/extracorporeal life support, toxemia of pregnancy, heart failure, oxygenation index ≤100, previous use of blood products, weight <1000 g at birth, and intubation in the delivery room. Presence of PDA or early-onset sepsis increases the risk in ELBW infants. **Significant risk factors for infants near term or term** are hypotension, requirement of positive-pressure ventilation in the delivery room, and meconium aspiration. **Significant risk factors for preterm infants** are thrombocytopenia and requirement for positive pressure ventilation in the delivery room.

G. **Did the infant receive prophylactic indomethacin?** Prophylactic indomethacin reduces the rate of early serious pulmonary hemorrhage by 35%, but only in the first few days after birth. It did not decrease the rate after the first week.

III. **Differential diagnosis.** Most cases of pulmonary hemorrhage are secondary to hemorrhagic pulmonary edema and not a true bleed. The differential diagnosis includes the following:

A. **Direct trauma to the airway** due to nasotracheal or endotracheal intubation, vigorous suctioning, bag-and-mask ventilation, mechanical ventilation, or lung trauma during chest tube insertion. Local trauma usually has a smaller amount of bleeding with no clinical deterioration.

   1. **Bleeding from the upper respiratory tract (nasal cavity, pharynx, larynx) or upper gastrointestinal tract,** which can mimic a pulmonary hemorrhage.

   2. **Aspiration of maternal blood after cesarean or vaginal delivery.** The majority of blood is usually obtained from the nasogastric tube, but blood may be seen in the ETT. An Apt test can be done on the blood to determine if it is maternal blood (see Chapter 60).

B. **Hemorrhagic pulmonary edema.** The fluid is not whole blood but a mixture of plasma and blood with a low Hct, usually 15% to 20% below the expected venous Hct. Its cause is not known and may be multifactorial: stress, injury to fragile pulmonary capillaries, inadequate surface tension, acute left ventricular failure caused by asphyxia, and severe acidosis or other conditions that lead to capillary endothelium injury. The most accepted theory is that a decrease in pulmonary vascular resistance causes an increase in left-to-right shunting through a patent ductus arteriosus (PDA), which increases the pulmonary blood flow. This causes an increase in capillary filtrate and red blood cells, which leak into the alveoli. It is essentially an extreme form of pulmonary edema. Other theories include surfactant dysfunction, role of surfactant in platelet function, or intrauterine neutrophil activation in premature infants with RDS causing pulmonary hemorrhage.

C. **Massive pulmonary hemorrhage** is a pulmonary hemorrhage that involves at least 2 lobes of the lungs. The presence of a PDA or early-onset sepsis is associated with an increased risk of massive pulmonary hemorrhage (MPH) in ELBW infants. A higher 5-minute Apgar score is associated with a decreased risk of MPH.

D. **Other disorders associated with pulmonary hemorrhage**

1. **Hypoxia/asphyxia.** Acute left ventricular failure due to asphyxia is a factor in pulmonary hemorrhage. Intrauterine and intrapartum asphyxia can be related to pulmonary hemorrhage. Resuscitation may exacerbate pulmonary hemorrhage.

2. **Hypervolemia.** Overtransfusion or fluid overload.

3. **Congenital heart disease or congestive heart failure (especially in pulmonary edema caused by patent ductus arteriosus).** A PDA can cause a rapid increase in pulmonary blood flow. In 1 series, 60% of infants with pulmonary hemorrhage had a clinical PDA, with >90% of those with a pulmonary hemorrhage having a PDA of >1.6 mm in size. Pulmonary hemorrhage occurred after corrective surgery in a neonate with transposition of the great arteries and intact ventricular septum with a postoperative computed tomography scan showing an aortopulmonary collateral artery arising from the descending aorta.

4. **Pulmonary related.** RDS, pulmonary interstitial emphysema, pneumothorax, meconium aspiration, aspiration, and pneumonia (usually caused by gram-negative organisms). Pulmonary congestion (severely reduced left ventricular function in an asphyxiated or septic infant) can also be a factor. Diffuse pulmonary emboli can be a predisposing factor. Extralobar pulmonary sequestration can cause recurrent pulmonary hemorrhage.

5. **Surfactant administration.** Pulmonary hemorrhage within hours of surfactant therapy may be related to a rapid increase in pulmonary blood flow due to improved lung function. There is a significant relationship between pulmonary hemorrhage and a clinical PDA in surfactant-treated infants. Rescue surfactant therapy did not increase the risk of pulmonary hemorrhage, but prophylactic surfactant did. Studies show that pulmonary hemorrhage inactivates surfactant due to contamination with red blood cell lipids and hemoglobin.

6. **Hematologic disorders.** Severe Rh incompatibility, thrombocytopenia, vitamin K deficiency bleeding (from failure to administer vitamin K), and coagulation protein disorders or congenital factors (von Willebrand disease). Coagulation abnormalities may not be the direct cause of pulmonary hemorrhage (as believed earlier) but have been found to exacerbate the degree of hemorrhage. DIC is not seen often in infants with pulmonary hemorrhage but can be seen after an MPH.

7. **Hypoplastic lung disease.** Because of the reduced size of the vascular bed in pulmonary hypoplasia, there is a higher chance of an increase in lung microvascular pressure that can cause a pulmonary hemorrhage.

8. **Prematurity, intrauterine growth restriction,** and/or multiple births.

9. **Cold injury syndrome.** Cold injury causes platelet aggregation, which causes thrombocytopenia, which is a major risk factor for pulmonary hemorrhage. In 1 study of hypothermic infants and newborns, pulmonary hemorrhage was a primary cause of death.

10. **Infection/sepsis.** Overwhelming sepsis is seen in many cases of pulmonary hemorrhage and may be associated with the DIC that accompanies sepsis and the increased microvascular permeability. Pulmonary hemorrhage can occur from coxsackievirus B infection and multiple infections with septicemia (eg, congenital cytomegalovirus, *Haemophilus influenzae, Escherichia coli, Candida, Staphylococcus epidermis*).

11. **Urea cycle defects with hyperammonemia.** These infants typically have hepatomegaly, coagulopathy, and usually normal liver function tests except for hyperammonemia. Pulmonary bleeding is usually a terminal event in these infants.

12. **High concentrations of oxygen or oxygen toxicity.** Histologic evidence of oxygen toxicity has been associated with MPH. It causes increased microvascular permeability.

13. **Airway hemangioma (rare).**

14. **Neonatal pulmonary hemosiderosis.** Idiopathic pulmonary hemosiderosis is a very rare disease that causes acute recurrent episodes of hemoptysis as a result of a pulmonary hemorrhage, iron deficiency anemia, abnormal amount of hemosiderin in the alveolar macrophages, and diffuse alveolar infiltrates.

IV. **Database**

A. **Physical examination.** Typically, the infant is premature and, on the second to fourth day of life, has a sudden cardiorespiratory deterioration and bloody secretions from the airway. Clinical signs may vary from the infant being pale, limp, and unresponsive, to fighting the ventilator (usually term infants), to looking well. The infant can be cyanotic, bradycardic, apneic, gasping, hypotensive, agitated, hypoxic, or hypercapnic or have an increased work of breathing and require more ventilatory support. Note the presence of other bleeding sites and signs of pneumonia, infection, or congestive heart failure. Look for peripheral edema, hepatosplenomegaly, and murmur of a PDA. Listen to the chest for decreased breath sounds and crepitations. There can be a **prodrome of frothy, reddish, blood-tinged tracheal secretions** before the pulmonary hemorrhage.

B. **Laboratory studies**

1. **Complete blood count with differential and platelet count.** With pneumonia, sepsis, or other infection, results of these studies may be abnormal. Thrombocytopenia may be seen. The Hct should be checked to determine whether excessive blood loss has occurred.

2. **Coagulation profile (prothrombin time, activated partial thromboplastin time, thrombin time, D-dimers, fibrinogen level)** may reveal coagulation disorders. Coagulation studies are not abnormal prior to the bleed but are usually abnormal after the bleed. Secondary DIC frequently occurs with a pulmonary hemorrhage.

3. **Arterial blood gas levels** detect a severe hypoxia, hypercarbia, and a metabolic acidosis. The oxygenation index can increase significantly after the hemorrhage.

4. **Sepsis evaluation.** Blood cultures should be drawn because many infants with a pulmonary hemorrhage have bacterial sepsis. Any other cultures that are appropriate should be done depending on the infant.

5. **Serum electrolytes** should be checked for hypoglycemia and hypocalcemia. Check blood urea nitrogen and creatinine for renal function because these infants can have renal failure.

6. **Apt test** if aspiration of maternal blood is suspected. (See Chapter 60.)

7. **Hematocrit of the aspirate** may differentiate between hemorrhagic pulmonary edema and a true bleed (see Section II.D).

8. **Ammonia level** to evaluate for urea cycle defects that can be associated with pulmonary hemorrhage.

9. **Metabolic workup.** Complete any of the state-mandated newborn screens before any blood is given, if possible.

C. **Imaging and other studies**

1. **Chest radiograph** can be variable and nonspecific. Pulmonary hemorrhage often looks like pneumonia on radiographs, and it is difficult to distinguish between the 2 conditions. With pulmonary hemorrhage, radiographic findings depend on whether the hemorrhage is focal (patchy, linear, ground-glass opacities; nodular densities; or fluffy opacities), lobar (hemorrhage in 1 lobe of the lung causing consolidation), or massive (the film shows a complete whiteout with just an air bronchogram visible or diffuse ground-glass opacities). The chest radiograph can also be clear in an early pulmonary hemorrhage.

2. **Lung ultrasonography** can be used to diagnose pulmonary hemorrhage. The main findings associated with pulmonary hemorrhage on ultrasound are lung consolidation with air bronchograms (83%), shred sign (92 %), pleural effusion (84%), and pleural line abnormalities and disappearing A lines (100 %). The shred sign demonstrated a sensitivity of 91% and a specificity of 100% for diagnosing pulmonary hemorrhage.

   a. **The shred sign was the most common and specific ultrasound finding of pulmonary hemorrhage.** It is a static sonographic sign observed in lung consolidation. The sign represents where the deeper border of the consolidated lung tissue that makes contact with the aerated lung is shredded and irregular.

   b. **Pleural line** is the parallel echogenic line under the superficial layers of the thorax that move during respiration.

   c. **A lines** are a series of horizontal, echogenic parallel lines below the pleural line that are equidistant from one another.

3. **Echocardiogram** to rule out left-to-right shunting through a PDA, assess ventricular function, identify intravascular fluid overload (dilatation of the left atrium, sometimes dilatation of the left ventricle), and evaluate the need for vasoactive medications.

V. **Plan**

A. **Emergency measures**

1. **Suction the airway initially (sometimes as often as every 15 minutes) until bleeding subsides.** This is critical to reduce the risk of secretions blocking the airway. Use a 6.5-F suction catheter for a 2.5-mm ETT and an 8.0-F suction catheter for a 3.0- or 3.5-mm ETT. **Percussion should be used with caution and has no primary role in pulmonary hemorrhage.**

2. **Oxygen therapy should be given.** If already given, increase the inspired oxygen concentration to maintain a normal saturation.

3. **If mechanical ventilation is not being used,** consider using it. Infants with a massive pulmonary hemorrhage should be intubated and ventilated.

4. **If already on a ventilator,** increase the mean airway pressure to reverse or slow down the hemorrhagic pulmonary edema.

   a. **Increase the positive end-expiratory pressure to 6 to 8 cm H_2O (or higher if needed).** This may cause tamponade of the capillaries, forces edema back into the pulmonary vascular bed, and improves ventilation and oxygenation. Risks of increasing positive end-expiratory pressure include hypercapnia and hyperventilation.

   b. **Consider increasing the inspiratory time.** Some will also use a long inspiratory time (0.4–0.5 seconds).

   c. **Consider increasing the peak inspiratory pressure.** Consider if bleeding does not subside to improve ventilation and raise the mean airway pressure.

B. Other measures
1. **Support and correct the blood pressure with volume expansion (colloids) and inotropes.** (See Chapter 70.) Vasoactive medications may be necessary.
2. **Blood volume and hematocrit** should be restored with slow administration of packed red blood cell transfusions after the infant has been stabilized. The majority of these infants are not volume depleted, and thus administering excessive fluid volume may only worsen the situation (increasing the left arterial pressure may increase the pulmonary edema).
3. **Correct acidosis** by correcting hypovolemia, hypoxia, and low cardiac output. Bicarbonate infusion in certain select cases may be considered **if metabolic acidosis persists** after ventilation is adequate and volume is restored but is not routinely recommended (*controversial*).
4. **Treat any underlying disorder.**
   a. **Early recognition and treatment of patent ductus arteriosus** is essential, especially in extremely premature infants. Pharmacologic or surgical treatment of the PDA should be considered. Surgical treatment is preferred because indomethacin can exacerbate the bleeding.
   b. **Treat sepsis/infection** with antibiotics if indicated. Get blood cultures and start antibiotics. The chest x-ray often looks like pneumonia, so antibiotics are usually started.
   c. **Correct any underlying disorders of coagulation** if present. Platelets and vitamin K may need to be given.
C. Other measures to consider if the preceding methods are not effective (*controversial*)
1. **Endotracheal tube administration of epinephrine or nebulized epinephrine (0.1 mL/kg of 1:10,000 dilution) (*controversial*).** This is used because of its vasoconstrictive effects (may cause constriction of the pulmonary capillaries which decreases bleeding) and inotropic effects (increases mean airway pressure). Eepinephrine or 4% cocaine (4 mg/kg) may be a useful adjunct in the management of pulmonary hemorrhage. Epinephrine is more often used clinically, even though the efficacy has not been proven in clinical trials.
2. **Consider high-frequency ventilation.** It is not known whether high-frequency ventilation has any benefits over conventional ventilation, but some studies suggest that high-frequency ventilation may improve survival. One review showed a 71% survival with the use of high-frequency ventilation (high-frequency jet ventilation, high-frequency oscillatory ventilation [HFOV], and high-frequency flow interrupter were used in the review) after conventional ventilation failed. HFOV has been used as rescue therapy in some infants with MPH; it decreased the oxygenation index in these infants and the infants showed dramatic improvement.
3. **Rescue surfactant.** Consider using a single dose of surfactant after the infant is stabilized on the ventilator. Although surfactant may be a contributing factor of pulmonary hemorrhage, a **single dose** has been reported to improve respiratory status based on the oxygenation index after the infant has been stabilized on the ventilator.
   a. **American Academy of Pediatrics Committee on Fetus and Newborn** states that surfactant treatment is plausible because blood inhibits surfactant function, but because of the lack of studies, the benefit has not been established. **The committee recommends that rescue surfactant may be considered in infants with hypoxic respiratory failure** caused by secondary surfactant deficiency in pulmonary hemorrhage.
   b. **Cochrane review (2012)** could not give a recommendation because there were no randomized trials done to evaluate the effect of surfactant in pulmonary hemorrhage. They feel more trials are needed.
4. **High-frequency oscillatory ventilation combined with pulmonary surfactant.** This combination was found to improve the oxygenation function and

shorten the duration of pulmonary hemorrhage and ventilation time in 1 study.

5. **Diuretics.** Some advocate diuretic therapy (furosemide 1 mg/kg) if there is evidence of significant fluid overload. Furosemide does have a beneficial effect on respiratory function in pulmonary edema (it decreases lung lymph flow and improves ventilation/perfusion mismatch), but there is no direct evidence that it is effective in pulmonary hemorrhage.

6. **Steroids.** Because chronic inflammation was found on lung biopsies of infants with pulmonary hemorrhage and more infants survived with pulmonary hemorrhage who had been on steroids, steroid use can be considered. Methylprednisolone (1 mg/kg every 6 hours during hospital stay and 1 mg/kg daily thereafter and discontinued after a 4-week period) has been reported to be beneficial.

7. **Recombinant factor VIIa.** Recombinant activated human factor VIIa (rFVIIa) is a vitamin K–dependent glycoprotein which is a low-volume alternative to blood products and is effective as a panhemostatic agent. It activates platelets, thereby causing thrombin formation and fibrin clotting. If platelets are given at the same time, the effect is enhanced. It is approved for use in life-threatening hemorrhages and perioperative prevention in patients with certain types of inherited or acquired hemophilia (A and B). It has been used in very low birthweight infants with a pulmonary hemorrhage when conventional ventilator management failed. There are a few positive studies, but the optimal dose has not been established. One dose of 50 mcg/kg twice per day 3 hours apart for 2 to 3 days was used successfully. A recent study on infants <30 weeks' gestation or with a birthweight of <1250 g with pulmonary hemorrhage who either did or did not get a dose of rFVIIa showed that rFVIIa administration was 67% effective in stopping pulmonary hemorrhage (single dose of 50 mcg was given), decreasing the blood product requirement, and improving coagulation test parameters with no increase in short-term complications. It did not decrease the intraventricular hemorrhage rate or mortality.

8. **Hemocoagulase** is a purified enzyme mixture from the venom of the Brazilian snake *Bothrops atrox*. It decreases bleeding time and helps with coagulation. A study of preterm infants treated with hemocoagulase (0.5 KU [Klobusitzky units]) through the ETT every 4 to 6 hours until the hemorrhage stopped plus mechanical ventilation for pulmonary hemorrhage showed promising results; the duration of ventilation, pulmonary hemorrhage, and mortality were all decreased compared with controls. Another study used it prophylactically, and it was associated with a decrease in incidence and duration of the hemorrhage, but had no effect on mortality. Due to potential risks of use and lack of quality studies, routine use is not recommended yet. **Use as a last resort.**

D. **Specific targeted therapy**

1. **Direct nasotracheal or endotracheal trauma.** If there is significant bleeding immediately after an endotracheal or nasotracheal intubation, trauma is the most likely cause; surgical consultation is indicated.

2. **Aspiration of maternal blood.** If the infant is stable, no treatment is needed because the condition is typically self-limited.

3. **Coagulopathy.** See Chapter 92.
   a. **Vitamin K deficiency bleeding.** Vitamin K, 1 mg, administered intravenously with fresh-frozen plasma with active bleeding.
   b. **Other coagulopathies.** Transfusion of blood products and correction of coagulopathies is necessary. Fresh-frozen plasma, 10 mL/kg every 12 to 24 hours, may be given. If the platelet count is low, transfuse 1 unit and monitor closely. Monitor prothrombin time/partial thromboplastin time, platelet count, and fibrinogen level. DIC is managed as noted in Chapter 92.

4. **Sepsis.** Appropriate antibiotics should be started immediately.

80 Rash and Dermatologic Problems

I. **Problem.** <u>A nurse calls you to tell you that an infant has a rash.</u> A rash is any change of skin that affects its color, appearance, or texture. **Although the majority of rashes in newborns are benign and require no treatment, certain rashes require a workup and intervention.**

II. **Immediate questions**

A. **What are the characteristics of the rash?** Morphology of the lesion aids differential diagnosis. **Is it macular** (flat lesion <1 cm), **papular** (raised up to 1 cm), **nodular** (raised up to 2 cm), **vesicular** (raised, <1 cm, filled with clear fluid), **bullous** (raised, >1 cm, with clear fluid), or **pustular** (raised with purulent fluid)?

B. **Are there petechiae (tiny pinpoint red dots from broken blood vessels), purpura (large, flat area of blood under tissue), or ecchymosis (very large bruised area)?** All can result from intradermal bleeding and need to be differentiated from **erythema** (redness of the skin). With erythema, the redness is cleared when pressed and returns when you release. With pressure, petechiae, purpura, and ecchymosis do not blanch. Petechiae on the lower body after a breech delivery or upper body with a vertex presentation can be normal. If widespread, petechiae are considered abnormal. **Petechiae and purpura can signify thrombocytopenia and require a workup.**

C. **Is there a history of a congenital infection?** Obtain a thorough maternal history. TORCH (toxoplasmosis, other, rubella, cytomegalovirus, herpes simplex virus) infections are known to cause rashes. The **"blueberry muffin baby"** has widespread purpura and papules and can be seen in rubella (the term was first used to describe infants infected with rubella in the epidemic of 1960), cytomegalovirus (most common viral infection), and syphilis. Cutaneous extramedullary hematopoiesis causes the "blueberry muffin" rash. The "blueberry muffin" rash has historically been associated with congenital viral infections but can also be seen in blood disorders (hemolytic disease of the newborn, twin-to-twin transfusion, hereditary spherocytosis), vascular disorders (multiple hemangiomas), and malignancies (neuroblastoma, congenital leukemia cutis, Langerhans cell histiocytosis, and congenital rhabdomyosarcoma). See Chapter 148 and disease-specific chapters.

D. **Is the infant ill appearing?** A well infant with a rash suggests a benign rash. A febrile or ill-appearing infant with a rash requires a thorough workup to search specifically for an infectious cause.

E. **What medications did the mother receive during pregnancy and delivery? Is the mother breast feeding and taking any medications?** Medications are a rare cause of rash in infants. Methimazole, an antithyroid medication, and also valproic acid during pregnancy have been associated with aplasia cutis, a localized absence of skin on the scalp (see Figure 80–1).

F. **Does the skin lesion make you think of a genetic disorder?** Skin lesions can be associated with genetic syndromes. **Blisters:** epidermolysis bullosa. **Brown, flat patches:** Neurofibromatosis. **Cutis marmorata:** Cornelia de Lange syndrome and in trisomies 18 (Edward syndrome) and 21 (Down syndrome). **Deficient hair and nails:** ectodermal dysplasias. **Scaly, thick skin:** ichthyoses. **Thin, fragile skin:** collagen disorders and hypoplasia of the dermis. **Unformed skin:** aplasia cutis congenita, Adams-Oliver syndrome, and epidermolysis bullosa. **White skin and hair:** piebaldism and tuberous sclerosis.

III. **Differential diagnosis**

A. **Absence of part of the skin. Aplasia cutis congenita** consists of 9 groups of disorders based on the location and presence of other malformations that involve absence of

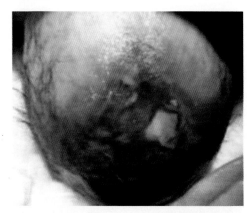

FIGURE 80–1. Aplasia cutis congenita on scalp. (*Used with permission from Andrew Bowe, DO, Pediatrix Medical Group.*)

part of the skin. It can be localized (most commonly on the scalp) or involve a large portion of the body (Figure 80–1).

B. **Skin and soft tissue infections in the neonatal intensive care unit.** These are common because preterm infants have fragile skin. Types of infections seen are **cellulitis, abrasions, and abscesses** and usually occur where the skin has been traumatized (diaper areas, surgical incision sites, fetal scalp electrodes, venipuncture sites, heel stick sites). The most common organism is *Staphylococcus aureus.* Methicillin-resistant strains are becoming more frequent. Skin and soft tissue infections involving surgical procedures (gastrointestinal [GI] tract) are caused more commonly by gram-negative rods and yeasts. **Omphalitis,** an infection of the umbilical stump and the area around it, can also occur and is usually caused by bacteria (gram negative or gram positive).

C. **Benign skin disorders/rashes that usually require no workup or intervention.** These rashes are very common.

1. **Erythema toxicum.** The most common newborn rash, it consists of erythematous macules with a central papule or pustule. It can be present at birth, typically appears within the first 48 hours, and resolves by 2 weeks of age. It is more common in full-term infants and more common on the trunk, extremities, and perineum. New lesions can appear after the initial onset and usually disappear after a week (Figure 80–2).

2. **Transient neonatal pustular melanosis.** These 2- to 5-mm pustules are usually present at birth on various sites, typically the face and sacrum of full-term infants. Pustules evolve and disappear within 48 hours, but can leave hyperpigmented macules that spontaneously resolve after a few months (Figure 80–3).

3. **Sebaceous gland hyperplasia.** Tiny yellow papules usually occurring on the cheeks and nose. Smaller and more yellow than milia.

4. **Milia.** Tiny (1-mm) white-yellow papules frequently present on the face, chin, forehead, and scalp. Caused by sebaceous retention cysts (Figure 80–4).

5. **Miliaria crystallina.** Obstruction of eccrine/sweat ducts. May appear on the scalp or face as vesicular or papular lesions with or without erythema. Exacerbated by heat and humidity, they resolve quickly when the infant is cooled.

6. **Miliaria rubra ("prickly heat").** One- to two-mm papules or papulopustules surrounded by small red areas. Miliaria pustulosis is a variant with more pustules and less erythema.

7. **Miliaria profunda.** Deep obstruction of the sweat ducts. White papules and edema that can prevent sweating, leading to hyperthermia.

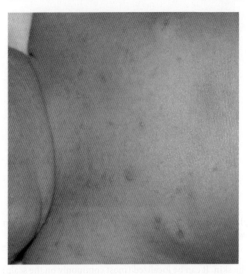

FIGURE 80–2. Erythema toxicum. (*Used with permission from Leslie Castelo-Soccio, MD, PhD, Children's Hospital of Philadelphia Division of Dermatology.*)

8. **Acropustulosis of infancy.** Recurrent areas of pruritic vesicopustules develop on the palmar surface of the hand and plantar surface of the feet. Usually last 7 to 14 days (Figure 80–5).
9. **Seborrheic dermatitis.** Patchy redness and scales on the scalp (**"cradle cap"**), face, skin folds, and behind the ears.
10. **Neonatal acne.** Erythematous comedones, papules, and pustules. May be present at birth or develop during early infancy; may take several weeks or months for complete resolution (Figure 80–6).
11. **Sucking blister.** Vesicular or bullous lesions present at birth on fingers, lips, or hands; no associated erythema (distinguishes these from herpetic lesions).
12. **Subcutaneous fat necrosis.** Erythematous nodules and plaques occurring during the first few weeks of life and resolving by 2 months of age. Usually on areas

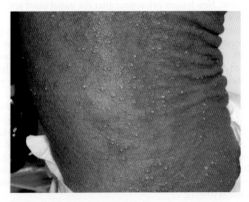

FIGURE 80–3. Transient neonatal pustular melanosis. (*Used with permission from Leslie Castelo-Soccio, MD, PhD, Children's Hospital of Philadelphia Division of Dermatology.*)

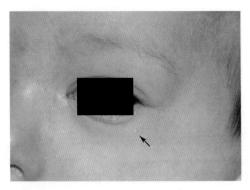

FIGURE 80–4. Milia. (*Used with permission from Leslie Castelo-Soccio, MD, PhD, Children's Hospital of Philadelphia Division of Dermatology.*)

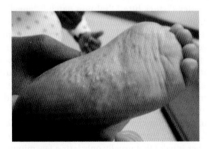

FIGURE 80–5. Acropustulosis of infancy. (*Used with permission from Leslie Castelo-Soccio, MD, PhD, Children's Hospital of Philadelphia Division of Dermatology.*)

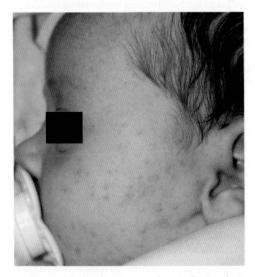

FIGURE 80–6. Neonatal acne. (*Used with permission from Leslie Castelo-Soccio, MD, PhD, Children's Hospital of Philadelphia Division of Dermatology.*)

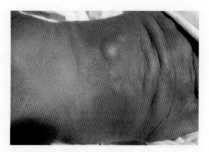

FIGURE 80–7. Subcutaneous fat necrosis. (*Used with permission from Leslie Castelo-Soccio, MD, PhD, Children's Hospital of Philadelphia Division of Dermatology.*)

of trauma (face, back, arms, legs, and buttocks). Hypercalcemia can occur if these lesions calcify (Figure 80–7).

13. **Nevus simplex ("stork bite," "salmon patch," "angel's kiss").** Pink macules that are dilated superficial capillaries, seen commonly at the nape of the neck, midforehead, and upper eyelids, but also on nose and upper lip, that usually fade within a year. The most common vascular malformation.

14. **Mongolian spot (congenital dermal melanocytosis).** A blue-black macular discoloration at the base of the spine and on the buttocks but can occur elsewhere. More common in blacks (>90%) and Asians (81%); usually fades over several years. Extensive spots have been described in infants with GM1 gangliosidosis (Figure 80–8).

15. **Harlequin sign (color change, not Harlequin fetus).** Secondary to vasomotor instability, there is a sharp demarcation of blanching (one side of the body is red and the other is pale) that usually only lasts a few minutes.

16. **Infantile hemangioma.** A common vascular tumor (3%–5% of all infants). More common in girls and preterm infants.

17. **Benign petechiae.** Nonblanching erythematous macules present on the lower body after a breech delivery or upper body with a vertex presentation.

D. **Rashes caused by infections.** These typically require intervention. The most common pathogens are *S aureus, Streptococcus* species, *Candida albicans,* and herpes simplex.

   1. **Bacterial infections causing rashes**
      a. *Staphylococcus aureus*

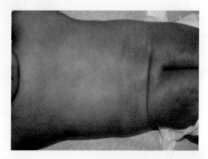

FIGURE 80–8. Mongolian spots (congenital dermal melanocytosis is preferred term). (*Used with permission from Leslie Castelo-Soccio, MD, PhD, Children's Hospital of Philadelphia Division of Dermatology.*)

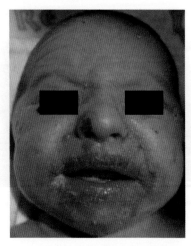

FIGURE 80–9. Staphylococcal scalded skin syndrome. (*Used with permission from Leslie Castelo-Soccio, MD, PhD, Children's Hospital of Philadelphia Division of Dermatology.*)

  i. **Impetigo (nonbullous and bullous).** Usually presents with intact vesicles, and then intact pustules rupture, erode, and dry out to form crusts often secondary to an infected umbilical wound.
  ii. **Staphylococcal scalded skin syndrome.** Toxin-mediated disease (exfoliative toxins A and B) with age-related presentations. In the first week of life, staphylococcal scalded skin syndrome (SSSS) presents as a tender scarlatiniform rash, with flaking and desquamation presenting in older infants and children (Figure 80–9). Bacteremia is rare; however, superinfection and significant dehydration can occur with severe presentations.
 b. **Cutaneous streptococcal infections.** Uncommon, group A streptococcal infections can have an erysipelas-like eruption. Skin infections caused by group B streptococci are very rare. Vesiculopustular lesions, abscesses, and cellulitis (most common) have been reported.
 c. **Syphilis.** This rash consists of small reddish-copper maculopapular eruptions that, like nasal secretions, are highly infectious. Hemorrhagic bullae on the palms and soles are characteristic of syphilis.
 d. ***Listeria monocytogenes.*** Small (2- to 3-mm) cutaneous pinkish-gray granulomas, termed *granulomatosis infantisepticum*, are characteristic of severe newborn infection.
 2. **Viral infections causing rashes**
 a. **Herpes simplex virus** (Figure 80–10). See also Chapter 137.
  i. **Congenital herpes simplex virus.** Transmitted perinatally and occurs in 3 forms (disseminated disease, localized central nervous system [CNS] disease, and skin, eyes, and/or mouth [SEM] disease). Infants with SEM disease present with erythematous papules or vesicles that progress to pustular clusters with intense erythema in 80% of cases. Typically associated with low birthweight, chorioretinitis, and microcephaly.
  ii. **Neonatal herpes simplex virus.** This type of herpes infection is often severe with high morbidity and mortality and can occur anytime between birth and 6 weeks of age.
 b. **Varicella-zoster virus.** See also Chapter 153.

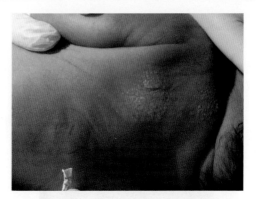

FIGURE 80–10. Herpes simplex virus. (*Used with permission from Leslie Castelo-Soccio, MD, PhD, Children's Hospital of Philadelphia Division of Dermatology.*)

      i. **Congenital/fetal varicella syndrome.** Acquired in utero in the first or second trimester (before 20 weeks' gestation). Infant is born with cicatricial scars.

     ii. **Congenital/perinatal/early neonatal varicella.** Acquired in utero late in third trimester (greater than 20 weeks' gestation) or in the first few days postpartum. Infant presents with centripetal rash similar to postnatal rash in the first 10 to 12 days of life.

    iii. **Postnatally acquired chickenpox.** No transplacental infection. Infant presents with symptoms on days 12 to 28 of life. Typical chickenpox rash with centripetal spreading first on trunk and then face and scalp. All stages appear (red macules, clear vesicles, crusting) (Figure 80–11).

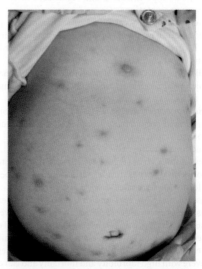

FIGURE 80–11. Varicella zoster on the abdomen. (*Used with permission from Leslie Castelo-Soccio, MD, PhD, Children's Hospital of Philadelphia Division of Dermatology.*)

    c. Cytomegalovirus. Most common congenital infection. The majority of cases are asymptomatic. If symptomatic, they can have multiorgan disease with petechiae (from thrombocytopenia), purpura, and jaundice.

    d. Rubella. Can have petechiae, but if severe, may have bluish red maculopapular rash ("blueberry muffin") that appears on the head and face and then becomes generalized in 1 to 3 days.

    e. Zika. Single-stranded RNA virus in the same family as dengue, yellow fever, and West Nile, among others, that was originally identified in Africa in 1947. Zika came to prominence recently following a large outbreak in 2015 in Brazil, the first known emergence in the Western Hemisphere. Approximately 50% of exposed adults and older children present with fever and maculopapular rash within 1 week of exposure to a mosquito bite within an endemic area. Further information regarding high-risk areas can be found at www.cdc.gov/zika/geo/index.html and wwwnc.cdc.gov/travel/page/zika-travel-information.

        i. Congenital Zika. Can cause fetal loss and severe brain abnormalities, such as microcephaly, subcortical calcifications, ventriculomegaly, abnormal gyral patterns, agenesis of the corpus callosum, and cerebellar hypoplasia.

        ii. Perinatal transmission of Zika. Occurs when the mother is infected with Zika virus within 2 weeks of delivery and the infant gets the virus at or around the time of delivery. Symptoms include maculopapular rash, conjunctivitis, arthragia, and fever.

3. Fungal infections causing rashes

    a. *Candida albicans.* The most common fungal infection in neonates is discussed here. Other species (eg, *Candida parapsilosis, Candida lusitaniae, Candida glabrata*) are less common.

        i. *Candida* diaper dermatitis/oral candidiasis (thrush). Most common presentation of *Candida* infections in a normal infant. The diaper rash is usually erythematous with satellite pustules. Oral candidiasis can present with fussiness and refusal to take oral feedings and is characterized by white patches in the oral cavity that cannot be easily scraped away.

        ii. Congenital candidiasis. Acquired in utero, infants can either have cutaneous or systemic disease (especially extremely preterm infants). **Congenital cutaneous candidiasis** presents with an extensive rash within 12 hours of birth. The rash consists of erythematous macules, diffuse papules, and pustules. Unlike erythema toxicum, this rash frequently involves the palms and soles. In term infants, there is desquamation of these lesions, which may mimic SSSS. Premature infants may present with a rash with variable presentation (pustules, vesicles, or a burn-like dermatitis with peeling) (Figure 80–12). In **congenital systemic candidiasis,** the majority of infants do not have a rash but can present with pneumonia, meningitis, or other presentations. This is a very invasive infection with a high mortality rate, especially in very low birthweight infants.

    b. Aspergillus. This has been reported to cause cutaneous fungal infections but is rare.

        i. Primary cutaneous aspergillosis. Characterized by lack of involvement of organs except the skin at the time of diagnosis. Preterm infants are at risk for primary cutaneous aspergillosis (PCA) because of vulnerability of their skin and immature host defenses. Risk factors include prematurity, neutropenia, prior use of antibiotics, and glucocorticoid administration. A plaque with an eschar is characteristic of PCA. Disruption of the skin occurs due to contaminated hand splints, skin maceration caused by oximeter sensor, or adhesive tape.

        ii. Secondary aspergillosis. Characterized by involvement of organs and a maculopapular eruption caused by thrombosis of small vessels.

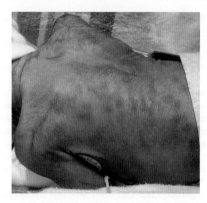

FIGURE 80–12. Congenital cutaneous candidiasis. (*Used with permission from Leslie Castelo-Soccio, MD, PhD, Children's Hospital of Philadelphia Division of Dermatology.*)

4. **Parasitic infections that can cause a rash**
    a. **Scabies.** An infestation with the mite *Sarcoptes scabiei* has been reported in infants as young as 2 weeks. Infants tend to have widespread lesions often on the face and scalp (usually not seen in older patients who present with intertriginous locations). They can have papules, nodules, vesicles, and pustules caused by burrowing of the adult female mites. Itching is intense, especially at night.
    b. *Toxoplasma gondii* **infections.** The classic triad for infection by *Toxoplasma gondii* is chorioretinitis, intracranial calcifications, and hydrocephalus. The infant may also present with a maculopapular rash and petechiae similar to other TORCH infections.
E. **Rashes that cause scaling.** Usually benign and self-limited. Infectious and dietary etiologies need to be ruled out because they need immediate treatment. Genetic and immune etiologies can be considered later in the differential.
    1. **Postmaturity.** The majority of term and postmature infants normally shed their skin. The skin appears similar to parchment paper and peels off. This is a normal physiologic finding that requires no medical treatment.
    2. **Seborrheic dermatitis.** Usually seen on the scalp and flexure areas. It is a red erythematous rash with yellow scaling. Can be seen in the diaper area and is self-limiting.
    3. **Fatty acid deficiency.** Superficial scaling and desquamation can occur. Can be seen in fatty acid deficiency syndrome (where infants have decreased fat stores) or in fat malabsorption. Fatty acid replacement is necessary.
    4. **Ichthyoses.** May present as "harlequin fetus" or "collodion baby." Many types of ichthyoses are present. These are genetic disorders that cause severe thick, scaly skin, sometimes with restricted movement. The infant can have a shiny, tight membrane covering at birth that can peel off. The skin is prone to cracking and secondary infection. Some of the ichthyoses are associated with sensorineural hearing defects; others are associated with neurologic problems including seizures (Figure 80–13).
    5. **Infantile eczema.** Scaling is present. Eczema is rarely seen in the newborn but is often seen in infants.
    6. **Atopic dermatitis.** Red scaly and itchy rash; rarely seen in the newborn.
    7. **Staphylococcal scalded skin syndrome.** See page 731 and Figure 80–9.

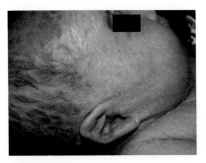

FIGURE 80–13. Lamellar ichthyosis. (*Used with permission from Leslie Castelo-Soccio, MD, PhD, Children's Hospital of Philadelphia Division of Dermatology.*)

8. **Psoriasis.** Seen as a diaper rash with dissemination (scaly patches beyond the diaper rash) or can present as erythroderma progressing to pustular psoriasis.
9. ***Candida* infections.** These can also cause redness and scaling (see earlier).
10. **Syphilis infections.** See page 731.
11. **Ectodermal dysplasias.** There are >150 subtypes, but the most common form is X-linked recessive hypohidrotic ectodermal dysplasia.
12. **Immunodeficiencies.** Infants with immunodeficiencies (acquired immunodeficiency syndrome [AIDS], severe combined immunodeficiency, diffuse cutaneous mastocytosis, Wiskott-Aldrich syndrome, Langerhans cell histiocytosis) can have a red scaly rash.
13. **Neonatal lupus.** An immune-mediated disorder that is caused by maternally transferred autoantibodies (SSA/Ro, SSB/La, and/or U1RNP). Major manifestations are skin and cardiac (primary cause of congenital heart block). Skin findings are transient and usually start at a few weeks of age but can be present at birth. Two variants are papulosquamous and annular. Fifteen to twenty-five percent of cases have cutaneous manifestations. Typical rash involves 0.5- to 3-cm annular erythematous papules with a central scale. Liver and hematologic involvement occurs in about 10% of cases (Figure 80–14).
F. **Rashes that cause blisters and bullae.** Infectious and dietary causes need to be ruled out because they require immediate treatment. Then less common causes can be evaluated.
1. **Epidermolysis bullosa.** A group of inherited diseases that cause blistering. Trauma induces the blisters. Congenital localized absence of skin is often noted at birth (Figure 80–15).
2. **Zinc deficiency dermatosis.** Presents as a blistering rash or more commonly an eczematous rash on the angle of the mouth, chin, or cheeks in a U-shaped distribution and on the diaper area. It can be red and scaly and can have a dark color at the periphery.
3. **Congenital herpes infection.** See Section III.D.2.a.i.
4. **Staphylococcal scalded skin syndrome.** See Section III.D.1.a.ii.
5. **Incontinentia pigmenti.** A rare X-linked dominant genetic disorder that is more common in females. It has 4 stages: stage 1 occurs at birth to 2 weeks—vesiculobullous (erythematous vesicles/bullae that occur linearly on the trunk, extremities, and scalp); stage 2 occurs 2 to 3 weeks after birth—verrucous; stages 3 and 4 occur later. Infants can also have neurologic, dental, and ophthalmologic abnormalities. *Note:* Stage 1 lesions can be confused with herpes simplex infection (Figure 80–16).

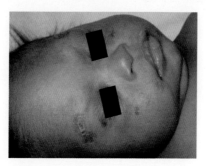

FIGURE 80–14. Neonatal lupus. (*Used with permission from Leslie Castelo-Soccio, MD, PhD, Children's Hospital of Philadelphia Division of Dermatology.*)

      6. Less common causes. Genetic disorders, epidermolytic hyperkeratosis, toxic epidermal necrolysis, and bullous mastocytosis.

  G. Birthmarks. The majority of birthmarks are benign and require no treatment. However, if there are many lesions present, this may signify an associated syndrome, or if very large, patients can be at risk for melanoma and have to be closely followed. Vascular lesions need to be evaluated because they may interfere with vital organs.

      1. Pigmented lesions

        a. Café-au-lait spots (macules). Benign lesions that are oval or irregular with a light brown color. If they are >5 mm in diameter and there are >6, suspect an associated syndrome (think neurofibromatosis, Albright syndrome, Turner or Noonan syndrome, tuberous sclerosis, ataxia-telangiectasia).

        b. Mongolian blue spot. See page 730.

        c. Nevus of Ota/Ito. A blue or grayish area involving the orbital and zygomatic area common in Asians that carries the risk of glaucoma. Unlike Mongolian spots, these do not fade.

      2. Diffuse hyperpigmentation. Not normal and can be secondary to Addison disease, biliary atresia, hepatic atresia, sprue, melanism, lentiginosis, porphyria, or Hartnup disease or idiopathic.

      3. Hypopigmentation/hypopigmented lesions

        a. Diffuse or localized loss of pigment. This can be secondary to phenylketonuria, Addison disease, trauma, postinflammation, or genetic.

        b. Ash-leaf macules. Small area of hypopigmentation, oval shaped, and similar to the leaf of an ash tree; a marker for tuberous sclerosis.

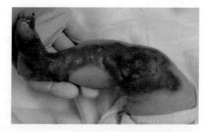

FIGURE 80–15. Congenital absence of skin in epidermolysis bullosa, dominant dystrophic. (*Used with permission from Leslie Castelo-Soccio, MD, PhD, Children's Hospital of Philadelphia Division of Dermatology.*)

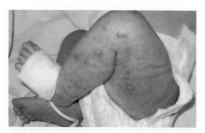

FIGURE 80–16. Incontinentia pigmenti. (*Used with permission from Leslie Castelo-Soccio, MD, PhD, Children's Hospital of Philadelphia Division of Dermatology.*)

    c. Hypomelanosis of Ito. Syndrome (primarily neurologic) with hypopigmented macule or linear/whorled pattern of hypopigmentation.

    d. Partial albinism (piebaldism). An autosomal dominant disorder of off-white macules on forehead, scalp, trunk, and extremities. This type of depigmentation can also be seen secondary to Addison disease, tuberous sclerosis, vitiligo, and Klein-Waardenburg syndrome.

    e. Albinism. Genetic disorders that cause abnormal melanin synthesis.

  4. Vascular lesions

    a. Port wine stain (nevus flammeus). This usually presents at birth on the face or extremities. It is a permanent capillary angioma. Rarely it is associated with Sturge-Weber syndrome, Klippel-Trenaunay syndrome, Parkes-Weber syndrome, or *RASA-1* mutations (Figure 80–17).

    b. Nevus simplex/salmon patch. See page 730.

    c. Hemangiomas. Most common benign tumors of vascular endothelium of infancy and are more frequent in premature infants. Females are more likely to be affected, and they occur most commonly on the head and neck, followed by the trunk and limb.

      i. Superficial ("strawberry") hemangioma. A bright red tumor (of dilated mass of capillaries) that protrudes above the skin and can appear anywhere on the body. Usually does not require treatment unless it interferes with vital functions.

      ii. Deep (cavernous) hemangioma. More deep into the skin and bluish red; usually benign unless it interferes with vital organs.

      iii. Mixed hemangioma. This has both deep and superficial components.

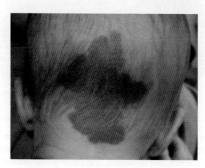

FIGURE 80–17. Port wine stain. (*Used with permission from Leslie Castelo-Soccio, MD, PhD, Children's Hospital of Philadelphia Division of Dermatology.*)

            iv. **Benign neonatal hemangiomatosis.** Multiple congenital cutaneous hemangiomas that appear at birth or shortly after with spontaneous regression of lesions within the first 2 years of life.

            v. **Diffuse neonatal hemangiomatosis.** Multiple cutaneous hemangiomas plus hemangiomas of at least 3 separate organ systems. This disorder has a grave prognosis if not recognized and treated.

H. **Rashes that cause petechiae/purpura.** These may relate to birth trauma (considered "normal") or, if generalized and recurring, can signify a serious infection or hematologic etiology that needs immediate evaluation and treatment.

    1. **Birth trauma.** Petechiae on the lower body after a breech delivery or on the upper body with a vertex presentation can be normal. They do not recur.

    2. **Autoimmune disorders.** Neonatal lupus with maternal transmission of autoantibodies.

    3. **Thrombocytopenia.** Usually generalized scattered petechiae, particularly in response to minor trauma.

    4. **Neonatal alloimmune thrombocytopenia.** An isoimmune reaction that can cause thrombocytopenia and severe bleeding, including intracranial bleeding.

    5. **Maternal idiopathic thrombocytopenic purpura.** Approximately 80% of cases of thrombocytopenia are caused by autoimmune form.

    6. **Coagulation factor deficiencies.** Petechiae and purpura are more common in thrombocytopenia, with large ecchymoses, muscle hemorrhages, and bleeding from heel sticks, venipuncture, and other sites more common with coagulation defects.

    7. **Sepsis/infection related.** Usually caused by gram-negative bacterial sepsis (*Escherichia coli*, *Pseudomonas*). Listeriosis and aspergillosis are also involved. Coxsackievirus can cause "blueberry muffin" lesions.

    8. **Disseminated intravascular coagulation.** Main causes are sepsis, birth asphyxia, necrotizing enterocolitis, and respiratory distress syndrome. One can see petechiae on the skin, and bleeding can occur from venipuncture sites and the GI tract.

    9. **Purpura fulminans.** Symmetrical and well-defined lakes of confluent ecchymosis without petechiae, with sudden onset and development of hemorrhagic bullae and sudden death. Characteristic of meningococcal sepsis or other life-threatening infection.

    10. **TORCH infections.** Toxoplasmosis, other infections (syphilis), rubella, cytomegalovirus, and herpes can all cause "blueberry muffin" lesions (widespread papules and purpura) (Figure 80–18).

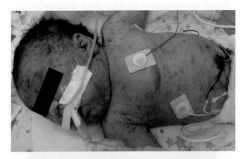

FIGURE 80–18. "Blueberry muffin" lesion of congenital leukemia. Can also be seen in congenital viral infections (TORCH [toxoplasmosis, other, rubella, cytomegalovirus, herpes simplex virus]), blood and vascular disorders, and other malignancies. (*Used with permission from Leslie Castelo-Soccio, MD, PhD, Children's Hospital of Philadelphia Division of Dermatology.*)

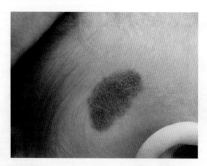

FIGURE 80–19. Congenital melanocytic nevus of the scalp. (*Used with permission from Leslie Castelo-Soccio, MD, PhD, Children's Hospital of Philadelphia Division of Dermatology.*)

11. **Maternal drugs.** Salicylates (especially during last 2 weeks of pregnancy).
12. **Congenital leukemia cutis.** A rare disorder. Cutaneous leukemic infiltrates occur in 25% to 30% of infants with congenital leukemia. Infants can present with petechiae, purpura, firm blue violaceous lesions, purple nodules, hepatosplenomegaly, lethargy, pallor, and fever. Chloromas (nodular infiltrations of the skin that are solid collections of myeloblasts) look like red-purple papules and nodules (**"blueberry muffin"** rash) (see Figure 80–18). Congenital leukemia can be associated with Down, Edward, and Patau syndromes. Can be confused with benign hemangiomatosis.

I. **Rashes that lead to malignant transformation**
1. **Congenital melanocytic nevus.** Nevi that are small (<1.5 cm) and intermediate (<20 cm) in size are common with a small risk of malignant melanoma (Figure 80–19). Large congenital nevi (>20 cm) and giant congenital nevi (>40 cm) have a higher risk of malignant transformation (5%–15% risk). Giant congenital nevi also have a risk of neurocutaneous melanosis (Figure 80–20).

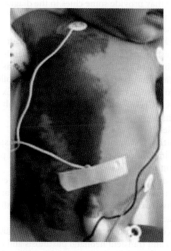

FIGURE 80–20. Congenital giant melanocytic nevus. (*Used with permission from Andrew Bowe, DO, Pediatrix Medical Group.*)

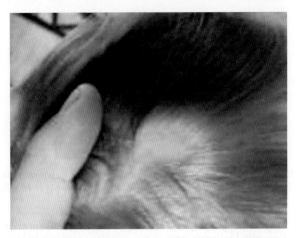

FIGURE 80–21. Sebaceous nevus of Jadassohn. (*Used with permission from Andrew Bowe, DO, Pediatrix Medical Group.*)

2. **Sebaceous nevus of Jadassohn.** Congenital hamartomatous lesion located on the scalp. It grows with age and most commonly transforms into malignant basal cell carcinoma or a benign trichoblastoma. Found in approximately 0.3% of newborns. (Figure 80–21).

IV. **Database**

A. **History.** Obtain thorough history from the mother and family and a detailed history from the obstetric department. Is there a family history of skin disorders? Many skin disorders are genetic (ichthyoses, immunodeficiency, albinism). Asking about recent infections (varicella), early infections during the pregnancy (congenital infections), sexual history (syphilis), unusual travel destinations, and pet history (*T gondii*) may provide some clues to the diagnosis. Does the mother have herpes? Did she have any unusual food products or undercooked food (*Listeria*)? What medications did the mother take?

B. **Physical examination.** Check vital signs. Is the infant febrile, or does the infant appear sick, suggesting an infection? Do not just examine the presenting rash, but check the entire body to see if there are signs of the rash anywhere else. The distribution of the rash may be characteristic. Frequent follow-up examinations may document any progression or resolution of the lesions. Examine the eye to check for chorioretinitis (TORCH infections). Hepatosplenomegaly may be seen in congenital TORCH infections.

C. **Laboratory studies**

1. **Sepsis evaluation** if systemic infection suspected. **Aspirate appropriate lesions** that contain fluid for bacterial culture, viral culture, polymerase chain reaction, and fungal culture.

2. **If active bleeding suspected,** send complete blood count (CBC) with differential, platelet and reticulocyte count, TORCH titers, and sepsis workup.

3. **Potassium hydroxide prep** if *Candida*/fungal infection suspected (reveals pseudohyphae).

4. **Wright stain** of lesion fluid can show polymorphonuclear neutrophils with bullous impetigo and transient neonatal pustulosis and eosinophils with erythema toxicum. Wright stain of milia shows keratinocytes.

5. **Mineral oil prep** can show mites and ova with scabies.

6. **Polymerase chain reaction or direct fluorescent antibody** of cutaneous lesion if herpes suspected.
7. **Skin biopsy** is sometimes indicated, especially if the lesion is atypical.
8. **Gram stain, culture** of the purulent material of cellulitis/abscess. Gram stain of staphylococcal pustulosis will show gram-positive cocci and neutrophils.
9. **Maternal and neonatal autoantibodies** for lupus.
10. **Coagulation studies.** Platelet count, fibrinogen, prothrombin time, and partial thromboplastin time.
11. **Molecular cytogenetic analysis of DNA of skin biopsy** if congenital leukemia suspected.

D. **Imaging and other studies (rarely needed)**
1. **Computed tomography scan or contrast-enhanced magnetic resonance image of the head** to rule out calcifications if Sturge-Weber syndrome is suspected.
2. **Ultrasound, echocardiography, and/or computed tomography scans** may be needed to manage hemangiomas.
3. **Imaging studies** may be necessary for larger defects of aplasia cutis congenita to rule out underlying bone or soft tissue defects.

V. **Plan.** As noted previously, the majority of rashes that occur in the neonate do not require treatment. **Pediatric dermatology consultation** is recommended for any unusual lesions. It is important to note that acyclovir is recommended early in cases of infants with a vesicular skin rash, even if the diagnosis of herpes is not confirmed.

A. **Aplasia cutis congenita.** Depending on the size and involvement, treatment includes medical (local includes cleaning, ointment, possible antibiotics), surgical (none if small; larger may require excision with closure, skin grafting, and other treatment), or both.

B. **Skin and soft tissue infections (abscesses and/or cellulitis, omphalitis).** Incision and drainage of **abscess** (if indicated) with local wound care. Send fluid for culture and sensitivity. An incision and drainage of the abscess may be adequate if the infant is not clinically ill. If the infant is clinically ill, a CBC with differential and blood culture are usually done. Antibiotics (usually nafcillin) are started to cover for skin flora, unless methicillin-resistant *S aureus* is suspected (use vancomycin). Lumbar puncture is done if the infant has any signs suspicious for meningitis. Infants with **cellulitis**, especially at intravenous (IV) sites, are usually treated with antibiotics based on culture or empirically with oxacillin or nafcillin and gentamicin. **Omphalitis** is treated with a full sepsis workup (including a lumbar puncture), and antibiotics (ampicillin and gentamicin) are started to cover both gram-positive and gram-negative organisms until the results of culture and sensitivities are available.

C. **Benign skin disorders.** No treatment is necessary.

D. **Rashes that are caused by infections.** See specific infectious disease chapters for more details where appropriate.
1. *Staphylococcus aureus.* Systemic antibiotics.
2. *Streptococcus.* Cutaneous infection is usually group A, which is treated by penicillin.
3. **Syphilis.** See Chapter 147.
4. *Listeria monocytogenes.* Ampicillin and an aminoglycoside such as gentamicin (cephalosporins are not active).
5. **Herpes simplex.** Acyclovir 60 mg/kg/d IV divided every 8 hours for 14 days for SEM disease only if there is no CNS involvement or disseminated disease.
6. **Varicella.** Acyclovir and VariZIG (varicella-zoster immune globulin; see doses in Chapter 155) may decrease the severity of the course and improve outcome. Treatment must begin early in the course of the illness.
7. **Cytomegalovirus.** Ganciclovir (Cytovene) in adults; limited data in pediatrics. Parenteral ganciclovir and oral valganciclovir are being used but are limited to use in those with symptomatic congenital cytomegalovirus disease with CNS disease. See Chapter 132.

8. **Rubella.** Supportive management. See Chapter 145.
9. *Candida albicans.* Systemic antifungal medications such as amphotericin B to treat disseminated infection. Topical antifungals are used to treat isolated skin lesions. Thrush is treated by oral nystatin, 0.5 mL inside each cheek twice daily, for 10 days.
10. *Aspergillus.* Voriconazole is the drug of choice. (In children age 2–12 years, load with 9 mg/kg IV every 12 hours for 2 doses, and then continue IV dosing of 8 mg/kg/dose every 12 hours.) Maintain drug levels between 2 and 6 mcg/mL.
11. **Scabies.** Apply 5% permethrin cream topically. (*Note:* Permethrin is off label in neonates and may not be safe in very low birthweight infants.)
12. **Toxoplasmosis.** See Chapter 149.

E. **Rashes that cause scaling**

1. **Postmaturity.** No treatment is necessary.
2. **Seborrheic dermatitis.** Usually resolves by 1 year; supportive care.
3. **Fatty acid deficiency.** Replacement of fatty acids through IV lipid solutions or diet is necessary.
4. **Ichthyoses.** Aggressive supportive care, close monitoring of fluid and electrolytes, and meticulous skin care with the goal of preventing infections. Collodion babies frequently have temperature instability and excessive fluid loss.
5. **Infantile eczema.** Avoid any irritants; use protective creams such as zinc oxide in the diaper area. Short-term topical steroids may be needed.
6. **Atopic dermatitis.** Emollients and mild topical steroids are used.
7. **Staphylococcal scalded skin syndrome.** Antibiotics (IV penicillinase resistant, antistaphylococcal [eg, Cloxacillin]), supportive care, and attention to fluid and electrolyte management.
8. **Psoriasis.** Topical steroids and sometimes wet dressings are used.
9. *Candida.* See Section V.D.9.
10. **Syphilis.** See Chapter 147.
11. **Ectodermal dysplasias.** Supportive care with artificial tears.
12. **Immunodeficiencies.** See specific entity.
13. **Neonatal lupus erythematosus.** Thorough cardiac examination, liver function tests, and CBC. Apply protective sunscreen and avoid direct sunlight for 4 to 6 months. Topical steroids may be necessary.

F. **Rashes that cause blisters and bullae**

1. **Epidermolysis bullosa.** Meticulous skin care, infection prevention, and special attention to nutrition and feedings because of the problems with dysphagia from scarring.
2. **Zinc deficiency dermatosis.** Zinc supplementation.
3. **Congenital herpes.** See Chapter 137.
4. **Staphylococcal scalded skin syndrome.** See Section V.D.1.
5. **Incontinentia pigmenti.** No specific treatment for the cutaneous lesions.

G. **Birthmarks**

1. **Hyperpigmented lesions.** Most of these lesions require no treatment. If the lesions are large (>3 cm), removal is recommended. Giant hairy nevi are removed to prevent cancer development.
2. **Hypopigmented lesions.** Piebaldism is treated with cosmetic camouflage. Those with albinism should follow sun restriction guidelines and use sunblock.
3. **Vascular lesions.** Many hemangiomas can be closely watched and left to regress. If treatment is necessary, steroid therapy, embolization, excision, occlusion, laser therapy, α-interferon, and radiotherapy are options. Port wine stains can be treated with laser therapy. Need to differentiate benign neonatal hemangiomatosis from diffuse neonatal hemangiomatosis because treatment is different.

H. **Rashes that cause petechiae and purpura.** These rashes usually require a thorough workup and treatment if there is a bleeding disorder. Infections are treated with antibiotics or antiviral agents. Platelet transfusion and replacement of coagulation factors may be necessary.
   1. **Birth trauma.** No treatment is necessary.
   2. **Autoimmune disorders such as maternal or neonatal lupus.** Cardiology examination to look for heart block is indicated.
   3. **Thrombocytopenia, neonatal isoimmune thrombocytopenia/maternal idiopathic thrombocytopenic purpura.** See Chapter 128.
   4. **Coagulation factor deficiencies.** See Chapter 92.
   5. **Sepsis/TORCH infections.** See Chapters 146 and 148.
   6. **Disseminated intravascular coagulation.** See Chapter 92.
   7. **Purpura fulminans.** Treat the underlying infection.
   8. **Congenital leukemia.** The optimum treatment plan is unclear. Treatment consists of intensive combination therapy plus supportive care.

81 Sedation and Analgesia

I. **Problem.** An infant with pulmonary hypertension with extreme lability needs sedation. Should this infant be sedated, and which agent is available to use? An infant is having a bedside procedure, should I use a local anesthetic? (See Chapter 15.)
II. **Immediate questions**
   A. **What is the indication for the sedation?** Agitation and movement by the infant during procedures such as extracorporeal life support (ECLS) can risk injury. Certain procedures (eg, magnetic resonance imaging [MRI]) mandate that the infant be immobilized, so sedation may be required. Infants with extreme lability on mechanical ventilation may benefit from sedation.
   B. **Why does the infant need analgesia?** If the newborn is to undergo minor procedures such as elective circumcision, local anesthesia is usually administered. For emergency procedures such as chest tube placement, the need for analgesia must be weighed against the delay of administering the analgesic agent.
   C. **If treating for agitation while an infant is on mechanical ventilation, is the infant adequately ventilated?** Hypoxia and inadequate ventilation can result in agitation, and sedation is dangerous in these situations.
   D. **Is sedation needed for a short period (eg, for a diagnostic procedure) or long term?** Certain medications are indicated for short-term sedation and should not be used long term.
III. **Differential diagnosis and indications**
   A. **Indications for analgesia.** Whether newborns can experience pain remains in the philosophical realm, but they undeniably react to painful stimuli (nociception). Such stimuli elicit both clinical symptoms (eg, tachycardia, hypertension, and decreased oxygenation) and complex behavioral responses in term and preterm infants. By 23 weeks' gestation, the nervous system has developed sufficiently to enable the conduction of nociceptive stimuli from peripheral skin receptors to the brain. The development of the descending inhibiting pathways occurs at a later stage; therefore, the more immature infant may have an even lower threshold for noxious stimulus than at a later age. Neonates possibly have an increased sensitivity to pain compared with

older age groups. During surgical interventions, the neonate, like the adult, mounts a hormonal response that consists of the release of catecholamines, β-endorphins, corticotropin, growth hormone, and glucagon as well as the suppression of insulin secretion. This response is reduced by prior administration of analgesia or anesthesia. Although we do not know whether the neonate experiences psychological distress and lasting psychological sequelae, it has been estimated that during their stay in the neonatal intensive care unit (NICU) infants experience an average of 14 painful procedures a day during the first 2 weeks of life. Thus, there are enough reasons to attempt to control exposure to pain as well as other unpleasant experiences.

1. **Major surgical procedures such as ligation of the ductus arteriosus or laparotomy require major anesthesia.** General anesthesia should be provided by inhalation of anesthetic gases or intravenous (IV) administration of narcotic agents. In all these conditions, **the use of paralytic agents without analgesia is absolutely contraindicated.**

2. Postoperative management
   a. **Narcotic agents should always be included in the immediate postoperative period.** Supplementary sedation is often provided by benzodiazepines, which are useful to combat agitation and potentiate the effect of opiates. It is important to remember that these sedative agents do not have any analgesic effect and, therefore, cannot be given alone to relieve pain.
   b. **Other pain-relieving agents.** IV paracetamol (acetaminophen) has been used in Europe for neonatal analgesia and is now available in the United States (Ofirmev). Its use may be helpful to reduce the dosage and frequency of opiate administration.

3. **Minor surgical procedures.** Analgesia for so-called "minor procedures" is mostly provided by local anesthesia, at times supplemented by small doses of opiates or sedative agents.
   a. **Unless the infant's condition requires extreme urgent action, provide analgesia for procedures** such as chest tube insertion and vascular cutdown.
   b. **The need for local analgesia for circumcision** is becoming less controversial and is now widely accepted.
   c. **The effectiveness of and need for analgesia for more minor procedures** such as lumbar puncture have not been demonstrated.

4. **"Stressful" conditions.** There is wide controversy with regard to providing analgesia or sedation in "stressful" conditions, akin to "anxiolysis" in the adult and pediatric populations. The period during which mechanical ventilation and its related routine procedures are provided has been identified as the most frequent time when infants are being "stressed."

5. **"Painful" conditions.** Pain scores and scales have been proposed to provide a rational approach for assessing the need for and monitoring the efficacy of pain management. Those scores are usually composites of measured behavioral, physiologic, and stress responses. Several pain scoring tools have found widespread use. Those used most commonly are the Neonatal Infant Pain Scale (NIPS); the Children's Revised Impact of Event Scale (CRIES); the Premature Infant Pain Profile (PIPP); the Neonatal Facial Coding System (NFCS); the Neonatal Pain, Agitation, and Sedation Scale (N-PASS); the Distress Scale for Ventilated Newborn Infants (DVSNI); the Pain Assessment Tool (PAT); the COMFORT scale; and the Échelle de Douleur et d'Inconfort du Nouveau-né Scale (EDIN). The wide variety of these scores exemplifies the lack of a gold standard.
   a. **The arguments in favor of analgesia or sedation for these situations are as follows:**
      i. **It reduces the level of various biochemical markers** of stress, such as blood levels of catecholamines, cortisol, and β-endorphin.
      ii. **It lessens the duration of hypoxemia** associated with endotracheal intubation and/or suctioning.

     iii. Additional argument for its use involves the difficulty in diagnosing discomfort and pain when the infant is under muscle paralysis.

  b. The arguments against such routine use of analgesia or sedation are as follows:

     i. The pharmacokinetic characteristics of narcotic agents in the preterm infant are variable and not always predictable.

     ii. The same assumed "safe" dose for some infants can, for others, result in severe toxicity (eg, hemodynamic and respiratory depression or toxic accumulation, leading to a transient comatose state).

     iii. The prolonged use (sometimes as little as 4 days) of narcotic and sedative agents is associated with the rapid development of tolerance, withdrawal, and encephalopathy and the requirement for higher ventilatory support in the early phase of respiratory distress syndrome. Furthermore, it often delays weaning from mechanical ventilation.

     iv. Treating for "agitation" by sedation can be dangerous when the former is the result of inadequate ventilation or hypoxemia. Therefore, before treating agitation, one must always ensure, by careful examination, that the endotracheal tube is not obstructed or misplaced and that adequate ventilating pressures are being used.

B. Indications for sedation

  1. Extreme respiratory lability. Infants who have demonstrated extreme respiratory lability develop hypoxemia rapidly with minimal handling. Infants with severe pulmonary hypertension and pulmonary vascular hyperreactivity are often candidates for sedation.

  2. Therapeutic procedures. When it is necessary to prevent the child from moving vigorously (eg, during ECMO/ECLS), sedation may be needed to prevent accidental dislodgment of the vascular cannulas.

  3. Diagnostic procedures. Procedures that require the child to be immobilized include imaging procedures such as MRI, cardiac catheterization, and occasionally computed tomography (CT).

  4. Elective endotracheal intubation and rapid sequence intubation. The question of premedicating neonates before nonemergent intubation has been debated in the past, and its use is on the rise. Various combinations of drugs have been proposed, including anticholinergic agents (to prevent reflex bradycardia), short-acting analgesics and/or hypnotic/sedatives (to prevent pain and hypertension), and muscle relaxants (to decrease the time and number of attempts for successful intubation). See Table 33–2.

IV. Database

  A. Physical examination. Before instituting any type of sedation or analgesia, there must be a clear diagnosis. The physical examination is directed at the underlying condition.

  B. Laboratory studies. These are usually not needed, except in the context of the underlying disease.

  C. Imaging and other studies. Such studies are usually not needed, except in the context of the underlying disease.

V. Plan

  A. General management. Prevention of distress and pain should be a priority in the neonatal unit and in newborn nurseries. Measures to prevent or minimize stress in the neonate should include the following:

    1. Reduce noise (eg, close the incubator door gently).

    2. Protect the infant from intense light.

    3. Cluster blood drawings as much as possible.

    4. Use spring-loaded lancets for heel sticks.

    5. Replace tape with a self-adhesive bandage.

    6. Perform intratracheal suctioning only if indicated.

    7. Use adequate medication before invasive procedures.

B. Specific agents
1. **Pharmacologic management provided by systemic analgesia**
   a. **Opiates.** All opiates may lead to respiratory depression and hypotension. Muscular rigidity is seen mostly with the synthetic opiates with rapid IV administration, such as fentanyl (>2 mcg/kg), sufentanil, and especially alfentanil. The risk of chest wall rigidity can be attenuated by slow administration (preferably over 3–5 minutes or at least 1–2 minutes). It can be treated with a muscle-relaxing agent (eg, rocuronium) and acutely reversed by naloxone (0.1 mg/kg).
      i. **Morphine sulfate.** The most commonly used opioid for sedation during mechanical ventilation. A loading IV dose of 50 to 200 mcg/kg is followed by IV infusion of 10 to 40 mcg/kg/h. The peak action occurs in 20 minutes and lasts for 2 to 4 hours in full-term infants and 6 to 8 hours in preterm infants. The use of morphine infusions reduces pain and stress in mechanically ventilated preterm infants at the expense of increasing the duration of mechanical ventilation. For shorter duration of sedation, only 50 to 100 mcg/kg (0.05 to 0.1 mg/kg) can be administered IV or intramuscularly (IM). The onset of action will occur only 5 to 10 minutes after IV administration of the drug and after 10 to 30 minutes when given IM.
      ii. **Fentanyl (Sublimaze).** Frequently used in neonates for its ability to provide rapid analgesia. It has a faster onset (3–4 minutes) and shorter duration of action (30 minutes) and is 13 to 20 times more potent than morphine. Fentanyl blocks endocrine stress responses and prevents pain-induced increases in pulmonary vascular resistance, while hemodynamic stability is better preserved than with morphine because it causes less histamine release. For anesthesia, use IV bolus 10 to 50 mcg/kg, and for analgesia, use 1 to 4 mcg/kg. In case of no IV access, it can be given IM, resulting in a slower onset of action (7–15 minutes). A continuous IV infusion of 1 to 3 mcg/kg/h may be used for ongoing sedation. Tolerance to opioid-induced analgesia and sedation occurs more rapidly than with morphine. A cumulative fentanyl dose of >2.5 mg/kg or a duration of infusion >9 days is predictive of opioid withdrawal syndrome.
      iii. **Remifentanil.** Has a chemical structure identical to that of fentanyl but has twice its analgesic potency. An IV administration of 1 to 3 mcg/kg gives nearly immediate analgesia that lasts only 3 to 15 minutes.
      iv. **Sufentanil.** Give 0.2 mcg/kg over 20 minutes, then continuous IV, 0.05 mcg/kg/h.
   b. **Ketamine.** It is an N-methyl-D-aspartate receptor antagonist with analgesic and amnesic effects. In addition to its analgesic efficacy, ketamine has the advantage of maintaining stable cardiovascular and respiratory function. Ketamine also exerts a bronchodilator effect and improves lung compliance. Infrequent transient laryngospasm and excessive salivation have been reported. At a dosage of 0.5 to 2 mg/kg IV, its onset of action is between 0.5 and 2 minutes, and the duration of action is 5 to 60 minutes. It can also be given IM or enterally. It does not affect cerebral blood flow and might be a good choice for unstable hypotensive neonates requiring procedures such intubation or ECMO cannulation. Primate studies have shown apoptotic and necrotic cell death after prolonged ketamine exposure in early postnatal life (day 5 of life), whereas this is not seen at a later age (day 35 of life) and with shorter duration of exposure (3 hours). Use in the NICU has been limited. It may be of value, possibly in combination with atropine sulfate, for sedation before endotracheal intubation. Infants with severe bronchopulmonary dysplasia and refractory bronchospasm may also benefit from the use of ketamine for its additional bronchodilatory effect.

    c. **Propofol.** A nonbarbiturate anesthetic used for induction of anesthesia. It is lipophilic and rapidly equilibrates between plasma and brain with quick loss of consciousness (within 30 seconds) and short duration of action after a single bolus dose (3–10 minutes). Possible adverse effects are histamine release, apnea, hypotension, bradycardia, and bronchospasm. It often causes pain at injection site. Neonatal dosing has not yet been well established.

2. **Pharmacologic management provided by sedative-hypnotics**

    a. **Benzodiazepines.** Activate γ-aminobutyric acid (GABA) receptors and produce sedation, anxiolysis, muscle relaxation, amnesia, and anticonvulsant effects. They may improve synchrony with assisted ventilation but offer little pain relief. Side effects include respiratory depression, hypotension, dependence, and occasional neuroexcitability or clonic activity resembling seizures.

      i. **Midazolam (Versed)** has a rapid onset of action (1–2 minutes) and can produce apnea if given too rapidly. Its very short half-life (30–60 minutes) makes it a good choice for brief rapid sedation. Midazolam is given as a single dose, 50 to 100 mcg/kg, or by continuous infusion at a rate of 0.4 to 0.6 mcg/kg/min. Withdrawal may occur when given continuously for >48 hours. Combining midazolam with opioids increases the incidence of adverse effects of both agents. Although it is the most commonly used benzodiazepine in the NICU, concern about its efficacy and safety has been raised recently. The lower number of GABA$_A$ receptors in neonates may contribute to neuroexcitability and myoclonic activity that resembles or progresses to convulsions.

      ii. **Lorazepam (Ativan)** has a longer duration of action (8–12 hours) and may require less frequent dosing (50–100 mcg/kg every 8 hours).

    b. **Chloral hydrate.** A sedative-hypnotic used primarily for short-term sedation but is not available in the United States. It is especially useful during diagnostic procedures such as CT and MRI. The onset of action is usually within 10 to 15 minutes. Administer 20 to 50 mg/kg every 6 to 8 hours rectally or orally for sedation. It should not be used long term.

    c. **Acetaminophen (Paracetamol)** inhibits the cyclooxygenase-2 enzymes in the brain. It is frequently used in conjunction with other pain relief to decrease opioid use, especially for postsurgical pain. IV acetaminophen decreases the amount of opioids needed after surgery and is particularly useful for routine postsurgical care with opioid-sparing effects. In contrast to its use in older children or adults, acetaminophen rarely causes hepatic or renal toxicity in newborns. In both preterm and term infants, the clearance of acetaminophen is slower than in older children, so oral or rectal dosing is required less frequently. Single oral doses of 10 to 15 mg/kg may be given every 6 to 8 hours; 20 to 25 mg/kg can be given rectally at the same time intervals. For IV acetaminophen in neonates, pharmacokinetic analysis suggests a loading dose of 20 mg/kg and maintenance dose of 7.5 mg/kg every 6 to 8 hours for neonates between 23 and 32 weeks of postmenstrual age (PMA). Total recommended daily dose is 20 to 30 mg/kg at 24 to 30 weeks PMA, 35 to 50 mg/kg at 31 to 36 weeks PMA, and 50 to 60 mg/kg at 37 to 42 weeks PMA. The administration of the repeated dose should not exceed 48 to 96 hours. The new IV formulation (Ofirmev) requires extreme caution because a 10-fold dosing error is facilitated by the preparation's concentration being formatted for adult use.

    d. **Dexmedetomidine (Precedex)** is a selective α$_2$-adrenoceptor agonist that, unlike traditional sedative agents, is reported to produce its sedative effect, at least in part, through an endogenous sleep-promoting pathway that does not produce clinically significant respiratory depression. Although not approved for use in children by the US Food and Drug Administration, it has gained popularity in pediatric critical care. The use of dexmedetomidine as a primary agent in low-criticality patients offers the benefit of rapid achievement of targeted sedation levels. The use of dexmedetomidine to facilitate extubation in children intolerant of an awake, intubated state may abbreviate ventilator weaning. For clinicians using this medication, initial loading doses in the range of 0.35 to 1 mcg/kg over 10 minutes and continuous infusion of 0.25 to 0.75 mcg/kg/h are used. The most common side effects of dexmedetomidine are hypotension and bradycardia, which generally resolve by decreasing the dose.

3. **Additional medications for premedication for nonemergency intubation (rapid sequence intubation)**

   a. **Muscle relaxants.** Given to facilitate intubation and minimize the increase in intracranial pressure that occurs during awake intubation. The adverse effects of muscle relaxants may include histamine release, tachycardia, hypertension/hypotension, and bronchospasm. Their effects can be reversed by atropine and neostigmine. **The use of a muscle relaxant for intubation should never be attempted without the presence of individuals well experienced with the bag-and-mask ventilation technique.** As an alternative to bag-and-mask ventilation, an appropriate-size laryngeal mask airway has been used successfully in late preterm and term newborns.

      i. **Vecuronium.** Vecuronium 0.1 mg/kg IV has a duration of action of 30 to 40 minutes.

      ii. **Rocuronium.** Rocuronium 0.6 to 1.2 mg/kg IV, a metabolite derivative of vecuronium, has a quicker onset to paralysis (1–2 minutes) and shorter duration of action (20–30 minutes).

      iii. **Succinylcholine.** Succinylcholine (1–2 mg/kg IV) is a neuromuscular depolarizing agent with the most rapid onset of action (20–30 seconds) and the shortest duration (4–6 minutes) of all muscle relaxants. If no IV access is available, it can be administered IM (2 mg/kg); this results in a longer onset of action (2–3 minutes) and duration of action (10–30 minutes) than when administered IV. **Succinylcholine is contraindicated in the presence of hyperkalemia or a family history of malignant hyperthermia.**

   b. **Vagolytic agents.** Prevent bradycardia during intubation and decrease bronchial and salivary secretions.

      i. **Atropine.** Dose is 0.02 mg/kg IV or IM. Its onset of action is 1 to 2 minutes, and the duration of action is 0.5 to 2 hours. Tachycardia occurs frequently.

      ii. **Glycopyrrolate.** Dose is 4 to 10 mcg/kg IV. Tachycardia occurs less frequently than with atropine.

4. **Pharmacologic management provided by local analgesia**

   a. **Subcutaneous infiltration with lidocaine, 0.5% to 1% concentration.** Always use solution without epinephrine. Maximum dose (subcutaneous infiltration): 5 mg/kg or 1 mL/kg of 0.5% concentration or 0.5 mL/kg of 1% concentration.

   b. **Buffered lidocaine.** One part sodium bicarbonate with 10 parts 1% lidocaine; typically prepared in the hospital pharmacy. The pain associated with anesthetic infiltration is reduced by buffering the pH from 7.0 to 7.4.

   c. **Topical local anesthetics**

      i. **Lidocaine 2.5% and prilocaine 2.5% (EMLA cream).** This is a eutectic anesthetic mixture (ie, liquid at room temperature). A single dose of 0.5 to 1.25 g of EMLA cream applied under an occlusive dressing provides adequate local anesthesia 60 to 80 minutes later. In the term infant, it is an alternative to penile dorsal block for anesthesia during circumcision. The risk of methemoglobinemia (from prilocaine) may restrict its use to the full-term infant, and repeated doses should be avoided.

      ii. **Tetracaine 4% gel (Ametop).** Apply 1.5 g 30 to 60 minutes before the procedure. It has no risk of methemoglobinemia, but its repeated use may lead to contact dermatitis.

      iii. **4% Liposomal lidocaine cream (L.M.X.4 or Ela-Max).** Increasingly used in pediatrics for its rapid onset of action (20–30 minutes) and can be applied with (preferred) or without an occlusive dressing.

5. **Oral sucrose.** A disaccharide composed of fructose and glucose shown to promote calming behaviors and reduce distress associated with acute painful events. Gustatory inputs from the taste buds lead to cholecystokinin release in the brainstem, which activates descending inhibitory opioid. It is effective for the management of procedural pain in the neonate. Analgesic effects are present with doses as low as 0.1 mL of 24% sucrose. The usual dose is 0.5 to 1.5 mL of a 24% sucrose solution given by syringe or pacifier 2 minutes before procedures such as heel stick or venipuncture. The potential risk for fluid overload, hyperglycemia, and necrotizing enterocolitis should limit this method to infants >34 weeks' gestation. Other sweet-tasting liquids such as glucose, mother's milk, and saccharin are reported to be equally effective.

6. **Nonpharmacologic management.** Physical measures such as the use of swaddling, containment, or facilitated tucking as well as skin-to-skin contact with the mother ("kangaroo care") are likely to be efficacious in decreasing the noxious effects of the routine procedures (eg, heel stick) needed for the management of the sick infant. Nonnutritive sucking may be helpful. (See page 215)

82 Seizure Activity: On Call

I. **Problem.** The nurse reports that an infant is having abnormal movements of the extremities consistent with seizure activity. **A seizure is an event** defined as "a transient occurrence of signs and/or symptoms due to abnormal excessive or synchronous neuronal activity in the brain." Further categories of a neonatal seizures include:

A. **Clinical-only seizure:** "A sudden paroxysm of abnormal clinical changes that occur without a definite EEG [electroencephalogram] seizure."

B. **Electroclinical seizure:** "Clinical signs that occur simultaneously with an electrographic seizure."

C. **Electrographic-only (subclinical) seizure:** "Presence of a definite EEG seizure that is not associated with any clinical signs of a seizure."

D. **Epilepsy:** Involves recurrent unprovoked seizures and is defined as "a disease of the brain defined by any one of the following conditions: at least two unprovoked seizures or reflex seizure occurring more than 24 hours apart, one unprovoked or reflex seizure and a probability of having another seizure similar to the general recurrence risk after two unprovoked seizures occurring over the next 10 years, or diagnosis of an epilepsy syndrome."

E. **Status epilepticus:** Seizures appear in close succession or do not stop. Status epilepticus is a serious condition that requires prompt medical attention. There is no real definition of status epilepticus in neonates. Three definitions that have been used in the literature are as follows: (1) continuous seizures for a minimum of 30 minutes or seizures that recur over at least 30 minutes that do not return to a baseline neurologic activity; (2) at least 30 minutes of seizure activity over a 1-hour defined period; and (3) EEG seizure activity of >50% of the recording time of approximately 30 minutes.

The incidence of seizures in the neonatal age group is higher than at any other time in life, about 2 to 3 per 100 live births (up to 13 per 100 live births in preterm infants and up to 58 per 100 live births in very low birthweight infants). Studies have reported there is a higher incidence in preterm infants (vs term), low birthweight infants (vs normal weight), male infants (vs females), and African American infants (vs white or other races or ethnicities).

The etiology and semiology of seizures are quite different in neonates compared to older age groups. Most seizures in neonates are symptomatic of an acute illness and caused by an underlying condition. Most neonatal seizures occur during the first 24 hours of life. Developmental immaturity of the neonatal brain (immature inhibitory systems and the predominance of excitatory neurotransmitters) leads to unique seizure tendency and seizure patterns, altered drug pharmacodynamics, and increased susceptibility to developmental effects of anticonvulsants. This makes it imperative that we are able to recognize seizures and differentiate seizures from the movements that mimic seizures. It is now known that neonates with seizures are not only at a higher risk of death, but also at an increased risk of developmental delay, cerebral palsy, and epilepsy. Additional information on seizures can be found in Chapter 120.

II. **Immediate questions**

A. **Is the infant really seizing? Is this a nonepileptic motor phenomenon seen in neonates? Is this a seizure mimic?** It has been recognized that seizures are only correctly identified by clinical observation in 50% of cases. Infants can have many unusual movements that may look like seizures but are not. It is important to distinguish between the 2 conditions because nonepileptic events do not require treatment with anticonvulsants. Seizure mimics might occur in healthy or sick neonates. Some seizure mimics are benign events, whereas others indicate an underlying brain dysfunction. It is sometimes difficult to distinguish these, and an EEG is often necessary to distinguish between seizures and seizure mimics. Seizures have associated autonomic changes, have abnormal ocular movements, and are sometimes associated with ictal EEG discharges that seizure mimics do not have. The ability to stop the movements by restraining the body part or changing the position of the infant and movements that are elicited by tactile stimulation are characteristic of nonseizure movements. The following are nonepileptic events that occur in neonates that may be confused with seizures.

1. **Jitteriness/tremors.** The most common abnormal movement in a neonate is a tremor; up to 44% of infants will be jittery. A **tremor** is "an involuntary rhythmical oscillatory movement of equal amplitude." **Jitteriness** is recurrent tremors. Etiology includes elevated levels of circulating catecholamines and immaturity of spinal inhibitory interneurons and can be benign or pathologic. In a jittery infant, eye movements are normal (no ocular deviation), limb movements are bilateral with both phases of movement having equal speed, movements can be stimulus sensitive and can be suppressed by holding the limb, and there are no associated autonomic changes. In an infant who is seizing, eye movements are usually abnormal (eg, staring, blinking, nystagmoid jerks, or tonic horizontal eye deviation); movements are not stimulus sensitive, are asymmetric with a faster contraction and slower relaxation phase, and cannot be suppressed by holding the limbs; and autonomic changes occur. **Transient neonatal jitteriness** can occur with maternal use of opiates, marijuana, inhaled volatile substances, and selective serotonin reuptake inhibitors (sertraline [Zoloft]). **Familial tremor of the chin** is an autosomal dominant condition that can be seen in an infant who is crying. **Neonatal hyperexcitability syndrome** is a coarse tremor that is seen in mildly asphyxiated neonates with increased tendon reflexes and excessive Moro response. **Persistent or worsening tremors** need to be evaluated, and the following need to be ruled out: seizures, hypoglycemia, hypocalcemia, hypomagnesemia, hypothermia, hyperthyroidism, intracranial hemorrhage (ICH), drug withdrawal, sepsis, and vitamin D deficiency.

2. **Nonepileptic myoclonus** is an irregular shock-like movement of a limb that is caused by the muscle contracting. It can be benign or pathologic. Note that during sleep an infant can have fragmentary myoclonic jerks or an isolated myoclonic jerk as the infant wakes up, which is considered normal.

a. **Benign neonatal myoclonus or benign neonatal sleep myoclonus.** This presents with rhythmic movements (myoclonic jerks of the extremities, whole body [usually not the face], or trunk) only during sleep. They occur from birth to 6 months, can last up to 1 hour (mistaken for status epilepticus), can be provoked, and stop when the infant is awakened.

   b. **Pathologic nonepileptic myoclonus.** Infants present with focal/multifocal or generalized myoclonic jerks secondary to a pathologic cause (hypoxic ischemic encephalopathy [HIE], infection, medications, cerebral vascular events, severe intraventricular hemorrhage [IVH], drug withdrawal, toxic metabolic disturbances [glycine encephalopathy, drugs], and others).

3. **Apnea.** Apnea as a seizure manifestation is not very common in infants. If it occurs, it happens more often in term infants than in premature infants. **Apneic episodes in an infant are associated with bradycardia, whereas apnea with a seizure is usually associated with tachycardia** and other manifestations such as eye opening, hypertension, stiffening, clonus, or mouth movements.

4. **Hyperekplexia (congenital stiff-person syndrome, familial startle disease).** Hyperekplexia is a rare, nonepileptic disorder. It may be caused by glycine receptor gene mutations, and in some infants, it is inherited as an autosomal dominant disorder. It has a minor and a major form. Often confused with a seizure, it can present only as the exaggerated startle (minor form), or it can present with a triad of symptoms: an exaggerated startle (tonic flexion of limbs and trunk, clenching of fists, and anxious stare) to external stimuli, nocturnal myoclonus, and a generalized stiffness with an increased risk of sudden infant death syndrome. Hallmark of this disease: Tap the nasal bridge, and the infant will elicit an exaggerated startle.

5. **Neonatal opsoclonus ("dancing eyes").** This is characterized by rapid, random, to-and-fro oscillations of the eyes. It can be continuous and occur during sleep. Note that nystagmus is rhythmic horizontal oscillations of both eyes, whereas opsoclonus is irregular and chaotic. It can be seen as a transient phenomenon in a healthy infant, in neonates with major neurologic or visual disabilities, or as an early sign of herpes simplex encephalitis or in HIE.

6. **Rapid eye movement–associated movements.** During rapid eye movement sleep, infants can have rapid vertical and horizontal eye movements, grimacing, sucking episodes, twitching of a limb, or movements of the entire body that look similar to a seizure.

7. **Excessive hiccups.** Hiccups are normal in neonates except in the case of glycine encephalopathy, where excessive hiccups can occur with apnea and seizures.

8. **Motor automatisms.** These are movements that include pedaling, swimming, and bicycling. They are not associated with EEG abnormalities and may be secondary to brainstem release.

9. **Oral-buccal-lingual movements.** These movements consist of tongue thrusting or lip smacking and can be normal or associated with seizure activity. If normal, usually no other manifestation of seizures occurs. Sucking and puckering movements are considered normal if no other signs are seen. **Tongue fasciculations in the neonate** are seen with lower motor neuron disease. Assess movements when the tongue is at rest.

10. **Sandifer syndrome.** Infants with gastroesophageal reflux can have spells of opisthotonic posturing and stiffening with staring, apnea, and jerking of extremities after feeding. This can be secondary to pain from acidic material refluxing into the esophagus or an effort to decrease reflux by increasing lower esophageal sphincter tone.

11. **Paroxysmal extreme pain disorder.** Presents at birth, this is an autosomal dominant condition that is caused by a sodium channelopathy involving SCN9A that can occur in the neonatal period. It features nonepileptic tonic attacks of excruciating pain that affect different parts of the body (eg, rectum, genitalia, face, limbs); skin flushing, infants who are red and stiff, harlequin color changes, and abnormalities in the pupil can be triggered by defecation. Often misdiagnosed as hyperekplexia/epilepsy.

12. **Neonatal dystonia/dyskinesia.** These abnormal movements (arching, fisting) can be associated with HIE, metabolic diseases, or maternal drug toxicity.

13. **Paroxysmal tonic downgaze or upgaze** can be seen rarely in neonates and is more common in infants. It is a sustained upward or downward deviation of the eyes that lasts for several hours or all day.

14. **Congenital nystagmus.** Congenital nystagmus presents at birth or few days after and is a rhythmic, horizontal oscillations of the eyes. A full ophthalmologic evaluation is needed because visual sensory abnormalities may occur with rare tumors or visual pathway defects.

15. **Bronchopulmonary dysplasia–associated extrapyramidal movement disorder.** Preterm infants with severe bronchopulmonary dysplasia can exhibit oral-buccal-lingual movements (darting tongue), restlessness, and chorea-like movements of the limbs, neck, trunk, and face. The presumed cause is chronic hypoxemia, most likely caused by injury to the basal ganglia.

B. **Are there vital sign changes?** The majority of vital sign changes are not manifestations of seizures, and those that are include oxygen desaturation and apnea, especially when accompanied by other signs of a seizure.

C. **How old is the infant?** The age of the infant is often the best clue to the cause of the seizures. Common causes of seizures for specific ages are as follows:

1. **At birth.** Maternal anesthetic agents injected into the neonate accidentally during delivery can cause severe tonic seizures typically in the first few hours of life. The neonate presents with apnea, flaccidity, asphyxia, and seizures.

2. **Within 30 minutes to 3 days after birth.** Pyridoxine deficiency (B6-dependent seizures). These infants can also have seizures in utero.

3. **Day 1 (first 24 hours).** Metabolic abnormalities such as hypoglycemia, hypocalcemia, or HIE (presenting at 6–18 hours after birth and becoming more severe in the next 24–48 hours); birth trauma (presents at ≥12 hours: primary subarachnoid hemorrhage, laceration of falx or tentorium with subdural hematoma); central nervous system (CNS) intrauterine infections and sepsis; drug withdrawal; inadvertent local anesthetic toxicity; and pyridoxine dependency.

4. **At 24 to 72 hours.** Cerebral dysgenesis, neonatal stroke (cerebral infarct, intracerebral hemorrhage, cortical vein/sinus thrombosis), IVH, subarachnoid hemorrhage with cerebral contusion from birth trauma, metabolic disorders (hypocalcemia, hypoglycemia, hyponatremia, hypernatremia), glycine encephalopathy, urea cycle disorders, aminoacidurias, organic aciduria, drug withdrawal, pyridoxine dependency, meningitis.

5. **At 72 hours to 1 week.** Familial neonatal seizures, cerebral malformations, cerebral infarction, hypoparathyroidism, vascular events, kernicterus, glycine encephalopathy, urea cycle disorders, aminoacidurias and organic aciduria, hypocalcemia, and TORCHZ (toxoplasmosis, other, rubella, cytomegalovirus, herpes simplex virus, and Zika virus) infections.

6. **At >1 week.** Late-onset hypocalcemia, peroxisomal disorders, cerebral dysgenesis, fructose dysmetabolism, Gaucher disease type 2, GM1 gangliosidosis, herpes simplex virus type 2 encephalitis, ketotic hyperglycinemia, maple syrup urine disease, tuberous sclerosis, urea cycle disorders, methadone withdrawal, and De Vivo syndrome (earliest seizures at 2 weeks of age, but typically in this range).

7. **Variable onset.** Stroke, sinus thrombosis, other developmental defects, epilepsy syndromes, ICH, intracranial infection, and hypocalcemia.

D. **Is the infant full term or preterm?** HIE is the most common cause of seizures in **full-term and premature infants.** In **term babies,** the second most common cause is a perinatal ischemic stroke. With ICH, term infants are more likely to have a subarachnoid hemorrhage or a subdural hemorrhage; **preterm babies** are more likely to have a germinal matrix hemorrhage–IVH. The prevalence of **hypoglycemia,**

hypocalcemia, and CNS infections is the same as for term and preterm infants. The following can cause seizures at any gestational age: meningitis, metabolic disorder, focal cerebral infarction, and congenital anomalies. Preterm infants with seizures are at higher risk for long-term adverse outcomes than term infants with neonatal seizures.

E. **What is the blood glucose level ? Is the infant at risk for hypoglycemia?** Hypoglycemia is the **most common metabolic problem in neonates** and is an easily treatable cause of seizures in the neonatal period. The incidence is 1 to 5 per 1000 live births but is higher in at-risk populations (late preterm infants, term small for gestational age [SGA] infants, infants of diabetic mothers [IDM]/large for gestational age [LGA] infants). A blood glucose should be obtained immediately to rule out low blood sugar.

F. **Is there a history of a sentinel hypoxic event occurring immediately before or during labor and delivery? Does the neonate have 1 of the 4 signs consistent with an acute peripartum or intrapartum event?** Because HIE is the most common cause of neonatal seizures in term and preterm infants, it is important to obtain a thorough prenatal and delivery history. Sentinel events include ruptured uterus, umbilical cord prolapse, maternal cardiovascular collapse, amniotic fluid embolus with maternal hypotension and hypoxemia that is severe and prolonged, and fetal exsanguination (fetomaternal hemorrhage/vasa previa). The American Academy of Pediatrics (AAP) list of neonatal signs consistent with an acute peripartum or intrapartum event include the following: fetal umbilical artery acidemia with pH <7 or base deficit >12 or both, Apgar score <5 at 5 and 10 minutes, presence of multiple-organ failure consistent with HIE, and evidence of acute brain injury on brain magnetic resonance imaging (MRI) or spectroscopy consistent with hypoxia-ischemia. Other factors include fetal heart rate monitor and MRI patterns that are consistent with an event.

G. **Is there a family history of seizures?** If so, a genetic or inherited syndrome may be present. There are many syndromes and causes of epilepsy that are genetic, with more genes discovered nearly every week. Examples include all the early infantile epileptic encephalopathies (Ohtahara syndrome), self-limited familial neonatal epilepsy, Zellweger syndrome, Smith-Lemli-Opitz syndrome, and others.

H. **Are there any risk factors for neonatal seizures?** Risk factors described vary by study and region.
   1. **Maternal risk factors:** Primiparity, grand multiparity, obesity, intrauterine growth restriction (IUGR), heavy cigarette smoking, maternal diabetes, preeclampsia, gestational diabetes, thyroid dysfunction, abnormal amniotic fluid volume, asthma, advanced maternal age, maternal age of 18 to 24 years, and suspicious or ominous fetal heart rate (FHR) tracing before labor.
   2. **Intrapartum risk factors:** Prolonged second stage of labor, fetal distress, cesarean or operative vaginal delivery, maternal fever, TORCHZ infections, history of rubella, ruptured uterus, umbilical cord prolapse, maternal cardiovascular collapse, amniotic fluid embolus with maternal hypotension and hypoxemia that is severe and prolonged, fetal exsanguination (fetomaternal hemorrhage/vasa previa), and suspicious or ominous FHR tracing before labor.
   3. **Infant risk factors:** Prematurity, postmaturity, low birthweight, high birthweight, male sex, birth in a private or university hospital, birth by cesarean section, SGA, infants of African American mothers, CNS and major systemic anomalies, cardiorespiratory failure, and congenital heart disease (CHD).

III. **Differential diagnosis** (see also Chapter 120 and Table 120-1). The majority of newborns (75%–90%) with seizures have an **underlying pathologic cause**, and few cases are idiopathic or part of an epileptic syndrome. Note that although the causes of neonatal seizures are extensive, **3 etiologies** account for almost 75% of all neonatal seizures: **HIE (40%–50%), perinatal arterial ischemic stroke (10%–15%), and ICH (10%–20%).** Other causes are noted later in this chapter. **Neonatal epilepsy genetics** is a rapidly expanding field involving many genetic disorders associated with neonatal-onset epilepsy. Seizure activity may be secondary to the following:

A. **Central nervous system abnormalities**
1. **Hypoxic etiologies.** **Hypoxic ischemic encephalopathy (HIE)** is the **most common cause** of neonatal seizures in both **full-term and preterm infants** and causes up to 50% of seizures in the first 48 hours of life (more common first 24 hours of life). The majority of cases occur because of an acute peripartum or intrapartum event. MRI studies suggest the period around birth accounts for >75% of the causative period. It can be secondary to prenatal, perinatal, and postnatal causes. Other hypoxic events can occur in the neonatal period that may cause seizures.
2. **Infarction/stroke.** **A perinatal arterial stroke is the second** most common cause of seizures in full-term infants, and up to 97% of infants diagnosed with a neonatal stroke present with seizures. These infants usually present with focal seizures in the first 18 to 36 hours of life and can be active and alert between seizures, unlike infants with HIE. **Cerebral sinus venous thrombosis** is less common than an arterial stroke and has an incidence of 1 in 8 to 38,000 children per year. It presents with seizures and diffuse and focal neurologic deficits. There are genetic risk factors and disorders predisposing to an ischemic stroke.
3. **Central nervous system hemorrhage.** ICH, including subarachnoid and subdural hemorrhage (more common in term infants), germinal matrix hemorrhage, periventricular-intraventricular hemorrhage, parenchymal hemorrhage (mainly in preterm), and intracerebral hemorrhage (traumatic or spontaneous), can cause seizures in the neonate. **Subarachnoid hemorrhage** in term infants can cause seizures on the second postnatal day, and infants may appear well during the interictal period. **Subdural hemorrhage** is usually associated with trauma (cerebral contusion) and can be asymptomatic in a less severe hemorrhage; in the most common type, the infant will present with focal seizures in the first 48 hours of life. **Germinal matrix hemorrhage–IVH** occurs in premature infants from hemorrhage in the small blood vessels in the subependymal germinal matrix and can be associated with parenchymal injury; infants present with seizures in the first 3 days of life. There are genetic risk factors and disorders that predispose an infant to fetal or neonatal IVH or intraparenchymal hemorrhage; one example is related to *COL4A1*, which encodes type IV collagen.
4. **Brain malformations.** Brain malformations cause seizures in 5% to 10% of neonates. The majority of these do not present with seizures in the neonatal period. For example, only 5% of infants with tuberous sclerosis present with seizures. Often the infant has obvious anomalies of the face or head if developmental abnormalities are present. Common malformations include lissencephaly, focal cortical dysplasia, subcortical band heterotopia, periventricular nodular heterotopia, schizencephaly, hemimegaloencephaly, polymicrogyria, and hydranencephaly, and many have a genetic basis. **Neurocutaneous syndromes** (tuberous sclerosis complex, association with hemimegaloencephaly, and incontinentia pigmenti) are also included and all have a genetic cause.
5. **Hypertensive encephalopathy** (very rare) can be secondary to neonatal thyrotoxicosis or renovascular disease.

B. **Transient metabolic disturbances**
1. **Hypoglycemia** is responsible for 3% to 7.5% of neonatal seizures, with the onset of seizures typically occurring on the second day. Hypoglycemia occurs more commonly in high risk infants who are term or late preterm SGA, LGA, and IDM infants. Seizures from hypoglycemia occur more commonly in SGA infants than in IDMs. A blood glucose should be obtained immediately to rule it out.
2. **Hypocalcemia** is responsible for approximately 2.3% to 9% of neonatal seizures. Most infants with hypocalcemia are asymptomatic. **Early hypocalcemia** (first 2–3 days of life) usually occurs in infants with prematurity, birth asphyxia, IUGR,

and low birth weight and in IDM infants. Early hypocalcemia is often associated with seizures and not the primary cause of seizures. **Late hypocalcemia** (5–14 days of life) usually occurs in full-term infants, and if moderate to severe, it is more common in male and Hispanic infants. It can occur from nutritional causes (unusual in the United States), genetic causes, maternal hyperparathyroidism or neonatal hypoparathyroidism, or vitamin D deficiency or with CHD (DiGeorge syndrome may or may not be present). Approximately 50% of infants with hypocalcemic seizures have hypomagnesemia.

3. **Hypomagnesemia** is a rare cause of seizures and often occurs along with hypocalcemia. It is frequently seen in premature infants or infants with respiratory distress syndrome, diarrhea, or neonatal hepatitis. Consider this if a neonate with hypocalcemia continues to seize after adequate calcium therapy. **Primary hypomagnesemia** (presents alone) is very rare and is caused by a defect of magnesium absorption or handling (**inherited hypomagnesemia** examples: congenital magnesium malabsorption, neonatal severe primary hyperparathyroidism, hypomagnesemia with secondary hypocalcemia) and presents with seizures at 2 to 6 weeks of age.

4. **Hyponatremia** is an uncommon cause of neonatal seizures. Causes include oxytocin administration, excessive fluid intake, syndrome of inappropriate antidiuretic hormone (ICH, HIE, bacterial meningitis), congenital adrenal hypoplasia, congenital hypothyroidism, and maternal water intoxication.

5. **Hypernatremia is also an uncommon cause** of neonatal seizures and can be caused by breast milk hypernatremia (more common in term infants), inadequate fluid replacement, excessive sodium bicarbonate administration, and rarely diabetes insipidus. Rapid correction of hypernatremia with fluid resuscitation can cause cerebral edema and seizures.

C. **Infectious etiology.** The incidence of infection causing seizures in newborns is equal in preterm and term infants and is the etiology in 5% to 20% of newborns with seizures. It is important to note that **early seizures** usually occur with nonbacterial infections (cytomegalovirus or toxoplasmosis) and that **late-onset seizures** occur with bacterial meningitis or herpes simplex encephalitis.

1. **Meningitis, encephalitis, or brain abscess.** Bacterial meningitis (most common pathogens are *Escherichia coli* and group B *Streptococcus*) usually presents with seizures at the end of the first week or later. Herpes simplex is the most common cause of nonbacterial encephalitis. **Brain abscesses** occur as a complication of bacterial meningitis and are very rare, and most cases are secondary to gramnegative organisms (*Pseudomonas, Serratia,* and *Proteus* species). **Encephalitis** is most commonly caused by viral infections but can be caused by bacteria.

2. **Sepsis.** Often due to gram-negative bacilli and group B *Streptococcus*. Sepsis without meningitis can present with seizures.

3. **Congenital infections.** Toxoplasmosis, cytomegalovirus, herpes simplex, rubella, and coxsackie B virus can all present with seizures in the neonate. Intrauterine toxoplasmosis or cytomegalovirus can present with seizures in the first 3 days of life. Seizures with herpes present after 7 days of life and are usually focal. Zika virus can cause seizures and trigger epilepsy in infants.

D. **Inborn errors of metabolism presenting as neonatal seizures (genetic metabolic causes)** (see also Chapter 100). Seizures are a common presenting symptom in metabolic disorders and present as medically intractable seizures. Seizure type or EEG findings are rarely specific for a particular metabolic disorder. Seizures caused by inborn errors of metabolism (IEM) usually start in the antepartum period and do not respond to anticonvulsants. Clinically, these infants get progressively worse and have worsening EEG abnormalities. EEG may show burst suppression or unexplained slowing of the background activity. MRI shows brain atrophy. Infants have clinical findings of HIE with no history of HIE. Other signs that an infant may have an IEM include family history, progressive myoclonic epilepsy, seizures related to eating, seizures get worse with some antiepileptic medications, and unexplained status epilepticus. IEMs presenting with seizures almost always have other extraneurologic signs and symptoms. They can also be seen in infants after feeding who are >72 hours of age. The IEMs presenting with seizures include aminoacidopathies, urea cycle disorders, and organic acidurias. The most common of these, which present with hyperammonemia or acidosis or both, include nonketotic hyperglycinemia, sulfite oxidase deficiency, multiple carboxylase deficiency, glutaric aciduria type II, and urea cycle defect. Other less common causes of neonatal seizures include mitochondrial (pyruvate dehydrogenase deficiency and cytochrome c oxidase deficiency) or peroxisomal disturbances (Zellweger syndrome or neonatal adrenoleukodystrophy). Other IEMs presenting with intractable seizures in the neonatal period include glycine encephalopathy, D-2-hydroxyglutaric aciduria, pyruvate carboxylase deficiency, γ-aminobutyric acid transaminase deficiency, dihydropyridine dehydrogenase deficiency, congenital disorders of glycosylation, mitochondrial glutamate transporter defect, Menkes disease, peroxisomal biogenesis defects, and mitochondrial encephalopathy. **Vitamin-responsive IEMs** include pyridoxine dependency, pyridoxal phosphate–dependent seizures, folinic acid–responsive seizures, and multiple carboxylase deficiency (biotin dependent). **Pyridoxine dependency**, a rare disease, is a pyridoxine metabolism disturbance whereby the infant can present with intrauterine seizures or seizures within the first few hours of life. The seizures are multifocal and clonic and do not respond to any medication. If they are not treated, the infant will progress to a progressive encephalopathy and death. Antiquitin deficiency is the main cause of pyridoxine-dependent epilepsy. **Pyridoxamine phosphate oxidase deficiency** is a disorder that involves a molecular defect involving pyridoxamine phosphate oxidase. The infant presents with fetal seizures and encephalopathy. In **folinic acid–responsive seizures,** infants presents with seizures in the first few hours of life and an EEG with multifocal sharp waves. **It is important to note treatable causes of IEMs because it is vital to recognize these early on so they can be treated** (pyridoxine-responsive seizures, pyridoxine 5′-phosphate oxidase deficiency, folinic acid–responsive seizures, multiple carboxylase deficiency, GLUT-1 deficiency [De Vivo syndrome], 3-phosphoglycerate dehydrogenase deficiency, primary hyperinsulinemic hypoglycemia, congenital magnesium malabsorption, cerebral creatine disorders, and congenital disorders of glycosylation).

E. **Congenital hypothyroidism** can present with neonatal seizures.

F. **Genetic epilepsy syndromes**

  1. **Inherited metabolic syndromes.** Those that can present with seizures include Zellweger syndrome spectrum, Smith-Lemli-Opitz syndrome, DEND syndrome, and microcephaly capillary malformation syndrome. **DEND syndrome** encompasses developmental delay, epilepsy, and neonatal diabetes. Hyperinsulinism/hyperammonemia syndrome is associated with hypoglycemia and neonatal seizures (20% present within the first 72 hours of life).

  2. **Syndromic genetic etiologies** that are associated with neonatal seizures include early-onset Aicardi-Goutieres syndrome (pseudo-TORCHZ syndrome), Charge syndrome, DiGeorge syndrome, Wolf-Hirschhorn syndrome, and trisomies 13, 18, and 21.

G. **Neonatal epileptic syndromes.** The following are early epileptic syndromes that can present in the newborn period (**rare cause of neonatal seizures**). These infants can have a normal examination and appear well with recurrent seizures. It is important to identify these infants because the treatment and long-term management are different.

  1. **Self-limited (benign) familial neonatal epilepsy.** Autosomal dominant inheritance and family history are required. Seizures start between days 4 and 7 of life, can occur over hours to days, and include initially unilateral clonic events involving the face and limbs and then tonic events with autonomic features, apnea, and cyanosis in up to 33% of infants. The most common genetic etiology is mutation in *KCNQ2*; mutations in *KCNQ3* have also been noted.

2. **Early myoclonic encephalopathy is a rare epileptic encephalopathy.** It can present within hours of birth or up to 10 days of life with frequent (almost continuous) seizures and early encephalopathy. Seizures begin as myoclonus, either localized or involving the face and limb. Focal seizures can then occur, followed by tonic seizures. EEG is characteristic (bursts of paroxysmal activity with lack of activity). There is usually no family history because this condition is usually sporadic, but genetic etiology (*ErbB4*) or underlying metabolic defect (eg, glycine encephalopathy) or cerebral malformation may exist. Infants have reduced life expectancy.

3. **Early infantile epileptic encephalopathies.** There are 3 of these, but only 1, Ohtahara syndrome, presents in the neonatal period. Ohtahara syndrome is a severe epileptic syndrome with frequent intractable seizures and severe early encephalopathy. All infants have frequent early-onset tonic seizures, and some have focal clonic or hemiclonic seizures. Etiologies include the following: structural brain malformation (most common), sporadic, metabolic (nonketotic hyperglycinemia, carnitine palmitoyl transferase deficiency, mitochondrial disorders, pyridoxine/pyridoxal 5′-phosphate disorders, and others), and genetic causes (most common associated genes are *STXBP1* and *KCNQ2*).

H. **Unknown and other causes.** In approximately 10% of seizures, the cause is either unknown or secondary to other causes.

1. **Unknown.** No identifiable etiology.

2. **Other causes**

a. **Infant of mother with substance use disorder** (see Chapter 102). Seizures are an uncommon manifestation of withdrawal, especially opiate withdrawal. Infants usually present with seizures in the first several days. Infants can also have an abnormal EEG without seizures (30% in opiate withdrawal). Seizures can also occur in nonnarcotic withdrawal (alcohol, antidepressants, tricyclic antidepressants, diazepam, propoxyphene, selective serotonin reuptake inhibitors, barbiturates, sedative-hypnotics, cocaine). Neonatal jitteriness can occur from maternal use of sertraline (Zoloft). Infants exposed to heroin present with signs of neonatal abstinence syndrome within 24 hours of birth; with methadone or buprenorphine exposure, they present with neonatal abstinence syndrome 2 to 6 days after delivery.

b. **Local anesthetic intoxication (rare cause).** If a local anesthetic (eg, mepivacaine) is accidentally injected into the infant's scalp during a pudendal or paracervical block (most common) or epidural block or during local anesthesia for an episiotomy, seizures can occur within the first 6 hours of birth. Transplacental transmission has also been reported. This occurrence is often mistaken for HIE, since both present with early occurrence of seizures. Seizures are most commonly tonic. Three diagnostic features of local anesthetic intoxication include the following: the infant has pupils fixed to light that are commonly dilated, the infant will exhibit the **"doll's eye" reflex** (oculocephalic reflex; when head is turned to the right side, the eyes turn to the left; when the head is turned to the left, the eyes move to the right), and the infant will improve over the first 24 to 48 hours with proper support. Look for needle marks on the scalp and confirm by sending the level of suspected agent in the blood, urine, or cerebrospinal fluid (CSF).

c. **Drug toxicity.** Toxic doses of theophylline or caffeine can cause jitteriness and seizures. Early high-dose caffeine therapy has been associated with an increase in seizures and total seizure burden in extremely premature infants.

d. **Polycythemia with hyperviscosity** rarely causes seizures.

e. **Acute bilirubin encephalopathy.** These infants can have mental status changes, hypertonia, retrocollis and opisthotonos, and rarely seizures.

f. **Extracorporeal life support-related seizures** occurred in 5% to 30% of neonates and children who underwent ECLS. One risk factor was low cardiac output syndrome.

g. **Congenital heart disease may result in seizures and epilepsy.** Congenital heart disease (CHD) with cyanotic right-to-left shunts (transposition of the great arteries and tetralogy of Fallot) accounts for the majority, but CHD with left-to-right shunts also causes seizures. Seizures also occur after hypothermic cardiopulmonary bypass surgery and repair of cyanotic CHD. CHD is also part of syndromes that predispose infants to seizures.

IV. **Database**

A. **History.** A detailed history (prenatal, natal, and postnatal history) may help diagnose seizure activity. Does the mother have gestational diabetes, maternal hyperparathyroidism, prolonged rupture of membranes, peripartum fever, or any sexually transmitted diseases/sexually transmitted infections? Does the mother use any medications or drugs? Is there maternal narcotic abuse? Does the mother have a bleeding disorder or any history of epilepsy in the family? Did the mother experience excessive fetal movements (intrauterine seizures)? A history of consanguinity and previous neonatal deaths in the family might suggest IEMs. The provider observing the activity should record a complete description of the event on the chart. Did the mother note hiccups in utero (nonketotic hyperglycemia)? Is there any history of birth trauma, difficult delivery, or perinatal asphyxia?

B. **Physical examination.** Pay close attention to the neurologic status. Look at the scalp for evidence of injection during delivery. Is there macro-/microcephaly? Does the cutaneous examination reveal a vesicular rash (herpes, incontinentia pigmenti)? Look for dysmorphic features seen in Zellweger syndrome or Smith-Lemli-Opitz syndrome. Is there hepatosplenomegaly, hypotonia, or dysmorphic features (suggests peroxisomal or lysosomal disorders)? Are there inverted nipples and abnormal fat pads (consider congenital disorders of glycosylation)? An ophthalmology examination is recommended because there are various abnormalities on the exam (retinitis pigmentosa, cataracts) that can be seen in metabolic diseases.

C. **Clinical classification of seizures.** In the evaluation of an infant, it is useful to use a defined classification system to clearly identify the clinical characteristics of the seizure. The clinical classification of neonatal seizures has historically been based on Volpe or Mizrahi and Kellaway. A new classification is being developed by the ILAE but has not been published yet. Note that >50% of neonatal seizures are seen only on EEG and are not clinically apparent.

1. **Volpe classification is based on clinical observations**

a. **Subtle:** Most common type of seizure in preterm and term infants. Involves any alterations in neonatal behavior, motor functions, and autonomic function that are usually difficult to recognize and are overlooked. Examples include **ocular movements** (blinking, staring, eye deviation), **oral movements** (chewing, sucking, smiling, mouthing), **body movements** (pedaling, swimming, limb posturing), and **autonomic phenomena** (central apnea [more common presentation of a subtle seizure in term infant], changes in blood pressure or heart rate, pallor, increased secretions). Many of these alterations may not represent seizure activity but brainstem release (automatic reflex behaviors released when the cerebral cortex is not functioning normally). If found in preterm infants, it is more common and more likely to be seizure activity than if found in term infants.

b. **Clonic:** Can be unifocal/multifocal; repetitive jerking typically seen in 1 extremity or only 1 side of body.

c. **Myoclonic:** Can be focal, multifocal, or generalized; rapid flexion/extension movements of extremities, twitching or jerking movements. Typically involves 1 extremity or several body parts.

d. **Tonic:** Focal (less common) or generalized (more common). Typically involves 1 extremity or whole body with extension of arms and legs or stiffening of body with decerebrate posturing. Eyes deviate upward, and infant may be apneic.

2. **Mizrahi and Kellaway classification is based more on pathophysiology**
   a. **Focal clonic:** Muscle contractions that are rhythmic.
   b. **Focal tonic:** Sustained limb/trunk posturing.
   c. **Myoclonic:** Single contractions that are random.
   d. **Spasms:** Flexor/extensor spasms; may occur in clusters.
   e. **Electrographic:** The majority of neonatal seizures are EEG-only seizures (no clinical correlate, subclinical, or nonconvulsive), would not be identified unless continuous EEG monitoring occurred, and are common in high-risk neonates. Only one-third of seizures are accompanied by clinical signs on a video EEG.
   f. **Generalized tonic:** Sustained symmetric posturing.
   g. **Motor automatism:** Oral-buccal-lingual, ocular, and limb movements.
3. **The International League Against Epilepsy is revising its classification, and it will be published shortly. This represents work available for public comment prior to publication.**
   a. **With clinical signs**
      i. **Motor**
         (a) **Automatisms:** Coordinated motor activity that occurs when cognition is impaired. In the neonate, these seizures are very common and are seen in HIE and preterm infants. It is usually oral and is associated with other features. Can be unilateral, bilateral asymmetric, or bilateral symmetric.
         (b) **Clonic:** Either symmetric or asymmetric jerking of the same muscle groups, usually repetitive. Most common seizure type recognized in the neonate. It is typically seen in vascular etiologies in term infants (neonatal stroke, cerebral hemorrhage) and in HIE. Can be focal, multifocal, or bilateral.
         (c) **Epileptic spasms:** Sudden extension, flexion, or mixed extension-flexion of mainly truncal and proximal muscles. May occur in clusters (eg, head nodding, subtle eye movements, grimacing). Can be unilateral, bilateral asymmetric, or bilateral symmetric. Seen most commonly in IEMs or Ohtahara syndrome.
         (d) **Myoclonic:** Brief (<100 millisecond), involuntary, multiple or single contractions of muscles/muscle groups of variable parts of the body. In the neonate, it is similar to nonepileptic myoclonus. Can be focal, multifocal, bilateral asymmetric, or bilateral symmetric. Typically seen in IEM, myoclonic encephalopathy, genetic epilepsy syndromes, preterm infants, and HIE.
         (e) **Sequential:** A type of seizure characterized by a sequence of signs, symptoms, and EEG changes at different times. In the neonate, it presents with a variety of clinical signs. Seen typically in genetic etiologies; often seen in channelopathies (benign familial neonatal epilepsy or *KCNQ2* encephalopathy)
         (f) **Tonic:** An increase in muscle contraction that is sustained and can last a few seconds to minutes. In the neonate, it is most commonly focal, unilateral, or bilateral asymmetric. Can be focal, bilateral asymmetric, or bilateral symmetric. Can be seen in HIE but is typically seen in genetic etiologies (early infantile epileptic encephalopathy, *KCNQ2* and *KCNQ3* mutations, other epileptic encephalopathies).
      ii. **Nonmotor**
         (a) **Autonomic:** Alteration of the autonomic nervous system including cardiovascular, gastrointestinal, vasomotor, thermoregulatory, and pupillary functions. Seen in IVH, temporal and occipital lobe lesions, and Ohtahara syndrome.

(b) **Behavior arrest:** Arrest of all activities. Rarely occurs in isolation and can include focal and motor seizures. Can include apnea and other autonomic manifestations.

iii. **Unclassified.** Unable to classify in a category.

b. **Without clinical signs (electrographic only).** Most common seizure type in preterm and term infants. Occurs in infectious causes and in HIE (thalamus/basal ganglia injury); also seen in neonates undergoing cardiac surgery.

D. **Laboratory studies.** It is important to rule out the most common etiologies that require immediate treatment. Blood glucose to rule out hypoglycemia and lumbar puncture once the seizures stabilize to rule out bacterial meningitis are important to do as early as possible since treatment is essential. Other laboratory tests should include arterial blood gas, serum electrolytes (sodium, potassium, calcium, magnesium, phosphorus), and complete blood count with differential. Check the newborn screening results for hypothyroidism and some IEMs.

1. **Metabolic workup**
   a. **Serum glucose.** If bedside testing is <40 mg/dL, obtain a central value.
   b. **Serum sodium.** To evaluate for hyponatremia or hypernatremia.
   c. **Serum ionized and total calcium levels.** Only an ionized calcium (most accurate) is necessary, but if this cannot be done stat, a total calcium should be ordered.
   d. **Serum magnesium.**

2. **Infection workup**
   a. **Complete blood count with differential.** A hematocrit also rules out polycythemia.
   b. **Inflammatory markers** such as C-reactive protein or procalcitonin.
   c. **Blood, urine, and cerebrospinal fluid cultures (for bacteria and viruses).** CSF polymerase chain reaction for herpes simplex virus if suspected.
   d. **Serum immunoglobulin M and immunoglobulin M–specific TORCHZ titers.** The serum immunoglobulin M titer may be elevated in TORCHZ infections.

3. **Urine drug screening.** If neonatal abstinence is suspected.

4. **Theophylline or caffeine level** if toxicity is suspected.

5. **Blood gas levels.** To rule out hypoxia or metabolic acidosis.

6. **Serum bilirubin** if indicated.

7. **Additional studies for inborn errors of metabolism.** Check newborn screening for any positive results. Include serum ammonia (increased in urea cycle and organic acid metabolism defects), lactic acid (elevated in organic acid metabolic disorders), pyruvate, CSF lactate, urine organic acids/serum amino acid assays, carnitine levels, and an acylcarnitine profile. Test serum and CSF for glycine (nonketotic hyperglycinemia) and serine (serine deficiency). Test plasma and urine α-aminoadipic semialdehyde and pipecolic acid levels (elevated in pyridoxine dependency). Test CSF for pyridoxal phosphate and biogenic amines, elevated CSF glycine (transient or true nonketotic hyperglycinemia), low CSF glucose with normal blood glucose (glucose transporter deficiency), elevated CSF lactate (mitochondrial disorder), and low CSF biogenic amine metabolites (neurotransmitter deficiency).

8. **Lumbar puncture.** To rule out bacterial or viral meningitis and encephalitis. If blood is in the CSF, it may suggest an IVH. Cultures and rapid testing of the fluid should be done to diagnose infection (see Chapters 38 and 140). Check CSF as noted earlier in Section IV.D.7. Additional analysis of CSF includes CSF neurotransmitters for folinic acid–responsive seizures, glycine for nonketotic hyperglycinemia, lactic acid for mitochondrial disorders, and neurotransmitters for 5-hydroxyindoleacetic acid and homovanillic acid. Elevated ammonia level may indicate a urea cycle or organic acid metabolism defect.

9. **Genetic testing.** Genetic testing is now recommended for neonates with epilepsy in order to diagnose the cause, which can guide management and targeted treatment plans as well as help in determining the prognosis and recurrence risk for families. Newborn epilepsy is often due to identifiable genetic causes. In 1 study of 29 infants with epilepsy not linked to another cause, 83% had a genetic cause. In another study, >75% had identifiable genetic etiologies. **Neonatal epilepsy genetics** is a rapidly expanding field. The genetic causes of seizures can be grouped into genetic vascular, genetic metabolic, genetic syndromic, genetic cellular, and malformations of cortical development. Genetic testing is now recommended as early as possible in neonates who have no identifiable cause for epilepsy based on initial and secondary testing. **Epilepsy gene panels (next-generation sequencing–based tests)** are recommended as the first-line genetic test for genetic epilepsies over chromosomal microarray tests because the diagnostic yield is better. One example is the epilepsy gene panel. The most common gene identified by a gene panel analysis is *SCN2A*. A genetic etiology may help in developing a treatment plan and in determining prognosis and recurrence risk for families. See genetic testing information at https://www.ncbi.nlm.nih.gov/gtr. **Pharmacogenomics of epilepsy** is of interest since it will focus on detecting genetic markers that identify infants who are refractory to medications, which will allow better medication selection. For example, **genetic testing for hyperekplexia** includes mutations in the *GLRA1* and *SLC6A5* genes, sequence analysis of the *ARHGEF9* gene, or mutations in the *GLRB* and *GPHN* genes. Do a single-gene test or multiple-gene panel that includes *ALDH7A1* for a mutation analysis (to rule out possible antiquitin deficiency in pyridoxine dependency).

E. **Imaging and other studies.** An ultrasound, computed tomography, or magnetic resonance imaging test may be performed as part of an evaluation to help determine the etiology of neonatal seizures. Each test has its strengths and weaknesses in diagnosing intracranial lesions. These tests should not be done to determine the presence or absence of clinical seizures.

1. **Ultrasound examination of the head.** First-line imaging test to rule out CNS malformations, confirm periventricular hemorrhage–IVH, intracerebral bleeds. Studies report an abnormal finding was found on head US in 10% to 43% of infants.

2. **Cranial magnetic resonance imaging.** A very sensitive test (seizure etiology detected in 88%–95% of cases) that is used to help determine the etiology of the seizures. It actually has greater sensitivity in identifying ischemic damage, ICH, and brain malformations than CT or ultrasound. Its disadvantage is that it is difficult to obtain in an unstable infant. MRI of an infant with an IEM will show prominent brain atrophy. **Magnetic resonance angiography and venography** is helpful in making the diagnosis of cerebral infarction. **Diffusion-weighted imaging** is helpful in early hypoxic injury. **Brain magnetic resonance spectroscopy** should be considered because it can help in the diagnosis of IEMs.

3. **Computed tomography scan of the head.** To diagnose subarachnoid or subdural hemorrhage. It may also reveal calcifications in a congenital malformation or cerebral infarction if suspected.

4. **Electroencephalography.** (See also Chapter 18.) The EEG gives important diagnostic and prognostic information and can also aid in the management of seizures in newborns. **The American Clinical Neurophysiology Society Guideline on continuous EEG monitoring in neonates recommends EEG testing** to clarify if a clinical event is a seizure, to detect seizures in high-risk neonates, to monitor for seizure recurrence during weaning of medications, to monitor burst suppression, and for other long-term monitoring indications. The World Health Organization (WHO), International League Against Epilepsy (ILAE), and the International Bureau of Epilepsy (IBE) recommend that all clinical seizures should be confirmed by an EEG if available. It should not be performed

for the purpose of determining the etiology of the seizures. AAP recommends that all newborns with HIE who receive therapeutic hypothermia need either an amplitude-integrated EEG (aEEG) or conventional EEG for identification of seizures. **Certain EEG patterns can suggest etiology (eg,** IEM: usually nonspecific, but burst suppression is seen in nonketotic hyperglycinemia, generalized bursts of bilaterally synchronous 1- to 4-Hz activity with spikes or sharp waves are seen in pyridoxine dependency, and high-voltage and rhythmic delta slow waves with myoclonus and paroxysmal responses during photic intermittent stimulation are seen in progressive myoclonic epilepsy). **The EEG also predicts neurologic sequelae in infants.** With a normal EEG, <10% of infants will have neurologic sequelae; with moderate abnormalities on EEG, approximately 50% of infants will have neurologic sequelae; with severe abnormalities on EEG, ≥90% of infants will have neurologic sequelae. There are several types of EEG used in the neonatal intensive care unit:

a. **Basic conventional electroencephalography** is done on infants at low risk for seizure activity. It is limited for capturing seizures because the usual duration is 60 minutes, but can be up to 8 hours. Most infants will have seizures if the recording is for a minimum of 24 hours.

b. **Continuous electroencephalography** (cEEG). The cEEG captures the electrical activity over a prolonged period of time (≥24 hours) Most infants will have seizures if the recording is for a minimum of 24 hours.

It is also used to aid in management of seizures. The American Clinical Neurophysiological Society states that the continuous EEG is superior to the aEEG (see Section IV.E.4.d) for monitoring and classifying neonatal seizures.

c. **Multichannel video EEG recording** is considered the **gold standard for diagnosis of seizures in neonates**. It is recommended to characterize clinical events and to assess for artifacts that may mimic electrographic seizures. It is recommended for 24 hours as most infants will have a seizure within the first day.

d. **Amplitude-integrated electroencephalography (aEEG).** Smaller portable units are used at the bedside with only 2 to 4 scalp electrodes, instead of the usual 12 to 16. These units also provide shorter, simpler readouts than the conventional EEG. These units detect most seizures in at-risk infants. aEEG has a high sensitivity and specificity when performed by experienced users. Use of aEEG is associated with a shorter time to diagnosis of seizures in encephalopathic infants. It has been stated it is a **"useful initial complementary tool"** because there are concerns of underdiagnosing seizures and neonatologists are not confident in their aEEG interpretations.

V. **Plan** Treatment consists of stabilizing the infant, ensuring adequate ventilation and circulation first, and then quickly sending stat labs for any underlying disorders that may be causing the seizures (eg, hypoglycemia, hypocalcemia, sepsis evaluation). Treat any acute transient metabolic conditions before starting an antiepileptic medication. **Neonatal seizures are considered the most common neurologic emergency. The workup should be begun as soon as possible.**

A. **General measures.** If an infant is actively seizing or is having repeated seizure activity, it is considered an emergency and the infant should be treated as soon as possible. If the infant is not actively seizing and is stable, one can attempt to confirm and verify the seizure with an EEG if possible. WHO, ILAE, and IBE guidelines strongly recommend that all clinical seizures be confirmed by an EEG. They also recommend that "any electrical seizure, even in the absence of a clinically apparent seizure, should be treated."

1. **Airway, breathing, circulation.** Assess the infant's airway, breathing, and circulation. Intubation and mechanical ventilation may be necessary to maintain oxygenation. Correct hypoxia and metabolic acidosis.

2. **Check laboratory studies for metabolic causes.** There is no evidence to support or reject giving empirical treatment prior to obtaining laboratory studies. Remember that treating infants empirically with glucose before lab results can cause worsening of hyperglycemia in HIE and that giving intravenous (IV) calcium can cause asystole or skin necrosis.

   a. **Check glucose level.** Hypoglycemia needs to be ruled out and treated before an antiepileptic drug is considered. A bedside glucose test should be done immediately to rule out hypoglycemia while a stat sample is sent to the laboratory for confirmation. If the paper-strip test shows low blood glucose, it is acceptable to give 10% glucose, 2 mL/kg IV push, before obtaining results from the laboratory. If one is unable to measure a serum glucose, consider empirical treatment with glucose. Unexplained or persistent hypoglycemia should be thoroughly evaluated (see Chapter 67).

   b. **Obtain stat serum calcium, magnesium, and sodium levels.** If these levels were low on earlier values and a metabolic disorder is strongly suspected as the cause of the seizures, it is acceptable to treat the infant before new laboratory values are available.

3. **Rule out sepsis/meningitis.** Sepsis evaluation is recommended and possible treatment with antibiotics. Some sources recommend all infants who have had a seizure be evaluated for sepsis/meningitis, others recommend to only do a work up if there are clinical signs or if they are considered a high risk for an infection. If the decision is made to begin antibiotics, preferably do it after obtaining a sepsis evaluation, including a blood culture and lumbar puncture. If this is not possible, empirical treatment with antibiotics if clinical signs are present can be considered. Do a lumbar puncture once the infant is stable enough to perform it. **Treat herpes encephalitis** with acyclovir or treat if there is a high index of suspicion of herpes infection.

4. **Some institutions will treat the infant with pyridoxine** before an antiepileptic drug is given (weak WHO recommendation), whereas others will give it after antiepileptic medications have been given. Follow your institution guidelines. **Only consider this** if all other obvious etiologies are ruled out.

5. **Pediatric neurology consultation is recommended,** especially if seizures persist, are prolonged, or are recurrent.

B. **Anticonvulsant therapy (Table 82–1).** The decision to treat with antiepileptic medication is very difficult because there are no clearly defined, evidence-based guidelines, the recommendations vary, and there is very little scientific evidence to support the best management of seizures in the neonate. In fact, Cochrane review states there is little evidence from randomized controlled trials to support the use of any of the anticonvulsants currently used in the neonatal period. **WHO, ILAE, and IBE guidelines recommend treatment** of any clinically apparent seizure in a neonate if it lasts >3 minutes or if the infant has brief serial seizures. They also recommend that all electrical seizures should be treated, even if there are no apparent clinical signs of a seizure. There is extensive experimental data on neonatal seizures in animal models but very little data on human newborns. The majority of evidence suggests that a single neonatal seizure does not cause any serious defects, but prolonged or brief recurrent seizures may be associated with worse outcomes since they can be damaging to the developing brain. Seizures can cause immediate and long-term adverse consequences, including developmental delay, cerebral palsy, cognitive impairment, epilepsy, and even death. Therefore, treatment of seizures is recommended. However, treatment of seizures with antiepileptic medications is not benign because of the associated risks of the medications (respiratory depression and others) and the effects on the immature brain, which are not well defined. **Seizure medications are often referred to as first-line, second-line, and third-line/emerging medications.** It is very difficult to categorize medications into these groups because it depends on the reference or study that is quoted. Follow your institutional guidelines on

Table 82–1. MEDICATIONS USED FOR NEONATAL SEIZURES

Drug	Drug Class	Dosing Regimens	Comments and Side effects
Phenobarbital	Barbiturate	LD: 15–20 mg/kg/dose IV; may repeat 5–10 mg/kg/dose every 15–20 minutes to a maximum total dose of 40 mg/kg MD: 3–5 mg/kg/d IV/PO in 1–2 divided doses	• Additional respiratory support may be required. • Therapeutic drug monitoring recommended with trough between 15 and 40 mcg/mL.
Phenytoin/ fosphenytoin	Hydantoin anticonvulsant	LD: 15–20 mg/kg/dose IV MD: 4–8 mg/kg/d IV/PO in 2–3 divided doses	• Fosphenytoin is a prodrug of phenytoin; dosing is per phenytoin equivalent (PE) and fosphenytoin is preferred over phenytoin due to better cardiac adverse effect profile and lower risk of extravasation (vesicant). • May cause blood dyscrasias, severe dermatologic reactions, and hepatotoxicity. • Hypotension and cardiac arrhythmias may occur with rapid infusion. • Therapeutic monitoring is recommended with troughs of 8–20 mcg/mL for total phenytoin and 1–2.5 mcg/mL for free phenytoin. • Hazardous agent; exercise appropriate handling precautions.
Levetiracetam	Miscellaneous anticonvulsant	LD: 10–50 mg/kg/dose IV MD: 10–80 mg/kg/d IV/PO in 2 divided doses	• May cause CNS depression, agranulocytosis, pancytopenia, thrombocytopenia, severe dermatologic reactions, and isolated elevation in diastolic blood pressure in young patients. • Abrupt discontinuation may increase seizure frequency. • Dosing adjustment may be required in renal impairment.
Lidocaine	Antiarrhythmic	LD: 2 mg/kg/dose IV over 10 minutes MD: 5–7 mg/kg/h × 4 hours, then 2.5–3.5 mg/kg/h × 6–12 hours, then 1.25–1.75 mg/kg/h × 12 hours	• Caution use in renal and/or hepatic impairment. • Contraindicated in severe heart block. • Therapeutic goal is 6–7 mcg/mL after continuous infusion for 4–6 hours.

Drug	Class	Dose	Comments
Diazepam	Benzodiazepine	0.1–0.3 mg/kg/dose IV; may repeat every 15–30 minutes to a maximum total dose of 2 mg	• **Not recommended as first-line agent;** use only after multiple agents have failed. • Vesicant; injection contains benzoic acid, sodium benzoate, and benzyl alcohol. • Caution use in renal and/or hepatic impairment.
Lorazepam	Benzodiazepine	0.05–0.1 mg/kg/dose IV; may repeat in 5–15 minutes as needed	• May cause CNS and respiratory depression and myoclonus (especially in premature neonates). • Injection formulation may contain polyethylene glycol and/or propylene glycol. Avoid high-dose and/or long-term use to prevent toxicity. • Caution use in renal and/or hepatic impairment.
Midazolam	Benzodiazepine	**LD:** 0.05–0.15 mg/kg/dose IV **MD:** 0.06–0.4 mg/kg/h continuous infusion	• May cause hypotension, respiratory depression, CNS depression, and myoclonus (especially in premature neonates). • Caution use in renal impairment.
Topiramate	Miscellaneous anticonvulsant	5–10 mg/kg/d PO once daily	• May cause hyperammonemia, encephalopathy, metabolic acidosis, hyperthermia, and nephrolithiasis. • Dosing adjustment may be required in renal and hepatic impairment. • Abrupt discontinuation may increase seizure frequency. • Hazardous agent; exercise appropriate handling precautions.

CNS, central nervous system; IV, intravenous; LD, loading dose; MD, maintenance dose; PO, oral.

Data from Vanden Hoek TL, Morrison LJ, Shuster M, et al. Part 12: Cardiac arrest in special situations: 2010 American Heart Association Guidelines for Cardiopulmonary Resuscitation and Emergency Cardiovascular Care. *Circulation.* 2010; 122(18 Suppl 3):829-861; and Lexi-Comp Online™. Pediatric & Neonatal Lexi-Drugs Online™, Hudson, Ohio: Lexi-Comp, Inc.; 2017; November 13, 2017.

which medications to use and when to use them. **First-line agents typically include** phenobarbital (most common), phenytoin, and benzodiazepines (lorazepam and midazolam); some units are now using levetiracetam. **Second-line agents typically include** phenytoin/fosphenytoin, levetiracetam, benzodiazepines, and lidocaine. **Third-line or emerging agents may include** clonazepam, lidocaine, topiramate, bumetanide, vigabatrin, and lamotrigine. **Medications reported but rarely used for neonatal seizures include** primidone, carbamazepine, lignocaine, valproic acid, pentobarbital, and thiopental. Phenobarbital and phenytoin are the most common antiseizure drugs used in the neonatal period even though their efficacy is poor (phenobarbital has approximately 43% seizure control, phenobarbital with phenytoin together has approximately 60% seizure control).

1. **Phenobarbital is the preferred first-line drug,** despite suboptimal efficacy. WHO, ILAE, and IBE strongly recommends this as the first-line agent because it is easier to administer, low cost, and readily available. Initially, 20 mg/kg IV is given as the loading dose, and if the seizures resolve, begin a maintenance dose of 3 to 4 mg/kg/d PO/IV divided twice a day. If seizures continue after 15 to 20 minutes, give an additional dose of 10 to 20 mg/kg IV, up to 40 to 50 mg/kg in 24 hours.

2. **If seizures persist after a maximum dose of phenobarbital, there is no real consensus on the second drug of choice.** Second-line drugs include phenytoin/ fosphenytoin, levetiracetam, lidocaine, and benzodiazepines. Most often, phenytoin is given as the second-line drug. **Give phenytoin** (Dilantin) 20 mg/kg/ dose at a rate of ≤1 mg/kg/min. **Fosphenytoin may be preferred** at some centers (see dosage in Chapter 155) because it has been associated with fewer side effects than phenytoin (less hypotension, fewer cardiac abnormalities, and less soft tissue injury). **As a second-line antiepileptic drug, WHO, ILAE, and IBE guidelines (2012) recommend either a benzodiazepine or phenytoin or lidocaine for control of seizures. WHO (2017) recommends either midazolam or lidocaine in any neonate who is continuing to have seizures.** Some clinicians will choose the second medication based on whether the infant has any cardiac abnormalities or cardiac instability. **With cardiac issues,** it may be better to choose midazolam or levetiracetam. **For infants without cardiac issues,** choose fosphenytoin or lidocaine. Remember if using phenytoin or lidocaine, cardiac monitoring is recommended.

3. **Levetiracetam used as second-line medication.** Over the past decade, there has been an increasing interest in using levetiracetam in neonatal seizures. Recently there are a few studies confirming its effectiveness as a first-line treatment with less side effects than phenobarbital (lethargy, feeding difficulty). It has been used off-label by pediatric neurologists for treating neonatal seizures for many years. According to the current research, it has a good safety profile, good efficacy, and favorable pharmacokinetics and seems to be a promising agent for seizure control in neonates. Loading dose is 20 mg/kg, and maintenance dose is 10 to 80 mg/kg/d in 2 divided doses.

4. **Lidocaine.** Used as a second- or third-line drug. Mechanism of action is uncertain as an anticonvulsant. Used more commonly in Europe. Full-term infants respond better than preterm infants. Avoid in infants with CHD. Reduce dose in premature infants and those undergoing therapeutic hypothermia. Stop after 36 hours because there is a risk of toxicity.

5. **Benzodiazepines.** Respiratory depression can occur with these medications but is usually not a problem because most infants are already on mechanical ventilation. Most institutions use lorazepam.

   a. **Lorazepam.** Used as second- or third-line drug. Given IV, dose can be repeated 4 to 6 times in a 24-hour period. It is advantageous to use over diazepam because its duration of action is longer and it causes less sedation, hypotension, and respiratory depression. Dose is 0.05 to 0.1 mg/kg every 8 to 12 hours.

    b. **Midazolam.** Useful in refractory neonatal seizures. A short-acting benzodi-azepine that can be given by continuous infusion. Less respiratory depression and sedation than with diazepam and lorazepam. See dose in Chapter 155.

    c. **Diazepam.** Effective anticonvulsant but used less often because of multiple issues (short duration of action, risk of circulatory collapse with respiratory failure, contains sodium benzoate, which can increase kernicterus risk).

6. **If seizures persist and other causes have been ruled out:** Three disorders need to be considered because they are treatable. First treat with pyridoxine. If that does not work, try pyridoxal 5′-phosphate. If that does not work, try folinic acid.

    a. **Pyridoxine (B6)-dependent seizures.** A trial dose of pyridoxine (vitamin B6), 50 to 100 mg, is given IV (with EEG monitoring) followed by a 30-minute observation period. If a response is seen, a maintenance dose of 50 to 100 mg/d orally is given. With pyridoxine dependency, the seizures stop quickly after the medication is given and the EEG normalizes.

    b. **Pyridoxine 5′-phosphate oxidase deficiency.** A trial of pyridoxal 5′-phosphate needs to be given. Dose is 30 mg/kg/d in 3 doses.

    c. **Folinic acid–responsive seizures (rare).** Obtain CSF neurotransmitter studies. Then folinic acid is given at 2.5 to 5 mg orally twice a day; dose may be increased to up to 8 mg/kg/d.

7. **If seizures still persist.** The following adjunctive agents may be used depending on institutional preference:

    a. **Bumetanide** is another novel neuroprotective agent. It was shown to be safe and had promising antiseizure activity in an early-phase trial. Can be given IV or intramuscularly.

    b. **Valproic acid.** Effective for recurrent seizures and status epilepticus, but because of the high risk of fatal hepatotoxicity in neonates, it is of limited value. Can be given orally, rectally, and IV.

    c. **Oral agents used in neonatal seizures** (however, because they are administered orally only, they are difficult to use because of dosing issues and variable blood levels)

        i. **Topiramate.** Although the research is limited, topiramate has been used as an add-on agent for refractory neonatal seizures and has been found to be effective. Furthermore, the benefit of topiramate lies in the fact that it is neuroprotective in hypoxic injury.

        ii. **Carbamazepine.** Has been used as an initial agent with success in a small study and as maintenance therapy as an alternative to phenobarbital or phenytoin.

        iii. **Primidone.** Another oral agent that has been used in small studies with success but had variable blood levels in another study. It can only be given orally.

        iv. **Clonazepam, felbamate, lamotrigine, and vigabatrin** are others reported.

8. **Medications used for refractory status epilepticus or seizures resistant to other medications. Pentobarbital anesthesia** has been used for refractory status epilepticus but has the potential for serious complications, and intense monitoring is required. **Thiopental** has been used in ventilated patients but is no longer available in the United States.

C. **Specific measures based on etiology of the seizure**

    1. **Hypoxic ischemic injury.** Therapeutic hypothermia is now the standard of care for hypoxic ischemic injury. Therapeutic hypothermia may decrease electrographic seizures in neonates with HIE. WHO, ILAE, and IBE do not recommend prophylactic treatment with phenobarbital in the absence of clinical seizures. Cochrane review states that prophylactic barbiturate therapy to infants following perinatal asphyxia did decrease the risk of seizures, but there was no decrease seen in mortality. See Chapter 43.

2. **Hypoglycemia.** Give 2 mL/kg IV of dextrose 10%; give a second dose if necessary. Make sure the infant is on maintenance glucose. Treat and determine the cause, as outlined in Chapter 67.
3. **Hypocalcemia.** Give 100 to 200 mg/kg of calcium gluconate slowly IV under cardiac monitoring. Make certain that the infant is receiving maintenance calcium therapy (usually 50 mg/kg every 6 hours). Confirm correct IV position. (See also Chapter 91.)
4. **Hypomagnesemia.** Give 0.2 mEq/kg of magnesium sulfate IV every 6 hours until magnesium levels are normal or symptoms resolve. (See Chapter 105.)
5. **Hyponatremia.** See Chapter 69.
6. **Hypernatremia.** If hypernatremia is secondary to decreased fluid intake, increase the rate of free water administration. The amount of sodium needs to be decreased; it should be reduced over 48 hours to decrease the possibility of cerebral edema.
7. **Infection.** If sepsis is suspected, a complete workup should be performed and empirical broad-spectrum antibiotic therapy initiated. Remember aminoglycosides have poor CSF penetration. Antiviral therapy (acyclovir) should be considered in infants >1 week of age or sooner if there was premature rupture of membranes for treatment of herpes simplex virus. Some institutions treat all infants with seizures empirically with acyclovir when there is a high index of suspicion for herpes infection.
8. **Local anesthetic intoxication.** Infants improve over 48 hours with prompt recognition, because the half-life of the medication is 8 to 10 hours. Vigorous support including ventilation and removal of the drug by diuresis, with acidification of the urine, is recommended and more effective than removal by exchange transfusion. Seizure medications are usually not needed. Outcome is favorable.
9. **Drug withdrawal syndrome.** Supportive therapy and anticonvulsants are used. (See Chapter 102.)
10. **Subarachnoid hemorrhage.** Only supportive therapy is necessary. (See Chapter 103.)
11. **Subdural hemorrhage.** Only supportive therapy is necessary, unless the infant has lacerations of the falx and tentorium, for which rapid surgical correction is necessary. Hemorrhage over cerebral convexities is treated by subdural taps. (See Chapter 103.)
12. **Polycythemia with hyperviscosity.** IV hydration and/or partial plasma exchange are often used. (See Chapters 34 and 116.)
13. *KCNQ2-* and *SCN2A*-related neonatal epilepsy. Use sodium channel blockers such as oral carbamazepine (drug of choice) or phenytoin.
14. **DEND syndrome.** Treat with oral hypoglycemic agents (sulfonylurea) because insulin does not work.
15. **Hyperinsulinism/hyperammonemia syndrome.** Treat with diazoxide.
16. **Treatable inborn errors of metabolism**
    a. **Pyridoxine-responsive seizures.** Treat with pyridoxine.
    b. **Pyridoxine 5′-phosphate oxidase deficiency.** Treat with pyridoxyl phosphate.
    c. **Folinic acid–responsive seizures.** Treat with folinic acid and pyridoxine.
    d. **Multiple carboxylase deficiency.** Treat with biotin.
    e. **GLUT-1 and pyruvate dehydrogenase deficiency.** Treat with ketogenic diet.
    f. **3-Phosphoglycerate dehydrogenase deficiency.** Treat with serine.
    g. **Primary hyperinsulinemic hypoglycemia.** Treat with glucose.
    h. **Congenital magnesium malabsorption.** Treat with magnesium.
    i. **Cerebral creatine disorders** (guanidinoacetate methyltransferase and arginine: glycine amidinotransferase deficiency). Treat with oral creatine

monohydrate. Guanidinoacetate methyltransferase deficiency also requires supplementation with ornithine and a restriction of arginine/protein.

    j. Congenital disorders of glycosylation type Ib. Treat with mannose.

D. Maintenance anticonvulsant therapy is not needed if 1 or 2 loading doses stop the seizures and it does not recur (controversial). If repeated doses are needed and seizures continue, a maintenance dose should be started 12 hours after the loading dose.

E. Duration of therapy. From 10% to 30% of neonates who have seizures will have subsequent epilepsy. Three factors should be considered in determining the duration of therapy: neonatal examination (if abnormal, the risk of having recurrent seizures is higher), cause of the neonatal seizure (risk after cortical dysgenesis is approximately 100%; after HIE, 30%–50%; after late-onset hypocalcemia, 0%), and the EEG results (normal or minimal depression showed no risk; marked depression showed a risk of 41%).

F. When to stop the antiepileptic medication. WHO, ILAE, and IBE guidelines state that if the infant has a normal neurologic examination and/or a normal EEG, one can consider stopping the medication if the infant is seizure free for 72 hours. For an infant on 1 medication, one can just discontinue the medication. For an infant on >1 medication, stop the medications 1 at a time, and stop phenobarbital last.

83 Traumatic Delivery

I. Problem. <u>An infant is noted to have severe bruises after birth, and a nurse observes that the infant is not using his right arm. The birth was noted to be traumatic, and the nurse calls you to evaluate the infant.</u> The terms **birth injuries** and **birth trauma** are used interchangeably. According to the National Vital Statistics Reports, **birth injury** is "the impairment of the infant's body function or structure due to adverse influences that occurred at birth." **Birth trauma** is defined as "a physical injury sustained by an infant in the process of birth." The rate of birth trauma has declined over the past 20 years, and the incidence is unclear, with study estimates ranging from approximately 6 to 8 per 1000 live births. The highest percentage of birth injuries occurs in mothers who were subjected to birthing instruments (eg, vacuum extraction, forceps). African Americans and Hispanics experience lower rates of birth injuries than whites and Asians/Pacific Islanders. Birth injuries occur from both vaginal and cesarean deliveries. Infants delivered by cesarean section are at risk for different types of birth trauma than infants delivered vaginally. Infants delivered by cesarean have a decreased risk of all birth trauma due to the decreased risk of clavicle fractures and injuries to the brachial plexus and scalp. Birth injuries can range from minor (petechiae) to severe (spinal cord injury resulting in death). The **most common birth injuries** are brachial plexus palsy (Erb palsy), bone fractures (fracture of the clavicle most common), cephalohematoma, caput succedaneum, intracranial hemorrhage, subconjunctival hemorrhage, facial paralysis, spinal cord injuries, and cerebral palsy. **Documentation of injuries** (rib fractures, clavicle fractures, retinal hemorrhages) is very important at the first physical examination because some of these injuries can be confused with nonaccidental trauma after discharge.

II. Immediate questions
    A. **Are there any risk factors for a birth injury?** Certain factors predispose the infant to birth injuries. **Macrosomia and instrumental deliveries** are major risk factors.
        1. **Risk factors**
            a. **Maternal:** Small maternal stature, primigravida, maternal pelvic abnormalities, maternal obesity, cephalopelvic disproportion, increased maternal age (clavicle fracture), maternal trauma 1 to 2 weeks before delivery (intra-abdominal injuries in infant), twin pregnancy (femur fracture).
            b. **Delivery:** Prolonged or very rapid labor, precipitous delivery, difficult fetal extraction, abnormal presentation (especially breech by vaginal delivery; 30 per 1000 live births), cephalopelvic disproportion, nuchal cord, oligohydramnios, instrumental deliveries (use of mid-forceps [4-fold increase] or vacuum extraction [3-fold increase]), excessive traction during delivery.
            c. **Infant:** Macrosomia irrespective of route of delivery The higher the degree of macrosomia the higher is the risk of birth injury (risk is increased by 2-fold with BW of 4000–4500 g, 3-fold with BW of 4500–4900 g, and 4.5-fold with BW >5000 g), very large fetal head, very low BW infant, fetal anomalies (osteogenesis imperfecta), prematurity, male gender (head and neck trauma), shoulder dystocia (brachial plexus injury, clavicular fracture, humerus fracture).
        2. **Injuries associated with risk factors**
            a. **Vacuum extraction:** Subgaleal hemorrhage, depressed skull fracture, iatrogenic encephalocele, cephalic hematoma, cephalohematoma, intracranial hematoma, subdural hemorrhage, retinal hemorrhage.
            b. **Forceps delivery:** Most common cause of injury to the facial nerve, cephalohematoma.
            c. **Forceps and vacuum extraction:** Shoulder dystocia, retinal hemorrhages, intracranial hemorrhage, cephalohematoma, subdural hemorrhage.
            d. **Breech presentation:** Long bone fractures, intracranial hemorrhage, brachial plexus palsy, lacerations of the buttocks.
            e. **Macrosomia:** Clavicle and rib fractures, shoulder dystocia, cephalohematoma, caput succedaneum.
            f. **Premature birth:** Intracranial and extracranial hemorrhage, bruising.
            g. **Precipitous delivery:** Retinal hemorrhage, bruising, intracranial or extracranial hemorrhage.
            h. **Abnormal presentation:** Lacerations, retinal hemorrhage, bruising.
            i. **Shoulder dystocia:** Brachial risk injury.
    B. **Is the injury so serious that it requires immediate attention?** The majority of birth injuries are not serious and do not require urgent treatment. Significant injuries are an emergency and require immediate intervention and close monitoring; significant injures include subgaleal hemorrhage (can be fatal), posterior fossa subdural hematoma (can cause brainstem compression resulting in respiratory compromise), spinal cord injuries (can be fatal), and abdominal organ injuries (present as shock secondary to bleeding and require immediate diagnosis).
III. **Differential diagnosis (based on site of injury)**
    A. **Skin trauma**
        1. **Petechiae. Petechiae are** small (<3 mm) bruises that do not blanch on pressure. They usually **occur with a precipitous delivery, breech presentation, or tight nuchal cord.** In birth trauma, petechiae are usually localized (eg, on the head, neck, upper chest area, and lower back). There is no associated bleeding, and no new lesions appear. If petechiae are diffuse and continue to progress, suspect coagulopathy, disseminated intravascular coagulation (with abnormal coagulation profiles, thrombocytopenia, oozing from bleeding sites such as venipuncture), infection (other signs such as temperature irregularity and cardiopulmonary distress are present), or other systemic disease.

2. **Ecchymosis/bruising.** A bruise is a superficial injury produced by trauma with extravasation of blood into the skin. Ecchymosis is a nonraised skin discoloration >1 cm caused by blood vessel rupture with blood leaking into the layer of skin tissues. Ecchymosis can be from a medical condition (thrombocytopenia), internal bleeding, or trauma. Bruising can occur after a traumatic delivery, especially when labor is rapid or the infant is premature or in a breech delivery. Extensive ecchymoses may indicate occult blood loss. The risk of hyperbilirubinemia (usually at 3–5 days) is increased in these injuries (increased bilirubin due to blood breakdown).

3. **Abrasions or lacerations** are more frequent in emergency cesarean deliveries for fetal distress. These can occur due to a scalpel or other instrument during delivery and are usually located on the scalp, buttocks, or thigh. Sometimes suturing is necessary for deep lacerations. Fetal scalp blood sampling can cause a scalp abrasion.

4. **Forceps injury/marks.** Frequently, reddish linear marks are seen across both sides of the face from the pressure of the blades.

5. **Scalp electrode injury.** The site of insertion of the scalp electrode can sometimes become infected (1% of cases), and in premature infants, it can rarely cause severe bleeding.

6. **Subcutaneous fat necrosis** is caused by localized pressure and ischemia to the fatty tissue in the subcutaneous space during the birth process and usually occurs in term or postterm infants. Typically involves the trunk, shoulders, arms, thighs, cheeks, and buttocks with a well-circumscribed firm lesion of the skin and underlying tissue. It usually appears between 6 and 10 days of age. Lesion size is 1 to 10 cm, lesions can be irregular and hard, the overlying skin can be deep red/purple or colorless, and the condition can cause hypercalcemia. (See Chapter 80 and Figure 80–7.)

7. **Neonatal alopecia** (hair loss) can occur associated with birth trauma. Neonatal alopecia needs to be differentiated from aplasia cutis congenital, which is localized congenital absence of the skin with loss of subcutaneous tissue, bone, or dura not usually related to birth trauma.

B. **Head trauma**

1. **Traumatic cyanosis.** Cyanosis of the head and face can occur from venous congestion, from a face presentation, or a tight umbilical cord around the neck.

2. **Soft tissue injury.** Bruising and petechiae.

3. **Iatrogenic encephalocele with enlarging subcutaneous cerebrospinal fluid collection** is a herniation of brain tissue (not involving the meninges) and is a rare complication of a vacuum extraction delivery. It presents similar to a caput succedaneum.

4. **Extracranial injury.** See also Chapter 7, Figure 7–3.

   a. **Caput succedaneum.** Relatively common, this accumulation of blood and serum (from increased pressure of the uterine and vaginal walls during labor on the fetal head) causes an edematous swelling at birth over the presenting part of the scalp during a vertex delivery. Associated with overlying erythema, bruising, and petechiae. This swelling is subcutaneous but exterior to the periosteum. **It crosses the midline of the skull and suture lines.** It is usually associated with molding. Hyperbilirubinemia rarely develops. **A vacuum caput** is a caput succedaneum that occurs during a delivery using a vacuum device. It typically has well-defined margins of the vacuum cup.

   b. **Cephalohematoma.** This is subperiosteal accumulation of blood that is caused by rupture of superficial veins between the skull and periosteum. Incidence is up to 2% of all live births. It is more common in males and in instrumental deliveries (4–5 times higher in forceps deliveries, 8–9 times higher in vacuum deliveries, and 11–12 times higher in forceps plus vacuum deliveries). The bleed is below the periosteum overlying 1 cranial bone, usually the parietal bone. **There is no crossing of the suture lines,** the scalp is not discolored, and the swelling sometimes takes ≥24 hours to become apparent because the bleeding is slow. The affected area is largest on postnatal day 3. An associated skull fracture is present in up to 25% of affected infants (often a linear fracture). Hyperbilirubinemia (sometimes significant if the lesion is extensive) may develop. The cephalohematoma can become infected with complications such as skull osteomyelitis (*Escherichia coli* most common), and sepsis or meningitis can occur. Two conditions that are similar and might be confused with cephalohematoma are cranial meningocele (associated with pulsations, increased pressure with crying) and caput succedaneum (crosses the midline, with discoloration of the skin).

   c. **Subgaleal hemorrhage** (also called subaponeurotic hemorrhage) is the least common extracranial injury but the most serious and is caused by rupture of the emissary veins that connect the scalp veins to the dural sinuses. It occurs in approximately 64 in 10,000 vacuum extraction deliveries and 4 in 10,000 noninstrumented deliveries. Blood collects in the soft tissue space between the epicranial aponeurosis and the periosteum of the skull. Diffuse swelling of the soft tissue, often spreading toward the neck and behind the ears, and periorbital swelling are also evident. **The "classic triad" is tachycardia, decreasing hematocrit, and an increasing occipital frontal circumference (OFC). The OFC can increase 1 cm for every 30 to 40 mL of blood.** Associated signs include hemorrhagic shock, severe blood loss (potential to hold >40% of the total blood volume), shock, anemia, hypotonia, seizures, and pallor. This can be a fatal complication (mortality rate up to 14 %) of a traumatic birth.

5. **Intracranial injury.** Most common is subdural hemorrhage (73%), then subarachnoid (20%), intracerebral (20%), intraventricular, and epidural hemorrhage. (See also Chapter 103.)

   a. **Subdural hemorrhage** is the **most common intracranial hemorrhage** in a term newborn (2.9 per 100,000 spontaneous deliveries; if vacuum or forceps are used, incidence is 5.8 per 100,000; if both vacuum and forceps are used, incidence is 29 per 100,000). It is caused by rupture of the bridging veins and causes blood between the arachnoid layer of the brain and dura mater. Infants usually present in the first 24 to 48 hours after birth with stupor, altered level of consciousness, seizures, respiratory depression, apnea, irritability, full fontanelle, unresponsive pupils, and coma. Posterior fossa subdural hemorrhage is rare (suspected if excessive fetal molding) but may result in death from compression of the respiratory center in the brainstem.

   b. **Subarachnoid hemorrhage** is the **second most common intracranial hemorrhage.** It is caused by rupture of the bridging veins in the subarachnoid space. Blood is located between the arachnoid membrane and pia mater. Usually asymptomatic, but signs can occur at 24 to 48 hours after birth: seizures, apnea, and other complications such as high bilirubin. Typical scenario is a well term baby with new-onset seizures; apnea is common in premature infants.

   c. **Intraparenchymal hemorrhage**

      i. **Intracerebellar hematoma/cerebellar hemorrhage.** Associated with traumatic delivery and can present with apnea, unexplained motor agitation in preterm infants, bulging fontanel, and decreased hematocrit.

      ii. **Intracerebral hemorrhage.** This can occur from cranial birth trauma but is more commonly associated with other causes.

   d. **Intraventricular hemorrhage** (IVH) is usually associated with preterm deliveries and not associated with birth trauma. IVH in term infants can occur secondary to birth trauma or asphyxia. Incidence is 4% in term infants and is highest in vacuum- and forceps-assisted delivery. IVH presents with apnea, lethargy, cyanosis, seizures, weak suck, and high-pitched cry.

   e. **Epidural hematoma (rare). This is injury to the middle meningeal artery.** Blood is between the skull and outside of the dura. One cause is the infant being dropped during delivery. Signs are similar to those of subdural hemorrhage (hypotonia, seizures, bulging fontanelles, change in level of consciousness), and it is diagnosed by head computed tomography (CT) or magnetic resonance imaging (MRI). Clinical manifestations are usually delayed, and it is often associated with linear skull fracture and cephalohematoma.

   f. **Contusion bruise (cerebral and cerebellum) of the brain.** Presents with nonspecific neurologic dysfunction. CT demonstrates punctate hemorrhages.

6. **Skull fracture** injuries are uncommon in neonates; most are linear and are associated with a cephalohematoma. Fractures at the base of the skull may result in shock. Occipital fractures are most commonly associated with breech deliveries. Evaluate for any **neurologic deficit** because this changes management.

   a. **Linear (nondepressed) fracture (most common).** A break that traverses the full thickness of the skull, is straight, and has no displacement. The parietal bone is usually involved. Usually without any signs, but bleeding can occur, most commonly extracranially. Rarely, intracranial bleeding can occur.

   b. **Depressed fracture** (also called "ping-pong fracture") of the skull is caused by the bone (most commonly the parietal or the frontal) being displaced inward. There is an increased incidence of an intracranial process in depressed fractures, especially those >1 cm. Depressed fractures are often visible and can result in seizures. They occur from birth trauma, but a congenital depressed fracture of the skull can also occur prenatally or in the absence of trauma. **Subdural hematoma** is the most common intracranial injury associated with a depressed skull fracture.

   c. **Occipital osteodiastasis.** This is usually a complication of breech deliveries but is rare now because the American Congress of Obstetricians and Gynecologists recommends cesarean delivery for term breech singletons. It is a traumatic separation of the cartilaginous joint between the squamous and lateral portions of the occipital bone that results in a posterior fossa subdural hemorrhage associated with laceration of the cerebellum. There are 3 types: a classic form, a fatal form, and a less severe variant compatible with survival.

C. **Facial trauma**
1. **Fractures of the nose, mandible, maxilla, lacrimal bones, and septal cartilage.** These can often present as respiratory distress or feeding problems and require treatment. Urgent plastic surgery/otorhinolaryngology consultation is recommended.

2. **Dislocations of the facial bones.** Nasal septal dislocation (the most common facial injury) can occur and presents as stridor and cyanosis. Facial bone and mandibular fractures can occur.

3. **Facial nerve injury.** This is the most **common peripheral nerve** (cranial nerve VII) injury secondary to birth trauma and is seen in up to 1% of live births. Most cases implicate forceps use, but approximately 33% occur in deliveries without instruments. The injury is secondary to the pressure of the forceps or the face lying on the maternal sacral promontory. The nerve is injured at the point where it emerges from the stylomastoid foramen. Rule out other causes of asymmetric crying face (congenital deficiency or absence of the depressor anguli oris muscle, which controls the downward motion of the lip) by observing that the eye and forehead muscles are unaffected in asymmetric crying face.

   a. **Peripheral facial nerve injury (more common)** involves the entire side of the face. At rest, the infant has an open eye on the affected side. The nasolabial fold is flattened, and the mouth droops. When the infant cries, the findings are similar to those with central paralysis.

   b. **Central facial nerve injury.** Involves the lower half or two-thirds of the contralateral side of the face. On the paralyzed side, the nasolabial fold is obliterated, the corner of the mouth droops, and the skin is smooth and full. When the infant cries, the wrinkles are deeper on the normal side, and the mouth is drawn to the normal side.

    c. **Peripheral nerve branch injury.** Only 1 group of facial muscles is involved (mouth, eyelid, or forehead), and injury results in paralysis of only that area.

D. Ocular trauma

    1. **Eyelids.** Edema and bruising can occur. Swollen eyelids should be forced open to examine the eyeball. Laceration of the eyelid can also occur.

    2. **Orbit fracture.** Rarely occurs. Immediate ophthalmologic evaluation is necessary if disturbances of the extraocular muscle movements and exophthalmos are evident. Severe injuries may result in death.

    3. **Horner syndrome.** Due to impaired sympathetic outflow with signs such as miosis, partial ptosis, enophthalmos, and anhidrosis of the ipsilateral side of the face. Delayed pigmentation of the ipsilateral iris can be seen as the child grows.

    4. **Subconjunctival hemorrhage.** A common finding that resolves without treatment.

    5. **Cornea.** Haziness can be secondary to edema or use of eye prophylaxis. With persistent cornea opacity (haziness/clouding) and prolonged corneal edema, suspect detachment of the Descemet membrane. A forceps injury can induce a tear in the Descemet membrane; it is usually unilateral with a vertical break.

    6. **External ocular muscle injuries** involving the third, fourth, and sixth cranial nerves.

    7. **Optic nerve injury.** Vision may be affected.

    8. **Intraocular hemorrhage**

        a. **Retinal hemorrhage.** It occurs most commonly in vacuum deliveries (75%) but can occur in spontaneous vaginal deliveries and cesarean deliveries. Cause is unknown, but it is believed to be due to the pressure exerted on the head through the birth canal. Most commonly, a flame-shaped or streak hemorrhage is found near the optic disk. It can be seen 3 to 4 weeks after birth. A subdural hemorrhage can cause preretinal and intraretinal hemorrhages.

        b. **Subconjunctival hemorrhage (under the conjunctiva)** is a common finding that resolves without treatment.

        c. **Hyphema** is gross blood in the anterior chamber and should be evaluated by ophthalmology.

        d. **Vitreous hemorrhage** is indicated by floaters, absent red reflex, and blood pigment seen on slit-lamp examination by ophthalmology.

E. Ear injuries (abrasions, bruising, hematomas, avulsion, or laceration of the auricle) can occur, often due to forceps. Fetal malposition also contributes to injuries to the ear. Hematomas of the pinna can lead to a "cauliflower ear" (an irreversible condition that occurs when the external portion of the ear is injured; a collection of fluid develops under the perichondrium, cartilage dies, fibrous tissue is formed, and the outer ear becomes deformed and swollen).

F. Nose injuries. Nasal fracture and dislocation of the nasal cartilage can occur. The most common is nasal dislocation; incidence is <1%. Nasal deformity without dislocation can also occur. Nasal fracture and dislocation are increased in prolonged delivery, with increased head circumference, and in vaginal delivery.

G. Vocal cord injuries/recurrent laryngeal nerve injury. Although rare, these injuries can occur as a result of excessive traction on the head during delivery and are caused by an injury to the recurrent laryngeal branch of the vagus nerve. Often associated with forceps in a difficult delivery, they can result in bilateral or unilateral vocal cord paralysis and may cause acute respiratory compromise.

    1. **Unilateral paralysis** involves the recurrent laryngeal branch of 1 of the vagus nerves in the neck. Asymptomatic at rest, but hoarse cry, weak cry, abnormal voicing, and mild to moderate stridor with inspiration are seen. Unilateral vocal cord paralysis is usually left sided because of the nerve's longer course and position for injury.

2. **Bilateral paralysis.** Caused by trauma to both recurrent laryngeal nerves. Signs include respiratory distress, stridor, and cyanosis.

H. **Neck, shoulder, and chest injuries**

1. **Shoulder dystocia.** Occurs when the head is delivered and the shoulder gets stuck during delivery. Trauma to the neck can occur when the baby is delivered. The most common injury is brachial plexus injury, but the clavicle can be broken or cord compression can occur.

2. **Clavicular fracture.** The **most common bone fracture during delivery** (~1%–1.5% from birth trauma). Risk factors include macrosomia, increased maternal age, shoulder dystocia, and use of instruments at delivery (forceps and vacuum). Most fractures are greenstick/incomplete type. If the fracture is complete, symptoms involve decreased or absent movement of the arm, gross deformity of the clavicle, pain response on palpation, localized crepitus and petechiae over affected side, and an absent or asymmetric Moro reflex. Nondisplaced fracture usually presents with no symptoms, and the diagnosis is made because of callus formation at 7 to 10 days. Bilateral clavicle fractures can occur but are rare. Brachial plexus injury or phrenic nerve palsy can be associated.

3. **Rib fractures.** Very rare.

4. **Brachial plexus injury.** Incidence is 0.5 to 2.5 per 1000 live births. Involves paralysis of upper arm muscles following trauma to spinal roots C5 to T1. Usually secondary to a prolonged delivery of a macrosomic infant with excessive strain on the head, neck, and arm. The spinal roots of the fifth cervical through the first thoracic spinal nerves (brachial plexus) are injured during birth. This is usually unilateral and occurs twice as often on the right as the left. Brachial plexus injury is diagnosed by **unilateral arm weakness.** Obstetrical shoulder dystocia training was associated with a lower incidence of brachial plexus injury. There are 4 forms of brachial plexus injury:

   a. **Erb palsy (Erb-Duchenne palsy)** caused by injury to nerve roots C5 and C6. Erb palsy is the most common form of brachial plexus injury and involves the upper arm (~90% of cases). The fifth and sixth cervical roots are affected, and the arm is adducted and internally rotated and fully extended at the elbow with pronation of the forearm and flexion of the wrist. (**"waiter's tip"** position). The deltoid muscle is paralyzed, which prevents the arm from being raised. The paralysis of the biceps brachii and brachialis muscle causes the arm to be limp and the forearm pronated. The Moro reflex is absent or weakened. The grasp reflex is intact, which rules out total arm paralysis. In some infants, a complete ossified cervical rib is found, and some feel that this anatomic variation (also including fibrous bands) is thought to cause narrowing of the supra-costoclavicular space, allowing the nerves to be more susceptible to trauma. If the infant with brachial palsy has tachypnea and needs oxygen, rule out phrenic nerve involvement because brachial palsy can be associated with phrenic nerve palsy.

   b. **Total brachial plexus injury** is present in almost 10% of cases, and all nerve roots are involved. Entire arm (global or total brachial plexus) paralysis is present. Because the entire brachial plexus is damaged, the patient has a flaccid arm that hangs limply with no reflexes. Horner syndrome can accompany this injury if the sympathetic fibers of T1 are damaged.

   c. **Klumpke palsy.** Occurs when there is damage to the C8 to T1 nerve roots and is isolated to the lower arm because the seventh and eighth cervical and first thoracic roots are injured; it is rare (<1% of cases). The hand is paralyzed, the wrist does not move, and the grasp reflex is absent (ie, "dropped hand"). Cyanosis and edema of the hand can also occur. An ipsilateral Horner syndrome (ptosis, miosis, and enophthalmos) can be seen because of injury involving the cervical sympathetic fibers of the first thoracic root.

   d. **Horner syndrome** is a preganglionic injury with damage to the sympathetic outflow via nerve root T1. The classic triad is miosis (a constricted pupil), (partial) ptosis (upper eyelid droops over the eye), and anhidrosis (loss of hemifacial sweating). Enophthalmos (posterior retrodisplacement of the eyeball in the orbit) can also be associated.

5. **Phrenic nerve paralysis** involves the C3, C4, and C5 nerve roots. Difficult breech delivery with lateral extension of the neck, with avulsion of C3 through C5 nerve roots, can cause **diaphragmatic paralysis** (75% of cases). It can be associated with brachial plexus injury. Signs include recurrent episodes of cyanosis, tachypnea, irregular respirations, and thoracic breathing with no bulging of the abdomen. It causes ineffective respirations and presents with difficulty breathing in the first few hours of life, with elevation of the diaphragm on x-ray.

6. **Sternocleidomastoid muscle injury** is also called congenital muscular torticollis and involves a well-circumscribed, immobile mass (1–2 cm) in the midportion of the sternocleidomastoid muscle (SCM) that enlarges, regresses, and disappears. This results in a transient torticollis after birth. The head tilts toward the involved side, the chin is elevated and rotated, and the infant cannot move the head into normal position. Usually occurs on the right side of the neck and is most apparent at 1 to 4 weeks of age. Facial asymmetry can be seen.

I. **Spinal cord injuries.** Rare (<0.2 per 10000 births) and are caused by lateral or longitudinal stretching force of the neck or hyperextension or torsion of the fetal neck. Signs vary depending on the location of the injury, and these injuries usually occur with breech deliveries or use of forceps. They can involve meningeal damage with epidural hemorrhage, spinal artery occlusion, vertebral artery injuries and occlusion, laceration of the spinal nerve roots and bruising, and laceration or complete transection of the cord. The higher the injury, the greater is the risk of respiratory problems. Suspect this in a neonate with severe respiratory compromise and profound hypotonia. Spinal shock can occur, which presents with paralyzed abdominal movements, diaphragmatic breathing, distended bladder, and extremities that are flaccid.

1. **Infants with a high cervical lesion or brainstem injury.** Usually born stillborn or with severe respiratory depression, shock, or hypothermia with paralysis at birth. Mortality is high. Death usually occurs within a few hours after birth.

2. **Upper or midcervical lesions.** Present with lower extremity paralysis, absent deep tendon reflexes, absent sensation in the lower half of the body, constipation, urinary retention, and respiratory depression.

3. **Lesions in the seventh cervical to first thoracic roots.** Injury may be reversible. Muscle atrophy, contractures, bony deformities, constant urinary leakage.

4. **Partial spinal cord injuries.** On neurologic examination, these infants have signs of spasticity.

J. **Abdominal organ injuries (uncommon and infrequent)** are associated with maternal trauma 1 to 2 weeks before delivery or trauma during the delivery process. **Most common is liver injury.** These injuries should be suspected with shock, increasing abdominal circumference, anemia, pallor, and irritability. These infants can be asymptomatic for hours and then deteriorate acutely. Risk factors for these injuries include macrosomia and breech presentation. **Intraperitoneal bleed needs to be ruled out in every infant who presents with shock and abdominal distension**, and paracentesis is essential for diagnosis.

1. **Liver hematoma/rupture/fracture.** The liver is the most commonly injured solid organ by direct pressure from birth trauma. **Subcapsular hematomas** are the most common lesion, are usually not easily diagnosed, and are usually asymptomatic at birth (subtle signs of blood loss include poor feeding, tachypnea, pallor, and onset of jaundice). **Rupture of the hematoma** presents with

sudden circulatory collapse and discoloration of the abdominal wall. Liver fracture can present with shock, anemia, pallor, and abdominal distension.

2. **Splenic hematoma/rupture.** Signs are similar to rupture of the liver; blood loss and hemoperitoneum may be seen. Less frequent than hepatic injury.
3. **Adrenal hemorrhage.** Usually right sided (70 %) and unilateral (90%). Presents with an abdominal mass. Symptoms vary depending on degree and rate of hemorrhage and include fever, tachypnea, flank mass, pallor, purpura, hypotension, cyanosis, poor feeding, shock, irritability, vomiting, and diarrhea. Hypoglycemia, early-onset hyperkalemia, and prolonged hyperbilirubinemia can be seen.
4. **Renal hemorrhage.** Suspect in a newborn with a flank mass and hematuria with a history of birth trauma.

K. **Extremity injuries.** See also Chapter 112. Besides the clavicle, the humerus and femur are the most common fractures during the birth process.
1. **Fractured humerus** is seen in 0.2 per 1000 deliveries and is the second most common fracture during birth trauma. The arm is immobile, and there can be swelling and localized crepitus, with pain on movement and palpation. Moro reflex is absent on the affected side.
2. **Fractured femur** occurs in 0.13 per 1000 deliveries and is the third most common fracture during birth trauma. Usually occurs secondary to breech delivery with a pop or snap sometimes heard at delivery. Infants with congenital hypotonia are at risk. Deformity is usually obvious; the affected leg does not move, there is swelling, and there is pain with assisted movement.
3. **Fractured radius.** Rare.
4. **Epiphyseal separation.** Rarely seen, this usually involves the radial head but can also involve the humeral or femoral epiphysis. Examination reveals adduction, internal rotation of the affected arm, and poor Moro reflex. Femoral separation exhibits more pain and tenderness with palpation.
5. **Sciatic nerve palsy.** Rare and can occur in breech deliveries. Prolonged labor and a forceful extraction of the leg are usually obtained from the history. Complete or partial paralysis can occur.
6. **Radial nerve palsy (rare).** Infants present with absent wrist and digital extension but good shoulder and elbow function. Ecchymosis and fat necrosis may support a compression injury during labor.
7. **Growth plate injuries** can occur in the long bones in the newborn. They are often misdiagnosed as joint fractures with dislocation. Birth injuries to the growth plates can occur and have been reported in the proximal humerus (shoulder) and the distal humerus (elbow).

L. **Genital injuries.** Neonatal genital trauma can occur in both males and females. It is a rare and uncommon complication of breech presentation. Males can have edema, bruising, and diffuse hematoma of the scrotum. Females may present with swollen and tender masses with diffuse hematoma of the labia majora and discoloration of both the labia majora and minora. Injury usually does not affect micturition.
1. **Testicular and epididymal injury.** Findings are scrotal swelling, with the infant experiencing vomiting and irritability. A **hematocele** can form if the tunica vaginalis testis is injured; the scrotum will not transilluminate and needs to be differentiated from a congenital hernia/hydrocele usually by ultrasound. **Scrotal rupture** has only been reported in case reports. Scrotal hematoma may be a sign of adrenal hemorrhage.
2. **Perineal/rectovaginal injury/tear.** Rare birth injury that has been reported usually with breech presentation delivered vaginally.

M. **Umbilical cord rupture.** This can occur from trauma from an operative vaginal delivery (forceps or vacuum device used). Hemorrhage with bradycardia and respiratory distress can occur.

IV. Database
  A. **Physical examination.** Details on the initial physical examination of the newborn are found in Chapter 7.
    1. **Skin.** Look for petechiae, bruising, and any lacerations. Check the side of the face for forceps marks. Look for and palpate any area that looks like fat necrosis.
    2. **Head.** Carefully examine the head for any evidence of a caput succedaneum, cephalhematoma, subgaleal hemorrhage, or fracture. Check to see whether the suture lines are crossed (differentiates between the caput succedaneum and cephalhematoma). Depressed skull fractures are obvious; others may require radiologic studies.
    3. **Face.** Examine the face at rest and during crying to look for any facial asymmetry (nerve palsy or facial fractures). Facial fractures can present with asymmetry of the face, ecchymoses, edema, poor feeding, or respiratory distress. Check for any signs of respiratory distress (stridor or cyanosis).
    4. **Eyes.** Examine the eyeball and the eyelid. Make sure that extraocular muscle movements are normal. Check for the red reflex. Check for corneal clouding and edema. Funduscopic examination within the first 24 hours of birth will increase the chance of finding a retinal hemorrhage.
    5. **Ears.** Examine the front and back of the ear, looking for lacerations, swelling, and hematomas.
    6. **Nose.** Check for dislocation versus deformation. Flatten the tip of the nose; with a deformation, no nasal deviation occurs, whereas with a dislocation, one can see the deviated septum and the nares collapse.
    7. **Vocal cords.** Signs may include high-pitched cry or stridor. If injury is suspected, examine the vocal cords by direct laryngoscopy or use a flexible fiberoptic laryngoscope.
    8. **Neck and shoulder injuries.** Carefully examine the neck and the shoulder. Check Moro and grasp reflexes. Examine the arm to see whether movement is normal. Check respirations, and note any thoracic breathing. Make sure the head rests in a normal position and is not tilted. Examine the hips in an infant with congenital torticollis, since 10% will have congenital hip dysplasia.
    9. **Spinal cord.** A careful and thorough neurologic examination should be done.
    10. **Abdomen.** Examine the abdomen, and check for ascites, masses, and increase in size.
    11. **Extremities.** Observe for movement and deformity. Check for pain with passive movement and palpation.
    12. **Genitalia.** Examine the testes and the penis in males; transilluminate the scrotum. Carefully look at labia for bruising or hematoma.
  B. **Laboratory studies based on site of trauma**
    1. **Skin**
      a. **Platelet count.** A normal platelet count excludes neonatal thrombocytopenia.
      b. **Serum bilirubin test.** Hyperbilirubinemia may result from reabsorption of blood from extensive ecchymoses.
      c. **Serum hematocrit.** Anemia may result from severe ecchymoses.
      d. **Calcium levels** should be followed with fat necrosis due to hypercalcemia risk.
    2. **Head**
      a. **Hematocrit.** Blood loss can occur, sometimes requiring transfusions, especially in subgaleal hemorrhage.
      b. **Serum bilirubin.** Significant hyperbilirubinemia may result from cephalohematoma or other traumatic bleeding event.
      c. **Coagulation studies** are required to detect the consumption coagulopathy associated with subgaleal hemorrhage.
    3. **Face.** Arterial blood gas may be indicated in infants with grunting. Nerve excitability or conduction tests are recommended if there is no improvement in the facial nerve palsy after 3 to 4 days.

4. **Eyes, ears, or vocal cords.** No laboratory tests are usually required.
5. **Neck and shoulder.** Arterial blood gas helps diagnose hypoxia associated with phrenic nerve paralysis.
6. **Spinal cord.** The usual laboratory tests required for respiratory depression and shock, if indicated.
7. **Abdomen.** Obtain hematocrit to rule out anemia and blood loss and urine dipstick to check for hematuria. Consider abdominal paracentesis with fluid sent to the laboratory for cell count with differential.
8. **Extremities and genitalia.** No laboratory tests are usually needed.

C. **Imaging and other studies**
1. **Head.** Skull radiographs should be obtained to rule out the possibility of skull fractures. Head ultrasonography can be performed at the bedside and can detect an intracranial hemorrhage if the image is high quality and the sonographer is experienced. It is used to detect IVH. A CT scan can also be obtained and can be useful in the diagnosis of an intracranial hemorrhage (epidural, subarachnoid). MRI should be obtained if neurologic symptoms occur or if an intracranial injury occurs with a cephalhematoma or a skull fracture. Imaging should be considered in any infant with a large caput succedaneum that does not decrease in 72 hours, if the swelling increases >24 hours after delivery, or if there are neurologic deficits.
2. **Face.** Radiographs should be considered if a significant injury is suspected. A cranial CT scan or MRI may be necessary to further delineate the fracture.
3. **Eyes.** Radiographs, to rule out orbit fracture, may be indicated. Ultrasound and handheld optical coherence tomography may be necessary to rule out Descemet membrane detachment.
4. **Neck and shoulder**
   a. **Ultrasound or radiograph of the clavicle** is necessary for confirmation of the diagnosis of fracture. Ultrasound is a satisfactory alternative to a radiograph for the diagnosis of fractures of the clavicle.
   b. **Radiograph of the chest for phrenic nerve paralysis** will show an elevated diaphragm. **Fluoroscopy** reveals elevation of the affected side and descent of the normal side on inspiration with phrenic nerve impairment. Opposite movements occur with expiration. **Dynamic ultrasound of the diaphragm for phrenic nerve evaluation** shows abnormal motion on the affected side.
   c. **Magnetic resonance imaging of the neck and spine** for nerve root avulsion.
   d. **Electroencephalogram.** Reveals the extent of the denervation weeks after the injury.
5. **Spinal cord**
   a. **Cervical and thoracic spine radiographs.**
   b. **Magnetic resonance imaging.** Most reliable method for diagnosing spinal cord injuries.
6. **Abdomen.** Abdominal ultrasound usually diagnoses liver rupture or subcapsular hematoma, splenic rupture, adrenal hemorrhage, and kidney damage. An abdominal radiograph may reveal a stomach bubble displaced medially in splenic rupture. CT scan and ultrasonography are the preferred modalities to diagnose an abdominal injury.
7. **Extremities.** A radiograph/ultrasound of the extremities usually confirms the diagnosis of bone injury. An **ultrasound** is diagnostic for epiphyseal separation because it can diagnose a growth plate injury since it can visualize the nonossified epiphysis.
8. **Genitalia.** Ultrasonography is usually diagnostic.

V. **Plan**
A. **Skin**
1. **Petechiae.** No specific treatment is necessary because traumatic petechiae usually fade in 2 to 3 days.

2. **Subcutaneous fat necrosis.** The lesions require observation only because they usually disappear within weeks to a few months without any cutaneous sequelae. Extensive calcification can occur within the lesions, and pain can occur, requiring analgesics. Hypercalcemia is a life-threatening complication of subcutaneous fat necrosis and can occur in approximately 35% to 56% of infants. Its exact cause is unknown. Closely monitor blood levels for up to 6 months after the onset of the fat necrosis for symptomatic hypercalcemia (vomiting, fever, and weight loss with high serum calcium), which can occur up to 6 months. This can usually be treated with restricting supplemental calcium and vitamin D, intravenous hydration, and furosemide. In severe cases, hydrocortisone therapy and bisphosphonates have been used.

3. **Ecchymoses.** No specific treatment is necessary because they usually resolve within 1 week. Monitor for hyperbilirubinemia (reabsorption of blood from a bruised area), anemia (blood loss from bruising), and hyperkalemia if extensive.

4. **Lacerations and abrasions.** For abrasions, cleaning the wound and observation are all that is needed. For lacerations, if superficial, the edges may be held together with butterfly adhesive or Steri-Strips. If deeper, they should be sutured with 7–0 nylon. Healing is usually rapid. Observe for infections, especially a scalp lesion and caput succedaneum.

B. **Head**

1. **Caput succedaneum.** No specific treatment is necessary because it resolves within the first several days after birth but can be present for up to 4 to 6 days. It rarely causes jaundice or significant blood loss. Rarely, scalp necrosis can occur. Consider imaging if there is a large caput succedaneum that does not go away in 48 to 72 hours after birth or if there is an increase in swelling 24 hours after birth, presence of neurologic deficits, or hemodynamic instability.

2. **Cephalhematoma.** Observation is usually all that is needed. Incision and aspiration are **not recommended**. The cephalohematoma usually resolves in 3 to 4 weeks, leaving a palpable subcutaneous nodule that is reabsorbed after 3 to 4 months. CT or skull radiography may be necessary if neurologic symptoms occur or underlying skull fracture needs to be ruled out. In some cases, blood loss and hyperbilirubinemia can occur and should be treated.

3. **Subgaleal hemorrhage.** Recommended treatment is close observation and aggressive management of hypovolemia and severe blood loss with shock.

   a. **Place an umbilical venous line for access;** place an arterial line for blood pressure management and labs.

   b. **Measure serial hematocrit and occipital frontal circumference.** Volume loss needs to be treated aggressively (10–20 mL kg bolus infusions) with normal saline, whole blood, fresh-frozen plasma, or packed red blood cells. Assume a 40-mL amount of blood loss for every 1-cm increase in occipital frontal circumference.

   c. **Consider treating metabolic acidosis,** provide adequate oxygenation and assisted ventilation, monitor serial hematocrits, and evaluate for coagulopathy.

   d. **Monitor fluid intake and urinary output.**

   e. **If hypovolemic shock develops,** treat immediately with volume resuscitation, and correct any coagulopathy.

   f. **Phototherapy** may be needed for indirect hyperbilirubinemia (see Chapters 63 and 99).

   g. **Observe any skin lesions** for infection and treat appropriately.

   h. **Surgical evacuation of the hematoma** may be required if there are signs of brain compression, if there is increased intracranial pressure, if bleeding does not subside, or if there is severe clinical deterioration.

4. **Intracranial hemorrhage.** Circulatory and ventilatory support is indicated in deteriorating conditions. Consultation with neurosurgery is recommended. (See also Chapter 103.)
   a. **Subarachnoid hemorrhage.** Resolution usually occurs without treatment. Observe for signs of herniation; if present, surgical evacuation is needed.
   b. **Epidural hemorrhage.** Close observation is usually all that is needed. Monitor for signs of herniation; if present, surgical evacuation may be necessary. Prompt surgical evacuation for large bleeds has good prognosis with early treatment.
   c. **Subdural hemorrhage.** Treatment depends on the location and how much bleeding has occurred. Most infants can be closely observed without surgical intervention. Surgical evacuation is necessary for infants who have signs of increased intracranial pressure. Posterior fossa subdual hemorrhage treatment is supportive with correction of coagulopathy. Consultation with neurosurgery is recommended if there is hydrocephalus, severe hemorrhage, or dysfunction of the brainstem.
5. **Skull fracture.** The majority of skull fractures are asymptomatic. If there is any evidence of any neurologic deficit or if the depression is >1 cm, further imaging is necessary.
   a. **Linear skull fractures.** Uncomplicated linear skull fractures usually require only close follow-up evaluation and monitoring.
   b. **Depressed skull fractures. Check for neurologic deficits.**
      i. **If the fracture is <1 cm with no neurologic deficit,** manage by close monitoring.
      ii. **If the fracture is >1 cm.** Imaging with CT is recommended to rule out other intracranial lesions. Neurosurgical consultation is recommended as soon as possible if there is evidence of an intracranial lesion. A vacuum extractor or breast pump (*controversial*) has been used to elevate the fracture but is not routinely recommended because not enough studies have been done to prove that it is safe and effective.
      iii. **If cerebrospinal fluid leakage is seen** (usually from the nose or ears), start antibiotic therapy and consult neurosurgery immediately.
      iv. **Follow-up imaging is recommended** to rule out leptomeningeal cyst formation.
C. **Face**
   1. **Facial nerve injury.** No specific therapy is necessary. Full resolution usually occurs by 2 to 3 weeks. Neurology consult should be obtained if no improvement after 3 weeks.
      a. **Complete peripheral paralysis.** Cover the exposed eye with an eye patch and instill synthetic tears (1% methylcellulose drops) every 4 hours. This will prevent irritation from the dryness.
      b. **Electrodiagnostic testing.** May be beneficial in predicting recovery.
      c. **Surgery.** May be necessary in severe cases.
   2. **Fractures.** Maxilla, lacrimal, mandible, and nasal fractures require immediate evaluation because healing begins as early as 7 to 10 days and untreated fractures can result in subsequent eating issues and malocclusion. An oral airway is required, and surgical consultation is needed. The fractures must be reduced and fixated immediately. Otorhinolaryngology and plastic surgery consultations are recommended. If the fracture involves the sinus or middle ear, antibiotics are recommended. Treated fractures usually heal with no evidence of complications.
D. **Eyes.** Hemorrhages (subconjunctival or retinal) can occur after a vaginal delivery because of increased pressure and venous congestion. Ocular and periorbital injury can occur from malpositioned forceps. Ophthalmology consultation is recommended.
   1. **Eyelids.** Edema and bruising usually resolve within 1 week. **Laceration of the eyelid** may require microsurgery.
   2. **Orbit fracture.** Immediate ophthalmologic consultation is required.

      3. Horner syndrome. No treatment is necessary, and resolution usually occurs.
      4. Subconjunctival hemorrhage. No treatment is necessary because the blood is usually absorbed within 1 to 2 weeks. No long-term complications occur.
      5. Cornea. Haziness disappears usually within 2 weeks. If persistent and if rupture of Descemet membrane has occurred, then a white opacity of the cornea will occur. This is usually permanent, and ophthalmologic input is essential.
      6. Intraocular hemorrhage
        a. Subconjunctival hemorrhages usually resorb and resolve within 1 to 2 weeks. No long-term complications occur.
        b. Retinal hemorrhage. Usually disappears within 1 to 7 days. No treatment is necessary. If there is an associated optic nerve injury, there is increased risk of visual impairment.
        c. Hyphema (in anterior chamber). Usually resolves without treatment within 1 week.
        d. Vitreous hemorrhage. If resolution does not occur within 1 year, surgery must be considered.
  E. Ears. Consult an otolaryngologist if the temporal bone or cartilage is involved.
      1. Abrasions and ecchymoses. These injuries are usually mild and require no treatment, except for keeping the area clean, because they resolve spontaneously.
      2. Hematomas. Incision and evacuation may be indicated. Hematomas of the pinna should be drained to prevent the development of "cauliflower ear."
      3. Avulsion of the auricle. Surgical consultation is required if cartilage is involved.
      4. Laceration of the ear. Most of these can be sutured with 7–0 nylon sutures.
  F. Nose
      1. Protection of airway is essential and consult with otorhinolaryngology.
      2. Treat fractures promptly because deformities can occur if fractures are not fixed. Nose fractures start to heal as early as 7 days.
      3. Treatment of nasal dislocation is important to make sure there is no long-term septal deformity.
  G. Vocal cords
      1. Unilateral paralysis. Observe these infants closely. Keeping them quiet and giving small, frequent feedings decrease the risk of aspiration. This condition usually resolves within 4 to 6 weeks.
      2. Bilateral paralysis. Intubation is required if there is airway obstruction. Otorhinolaryngology consultation and tracheostomy are usually required. The prognosis is variable.
  H. Neck and shoulder
      1. Clavicular fracture. No specific treatment is necessary. Immobilization (pinning the infant's sleeve to the shirt) is sometimes done to help decrease pain, and the prognosis is excellent. Pain medication (acetaminophen) can be given. Once a callus is formed, the pain subsides.
      2. Brachial plexus injury/palsy. Once the diagnosis is made, physical therapy is started and continued weekly for at least 3 months. Immobilization and physical therapy help prevent contractures until the brachial plexus recovers. Recovery depends on the extent of the lesions and is usually good but may take many months. In Erb-Duchenne paralysis, one can see improvement in 2 weeks, and recovery is usually complete by 3 to 4 months. Orthopedic consultation is recommended early on, especially if no improvement of range of motion is seen; brachial plexus nerve root avulsion needs to be ruled out. Nerve reconstruction is ***controversial***; infants with brachial plexus nerve root avulsion are eligible, and if done, it is performed around age 6 months or older. Botulinum toxin has been used in older infants with contractures. Pain management is important, and infants tend to self-splint. Prognosis varies from 0% to 90% recovery. In Klumpke paralysis, the prognosis is poorer, and sometimes recovery is never complete. Muscle atrophy and contractures can occur.

3. **Phrenic nerve paralysis.** Treatment is close observation, usually supportive and nonspecific, and the prognosis is usually good, with recovery usually by 1 month. Some infants may require continuous positive airway pressure or mechanical ventilation. Surgical plication or diaphragmatic pacing may be pursued if recovery is not made.

4. **Sternocleidomastoid muscle injury.** Most recover spontaneously. Passive exercise (stretching of the muscle) should be started and done several times a day. It usually resolves by 3 to 4 months of age. Approximately 20% of cases do not resolve, and if it is not resolved within 6 months after physical therapy, surgery should be considered. Rule out hip dysplasia because 10% of SCM injuries will have it as well.

I. **Spinal cord.** Prognosis depends on the level and severity of the injury. Most infants with a severe spinal cord injury do not survive. Treatment is supportive, and some require intubation for respiratory problems. Specific therapy needs to be directed at the bladder, bowel, and skin because these present as ongoing problems. Neurology and neurosurgical consultations are recommended.

J. **Abdomen.** Surgical consultation is needed, and the prognosis for all of these injuries depends on early recognition and treatment. Early management strategies that increase survival include volume replacement and identifying and correcting coagulation disorders.

1. **Liver rupture.** Fluid resuscitation, transfusion to replace blood loss and clotting factors, possible surgery (laparotomy) with evacuation of hematomas, and repair of any laceration.

2. **Splenic rupture.** Volume replacement with transfusion of whole blood and correction of coagulation disorders. Exploratory laparotomy with preservation of the spleen, if possible.

3. **Adrenal hemorrhage.** Management is supportive, with blood transfusion and intravenous steroids for adrenal insufficiency. Surgery is rarely needed.

K. **Extremities**

1. **Fractured humerus.** Obtain an orthopedic consultation. Immobilize the arm with the elbow in 90 degrees for usually 2 weeks. Displaced fractures may require closed reduction and casting; the prognosis is excellent.

2. **Fractured femur.** Obtain an orthopedic consultation. Splinting and strict immobilization are necessary. For a stable undisplaced fracture, a splint is used. Unstable fractures require Pavlik harness or a spica cast. Overall, the prognosis is excellent.

3. **Epiphyseal separation.** Treatment is immobilization of the extremity for 10 to 14 days.

L. **Genitalia**

1. **Edema and bruising.** These usually resolve within 4 to 5 days, and no treatment is necessary.

2. **Testicular injury.** Urgent urologic or pediatric surgical consultation is necessary because rupture may require surgical repair.

3. **Hematocele.** Elevate the scrotum with cold packs. Resolution occurs without other treatment, unless there is a severe underlying testicular injury.

4. **Perineal lesions.** Pressure with a moist saline pack can control vulvar hematomas. A more serious injury (eg, perineal or rectovaginal injury or tear) may require multilayer primary repair.

84 Vasospasms and Thromboembolism

I. **Problem.** <u>An infant with an indwelling umbilical artery catheter develops a vaso-spasm in 1 leg. The nurse notifies you that another infant with an indwelling umbilical line has no pulses in the lower legs with severely decreased perfusion.</u> **Infants during the first month of life are at much higher risk of thrombosis and its complications when compared to any other pediatric age.** This is due to many factors: an immature coagulation and fibrinolytic system (hypofibrinolytic state, decreased synthesis and altered function of some coagulation proteins, accelerated clearance of factors, platelet function differences, more active coagulation mechanism), smaller vessel size, and frequent indwelling catheter use (thrombogenic material in catheter, catheter slows blood flow and may damage the vascular endothelium, frequent medications may damage vessel wall). Other risks include maternal, delivery, neonatal, acquired, and inherited prothrombotic abnormalities. Incidences vary depending on the source, type of thrombosis, and screening methods used, but overall incidence of a symptomatic thromboembolic event is 5.1 per 100,000 live births and 2.4 to 6.8 per 1000 neonatal intensive care unit (NICU) admissions, affecting term and preterm male and females equally.

II. **Immediate questions**

A. **Is there a catheter in place? Can the catheter be removed?** Catheters involved include central venous catheters, arterial and venous umbilical catheters, and other arterial catheters. The **most prevalent risk factor for an arterial or venous thrombosis** is an **indwelling vascular catheter.** It has been stated that "90% of thromboembolic events are catheter related." Evaluate the need for the catheter. If the catheter can be removed, this is the treatment of choice. **Vasospasm** is most commonly related to the use of umbilical artery catheters (UACs), but it can also occur in other catheters such as radial artery catheters. Over 90% of **venous thromboembolisms** in newborns are secondary to central venous lines. **Portal venous thrombosis** is often associated with the placement of an umbilical venous catheter (UVC). **Arterial thromboses** are almost always secondary to arterial vascular catheterization of central or peripheral arteries (UAC: renal artery thrombosis, aortic thrombosis). In some cases of thrombosis, **the catheter should not be removed so thrombolytic medication can be given** into the line. *Note:* **Renal vein thrombosis** is the most common type of venous thrombosis **not related to a central venous catheter.**

B. **Was a medication given recently through the catheter?** Most medications, if given too rapidly, can cause a vasospasm.

C. **How severe is the vasospasm?** Deciding on the severity of the vasospasm may dictate treatment choices (see Sections IV.B.1 and IV.B.2).

D. **Is there a pulse in the affected extremity?** A loss of pulse with a thrombus is a medical emergency.

E. **Does the infant have any risk factors for thromboembolism?**

1. **Maternal.** Advanced maternal age, hypertension, autoimmune disorders, premature rupture of membranes, maternal diabetes, maternal obesity, maternal lupus, preeclampsia, infertility, oligohydramnios, prothrombotic disorder, intrauterine growth restriction (IUGR), chorioamnionitis, family history of thrombosis, antiphospholipid or anticardiolipin antibodies.

2. **Delivery.** Instrumentation, fetal heart rate abnormalities, emergency delivery/cesarean section, traumatic delivery, induction with prolonged labor.

3. **Neonate.** Central arterial catheters (most common risk factor for arterial thromboembolism), central venous catheters (one of the most common risk factors for venous thromboembolism), cyanotic congenital heart disease, birth asphyxia,

sepsis, small for gestational age, IUGR, patent ductus arteriosus, respiratory distress syndrome, polycythemia, necrotizing enterocolitis (NEC), meconium staining, pulmonary hypertension, dehydration, major surgery, extracorporeal life support (ECLS), congenital renal vein defects, congenital nephrotic syndrome (increased venous thromboembolism risk) or nephritic syndrome, prematurity, hypotension, disseminated intravascular coagulation (DIC), impaired liver function, fluctuations in cardiac output, low cardiac output, prothrombotic disorders and elevated hematocrit (increases risk of UVC-associated thrombosis), postnatal steroid use in premature infants.

4. **Inherited factors.** Protein C (most common thrombophilic risk factor) or protein S deficiency, plasminogen deficiency, factor V Leiden mutation, antithrombin deficiency, elevated fasting homocysteine, prothrombin gene G20210A mutation, elevated lipoprotein(a) levels, and others.

III. **Differential diagnosis**

A. **Vasospasm is a muscular contraction (spasm) of an arterial vessel,** manifested by an acute color change (white or blue) in the perfused extremity (upper or lower extremity, sometimes only on the toes or fingers). Occasionally, the color change extends to the buttocks and the abdomen. The change in color is usually transient (usually <4 hours). It may be caused by prior injection of medication, intravascular arterial catheterization, or arterial blood sampling. A vasospasm can be a manifestation of a thromboembolism, but a thromboembolism will have discoloration of the skin that will not recover in 4 hours with other signs unique to the thromboembolism.

B. **Thromboembolism.** A **thrombosis** is the condition where a blood clot forms (a **thrombus**) in an artery or vein and can cause partial or complete obstruction. An **embolism** is the condition where part of the blood clot detaches, becomes mobile, and moves and lodges in a blood vessel and may cause obstruction or vasospasm. **Thromboembolism** is "blocking of a blood vessel by a particle that has broken away from a blood clot at its site of formation." A **thrombosis can be iatrogenic (catheter related) or spontaneous (non–catheter related) and can be arterial or venous.**

1. **Arterial thrombosis includes:** Aortic thrombosis, peripheral arterial thrombosis, mesenteric artery thrombosis, renal artery thrombosis, pulmonary embolism, neonatal arterial perinatal stroke.

2. **Venous thrombosis includes:** Limb thrombosis, renal vein thrombosis, inferior vena cava thrombosis, superior vena cava thrombosis, right atrial thrombosis, cerebral sinovenous thrombosis (CSVT), neonatal portal vein thrombosis, mesenteric venous thrombosis, umbilical vein thrombosis.

3. **Venous and arterial:** A **systemic air embolism** or **stroke** can occur from a venous or arterial embolism.

C. **Inherited/congenital thrombophilias.** Less commonly, thromboembolic phenomena are due to inherited or acquired thrombophilias. **Thrombophilia describes inherited or congenital blood coagulation disorders that predispose the infant to thrombosis.** Positive family history, early onset of disease, and >1 thromboembolism are clues to an inherited thrombophilia. **Prothrombotic genetic mutations** do not appear to increase the risk of umbilical catheter–associated thrombosis. The presence of inherited thrombophilias is increased in neonates with renal, portal, or hepatic venous thrombosis and stroke.

1. **Inherited/congenital.** Established genetic factors are factor V Leiden mutation, prothrombin G20210A mutation, protein C deficiency, protein S deficiency, and antithrombin deficiency. Rare genetic factors are hyperhomocystinemia (MTHR enzyme gene mutation) and dysfibrinogenemias. Other **indeterminate factors** include elevated factor VIII or IX or XI, tissue plasminogen activator, plasminogen deficiency, elevated lipoprotein (a), factor VII or XII, and others.

2. **Acquired.** Severe illness, sepsis, asphyxia, maternal lupus, maternal diabetes, and poor cardiac output are some of the risk factors of acquired thromboembolism. **All of these conditions can cause** deficiencies of protein C, protein S, or antithrombin III which can cause acquired thrombophilia. Elevated factor VIII activity, antiphospholipid antibodies, and lupus anticoagulant and anticardiolipin antibody can also cause it. Placental transfer of antibodies can cause an acquired thrombophilia in the newborn. Newborns with sepsis have an increased and ongoing consumption of coagulation factors and platelets, with reduced levels of protein C.

3. **Neonatal purpura fulminans is a rare but very severe condition that should be treated as a medical emergency** as it can cause loss of limbs from necrotic/gangrenous affected areas or be fatal. It can be inherited or acquired. If inherited, it is caused by a deficiency in protein C (more common) or a deficiency in protein S (less common) and presents after birth (2–12 hours) with ecchymosis, venous and arterial thromboses, and DIC. Severe protein C deficiency can cause severe complications (sometimes antenatally) such as thrombosis of cerebral vasculature and retinal detachment resulting in blindness. The **acquired form** is more common and usually occurs in older infants but has been described in neonates. It is secondary to a consumptive coagulopathy (infection such as eg group B *Streptococcus*, DIC, antiphospholipid antibodies, acute venous thrombosis, or cardiac bypass) or decreased synthesis (galactosemia, warfarin therapy, severe hepatic dysfunction, or severe congenital heart disease).

IV. **Database**

A. **History**

1. **For vasospasm:** Ask about what happened prior to the vasospasm. Was a medication given? Was an umbilical or percutaneous arterial line placed?

2. **For thrombosis:** Ask about risk factors (see earlier) and what signs the infant is showing. Obtain a detailed family history of any inherited clotting or other hematologic disorder.

B. **Physical examination.** The severity of the vasospasm and thrombosis must be assessed because it dictates treatment. Early clinical signs are similar in both vasospasm and thrombosis (pallor, cyanosis, weak peripheral pulses), and it may be difficult to differentiate a vasospasm from early signs of a thrombosis. The areas of involvement, appearance of the skin over the involved areas, and pulses of the affected extremity are measures of severity. Compare the affected extremity with the other extremity. A handheld Doppler is useful to assess peripheral arterial flow. Determine if the thrombosis is arterial or venous.

1. **Severe vasospasm.** Involves a large area of 1 or both legs, the abdomen, or the buttocks. In the upper extremity, a severe vasospasm includes most of the arm and all of the fingers. The skin may be completely white. Decreased perfusion is present, and pulses of the affected extremity are weak but detectable.

2. **Less severe vasospasm.** Involves a small area of 1 or both legs (usually some of the toes and part of the foot). In the arm, it can involve part of the extremity and some fingers. The skin has a mottled appearance, and pulses are present but can be diminished.

3. **Thrombosis.** A thrombosis can be arterial or venous. If pulses are completely absent, an arterial thrombosis, which is a medical emergency, is likely. Venous thrombosis is more common. Iatrogenic venous thrombosis in the newborn occurs most commonly from an indwelling venous catheter (90% central venous pressure or UVC) or from a non–catheter-related reason (most commonly renal vein thrombosis). **If catheter related,** presentation may include difficulty infusing and withdrawing from the line. Other signs are persistent thrombocytopenia and persistent infection. See Table 84–1 for clinical signs and symptoms of thromboembolism in critically ill neonates.

Table 84–1. CLINICAL SIGNS AND SYMPTOMS OF THROMBOEMBOLISM IN CRITICALLY ILL NEONATES

	Extremities	Intestine	Kidney	Aorta/Inferior Vena Cava	Central Nervous System	Lung
Arterial early signs	Extremities pale and/or cold Pulse weak or absent Blood pressure reduced	Mesenteric artery infarction: Feeding intolerance Gastric aspirates: bilious Stools: bloody Bowel wall pneumatosis	Renal artery thrombosis: Blood pressure elevated	Aorta: Blood pressure higher in arms than in legs	Arterial ischemic stroke: Lethargy Seizures (no hemiplegia)	Pulmonary embolism: Right heart failure Oxygen saturation low Ventilation/perfusion mismatch
Venous early signs	Venous thrombosis: Limb swelling Pain Cyanosis Hyperemic color	Portal vein: Impaired liver function Splenomegaly Hepatomegaly	Renal vein thrombosis: Hematuria Proteinuria Abdominal mass	Inferior vena cava: Hematuria Lower limb edema Both kidneys palpable Respiratory distress	Lethargy Seizures	
Late signs	Venous collaterals Reduced limb growth Postthrombotic syndrome (edema, pruritus, cellulitis, purpura, eczematous dermatitis)	Portal vein: Portal hypertension Gastrointestinal hemorrhage Hepatic atrophy Splenomegaly	Blood pressure abnormalities Renal insufficiency	Inferior vena cava: Leg and abdominal pain Varicose veins Postthrombotic syndrome	Neurodevelopmental delay Cognitive impairment Cerebral palsy	Right heart hypertrophy

Reproduced with permission from Veldman A, Nold MF, Michel-Behnke I: Thrombosis in the critically ill neonate: incidence, diagnosis, and management, *Vasc Health Risk Manag.* 2008;4(6):1337-1348.

4. Specific thromboses

  a. Venous thrombosis. Premature infants are more likely to have a venous thromboembolism than term infants. Most venous thromboses occur secondary to a central venous line. Sites in which a venous thrombosis can occur are limb (peripheral veins in limb), renal vein, inferior vena cava, superior vena cava, right atrium, cerebral sinovenous system, portal vein, mesenteric vein, umbilical vein, and less commonly adrenal and hepatic veins. Catheter-associated venous thrombosis in an infant usually presents with difficulty using the central venous line. Infants can have pulmonary embolism, organ impairment, or superior vena cava syndrome.

   i. Central venous line–associated venous thrombosis (peripheral/limb thrombosis). Malfunction of the central venous line. Symptoms include swollen and edematous extremities, pain, elevated temperature, cyanosis, hyperemia, and discoloration with distended superficial veins. Superior vena cava syndrome can develop in upper limb involvement.

   ii. Renal vein thrombosis is the most common type of spontaneous venous thrombosis (not related to a central venous catheter). Classic triad (seen in ~13%) includes gross hematuria, thrombocytopenia, and a palpable flank mass (unilateral or bilateral enlargement of the kidneys). Acute hypertension, proteinuria, and renal dysfunction can also occur. There is a higher male prevalence, it is usually unilateral (75%) or involves the left kidney (64%), and it is increased in premature infants, with a high level of thrombophilia. The majority of cases present in the first 3 days of life, but it can also develop in utero. In 50% of cases, the thrombosis reaches the vena cava (with lower limb cyanosis, edema, hypothermia); 25% of cases are bilateral. An acute scrotum (discoloration and pain upon palpation) can be caused by renal vein thrombosis.

   iii. Inferior vena cava thrombosis. Edematous, cool, cyanotic lower limbs, respiratory distress, and hypertension can also be seen. If renal vein is involved, obstruction of the renal vein (palpable kidneys and hematuria) can be seen.

   iv. Superior vena caval thrombosis. Common after repair of complex congenital heart disease. It can be asymptomatic or symptomatic (edema/swelling in upper limbs and head, chylothorax, heart failure).

   v. Right atrial thrombosis is a thrombosis of the superior vena cava with extension into the right atrium. The majority of patients have had a central venous catheter (most important risk factor), with an increased association of the catheter tip in the right atrium. Also occurs in infants with complex congenital heart disease undergoing repair. It can be asymptomatic (detected on echocardiography), or symptoms may include signs of congestive heart failure or right-sided heart failure (new murmur, bradycardia, tachyarrhythmia, respiratory distress, persistent sepsis, pericardial tamponade). Right atrial thrombi can be life threatening and disseminate into lungs or obstruct the right pulmonary artery (infant has acute onset of respiratory distress and stroke).

   vi. Cerebral sinovenous thrombosis is a multifactorial rare disease (2.6 per 100,000 newborns per year) and usually presents with generalized (most common) or focal seizures. Clinical symptoms include apnea, agitation, sepsis-like depressed consciousness, poor tone, respiratory distress, fetal distress, lethargy, and poor feeding. Most common sites are sinuses (multiple), superior sagittal sinus, straight sinus, and transverse sinus. **Thalamic hemorrhage suggests CSVT.**

    vii. **Portal vein thrombosis** is uncommon but is increasing in incidence. Risk is higher in neonates than in children. Clinical presentation is nonspecific or asymptomatic in 90%. Impaired liver function with elevations of liver enzymes, portal hypertension, hepatomegaly, and splenomegaly can be seen. UVC, exchange transfusion, omphalitis, sepsis, and thrombophilia are all risk factors. **UVC position** (unless placed in the portal vein) is not significantly associated with portal vein thrombosis.

    viii. **Mesenteric venous thrombosis** is very rare and presents with gradual onset of abdominal pain with vomiting, diarrhea, and hematochezia and with later signs once necrosis develops. Heme-positive stool is seen.

    ix. **Umbilical vein thrombosis.** Very rare but life threatening. The majority of cases have umbilical cord abnormalities (knot in cord, stretching of cord, obstetrical complications due to a systemic fetal condition such as maternal diabetes, hemolytic disease, fetomaternal transfusion). Portal vein thrombosis should be ruled out.

b. Arterial thrombosis. Less common than venous thrombosis, this occurs more commonly in the iliac, femoral, or cerebral arteries. Almost always related to arterial vascular catheterization of UAC (descending tract and renal arteries), peripheral arterial line, or femoral artery catheters. Symptoms depend on the location and size of the thrombus (line dysfunction, blanching, ischemia and cyanosis of the extremity, arterial hypertension, NEC, sepsis, persistent thrombocytopenia, and stroke). Incidence varies; one report indicated 1% to 3% based on clinical signs, 14% to 35% based on ultrasonogram findings, and 64% based on angiography. **Spontaneous (not catheter related)** arterial thromboses are rare but usually involve the iliac artery, left pulmonary artery, aortic arch, and descending aorta, and symptoms depend on the location. Neonatal arterial thrombosis can occur in the aorta and present as cyanotic heart disease such as coarctation of the aorta. Sites in which arterial thrombosis can occur include aorta, peripheral arteries, mesenteric arteries, renal arteries, and pulmonary arteries. Infants can have renal failure, hypertension, organ failure, peripheral gangrene, intestinal necrosis, and death.

    i. **Aortic thrombosis.** Rare in newborns. UAC will stop working, and blood pressure will be higher in the arms than in the legs. Decreased or no pulses in the lower extremities with color change and a decrease in perfusion. Oliguria, microscopic or gross hematuria, signs of NEC, systemic hypertension, or congestive heart failure can be seen. Congenital cytomegalovirus infection has been implicated as a cause of **aortic arch thrombosis** since it can infect and damage vascular endothelium. *Note:* Aortic thrombosis can mimic NEC (bowel ischemia) and coarctation of the aorta (blood pressure differences in the upper and lower body).

    ii. **Peripheral arterial thrombosis.** Radial, posterior tibial, and dorsalis pedis arterial lines are rarely associated with thrombosis. Signs include weak or absent peripheral pulse, pallor of the extremities, coldness, and decreased perfusion of the extremity. Acute arterial occlusion in a limb in a newborn is rare.

    iii. **Mesenteric artery thrombosis.** Similar to signs of NEC. (Bloody stools, bilious aspirates, abdominal pain, feeding intolerance, pneumatosis).

    iv. **Renal artery thrombosis.** Causes elevated blood pressure, with or without renal failure.

v. **Umbilical artery catheter–associated thromboses.** Asymptomatic or presents with poor perfusion and blanching of ≥1 toe, 1 or both limbs, or buttocks. Occlusion of the renal arteries (hypertension, renal failure), occlusion of the mesenteric arteries (NEC), or occlusion of the spinal arteries (spinal cord infarction) can occur.

vi. **Pulmonary embolism.** Very rare with only a few cases reported in neonates. Clinical signs include respiratory failure. It can be seen in infants with congenital heart disease with right heart failure, poor oxygenation, and ventilation/perfusion mismatch.

vii. **Spontaneous arterial thromboembolism.** Very rare in infancy. Most common thrombotic sites include, in descending frequency: umbilical, aorta, extremities, cerebral, subclavian, pulmonary, and placental. Risk factors include congenital, acquired, inherited prothrombotic risk, and maternal. Evaluate for prothrombotic disorder.

c. **Venous or arterial embolism/occlusion.** These include systemic air embolism or a stroke.

i. **Systemic air embolism.** In neonates, it is devastating and usually fatal. Most iatrogenic air emboli are venous and occur from central venous catheters (UVC, peripherally inserted central catheter [PICC]), but rarely can also occur from peripheral venous or arterial lines. A disconnected line is a common cause. Air embolism secondary to mechanical ventilation (barotrauma leads to systemic gas embolism) is rare but can occur in premature infants. Suspect embolism if air bubbles are in the infusion line. Clinical signs of systemic air embolism are usually sudden and dramatic and can include pallor, cyanosis, hypoxemia, seizures, shock, bradycardia, respiratory distress, mottling of the skin, or neurologic deficits (if central nervous system [CNS] emboli) such as paraplegia. Infants with cyanotic congenital heart disease are at a risk for **cerebral arterial gas embolism** from infusion lines.

ii. **Neonatal and perinatal stroke.** This is classified as a cerebrovascular accident that occurs from 20 weeks' gestation up to 28 days of life after birth and includes ischemic (blockage of vessel) and hemorrhagic (blood vessel ruptures and bleeds) event. These include perinatal arterial ischemic stroke, hemorrhagic stroke, and CSVT. Incidence is 1 in 1600 to 4000 live births. Ischemic stroke accounts for 80%, and 20% are CSVT or hemorrhage. **Ischemic strokes are either arterial (thromboembolism/thrombosis) or venous. Neonates present with seizures (focal or generalized)** 12 to 72 hours after birth with nonspecific neurologic signs including lethargy, temperature instability, feeding difficulties, respiratory failure, and encephalopathy (hypertonic/irritable or hypotonic/lethargic). With CSVTs, a tense anterior fontanel, engorged scalp veins, and diastasis of the cranial sutures may be seen. They rarely present with a unilateral motor deficit (hemiparesis), as seen in older children.

(a) **Perinatal arterial ischemic stroke** is occlusion of the cerebral arterial flow entering the brain that most commonly occurs from arterial infarction in the left hemisphere. Most (89%) present with an isolated lesion in anterior circulation (internal carotid artery, anterior cerebral artery, and middle cerebral artery), most often left sided. Usually secondary to embolism (indwelling intravascular catheters) but can also be secondary to lupus anticoagulant. Placental pathology may play a role in the etiology. Most infants present within the first 3 days of life with seizures (95%), abnormal tone, or altered mental status. Other symptoms are nonspecific (feeding difficulties, respiratory problems, hemiparesis).

    (b) **Hemorrhagic stroke (includes parenchymal, subarachnoid, or intraventricular hemorrhage).** Secondary from intracranial hemorrhage from ischemic infarction of arterial/venous or primary intraparenchymal hemorrhage. Causes include idiopathic, bleeding diatheses or vascular anomalies, ECMO, vitamin K deficiency, coarctation of the aorta, and venous thrombosis. Presents with seizures, apnea, poor feeding, hypotonia, encephalopathy, and focal weakness.

    (c) **Cerebral sinovenous thrombosis is very rare and occurs when there is occlusion of the venous blood flow in a major sinus.** It can cause hemorrhagic infarction and bleeding and usually involves the superior sagittal and lateral sinuses. Majority of cases are secondary to preeclampsia, diabetes, and chorioamnionitis in the mother or systemic illness and inherited thrombophilia in the neonate. Presents with focal/generalized seizures, lethargy, irritability, poor feeding, jitteriness, cranial nerve palsies, hemiparesis, and decreased level of consciousness.

    (d) **Inherited thrombophilias.** See Chapter 92.

C. **Laboratory studies.** Not usually needed for vasospasm. Infants with non–catheter-related thromboses or severe, recurrent, or spontaneous thromboses should undergo further laboratory testing. A baseline coagulation profile should be obtained if a thrombosis is suspected and clot-dissolving medication is to be used.

    1. **Baseline coagulation profile.** Prothrombin time (PT), activated partial thromboplastin time (aPTT), thrombin time, international normalized ratio (INR), plasma fibrinogen concentration.

    2. **Complete blood count with peripheral blood smears.**

    3. **Platelet count.** Thrombocytopenia usually accompanies thrombosis in neonates and is one of the most sensitive indicators of thrombosis. The thrombus itself and the use of heparin can cause thrombocytopenia.

    4. **D-dimer measurement.** Negative D-dimers can rule out thrombosis.

    5. **Genetic tests.** May be done at some point to evaluate congenital thrombophilia.

    6. **Cytomegalovirus workup if suspected.** See Chapter 132.

    7. **Workup for a suspected prothrombotic disorder.** Includes antithrombin, protein S, and protein C concentrations; activated protein C resistance; factor V Leiden mutation; prothrombin gene 20210A mutation; lipoprotein levels; and plasma homocysteine values. Maternal testing for lupus anticoagulant and anticardiolipin antibody. See Chapter 92 for more details.

D. **Imaging and other studies.** Imaging confirms the diagnosis of a vascular thrombosis, but the best imaging modality is *controversial*. Catheter angiography is the most accurate imaging technique but is invasive and has high radiation exposure; therefore, it is used selectively and usually as a last test. Common approach is to start with a Doppler ultrasound and, if negative, go on to magnetic resonance imaging (MRI) or computed tomography (CT) or a more invasive test. **Cranial ultrasound prior to starting any antithrombotic therapy is essential.**

    1. **Doppler ultrasound (real-time ultrasonography with color Doppler flow imaging).** Commonly the first imaging test used, it can evaluate blood flow through arteries and veins. It is readily available and noninvasive with no exposure to radiation. It can also be used to monitor progress over time. In renal vein thrombosis, ultrasound shows enlarged echogenic kidneys with a loss of renal corticomedullary differentiation, and in color Doppler ultrasound studies, there is absence of flow in the involved veins. Transfontanellar Doppler ultrasound can help diagnose an ischemic stroke.

    2. **Magnetic resonance angiography.** Usually performed under sedation or general anesthesia (to limit motion artifact). Recommended to diagnose perinatal ischemic stroke in term infants.

3. **Computed tomography angiography.** Injection of contrast material with CT scanning to diagnose arterial and venous vessel disease. Quicker test than MRI, and sedation not always required.

4. **Ultrasound of the head.** To evaluate for intraventricular hemorrhage (IVH) before initiating thrombolytic therapy.

5. **Computed tomography of the head.** To evaluate for CSVT or to identify intracranial air bubbles in air embolism.

6. **"Linograms."** Injecting radiopaque dye directly into the catheter to detect an intraluminal clot.

7. **Contrast venography/magnetic resonance venography** is considered the gold standard for diagnosing neonatal catheter-induced thromboembolism. Done by injection of contrast through peripheral vessels.

8. **Catheter angiography uses magnetic resonance imaging, computed tomography, or plain x-ray.** Contrast is injected in a catheter to produce images of a major blood vessel. Can be performed through the UAC and can be used to diagnose aortoiliac thrombosis. In several studies, this procedure was found to be the most effective diagnostic technique. It can be used to diagnose an ischemic neonatal stroke. A contrast study should be considered before administrating a fibrinolytic agent. Remember, this test is difficult to perform in sick neonates. MRI angiography can also be used to diagnose pulmonary embolism.

9. **Magnetic resonance imaging/diffusion magnetic resonance imaging** to diagnose a stroke from a venous sinus thrombosis.

10. **Echocardiography (transthoracic)** is used to diagnose right atrial thrombosis. An echocardiogram of venous air embolism shows an acute obstruction of the right ventricular outflow tract secondary to air embolism (known as an "air lock").

11. **Ventilation/perfusion scan** to diagnose rare pulmonary embolism.

V. **Plan.** Management of vasospasms is *controversial*, whereas the management of thrombosis is largely based on treatment plans for older children and adults. Current management protocols for thrombophilia can be obtained from the International Children's Thrombophilia Network (phone: 1-800-NO-CLOTS). The network was established as a free consultative service and to develop collaborative research studies.

A. **Key management points**

1. **Monitor for potential signs of vasospasm or thromboembolic complications** in all infants with any intravascular catheter.

2. **Thromboembolism can occur in newborns** and produce little or no clinical symptoms.

3. **Heparin is often added to neonatal infusions** because it prolongs patency, extends catheter life (UACs, UVCs, PICCs, peripheral arterial catheters), and may also decrease the incidence of thromboembolic occlusions. For extremely low birthweight infants, use the lowest dose. There are no randomized trials of heparin use in PICCs, but its use is common in NICUs. Heparin use in UVCs is *controversial*, but the majority of NICUs use heparin in UVCs. Heparin is not used in peripheral intravenous (IV) lines. **Common recommendations include the following:**

a. **Central venous lines** (UVC, PICC, percutaneous central venous catheter). The American College of Chest Physicians Evidence-Based Clinical Practice Guidelines study recommends heparin in central venous access devices (CVADs) to maintain patency. They recommend unfractionated heparin (UFH) continuous infusion at 0.5 U/kg/h or intermittent local thrombolysis to maintain CVAD patency. Cochrane review supports the prophylactic use of heparin in peripherally placed percutaneous central venous catheters in neonates and recommends monitoring for side effects. For a blocked CVAD, local thrombolysis after clinical assessment is recommended.

    b. **Peripheral arterial catheters.** The American College of Chest Physicians Evidence-Based Clinical Practice Guidelines study recommends UFH continuous infusion at 0.5 U/mL at 1 mL/h.

    c. **Umbilical artery catheters.** Heparin (0.25–1 U/mL) for a total heparin dose of 25 to 200 U/kg/d to maintain patency. Per the Perinatal Continuing Education Program, 12 U/kg body weight/h is recommended for continuous infusion. Cochrane review notes the use of heparin (as low as 0.25 U/mL) is recommended to prolong the life of the catheter by decreasing the incidence of catheter occlusion. It does not decrease the incidence of UAC-related aortic thrombosis. Heparinization of intermittent flushes alone is ineffective in preventing catheter occlusion. The **American Academy of Pediatrics** recommends low doses of heparin (0.25–1.0 U/L) through the UAC. The **American College of Chest Physicians Evidence-Based Clinical Practice Guidelines** (2012) recommend prophylaxis with a low-dose UFH infusion via the UAC (heparin concentration of 0.25–1 U/mL; total heparin dose of 25–200 U/kg/d to maintain patency).

    d. **Congenital nephrotic syndrome.** Because infants with congenital nephrotic syndrome are at risk of venous thromboembolism, some advocate giving prophylactic anticoagulant therapy depending on the severity. Infants who develop venous thromboembolism should be treated with anticoagulant therapy for the duration of the nephrotic syndrome.

4. **Umbilical lines should be removed as soon as possible when they are no longer needed** because duration of both UACs and UVCs is a significant risk factor for thrombosis. The Centers for Disease Control and Prevention recommends that UACs should not be left in place >5 days after insertion and that UVCs should be removed as soon as possible but can be used for up to 14 days.

5. **High umbilical artery catheters** have a lower incidence of thrombotic complications and a longer catheter life. Low UACs are associated with an increased incidence of vasospasms and cyanosis of the extremities. Cochrane review and the American College of Chest Physicians Evidence-Based Clinical Practice Guidelines recommend **high position** for UACs. Some advocate abandoning low UACs due to the risks involved (see Chapter 28).

6. **Use a peripheral arterial line over a UAC.** Choose a safer site for a peripheral arterial line that has collateral circulation (radial, dorsalis pedis, posterior tibial arteries, ulnar arteries).

7. **If there is difficulty infusing into the line,** consider a thrombotic event.

8. **Heparinization of flush solution** without heparinization of the infusate is inadequate. Use of intermittent heparin flushes has no benefit over normal saline (NS) flushes.

9. **Always use umbilical artery catheters** with a hole at the end and not the side, as the side hole may increase aortic thrombosis risk. Single-lumen construction is associated with a decrease in thrombosis. Cochrane review states that side hole catheters should be avoided for UACs in neonates.

10. **The use of multiple-lumen umbilical venous catheters** is associated with a decrease in the need for peripheral IV lines in the first week of life but with an increase in catheter malfunctions.

11. **Heparin-bonded catheters versus polyvinyl chloride catheters** showed no difference in the incidence of aortic thrombosis or duration of patency.

12. **A peripherally inserted central catheter line** has a lower incidence of thrombosis when compared to a central line. The highest incidence is in femoral lines.

13. **Papaverine, an opium alkaloid with vasodilatory and spasmolytic action,** was found to prolong the patency of peripheral arterial catheters in a study of neonates, with no difference in the incidence of IVH (*controversial*).

14. **Peripheral nerve block (case reports only)** has successfully been used as an effective treatment for neonatal vascular spasm and/or thrombosis causing limb ischemia. The mechanism is induction of vasodilatation of the peripheral vessels (sympathetic blockade) and inhibition of peripheral vasoconstriction (decreased pain release of antidiuretic hormone, cortisol, and catecholamines).

15. **Hyperbaric oxygen therapy** (*experimental and controversial*). Anecdotal evidence in a case report of **hyperbaric oxygen therapy combined with anti-coagulant therapy** demonstrated improved outcome of neonatal arterial thromboembolism of lower extremities.

B. **Vasospasm.** This can be secondary to a **peripheral arterial line or UAC.** Treatment is *controversial*, and guidelines vary extensively. Check your institution's guidelines before initiating treatment. Rapid intervention is recommended. Noninvasive treatments include removal of the catheter and warming the contralateral extremity. Secondary treatments include topical vasodilators and other medications (papaverine, lidocaine). Use of heparin and thrombolytics is not recommended. If the vasospasm does not resolve with treatment and the tissue ischemia persists, this could represent the primary event leading to thrombosis and a change in management.

1. **Severe vasospasm of the leg or arm**

   a. **If possible, remove the catheter.** Spontaneous resolution is likely with some success in warming the contralateral extremity before removing the catheter. If warming does not resolve the vasospasm, remove the catheter. If warming does resolve the vasospasm, closely follow the infant, and if the vasospasm returns, remove the catheter.

   b. **Warming the contralateral leg/arm.** Wrap the entire *unaffected* leg in a warm (not hot) washcloth. This measure dilates the blood vessels in the unaffected arm and causes a sympathetic **reflex vasodilatation** response in the affected arm. Treatment should continue for 15 minutes before a beneficial effect is seen. Do not wrap the affected arm or leg, as this will increase the metabolic demand and blood flow to an area that is already compromised.

   c. **If symptoms persist after warming contralateral extremity and removing the catheter:**

      i. **Topical nitroglycerin therapy** (*controversial*) (2% ointment, 4 mm/kg, applied as a thin film over the area). Nitroglycerin has a direct vasodilating effect on vascular smooth muscle, is readily absorbed through the skin, and improves circulation. Reports note 1 application, but some repeat it every 8 hours for 2 to 27 days. Improvement was usually seen within 15 to 45 minutes. Observe for hypotension.

      ii. **Papaverine** (*controversial*). A spasmolytic and mild vasodilator with direct action on vascular smooth muscle. Dosing is 1 mg intramuscularly in the unaffected leg; the effect is apparent within 30 minutes.

      iii. **Lidocaine** has been used intra-arterially for vasospasm. It has a vasodilating effect with questionable results (*controversial*).

      iv. **Intra-arterial lidocaine and papaverine** have been used successfully to treat a catheter-induced vasospasm during arterial catheterization (*controversial*, case reports only).

   d. **If it is not possible to remove the catheter (as in a tiny infant) and this is the only catheter.** Consider a papaverine-containing solution (60 mg/500 mL in 1/2 NS with 1.0 U/mL heparin) through the catheter as a continuous infusion for 24 to 48 hours (*controversial*). If the vasospasm resolves, the infusion may be stopped. If the vasospasm does not resolve, remove the catheter. **Exercise caution using this technique** in premature infants in the first few days of life where the incidence of developing an intracranial hemorrhage is high.

2. **Less severe vasospasm of the leg/arm.** Follow recommendations in Sections V.B.1.a and V.B.1.b for severe spasm.

C. **Problems with vasospasm and peripheral tissue ischemia.** Ischemia can some-times occur after a vasospasm. Even after a catheter has been removed, a persis-tent vasospasm or small emboli in distal end arteries can cause poor perfusion of an extremity. **Topical 2% nitroglycerin ointment** (4 mm/kg of body weight) can be applied to the ischemic area with no adverse effects except mild episodes of decreased blood pressure (*controversial*). One small study found that **intra-arterial papaverine** before removal of the patent arterial line was effective in preventing residual damage in arterial catheterization–induced ischemia in extremely low birthweight neonates.

D. **Thromboembolism.** If suspected and there is loss of pulses in the affected extremity, it is a **medical emergency.** Symptomatic thrombosis can lead to irreversible organ damage or loss of limbs or digits. The most common treatments are observation with supportive care, anticoagulation therapy with heparin or low molecular weight hepa-rin (LMWH), thrombolytic agents (clot-dissolving drugs, streptokinase, and tissue plasminogen activator), or surgery. Clot-dissolving drugs can cause severe bleeding, and there are no current randomized trials comparing these treatments. Manage-ment is *controversial.* Treatment depends on the extent and severity of the thrombus (occlusive or nonocclusive thrombosis, life-threatening thrombosis, thrombosis that can lead to loss of limb or organ). Management is similar for peripheral arterial thrombosis, venous thrombosis, and aortic thrombosis.

1. **Asymptomatic thrombosis.** Supportive care and monitoring of the size of the thrombus. If the thrombus advances, therapy with an anticoagulant may be necessary.
2. **Mild or minor thrombosis.** This can present with decreased limb perfusion, hypertension, and hematuria and can usually be treated with removal of the catheter, supportive care, and close ultrasonographic follow-up. Many of these resolve spontaneously.
3. **Moderate thrombosis.** This has all the findings of mild/minor thrombosis plus oliguria and congestive heart failure. Can be treated with systemic heparin therapy and with management of systemic hypertension.
4. **Major thrombosis.** Presents with all of the above plus major multiorgan failure. Should be treated aggressively with systemic heparin therapy, antithrombolytic agents, and supportive care. May require further evaluation for underlying hypercoagulative disorder.

E. **General guidelines for thrombosis treatment.** Treatment involves supportive care, observation only, thrombolytic and/or anticoagulant therapy, and surgery. (See also Chapter 92.) It is best to consult a pediatric hematologist experienced in treating thrombosis prior to starting therapy and have the hematologist manage the patient.

1. **Supportive care**
   a. **Prompt removal of the catheter is indicated** unless it is needed to facilitate arteriography or thrombolytic drug infusion. A CVAD or UVC should be removed after 3 to 5 days of thrombolytic therapy. Peripheral arterial catheters should be removed immediately; this is mandatory in their management except in rare isolated cases.
   b. **Prior to starting antithrombotic therapy,** obtain PT, aPTT, and platelet and fibrinogen levels.
   c. **Treatment of volume depletion, electrolyte abnormalities, sepsis, thrombocytopenia, and anemia is essential.** Control hypertension and any coagulation deficiency or hypofibrinogenemia before initiation of treatment.
   d. **Emergency consultation** with vascular surgery and pediatric hematology is recommended.
   e. **Evaluate patients for intraventricular hemorrhage** before initiating thrombolytic therapy. A cranial ultrasound is a must. During treatment, ultrasounds of the head should be obtained at regular intervals.

    f. **Absolute contraindications for thrombolytic therapy.** Contraindications include the following: CNS surgery in the previous 3 weeks, major surgery or bleeding in the past 10 days or birth asphyxia in the past 7 days, evidence of active bleeding, invasive procedures within previous 3 days, seizures within the past 48 hours, gestational age <32 weeks, and thrombolytic therapy.

    g. **Relative contraindications** for anticoagulant and thrombolytic therapy are hypertension, severe coagulation deficiency, platelet count <50 × 10^4/mm^3 (<100 × 10^4/mm^3 for ill neonates), fibrinogen concentration <100 mg/dL, and INR >2.

    h. **The Neonatal Central Venous Line Observational Study on Thrombosis (NEOCLOT)** is being conducted in the Netherlands to address catheter-related thrombosis (central venous catheter thrombosis) management in a clinical trial (*BMC Pediatrics*, February 23, 2018).

2. **Heparin therapy is recommended** for clinically significant thrombosis with the purpose of preventing embolism or expansion of the clot. **LMWHs** are best because of the following advantages: reduced need for laboratory monitoring, subcutaneous dosing, longer half-life (dose every 12–24 hours), more predictable response, decreased risk of osteopenia and heparin-induced thrombocytopenia, and decreased risk of bleeding. **Advantages of UFH** are the fast reversibility and low cost. Cochrane review found no evidence to recommend or refute the use of heparin for the treatment of neonates with thrombosis. Monitor platelet counts if heparin is used. Obtain daily complete blood count with platelets and aPTT. **General recommendations are as follows:**

    a. **Low molecular weight heparin therapy using enoxaparin (Lovenox)** is the treatment of choice in neonates with symptomatic thrombosis. Other LMWH preparations include dalteparin and reviparin. For therapeutic treatment in infants <2 months of age, use enoxaparin 1.5 mg/kg/dose every 12 hours subcutaneously; if >2 months, use 1.0 mg/kg/dose subcutaneously. Recent studies reinforce the necessity and safety of higher doses to achieve target anti–factor Xa levels (1.7 mg/kg in term infants, 2 mg/kg in preterm infants every 12 hours subcutaneously). Follow anti–factor Xa activity levels 4 to 6 hours after subcutaneous dose (target anti–factor Xa range of 0.5–1 U/mL; or target anti–factor Xa range of 0.5– 0.8 U/mL in a sample taken 2–6 hours after subcutaneous injection). Adjust as needed.

    b. **Unfractionated (standard) heparin is preferred over low molecular weight heparin in patients with renal insufficiency.** Load 75 U/kg IV over 10 minutes, then 28 U/kg/h maintenance through a dedicated IV line. (Premature infants: 25–50 U/kg/h over 10 minutes, then 15–20 U/kg/h.) **Adjust based on aPTT 4 hours after initiation of each dosing change** (target aPTT 60–85 seconds). Duration of therapy is generally 5 to 14 days. Always increase or decrease the infusion amount by 10%, depending on the aPTT. If the aPTT is >96 seconds, hold the heparin for 30 to 60 minutes and start at a lower infusion rate. Avoid long-term use of therapeutic UFH in children.

    c. **If urgent reversal of unfractionated heparin effect is needed due to bleeding or heparin-induced thrombocytopenia,** IV protamine can be given based on the total amount of heparin administered in the previous 2 hours. Stopping the infusion is usually sufficient for LMWH, and protamine is only partially effective. Dosing is 1 mg of protamine per 100 U of heparin via IV infusion over 10 minutes.

    d. **Duration of thrombosis treatment.** This has not been established; guidelines include between 6 weeks and 3 months.

    e. **During anticoagulant therapy,** maintain the platelet count >50 × 10^9/L and the fibrinogen >100 mg/dL.

3. **Oral anticoagulants.** Not recommended in neonates (bleeding risk, difficulty in maintaining therapeutic doses, drug interactions including vitamin K content of the diet, tablet formulation). May be indicated for some cases of long-term management. Two therapies are used: warfarin or acenocoumarol. Initial dose is 0.2 mg/kg/d to achieve an INR between 2 and 3. Other dose reported is 0.33 mg/kg/d. If bleeding occurs from an excessive dose, give vitamin K.

4. **Thrombolytic drugs.** These medications break down fibrin by converting plasminogen to plasmin. Do not use in milder cases, and few studies have been done in very preterm infants. With life-threatening thrombosis the possibility of limb loss or organ damage, 1 of these drugs may be used. Treatment with thrombolytics is ***controversial***, and it is best to follow institutional guidelines. When using thrombolytic therapy, maintain a platelet count >50 × 10^4/mm^3 (50 × 10^9/L) and fibrinogen >100 mg/dL using selected platelet transfusion and cryoprecipitate. Monitor PT/INR, partial thromboplastin time (PTT), and fibrinogen every 4 hours. If the catheter is still patent, the medications can be given through it. If the catheter is obstructed and needs to be removed, systemic therapy is used. Recombinant tissue plasminogen activator (tPA) is more effective near the thrombus than streptokinase or urokinase).

   a. **Recombinant tissue plasminogen activator (alteplase)** has become the **drug of choice** over the older agents streptokinase or urokinase (lower risk of allergies, the shortest half-life, fewer manufacturing concerns). It has an increased affinity for fibrin-bound plasminogen, making it more effective near the thrombus. See Chapter 155 for dosage.

   b. **Infusion of intra-arterial streptokinase** has been successful in some infants. One study found the efficacy and safety were similar to tPA. Dosing is 2000 U/kg IV over 30 to 60 minutes or 1000 to 2000 U/kg/h as continuous infusion for 6 to 12 hours. Lower doses (500 U/kg/h) have been effective. In 1 study of aortoiliac thrombosis, a dose of 50 U/kg/h given directly into the clot was effective. Because of systemic side effects (allergic and toxic reactions and bleeding), its use has declined.

   c. **Urokinase** is no longer available in the United States but may be used in other countries; it is not formally approved for use in children. Dose reported has been 4400 U/kg initial bolus dose IV over 10 minutes, then 4400 U/kg/h for 6 to 12 hours.

   d. **The newer thrombolytic agents argatroban, bivalirudin, and fondaparinux have limited data in pediatrics.** Argatroban (direct thrombin inhibitor) has been used for heparin-induced thrombocytopenia in adults. There is not enough evidence to warrant its use. Bivalirudin (direct thrombin inhibitor) has had 1 study in pediatric patients and 1 in infants. Fondaparinux is a selective antithrombin-dependent factor Xa inhibitor with no studies in patients <1 year of age. The **target-specific oral anticoagulants**/direct oral anticoagulants (direct factor Xa inhibitors and direct factor IIa inhibitors) dabigatran, rivaroxaban, and apixaban may be promising because they have high bioavailability and rapid onset of action, limit the need for monitoring, have minimal interactions and foreseeable anticoagulant effects, and are under study in children.

5. **Catheter-directed thrombolysis.** A method in which the thrombolytic agent is injected directly into the thrombus. In some reports, it is superior to systemic thrombolytic therapy with fewer side effects. It has also been used if neonates fail to respond to UFH therapy. **For a blocked CVAD**, local thrombolysis is recommended after clinical assessment. **For neonates with limb-threatening or organ-threatening femoral artery thrombosis** who fail initial UFH therapy, thrombolysis is recommended. Drug of choice is tPA with a dose of 0.01 to 0.05 mg/kg/h.

6. **Surgery.** Microsurgery has been successfully performed in a small subset of neonates and may be indicated in the presence of an occluding embolism if thrombolysis is contraindicated for peripheral arterial occlusion, but it is rarely recommended because of the small caliber of their blood vessels, frequent reocclusion, and the poor clinical status of the infant with the thrombosis. Guidelines are not well established. Surgical options include thrombectomy, microvascular reconstruction, vascular decompression through the use of a fasciotomy, mechanical disruption of the thrombus (medical thrombectomy), and amputation. If antithrombotic therapy is contraindicated, arteriotomy, embolectomy, and microvascular reconstruction are options.

7. **Specific treatments**

   a. **Peripheral arterial catheter–related thromboembolism.** Remove the catheter immediately. In symptomatic peripheral arterial catheter–related thromboembolism, UFH anticoagulation with or without thrombolysis or surgical thrombectomy with microvascular repair with heparin therapy is recommended. Surgical consult is recommended. Thrombolytic therapy is recommended if viability of the limb or organ is compromised.

   b. **Central venous access devices or umbilical venous catheters with confirmed thrombosis.** Remove CVAD or UVC after 3 to 5 days of therapeutic anticoagulation. Recommendation: initial anticoagulation or supportive care with radiologic monitoring for extension of the thrombosis. In infants who have not been treated, start anticoagulation if extension occurs. Start with either LMWH or UFH, and then administer LMWH for a total duration of 6 weeks to 3 months. Give a prophylactic dose of anticoagulation if either the CVAD or UVC is still in after completion of therapeutic anticoagulation until it is removed. If the VTE is causing major occlusion, resulting in critical compromise of limbs or organ, use tPA and fresh-frozen plasma (FFP) prior to finishing treatment.

   c. **Acute femoral artery thrombosis.** Therapeutic doses of IV UFH as initial therapy or LMWH for a total of 5 to 7 days of anticoagulation. For infants with limb-threatening or organ-threatening femoral artery thrombosis who fail to respond to UFH therapy and in whom there are no contraindications: thrombolysis. With contraindications and when organ or limb death is imminent: surgical intervention.

   d. **Renal vein thrombosis.** Treatment is ***controversial***. Outcomes are similar between supportive care and anticoagulation. Anticoagulant therapy with heparin has improved survival and prevents renal atrophy. Remove the central catheter in the inferior vena cava if present.

      i. **Supportive care.** Correction of fluid and electrolyte disturbances and treatment of infection. If DIC, consider UFH/LMWH.

      ii. **Unilateral (no renal impairment, no inferior vena cava extension).** Either supportive care with close observation and follow-up by radiology for extension of thrombosis or start on anticoagulation therapy with UFH/LMWH or LMWH in therapeutic doses for total duration between 6 weeks and 3 months. **Unilateral (with extension into inferior vena cava):** anticoagulation for 6 weeks to 3 months. Possible surgery.

      iii. **Bilateral renal vein thrombosis with evidence of renal impairment:** Anticoagulation with UFH/LMWH or initial thrombolytic therapy with tPA, followed by anticoagulation with UFH/LMWH.

      iv. **Patients with renal insufficiency:** UFH is preferred over LMWH. If using LMWH, use a lower dose.

e. Stroke. Anticoagulant therapy is usually not recommended; the exception is a cardioembolic stroke where anticoagulant therapy is used. Treatment should consist of avoiding or managing seizures.

    i. **Venous sinus thrombosis (without significant intracerebral hemorrhage).** Heparinization is recommended for 6 weeks to 3 months. **With significant intracerebral hemorrhage:** anticoagulation or supportive care with radiologic monitoring, and anticoagulation if extension of the thrombus occurs.

    ii. **First arterial ischemic stroke with no documented ongoing cardioembolic source.** Supportive care is recommended over anticoagulation. **With documented cardioembolic source,** anticoagulation recommended with UFH or LMWH.

    iii. **Recurrent arterial ischemic stroke.** Anticoagulant or aspirin therapy.

    iv. **Cerebral sinovenous thrombosis without significant intracranial hemorrhage.** Anticoagulation, initially with UFH or LMWH and then LMWH for 6 weeks to 3 months.

f. **Cerebral sinovenous thrombosis with significant hemorrhage.** Either anticoagulation or supportive care with monitoring by radiology of the thrombosis at 5 to 7 days and anticoagulation if the thrombus extends.

g. **Right atrial thrombosis.** Remove central venous catheter. Small thrombi possibly can be treated conservatively (*controversial*). Start anticoagulation therapy with UFH or LMWH. If compromised cardiac function, start tPA.

h. **Systemic air embolism.** Use caution in setting up infusion lines with complex parts; use of IV fluid filters may decrease air embolism. Treatment is supportive cardiac care and supportive respiratory care, with 100% oxygen therapy. Hyperbaric oxygen has been used in some cases.

i. **Neonatal purpura fulminans.** Treatment of neonatal purpura fulminans includes the following:

    i. **For initial management of homozygous protein C deficiency:** Either 10 to 20 mL/kg of FFP every 12 hours or protein C concentrate when available at 20 to 60 U/kg until the clinical lesions resolve. After initial stabilization: long-term treatment with vitamin K antagonists, LMWH, protein C replacement, or liver transplantation.

    ii. **For initial management for protein S deficiency:** FFP is used.

    iii. **Long-term management:** Anticoagulation therapy with heparin or oral warfarin.

    iv. **Other treatments:** Include case reports of subcutaneous protein C concentrate and liver transplantation.

Diseases and Disorders, General

85 ABO Incompatibility

I. **Definition.** Isoimmune hemolytic anemia may result when ABO incompatibility occurs between the mother and the newborn infant. This disorder is **most common with blood type A or B infants born to type O mothers.** The hemolytic process begins in utero and is the result of active placental transport of maternal isoantibody. In type O mothers, isoantibody is predominantly 7S-IgG (immunoglobulin G) and is capable of crossing the placental membranes. Because of its larger size, the mostly 19S-IgM (immunoglobulin M) isoantibody found in type A or type B mothers cannot cross. Symptomatic clinical disease, which usually does not present until after birth, is a compensated mild hemolytic anemia with reticulocytosis, microspherocytosis, and early-onset unconjugated hyperbilirubinemia.

II. **Incidence.** Risk factors for ABO incompatibility are present in 12% to 15% of pregnancies, but evidence of fetal sensitization (positive direct Coombs test) occurs in only 3% to 4%. Symptomatic ABO hemolytic disease occurs in <1% of all newborn infants but accounts for approximately two-thirds of observed cases of hemolytic disease in the newborn.

III. **Pathophysiology.** Transplacental transport of maternal isoantibody results in an immune reaction with the A or B antigen on fetal erythrocytes, which produces characteristic **microspherocytes.** This process eventually results in complete extravascular hemolysis of the end-stage spherocyte. The ongoing hemolysis is balanced by compensatory reticulocytosis and shortening of the cell cycle time, so that there is overall maintenance of the erythrocyte indices within physiologic limits. A paucity of A or B antigenic sites on the fetal (in contrast to the adult) erythrocytes and competitive binding of isoantibody to a myriad of other antigenic sites in other tissues may explain the often mild hemolytic process that occurs and the usual absence of progressive disease with subsequent pregnancies.

IV. **Risk factors**

   A. **A₁ antigen in the infant.** Of the major blood group antigens, the A_1 antigen has the greatest antigenicity and is associated with the greater risk of symptomatic disease. However, the hemolytic activity of anti-B antibodies is higher than that of anti-A antibodies and may produce a more severe disease, in particular among infants of African American descent.

   B. **Elevated isohemagglutinins.** Antepartum intestinal parasitism or third-trimester immunization with tetanus toxoid or pneumococcal vaccine may stimulate isoantibody titer to A or B antigens.

   C. **Maternal immune serum globulin anti-A/B titers.** Anti-A/B titers >512% are significantly associated with the risk of ABO hemolytic disease of the newborn and may be an early indicator for therapy.

   D. **Birth order.** Birth order is not considered a risk factor. Maternal isoantibody exists naturally and is independent of prior exposure to incompatible fetal blood group antigens.

V. **Clinical presentation**

   A. **Jaundice.** Icterus is often the sole physical manifestation of ABO incompatibility with a clinically significant level of hemolysis. The onset is usually within the first 24 hours of life. The jaundice evolves at a faster rate over the early neonatal period than nonhemolytic physiologic pattern jaundice.

B. **Anemia.** Because of the effectiveness of compensation by reticulocytosis in response to the ongoing mild hemolytic process, erythrocyte indices are maintained within a physiologic range that is normal for asymptomatic infants of the same gestational age. Additional signs of clinical disease (eg, hepatosplenomegaly or hydrops fetalis) are extremely unusual but may be seen with a more progressive hemolytic process (see Chapter 119). Exaggerated physiologic anemia may occur at 8 to 12 weeks of age, particularly when treatment during the neonatal period required phototherapy or exchange transfusion.

VI. **Diagnosis.** Obligatory screening for infants with unconjugated hyperbilirubinemia includes the following studies:

A. **Blood type and Rh factor in the mother and the infant.** These studies establish risk factors for ABO incompatibility. Noninvasive prenatal typing can now be done using cell-free fetal DNA genotyping.

B. **Reticulocyte count.** Elevated values after adjustment for gestational age and degree of anemia, if any, support the diagnosis of hemolytic anemia. For term infants, normal values are 4% to 5%; for preterm infants of 30 to 36 weeks' gestational age, values are 6% to 10%. In ABO hemolytic disease of the newborn, values range from 10% to 30%.

C. **Direct Coombs test (direct antiglobulin test).** Because there is very little antibody on the red blood cell (RBC), the direct Coombs test is often only weakly positive at birth and may become negative by 2 to 3 days of age. A strongly positive test is distinctly unusual and would direct attention to other isoimmune or autoimmune hemolytic processes.

D. **Blood smear.** The blood smear typically demonstrates **microspherocytes, polychromasia** proportionate to the reticulocyte response, and **normoblastosis** above the normal values for gestational age. An increased number of nucleated RBCs in the cord blood could be a sign of ABO incompatibility.

E. **Bilirubin levels (fractionated or total and direct).** Indirect hyperbilirubinemia is mainly present and provides an index of the severity of disease. The rate at which unconjugated bilirubin levels are increasing suggests the required frequency of testing, usually every 4 to 8 hours until values plateau.

F. **Additional laboratory studies.** Supportive diagnostic studies may be indicated on an individual basis if the nature of the hemolytic process remains unclear.

   1. **Antibody identification (indirect Coombs test).** The indirect Coombs test is more sensitive than the direct Coombs test in detecting the presence of maternal isoantibody and identifies antibody specificity. The test is performed on an eluate of neonatal erythrocytes, which is then tested against a panel of type-specific adult cells.

   2. **Maternal IgG titer.** The absence in the mother of elevated IgG titers against the infant's blood group tends to exclude a diagnosis of ABO incompatibility.

VII. **Management**

A. **Antepartum treatment.** Because of the low incidence of moderate to severe ABO hemolytic disease, invasive maneuvers before term is reached (eg, amniocentesis or early delivery) are usually not indicated.

B. **Postpartum treatment**

   1. **General measures.** The maintenance of adequate hydration and evaluation for potentially aggravating factors (eg, sepsis, drug exposure, or metabolic disturbance) should be considered.

   2. **Phototherapy.** Once a diagnosis of ABO incompatibility is established, phototherapy may be initiated before exchange transfusion is given. Because of the usual mild to moderate hemolysis, phototherapy may entirely obviate the need for exchange transfusion or may reduce the number of transfusions required. For guidelines on phototherapy, see Table 63–1 and Figure 99–2.

   3. **Exchange transfusion.** See Table 63–1 and Figure 99–3 for guidelines on exchange transfusion and Chapter 34 for exchange transfusion procedure.

4. **Tin porphyrin.** This can decrease the production of bilirubin and reduce the need for exchange transfusion and duration of phototherapy. It is an inhibitor of heme oxygenase, which is the enzyme that allows the production of bilirubin from heme. The dose of stannsoporfin is 6 μmol/kg intramuscularly as a single dose given within 24 hours of birth with severe hemolytic disease, and it is available via compassionate use protocol. (***Note:*** In May 2018, the US Food and Drug Administration advisory committee recommended that the risk–benefit profile of stannsoporfin does not support the approval for treatment of newborns ≥35 weeks of gestational age at risk for hyperbilirubinemia.)

5. **Intravenous immunoglobulin.** By blocking neonatal reticuloendothelial Fc receptors and thus decreasing hemolysis of the antibody-coated RBCs, high-dose intravenous immunoglobulin (IVIG; 1 g/kg over 4 hours) reduces serum bilirubin levels and the need for blood exchange transfusion with ABO or Rh hemolytic diseases. AAP recommends IVIG 0.5 to 1 g/kg over 2 hours if the TSB is rising despite intensive phototherapy or if the TSB level is within 2 to 3 mg/dL of the exchange level, can be repeated in 12 hours. Cochrane review (2018) does not recommend routine use of IVIG in alloimmune HDN because of low quality of evidence. Caution should be used when considering treatment with IVIG as there are emerging reports of increased incidence of necrotizing enterocolitis in term and late preterm infants with hemolytic disease of the newborn and isoimmune neonatal thrombocytopenia who were treated with IVIG.

VIII. **Prognosis.** For infants with ABO incompatibility, the overall prognosis is excellent. Timely recognition and appropriate management of the rare infant with aggressive ABO hemolytic disease may avoid any potential morbidity or severe hemolytic anemia and secondary hyperbilirubinemia and the inherent risks associated with exchange transfusion with the use of blood products.

86 Acute Kidney Injury

I. **Definition.** There is no unified definition of acute kidney injury (AKI), previously termed acute renal failure, in neonates. Historically, neonatal AKI is defined as absolute serum creatinine ≥1.5 mg/dL, regardless of age or urine output, with normal maternal renal function. In 2013, a panel of experts at a National Institutes of Health-sponsored workshop proposed the adaptation of the categorical modified Kidney Disease: Improving Global Outcomes (KDIGO) definition to predict neonatal clinical outcomes (Table 86–1). According to neonatal KDIGO definition, AKI is defined as an absolute rise of ≥0.3 mg/dL or a ≥50% rise from lowest baseline serum creatinine. AKI can be **anuric** (absence of urinary output by 24–48 hours of age), **oliguric** (urine output of <1.0 mL/kg/h over 24 hours), or **nonoliguric** (>1.0 mL/kg/h). AKI can present with normal urinary output (seen in asphyxiated neonates). Normal urine output is approximately 1 to 3 mL/kg/h with almost all infants voiding within 24 hours of birth. See Table 73–1.

II. **Incidence.** In some studies, as many as 30% of neonatal intensive care unit–admitted neonates have some degree of renal failure. **Prerenal is the most common type in the neonate**, which may be identified in up to 85% of cases. Intrinsic renal disease incidence is 11%, and postrenal incidence is 3% to 5%.

III. **Pathophysiology.** The normal newborn kidney has poor concentrating ability (maximum urine concentration is approximately 700 mOsm/L in the first few days after birth as compared to 1200 mOsm/L at 1 year of age). Renal injury leads to problems

Table 86–1. NEONATAL KDIGO (KIDNEY DISEASES: IMPROVING GLOBAL OUTCOMES) ACUTE KIDNEY INJURY DEFINITION

Stage	Serum Creatinine (SCr)	Urine Output Over 24 Hours
0	No change in SCr or rise <0.3 mg/dL	>1 mL/kg/h
1	SCr rise ≥0.3 mg/dL within 48 hours or SCr rise ≥1.5 to 1.9× reference SCr within 7 days	>0.5 and ≤1 mL/kg/h
2	SCr rise ≥2 to 2.9× reference SCr	>0.3 and ≤0.5 mL/kg/h
3	SCr rise ≥3× reference SCr or SCr ≥2.5 mg/dL or Receipt of dialysis	≤0.3 mL/kg/h

Reference SCr is the lowest prior SCr measurement (serving as baseline SCr).

with volume overload, hyperkalemia, acidosis, hyperphosphatemia, and hypocalcemia. Neonatal AKI is traditionally divided into 3 categories:

A. **Prerenal failure is due to decreased renal blood flow/perfusion, which leads to a decreased renal function in a normal kidney.** Any condition that causes inadequate renal perfusion can cause prerenal AKI. **Common causes include:** hemorrhage, dehydration, septic shock, congestive heart failure, patent ductus arteriosus, and necrotizing enterocolitis. Other causes include respiratory distress syndrome, hypoxia, congenital heart disease, hypoalbuminemia, perinatal asphyxia, ECLS, and hypotension. Medications in neonates that can decrease renal blood flow include indomethacin, ibuprofen, angiotensin-converting enzyme (ACE) inhibitors, and phenylephrine eye drops. Maternal use of nonsteroidal anti-inflammatory drugs (NSAIDs), ACE inhibitors, or cyclooxygenase-2 inhibitors can also decrease renal blood flow.

B. **Intrinsic renal failure refers to direct damage to the glomeruli, renal tubules, vessels, or interstitium of the kidneys.** Prolonged prerenal and postrenal AKI often results in some degree of intrinsic renal dysfunction. **Etiologies of intrinsic renal failure include:** acute tubular necrosis (ATN), congenital anomalies, vascular lesions, and infections/ exogenous toxins. **ATN** is the most common cause, and it can be due to prolonged poor renal perfusion, ischemia or hypoxia, sepsis, cardiac surgery (blood product transfusions), or nephrotoxins (aminoglycosides, NSAIDs, amphotericin B, contrast agents, or acyclovir). **Congenital anomalies** (eg, bilateral renal agenesis, polycystic kidney disease, congenital nephrotic syndrome of the Finnish type, renal hypoplasia/ dysplasia), **vascular lesions** (eg, bilateral renal vein/artery thrombosis, cortical necrosis, disseminated intravascular coagulation [DIC]), **infections** (congenital: syphilis, toxoplasmosis; candidiasis, pyelonephritis), and **exogenous toxins** (eg, uric acid nephropathy, myoglobinuria, hemoglobinuria) are the other causes.

C. **Postrenal/obstructive uropathy involves obstruction of urinary outflow secondary to intrinsic obstruction, extrinsic compression, or congenital anomalies of the urinary tract.** Congenital causes include posterior urethral valves, prune belly syndrome, bilateral ureteropelvic junction obstruction, unilateral obstruction of a solitary kidney, and large ureterocele. Other postnatal causes include urethral strictures, meatal stenosis, neurogenic bladder, such as due to myelomeningocele, and blocked urinary drainage catheters. Rare causes in neonates include intrinsic obstruction (nephrolithiasis, bilateral fungal bezoar) and extrinsic tumor compression of the bladder or ureters (sacrococcygeal teratoma, neurofibromatosis).

IV. **Risk factors.** Include dehydration; sepsis; perinatal asphyxia; administration of nephrotoxic drugs; prematurity; very low birthweight (<1000 g) infants; congenital heart disease affecting systemic circulation, especially those undergoing cardiopulmonary bypass; and ECLS. Maternal diabetes may increase the risk for renal vein thrombosis and subsequent renal insufficiency.

V. **Clinical presentation**

   A. **Decreased or absent urine output.** Low or absent urine output is usually the presenting problem. Virtually all infants with normal renal function void by 24 hours after birth.

   B. **Family history.** History of urinary tract disease in other family members; history of oligohydramnios, which frequently accompanies urinary outflow obstruction or severe renal dysplasia or agenesis; and history of maternal diabetes should be obtained.

   C. **Physical examination**

      1. **Abdominal mass** may be due to a distended bladder, polycystic kidneys, hydronephrosis, or tumors.

      2. **Potter facies** is associated with renal agenesis.

      3. **Meningomyelocele** is associated with neurogenic bladder.

      4. **Pulmonary hypoplasia** is due to severe oligohydramnios in utero.

      5. **Urinary ascites** may be seen with posterior urethral valves and severe upper urinary tract obstruction.

      6. **Prune belly syndrome.** Hypoplasia of the abdominal wall musculature, cryptorchidism, and dilated upper urinary tracts.

      7. **Edema,** anasarca, or unexpected weight gain.

VI. **Diagnosis**

   A. **Urethral catheterization.** Use a urethral catheter to measure volume of retained urine to monitor output (see Chapter 30).

   B. **Laboratory studies**

      1. **Blood urea nitrogen and creatinine**

         a. **Blood urea nitrogen.** A level of 15 to 20 mg/dL suggests dehydration or renal insufficiency.

         b. **Creatinine.** Normal serum creatinine values are 0.8 to 1.0 mg/dL at 1 day, 0.7 to 0.8 mg/dL at 3 days, and <0.6 mg/dL by 7 days of life. Higher values suggest renal disease except in low birthweight infants, in whom a creatinine level of <1.6 mg/dL is considered normal. (Rule of thumb: for every doubling of the creatinine, renal function is reduced by 50 %.)

      2. **Urinary indices** (Table 86–2) are used to assess prerenal versus intrinsic renal disease. Due to the immaturity of newborn kidney, particularly in the preterm

Table 86–2. **URINARY INDICES IN THE NEONATE USED IN THE EVALUATION OF ACUTE KIDNEY INJURY**

Urinary Indices	Prerenal	Intrinsic
Urine osmolality (mOsm/L)	>1400	≤400
Urine sodium (mEq/L)	<30	>60
Urine specific gravity	>1.020	<1.010
Urine/plasma creatinine ratio	29 ± 16	10 ± 4
Blood urea nitrogen/creatinine ratio	>30	<20
Fractional excretion of sodium (FE_{Na}) (%)[a]	<2	>2.5
Fractional excretion of urea (FE_{Urea}) (%)	<35	>50
Renal failure index (RFI)	<3.0	>3.0
Response to volume challenge	UO >2 mL/kg/h	No change in UO

UO, urinary output.

[a]FE_{Na} cutoff values are gestational age (GA) dependent. The following cutoff values indicate intrinsic acute kidney injury: >3% in infants >30 weeks' GA, >6% in infants 29 to 30 weeks' GA. FE_{Na} is not used in infants <28 weeks' GA. In the presence of diuretics, FE_{Urea} is used instead of FE_{Na}.

infant, urine indices are less useful than in older infants; urine indices may suggest intrinsic disease even with prerenal etiology. A spot urine osmolality, serum and spot urine sodium, and serum and urine creatinine are used to calculate the fractional excretion of sodium (FE_{Na}). These indices are of limited value if measured while the effects of diuretics, such as furosemide, are present. In the presence of diuretics, fractional excretion of urea (FE_{Urea}) may be helpful instead.

$$FE_{Na} = \frac{(\text{Urine sodium} \times \text{Plasma creatinine})}{(\text{Plasma sodium} \times \text{Urine creatinine})} \times 100$$

$$FE_{Urea} = \frac{(\text{Urine urea} \times \text{Plasma creatinine})}{(\text{Plasma urea} \times \text{Urine creatinine})} \times 100$$

3. **Complete blood count and platelet count.** May reveal thrombocytopenia, which is seen with sepsis or renal vein thrombosis.
4. **Serum potassium.** May be increased with renal insufficiency.
5. **Urinalysis.** May reveal hematuria (associated with renal vein thrombosis, tumors, or DIC); pyuria, suggesting urinary tract infection; or muddy brown casts suggestive of ATN.
6. **Biomarkers.** Biomarkers allow for earlier identification of neonates with AKI, before the 48 hours it takes serum creatinine to rise. Neutrophil gelatinase–associated lipocalin (NGAL) and cystatin C (CysC) are most studied in neonates and both show higher sensitivity than creatinine. These are usually abnormally expressed proteins in renal injury. Other biomarkers studied include serum CysC, urinary interleukin-18 (IL-18), serum and urinary NGAL, kidney molecule-1 (KIM-1), osteopontin, β_2-microglobulin, and angiotensinogen. Some of these markers in the urine are higher in those with AKI (NGAL, osteopontin, CysC, β_2-microglobulin, KIM-1, epithelial growth factor, osteopontin, uromodulin, clusterin, α-glutathione S-transferase). Some of the serum and urine levels are early predictive biomarkers for AKI (serum and urine NGAL and CysC, urinary IL-18, KIM-1). These markers in the urine and/or serum are higher in AKI and may be predictive for AKI. Some of the biomarkers correlate with drug-induced AKI. The use of omics (genomics, proteomics, metabolomics) in neonatal nephrology is increasing.

C. **Diagnostic fluid challenge.** If the patient does not have clinical volume overload or congestive failure, give a fluid challenge. Administer normal saline or colloid solution, 5 to 10 mL/kg as an intravenous (IV) bolus, and repeat once as needed. If there is no response, give furosemide 1 mg/kg IV. If there is still no increase in urine output, obstruction above the level of the bladder must be ruled out by ultrasound examination. If there is no evidence of obstruction, and the patient does not respond to these maneuvers, the most likely cause of anuria or oliguria is intrinsic renal failure.

D. **Imaging studies**
1. **Abdominal ultrasonography.** May identify urinary tract dilation, renal vein thrombosis, abdominal masses, or a distended bladder.
2. **Abdominal radiograph studies.** May show spina bifida or sacral agenesis, which may be associated with a neurogenic bladder. Displaced bowel loops suggest the presence of a space-occupying mass.
3. **Radionuclide scanning.** May be used to assess function of renal parenchyma but is less accurate in infants <6 weeks old due to immature kidneys.

VII. **Management.** See also Chapter 73.
A. **General management**
1. **Keep strict intake and output and frequent weights.**
2. **Total fluid goal should be insensible fluid losses** (preterm, 50–70 mL/kg/d; term, 30 mL/kg/d) plus fluid output (urine and gastrointestinal tract) replacement.
3. **Monitor serum sodium and potassium levels frequently.** Hyponatremia in setting of AKI is often due to dilutional factors and is best treated with fluid restriction rather than sodium supplementation. Acute hyperkalemia can be

a lethal complication of AKI. Correction of acidosis can be helpful to improve hyperkalemia.

4. **Nutrition.** Breast milk and Similac PM 60/40 are ideal because of the low phosphorus and potassium content and reduced osmotic load for those with polyuric renal failure.

5. **Hyperphosphatemia and hypocalcemia frequently coexist.** To control hyperphosphatemia, nutrition can be switched to Similac PM 60/40. Once phosphate is normalized, calcium (with or without vitamin D supplementation) is usually needed.

6. **For tetany or convulsions, acute intravenous calcium replacement** with 10% calcium gluconate, 40 mg/kg, or 10% calcium chloride will increase the serum calcium 1 mg/dL. Monitor ionized calcium.

7. **Metabolic acidosis may require chronic oral bicarbonate supplementation.** The immature or injured kidney is unable to reclaim bicarbonate effectively. Serum bicarbonate should be kept in the normal range with supplementation provided as necessary to offset renal losses.

$$\text{Bicarbonate deficit} = (24 - \text{observed})\, 0.5 \times \text{body weight (kg)}$$

8. **Hypertension** can be seen with AKI, particularly in the setting of volume overload. Blood pressure should be monitored serially because these infants are always at risk for chronic hypertension.

B. **Definitive management**

1. **Prerenal failure.** Treated by providing volume to increase and restore renal perfusion and to treat the underlying cause.

2. **Postrenal failure.** Acute management involves bypassing the obstruction with a bladder catheter or by percutaneous nephrostomy drainage, depending on the level of the obstruction. Urinary tract infection prophylaxis may be indicated. Consult with pediatric urology early for evaluation and potential surgical intervention. Watch for the development of polyuria once obstruction is relieved.

3. **Intrinsic renal disease.** Stop or adjust doses of any nephrotoxic medications if possible. Supportive therapy is indicated (see previous text). Diuretics (furosemide, 1–2 mg/kg/dose) may increase urine output and aid in fluid management, but studies show that it does not improve the course of kidney injury. Observe for hyponatremia, hyperkalemia, hyperphosphatemia, hypocalcemia, and metabolic acidosis as they can occur frequently in intrinsic renal disease. Follow blood pressure because hypertension can occur (more common in renal artery/venous thrombosis). Renal feeding formulas that have a low renal solute and phosphorus should be considered. Pediatric nephrology should be consulted.

4. **Renal replacement therapy (peritoneal dialysis, hemodialysis, hemofiltration with or without dialysis).** This is used if other measures fail. Modality of choice is often center based and dependent on stability of the patient. Peritoneal dialysis is often technically easiest because of the difficulty in securing large-caliber IV dialysis catheters in newborns.

VIII. **Prevention.** In preterm infants at risk of AKI, the follow measures should be taken:

A. **Avoidance of nephrotoxic agents.**

B. **Strict fluid management.**

C. **Avoidance of intravascular volume depletion.**

D. **The Kidney Disease: Improving Global Outcomes acute kidney injury guidelines** suggest that a single dose of theophylline at a dose of 5 to 8 mg/kg may be given in neonates in the first hour of life with severe perinatal asphyxia who are at high risk of AKI.

E. **Early administration of caffeine** is associated with decreased incidence and severity of AKI in preterm neonates. However, the optimal timing and dosage of caffeine are still under investigation.

IX. **Prognosis.** The prognosis for AKI depends on the underlying cause, the extent of damage, and gestational age. If renal disease is caused by toxins or ATN, renal function may recover to some extent with time. Chronic renal failure may ensue in 16.6% of neonates with AKI. Factors that increase morbidity and mortality in newborns include hypotension, need for mechanical ventilation, dialysis, use of vasopressors, hemodynamic instability, and multiorgan failure. Follow-up by a pediatric nephrologist with monitoring of urine, blood pressure, and renal function is necessary for early detection of long-term complications such as proteinuria, hypertension, and chronic kidney disease, respectively.

87 Air Leak Syndromes

I. **Definition.** **The pulmonary air leak syndromes** (pneumomediastinum, pneumothorax, pulmonary interstitial emphysema [PIE], pneumatocele, pneumopericardium, pneumoperitoneum, and pneumoretroperitoneum) compose a spectrum of diseases with the same underlying pathophysiology. Overdistention of alveolar sacs or terminal airways leads to disruption of airway integrity, resulting in dissection of air into extra-alveolar spaces. Very rarely, air can enter pulmonary vasculature (pulmonary veins) and cause air embolus. Air can also leak into the subcutaneous layers of the skin, especially skin of the chest, neck, and face, causing subcutaneous emphysema.

II. **Incidence.** The exact incidence of the air leak syndromes is difficult to determine. **Pneumothorax is the most common of the air leak syndromes**, reported to occur spontaneously in 1% to 2% of all neonates. The incidence increases in preterm infants to about 6%. The incidence also increases to 9% to 10% in infants with underlying lung disease (eg, respiratory distress syndrome [RDS], meconium aspiration, pneumonia, and pulmonary hypoplasia) who are on ventilatory support and in infants who had vigorous resuscitation at birth.

III. **Pathophysiology.** Overdistention of terminal air spaces or airways can result from uneven alveolar ventilation, air trapping, or injudicious use of alveolar-distending pressure in infants on ventilatory support. As lung volume exceeds physiologic limits, mechanical stresses occur in all planes of the alveolar or respiratory bronchial wall, with eventual tissue rupture. Air can track through the perivascular adventitia, causing **PIE**, or dissect along vascular sheaths toward the hilum, causing a pneumomediastinum. Rupture of the mediastinal pleura and into the thoracic cavity results in a **pneumothorax. Pneumoretroperitoneum and pneumoperitoneum** may occur when mediastinal air tracks downward to the extraperitoneal fascial planes of the abdominal wall, mesentery, and retroperitoneum and eventually ruptures into the peritoneal cavity. The mechanism by which **pneumopericardium** develops is probably due to passage of air along vascular sheaths.

A. **Barotrauma. The common denominator of the air leak syndromes is barotrauma/volutrauma.** Barotrauma results whenever positive pressure is applied to the lung. It cannot be avoided in the ill newborn infant needing ventilatory support, but its effects should be minimized. Peak inspiratory pressure (PIP), positive end-expiratory pressure (PEEP), inspiratory time (IT), respiratory rate, and the inspiratory waveform play important roles in the development of barotrauma. Contributing factors include high PIP, large tidal volume, and a long IT. It is difficult to determine which of these parameters is the most damaging and which plays the largest role in the development of the air leaks.

B. **Other causes of lung overdistention.** Barotrauma is not the only cause of lung overdistention. Atelectatic alveoli in RDS may cause uneven ventilation and subject the more distensible areas of the lung to receive high pressures, placing them at risk for rupture. Small mucous plugs in the airway in meconium aspiration may cause gas trapping secondary to a ball-valve effect. Other events, such as inappropriate intubation of the right mainstem bronchus, failure to wean after surfactant replacement therapy, and vigorous resuscitation or the development of high opening pressures with the onset of air breathing, can also lead to overdistention, with rupture of airway integrity at birth.

C. **Lung injury**
   1. **Large tidal volume.** It has long been considered that lung injury is primarily a result of high-pressure ventilation (barotrauma). Although reports show variable relationships between airway pressures and lung injury, more recent studies support the concept that lung overdistention resulting from high maximal lung volume ("volutrauma") and transalveolar pressure, rather than high airway pressure, is the harmful factor.
   2. **Atelectasis.** The alveolar units in patients with RDS are subjected to a cycle of recruitment and derecruitment. Strategies to decrease this mechanism of atelectatic trauma, optimizing lung recruitment and decreasing lung injury and severity of lung disease, lessen the risk for pulmonary air leak.

IV. **Risk factors**
   A. **Ventilatory support.** Infants on ventilatory support, such as preterm infants and infants with underlying pulmonary disease, have an increased risk of developing one of the air leak syndromes. Various reports have indicated an incidence as high as 41%, and as low as 9% for infants receiving some form of mechanical ventilatory assistance. Factors that contribute to the development of air leak include high inspiratory pressure, large tidal volume, long IT, excessive PEEP, and high-frequency ventilation with resultant insufficient expiratory time.
   B. **Meconium staining.** Other infants at risk include those who are meconium stained at birth. In these infants, meconium may partially plug the airways, with resultant air trapping. During inspiration, the airway expands, allowing air to enter; however, during exhalation, the resultant smaller airway diameter will lead to alveolar gas being trapped behind the meconium plugs.
   C. **Failure to wean after surfactant therapy.** Studies have shown that prophylactic use of surfactant therapy in infants at risk for RDS is associated with a decrease in the incidence of pneumothorax and PIE. Similar findings were noted in treating premature newborns with established RDS. With the return of pulmonary compliance after receiving surfactant, appropriate decreases in pressure support and more cautious ventilatory management of these infants are necessary immediately after therapy. The clinician must closely watch for improvement in the infant's arterial blood gas levels and must wean ventilatory support as required.

V. **Clinical presentation.** Air leak syndromes are potentially lethal, and a high index of suspicion is necessary for the diagnosis. On clinical grounds, respiratory distress or a deteriorating clinical course strongly suggests air leak. See Section IX below for clinical presentation of specific air leak syndromes.

VI. **Diagnosis.** The **definitive diagnosis** of all of these syndromes is made **radiographically**. An anteroposterior (AP) chest radiograph along with a cross-table lateral film is essential in diagnosing an air leak (see Chapter 12 for various radiographic examples). Ultrasound may be useful in diagnosing air leaks in the neonate (eg, lung ultrasound to diagnose a pneumothorax and abdominal ultrasound can diagnose a pneumoperitoneum.) (See Chapter 44.)

VII. **Management.** The best mode of treatment for all of the air leak syndromes is prevention and judicious use of ventilatory support, with close attention to distending pressure, PEEP, and IT. Barotrauma remains a prominent disadvantage to ventilatory support. The careful use of ventilatory pressures and the adjustment of ventilator settings to provide a minimum of barotrauma are extremely important in the neonatal intensive care unit. The use of surfactant therapy for RDS substantially decreases the incidence of pneumothorax and PIE. Earlier treatment is more beneficial than later treatment. A review of 6 randomized trials found that early surfactant administration with extubation to nasal continuous positive airway pressure (CPAP) was associated with significant reductions in the need for mechanical ventilation and fewer air leak syndromes compared with later selective surfactant administration and continued mechanical ventilation in infants with RDS. In infants with established PIE, high-frequency jet ventilation (HFJV) can facilitate resolution of the air leak.

VIII. **Prognosis.** The prognosis for the infant in whom an air leak develops depends on the underlying condition. In general, if the air leak is treated rapidly and effectively, the long-term outcome should not change; however, it must be remembered that early-onset PIE (<24 hours of age) is associated with a high mortality rate. Chronic lung disease of the newborn (bronchopulmonary dysplasia) is also associated with severe pulmonary air leak syndromes. Pneumothorax is also described as a risk factor for intraventricular hemorrhage, cerebral palsy, and delayed mental development.

IX. **Specific air leaks**

A. **Pneumomediastinum**

1. **Definition.** A pneumomediastinum is air in the mediastinum from ruptured alveolar air that enters the perivascular sheaths dissecting into the hilum, through the visceral pleura, into the loose connective tissue spaces of the mediastinum.

2. **Incidence.** The actual incidence of pneumomediastinum is uncertain because it is usually asymptomatic and may go undetected. It has been reported to occur spontaneously in 25 of 10,000 live births in asymptomatic infants; otherwise, the exact incidence varies with the degree of ventilatory support and other associated air leaks (eg, pneumothorax or PIE).

3. **Pathophysiology.** Pneumomediastinum is preceded by alveolar air rupture. After alveolar rupture, air traverses the fascial planes and passes into the mediastinum.

4. **Risk factors.** See Section IV earlier in this chapter.

5. **Clinical presentation.** Unless accompanied by a pneumothorax, a pneumomediastinum may be totally asymptomatic. **Spontaneous pneumomediastinum** may develop in term infants not on ventilatory support and may be accompanied by mild respiratory distress. Physical findings in addition to respiratory distress may include an increase in AP diameter of the chest and distant heart sounds.

6. **Diagnosis.** (See Figure 12–22.) Radiographically, a pneumomediastinum may present in several ways. The **classic description** is that of a **"wind-blown spinnaker sail"** (a lobe or lobes of the thymus being elevated off the heart), most likely to be seen on a left lateral oblique view. In other cases, a halo may be seen around the heart in the AP projection. This must be distinguished from a pneumopericardium in which air completely surrounds the heart, including the inferior border. The cross-table lateral projection will show an anterior collection of air that may be difficult to distinguish from a pneumothorax.

7. **Management.** In isolated pneumomediastinum, close observation is required because it can progress to a pneumothorax. One should resist the temptation to insert a drain into the mediastinum because it will not be beneficial and may cause more problems than it will solve.

8. **Prognosis.** The prognosis is good because recovery is frequently spontaneous without treatment.

B. **Pneumothorax.** See also Chapter 75 on-call problem discussing pneumothorax.

1. **Definition.** A pneumothorax is air between the visceral pleura of the lungs and the parietal pleura of the chest wall.

2. **Incidence.** The incidence of pneumothorax varies between units. It occurs more frequently in the neonatal period than in any other time of life with an incidence of 1% to 2%. With the advent of neonatal ventilator care, however, the incidence

has risen dramatically. Although the exact incidence is difficult to determine, it is directly related to the degree of ventilatory support delivered. The incidence has been as high as 30% to 40%, but in recent years, the incidence has declined to a range of 9% to 11% and is reflective of the underlying pulmonary disease, especially in patients who require mechanical ventilation. In a population of 288 infants with birthweights of 1000 to 1600 g (circa 2004–2008) who received surfactant therapy and/or early CPAP, the overall incidence of pneumothorax or PIE was 5.4%.

3. **Pathophysiology**

   a. **Term infant not on ventilatory support.** A pneumothorax may develop spontaneously. It usually occurs at delivery, when a large initial opening pressure is necessary to inflate fluid-filled alveolar sacs. It is thought to result from uneven inflation of alveoli throughout the lung, combined with the high negative intrathoracic pressure that occurs during the first breath.

   b. **Infant on ventilatory support** has alveolar overdistention secondary to either injudicious use of distending pressure or failure to wean ventilatory pressure when compliance begins to return. A pneumothorax is usually preceded by rupture of the alveoli, with the interstitial air traversing via fascial planes into the mediastinum. Air breaks through the mediastinal pleura to form a pneumothorax.

4. **Risk factors.** See Section IV earlier in this chapter.

5. **Clinical presentation.** The clinical presentation of the neonate with a pneumothorax depends on the setting in which it develops.

   a. **Term infants with a spontaneous pneumothorax** may be asymptomatic or only mildly symptomatic. These infants usually have tachypnea and mild oxygen needs early, but they may progress to the classic signs of respiratory distress (grunting, flaring, retractions, and tachypnea).

   b. **Infant on ventilatory support** generally has a sudden, rapid clinical deterioration characterized by cyanosis, decreased oxygen saturation, hypotension, bradycardia, hypoxemia, hypercarbia, and respiratory acidosis. Other clinical signs may include decreased breath sounds on the involved side, shifted heart sounds, asynchrony of the chest, and abdominal distention from displaced diaphragm. When compression of major veins and decreased cardiac output occur because of downward displacement of the diaphragm, signs of shock may be evident.

6. **Diagnosis.** A high index of suspicion is necessary for the diagnosis of pneumothorax.

   a. **Transillumination of the chest.** (See Chapters 44 and 75.) With the aid of transillumination, the diagnosis of pneumothorax may be made without a chest radiograph. A fiberoptic light probe placed on the infant's chest wall will illuminate the involved hemithorax. Although this technique is beneficial in an emergency, it should not replace a chest radiograph as the means of diagnosis.

   b. **Chest radiograph.** (See Figure 12–23.) Radiographically, a pneumothorax is diagnosed based on the following characteristics:

      i. **Presence of air in the pleural cavity** separating the parietal and visceral pleura. The area appears hyperlucent with absence of pulmonary markings.

      ii. **Collapse of the ipsilateral lobes.**

      iii. **Displacement of the mediastinum** toward the contralateral side.

      iv. **Downward displacement of the diaphragm.** In infants with RDS, the compliance may be so poor that the lung may not collapse, with only minimal shift of the mediastinal structures. The AP radiograph may not demonstrate the classic radiographic appearance if a large amount of the intrapleural air is situated just anterior to the sternum. In these situations, the cross-table lateral radiograph will show a large lucent area immediately below the sternum, or the lateral decubitus radiograph (with the suspected side up) will show free air.

7. **Management.** Treatment of a pneumothorax depends on the clinical status of the infant. In infants without respiratory distress, continuous air leak, or need for assisted ventilation, close monitoring and observation may be all that is needed. The pneumothorax typically resolves in 1 to 2 days. If the pneumothorax affects <15% of a patient's hemithorax, the pneumothorax most likely will resolve spontaneously; otherwise, the air must be removed.

   a. **Oxygen supplementation.** In the term infant who is mildly symptomatic, an oxygen-rich environment is often all that is necessary. The inspired oxygen facilitates nitrogen washout of the blood and tissues and thus establishes a difference in the gas tensions between the loculated gases in the chest and those in the blood. A diffusion gradient results for resorption of the loculated gas and resolution of the pneumothorax. The pneumothorax usually resolves within 1 to 2 hours. This mode of therapy is not appropriate in the preterm infant because of the high oxygen levels needed for washout and the resulting increase in oxygen saturation, making it unsuitable for premature infants with a high risk for retinopathy of prematurity. Recent reviews show that high concentration of oxygen does not show any benefit over targeted oxygen therapy.

   b. **Decompression.** In the symptomatic neonate or the neonate on mechanical ventilatory support, immediate evacuation of air is necessary. The technique is described in Chapter 75. Placement of a chest tube of appropriate size will eventually be necessary (see Chapter 31 on chest tube placement).

8. **Prognosis.** See Section VIII earlier in this chapter.

C. **Pulmonary interstitial emphysema**

1. **Definition.** PIE is dissection of air into the perivascular tissues of the lung from alveolar overdistention or overdistention of the smaller airways.

2. **Incidence.** This disorder arises almost exclusively in the very low birthweight infant on ventilatory support. It may also emerge in the extremely low birthweight infant without mechanical ventilation but receiving ventilatory support by CPAP. Although localized persistent PIE is rarely reported in infants not receiving ventilatory support, it must be considered in any infant with cystic lung lesions. PIE has been reported to occur in at least a third of infants <1000 g who have RDS on the first day of life and are receiving mechanical ventilator support. PIE frequently develops in the first 48 to 72 hours of life.

3. **Pathophysiology.** PIE may be the precursor of all other types of pulmonary air leaks. With overdistention of the alveoli or conducting airways, or both, rupture may occur, and there may be dissection of the air into the perivascular tissue of the lung. The interstitial air moves in the connective tissue planes and around the vascular and lymphatic axes, particularly the venous ones. Once in the interstitial space, the air moves along bronchioles, lymphatics, and vascular sheaths or directly through the lung interstitium to the pleural surface. The extrapulmonary air is trapped in the interstitium (PIE), or it may extend and cause pneumomediastinum, pneumopericardium, or pneumothorax. PIE may exist in 2 forms, either localized (which involves 1 or more lobes) or diffuse (bilateral).

4. **Risk factors.** See Section IV earlier in this chapter.

5. **Clinical presentation.** The patient in whom PIE develops may have sudden deterioration accompanied by bradycardia and hypotension. More commonly, however, the onset of PIE is heralded by slow, progressive deterioration of arterial blood gas levels (hypoxemia, hypercarbia, acidosis) and the apparent need for increasing ventilatory support. The response to increased ventilatory support in the face of poor arterial blood gas levels may lead to worsening of PIE and further clinical deterioration.

6. **Diagnosis.** In infants with PIE, the chest radiograph generally reveals radiolucencies that are either linear or cyst like. The linear radiolucencies vary in
length and do not branch. They are seen in the periphery of the lung as well as
medially and may be mistaken for air bronchograms. The cyst-like lucencies
vary from 1.0 to 4.0 mm in diameter and can be lobulated. (See Figure 12–24.)
In severe cases, chest radiograph film may also reveal overexpanded lung fields
and a decreased heart shadow.
7. **Management**
   a. **Lessening lung injury.** In general, once PIE is diagnosed, an attempt should
   be made to decrease ventilatory support and lessen lung trauma. Decreasing
   the PIP, decreasing the PEEP, or shortening the IT may be required. When
   decreasing these settings, some degree of hypercarbia and hypoxia may have
   to be accepted.
   b. **Positioning of the infant with the involved side down.** This has also proved
   beneficial in some cases of unilateral PIE.
   c. **Other treatments.** Suctioning of the endotracheal tube and manual positive-
   pressure ventilation should be minimized. More invasive measures include
   selective collapse of the involved lung on the side with the worse involvement, with selective intubation or even the insertion of chest tubes before
   the development of pneumothorax. In cases of severe PIE, surgical resection
   of the affected lobe may be considered.
   d. **High-frequency ventilation.** Both high-frequency oscillatory ventilation
   (HFOV) and mostly HFJV are used effectively in the treatment of PIE and
   other types of air leak syndromes. Although these treatment modalities may
   improve survival of the infant with PIE, the long-term outcome remains
   uncertain.
8. **Prognosis.** See Section VIII earlier in this chapter.
D. **Pneumopericardium**
   1. **Definition.** A pneumopericardium is air in the pericardial sac, which is usually
   secondary to passage of air along pulmonary vascular sheaths. It is most often a
   complication of mechanical ventilation and often results in fatal cardiac tamponade.
   2. **Incidence.** A pneumopericardium is a rare occurrence and the least common
   form of pulmonary air leak in the neonatal period. The incidence in a study
   involving very low birthweight neonates was reported at 2%.
   3. **Pathophysiology.** A pneumopericardium is usually preceded by pneumomediastinum or other air leaks such as PIE or pneumothorax. It is associated with
   the use of extremely high PIPs or a catastrophic sudden obstruction of the expiratory part of the mechanical respiratory circuit. The mechanism by which a
   pneumopericardium develops is probably due to passage of air along vascular
   sheaths. From the mediastinum, air can travel along the fascial planes in the
   subcutaneous tissues of the neck, chest wall, and anterior abdominal wall and
   into the pericardial space, causing a pneumopericardium.
   4. **Risk factors.** See Section IV earlier in this chapter.
   5. **Clinical presentation.** A pneumopericardium is rarely asymptomatic and more
   often presents as a full picture of cardiac tamponade. The first sign of a pneumopericardium may be a decrease in blood pressure or a decrease in pulse pressure.
   There may also be an increase in heart rate with distant heart sounds. Absent
   peripheral pulses, marked abdominal distention due to massive hepatomegaly,
   and severe hypoxemia, with breath sounds that are adequate and equal on both
   sides of the chest, are likely to develop shortly thereafter.
   6. **Diagnosis.** A pneumopericardium has the most classic radiographic appearance
   of all the air leaks (see Figure 12–21). **A broad radiolucent halo completely surrounds the heart, including the diaphragmatic surface.** This picture is easily
   distinguished from all the other air leaks by its extension completely around the
   heart in all projections.

7. **Management.** Treatment of a pneumopericardium requires the urgent placement of a pericardial drain or repeated pericardial taps. Tube drainage is recommended for all neonates because of a high rate of reaccumulation (as much as 50% of the time). The procedure is described in Chapter 41. Successful pericardiocentesis in most instances should result in 75% to 80% survival.

8. **Prognosis.** See Section VIII earlier in this chapter.

E. **Pneumoperitoneum.** See also Chapter 74.

1. **Definition.** A pneumoperitoneum is air in the peritoneal cavity that is usually caused by gastrointestinal perforation, but it can also be caused by air that has ruptured from the mediastinum into the peritoneum.

2. **Incidence.** A pneumoperitoneum from passage of air into the chest is rare. It has been reported to occur in approximately 1% of mechanically ventilated children in intensive care units.

3. **Pathophysiology.** A pneumoperitoneum in the newborn most commonly arises from a perforated hollow viscus or a preceding abdominal operation. It can also be secondary to ventilator-assisted pulmonary air leakage. Air from ruptured alveoli can flow transdiaphragmatically along the great vessels and esophagus into the retroperitoneum. When air accumulates in the retroperitoneum, rupture into the peritoneal cavity can occur.

4. **Risk factors.** See Section IV earlier in this chapter.

5. **Clinical presentation.** Depending on the cause and severity, a pneumoperitoneum can present with or without associated abdominal findings. Because a pneumoperitoneum can occur as a result of pneumothorax, pneumomediastinum, and PIE, infants generally present with increasing signs of respiratory distress.

6. **Diagnosis.** A pneumoperitoneum can be detected in radiographic films as free air under the diaphragm. (See Figure 12–25.)

7. **Management.** Conservative management may be strongly considered if evidence of pulmonary air leak precedes or simultaneously appears with pneumoperitoneum. See Chapter 40 for air removal technique.

8. **Prognosis.** See Section VIII earlier in this chapter.

F. **Pneumoretroperitoneum.** A pneumoretroperitoneum is the presence of air in the retroperitoneal space. **An isolated pneumoretroperitoneum is rare in neonates.** It can occur when massive intrathoracic pressure from a pneumothorax or pneumomediastinum causes free air to dissect into the retroperitoneal space from the chest. On radiograph, one sees air around the kidneys and in the perinephric space.

G. **Pneumatocele.** A pneumatocele represents subpleural or intraparenchymal cystic lesions in the lungs. They are thin-walled, air-filled cysts and mainly result from ventilator-induced lung injury in preterm infants. Pneumatoceles also can occur as a sequela of acute pneumonia. Causative agents include *Staphylococcus aureus*, *Streptococcus pneumoniae*, *Haemophilus influenzae*, and *Escherichia coli*. Most pneumatoceles are asymptomatic. They rarely require any surgical intervention. Traumatic pneumatoceles caused by positive-pressure ventilation commonly resolve spontaneously; however, it is important to follow them closely, because high pressures during mechanical ventilation can cause a sudden increase in their size and result in a pneumothorax.

H. **Subcutaneous emphysema.** Subcutaneous emphysema occurs when an air leak dissects into tissues beneath the skin (tissue planes of the face, neck, and upper chest). It can be seen as a smooth bulging of the skin and detected by palpation of crepitus in the involved area. Usually it does not cause any clinical deterioration, but in extremely low birthweight infants, subcutaneous emphysema can result in compression of the airway. Subcutaneous emphysema is of clinical importance as it may signify a more serious underlying air leak.

88 Anemia

I. **Definition.** Anemia developing during the neonatal period (0–28 days of life) in infants >34 weeks of gestational age is indicated by a central venous hemoglobin <13 g/dL or a capillary hemoglobin <14.5 g/dL.

II. **Incidence.** Anemia is the **most common hematologic abnormality** in the newborn. Specific incidence depends on the cause of the anemia.

III. **Pathophysiology**

A. **Normal physiology.** At birth, normal values for the central venous hemoglobin in infants of >34 weeks of gestational age are 14 to 20 g/dL, with an average value of 17 g/dL. Reticulocyte count in the cord blood of infants ranges from 3% to 7%. The average mean corpuscular volume of red blood cells (RBCs) is 107 fL (femtoliters). Premature infants have slightly lower hemoglobin and higher mean corpuscular volume and reticulocyte counts. In healthy term infants, **hemoglobin values remain unchanged until the third week of life and then decline, reaching a mean nadir of 11 g/dL** (but may be as low as 9 g/dL) **at 8 to 12 weeks.** This is known as the **"physiologic anemia of infancy."** In preterm infants, this decline is more profound, reaching a nadir of 7 to 9 g/dL at 4 to 8 weeks. This exaggerated physiologic anemia of prematurity is related to a combination of decreased RBC mass at birth, increased iatrogenic losses from laboratory blood sampling, shorter RBC life span, inadequate erythropoietin production, and rapid body growth. In the absence of clinical complications associated with prematurity, infants remain asymptomatic during this process.

B. **Etiologies of anemia.** Anemia in the newborn infant results from 1 of 3 processes: **loss of RBCs, or hemorrhagic anemia,** the most common cause; **increased destruction of RBCs, or hemolytic anemia;** or **underproduction of RBCs, or hypoplastic anemia.**

1. **Hemorrhagic anemia**

a. **Antepartum period** (1 in 1000 live births)

   i. **Loss of placental integrity.** Abruptio placentae, placenta praevia, or traumatic amniocentesis (acute or chronic) may result in loss of placental integrity.

   ii. **Anomalies of the umbilical cord or placental vessels.** Velamentous insertion of the umbilical cord occurs in 10% of twin gestations and almost all gestations with >3 fetuses. Communicating vessels (vasa praevia), umbilical cord hematoma (1 in 5500 deliveries), or entanglement of the cord by the fetus may also cause hemorrhagic anemia.

   iii. **Twin-twin transfusion.** This is observed only in monozygotic (MZ) multiple births. MZ twin pregnancies account for approximately 30% of spontaneously conceived twins. The occurrence of MZ twins is 0.4% to 0.45% of nonstimulated in vivo conceptions. The incidence of monochorionic twins is rising due to the increase in the use of assisted reproductive technology (ART). The use of ART has been associated with a 2- to 12-fold increase in the conception of MZ twins. In the presence of a monochorionic placenta, 5% to 30% of twin pregnancies are associated with twin-twin transfusion leading to a hemoglobin concentration difference in excess of >5 g/dL. The anemic donor twin may develop congestive heart disease, whereas the recipient plethoric twin may manifest signs of the hyperviscosity syndrome. In utero laser photocoagulation, which interrupts the vascular connections on the chorionic plate, has improved the low survival rate for twin-twin transfusion diagnosed before 26 weeks' gestation.

b. Intrapartum period

   i. Fetomaternal hemorrhage. Fetomaternal hemorrhage (FMH) is a common event during pregnancy, demonstrable in approximately 75% of gestations. The risk is increased with preeclampsia, with the need for instrumentation, and with cesarean delivery. In approximately 8% of pregnancies, the volume of the hemorrhage is >10 mL. Clinically significant FMH has traditionally been set at a cutoff of 30 mL. At this cutoff, the incidence of FMH has been estimated to be 3 per 1000 births. One in 2000 pregnancies is associated with FMH of ≥100 mL, which carries a 70% perinatal mortality rate. The severity of the FMH is related to the size of the bleed in relation to the overall fetal blood volume, as well as the rate at which this blood is lost, and whether the event is acute or chronic.

   ii. Cesarean delivery. In elective cesarean deliveries, there is a 3% incidence of anemia. The incidence is increased in emergency cesarean deliveries.

   iii. Traumatic rupture of the umbilical cord. Rupture may occur if delivery is uncontrolled or unattended.

   iv. Failure of placental transfusion. Failure is usually caused by umbilical cord occlusion (eg, a nuchal cord or an entangled or prolapsed cord) during vaginal delivery. Blood loss may be 25 to 30 mL in the newborn.

   v. Obstetric trauma. During a difficult vaginal delivery, occult visceral or intracranial hemorrhage may occur. It may not be apparent at birth. Difficult deliveries are more common with large for gestational age infants, breech presentation, or difficult extraction.

c. Neonatal period

   i. Enclosed hemorrhage. Hemorrhage severe enough to cause neonatal anemia suggests obstetric trauma, severe perinatal distress, or a defect in hemostasis. See Figure 7–3 for examples of intracranial hemorrhages in a newborn.

   (a) Caput succedaneum is relatively common and may result in benign hemorrhage.

   (b) Cephalhematoma is found in up to 2.5% of births. It is associated with vacuum extraction and primiparity (5% risk of associated linear nondepressed skull fracture).

   (c) Subgaleal (subaponeurotic) hemorrhage is a rare but potentially lethal medical emergency caused by a rupture of the emissary veins, which are connections between the dural sinuses and the scalp veins. Blood accumulates between the epicranial aponeurosis of the scalp and the periosteum. This potential space extends forward to the orbital margins, backward to the nuchal ridge, and laterally to the temporal fascia. In term infants, this subaponeurotic space may hold as much as 260 mL of blood (40 mL per every 1-cm increase in head circumference). Subgaleal hemorrhage is most often associated with vacuum extraction and forceps delivery, but it may also occur spontaneously from an associated coagulopathy.

   (d) Intracranial hemorrhage may occur in the subdural, subarachnoid, or subependymal space.

   (e) Visceral parenchymal hemorrhage is uncommon. It is usually the result of obstetric trauma (eg, difficult breech extraction) to an internal organ, most commonly the liver, but it also can involve the spleen, kidneys, or adrenal glands.

    ii. Defects in hemostasis. Defects in hemostasis may be congenital, but more commonly, hemorrhage occurs secondary to consumption coagulopathy, which may be caused by the following:

    (a) Congenital coagulation factor deficiency

    (b) Consumption coagulopathy

      (i) Disseminated congenital or viral infection

      (ii) Bacterial sepsis

      (iii) **Intravascular embolism of thromboplastin** (as a result of a dead twin, maternal toxemia, necrotizing enterocolitis, or others)

    (c) **Deficiency of vitamin K–dependent coagulation factors** (factors II, VII, IX, and X)

      (i) **Failure to administer vitamin K at birth** usually results in a bleeding diathesis at 3 to 4 days of age.

      (ii) **Use of antibiotics** may interfere with the production of vitamin K by normal gastrointestinal flora.

      (iii) **Maternal ingestion of anticonvulsants** (carbamazepine, phenytoin, and barbiturates but not valproic acid), antituberculosis agents (isoniazid, rifampicin), and vitamin K antagonists.

    (d) **Thrombocytopenia.** See Chapter 128.

      (i) **Immune thrombocytopenia** may be isoimmune or autoimmune.

      (ii) **Congenital thrombocytopenia with absent radii** is a syndrome frequently associated with hemorrhagic anemia in the newborn.

      (iii) **Iatrogenic blood loss.** Anemia may occur if blood loss resulting from repeated venipuncture is not replaced routinely. Symptoms may develop if a loss of >20% occurs within a 48-hour period.

2. Hemolytic anemia

  a. Immune hemolysis

    i. Isoimmune hemolytic anemia. Caused mostly by Rh incompatibility.

    ii. Autoimmune hemolytic anemia.

  b. Nonimmune hemolysis

    i. Bacterial sepsis may cause primary microangiopathic hemolysis.

    ii. Congenital TORCH (*t*oxoplasmosis, *o*ther, *r*ubella, *c*ytomegalovirus, and *h*erpes simplex virus) infections (see Chapter 148).

  c. Congenital erythrocyte defect

    i. Metabolic enzyme deficiency

      (a) **Glucose-6-phosphate dehydrogenase deficiency**

      (b) **Pyruvate kinase deficiency**

    ii. Thalassemia. Hemolytic anemia secondary to thalassemia is invariably associated with homozygous α-thalassemia and presents at birth. The disorders in β-thalassemia become apparent only after 2 to 3 months of age.

    iii. Hemoglobinopathy. May be characterized as unstable hemoglobins or congenital Heinz body anemia.

    iv. Membrane defects. Usually autosomal dominant.

      (a) **Hereditary spherocytosis** (1 in 5000 neonates) commonly presents with jaundice and less often with anemia.

      (b) **Hereditary elliptocytosis** (1 in 2500 neonates) rarely presents in the newborn infant.

  d. Systemic diseases

    i. Galactosemia

    ii. Osteopetrosis

  e. Nutritional deficiency. Vitamin E deficiency occurs with chronic malabsorption but usually does not present until after the neonatal period.
 3. Hypoplastic anemia
  a. Congenital disease
   i. Diamond-Blackfan syndrome (congenital hypoplastic anemia)
   ii. Atransferrinemia
   iii. Congenital leukemia
   iv. Sideroblastic anemia
  b. Acquired disease
   i. Infection. Rubella and syphilis are the most common causes.
   ii. Aplastic crisis.
   iii. Aplastic anemia.
IV. Risk factors. Prematurity, certain race and ethnic groups, and hereditary blood disorders (see Section III earlier in this chapter).
V. Clinical presentation
 A. Symptoms and signs. The 4 major forms of neonatal anemia may be demonstrated by determination of the following factors: age at presentation of anemia, associated clinical features at presentation, hemodynamic status of the infant, and presence or absence of compensatory reticulocytosis.
  1. Hemorrhagic anemia. Often dramatic in clinical presentation when acute but may be more subtle when chronic. Both forms have significant rates of perinatal morbidity and mortality if they remain unrecognized. Neither form has significant elevation of bilirubin levels or hepatosplenomegaly.
   a. Acute hemorrhagic anemia. Presents at birth or with internal hemorrhage after 24 hours. There is pallor not associated with jaundice and often without cyanosis (<5 g of deoxyhemoglobin) and unrelieved by supplemental oxygen. Tachypnea or gasping respirations are present. Vascular instability ranges from decreased peripheral perfusion (a 10% loss of blood volume) to hypovolemic shock (20%–25% loss of blood volume). There is also decreased central venous pressure and poor capillary refill. Normocytic or normochromic RBC indices are present, with reticulocytosis developing within 2 to 3 days of the hemorrhagic event.
   b. Chronic hemorrhagic anemia. Presents at birth with unexplained pallor, often without cyanosis (<5 g of deoxyhemoglobin), and unrelieved by supplemental oxygen. Minimal signs of respiratory distress are present. The central venous pressure is normal or increased. Microcytic or hypochromic RBC indices are present, with compensatory reticulocytosis. The liver is often enlarged because of compensatory extramedullary erythropoiesis. Hydrops fetalis or stillbirth may occur with failure of compensatory reticulocytosis or intravascular volume maintenance.
   c. Asphyxia pallida (severe neonatal asphyxia). Not associated with hemorrhagic anemia at presentation. This disorder must be distinguished clinically from acute hemorrhage because specific immediate therapy is needed for each disorder. Asphyxia pallida presents at birth with pallor and cyanosis which improves with supplemental oxygen delivery, respiratory failure, bradycardia, and normal central venous pressure.
  2. Hemolytic anemia. Jaundice is often seen before diagnostic levels of hemoglobin are obtained, in part because of the compensatory reticulocytosis that is invariably present. The infant usually presents with pallor after 48 hours of age. However, severe Rh isoimmune disease or homozygous α-thalassemia presents at birth with severe anemia and, in many cases, hydrops fetalis. Unconjugated hyperbilirubinemia of >10 to 12 mg/dL, tachypnea, and hepatosplenomegaly may be seen with hemolytic anemia.
  3. Hypoplastic anemia. Uncommon and characterized by presentation after 48 hours of age, absence of jaundice, and reticulocytopenia.

4. **Other forms of anemia**
   a. **Anemia associated with twin-twin transfusion.** If chronic hemorrhage is occurring, there is often a >20% difference in the birthweights of the 2 infants, with the donor being the smaller twin.
   b. **Occult (internal) hemorrhage**
      i. **Intracranial hemorrhage.** Signs include a bulging anterior fontanel and neurologic signs (eg, a change in consciousness, apnea, or seizures).
      ii. **Visceral hemorrhage.** Most commonly, the liver has been injured. An abdominal mass or distention is seen.
      iii. **Pulmonary hemorrhage.** Partial or total radiographic opacification of a hemithorax and bloody tracheal secretions are seen. (See Chapter 79.)

B. **History**
   1. **Anemia at birth**
      a. **Hemorrhagic anemia.** There may be a history of third-trimester vaginal bleeding or amniocentesis. Hemorrhagic anemia may be associated with multiple gestation, maternal chills or fever postpartum, and nonelective cesarean delivery.
      b. **Hemolytic anemia.** May be associated with intrauterine growth restriction (IUGR) and Rh-negative mothers.
   2. **Anemia presenting after 24 hours of age** is often associated with obstetric trauma, unattended delivery, precipitous delivery, perinatal fetal distress, or a low Apgar score.
   3. **Anemia presenting with jaundice** suggests hemolytic anemia. There may be evidence of drug ingestion late in the third trimester; IUGR; a family member with splenectomy, anemia, jaundice, or cholelithiasis; maternal autoimmune disease; or Mediterranean or Asian ethnic background.

VI. **Diagnosis**
A. **Obligatory initial studies**
   1. **Hemoglobin**
   2. **Red blood cell indices**
      a. **Microcytic or hypochromic red blood cell indices** suggest FMH, twin-twin hemorrhage, or α-thalassemia (mean corpuscular volume <90 fL; normal 107 fL).
      b. **Normocytic or normochromic red blood cell indices** are suggestive of acute hemorrhage, systemic disease, intrinsic RBC defect, or hypoplastic anemia.
   3. **Reticulocyte count (corrected).** An elevated reticulocyte count is associated with antecedent hemorrhage or hemolytic anemia. A low count is seen with hypoplastic anemia. The following formula is used:

$$\text{Corrected reticulocyte count} = \frac{\text{Observed reticulocyte count} \times \text{Observed hematocrit}}{\text{Normal hematocrit for age}}$$

   4. **Blood smear**
      a. **Spherocytes** are associated with ABO isoimmune hemolysis or hereditary spherocytosis.
      b. **Elliptocytes** are seen in hereditary elliptocytosis.
      c. **Pyknocytes** may be seen in glucose-6-phosphate dehydrogenase deficiency.
      d. **Schistocytes or helmet cells** are most often seen with consumption coagulopathy.
   5. **Direct antiglobulin test (direct Coombs test).** This test is positive in isoimmune or autoimmune hemolysis.

B. **Other selected laboratory studies**
   1. **Isoimmune hemolysis.** The blood type and Rh type should be determined, and an eluate of neonatal cells prepared.
   2. **Fetomaternal hemorrhage.** The **Kleihauer-Betke test** should be performed. Using an acid elution technique, a maternal blood smear is stained with eosin. Fetal RBCs containing hemoglobin F are resistant to acid elution stain darkly. Adult

RBCs voided of their acid-sensitive hemoglobin A do not stain and appear as "ghost cells." A 50-mL loss of fetal blood into the maternal circulation shows up as 1% fetal cells in the maternal circulation. **ABO incompatibility between mother and infant results in an increased clearance rate of fetal cells from the maternal circulation, giving a falsely low result.** Conversely, the Kleihauer-Betke test may overestimate the extent of the hemorrhage, with maternal conditions leading to the overproduction of maternal hemoglobin F such as hereditary sickle cell anemia and β-thalassemia trait. Immunofluorescence flow cytometry is an alternative diagnostic test that circumvents some of the problems associated with the Kleihauer-Betke screen. This technology quantifies the number of fetal cells present by measuring the fluorescence intensity of monoclonal antibodies binding to hemoglobin F or to other surface antigens (eg, carbonic anhydrase) differentially expressed in fetal compared with adult erythrocytes. **The College of American Pathologists has published a tool, accessible online at http:// capatholo.gy/RHIG (accessed September 9, 2018), that allows users to plug in the percentage of fetal cells observed by the Kleihauer-Betke test or flow cytometry and the maternal height and weight to calculate the FMH volume.**
3. **Congenital hypoplastic or aplastic anemia.** Bone marrow aspiration is usually indicated.
4. **TORCH infection**
   a. **Skull and long-bone films**
   b. **Immunoglobulin M levels**
   c. **Acute or convalescent serology**
   d. **Urine culture for cytomegalovirus**
5. **Consumption coagulopathy**
   a. **Prothrombin time and partial thromboplastin time**
   b. **Platelet count**
   c. **Thrombin time or fibrinogen assay**
   d. **Factor V and factor VIII levels**
   e. **Fibrin split products (D-dimers)**
6. **Occult hemorrhage**
   a. **Pathologic examination of the placenta**
   b. **Cranial or abdominal ultrasonography will help identify the site of bleeding**
7. **Intrinsic red blood cell defect**
   a. **Red blood cell enzyme studies**
   b. **Analysis of the globin chain ratio**
   c. **Studies of red blood cell membrane**
VII. **Management.** Treatment of neonatal anemia may involve, individually or in combination, simple replacement transfusion, exchange transfusion, nutritional supplementation, or treatment of the underlying primary disorder.
   A. **Simple replacement transfusion**
      1. **Indications**
         a. **Acute hemorrhagic anemia.**
         b. **Ongoing deficit replacement.**
         c. **Maintenance of effective oxygen-carrying capacity.** There are no universally accepted guidelines; however, those presented next are fairly representative of most common practice.
            i. **Hematocrit <35% with severe cardiopulmonary disease** (eg, intermittent positive-pressure ventilation with mean airway pressure >6 cm H_2O).
            ii. **Hematocrit <30%.**
               (a) **With mild to moderate cardiopulmonary disease** (FiO_2 >35%, continuous positive airway pressure).
               (b) **With significant apnea** (>9–12 hours or apnea requiring bag-and-mask ventilation).

       (c) **"Symptomatic anemia"**: Weight gain <10 g/kg/d at full caloric intake and heart rate >180 beats/min persisting for 24 hours.

       (d) **If undergoing major surgery.**

     iii. **Hematocrit <21%.** Asymptomatic but with low reticulocyte count (<2%).

  2. **Emergency transfusion at birth only. Use type O, Rh-negative packed RBCs.**

    a. **Adjust the hematocrit to 50%.**

    b. **If a medical emergency exists,** blood that has not been cross-matched may be given; if time permits, blood may be cross-matched to the mother's blood.

    c. **Alternative replacement fluids** include normal saline, fresh-frozen plasma, and 5% albumin in saline. Timely infusion of packed RBCs or partial exchange transfusion should follow.

    d. **Perform umbilical vein catheterization** to a depth of 4 to 5 cm or until free blood flow is established (see Chapter 48).

    e. **Draw initial blood samples for diagnostic studies.** Obtain a complete blood count and differential, blood type and Rh type, direct Coombs test, and, if indicated, total bilirubin levels. In a medical emergency, transfusion may be started before the results of laboratory testing are known.

    f. **Infuse 10 to 15 mL/kg of replacement fluid over 10 to 15 minutes if emergency measures are needed.** Once the infant's status is stable, reassess the diagnostic studies, physical examination, and obstetric history.

    g. **Calculate the red blood cell volume.** Under controlled circumstances or if simple transfusion is indicated, calculate the volume of packed RBCs needed to achieve the desired increase in RBC mass (see page 624). **The volume of a single transfusion should not exceed 10 to 20 mL/kg.**

B. **Exchange transfusion**

  1. **Indications**

    a. **Chronic hemolytic anemia or hemorrhagic anemia** with evidence of tissue hypoxia (poor perfusion, metabolic acidosis, oliguria).

    b. **Severe isoimmune hemolytic anemia** with circulating sensitized RBCs and isoantibody.

    c. **Consumption coagulopathy.**

  2. **Technique.** See Chapter 34 for the technique of exchange transfusion in neonates.

C. **Nutritional replacement**

  1. **Iron.** Iron replacement is useful in the following situations:

    a. **Fetomaternal hemorrhage** of significant volume.

    b. **Chronic twin-twin transfusion** (in the donor twin).

    c. **Incremental external blood loss** (if unreplaced).

    d. **Preterm infant** (<36 weeks' gestational age).

  2. **Folate.** Especially with serum levels <0.5 ng/mL.

    a. **Premature infants weighing** <1500 g or <34 weeks' gestational age.

    b. **Chronic hemolytic anemias** or conditions involving "stress erythropoiesis."

    c. **Infants receiving phenytoin (Dilantin).**

  3. **Vitamin E.** Preterm infants of <34 weeks' gestational age, unless they are being breast fed.

D. **Prophylactic**

  1. **Recombinant human erythropoietin (*controversial*).** High doses of erythropoietin are capable of increasing neonatal erythropoiesis and have very few adverse side effects. It decreases the requirement for "late" transfusions (those required past the age of 2–3 weeks); it will not compensate for the anemia secondary to phlebotomy losses. Its use in the very low birthweight infant continues to be ***controversial*** because the severity of anemia in this group can be more effectively minimized by a restrictive policy for blood sampling and the use of micromethods in the laboratory. The need for transfusions is also reduced when

a consistent "protocolized" approach for transfusions is available in the neonatal intensive care unit. It has been also argued that what needs to be avoided, more than the transfusion itself, is the exposure to multiple donors. The allocation of a single donor for each high-risk infant, for a 42-day period, is the most effective way to reach that former goal. Early and late strategies have been used for erythropoietin treatment. (See doses in Chapter 155.)

- a. **Early.** Starting on day 1 or 2, 1200 to 1400 U/kg/wk. Recombinant human erythropoietin is added to the total parenteral nutrition solution, and 1 mg/kg/d of iron is added.
- b. **Late.** 500 to 700 U/kg/wk given 3 to 5 times per week subcutaneously. Supplemental oral iron needs to be provided at 3 mg/kg/d in 3 divided doses. The iron dose is increased to 6 mg/kg/d as soon as the infant is tolerating full enteral feeds.
- c. **Darbepoetin.** This new molecule was more recently created by biologically modifying 5 amino acids of the original protein in order to generate 5 carbohydrate binding sites compared with 3 in recombinant erythropoietin. This modification resulted in a half-life more than twice that of recombinant erythropoietin and increases the erythropoietin activity of recombinant erythropoietin with less frequent dosing.

2. **Nutritional supplementation**
   - a. **Elemental iron.** 1 to 2 mg/kg/d, beginning at 2 months of age and continuing through 1 year of age.
   - b. **Folic acid.** 1 to 2 mg/wk for preterm infants; 50 mcg/d for term infants.
   - c. **Vitamin E.** 25 IU/d until a corrected age of 4 months is reached.

E. **Treatment of selected disorders**
   1. **Consumption coagulopathy**
      - a. **Treat the underlying cause (eg, sepsis).**
      - b. **Give blood replacement therapy.** Perform exchange transfusion or give fresh-frozen plasma, 10 mL/kg every 12 to 14 hours. Platelet concentrate, 1 U, may be used as a substitute for plasma transfusion.
      - c. **Perform coagulation studies.** Monitor the partial thromboplastin time, prothrombin time, and fibrinogen and D-dimers levels and the platelet count.
   2. **Immune thrombocytopenia**
      - a. **Isoimmune thrombocytopenia**
        - i. **Consider performing cesarean delivery if the diagnosis has been confirmed** and there is an older sibling with immune thrombocytopenia (75% risk of recurrence).
        - ii. **Give maternal washed platelets when indicated for bleeding diathesis** in an infant with a platelet count <20,000 to 30,000/mm^3. Exchange transfusion may be used as an alternative.
        - iii. **Corticosteroid therapy and intravenous immune globulin are _controversial_.**
      - b. **Autoimmune thrombocytopenia**
        - i. **Cesarean delivery.** Consider if the maternal platelet count is <100,000/mm^3 or the fetal platelet count is <50,000/mm^3.
        - ii. **Use of corticosteroids is _controversial_.** Under the conditions just mentioned, consider giving corticosteroids to the mother several weeks before delivery. Transfusion of random donor platelets may be given when indicated.

VIII. **Prognosis.** Depends on the underlying cause, its severity, and how acutely the anemia develops.

89 Apnea

Apnea is common and a significant clinical problem in preterm neonates. It is manifested by an unstable respiratory rhythm, reflecting the immaturity of the respiratory control system. Apnea can also be secondary to other pathologic conditions that need to be excluded before the diagnosis of apnea of prematurity (AOP) is assumed. In contrast, periodic breathing is a benign condition and does not merit any treatment. (See also on-call problem Apnea and Bradycardia in Chapter 52.)

I. **Definition.** AOP is most widely defined as cessation of breathing for >20 seconds or a shorter respiratory pause if associated with hypoxemia and/or bradycardia in infants who are younger than 37 weeks' gestation. Apnea that lasts for <10 seconds is considered "significant" if it is associated with a decrease in oxygen saturation (SpO_2) to ≤80% or 85%, whereas "significant" bradycardia has been defined as a decrease in heart rate to <80 beats/min or less than two-thirds of baseline.

A. **Central apnea:** Related to immaturity of the central nervous system, central apnea is characterized by total cessation of inspiratory effort with no evidence of obstruction to airflow.

B. **Obstructive apnea:** Presents clinically with the preservation of chest wall movement while airflow is obstructed. The primary site of airway obstruction is the pharynx. Lack of coordination of respiratory musculature, neck flexion, or nasal obstruction may further enhance the severity of this impairment of airway airflow.

C. **Mixed apnea:** Consists of both obstructive and central apnea, with 1 type triggering the onset of the second type of apnea.

D. **Periodic breathing:** Periodic breathing is a normal breathing pattern characterized by ventilatory cycles of 10 to 15 seconds followed by respiratory pause for 5 to 10 seconds without change in heart rate or skin color. It is due to an imbalance between the opposite response of peripheral and central chemoreceptors on ventilatory drive stimuli. Periodic breathing in premature infants is often due to excessive stimulation by the peripheral chemoreceptors promoting a breathing instability. Prevalence of periodic breathing approaches 100% in preterm infants <1000 g. It is more frequent during active sleep. The prognosis is good, although severe hypoxic events are noted to be often preceded by hypoventilation or arterial oxygen saturations of ≤90% associated with a short apneic pause or periodic breathing.

II. **Incidence.** The incidence of apnea increases with decreasing gestational age. Practically all infants born at <29 weeks will develop apnea, whereas by 30 weeks, this proportion will decrease to 85% and is further reduced to 20% among those born at 34 weeks. **Mixed is the most common type of apnea (50%), followed by central (40%) and then obstructive (10%).**

III. **Pathophysiology.** AOP is a developmental disorder and generally resolves by 36 to 37 weeks in infants born beyond 27 weeks' gestation. Among more immature infants, apnea can often persist past term gestation. It reflects a "physiologic" rather than "pathologic" immature state of respiratory control.

A. **Fetal to neonatal transition.** Peripheral chemoreceptors are active only at the low oxygen levels in the fetal life and thus become essentially silent in the immediate postnatal period following the increase in partial pressure of oxygen from <30 mm Hg to 50 to 70 mm Hg. Peripheral chemoreceptors undergo a progressive reset postnatally, and chemoreceptor drive is significant at the relatively hypoxic level of 50 to 70 mm Hg. This postnatal adjustment may be delayed when neonates are exposed to 100% oxygen during resuscitation. These infants can become apneic when their inspired oxygen is increased sufficiently to produce a physiologic denervation of peripheral chemoreceptors, resulting in a brief delay in the onset of spontaneous breathing.

B. **Ventilatory response to hypoxia.** In contrast to adults who show a sustained increase in ventilation in response to hypoxia, preterm infants exhibit a biphasic ventilatory response where the initial increase in ventilation is transient (approximately 1 minute) and is followed by a late sustained decrease in spontaneous breathing. This unique response to hypoxia may last for several weeks in response to hypoxic episodes after birth. This late ventilatory depression is likely an expression of delayed synaptogenesis or myelination within the brainstem and the reticular activated system.

C. **Ventilatory response to laryngeal chemoreflex.** The laryngeal chemoreflex is mediated through the superior laryngeal nerve afferents and is assumed to be a protective reflex. An exaggerated response brought about during feedings may also contribute to apneic episodes.

D. **Neurotransmitters and apnea.** Increased sensitivity to inhibitory neurotransmitters such as γ-aminobutyric acid (GABA), adenosine, serotonin, and prostaglandins may be related to apnea.

E. **Genetic variability and apnea.** Genetic and environmental factors may lead to apnea. Heritability of AOP was 87% among same-gender twins. The congenital hypoventilation syndrome, defined by a lack of carbon dioxide (CO_2) responsiveness during sleep, is thought to occur due to the mutation of the developmental transcription factor PHOX2b.

F. **Sleep-related apnea.** Most apnea occurs during active sleep. Preterm infants are asleep 80% of time, and 50% of sleep is active. This relationship lasts until 6 months of age. During active sleep, there is low-voltage electrocortical activity, decreased arousal from sleep, decreased muscular tone, absence of upper airway adductor activity, and decreased respiratory drive. Irregular breathing and inspiratory chest wall distortion associated with decreased ventilatory drive cause slight elevation in arterial partial pressure of CO_2. The ventilatory response to hypoxia and ventilatory sensitivity to CO_2 are more depressed during active sleep. Activation of serotonin-containing neurons, which are part of the arousal system of the brainstem, decreases by nearly half during slow-wave sleep and becomes nearly silent during rapid eye movement sleep via activation of GABAergic inputs.

G. **Siblings of infants with sudden infant death.** The Collaborative Home Infant Monitoring Evaluation (CHIME) study showed that the incidence of apnea was the same in siblings of infants with sudden infant death syndrome and normal term infants.

H. **Gastroesophageal reflux and apnea.** Most studies have shown no clear temporal relationship between gastroesophageal reflux (GER) and apnea. A decreased lower esophageal sphincter tone and increased GER following apnea have been documented. Apnea with desaturation events can lead to relaxation of the gastroesophageal junction and may explain the presence of formula often found in the pharynx of infants suctioned during an apneic event. Only a small minority of apneic preterm infants are likely to benefit from antireflux therapy. If therapy is started, it should only be continued in the face of clear benefit and discontinued if symptoms fail to improve.

IV. **Risk factors**

A. **Physiologic immaturity of the respiratory center.** This condition is usually present after 1 to 2 days of life and is often referred to as AOP.

B. **Secondary causes**

1. **Neurologic:** Birth trauma, meningitis, intracranial hemorrhage, seizures, perinatal asphyxia, congenital myopathies or neuropathies, placental transfer of narcotics, magnesium sulfate, or general anesthetics.

2. **Pulmonary:** Surfactant deficiency, pneumonia, pulmonary hemorrhage, obstructive airway lesions, pneumothorax.

3. **Cardiac:** Cyanotic congenital heart disease, hyper- or hypotension, congestive heart failure, patent ductus arteriosus, increased vagal tone, and prostaglandin therapy.

4. **Gastrointestinal:** Necrotizing enterocolitis (NEC), GER.
5. **Hematologic:** Anemia.
6. **Hypothermia or hyperthermia.**
7. **Metabolic:** Acidosis, hypoglycemia, hypocalcemia, and hypo- or hypernatremia.
8. **Inborn errors of metabolism.**
9. **Sepsis.**

V. **Clinical manifestations.** It is difficult to separate clinical manifestations of apnea from its consequences. Symptoms and signs depend on the duration and frequency of apnea and most are related to hypoxia. Other clinical manifestations depend on the etiology of apnea such as feeding intolerance, lethargy, temperature instability, jitteriness, poor feeding, central nervous system depression, irritability, desaturation tachypnea, bradycardia, hypotonia, and seizures.

VI. **Diagnosis**

A. **History and physical examination** must include a review of maternal risk factors, medications, birth history, and feeding intolerance. Physical examination should include a search for abnormal neurologic signs and signs of sepsis.

B. **Laboratory studies**

1. **Complete septic workup.**
2. **Screening for metabolic disorders.**
3. **Imaging** to look for pneumonia, air leak, and NEC and cranial ultrasound to detect intracranial hemorrhage or congenital abnormalities.
4. **Electroencephalogram to rule out seizures,** because apnea may be the sole presentation of seizures.

VII. **Management.** Treatment strategies for AOP should be based on modulating an unstable respiratory rhythm into a more stable one.

A. **Pharmacologic management**

1. **Methylxanthines.** Methylxanthines have been the mainstay of pharmacologic treatment of apnea for decades. The primary mechanism of action is thought to be blockade of inhibitory adenosine A_1 receptors with resultant excitation of respiratory neural output. Initially, theophylline (aminophylline) was the standard of treatment, and it required close monitoring of serum levels. **Caffeine citrate has largely replaced theophylline as the first drug for AOP.** Its longer half-life makes for a convenient once-a-day dosing regimen without the need for monitoring blood levels at the recommended dosing.

   Methylxanthines increase minute ventilation, improve CO_2 sensitivity, decrease hypoxic depression, enhance diaphragmatic activity, and decrease periodic breathing. Common side effects include tachycardia, feeding intolerance, emesis, jitteriness, restlessness, and irritability. Toxic effects may produce arrhythmias and seizures. Methylxanthines increase metabolic rate and oxygen consumption and have a mild diuretic effect. In general, caffeine is recommended for all infants born at ≤28 weeks' gestation. Some recommend treating all infants born between 29 and 32 weeks, since most of them have apnea. In a large multicenter randomized study, caffeine treatment was associated with a significant reduction in the incidence of bronchopulmonary dysplasia and retinopathy of prematurity, as well as the duration of mechanical ventilation. Furthermore, a significant decrease in the incidence of cerebral palsy in the caffeine-treated group was observed by 2 years of age. The early beneficial effect on cognitive function was not sustained, but caffeine exposure was associated with a sustained beneficial effect on developmental coordination disorders at 5 years of age and a lesser frequency of motor impairment by 11 years of age. See Chapter 155 for dosing.

2. **Doxapram.** Doxapram is a potent nonspecific respiratory stimulant. It stimulates peripheral chemoreceptors at low dose and central chemoreceptors at high dose. Doxapram increases tidal volume and minute ventilation. Studies have shown effectiveness of doxapram in reducing apnea when refractory to

methylxanthines. As a result of its poorly defined enteral absorption, it is generally administered as a continuous intravenous infusion. Side effects include increases in blood pressure, abdominal distension, irritability, jitteriness, gastric residuals, and emesis. See Chapter 155 for dosing.

B. **Nonpharmacologic management**

1. **Evidence based**

   a. **Prone head-elevated positioning.** The chest wall is stabilized and thoracoabdominal asynchrony is reduced in the prone position. Prone position along with the head elevated in a tilt position showed reduction in apnea and bradycardia.

   b. **Continuous positive airway pressure.** Continuous positive airway pressure (CPAP) at 4 to 6 cm H_2O has proven to be a safe and effective therapy of AOP. It is effective primarily against the obstructive components of apneic episodes. CPAP appears to be effective by "splinting" the upper airway with positive pressure and decreasing the risk of pharyngeal or laryngeal obstruction. Lung functional residual capacity, often reduced in preterm infants, increases with the application of CPAP. As such, an increase in pulmonary oxygen stores may reduce the severity and duration of apnea-induced hypoxemia. Devices that provide high-flow delivery of gas through nasal cannula can produce a similar benefit while enhancing the mobility of the infant. The safety of high-flow delivery devices is of concern because the resultant airway pressures generated are relatively unregulated.

   c. **Synchronized nasal ventilation.** An extension of CPAP is administration of nasal intermittent positive-pressure ventilation, which delivers intermittent lung inflations set to a peak pressure delivered through nasal prongs or mask. Its use has been shown to decrease the need for and duration of endotracheal (invasive) mechanical ventilation.

2. **Other interventions with unclear efficacy**

   a. **Orogastric versus nasogastric feeding tube placement.** A nasogastric tube increases nasal resistance by 50%; therefore, orogastric feeding tubes are sometimes preferred in preterm infants with apnea.

   b. **Kangaroo mother care.** Studies have shown that infants receiving kangaroo mother care had decreased episodes of apnea and bradycardia. The effect of kangaroo mother care in improvement of apnea and bradycardia is the same as that seen with prone positioning.

   c. **Stable environmental temperature.** Provision of a stable thermal environment avoids temperature fluctuations, which can precipitate apneic episodes.

   d. **Tactile stimulation.** Synchronization of respiration may be achieved between the infant's own breathing rhythm and an external rhythm generator (eg, inflatable mattress connected to a respirator). Recently, stochastic mechanosensory stimulation using actuators embedded in a specially designed mattress for subcutaneous stimulation has been shown to decrease the duration of oxygen desaturation.

   e. **Red blood cell transfusion.** An increase in respiratory drive resulting from an increased tissue oxygenation is one of the proposed mechanisms for red blood cell transfusion to ameliorate AOP. Over the past 30 years, there have been few and often conflicting studies on the association between red blood cell transfusions and apnea. Many of these studies defined apnea events from nursing charts, which have been demonstrated to underreport and inaccurately identify apnea events. Its potential beneficial effect on the frequency of apnea is mitigated by the concern that blood transfusion may be associated with an increased risk for NEC.

   f. **Oxygen administration.** Supplemental oxygen should be provided as needed to avoid hypoxia and maintain SpO_2 between 88% and 94%, because hypoxia can lead to severe desaturation episodes. Risk of hyperoxia and retinopathy of prematurity should limit this modality of treatment.

      g. **Treating gastroesophageal reflux.** Some treat GER due to the belief that GER precipitates episodes of apnea. The mechanism could be secondary to the laryngeal chemoreflex. Studies on pharmacologic treatment have not shown any association or benefit.

VIII. **Discharge planning and follow-up**
  A. **Consider stopping caffeine at 34 weeks of postmenstrual age.**
  B. **A more aggressive approach is to stop when the infant is apnea free** for a period of 5 to 7 days irrespective of age.
  C. **If asymptomatic for 5 to 7 days after stopping methylxanthines,** the infant may be discharged without further therapy. Measurement of serum caffeine levels may be necessary beforehand as these levels may not become subtherapeutic until 11 to 12 days after cessation of treatment.
  D. **Considerations for home apnea monitoring**
    1. Persistent, symptomatic apnea at >36 weeks of postmenstrual age.
    2. History of severe apparent life-threatening event and abnormal polysomnography.
    3. Technology-dependent infant (eg, home mechanical ventilation).
    4. Home oxygen administration.
    5. Central hypoventilation syndromes.

IX. **Prognosis.** AOP resolves with maturation. Physiologic basis for resolution of apnea is believed to be myelination of the brainstem. Poor neurodevelopmental outcome is associated with a delay in myelination in infants with AOP. Otherwise, in most infants, apnea resolves without the occurrence of long-term deficiencies.

90 Bronchopulmonary Dysplasia/Chronic Lung Disease

I. **Definition.** Classic bronchopulmonary dysplasia (BPD) is a neonatal form of chronic pulmonary disorder. BPD was solely defined as persistent oxygen dependency up to 28 days of life. The severity of BPD-related pulmonary dysfunction and neurodevelopmental impairment in early childhood is more accurately predicted by an oxygen dependence at 36 weeks' postmenstrual age (PMA) in infants <32 weeks' gestational age (GA) and at 56 days of age in infants with older GA. **BPD is thus classified at this later postnatal age according to the type of respiratory support required to maintain a normal arterial oxygen saturation (>89%) among infants who had been requiring supplemental oxygen during the first 28 days of life.**
  A. **Mild bronchopulmonary dysplasia.** Infants who have been weaned from supplemental oxygen.
  B. **Moderate bronchopulmonary dysplasia.** Infants who continue to need up to 30% oxygen.
  C. **Severe bronchopulmonary dysplasia.** Infants whose requirements exceed 30% and/or include continuous positive airway pressure (CPAP) or mechanical ventilation. However, recently, it has been suggested to further classify severe BPD (sBPD) into **type 1 sBPD**, which consists of oxygen dependency of >30% or need for nasal CPAP/high-flow nasal cannula, and **type 2 sBPD** if mechanical ventilation was needed, regardless of the degree of oxygen dependency, at or beyond 36 weeks' PMA.

II. **Evolution.** The old or "classic" form of BPD was described by Northway in 1967 during the presurfactant era and prior to the use of "gentler" mechanical ventilation strategies. It consisted of tissue damage in both airways and alveoli. In contrast, the recent and new form of BPD consists of no injuries but rather arrested lung growth and lack of both alveolar septation and vascular simplification (remodeling).

III. **Incidence.** The incidence of BPD is influenced by many risk factors, the most important of which is degree of immaturity. The incidence of BPD increases with decreasing birthweight and affects approximately 30% of infants with birthweights <1000 g. The large variability in rates among centers is partly related to differences in clinical practices, such as criteria used for the management of mechanical ventilation.

IV. **Pathophysiology.** A primary lung injury is not always evident at birth. The secondary development of a persistent lung injury is the result of abnormal repair process of recurrent injuries occurring during a critical window of lung development.

  A. **The major factors contributing to bronchopulmonary dysplasia are as follows:**

    1. **Inflammation.** Central to the development of BPD. An exaggerated inflammatory response (alveolar influx of numerous proinflammatory cytokines as well as macrophages and leukocytes) occurs in the first few days of life in infants in whom BPD subsequently develops.

    2. **Mechanical ventilation.** Volutrauma/barotrauma is 1 of the key risk factors for the development of BPD. Minimizing the use of mechanical ventilation by the use of early nasal CPAP, noninvasive ventilatory support (nasal intermittent positive-pressure ventilation), and early use of methylxanthines (caffeine) has led to fewer days of mechanical ventilation, lesser use of postnatal steroids, and lower rates of sBPD.

    3. **Oxygen exposure.** Classic BPD observed before the availability of exogenous surfactant treatment was always associated with prolonged exposure (>150 hours) to a fraction of inspired oxygen >60%. Today, in the postsurfactant era, exposure to prolonged high oxygen is limited, and a new form of BPD has been reported. For this **"new" BPD**, the association between persistent need for mechanical ventilation and supplemental oxygen in the first 2 weeks of life is not as strong as it was in the past. For instance, a third of the preterm infants receiving either supplemental oxygen or intermittent positive-pressure ventilation at 14 days did not develop BPD, whereas 17% of the infants on room air at 14 days of age did.

  B. **Pathologic changes.** Compared with the presurfactant era, lungs of infants currently dying from BPD have normal-appearing airways, less fibrosis, and more uniform inflation. However, these lungs have deficient septation, leading to fewer and larger alveoli with possible reduced pulmonary capillarization that may lead to pulmonary hypertension.

V. **Risk factors.** Major risk factors are prematurity, white race, male sex, chorioamnionitis, tracheal colonization with *Ureaplasma*, and the increased survival of the extremely low birthweight infant. Other risk factors are chorioamnionitis, respiratory distress syndrome (RDS), small for gestation, excessive early intravenous fluid administration, symptomatic patent ductus arteriosus (PDA), sepsis, oxygen therapy, and vitamin A deficiency.

VI. **Clinical presentation.** BPD is usually suspected in infants with progressive and idiopathic deterioration of pulmonary function. Infants in whom BPD develops often require oxygen therapy or mechanical ventilation beyond the first week of life. Severe cases of BPD are usually associated with poor growth, pulmonary edema, and a hyperreactive airway.

VII. **Diagnosis**

  A. **Physical examination**

    1. **General signs.** Worsening respiratory status is manifested by an increase in the work of breathing, in oxygen requirement, in apnea-bradycardia, or in a combination of these signs.

   2. **Pulmonary examination.** Retractions and diffuse fine rales are common. Wheezing or prolongation of expiration may also be noted.
   3. **Cardiovascular examination.** A right ventricular heave, single S_2, or prominent P_2 may accompany cor pulmonale.
   4. **Abdominal examination.** The liver may be enlarged secondary to right-sided heart failure or may be displaced downward into the abdomen secondary to lung hyperinflation.
   B. **Laboratory studies.** These studies are intended to rule out the differential diagnosis such as sepsis or PDA during the acute nature of the disease and to detect problems related to BPD or its therapy.
   1. **Arterial blood gas levels.** Frequently reveal carbon dioxide retention. However, if the respiratory difficulties are chronic and stable, the pH is usually subnormal (pH ≥7.25).
   2. **Electrolytes.** Abnormalities of electrolytes may result from chronic carbon dioxide retention (elevated serum bicarbonate), diuretic therapy (hyponatremia, hypokalemia, or hypochloremia), or fluid restriction (elevated urea nitrogen and creatinine), or all 3.
   3. **Complete blood count and differential.** To diagnose neutropenia or an elevated white blood count in sepsis.
   4. **B-type natriuretic peptide.** After 6 weeks of age, monitoring B-type natriuretic peptide (BNP) levels biweekly may help in an early detection of pulmonary hypertension, which if unrecognized will lead to cor pulmonale. A rise in BNP plasma levels suggests a need to perform an echocardiogram.
   5. **Urinalysis.** Microscopic examination may reveal the presence of red blood cells, which might suggest nephrocalcinosis as a result of prolonged loop diuretic treatment.
   C. **Imaging and other studies.** To detect problems related to BPD or its therapy.
   1. **Chest radiograph.** Radiographic findings may be quite variable. Most frequently, BPD appears as diffuse haziness and lung hypoinflation in infants who were very immature at birth and have persistent oxygen requirements. In other infants, a different picture is seen, reminiscent of that originally described by Northway: streaky interstitial markings, patchy atelectasis intermingled with cystic area, and severe overall lung hyperinflation. Because those findings persist for a prolonged period, new changes (eg, a secondary infection) are difficult to detect without the benefit of comparison to previous radiographs. (See Figure 12–20 for an example of BPD.)
   2. **Renal ultrasonography.** Radiologic studies of the abdomen should be considered during loop diuretic therapy to detect the presence of nephrocalcinosis. It should be performed when red blood cells are present in the urine.
   3. **Echocardiography.** Screening echocardiograms are indicated monthly in non-improving or weekly in worsening BPD. Echocardiograms can detect pulmonary hypertension, manifested by right ventricular hypertrophy and elevation of pulmonary artery pressure (increased tricuspid regurgitant jet velocity), increased right systolic time intervals, thickening of the right ventricular wall, and abnormal right ventricular geometry (ventricular septal wall flattening).
VIII. **Management**
   A. **Prevention of bronchopulmonary dysplasia**
   1. **Prevention of prematurity and respiratory distress syndrome.** Therapies directed toward decreasing the risk of prematurity and lowering the incidence of RDS include improved prenatal care and antenatal corticosteroids.
   2. **Reducing exposure to risk factors.** Successful measures should include minimizing exposure to oxygen by limiting arterial oxygen saturation to 90% to 95%, ventilation strategies that minimize the use of excessive tidal volume (>4–6 mL/kg), prudent administration of fluids, aggressive closure of PDA (***controversial***), and adequate nutrition. **Early surfactant replacement therapy may be**

beneficial, but the avoidance of intubation and mechanical ventilation with the initiation of CPAP shortly after birth may prove to be an effective preventive strategy. Lesser invasive methods of pulmonary administration of surfactant through methods such as **LISA** (less invasive surfactant administration: surfactant via thin diameter tubes under direct vision using laryngoscopes) **or INSURE** (intubation and surfactant administration followed by immediate extubation) **both in conjunction with CPAP are associated with the lowest likelihood of the composite outcome of death or BPD at 36 weeks.** A similar beneficial effect has been reported when surfactant is intratracheally co-administered with budesonide.

3. **Vitamin A.** Low blood levels of vitamin A seen in extremely low birthweight infants have been associated with increased risk of BPD. Vitamin A supplementation, 5000 IU administered intramuscularly 3 times per week for 4 weeks, showed modest reduction in the rate of BPD. The number needed to treat to prevent 1 BPD was 15; however, no long-term beneficial respiratory or neurodevelopmental outcomes have been found.

4. **Caffeine.** Methylxanthines decrease the frequency of apnea and allow for shorter duration of mechanical ventilation, leading to a reduced rate of BPD.

5. **Inhaled nitric oxide.** At present, routine use of inhaled nitric oxide (iNO) for preterm infants at risk for BPD is not recommended.

B. **Treatment of bronchopulmonary dysplasia.** Once BPD is present, the goal is to prevent further injury by minimizing respiratory support, improving pulmonary function, preventing cor pulmonale, and emphasizing growth and nutrition.

1. **Respiratory support**

   a. **Supplemental oxygen.** Maintaining adequate oxygenation (oxygen saturation 90%–95%) is important in the infant with BPD to prevent alveolar hypoxia-induced pulmonary hypertension, bronchospasm, cor pulmonale, and growth failure. However, the least-required oxygen should be delivered to minimize oxygen toxicity. Routine blood gas measurements are important for the assessment of trends in pH, arterial partial pressure of carbon dioxide ($PaCO_2$), and serum bicarbonate, but they are of limited use in monitoring oxygenation because they provide information about only 1 point in time.

   b. **Positive-pressure ventilation.** Mechanical ventilation should be used only when clearly indicated. Similarly, inspiratory pressure needs to be limited at the expense of tolerating $PaCO_2$ of 50 to 60 mm Hg (*controversial*). Nasal CPAP and noninvasive nasal ventilation can be useful as an adjunctive therapy after extubation.

2. **Improving lung function**

   a. **Fluid restriction.** Restricting fluid to 120 mL/kg/d is often required. It can be accomplished by concentrating proprietary formulas to 24 kcal/oz. Increasing the caloric density further to 27 to 30 kcal/oz may require the addition of fat (eg, medium-chain triglyceride oil or corn oil) and carbohydrate (eg, Polycose) to avoid excessive protein intake.

   b. **Diuretic therapy.** See Chapter 155 for dosing.

      i. **Furosemide.** Furosemide (1–2 mg/kg every 12 hours, orally or intravenously) is a potent diuretic that is particularly useful for rapid diuresis and acute improvement in lung mechanical properties. There is less evidence for its long-term pulmonary benefit. Its chronic use is associated with side effects such as electrolyte abnormalities, calciuria with bone demineralization, renal stone formation, and ototoxicity. When used as a chronic medication, Na^+ and K^+ supplementation is often required.

      ii. **Bumetanide.** Bumetanide 0.015 to 0.1 mg/kg daily or every other day, orally or intravenously. When administered orally, 1 mg of bumetanide (Bumex) has a diuretic effect similar to that of 40 mg of furosemide. Whereas furosemide's bioavailability is 30% to 70%, bumetanide's bioavailability is >90%. Bumetanide produces side effects similar to those of furosemide, except that it may produce less ototoxicity and less interference with bilirubin-albumin binding.

   iii. **Chlorothiazide and spironolactone.** When used in doses of 20 mg/kg/d (chlorothiazide) and 2 mg/kg/d (spironolactone), a good diuretic response can often be achieved. Although less potent than furosemide, this combination is often better suited for chronic management because it has relatively fewer side effects. In the absence of the need for sodium supplementation, it may be the diuretic combination of choice when the calciuric effect of furosemide has led to the development of nephrocalcinosis.

c. **Bronchodilators.** See doses in Table 9–3.

   i. **β_2-Agonists.** Inhaled β_2-agonists (eg, albuterol, levalbuterol) produce acute improvements in lung mechanics and gas exchange in infants with BPD exhibiting symptoms of increased airway tone. Their effect is usually time limited. Because of their side effects (eg, tachycardia, hypertension, hyperglycemia, and possible arrhythmia), their use should be limited to the management of acute exacerbations of BPD. **Levalbuterol (Xopenex)** is a nonracemic form of albuterol. The difference between levalbuterol and albuterol is modest, but levalbuterol has fewer side effects. If bronchodilators are being used long term, a frequent reevaluation of their benefits is essential.

   ii. **Anticholinergic agents.** The best studied and most widely available inhaled quaternary anticholinergic is **ipratropium bromide** (nebulized Atrovent). Its bronchodilatory effect is more potent than that of atropine and similar to that of albuterol. Combined albuterol and ipratropium therapy has a greater effect than either agent alone. Unlike atropine, systemic effects do not occur because of its poor systemic absorption.

d. **Corticosteroids.** Several randomized controlled trials have demonstrated that among infants at risk for BPD, treatment with systemic corticosteroids facilitates extubation and improves lungs mechanical properties. There is a significant heterogeneity regarding the type, dose, and duration of corticosteroid treatment. Although very efficient, the use of postnatal steroids should be limited to infants who are at high risk for mortality secondary to severe lung disease. There are concerns regarding the short- and long-term side effects of systemic steroids. These include hyperglycemia, hypertension, hypertrophic cardiomyopathy, gastrointestinal hemorrhage and perforation (in conjunction with prostaglandin inhibitors such as indomethacin), enhanced catabolism and growth failure, nephrocalcinosis, poor bone mineralization, and susceptibility to infection. Parents should be informed that the use of postnatal steroids could be associated with impaired brain and somatic growth and increased incidence of cerebral palsy. Although dexamethasone has been the most studied postnatal steroid in the treatment of BPD, various therapy regimens and using milder types of steroids have been proposed, in hopes of decreasing the observed adverse effects.

   i. **Dexamethasone.** Initiate at >7 days of age at 0.25 mg/kg twice daily for 3 days and then gradually taper by 10% every 3 days for a total course of 42 days. It is one of the original regimens that have been proven efficacious in the treatment of BPD. When the risk of BPD is less than approximately 33%, this treatment significantly increased the risk of death or cerebral palsy. At a higher probability to develop BPD (approximately >60%), the same therapy reduced the risk of death or cerebral palsy. Lower doses and shorter duration of dexamethasone have been attempted to decrease its undesirable effects such as a 10-day tapering course of dexamethasone for a total of 0.89 mg/kg over 10 days.

ii. **Hydrocortisone.** 5 mg/kg/d divided every 6 hours for 1 week, and then gradually tapered for the following 2 to 5 weeks (>7 days of age). In contrast to infants treated with dexamethasone, when compared with controls, hydrocortisone therapy has not been associated with adverse neurodevelopmental outcome or with brain abnormalities on magnetic resonance imaging in long-term follow-up studies of patients up to 5 to 8 years of age. Recently, early (first 10 days of age) low-dose hydrocortisone (1 mg/kg/d for 7 days, then 0.5 mg/kg/d) was found to be helpful and safe.

iii. **Prednisolone and methylprednisolone (Solu-Medrol)** have also been used.

iv. **Nebulized corticosteroids.** Nebulized corticosteroids (beclomethasone or budesonide) produced fewer side effects than oral or parenteral forms but are much less efficacious in the treatment of BPD when given at a late stage. Earlier onset of treatment has been shown to be more efficient, but concern about a possible poorly explained increase in mortality has been raised.

e. **Tracheostomy.** For infants who have failed several attempts at extubation and have become large enough for their head movements to interfere with artificial ventilation. It provides respiratory stability, helps in involving families in infant care, and facilitates home discharge

3. **Pulmonary hypertension**

a. **The "new" bronchopulmonary dysplasia** is characterized by defects in alveolarization as well as a defect in angiogenesis, leading to the development of pulmonary hypertension. Pulmonary hypertension has been reported to be associated with BPD in nearly 20% of extremely preterm babies overall and in 50% of those with severe chronic lung disease (sBPD). A high index of suspicion needs to be present whenever a progressive increase in the level of respiratory support is noticed. Screening echocardiograms for evidence of pulmonary hypertension by echocardiography should be performed in all patients with sBPD. Subsequent echocardiograms should be performed in patients with sBPD at 1- to 2-month intervals until the respiratory status of the patient is significantly improved. Changes in serial blood BNP and N-terminal pro-BNP levels may provide additional guides.

b. **Treatment.** Periods of acute hypoxemia, whether intermittent or prolonged, contribute to the pathogenesis of late pulmonary hypertension in sBPD; therefore, oxygen saturation limits may need to be changed to avoid intermittent or sustained hypoxemia with targets generally between 92% and 95%.

c. **Current therapies used for pulmonary hypertension therapy in infants with BPD** generally include iNO, phosphodiesterase type 5 inhibitors, endothelin receptor antagonists, calcium channel blockers, endothelin receptor antagonists, and prostacyclin analogs (see Chapter 115 on pulmonary hypertension).

4. **Growth and nutrition.** Because growth is essential for recovery from BPD, adequate nutritional intake is crucial. Infants with BPD frequently have high caloric needs (≥120–150 kcal/kg/d) because of increased metabolic expenditures. Concentrated formula is often necessary to provide sufficient calories and prevent pulmonary edema. In addition, specific micronutrient supplementation, such as antioxidant therapy, may also enhance pulmonary and nutritional status. Enteral docosahexaenoic acid supplementation may increase the risk for BPD.

C. **Discharge planning.** Care plans for older infants with BPD should include adapting their routine for home life and involving the parents in their care. All parents should be instructed in cardiopulmonary resuscitation.

1. **Oxygen therapy** can often be discontinued before discharge from the neonatal intensive care unit. However, home oxygen therapy can be a safe alternative

to long-term hospitalization. The need for home respiratory, heart rate, and oxygen monitoring must be decided on an individual basis but is generally recommended for infants discharged home on oxygen.

2. **Immunizations.** Immunizations should be given at the appropriate chronologic age. Synagis (palivizumab, humanized monoclonal antibodies against respiratory syncytial virus [RSV]) should be given monthly (15 mg/kg administered intramuscularly) throughout the RSV season. All parents should be instructed in cardiopulmonary resuscitation. **Periodic screening** for chemical evidence of rickets and echocardiographic evidence of pulmonary hypertension is recommended

3. **Assessment by a developmental specialist** and occupational or physical therapist, or both, can be useful for prognostic and therapeutic purposes.

IX. **Prognosis.** The prognosis for infants with BPD depends on the degree of pulmonary dysfunction and the presence of other medical conditions. Most deaths occur in the first year of life as a result of cardiorespiratory failure, sepsis, or respiratory infection or as a sudden, unexplained death.

A. **Pulmonary outcome.** The short-term outcome of infants with BPD, including those requiring oxygen at home, is surprisingly good. Weaning from oxygen is usually possible before their first birthday, and infants demonstrate catch-up growth as their pulmonary status improves. However, in the first year of life, rehospitalization is necessary for approximately 30% of patients for treatment of wheezing, respiratory infections, or both. Although upper respiratory tract infections are probably no more common in infants with BPD than in normal infants, they are more likely to be associated with significant respiratory symptoms. Most adolescents and young adults who had moderate to severe BPD in infancy have some degree of pulmonary dysfunction, consisting of airway obstruction, reactive airway disease, and hyperinflation.

B. **Neurodevelopmental outcome.** Children with moderate to severe BPD appear to be at an increased risk for adverse neurodevelopmental outcome compared with comparable infants without BPD. Neuromotor and cognitive dysfunction appears to be more common. In addition, children with BPD may be at higher risk for significant hearing impairment and retinopathy of prematurity. They are also at risk for later problems, including learning disabilities, attention deficits, and behavior problems.

91 Calcium Disorders (Hypocalcemia, Hypercalcemia)

Abnormalities of calcium (Ca^{2+}) and magnesium (Mg^{2+}) metabolism are not infrequent occurrences among infants admitted for neonatal intensive care. Moreover, the disturbances of Ca^{2+} may be mirrored by Mg^{2+}, or conversely, as in hypocalcemia and hypomagnesemia. Infants of diabetic mothers (IDMs) and infants with fetal growth restriction (FGR) may present with low serum levels of either Ca^{2+} or Mg^{2+} or both. Serum values for Ca^{2+} and Mg^{2+} above or below accepted normal values are of concern in any infant and warrant further clinical studies. Magnesium disorders are discussed in Chapter 105.

I. **Hypocalcemia**

A. **Definition.** Hypocalcemia is determined by either **total serum calcium (tCa) or ionized calcium (iCa) values.** Clinical chemistry values for serum levels vary by units (ie, mEq/L, mmol/L, or mg/dL), by gestational age, and by day of age following the immediate newborn period. Reference textbooks reflect considerable variance of serum values for Ca^{2+} and Mg^{2+}. Interpretation of serum values for any given patient is dependent on recognition of one's institution laboratory values and range of acceptable values.

A generally accepted value for hypocalcemia is <2.0 mmol/L (<8.0 mg/dL) for a term infant or <1.75 mmol/L (<7.0 mg/dL) for a preterm infant. A typical range of normal values for a term newborn can be 2.25 to 2.65 mmol/L (9.0–10.6 mg/dL) throughout the first week of life. Preterm infant tCa levels closely parallel those for term infants. Of greater significance is the ionized fraction of Ca^{2+}. It is the active physiologic component and is dependent on the interaction of tCa^{2+}, acid-base status, and serum albumin. Typical iCa^{2+} values for term infants over the first 72 hours of life are 1.22 to 1.24 mmol/L (4.88–4.96 mg/dL). Preterm infant mean values are similar for 24 to 72 hours: 1.21 to 1.28 mmol/L (4.84–5.12 mg/dL). Thereafter, preterm infants have slightly increased iCa^{2+} levels, whereas term infants experience a slight decline. **iCa levels of <1.2 mmol/dL (4 mg/dL) are considered hypocalcemic.**

B. **Incidence.** Hypocalcemia is likely the most common disorder of either Ca^{2+} or Mg^{2+} in newborn infants, and it affects both preterm and term infants. It occurs in up to 30% of infants with birthweight <1500 g. Late-onset hypocalcemia is more common in developing countries where cow's milk or formulas with phosphate concentrations are used.

C. **Pathophysiology.** iCa^{2+} is the biologically important form of calcium. The tCa^{2+} levels have been repeatedly shown to not be predictive of iCa^{2+} levels. Therefore, tCa^{2+} levels are unreliable as criteria for true hypocalcemia. In premature infants, it has been shown that tCa^{2+} levels as low as ≤6 mg/dL correspond to iCa^{2+} levels >3 mg/dL.

D. **Risk factors**

   1. **Early-onset neonatal hypocalcemia.** During the third trimester of pregnancy, the human fetus receives at least 120 to 150 mg/kg/d of elemental Ca^{2+} via the umbilical cord. Most of this Ca^{2+} is readily incorporated into the newly forming bones. After delivery, this massive supply of Ca^{2+} is suddenly stopped, and Ca^{2+} must be given enterally.

      a. **A full-term infant receiving 100 to 120 mL of normal formula** would be receiving 50 to 60 mg/kg/d of Ca^{2+} orally. Despite this drop in supply, full-term infants tolerate the change well and do not become hypocalcemic.

      b. **Premature (especially <28 weeks) or sick infants** often become hypocalcemic during the first 3 days of life. Total serum Ca^{2+} levels can drop to <7 mg/dL and occasionally fall below 6 mg/dL.

      c. **Calcium levels** (both iCa^{2+} and tCa^{2+}) usually return to normal within 48 to 72 hours regardless of whether supplemental Ca^{2+} is given. Immunoreactive parathyroid hormone is often low at birth but rises to higher levels within 24 to 72 hours after delivery. Intravenous (IV) Ca^{2+} supplementation suppresses this increase in immunoreactive parathyroid hormone; thus, some centers for neonatal care do not use early IV calcium supplementation.

   2. **Perinatal stress.** Term or preterm infants who have perinatal asphyxia can present with hypocalcemia secondary to elevated blood calcitonin level. Resuscitation and the use of alkali to correct acidosis (bicarbonate therapy), even though used less frequently since the new Neonatal Resuscitation Program guidelines, may result in alkalosis that increases the affinity of albumin for calcium and thereby decreases the concentration of ionized calcium.

   3. **Infant of diabetic mother.** Onset of hypocalcemia is usually early (1–3 days) and may recur throughout the first week. The mechanism for IDM hypocalcemia is unknown. Related factors that have been identified are increased calcitonin levels, decreased bone Ca^{2+} flux, hypomagnesemia, hypoparathyroidism, and hyperphosphatemia. The occurrence and severity of IDM hypocalcemia follow the severity of maternal diabetes and the prenatal management for euglycemic control.

4. **Intrauterine growth restriction.** Sporadic hypocalcemia occurs and may be associated with ≥1 of the known complications of IUGR (eg, hypoglycemia, asphyxia, hypothermia, polycythemia, or placental insufficiency).

5. **Nutritional deprivation.** Infants unable to take enteral feeds by 3 days of age will need calcium supplementation. Breast milk or calcium-enriched formulas provide adequate Ca^{2+} intake. Because hypocalcemia is related to hypomagnesemia, both elements require supplementation to prevent a secondary suppression of parathormone leading to the recurrence of hypocalcemia.

6. **Hypomagnesemia.** May be secondary to maternal gestational magnesium losses or to impaired intestinal uptake. Hypomagnesemia frequently occurs with hypocalcemia and must be looked for in any at-risk infant.

7. **Congenital abnormalities.** The DiGeorge sequence with absence of parathyroid glands and related craniofacial and cardiac anomalies often presents with hypocalcemia. Other rare conditions may include familial isolated hypoparathyroidism.

8. **Maternal hyperparathyroidism.** This causes transient hypoparathyroidism in the infant due to fetal parathyroid suppression.

9. **Other therapeutic modalities.** These include furosemide-induced hypercalciuria; citrated blood transfusions, which reduce iCa^{2+} due to a citrate-calcium complex and alkalosis following metabolism of citrate; and inadequate prenatal vitamin D supplementation of the mother or the infant during the first 6 months of life. Maternal use of anticonvulsants such as phenobarbital can cause increased hepatic catabolism of vitamin D, resulting in maternal vitamin D deficiency and subsequent neonatal hypocalcemia.

E. **Clinical presentation**
   1. **Early-onset hypocalcemia (first week of life)**
      a. Apnea
      b. Stridor
      c. Irritability, jitteriness, tremors, or hyperreflexia
      d. Clonus, tetany, or seizures
      e. Arrhythmia secondary to prolonged QT interval
   2. **Late-onset hypocalcemia (any time after first week)**
      a. Lethargy, apnea
      b. Feeding intolerance
      c. Abdominal distention
      d. Bone demineralization, increased alkaline phosphatase
      e. Skeletal fractures
   3. **Paradoxically, neonatal hypocalcemia is often asymptomatic.** Only an index of suspicion based on risk factors will lead to a correct diagnosis.

F. **Diagnosis**
   1. **Laboratory studies**
      a. **Total and ionized calcium levels** should be available for the neonatal intensive care unit patient. Serum tCa levels of <1.75 mmol/L (7.0 mg/dL) are diagnostic and iCa levels of <1.10 mmol/L (4.4 mg/dL) are confirmatory of hypocalcemia.
      b. **Serum magnesium levels** of <1.5 mg/dL are indicative of hypocalcemia because they often coexist.
      c. **Elevated alkaline phosphatase levels.**
      d. **Urinary calcium losses** of >4 mg/kg/24 h are indicative of hypercalciuria.
      e. **Testing for vitamin D** metabolites, parathyroid hormone level, calcitonin, and genetic screening (eg, microarray for 22q deletion) should also be considered to determine the etiology of hypocalcemia.
   2. **Imaging studies for bone demineralization, metaphyseal lucencies, and rib and long bone fractures** may be helpful for late hypocalcemia. More acutely, the absence of a thymic shadow on chest radiograph will suggest the DiGeorge sequence. For late-onset hypocalcemia and rickets, dual-energy X-ray

absorptiometry scan and quantitative ultrasonography using broadband ultrasonographic measurement, speed of sound, or bone transmission time have been employed to assess bone density.

3. **Electrocardiographic studies** will identify arrhythmias due to QT interval changes.

G. **Management**

1. **Acute treatment.** Reserved for the symptomatic hypocalcemic infants with apneic spells, seizures, or cardiac failure with arrhythmia. Dosage is 100 to 200 mg/kg of 10% calcium gluconate *slowly* by peripheral IV over 15 to 20 minutes with constant cardiac monitoring (see Chapter 155 for dosing information).

2. **Maintenance treatment.** For infants with limited enteral intake or who are dependent on parenteral calcium intake, an IV dosage of 20 to 60 mg/kg/d of elemental calcium with a calcium-to-phosphate ratio ranging from 1.3:1.0 to 2:1 is adequate for promoting both calcium and phosphate retention. Parenteral fluids cannot approximate the intrauterine level of Ca^{2+} intake (~140 mg/kg/d of elemental calcium) without some precipitation in solution. Therefore, early and continuous maintenance treatment is essential until milk or formula feeds can be successfully initiated.

3. **Vitamin D supplementation.** Should be started along with parenteral nutrition at 400 IU/d.

4. **Intravenous calcium administration.** This is not without some risk for complications. The potential problems include extravasation of calcium solution and resulting subcutaneous calcium deposition with limited joint movement, sloughing of skin, nephrocalcinosis, cardiac arrhythmias with prolonged QT intervals, or bradycardia if Ca^{2+} gluconate is given too quickly.

5. **Hypocalcemia secondary to blood/exchange transfusions.** This may require supplementation with Ca^{2+} gluconate but may result in rebound hypercalcemia.

6. **Hypocalcemia secondary to diuretic therapy.** Infants receiving loop diuretics have an increased urinary loss of calcium. This loss can be demonstrated by the urine calcium-to-creatinine ratio (>0.21–0.25). If hypercalciuria exists, an attempt should be made to substitute furosemide or bumetanide with chlorothiazide. Thiazide diuretics cause calcium retention and tend to offset the calciuric effect of loop diuretics in the absence of sodium supplementation.

H. **Prognosis.** No long-term effects of neonatal hypocalcemia are seen as attributable to known adverse neurobehavioral or neurologic outcomes of preterm or sick term infants. Both hypocalcemia and hypomagnesemia have a generally good outcome if diagnosed promptly and treated adequately. The exception is a clinical presentation that includes seizures for either hypocalcemia or hypomagnesemia associated with asphyxia or an underlying endocrine or genetic disorder.

II. **Hypercalcemia**

A. **Definition. Hypercalcemia is defined as an iCa^{2+} serum level >1.35 mmol/L (5.4 mg/dL) for any infant, irrespective of a tCa serum level.** The iCa^{2+} level is the physiologically active component of serum Ca^{2+} and thus the most important determination. Although tCa^{2+} is indicative of hypercalcemia at levels >2.75 mmol/L (11 mg/dL), it is not a reliable measure.

B. **Incidence.** Uncommon and a specific occurrence rate is unknown. It occurs much less often in infants than adults.

C. **Pathophysiology.** Hypercalcemia may be due to parathyroid-related causes or to mechanisms unrelated to the parathyroid. A number of cases of hypercalcemia have recently been reported in neonatal units due to subcutaneous fat necrosis following therapeutic hypothermia as treatment for hypoxic ischemic encephalopathy. A number of cases of hypercalcemia are related to clinical management due to excessive supplementation of vitamin A or D, calcium salts, or thiazide diuretics. A rare condition due to polymorphisms of calcium-sensing receptors can also result in hypercalcemia. Two forms involving calcium receptors are familial hypocalciuric hypercalcemia and neonatal hyperparathyroidism.

D. Risk factors
   1. **Congenital hyperparathyroidism**
      a. **Primary.** Due to genetic defects as either familial hypocalciuria, hypercalcemia, or severe neonatal hyperparathyroidism.
      b. **Secondary.** Due to maternal hypoparathyroidism.
   2. **Maternal hypocalcemia**
   3. **Subcutaneous fat necrosis**
   4. **Therapeutic hypothermia**
   5. **Idiopathic infantile hypercalcemia**
   6. **Williams syndrome**
   7. **Hypophosphatasia**
   8. **Hyper- or hypothyroidism**
   9. **Malignancy (very rare in the newborn)**
   10. **Distal renal tubular acidosis, Jansen metaphyseal chondrodysplasia**
   11. **Iatrogenic**
      a. Hypophosphatemia due to inadequate dietary intake of phosphorus, especially in preterm infants
      b. Excessive vitamin D intake
      c. Excessive calcium intake
      d. Thiazide diuretics
      e. Extracorporeal life support
E. Clinical presentation. Mostly hypercalcemia is asymptomatic unless severe hypercalcemic levels have been reached and signs as described below appear.
   1. Feeding intolerance, constipation, failure to thrive
   2. Polyuria, dehydration
   3. Hematuria, nephrocalcinosis, nephrolithiasis
   4. Lethargy, hypotonia, seizures (rare, only in the most severe hypercalcemia)
   5. Bradycardia, short QT interval, hypertension
F. Diagnosis
   1. **Laboratory studies**
      a. Serum calcium for levels as given previously
      b. Serum total protein and albumin-globulin ratio for hypoproteinemia
      c. Blood gases for acid-base status
      d. Serum phosphorus for hypophosphatemia
      e. Urine calcium and phosphorus
      f. Parathyroid hormone, 25-hydroxy (OH) vitamin D, 1, 25-OH vitamin D
      g. Thyroid studies
      h. Alkaline phosphatase for hypophosphatasia
      i. Serum creatinine
   2. **Imaging studies**
      a. Renal ultrasound for calcifications
      b. Long bone x-rays for demineralization secondary to hyperparathyroidism or osteosclerotic lesions secondary to hypervitaminosis
G. Management. Treatment depends on the cause and severity of hypercalcemia. Hypercalcemia is usually mild, and a conservative approach is prudent. Immediate steps are to calculate calcium and vitamin D intake and correct excess doses or discontinue. After hypercalcemia has been resolved, dietary calcium, phosphorus, and vitamin D intakes can be recalculated and administered according to basic daily requirements. An endocrine consult is recommended.
   1. **Acute symptomatic hypercalcemia**
      a. **Discontinue any parenteral intake of calcium.**
      b. **Increase fluid intake as intravenous normal saline.**
      c. **Augment calcium loss** (calciuria) using furosemide with IV saline intake; exercise caution to monitor urine output and serum electrolytes.

2. **Less acute but severe hypercalcemia.** Consider:
   a. **Calcitonin** (limited newborn/neonatal experience).
   b. **Glucocorticoids** are effective on a short-term basis but are not recommended.
   c. **Intravenous bisphosphonates** are promising (limited newborn/neonatal experience). Recently, there have been some case reports of successful use of bisphosphonates in neonates for therapy of hypercalcemia occurring in infants receiving therapeutic hypothermia due to hypoxic ischemic encephalopathy.
3. **Refractory hypercalcemia.** In extreme situations, parathyroidectomy has been the last resort.

H. **Prognosis.** Hypocalcemia generally has a good outcome if diagnosed promptly and treated adequately. The exception is a clinical presentation that includes seizures. Follow-up studies have suggested 20% or greater incidence of neurologic abnormalities. If unrecognized and not treated, it may result in renal and central nervous system damage.

92 Coagulation Disorders

Bleeding and thrombosis are the 2 extremes of the physiologic process of coagulation disorders. Despite major differences in the levels of individual components of the hemostatic system, neonatal coagulation is equal to or somewhat more rapid than that observed in adults. This suggests the existence of a delicately balanced hemostatic system in neonates, with uncommon bleeding or thrombosis in healthy term infants. However, a number of perinatal or neonatal conditions can disrupt this balance and increase the risk for either hemorrhage or thrombus formation. The presence of bleeding in a healthy term or late preterm infant, especially in an infant with a normal platelet count, is strongly suggestive of a congenital bleeding disorder.

In general, coagulation disorders in the neonate can be classified as **inherited bleeding disorders** (hemophilia A and B, von Willebrand disease, or isolated factor II, VII, X, VIII, or XIII deficiencies) **or acquired bleeding disorders** (vitamin K deficiency bleeding, disseminated intravascular coagulation [DIC], liver disease, or extracorporeal life support related). The inherited disorders **hemophilia A and B and von Willebrand disease** account for 95% to 98% of congenital bleeding disorders.

PRINCIPLES OF HEMOSTASIS

I. **Normal physiology of hemostasis**
   A. **The primary phase.** This is the production of the platelet plug. It involves platelet adhesion (to the injured vessel's subendothelium) and their activation mediated by platelet surface glycoprotein (Ib, IIb/IIa) and von Willebrand factor (vWF).
   B. **The secondary phase.** Results in the formation of a cross-linked fibrin clot. Coagulation proteins (factors XII to V) circulating as inactive precursor forms (zymogens) are converted to active forms through limited proteolysis. These activated proteins then further activate other zymogen factors in a chain reaction. Ultimately, the activation of factors V and X leads to cleavage of prothrombin (factor II) to thrombin (factor IIa). Cleavage of fibrinogen (factor I) to fibrin (factor Ia) by thrombin results in the formation of the blood clot.
   C. **The third phase.** Modulates and limits the interactions of activated platelets and the clotting cascade (and Ca^{2+}) that give rise to a clot. This includes the removal of activated factors (through the reticuloendothelial system) and the control of

activated procoagulants by natural antithrombotic pathways (antithrombin III, protein C, protein S). Furthermore, restoration of vessel patency is triggered by the fibrinolytic pathway that generates plasmin from plasminogen. This is stimulated by tissue plasminogen activator (tPA) and limited by α_2-antiplasmin and plasminogen activator inhibitor. Plasmin is a proteolytic enzyme that degrades fibrin into fibrin split products such as D-dimers. Defects in fibrinolytic factors that result in excessive plasmin generation can lead to bleeding.

II. **Newborn hemostasis**
   A. **Neonatal platelets are reported to be hyporeactive;** however, this deficiency is balanced by increased vWF activity, resulting in overall normal platelet function.
   B. **Factor VIII, factor V, fibrinogen, and factor XIII levels are normal at birth.**
   C. **Vitamin K–dependent factors (II, VII, IX, and X) and contact factors (XI and XII) are reduced to about 50% of normal adult values** and are further reduced in preterm infants. Similarly, concentrations of the naturally occurring anticoagulants antithrombin, protein C, and protein S are low at birth. As a consequence, both thrombin generation and thrombin inhibition are reduced in the newborn period.
   D. **Neonatal fibrinolytic activity is intact,** despite the decreased concentrations and functional activity of plasminogen. Very low levels of histidine-rich glycoprotein (a physiologic inhibitor of plasminogen binding) and delayed inactivation of neonatal plasmin partially compensate for the reduced plasmin capacity. On the other hand, the increased plasma levels of plasminogen activator inhibitor may explain the high rate of thromboembolic phenomena associated with intravascular devices in newborns. Most coagulation factors reached adult levels by 6 months of life with the exception of protein C levels, which remain low until later in childhood.

III. **Hemostatic testing in neonates.** Correct interpretation of coagulation tests in the newborn is fraught with difficulties. The following precautions are needed for the appropriate interpretation of neonatal coagulation testing.
   A. **Gestational and postnatal age reference ranges.** Vital to adequately interpret coagulation results in preterm and term neonates (Table 92–1).
   B. **A free-flowing blood specimen.** Specimens must be obtained from an atraumatic venipuncture. Samples obtained through intravascular catheters may be contaminated with heparin as it adheres tightly to the walls of the tubing. This sample contamination with trace amounts of heparin will result in a prolonged activated partial thromboplastin time (aPTT) and sometimes prothrombin time (PT), unless heparin is degraded in the specimen. Additionally, small clots can form within the catheter or at the tip, resulting in consumption of clotting factors and alteration of coagulation testing. A difficult venipuncture can hamper sample integrity and lead to platelet clumping that produces a falsely low platelet count.
   C. **Special sample tubes should be prepared for coagulation testing in infants with a hematocrit >55% or <25%.** This allows for a correct amount of anticoagulant to be added to the blood sample (citrate-to-blood ratio of 1:9). Similarly, an insufficient filling of adequately citrated tube (<80%) can produce falsely prolonged coagulation time.
   D. **A stepwise approach to the neonate with suspected coagulation disorders is key to a correct diagnosis.**
      1. **Initial screening.** Consists of a complete blood count (CBC) with platelets, PT/international normalized ratio (INR), aPTT, and fibrinogen level.
      2. **Prolonged prothrombin time.** Reflects decreased plasma concentrations of vitamin K–dependent factors.
      3. **Prolonged activated partial thromboplastin time.** Results from decreased plasma levels of contact factors (V and VIII to XI) as well.
      4. **Bleeding neonate who has no laboratory abnormality.** Factor XIII and α_2-antiplasmin activity should be assessed.

Table 92–1. REFERENCE VALUES FOR COAGULATION STUDIES IN HEALTHY FULL-TERM AND PRETERM INFANTS DURING THE FIRST 30 DAYS OF LIFE

Tests	Healthy Full Term (Mean ± SD)			Healthy Preterm (30–36 wks) Infant: Mean (range)		
	Day 1	Day 5	Day 30	Day 1	Day 5	Day 30
PT (seconds)	13.0 ± 1.43	12.4 ± 1.46	11.8 ± 1.25	13 (10.6–16.2)	12.5 (10.0–15.3)	11.8 (10.0–13.6)
aPTT (seconds)	42.9 ± 5.80	42.6 ± 8.62	40.4 ± 7.42	53.6 (27.5–79.4)	50.5 (26.9–74.1)	44.7 (26.9–62.5)
TCT (seconds)	23.5 ± 2.38	23.1 ± 3.07	24.3 ± 2.44	24.8 (19.2–30.4)	24.1 (18.8–24.4)	24.4 (18.8–29.9)
Fibrinogen (g/mL)	2.83 ± 0.58	3.12 ± 0.75	2.70 ± 0.54	2.43 (1.50–3.73)	2.8 (1.60–4.18)	2.54 (1.50–4.14)
Factor II (U/mL)	0.48 ± 0.11	0.63 ± 0.15	0.68 ± 0.17	0.45 (0.20–0.77)	0.57 (0.29–0.85)	0.57 (0.36–0.95)
Factor V (U/mL)	0.72 ± 0.18	0.95 ± 0.25	0.98 ± 0.18	0.88 (0.41–1.44)	1 (0.46–1.54)	1.02 (0.48–1.56)
Factor VII (U/mL)	0.66 ± 0.19	0.89 ± 0.27	0.90 ± 0.24	0.67 (0.21–1.13)	0.84 (0.30–1.38)	0.83 (0.21–1.45)
Factor VIII (U/mL)	1.00 ± 0.39	0.88 ± 0.33	0.91 ± 0.33	1.11 (0.50–2.13)	1.15 (0.53–2.05)	1.11 (0.50–1.99)
vWF (U/mL)	1.53 ± 0.67	1.40 ± 0.57	1.28 ± 0.69	1.36 (0.78–2.10)	1.33 (0.72–2.19)	1.36 (0.66–2.16)
Factor IX (U/mL)	0.53 ± 0.19	0.53 ± 0.19	0.51 ± 0.15	0.35 (0.19–0.65)	0.42 (0.14–0.74)	0.44 (0.13–0.80)
Factor X (U/mL)	0.40 ± 0.14	0.49 ± 0.15	0.59 ± 0.14	0.41 (0.11–0.71)	0.51 (0.19–0.83)	0.56 (0.20–0.92)
Factor XI (U/mL)	0.38 ± 0.14	0.55 ± 0.16	0.63 ± 0.13	0.3 (0.08–0.52)	0.41 (0.13–0.69)	0.43 (0.15–0.71)
Factor XII (U/mL)	0.53 ± 0.29	0.47 ± 0.18	0.49 ± 0.16	0.38 (0.10–0.66)	0.39 (0.09–0.69)	0.43 (0.11–0.75)
Prekallikrein (U/mL)	0.37 ± 0.16	0.48 ± 0.14	0.57 ± 0.17	0.33 (0.09–0.57)	0.45 (0.26–0.75)	0.59 (0.31–0.87)
HMW-K (U/mL)	0.54 ± 0.24	0.74 ± 0.28	0.77 ± 0.22	0.49 (0.09–0.89)	0.62 (0.24–1.00)	0.64 (0.16–1.12)
Factor XIIIa (U/mL)	0.79 ± 0.26	0.94 ± 0.25	0.93 ± 0.27	0.7 (0.32–1.08)	1.01 (0.57–1.45)	0.99 (0.51–1.47)
Factor XIIIb (U/mL)	0.76 ± 0.23	1.06 ± 0.37	1.11 ± 0.36	0.81 (0.35–1.27)	1.1 (0.68–1.58)	1.07 (0.57–1.57)
Plasminogen (U/mL)	1.95 ± 0.35	2.17 ± 0.38	1.98 ± 0.36	1.7 (1.12–2.48)	1.91 (1.21–2.61)	1.81 (1.09–2.53)

aPTT, activated partial thromboplastin time; HMW-K, high molecular weight kininogen; PT, prothrombin time; SD, standard deviation; TCT, thrombin clotting time; vWF, von Willebrand factor.

Adapted with permission from Andrew M, Monagle PT, Brooker L. *Thromboembolic Complications During Infancy and Childhood.* Hamilton, Ontario: BC Decker; 2000.

5. **D-dimers.** Elevated as an acute-phase reaction in all patients with infection or systemic inflammatory response syndrome (SIRS). A negative D-dimer assay is relatively accurate in ruling out thrombosis.

IV. **Bleeding disorders in neonates**

A. **Clinical presentation.** Persistent oozing from the umbilical stump, excessive bleeding from peripheral venipuncture/heel stick sites, large caput succedaneum and cephalhematoma or subgaleal hemorrhage occurring without significant birth trauma history, and prolonged bleeding following circumcision are common presentations of neonatal bleeding disorders. The presence of an intracranial hemorrhage in a term or late preterm infant without history of birth trauma should be investigated for possible coagulation defect. Gastrointestinal bleeding must be distinguished from swallowed maternal blood (see page 528). Pulmonary hemorrhages are most frequently hemorrhagic pulmonary edema not associated with specific coagulation anomaly. Similarly, major abdominal organ bleeding such as from the liver or spleen is more often related to a traumatic injury or local lesion (eg, teratoma) than any coagulopathy.

B. **Maternal, family, and neonatal history.** A history of any prior pregnancies and their outcomes can be a clue for disorders such as neonatal alloimmune thrombocytopenia. Maternal medication use can also lead to immune-mediated thrombocytopenia. Parental ethnic background and whether there is consanguinity are significant. However, absence of family history for a bleeding disorder cannot exclude occurrence of severe bleeding disorders. Perinatal complications can result in coagulation activation and DIC. Although giving vitamin K to neonates is almost a universal routine, it is still important to ascertain that the vitamin K was indeed administered.

C. **Physical examination.** An otherwise normal neonate with thrombocytopenia is suggestive of alloimmune thrombocytopenia. Skeletal abnormalities such as absence of thumb or radii are important clues for conditions such as thrombocytopenia with absent radii or Fanconi anemia. Cardiac defects may be associated with factor V deficiency. Delayed cord separation and persistent oozing from the umbilical stump are typical for infants with defective fibrinogen production or function and factor XIII deficiency. Acquired consumptive coagulopathy is generally a secondary event in a "sick" acting infant. Bacterial or viral infection and metabolic disorders (eg, tyrosinemia) are a few of the conditions that then need to be considered.

INHERITED BLEEDING DISORDERS: HEMOPHILIA A AND B

I. **Definition.** Hemophilia A and B are inherited as sex-linked (X chromosome) recessive traits and are characterized by deficiencies of factor VIII or IX. However, one-third of cases will occur in the absence of a positive family history. Factor VIII deficiency is 5 times as common as factor IX deficiency.

II. **Incidence.** Hemophilia A occurs in 1 per 5000 males, and hemophilia B occurs in 1 per 25,000 males; it is very rare in females.

III. **Pathophysiology.** Deficiency of factor VIII or IX interferes with coagulation cascade.

IV. **Risk factors.** Male sex, family history of hemophilia or bleeding disorders.

V. **Clinical presentation.** The pattern of hemophilia-associated bleeding differs from that seen in older children. Hemarthroses are rare, and many bleeds are iatrogenic in origin (eg, oozing or hematoma following venipuncture or vitamin K intramuscular [IM] administration, prolonged bleeding following circumcision). Major bleeding, both intracranial (mostly subdural) and extracranial, is also occasionally seen. **Severe factor VIII deficiency (factor VIII activity <1%)** is the most common congenital coagulation disorder to present in the neonatal period. A third of cases will present with bleeding manifestations during the first month of life.

VI. **Diagnosis.** Screening coagulation test shows a prolonged aPTT, whereas PT and platelet counts are within normal range. Factor VIII normally approaches adult level at birth; thus, a low level reliably diagnoses hemophilia A. On the other hand, the diagnosis of moderate hemophilia B requires testing beyond the neonatal age because factor IX levels are low at birth ($\approx$15%), reaching adult values at 2 to 6 months.

VII. **Management**

    A. **The treatment for hemophilia A or B is recombinant factor VIII or factor IX concentrate, respectively.** Fresh-frozen plasma (FFP) should be used only in the instance of acute hemorrhage when confirmatory testing is not yet available.

    B. **Desmopressin has been used for mild hemophilia A and for von Willebrand disease type 1 or 2 to increase release of factor VIII and von Willebrand factor from endothelial stores.** The antifibrinolytic agents α-aminocaproic acid (Amicar) and tranexamic acid can be used in mucocutaneous bleeding to stabilize the fibrin clot and retard fibrinolysis. These agents are contraindicated in hematuria because of concerns about obstruction of urine flow by thrombi.

VIII. **Prognosis.** In most Western countries, people with hemophilia have a life expectancy not different from that of the male population without hemophilia. The optimal schedule for lifelong prophylaxis treatment continues to be *controversial* and onerous, and the development of inhibitors to factor VIII is still a major unresolved problem.

INHERITED BLEEDING DISORDERS: VON WILLEBRAND DISEASE

von Willebrand disease rarely presents during the neonatal period, because healthy neonates have higher plasma concentrations of vWF activity and an increased proportion of high molecular weight vWF multimers compared with adults. The condition is divided into 3 types. Type 3, an autosomal recessive disorder where vWF concentrations are almost absent, is the only type presenting with severe neonatal bleeding.

INHERITED BLEEDING DISORDERS: ISOLATED FACTOR II, VII, X, VIII, OR XIII DEFICIENCIES

Isolated factor II, VII, X, VIII, or XIII deficiencies can present in the neonatal period. These rare coagulation deficiencies have an autosomal recessive inheritance (except factor XIII) and present with abnormal coagulation screening tests.

ACQUIRED BLEEDING DISORDERS: VITAMIN K DEFICIENCY BLEEDING

    I. **Definition.** Vitamin K deficiency bleeding (VKDB) in the newborn.

    II. **Incidence.** Rare in the United States with routine administration of vitamin K.

    III. **Pathophysiology.** Vitamin K, a fat-soluble vitamin, is required for carboxylation of glutamic acid residues on precursors of vitamin K–dependent coagulation proteins (factors II, VII, IX, and X and proteins C and S). Vitamin K exists in 2 forms: vitamin K1 or phylloquinone (the plant form of the vitamin) and vitamin K2, a series of compounds synthesized by bacteria and referred to as menaquinones. In contrast to human milk, infant formula contains large amounts of vitamin K (10 vs 65–100 mcg/L). Newborn infants are at risk for vitamin K deficiency because of vitamin K's poor placental transfer, insufficient endogenous production from the intestinal bacterial flora prior to complete colonization of the neonatal colon, and inadequate dietary intake among solely breast-fed infants.

    IV. **Risk factors.** Additional risk factors are liver disease, cholestasis, and maternal short-gut syndrome.

    V. **Clinical presentation**

        A. **Mild vitamin K deficiency.** Manifests as an isolated prolongation of PT, with more severe deficiency characterized by prolongation of aPTT. The diagnosis can be confirmed by high serum level of an abnormal form of prothrombin (protein induced by vitamin K absence-II [PIVKA-II]).

B. **Early vitamin K deficiency bleeding.** Occurs in the first 24 hours among infants born to mothers on oral anticoagulants, anticonvulsants, or antituberculosis therapy and presents generally as serious bleeding such as intracranial hemorrhage (ICH).

C. **Classic disease.** Presents between days 1 and 7 with gastrointestinal bleeding, ICH, skin bruising, and bleeding following circumcision and tends to occur in infants who did not receive vitamin K at birth and are breast fed or receiving inadequate overall milk intake. In the absence of vitamin K prophylaxis, the incidence of classic VKDB is 0.25% to 1.7%.

D. **Late vitamin K deficiency bleeding.** Presents between 2 and 12 weeks of life. These infants are exclusively breast-fed infants who received no or only 1 oral dose of vitamin K or have an associated disease process that interferes with the absorption or supply of vitamin K (intestinal malabsorption defects, cholestatic jaundice, cystic fibrosis, biliary atresia, α_1-antitrypsin deficiency). The majority of cases of late VKDB, the incidence of which is 4 to 7 per 100,000 births, present with ICH.

VI. **Diagnosis.** No routine test is diagnostic. Increased PT with normal platelet and fibrinogen levels is typical.

VII. **Management**

A. **Infants who present with a non–life-threatening bleed only need to be treated with vitamin K1** given slowly intravenously (IV) or subcutaneously (no IM injection) at a dose of 250 to 300 mcg/kg to restore PT to 30% to 50% of its normal value within an hour.

B. **Treatment of serious bleeding** includes FFP (20 mL/kg), a prothrombin complex concentrate (50 U/kg), or recombinant factor VIIa (100 mcg/kg).

C. **The American Academy of Pediatrics recommends** that all infants receive 1 mg of IM vitamin K on the first day of life (0.3 mg for infants <1000 g and 0.5 mg for infants >1000 g but <32 weeks). This single parenteral dose prevents both classic and late VKDB.

D. **The safety of intramuscular vitamin K was questioned** because of its reported possible association with increased incidence of childhood cancer. Subsequent studies have disproved this risk. Nevertheless, an alternative oral regimen of a 2-mg dose at birth followed by a 1-mg dose given weekly for 3 months has been suggested. Its efficacy has not been well established.

VIII. **Prognosis.** Depends on the severity and location of the bleeding.

ACQUIRED BLEEDING DISORDERS: DISSEMINATED INTRAVASCULAR COAGULATION

I. **Definition.** DIC is the result of excessive and inappropriate activation of the hemostatic system related to exposure of blood to a source of tissue factor. It is a secondary manifestation of an underlying problem such as bacterial or viral infection, asphyxia, or necrosis.

II. **Incidence.** The most common causes of DIC in the newborn are sepsis, severe respiratory distress syndrome, asphyxia, and necrotizing enterocolitis.

III. **Pathophysiology.** Massive thrombin generation with widespread fibrin deposition and consumption of coagulation proteins and platelets leads to multiple organ dysfunction.

IV. **Risk factors.** Concurrent bacterial or viral infection, asphyxia, or necrosis.

V. **Clinical presentation.** The presence of DIC in a neonate without any evidence of sepsis or history of asphyxia should warrant the evaluation for a capillary hemangioma.

VI. **Diagnosis.** The diagnosis of DIC is made in an ill neonate with thrombocytopenia, prolonged PT and aPTT, reduced fibrinogen, and increased D-dimers.

VII. **Management**
   A. **The most important therapeutic intervention** is to treat the underlying cause of the disseminated intravascular coagulation.
   B. **Focus on the acute hematologic management is to support adequate hemostasis to limit hemorrhage.** This is usually achieved with platelet transfusions, FFP, or cryoprecipitate, with a goal of maintaining platelets >50,000 to 100,000/mm^3, PT <3 seconds above the upper limit of normal, and fibrinogen >100 mg/dL.
   C. **Anticoagulant therapy is not generally used.** The benefit has not proved to outweigh the added risk for hemorrhage.
   D. **The use of activated protein C is** *controversial* **(may increase risk of intracerebral hemorrhage).**
   E. **Recombinant factor VIIa (40–300 mcg/kg).** This has been used successfully to treat severe bleeding in infants with DIC. In the presence of endothelial damage, recombinant factor VIIa (rFVIIa) binds to exposed tissue factor to activate factor X and thus generate thrombin. The potential for thrombotic complications makes its use limited to life-threatening hemorrhagic situations.
VIII. **Prognosis.** Related to the underlying cause of the DIC.

ACQUIRED BLEEDING DISORDERS: LIVER DISEASE

Vitamin K–dependent factors (II, VII, IX, and X) as well as factor V are synthesized by the liver, and hepatic damage can result in lower levels. The diagnosis of acute liver disease should include elevated liver enzymes, direct hyperbilirubinemia, and elevated ammonia concentration. A low factor VII associated with low factor V will distinguish between vitamin K deficiency and hepatic dysfunction. A normal factor VIII may differentiate between liver disease and DIC where all clotting factors are depleted. On the other hand, liver disease may trigger DIC, and ascites may lead to a loss of all clotting factors.

ACQUIRED BLEEDING DISORDERS: EXTRACORPOREAL LIFE SUPPORT RELATED

Systemic anticoagulation with heparin is performed during the duration of ECLS to minimize the potential for clotting within the circuit. Monitoring to prevent bleeding complications is essential. This is done by the activated coagulation time, a rapid, whole blood point-of-care test. Patients are usually maintained close to a target time of 200 seconds.

THROMBOEMBOLIC DISEASE IN NEONATES

Thrombotic complications are more frequent in neonates than in any other pediatric age group. Depending on the type of thrombosis and screening methods used, incidences of 0.5 events per 10,000 live births or 2.4 clinically apparent events (excluding stroke) per 1000 neonatal intensive care unit (NICU) admissions have been reported.

ARTERIAL THROMBOSIS: PERINATAL AND PRENATAL ARTERIAL ISCHEMIC STROKE

   I. **Definition.** An arterial ischemic stroke (AIS) is a cerebrovascular event occurring between 28 weeks of gestation and 28 days of birth with radiologic or pathologic evidence of focal arterial infarction of the brain.
   II. **Incidence.** The incidence of cerebral arterial occlusion may range from 0.5 to 1 per 1000 live births. Most occur within the middle cerebral artery of the left hemisphere.

III. **Pathophysiology.** Paradoxical embolism (through the foramen ovale) from the fetal placental circulation is believed to be the most common etiology. Clotting activation originating from the placenta could release thrombin or small fibrin clots into the fetal circulation.

IV. **Risk factors.** Twin-to-twin transfusion syndrome, fetal heart rate abnormality, and hypoglycemia are independent risk factors.

V. **Clinical presentation.** Approximately 60% of the cases are perinatal AIS and present with symptoms in the first few days of life, chiefly seizures and apnea. **AIS is the second most common underlying etiology of neonatal seizures in the full-term newborn.** Presumed prenatal stroke, asymptomatic at birth, presents with asymmetrical motor development, hemiplegia, or seizures several months postnatally.

VI. **Diagnosis.** Magnetic resonance imaging (MRI) with diffusion-weighted imaging is the most sensitive technique for the early detection of acute cerebral infarction. Magnetic resonance angiography allows for the detection of thrombosed cerebral vessels. Cranial ultrasound has a poor sensitivity for the detection of AIS.

VII. **Management.** In adults with AIS, recombinant tissue plasminogen activator (rTPA) has shown efficacy in restoring cerebral blood flow when delivered within 3 hours of its onset. In the neonate with AIS, the determination of time of onset is challenging, and there is currently no evidence for the efficacy of any form of anticoagulation treatment.

VIII. **Prognosis.** Many newborns with symptomatic AIS appear clinically normal after recovery from the acute event. On follow-up, one-third will exhibit hemiparesis, and another third will exhibit cognitive abnormalities affecting speech and language.

ARTERIAL THROMBOSIS: IATROGENIC/SPONTANEOUS ARTERIAL THROMBOSIS

I. **Definition.** An arterial thrombosis is classified as catheter related or non–catheter related.

II. **Incidence.** Spontaneous arterial thrombosis is extremely rare. The incidence of catheter-related (mostly umbilical arterial catheter [UAC]) thrombosis has been reported as being as high as 30% depending on the method used for diagnosis (eg, ultrasound, angiography). The incidence of major clinical symptoms attributable to UAC thrombus is approximately 1% to 5% of catheterized infants.

III. **Pathophysiology.** An arterial thrombosis usually involves the aorta and tends to mimic congenital heart disease (eg, coarctation). Iatrogenic arterial thrombosis is mainly related to complications from indwelling catheters.

IV. **Risk factors.** Presence of UACs and peripheral arterial catheters.

V. **Clinical presentation.** Findings suggestive of an acute thrombosis include line dysfunction, extremity blanching and/or cyanosis, decreased pulse, and persistent thrombocytopenia.

VI. **Diagnosis.** Ultrasound Doppler is the method more frequently used in sick preterm infants, although contrast angiography may be more accurate when feasible.

VII. **Management**

A. **Suspicion or confirmation of an arterial thrombosis.** Warrants prompt removal of the catheter unless local instillation of tPA into the thrombus is contemplated.

B. **Recommendations for umbilical artery catheter–related thrombosis.** Treat with heparin. rTPA thrombolysis may be attempted for life-, limb-, or organ-threatening conditions (see pages 849–850).

VIII. **Prognosis.** Most symptomatology attributed to thrombus formation will resolve with prompt removal of the catheter.

ARTERIAL THROMBOSIS: PURPURA FULMINANS

I. **Definition.** Purpura fulminans (PF) is a rare syndrome of diffuse intravascular thrombosis and hemorrhagic infarction of the skin that is rapidly progressive and often fatal.

II. **Incidence.** The incidence of severe protein C deficiency is 1 per 1,000,000 live births.

III. **Pathophysiology.** Based on severe genetic (or acquired) protein C and/or protein S deficiency. Acquired PF may result from conditions triggering acute reduction of protein C activity such as bacterial infection.

IV. **Risk factors.** Protein C deficiency.

V. **Clinical presentation.** Extensive venous and arterial thrombosis with ecchymosis is present soon after delivery and can result in skin necrosis.

VI. **Diagnosis.** Laboratory tests yield results consistent with DIC (thrombocytopenia, hypofibrinogenemia, and increased PT and aPTT) and show no measurable protein C or S.

VII. **Management.** Early treatment is paramount for successful outcome and consists of FFP, protein C concentrate, or activated protein C and lifelong anticoagulation.

VIII. **Prognosis.** PF is associated with a high mortality rate.

VENOUS THROMBOSIS: CEREBRAL SINOVENOUS THROMBOSIS

I. **Definition.** Cerebral sinovenous thrombosis (CSVT) typically involves the thrombosis of cerebral veins or the dural sinus with cerebral parenchymal lesions or central nervous system (CNS) dysfunction.

II. **Incidence.** The incidence of CSVT has been reported as 0.4 per thousand live births.

III. **Pathophysiology.** Thrombophilic factors (Table 92–2) may play a role in perinatal stroke. The superior and lateral sinuses are the most frequently involved vessels, and up to 30% of cases have venous infarction with subsequent hemorrhage.

IV. **Risk factors.** Often associated with perinatal asphyxia, coagulopathy, maternal diabetes, and infection.

V. **Clinical presentation.** The symptoms of CSVT are those of a perinatal stroke and include seizures, apnea, and lethargy.

Table 92–2. **THROMBOPHILIC CONDITION MARKERS FOR THROMBOPHILIA AND PREVALENCE IN HEALTHY POPULATION**

Condition/Marker	Testing Methods	Prevalence (%)
Genetic		
Factor V Leiden mutation	PCR	4–6
Prothrombin G20210A mutation	PCR	1–2
Elevated plasma lipoprotein(a)	ELISA	
Acquired or genetic		
Antithrombin deficiency	Chromogenic (functional) assay	0.019
Protein C deficiency	Chromogenic (functional) assay	0.023
Protein S deficiency	ELISA for free protein S antigen	0.037
Elevated factor VIII	One-stage clotting assay (aPTT based)	
MTHR enzyme gene mutation	Hyperhomocysteinemia	9
Maternal lupus	ELISA for antiphospholipid antibodies	
Activate protein resistance	Clotting assay (aPPT based)	

aPTT, activated partial thromboplastin time; ELISA, enzyme-linked immunosorbent assay; PCR, polymerase chain reaction.
Modified with permission from Goldenberg NA, Bernard TJ: Venous thromboembolism in children, *Hematol Oncol Clin North Am.* 2010 Feb;24(1):151-166.

VI. **Diagnosis.** Diagnosis of CSVT is best made through diffusion MRI and magnetic resonance venography.

VII. **Management.** Heparin anticoagulation is indicated only when there is evidence of thrombus propagation, multiple emboli, or a severe prothrombotic state, but is contraindicated in the presence of intracerebral hemorrhage.

VIII. **Prognosis.** Based on extent of cerebral defect.

VENOUS THROMBOSIS: UPPER AND LOWER VENOUS SYSTEM DEEP VEIN THROMBOSIS

I. **Definition.** Thrombus in a major vein in the upper or lower extremity with or without central extension.

II. **Incidence.** The true incidence of neonatal deep vein thrombosis (DVT) is difficult to determine, and many central venous lines (CVLs) related to venous thrombosis are clinically "silent." Thrombosis and infection have been reported to occur in 2% to 22% of neonates with indwelling CVLs, with a higher incidence reported in studies applying regular ultrasound screening.

III. **Pathophysiology.** Infants are at increased risk of thrombosis, with indwelling catheters further increasing the risk of venous thrombosis.

IV. **Risk factors.** Nearly one-third of cases are associated with systemic infection, whereas prematurity is also correlated with higher prevalence of DVT. Other risk factors may include polycythemia, dehydration, repair of congenital heart disease, hypoxia, and parenteral nutrition.

V. **Clinical presentation.** Upper or lower venous DVT in neonates may present as swelling and discoloration of the associated limb, swelling of the face and head, chylothorax, and superior vena cava syndrome. Thrombocytopenia may be present.

VI. **Diagnosis.** Doppler ultrasound is the technique most frequently used for confirmation of neonatal DVT, although a venogram might be a more sensitive diagnostic method.

VII. **Management**
   A. **Suspicion or confirmation of a venous thrombus.** This warrants prompt catheter removal. However, due to the risk for emboli, delaying CVL removal until 3 to 5 days after the start of anticoagulant therapy may be considered (*controversial*).
   B. **Anticoagulation and thrombolytic treatment are equally** *controversial.* The decision needs to take into account the degree of threat to limbs or vital organs.
   C. **Role of thrombophilia screening in neonatal deep vein thrombosis.** In light of its poor yield and the low risk and predictability of DVT recurrences, this remains *controversial* as well.

VIII. **Prognosis.** Short-term morbidities include pulmonary embolism and neonatal stroke from emboli or brain hemorrhagic infarction.

VENOUS THROMBOSIS: RIGHT ATRIAL THROMBOSIS

I. **Definition.** Thrombosis of the superior vena cava with extension into the right atrium.

II. **Incidence.** Right atrial thrombosis (RAT) accounts for 6% of all neonatal thromboses.

III. **Pathophysiology.** Despite early administration of aspirin, this has become a common complication in infants undergoing repair of complex congenital heart disease. There is a strong association of the location of the catheter tip in the right atrium and the development of RAT.

IV. **Risk factors.** The most important risk factor is an indwelling CVL. Other associated risk factors include prematurity, administration of parenteral nutrition, sepsis, and congenital heart disease.

V. **Clinical presentation.** More than half of the cases are asymptomatic and are detected incidentally during echocardiography performed for other reasons such as investigation for a persistent infection focus. The remaining cases may present with respiratory distress, new heart murmur, heart failure symptoms, or tachyarrhythmia.

VI. **Diagnosis.** The diagnostic method of choice for RAT is echocardiography. Documentation of the size, mobility, and shape of the thrombus, as well as the concomitant cardiac function, is essential in helping to decide on treatment and predict outcome.

VII. **Management**

A. **Asymptomatic and hemodynamically stable infants with small, immobile right atrial thromboses** may need no treatment except close echocardiography follow-up.

B. **For symptomatic patients or RATs that are large,** mobile, pedunculated, or snake shaped, treatment should include systemic anticoagulation therapy.

C. **Thrombolytic therapy or surgical embolectomy** may be indicated in life-threatening conditions.

VIII. **Prognosis.** Thrombolytic therapy in preterm infant with infective endocarditis carries a high risk for ICH.

VENOUS THROMBOSIS: RENAL VEIN THROMBOSIS

I. **Definition.** Renal vein thrombosis (RVT) is the most common cause of non–catheter-associated thrombosis and usually presents in the first week of life.

II. **Incidence.** RVT accounts for up to 10% of venous thromboses in newborns.

III. **Pathophysiology.** Unilateral left-sided RVTs are the most common.

IV. **Risk factors.** Risk factors for the development of RVT include perinatal asphyxia, dehydration, maternal diabetes, and male sex.

V. **Clinical presentation.** The **classic clinical triad of RVT** includes hematuria, palpable abdominal mass, and thrombocytopenia. Other features include hypertension, proteinuria, and renal impairment. Patients with thrombus extension and caval occlusion may also develop bilateral lower limb edema.

VI. **Diagnosis.** The diagnosis of RVT is usually made via ultrasound with Doppler. Ultrasonographic features of RVT include enlarged, echogenic kidneys with attenuation or loss of corticomedullary differentiation. Color flow Doppler shows absence of flow in the main or arcuate renal veins.

VII. **Management.** The treatment for RVT is ***controversial***. Renal outcomes appear to be similar between supportive treatment and anticoagulation therapy. Similar proportions of affected kidneys that received supportive care or received anticoagulation became atrophic on follow-up. Possible exceptions to exclusive supportive treatment may include the following:

A. **Low molecular weight heparin therapy** for unilateral RVT with inferior vena cava extension for 6 weeks to 3 months. (See page 851.)

B. **Bilateral renal vein thrombosis with caval extension** may warrant thrombolytic therapy. (See page 852.)

VIII. **Prognosis.** Acute complications of RVT include adrenal hemorrhage, extension of the clot into the inferior vena cava, renal failure, hypertension, and death. Chronically, cortical or segmental infarction of the affected kidney and/or hypertension is common.

VENOUS THROMBOSIS: PORTAL VEIN THROMBOSIS

I. **Definition.** Thrombus in the portal vein usually associated with umbilical vein catheterization.

II. **Incidence.** The incidence of portal vein thrombosis (PVT) has been reported as 3.6 per 1000 NICU admissions. The incidence of PVT in neonates associated with the insertion of umbilical venous catheters (UVCs) varies between 1% and 43%, depending on imaging protocols.

III. **Pathophysiology.** Hypercoagulability of the newborn coupled with UVC entering the liver in an area of relatively low flow.

IV. **Risk factors.** Risk factors include umbilical infection as well as position of the tip of the UVC. The UVC tip should be kept outside the low-flow portal venous system and placed at the level of inferior vena cava/right atrium, or below the level of the umbilical-portal confluence. Its position needs to be ascertained by imaging.

V. **Clinical presentation.** Most thromboses in the portal venous system are clinically silent and spontaneously resolve within a short period of time after catheter removal.

VI. **Diagnosis.** Large studies have shown that PVT can usually be detected by ultrasound within the first week of a UVC insertion.

VII. **Management.** Use of anticoagulation is *controversial* (see Prognosis). For dosing, see page 850.

VIII. **Prognosis.** Long-term outcome of neonatal PVT and whether anticoagulation has any benefit in the outcome is unknown. Left lobe atrophy and portal hypertension are the most important sequelae. PVT is the major cause of extrahepatic portal hypertension in children, and a history of neonatal umbilical venous catheterization is frequently found among those children.

VENOUS THROMBOSIS: THROMBOPHILIA

I. **Definition.** Thrombophilia is a term used to describe known inherited or congenital blood coagulation disorders that may predispose to thrombosis.

II. **Incidence.** Rare.

III. **Pathophysiology.** Conditions that predispose to thrombophilia are noted in Table 92–2. Despite a high prevalence of multiple thrombophilic gene mutations, the majority of neonates with these traits do not develop thrombosis.

IV. **Risk factors.** Central venous and arterial catheters constitute the greatest acquired risk for the development of thromboembolic events in neonates, in addition to those noted in Table 92–2.

V. **Clinical presentation.** Thrombophilia should be considered in any neonate who presents with thrombotic events or extensive thrombosis in the absence of identifiable environmental risk factors (intravascular catheter, neonatal sepsis, or shock).

VI. **Diagnosis.** The evaluation of a neonate with a significant thromboembolic event for a prothrombotic disorder is *controversial*.

VII. **Management.** See Management of Thrombosis section that follows.

VIII. **Prognosis.** Neonates with multiple traits of thrombophilia and symptomatic thrombosis are at an increased risk for thrombus recurrence, although recurrences usually occur in the setting of other comorbidities, such as infection, surgery, or trauma.

MANAGEMENT OF THROMBOSIS: GENERAL GUIDELINES

The optimal treatment modality for neonates with thrombosis is *controversial*. Information on treatment of neonatal thrombosis is limited to case reports and small case series. Dosing information is often extrapolated from children or adult data. Available options include observation, anticoagulation (unfractionated heparin [UFH] or low molecular weight heparin [LMWH]), thrombolytic therapy, and surgical thrombectomy. Treatment should be limited to clinically significant thrombosis with the goal of preventing clot expansion or embolism.

I. **Unfractionated heparin**

A. **Pharmacology**

1. **Unfractionated heparin is a heterogeneous mixture** of negatively charged glycosaminoglycans with a molecular weight ranging from 5000 to 30,000 kDa. The anticoagulant properties are via conformational change in antithrombin, converting it to a more efficient (1000-fold) inhibitor of factors IIa, IXa, Xa, XIa, and XIIa.

Table 92–3. **DOSAGE OF UNFRACTIONATED HEPARIN IS MODULATED ACCORDING TO POSTCONCEPTIONAL AGE**

Postconceptional Age	<28 Weeks	28–37 Weeks	>37 Weeks
Loading dose IV over 10 minutes	25 U/kg	50 U/kg	10 U/kg
Maintenance dose IV	15 U/kg/h	15 U/kg/h	28 U/kg/h

IV, intravenous.

2. **The anticoagulant activity of heparin** is variable because of the differential clearance of the various sizes of heparin moieties, as well as its propensity to bind to other positively charged noncoagulation proteins, as well as to platelets and endothelial surfaces.

3. **The most important anticoagulant actions of heparin** are the potentiation of antithrombin inhibition of thrombin (IIa) and factor Xa.

B. **Dosage.** See Table 92–3.

1. **The half-life of unfractionated heparin, secondary to increased clearance, is short in neonates.** Infants with the most significant thromboses demonstrate the highest clearance.

2. **The efficacy of unfractionated heparin might be decreased in neonates because of the physiologically low antithrombin plasma concentration.** Antithrombin supplementation with FFP is sometimes suggested.

3. **Neonates require continuous intravenous therapy.** Higher doses than those used in older patients are required to achieve therapeutic adult aPTT levels. Anticoagulation is recommended for 10 to 14 days.

C. **Monitoring**

1. The goal for anticoagulation is to maintain activated partial thromboplastin time at 1.5 to 2 times the upper limit of age values. When feasible, anti–factor Xa level monitoring is preferable, with its level kept at 0.3 to 0.7 U/mL.

2. Following the initial dose, anti–factor Xa or activated partial thromboplastin time level is assessed 4 or 6 hours later, respectively, and once daily thereafter. If the level of anticoagulation is below or above target values, the test is repeated 4 to 6 hours after appropriate dose adjustment. In general, a 10% rate adjustment is made when levels are inappropriate. An additional 50 U/kg may be given if aPTT is <50 seconds.

3. A complete blood count, platelet count, and coagulation screening (including activated partial thromboplastin time, prothrombin time, and fibrinogen) should be performed before starting unfractionated heparin therapy. Platelet count and fibrinogen levels should be repeated daily for 2 to 3 days once therapeutic levels are achieved and twice weekly thereafter.

D. **Complications**

1. **The most important adverse effect from heparin therapy is bleeding.** A 2% risk has been reported in term infants, and the risk is higher among preterm infants.

2. **Accidental overdose of unfractionated heparin is a major safety issue.** This occurs when an inappropriately diluted, supposedly low-dose UFH is used to flush a vascular access device.

3. **Heparin-induced thrombocytopenia rarely occurs in neonates.**

4. **Treatment of hemorrhage**

a. **Usually, due to unfractionated heparin's short half-life, it only requires cessation of the infusion.**

b. **If bleeding continues following cessation of the infusion.** A full coagulation assessment should be performed, and hemostatic deficiencies should be replaced as indicated.

      c. Protamine. One milligram of protamine will neutralize 100 U of UFH. The amount to be administered is based on the time elapsed since the last heparin injection. A full neutralizing amount is to be given if that time was <30 minutes. This dose is reduced by 50% for every hour past the last time heparin had been given. A repeat aPTT is required 15 minutes later.

  E. Advantages over low molecular weight heparin

      1. **Because of its short half-life,** it can be used as the first-line agent in patients whose anticoagulation may need to be stopped rapidly.

      2. **Antidote (protamine sulfate) is available.**

      3. **At doses <100 U/kg,** its elimination is unaffected by renal dysfunction.

II. Low molecular weight heparin

  A. Pharmacology

      1. **Low molecular weight heparin is a glycosaminoglycan of smaller molecular weight (2000–8000 kDa) than unfractionated heparin.** As such, it lacks a binding site for thrombin.

      2. **Primary action of low molecular weight heparin** is to potentiate the antithrombin inhibition of factor Xa with little effect on the antithrombin inhibition of thrombin. Consequently, aPTT is unaffected at therapeutic LMWH doses.

  B. Dosage of low molecular weight heparin (enoxaparin)

      1. **Dosing recommendations for enoxaparin:** 1.7 mg/kg every 12 hours in term neonates and 2.0 mg/kg every 12 hours in preterm neonates.

      2. **Low molecular weight heparin can be administered by subcutaneous injection.** Frequent needle pricks can be minimized with the use of an extremely low dead space subcutaneous catheter (Insuflon, Unomedical/ConvaTec). Local bruising, induration, and leakage occur in 10% of neonates.

  C. Monitoring. See Table 92–4.

      1. **Low molecular weight heparin works largely by inhibiting factor Xa;** thus, dosing must be titrated to anti–factor Xa activity and not to the aPTT.

      2. **The goal of treatment is to maintain an anti–factor Xa level of 0.5 to 1.0 U/mL.**

      3. **Levels should be obtained 4 hours after the second dose and then weekly.**

  D. Advantage over unfractionated heparin. LMWH (specifically, enoxaparin) has become an increasingly popular alternative to UFH following studies in adults that demonstrated at least comparable efficacy and safety.

      1. **Pharmacokinetics** of LMWH are more predictable, making the need for monitoring less frequent.

      2. **Lesser risk of bleeding complications.**

      3. **Low molecular weight heparin is given subcutaneously,** which eliminates the requirement for IV access.

Table 92–4. LOW MOLECULAR WEIGHT HEPARIN (ENOXAPARIN) ADJUSTMENT[a]

Anti–Factor Xa Level (U/mL)	Hold Next Dose	Dose Change
>0.35	No	Increase by 25%
0.35–0.49	No	Increase by 10%
0.5–1.0	No	No change
1.1–1.5	No	Decrease by 20%
1.6–2.0	3 hours	Decrease by 30%
>2.0	Until anti–factor Xa 0.5 U/mL	Decrease by 40%

[a]A repeat anti–factor Xa needs to be measured after every individual adjustment.
Modified with permission from Andrew M, de Veber G. *Pediatric Thromboembolism and Stroke Protocols.* Hamilton, Ontario: BC Decker; 1997.

   4. **Low molecular weight heparin has a lesser risk of heparin-induced throm-bocytopenia** as well a reduced risk of osteoporosis that is associated with long-term use of UFH.
III. **Thrombolytic therapy.** The goal of thrombolytic therapy is to degrade fibrin and dissolve the fibrin clot. Systemic thrombolytic therapy should be strongly considered for clots that have a high risk of morbidity and mortality. The rate of vascular patency following anticoagulant therapy in older children has been reported at 50%; following thrombolysis, it is >90%.
   A. **Pharmacology**
      1. **Recombinant tissue plasminogen activator** facilitates conversion of plasminogen to plasmin to enhance degradation of fibrin, fibrinogen, and factors V and VII; it is the most commonly used agent.
      2. **Systemic tissue plasminogen activator is effective** when administered within 2 weeks of symptomatic clot onset and is only partially effective beyond 2 weeks.
      3. **Direct instillation of potent thrombolytic agents into clots via an infusion catheter** has been shown to result in significant increases in vessel patency rates in adults. It also carries the potential advantage of less exposure to the bleeding risks of systemic thrombolysis.
   B. **Dosage.** Based on a limited number of studies, the following protocol is proposed:
      1. **Systemic low doses.** Starting dose of 0.06 mg/kg/h with possible escalation up to 0.24 mg/kg/h over the next 48 to 96 hours.
      2. **Alternatively, use 1 of the following local treatments:**
         a. **Bolus.** Initial dose of 0.25 to 0.5 mg/kg for 15 minutes to be followed by 0.1 to 0.4 mg/kg/h for a maximal period of 72 hours.
         b. **Single dose.** A dose of 0.7 mg/kg over 30 to 60 minutes.
      3. **Repeat echocardiogram/Doppler** every 6 to 8 hours to assess the presence of the clot to guide the escalation of thrombolytic treatment or its cessation.
      4. **Heparin.** Because thrombolysis does not inhibit clot propagation or directly affect hypercoagulability, simultaneous treatment with low-dose UFH (5–10 U/kg/h) or LMWH (0.5 mg/kg twice a day) is recommended.
      5. **Plasminogen supplementation.** Prolonged thrombolytic therapy is likely to exhaust the low plasminogen neonatal supplies more readily than in adults. With thrombolytic therapy lasting >24 hours, consideration should be given to either monitoring plasminogen concentrations or empiric infusion of FFP (10–20 mL/kg) to optimize thrombolysis.
      6. **Fibrinogen.** Fibrinogen concentration decreases by 25% to 50% in response to systemic thrombolytic therapy. If fibrinogen concentrations are <100 mg/mL, dose reductions of the thrombolytic agent and infusion of replacement therapy in the form of cryoprecipitate or FFP should be considered.
      7. **Platelet counts.** Need to be maintained over 50,000/mm^3.
      8. **D-Dimer and fibrinogen degradation product** plasma concentrations are expected to increase as a response to effective thrombolytic action.
      9. **Daily head sonograms.**
      10. **Avoid intramuscular injections and urinary catheterizations.**
   C. **Exclusion criteria for tissue plasminogen activator thrombolysis**
      1. **Major surgery or central nervous system bleeding within 10 days.**
      2. **Major asphyxial event within 7 days (usually birth asphyxia).**
      3. **An invasive procedure within 72 hours.**
      4. **Seizures within 48 hours.**
   D. **Adverse effects**
      1. **Bleeding complications** have been reported in nearly two-thirds of pediatric patients; half of those patients required replacement blood transfusions.
      2. **Most frequently, bleeding is at sites of invasive procedures.** Gastrointestinal, pulmonary, and intraventricular hemorrhages are reported in about 1% of term infants and 14% of preterm infants.

3. **The frequency and severity of bleeding** may be dose and duration (<6 hours) dependent.

4. **Concurrent low-dose heparin treatment and fresh-frozen plasma (10 mL/kg)** given a half hour before each tPA infusion may lessen those bleeding risks.

IV. **Surgical thrombectomy.** The small size of neonatal blood vessels, the rarity of thrombosis in neonates, and the severity of illness in neonates with thrombosis preclude the use of surgical thrombectomy in the majority of neonates. However, with the use of microsurgical techniques combined with thrombolytic regimens, thrombectomy has been successfully used in neonates in isolated cases.

93 Common Multiple Congenital Anomalies: Syndromes, Sequences, and Associations

I. **Definition.** A congenital anomaly (also called birth defect, congenital malformation, or congenital abnormality) is defined as a **structural or functional defect** that is present at birth and different from what is considered normal. A **structural defect** is an abnormality in the structure of the parts of the body (skeleton and organs). Structural defects most often occur during the critical period of fetal development in the first trimester. Structural defects include heart defects, cleft palate, neural tube defects, club foot, and others. A **functional defect** is defined as a defect in how the body system works (eg, metabolic disorders, brain and nervous system problems, degenerative disorders, immune disorders, sensory disorders). This chapter will discuss only structural defects; functional defects are discussed elsewhere.

II. **Classification of anomalies**

A. **Classification based on major and minor anomalies.** An anomaly can be further divided into **major anomalies** that require medical and surgical care (eg, congenital heart defects, anencephaly, gastroschisis, cleft lip/palate, meningomyelocele) and **minor anomalies** that do not have medical significance (eg, single palmar crease, epicanthal folds, fifth digit clinodactyly). Approximately 75% of newborns with major congenital anomalies present with an isolated anomaly, and approximately 25% have more than 1 major anomaly. Neonates can have both major and minor anomalies.

B. **Classification based on developmental process.** Congenital anomalies can be classified based on the **developmental process** involved in their formation and may be described as **malformations, deformations, disruptions, dysplasias, syndromes, associations, or sequences** (see Table 93–1 for definitions). It is also important to understand that these may not be entirely mutually exclusive.

III. **Incidence.** Approximately 3% of all newborns have a congenital anomaly in the United States, and worldwide, approximately 6% of all newborns have a congenital anomaly. Approximately 0.7% of infants have multiple major anomalies. The **most common congenital anomalies** are congenital heart defects, neural tube defects, and Down syndrome. Congenital malformations account for 20% of the cases of neonatal deaths.

IV. **Causes of congenital anomalies** include **genetic causes** (chromosomal disorders, single-gene defects, autosomal dominant or recessive inheritance, and others), **maternal conditions during pregnancy** (infections, chronic maternal diseases, smoking,

Table 93–1. TYPES OF CONGENITAL ANOMALIES

Malformation: The morphologic defect of an organ or larger region of the body resulting from an intrinsically abnormal developmental process. A primary defect.

Deformation: An alteration in shape and/or structure caused by biomechanical forces that distort an otherwise normally developing structure. A secondary defect.

Disruption: A structural defect resulting from an extrinsic insult to an originally normal developmental process.

Dysplasia: An abnormality in the organization or differentiation of cells within a specific tissue type that results in clinically apparent structural changes.

Syndrome: A recognizable pattern of anomalies considered to have a specific cause.

Association: A nonrandom, statistically significant association of multiple anomalies for which no specific etiology has been described.

Sequence: A pattern of multiple anomalies derived from a single abnormality followed by a cascade of secondary effects.

medications, poor nutrition, environmental factors, TORCHZ (toxoplasmosis, other, rubella, cytomegalovirus, herpes simplex virus, and Zika virus), hyperthermia, alcohol and drug use), **multifactorial causes** (genetic plus environment), and **unknown etiologies.**

V. **General approach to diagnosis.** In the management of congenital anomalies, the neonatologist must deal with complex clinical issues calling for a wide range of diagnostic skills. Identifying the correct unifying diagnosis related to the congenital anomaly can help guide management, ensuring that interventions are appropriate and effective. This also facilitates realistic counseling about prognosis and recurrence risk. Only a few common syndromes associated with **multiple congenital abnormalities** are life-threatening in the neonatal period. It is important to note, however, that **congenital malformations are the most common cause of death at this critical point** in the life span. When overt malformations are present, a **syndromic association** will be suspected much earlier, and diagnostic efforts will start sooner. However, if external features of the disorder are subtle or nonspecific and the usual procedures associated with intensive newborn support have been started, a syndromic diagnosis may not be recognized until later. The diagnostic approach to congenital anomalies in neonates is no different from that in older children. Many of these affected children are intubated with multiple lines and tubes, which often makes a detailed assessment of physical characteristics challenging. Clinical photographs are extremely helpful, especially when a clinical geneticist is not available locally. If specialists in these fields are not available, a telephone call to a university medical center for expert advice is often useful. If the infant is critically ill and suspicion for a syndromic association is present, looking for other major malformations is important (eg, echocardiogram, renal/abdominal ultrasound, brain imaging). **The basis for diagnosis of a genetic syndrome in a neonate involves a combination of defining the physical manifestations and diagnostic genetic testing.** It is important to note that approximately 25% of all congenital anomalies may have a genetic cause. Identifying an underlying diagnosis may be delayed because immediate efforts tend to emphasize therapy. Nevertheless, clarifying the complete clinical picture often facilitates or guides therapy more efficiently. One study revealed that molecular diagnoses in congenital malformations directly affected medical management in approximately 50% of neonates.

VI. **Diagnosis**

A. **Prenatal diagnosis.** There are multiple screening evaluations available prenatally that can help with early detection of a congenital anomaly. Prior to and during early pregnancy, carrier screening can be used to determine risk for disorders, often based on ethnic background. These include noninvasive and invasive testing.

1. **Noninvasive testing** includes ultrasound, standard anomaly scan at 18 to 20 weeks, fetal echocardiography, magnetic resonance imaging, and screening tests (noninvasive prenatal screening using cell-free fetal DNA analysis, multiple marker screening for aneuploidy [nuchal translucency measurement, pregnancy-associated plasma protein A, and β-human chorionic gonadotropin], and screening for neural tube defects [maternal α-fetoprotein]). A sequential screen can determine risk of Down syndrome, trisomy 18, and open neural tube defects.

2. **Invasive techniques** include embryoscopy, fetoscopy during the second trimester, amniocentesis, chorionic villus sampling, percutaneous umbilical blood sampling, and fetal tissue sampling. Chromosomal analysis (karyotyping), fluorescence in situ hybridization (FISH), and chromosomal microarray analysis can be done prenatally. Molecular genetic testing can be done prenatally using amniocytes, chorionic villi, or fetal blood cells looking for genetic mutations/deletions.

B. **Detailed family history is of utmost importance.** Any consanguinity? Stillborn? Miscarriage? Other family members with anomaly? Ethnic origin? Doing a pedigree is recommended.

C. **Detailed pregnancy history.** Were there any exposures to drugs, toxins, or chemicals? Did the mother have any chronic medical condition? Did the infant grow normally?

D. **Detailed physical examination** to rule out multiple malformations and to look for clues to help diagnose a syndrome or a sequence. See Table 93–2 to for symptoms and signs that might indicate a congenital anomaly and Chapter 7. Look for clues for specific syndromes such as webbed or wide neck (Turner/Noonan

Table 93–2. **SYMPTOMS AND SIGNS IN NEONATES THAT MIGHT INDICATE A MULTIPLE CONGENITAL ANOMALY SYNDROME**

Prenatal

Oligohydramnios
Polyhydramnios
Decreased or unusual fetal activity
Abnormal fetal problem/position

Postnatal

Abnormalities of size: small for gestational age or large for gestational age, microcephaly or macrocephaly, large or irregular abdomen, small chest, limb-trunk disproportion, asymmetry
Abnormalities of tone: hypotonia, hypertonia
Abnormalities of position: joint contractures, fixation of joints in extension, hyperextension of joints
Midline aberrations: hemangiomas, hair tufts, dimples or pits
Problems of secretion, excretion, or edema: no urination, no passage of meconium, chronic nasal or oral secretions, edema (nuchal, pedal, generalized, ascites)
Symptoms: unexplained seizures, resistant or unexplained respiratory distress
Metabolic disorders: resistant hypoglycemia, unexplained hypo- or hypercalcemia, polycythemia, hyponatremia, thrombocytopenia

syndrome), redundant nuchal folds, tongue protrusion (Down syndrome), microcephaly (TORCHZ infection), hypotelorism and polydactyly (trisomy 13, Down syndrome), pectus excavatum, and arachnodactyly (Marfan syndrome).

E. **Laboratory evaluation**

1. **Evaluate for infections if indicated** (TORCHZ). Serologic testing (specific immunoglobulin [Ig] G, IgM, IgA) and polymerase chain reaction assays can be performed.

2. **Diagnostic genetic testing is recommended if a genetic defect is suspected.**

   a. **Array comparative genomic hybridization or chromosomal microarray analysis** is the **initial (first-tier) test** recommended for infants with ≥1 congenital anomalies, without an obvious single-gene syndromic diagnosis. It is a cytogenetic technique used to detect chromosomal deletions or duplications and assesses all regions of the chromosomes including subtelomeric and pericentromeric regions.

   b. **High-resolution karyotype.** Analysis of chromosomes obtained from white blood cells present in the peripheral blood sample. This test can take up to 2 weeks for completion. Used to detect differences in the number of whole chromosomes (aneuploidy), large chromosomal deletions/duplications, and translocations. This test remains the standard for confirming a well-recognized syndrome associated with aneuploidy, such as trisomies (Down syndrome) and monosomy X (Turner syndrome).

   c. **Fluorescence in situ hybridization.** A cytogenetic technique in which a fluorescently labeled probe can be used to detect specific DNA sequences. This test can detect small submicroscopic chromosomal deletions. The turnaround time is much faster than high-resolution karyotyping with results typically available in about 48 hours. FISH is often used to quickly confirm a diagnosis in a critically ill infant with trisomy 13, 18, or 21 or Turner syndrome or to confirm genetic sex in an infant with a suspected disorder of sexual development.

   d. **Multigene panel** is used for disorders where variants occur in multiple genes (eg, Noonan syndrome).

   e. **Genomic sequencing. Whole-exome sequencing and whole-gene sequencing** may be considered for infants with multiple congenital anomalies with suspected monogenic disorders, typically after nondiagnostic cytogenetic testing. This is a rapidly evolving field and is reviewed in detail in Chapter 17.

F. **Imaging.** The following tests may be required: computed tomography scan, magnetic resonance imaging, magnetic resonance angiography, skeletal survey, bone age, abdominal ultrasound, and echocardiogram.

G. **Subspecialty consultations.** Ophthalmology evaluation is important to rule out ocular abnormalities. An audiology evaluation is needed to rule out hearing loss. Any other consults depending on the specific need of the infant (eg, cardiology, orthopedics, endocrinology, pediatric surgery, pediatric urology)

VII. **Genetic counseling.** For infants with congenital anomalies, counseling can be complex and requires a great deal of sensitivity. Appropriate genetic counseling is reliant on having a specific diagnosis, if possible. The next step is to establish the parents' understanding of the entire situation and what information they have received from other professionals or gathered on their own. Be sure you know what questions the parents want answers to before the factual counseling begins. Do not give excessive details, and avoid specific predictions regarding timing and the presence or absence of certain future problems. Leave some degree of hope, but be honestly realistic, particularly if the parents clearly demand it. Be sure to offer follow-up counseling sessions, and outline a long-term program for the child's care and evaluations. Recurrence risk figures and the availability of prenatal diagnosis for subsequent pregnancies should also be discussed. Remember, medical providers may view the child's problems much differently than the parents, and it is important to work with the family from their perspective.

VIII. Selected examples of congenital anomalies based on their causes

  A. Chromosomal syndromes. The most common causes of syndromes associated with multiple congenital abnormalities diagnosed in the neonatal period are chromosomal abnormalities. Chromosomal abnormalities (extra or missing chromosomes or pieces of chromosomes) are identified in approximately 10% of children with congenital anomalies. Common chromosomal syndromes seen in the neonatal period include the following:

  1. Trisomy 21 (Down syndrome)

  a. Incidence. Trisomy 21 is one of the most common syndromes, occurring in about 1 in 800 live births.

  b. Neonatal mortality. This has decreased significantly with time but is relatively high for neonates who are very low birthweight and have severe congenital heart defects.

  c. Physical findings. Findings include hypotonia, a poor or absent Moro reflex, flat facial profile, upslanting palpebral fissures, Brushfield spots, small, unusual ears, protruding tongue, excess nuchal skin, fifth-digit brachydactyly/clinodactyly, and a single transverse palmar crease.

  d. Associated anomalies. Include congenital heart defects (~50%), most commonly an atrioventricular canal defect or ventricular septal defect. Major gastrointestinal malformations include Hirschsprung disease, duodenal or esophageal atresia, imperforate anus, and renal and urinary tract anomalies.

  2. Trisomy 18 (Edwards syndrome)

  a. Incidence. Approximately 1 in 5000 live births. There is a 3:1 female-to-male ratio.

  b. Neonatal mortality. Median survival time is about 14 days, and 50% of infants die in the first month. Survival beyond the first year is rare; however, there are reports of affected children living older than 10 years of age.

  c. Physical findings. Common findings include prenatal and postnatal growth deficiency, decreased subcutaneous fat, initial hypotonia followed by hypertonia, microcephaly, dolichocephaly with a prominent occiput, micrognathia, malformed auricles, short sternum with widely spaced nipples, overlapping digits with hypoplastic nails, and clubbed or rocker-bottom feet.

  d. Associated anomalies. Congenital heart disease is typically present (95% incidence) and is usually complex. Less frequent anomalies include cryptorchidism, horseshoe kidney, umbilical or inguinal hernia.

  3. Trisomy 13 (Patau syndrome)

  a. Incidence. Approximately 1 in 16,000 live births.

  b. Neonatal mortality. Median survival is about 7 days, and 90% die within the first year. Survival beyond the first year is rare. Individuals with trisomy 13 mosaicism are often more mildly affected, and survival is usually longer.

  c. Physical findings. Common findings include low birthweight, microcephaly with sloping forehead, scalp cutis aplasia, microphthalmia, cleft lip and palate, dysplastic ears, redundant nuchal skin, postaxial polydactyly, and overlapping and flexed fingers with hyperconvex nails.

  d. Associated anomalies. Congenital heart disease is typically present (80% incidence) and usually complex. Renal abnormalities are common and can include polycystic kidneys, hydronephrosis, hydroureters, or horseshoe kidney. Holoprosencephaly, cryptorchidism, a single umbilical artery, and inguinal or umbilical hernias are common.

  4. Monosomy X (Turner syndrome)

  a. Incidence. Approximately 1 in 2500 live-born females.

  b. Neonatal mortality. Turner syndrome is usually compatible with survival if the child reaches term. Approximately 98% to 99% of pregnancies in which a fetus has Turner syndrome end as miscarriages or stillbirths.

    c. **Physical findings.** Epicanthal folds, prominent ears, micrognathia, low posterior hairline, excess nuchal skin, webbed neck, broad chest with wide-spaced nipples, hypoplastic nails, peripheral lymphedema of the hands and feet, and pigmented nevi.

    d. **Associated anomalies.** Include congenital heart defects, typically a bicuspid aortic valve or aortic coarctation, horseshoe kidney, and gonadal dysgenesis.

  5. **22q11.2 Deletion syndrome (DiGeorge syndrome, velocardiofacial syndrome).** It is now understood that the phenotypes of DiGeorge syndrome (congenital heart disease, hypocalcemia, and immunodeficiency), velocardiofacial syndrome (velopharyngeal incompetence, congenital heart disease, and characteristic facial features), and conotruncal anomaly facial syndrome are all encompassed by and result from the chromosome 22q11.2 microdeletion.

    a. **Incidence.** Approximately 1 in 4000 live births.

    b. **Neonatal mortality.** Neonatal deaths occur in about 8% of cases and are almost exclusively due to cardiac defects.

    c. **Physical findings.** Include a range of malformations including:

      i. **Congenital heart disease** (~75%). Conotruncal malformations including tetralogy of Fallot, interrupted aortic arch, ventricular septal defects, or truncus arteriosus.

      ii. **Palatal abnormalities** (~70%). Velopharyngeal incompetence, submucosal cleft palate, and cleft palate.

      iii. **Immune function** (~75%). Immunodeficiency occurs because of thymic hypoplasia and secondary T-cell abnormalities.

      iv. **Craniofacial features.** Include microcephaly, malar flattening, mandibular retrusion, overfolded or squared-off helices, prominent nasal root, bulbous nasal tip, hooded eyelids, and hypertelorism. However, the facial features are not typically suggestive of the diagnosis during the neonatal period, especially in persons not of Caucasian ancestry.

    d. **Associated anomalies.** Hypocalcemia (~50%), significant feeding problems (~30%), renal anomalies (~33%), hearing loss (both conductive and sensorineural), and hyperextensibility of hands and fingers.

  6. **Williams syndrome (7q11.23 deletion)**

    a. **Incidence.** Approximately 1 in 7500 to 1/20,000 live births.

    b. **Neonatal mortality.** Quite small and mostly due to severe cardiac anomalies.

    c. **Physical findings.** Flat midface, medial eyebrow flare, short palpebral fissures, epicanthal folds, depressed nasal bridge, anteverted nostrils, long philtrum, thick lips, and blue irides with a stellate pattern.

    d. **Associated anomalies.** Include congenital heart defects (~80%), inguinal or umbilical hernias, hypercalcemia, and feeding difficulties.

B. **Common sequences seen in the neonatal period**

  1. **Oligohydramnios sequence (Potter sequence)**

    a. **Incidence.** Approximately 1 in 4000 live births.

    b. **Neonatal mortality.** Almost all of these infants die.

    c. **Pathophysiology.** The initial malformations in this sequence are varied, but all lead to oligohydramnios. Primary malformations can include bilateral renal agenesis, severe polycystic kidneys, or a urinary tract obstruction. The resultant oligohydramnios then results in deformations and disruptions including compression deformities of the face and limbs, pulmonary hypoplasia with pneumothoraces, wrinkled skin, and growth restriction. Absent abdominal musculature (prune belly) and cryptorchidism may also be present.

    d. **Associated anomalies.** Include congenital heart defects, esophageal and duodenal atresia, imperforate anus, sirenomelia, hypoplastic nails, Pierre

Robin sequence, large fontanelles, wide sutures, flexion contractures, and clubfeet.

2. **Amniotic band sequence**
   a. **Incidence.** Approximately 1 in 1200 to 15,000 live births.
   b. **Neonatal mortality.** Variable based on affected tissues and organs.
   c. **Pathophysiology.** The effects of early amnion rupture with entanglement of body parts in bands or strands of amnion is the primary event. The resulting biomechanical forces can lead to disruptions, deformations, and malformations. Viscera that are normally outside the fetus in early embryonic development may be hindered in their return, giving rise to an omphalocele and other anomalies.
   d. **Physical findings.** Examination of the placenta and amniotic membranes is diagnostic. Aberrant bands or strands are noted, and remnants of the amnion may be tangled within the umbilical cord.
      i. **Extremities.** Anomalies of the extremities include congenital amputations, constrictions, and distal swellings (Figure 93–1).
      ii. **Craniofacies.** Craniofacial anomalies include microcephaly, encephaloceles, and facial clefts.
      iii. **Viscera.** Visceral anomalies include omphaloceles, ectopia cordis, thoracoschisis, and abdominoschisis.
3. **Arthrogryposis multiplex congenita (multiple joint contractures)**
   a. **Incidence.** Approximately 1 in 3000 to 1 in 5000 live births.
   b. **Neonatal mortality.** Variable based on etiology.
   c. **Pathophysiology.** Arthrogryposis is essentially a descriptive diagnosis related to hundreds of diseases with varying etiologies. Factors that lead to reduced movement, including primary neurologic, muscular, or orthopedic problems, can all lead to arthrogryposis. Joint contractures can also be secondary to factors that are extrinsic to the developing fetus, such as fetal crowding and constraint. Neurologic abnormalities include meningomyelocele, prenatal

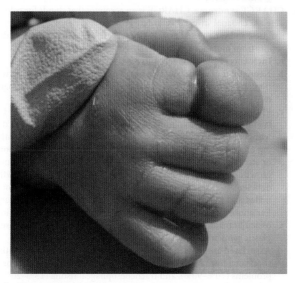

FIGURE 93–1. Amniotic band syndrome. (*Used with permission from Leslie Castelo-Soccio, MD, PhD, Children's Hospital of Philadelphia Division of Dermatology.*)

spasticity, anencephaly, and hydranencephaly. Muscle abnormalities include muscle agenesis and fetal myopathies. Orthopedic abnormalities include synostosis, joint laxity with dislocations, and aberrant soft tissue fixations.

    d. **Clinical presentation.** The newborn infant may present with a combination of joint contractures and/or dislocations. Those with arthrogryposis of central nervous system origin are at increased risk for aspiration and inadequate respiratory movement. (See also Chapter 112.)

  4. **Pierre Robin sequence.** This sequence can occur in isolation or as part of a larger multiple congenital abnormality syndrome. The most common associated syndrome is Stickler syndrome.

    a. **Incidence.** Approximately 1 in 8500 to 14,000 live births.

    b. **Neonatal mortality.** Small and mostly due to severe upper airway obstruction at birth.

    c. **Pathophysiology.** The primary event of this sequence is hypoplasia of the mandible, which results in secondary glossoptosis. The glossoptosis then leads to both upper airway obstruction and the development of a cleft palate.

    d. **Clinical presentation.** Infants have micrognathia or a receding chin with a cleft palate. Respiratory distress can occur because of upper airway obstruction. Low-set ears may also be present.

C. **Miscellaneous associations and syndromes seen in the neonatal period**

  1. **VATER/VACTERL association.** VATER is an acronym that stands for *v*ertebral defects, *a*nal atresia, *t*racheoesophageal fistula, and *r*adial or *r*enal dysplasia. VACTERL is an acronym that stands for *v*ertebral defects, *a*nal atresia, *c*ardiac malformations, *t*racheoesophageal fistula, *r*enal dysplasia, and *l*imb abnormalities.

    a. **Incidence.** Estimated at 1 in 10,000 to 40,000 live births.

    b. **Neonatal mortality.** Small and mostly due to severe cardiac or renal anomalies.

    c. **Clinical presentation.** Aside from the defects described in the acronyms, other features of these disorders include a single umbilical artery and prenatal growth deficiency.

  2. **CHARGE syndrome.** CHARGE is an acronym that stands for *c*oloboma, *h*eart defects, choanal *a*tresia, *r*etarded growth and development, *g*enital abnormalities, and *e*ar anomalies. CHARGE is an autosomal dominant disorder that results from mutations in the *CHD7* gene.

    a. **Incidence.** Approximately 1 in 8500 to 10,000 live births.

    b. **Neonatal mortality.** Variable based on the degree of upper airway obstruction and congenital heart disease. Feeding difficulties are a major cause of morbidity in all age groups.

    c. **Physical findings.** The major features of CHARGE syndrome include unilateral or bilateral coloboma of the iris, retina, choroid, and/or discs with or without microphthalmos (80%–90%); cardiovascular malformations including conotruncal defects (75%–85%); unilateral or bilateral choanal atresia or stenosis (50%–60%); and developmental delay and hypotonia (~100%); growth deficiency is typically postnatal with or without growth hormone deficiency (70%–80%). Genital abnormalities include cryptorchidism in males and hypogonadotropic hypogonadism in both males and females. Ear anomalies are both external with anomalous auricles and internal with ossicular malformations, Mondini defect of the cochlea, and absent or hypoplastic semicircular canals.

    d. **Associated anomalies.** Include cranial nerve dysfunction resulting in hyposomia or anosmia, unilateral or bilateral facial palsy (40%) and/or swallowing problems (70%–90%), and tracheoesophageal fistula (15%–20%).

  3. **Beckwith-Wiedemann syndrome**

    a. **Incidence.** Approximately 1 in 137,000 live births.

   b. Neonatal mortality. Infants have an approximately 20% mortality rate, mainly caused by complications of prematurity.

   c. Physical findings. Perinatal findings include polyhydramnios, premature birth, macroglossia, linear ear creases, and macrosomia. Hemihyperplasia may be present at birth but can develop over time. Neonatal hypoglycemia is often present and clinically important. Anterior abdominal wall defects, including omphalocele and umbilical hernia, are common.

   d. Associated anomalies. Include renal anomalies and an increased risk of mortality associated with Wilms tumor and hepatoblastoma. The estimated risk for tumor development in children with Beckwith-Wiedemann syndrome is 7.5%. This increased risk for neoplasia seems to be concentrated in the first 8 years of life. Tumor development is uncommon in affected individuals >8 years of age.

D. Teratogenic malformation syndromes. Few drugs have a known teratogenic effect on the infant. These include alcohol, phenytoin (Dilantin), valproic acid, retinoic acid, warfarin, cocaine, thalidomide, lithium, and antifolates. (See also Table 94–2 for teratogens associated with heart defects.)

   1. Fetal alcohol syndrome. In the United States, the incidence is approximately 0.5 to 2 per 1000 live births, but it is estimated to be more common in certain areas of the United States and in other countries (1%–5%). Features include prenatal and postnatal growth deficiency, irritability in infancy, microcephaly, short palpebral fissures, smooth philtrum with thin and smooth upper lip, joint anomalies, and congenital cardiac defects. Brain development and function are the most serious consequences of prenatal alcohol exposure. (See also Chapter 102.)

   2. Fetal hydantoin (Dilantin) syndrome. When phenytoin is taken during pregnancy, it results in a 2- to 3-fold increased risk for congenital malformations. Approximately 5% to 10% of exposed fetuses manifest the embryopathy. Features include mild to moderate prenatal growth deficiency, microcephaly, wide anterior fontanelle, low-set hairline, hirsutism, hypertelorism, strabismus, broad and depressed nasal bridge, cleft lip and palate, digit and nail hypoplasia, and umbilical and inguinal hernias. Similar craniofacial features are also associated with prenatal exposure to carbamazepine, mysoline, and phenobarbital.

   3. Fetal valproate syndrome was described when an association was recognized between maternal ingestion of valproic acid during the first trimester and neural tube defects. Additional anomalies of fetal valproate syndrome include narrow bifrontal diameter; epicanthal folds; telecanthus; midface hypoplasia; broad, low nasal bridge with a short nose; long philtrum; micrognathia; long, thin fingers; congenital heart defects; genitourinary anomalies; and clubfeet.

   4. Fetal retinoid syndrome. The most common cause is maternal use of isotretinoin, an active metabolite of vitamin A, for severe cystic acne. An estimated 20% to 35% of fetuses exposed to isotretinoin have a major malformation. Fetal anomalies include congenital heart defects, hydrocephalus, microcephaly, cranial nerve deficits, microtia, and a cleft palate. Pregnancy should wait until 2 years after treatment with isotretinoin. Ingestion of large amounts of vitamin A may result in the same adverse effects to the fetus.

   5. Fetal warfarin syndrome causes eye abnormalities, nasal hypoplasia, stippled epiphyses, and intellectual disability.

   6. Fetal cocaine syndrome causes microcephaly, fetal growth restriction (FGR), neurobehavioral disorders prematurity, and cerebral infarction. (See also Chapter 102.)

   7. Other medications that cause malformations: Thalidomide (abnormal development of limbs), **lithium carbonate** (neural tube defects, cardiovascular

anomalies [Ebstein anomaly]), **antifolates** (IUGR; skeletal defects; central nervous system malformations; neural tube, cardiovascular, and urinary tract defects), **angiotensin-converting enzyme inhibitors** (renal hypoplasia/agenesis, skull defects), **methotrexate/aminopterin** (skeletal defects, craniosynostosis, syndactyly, cleft, growth restriction, dysmorphic features).

E. **Maternal conditions that can cause congenital malformations in the neonate**
  1. **Diabetic embryopathy.** Children born to insulin-dependent diabetic mothers have a 2- to 3-fold risk for congenital malformations. The cardiovascular, genitourinary, and central nervous systems are the most frequently affected systems. Cardiovascular anomalies include ventricular septal defect, transposition of great arteries, single umbilical artery, and situs inversus. Anomalies of the genitourinary system consist of renal agenesis and hypospadias, and anomalies of the central nervous system include spina bifida and anencephaly.
  2. **Infants of mothers with myotonic dystrophy** vary in their clinical presentation from mild hypotonia and feeding problems to severe respiratory insufficiency causing death. Other abnormalities include a history of polyhydramnios and decreased fetal movement, multiple joint contractures, clubfeet, and facial weakness. The mutation identified to be the cause of myotonic dystrophy is a trinucleotide-containing cytosine-thymidine-guanosine that undergoes expansion in females with each transmission from an affected mother to a child. The severity of symptoms and onset of disease increase with transmission of this disorder to family members in subsequent generations.
  3. **Maternal phenylketonuria.** If the mother has an elevated serum phenylalanine level during pregnancy, the infant can have microcephaly, severe heart defects, and intellectual disability.
  4. **Maternal systemic lupus.** The infant can have cardiac conduction abnormalities.
  5. **Elevated maternal temperature.** Can cause growth retardation and developmental defects.
  6. **Maternal thyroid disease** (see Chapter 129).

F. **Infectious agents that can cause congenital malformations**. TORCHZ infections are the first thought when discussing infections and congenital anomalies. Besides toxoplasmosis, rubella, cytomegalovirus, herpes, and now Zika, the "other" infections of TORCHZ include syphilis, parvovirus B19 (case reports only of congenital anomalies), varicella-zoster, and human immunodeficiency virus. Syphilis and rubella are major causes of congenital anomalies in low-income countries. Congenital Zika syndrome is a new syndrome that has been described and can cause multiple anomalies. Intracerebral calcifications seen on ultrasound are suspicious for an intrauterine infection. Details are found in other chapters in this book.
  1. **Toxoplasmosis:** Microcephaly, intellectual disability, microphthalmia.
  2. **Rubella:** Microcephaly, IUGR, congenital cataracts, deafness, congenital heart disease, intellectual disability, microphthalmia.
  3. **Herpes simplex virus:** Hydranencephaly, chorioretinitis.
  4. **Syphilis:** Hydrocephalus, congenital deafness, intellectual disability.
  5. **Varicella:** Hydrocephalus, eye malformations, limb scarring and paresis, intellectual disability.
  6. **Human immunodeficiency virus:** Microcephaly, hypertelorism, growth failure, prominent forehead, microphthalmia.
  7. **Cytomegalovirus:** microcephaly, chorioretinitis, sensorineural hearing loss, hydrocephaly, intellectual disability.
  8. **Zika virus;** Severe microcephaly, hypertonia, congenital contractures, ocular abnormalities, decreased brain tissue and brain damage.

94 Congenital Heart Disease

The diagnostic dilemma of the newborn with congenital heart disease (CHD) must be resolved quickly because therapy may prove lifesaving for many of these infants. CHD occurs in approximately 1% of live-born infants. Nearly half of all cases of CHD are diagnosed during the first week of life, or now that fetal echocardiogram is becoming so widespread and available, diagnosis is made in utero (up to 70%). In patients with complex CHD, neonatal hospital mortality can be as high as 7%. These patients have a high frequency of multiple congenital anomalies, genetic syndromes, low birthweight, and prolonged length of stay. The most frequently occurring anomalies seen during this first week are patent ductus arteriosus, dextro-transposition of the great arteries, hypoplastic left heart syndrome (HLHS), tetralogy of Fallot, and pulmonary atresia.

I. **Classification.** Symptoms and signs in newborns with heart disease permit grouping according to levels of arterial oxygen saturation based on the hyperoxia test (see later in this chapter). Further classification (based on other physical findings, laboratory testing) facilitates delineation of the exact cardiac lesion present.

    A. **Cyanotic heart disease.** Infants with cyanotic heart disease are usually unable to achieve a partial pressure of oxygen (PaO_2) of >100 mm Hg after breathing 100% inspired oxygen for 10 to 20 minutes (hyperoxia test).

    B. **Acyanotic heart disease.** Infants with acyanotic heart disease achieve PaO_2 levels of >100 mm Hg under the same conditions as noted in Section I.A.

II. **Cyanotic heart disease.** See Figure 94–1. (See also Chapter 56, "Cyanosis.")

    A. **Hyperoxia test.** (See Chapter 56, pages 489 and 490.) Because of obligate total mixing, the newborn with cyanotic CHD (in contrast to the infant with pulmonary disease) is unable to raise the arterial saturation, even in the presence of increased ambient oxygen.

        1. **Determine partial pressure of oxygen** while the infant is on room air by arterial blood gas.

        2. **Give 100% oxygen for 10 to 20 minutes** by mask, hood, or endotracheal tube.

        3. **Obtain an arterial blood gas level** while the infant is breathing 100% oxygen.

        4. **Interpret results.** See page 490 for hyperoxia test interpretation.

    B. **Pulse oximetry screen.** See also Chapter 7 and Figure 7–1, page 61. This is the test to screen for critical CHD that will require early intervention. It was endorsed by the US Department of Health and Human Services and American Academy of Pediatrics in 2011 as part of routine universal screening.

        1. **Determine pulse oximetry in right hand and foot in infants 24 to 48 hours of age.**

            a. If pulse oximetry is <90% in right hand or foot, this is a **positive screen** and further evaluation is needed.

            b. If pulse oximetry is >95% in right hand or foot or there is a ≤3% difference between right hand and foot, this is a **negative screen.**

            c. If pulse oximetry is between 90% and 95% in right hand and foot or there is a >3% difference between right hand and foot, repeat in 1 hour. Can repeat up to 3 times; if these findings continue, further evaluation is needed.

    C. **Cyanosis.** Care must be taken in evaluating cyanosis by skin color because polycythemia, jaundice, racial pigmentation, or anemia may make clinical recognition of cyanosis difficult (see Chapter 56).

    D. **Murmur.** The infant with cyanotic CHD often does not have a distinctive murmur. The most serious of these anomalies may not be associated with a murmur at all.

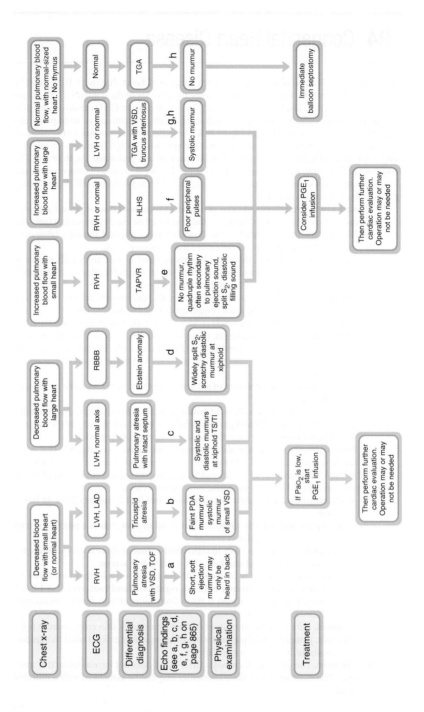

Chest x-ray	Decreased blood flow with small heart (or normal heart)		Decreased pulmonary blood flow with large heart		Increased pulmonary blood flow with small heart	Increased pulmonary blood flow with large heart		Normal pulmonary blood flow, with normal-sized heart. No thymus
ECG	RVH	LVH, LAD	LVH, normal axis	RBBB	RVH	RVH or normal	LVH or normal	Normal
Differential diagnosis	Pulmonary atresia with VSD, TOF	Tricuspid atresia	Pulmonary atresia with intact septum	Ebstein anomaly	TAPVR	HLHS	TGA with VSD, truncus arteriosus	TGA
Echo findings (see a, b, c, d, e, f, g, h on page 865)	a	b	c	d	e	f	g,h	h
Physical examination	Short, soft ejection murmur may only be heard in back	Faint PDA murmur or systolic murmur of small VSD	Systolic and diastolic murmurs at xiphold TS/TI	Widely split S_2; scratchy diastolic murmur at xiphold	No murmur, quadruple rhythm often secondary to pulmonary ejection sound, split S_2; diastolic filling sound	Poor peripheral pulses	Systolic murmur	No murmur
Treatment	If Pao_2 is low, start PGE_1 infusion. Then perform further cardiac evaluation. Operation may or may not be needed					Consider PGE_1 infusion. Then perform further cardiac evaluation. Operation may or may not be needed		Immediate balloon septostomy

a: **Tetralogy of Fallot/Pulmonary Atresia with VSD**– A large VSD with an overriding aorta. The right ventricular outflow tract will be narrow with obstruction (complete in the case of pulmonary atresia with VSD). The branch pulmonary arteries will be small.

b: **Tricuspid Atresia**– linear density in the location of the tricuspid valve.

c: **Pulmonary Atresia with intact septum**– Imperforated polmonary valve with no defect in the ventricular septum. These patients often have connections between the coronary arteries and ventricle which need to be delineated with angiography.

d: **Ebstein Anomaly**– displacement of the tricuspid valve toward the apex, atrialization of the right ventricle so one may see dilation of the right atrium and a smaller right ventricle.

e: **Total Anomalous Pulmonary Venous Connection (TAPVC)**– pulmonary veins do not drain to the left atrium. The pulmonary veins will drain to a confluence and can drain back to the right atrium in different ways: the confluence may drain directly to the right atrium through the coronary sinus (cardiac), to a vertical vein that drains to the left innominate vein and then to the SVC (supracardiac), or to a vein that then joins the portal vein, hepatic veins, or IVC (infracardic). The pulmonary veins can be obstructed or nonobstructed which can give different findings on echo (beyond the scope of this text).

f: **HLHS**– small left ventricle that does not extend to the apex. The endocardium often appears echo bright. The aortic valve may be patent. The mitral valve is often imperforate. The ascending aorta is small.

g: **Truncus Arteriosus**– A single vessel arising from the heart. The pulmonary arteries can be seen originating from this single vessel as it is further examined. A ventricular septal defect can also be seen.

h: **Transposition of the Great Vessels**– The great vessels will be in parallel with the posterior vessel demonstrating early branching typical of the pulmonary artery.

i: **Aortic Stenosis/Pulmonic Stenosis**– thickened aortic/pulmonic valve leaflets. There will be restricted motion of the valve during systole and doming of the valve leaflets. One can measure the velocity of blood flow through the valve to quantify the severity of stenosis.

j: **Coarctation of the Aorta**– Narrowing of the descending aorta just distal to the left subclavian artery.

k: **AtrioVentricular Canal**– There are many variants but one should always see a defect in the inlet ventricular septum and inferior displacement of atrioventricular valves so valves are at the same level. The 4 chamber view will also allow visualizing the defect in the lower atrial septum. (there are many other echo characteristics noted in this defect but beyond the scope of this text.)

FIGURE 94–1. Cyanotic congenital heart disease (PaO$_2$ <100 mm Hg in 100% FiO$_2$). ECG, electrocardiography; HLHS, hypoplastic left heart syndrome; LAD, left axis deviation; LVH, left ventricular hypertrophy; PDA, patent ductus arteriosus; PGE$_1$, prostaglandin E$_1$; RBBB, right bundle branch block; RVH, right ventricular hypertrophy; TAPVR, total anomalous pulmonary venous return; TGA, transposition of the great arteries; TI, tricuspid incompetence; TOF, tetralogy of Fallot; TS, tricuspid stenosis; VSD, ventricular septal defect.

E. **Other studies.** Cyanotic infants may be further classified based on pulmonary circulation on chest radiograph and electrocardiographic and echocardiographic findings.

F. **Diagnosis and treatment.** Figure 94–1 outlines the diagnosis and treatment of cyanotic heart disease.

G. **Specific cyanotic heart disease abnormalities**

1. **Dextro-transposition of the great arteries.** This is the most common cardiac cause of cyanosis in the first year of life, with a male-to-female ratio of 1.5:1 to 3.2:1. The aorta comes from the right ventricle and the pulmonary artery from the left ventricle, with resultant separate systemic and pulmonary circuits. With modern newborn care, the 1-year survival rate is >90%.

   a. **Physical examination.** Typical infant is large and vigorous, with cyanosis but little or no respiratory distress. There may be no murmur or a soft, systolic ejection murmur.

   b. **Chest radiograph.** This study may be normal, but typically, it reveals a very narrow upper mediastinal shadow ("egg on a stick" appearance).

   c. **Electrocardiography.** There are no characteristic electrocardiography (ECG) findings.

   d. **Echocardiography is diagnostic.** Typical findings include branching of the anterior great vessel into the innominate, subclavian, and carotid vessels and branching of the posterior great vessel into the right and left pulmonary arteries.

   e. **Cardiac catheterization.** Like echocardiography, this study is diagnostic and often therapeutic, as outlined next.

   f. **Treatment.** If severe hypoxia or acidosis occurs, urgent balloon atrial septostomy can be done under echocardiogram guidance in the nursery. Cardiac catheterization with balloon septostomy and subsequent arterial switch operation are methods of treatment. Prostaglandin E_1 (PGE_1) may increase shunting and should still be initiated while awaiting definitive treatment.

2. **Tetralogy of Fallot.** Tetralogy of Fallot is characterized by 4 anomalies: pulmonary stenosis, ventricular septal defect, overriding aorta, and right ventricular hypertrophy (RVH). There is a slight male predominance. Cyanosis usually signifies complete or partial atresia of the right ventricular overflow tract or extremely severe pulmonary stenosis with hypoplastic pulmonary arteries. The degree of right ventricular outflow obstruction is inversely proportional to pulmonary blood flow and directly proportional to the degree of cyanosis. Tetralogy of Fallot with an absent pulmonary valve may present with respiratory distress or poor feeding (because of compression of the esophagus or bronchi by the large pulmonary arteries).

   a. **Physical examination.** The patient is cyanotic with a systolic ejection murmur along the left sternal border. Loud murmurs are associated with more flow across the right ventricular outflow tract and milder degrees of desaturation. Softer murmurs are associated with less flow and more hypoxia.

   b. **Chest radiograph.** The chest radiograph film reveals a small, often "boot-shaped" heart, with decreased pulmonary vascular markings. A right aortic arch is seen in approximately 20% of these infants, often associated with 22q11 microdeletion.

   c. **Electrocardiography.** The ECG may be normal or may demonstrate RVH. The only sign of RVH may be an upright T wave in V_4R or V_1 after 72 hours of age.

   d. **Echocardiography.** Usually diagnostic, with an overriding aorta, ventricular septal defect (VSD), and small right ventricular outflow tract.

   e. **Treatment.** Pulmonary blood flow may be ductal dependent with severe cyanosis and may respond to ductal dilation using PGE_1 (see dosing information in Chapter 155). This measure allows more flexibility for planning cardiac catheterization and surgical correction. Surgery (possibly initially with shunting followed by total correction or just total correction) may be considered. Total surgical correction involves closure of the VSD and ensuring pulmonary blood flow is adequate through different methods (beyond the scope of this chapter).

3. **Truncus arteriosus.** Truncus arteriosus is characterized by a single artery that gives rise to systemic, pulmonary, and coronary arteries. There are different classifications based on how the pulmonary arteries originate from the single vessel (beyond the scope of this chapter). There is almost always a VSD associated with this defect, and the truncal valve is often abnormal.

    a. **Physical examination.** Depends on the amount of pulmonary blood flow. If there is increased pulmonary blood flow, the infant will present with symptoms of heart failure (tachycardia, dyspnea, diaphoresis) and be acyanotic. If pulmonary blood flow is limited, then the infant will be cyanotic. Patients will usually have bounding pulses. A click followed by a systolic murmur is often heard with a loud single S_2. A diastolic murmur may be appreciated if there is significant truncal insufficiency.

    b. **Chest radiograph.** The chest radiograph typically reveals moderate cardiomegaly and increased pulmonary vascular markings. A right aortic arch is seen in up to 30% of these infants, often associated with 22q11 microdeletion.

    c. **Electrocardiography.** There is usually a normal QRS axis, with possibly a minimal rightward axis and biventricular hypertrophy.

    d. **Echocardiography.** Usually diagnostic with a single arterial vessel giving rise to all 3 blood supplies and a VSD.

    e. **Treatment.** Surgical correction is necessary and is performed preferably in the first few weeks of life. If surgery is delayed, early pulmonary vascular disease and death can result. Surgical correction involves closure of the VSD, connection between the right ventricle and pulmonary arteries with a conduit, and potentially intervention on the truncal valve.

4. **Total anomalous pulmonary venous return.** Total anomalous pulmonary venous return is characterized by the pulmonary veins having no connection with the left atrium. There are different classifications based on how pulmonary venous flow returns to the heart (beyond the scope of this chapter) and whether or not the pulmonary veins are obstructed. For the majority of cases, there is no sex predilection. These patients can have associated syndromes including asplenia, polysplenia, and cat's eye syndrome.

    a. **Physical examination.** Depends on whether there is associated pulmonary venous obstruction. Infants can be asymptomatic at birth with mild cyanosis that is difficult to assess (unobstructed) versus cyanotic and tachypneic (obstructed).

    b. **Chest radiograph.** There is evidence of increased pulmonary blood flow. A "figure 8" or "snowman" appearance can be present when the pulmonary veins drain to the innominate vein (supracardiac), although this may not be seen in the neonate. The right heart can be enlarged in unobstructed venous return.

    c. **Electrocardiography.** RVH is usually present. Rightward axis and right atrial enlargement may be seen.

    d. **Echocardiography** will demonstrate no pulmonary venous return to the left atrium. Determining the pulmonary vein confluence and where this confluence drains to the heart can sometimes be a challenge.

    e. **Treatment.** Surgical correction in infancy should be performed with redirection of pulmonary venous flow to the left atrium (technique depends on where pulmonary veins drain into).

5. **Single ventricle.** Because single-ventricle physiology is a complete mixing lesion, it can be considered as a cyanotic lesion, although infants may not be

obviously cyanotic. There are many variants including tricuspid atresia, unbalanced atrioventricular (AV) canal, and HLHS. Most of this discussion is beyond the scope of the chapter, but see later section on HLHS for more information on single-ventricle management/palliation.

III. **Acyanotic heart disease (Figure 94–2)**

   A. **Hyperoxia test.** See Section II.A.

   B. **Murmur.** The infant who is not cyanotic may have either a heart murmur or symptoms of congestive heart failure, or these may develop over time.

   C. **Diagnosis and treatment.** See Figure 94–2.

   D. **Specific acyanotic heart disease abnormalities**

   1. **Ventricular septal defect.** The second most common congenital heart abnormality with equal sex distribution. Murmurs may be heard at birth but typically appear between 3 days and 3 weeks of age. Congestive heart failure is unusual before 4 weeks of age but may develop earlier in premature infants. Symptoms and physical findings vary with patient age and defect size. Spontaneous closure occurs in half of the patients. Surgical correction is reserved for large, symptomatic VSDs only.

   2. **Atrial septal defect.** Not an important cause of morbidity or mortality in infancy. Occasionally, congestive heart failure can occur in infancy but not usually in the neonatal period, and rarely without additional cardiac or pulmonary abnormalities. Surgical correction is reserved for only large atrial septal defects (ASDs) and is usually not performed in the newborn period.

   3. **Endocardial cushion defects.** Includes ostium primum–type ASD with or without a cleft mitral valve and an AV canal. These defects are commonly associated with multiple congenital anomalies, especially Down syndrome. If marked AV valve insufficiency is present, the patient may have congestive heart failure at birth or in the neonatal period.

      a. **Physical examination.** On physical examination, a systolic murmur resulting from AV valve insufficiency may be heard. Cyanosis may be present but is often not severe. Infants with severe pulmonary arterial hypertension may have little or no murmur.

      b. **Chest radiograph.** Variable findings may include a dilated pulmonary artery or a large heart secondary to atrial dilatation.

      c. **Electrocardiography.** Left axis deviation (left superior vector) is *pathognomonic*; the PR interval may be long, or there may be an RSR′ pattern in V_4R and V_1.

      d. **Echocardiography.** Usually diagnostic; the echocardiogram usually demonstrates a common AV valve with inlet VSD or a defect in the septum primum with an abnormal mitral valve. Subtype classifications exist but are beyond the scope of this text.

      e. **Treatment.** Congestive heart failure is treated primarily with diuretics or angiotensin-converting enzyme inhibitors (or angiotensin receptor blockers), (for dosages, see Chapter 155); early cardiac catheterization with corrective surgery may be needed to prevent pulmonary vascular obstructive disease. Surgical correction involves closure of the ASDs and VSDs with creation of 2 AV valves (in the complete form; other forms may include reconstruction of the left AV valve).

   4. **Bicuspid aortic valve. The most common congenital heart defect.** A click and a murmur may be appreciated. Unless there is significant stenosis or insufficiency associated with the valve, it rarely presents with complications in the neonatal period. However, it is heavily associated with 2 more severe congenital heart defects: coarctation of the aorta and Shone complex.

   5. **Coarctation of the aorta.** Usually a discrete stenosis of the proximal thoracic aorta, although more widespread narrowing of the arch can occur. Clinical presentation will depend on severity and extent of narrowing.

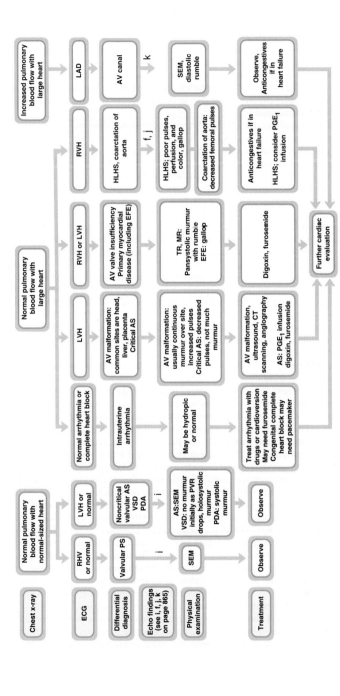

FIGURE 94–2. Acyanotic congenital heart disease (PaO₂ >100 mm Hg in 100% FiO₂). AS, aortic stenosis; AV canal, atrioventricular canal; AV malformation, arteriovenous malformation; AV valve, atrioventricular valve; CT, computed tomography; ECG, electrocardiogram; EFE, endocardial fibroelastosis; HLHS, hypoplastic left heart syndrome; LAD, left axis deviation; LVH, left ventricular hypertrophy; MI, myocardial infarction; PDA, patent ductus arteriosus; PGE₁, prostaglandin E₁; PS, pulmonary stenosis; RVH, right ventricular hypertrophy; TI, tricuspid incompetence; VSD, ventricular septal defect.

869

      a. **Physical examination.** A systolic murmur resulting from the narrowing of the aorta will be present with radiation toward the back. Patients will have decreased pulses in the lower extremities. Pulse oximetry will have an increased difference between lower and upper extremity. If severe, newborns can present with heart failure with associated symptoms including tachycardia, dyspnea, diaphoresis, and hepatomegaly.

      b. **Chest radiograph.** In infancy, this is nonspecific with findings of cardiomegaly and increased pulmonary vascular markings. Typical rib notching seen in older children is not seen in infants because collateral circulation is not yet developed.

      c. **Electrocardiography.** Generally normal. In infancy, there may be increased right-sided forces and RVH. If the ECG shows left ventricular hypertrophy with a strain pattern, then aortic stenosis should be considered.

      d. **Echocardiography.** Usually diagnostic; the echocardiogram usually demonstrates a narrowing of the arch just distal to the left subclavian artery.

      e. **Treatment.** There are 3 different options for treatment including surgery, balloon angioplasty, or stent placement. In the newborn period, however, surgical intervention is standard.

IV. **Hypoplastic left heart syndrome.** Occurs in both cyanotic and acyanotic forms. In 15% of cases, the foramen ovale is intact and thus prevents mixing at the atrial level, causing cyanosis. Infants with mixing at the atria are acyanotic. HLHS accounts for 25% of all cardiac deaths during the first week of life.

    A. **Physical examination.** The infant is typically pale and tachypneic, with poor perfusion and poor to absent peripheral pulses. A loud single S_2 is present, usually with a gallop and no murmur. There is hepatomegaly, and metabolic acidosis is usually present by 48 hours of age.

    B. **Electrocardiogram.** Demonstrates small or absent left ventricular forces.

    C. **Chest radiograph.** Moderate cardiomegaly is present, often with a large main pulmonary artery shadow.

    D. **Echocardiography.** A diagnostic study demonstrates a small or slit-like left ventricle with a hypoplastic ascending aorta.

    E. **Treatment.** Systemic blood flow is ductal dependent; therefore, PGE_1 is of value. Oxygen should not be given, as the resultant dilatation of the pulmonary vessels increases pulmonary blood flow. Respiratory compromise and subsequent dilatation and reduced right ventricular function are undesired effects of oxygen administration. In fact, infants with HLHS and pulmonary overcirculation may require oxygen concentrations <21%. Frequent monitoring of blood gases and lactate is required preoperatively. Surgical correction is done in 3 stages. The first is palliation (the Norwood procedure), redirecting the blood flow so that the right ventricle serves as the "systemic ventricle" and a surgically constructed "shunt" provides pulmonary blood flow. Some surgeons prefer to do a Sano modification of the Norwood, which involves placing a Gore-Tex tube from the right ventricle to the main pulmonary artery. The second stage usually consists of a hemi-Fontan or bidirectional Glenn operation, routing superior vena cava blood to the lungs and closing the systemic-to-pulmonary artery shunt. The third stage (the Fontan procedure) directs the remaining systemic venous return directly to the pulmonary circulation. In the past decade, the "hybrid procedure" has become possible as an alternative to the stage I Norwood procedure for infants with HLHS or single-ventricle equivalent with multiple areas of left heart obstruction. Time will tell which procedure will become the operation of choice for these babies. Neonatal cardiac transplantation is another option, but shortage of organs is a significant deterrent. Compassionate care (keeping the infant comfortable until death) may be appropriate in select instances.

V. **Associated anomalies and syndromes (Table 94–1).** A discussion of heart disease in neonates would not be complete without the inclusion of common multiple congenital

Table 94–1. CONGENITAL ANOMALIES ASSOCIATED WITH HEART DEFECTS

Congenital Anomaly	Heart Defect
Chromosomal anomaly	
Trisomy 21 (Down syndrome)	Atrioventricular canal, ventricular septal defect
Trisomies 13, 15, and 18	Ventricular septal defect, patent ductus arteriosus
Syndrome associated with 4p–	Atrial septal defect, ventricular septal defect
Syndrome associated with 5p– (cri du chat syndrome)	Variable
XO (Turner syndrome)	Coarctation of aorta, aortic stenosis
Syndromes with predominantly skeletal defects[a]	
Ellis-van Creveld syndrome	Atrial septal defect, single atrium
Laurence-Moon-Biedl syndrome	Tetralogy of Fallot, ventricular septal defect
Carpenter syndrome	Patent ductus arteriosus, ventricular septal defect
Holt-Oram syndrome	Atrial septal defect, ventricular septal defect
Fanconi syndrome	Patent ductus arteriosus, ventricular septal defect
Thrombocytopenia–absent radius syndrome	Atrial septal defect, tetralogy of Fallot
Syndromes with characteristic facies[a]	
Noonan syndrome (long arm of chromosome 12)	Pulmonary stenosis, atrial septal defect, hypertrophic cardiomyopathy
Chromosome 22q11 deletion (DiGeorge syndrome)	Tetralogy of Fallot, aortic arch anomalies, right aortic arch, vascular rings
Smith-Lemli-Opitz syndrome	Ventricular septal defect, patent ductus arteriosus
Cornelia de Lange syndrome	Tetralogy of Fallot, ventricular septal defect
Goldenhar syndrome	Tetralogy of Fallot, variable
Williams syndrome	Supravalvular aortic stenosis, peripheral pulmonary artery stenosis
Asymmetric crying facies	Variable

[a]Not all infants with these syndromes have heart defects.

anomaly syndromes associated with heart defects. Often, recognition of multiple congenital anomaly syndromes facilitates identification of the heart defect. Syndromes that tend to present after the newborn period have not been included. See Chapter 93 for a complete discussion of anomalies and syndromes.

VI. **Teratogens and heart disease.** Several teratogens associated with CHD have been identified (Table 94–2), although there is not a 100% relationship between exposure and heart defects. A history of teratogen exposure may help in the diagnosis.

VII. **Abnormal situs syndromes.** Syndromes of abnormal situs are associated with CHD. For example, an infant with situs inversus totalis and dextrocardia has the same incidence of CHD as the general population. If, however, there is disparity between thoracic and abdominal situs, the incidence of CHD is >90%. (Check the chest radiograph to see that the cardiac apex and the stomach bubble are on the same side. Both should

Table 94–2. TERATOGENS ASSOCIATED WITH HEART DEFECTS

Teratogen	Heart Defect
Drugs	
Alcohol	Ventricular septal defect, tetralogy of Fallot, atrial septal defect
Anticonvulsants	Variable, ventricular septal defect, tetralogy of Fallot
Retinoic acid	Aortic arch anomalies
Lithium	Ebstein anomaly of the tricuspid valve
SSRIs	Slightly increased risk septal defects
Environmental agents	
Irradiation	Variable
High altitude	PDA; others variable
Maternal factors	
Diabetes	Variable
Maternal lupus	Complete (third-degree) AV block
Maternal PKU	Ventricular septal defect, coarctation
Infections	
Rubella syndrome	PDA, peripheral pulmonary stenosis
Parvovirus, coxsackie	Cardiomyopathy
Other viruses	Variable

AV, atrioventricular; PDA, patent ductus arteriosus; PKU, phenylketonuria.

be on the left.) Some of these syndromes involve bilateral left-sidedness (2 bilobed lungs or multiple spleens) and complex cyanotic CHD, whereas others have bilateral right-sidedness (2 trilobed lungs or an absent spleen) and complex cyanotic CHD.

VIII. **Other imaging modalities**

    A. **Fetal echocardiography**

        1. **General considerations.** Fetal echocardiography is now possible in many centers. The optimal gestational age to perform echocardiography is between 18 and 20 weeks when structural abnormalities and arrhythmias can be detected. This is being pushed earlier with developing technology. Some centers are performing fetal echocardiograms as early as 8 to 12 weeks. With early detection of cardiac abnormalities, arrangements can be made for delivery at a center with pediatric cardiac and surgical facilities that can possibly affect neonatal mortality. If the anomaly is not consistent with life, some families may elect termination of pregnancy.

        2. **Indications for fetal echocardiography**

            a. **Maternal factors.** Oligohydramnios or polyhydramnios, diabetes, collagen vascular disease, maternal drug/teratogen exposure, or a previous child with CHD.

            b. **Fetal factors.** Suspected cardiac abnormality on obstetric ultrasound examination, pleural fluid, pericardial fluid, fetal hydrops, heart rate abnormalities, fetal growth restriction, or other abnormality on obstetric ultrasound examination.

            c. **Genetic factors.** Familial history of chromosomal disorders or CHD.

B. **Magnetic resonance imaging/computed tomography.** Although magnetic resonance imaging (MRI) is enjoying increasing utility in the identification of CHD in children, MRI of the neonatal heart is of limited availability. The rapid heart rate of neonates makes gaiting for image acquisition difficult but not impossible. It does require intubation and anesthesia. Computed tomography (CT) and CT angiography (CTA) may help identify anomalies of pulmonary venous return. CTA has become the gold standard of evaluation of vascular rings, but these do not usually present in the immediate neonatal period.

IX. **General principles of management**

A. **Emergency therapy.** Once the specific lesion has been identified as emergent, a decision about therapy must be made. As an example, if confronted with a very cyanotic infant with no murmur, a normal chest radiograph, and a normal ECG and it is believed that the diagnosis of dextro-transposition of the great arteries is likely, it is necessary to prepare for a **balloon septostomy.**

B. **Prostaglandins.** As a general principle, if an infant is cyanotic and has decreased pulmonary blood flow, the PaO_2 will be improved by promoting flow through the ductus arteriosus via a drip of **prostaglandin E_1** (alprostadil or Prostin VR Pediatric). Maintaining patency of the ductus may enable stabilization of the infant and subsequent catheterization or surgery to be planned on an urgent rather than emergent basis. Similarly, if poor peripheral pulses and acidosis from poor perfusion are present, infusion of prostaglandin, using the same dose, may reopen the ductus arteriosus and allow right ventricular blood flow to augment the systemic circulation. This measure is beneficial in critical aortic stenosis, coarctation of the aorta, and HLHS. (For dosage information, see Chapter 155.)

C. **Antiarrhythmic drugs.** Rapid arrhythmias may occur during intrauterine life or after delivery (see full discussion in Chapter 53). Arrhythmias are a cause of fetal hydrops and intrauterine death; most often, the rhythm disturbance is a rapid supraventricular tachycardia with a 1:1 ventricular response. Occasionally, atrial flutter with 2:1 block presents before or just after birth. Some antiarrhythmia medications given to mothers can cross the placenta, enabling fetal treatment. **Digoxin, flecainide, sotalol,** and **propranolol** have been successful antiarrhythmic agents in newborns, but treatment with adenosine or electrical cardioversion (see Chapter 32) is also sometimes necessary. Digoxin is contraindicated in Wolff-Parkinson-White syndrome.

D. **Pacemaker.** Fetal hydrops can result from congenital complete heart block. If cardiovascular demise is imminent, delivery and **temporary transvenous ventricular pacing may be lifesaving.** It should be followed by urgent surgical placement of a permanent pacemaker. Mothers may have anti-Rho or anti-LA antibodies.

E. **Other considerations.** Optimal care of the infant prior to and immediately after heart surgery determines overall outcome. A perfectly executed corrective procedure cannot succeed without support of the infant postoperatively. Drugs that manipulate pulmonary vascular resistance (nitric oxide, sildenafil, oxygen) and have a favorable influence on cardiac output and its distribution are required more often than not. Milrinone as an afterload reducer is often used and can be transitioned to the oral enalapril. Nesiritide (Natrecor), a recombinant form of human B-type natriuretic peptide, has both vasodilation and diuretic properties and can be safely used for shorter periods of time than milrinone. Levosimendan, a calcium-sensitizing agent, has inotropic and vasodilator effects. Studies with small numbers of infants/neonates have, to date, shown no advantage of levosimendan over milrinone in low cardiac output states following open-heart surgery. Milrinone use after surgical ductal ligation treats hemodynamic instability, facilitating central nervous system and gut perfusion.

95 Disorders of Sex Development

I. **Definition.** Atypical genitalia are present when the sex of an infant is not readily apparent after examination of the external genitalia. If the appearance resembles neither a male with a normal phallus and palpable testes nor a female with an unfused vaginal orifice and absence of an enlarged phallic structure, the genitalia are atypical, and investigation before gender assignment is indicated. These conditions are now referred to as **disorders of sex development** (DSDs, more recently also as **differences in sex development**). The term **atypical genitalia** instead of *ambiguous genitalia* has been suggested. Definitions and classifications are very complex; for the purpose of this on-call manual, the embryology and pathophysiology are only reviewed as relevant to the initial evaluation and treatment of neonatal patients.

II. **Incidence.** The quoted incidence of atypical genitalia varies according to the source and definition, and it can vary for different ethnic groups; it appears to be around 1 in 5000. Congenital adrenal hyperplasia is often considered the most common cause, followed by androgen insensitivity and mixed gonadal dysgenesis. Hypospadias has a frequency of about 1 in 300 births, but only a minority of these patients have DSDs (usually presenting with hypospadias in combination with cryptorchidism).

III. **Embryology.** The early fetus, regardless of the genetic sex (XX or XY), is bipotential and can undergo either male or female differentiation. The innate tendency of the embryo is to differentiate along female lines.

   A. **Development of the gonads.** Gonadal development occurs during the embryonic period (the third through the eighth week of gestation).

      1. **Testicular differentiation.** Gonadal differentiation is determined by the absence or presence of the Y chromosome. If the **Y chromosome** (more specifically, the sex-determining region of the Y or *SRY* gene) is present, the gonads differentiate as testes. The testes then produce and release testosterone, which is converted to dihydrotestosterone (DHT) in the target organ cells by 5α-reductase. DHT induces male differentiation of the external genitalia (see Section III.B.1). The testes descend behind the peritoneum and normally reach the scrotum by the eighth or ninth month.

      2. **Ovarian differentiation.** In the female fetus, where the Y chromosome/*SRY* gene is absent, the gonads form ovaries (even in 45,X Turner syndrome, histologically normal ovaries are present at birth). As ovaries do not produce testosterone, female differentiation proceeds. Two X chromosomes are needed for differentiation of the primordial follicle. If part or all of the second X chromosome is missing, ovarian development fails, resulting in atrophic streaky gonads by 1 to 2 years of age.

   B. **Development of external genitalia.** This part of sexual differentiation occurs in the fetal period, beginning in the eighth week of gestation, and proceeds up to the 14th week.

      1. **Normal male.** At approximately 9 weeks of postconceptional age, in the presence of systemic androgens (especially DHT), masculinization begins with lengthening of the anogenital distance. The urogenital and labioscrotal folds fuse in the midline (beginning caudally and progressing anteriorly), leading to the formation of the scrotum and the penis.

      2. **Normal female.** In the female fetus, the anogenital distance does not increase. The urogenital and labioscrotal folds do not fuse and instead differentiate into the labia majora and minora. The urogenital sinus divides into the urethra and the vagina.

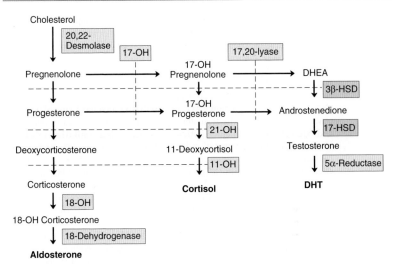

FIGURE 95–1. Adrenal metabolic pathways relevant to normal sex development. 11-OH, 11-hydroxylase; 17-OH, 17-hydroxylase; 18-OH, 18-hydroxylase; 21-OH, 21-hydroxylase; 3β-HSD, 3β-hydroxysteroid dehydrogenase; 17-HSD, 17-hydroxysteroid dehydrogenase (17-ketosteroid reductase); DHEA, dehydroepiandrosterone; DHT, dihydrotestosterone.

IV. Pathophysiology

    A. **Virilization of female infants (female pseudohermaphroditism).** Many neonates with DSDs belong to this group. They have a 46,XX karyotype, are *SRY* negative, and have exclusively ovarian tissue. The degree of masculinization depends on the potency of the androgenic stimulation, the stage of development at the time of initial exposure, and the duration of exposure.

        1. **The most common cause of excess fetal androgens** is an autosomal recessively inherited **enzymatic deficiency in the cortisol pathway,** leading to excessive corticotropin (adrenocorticotropic hormone [ACTH]) stimulation with **congenital adrenal hyperplasia (CAH)** and excessive production of adrenal androgens (dehydroepiandrosterone and androstenedione) and testosterone (Figure 95–1). Most common is **21-hydroxylase deficiency,** which causes inadequate cortisol levels, leading to excessive ACTH stimulation (through feedback to the hypothalamus and pituitary), adrenal hyperplasia, and excessive production of adrenal androgens (dehydroepiandrosterone and androstenedione) and testosterone, producing virilization. **Two forms of CAH are seen in neonates, depending on the associated relative or absolute aldosterone deficiency: a simple virilizing form and a salt-losing form.** In the first form, the salt loss is mild and adrenal insufficiency tends not to occur, except in stressful circumstances. In the second, adrenal insufficiency occurs under basal conditions and tends to manifest in the neonatal period or soon thereafter as an adrenal crisis. The electrolyte status of all infants with 21-hydroxylase deficiency should be monitored because the extent of virilization is not a reliable indicator of the degree of adrenal insufficiency. **11-Hydroxylase enzyme deficiency** is less common and associated with salt retention, volume expansion, and hypertension.

        2. **Other, less common causes.** Virilizing maternal or fetal tumors or maternal androgen ingestion or topical use.

B. **Inadequate virilization of male infants (male pseudohermaphroditism).** This condition is caused by inadequate androgen production or incomplete end-organ response to androgen. These patients have a 46,XY karyotype and exclusively testicular tissue. These abnormalities are rare, and most require extensive laboratory investigation before an exact diagnosis can be determined.

   1. **Decreased androgen production.** This can be caused by 1 of several rare enzyme defects that are inherited (autosomal recessive). Some of these defects also cause cortisol deficiency and **nonvirilizing adrenal hyperplasia**, and others are specific to the testosterone pathway. Other causes of decreased androgen production include **deficiency of Müllerian-inhibiting substance** (the most common presentation is a male infant with inguinal hernias that contain a uterus or fallopian tubes); **testicular unresponsiveness to human chorionic gonadotropin (hCG) and luteinizing hormone (LH);** and **anorchia** (absent testes caused by loss of vascular supply to the testis during fetal life). Presence of **microphallus/micropenis** and **hypoglycemia** suggests a **pituitary deficiency** with absence of gonadotropins, ACTH, and/or growth hormone.

   2. **Decreased end-organ response to androgen.** Also referred to as **testicular feminization,** can be caused by a defect in the androgen receptor or an unknown defect with normal receptors. It can be total (labial testes with otherwise normal-appearing female genitalia) or, more commonly, partial (incomplete virilization of a male).

   3. **5α-Reductase deficiency.** Results in failure of the external genitalia to undergo male differentiation because of the lack of DHT (see Figure 95–1). The outcome is a neonate with a 46,XY karyotype and female or atypical genitalia with internal testes and male ducts.

C. **Disorders of gonadal differentiation**

   1. **True hermaphroditism.** The presence of both a testis and an ovary (or ovotestes) in the same individual is a rare cause of atypical genitalia. Most individuals with true hermaphroditism have a 46,XX karyotype, but mosaics of 46,XX/45,X/46,XY/multiple X/multiple Y have all been reported. The appearance of the genitalia is variable.

   2. **Gonadal dysgenesis**

      a. **Pure gonadal dysgenesis.** Characterized by the presence of a streak gonad bilaterally (complete gonadal dysgenesis) or unilaterally (partial gonadal dysgenesis). It is important to distinguish the X-chromosomal from the Y-chromosomal form because the streak gonads in Y-positive patients carry a significant **risk for tumor development**.

      b. **Mixed gonadal dysgenesis.** Characterized by the presence of a unilateral functioning testis and a contralateral streak gonad. All patients have a Y chromosome and some degree of virilization of the external genitalia; there is a high risk of **gonadal malignancy** in mid to late childhood.

D. **Chromosome abnormalities, syndromes, and associations.** Chromosomal abnormalities infrequently lead to atypical genitalia. However, disruption of normal sex development has been reported occasionally in **trisomies 13 and 18, triploidy, and a number of other chromosomal anomalies.** Note that Klinefelter and Turner syndromes (47,XXY, 45,X, and variants) are DSDs but are asymptomatic in newborns in regard to genital appearance. At least 90 single-gene disorders and syndromes have been associated with atypical genitalia. The list includes **Smith-Lemli-Opitz syndrome, Rieger syndrome, CHARGE syndrome** (*c*oloboma, *h*eart defects, choanal *a*tresia, *r*etarded growth and development, *g*enital abnormalities, and *e*ar anomalies), and **camptomelic/campomelic dysplasia;** atypical genitalia can be present in patient with **VATER/VACTERL association** (*v*ertebral, *a*nal, *t*racheal, *e*sophageal, *r*enal dysplasia, *c*ardiac malformations, and *l*imb abnormalities).

V. **Risk factors.** The etiology of DSDs is mainly developmental/genetic. Behavioral risk factors (eg, excessive exposure to androgens) are rare; a history of relatives with genital anomalies, abnormal pubertal development, infertility, or neonatal/infant deaths could be relevant. The potential association of assisted reproduction, especially in vitro fertilization with intracytoplasmic sperm injection, with DSDs and other birth defects remains *controversial*; the underlying cause of infertility may be more pertinent than the process of assisted reproduction.

VI. **Clinical presentation.** In 2006, after an International Consensus Conference on Intersex, a "Consensus Statement on the Management of Intersex Disorders" was published; there have been recent revisions and updates (see Selected References).

 A. **History.** Any **family history** of neonatal or early infancy deaths (death accompanied by vomiting and dehydration may be secondary to CAH) or female relatives with amenorrhea and infertility (male pseudohermaphroditism or chromosomal anomalies) is relevant, as are **consanguinity** of the parents (increased risk for autosomal recessive disorders) and **maternal history** of virilization or CAH and ingestion or topical use of drugs during pregnancy (particularly androgens or progestational agents).

 B. **Physical examination**

  1. **General examination.** Note presence of any of the following: dysmorphic features (syndromes and chromosomal abnormalities), hypertension or hypotension, areolar hyperpigmentation, and signs of dehydration (as signs of CAH).

  2. **Genitalia.** The number, size, and symmetry of gonads should be evaluated. Palpable gonads below the inguinal canal are usually testes. Ovaries are not found in scrotal folds or in the inguinal region. However, testes may be intraabdominal. **Phallus length:** Measured from the pubic ramus to the tip of the glands, a stretched penile length in a full-term infant should be ≥2.0 cm. Reference values for premature infants have been established; ethnic background may influence penile length. **Urethral meatus:** Look for hypospadias (usually accompanied by chordee). **Labioscrotal folds:** Labia majora are normally unfused but may show variable degrees of posterior fusion; the presence of a vaginal opening or urogenital sinus should be determined. The scrotum is normally fused or may be bifid.

VII. **Diagnosis**

 A. **Laboratory studies**

  1. **Initial evaluation.** An important test in the initial evaluation is the **chromosome analysis** (traditional cytogenetic analysis or array technology). **Fluorescent in situ hybridization techniques** allow for fast determination of the sex chromosome status using X- and Y-specific probes. Buccal smears are unreliable and obsolete. Further diagnostic evaluation depends on the sex chromosome status. Blood for **basic biochemical studies** can be obtained at the same time as the karyotype, including 17-hydroxyprogesterone (17-OHP), testosterone, DHT, sodium, and potassium levels. Further tests may be indicated and are discussed below in the context of the different chromosomal constellations.

  2. **Normal 46,XX karyotype.** This finding implies virilization of a genetic female and is caused by excessive maternal or fetal androgen. If the mother is not virilized, the infant most likely has **virilizing adrenal hyperplasia;** to confirm the diagnosis, measure:

   a. **17-Hydroxyprogesterone.** This is the immediate precursor to the enzyme defect in 21-hydroxylase enzyme deficiency and a precursor 1 step further removed in 11-hydroxylase enzyme deficiency. In infants with either defect, serum or plasma levels of 17-OHP will be 100 to 1000 times the normal infant level. Because 17-OHP levels may be elevated some in normal infants within the first 24 hours of life, a repeat level several days later may be indicated while fluid status and electrolytes are monitored. Newborn screening programs in the United States and elsewhere use 17-OHP for CAH screening.

b. **Electrolyte monitoring.** Infants with 21-hydroxylase enzyme deficiency usually have relative or absolute aldosterone deficiency and begin to demonstrate hyperkalemia at days 3 to 5 and hyponatremia 1 to 2 days later. If hyperkalemia becomes clinically significant before the 17-OHP result is available, empirical treatment with intravenous saline, cortisol, and fludrocortisone may be needed (for dosages, see Section VIII.B.1.a and b).

c. **Serum testosterone.** About 3% of infants with atypical genitalia are true hermaphrodites (most have a 46,XX karyotype). Without elevation of 17-OHP and in absence of maternal virilization, a high testosterone level suggests hermaphroditism or a fetal testosterone-producing tumor.

3. **Normal 46,XY karyotype.** The differential diagnosis of an **incompletely virilized genetic male** is extremely complex and includes in utero testicular damage, defects of testosterone synthesis, end-organ resistance, and an enzymatic defect in the conversion of testosterone to DHT. The laboratory evaluation is correspondingly complex and usually proceeds through a number of steps.

a. **Testosterone and dihydrotestosterone.** These hormone levels should be measurable and are higher in newborns than later in childhood. In the male pseudohermaphrodite, testosterone is low in any defect in testosterone production. The testosterone-to-DHT ratio should be between 5:1 and 20:1 when expressed in similar units. A high testosterone-to-DHT ratio suggests 5α-reductase deficiency (see also Section VII.A.3.c). **Androstenedione** levels are measured to diagnose **17-ketosteroid reductase deficiency.**

b. **Luteinizing hormone and follicle-stimulating hormone.** These hormones are also higher in infancy than they are in childhood. A diagnosis of gonadotropin deficiency is suspected if these values are low in a reliable assay but can be confirmed in infancy only if there are **other pituitary hormone deficits** (see Section VII.A.3.d). Note that growth hormone and ACTH deficiency may manifest in the newborn period as **hypoglycemia.** In primary gonadal defects and some androgen-resistant states, LH and follicle-stimulating hormone are elevated.

c. **Human gonadotropin stimulation test.** Administration of hCG to assess the stimulation of gonadal steroid production when testosterone values are low (as in gonadotropin deficiency or a defect in testosterone synthesis). Specifics are beyond the scope of this manual; the test should be performed under the guidance of a specialist. Gonadal response to hCG is assessed: a rise in the testosterone level confirms the presence of Leydig cells and, by implication, testicular tissue. In patients with 5α-reductase deficiency, the basal testosterone-to-DHT ratio may be normal but elevated after hCG stimulation. Other steroid intermediates may be measured as per request of the specialist involved.

d. **Assessment of pituitary function.** If gonadotropin deficiency due to impairment of pituitary function is suspected (eg, microphallus/micropenis combined with hypoglycemia), thyroid function tests, growth hormone levels, ACTH stimulation test, and imaging studies of the pituitary gland may be indicated.

4. **Abnormal karyotype.** Mixed gonadal dysgenesis with a dysplastic gonad may be present in infants with abnormal karyotype and atypical genitalia. Hormone studies are unlikely to be revealing in this scenario. **Conventional karyotypes, fluorescent in situ hybridization, and microarray analysis** are often used initially; note that a normal karyotype from peripheral white blood cells does not

exclude tissue mosaic chromosomal abnormalities. Recently, **DNA panels and genomic analysis** play an increasing role in the diagnosis of DSDs. Genetic analysis allows detection of *SRY* gene material in 46,XX phenotypic males and can determine whether Y material is present in a 45,X individual, placing the patient at risk for gonadoblastoma.

- B. **Radiographic studies**
    1. **Ultrasonography** to evaluate adrenal and pelvic structures. Although a uterus is sometimes palpable on rectal examination shortly after birth (because of enlargement in response to maternal estrogen), ultrasonography is more reliable and less invasive. Although ultrasonography does not always provide definitive answers, when the structures are found, it can confirm the presence and localization of gonads. Adrenal ultrasonography is sufficiently sensitive to determine adrenal abnormalities in the majority of patients with untreated adrenal hyperplasia.
    2. **Contrast studies** to outline the internal anatomy (sinography, urethrography, vesico-cysto-ureterography, and intravenous urography) may be indicated in complex cases and before reconstructive surgery.
    3. **Magnetic resonance imaging** has been used to evaluate patients with DSDs, but, at least in the neonatal period, sensitivity may only be marginally improved over ultrasound.

VIII. **Management**
- A. **General considerations.** The presence of any DSD is likely to cause significant emotional and social stresses and anxieties for the family. It is very important to protect the privacy of child and parents while diagnostic studies are in progress. A multidisciplinary team should assist the patient and family throughout the diagnostic process and beyond. Once a diagnosis has been established, gender should be assigned (see Section IX) and a team of specialists should supervise medical treatment (eg, steroid replacement, gonadal removal, reconstructive surgery) and treatment of psychosocial aspects. **Circumcision should be delayed in any infant with a DSD until completion of multidisciplinary evaluation and gender assignment.**
    1. **Early interactions with the parents and general care.** As soon as atypical genitalia are noted, a senior physician responsible for the infant should be notified and the parents should be informed. During the initial counseling of the family, gender-neutral terms such as "your infant" should be used; gender-specific pronouns should be avoided. A phrase often recommended in this situation is to refer to the genitalia as "incompletely developed." Parents should be informed that it is not possible without further tests to identify the sex of their child. Meet with the parents as soon as possible to discuss the situation in more detail (the delivery room is usually not appropriate for an in-depth discussion). The feelings, impressions, and biases perceived at the time parents first learn about the diagnosis of a sex differentiation disorder often persist. Examining the infant together with the parents may be beneficial, but any attempts to identify the sex of the child on the basis of appearance should be resisted, although there may be pressures to do so from parents, relatives, and hospital personnel. It is important not to complete the birth certificate or make any reference to gender in any of the permanent medical records of the mother or the child. It may be advisable to isolate the child and parents from the inquiries of certain nonessential hospital personnel and the community, but any actions implying that the condition is shameful or should be "hidden" must be avoided. Parents may want to delay sending out birth announcements and telling anyone outside the immediate family that the infant has been born until a gender assignment has been made. Be aware that many children live the majority of their lives in the community of their birth, and confusion about gender assignment because of premature release of information may

have long-term consequences. Parents should be reassured that in most cases the gender will be determined as soon as test results are available, and some specialists discourage the assignment of unisex/epicene names in the early neonatal period.

   2. **Early referral.** It is advisable to seek consultation from a specialist in the evaluation of children with DSDs (the first specialist involved is often a pediatric endocrinologist) as soon as feasible. It is usually not appropriate to discharge a child from the nursery before a detailed evaluation is done. In most cases, a complete diagnosis, assignment of the sex of rearing, and a plan for future treatment can be accomplished before discharge.

B. **Medical management in the neonatal period and early infancy**

   1. **Congenital adrenal hyperplasia.** The question of whether a neonate with atypical genitalia has CAH needs to be addressed quickly as the onset of adrenal insufficiency occurs between days 3 and 14 in 50% of affected patients. All forms of adrenal hyperplasia have absolute or relative cortisol deficiency and require early diagnosis and replacement therapy to prevent potential life-threatening complications such as vascular collapse.

      a. **Glucocorticoid therapy.** Should be initiated as soon as possible. Maintenance cortisol replacement therapy is often given orally. **Hydrocortisone** is the oral preparation of choice. Initial doses usually range from 10 to 20 mg/m^2/d given as 3 divided doses and often require adjustments for growth and during periods of stress. Alternatively, intramuscular **cortisone acetate** is sometimes used in children <6 months of age out of concern that oral hydrocortisone may be absorbed erratically in young infants. Supervision of replacement therapy and long-term follow-up with a pediatric endocrinologist are advised; institutional practices may vary.

      b. **Mineralocorticoid therapy.** Fludrocortisone acetate at a dose of 0.05 to 0.1 mg daily (given orally) is often used. Unlike hydrocortisone, the dose of fludrocortisone does not change with increase of body size or during stress. Some endocrinologists also recommend sodium supplementation (1–5 mEq/kg/d).

      c. **Incompletely virilized genetic male.** Treatment with **depo-testosterone** might be considered by the team of specialists depending on the results of the diagnostic evaluation.

IX. **Prognosis, gender assignment, long-term care.** Discussion surrounding issues of gender assignment are beyond the scope of this book. In general, the sex of rearing should be determined only after diagnostic evaluation by a specialist team. In the past, gender assignment had been approached as though individuals are psychosexually neutral at birth and as though healthy psychosexual development is related to the appearance of the external genitals. It is now believed that prenatal and early exposure of the brain to androgens, if present, influences gender-specific behavioral patterns and sexual identity in addition to the external appearance of the genitalia or their future function. Considering the significance of the decision for the affected patient's emotional, physical, and reproductive health, a highly specialized multidisciplinary team of pediatricians, urologists, endocrinologists, geneticists, psychiatrists, and others is needed, and each case must be approached individually. Specialized treatment centers should provide long-term care to optimize care and prognosis. The Consortium on Disorders of Sex Development maintains a website with clinical guidelines and information for families (www.dsdguidelines.org; accessed September 14, 2018), as do many other support groups such as the Intersex Society of North America (www.isna.org; accessed September 14, 2018), the Congenital Adrenal Hyperplasia Support and Education Foundation (www.caresfoundation.org; accessed September 14, 2018), and others.

96 Eye Disorders of the Newborn

I. **Visual development.** Newborns are born with poor visual acuity, measuring 20/600 at birth, which then improves to 20/120 by 3 months and to 20/60 by 6 months of age. Binocularity begins developing by 3 to 4 months of age, and the ability to distinguish color begins at 5 months. The visual system does not reach maturity until 9 to 10 years of age. The time of development and plasticity between birth and visual maturity is known as the critical period, the time during which proper vision must develop in order to have normal visual acuity and binocular vision. Alterations or impediments to the image projected onto the retina profoundly affect visual development and can lead to vision-threatening and blinding diseases. It is, therefore, essential to identify such degradations early to prevent poor visual outcomes. Most vision loss is preventable or reversible with the right intervention for the individual etiology. The recovery depends on the maturity of the visual connections, the length of deprivation, and the age at which therapy is begun.

II. **Eye examination.** The newborn eye examination is essential for identifying potentially blinding eye diseases early in life and to prevent permanent vision loss or impairment. The goal of the examination is to identify sight- and eye-threatening conditions such as orbital tumors, abnormal eyelid position or function, strabismus, cataracts, corneal opacities, congenital malformations, and retinal abnormalities, prompting referral to a pediatric ophthalmologist (see also Chapter 7).

   The American Academy of Pediatrics recommends an age-appropriate assessment in the newborn period. Infants at high risk of eye problems (eg, those with prematurity, significant neurologic or developmental delays, metabolic or genetic diseases, positive family history of blinding eye diseases, any systemic diseases associated with eye abnormalities) should be referred for a specialized eye examination by a pediatric ophthalmologist. Normal findings that resolve include edema, lid eversion, bruising, subconjunctival hemorrhage, and nevus simplex. Any unexpected abnormalities on examination should be referred.

   A. **Ocular and family history.** A full history of family eye diseases should be obtained, including history of congenital cataracts, retinoblastoma, and hereditary retinopathies.

   B. **Vision assessment.** Even as a newborn, an infant will blink in response to a penlight; this reflex should be equal in both eyes. The ability to fixate on and follow an object, however, may not be present for the first few months of life.

   C. **External exam.** External inspection of the eyes (conjunctiva, sclera, cornea, and iris) and lids should be performed to identify congenital or acquired anomalies. The lids should be completely formed without deformity, ptosis, or retraction. The cornea should be clear and 9.5 to 10.5 mm in diameter. The iris should be present, and the color should be uniform and equal in both eyes. Subconjunctival hemorrhage and eyelid edema and ecchymosis may be present and usually resolve without intervention.

   D. **Motility.** Transient binocular nystagmus is common in infants <6 months, but monocular or constant nystagmus should prompt referral. Intermittent strabismus is also common in infants <6 months, but poor motility of the eye muscles or large, constant eye deviations should prompt referral.

   E. **Pupil examination.** The pupillary light response is present in newborns of 31 or more weeks' gestation. Newborn pupils are small as the pupillary reflex is still underdeveloped until age 5 months, but they should be equal, round, and reactive to light.

   F. **Red reflex.** A bright direct ophthalmoscope should be used to evaluate the red reflex of both eyes simultaneously in a darkened room. The reflex should be equal, bright reddish-yellow, or light gray in brown-eyed infants, with no opacifications.

III. **Eye disorders**
 A. **Anophthalmos/microphthalmos**
   1. **Definition.** Anophthalmos is absence of ocular tissue in the orbit. Microphthalmos describes an eye that measures <15 mm in diameter after birth.
   2. **Incidence.** The prevalence of anophthalmos and microphthalmos is generally estimated to be 3 and 14 per 100,000 births, respectively. The combined prevalence may be up to 30 per 100,000 births.
   3. **Pathophysiology.** Anophthalmos is caused by either failure of development of optic vesicle or regression after initiation of vesicle development and may occur in isolation or as part of a syndrome.
   4. **Risk factors.** Advanced maternal age, multiple births, prematurity, and low birthweight.
   5. **Clinical presentation.** Either the presence of no eye tissue or a small orbit defines the condition. Diagnosis is made by inspection, palpation, and imaging. Ultrasound is commonly used to determine length of the globe in microphthalmia. Computed tomography and magnetic resonance imaging can facilitate diagnosis of anophthalmia. Detectable function may be present in microphthalmic cases.
   6. **Management.** Conservative approaches include refraction and treating any underlying amblyopia. In unilateral cases, the "good" eye must be protected and any visual deficit managed appropriately. Reconstructive surgical interventions allow for growth of the orbit and prevention of orbital hypoplasia.
   7. **Prognosis.** Visual development depends on the degree of retinal development and other ocular characteristics in microphthalmic patients. Therapy is aimed at maximizing existing vision and enhancing cosmetic appearance rather than improving sight.
 B. **Coloboma**
   1. **Definition.** Colobomas are cleft-shaped fissures in the eyelid, iris, lens, ciliary body, retina, choroid, or optic nerve.
   2. **Incidence.** Ocular colobomas occur in 1 per 2077 live births.
   3. **Pathophysiology.** The condition results from incomplete embryologic closure of fetal fissures that may be associated with persistence of hyaloid vessels and pupillary membrane.
   4. **Risk factors.** The majority are sporadic, but there is an increased incidence in infants with trisomy 13 and infants with CHARGE syndrome (*c*oloboma, *h*eart defects, choanal *a*tresia, *r*etarded growth and development, *g*enital abnormalities, and *e*ar anomalies), or as a result of maternal ingestion of d-lysergic acid diethylamide or thalidomide. Eyelid colobomas are associated with Goldenhar syndrome and Treacher Collins syndrome. Familial colobomas are autosomal dominant.
   5. **Clinical presentation.** A keyhole-shaped defect that may be seen in the ocular and adnexal structures listed earlier.
   6. **Management.** Surgical intervention is indicated when an eyelid coloboma prevents adequate lid closure. In addition, if there is anisometropia (difference in the refractive error between the 2 eyes), eyeglasses should be prescribed. Patching the good eye may also help to rehabilitate the affected eye.
   7. **Prognosis.** Visual potential is dependent on the location of the coloboma. A coloboma of the iris does not affect vision. A coloboma that includes the optic nerve, the macula, or other parts of the retina can cause legal blindness.
 C. **Congenital cataracts**
   1. **Definition.** Cataracts are an opacification of the crystalline lens that is present at birth.
   2. **Incidence.** Estimates are 1.2 to 6.0 cases per 10,000 in the United States.
   3. **Pathophysiology.** Any process that alters the glycolytic pathway or epithelial cell mitosis of the avascular lens causes cataracts.

4. **Risk factors.** About 25% of the cases are hereditary; the most frequent mode of transmission is autosomal dominant. About one-third of cases occur sporadically.
   a. **Metabolic causes.** Hypoglycemia, hypoparathyroidism, mannosidosis, maternal diabetes, galactosemia, hypocalcemia, and vitamin A or D deficiency.
   b. **Congenital infections.** Infants with rubella, cytomegalovirus, syphilis, toxoplasmosis, herpes simplex, and varicella can have congenital cataracts.
   c. **Other causes.** In utero radiation exposure and associations with specific genetic syndromes (trisomy 21; Lowe, Alport, or Smith-Lemli-Opitz syndrome) can cause opacification.
5. **Clinical presentation.** The newborn presents with leukocoria (opacification of the red reflex). Lens opacities may be isolated or associated with other eye anomalies or systemic conditions.
6. **Management.** The initial workup includes the many causes and associations. Maternal and infant histories direct laboratory evaluation. An ophthalmologic slit lamp confirms the presence of a cataract. If the cataract directly threatens vision, then prompt surgical removal is indicated to avoid legal blindness from deprivation amblyopia. Infants will require significant visual rehabilitation after cataract extraction.
   a. **Contact lenses or glasses are used to correct refractive error.**
   b. **Occlusion therapy of the better eye to reverse amblyopia** may be necessary. Length of treatment depends on visual rehabilitation.
7. **Prognosis.** Cataracts lead to varying degrees of visual impairment from blurred vision to blindness, depending on the extent and location of the opacity and the promptness of and adherence to treatment.
D. **Congenital glaucoma**
   1. **Definition.** Increased intraocular pressure due to impaired drainage of the aqueous humor that causes damage to the optic nerve and permanent vision loss.
   2. **Incidence.** Occurs in 1 out of 10,000 births.
   3. **Pathophysiology.** Primary congenital glaucoma is caused by structural abnormalities of the aqueous humor drainage channels. Secondary causes include aniridia, anterior segment dysgenesis, Sturge-Weber syndrome, retinopathy of prematurity, persistent fetal vasculature, congenital rubella, and homocystinuria.
   4. **Risk factors.** In primary congenital glaucoma, males are found to have a higher incidence of the disease, composing approximately 65% of cases. The disease is typically sporadic or autosomal recessive. Secondary glaucomas can be inherited in a variety of patterns, including autosomal dominant, autosomal recessive, and sporadic. Infants with galactosemia, lysosomal storage disorders, and peroxisomal disorders can all present with glaucoma.
   5. **Clinical presentation.** Signs and symptoms include corneal haze, photophobia, epiphora, buphthalmos, blepharospasm, and eye rubbing. The diagnosis is made by measuring intraocular pressure and inspecting the optic nerve.
   6. **Management.** Infants usually require surgery to improve drainage.
   7. **Prognosis.** Early intervention is essential to prevent blindness, which occurs in 2% to 15% of cases.
IV. **Congenital ptosis**
   A. **Definition.** Ptosis is a unilateral or bilateral decrease in the vertical distance between the upper and lower eyelids.
   B. **Incidence.** Congenital ptosis occurs in 1 in 842 births.
   C. **Pathophysiology.** It usually occurs due to dysfunction of the levator palpebrae muscle but can sometimes be due to denervation of the superior tarsal muscle (Müller muscle) as in Horner syndrome.

    D. **Risk factors.** It may be transmitted as an autosomal dominant condition or caused by third-nerve palsy.

    E. **Clinical presentation.** Ptosis can affect 1 or both eyes. With partial dysfunction, the eyelid droops; with complete dysfunction of the muscle, there is no elevation of the eyelid. Infants with mild unilateral ptosis should be evaluated for Horner syndrome.

    F. **Management.** Infants should be monitored for signs of amblyopia. Surgical correction of congenital ptosis can be undertaken at any age depending on the severity of visual impairment. Earlier intervention may be required if potential for significant amblyopia or torticollis is present.

    G. **Prognosis.** Repair of congenital ptosis can produce excellent functional and cosmetic results. Of patients who require surgical intervention, 50% or more may require repeat surgery in 8 to 10 years following the initial surgery. With careful observation and treatment, amblyopia can be treated successfully.

  V. **Conjunctivitis.** See Chapter 58.

 VI. **Congenital nasolacrimal duct obstruction or congenital dacryocele.** See also Chapter 58.

    A. **Definition.** Congenital obstruction of the nasolacrimal duct.

    B. **Incidence.** Congenital nasolacrimal duct obstruction (CNLDO) is found in 2% to 6% of all newborns. Congenital dacryocele occurs in 1 in 3884 live births and has a female predominance.

    C. **Pathophysiology.** The obstruction is caused by an imperforate membrane at the valve of Hasner in the nasolacrimal duct. In a dacryocele, the lacrimal sac becomes distended and is blocked both at the common canaliculus superiorly and at the valve of Hasner inferiorly.

    D. **Risk factors.** Children with Down syndrome, craniosynostosis, Goldenhar sequence, clefting syndromes, hemifacial microsomia, or any midline facial anomaly are at an increased risk.

    E. **Clinical presentation.** Symptoms include increased mucus or mucopurulent discharge and epiphora. The periocular skin is sometimes irritated and erythematous. The eye is usually white. Pressure over the lacrimal sac produces a reflux of mucoid or mucopurulent material from the punctum. Newborns do not produce tears until 4 to 6 weeks of age; therefore, obstruction often does not become apparent until then.

       A congenital dacryocystocele presents as a bluish swelling inferior and nasal to the medial canthus. The nose should also be inspected to assess for concurrent intranasal mucocele.

    F. **Management.** Treatment of CNLDO consists of initial observation for resolution followed by surgical probing of children with persistent duct obstruction past 12 months of age. Medical management includes observation, lacrimal massage, and treatment with topical antibiotics. A dacryocele often requires decompression to relieve obstruction as infection and local inflammation usually develop within the first week of life. In addition, marsupialization of concurrent nasal mucocele is often required to prevent respiratory problems.

    G. **Prognosis.** Ninety-five percent of CNLDOs will resolve spontaneously by the first birthday. Surgical intervention of both persistent CNLDO and congenital dacryocele has a high rate of success.

 VII. **Retinopathy of prematurity.** See Chapter 118.

VIII. **Retinoblastoma**

    A. **Definition.** A cancerous tumor of the retina.

    B. **Incidence.** Retinoblastoma affects 1 in every 15,000 to 30,000 live babies who are born in the United States. It is the most common primary cancer of the eye in children.

    C. **Pathophysiology.** In all cases, it is caused by an abnormality in chromosome 13, which is responsible for controlling cell division.

    D. **Risk factors.** Sixty percent of cases are due to somatic mutations, whereas approximately 33% are due to germline mutations. The mutation is transmitted

in an autosomal dominant fashion. It affects children of all races and both boys and girls.
E. **Clinical presentation.** The majority of infants present with leukocoria. Other signs are strabismus, poor vision, enlarged pupils, or inflammation of tissue around the eye. Most cases (75%) involve only 1 eye. Bilateral cases are usually due to germline mutations.
F. **Management.** Diagnosis is made during an ophthalmologic examination under general anesthesia. Treatment is customized for each patient. Systemic and intra-arterial chemotherapy are the treatment modalities currently in use. Radiation, laser therapy, and cryotherapy are also used in some cases. Enucleation is reserved for advanced disease in which there is high chance of metastases, and there is poor prognosis for visual recovery.
G. **Prognosis.** Long-term prognosis is good. In the United States, nearly 98% of children survive. Long-term ocular and pediatric examinations are necessary because recurrence is common.

97 Hydrocephalus and Ventriculomegaly

I. **Definition. Hydrocephalus** is the progressive enlargement of the ventricular system secondary to excessive cerebrospinal fluid (CSF) volume. It is caused by an imbalance between CSF production, absorption, and impaired CSF circulation. Hydrocephalus is associated with increased intracranial pressure (ICP) and an enlarging head. Typically, an occipitofrontal head circumference of >2 standard deviations of normal is consistent with macrocephaly due to hydrocephalus. Hydrocephalus occurs when the ventricles are >15 mm wide. Occasionally, hydrocephalus can present with normal head size but with marked ventricular dilatation.

Ventriculomegaly (VM) is an enlargement of the cerebral ventricles. In a normal fetal brain the ventricles are <10 mm wide (mean diameter of normal atrium is 7.6 mm). In mild VM, ventricles are between 10 and 15 mm wide; in severe VM, ventricles are >15 mm wide. VM may or may not be associated with macrocephaly. Increased ventricular dimension can be due to increased intraventricular pressure (as in hydrocephalus) or the result of passive ventricular enlargement caused by loss of periventricular white matter (such as diffuse leukomalacia). **Early diagnosis of fetal VM and hydrocephalus remains a diagnostic dilemma.**

Cerebrospinal fluid is primarily produced in the choroid plexus that lines the ventricles (mostly by lateral ventricles in humans). Approximately 80% is choroid plexus in origin, and the remainder is contributed from substances of the brain and spinal cord. Cerebral fluid acts as a buffer between the brain and the skull. Normally secretion of CSF occurs at a rate of 0.3 to 0.4 mL/min (500 mL/d). Total volume of CSF ranges from 10 to 30 mL for preterm infants and 40 mL for full-term infants; 99% of CSF is water. Sodium is a major cation. Replacement occurs every 4 to 6 hours. The mean CSF opening pressure in neonates and preterm infants is typically lower (100 mm H_2O and 95 mm H_2O, respectively). CSF values for cell count, protein, and glucose concentrations vary with gestational age (GA) and postmenstrual age (PMA). CSF protein concentrations decrease with both advancing PMA and postnatal age. The white blood cell count is higher in the CSF of neonates as compared with older children. CSF drains from lateral ventricles via the foramen of Monro into the third ventricle, via the aqueduct of Sylvius into the fourth ventricle, and then into the subarachnoid space via the foramina of Luschka and Magendie. CSF enters the venous circulation by way of the absorptive arachnoid villi that line the superior sagittal sinus. Disruption in this pathway can cause hydrocephalus. **Two mechanisms exist to explain the pathologic accumulation of CSF:**

    A. **Noncommunicating (or obstructive) hydrocephalus.** This may be any blockage along the ventricular CSF pathway that keeps it from reaching the subarachnoid space or disrupts the normal resorptive function of the arachnoid villi. For example, blockage may be from aqueductal stenosis, ventriculitis, or a clot following an extensive intraventricular hemorrhage resulting in noncommunicating hydrocephalus.

    B. **Communicating (absorptive) hydrocephalus.** Results when CSF is able to pass through all the foramina, including the foramina at the base of the skull (cisterna magna), but is not absorbed into the venous drainage of the cerebral circulation because of the obliteration of the arachnoid villi, as in bacterial meningitis or following an extensive subarachnoid hemorrhage.

  II. **Incidence.** The incidence of neonatal hydrocephalus alone is unknown. When included in the diagnosis of spina bifida, it occurs in 2 to 5 births per 1000. The incidence of VM is between 0.3 and 1.5 per 1000 births.

III. **Pathophysiology**

    A. **Congenital hydrocephalus.** Congenital hydrocephalus (CH) is a state of progressive ventricular enlargement that starts before birth and is apparent on the first day of life. CH is noncommunicating (obstructive) in presentation and results from developmental malformations of the brain that disturb CSF pathways. Most malformations occur between 6 and 17 weeks of gestation. CH is usually accompanied by other anomalies of the brain, namely holoprosencephaly or encephalocele. Fifty percent of CH cases presenting as fetal hydrocephalus are associated with myelomeningocele, Arnold-Chiari malformation, aqueduct stenosis, or Dandy-Walker malformation.

    B. **Postinfectious hydrocephalus.** May be either communicating or noncommunicating. Bacterial meningitis (eg, group B *Streptococcus*, *Escherichia coli*, or *Listeria monocytogenes*) and subsequent arachnoiditis cause communicating hydrocephalus due to loss of the CSF absorptive sites. However, a ventriculitis leads to obstruction within the ventricular system, usually the floor of the third ventricle and within the aqueduct of Sylvius (tuberculosis or toxoplasmosis). Indirectly related to the CSF circulatory disturbance can be the formation of postinfectious subdural effusion with increased ICP and subsequent hydrocephalus.

    C. **Posthemorrhagic ventricular dilation and posthemorrhagic hydrocephalus.** It is important to distinguish between posthemorrhagic ventricular dilation (PVD) and posthemorrhagic hydrocephalus (PHH). Progression of ventricular enlargement and evidence of increased ICP are major factors. PVD follows more severe germinal matrix/intraventricular hemorrhage (GM/IVH) in nearly one-third of all cases and presents as asymmetric or symmetric dilation of the lateral ventricles.

      1. **Posthemorrhagic ventricular dilation.** PVD may present early as an acute ventricular dilation within the first week of hemorrhage or develop slowly over ≥2 weeks. By definition, hydrocephalus must present with some signs of increased ICP. PVD does not present with signs of increased pressure; moreover, recognizing PVD and following it closely will reveal whether it is self-limiting and possibly self-resolving without intervention. It may simply represent VM due to disturbed CSF flow after hemorrhage. Hemorrhagic blood and clots may dissipate and allow resumption of CSF circulation.

      2. **Posthemorrhagic hydrocephalus.** PHH may acutely complicate a massive IVH, but more typically, it evolves after hemorrhage and presents as either communicating or noncommunicating hydrocephalus with ICP. A helpful overview by Goddard-Feingold et al suggests the following outcomes of VM after GM/IVH:

        a. **Posthemorrhagic ventricular dilation that resolves,** leaving normal ventricles.

        b. Transient posthemorrhagic hydrocephalus that resolves, leaving some residual, but a static VM, and may also be referred to as an arrested hydrocephalus.

        c. Posthemorrhagic hydrocephalus that is progressive and requires intervention to maintain a stable ICP.

        d. Ventriculomegaly with cerebral atrophy and no ICP.

  D. **Ventriculomegaly.** Fetal VM can be caused by an abnormal turnover of CSF (obstructive and nonobstructive), agenesis of corpus callosum, neuronal migration disorders (lissencephaly, schizencephaly), neuronal proliferation disorders (megalencephaly, microcephaly), holoprosencephaly, and cerebral vascular abnormalities. VM is frequently associated with syndromes caused by chromosomal abnormalities. Clinical presentation and management of neonatal VM depend on the etiology, type of parenchymal malformation, and whether the VM is associated with increased CSF volume and pressure.

        1. **Ventriculomegaly that reflects cortical atrophy** has been called hydrocephalus ex vacuo; the term is no longer used because the condition is not a true hydrocephalus.

        2. **Ventriculomegaly with loss of periventricular white matter** may be a complication of periventricular hemorrhagic infarction (PVHI). It can present as either unilateral or bilateral and be decidedly asymmetric. PVHI with loss of periventricular white matter may present as a large extended porencephalic cyst. Increasing ICP is not a factor in either VM with cortical atrophy or periventricular white matter loss.

        3. **Ventriculomegaly associated with hydrocephalus** should not be confused with **hydranencephaly.** An infant with hydranencephaly has an absence of the cerebral hemispheres, but the midbrain and brainstem are relatively intact. It may be caused by herpes simplex cerebritis, congenital toxoplasmosis, or ischemic brain necrosis; however, in many cases, the cause is unknown. These infants may have normal or enlarged head size at birth, but progressive enlargement soon becomes apparent and readily transilluminates with a head lamp. See Table 97–1 for other causes of VM.

IV. **Risk factors.** Congenital malformations (eg, aqueductal stenosis), central nervous system hemorrhages, and infections are the more common risk factors for the development of hydrocephalus.

V. **Clinical presentation**

  A. **Head circumference.** Daily head circumferences (HC) performed by a primary medical caregiver improve the reliability of the measurements. Normal head growth is 0.5 to 1 cm/wk. An abnormally increased HC remains a hallmark of clinical findings. In addition, distended scalp veins, separating scalp sutures, a full or bulging fontanel, and cerebral bruit are signs of significantly increased ICP and PHH.

  B. **Apnea.** Apnea with bradycardia in association with post-GM/IVH monitoring is a strong clinical sign of increasing ICP.

  C. **Bradycardia, hypertension, and widening of pulse pressure** are known as Cushing's triad and are signs of increased ICP.

  D. **Gastrointestinal.** Feeding intolerance, with or without vomiting, is associated with PHH.

  E. **Eye findings.** The "setting-sun sign" of the eyes shows increased appearance of sclera above the iris and is suggestive of increased ICP. It is an important but inconsistent sign in preterm and term infants.

  F. **Behavioral state changes.** Irritability or lethargy not previously attributed to the infant's day-to-day behavior is noteworthy when seen with any of the preceding signs.

  G. **Seizures.** Seizures may develop but are not of any particular presentation or of any specific electroencephalographic character.

Table 97–1. CAUSES OF HYDROCEPHALUS/VENTRICULOMEGALY

Communicating

Achondroplasia

    Basilar enlargement of subarachnoid space

    Choroid plexus papilloma

    Meningeal malignancy

    Meningitis

    Posthemorrhagic

Noncommunicating

Aqueductal stenosis

    Infectious

    X-linked

Chiari malformation

Dandy-Walker malformation

Klippel-Feil syndrome

Mass lesions

    Abscess

    Hematoma

    Tumors of neurocutaneous disorders

    Vein of Galen malformation

    Walker-Warburg syndrome

Hydranencephaly

    Holoprosencephaly

    Massive hydrocephalus

    Porencephaly

Adapted with permission from Fenichel GM: *Clinical Pediatric Neurology*, 5th ed. Philadelphia, PA: Elsevier; 2005.

VI. **Diagnosis**

  A. **Antenatal diagnosis.** Fetal hydrocephalus may be detected by fetal ultrasound as early as 15 to 18 weeks' gestation. Amniocentesis is advisable to evaluate chromosomal abnormalities (trisomy 13 and 18), fetal sex (X-linked aqueductal stenosis), and α-fetoprotein levels. Maternal serology may establish a suspected intrauterine infection (toxoplasmosis, syphilis, or cytomegalovirus).

  B. **Newborn physical examination.** Head growth of 2 cm/wk is a sign of progressive ventricular dilation.

    1. **Make a note of the parents' head sizes.** Some parents may have a constitutionally large head size, and so might their infant. Normal HC for adult women is 54 ± 3 cm, and for men, it is 55 ± 3 cm. No further evaluation of the infant is needed unless there are risk factors for an enlarging head or signs of increasing ICP.

    2. **Infants with X-linked aqueductal stenosis** may have a characteristic flexion deformity of the thumb.

3. **Infants with Dandy-Walker malformation** have occipital cranial prominence.
4. **Funduscopic evaluation** may reveal chorioretinitis indicative of intrauterine infection.

C. **Cerebral bruit.** May be a sign of arteriovenous malformation of the vein of Galen or a transmitted sound from a cardiac murmur.

D. **Cranial ultrasound.** The most important screening tool for premature infants at risk for VM or hydrocephalus (see Figures 12–4D, E, and F). Ventricular dilation may precede clinical signs of hydrocephalus by days and weeks. Clearly, signs of increasing HC dictate a screening cranial ultrasound (CUS). Likewise, infants with difficult labor and delivery or those who may have needed resuscitation measures are candidates for screening CUS. Ventricular size, change in shape, rate of posthemorrhagic ventricular dilation, and the clinical picture guide the management.

1. **In our institution, initial cranial ultrasound** is obtained for every infant ≤32 weeks' GA between days 10 and 14.
2. **Cranial ultrasound can be considered sooner than 10 days** under certain conditions (eg, infant with multiple clinical complications).
3. **If initial cranial ultrasound is normal,** a second CUS is obtained at 36 weeks' GA or at discharge, whichever comes sooner.
4. **If initial cranial ultrasound is abnormal,** consider weekly CUS to monitor progression of hemorrhage and posthemorrhagic hydrocephalus. Continue weekly monitoring until the injury is stable.

E. **Computed tomography** cranial scanning remains useful for image studies in selected patients. It provides the following information:
1. **Ventricular dilation identification**
2. **Determination of size of the cerebral mantle**
3. **Detection of associated central nervous system anomalies**
4. **Detection of parenchymal destruction (calcification or cyst)**
5. **Determination of a likely site of disturbance of cerebrospinal fluid dynamics**

F. **Magnetic resonance imaging.** Magnetic resonance imaging (MRI) has become the most effective means of detailing brain injury, hypoxic ischemic events, hemorrhage, malformations, and VM. Fetal brain imaging with new ultrafast MRI studies negates the motion artifact of the fetus. Ultrafast MRI now lends itself to in utero imaging for congenital anomalies of the brain and fetal hydrocephalus. For infants with GM/IVH and at risk for PVHI, studies by MRI are more accurate at documenting parenchymal loss and the formation of porencephalic cysts. Disadvantages of MRI are poor identification of calcifications and possible requirement of sedation and transport.

VII. **Management**
A. **Fetal hydrocephalus**
1. **If fetal pulmonary maturity can be assured,** consider prompt cesarean delivery.
2. **If the lungs are immature,** there are 3 options:
   a. **Immediate delivery with the risk of prematurity.**
   b. **Delayed delivery until the lungs are mature** with the risk of persistently increasing ICP. Antenatal steroids can be administered for induction of lung maturity, with delivery of the infant as soon as lung maturity is established.
   c. **Fetal surgery options** of in utero ventricular drainage with ventriculoamniotic shunt or transabdominal external drainage.
3. **Consultation.** Ideal management calls for a team approach with the obstetrician, neonatologist, neurosurgeon, ultrasonographer, geneticist, ethicist, and family members.
B. **Congenital aqueductal stenosis or neural tube defects.** Decompress by prompt placement of a ventricular bypass shunt into an intracranial or extracranial compartment.

C. **Posthemorrhagic hydrocephalus**
  1. **Mild hydrocephalus.** Usually arrests within 4 weeks of progressive ventricular dilation or returns to normal within the first few months of life.
  2. **Temporizing measures**
     a. **Serial lumbar punctures** may be instituted if there is communicating hydrocephalus. Removal of 10 to 15 mL/kg CSF is frequently necessary. Approximately two-thirds of infants undergo arrest with partial or total resolution, and one-third still require extracranial shunting of CSF.
     b. **Drainage, irrigation, and fibrinolytic therapy** is advocated as another means of minimizing clot obstruction with improved outcomes of neurodevelopmental function at 2 years of age.
     c. **Ventricular drainage.** This can be done by direct or tunneled external ventricular drain or by a subcutaneous ventricular catheter that drains to a reservoir or to subgaleal or supraclavicular spaces. This is indicated for infants who have not responded adequately to lumbar puncture and who are not good candidates for placement of extracranial shunt. The incidence of infection with these devices is approximately 5%.
     d. **Ventriculostomy.** Of more recent development has been the success of a third ventricle ventriculostomy. It is an endoscopic procedure that creates a communication (stoma) from the floor of the third ventricle directly into the subarachnoid space at the level of the foramina of the cistern magna. It is a redirection of CSF and a preservation of the subarachnoid to venous pathway for CSF resorption. It has been particularly promising for obstructive PHH with occlusion of the aqueduct of Sylvius.
  3. **Surgical management.** The method of choice is placement of a ventriculoperitoneal (VP) shunt. The outcome may be better with "early" shunting. It remains ***controversial*** whether elevated CSF protein level increases the risk of shunt complications and whether shunting should be delayed in patients with a high CSF protein content. VP shunt placement is indicated in nearly all cases to facilitate control of occipital frontal circumference, improved head control, skin care, general nursing care, and patient comfort. VP shunt function depends on shunt valve integrity. The Holter valve was a standard device for almost 50 years, but its limitations included overdrainage of CSF, causing symptoms of headache and dizziness, and renewed obstruction because of collapse of the ventricles (the slit ventricle syndrome). Newer shunts combine programmable magnetic valves with added antisiphon controls for protection against overdrainage when the patient is in the upright position. In many institutions, VP shunts usually are placed when the patient reaches 2 kg of body weight.
  4. **Long-term complications of shunts.** Include scalp ulceration, infection (usually staphylococcal), arachnoiditis, occlusion, development or clinical worsening of an inguinal hernia or hydrocele, organ perforation (secondary to intraperitoneal contact of a catheter with a hollow viscus), blindness, endocarditis, and renal and heart failure. The age of <6 month appears to be a major risk factor for shunt infection in infants.

VIII. **Prognosis**
  A. **Outcomes have significantly improved with modern neurosurgical techniques for posthemorrhagic hydrocephalus.** Long-term survival now approaches 90% with functioning shunts in place.
  B. **Predictors of unfavorable outcome**
     1. **Cerebral mantle with <1 cm before shunt placement.**
     2. **Regarding the cause of hydrocephalus, prognosis decreases in the following order:** communicating hydrocephalus and myelomeningocele > aqueduct stenosis > Dandy-Walker malformation.
     3. **Reduced size of the corpus callosum** is associated with decreased nonverbal cognitive skills and motor abilities.

4. **Mean intelligence quotient is low** compared with that of the general population.
5. **Accelerated pubertal development** is noted in patients with meningocele or shunted hydrocephalus due to increased gonadotropin production.
6. **Visual problems,** such as strabismus, visual field defects, visuospatial abnormalities, and optic atrophy with decreased acuity due to increased ICP, are common.
7. **In preterm infants with posthemorrhagic hydrocephalus,** poor long-term outcome is directly correlated with the severity of IVH, the presence of PVHI or cystic periventricular leukomalacia, the need for VP shunt, shunt infections, and a high number of shunts.

98 Hyperbilirubinemia: Conjugated

Hyperbilirubinemia presents as either unconjugated hyperbilirubinemia or conjugated hyperbilirubinemia. The two forms involve different pathophysiologic causes with distinct potential complications. In contrast to unconjugated hyperbilirubinemia, which can be transient and physiologic in the newborn period, **conjugated hyperbilirubinemia is always pathologic and requires thorough investigation.** See Chapter 99 for a discussion of unconjugated hyperbilirubinemia and Chapters 62 and 63 for rapid "on-call" assessment and management.

Bilirubin is the end product of the catabolism of heme derived primarily from the breakdown of red blood cell hemoglobin in the reticuloendothelial system. Bilirubin circulates in the blood predominantly bound to serum albumin (unconjugated) before uptake in the liver where it becomes conjugated. Inside liver cells, unconjugated bilirubin is bound immediately to intracellular proteins, the most important one being ligandin. It is then converted into an excretable and soluble form through the process of conjugation that consists of transfer of 1 or 2 glucuronic acid residues from uridine diphosphate glucuronic acid to form a monoglucuronide or diglucuronide conjugate. Uridine diphosphate glucuronyl transferase (UDPGT) is the major enzyme involved in this process. Conjugation is impaired in newborns due to reduced UDPGT activity and a relatively low level of uridine diphosphate glucuronic acid. Conjugated bilirubin is water soluble and can be excreted in the urine, but most of it is rapidly excreted as bile into the intestine. Conjugated bilirubin is further metabolized by bacteria in the intestine into urobilin/stercobilin and excreted in feces (and urine).

I. **Definition. Conjugated hyperbilirubinemia** is defined as direct reacting bilirubin of >1.0 mg/dL (>17 μmol/L) if the total serum bilirubin is ≤5 mg/dL, or >20% of total serum bilirubin when the total bilirubin is >5 mg/dL. It is a biochemical marker of reduced bile flow/formation leading to biliary substance retention within the liver, a condition called **cholestasis**.

II. **Incidence.** Conjugated hyperbilirubinemia affects approximately 1 in every 2500 infants and is much less common than unconjugated hyperbilirubinemia.

III. **Pathophysiology.** Normal bile production involves 2 main processes: bile acid uptake by the hepatocytes from the blood and bile excretion into the biliary canaliculus. Bile uptake from the blood is an active process facilitated by 2 main receptors at the basolateral membranes, whereas bile secretion at the canalicular membrane is mediated largely by the bile salt export pump. In healthy newborns, the cellular processes that regulate bile flow are immature and do not function at the normal adult level, making them more susceptible to cholestasis.

IV. **Risk factors.** Well-known risk factors include congenital infections, sepsis, neonatal hepatitis, hemolysis (biliary sludging), trisomy 21, and the use of parenteral nutrition (PN).

V. **Clinical presentation.** Prolonged clinical jaundice is the main presenting feature of conjugated hyperbilirubinemia, along with pale (acholic) stools and dark urine. The North American Society for Pediatric Gastroenterology, Hepatology, and Nutrition (NASPGHAN) and European Society for Paediatric Gastroenterology, Hepatology, and Nutrition (ESPGHAN) guideline for the evaluation of cholestatic jaundice in infants recommends that any infant noted to be jaundiced at 2 weeks of age be evaluated for cholestasis with fractionated bilirubin. Breast-fed infants who have a normal history and physical examination and can reliably be monitored could be evaluated for cholestasis at 3 weeks of age, if jaundice is persistent. No single screening test can predict which infant will develop cholestasis; however, various screening tools have been implemented in some countries. In Taiwan, use of a stool color card proved to be effective with 95% sensitivity for pale stools. Similar findings were reported from Japan and Canada. Very few cholestatic disorders (galactosemia, fatty acid oxidation defects, cystic fibrosis) are picked up through the newborn metabolic screen

The differential diagnosis of cholestasis is extensive. It can be classified based on the anatomic location of the pathologic process (extrahepatic vs intrahepatic causes), or it can be categorized into broad etiologic causes, such as infectious, familial, metabolic, toxic, chromosomal, vascular, and bile duct anomalies. The recent understanding in molecular genetics has pointed to new directions of investigations that resulted in identification of the molecular mechanisms of a subset of hepatobiliary diseases that often can lead to ongoing liver dysfunction. The most common differential diagnoses of neonatal cholestasis are listed in Table 98–1.

A. **Specific diseases**

1. **Biliary atresia.** Biliary atresia (BA) is the most common cause of cholestasis in the first 3 months of life and remains the single most common reason for liver transplantation in children. It is a progressive idiopathic inflammatory process that leads to chronic cholestasis and fibrosis of both the intrahepatic and extrahepatic bile ducts and subsequent biliary cirrhosis. Estimated worldwide incidence is 1 in 15,000 live births, with the highest incidence in Taiwan and French Polynesia (1 in 3000 live births). BA is classified into:

   a. **Nonsyndromic form.** It is the most common and occurs in approximately 84% of cases;

   b. **Syndromic form with laterality defects (10%).** The syndromic form with laterality defects is commonly associated with splenic abnormalities.

   c. **Biliary atresia with at least 1 malformation identified but without laterality (6%).** The most common anomalies found include cardiovascular, gastrointestinal, and genitourinary. The etiology of BA is not known; theories of pathogenesis include bile duct dysmorphogenesis due to genetic predisposition, viral infections, toxins, and chronic inflammatory or autoimmune bile duct injury. It is critical to confirm or exclude the diagnosis of BA as the cause of conjugated hyperbilirubinemia by 45 to 60 days of age. Evidence suggests that early surgical intervention with Kasai hepatic portoenterostomy (KHPE) leads to a better outcome and prognosis. If the KHPE is performed within the first 60 days of life, approximately 70% of patients will establish bile flow; after 90 days of life, <25% of patients will have bile flow. "Red flags" that mandate evaluation for BA include acholic stools, high γ-glutamyl transpeptidase (GGTP), cholestasis without alternative etiology, and abnormal or absence of gallbladder on ultrasound.

2. **Choledochal cysts/biliary cysts** usually present with cholestasis, but sometimes infants develop cholangitis and present with fever, elevation of GGTP, and direct hyperbilirubinemia. They can be easily diagnosed with ultrasonography; as opposed to BA, the intrahepatic bile ducts are normal or dilated rather than sclerosed and the gallbladder appears normal. However, a diagnosis of a choledochal cyst in a cholestatic neonate should always prompt careful evaluation for BA (atresia of the distal common bile duct

Table 98–1. SELECTED CAUSES OF CONJUGATED HYPERBILIRUBINEMIA

Extrahepatic biliary disease

Biliary atresia[a]

Biliary cysts/choledochal cysts

Bile duct stenosis

Spontaneous perforation of the bile duct

Cholelithiasis

Neoplasms/masses

Intrahepatic biliary disease

Intrahepatic bile duct paucity (syndromic [Alagille] or nonsyndromic)

Progressive familial intrahepatic cholestasis

Inspissated bile

Neonatal sclerosing cholangitis

Hepatocellular disease

Metabolic and genetic defects

  α_1-Antitrypsin deficiency, cystic fibrosis, mitochondrial hepatopathies, Dubin-Johnson syndrome, Rotor syndrome, galactosemia, progressive familial intrahepatic cholestasis (Byler disease), hereditary fructose intolerance, tyrosinemia, recurrent cholestasis with lymphedema, cerebro-hepatorenal syndrome (Zellweger syndrome), congenital erythropoietic porphyria, Niemann-Pick disease, Menkes kinky hair syndrome

Infections

  Viral: Adenovirus; cytomegalovirus; toxoplasmosis, syphilis, herpes simplex virus; enterovirus; rubella, coxsackie B, echovirus; HIV, adenovirus, parvovirus B19
  Bacterial: Urinary tract infection; syphilis; sepsis (*Escherichia coli,* group B *Streptococcus, Staphylococcus aureus, Listeria*)
  Other: *Toxoplasma gondii*

Total parenteral nutrition: Parenteral nutrition–associated liver disease

Endocrine disorders: Hypopituitarism and hypothyroidism

Idiopathic neonatal hepatitis[a]

Gestational alloimmune liver disease (neonatal hemochromatosis)

Drugs (eg, carbamazepine, ceftriaxone, isoniazid, trimethoprim-sulfamethoxazole)

Miscellaneous

Shock; hypoxic ischemic liver injury

Extracorporeal life support

[a]Biliary atresia and idiopathic neonatal hepatitis are the 2 most common causes; each accounts for approximately 25% of the cases.

accompanied by cystic dilation: type 1 BA). Rarely, choledochal cysts can coincide with BA.

3. **Genetic intrahepatic cholestasis.** There are multiple forms of genetic intra-hepatic cholestasis, each with different clinical features and variable clinical

presentation and prognosis. Some progressive familial forms (eg, progressive familial intrahepatic cholestasis [PFIC]) are potentially fatal; the syndromic paucity of intrahepatic bile ducts (Alagille syndrome [ALGS]) tends to have a more favorable prognosis. The pathogenetic mechanisms of this group of disorders have been defined only partially, and molecular genetics diagnostic techniques have only been recently applied.

a. **Alagille syndrome.** Also known as arteriohepatic dysplasia, ALGS is an autosomal dominant disorder with multisystem involvement characterized by paucity of the intrahepatic bile ducts (chronic cholestasis), cardiovascular anomalies (peripheral pulmonic stenosis), skeletal abnormalities (butterfly vertebrae), ophthalmologic finding (posterior embryotoxon), and "typical facies" (facial shape of an inverted triangle, with broad forehead, deep-set eyes, mild hypertelorism, straight nose with flattened tip, prominent chin, and small low-set malformed ears). It occurs secondary to defects in components of the Notch signaling pathway, most commonly due to mutation in *JAG1* (ALGS type 1) but in a small proportion of cases due to mutation in *NOTCH2* (ALGS type 2). The abnormality of bile ducts is considered to be the most consistent finding in ALGS; repeat liver biopsies may be needed in patients with clinically suspected diagnosis but not confirmed on initial histologic diagnosis. Long-term prognosis depends on severity and duration of cholestasis, severity of cardiovascular defect, and liver status as it relates to need for liver transplantation.

b. **Progressive familial intrahepatic cholestasis.** PFIC is a group of genetic disorders with autosomal recessive inheritance and characterized by progressive intrahepatic cholestasis. The predominant mechanism for the intrahepatic cholestasis is altered canalicular transport. Three types of PFIC are recognized:

    i. **PFIC-1 was originally called Byler disease.** It is caused by *ATP8B1* gene deficiency, and GGTP is characteristically normal or low. It presents with conjugated hyperbilirubinemia early in life, typically within the first 3 months. Diarrhea, pancreatitis, and deficiency of fat-soluble vitamins are seen. Cirrhosis is seen by the first decade of life, and liver transplantation is usually needed by the second decade of life.

    ii. **PFIC-2 is caused by *ABCB11* gene defect resulting in bile salt export pump deficiency** and altered bile acid transport. It has a presentation similar to PFIC-1 with no evidence of pancreatitis. As in PFIC-1, serum GGTP is not elevated despite severe cholestasis.

    iii. **PFIC-3 is due to multidrug resistance protein 3 (MDR3, also called ABCB4) gene deficiency,** resulting in altered phospholipid transport into the canaliculus. It is clinically similar to PFIC-1 and PFIC-2 but seems to present later in infancy or in early childhood, and GGTP level is elevated.

c. **Bile acid synthesis disorders.** Several enzymes are involved in the synthesis of bile acids from cholesterol precursor molecules. Bile acid synthesis disorders (BASDs) are rare but in many cases treatable. They present with variable cholestasis and normal or low GGTP. In contrast to other cholestatic disorders, total serum bile acids are usually low. They respond well to treatment with cholic acid and chenodeoxycholic acid.

4. **Metabolic disorders.** The most common metabolic disease that presents as cholestasis is α_1-antitrypsin (A1AT) deficiency. Metabolic diseases that can present with rather fulminant liver dysfunction include galactosemia, tyrosinemia, and hereditary fructose intolerance. Hereditary fructose intolerance does not present in the neonatal period unless the infant was exposed to a fructose-containing diet.

a. **Galactosemia.** An autosomal recessive disorder of galactose metabolism that is caused by deficiencies in 1 of 3 enzymes involved in the metabolism of galactose: galactose-1-phosphate uridylyltransferase (GALT), galactokinase (GALK), and uridine diphosphate galactose-4-epimerase (GALE).

   i. **Classical galactosemia** is the most common and most severe. It is caused by deficiency of the GALT enzyme. It affects approximately 1 in 10,000 to 1 in 30,000 live births. Deficiency of the GALT enzyme results in accumulation of galactose-1-phosphate and other metabolites that are thought to be toxic to the liver and other organ systems. The gold standard for diagnosis is measurement of GALT activity in erythrocytes. Clinical presentation is variable and nonspecific in the neonatal period (occurs after ingestion of galactose-containing formula) and includes vomiting, loose stools, prolonged jaundice, irritability, and poor weight gain. Continued ingestion of galactose results in multiorgan toxicity with hepatomegaly, worsening liver dysfunction, splenomegaly, renal dysfunction, and central nervous system involvement. While on lactose-containing formula, these infants have galactose in the urine, resulting in a positive reducing substance (Clinitest) but negative urine test for glucose (glucose oxidase). A cataract may be detected on examination. "Oil-drop" cataracts are highly typical of galactosemia and may resolve with treatment if diagnosed early. Neonatal sepsis due to *Escherichia coli* and other gram-negative organisms is more frequent in galactosemic infants. The reason for this unique predisposition remains unclear. Treatment for galactosemia consists of immediate removal of galactose from the diet as soon as diagnosis is suspected. Liver disease usually improves, but long-term neurodevelopmental complications may develop later despite good dietary control.

   ii. **GALK deficiency** results in accumulation of galactose, galactitol, and galactonate and leads to early onset of juvenile bilateral cataract. Although uncommon, pseudotumor cerebri, mental retardation, hepatosplenomegaly, hypoglycemia, and seizures have been described in GALK-deficient patients.

   iii. **GALE deficiency.** The rarest and most poorly understood among the 3 types of galactosemia is GALE deficiency. Natural history of GALE deficiency galactosemia is limited due to small number of patients reported to date. When a diet containing lactose is not removed immediately, infants typically present with generalized hypotonia, poor feeding, vomiting, weight loss, progressive cholestatic jaundice, hepatomegaly, liver dysfunction, aminoaciduria, and cataracts. Prompt removal of galactose from their diet resolves or prevents acute symptoms.

b. **Tyrosinemia.** Biochemical basis for this disorder is a defect in tyrosine metabolism due to lack of fumarylacetoacetate hydrolase. It is inherited as an autosomal recessive disorder that clinically presents with hepatocellular damage, renal tubular dysfunction, and neuropathy. Neonates with tyrosinemia may present with failure to thrive, vomiting, ascites, coagulopathy, hypoglycemia, and hyperbilirubinemia. One characteristic pattern of tyrosinemia is a very high α-fetoprotein. Patients who survive infancy are at high risk of developing hepatocellular carcinoma.

c. **Zellweger or cerebrohepatorenal syndrome.** This is a peroxisomal disorder characterized by the absence of peroxisomes and deranged mitochondria; it is inherited as an autosomal recessive trait and presents in the neonatal period with cholestasis, hepatomegaly, profound hypotonia, and dysmorphic features. Diagnosis is confirmed by the presence of abnormal levels of very-long-chain fatty acids in the serum. Most infants die within 1 year. Survivors beyond 1 year of age have severe mental retardation and seizures.

    d. **α_1-Antitrypsin deficiency.** The **most common genetic cause of liver disease**, inherited as autosomal dominant disorder, with an incidence of 1 in 1600 to 1 in 2000 live births in North American and European populations. A1AT is the most abundant proteinase inhibitor, and it acts by inhibiting destructive proteases. Clinical phenotypes include both liver and pulmonary manifestations with variable penetrance. Liver disease commonly presents in the newborn period. Diagnosis is made by protein phenotyping since serum level of A1AT is less reliable. A1AT is an acute-phase reactant; it can be elevated into the normal range during times of systemic inflammation and/or infection. A1AT phenotyping (Pi type) is the most specific and preferred diagnostic serum test. A1AT variants are named according to their isoelectric point pattern, with M normal and Z most deficient. The homozygous variant, PiZZ, is the most likely associated with neonatal liver disease and adult emphysema. Despite carrying the same mutation, only 10% to 15% of newborns present clinically. Treatment is mostly supportive or liver transplantation if cirrhosis is progressive. Outcome is related to severity of neonatal liver disease; 50% of children are clinically normal by 10 years of age, 5% to 10% require liver transplantation, and in 20% to 30% of patients, cholestasis resolves with residual evidence of cirrhosis that may eventually require liver transplantation.

    e. **Mitochondrial hepatopathies.** Usually presents as metabolic crises with associated multiorgan dysfunction. However, mitochondrial disorders can be organ specific with subtle clinical findings to frank liver failure with or without signs of other organ involvement. Infants presenting with features suggestive of liver dysfunction, such as lactic acidosis, hypoglycemia, cholestasis, and coagulopathy, should be worked up for mitochondrial hepatopathies. Routine diagnosis from muscular biopsies and fibroblast may not reveal diagnosis if the dysfunction is primarily in the liver; 80% to 95% of patients with clinically suspected mitochondrial disease do not have a detectable pathogenic DNA mutation. Treatment is mainly supportive and, in some cases, liver transplantation.

  5. **Infection**

    a. **Congenital infections.** Congenitally acquired infections such as TORCH (*t*oxoplasmosis, *o*ther infections, *r*ubella, *c*ytomegalovirus, and *h*erpes simplex virus) infections have a spectrum of manifestations including cholestasis but are usually asymptomatic. They share similar findings such as hepatosplenomegaly, jaundice, petechial rash, and intrauterine growth restriction. Liver dysfunction can occur with any of them, but it is most common with herpes simplex infection. Vertical transmission of hepatitis viruses (B and C) is generally asymptomatic, but clinical hepatitis, including hepatic failure, may develop later.

    b. **Bacterial infections.** Inflammation-induced cholestasis has been linked predominantly with gram-negative infections (particularly *E coli*), although gram-positive infections can also lead to cholestasis. Studies point to lipopolysaccharide or endotoxins with subsequent release of cytokines during infections as the major factors in sepsis-associated cholestasis. **Disproportionate elevation of serum bilirubin in comparison with serum transaminases should make a clinician think of an underlying infection.** Infection should be part of the differential diagnosis of new-onset or worsening jaundice in any infant. Urinary tract infection in particular has been reported to be associated with persistent hyperbilirubinemia (both indirect and direct).

  6. **Parenteral nutrition–associated liver disease.** The frequency, not necessarily the severity, of cholestasis associated with PN is partly a function of the degree of prematurity. Cholestasis develops in >50% of infants with birthweight of <1000 g and <10% of term infants after prolonged hyperalimentation.

Of infants who require long-term PN for intestinal failure, 40% to 60% develop PN-associated liver disease (PNALD). Pathogenesis is unknown but thought to be multifactorial and directly related to prematurity, low birthweight, being small for gestational age, episodes of sepsis, and duration of PN use. One of the most important contributing factors is lack of enteral feeding leading to decreased gut hormone secretion, reduction of bile flow, and biliary stasis. Even small amounts oral feedings (continuous or bolus) during hyperalimentation may prevent or ameliorate PNALD. The resumption of normal enteral feeds is associated with improvement of cholestasis in 1 to 3 months, with minimal or no residual fibrosis and normal hepatic function. Hepatic complications are potentially reversible if PN is discontinued before significant liver damage has ensued. Not a single component of PN solution has been definitely identified as the cause of cholestasis; however, evidence suggests that soy bean lipid emulsion (predominantly omega-6 polyunsaturated fatty acids) contributes to hepatotoxicity. Evidence suggests that using fish oil–containing lipid may decrease bilirubin levels in children with intestinal failure on prolonged PN. Two approaches have been proposed for the treatment of PNALD: lipid restriction and lipid modification. Lipid restriction ($\leq$1 g/kg/d) reduces exposure to parenteral soybean oil and may attenuate the deleterious effects. Lipid modification replaces parenteral soybean oil with parenteral fish oil. It is important to note that a diagnosis of BA has been made in infants thought to have PNALD initially; therefore, vigilance and exclusion of other diagnoses are needed when diagnosing PNALD.

7. **Inspissated bile.** The *inspissated bile syndrome* is the term traditionally used for conjugated hyperbilirubinemia resulting from severe jaundice associated with hemolysis due to Rh or ABO incompatibility, although a multifactorial cause cannot be entirely excluded. Intrahepatic cholestasis is found on liver biopsy, and cholestasis is probably related to direct hepatocellular damage produced by unconjugated hyperbilirubinemia. Prognosis is generally good.

8. **Gestational alloimmune liver disease (GALD)** was previously known as neonatal hemochromatosis or neonatal iron storage disease. It is a disorder characterized by hepatic failure and hepatic/extrahepatic iron accumulation (hemosiderosis) during the fetal and neonatal period. Newborns present with signs of severe liver failure, including coagulopathy, ascites, and hypoalbuminemia as well as hyperbilirubinemia. Hepatic cirrhosis is common, underscoring the antenatal timing of the hepatic insult. The diagnosis may be suspected on the basis of the iron studies (very high serum ferritin level) and early hypoalbuminemia. GALD occurs as a result of maternal alloimmune injury (analogous to erythroblastosis fetalis) resulting from transplacental passage of specific reactive immunoglobulin G that activates fetal complement cascade resulting in fetal liver injury. A high level of immunostaining for the anti-human C5b-9 complex (the terminal complement cascade) is a characteristic feature. The rate of recurrence of GALD in pregnancies subsequent to the index case is close to 90%. Maternal high-dose intravenous immunoglobulin (IVIG) is the treatment of choice if diagnosis is made antenatally followed by a combination of exchange transfusion and IVIG for symptomatic newborns postnatally.

9. **Idiopathic neonatal hepatitis.** This is defined as presence of prolonged conjugated hyperbilirubinemia with liver histology showing giant-cell multinucleated hepatocytes; no known infectious or metabolic/genetic cause has been found. Diagnosis is one of exclusion and appears to be declining with advancements in diagnostic evaluation and discovery of new etiologies with the use of available next-generation DNA sequencing technologies. Management is mostly supportive. Overall prognosis is difficult to estimate but generally good for infants whose liver disease resolves in the first year.

VI. Diagnosis. Infants who have persistent jaundice at 2 weeks of age should have complete evaluation that includes family history and gestational history of the mother, physical examination, inspection of stool color, and obtaining a fractionated bilirubin measurement. Although presence of jaundice is common in newborns and most likely physiologic in nature, continued presence of jaundice at this age should alert clinicians to the possibility of a pathologic process. Evaluation of cholestasis can be extensive; therefore, it should be individualized to establish a diagnosis efficiently and promptly. The presence of elevated serum direct/conjugated bilirubin levels is considered abnormal when values are >1.0 mg/dL (17 mmol/L). When cholestasis is suspected, immediate focused investigations are recommended (tier 1). Once cholestasis is confirmed, consultation with a pediatric gastroenterologist/hepatologist is a must for a disciplined and stepwise approach of targeted diagnostic workup (tier 2) (Figure 98–1).

A. Laboratory studies

1. **Bilirubin levels (total and direct).** The most important initial investigation in a persistently jaundiced infant is determining the fractionated serum bilirubin levels. Presence of direct reacting bilirubin of >1.0 mg/dL is consistent with conjugated hyperbilirubinemia.

2. **Liver enzymes.** Serum transaminases (alanine aminotransferase [ALT] and aspartate aminotransferase [AST]) are sensitive indicators of hepatocellular inflammation but are neither specific nor of any prognostic value. ALT is more specific for liver; an elevated serum AST without substantial increase in ALT, total bilirubin, or direct bilirubin may point to a hematologic or muscular process because AST is an enzyme present in red blood cells and myocytes. ALT/AST may be helpful in monitoring the course of the disease. Alkaline phosphatase is nonspecific because it is found in the liver, kidney, and bone.

3. **Prothrombin time and partial thromboplastin time** are reliable indicators of liver synthetic function.

4. **γ-Glutamyl transpeptidase** is an enzyme released from biliary epithelium. Elevated levels are a very sensitive marker of biliary obstruction or inflammation. A normal level makes BA an unlikely diagnosis. Normal levels of GGTP in the presence of cholestasis indicate failure of bile excretion at the canalicular level and can be seen with PFIC type 1 (*ATP8B1* deficiency) and 2 (*ABCB11* deficiency), BASDs, and tight-junction protein type 2 deficiency.

5. **Complete blood count, C-reactive protein, and blood and urine bacterial cultures** should be considered as screening tools for infection.

6. **Serum cholesterol, triglycerides, and albumin levels.** Triglyceride and cholesterol levels may aid in nutritional management and assessment of liver failure. Albumin is a long-term indicator of hepatic function.

7. **Ammonia level** should be checked if liver failure is suspected.

8. **Serum glucose level** should be checked if the infant appears ill. Metabolic disorders may present with hypoglycemia along with conjugated hyperbilirubinemia.

9. **Urine testing for reducing substances.** A simple screening test that should always be performed to screen for metabolic disease, especially for galactosemia. Galactose results in a positive reducing substance in the urine on a Clinitest reagent tablet but has a negative urine test for glucose (glucose oxidase).

10. **TORCH titers and urine cytomegalovirus culture or polymerase chain reaction.** The use of TORCH titers is less preferable; direct identification of viral infection or measurement of specific immunoglobulin M antibodies should be done for rapid diagnosis. Polymerase chain reaction–based diagnostic studies are extremely helpful and specific.

11. **The Jaundice Chip resequencing array.** The advances in next-generation sequencing technology have produced newer and expanding cholestasis panels with a comprehensive genetic test menu for a wide range of heritable liver diseases. Diseases intended for screening include ALGS, A1AT deficiency, citrin

Presence of jaundice at 2 weeks of age
Normal physical exam; no history of dark urine or acholic stool

→ **Exclusively breast fed**

→ **Formula fed or ill-appearing or poor growth**
Presence of dysmorphic features or other "red flags"

Follow-up in 1 week

- **No jaundice** → **No further workup**
- **+ jaundice** → **Obtain total and direct bilirubin**

Elevated direct bilirubin (>1 mg/dL) indicates cholestasis

Tier 2: Aim to complete a targeted elevation in concert with pediatric gastroenterologist/hepatologist.

General—TSH and T_4 values, serum bile acids, cortisol
Consideration of specific etiologies:
Metabolic—serum ammonia, lactate level, cholesterol, red blood cell galactose-1-phosphate uridyltransferase, urine for succinylacetone and organic acids. Consider urine for bile salt species profiling
ID—direct nucleic acid testing via PCR for CMV, HSV, Listeria
Genetics—in discussion with pediatric gastroenterologist/hepatologist, with a low threshold for gene panels or exome sequencing Sweat chloride analysis (serum immunoreactive trypsinogen level or CFTR genetic testing) as appropriate
Imaging
CXR—lung and heart disease
Spine—spinal abnormalities (such as butterfly vertebra)
Echocardiogram—evaluating for cardiac anomalies seen in Alagille syndrome
Cholangiogram
Liver biopsy (timing and approach will vary according to institution and expertise)
Consideration for consultations:
 Ophthalmology
 Metabolic/genetic: Consider when to involve, especially when there is consideration for gene panels or whole exome sequencing
 Cardiology: ECHO if murmur present or has hypoxia, poor cardiac function
 General pediatric surgery
 Nutrition/dietician

Tier 1: Aim to evaluate after cholestasis has been established in order to both identify treatable disorders as well as to define severity of the liver involvement.

Blood—CBC and differential, INR, AST, ALT, AP, GGTP, TB, DB (or conjugated bilirubin), albumin, and glucose. Check α_1-antitrypsin phenotype (Pi typing) and level; TSH, T_4 if newborn screen results not readily available
Urine—urinalysis, culture, reducing substances (rule out galactosemia)
Consider bacterial cultures of blood, urine, and other fluids especially if infant is clinically ill
Verify results of treatable disorders (such as galactosemia and hypothyroidism) from newborn screen
Obtain fasting ultrasound

ALT = alanine aminotransferase; AP = akaline phosphatase; AST = aspartate aminotransferase; CBC = complete blood count; CFTR = cystic fibrosis transmembrane receptor; CMV = cytomegalovirus; CXR = chest x-ray; DB = conjugated (direct) bilirubin; ECHO = echocardiogram; GGTP = γ-glutamyl transferase; HSV = herpes simplex virus; ID = infectious diseases; INR = international normalized ratio; PCR = polymerase chain reaction; TB = total bilirubin; TSH = thyroid-stimulating hormone.

FIGURE 98–1. Approach in evaluation of infant with persistent neonatal jaundice and cholestasis. (*Data from Fawaz R, Baumann U, Ekong U, et al: Guideline for the Evaluation of Cholestatic Jaundice in Infants: Joint Recommendations of the North American Society for Pediatric Gastroenterology, Hepatology, and Nutrition and the European Society for Pediatric Gastroenterology, Hepatology, and Nutrition,* J Pediatr Gastroenterol Nutr. *2017 Jan;64(1):154-168.*)

deficiency, PFIC, arthrogryposis–renal dysfunction–cholestasis, neonatal ichthyosis and sclerosing cholangitis, and BASD.

12. **Other tests.** More specific tests are indicated in the investigation of the specific causes of conjugated hyperbilirubinemia.

   a. **Urine organic acids and plasma amino acids.** Screen for inborn errors of metabolism as a cause of neonatal liver dysfunction. High concentrations of tyrosine and methionine, and their metabolic derivatives, are seen in the urine in cases of tyrosinemia.

   b. **α_1-Antitrypsin serum level.** Decreased serum A1AT concentration and/or presence of PiZZ, PiSZ, or rarely, PiSS phenotype confirms the diagnosis of A1AT deficiency. The classic histologic finding, although not pathognomonic in A1AT deficiency, is periodic acid-Schiff–positive, diastase-resistant, eosinophilic globules within the hepatocytes.

   c. **Sweat chloride test** is done for confirmatory diagnosis of cystic fibrosis (CF) in infants older than 4 months. If CF is suspected before 4 months, genetic testing (mutation analysis) for common CF mutations can be done. Serum immunoreactive trypsinogen level can be used before 8 weeks of age and is approximately 80% sensitive.

B. **Diagnostic imaging**

   1. **Chest radiograph.** Presence of cardiovascular or situs anomalies may be suggestive of BA. Skeletal abnormalities, such as butterfly vertebrae, may be consistent with a diagnosis of ALGS.

   2. **Fasting abdominal ultrasonography.** A simple and noninvasive test that should be done in all infants presenting with cholestasis after a 4-hour fast; a small or absent gallbladder, triangular cord sign, and nonvisualization of the common bile duct are suggestive of BA. Findings such as abdominal heterotaxy, midline liver, polysplenia, asplenia, and preduodenal portal vein increase the concern for BA with malformations. However, it is imperative to remember that a normal ultrasound does not rule out nonsyndromic BA. Ultrasound is a sensitive method for recognizing other surgical causes of neonatal cholestasis, such as a choledochal cyst or structural abnormalities of the biliary tree.

   3. **Hepatobiliary scintigraphy.** Contrast agents are taken up by the liver and excreted into the bile; they are technetium labeled and provide a clear image of the biliary tree after intravenous injection. Serial images are taken for up to 24 hours or until gut activity is visualized. Nonvisualization of contrast material within the intestine in 24 hours is considered an abnormal finding indicative of biliary obstruction or hepatocellular dysfunction. Sensitivity of this test for BA is high, but specificity is low because patients without an anatomic obstruction may not excrete the tracer. Neonatal hepatitis, hyperalimentation, and septo-optic dysplasia are reported causes of absent gastrointestinal contrast excretion and must be considered in the differential diagnosis. Administration of phenobarbital for few days prior to the study may improve the precision of the test.

   4. **Endoscopic retrograde cholangiopancreatography.** Sensitivity and specificity are excellent. This procedure can be both diagnostic and therapeutic in cases of cholestasis caused by bile duct stones. It is technically demanding and currently has a limited role in the evaluation of cholestasis in neonates.

   5. **Magnetic resonance cholangiopancreatography.** The few reports available to date regarding the use of magnetic resonance cholangiopancreatography in children are encouraging. The procedure requires deep sedation or general anesthesia. Based on current available data, this modality is not routinely recommended in the evaluation of cholestasis in neonates.

C. **Histopathology. Liver biopsy** remains the single most definitive procedure in the evaluation of neonatal cholestasis; interpretation by an experienced pathologist will provide correct diagnosis in 90% to 95% of cases. If a liver biopsy is obtained early in the course of BA, findings may be indistinguishable from hepatitis. The classic histologic features of biliary obstruction are bile duct proliferation, bile plugs, portal or perilobular fibrosis, and edema, with preservation of the basic hepatic lobular architecture. In addition to its role in diagnosis, the liver biopsy may also reveal histologic features significant for prognosis such as the degree of fibrosis, which may help predict outcome following KHPE. Evidence supports that liver biopsy can be performed safely in young infants; therefore, it is recommended to be performed when noninvasive evaluation of persistent cholestasis is nonconclusive. In infants with histologic findings suggestive of biliary obstruction (ie, BA), **intraoperative cholangiogram** is typically performed to confirm nonvisualization of a patent extrahepatic biliary tree; when confirmed, this is typically followed by performing KHPE.

VII. **Management.** Rapid "on-call" assessment and management are discussed in Chapter 62.
  A. **Supportive medical management.** Few conditions causing neonatal cholestasis are treatable, and these conditions (ie, BA and choledochal cyst) need timely diagnosis and management. Medical treatment is mostly supportive and should be directed toward promoting growth and development and in treating the other complications of chronic cholestasis, such as pruritus, malabsorption, nutritional deficiencies, and portal hypertension. Management involves dietary manipulation and fat-soluble vitamin support.
    1. **Special formula.** Elemental formula containing medium-chain triglycerides is preferable because it can be better absorbed regardless of luminal concentration of bile acids. Infants with cholestasis must be given a caloric intake of approximately 125% more than the recommended dietary intake for healthy infants.
    2. **Medium-chain triglycerides.** Infants with cholestasis often require a diet that includes medium-chain triglycerides (MCTs), which can be absorbed without the action of bile salts. Some formulas containing MCTs include Enfaport and Pregestimil. Breast-fed cholestatic infants should be given supplemental MCT.
    3. **Vitamin supplementation.** Fat malabsorption interferes with maintenance of adequate levels of fat-soluble vitamins. Supplementation of vitamins A, D, E, and K is needed. Extra vitamin K supplementation may be necessary if a bleeding tendency develops.
    4. **Dietary restrictions.** Removal of galactose and fructose from the diet may prevent the development of cirrhosis and other manifestations of galactosemia and hereditary fructose intolerance, respectively. Dietary restrictions may also be used to treat tyrosinemia but usually are less successful. Most other metabolic causes of cholestatic jaundice have no specific therapy.
  B. **Pharmacologic management.** See Chapter 155 for drug dosages.
    1. **Ursodiol (ursodeoxycholic acid, Actigall).** A naturally occurring dihydroxy bile acid that appears to help cholestasis in 2 ways: substitution in the bile acid pool for more hydrophobic bile acids, and stimulation of bile flow. It was found to lower levels of aminotransferases in patients with viral hepatitis and to lower biochemical markers and slow the progression of hepatic fibrosis in PFIC. Recommended dose is 20 mg/kg/d in divided doses. The only common side effect is diarrhea, which usually responds to dose reduction.
    2. **Phenobarbital.** Its use is controversial. Presumed mode of action is enhancing bile acid synthesis, increasing bile flow, and inducing hepatic microsomal enzymes. Recommended dose is 3 to 5 mg/kg/d. Use is limited by its behavioral and sedative side effects.
    3. **Cholestyramine.** It binds bile acids in the intestinal lumen, thereby decreasing enterohepatic circulation of bile acids, which leads to increased fecal excretion and increased hepatic synthesis of bile acids from cholesterol, which may lower serum cholesterol levels. Side effects include binding of fat-soluble vitamins, metabolic acidosis, and constipation.
    4. **Rifampin.** It is effective in the management of pruritus due to cholestasis, but experience is very limited in neonates. Patients should be monitored for

hepatotoxicity and idiosyncratic hypersensitivity reaction, such as renal failure, hemolytic anemia, and thrombocytopenia.

C. **Surgical management**

1. **Kasai procedure.** Surgical procedures such as KHPE should be done to establish biliary drainage in patients diagnosed with BA. Optimal results are obtained if the procedure is done before 8 weeks of age. The most significant predictor of long-term outcome is resolution of jaundice. The procedure is usually used as a bridge to transplantation.

2. **Liver transplantation.** When end-stage liver disease is inevitable, liver transplantation is the last resort. BA remains the most common indication for liver transplantation in the United States. Overall, the success of liver transplantation has improved significantly. Due to continuing improvements in surgical and interventional techniques as well as neonatal and pediatric postoperative care, the number of patients transplanted within the first year of life continues to increase. According to the Studies of Pediatric Liver Transplantation registry of 1611 pediatric patients, the 1-year patient and graft survival rates were 88% and 82%, respectively, whereas the 4-year patient and graft survival rates were 83% and 74%, respectively. Long-term complications include immunosuppression, infection, renal failure, and growth retardation.

VIII. **Prognosis** depends on individual etiologies (see Section V). Diseases with relatively favorable prognosis include choledochal cyst, inspissated bile syndrome, ALGS, BASD, and PNALD. Infant with BA do better when KHPE is done before 2 months of age. In most patients, KHPE is used as a bridge to liver transplantation. A recent publication showed that among 1107 patients diagnosed with BA between 1986 and 2009 in France, 94% underwent the KHPE. Survival with the native liver (no transplantation) was 40% at 5 years, 36% at 10 years, and 30% at 20 years of age. Overall patient survival was 81% at 5 years, 80% at 10 years, and 77% at 20 years of age.

99 Hyperbilirubinemia: Unconjugated

I. **Definition.** When the rate of bilirubin production exceeds the rate of elimination, the end result is a rise in the total serum bilirubin (TSB), a clinical condition called **hyperbilirubinemia.** The accumulation of bilirubin manifests as yellow discoloration of the skin, sclera, and mucosa called jaundice. Neonates with severe hyperbilirubinemia (defined as a TSB >25 mg/dL in late preterm and term infants) are at risk for **bilirubin-induced neurologic dysfunction (BIND),** which occurs when bilirubin crosses the blood–brain barrier and binds to targeted brain tissues. Hyperbilirubinemia presents as either **unconjugated hyperbilirubinemia** or **conjugated hyperbilirubinemia**. The 2 forms involve different causes and complications. In contrast to unconjugated hyperbilirubinemia, which can be transient and physiologic in the newborn period, conjugated hyperbilirubinemia is always pathologic and requires thorough investigation. See Chapter 98 for a discussion of conjugated hyperbilirubinemia (direct) and Chapters 62 and 63 for rapid "on-call" assessment and management of the 2 conditions.

II. **Incidence.** Neonatal hyperbilirubinemia is a common problem to address in the newborn period. It occurs in approximately 60% to 70% of term and approximately 80% of preterm infants in the first week of life. The incidence of severe hyperbilirubinemia is approximately 0.14%. Incidence is higher in populations living at higher altitudes and varying ethnicities such as East Asians, Greeks, and Native Americans; it is generally lower in African Americans.

III. **Pathophysiology.** Bilirubin is a product of heme degradation (80%–90% derived from hemoglobin found in red blood cells [RBCs]). The enzyme heme oxygenase catalyzes the breakdown of heme in reticuloendothelial system, resulting in the formation of equimolar quantities of carbon monoxide (CO) and biliverdin. Biliverdin then is converted to bilirubin by the enzyme biliverdin reductase. Bilirubin is carried bound to albumin for uptake in the liver, followed by conjugation and then excretion in the bile. Gut bacteria convert conjugated bilirubin into urobilin and stercobilin. There are 3 main basic pathophysiologic mechanisms responsible for development of unconjugated hyperbilirubinemia: overproduction, decreased uptake, and impaired conjugation.

A. **"Physiologic" unconjugated hyperbilirubinemia.** The pathophysiologic mechanisms of neonatal jaundice involve 2 major contributing factors. First is the greater production of bilirubin secondary to increased heme turnover. The other is decreased ability of the newborn liver to conjugate bilirubin. Both factors are interrelated and important. Because all newborns have transient immaturity of the conjugating enzyme uridine diphosphate glucoronyl transferase (UDPGT), overproduction becomes the determining factor of exaggerated physiologic or pathologic jaundice. Bilirubin can function as an antioxidant, and some degree of hyperbilirubinemia may be physiologic and beneficial. Accepted "normal" or physiologic ranges of TSB levels vary widely because levels are influenced by many diverse factors such as gestational age, birthweight, disease state, degree of hydration, nutritional status, racial background, breast feeding, and other genetic and epidemiologic factors. Although most of these infants are healthy and will not need therapy, they need to be monitored closely as severe unconjugated hyperbilirubinemia can become potentially toxic to the neurons. Published data suggest that upper limits of TSB levels (95th percentile) can be as high as 17 to 18 mg/dL. Preterm infants have no established "physiologic" bilirubin guidelines. Meaningful interpretation of bilirubin levels in the first several days of life has to be made in relationship to the infant's age in hours.

1. **Exclusion criteria for diagnosis of "physiologic" jaundice**
   a. Jaundice appearing within the first 24 hours of life.
   b. Total serum bilirubin level >95th percentile for age in hours based on a nomogram for hour-specific serum bilirubin concentration (Figure 99–1).
   c. Bilirubin level increasing at a rate >0.2 mg/dL/h or >5 mg/dL/d.
   d. Direct serum bilirubin level >1.5 to 2.0 mg/dL or >20% of the TSB.
   e. Jaundice persisting for >2 weeks in full-term infants.

2. **Mechanisms that predispose newborn infants to hyperbilirubinemia**
   a. **Increased bilirubin synthesis** due to larger RBC mass, increased hemoglobin breakdown (2–3 times adult's rate) due to shorter RBC life span in neonates, and increased rate of RBC degradation within the bone marrow before release to the circulation (ineffective erythropoiesis).
   b. **Decreased binding and transport.** Decreased hepatic uptake of bilirubin from plasma due to decreased plasma albumin and the liver transfer protein ligandin.
   c. **Impaired conjugation and excretion.** Reduced UDPGT activity (1% of adult level at 7 days of age) in the newborn liver results in decreased mono- and diglucuronide bilirubin conjugates that can be excreted in the bile.
   d. **Enhanced enterohepatic circulation.** Conjugated bilirubin is unstable and can be hydrolyzed by the intestinal enzyme β-glucuronidase to its unconjugated form; this can be readily absorbed through the intestinal mucosa and move back to the liver (enterohepatic circulation). Sterility of intestinal mucosa prevents further formation of the more excretable products namely, urobilin and stercobilin.

B. **Breast milk and jaundice.** The association between breast milk (BM) and hyperbilirubinemia has been well documented; it can be classified into 2 types

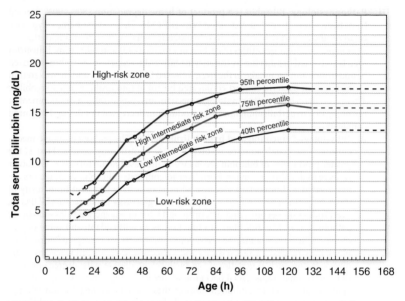

FIGURE 99–1. Nomogram for designation of risk in well newborns at ≥36 weeks' gestation with birthweight ≥2000 g or ≥35 weeks' gestational age with birthweight ≥2500 g based on the hour-specific serum bilirubin values. (*Reproduced with permission from Bhutani VK, Johnson L, Sivieri EM: Predictive ability of a predischarge hour-specific serum bilirubin for subsequent significant hyperbilirubinemia in healthy term and near-term newborns,* Pediatrics. *1999 Jan;103(1):6-14.*)

based on the age of onset: **early-onset breast-feeding failure jaundice** and **late-onset BM jaundice.** Demographic, environmental, and genetic factors are involved in the development of hyperbilirubinemia in breast-fed neonates. Polymorphism and common mutations/variants in the *UGT1A1* gene as well as glucose-6-phosphate dehydrogenase (G6PD) deficiency (homo- or heterozygous) result in high risk for hyperbilirubinemia in breast-fed infants, especially if born via vaginal delivery.

1. **Breast-feeding failure jaundice.** Begins in the first week of life due to dehydration, caloric deprivation, and increased enterohepatic circulation, and may occur in >1 in 10 exclusively breast-fed infants. The exact mechanism is unclear but may involve shifts in bilirubin pools, less efficient conjugation, and enhanced bilirubin absorption in the intestine.

2. **Breast milk jaundice.** Breast-fed infants are much more likely than formula-fed infants to have jaundice that can extend beyond 3 to 4 weeks of life. Prolonged indirect hyperbilirubinemia has been reported to occur in up to 30% of breast-fed infants. Current literature supports genetic pathogenesis characterized by polymorphism of the *UGT1A1* gene. Some infants with prolonged BM jaundice have been found to have Gilbert syndrome. A high level of β-glucuronidase in BM is found in 20% to 40% of women; this can be a contributing factor. Although BM jaundice was considered by some experts as an extension of physiologic jaundice, it cannot be considered totally benign. Kernicterus has been reported in apparently healthy term and late preterm infants as a complication of BM jaundice.

C. **Pathologic unconjugated hyperbilirubinemia**
  1. **Disorders of production**
     a. **Immune-mediated hemolytic disease is the most common cause of pathologic hyperbilirubinemia in the newborn period.** The process may begin in fetal life or immediately after birth depending on the etiology.
        i. **Rh (D antigen) incompatibility** as well as other antigens in the Rh blood-group system (c, C, e, E, cc, and Ce) can cause immune-mediated hemolytic disease. Alloimmunization occurs when as little as 0.1 mL of RBCs from an Rh(D)-positive fetus cross the placenta into the circulation of an Rh(D)-negative mother. The initial response in the maternal circulation is the production of immunoglobulin (Ig) M that does not cross the placenta, which is then later followed by IgG, which in subsequent pregnancies crosses the placenta and causes a hemolytic process that can begin in utero. The severe form of this process can result in erythroblastosis fetalis with hydrops.
        ii. **ABO incompatibility** occurs in 3% of all infants. Antigens present on the surface of RBCs react with antibodies in the plasma of opposing blood types, resulting in ABO incompatibility with sensitization. Hemolysis is generally limited to group A or B infants born to group O mothers. Risk of recurrence can be as high as 88% in infants with the same blood type as their index sibling. ABO incompatibility is somewhat protective of Rh sensitization because the fetal ABO-incompatible RBCs are rapidly destroyed in the maternal circulation, thereby decreasing the opportunity of Rh antigen to mount an immune response (see Chapter 85).
     b. **Red blood cell enzyme deficiencies**
        i. **Glucose-6-phosphate dehydrogenase deficiency** is the most common RBC enzyme deficiency and affects millions of people. The major function of G6PD is preventing oxidative damage of cells. The G6PD gene is located on the X chromosome. Prevalence of hyperbilirubinemia is twice that of general population in males who carry the defective gene and in homozygous females. Although it is more common in the African, Middle Eastern, southern European, and Asian populations, the ease of migration and intermarriage has transformed G6PD deficiency into a global problem. The rapid rise in TSB in infants with this enzyme deficiency may not be accompanied by evidence of a hemolytic process.
        ii. **Pyruvate kinase deficiency** is inherited in an autosomal recessive manner and most common in northern European descendants. It presents in the newborn period with jaundice, anemia, and reticulocytosis. This condition needs to be considered in a newborn with a nonspherocytic and direct antiglobulin test (DAT)-negative hemolytic anemia.
     c. **Red blood cell membrane defects**
        i. **Hereditary spherocytosis.** Hereditary spherocytosis (HS) is a result of heterogeneous alterations in 1 of 6 genes that encode for proteins involved in vertical associations that tie the RBC membrane skeleton to the lipid bilayer. It is characterized by spherical, doughnut-shaped RBCs in the peripheral blood. HS is mostly found in patients of northern European ancestry, but can be seen worldwide, with a prevalence of 1 in 2000 to 5000 births. The inheritance is dominant in 75% of the cases, but some cases of de novo mutations have also been reported. Jaundice associated with HS can range from mild to severe, causing kernicterus. A simple way to screen for HS in neonates is the ratio of mean corpuscular hemoglobin concentration (MCHC) to mean corpuscular volume (MCV), also called HS ratio (MCHC/MCV). A recent study found that an HS ratio >0.36 was 97% sensitive and 99% specific and had a negative predictive

value of 99%. The incubated osmotic fragility test is considered the gold standard for making the definitive diagnosis of HS.

  ii. **Hereditary elliptocytosis** is an autosomal dominant, clinically heterogeneous group of disorders that are characterized by the presence of elongated, oval, or elliptically shaped RBCs on the peripheral blood smear. It is caused by mutations of the RBC membrane cytoskeletal proteins (usually spectrin or protein 4.1). Hereditary elliptocytosis rarely causes hemolysis and jaundice except in cases of homozygotes or compound heterozygotes.

  d. **Hemoglobinopathies.** Developmental differences in globin chain synthesis are responsible for the different clinical manifestations of α-chain and β-chain defects in the perinatal period. Although these conditions generally do not present in the newborn period, patients with deletion of 3 α-globin genes (hemoglobin H) are often born with hypochromic hemolytic anemia and are at risk for developing severe hyperbilirubinemia.

  e. **Infection** causes hyperbilirubinemia by increasing bilirubin concentrations via hemolysis, and it may impair conjugation, leading to decreased excretion of bilirubin. Both early- and late-onset jaundice are reported to be some of the more common clinical manifestations of urinary tract infection.

  f. **Increased erythrocyte load**
    i. **Blood sequestration.** Extravascular blood can result in increased bilirubin production due to breakdown of RBCs. The catabolism of 1 g of hemoglobin yields 35 mg of bilirubin. Occult hemorrhages, such as bruising, cephalohematomas, and intracranial bleeding, can cause severe hyperbilirubinemia.
    ii. **Polycythemia.** Increased RBC mass is a known risk factor for hyperbilirubinemia due to an increase in the bilirubin load presented to the liver for conjugation and excretion.
    iii. **Infants of diabetic mothers.** Infants of diabetic mothers have high erythropoietin levels causing increased erythropoiesis, leading to polycythemia that contributes to hyperbilirubinemia.

2. **Disorders of bilirubin clearance**
  a. **Crigler-Najjar syndrome type I.** Autosomal recessive disease characterized by almost complete absence of hepatic UDPGT activity. TSB is commonly >20 mg/dL. The diagnosis of Crigler-Najjar syndrome type I (CNS-I) can usually be made by microassay of UDPGT activity or by measurement of menthol glucuronide in urine after oral menthol. Treatment consists of exchange transfusion soon after birth, followed by daily phototherapy for 12 to 24 hours and liver transplantation later on. The use of tin protoporphyrin may help decrease the bilirubin level temporarily and may shorten the need for daily phototherapy. Oral calcium phosphate supplementation makes phototherapy more efficient (amorphous calcium phosphate traps unconjugated bilirubin in the gut). TSB is unresponsive to phenobarbital therapy.
  b. **Crigler-Najjar syndrome type II**, also known **Arias disease**, is more common than CNS-I and typically benign. Crigler-Najjar syndrome type II (CNS-II) can occur as a result of autosomal recessive and dominant inheritance. It is caused by a single base pair mutation leading to decreased but not totally absent UDPGT enzyme activity. TSB rarely exceeds 20 mg/dL and is lowered by phenobarbital administration. A definitive diagnosis is made by identifying the genetic defect.

    For routine clinical practice, CNS-I and CNS-II can be differentiated by their response to phenobarbital therapy and bile analysis. In CNS-I, bile is totally devoid of bilirubin conjugates, whereas bilirubin monoconjugates are present in CNS-II, and some diconjugates may be detectable after phenobarbital treatment.

    c. **Gilbert syndrome** is a relatively common (~9% of whites) disorder characterized by mild, lifelong, unconjugated hyperbilirubinemia in the absence of hemolysis or evidence of liver disease. Autosomal dominant and recessive patterns of inheritance have been suggested. Hepatic glucuronidation activity is 30% of normal, resulting in an increased proportion of monoglucuronide. Studies have shown that neonates who carry the genetic marker for Gilbert syndrome have a more rapid rise and duration of neonatal jaundice. It is important to remember that Gilbert syndrome is a condition with no consequences for adults, but it can put a neonate at significant risk for hyperbilirubinemia and the potential for complications of bilirubin encephalopathy

    d. **Lucey-Driscoll syndrome** , also known as **transient familial neonatal hyperbilirubinemia**, is associated with TSB concentrations that usually reach ≥20 mg/dL. The sera of affected neonates and their mothers are found to contain a high concentration of an unidentified UDPGT inhibitor when tested in vitro.

  3. **Metabolic and endocrine disorders**

    a. **Galactosemia.** Jaundice may be 1 of the presenting signs; however, infants with significant hyperbilirubinemia due to galactosemia typically have other presenting signs and symptoms such as poor feeding, vomiting, and lethargy. Hyperbilirubinemia during the first week of life is almost always unconjugated, and then it becomes mostly conjugated during the second week, reflective of developing liver disease.

    b. **Hypothyroidism.** Prolonged jaundice is found in up to 10% of newborns diagnosed with hypothyroidism. It is due to a deficient activity of UDPGT. Early-onset hyperbilirubinemia has been reported as the only presenting sign of congenital hypothyroidism. Treatment with thyroid hormone improves hyperbilirubinemia.

  4. **Increased enterohepatic circulation of bilirubin**

    a. **Conditions that cause gastrointestinal obstruction** (eg, pyloric stenosis, duodenal atresia, annular pancreas) or a decrease in gastrointestinal motility may result in exaggerated jaundice due to increased enterohepatic recirculation of bilirubin. Blood swallowed during delivery and decreased caloric intake may also be contributing factors.

    b. **Breast-feeding jaundice and breast milk jaundice (discussed earlier).**

  5. **Substances affecting binding of bilirubin to albumin.** Certain drugs occupy bilirubin-binding sites on albumin and increase the amount of free unconjugated bilirubin that can cross the blood–brain barrier. Drugs in which this effect may be significant include aspirin, moxalactam, ceftriaxone, sulfisoxazole, and other sulfonamides. Chloral hydrate competes for hepatic glucuronidation with bilirubin and thus increases serum unconjugated bilirubin. Common drugs used in neonates such as penicillin and gentamicin also compete with bilirubin for albumin-binding sites.

IV. **Risk factors.** Sepsis, acidosis, lethargy, asphyxia, temperature instability, G6PD deficiency, hemolytic disease (ABO or G6PD deficiency), late preterm (34–36 weeks) and early term gestation (37–38 weeks), exclusive breast feeding, East Asian ethnicity, cephalohematoma or significant bruising, male sex, Native American infants, maternal diabetes, family history of neonatal jaundice, and use of oxytocin in labor.

V. **Clinical presentation**

A. **Clinical assessment**

  1. **Monitor for jaundice.** Each nursery must have an established guideline for routine assessment of jaundice. Jaundice is clinically visible when the serum bilirubin level approaches 5 mg/dL. The yellow color is seen more easily in the "fingerprint" area than in the surrounding skin. Progression is cephalocaudal,

so that for a given bilirubin level, the face appears more yellow than the rest of the body.

2. **Clinical history.** Family history of jaundice, anemia, splenectomy, or metabolic disorder is significant and may suggest underlying etiology for jaundice. Maternal history of infection or diabetes may increase the newborn's risk for jaundice. Breast feeding and factors affecting normal gastrointestinal function in the newborn period increase the tendency for more severe jaundice.

3. **Physical examination.** Areas of bleeding such as cephalhematoma, petechiae, or ecchymoses indicate blood extravasations. Hepatosplenomegaly may signify hemolytic disease, liver disease, or infection. Physical signs of prematurity, plethora with polycythemia, pallor with hemolytic disease, and macrosomia with maternal diabetes all can be associated with jaundice. Omphalitis, chorioretinitis, microcephaly, petechiae, and purpuric lesions suggest infectious causes of increased serum bilirubin.

4. **Neurologic examination.** Severe hyperbilirubinemia can be toxic to the auditory pathways and to the central nervous system and can result in hearing loss and encephalopathy. The appearance of subtle abnormal neurologic signs heralds the onset of early bilirubin encephalopathy. Clinical signs may include lethargy, poor feeding, vomiting, hypotonia, and seizures. The progression of neurologic changes parallels the stages of bilirubin encephalopathy from acute to chronic and irreversible changes.

VI. **Diagnosis**
  A. Basic laboratory studies
    1. **Total and direct serum bilirubin**
      a. **Total serum bilirubin level determination** is indicated in all infants who develop jaundice in the first 24 hours of life. Jaundice appearing this early is almost always associated with a pathologic process.
      b. **Direct (conjugated) bilirubin fraction** has to be obtained as well, especially for those with progressive and/or prolonged jaundice.
      c. **During the first few days of life,** bilirubin levels should be interpreted based on age in hours (refer to nomogram Figure 99–1). This can also be determined online (**bilitool.org;** accessed September 14, 2018).
    2. **Blood type and Rh status in both mother and infant**
      a. **ABO and Rh incompatibility** can be easily diagnosed by comparing infant and maternal blood types.
      b. **Cord blood** can be sent for DAT and routine blood typing.
    3. **Direct antiglobulin test is also known as direct Coombs test**
      a. **Detects antibodies** bound to the surface of RBCs.
      b. **Usually positive in hemolytic disease** resulting from isoimmunization.
      c. **Does not correlate with severity** of jaundice.
      d. **Can be obtained from the cord blood.**
    4. **Complete blood count and differential**
      a. **Presence of anemia** may be suggestive of a hemolytic process; polycythemia increases risk for exaggerated jaundice.
      b. **Evaluate red blood cell morphology;** spherocytes suggest ABO incompatibility or HS.
      c. **Look for mean corpuscular hemoglobin concentration and mean corpuscular volume;** MCHC/MCV ratio >0.36 is highly suggestive of congenital spherocytosis
      d. **Evaluate for indices suggestive of infection** (eg, leukopenia, neutropenia, and thrombocytopenia).
    5. **Reticulocyte count**
      a. **Elevation suggests hemolytic disease.**
      b. **Can also be elevated in cases of chronic occult or overt hemorrhage.**

6. **Other laboratory tests**
   a. **Urine should be tested** for reducing substances (to rule out galactosemia if the infant is receiving a galactose-containing formula) and for infectious agents.
   b. **If evidence of hemolysis is present,** in the absence of ABO or Rh incompatibility, further testing by hemoglobin electrophoresis, G6PD level, or osmotic fragility testing may be required.
   c. **Prolonged jaundice** (>2 weeks of life) may require additional tests for thyroid and liver function, blood and urine cultures, and metabolic screening workup, such as plasma amino acid and urine organic acid measurements.
7. **Measurement of serum albumin.** Bilirubin is mostly bound to albumin in the circulation; evidence suggests that neurotoxicity is caused by unbound bilirubin fraction. Therefore, **measurement of serum albumin** may help assess the fraction of unbound bilirubin in the circulation and thereby determine the need of an albumin infusion. It may be useful in the determination of exchange transfusion.

B. **Transcutaneous bilirubinometry** (TcB) is a portable instrument that uses reflectance measurements on the skin to determine the amount of yellow color present in the skin. Several studies have shown that TcB measurement correlates well with laboratory TSB measurement and is a reasonable tool to provide an estimate of TSB levels in healthy newborns. However, a potential clinically relevant issue is that TcB levels may underestimate TSB at higher serum bilirubin levels, in contrast to the tendency to overestimate at lower bilirubin levels. A TcB value of >15 mg/dL should be correlated with TSB. TcB results should be interpreted with caution in newborns with birthweight <2500 g, particularly in the first 48 hours of life. Any jaundice noticeable within the first 24 hours of life should be confirmed with TSB level.

C. **Expired carbon monoxide** breath measurement. An equimolar amount of CO is produced for every molecule of bilirubin formed from the degradation of heme. **Measurement of end-tidal CO (corrected for ambient CO) or end-tidal CO concentration (ETCOc) is an index of total bilirubin production.** This method can alert the attending physician to the presence of hemolysis irrespective of the timing of jaundice. Simultaneous measurement of ETCOc and bilirubin level in high-risk patients prior to discharge from the nursery may accurately identify patients with hemolysis. A commercial ETCOc instrument is now available and has been used at a number of institutions; however, adding ETCOc to hour-specific TSB does not improve the predictive ability of hour-specific TSB testing alone.

VII. **Management of indirect hyperbilirubinemia in infants ≥ 35 weeks' gestation.** Three methods of treatment are commonly used to decrease the level of unconjugated bilirubin: phototherapy, pharmacologic therapy, and exchange transfusion. The American Academy of Pediatrics (AAP) has published guidelines on risk designation and when to start phototherapy for infants >35 to 36 weeks' gestation. Low birthweight and preterm infants are excluded from these guidelines. The authors suggest that each institution and its practicing physicians establish their criteria for phototherapy and exchange transfusion by gestational age, weight groups, postnatal age, and the infant's condition consistent with current standard of pediatric practice

A. **Practice guidelines.** In 2004, the AAP put together evidence-based recommendations to reduce the incidence of severe hyperbilirubinemia and bilirubin-induced encephalopathy in infants ≥35 weeks' gestation (*Pediatrics.* 2004;114(1):297-316) that have become widely accepted. The recommendations include the following: to promote and support successful breast feeding, to perform a systematic risk assessment for severe hyperbilirubinemia prior to discharge, to provide early and focused follow-up for the high-risk patient, and to initiate immediate therapeutic intervention when indicated.

B. **Phototherapy** reduces serum bilirubin level through structural (irreversible) isomerization to lumirubin, which is a more soluble substance that is excreted without conjugation into bile and urine. This is probably the principal mechanism by which

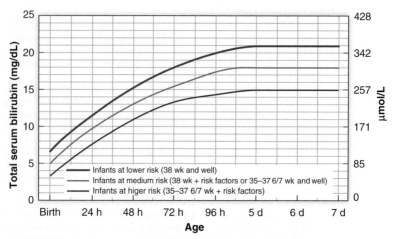

- Use total bilirubin. Do not subtract direct reacting or conjugated bilirubin.
- Risk factors–isoimmune hemolytic disease, G6PD deficiency, asphyxia, significant lethargy, temperature instability, sepsis, acidosis, or albumin <3.0 g/dL (if measured).
- For well infants 35–37 6/7 wk can adjust TSB levels for intervention around the medium risk line. It is an option to intervene at lower TSB levels for infants closer to 35 wks and at higher TSB levels for those closer to 37 6/7 wk.
- It is an option to provide conventional phototherapy in hospital or at home at TSB levels 2–3 mg/dL (35–50 mmol/L) below those shown, but home phototherapy should not be used in any infant with risk factors.

FIGURE 99–2. Guidelines for phototherapy in hospitalized infants of ≥35 weeks' gestation. G6PD, glucose-6-phosphate dehydrogenase; TSB, total serum bilirubin. (*Reproduced with permission from American Academy of Pediatrics Subcommittee on Hyperbilirubinemia: Management of hyperbilirubinemia in the newborn infant 35 or more weeks of gestation,* Pediatrics. *2004 Jul;114(1):297-316.*)

phototherapy works. Other mechanisms include photoisomerization (reversible) and photo-oxidation of bilirubin to less toxic and more soluble forms that can be eliminated in bile and urine.

1. **Indication.** Most infants with increasing jaundice are treated with phototherapy when it is believed that bilirubin levels could enter the toxic range (Figure 99–2).
2. **Factors influencing effective phototherapy**
   a. **Spectrum of light delivered.** Bilirubin absorbs light most effectively in the blue region of the spectrum (460–490 nm). High-intensity light-emitting diodes (LEDs) are most effective in degrading bilirubin compared to conventional phototherapy devices.
   b. **Energy output.** Conventional phototherapy has an irradiance of 6 to 12 μW/cm²/nm, whereas an intensive phototherapy has an irradiance of at least 30 μW/cm²/nm. Because light intensity is affected by distance, the recommended distance of an infant from the light source is approximately 12 to 16 inches (~30–40 cm).
   c. **Surface area exposed.** To maximize skin exposure, systems that provide light above and under the infant are recommended; the infant should be naked in servo-controlled incubators.
3. **Side effects.** Phototherapy is relatively safe and easy to use. Minor side effects include rashes, dehydration, and ultraviolet light irradiation. No changes in growth, development, and infant behavior have been reported.

a. **Bronze baby syndrome.** With conjugated hyperbilirubinemia, phototherapy causes photodestruction of copper porphyrins, causing urine and skin to become bronze in color. Clinical significance is unknown, and bronze baby syndrome (BBS) is generally regarded as harmless; however, a recent report has indicated that BBS may pose an additional risk to development of kernicterus.

b. **Congenital erythropoietic porphyria** is a rare disease in which phototherapy is contraindicated. Exposure to visible light of moderate to high intensity produces severe bullous lesions on exposed skin and may lead to death.

c. **Retinal effects.** The retinal effects of phototherapy to the exposed infant's eyes are unknown; however, animal studies suggest that retinal degeneration may occur. Eye shields must be used. The infant's eyes should be covered with opaque patches for overhead lamp phototherapy.

d. **Potential long-term effects**. Some reports linked phototherapy exposure to an increased (albeit small) risk for childhood cancer.

C. **Exchange transfusion.** (See also Chapter 34.) **Double-volume exchange transfusion (DVET)** is used when the risk of kernicterus is significant. DVET replaces approximately 85% of the circulating RBCs and decreases the bilirubin level to about half of the pre-exchange value. Patient-to-patient variations for the permeability of the blood–brain barrier exist; this is affected by several factors including isoimmune hemolysis, asphyxia/acidosis, significant lethargy, temperature instability, sepsis, hypoalbuminemia, and prematurity. There is no specific elevated bilirubin level that can be considered safe. Clinical practice parameters published by the AAP in July 2004 provide guidelines for exchange transfusions in healthy newborns ≥35 weeks of gestation (Figure 99–3). Direct or conjugated fraction should not be subtracted from the TSB when considering exchange transfusion.

1. **Indications.** DVET should be considered in the following circumstances:

a. **There is evidence of an ongoing hemolytic process** and high TSB (exchange threshold) failed to decline by 1 to 2 mg/dL with 4 to 6 hours of intensive phototherapy.

b. **Rate of rise** indicates that the level will reach 25 mg/dL within 48 hours.

c. **High concentration of total serum bilirubin** and early signs of bilirubin encephalopathy.

d. **Hemolysis** causing anemia and hydrops fetalis.

2. **General guidelines for exchange transfusion**

a. **Generally, type O Rh-negative blood** is used for ABO or Rh incompatibility. If the infant is type A or B and the mother is of the same blood type, then type-specific, Rh-negative donor blood can be used.

b. **Donor blood must always be crossmatched** with maternal serum.

c. **Donor blood should be warmed** to approximately 37°C.

d. **Use fresh blood** that is no more than 4 days old.

e. **Consider calcium gluconate** infusion during the course of the exchange transfusion because citrate (blood preservative) chelates calcium.

f. **Obtain parental consent.**

3. **Bilirubin levels.** TSB can be decreased by 50% of the pre-exchange level. Rebound increase in TSB is expected after an exchange transfusion as bilirubin in tissues "migrates" back into circulation.

4. **Adverse events.** Exchange transfusion is not risk free; therefore, the procedure should only be done after intensive phototherapy has failed and the risk of bilirubin encephalopathy outweighs the risk of the procedure. Adverse events include bloodborne infections (eg, cytomegalovirus), thrombocytopenia and coagulopathy, graft-versus-host disease, necrotizing enterocolitis, portal vein thrombosis, electrolyte abnormalities (eg, hypocalcemia and hyperkalemia), and cardiac arrhythmias. Risk of mortality is 0.5% to 2%.

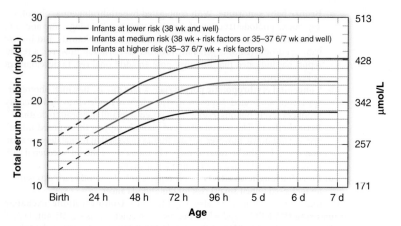

- The dashed lines for the first 24 h indicate uncertainty due to a wide range of clinical circumstances and a range of responses to phototherapy.
- Immediate exchange transfusion is recommended if infant shows signs of acute bilirubin encephalopathy (hypertonia, arching, retrocollis, opisthotonos, fever, high-pitched cry) or if TSB is 5 mg/dL (85 μmol/L) above these lines.
- Risk factors: isoimmune hemolytic disease, G6PD deficiency, asphyxia, significant lethargy, temperature instability, sepsis, acidosis.
- Measure serum albumin and calculate B/A ratio (see legend).
- Use total bilirubin. Do not subtract direct reacting or conjugated bilirubin.

Note that these suggested levels represent a consensus of most of the committee but are based on limited evidence, and the levels shown are approximations. During birth hospitalization, exchange transfusion is recommended if the TSB rises to these levels despite intensive phototherapy.

The following B/A ratios can be used together with but not in lieu of the TSB level as an additional factor in determining the need for exchange transfusion:

	B/A Ratio at Which Exchange Transfusion Should Be Considered	
	Risk Category	TSB mol/L/Alb, mol/L
Infants 38 0/7 wk	8.0	0.94
Infants 35 0/7–36 6/7 wk and well or 38 0/7 wk if higher risk or isoimmune hemolytic disease or G6PD deficiency	7.2	0.84
Infants 35 0/7–37 6/7 wk if higher risk or isoimmune hemolytic disease or G6PD deficiency	6.8	0.80

If the TSB is at or approaching the exchange level, send blood for immediate type and crossmatch. Blood for exchange transfusion is modified whole blood (red cells and plasma) crossmatched against the mother and compatible with the infant.

FIGURE 99–3. Guidelines for exchange transfusion in infants ≥35 weeks' gestation. B/A, bilirubin/albumin ratio; G6PD, glucose-6-phosphate dehydrogenase; TSB, total serum bilirubin. (*Reproduced with permission from American Academy of Pediatrics Subcommittee on Hyperbilirubinemia: Management of hyperbilirubinemia in the newborn infant 35 or more weeks of gestation,* Pediatrics. *2004 Jul;114(1):297-316.*)

D. **Pharmacologic therapy**

1. **Phenobarbital** affects the metabolism of bilirubin by increasing the concentration of ligandin in liver cells, inducing production of UDPGT and enhancing bilirubin excretion. It is used for treatment of CNS-II and Gilbert syndrome. It can also be used as an adjunct therapy for treatment of exaggerated unconjugated hyperbilirubinemia in the newborn period, but it takes 3 to 7 days to be effective; therefore, it is not helpful in acute management.

2. **Metalloporphyrins.** Synthetic metalloporphyrins are structural analogs of heme; they reduce bilirubin production by competitive inhibition of **heme oxygenase,** the rate-limiting enzyme in the catabolism of heme. Evidence suggests that a single dose of **tin mesoporphyrin (SnMP)** reduces the need for phototherapy and exchange transfusion. A recent (2016) clinical trial showed that prophylactic predischarge administration of a single intramuscular injection of 4.5 mg/kg of SnMP decreased the duration of phototherapy, reversed total bilirubin trajectory, and reduced the severity of subsequent hyperbilirubinemia. A reported untoward effect noted was a non–dose-dependent transient erythema when used in conjunction with phototherapy. Long-term safety of SnMP remains to be studied. It remains an unlicensed drug and is available on an investigational or "compassionate" use basis in the United States.

3. **Albumin.** Neurotoxicity is caused by the unconjugated fraction of bilirubin not bound to albumin (**free bilirubin**). Administration of intravenous albumin (1 g/kg over 2–3 hours) increases bilirubin-binding capacity, resulting in reduced free bilirubin. An albumin level <3.0 g/dL can be considered as 1 risk factor for lowering the threshold for phototherapy. Albumin infusion may be considered when albumin level is <3.0 g/dL, when TSB/albumin ratio is >6, and prior to DVET.

4. **Intravenous γ-globulin.** Intravenous immunoglobulin (IVIG) works by competing with sensitized neonatal RBCs at the Fc receptors in the reticuloendothelial system thus preventing further hemolysis. It is recommended in patients with isoimmune hemolysis when TSB is rising despite intensive phototherapy. Dose is 1 g/kg given over 2 to 4 hours; it can be repeated if needed in 12 to 24 hours (2 doses). Studies have shown that the use of IVIG has decreased the use of exchange transfusion in hemolytic disease of the newborn.

VIII. **Prognosis**

A. **General.** Outcome of hyperbilirubinemia is generally excellent, with minimal to no additional risk of adverse outcome if identified and treated appropriately. Unconjugated bilirubin in high concentration can cross the blood–brain barrier and lead to neuronal dysfunction and death. The exact mechanism of bilirubin-induced neuronal cell injury is not completely understood; high concentrations of unconjugated bilirubin can have neurotoxic effects on cellular membranes and intracellular calcium homeostasis, resulting in neuronal excitotoxicity and mitochondrial energy failure. Bilirubin concentrations that put a preterm infant at risk for kernicterus have not been identified; incidence of kernicterus in this group is unknown, and the relationship of serum bilirubin and neurodevelopmental outcome in the very low birthweight (VLBW) infant remains unclear.

B. **Encephalopathy**

1. **Transient.** Early BIND is transient and reversible. The auditory system serves as an objective window to assess the central nervous system in cases of severe hyperbilirubinemia. Auditory brainstem responses show significant prolongation of latency of specific wavelengths, it can be used as an early predictor of bilirubin encephalopathy. These changes may be reversed with either exchange transfusions or spontaneous decrease in bilirubin levels. TSB level of ≥22 mg/dL, Rh incompatibility, and early jaundice have been reported as independent predictors of abnormal development.

2. **Acute bilirubin encephalopathy** is a preventable neurologic sequela of untreated severe hyperbilirubinemia. It is an evolving encephalopathy that can progress in 3 clinical phases over several days. The major clinical features involve disturbances in level of consciousness, tone and movement, and brainstem function, especially relating to feeding and cry. The severity of abnormalities appears to correlate with both the severity and duration of hyperbilirubinemia.

   a. **Initial phase.** Initial phase is noted by lethargy, hypotonia, decreased movement, and poor suck. Clinical findings are nonspecific. A high index of suspicion is needed to recognize these signs as a signal of impending acute bilirubin encephalopathy. Prompt therapeutic intervention is critical to prevent deterioration and poor prognosis.

   b. **Intermediate phase** has cardinal signs of moderate stupor, irritability, and increased tone. Infant may exhibit backward arching of the neck (retrocollis) or of the back (opisthotonos). Fever has been reported to occur during this phase of the syndrome.

   c. **Advanced phase** is characterized by deep stupor or coma, increased tone, inability to feed, and a shrill cry. Seizures may occur. This is an ominous stage of acute bilirubin encephalopathy, suggesting irreversible central nervous system injury and the later development of chronic bilirubin encephalopathy (kernicterus) in most infants.

3. **Chronic bilirubin encephalopathy (kernicterus)** is a devastating and disabling neurologic disorder characterized by the following clinical tetrad: choreoathetoid cerebral palsy; high-frequency sensorineural hearing loss; palsy of vertical gaze; and dental enamel hypoplasia. **Kernicterus** is a pathologic diagnosis, describing the yellow discoloration of the deep nuclei of the brain. Brain regions that are typically affected are the globus pallidus, subthalamic nucleus, metabolic sector of the hippocampus, oculomotor nuclei, ventral cochlear nuclei, and Purkinje cells of the cerebellar cortex. The pattern of involvement is similar across different ages of affected individuals. Clinical terminology is bilirubin encephalopathy. To simplify and unify the diagnosis of bilirubin toxicity based on pathophysiologic and clinical criteria, a new designation called **kernicterus spectrum disorder (KSD)** has been proposed, acknowledging that kernicterus is symptomatically broad and diverse. Severity varies from mild to severe in children and adults. Mildly affected individuals remain highly functional; moderately affected individuals have more prominent dystonia and are likely to have athetoid movements. Severely affected individuals have speech difficulty and a more disabling dystonia to the point of not being ambulatory. This is a form of static encephalopathy, in which the degree of disability may change slightly over time but only within limits and never dramatically. Bilirubin encephalopathy is not a reportable condition in the United States; therefore, its true prevalence is not known.

IX. **Prematurity and hyperbilirubinemia.** Premature infants are at greater risk for developing severe hyperbilirubinemia and BIND because they are more likely to be sicker and have lower serum albumin level than their term newborn counterparts. Since there has been no definitive evidence-based recommendation as to what level of bilirubin necessitates treatment in premature infants, it is a common practice to use a lower TSB level to initiate phototherapy and not uncommon to use of prophylactic phototherapy in extremely low birthweight (ELBW) infants. A post hoc analysis from the National Institute of Child Health and Human Development (NICHD) Neonatal Research Network trial of aggressive versus conservative use of phototherapy in ELBW infants showed that at 18 to 22 months of corrected age, phototherapy was associated with a reduction in significant neurodevelopmental impairment (mental development index <50) for infants with birthweight of 501 to 750 g; however, marginal increased mortality was noted among the smallest infants. A consensus-based recommendation that provides a gestational age–guided approach to the use of phototherapy and exchange transfusion in preterm infants has been published (see Table 63–1).

Emerging evidence suggests that intermittent phototherapy is equally effective in lowering bilirubin level with potentially fewer side effects.

It is recommended that clinicians use the lower level of TSB from this guideline in initiating management of infants at greater risk of bilirubin toxicity. The following conditions increase risk of BIND:

A. **Lower gestational age**
B. **Serum albumin levels <2.5 g/dL**
C. **Rapidly rising total serum bilirubin levels, suggesting hemolytic disease**
D. **Evidence of hemolytic process**
E. **Presence of overwhelming infection and clinical instability**
   Recommendations for exchange transfusion apply to infants in whom intensive phototherapy failed to control a rapid rise in TSB or infants who are showing evidence of bilirubin toxicity (see part B of Section VIII). Clinical signs and symptoms of bilirubin toxicity may not be easily recognizable in VLBW infants.

100 Inborn Errors of Metabolism with Acute Neonatal Onset

Inborn errors of metabolism (IEMs) are a group of disorders highly relevant to practitioners treating newborns; immediate diagnosis and appropriate treatment of these conditions can be directly linked to patient outcome to the extremes of avoiding death or irreversible brain damage. Pediatricians may feel overwhelmed by the number and complexity of these disorders (Table 100–1) and the interpretation of laboratory tests needed to establish the diagnosis. To assist clinicians, this chapter focuses on the symptom patterns, laboratory tests and their interpretation, and the initial stabilization of the patient rather than discussing details of the specific biochemical and genetic defects or special treatment measures of IEMs. Usually, the patient's ongoing treatment is supervised by a geneticist specially trained in biochemical genetics.

I. **Classification**
   A. **Classification by time of onset.** In this neonatal manual, we concentrate on metabolic disorders with onset in the neonatal period and early infancy, but some IEMs may present later in infancy, childhood, or even adolescence and adulthood. Even with comprehensive and well-executed newborn screening programs, a number of IEMs may present clinically before they are detected by screening tests or before the test result is available to the treating physicians. The use of **tandem mass spectrometry (MS/MS)** in newborn screening is now common practice. Due to the large amount of biochemical information obtained through MS/MS analysis, physicians involved in newborn care are often involved in follow-up evaluations and referrals of patients with a positive screening test.
   B. **Classification by clinical presentation.** Categorizing IEMs by clinical presentation has great utility when establishing the diagnosis. It is noted that some **syndromes with dysmorphic features** are now known to be IEMs (eg, Smith-Lemli-Opitz syndrome or Zellweger syndrome [see Section IX.A and B]). Other classic examples of IEMs are discussed only briefly because they are clinically asymptomatic in the neonatal period (see Section XI; phenylketonuria [PKU]). Note that some **skeletal dysplasias** and disorders affecting bone and cartilage formation (not discussed here) are, strictly speaking, also IEMs (eg, rhizomelic chondrodysplasia punctata and hypophosphatasia). The following classification

Table 100–1. INBORN ERRORS OF METABOLISM PRESENTING IN THE NEONATAL PERIOD AND INFANCY

Disorders of carbohydrate metabolism	Argininosuccinate lyase deficiency
Galactosemia	Arginase deficiency
Fructose-1,6-bisphosphatase deficiency	N-Acetylglutamate synthetase deficiency
Glycogen storage disease (types IA, IB, II, III, and IV)	**Lysosomal storage disorders**
Hereditary fructose intolerance	GM$_1$ gangliosidosis type I (β-galactosidase deficiency)
Disorders of amino acid metabolism	
Maple syrup urine disease	Gaucher disease (glucocerebrosidase deficiency)
Nonketotic hyperglycinemia	Niemann-Pick disease types A and B (sphingo-myelinase deficiency)
Hereditary tyrosinemia	
Pyroglutamic acidemia (5-oxoprolinuria)	Wolman disease (acid lipase deficiency)
Hyperornithinemia-hyperammonemia-homo citrullinemia syndrome	Mucopolysaccharidosis type VII (β-glucuronidase deficiency)
Lysinuric protein intolerance	I-cell disease (mucolipidosis type II)
Methylene tetrahydrofolate reductase deficiency	Sialidosis type II (neuraminidase deficiency)
	Fucosidosis
Sulfite oxidase deficiency	**Peroxisomal disorders**
Disorders of organic acid metabolism	Zellweger syndrome
Methylmalonic acidemia	Neonatal adrenoleukodystrophy
Propionic acidemia	Single enzyme defects of the peroxisomal β-oxidation
Isovaleric acidemia	
Multiple carboxylase deficiency	Rhizomelic chondrodysplasia punctata
Glutaric acidemia type II (multiple acyl-CoA dehydrogenase deficiencies)	Infantile Refsum disease
HMG-CoA lyase deficiency	**Miscellaneous disorders**
3-Methylcrotonoyl-CoA carboxylase deficiency	Adrenogenital syndrome (21-hydroxylase and other deficiencies)
3-Hydroxyisobutyric aciduria	Disorders of bilirubin metabolism (Crigler-Najjar syndrome and others)
Disorders of pyruvate metabolism and the electron transport chain	
Pyruvate carboxylase deficiency	Pyridoxine-dependent seizures
Pyruvate dehydrogenase deficiency	α_1-Antitrypsin deficiency
Electron transport chain defects	Fatty acid oxidation disorders (short, medium, and long chain)
Disorders of the urea cycle	Cholesterol biosynthesis defects (Smith-Lemli-Opitz syndrome)
Ornithine transcarbamylase deficiency	
Carbamyl phosphate synthetase deficiency	Congenital disorders of protein glycosylation (carbohydrate-deficient glycoprotein syndromes)
Transient hyperammonemia of the neonate	
Argininosuccinate synthetase deficiency (citrullinemia)	Neonatal hemochromatosis

CoA, coenzyme A; HMG, 3-hydroxy-3-methylglutaryl.

system forms the basis for the more detailed sections of this chapter; IEMs may present with the following:

1. **Encephalopathy with or without metabolic acidosis** (see Section VI)
2. **Impairment of liver function** (see Section VII)
3. **Impairment of cardiac function** (see Section VIII)
4. **Dysmorphic syndromes** (see Section IX)
5. **Nonimmune hydrops fetalis due to inborn errors of metabolism (less common)** (see Section X)

C. **Classification according to the biochemical basis of the disease.** Subdividing IEMs according to their biochemical characteristics assists with understanding of the pathogenesis and different treatment approaches but is of limited utility for those providing patient care.

II. **Incidence.** By some estimates, IEMs may account for as much as 20% of disease among severely ill full-term infants not known to have been born at any risk. Cumulatively, an IEM may be present in >1 in 500 live births.

III. **Pathophysiology.** Metabolic processes are catalyzed by genetically encoded enzyme proteins. The classical mechanism of a metabolic defect is lack or deficiency of a functioning enzyme resulting in **substrate accumulation** and conversion of intermediary metabolites to products not usually present. In addition, end products of the normal pathway will be deficient. Symptoms may result from an increased level of the normal substrate (eg, in urea cycle disorders, the substrate ammonia is toxic and leads to cerebral edema, central nervous system [CNS] dysfunction, and eventually death). Additionally, a **lack of normal end products** of metabolism can lead to symptoms (eg, lack of cholesterol in Smith-Lemli-Opitz syndrome [see Section IX.A]). **Alternative products may interfere with normal metabolic processes** (eg, accumulated propionyl-coenzyme A [CoA] may be used as substrate instead of acetyl-CoA in propionic acidemia). Finally, an **inability to degrade end products of a metabolic pathway** may lead to symptoms (eg, myocardial dysfunction in glycogen storage disease type II or hepatomegaly in glycogen storage disease type I). The time of clinical presentation may be related to the question of whether metabolites can be transported across the placenta; metabolites of low molecular weight can transport across and are therefore prenatally removed from the fetus and cleared by the maternal metabolism.

IV. **Risk factors. IEMs are genetic disorders.** Therefore, behavioral or environmental factors are not causative for IEMs, but environment and especially nutrition may affect presentation. A history of relatives with intellectual disability, protein avoidance, and, for many disorders, neonatal or childhood deaths or severe illness (liver disease, abnormal heart function, mental and/or physical decline, episodic illness) could indicate an increased risk for IEMs. A history of protein avoidance, liver dysfunction/failure, or mental changes in pregnancy and labor may be seen in female carriers of X-linked inherited urea cycle defects. Presence of consanguinity and, for a number of inborn errors, ethnic background are also risk factors.

V. **Clinical presentation.** Although there are several specific presentations (listed next) in which an IEM must be considered, the best assumption in clinical practice is that **an IEM should be considered in any sick newborn.** The newborn has a "limited repertoire" of symptoms that are often nonspecific. The differential diagnosis of symptoms such as **poor feeding, lethargy, hypotonia, vomiting, hypothermia, seizures, and disturbances of breathing** is extensive. Because it is common, the diagnosis of sepsis often tops the differential diagnosis list. But it is in the best interest of the patient to consider and evaluate for other causes, including IEMs, at the same time that laboratory investigations are initiated to rule out infection. This is essential for a timely diagnosis and can be accomplished with a relatively small number of laboratory tests of moderate cost that are readily available in most hospitals, as discussed in the following sections.

A. **An inborn error of metabolism must be strongly considered under the following circumstances:**

1. **History of unexplained neonatal deaths in the family** (prior siblings or male infants on the mother's side of the family).
2. **Infants who are the offspring of consanguineous mating** (because of higher incidence of autosomal recessive conditions; autosomal recessive inheritance is common among IEMs).
3. **Onset of signs and symptoms after a period of good health** that may be as short as a few hours.
4. **Infants who are quite ill with a lack of perinatal events or birth history** explaining their presentation.
5. **Symptoms are related to the introduction and progression of enteral feedings.**
6. **Failure of usual therapies to alleviate the symptoms or inability to prove a suspected diagnosis** such as sepsis, CNS hemorrhage, or other congenital or acquired conditions.
7. **Progression of symptoms.**
8. **Although patients with an inborn error of metabolism might be born prematurely, they are typically full-term infants.** An exception is the diagnosis of transient hyperammonemia of the neonate, a condition that typically affects preterm infants. While the exact cause of the hyperammonemia in these patients remains unclear, it is related to prematurity rather than being a genetic IEM.

B. **Signs and symptoms.** See Table 100–2 for a summary of signs and symptoms of IEMs. Table 100–3 lists common misdiagnoses of infants with IEMs. **Symptoms may overlap with frequent neonatal conditions**; for example, a child with an IEM may have transient tachypnea of the newborn or be at risk for sepsis for unrelated reasons. Occasionally, 2 seemingly unrelated conditions may be associated for unclear reasons; an example is the increased incidence of *Escherichia coli* sepsis in infants with galactosemia.

C. **Asymptomatic inborn errors of metabolism in the newborn.** Untreated PKU does not cause any symptoms in the newborn. It causes irreversible brain damage while the patient appears clinically well. Thus, newborn screening testing with prompt follow-up of abnormal results is essential. Early detection of PKU in the newborn allows for treatment that prevents extreme intellectual disability. (See Section XI.)

D. **To guide the clinician in the diagnostic workup, signs and symptoms are discussed in the following sections for 5 different major clinical presentations:** IEM presenting with encephalopathy, IEM presenting with liver disease, IEM presenting with impairment of cardiac function, IEM presenting as dysmorphic syndromes, and IEM presenting as nonimmune hydrops (see Sections VI to X). Flow diagrams in Figures 100–1 and 100–2 are designed to assist in the diagnostic workup. Details regarding the different **laboratory tests** are outlined in Section XII.

VI. **Major clinical presentation: inborn errors of metabolism presenting with encephalopathy.** Encephalopathies associated with IEMs are clinically often indistinguishable from those caused by a hypoxic-ischemic insult or other CNS insult (hemorrhage or infectious disease). **Abnormal tone** (hypotonia as well as hypertonia may be of central origin) and **abnormal movements and seizures** clearly indicate CNS involvement. Clinically, seizures may present as lip smacking, tongue thrusting, bicycling movements of the lower extremities, opisthotonos, tremors, or generalized tonic-clonic movements. In severe encephalopathy, burst suppression pattern may be seen on **electroencephalography (EEG) using conventional multilead EEG or bedside monitoring with amplitude-integrated EEG (aEEG)**. Discontinuous patterns detected by aEEG may be seen with less severe encephalopathy.

A. **Laboratory evaluation**
   1. **Acute evaluation. In any patient with encephalopathy of any degree,** careful **evaluation of the acid-base status** is advisable. Some IEMs present with

Table 100–2. **SIGNS AND SYMPTOMS AND ASSOCIATED METABOLIC DISORDERS**

Neurologic (hypotonia, lethargy, poor sucking, seizures, coma)

Glycogen storage disease, galactosemia, organic acidemias, hereditary fructose intolerance, maple syrup urine disease, urea cycle disorders, hyperglycinemia, pyridoxine dependency, peroxisomal disorders, congenital disorders of glycosylation, fatty acid oxidation disorders, and respiratory chain defects

Hepatomegaly/liver dysfunction

Lysosomal storage diseases, galactosemia, hereditary fructose intolerance, glycogen storage disease, tyrosinemia, α_1-antitrypsin deficiency, Gaucher disease, Niemann-Pick disease, Wolman disease, fatty acid oxidation defects, and respiratory chain defects

Hyperbilirubinemia

Galactosemia, hereditary fructose intolerance, tyrosinemia, α_1-antitrypsin deficiency, Crigler-Najjar syndrome, and other disorders of bilirubin metabolism

Nonimmune hydrops

Gaucher disease, Niemann-Pick disease, GM_1 gangliosidosis, congenital disorders of glycosylation

Cardiomegaly/cardiomyopathy

Glycogen storage disease type II, fatty acid oxidation defects, and respiratory chain defects

Macroglossia

GM_1 gangliosidosis, glycogen storage disease type II

Abnormal odor

Maple syrup urine disease (odor of maple syrup or burnt sugar)

Isovaleric acidemia, glutaric acidemia (odor of sweaty feet)

HMG-CoA lyase deficiency (odor of cat urine)

Abnormal hair

Argininosuccinic acidemia, lysinuric protein intolerance, Menkes kinky hair syndrome

Hypoglycemia

Galactosemia, hereditary fructose intolerance, tyrosinemia, maple syrup urine disease, glycogen storage disease, methylmalonic acidemia, propionic acidemia, fatty acid oxidation defects, and respiratory chain defects

Ketosis

Organic acidemias, tyrosinemia, methylmalonic acidemia, maple syrup urine disease

Metabolic acidosis

Galactosemia, hereditary fructose intolerance, maple syrup urine disease, glycogen storage disease, organic acidemias

Hyperammonemia

Urea cycle defects, transient hyperammonemia of the neonate, organic acidurias, HMG-CoA lyase deficiency, fatty acid oxidation disorders

Neutropenia

Organic acidemias, especially methylmalonic acidemia and propionic acidemia; nonketotic hyperglycinemia, carbamyl phosphate synthetase deficiency

(*Continued*)

Table 100–2. SIGNS AND SYMPTOMS AND ASSOCIATED METABOLIC DISORDERS (*CONTINUED*)

Thrombocytopenia

Organic acidemias, lysinuric protein intolerance

Dysmorphic features

Glutaric aciduria type II, 3-hydroxyisobutyric aciduria, Smith-Lemli-Opitz syndrome, peroxisomal disorders, congenital disorders of glycosylation

Renal cysts

Glutaric aciduria type II, peroxisomal disorders

Abnormalities of the eye (eg, glaucoma, retinopathy)

Galactosemia, lysosomal storage disorders, peroxisomal disorders

Abnormal fat distribution/inverted nipples

Congenital disorders of glycosylation

Epiphyseal stippling in radiograph

Peroxisomal disorders (Zellweger syndrome, neonatal adrenoleukodystrophy, rhizomelic chondrodysplasia punctata)

CoA, coenzyme A; HMG, 3-hydroxy-3-methylglutaryl.

quite pronounced metabolic acidosis. The following tests (for details, see Section XII) should be performed as part of the **acute evaluation** of patients with encephalopathy:

a. **Arterial or venous blood gas**
    i. **When interpreting the venous or arterial blood gas of a newborn, alterations in respiratory status**, which are frequent in this patient group, must be taken into consideration. An isolated respiratory acidosis is likely pulmonary or related to disturbed respiratory drive. A metabolic or mixed acidosis, especially shortly after delivery, may be related to perinatal events.

Table 100–3. MISDIAGNOSES OF METABOLIC DISEASE IN THE NEWBORN INFANT

Bacterial sepsis
Acute viral infection
Asphyxia
Gastrointestinal tract obstruction
Hepatic failure, hepatitis
Central nervous system catastrophe
Persistent pulmonary hypertension
Cardiomyopathy
Neuromuscular disorder

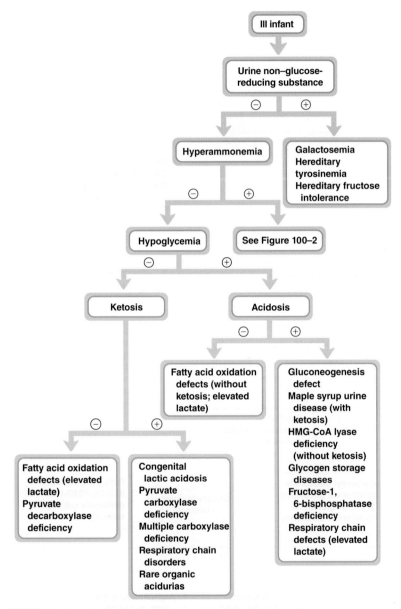

FIGURE 100–1. Algorithm for the diagnosis of metabolic disorders of acute onset in an ill infant (guideline only; for details, see text and references). CoA, coenzyme A; HMG, 3-hydroxy-3-methylglutaryl.

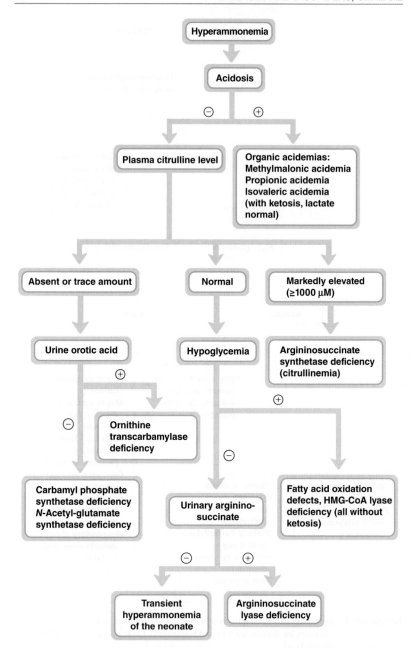

FIGURE 100–2. Algorithm for the differential diagnosis of hyperammonemia (guideline only; for details, see text and references). CoA, coenzyme A; HMG, 3-hydroxy-3-methylglutaryl.

ii. **In case of a severe and prolonged metabolic acidosis** without the presence of an underlying condition (eg, septic or hypovolemic shock and malperfusion) explaining the finding, it is mandatory to evaluate whether **acidic metabolites** (eg, the excessive production of lactic acid or other compounds) could be the cause of the imbalance. When considering compensatory mechanisms (eg, respiratory correction of a metabolic acidosis), remember that the resulting blood gas should reflect a mixed acid-base status.

iii. **Presence of an isolated respiratory alkalosis** is suspicious for central disturbance of the respiratory pattern (hyperpnea), and **hyperammonemia** should be ruled out in this situation. Ammonia directly stimulates the respiratory center, resulting in primary hyperventilation, which in turn leads to respiratory alkalosis.

b. **Serum electrolytes** with calculation of the anion gap.

c. **Ammonia level.**

d. **Lactate and pyruvate levels and ratio.**

e. **Urine collection** should be initiated, and the urine collected should be refrigerated or, ideally, frozen.

2. **Other causes of encephalopathy should be assessed by appropriate studies** (eg, imaging studies, sepsis evaluation, lumbar puncture) as indicated and outlined in other sections of this manual. If cerebrospinal fluid (CSF) is obtained, it is advisable to freeze a sample for possible future testing (eg, ~1–2 mL for tests such as CSF amino acid analysis to rule out nonketotic hyperglycinemia [NKH]; a matching plasma sample has to be obtained simultaneously and should be stored frozen). If an IEM remains a diagnostic possibility after the initial evaluation, plasma amino acids and urine organic acids should be analyzed.

B. **Differential diagnosis.** Although the **differential diagnosis** of IEMs associated with encephalopathy is extensive, the following conditions are discussed in more detail because of either their frequency or clinical significance. (Items 1–4 are typically without severe metabolic acidosis at presentation; items 5 and 6 are typically associated with a severe metabolic acidosis.)

1. **Urea cycle defects (and transient hyperammonemia of the neonate)**

a. **Clinical presentation.** In encephalopathy with hyperammonemia (not caused by liver dysfunction), consider 3 major diagnostic possibilities:

i. **A primary defect of 1 of the enzymes of the urea cycle** (which degrades ammonia produced in the metabolism of amino acids). The most common urea cycle defect is **ornithine transcarbamylase (OTC) deficiency**, which is transmitted in an X-linked recessive fashion. Newborn patients, therefore, are usually male. **Female heterozygotes** can be symptomatic, depending on the X-chromosome inactivation pattern in the liver, but affected females usually present later in life. It is important to note that a mother heterozygous for OTC deficiency may develop symptoms (hyperammonemia) at the time of delivery because of the metabolic stresses surrounding birth. The other urea cycle defects are inherited in an autosomal recessive fashion, with **carbamyl phosphate synthetase deficiency** being the second most common.

ii. **An organic acidemia as an underlying cause** with secondary impairment of the urea cycle (see Section VI.B.5).

iii. **Transient hyperammonemia of the neonate** (THAN), a condition usually seen in premature infants. The frequency of THAN seems to have declined over recent decades.

b. **Diagnosis.** Information regarding the diagnostic workup of patients with hyperammonemia is outlined in Figure 100–2. Quantitative measurement of plasma amino acids and orotic acid is necessary to establish the exact diagnosis. Urine organic acids should also be examined.

c. **Treatment.** Initial treatment is similar, independent of the final diagnosis (see Section XIII.A). Immediate transfer to a facility able to perform hemodialysis is strongly advised when hyperammonemia is detected. The use of medication such as sodium phenyl acetate and butyrate should be supervised by a biochemical geneticist. In some defects (eg, argininosuccinate lyase deficiency), substitution of arginine (intravenous arginine hydrochloride) may alleviate symptoms; arginine is a metabolite of the cycle and can be low if downstream from the deficient reaction. Long-term **protein restriction** is necessary (see Section XIII.B.1). Acute treatment of THAN is similar to that of inborn errors of the urea cycle, but deficiency of the metabolic pathway is temporary and normal protein intake is tolerated later in life.

d. **Outcome.** Outcome (especially in regard to CNS injury) depends on diagnosis and severity and duration of hyperammonemic episodes; outcome is more favorable for THAN compared with inherited urea cycle defects.

2. **Maple syrup urine disease.** Accumulation of **branched-chain amino acids (leucine, isoleucine, and valine)** is secondary to a defect in the decarboxylase involved in the catabolism of these amino acids. 2-Keto metabolites of the 3 amino acids also accumulate. Leucine is the amino acid that may be the most neurotoxic.

a. **Clinical presentation.** Symptoms typically develop after the second week of life but may manifest as early as at 24 hours of age and, therefore, may precede the report of the neonatal screening test result. **Typical symptoms** are feeding intolerance, lethargy, signs of encephalopathy such as hypotonia or posturing, abnormal movements, or frank seizures (late in the course). **Typical odor** (maple syrup or "burnt sugar") may not be prominent; metabolic acidosis is a late presentation.

b. **Diagnosis.** Maple syrup urine disease (MSUD) is diagnosed by quantitative amino acid analysis (leucine, isoleucine, valine, and glycine are elevated) and detection of 2-keto metabolites in urine organic acid analysis. The 2,4-dinitrophenylhydrazine (2,4-DNPH) test detects 2-keto acids (usually offered by specialized laboratories only).

c. **Treatment.** Restrict protein intake acutely while providing high amounts of glucose and fluid (see Section XIII.A). Later, provide formula low in leucine, valine, and isoleucine with restriction of natural protein. **Dialysis** may be needed as acute therapy if severe encephalopathy has developed. Some patients may show response to thiamine (see Section XIII.B.3).

3. **Nonketotic hyperglycinemia (glycine encephalopathy)**

a. **Clinical presentation.** A **typical presentation** for NKH is a patient suffering from a severe encephalopathy that is rapidly progressing and may eventually result in respiratory arrest. Standard evaluations for IEMs and other causes of this presentation do not reveal any abnormalities (no acidosis, hypoglycemia, or hyperammonemia and no other organ system affected). **Pronounced and sustained "hiccoughs"** in an encephalopathic infant have been associated with NKH.

b. **Diagnosis. Hyperglycinemia** in plasma is typical but may not be pronounced in young infants because of decreased renal reabsorption of this amino acid. In addition, other IEMs also result in increased blood glycine levels, such as MSUD (sometimes referred to as "ketotic hyperglycinemia"). Indications for **urine amino acids** are few, but in NKH, they can be of value because they detect the typical high renal glycine excretion. The diagnostic test for NKH is simultaneous measurement of CSF and plasma glycine levels to determine the **CSF-to-plasma glycine ratio.** Elevation of glycine in the

CSF is specific for NKH; a ratio of >0.08 is considered diagnostic (0.02–0.08 is equivocal; <0.02 is normal).

c. **Treatment.** Restoration of normal glycine levels in blood may be achieved through hydration or the use of sodium benzoate (see Section XIII.A.5), but the glycine accumulation in CSF remains unaffected. Several medications (eg, dextromethorphan) have been tried in attempts to favorably affect the CNS symptomatology but have achieved only limited success.

d. **Outcome.** Patients may survive because the respiratory depression has the potential to improve, but brain injury results in poor long-term outcome; patients with a rare transient form of NKH may do slightly better.

4. **Peroxisomal disorders**

a. **Clinical presentation.** Defects of peroxisome biogenesis (eg, Zellweger syndrome and neonatal adrenoleukodystrophy) and some of the peroxisomal single-enzyme defects (eg, multifunctional enzyme deficiency) present with encephalopathy in the neonatal period. Patients display **severe central hypotonia** ("floppy babies") and develop **seizures** (usually within the first week of life). Hepatomegaly, renal and hepatic cysts, and skeletal or retinal abnormalities may also be found.

b. **Diagnosis.** Most peroxisomal defects can be detected by analysis of plasma **very-long-chain fatty acids (VLCFAs)** (with carbon chains of ≥24 carbons). Other peroxisome function tests (see Section XII.C.8) and DNA analysis help define the exact peroxisomal defect.

5. **Organic aciduria/acidemias.** This group of IEMs is complex; because clinicians often feel overwhelmed by biochemical details regarding these conditions, the focus will be on clinical characteristics:

a. **Clinical presentations.** Many organic aciduria/acidemias (OAs) present later in infancy. Three conditions commonly present in the neonatal period and are clinically nearly indistinguishable: **methylmalonic acidemia, propionic acidemia**, and **isovaleric acidemia**. Affected newborns typically develop encephalopathy with severe acidosis, hyperammonemia, and seizures; an unusual **odor** (most noticeable in urine [see Table 100–2]) may be noted; **neutropenia** and **thrombocytopenia** may occur. More OAs are listed in Table 100–1.

b. **Diagnosis.** Analysis of plasma amino acids and urine organic acids is essential to diagnose OAs. These tests are best interpreted by an experienced biochemical geneticist familiar with the clinical presentation of the patient.

c. **Treatment.** If OAs are suspected, enteral feedings should be withheld. In addition to hydration and glucose infusion (both at least 1.5 times the maintenance level), hyperammonemia should be treated (see Section XIII.A) and the metabolic acidosis corrected with bicarbonate while ensuring appropriate ventilation. Involvement of a metabolic geneticist in diagnostic workup and treatment is advisable. Some OAs may partially respond to vitamins (see Section XIII.B.3).

6. **Congenital lactic acidosis.** Some possible causes of lactic acidosis (LA) in a neonate are **pyruvate dehydrogenase (PDH) defect, pyruvate carboxylase defect**, and **mitochondrial respiratory chain defects** (most common are defects of complex I and/or IV).

a. **Clinical presentation.** Congenital LA may be difficult to differentiate clinically from hypoxic ischemic encephalopathy, sepsis, and other conditions that result in metabolic acidosis, poor perfusion, and shock. LA is more likely a genetic congenital LA if **severe** (especially if unexpected or more severe than clinical history explains) and in infants who are **growth restricted** or who have mild **dysmorphic features** and/or anatomic anomalies of the brain. **Multiorgan disease** unexplained by other causes (eg, hypertrophic cardiomyopathy or cataracts) may occur. **Hypoglycemia** is common (but may also be a presentation of a glycogen storage disease; see Section VII.F).

   b. **Diagnosis.** Once an increase of lactic acid is found, determination of the **lactate-pyruvate ratio** further guides the diagnostic process (see Section XII.C.1). LA is a consequence of deficient energy production through aerobic metabolism, which depends on conversion of pyruvate to metabolites of the citrate cycle and an intact mitochondrial respiratory chain. In congenital LA, muscle and/or liver biopsies (Section XII.C.10) or sequencing of mitochondrial and/or genomic DNA (Section XII.C.11) may be needed to establish a diagnosis.

   c. **Treatment.** Although hydration and glucose at 1.5 times maintenance is beneficial to most patients with suspected IEMs, PDH deficiency is a rare exception as the LA may worsen with high glucose infusion.

7. **Other rare but relevant inborn errors of metabolism that can present with neonatal encephalopathy and/or seizures:**

   a. **Fatty acid oxidation disorders with dicarboxylic aciduria.** Although the most common fatty acid oxidation (FAO) defect (medium-chain acyl-CoA dehydrogenase [MCAD] deficiency) rarely causes illness in a neonate, short- and long-chain acyl-CoA dehydrogenase deficiencies (SCAD and LCAD, respectively) or other very rare FAO disorders may present in the neonatal period.

   b. **Multiple carboxylase deficiency.**

   c. **Holocarboxylase synthetase deficiency.**

   d. **Glutaric acidemia type II.** A defect of the electron transport flavoprotein or its dehydrogenase.

   e. **Pyroglutamic acidemia.** 5-Oxoprolinuria, a defect in glutathione synthetase.

   f. **Molybdenum cofactor deficiency** (xanthine oxidase deficiency or sulfite oxidase deficiency). One diagnostic clue to xanthine oxidase deficiency may be a **low plasma uric acid level**. A commercial test is available to determine urine sulfite excretion in urine.

   g. **3-Hydroxy-3-methylglutaryl–CoA lyase deficiency.**

   h. **Pyridoxine-dependent seizures.** Patients present with seizures in the neonatal period or in early infancy that are refractory to treatment with anticonvulsants but resolve with administration of vitamin B6 (100 mg of pyridoxine intravenously). Note that diagnostic markers such as α-aminoadipic semialdehyde, piperideine-6-carboxylate, and pipecolic acid need to be obtained prior to administration of vitamin B6.

   i. **Congenital disorders of glycosylation.** Although typically presenting later, congenital disorders of glycosylation (CDGs) may also present in neonates with acute encephalopathy, seizures, and stroke-like episodes. Many types of CDGs have been described in recent years. CDG type Ia is the most common, and if neonates are symptomatic, they are usually hypotonic. **Cerebellar atrophy** may be noted on pre- or postnatal imaging studies. Psychomotor development is delayed later in life; ataxia, dyskinesia, and muscle weakness become prominent. **Severe feeding problems and failure to thrive** are typical; intractable diarrhea in a neonate has been reported. **Unusual fat pads in the buttock area and inverted nipples** are believed to be quite characteristic findings.

   j. **These autosomal recessive conditions are characterized by defects in the glycosylation of proteins (see Section XII.C.9 for diagnostic testing).** They are multisystem disorders. Other than neurologic involvement, hepatic dysfunction with abnormal liver enzymes, pericardial effusions, nephrotic syndrome, nonimmune hydrops, and facial dysmorphic features (broad nasal bridge, prominent jaw and forehead, large ears, strabismus) have been described in infants.

VII. **Major clinical presentation: inborn errors of metabolism presenting with liver disease.** Several IEMs result in neonatal liver disease that may present with **hepatomegaly, jaundice, hepatocellular dysfunction, and/or hypoglycemia.** In addition to routine diagnostic testing (eg, bilirubin levels, liver enzyme levels, and liver imaging), glucose, cholesterol, coagulation studies, total protein, and albumin levels can assess the synthetic function of the liver. Because the liver is a main organ of amino acid metabolism, analysis of plasma amino acid can be of interest but requires interpretation by a metabolic geneticist (who may also recommend further disease-specific testing as indicated). The following conditions are discussed because of either their frequency or clinical significance.

A. **Galactosemia.** Does not present in an affected newborn until the patient is receiving galactose. Breast milk and most formulas contain **lactose** (a disaccharide of glucose and galactose); most soy formulas do not. Typical symptoms are **hyperbilirubinemia** (which may be unconjugated initially but later becomes mainly conjugated) and then signs of **liver dysfunction** (which may include **coagulopathy, hypoglycemia, hypoalbuminemia,** and **ascites**) and **hepatomegaly.** If untreated, symptoms may worsen to encephalopathy with cerebral edema, metabolic acidosis (hyperchloremia and hypophosphatemia), and renal dysfunction. Patients with galactosemia may have **congenital cataracts** and have an increased risk of *E coli* **sepsis. Testing urine for reducing substances** is an initial screening test (see Section XII.B.7). If galactose has been discontinued, reducing substance testing may be falsely negative and blood tests are essential to make a diagnosis. Galactosemia is due to a defect in either **galactose-1-phosphate uridyltransferase (GALT)** (classic galactosemia) or uridine 5′-diphosphate galactose 4-epimerase (rare variant). Red blood cells are used to measure GALT activity and/or accumulation of galactose-1-phosphate. Treatment consists of galactose restriction in the diet; the diet is relatively strict and difficult to follow. Even if compliance with the diet is good, many patients show **developmental delays**; females suffer **ovarian failure** later in life.

B. **Hepatorenal tyrosinemia.** Tyrosinemia type I, or hepatorenal tyrosinemia, usually presents in infancy, but some affected neonates may develop **severe liver dysfunction**, including hyperbilirubinemia, hypoglycemia, hyperammonemia, coagulopathy, hypoalbuminemia with ascites, and anasarca. This IEM also causes renal disease with mainly tubular dysfunction (amino aciduria or glucosuria) and results in hypophosphatemia and hyperchloremic metabolic acidosis. **Cardiomyopathy** can also develop; clinical presentation may thus overlap with disorders of fatty acid metabolism and respiratory chain defects. While tyrosine levels may be abnormal with liver dysfunction due to other causes, the presence of **succinylacetone** in urine is specific for tyrosinemia (see Section XII.C.4). Plasma cysteine might be low; plasma α-fetoprotein may be markedly increased. The only long-term treatment option is liver transplantation.

C. **α₁-Antitrypsin deficiency.** This IEM may present in neonates and infants as **hyperbilirubinemia**, which is usually prolonged and conjugated (with signs of cholestasis) but may resolve spontaneously within the first 6 months of life. These children may then not present again clinically until **liver cirrhosis** with portal hypertension has developed. **Emphysema** is the adult manifestation and may develop as early as the third decade of life and is much accelerated by smoking. The destruction of pulmonary and hepatic tissue in α₁-antitrypsin deficiency (AATD) is a consequence of a mutation in the *AATD* gene (designated as **Z mutation**), which, in homozygous carriers, results in deficiency of AAT, which is an inhibitor of an elastase, a degrading enzyme of neutrophils. Diagnosis is confirmed by **genotyping**, which is routinely available in most hospitals as a common test done in adults with emphysema. Although the symptoms during early life may resolve spontaneously and not all patients develop liver and lung manifestations, a diagnosis early in life allows patients to favorably affect their risk of serious adult disease through early behavior modification.

D. Inborn errors of bilirubin metabolism. Inherited defects in the metabolism of bilirubin include defects in conjugation (**Crigler-Najjar syndrome**) and uptake and excretion of bilirubin (**Dubin-Johnson and Rotor syndromes**). These conditions result in either indirect or direct hyperbilirubinemia. Dubin-Johnson and Rotor syndromes are rarely diagnosed in the newborn period.

E. Fatty acid oxidation disorders. FAO disorders may present with a combination of encephalopathy with cardiac and liver dysfunction; see Section VIII.A for more detailed information. The **liver dysfunction** may be milder than in other IEMs; **hyperammonemia** develops only with progression to significant liver dysfunction. The main clinical presentation may include generalized hypotonia and cardiomyopathy. Succinylacetone will be negative, whereas tyrosine metabolites may be present in urine organic acids. **Acylcarnitine profile** abnormalities may establish the diagnosis (see Section XII.C.5).

F. Glycogen storage disease type I (von Gierke disease). The clinical presentation of glycogen storage disorders in the newborn period may be limited to **hypoglycemia**, which can be severe and may be accompanied by LA. In von Gierke disease, the hypoglycemia is unresponsive to glucagon injection. **Liver enlargement and dysfunction** usually develop shortly thereafter (as soon as within 1–2 weeks). **Hyperlipidemia** may be present. Liver biopsy with enzyme analysis may be needed for diagnosis (see Section XII.C.10).

G. Peroxisomal disorders. Patients with disorders of peroxisomal biogenesis such as Zellweger syndrome and neonatal adrenoleukodystrophy develop **hepatomegaly** early in life which may progress to fibrosis and cirrhosis. The clinical presentation is usually dominated by **central hypotonia and seizures** (see Section VI. B.4.a). **Dysmorphic features** are present (Section IX.B). See Section XII.C.8 for specific diagnostic tests.

H. Others. Other inherited conditions that may present with hepatocellular dysfunction, sometimes as early as in the neonatal period, are as follows:

1. **Neonatal hemochromatosis.**
2. **Hereditary fructose intolerance.**
3. **Defects in carnitine metabolism.**
4. **Other glycogen storage diseases.**
5. **Lysosomal storage disorders.** Niemann-Pick disease may present with neonatal hepatitis.
6. **Congenital disorders of glycosylation.** See Section VI.B.7.i.

VIII. Major clinical presentation: inborn errors of metabolism presenting with impairment of cardiac function

A. Fatty acid oxidation disorders. Suspect in any neonate with impairment of cardiac function without clear etiology; cardiac arrhythmias occur in some. Additional symptoms such as encephalopathy (see Section VI.B.7.a) or impaired liver function (see Section VII.E), rhabdomyolysis and muscle weakness, and/or retinopathy may be present. FAO disorders affecting the dehydrogenase steps of β-oxidation are subdivided according to the length of the carbon chain of the fatty acids that accumulate: SCAD, MCAD, and LCAD deficiency. In addition, deficiency of long-chain 3-hydroxyacyl-CoA dehydrogenase (LCHAD) or other enzymes of the trifunctional enzyme complex and defects resulting in an inability to metabolize fatty acids properly due to defects of the plasma membrane carnitine transporter or carnitine palmitoyl transferase I or II have been described. In addition to **cardiomyopathy** usually resulting in cardiac failure, **encephalopathy, myopathy,** and **hepatomegaly** also occur. With low glucose intake or intercurrent illnesses, patients characteristically develop **hypoketotic hypoglycemia.** Maternal fatty liver of pregnancy and HELLP (*h*emolysis, *e*levated *l*iver enzymes, and *l*ow *p*latelets) syndrome have been associated with FAO defects, especially LCHAD and SCAD.

Acylcarnitine profile analysis by mass spectrometry (see Sections XII.C.5 and XII.C.6) helps to establish the diagnosis, which is then confirmed by enzyme assays in cultured fibroblasts. Newborn screening using the MS/MS will detect some FAO defects. Total and free **carnitine levels** should be determined (see Section XII.C.5). Treatment of FAO disorders consists of avoidance of prolonged periods without carbohydrate intake. Intravenous or oral carnitine may be indicated. Although medium-chain triglycerides (MCTs) are contraindicated in MCAD, they may be a good source of energy in the other conditions and can be given as commercially available MCT oil or through formulas with high levels of MCT oil as the predominant fat source.

B. **Pompe disease.** The cardiomyopathy of Pompe disease may (although not typically) present as early as in the neonatal period. Of diagnostic help are **electrocardiographic changes**, some of which are fairly characteristic: shortening of the PR interval, marked left-axis deviation, T-wave inversion, and enlarged QRS complexes. The diagnosis is confirmed by measurement of the deficient enzyme (α-glucosidase or acid maltase) in leukocytes or cultured fibroblasts (see Section XII.C.10).

C. **Hepatorenal tyrosinemia.** Type I tyrosinemia may present with cardiomyopathy in addition to liver and renal tubular dysfunction (see Section VII.B).

D. **Congenital disorders of glycosylation.** (See Section VI.B.7.i.) Pericardial effusions have been observed in affected patients.

IX. **Major clinical presentation: inborn errors of metabolism presenting as dysmorphic syndromes.** Several dysmorphic syndromes are now known to be IEMs. It is likely that more conditions initially described as syndromes will eventually be found to be IEMs or genetic conditions secondary to specific molecular mechanisms. Examples of disorders in this category include the following:

A. **Smith-Lemli-Opitz syndrome.** The metabolic basis of Smith-Lemli-Opitz syndrome is a defect in 7-dehydrocholesterol dehydrogenase, resulting in an **accumulation of 7-dehydrocholesterol** and typically low cholesterol levels in plasma. The main clinical signs of this relatively common syndrome (estimated frequency of 1 in 20,000) are as follows:

   1. **Growth deficiency** (usually postnatal) and microcephaly.
   2. **Dysmorphic features** including a high forehead, ptosis, epicanthal folds, strabismus, rotated and low-set ears, a nose with a wide tip, and micrognathia.
   3. **Hypospadias** in males.
   4. **Syndactyly** of the second and third toes (typically Y-shaped).
   5. **Other common findings** include cataracts, hypotonia, and significant psychomotor developmental delay.

B. **Zellweger spectrum disorders.** Initially defined by clinical characteristics, **Zellweger syndrome, neonatal adrenoleukodystrophy,** and **infantile Refsum disease** are all clinical phenotypes of defects in peroxisomal biogenesis and function. The diagnosis is established by measurement of VLCFAs and other biochemical parameters affected by peroxisomal dysfunction (see Section XII.C.8). Typical findings are as follows:

   1. **Dysmorphic features.** A high forehead, a wide and flat nasal bridge, epicanthal folds, and dysplastic ears; the fontanelles are wide open.
   2. **Severe hypotonia, seizures, and lack of psychomotor development.**
   3. **Hepatomegaly with fibrosis.**
   4. **Ocular abnormalities.** Corneal clouding, cataract, and retinal changes.
   5. **Punctate calcifications of the skeleton.**
   6. **Small renal cortical cysts.**

C. **Pyruvate dehydrogenase deficiency.** Patients with congenital LA (see Section VI.B.6) resulting from PDH deficiency often display dysmorphic features, including a high and prominent forehead, a widened nasal bridge, a small anteverted nose, and dysmorphic and enlarged ears.

D. **Congenital defects of glycosylation.** (See Section VI.B.7.i.) Dysmorphic features include broad nasal bridge, prominent jaw and forehead, large ears, and strabismus.

Unusual fat pads in the buttock area and inverted nipples are characteristic findings.

X. **Major clinical presentation: inborn errors of metabolism presenting as nonimmune hydrops.** The differential diagnosis of nonimmune hydrops is extensive. Although 3 groups of conditions are mentioned in the following sections, the list of possible genetic diagnoses is long; geneticists should be consulted and genome or exome sequencing should be considered.

  A. **In inherited hematologic conditions** (eg, glucose-6-phosphate dehydrogenase deficiency and pyruvate kinase deficiency), the hydrops is due to anemia and heart failure.

  B. **Genetic conditions with disturbed lysosomal function.** Cases of hydrops have been reported in **GM$_1$ gangliosidosis, Gaucher disease, Niemann-Pick disease**, and lysosomal disorders. The presence of **hepatomegaly, dysostosis multiplex**, and abnormal **vacuolated mononuclear cells** in the peripheral blood smear is a diagnostic clue.

  C. **Congenital disorders of glycosylation** rarely present with nonimmune hydrops fetalis (based on a small number of case reports).

XI. **An important inborn error of metabolism lacking neonatal symptoms: phenylketonuria.** Untreated PKU **does not cause symptoms in the neonate.** Even though the patient is clinically well, **irreversible brain damage** occurs as a result of accumulating phenylalanine and its metabolites. Therefore, patients benefit enormously from detection by neonatal screening for PKU.

  A. **If neonatal screening shows elevation of phenylalanine,** formula or breast milk must be discontinued and hydration provided (short-term enteral feedings with electrolyte solutions are feasible; intravenous therapy is usually not mandated). The patient should immediately (within hours) be referred to a geneticist for further evaluation (including differentiation between classic PKU and hyperphenylalaninemia), initiation of diet, and family education, training, and counseling.

  B. **A child of a mother with phenylketonuria** is an obligate heterozygote for the disease, and the PKU allele is frequent in the general population (1:20); the child has a 1 in 80 risk of being affected. Thus, measurement of phenylalanine levels after enteral feedings are established is mandatory. Although institutional practices vary, many geneticists recommend early quantitative amino acid analysis rather than routine newborn screening in this scenario. Newborns of affected mothers with insufficient treatment may manifest with **microcephaly, congenital heart disease**, and **intellectual disability** (even if the infant is not homozygous for PKU).

XII. **Diagnosis**

  A. **Prenatal.** Biochemical methods (eg, detection of metabolites in amniotic fluid and enzyme assays using cultured cells) and DNA analysis (specific mutation detection, genomics) are used for prenatal testing. Diagnostic procedures routinely available are **chorionic villus sampling** or **amniocentesis.** Newer methods such as **analysis of fetal cells in maternal circulation** or **preimplantation testing of the embryo with in vitro fertilization** may also be offered. Some in utero interventions may be available (eg, dietary control in maternal PKU or experimental fetal stem cell treatment); prenatal counseling is essential because, per local legislation, parents may be able to make an informed decision regarding continuation of pregnancy.

  B. **Postnatal.** Emphasis is on the detection of a metabolic disorder with a quick turnaround time and targeted secondary testing; cost and limitation in the blood volume that can safely be obtained from a neonate are concerns. Although some of the laboratory tests have already been discussed earlier, details regarding the specifics of these tests and their interpretations are outlined here. Refer also to Table 100–4.

    1. **Complete blood count with differential, hemoglobin, and platelets.** Note that neutropenia (often combined with metabolic acidosis) is not only typically found in sepsis and poor perfusion but may also be present in patients with organic acidopathy (especially propionic acidemia, methylmalonic acidemia,

Table 100–4. LABORATORY FINDINGS SUGGESTIVE OF METABOLIC DISEASE

Variable	Galactosemia	Glycogen Storage Disease	Maple Syrup Urine Disease	Nonketotic Hyperglycinemia	Glutaric Acidemia Type II	Organic Acidemia	Disorders of Pyruvate Metabolism	Disorders of the Urea Cycle	Transient Hyperammonemia of the Newborn
Hypoglycemia	+	+	±	–	±	±	+	–	–
Metabolic acidosis with or without elevated anion gap	+	±	+	–	±	+	±	±	±
Respiratory alkalosis	–	–	–	–	–	–	–	+	±
Hyperammonemia	–	–	–	–	–	+	–	+	+
Urine ketones	–	±	+	–	–	+	±	–	–
Urine abnormal odor or color	–	–	+	–	+	+	–	–	–
Neutropenia or thrombocytopenia	–	–	–	–	–	+	–	–	–

Note: Guidelines only; for details, see text and references.

931

and isovaleric acidemia). Thrombocytopenia may be present. Because patients are often typically also hyperammonemic, measurement of an ammonia level is essential in newborns with acidosis, leukopenia, or thrombocytopenia of unclear etiology.

2. **Blood gas.** Interpretation of the acid-base status is important (see Section VI.A.1.a). IEMs must be especially considered in the scenario of either a **severe metabolic acidosis** or a **respiratory alkalosis** (note that hyperventilation may be induced by a painful stimulus, such as blood sampling, but a pure respiratory alkalosis should not easily be dismissed as artifact). Ammonia measurement is indicated to rule out an organic aciduria with secondary hyperammonemia or a urea cycle defect causing a respiratory alkalosis as a result of hyperventilation due to direct stimulation of the respiratory center by ammonia. Be aware that excess heparin in a blood gas specimen may mimic a metabolic acidosis; specimens not instantly processed should be stored in ice water.

3. **Electrolyte determination.** In addition to the interpretation of the different electrolyte component levels, the **anion gap** should be calculated. The concentration of negatively and positively charged electrolytes is compared: Add the sodium and potassium levels (in mEq/L) and subtract the sum of the chloride and bicarbonate concentrations. An anion gap >17 mEq/L (consult with your local laboratory as cutoffs may vary depending on assays used) suggests an excess of negatively charged ions (eg, lactate or metabolites found in an organic acidopathy). If specimens are hemolyzed, potassium is released from cells that will distort the anion gap calculation (artificially increased). Disturbance of electrolytes is also found in other inherited conditions (eg, adrenogenital diseases).

4. **Ammonia level.** Measurement of ammonia levels can be of foremost importance in making the diagnosis of an IEM; unfortunately, the test is susceptible to artifacts, resulting in a false elevation of ammonia levels. Several precautions must be taken to avoid incorrect test results:

    a. **The specimen must be placed on ice** at the bedside.

    b. **Timely transfer to the laboratory** with instant preparation of the sample for analysis. If samples have to be stored, the blood must be separated and plasma frozen (at least −20°C). Without strict adherence to these precautionary measures, false elevation by as much as 60 to 100 mcg/dL may occur. Normal neonatal levels are up to 80 mcg/dL. IEMs typically result in levels in the hundreds and thousands. If a result is equivocal, a repeat measurement must be done; the hyperammonemia in IEM will most likely be worsening.

5. **Liver function tests.** Transaminases (aspartate aminotransferase and alanine aminotransferase) are released from hepatocytes with cell damage. γ-Glutamyl transferase (**GGT**) is produced in the liver cell but also is present in bile ducts. It is a very sensitive indicator of liver dysfunction and/or cholestasis; GGT may be elevated even with fairly minor exposures to medications/toxins. Raised **conjugated bilirubin** levels should always be considered abnormal (especially if >5% of total bilirubin) and can be due to a number of diseases including cholestasis. Cholesterol, albumin, and coagulation factor levels reflect the **synthetic function** of the liver. The **plasma amino acid pattern** is affected by IEMs and liver dysfunction. **Ammonia** levels are increased in IEMS and liver failure.

6. **Urine testing for ketones.** The presence of ketones in the urine of a neonate should always be considered abnormal. One of the IEMs that typically results in elevated urine ketones is MSUD.

7. **Urine testing for reducing substances.** Main indication in the neonate is suspected galactosemia. It is important that a nonenzymatic assay is done. A negative test does not rule out the diagnosis because even a few hours of galactose

restriction may result in a negative test. Consider which enteral nutrition the patient is receiving: soy formulas are often galactose free, whereas breast milk is not (lactose ["milk sugar"] is a disaccharide of glucose and galactose).

8. **Lipid levels and profile.** Low cholesterol may be noted in patients with Smith-Lemli-Opitz syndrome. Hyperlipidemia may be present in some glycogen storage disorders.

C. **Laboratory testing more specific for inborn errors of metabolism.** Although many of the following tests might be available through routine laboratories or through reference laboratories, we consider them second-line testing for IEM; involvement of a genetics service in their interpretation is recommended. Select tests may be needed to further evaluate a specific clinical presentation, to evaluate abnormalities found on initial testing, or to confirm a clinically suspected diagnosis of an IEM.

1. **Lactic acid level and lactate-to-pyruvate ratio.** Determination of lactate and pyruvate levels may be indicated in the evaluation of patients with severe metabolic acidosis. When excess lactate is present, the anion gap (see Section XII.B.3) is elevated. Blood to measure lactic acid is best obtained from a central line or as arterial specimen because even short stasis of blood (venous sampling using a tourniquet) increases lactate levels. The lactate-to-pyruvate ratio is normal (15–20) in PDH deficiency and defects of gluconeogenesis (glycogen storage diseases) and elevated to >25 in pyruvate decarboxylase deficiency and defects of the respiratory/electron transport chain.

2. **Amino acid analysis.** Amino acid analysis must be quantitative to aid in the diagnosis of IEMs. Urine amino acid analysis is not indicated with 2 exceptions: suspected NKH with high glycine excretion (see Section VI.B.3) or to rule out cystinuria with renal calculi. **Plasma amino acid results** are best evaluated after a 3-hour fast. Usually patterns of abnormalities are diagnostic as single amino acid abnormalities may be nutritional or artifacts (eg, taurine is often increased with delayed analysis of samples). Discussion of the many diagnostic patterns of plasma amino acid abnormalities is beyond the scope of this manual. Interpretation of results by an experienced biochemical geneticist who is aware of the clinical presentation and nutritional status of the patient is strongly recommended.

   Plasma amino acid analysis is not only indicated in classic IEMs of amino acid metabolism (eg, MSUD or PKU) but also helps evaluate urea cycle defects because several urea cycle metabolites are chemically amino acids (eg, citrulline, arginine, and ornithine; see Figure 100–2); in hyperammonemia, glutamine levels are often elevated as glutamine synthesis incorporates ammonia.

   At least 1 to 2 mL of blood should be obtained. Laboratories usually request heparinized blood or samples without additives. Samples should be cooled; if analysis is deferred to a later time, serum or plasma should be separated and frozen.

3. **Urine organic acid analysis.** This complex analytic test is usually performed by laboratories specializing in biochemical genetics. In expert hands, this test can provide an enormous amount of information. Urine organic acid analysis helps establish the diagnosis of organic acidemias. The most common of this large group of disorders are methylmalonic acidemia, propionic acidemia, and isovaleric acidemia (see Section VI.B.5). Most laboratories request at least 5 to 10 mL of fresh urine. As soon as the specimen is collected, it should cooled or, preferably, frozen until analysis.

4. **Succinylacetone in urine.** This test is specific for hepatorenal tyrosinemia. A sample is collected and used to wet a filter paper (as used for the routine neonatal screening tests). After air drying, the sample can be forwarded to the testing laboratory by mail or courier services.

5. **Acylcarnitine profile.** Fatty acids are conjugated with carnitine to facilitate their transport into the mitochondria. The acylcarnitine profiles allow for the recognition of diagnostic patterns of fatty acid metabolites typical for different FAO defects (note that VLCFAs with carbon chains of ≥24 carbons are metabolized in the peroxisome; see Section XII.C.8). Dried whole-blood samples placed on filter paper cards are used. As newborn screening by tandem mass spectrometry will assist in detection of FAO defects, an acylcarnitine profile should only be ordered after discussion with a biochemical geneticist; determination of **total and free carnitine plasma levels** (measured in heparinized blood) might also be indicated.

6. **Tandem mass spectrometry.** MS/MS detects a large number of disorders of amino and organic acid metabolism as well as FAO defects. This makes it a valuable tool for newborn screening, and MS/MS is **now used routinely by many neonatal metabolic screening programs**; many laboratories also accept samples obtained beyond the neonatal period from infants presenting with symptoms suggestive of an inborn error of metabolism. Samples are easy to obtain (blood spot samples mailed to laboratories), and testing is usually quite cost-effective. In symptomatic babies, the laboratory should be alerted to the possibility of an IEM as it might be possible to fast track selected samples.

7. **Galactosemia testing.** To measure galactose-1-phosphate levels and GALT activity, whole blood is usually requested by the laboratory because the metabolites and enzyme are localized in the erythrocytes. Blood must therefore be obtained before blood transfusions. An alternative in already transfused patients is testing of the parents as heterozygote detection is possible with the enzymatic assay.

8. **Peroxisomal function tests.** VLCFAs are measured by gas chromatography (GC) or GC/MS; normally, only trace amounts of fatty acids with carbon chains of ≥24 carbons are detectable. This test detects all peroxisomal disorders that affect the degradation of these compounds. Note that VLCFAs will be normal in a small subgroup of patients with peroxisomal defects (eg, rhizomelic chondrodysplasia punctata). Tests assessing other aspects of peroxisomal function (eg, plasmalogens, phytanic acid, or pipecolic acid measurements) may be necessary. Most of these analyses are done on plasma obtained from ethylenediaminetetraacetic acid (EDTA) blood. The red blood cell pellet of the sample should also be sent to the laboratory (separated) as plasmalogen levels are evaluated in red blood cells. Samples do not need to be frozen.

9. **Transferrin electrophoresis analysis.** A suspected diagnosis of carbohydrate-deficient glycoprotein syndromes (see Section VI.B.7.i) is initially evaluated by electrophoresis analysis of a glycoprotein, usually transferrin. The measurement of transferrin levels is inappropriate as a diagnostic test for these conditions (levels usually are normal). Involvement of a geneticist is essential as electrophoresis patterns are not abnormal in all patients and further specialized testing may be indicated. If electrophoresis of a patient of <2 months of age is normal, repeat testing beyond 2 months of age is recommended.

10. **Muscle, liver, and skin biopsies.** In patients with LA, **skeletal muscle biopsies** may be needed to establish diagnosis of a mitochondrial respiratory chain defect. Examination by electron microscopy, special stains, and enzyme essays may also be needed. Certain IEMs may require determination of enzyme activities in **cultured skin fibroblasts**. Glycogen storage disorders may require **liver biopsies** to establish the exact diagnosis.

11. **DNA analysis and sequencing.** Molecular defects are known for many IEMs. Although diagnoses can usually be established through biochemical testing, sequencing of **genomic or mitochondrial DNA** may be indicated in certain scenarios. Considering the complexity of these tests and the associated cost, DNA testing should usually be initiated and supervised by a geneticist. As

genome and exome sequencing is becoming more cost effective, it is increasingly used as first-line genetic testing. Cytogenetic arrays can identify segments of the genome with duplications, deletions, or loss of heterozygosity (LOH); patients with LOH are at higher risk for recessive disorders located in these areas.

D. **Postmortem evaluation when an inborn error of metabolism is suspected.** If an IEM is suspected as a possible cause of death in a newborn or young infant, we recommend obtaining the following samples postmortem:

1. **Blood.** Blood should be collected. If no central access was established, a postmortem cardiac puncture may be necessary to obtain a sufficient volume of blood. Serum and plasma should be frozen. In addition, keep the red blood cell pellets (not frozen). EDTA blood (nonseparated) and blood spots on filter paper should be kept to allow for later isolation and analysis of DNA.

2. **Urine.** Collect urine, if possible, and freeze it at –20°C. If no urine can be obtained but urine organic acid analysis is indicated, swabs of the bladder surface can be obtained on autopsy to attempt urine organic acid analysis.

3. **Skin.** A full-thickness sterile skin biopsy should be obtained (skin to be cleansed with alcohol, not iodine). Store in a sterile culture medium (if not available, store the sample in the patient's serum). Do not freeze the specimen, and transport it immediately to a tissue culture laboratory for fibroblast culture and storage.

4. **Cerebrospinal fluid.** If a lumbar puncture was not performed before death, a lumbar or ventricular puncture can be obtained postmortem. This procedure may be indicated to rule out infection or an IEM. In addition to obtaining cultures, we recommend freezing a 1- to 2-mL CSF specimen at –20°C.

5. **Percutaneous or open liver biopsy.** May be performed to obtain a specimen soon after death especially if the family did not consent to a full autopsy. Discuss the treatment of samples with the geneticist (frozen and/or formalin vs special solutions to preserve for assays and electron microscopy).

6. **Full autopsy and consultation with a geneticist (even postmortem).** The geneticist may give special recommendations for postmortem specimens to be obtained on autopsy (eg, frozen or specially prepared samples rather than standard formalin processing); genetic counseling may be indicated.

XIII. **Management.** For most IEMs, therapy consists often of dietary measures and/or special medications and vitamin supplementation. In some metabolic disorders, **liver, bone marrow, or stem cell transplantation** may be an option.

A. **Acute care while awaiting results of diagnostic studies**

1. **Supportive care.** Follow principles of neonatal and intensive care including provision of a secure **airway**, supporting **respiration** and **circulation**, and establishing **intravenous access**. General measures may also include correction of the acid-base balance, hypoglycemia, electrolyte abnormalities, and hydration status. Assisted ventilation may be required in severely affected neonates, and **antibiotic therapy** is frequently indicated because of the overlap in symptomatology with bacterial infection.

2. **Nutritional measures.** An acutely ill newborn should be NPO. For almost all IEMs, a **supply of sufficient glucose** to avoid a catabolic state is strongly indicated. Try to achieve a caloric intake of 80 to 100 kcal/kg/d. **Eliminate protein** acutely (24–48 hours) but not over prolonged periods because breakdown of endogenous protein may otherwise occur and may worsen the patient's clinical status. **Intravenous lipids may be contraindicated** in certain FAO defects.

3. **Hemodialysis or peritoneal dialysis.** May be needed to remove toxic metabolites. Exchange transfusions are not effective, and early transfer to a facility where hemodialysis is possible is mandatory in these situations (eg, hyperammonemia).

4. **Vitamin treatment.** Several IEMs have vitamin-responsive forms. Often, a combination of vitamin cofactors (vitamin B12, biotin, riboflavin, thiamine, pyridoxine, and folate) is considered while specific test results are still outstanding. Give vitamins only after appropriate specimens have been obtained for metabolic investigations and after consultation with a geneticist. **Carnitine substitution** may be indicated in some patients (eg, FAO defects or OAs). Carnitine (L-carnitine) may be given intravenously (30–50 mg/kg/d, some recommend giving a loading dose followed by divided doses; some patients may need higher doses) or orally (usually at higher doses than intravenously).

5. **Medications to treat hyperammonemia.** In patients with hyperammonemia, several medications can be used to provide an alternative pathway for ammonia excretion. These include **sodium phenyl acetate**, **sodium phenyl butyrate**, and **sodium benzoate**. A sodium phenyl acetate/sodium benzoate 10%/10% preparation is commercially available in the United States. Because of the intrinsic side effects, different indications, coordination with nutritional interventions, and frequent dosage adjustments necessary, the use of these medications should be initiated and supervised by an experienced biochemical geneticist.

6. **Other medications.** In tyrosinemia, NTBC (2-[2-nitro-4-trifluoromethylbenzoyl]-1,3-cyclohexanedione) may be used to prevent tyrosine degradation and production of succinylacetone.

B. **Long-term therapy**

1. **Diet.** One of the classic principles for the treatment of IEMs is the restriction of the substance leading to the accumulation of a toxic metabolite (eg, phenylalanine in PKU). In some disorders (eg, urea cycle defects), the overall protein intake is restricted. Careful monitoring is necessary to avoid essential amino acid deficiencies.

2. **Provision of a deficient substance** is effective when the deficient product is readily available and can reach the appropriate tissue (eg, cortisol and mineralocorticoid in 21-hydroxylase deficiency). Carnitine replacement may be needed in organic acidurias because carnitine is lost through renal excretion of metabolites bound to carnitine. Patients with urea cycle defects (with the exception of arginase deficiency) require arginine (and/or citrulline in some defects) replacement due to decreased synthesis.

3. **Vitamin, cofactor, and other disease-specific therapy.** Large doses of specific cofactors may increase the activity of partially deficient enzymes: vitamin B6 (homocystinuria), vitamin B12 (methylmalonic acidemia), biotin (multiple carboxylase deficiency), thiamine (MSUD), and riboflavin (glutaric acidemia II). A subgroup of patients with **PKU** may respond to **sapropterin dihydrochloride** with a reduction of phenylalanine levels. For a number of lysosomal storage disorders, **enzyme replacement** therapies are available.

4. **Supportive therapy** may help to reduce the morbidity associated with specific IEMs. **Splinting** may reduce deformities in mucopolysaccharidoses. **Splenectomy** may be indicated for thrombocytopenia associated with Gaucher disease.

5. **Long-term therapy.** Genetic disorders require lifelong nutritional, medical, and laboratory monitoring by a team of specialists in these disorders. Intercurrent illnesses and stress often precipitate the recurrence of symptoms.

6. **Early intervention and special education programs** may be beneficial in those disorders characterized by intellectual impairment. Families may find a forum for their concerns and stresses, and resources for valuable information can be found in **family support groups** such as the Genetic Alliance (www.geneticalliance.org; accessed September 18, 2018), the National Organization for Rare Disorders (NORD; www.rarediseases.org; accessed September 18, 2018), and numerous other disease- and syndrome-specific support groups.

7. **Liver, bone marrow, or stem cell transplantation** may be a treatment option for selected IEMs.

Table 100–5. USEFUL RESOURCES FOR THE CLINICIAN IN THE EVALUATION, DIAGNOSIS, AND TREATMENT OF NEWBORNS WITH INBORN ERRORS OF METABOLISM

- **Genetics Home Reference** (ghr.nlm.nih.gov; accessed September 18, 2018) maintained by the National Library of Medicine of the United States.
- **Multiple databases at the National Center for Biotechnology Information (NCBI)** (www.ncbi .nlm.nih.gov; accessed September 18, 2018), which includes Online Mendelian Inheritance of Man (OMIM), GeneTests, and GeneReviews.
- **Information through support and family organizations:** Genetic Alliance (www.geneticalliance.org; accessed September 18, 2018), the National Organization for Rare Disorders (NORD; www .rarediseases.org; accessed September 18, 2018), and numerous other disease- and syndrome-specific support groups.
- **Laboratory resources:** GeneTests (available via the National Center for Biotechnology Information [NCBI] at www.ncbi.nlm.org; accessed September 18, 2018), a helpful resource to localize a laboratory for a specific genetic test. (*Note:* Published test catalogs or websites of major healthcare providers and/or regional referral laboratories are often also helpful resources.)

XIV. **Prognosis.** Due to the great number of IEMs, prognosis ranges from extremely favorable with normal development and life expectancy to severe physical and/or intellectual disability and death. In general, early diagnosis and, if available, treatment are associated with more favorable outcomes.

XV. **Additional resources.** In order to assist the clinician with the care of newborns with IEMs, Table 100–5 provides a listing of useful resources.

101 Infant of a Diabetic Mother

Diabetes in pregnancy can cause many complications starting with major congenital anomalies and fetal growth restriction in the first trimester and chronic hyperinsulinism in the second to third trimester causing multiple disorders/diseases presenting after delivery; it can then continue to cause transgenerational effects (increased risk of type 2 diabetes mellitus [T2DM], obesity, and kidney disease) later on in life. Because of an improved understanding of the pathophysiology of diabetic pregnancies, these complications can be recognized and treated. Data indicate that perinatal morbidity and mortality rates in **infants of diabetic mothers (IDM)** have improved with dietary management and insulin therapy.

I. **Classification**

   A. **Definitions.** Any form of **diabetes mellitus (DM)** may require insulin. It is important to note, as stated by the American Diabetes Association, that "insulin use does not classify the patient." Types of diabetes during pregnancy are:

   1. **Pregestational diabetes mellitus (PGDM)** is diabetes that is diagnosed before pregnancy; 15% of pregnancies are complicated by PGDM.

      a. **Type 1 diabetes (T1DM)** occurs due to autoimmune B-cell destruction, which causes an insulin deficiency.

      b. **Type 2 diabetes (T2DM)** is caused by a progressive loss of B-cell insulin secretion with a background of insulin resistance.

   2. **Preexisting pregestational diabetes** is diabetes diagnosed in women by standard diagnostic criteria in the first trimester. The diabetes is usually type 2; rarely is it type 1 or monogenic diabetes.

Table 101–1. **WHITE'S MODIFIED CLASSIFICATION OF DIABETES IN PREGNANCY**

Class	Description
A_1	Gestational diabetes; diet controlled
A_2	Gestational diabetes; insulin controlled
B	Onset after age 20 years; <10 years in duration
C	Onset between 10 and 19 years or 10 to 19 years in duration
D	Onset before 10 years or duration >20 years
F	Nephropathy
R	Retinopathy
H	Ischemic myocardial disease
T	Prior renal transplantation

Data from White P: Diabetes mellitus in pregnancy, *Clin Perinatol.* 1974 Sep;1(2):331-347.

3. **Gestational diabetes** (GDM) is diabetes diagnosed in the second or third trimester of pregnancy with no signs of preexisting T1DM or T2DM prior to the pregnancy. When present, GDM results in complications in 85% of pregnancies.

B. **White classification.** The White classification is a list of alphabetically assigned categories of diabetes and their severity in pregnancy. It is based on age of onset, duration of the disease, and presence or absence of vascular complications. The original White classification (1949) was most likely based on T1DM and was used to assess maternal and fetal risk. There have been multiple revisions, each adding more detail, with the latest 1980 revision including the addition of GDM as a separate class and hypertension risks. See Table 101–1.

C. **American Diabetes Association classification** (2014) presents 4 categories of diabetes. T1DM and T2DM are based on pathophysiology of the disease, and the other category is based on specific types of diabetes due to other causes. GDM is based on the time of diagnosis and the glucose tolerance results. See Table 101–2.

II. **Incidence.** Globally, the incidence of diabetes is increasing. The International Diabetic Federation estimated that approximately 16% of babies born in 2015 were exposed to hyperglycemia, approximately 85% due to GDM, approximately 7.5% due to PGDM (type 1 or type 2), and 7.4% due to other types of diabetes.

A. **Gestational diabetes.** The incidence of GDM varies greatly depending on population characteristics, diagnostic criteria, genetic factors, and screening methods. Globally, the incidence varies from 1% to 28%. The incidence has risen in the past 10 to 20 years and often reflects the underlying rate of T2DM in the population. Incidence of GDM made by various US organizations:

1. **Centers for Disease Control and Prevention:** 2% to 10% of pregnancies.
2. **American Diabetes Association:** Up to 9.2% of pregnancies.
3. **US Preventive Services Task Force:** 1% to 25% of pregnancies.

B. **Type 1 and 2 diabetes.** Incidence of pregnant women with T1DM or T2DM is approximately 1% to 2%.

III. **Pathophysiology.** Most of the problems with IDM are related to fetal hyperglycemia and the resulting increase in production of insulin by the fetal pancreas, which causes chronic hyperinsulinism.

A. **Timing of poor diabetic control.** Maternal diabetic control is a key factor in determining fetal outcome and can be related to key periods in pregnancy.

Table 101–2. AMERICAN DIABETES ASSOCIATION CLASSIFICATION SYSTEM

Classification	Description
Type 1 diabetes (T1DM)	Due to β-cell destruction, usually leading to absolute insulin deficiency. It is either immune mediated or idiopathic.
Type 2 diabetes (T2DM)	Range of predominantly insulin resistance with relative insulin deficiency to a predominantly secretory defect with insulin resistance.
Other specific types	Genetic defects of the β-cell function, genetic defects in insulin action, diseases of the exocrine pancreas, endocrinopathies, drug or chemical induced, infections, uncommon forms of immune-mediated diabetes, other genetic syndromes sometimes associated with diabetes (eg, Down, Klinefelter, Turner, Prader-Willi).
Gestational diabetes mellitus (GDM)	Diabetes diagnosed in the second or third trimester of pregnancy that was not clearly overt diabetes prior to gestation. Diagnosis depends on either the **1-step** or **2-step strategy**, both of which test women with no prior diagnosis of diabetes, and at 24–28 weeks' gestation.
	1-step strategy: Perform a fasting 75-g OGTT in a 24- to 28-week gestational woman. Diagnosis of GDM if any of the following plasma levels are met or exceeded: Fasting: 92 mg/dL; 1 hour: 180 mg/dL; 2 hour: 153 mg/dL
	2-step strategy: Diagnosis of GDM made if at least 2 of the following 4 plasma glucose levels are met or exceeded: **Step 1:** Perform a nonfasting 50-g GLT. If the plasma glucose measured 1 hour after the load is >130 mg/dL, 135 mg/dL, or 140 mg/dL: **Step 2:** Perform a fasting 100-g OGTT. **Carpenter-Coustan or National Diabetes Data Group** **Fasting:** 95 mg/dL — 105 mg/dL **1 hour:** 180 mg/dL — 190 mg/dL **2 hour:** 155 mg/dL — 165 mg/dL **3 hour:** 140 mg/dL — 145 mg/dL

Patients with any form of diabetes may require insulin treatment at some stage of their disease. Such use of insulin does not, of itself, classify the patient.
GLT, glucose loading test; OGTT, oral glucose tolerance test.
Data from American Diabetes Association: 2. Classification and Diagnosis of Diabetes: Standards of Medical Care in Diabetes-2018, *Diabetes Care.* 2018 Jan;41(Suppl 1):S13-S27.

1. **Poor control prior to conception, at the time of conception, and in early first trimester.** Major congenital malformations, spontaneous early abortion, and fetal growth restriction.
2. **Poor control in the second trimester.** Hypertrophic cardiomyopathy with septal hypertrophy, polyhydramnios, preeclampsia, placental insufficiency, low intelligence quotient (IQ), pregnancy-induced hypertension, minor congenital anomalies, fetal loss, macrosomia.
3. **Poor control in the third trimester.** Macrosomia/large for gestational age (LGA) leading to cesarean delivery, birth trauma, fetal dystocia, neonatal hypoglycemia, respiratory distress syndrome, hypertrophic cardiomyopathy with septal hypertrophy, decreased oxygenation in the fetus, neonatal hypocalcemia, hypomagnesemia, hyperbilirubinemia, polycythemia/hyperviscosity, thrombocytopenia, intrauterine death.

    4. **Maternal hyperglycemia in labor.** Hypoglycemia in the infant and poor Apgar scores.

    5. **Long-term transgenerational effects.** Obesity, diabetes, hypertension, and kidney disease in children born to mothers with diabetes in pregnancy.

B. **Examples of complications and their pathophysiology**

    1. **Congenital anomalies.** Early in pregnancy during embryogenesis (before 7 weeks of gestation; **diabetic embryopathy**) with poorly controlled maternal insulin-dependent diabetes, some mechanism occurs to cause an increase in congenital anomalies. There are multiple factors in the diabetic mother that contribute to congenital anomalies, but the true teratogenic mechanism is not known. Hyperglycemia is thought to be the primary teratogen. It causes a deficiency of myoinositol, which is required in embryonic development. Other factors that have been suggested include hypoglycemia, insulin, vascular disease, oxygen free radicals, hypoxia, fetal zinc depletion, low maternal magnesium, hormone imbalances, amino acid/ketone abnormalities, protein glycosylation, and others.

    2. **Fetal growth restriction.** This has been attributed to maternal vascular disease causing uteroplacental insufficiency or lack of nutrients and oxygen required for growth. Ketosis and hypoglycemia may also contribute.

    3. **Perinatal asphyxia** is secondary to macrosomia and cardiomyopathy.

    4. **Prematurity.** Occurs secondary to maternal complications requiring early delivery (eg, hypertension, preeclampsia, intrauterine growth restriction) and a higher rate of preterm labor in diabetic mothers.

    5. **Macrosomia/large for gestational age.** It is the result of biochemical events along the maternal hyperglycemia–fetal hyperinsulinemia pathway, as described by Pedersen. This occurs because increased glucose and amino acids from the mother cross the placenta into the infant and the infant produces an increase in insulin to compensate. Insulin is actually a growth hormone and causes accelerated fetal growth in the infant. Other mechanisms contributing to macrosomia include maternal obesity, disturbances in lipid pathways in the placenta, and certain insulin-like growth factor hormones. Macrosomia causes birth trauma (fractured clavicle, brachial plexus injury).

    6. **Transient hypertrophic cardiomyopathy is hypertrophy of the left and/or right ventricle, and asymmetric septal hypertrophy** is thickening of the interventricular septum. Infants with hypertrophic cardiomyopathy associated with diabetes usually have asymmetric septal hypertrophy with a decrease in the ventricular chambers, which causes an obstruction of the left ventricular outflow tract. It is caused by hyperinsulinemia, which increases the fetal cardiac muscle mass by depositing glycogen and fat in the cells of the myocardium.

    7. **Respiratory distress syndrome.** Hyperinsulinemia causes a decrease in the production and secretion of surfactant by interfering with the glucocorticoid induction of the synthesis of surfactant. This increased risk even occurs in infants up to 38 weeks' gestation.

    8. **Hypocalcemia and hypomagnesemia.** Magnesium depletion occurs in mothers with diabetes secondary to increased renal loss and causes hypomagnesemia in the infant, which causes insufficient parathyroid to be released, resulting in hypocalcemia in the infant. Decreased parathyroid maturation/function may also contribute.

    9. **Hypoglycemia at delivery.** According to the Pedersen hypothesis, at birth, the transplacental glucose supply is terminated, and because of high concentrations of plasma insulin, blood glucose levels fall.

  10. **Polycythemia, hyperbilirubinemia, and thrombosis.** Chronic fetal hyperinsulinemia increases the metabolic rate and oxygen consumption. Relative hypoxemia occurs in utero, and the fetus produces more erythropoietin, which increases red blood cells (RBCs; polycythemia) to transport

oxygen. Hyperbilirubinemia occurs because of the increased breakdown of the increased RBCs. Increased RBCs mean sluggish blood flow and a prothrombotic state (renal vein thrombosis).

IV. **Specific disorders frequently encountered in the infant of a diabetic mother.** All of these disorders/diseases occur in GDM, T1DM, and T2DM, with the exception of congenital malformations (does not occur in GDM because it presents after the first trimester). Fetal risk is significantly higher in mothers with T1DM and T2DM than mothers with GDM.

A. **Disorders of growth**

1. **Macrosomia.** Macrosomia is the classic presentation of the infant of a poorly controlled diabetic mother. After 20 weeks' gestation, maternal hyperglycemia leads to macrosomia. Macrosomia occurs in >25% of diabetic pregnancies and plays a role in birth injuries.

2. **Fetal growth restriction.** Mothers with renal, retinal, or cardiac diseases are more likely to have small for gestational age (SGA) or premature infants, poor fetal outcome, fetal distress, or fetal death.

B. **Birth injuries** are increased in IDM because of macrosomia. They include the following:

1. **More common:** Shoulder dystocia, brachial plexus injury, clavicle/humerus fracture, perinatal asphyxia (difficult delivery, intrauterine hypoxia).

2. **Less common:** Facial palsy, subdural hemorrhage, cephalohematoma.

C. **Metabolic disorders**

1. **Hypoglycemia.** Hypoglycemia is defined as a blood glucose level <45 mg/dL in a preterm or term infant. This value continues to be a debated topic in pediatric medicine. The most recent American Academy of Pediatrics (AAP) policy statement, published in 2011 and reaffirmed in 2015, supports this level in the first days of life. It is present in up to 40% of IDMs, most commonly in macrosomic infants. It usually presents within 1 to 2 hours after delivery. Mothers with well-controlled blood glucose levels have fewer infants with hypoglycemia. Hypoglycemia in SGA infants born to mothers with diabetic vascular disease is caused by decreased glycogen stores; it appears 6 to 12 hours after delivery.

2. **Hypocalcemia.** Hypocalcemia has varying definitions, but serum levels of <7 mg/dL and ionized calcium levels <4 mg/dL are considered to be hypocalcemic. It is found in up to 50% of IDMs. The severity of hypocalcemia is usually related to the severity of maternal DM. Serum calcium levels are lowest at 24 to 72 hours of age.

3. **Hypomagnesemia.** A serum magnesium level <1.52 mg/dL in any infant indicates hypomagnesemia. It is related to maternal hypomagnesemia and the severity of maternal DM.

D. **Cardiorespiratory disorders**

1. **Perinatal asphyxia.** In a prospective study, 27% of IDMs, White class B-R-T, suffered asphyxia. Nephropathy appearing in pregnancy, maternal hyperglycemia before delivery, and prematurity were found to be significant risk factors.

2. **Respiratory distress syndrome**

   a. **Incidence.** The incidence of respiratory distress syndrome (RDS) has decreased to only 3% of IDMs because of better management of diabetes during pregnancy. Most cases are the result of premature delivery, delayed maturation of pulmonary surfactant production, or delivery by elective cesarean section.

   b. **Fetal lung maturity.** Pulmonary surfactant production in the IDM is deficient or delayed principally in class A, B, and C diabetics. Fetal hyperinsulinism may adversely affect the lung maturation process in the IDM by interfering with the incorporation of choline into lecithin. More recent evidence suggests that a change in insulin signaling leads to a decrease in the amount of surfactant production.

      c. Cesarean section. Infants delivered by elective cesarean section are at risk for RDS because of lack of appropriate surfactant production, decreased prostaglandin production, and increased pulmonary vascular resistance.

   3. Other causes of respiratory distress in infants of diabetic mothers

      a. Transient tachypnea of the newborn (TTN) is up to 3 times more common in IDM, especially after elective cesarean section. TTN may or may not require oxygen therapy and usually responds by 72 hours of age.

      b. Hypertrophic cardiomyopathy/asymmetric septal hypertrophy occurs in up to 30% to 50% of IDMs, although most are without signs of disease. Infants with inadequate ventricular filling and decreased intraventricular volume can present with congestive heart failure, cyanosis, tachypnea, cardiomegaly, and tachycardia.

E. Hematologic disorders

  1. Hyperbilirubinemia. Bilirubin production is increased in the IDM. The causes include prematurity, macrosomia, hypoglycemia, polycythemia, and delayed bilirubin clearance.

  2. Polycythemia and hyperviscosity. The cause of polycythemia is unclear but may be related to increased levels of erythropoietin in the IDM and increased RBC production secondary to chronic intrauterine hypoxia in mothers with vascular disease. Intrauterine placental transfusion resulting from acute hypoxia during labor and delivery may also contribute.

  3. Renal venous thrombosis (RVT) is a rare complication. The most likely causes include hyperviscosity, hypotension, or disseminated intravascular coagulation. RVT may present with hematuria and an abdominal mass and is usually diagnosed by ultrasonography.

F. Congenital malformations occur more frequently in IDMs than in the general population. These malformations account for a significant portion of perinatal deaths. Risk of a major malformation is approximately 5% to 6% in mothers with hyperglycemia and 10% to 12% in mothers requiring insulin therapy. The majority of anomalies involve either the cardiovascular system (approximately 8.5 in 100 live births) or the central nervous system (5.3 in 100 live births). Caudal regression, although rare, is strongly associated with DM. A recent study noted the following malformations as the most common: anencephaly, transposition of the great vessels, bilateral renal agenesis/dysgenesis, and hemivertebrae.

  1. Cardiac defects: Transposition of the great vessels, ventricular septal defect, truncus arteriosus, aortic stenosis, double outlet right ventricle, tricuspid atresia, hypoplastic left heart syndrome, and patent ductus arteriosus.

  2. Renal defects: Renal agenesis, ureteral duplication, hydronephrosis.

  3. Gastrointestinal tract defects: Small left colon syndrome, duodenal atresia, imperforate anus, anorectal atresia, situs inversus.

  4. Neurologic defects: Anencephaly, microcephaly, neural tube defects.

  5. Skeletal defects: Hemivertebrae, flexion contractures, caudal regression syndrome, unusual facies.

  6. Eye malformations: Microphthalmos, optic nerve hypoplasia, tear duct obstruction, ocular lipomas, lens opacity.

V. Risk factors. The following factors or conditions may be associated with an increased risk for problems in IDMs:

A. Maternal class of diabetes

  1. In gestational diabetes and class A diabetes controlled by diet alone, infants have few complications.

  2. Women with class A diabetes controlled with insulin and class B, C, and D diabetes are prone to deliver macrosomic infants if diabetes is inadequately controlled.

  3. Diabetic women with renal, retinal, cardiac, and vascular disease have the most severe fetal problems.

B. **Hemoglobin A1c.** To decrease perinatal morbidity and mortality, the diabetic woman should attempt to achieve good metabolic control before conception. Elevated hemoglobin A1c (normal <5.7%) levels during the first trimester appear to be associated with a higher incidence of congenital malformations. For example, with a hemoglobin A1c level of >11%, the risk of having an infant with a congenital malformation is 25%.

C. **Diabetic ketoacidosis.** Pregnant women requiring insulin are apt to develop diabetic ketoacidosis. The onset of this complication may be life threatening for the mother and fetus or may lead to preterm delivery.

D. **Preterm labor.** Preterm delivery occurs more frequently in diabetic pregnancies. Premature onset of labor in a diabetic woman is a serious problem because of the increased likelihood of RDS in the fetus. Furthermore, sympathomimetic agents used to prevent preterm delivery may be associated with maternal hyperglycemia, hyperinsulinemia, and acidosis.

E. **Immature fetal lung profile.** Fetal lung maturity tests are not recommended to guide the timing of delivery. Medical indications for late preterm and early term deliveries include PGDM with vascular disease and PGDM or GDM that is poorly controlled. Infants delivered during the late preterm and early term have an increased rate of respiratory morbidity. A course of antenatal steroids if indicated in the mother is associated with a decrease in RDS and respiratory support. In diabetic mothers who receive steroids, it is important that they are followed more closely and have frequent blood glucose levels. Supplementary insulin may be necessary.

VI. **Clinical presentation of the infant of a diabetic mother**

A. **During birth,** the infant may be LGA or, if the mother has vascular disease, SGA. The size of most infants is appropriate for gestational age; however, if macrosomia is present, birth trauma may occur. Any signs of respiratory distress in the delivery room need to be addressed immediately.

B. **After birth,** hypoglycemia can present as lethargy, poor feeding, apnea, or jitteriness in the first 6 to 12 hour after birth. Jitteriness that occurs after 24 hours of age may be the result of hypocalcemia or hypomagnesemia. Signs of respiratory distress secondary to immature lungs can be noted on examination. Cardiac disease may be present as an enlarged cardiothymic shadow on a chest x-ray film or by physical evidence of heart failure. Gross congenital anomalies may be noted on physical examination. Check for abdominal distension and passage of meconium (small left colon syndrome).

VII. **Diagnostic testing of the infant of a diabetic mother**

A. **Laboratory studies.** The following tests must be closely monitored in the IDM:

1. **Serum glucose levels** should be checked at delivery and may be needed frequently over the first 48 hours. Often values are checked hourly initially and then spaced out thereafter. Glucose levels should be checked with bedside measurement tools. Readings <45 mg/dL at the bedside should be verified by serum glucose measurements.

2. **Serum calcium levels** are often checked in the first day of life, and subsequent values are obtained as needed. If serum calcium levels are low, **serum magnesium levels** should be obtained because they may also be low.

3. **The hematocrit** is often checked at birth and again at 24 hours of life.

4. **Serum bilirubin levels** should be checked as indicated by physical examination.

5. **Other tests.** Arterial blood gas levels, complete blood cell counts, cultures, and Gram stains should be obtained as clinically indicated.

B. **Radiologic studies** are not necessary unless there is evidence of cardiac, respiratory, gastrointestinal, or skeletal problems. Any IDM with respiratory symptoms should undergo a chest x-ray. If there is abdominal distension and suspicion of small left colon syndrome, a contrast enema should be done. It will show a small left colon and abrupt transition zone at the splenic flexure.

    C. **Electrocardiography and echocardiography** should be performed if hypertrophic cardiomyopathy or a cardiac malformation is suspected. Echocardiography shows a hypercontractile thickened myocardium with septal hypertrophy.

VIII. **Management of the infant of a diabetic mother**

    A. **Initial evaluation.** Upon delivery, the infant should be closely evaluated by a trained provider as soon as possible, with close attention to specific complications due to birth trauma and major malformations the infant. In the nursery, blood glucose levels and a hematocrit may be obtained. The infant should be observed for jitteriness, tremors, convulsions, apnea, weak cry, and poor sucking. A physical examination should be performed, paying particular attention to the heart, kidneys, lungs, and extremities. Look for any evidence of birth trauma and closely look for any major or minor malformations.

    B. **Continuing evaluation.** Over the first several hours after delivery, the infant should be screened for hypoglycemia and assessed for signs of respiratory distress. During the first 48 hours, observe for signs of jaundice and for renal, cardiac, neurologic, and gastrointestinal tract abnormalities.

    C. **Metabolic management**

        1. **Hypoglycemia.** AAP recommends screening for late preterm and term IDM/LGA infants and has specific guidelines for management of hypoglycemia in those groups. The Pediatric Endocrine Society has published new recommendations for hypoglycemia in neonates. See Chapter 67 for the specific recommendations.

        2. **Hypocalcemia**

           a. **Calcium therapy.** Symptomatic infants should receive 10% calcium gluconate intravenously. The infusion should be given slowly to prevent cardiac arrhythmias, and the infant should be monitored for signs of extravasation. After the initial dose, a maintenance dose is given by continuous intravenous infusion. The hypocalcemia should respond in 3 to 4 days; until then, serum calcium levels should be monitored every 12 to 24 hours. Management is discussed in Chapter 91.

           b. **Magnesium maintenance therapy.** Magnesium is usually added to intravenous fluids or given orally as magnesium sulfate. See dose in Chapter 155.

    D. **Management of cardiorespiratory problems**

        1. **Perinatal asphyxia.** Close observation for fetal distress should continue throughout labor and delivery. See Chapter 110.

        2. **Respiratory distress.** Management of respiratory distress depends on the etiology. RDS, TTN, and other conditions are more common in the IDM. However, other causes should also be considered (eg, pneumonia or spontaneous pneumothorax). Provide oxygen and ventilator support as needed initially. Treatment depends on the etiology and is discussed further in Chapter 117.

        3. **Hypertrophic cardiomyopathy** associated with DM is self-limited and usually resolves within 6 months. Therapy includes possible mechanical ventilation, maintenance fluids, and correction of hypoglycemia and hypomagnesemia; if medication is necessary, the treatment of choice is short-acting β-blockers (esmolol, propranolol). Digoxin or other positive inotropic agents are contraindicated and can make the infant worse because of possible ventricular outflow obstruction and are only indicated if there is a decrease in cardiac contractility. Diuretics are not necessary unless there is fluid overload. If pulmonary hypertension is present, inhaled nitric oxide should be considered.

    E. **Hematologic management**

        1. **Hyperbilirubinemia.** Frequent monitoring of serum bilirubin levels may be necessary. Phototherapy and exchange transfusion for infants with hyperbilirubinemia are discussed in Chapters 63 and 99.

        2. **Polycythemia.** Observation and/or fluids and/or partial exchange transfusion depending on the hematocrit and clinical symptoms. See Chapters 76 and 116.

3. **Renal venous thrombosis.** Treatment consists of appropriate fluid management and close monitoring of electrolytes and renal status. Supportive therapy is indicated to ensure adequate blood circulation. Both anticoagulation and antithrombotic therapies are considered, and in unilateral disease, nephrectomy is usually only a last resort.

F. **Management of morphologic and functional problems**

1. **Macrosomia and birth injury**
   a. **Fractures of the extremities** should be treated with immobilization.
   b. **Brachial plexus injuries** are usually treated with physical therapy involving range-of-motion and strengthening exercises or possible reconstruction surgery if not resolved.

2. **Congenital malformations.** If a gross malformation is discovered, a specialist should be consulted.

IX. **Prognosis.** Less morbidity and mortality occur with adequate control during the diabetic pregnancy. Preconceptual counseling is used as an adjunct to preventive healthcare of the diabetic patient. The known pregnant diabetic woman is currently receiving better healthcare than before, but the challenge is early identification of women with biochemical abnormalities of GDM. The increased risk of subsequent diabetes in the infants of these women is at least 10 times greater than in the general population, suggesting the need for lifelong follow-up.

102 Infant of a Mother with Substance Use Disorder

Existing studies on the neonatal effects of drug exposure in utero are subject to many confounding factors. Many studies have relied on the history obtained from the mother, which is notoriously inaccurate. In addition to recall bias, there is a considerable incentive to withhold information. Testing of urine for drugs of abuse does not reflect drug exposure throughout pregnancy and does not provide quantitative information. Many women who abuse drugs are multiple drug abusers and also drink alcohol and smoke cigarettes. It is thus difficult to isolate the effects of any 1 drug. Social and economic deprivation is common among drug abusers, and this factor not only confounds perinatal data but also has a major effect on long-term studies of infant outcome.

I. **Definition. An infant of mother with substance use disorder** (formerly referred to as infant of substance-abusing mother) is one whose mother has taken drugs that may potentially cause neonatal withdrawal symptoms. The **constellation of signs and symptoms associated with withdrawal,** often polysubstance exposure that includes opioids, is called the **neonatal abstinence syndrome (NAS).** Table 102–1 lists the drugs associated with this syndrome.

II. **Incidence.** Maternal substance abuse has increased over the past decade. In the United States, the incidence of NAS increased nearly 5-fold between 2000 and 2012 and is continuing to increase, with the incidence of NAS being approximately 6 per 1000 hospital births. The incidence is subject to wide geographic variation.

III. **Pathophysiology.** Drugs of abuse are of low molecular weight and usually water soluble and lipophilic. These features facilitate their transfer across the placenta and accumulation in the fetus and amniotic fluid. The half-life of drugs is usually prolonged in the fetus compared with an adult. Most drugs of abuse either bind to

Table 102–1. **DRUGS CAUSING NEONATAL WITHDRAWAL SYNDROME**

Opiates	Barbiturates	Miscellaneous
Codeine	Butalbital	Alcohol
Heroin	Phenobarbital	Amphetamine
Meperidine	Secobarbital	Chlordiazepoxide
Methadone		Clomipramine
Morphine		Cocaine
Pentazocine		Desmethylimipramine
Propoxyphene		Diazepam
		Diphenhydramine
		Ethchlorvynol
		Fluphenazine
		Glutethimide
		Hydroxyzine
		Imipramine
		Meprobamate
		Phencyclidine
		Selective serotonin reuptake inhibitors (SSRIs)

various central nervous system (CNS) receptors or affect the release and reuptake of various neurotransmitters. This may have a long-lasting trophic effect on developing dendritic structures. Drugs of abuse have also been suggested to alter in utero or perinatal programming through either epigenetic or other factors. In addition, some drugs are directly toxic to fetal cells. The developing fetus may also be affected by the direct physiologic effects of a drug. Many of the fetal effects of cocaine, including its putative teratogenic effects, are thought to be due to its potent vasoconstrictive property.

Some drugs appear to have a partially beneficial effect. The incidence of respiratory distress syndrome (RDS) is decreased after maternal use of heroin and possibly also with cocaine use. These effects are probably a reflection of fetal stress rather than a direct maturational effect of these drugs. Particularly in the case of cocaine, the decreased incidence of RDS is more than offset by the considerable increase in preterm deliveries after its use. The major concern in these drug-exposed infants is the long-term outcome. The importance of direct and indirect effects of drugs on the developing CNS predominates, and the risks of drug abuse far outweigh the benefits. Pathophysiology of specific drugs is noted in the following text.

A. **Opiates.** Opiates bind to opiate receptors in the CNS; part of the clinical manifestations of narcotic withdrawal result from α_2-adrenergic supersensitivity (particularly in the locus coeruleus).

B. **Cocaine.** Cocaine prevents the reuptake of neurotransmitters (epinephrine, norepinephrine, dopamine, and serotonin) at nerve endings and causes a supersensitivity or exaggerated response to neurotransmitters at the effector organs. Cocaine is a CNS stimulant and a sympathetic activator with potent vasoconstrictive properties. It causes a decrease in uterine and placental blood flow with consequent fetal hypoxemia. It causes hypertension in the mother and the fetus with a reduction in fetal cerebral blood flow.

   C. **Alcohol.** Ethanol is an anxiolytic-analgesic with a depressant effect on the CNS. Both ethanol and its metabolite, acetaldehyde, are toxic. Alcohol crosses the placenta and also impairs its function. The risk of affecting the fetus is related to alcohol dose, but there is a continuum of effects and no known safe limit.

IV. **Risk factors.** Associated with an increased incidence of maternal drug abuse are the following:

   A. **Maternal history**
      1. **Poor social and economic circumstances.**
      2. **Poor antenatal care.**
      3. **Teenage or unwed mothers.**
      4. **Poor education.**
      5. **Associated conditions include infectious diseases** (hepatitis B, syphilis, and other sexually transmitted diseases/sexually transmitted infections), human immunodeficiency virus (HIV)-positive serology, multiple drug abuse, poor nutritional status, and anemia.

   B. **Obstetric complications**
      1. **Premature delivery.**
      2. **Premature rupture of membranes.**
      3. **Chorioamnionitis.**
      4. **Fetal distress.**
      5. **Intrauterine growth restriction.**
      6. **With cocaine use,** the following may be present (in addition to the conditions just noted):
         a. **Hypertension.**
         b. **Abruptio placentae.**
         c. **Cardiac.** Arrhythmias, myocardial ischemia, and infarction.
         d. **Cerebrovascular accident.**
         e. **Respiratory arrest.**
         f. **Fetal demise.**

V. **Clinical presentation.** Signs and symptoms of drug withdrawal are listed in Table 102–2. These signs essentially reflect CNS "irritability," altered neurobehavioral organization, and abnormal sympathetic activation. Although each drug may have its own effects, these signs and symptoms must be noted for every mother who may have polydrug use; conversely, drug abuse should be suspected in infants exhibiting these signs and symptoms. Signs and symptoms for specific drugs are as follows:

   A. **Opiates.** Infants born to opiate-addicted mothers show an increased incidence of fetal growth restriction (FGR) and perinatal distress. Even when these infants are not small for gestational age, they have lower weight and a smaller head circumference compared with drug-free infants.
      1. **Signs and symptoms of withdrawal occur in 60% to 90% of exposed infants.** The onset of symptoms may be minutes after delivery up to 1 to 2 weeks of age, but most infants exhibit signs by 2 to 3 days of life. The onset of withdrawal may be delayed beyond 2 weeks in infants exposed to methadone (parents should be appropriately informed).
      2. **The clinical course is variable, ranging from mild symptoms of brief duration to severe symptoms.** The clinical course may be protracted, with exacerbations or recurrence of symptoms after discharge. Restlessness, agitation, tremors, wakefulness, and feeding problems may persist for 3 to 6 months. There is a reduced incidence of both RDS and hyperbilirubinemia.

   B. **Cocaine**
      1. **Symptoms seen in neonates exposed to cocaine in utero.** Irritability, tremors, hypertonia, a high-pitched cry, hyperreflexia, frantic fist sucking, feeding

Table 102–2. SIGNS AND SYMPTOMS OF NEONATAL ABSTINENCE

Hyperirritability
  Increased deep-tendon and primitive reflexes
  Hypertonus, hyperacusis
  Tremors
  High-pitched cry

Seizures

Wakefulness

Increased rooting reflex

Uncoordinated or ineffectual sucking and swallowing

Regurgitation and vomiting

Loose stools and diarrhea

Tachypnea, apnea

Yawning, hiccups

Sneezing, stuffy nose

Mottling

Fever

Failure to gain weight

Lacrimation

problems, sneezing, tachypnea, and abnormal sleep patterns. A specific cocaine withdrawal syndrome has not been described. The symptoms just mentioned may be a reflection of cocaine intoxication rather than withdrawal, and after an initial period of irritability and overactivity, a period of lethargy and decreased tone has been described.

2. *Controversial* cocaine associations
   a. **In the neonate, the following have been described.** Necrotizing enterocolitis, transient hypertension, reduced cardiac output (on the first day of life), intracranial hemorrhages and infarcts, seizures, apneic spells, periodic breathing, abnormal electroencephalogram, abnormal brainstem auditory evoked potentials, abnormal response to hypoxia and carbon dioxide, and ileal perforation. These reports were mostly case reports or insufficiently controlled case series with numerous confounding factors and large case-control studies that have found no association between cocaine exposure and intraventricular hemorrhage. Despite earlier concerns, there does not appear to be an increased risk of sudden infant death syndrome (SIDS).
   b. **Cocaine has been suggested as a teratogen.** Its teratogenic potential is presumed to be due to its vascular effects, although direct toxicity on various cell lines may also play a role. Numerous CNS anomalies, as well as cardiovascular abnormalities, limb reduction defects, intestinal atresias, and other malformations, have been attributed to cocaine. However, most of these associations were derived from case reports, case series, or poorly controlled studies, and a detailed examination of the data does not substantiate most of these teratogenic associations. An exception appears to

be an increased risk of genitourinary tract defects associated with cocaine exposure during gestation. Moreover, there does not appear to be a dysmorphism recognizable as a "cocaine syndrome." Cocaine is associated with an increased incidence of spontaneous abortion, stillbirth, abruptio placentae, premature labor, and FGR.

C. **Alcohol.** Probably the foremost drug of abuse today. **The risk that an alcoholic woman will have a child with fetal alcohol syndrome (FAS) is approximately 35% to 40%.** However, even in the absence of FAS, and also with lower alcohol intake, there is an increased risk of congenital anomalies and impaired intellect. It is estimated that alcohol is the major cause of congenital intellectual disability today. **FAS consists of the following:**

1. **Prenatal or postnatal growth retardation** , CNS involvement such as irritability in infancy or hyperactivity in childhood, developmental delay, hypotonia, or intellectual impairment.

2. **Facial dysmorphology.** Microcephaly, microphthalmos, or short palpebral fissures; a poorly developed philtrum; a thin upper lip (vermilion border); and hypoplastic maxilla.

3. **Other congenital anomalies.** These have been described after exposure to alcohol in utero both with and without full-blown FAS. CNS symptoms may appear within 24 hours after delivery and include tremors, irritability, hypertonicity, twitching, hyperventilation, hyperacusis, opisthotonos, and seizures. Symptoms may be severe but are usually of short duration. Abdominal distention and vomiting are less frequent than with most other drugs of abuse. In premature infants of women who were heavy alcohol users (>7 drinks/wk), there is an increased risk of both intracranial hemorrhage and white matter CNS damage. (See also Chapter 93.)

D. **Barbiturates.** Symptoms and signs of withdrawal are similar to those observed in narcotic-exposed infants, but symptoms usually appear later. Most infants become symptomatic toward the end of the first week of life, although onset may be delayed up to 2 weeks. The duration of symptoms is usually 2 to 6 weeks.

E. **Benzodiazepines.** Symptoms are indistinguishable from those of narcotic withdrawal, including seizures. The onset of symptoms may be shortly after birth.

F. **Phencyclidine.** Symptoms usually begin within 24 hours of birth, and the infant may show signs of CNS "hyperirritability" as in narcotic withdrawal. Gastrointestinal symptoms of withdrawal are less common.

G. **Marijuana.** Studies have suggested a slightly shorter duration of gestation and somewhat reduced birthweight, but the extent of these differences does not seem to be clinically important. Marijuana may have some mild effect on a variety of newborn neurobehavioral traits.

H. **Selective serotonin reuptake inhibitors.** Selective serotonin reuptake inhibitors (SSRIs) are typically used as antidepressants, with symptoms occurring in up to 30% of exposed infants. Symptoms may include irritability, seizures, myoclonus, hyperreflexia, jitteriness, persistent crying, shivering, increased tone, feeding difficulties, tachypnea, and temperature instability. It may be difficult to make a clinical distinction between symptoms of withdrawal and those of a neonatal variant of the serotonin syndrome.

I. **Buprenorphine.** This drug, a partial μ-receptor opiate agonist, is being increasingly used as an alternative to methadone in the treatment of pregnant opiate users. Its short-term effects on the neonate are similar to that of methadone, although duration of symptoms appears to be decreased. Symptoms of withdrawal usually occur within the first 3 days of life.

VI. **Diagnosis**

A. **History.** Many, if not most, drug abusers withhold this information. Details of the extent, quantity, and duration of abuse are unreliable. However, the history is the simplest and most convenient means of diagnosis.

B. **Laboratory tests.** The most commonly used tests to detect drugs of abuse are immunoassays (enzymatic assays or radioimmunoassays). However, they are subject to a low rate of false-negative results and, because of cross-reactivity, false-positive testing. Thus, they are viewed as screening tests. When it is either medically or legally important, these tests should be supplemented by the more sensitive and specific chromatographic or mass spectrometric tests.

1. **Urine.** Easily obtained and is the most common substance used for drug testing. It reflects intake only in the last few days before delivery. Urine may be obtained from both the mother and the infant (in whom the substance may persist for a longer time).

   a. **False-negative immunoassays.** May be due to dilution (low specific gravity) or high sodium chloride content (detected by high specific gravity). Various adulterants may also affect detection; this is unlikely in the neonate but may occur in maternal urine.

   b. **False-positive immunoassays.** Although these depend on the specific assay used, the following have been reported:

      i. **Detected as morphine.** Codeine (found in many cold and cough medications and in analgesics). About 10% of codeine is metabolized to morphine in the liver. The consumption of baked goods containing poppy seeds (eg, bagels) can result in detectable amounts of morphine in the urine. These are "physiologic" false-positive results, but chromatography or mass spectrometry may determine the source by quantitative assays of other metabolites.

      ii. **Detected as amphetamines.** Ranitidine, chlorpromazine, ritodrine, phenylpropanolamine, ephedrine, pseudoephedrine, phenylephrine, phentermine, and phenmetrazine. Some of these (eg, pseudoephedrine) are found in many over-the-counter preparations.

2. **Meconium.** Easily obtained, and drugs may be detected up to 3 days after delivery. It reflects drug use after the first trimester, has a lower rate of false negatives, is a more sensitive test than urine for detecting drug abuse, and reflects usage over a longer period than is detectable by urine testing. Its main disadvantage is that the specimen requires processing before testing and hence places an additional burden on the laboratory. The ability to detect drugs is reduced after formation of fed stools.

3. **Hair.** This is by far the **most sensitive test** available for detection of drug abuse. Hair grows at 1 to 2 cm/mo; hence, maternal hair can be segmented and each segment analyzed for drugs. Thus, details of drug abuse throughout pregnancy may be obtained. There is a quantitative relationship between amounts of drug used and amounts incorporated in growing hair. Hair may be obtained from the mother or the infant (in whom it will reflect usage only during the last trimester). Hair may also be obtained from the infant a long time after delivery should symptoms occur that suggest in utero drug exposure that was previously unsuspected. The test requires processing before assay, is more expensive, and is currently not as widely available as other test methods.

4. **Routine laboratory testing.** Routine laboratory tests are usually not required in infants of mothers with substance use disorder (other than tests to confirm the diagnosis). Laboratory tests are required to rule out other causes of particular signs and symptoms (eg, calcium and glucose for cases of jerky movements) or to follow up and manage some particular complication of drug abuse appropriately.

C. **Other studies.** A **scoring system** has been devised for assessment of withdrawal signs. Commonly called the **Finnegan score**, after its originator, the score was devised for neonates exposed to opiates in utero. Its usefulness for assessing

Table 102–3. MODIFIED FINNEGAN'S SCORING SYSTEM FOR NEONATAL WITHDRAWAL

Signs and symptoms are scored between feedings.

Cry:	High-pitched	2
	Continuous	3
Sleep hours after feed:	1 h	3
	2 h	2
	3 h	1
Moro reflex:	Hyperactive	2
	Marked	3
Tremors when disturbed:	Mild	2
	Marked	3
Tremors when undisturbed:	Mild	3
	Marked	4
Muscle tone increased:	Mild	3
	Marked	6
Convulsions:		8
Feedings:	Frantic sucking of fists	1
	Poor feeding ability	1
	Regurgitation	1
	Projectile vomiting	1
Stools:	Loose	2
	Watery	3
Fever:	100–101°F	2
	>101°F	2
Respiratory rate:	>60/min	1
	Retractions	2
Excoriations:	Nose	1
	Knees	1
	Toes	1
Frequent yawning:		1
Sneezing:		1
Nasal stuffiness:		1
Sweating:		1
Total scores per day		( )

Once an objective score has been attained, a dose for treatment can be decided on.

Reproduced with permission from Morselli PL, Garattini S, Sereni F: *Basic and Therapeutic Aspects of Perinatal Pharmacology.* New York, NY: Raven Press; 1975.

signs after exposure to other drugs or for guiding management in these cases has not been established, but it can be used as a guide. The scoring system is shown in Table 102–3. Other tools for assessing neonatal abstinence are the **Lipsitz tool, Neonatal Narcotic Withdrawal Index, and the Neonatal Withdrawal Inventory**, but these are less commonly used.

VII. **Management.** Manifestations of drug withdrawal in many infants resolve within a few days, and drug therapy is not required. Supportive care suffices in many, if not most, infants. It is not appropriate to treat prophylactically infants of drug-dependent mothers. The infant's withdrawal score should be assessed to monitor the progression of symptoms and the adequacy of treatment.

A. **Supportive care**

1. **Minimal stimulation.** Attempt to keep the infant in a darkened, quiet environment. Reduce other noxious stimuli.

2. **Swaddling and positioning.** Use gentle swaddling with positioning that encourages flexion rather than extension.

3. **Prevent excessive crying with a pacifier, cuddling, and so on.** Feedings should be on demand if possible, and treatment should be individualized based on the infant's level of tolerance.

B. **General drug treatment.** *Warning:* **Naloxone (Narcan) may precipitate acute drug withdrawal in infants exposed to narcotics. It should not be used in infants born to mothers suspected of abusing opiates.**

The general aim of treatment is to allow sleep and feeding patterns to be as close to normal as possible. When supportive care is insufficient to do this, or if symptoms are particularly severe, drugs are used. Indications for drug treatment are progressive irritability, continued feeding difficulty, and significant weight loss. A score >7 on the Finnegan score for 3 consecutive scorings (done every 4 hours during the first 2 days) may also be regarded as an indication for treatment. However, the Finnegan score should not be followed slavishly and treated as a definitive laboratory value. Many centers use the Finnegan score only every 12 hours and increase the frequency of its application if the infant's scores rapidly escalate. Drugs used for withdrawal are discussed next. Additional treatment may be required for some symptoms (eg, dehydration or convulsions). There have been very few clinical trials in this area, and drug therapy is based largely on anecdotal evidence and hence is variable. Cumulative reports suggest that drugs that act on the relevant receptors are superior to sedatives. When compared with opiates, phenobarbital, at doses required to suppress symptoms of withdrawal, may impair sucking in infants withdrawing from maternal opiates and may require a more protracted duration of treatment.

1. **Morphine.** A recent randomized trial comparing morphine with tincture of opium showed that infants treated with morphine required a somewhat longer duration of treatment but had better weight gain. An appropriate schedule of treatment would be to start at a morphine dose of 0.04 mg/kg every 3 to 4 hours. Dosage may be increased every 4 hours at increments of 0.04 mg/kg until symptoms are under control (absent side effects) or a (recommended) total maximum of 1.3 mg/kg/d is reached. If the baby is still symptomatic after a maximal dose is given, an additional adjunct drug is used (see Section VII.B.10). Once the symptoms are under control (eg, Finnegan score <8), treatment is maintained at that dosage for 72 hours and then weaning is commenced. Weaning is done by decreasing the daily dose by 10% every day, as long as symptoms do not relapse. If the infant becomes symptomatic during weaning, the dose is increased back to the last previous dose that had controlled the symptoms. There are no reports of any maximal dose of morphine used for withdrawal, but prudence suggests that infants be closely watched for side effects, and some centers recommend cardiorespiratory monitoring if morphine dosage exceeds 0.8 mg/kg/d. As mentioned, there is a paucity of controlled trials on this topic, and treatment schedules are highly variable between institutions. The schedule just suggested is within the range of common practice but is not carved in stone.

2. **Methadone.** This has the advantage of a longer half-life and hence requires less frequent administration. However, there is large individual pharmacokinetic

variability and response in NAS patients. Many formulations also contain ethanol. There is no overall consensus as to the relative superiority of morphine and methadone as primary drug treatments for NAS. Typical dosage is 0.2 mg/kg/d divided into 2 to 6 doses.

3. **Paregoric (camphorated opium tincture).** This has 0.4 mg/mL morphine equivalents and is thought to be more "physiologic" than nonnarcotic agents but is no longer recommended due to other constituents present in the preparation (eg, camphor, alcohol, benzoic acid).

4. **Opium tincture, also called tincture of opium.** This is similar to paregoric and has the advantage of fewer additives. It has 10 mg/mL morphine equivalents and should be diluted to provide the same morphine dosage as in Section VII.B.1.

5. **Phenobarbital.** An adequate drug for controlling withdrawal from narcotics, especially signs of irritability, fussiness, and hyperexcitability. It is not as effective as morphine for control of gastrointestinal symptoms. It is not suitable for dose titration because of its long half-life. It is mainly useful for treatment of withdrawal from nonnarcotic agents. Anecdotally, phenobarbital is reportedly useful in the management of NAS following polydrug exposure. The dosage is a 10- to 20-mg/kg loading dose, followed by 2 to 4 mg/kg/d maintenance. Once symptoms have been controlled for 1 week, decrease the daily dose by 25% every week.

6. **Chlorpromazine** is quite effective in controlling symptoms of withdrawal from both narcotics and nonnarcotics. It has multiple untoward side effects (it reduces seizure threshold and can cause cerebellar dysfunction and hematologic problems) that make it **potentially undesirable** for use in neonates when alternatives can be used. The dosage is 3 mg/kg/d, divided into 3 to 6 doses per day.

7. **Clonidine.** This has been used for withdrawal from both narcotic and nonnarcotic agents. The dosage is 3 to 4 mcg/kg/d, divided into 4 doses per day.

8. **Diazepam.** This has been used to treat withdrawal from narcotics. One study showed a greater incidence of seizures after methadone withdrawal when infants were treated with diazepam rather than paregoric. When used to treat methadone withdrawal, it also impairs nutritive sucking more than methadone does alone. It may produce apnea when used with phenobarbital. It may be used for treatment of withdrawal from benzodiazepines and possibly also for the hyperexcitable phase after cocaine exposure. The dosage is 0.5 to 2 mg every 6 to 8 hours.

9. **Buprenorphine.** In a randomized trial, sublingual buprenorphine was found to reduce the duration of pharmacotherapy and length of stay in NAS when compared to morphine. Results are promising, but further trials are required before its widespread use. Also of concern is that the drug contains ethanol. Initial dosage is 4 to 5 mcg/kg/dose given every 8 hours, with doses increased up to a maximum of 60 mcg/kg/d.

10. **Combination therapy (failure of monotherapy).** When maximal dosage of a drug of choice has been reached and symptoms of NAS are still of concern, an adjunct drug is used. When morphine has been the initial first-line medication, either phenobarbital or clonidine is often use as an adjunct medication. Results of several studies yield contradictory results; however, a 2010 Cochrane review concluded that the addition of either phenobarbital or clonidine may reduce duration of treatment for NAS.

C. **Long-term management.** If the infant is discharged after 4 days, an early appointment with the pediatrician should be arranged and the parents should be informed as to possible signs of delayed-onset withdrawal. Minor signs and symptoms of drug withdrawal may continue for a few months after discharge. This places a difficult infant in a difficult home situation. There are a few reports of an increased incidence of child abuse in these circumstances. Thus, frequent follow-up visits and close involvement of social services may be required.

D. **Breast feeding.** The various drugs of abuse may be presumed to enter breast milk, and there have been case reports of intoxication in breast-fed infants whose mothers had continued to abuse drugs. Mothers on low-dose methadone have been allowed to breast feed, but this required close supervision, and there was a constant concern that unsupervised weaning would precipitate withdrawal. A recent study demonstrated that concentration of methadone in breast milk, even at peak maternal plasma levels, was low in the perinatal period. The mothers had been receiving methadone doses of 76 ± 22 mg. The data support recommendations of breast feeding for women on methadone maintenance. However, methadone-dependent women require special considerations and support and should also be counseled as to the unknown CNS effects of long-term exposure to small amounts of methadone present in breast milk. Similarly, there is no evidence that breast feeding should not be discouraged in mothers who are receiving treatment with SSRIs. However, pending definitive evidence, caution suggests that breast feeding might be discouraged in the particular case of fluoxetine use due to its long elimination half-life and risk of accumulation.

VIII. **Prognosis.** During the first few years of life, infants exposed to drugs in utero may have various neurobehavioral problems. Prognosis is largely dependent on the drug used.

A. **Opiates.** There are increased risks of SIDS and strabismus. A substantial proportion of children demonstrate good catch-up growth by 1 to 2 years of age, although they may still be below the mean. There are limited data on long-term follow-up, but at 5 to 6 years of age, these children appear to function within the normal range of mental and motor development. Some differences have been found in various behavioral, adaptive, and perceptual skills. At 9 years of age, there is a trend, in opiate-exposed children, to score lower than controls in some measures of language processing. Some children require special education classes. A positive and reinforcing environment can improve infant outcome significantly.

B. **Cocaine.** No major deficits in motor development have been found after gestational exposure to cocaine. By 1 to 6 years of age, there are no significant differences in weight, height, and head circumference between cocaine-exposed and nonexposed children. Gestational cocaine exposure may, however, be associated with long-term effects on behavior. Cocaine-exposed children exhibited more behavioral problems (both internalizing and externalizing) on follow-up to age 7 years, and these issues were related to degree of cocaine exposure during gestation. A long-term study found a 4.4-point decrease in intelligence quotient (IQ) at 4.5 to 7 years of age after gestational exposure to cocaine. In addition, cocaine-exposed children are more likely to be referred for special education services at school when compared with unexposed children.

C. **Phencyclidine.** Very few studies have been done, but at 2 years of age, these infants appear to have lower scores in fine motor, adaptive, and language areas of development. Although weight, length, and head circumference are somewhat reduced at birth, most children demonstrate adequate catch-up growth.

D. **Marijuana.** There is no definitive evidence of long-term dysfunction. Some scientific studies have found that infants born to women who used marijuana during their pregnancy display altered responses to visual stimulation, increased tremors, and a high-pitched cry, which may indicate problems with nervous system development. During preschool and early school years, marijuana-exposed children have been reported to have more behavioral problems and difficulties with sustained attention and memory than unexposed children.

103 Intracranial Hemorrhage

An **intracranial hemorrhage (ICH)** can occur in term and preterm infants and is the most common central nervous system (CNS) acute complication of a preterm birth. Types of ICH include subdural hemorrhage, epidural hemorrhage, subarachnoid hemorrhage, intracerebral intraparenchymal hemorrhage, intracerebellar parenchymal hemorrhage, and germinal matrix and intraventricular hemorrhage. An **ICH in term infants** tends to be extra-axial (subdural, subarachnoid, or subtentorial) and is most related to birth trauma, hypoxic ischemic events, and coagulopathies (eg, thrombophilias or thrombocytopenia). The **most common ICH in preterm infants** is bleeding from the subependymal germinal matrix and may result in intraventricular or periventricular hemorrhage, either of which can potentially cause hemorrhagic infarctions of the cerebral white matter. With the spread of improved neuroimaging techniques, cerebellar hemorrhage has been detected with increasing frequency, in particular among very immature preterm infants.

SUBDURAL HEMORRHAGE

I. **Definition.** A **subdural hemorrhage (SDH)** is an accumulation of blood between the dura and the arachnoid membrane and involves tears of bridging veins of the subdural compartment (see Figure 7-3). The vascular structures most affected are superficial cerebral veins, infratentorial posterior fossa venous sinuses, the inferior sagittal sinus, and tentorial sinuses and veins (eg, vein of Galen). Blood from an infratentorial hemorrhage in the posterior fossa may accumulate and cause acute symptoms of increased intracranial pressure (ICP) or reside as a hematoma that slowly evolves as a chronic subdural hematoma with increasing fluid accumulation and increasing ICP.

II. **Incidence.** Up to 45% of term newborns may have asymptomatic SDH. Symptomatic SDH usually follows a traumatic delivery of a late preterm or term infant. Only on rare occasions does SDH become clinically critical. Symptomatic SDH occurred in 2.9 per 10,000 spontaneous deliveries, as compared with 8.0 and 9.8 per 10,000 vacuum-assisted and forceps-assisted deliveries, respectively. When both vacuum and forceps are used in delivery, the rate goes up to 21.3 per 10,000.

III. **Pathophysiology.** An SDH is typically related to traumatic birth events involving labor and delivery. Undue pressure on the skull and torsion may produce shear forces resulting in rupture of superficial cerebral bridging veins (carrying blood through the dura mater to the arachnoid mater of the meninges) or tears in the dura or dural reflections (eg, either the falx cerebri or tentorium and associated venous sinuses), causing blood to collect below the dura and superior to the subarachnoid villi. These events are usually found over the cerebrum or within the posterior fossa. Occasionally, skull fractures accompany these findings. Timing of the onset of SDH and clinical findings may be acute or delayed. Clinical signs may be minimal to none, with the SDH self-resolving, or subtle findings of slight irritability or a seemingly hyperalert state may foretell an underlying accumulating SDH with delayed onset of more serious neuropathic circumstances. Latent SDH can lead to a subdural hematoma and subdural effusion with increasing ICP.

IV. **Risk factors.** Include precipitous labor and delivery, instrumented deliveries using forceps or vacuum-assist devices, a large for gestational age infant with cephalopelvic disproportion, abusive head trauma, blunt prenatal trauma, glutaric aciduria type 1, and coagulopathies including familial thrombophilias, vitamin K deficiency, and maternal ingestion of hydroxycoumarin derivatives (eg, warfarin).

V. **Clinical presentation.** Neonates with SDH may present similarly to those with hypoxic ischemic encephalopathy. Signs include lethargy alternating with irritability or asymmetric hypotonia of upper and lower extremities on the contralateral side of the SDH.

More specific to SDH is impaired third cranial nerve function ipsilateral to the SDH. Focal seizures may present at any time and are much more likely to occur in low birth-weight infants. Signs of increasing ICP may include a bulging fontanel, deviations of eye movements, and increasing occipital-frontal head circumference. Additional clinical signs can be poor feeding, intermittent vomiting, and failure to thrive, all of which are more often related to late post-SDH neuropathic events.

VI. **Diagnosis**
  A. **Laboratory**
    1. **Serial hematocrit.** Unexplained anemia.
    2. **Total serum bilirubin.** Persistent newborn jaundice.
    3. **Cerebrospinal fluid studies** are indicative but not diagnostic of SDH. Suggestive of an ICH hemorrhage is the cerebrospinal fluid (CSF) analysis combination of a large numbers of red bloods cells (especially if crenated), xanthochromia, elevated protein content, and hypoglycorrhachia (ie, CSF glucose <50% of concomitant blood glucose).
  B. **Imaging studies**
    1. **Computed tomography (CT)** readily identifies most SDH.
    2. **Magnetic resonance imaging (MRI)** is superior and currently recommended. It is best for detailing posterior fossa lesions and accumulations of blood or effusion. Routine use of MRI has shown that small asymptomatic SDHs are common.
    3. **Ultrasound (US)** does not readily lend itself to SDH identification, except for possible midline shifts.

VII. **Management.** Documentation of risk factors and appropriate cogent observation are the most important first clinical steps. Careful and repeated neurologic examinations will reveal neurologic signs that should be followed by laboratory and imaging studies. In most cases, blood collections will gradually resorb over the weeks and months following the initial hemorrhage. Rarely, in the case of a large SDH causing increased ICP or mass effect, neurosurgical drainage may be required.

VIII. **Prognosis.** The outcome of SDH ranges from early death to minimal or no disabling conditions. Much of the neurologic outcome of SDH depends on accompanying conditions soon after birth (eg, prematurity, birth asphyxia, shock, hypoxic ischemic encephalopathy, or infection). Up to 80% of infants with SDH show no disability. Massive tentorial tears and hemorrhage can result in death or severe and long-term handicap. Infants with major SDH can have mortality rates upward of 45%. Conversely, in most cases, SDH can be limited, produce few clinical signs, and have a good outcome. More than 50% of infants with minimal early clinical findings and later good outcomes have been largely found to have had small cerebral convexity SDH hemorrhages.

EPIDURAL HEMORRHAGE

An **epidural hemorrhage**, blood between the inner skull and dura, is extremely rare in newborns. It is usually caused by injury to the middle meningeal artery, which is less susceptible to injury because it moves freely (see Figure 7–3). Trauma is the most likely etiology, including birth trauma, an infant being dropped at delivery, or abusive head trauma. Diagnosis is typically by CT or MRI. Affected infants may also have a skull fracture and cephalohematoma, and treatment is supportive with possible surgical/needle aspiration.

SUBARACHNOID HEMORRHAGE

I. **Definition.** A **subarachnoid hemorrhage (SAH)** is an accumulation of blood between the arachnoid mater and the pia mater. The arachnoid mater is an avascular membrane situated below the dura mater and, together with the pia mater, constitutes what is known as the leptomeninges. Unlike adult SAH, which is arterial, infant SAH is venous in origin, coming from bridging veins within the subarachnoid space; however, on rare occasions, it may be arterial, coming from leptomeningeal arteries of the subarachnoid space. SAH may be primary, coming from the vessels of the subarachnoid space, or secondary, occurring when the blood extends from existing intraventricular, cerebral, or cerebellar hemorrhages.

II. **Incidence.** A small asymptomatic SAH is commonly seen in preterm and term newborn infants. It is of limited significance unless other conditions are present, such as prematurity, coagulopathies, birth trauma, or asphyxia. Primary bleeding within the subarachnoid space is usually self-limited, and it is the second most common ICH seen in newborns.

III. **Pathophysiology.** Rupture of the small vessels of the subarachnoid space can be associated with trauma in term infants or birth asphyxia in preterm infants and is most often idiopathic and insignificant.

IV. **Risk factors.** See Pathophysiology.

V. **Clinical presentation.** In term infants, an SAH is mostly asymptomatic. Mild to intermittent irritability or lethargy may herald the onset of seizures on the second to third day of life.

VI. **Diagnosis**
   A. **Laboratory.** CSF findings in SAH mirror those already discussed for SDH.
   B. **Imaging studies.** CT and MRI studies establish the existence of primary SAH or identify other lesions that may be the source of secondary SAH.

VII. **Management.** Close observation and repeated neurologic examinations suffice for those infants at risk but without signs of SAH. Anticonvulsant medication and intravenous fluid therapy are needed if the infant has lethargy and/or seizure activity. Serum electrolyte and urine output monitoring for possible syndrome of inappropriate antidiuretic secretion is recommended if a significant amount of SAH has been identified. Regular sequential head circumference measurements and, in some cases, serial head US will identify suspected cases of posthemorrhagic hydrocephalus. The latter is due to obliteration of CSF resorption sites by the organizing blood. Follow-up cranial imaging studies will also be needed.

VIII. **Prognosis.** The location and extent of the hemorrhage may play a role. A primary isolated SAH is mostly uncomplicated. Infants who have seizures that resolve before discharge from the hospital have an expected 90% uncomplicated outcome. Infants who develop long-term complications are mostly those who had coexisting problems associated with birth trauma or perinatal asphyxia. SAH in the frontal lobe is associated with higher rates of disability.

INTRACEREBRAL INTRAPARENCHYMAL HEMORRHAGE/ PERIVENTRICULAR HEMORRHAGIC INFARCTION

I. **Definition.** An **intracerebral parenchymal hemorrhage** occurs deep within the brain tissue after venous infarction and is commonly referred to as **periventricular hemorrhagic infarction (PVHI).** Porencephalic cysts and periventricular necrotic cystic lesions are not uncommon complications of PVHI.

II. **Incidence.** The occurrence of PVHI may be as high as 10% to 15% among infants with ICH.

III. **Pathophysiology.** It is postulated that venous thrombosis and/or venous congestion causes PVHI through increased intravascular pressure that leads to rupture of parenchymal vessels and ischemic necrosis secondary to impaired arterial perfusion. Affected preterm infants have hemorrhagic venous infarction of subcortical and periventricular white matter, whereas affected term infants develop subcortical hemorrhage with infarction of overlying cortex.

IV. **Risk factors.** PVHI is seen most often after a perinatal hypoxic ischemic event.

V. **Clinical presentation.** Clinical signs of PVHI follow those of severe neonatal encephalopathy and overlap with clinical signs as seen with SDH, SAH, or intraventricular hemorrhage (IVH).

VI. **Diagnosis**
  A. **Computed tomography** can be useful for detecting recent hemorrhage.
  B. **Magnetic resonance imaging** findings of hypodensities suggest evolving areas of brain injury.
  C. **Cranial ultrasound** is particularly useful in identifying PVHI. An echodense lesion of periventricular white matter with an associated germinal matrix (GM) hemorrhage or IVH usually identifies coexisting PVHI.
VII. **Management.** PVHI requires observational and supportive care, much as severe SDH or SAH. If imaging studies suggest a midline shift, neurosurgical consultation should follow. Subsequent posthemorrhagic hydrocephalus is always a threat, which also requires neurosurgical consultation.
VIII. **Prognosis.** Developmental studies of preterm infants with PVHI have shown that significant cognitive and/or motor delays complicate overall recovery in at least two-thirds of survivors. Careful follow-up is thus indicated in every case of PVHI.

INTRACEREBELLAR PARENCHYMAL HEMORRHAGE

  I. **Definition.** An **intracerebellar parenchymal hemorrhage (ICPH)** is a cerebellar hemorrhage that is increasingly detected and is more common in premature infants compared with term newborns. Cerebellar hemorrhage is now recognized as an important complication of preterm birth. Cerebellar hemorrhage can occur in isolation but more commonly occurs in combination with supratentorial brain injury and can range from small punctate hemorrhagic lesions to very large cerebellar hemorrhages.
  II. **Incidence.** Reports vary by gestational age and by the method of detection. By cranial US that includes an additional mastoid view, an incidence of 9% was reported among infants <33 weeks' gestation, of whom 60% weighed <750 g. Using brain MRI with specific MRI sequences (eg, susceptibility-weighted imaging), the incidence was reported to be 37% among a similar-age population.
  III. **Risk factors.** Traumatic delivery.
  IV. **Pathogenesis.** Four mechanisms for intracerebellar parenchymal hemorrhage are possible:
    A. **Primary hemorrhage into either cerebellar hemisphere or into the vermis.**
    B. **Venous infarction.**
    C. **Supratentorial intraventricular hemorrhage and subarachnoid hemorrhage** are associated with reduction of preterm cerebellar growth, which may reflect concurrent cerebellar injury or direct effect of the blood on cerebellar development.
    D. **Direct trauma to the posterior fossa with rupture of cerebellar bridging veins or the occipital sinuses.** This is seen primarily in term infants. Most ICPH is unilateral and focal with a predilection to the right cerebellar hemisphere.
  V. **Clinical presentation.** An ICPH is unique in causing unexplained motor agitation, in addition to respiratory compromise, apnea, and breathing irregularities. Otherwise, the general symptoms of ICH are present as well.
  VI. **Diagnosis.** CT and MRI have superior ability over US in diagnosing ICPH. However, US done via the mastoid fontanel can provide additional information.
  VII. **Management.** All management modalities presented for other ICH patients apply to infants with confirmed or suspected ICPH. For infants at risk for ICPH, the added combination of shock and acidosis is closely related and warrants diagnostic efforts specific for ICPH.
  VIII. **Prognosis.** Infants with ICPH usually require longer periods of mechanical ventilation. They will need close neurodevelopmental assessment, much as required with other types of ICH. In general, cerebellar hemorrhages seen only on MRI have much better prognosis than those detectable by US.

GERMINAL MATRIX AND INTRAVENTRICULAR HEMORRHAGE

I. **Definition.** IVH is the most common CNS acute complication of a preterm birth. The occurrence is greatly associated with the persistent presence of the GM. Chorioamnionitis, acidosis, birth asphyxia, shock, blood pressure fluctuations, and respiratory distress associated with hypocapnia, hypercapnia, hypoxemia, or mechanical ventilation are common related problems.

The GM, located between the caudate nucleus and the ependymal lining of the lateral ventricle, is normally not seen on cranial US. When GM hemorrhage occurs, it becomes readily identified by US and is seen as subependymal bleeding originating between the groove of the thalamus and the head of the caudate nucleus. Bleeding may be confined to the GM, or it may rupture into either lateral ventricle and thereby become a unilateral or bilateral GM/IVH.

By 36 weeks' postconceptional age, the GM has involuted for most infants. If IVH occurs in term infants, it originates most often in the choroid plexus; however, residual subependymal GM may also be a point of origin. Following IVH, further insult by venous thromboses may result in thalamic infarction.

II. **Incidence.** The overall occurrence of IVH in preterm infants <1500 g is about 18% to 25%. Rates vary by gestation, with the greatest risk of GM/IVH in preterm infants with birthweights <750 g. Because IVH is rarely seen in term infants, their incidence rates are exceptionally low and associated with birth-related injury or asphyxia. Curiously, 2% to 3% of seemingly normal term infants, when studied prospectively, have been noted to have asymptomatic IVH.

III. **Pathophysiology.** The GM is a highly vascularized area. The GM vessels exhibit a variety of characteristics that underlie the fragility and propensity to hemorrhage such as absence of a complete basal lamina, a fenestrated lining, and high morphometric ratio of diameter to wall thickness. The GM begins to involute after 34 weeks' postconceptional age, and thus, the peculiar vulnerability and predilection for GM/IVH for preterm infants lessens but is not totally removed. Late preterm infants (34–37 weeks' gestation) may have IVH that reflects those of early preterm infants. **Fluctuations in cerebral blood flow (CBF)** play an important role in the pathogenesis of GM/IVH because sick premature infants have **pressure-passive cerebral circulation.** A sudden rise or fall in systemic blood pressure can result in an increase in CBF with subsequent rupture of the GM vessels. Decreases in CBF can also result in ischemic injury to the GM vessels and surrounding tissues, making them prone to secondary rupture following reperfusion.

The unique deep venous anatomy at the level of the foramen of Monroe and the open communication between the GM vessels and the venous circulation contribute to the danger of abrupt or sharp fluctuations in cerebral venous pressure. Given this anatomic proximity, rupture through the GM subependymal layer results in entrance of blood into the lateral ventricles in nearly 80% of affected infants.

A. **Neuropathologic consequences of intraventricular hemorrhage**

1. **Germinal matrix ventricular-subventricular zone contains the migrating cells of origin for the cerebral cortex.** It is the site of production of neurons and glial cells of the cerebral cortex and basal ganglia. GM destruction may result in impairment of myelination, brain growth, and subsequent cortical development. Moreover, in preterm infants, GM/IVH leads to reduction of cerebral perfusion in the first 2 weeks after the hemorrhage. The reduction was found to be most severe around day 5 and was irrespective of the IVH grade.

2. **Periventricular hemorrhagic infarction** is venous in origin, associated with severe and usually asymmetric IVH, and invariably occurs on the side with the larger amount of intraventricular blood. It is a distinct pathologic event following venous stasis; it is often mistakenly described as an "extension" of IVH, of which it is not. Moreover, PVHI is neuropathologically distinct from periventricular leukomalacia (PVL). See preceding discussion under PVHI.

3. **Posthemorrhagic hydrocephalus** is more common in infants with the highest grade of hemorrhage. It is most frequently attributable to obliterative arachnoiditis either over the convexities of the cerebral hemispheres with occlusion of the arachnoid villi or in the posterior fossa with obstruction of outflow of the fourth ventricle. Rarely, aqueductal stenosis is caused by an acute clot or reactive gliosis.

4. **Periventricular leukomalacia** is a frequent accompaniment of IVH but is not directly caused by IVH. PVL is an ischemic brain injury followed by necrosis of periventricular white matter adjacent to the lateral ventricles. It is usually a nonhemorrhagic event resulting from hypotension, apnea, and other hypoxic ischemic events known to decrease CBF. Most PVL lesions are symmetrical in distribution.

IV. **Risk factors. Prematurity and respiratory distress syndrome have remained as the most closely related clinical circumstances to GM/IVH.** Other risk factors associated with the development of IVH include small for gestational age, male sex, and hypercarbia. As mentioned earlier, the immature cerebrovascular structures of preterm infants are extremely vulnerable to volume and pressure changes and to hypoxic and acidotic changes. Secondarily, respiratory distress and its attendant limitations for oxygenation further attenuate the immature vasculature of the preterm brain. The possible "overzealous" ventilatory maneuver performed to correct for the respiratory failure may adversely affect cerebral perfusion leading to GM venous congestion. Birth asphyxia, pneumothorax, shock/hypotension, acidosis, hypothermia, and therapeutic volume and/or osmolar overloads all serve to multiply the risk for GM/IVH. Even procedures that we perceive as routine in the care of premature infants may also be contributory, such as tracheal suctioning, abdominal examination, and handling to reposition or to instill mydriatics for an eye examination.

Of growing importance for the understanding of preterm GM/IVH is the possible role of fetal and neonatal inflammatory responses. Chorioamnionitis and funisitis may be harbingers of postnatal cerebral vascular events leading up to GM/IVH. Fetal inflammatory responses and subsequent neonatal hypotension and sepsis are closely related processes to IVH. Mediators of an inflammatory response, such as cytokines, have vasoactive properties that may be the source of exaggerated blood pressure changes that overwhelm the pressure-passive state of the GM.

V. **Clinical presentation.** The clinical presentation is diverse, and diagnosis requires neuroimaging for confirmation. The clinical symptoms may mimic those of other ICH or common neonatal disorders such as metabolic disturbances, asphyxia, sepsis, or meningitis. IVH may be totally asymptomatic, or there may be subtle symptoms, for example, a bulging fontanel, a sudden drop in hematocrit, apnea, bradycardia, acidosis, seizures, changes in muscle tone, or changes in level of consciousness. A catastrophic syndrome may accompany an extensive IVH. It is characterized by a precipitous decrease in hematocrit, a rapid onset of stupor or coma, respiratory failure, seizures, decerebrate posturing or a profound flaccid quadriparesis, and fixed pupils.

VI. **Diagnosis**

A. **Cranial ultrasound.** Cranial US (see Chapter 12 for imaging examples) is the procedure of choice for screening and diagnosis. CT and MRI are acceptable alternatives but are more expensive and require transport to the imaging service. They are valuable for a more definitive diagnosis or documentation of static brain injury before discharge from the hospital. Two systems for classifying GM/IVH have been advanced for clinical use. The older and most time honored has been that of Papile, based originally on CT but adapted for interpretation of cranial US. The second is the classification promulgated by Volpe, based also on cranial US. The utility of classification schema resides in the ability of clinicians to communicate degrees of severity and to have a source of information for comparison of lesions as well as having a means to follow progression or regression and recovery of the initial insult of IVH. **The GM/IVH classification by Papile** (updated in 2002) gives grades I to IV. Grades I and II are small hemorrhages. **Grade I** is hemorrhage only seen in the GM (~40% of all IVHs). **Grade II** shows hemorrhage from the GM extending into the lateral ventricles but without ventricular dilation (~25% of all IVHs). **Grade III** shows hemorrhage filling >50% of the lateral ventricles that are consequently enlarged (~20% of all IVHs). **Grade IV** is marked by extension of the hemorrhage into the surrounding brain white matter parenchyma (~15% of all IVHs).

A cranial US is indicated for screening sick preterm infants for IVH from the first day of life and throughout the hospitalization. Typically, a cranial US is done between day 1 and day 7, depending on the clinical presentation and institutional protocols, keeping in mind that 50% of GM/IVH may occur on day 1, but 90% have occurred by day 4 of life. Of all GM/IVH identified by day 4 of life, 20% to 40% will progress to more extensive hemorrhage during the first 7 to 10 days of life. Most clinicians obtain a final cranial US, CT, or MRI before discharge, or at 36 weeks' postconceptional age.

B. **Near-infrared spectroscopy** is a bedside monitor that measures real-time brain tissue oxygenation, which can reflect CBF and loss of autoregulation. Studies have correlated changes on the near-infrared spectroscopy monitor with increased IVH in preterm neonates.

C. **Amplitude electroencephalogram** may be associated with a depression in the background activity as well as dissimilarity between right and left waves in the case of unilateral IVH.

D. **Laboratory studies.** CSF initially shows elevated red and white blood cells, with elevated protein concentration. The degree of elevation of CSF protein correlates approximately with the severity of the hemorrhage. It is frequently difficult to distinguish IVH from a "traumatic tap." Within a few days after hemorrhage, the CSF becomes xanthochromic, with a decreased glucose concentration as in other forms of ICH. Often, the CSF shows a persistent increase in white blood cells and protein and a decreased glucose level, making it difficult to rule out meningitis.

VII. **Management**

A. **Prenatal prevention**

1. **Avoidance of premature delivery.**

2. **Transportation in utero.**

3. **Data suggest that active preterm labor may be a risk factor for early intraventricular hemorrhage and there may be a protective role for cesarean delivery.** However, Anderson et al showed that cesarean birth before the active phase of labor resulted in a lower frequency of severe IVH and less progression to severe IVH, although it did not affect the overall incidence of IVH. In a study by Durie et al, there was no correlation between mode of delivery and the incidence of IVH in very low birthweight infants who are presenting by the vertex.

4. **Antenatal steroid therapy.** Several large multicenter trials have shown a clear efficacy of antenatal steroids in reducing IVH. In 1 study, the incidence of GM/IVH was 2- to 3-fold lower in infants whose mothers received a complete course of antenatal steroids compared with those whose mothers received no steroids or an incomplete course (<48 hours). Moreover, this beneficial effect appears to be independent of the improvement in respiratory status. The prevention of IVH may be a composite effect of enhanced vascular integrity, decreased respiratory distress, and possibly altered cytokine production. Blickstein and coworkers have reported that antenatal steroids (given between 24 and 32 weeks' gestation) as a completed course (48 hours) resulted in a 2.5 times lower incidence of GM/IVH (7.7% vs 19.4%) for singleton and multiple births.

B. **Postnatal prevention**

1. **Avoid birth asphyxia.**

2. **Avoid large fluctuations in blood pressure.**

3. **Avoid rapid infusion of volume expanders or hypertonic solutions.**

4. Use prompt but cautious cardiovascular support to prevent hypotension.
5. Correct acid-base abnormalities.
6. Correct abnormalities of coagulation.
7. Avoid poorly synchronized mechanical ventilation. Consider sedation and, in difficult situations, pharmacologic paralysis.
8. Maintaining a midline head position for premature neonates can be beneficial because it allows for unobstructed drainage of the jugular veins, which prevents cerebral venous congestion that may make neonates prone to IVH.
9. Postnatal pharmacologic intervention with indomethacin. Ment et al reported in 1994 that low-dose prophylactic indomethacin significantly lowered the incidence and severity of IVH but did not appear to be of benefit in the prevention or extension of early IVH. Subsequent reports over the ensuing years have confirmed that on balance, in the total experience with indomethacin, a generally favorable preventive effect of the drug on IVH seems apparent, particularly in male patients. The use of "prophylactic" indomethacin remains *controversial because the IVH protective effect does not translate generally into a better neurodevelopment*. However, on long-term follow-up of school-age preterm infants when male and female patients are analyzed separately, a clear cognitive benefit is apparent in male but not female patients. Much of the controversy today surrounding low-dose prophylactic indomethacin therapy for the prevention or amelioration of GM/IVH involves the continuing concerns for indomethacin-related complications of necrotizing enterocolitis, spontaneous intestinal perforation, and decreased renal function (albeit transient in most cases). The use of other prostaglandins inhibitors, such as ibuprofen, for patent ductus arteriosus closure is not associated with a likewise neuroprotective action.

C. Management of acute hemorrhage
1. General supportive care to maintain a normal blood volume and a stable acid-base status.
2. Avoid fluctuations of arterial and venous blood pressures.
3. Follow-up serial imaging (cranial US or CT) to detect progressive hydrocephalus (see Chapter 97).

VIII. Prognosis
A. Short-term outcome of GM/IVH is directly related to birthweight, gestational age, and the ensuing severity of the hemorrhagic insult to the immature brain. The early mortality rates (first 14 days) are 12%, 24%, 32%, and 45% for grade I, II, III, and IV hemorrhages, respectively, among infants whose birthweight is <750 g. Posthemorrhagic ventricular dilation is mostly observed among infants with grade III (75% and 77%) and grade IV (83% and 66%) hemorrhage whose birthweight is below or above 750 g, respectively.
B. Long-term major neurologic sequelae of GM/IVH depend primarily on the extent of associated parenchymal injury, laterality, and any added effects of the short-term complications. The incidence of major neurologic sequelae (spastic motor deficits, major cognitive deficits) after minor degrees of hemorrhage is slightly higher than that in infants without hemorrhage and increases to approximately 50% in infants with severe hemorrhage; a higher incidence occurs in infants with IVH complicated by periventricular hemorrhagic infarction or cystic PVL, or both.

The rate of disability rises with immaturity. As an illustration, in the multicenter EPIPAGE study that enrolled 1954 infants, it was reported that <32 weeks' gestation cerebral palsy rates with isolated grade I to III IVH increased with immaturity, from 5% in infants born at 31 to 32 weeks to 10% to 15% in those born at 27 to 30 weeks and 33% in those born at 24 to 26 weeks.

The major determinant of outcome is the presence and severity of associated periventricular hemorrhagic infarction. In a recent study, the mortality rate for such infants was 59%, whereas it was only 8% for infants with the IVH grade III. Among the survivors, 87% exhibited major motor deficits, and 68% had cognitive function <80% of normal. The motor deficits correlated with the topography of the parenchymal lesions and thus consisted of either spastic hemiparesis or asymmetrical spastic quadriparesis. In more recent reports, the incidence of major motor deficits has been lower (ie, ~50% in 36 surviving infants <32 weeks of gestational age and 60% in 30 surviving infants <2500 g birthweight).

104 Intrauterine (Fetal) Growth Restriction

I. **Definitions.** Fetal growth restriction (FGR)/intrauterine growth restriction (IUGR) and small for gestational age (SGA) are sometimes used interchangeably but are not synonymous. **FGR and IUGR are the same conditions** where intrinsic fetal pathology exists or when placental support for the fetus is compromised, resulting in fetal hypoxia and undernourishment, and a pathologic restriction of the fetal genetic potential for growth. **SGA** describes an infant whose weight is lower than the population norms or a predetermined cutoff weight. Most commonly, **SGA infants** are defined as having a birthweight below the 10th percentile for gestational age and gender, or >2 standard deviations below the mean for gestational age. It can occur following a pathological process (FGR/IUGR) or just represent a small infant based on constitiutional factors (maternal weight, height, ethnicity, parity), known as **constitutional SGA**. FGR/IUGR infants are not all SGA, and SGA infants are not all FGR. It has been proposed that "SGA should be based on growth percentiles, and FGR be based on evidence of pathologic growth." This distinction between constitutional SGA and pathologic FGR has important implications for fetal monitoring, risks of perinatal morbidity and mortality, and the optimal timing of delivery. FGR increases the risk of fetal mortality 10- to 20-fold compared to an appropriately grown fetus. Constitutionally small infants are not at an increased risk of perinatal mortality or morbidity.

FGR (as opposed to IUGR) is used more often recently, especially in the obstetric literature. **The American College of Obstetrics and Gynecology defines FGR as a fetus with an estimated fetal weight (EFW) <10% of gestational age.** It is the condition where infants have not achieved their optimal intrauterine growth potential. FGR infants are further classified as **symmetric or asymmetric** based on anthropometric measurements and by **onset as early or late onset**.

A. **Symmetric or asymmetric FGR**

1. **Symmetric fetal growth restriction** (head circumference, height, and weight all <10th percentile). The head circumference, length, and weight are all proportionately reduced for gestational age. Symmetric FGR is due to either decreased growth potential of the fetus (congenital infection or genetic disorder) or extrinsic conditions that are active very early in pregnancy. Features include: earlier insult in gestation, less common than asymmetric, accounts for approximately 30% of FGR cases, ponderal index (see Section VI.E.4 for definition) normal, malnutrition less pronounced, normal cell size with reduced cell number, and poor prognosis.

2. **Asymmetric fetal growth restriction (more common).** Fetal weight is reduced out of proportion to the length and head circumference. The head circumference and length are closer to the expected percentiles for gestational age than is the weight. In these infants, brain growth is usually spared. Common etiologies

include uteroplacental insufficiency, maternal malnutrition, and extrinsic conditions appearing late in pregnancy. Features include: occurs later in gestation, more common than symmetric growth restriction (70%–80% of cases), normal cell number but cell size is reduced, low ponderal index, more pronounced malnutrition, and good prognosis.

B. **Early or late onset FGR.** Early detection of FGR identifies infants at risk of mortality in utero, but is difficult based on fetal anthropometry (by measuring crown-rump length) alone. Estimation of fetal growth velocity with serial measurements may be useful to identify FGR. For example, a fetus with weight >10th percentile may be growth restricted if fetal growth velocity declines.

1. **Early onset FGR (<32 weeks' gestation).** Early onset is associated with sequential changes in Doppler studies that parallel worsening placental function. Typically, umbilical artery Doppler changes precede biophysical profile parameters. Early FGR is associated with more severe placental disease, fetal hypoxia and undernutrition, systemic cardiovascular adaptation, increased risks of preeclampsia in the mother, and increased risks of fetal mortality and neonatal morbidity.

2. **Late onset (>32 weeks' gestation).** Late FGR is more difficult to identify and has less characteristic Doppler changes (see further discussion later in the chapter).

II. **Incidence.** About 3% to 10% (up to 15% in some studies) of all pregnancies are associated with FGR, and 20% of stillborn infants are growth restricted. The prevalence of early FGR is 1% to 2%, and that of late FGR is 3% to 5%. The perinatal mortality rate is 5 to 20 times higher for growth-restricted fetuses, and serious short- and long-term morbidities are noted in half of the affected surviving infants. FGR is estimated to be the predominant cause for low birthweight in developing countries. It is estimated that a third of infants with birthweights <2500 g are in fact growth restricted and not premature. Term infants with birthweights less than the third percentile have a 10 times higher mortality than appropriate for gestational age (AGA) infants. In the United States, uteroplacental insufficiency is the leading cause of FGR. An estimated 5% to 10% of cases are secondary to congenital infection. Chromosomal and other genetic disorders are reported in 5% to 20% of FGR infants.

III. **Pathophysiology.** Fetal growth is influenced by fetal, maternal, and placental factors.

A. **Fetal factors**

1. **Fetal genotype.** Approximately 20% of birthweight variability in a given population is determined by fetal genotype. Genetic determinants of fetal growth have their greatest impact in early gestation during the period of rapid cell development. Racial and ethnic backgrounds influence size at birth irrespective of socioeconomic status. Males weigh an average of 150 to 200 g more than females at birth. This weight increase occurs late in gestation. Birth order affects fetal size; infants born to primiparous women weigh less than subsequent siblings.

2. **Genetic causes.** Five to twenty percent of FGR is caused by genetic factors which include chromosomal anomalies, single gene disorders, and other genetic factors. **Chromosome anomalies** include: Aneuploidy (like Trisomy 21, 18, 13, and 16), uniparental disomy (of chromosomes 6, 14, 16), partial deletions or duplications (Cri du chat syndrome, Wolf Hirschhorn syndrome), ring chromosome, and aberrant genomic imprinting. The finding of symmetric FGR prior to 20 weeks of gestation suggests aneuploidy as the cause, most commonly trisomy 18. **Single gene disorders** such as Russell Silver syndrome, Bloom syndrome, Cornelia de Lange syndrome, and Fanconi anemia have been associated with FGR.

3. **Congenital malformations.** Congenital diaphragmatic hernia, abdominal wall defects (omphalocele and gastroschisis), renal agenesis or dysplasia, anencephaly, tracheoesophageal fistula, single umbilical artery, gastrointestinal atresia, Potter syndrome, anorectal malformation, and pancreatic agenesis are examples of

congenital anomalies associated with FGR. The frequency of FGR increases as the number of congenital defects increases.

4. **Cardiovascular anomalies may lead to abnormal fetal growth** (with the possible exception of transposition of the great vessels and tetralogy of Fallot). Greatest risk is in fetuses with major CHD (FGR is found in one-fifth of infants with major CHD). Abnormal hemodynamics are thought to be the basis of some cases of FGR.

5. **Congenital infection.** TORCHZ infections (*t*oxoplasmosis, *o*ther [syphilis, HIV, malaria], *r*ubella, *c*ytomegalovirus, *h*erpes simplex virus, and *Z*ika virus) are often associated with FGR and account for 5% to 10% of FGR fetuses. The incidence of FGR is highest when infection occurs in the first trimester. The clinical findings in different congenital infections are nonspecific and overlap considerably. Cytomegalovirus and rubella are associated with severe FGR. The most common infectious etiology of FGR in developed countries is CMV. Rubella causes damage during organogenesis and results in a decreased number of cells, whereas cytomegalovirus infection results in cytolysis and localized necrosis within the fetus. Zika virus is associated with severe microcephaly.

6. **Inborn errors of metabolism.** Transient neonatal diabetes, galactosemia, and phenylketonuria are other disorders associated with FGR. Single-gene defects affecting insulin-like growth factors or their receptors, or associated with impaired insulin secretion or action are often associated with impaired fetal growth (see Chapter 100).

B. **Maternal factors** (Table 104–1)

1. **Reduced uteroplacental blood flow.** Maternal disorders such as preeclampsia-eclampsia, chronic renal vascular disease, and chronic hypertensive vascular disease often result in decreased uteroplacental blood flow and result in FGR. Impaired delivery of oxygen and other essential nutrients is thought to limit organ growth and musculoskeletal maturation. Risk of placental thrombi is increased in conditions of inherited thrombophilias.

2. **Maternal malnutrition.** Small maternal size (height and prepregnancy weight) and minimal maternal weight gain during pregnancy increase the risk of FGR. Low maternal body mass index, defined as (weight [kg]/height [m^2])/100, and maternal malnutrition (particularly decreased intake) influence fetal growth and birthweight. A balanced protein energy supplementation during pregnancy decreases the risk of FGR.

3. **Multiple pregnancies.** Impaired growth results from failure to provide optimal nutrition for >1 fetus in utero. In total, 15% to 30% of multiple pregnancies develop FGR; the condition is more common in monochorionic twins affected by twin-to-twin transfusion syndrome. Up until the 28th to 30th week of pregnancy, fetuses in multiple pregnancies have growth rates similar to singletons; however, after this period, there is a 15% to 20% decrease in the growth rate. The degree of FGR increases with increasing number of fetuses.

4. **Maternal substance use.** See also Chapter 102.

   a. **Cigarettes and alcohol.** Chronic abuse of cigarettes or alcohol is demonstrably associated with FGR. The effects of alcohol and tobacco seem to be dose dependent, with FGR becoming more serious and predictable with heavy abuse.

   b. **Heroin and cocaine.** Maternal heroin and cocaine addictions are associated with FGR mediated by placental insufficiency or direct toxic effect on the fetus.

   c. **Others.** Other drugs and chemical agents causing FGR include known teratogens, antimetabolites, and therapeutic agents such as trimethadione, warfarin, valproic acid, and phenytoin. Each of these agents causes characteristic malformation syndromes. Repeated use of antenatal steroids and lithium use are also associated with low birthweight.

Table 104–1. **MATERNAL FACTORS IN FETAL GROWTH RESTRICTION**

Pregnancy-induced hypertension (>140/90 mm Hg)
Weight gain (<0.9 kg every 4 weeks)
Uterus fundus growth lag (<4 cm for gestational age)
Cyanotic heart disease
Heavy smoking
Residing at high altitude
Substance abuse and drugs
Maternal medication (warfarin, steroids, anticonvulsants)
Short stature
Low socioeconomic class
Anemia (hematocrit <30%)
Asthma
Prepregnancy weight and height (<50 kg, body mass index <20 kg/m^2)
Prior history of FGR
Chronic hypertension, diabetes mellitus
Collagen vascular disorders such as lupus
Renal disease
Severe maternal malnutrition
Multiple pregnancy
Low or advanced maternal age (<16 years, >35 years)
Preeclampsia
Inherited thrombophilias
Maternal infections (TORCHZ, malaria, tuberculosis)

FGR, fetal growth restriction; TORCHZ, toxoplasmosis, other, rubella, cytomegalovirus, herpes simplex virus, and Zika virus.

5. **Maternal hypoxemia.** Hypoxemia is seen in mothers with hemoglobinopathies, especially sickle cell disease, and they often have growth-restricted births. Chronic hypertension, preeclampsia, chronic renal insufficiency, SLE, and pregestational diabetes (classes C, D, R, F) can decrease fetal perfusion and lead to hypoxia. Infants born at high altitudes tend to have lower mean birthweights for gestational age.

6. **Other maternal factors.** Young maternal age, advanced maternal age, short interpregnancy interval, uterine anomalies, maternal race, lower socioeconomic status, living in a developing country, primiparous, grand multiparous, low prepregnancy weight, and poor weight gain during pregnancy are associated with subnormal birthweight. Maternal hyperhomocysteinemia is also associated with low birthweight.

7. **DNA damage** measured by micronucleus (MN) formation may play a role in FGR. MNs are formed by the lagging chromosomal fragments during anaphase in both mitosis and meiosis. Increased MN count in maternal

lymphocytes at 20 weeks' gestation is associated with increased risks of FGR and preeclampsia.

C. Placental factors

1. **Placental insufficiency.** In the first and second trimesters, fetal growth is determined mostly by inherent fetal growth potential. By the third trimester, placental factors (ie, an adequate supply of nutrients) assume major importance for fetal growth. When the duration of pregnancy exceeds the nurturing capacity of the placenta, placental insufficiency results with subsequent impaired fetal growth. This phenomenon occurs mostly in postterm gestations but may occur at any time during gestation. Presence of asymmetrically grown fetus, low amniotic fluid index, and umbilical artery abnormalities (abnormal waveforms, absent or reversed end-diastolic flows) together suggests placental insufficiency.

2. **Uteroplacental insufficiency.** It is the most common reason for FGR and occurs in almost 70% of infants with FGR. Impaired oxygen extraction and nutrient delivery (glucose and amino acids) leads to fetal hypoglycemia and hypoxia. The latter is associated with decrease in cell size and number, lighter brain weight, and lower DNA content. Small placental volume and a reduction in terminal villi are seen in FGR placentas.

3. **Placenta structural abnormalities.** Various anatomic factors, such as multiple infarcts, velamentous umbilical cord insertion, marginal cord insertion, bilobate placenta, circumvallate placenta, umbilical vascular thrombosis, and hemangiomas, are described in FGR placentas. FGR is twice as common with a 2-vessel-cord pregnancy as compared with 3-vessel-cord pregnancies. Premature placental separation may reduce the surface area exchange, resulting in impaired fetal growth. An adverse intrauterine environment is apt to affect placental and fetal development; hence, FGR infants usually have small placentas. One study noted that those with abnormal umbilical artery waveform abnormalities but normal uterine artery waveforms were more likely to deliver at higher gestational age, have higher risks of aneuploidy, and have chronic intervillositis and perivillous fibrin deposition, both of which carry high recurrence risks.

4. **Placental metabolic derangements.** FGR is associated with downregulation of placental amino acid and lipoprotein lipase transporter expression and activity at birth. These derangements lead to lower plasma amino acid levels and decreased fatty acid transfer. It is unknown whether these changes are a cause or a consequence of FGR. Placental genetic imprinting may also play a role in some cases of FGR (eg, alterations of the placenta-specific *IGF-2* gene in knockout mice have produced FGR).

5. **Fetal endocrine responses.** Include alterations in the hypothalamic-pituitary axis, resulting in elevated corticotropin-releasing hormone, adrenocorticotropic hormone, and cortisol with a decrease in insulin-like growth factor-1 (IGF-1). Thyroid-stimulating hormone is high, but thyroxine and triiodothyronine are low, as are serum vitamin D and osteocalcin. High cortisol levels are associated with decreased postnatal catch-up growth and delayed neurodevelopmental outcomes.

6. **Confined placental mosaicism.** Confined placental mosaicism (CPM) refers to chromosomal mosaicism in the placenta, but not in the fetus. It usually involves a trisomy and is strongly associated with FGR. CPM has been identified in about 10% of otherwise idiopathic FGR cases and in one-third of FGR cases associated with placental infarction and decidual vasculopathy. The severity of CPM-associated FGR depends on the chromosomes involved, the proportion of mosaic cells, and the presence of uniparental disomy.

IV. **Risk factors.** Related to fetal, maternal, or placental pathophysiologic factors (see previous text) (Table 104–2).

V. **Clinical presentation.** The maternal history may raise the index of suspicion regarding suboptimal fetal growth. The infant will have a reduced birthweight for gestational

Table 104–2. **PLACENTAL FACTORS IN FETAL GROWTH RESTRICTION**

Two-vessel cord (single umbilical artery)
Abruptio placentae, placental hematoma, placenta previa, chronic abruption
Hemangioma
Placental weight (weight <350 g)
Infarction
Aberrant cord insertion (velamentous cord)
Umbilical vessel thrombosis
Circumvallate placentation
Confined placental mosaicism
Massive perivillous fibrin deposition (immune mediated)
Chronic villitis of unknown etiology
Placental mesenchymal dysplasia
Placental infections (tuberculosis, malaria)

age. Using growth charts and the Ballard score can help assess gestational age and intrauterine and postnatal growth. See Figures 6–2 through 6–6.

VI. **Diagnosis**

A. **Establishing gestational age.** Determining the correct gestational age is imperative. The last menstrual period, size of the uterus, time of quickening, and early ultrasound measurements are used to determine gestational age. (See Chapter 6.)

B. **Fetal assessment.** FGR evolves from a preclinical phase to clinically apparent growth delay and fetal compromise before the onset of labor. Liver size (hence a decrease in abdominal circumference) is affected before head and body growth are affected. Abnormalities in placental perfusion in the maternal compartment increase uterine artery flow resistance. When fetal villi are affected, umbilical artery end-diastolic flow patterns get altered (see below). Finally, when fetal arterial partial pressure of oxygen is compromised, middle cerebral artery (MCA) Doppler flow velocities are affected. When FGR develops early, there is a greater degree of vascular abnormality in the maternal and fetal compartments of the placenta and a 40% to 70% rate of associated preeclampsia. Umbilical artery pulsatility index is elevated. When FGR develops late, cerebral and umbilical Doppler abnormalities may occur independently of each other. Failure of diagnosis or surveillance in late-onset FGR increases risks of stillbirth.

1. **Clinical diagnosis.** Manual estimations of weight, serial measurements for uterine fundus height, and maternal estimates of fetal activity are simple clinical measures.

2. **Ultrasonography.** Because of its reliability to date pregnancy and to detect impaired fetal growth by anthropomorphic measurements and fetal anomalies, ultrasonography currently offers the greatest promise for diagnosis. The following anthropomorphic measurements are used in combination to predict growth impairment with a high degree of accuracy.

a. **Estimated fetal weight.** To assess for FGR, 4 biometric measures are commonly used: biparietal diameter, head circumference, abdominal circumference, and femur length. The biometric measurements can be combined to generate an EFW. The estimate may deviate from the birthweight by up to 20%. The liver is the first organ to suffer the effects of growth restriction due to redistribution of ductus venosus blood flow to the heart and a decrease in glycogen deposition in the liver. Reduced growth of the abdominal circumference (<5 mm/wk) is the earliest sign of asymmetric growth restriction and diminished glycogen storage. A recent study noted a >17-fold higher risk of morbidity if the fetus was growth restricted (<10th percentile for age) and the abdominal circumference growth velocity was in the lowest decile.

Nomograms exist to monitor fetal growth using EFW. An EFW <10th percentile can identify FGR but may not distinguish it from a constitutionally SGA fetus. An EFW less than the third percentile and the abdominal circumference growth rate together are more likely to identify true FGR, and EFW estimates with abnormal Doppler studies can identify the fetus at increased risk of adverse outcomes (see later discussion). The World Health Organization (WHO) fetal growth charts for EFW and ultrasound biometric measurements are based on data from low-risk healthy pregnancies in 10 countries. Individualized growth charts taking into account maternal physiologic characteristics such as race, ethnicity, parity, and height, and fetal characteristics such as gender are also now available (INTERGROWTH-21st Project).

Term optimal weight (TOW) is defined as the optimal weight based on fetal weight curves of healthy infants born at term. For an individual pregnancy, fetal growth can be combined with TOW to show the **gestation-related optimal growth (GROW)** curve. GROW charts adjusted for maternal height, weight, parity, and ethnicity are available at www.gestation.net (accessed September 14, 2018).

b. **Ratio of head circumference to abdominal circumference.** This ratio normally changes as pregnancy progresses. In the second trimester, the head circumference is greater than the abdominal circumference. At about 32 to 36 weeks' gestation, the ratio is 1:1, and after 36 weeks, the abdominal measurements become larger. Persistence of a head-to-abdomen ratio <1 late in gestation is predictive of late-onset FGR.

c. **Femur length.** Femur length appears to correlate well with crown-heel length and provides an early and reproducible measurement of length. Serial measurements of femur length are as effective as head measurements for detecting early-onset FGR.

d. **Placental morphology and amniotic fluid assessment** may help in distinguishing a constitutionally small fetus from a growth-restricted fetus. For example, placental aging with oligohydramnios suggests FGR and fetal jeopardy, whereas normal placental morphology with a normal amount of amniotic fluid suggests a constitutionally small fetus.

e. **Placental volume measurements** may be helpful in predicting subsequent fetal growth. Placental weight and/or volume is decreased before fetal growth decreases. FGR with decreased placental size is more likely to be associated with fetal acidosis. Placental volume correlates with placental flow indices.

3. **Doppler measurements** in both maternal and various fetal vascular beds are increasingly used to detect, monitor, and optimize time of delivery in FGR infants. Doppler studies are more helpful in diagnosing moderate to severe FGR than mild FGR. The various groups of vessels used are as follows:

a. **Uterine artery flow abnormalities.** Used to predict FGR as early as 12 to 14 weeks. A persistent abnormality at 23 to 24 weeks has an approximate 75% sensitivity in predicting early FGR.

b. **Umbilical artery flow abnormalities.** Used to evaluate placental insufficiency, particularly in high-risk pregnancies. Normally, the umbilical artery (UA) resistance declines with pregnancy. Increased pulsatility index (PI), decreased end-diastolic velocity (EDV), and absent EDV (AEDV) or reversed EDV (REDV) occur with worsening fetal compromise. AEDV and REDV are associated with 20% to 68% mortality. Decreased EDV is seen when 30% of placental flow is attenuated, and AEDV/REDV is noted when 60% to 70% of placental flow is affected. AEDV and REDV are associated with a 4.0- and 10.6-fold increased risk of mortality, respectively, compared to those with normal Doppler.

c. **Fetal cerebral arterial flow.** Usually studied in the MCA as a PI (MCA PI) and MCA peak systolic velocity (MCA PSV). With worsening FGR, MCA PSV increases. Abnormal MCA PI precedes MCA PSV changes. Changes in MCA PI are not as consistent in predicting mortality, although decreased MCA resistance is associated with worse perinatal outcomes. MCA Doppler changes better identify late-onset FGR when the predictive ability of cerebroplacental ratio (CPR) decreases (see Section VI.B.3.e).

d. **Doppler venous flow studies** of the vena cava, umbilical vein (UV), and ductus venosus (DV) provide information about fetal cardiovascular and respiratory responses. Decreased venous blood flow in the UV and an abnormal deep or retrograde "a" wave in DV are suggestive of ventricular decompensation. Changes in venous flow are usually late and represent more severe decompensation. Absent or reversed DV flow correlates with acidosis and is associated with 63% to 100% mortality.

e. **Cerebroplacental ratio .** The CPR quantifies the redistribution of cardiac output by dividing the Doppler PI of the MCA with that of the UA: CPR = MCA PI/UA PI. Adverse outcomes have been associated with a CPR ratio of <1 or <1.08. CPR can be affected in about 25% of term SGA fetuses. The CPR seems to be more sensitive to hypoxia than its individual components. Gestational age–specific CPR nomograms are available and can accurately identify brain sparing in late FGR and those at risk of adverse outcomes. Adverse outcomes with FGR are rare when UA Doppler flows are normal, whereas abnormal CPR regardless of fetal size or the time of onset of FGR (early vs late onset) increases the need for operative delivery, admissions to the neonatal intensive care unit, perinatal mortality, and postnatal neurologic deficits. CPR abnormalities precede abnormalities in biophysical profile and UA or MCA abnormalities. An online CPR calculator is also available at https://fetalmedicine.org/research/thirdTrimesterDoppler (accessed September 18, 2018). A decrease in expected CPR measurement after 28 weeks' gestation is highly sensitive in diagnosing late-onset FGR.

Doppler study abnormalities outlined earlier correlate with fetal acid-base status and need for intervention. The frequencies of monitoring are shown in Table 104–3.

4. **Biophysical profile score.** Used for noninvasive fetal monitoring. The 5 components biophysical profile (BPP) scoring show a reliable and reproducible relationship with fetal pH irrespective of gestational age. A BPP <4 is associated with pH <7.20, and BPP <2 is 100% sensitive to detect fetal academia. However, BPP is less sensitive to detect longitudinal deterioration.

5. **Cardiotocography.** Used more commonly in Europe to assess the timing of delivery for situations wherein significant fetal acidosis is suspected. It is a component of BPP and is limited when used alone. In an FGR fetus, a short-term variability of <3.5 milliseconds predicts UA pH <7.20.

6. **Placental magnetic resonance imaging.** This can assess the severity of FGR on the basis of decreased placental volume and changes in placental thickness-to-volume ratio. Fetal demise can also be predicted by abnormal signal intensity.

C. **Diagnosing compensated versus decompensated fetus.** Persistence of uteroplacental insufficiency results in fetal adaptation to maintain adequate cerebral oxygenation and growth.

1. **Uteroplacental insufficiency results in increased placental vascular resistance and fetal hypoxemia by reducing umbilical blood flow.** The fetus responds by redistribution of blood to the brain (brain sparing) through cerebral

Table 104–3. **FREQUENCY OF MONITORING IN EARLY AND LATE FGR**

	Doppler Studies	Frequency of Monitoring
Early-onset FGR	Elevated UA Doppler indices (>2 SD for age)	Biweekly Weekly BPP
	Low MCA PI or CPR	Weekly Doppler + BPP
	UA absent EDV (AEDV)	Doppler 2×/week + BPP
	UA reversed EDV (REDV), increased Doppler indices, and/or oligohydramnios	3×/week Doppler + BPP, daily CTG
	Absent/reversed DV a-wave	Daily monitoring + BPP
Late-onset FGR	Elevated Doppler	Weekly Doppler + BPP
	Low MCA PI or CPR	2–3×/week Doppler + BPP

BPP, biophysical profile; CPR, cerebroplacental ratio; CTG, cardiotocography; DV, ductus venosus; EDV, end-diastolic flow; FGR, fetal growth restriction; FHR, fetal heart rate; MCA, middle cerebral artery; PI, pulsatility index; SD, standard deviation.

vasodilatation, mesenteric vasoconstriction, preferential shunting through the foramen ovale, increased fractional extraction of oxygen, polycythemia, and a relative decrease in fetal oxygen consumption. Fetal growth velocity and weight gain are decreased. Nonstress test (NST), BPP, and cardiotocography are normal. Decreased diastolic flow in the UA and increased diastolic component in the MCA may be seen. The fetus is hypoxemic but does not have cerebral hypoxemia at this stage.

2. **With worsening placental dysfunction,** fetal compromise may occur with cerebral hypoxemia and acidemia associated with no fetal weight gain, oligohydramnios, decreased fetal heart rate variability, and abnormal NST, cardiotocography, and BPP. UAs show AEDV followed by REDV. Deep "a" wave is seen in the DV, suggestive of ventricular dysfunction. With severe acidosis, MCA PI and MCA PSV decrease, suggesting the imminent collapse of the fetus.

3. **Acute fetal decompensation.** AEDV/REDV in UAs in early-onset FGR babies can be present up to 1 week before acute decompensation. Approximately 40% of fetuses with acidosis have AEDV/REDV pattern. MCA vasodilation with abnormal PI may be present for up to 2 weeks before acute deterioration in 50% to 80% of infants. MCA vasodilation may be independently associated with abnormal outcomes in late-onset FGR. Oligohydramnios develops in 20% to 30% of FGR infants about 1 week before acute deterioration (Table 104–4).

D. **Staging of fetal growth restriction and optimal timing of delivery.** No treatment has been shown to improve FGR. The assessment of fetal well-being and timely delivery are the major goals of management. Early delivery versus expectant management showed more disabilities in survivors delivered early. In term SGA infants as well, early delivery does not improve outcomes compared to expectant management. The optimal timing of delivery with FGR is determined by the severity of fetal compromise and the risk of stillbirth. Some have stratified FGR into stages as provided below to help determine the optimal time of delivery, whereas others have used Doppler studies for monitoring of fetal well-being (Table 104–3):

1. **Stage I (mild placental insufficiency):** Abnormal Doppler studies including CPR ratios.

2. **Stage II (severe uteroplacental insufficiency):** There is absent EDV in the UA. Delivery should be after 34 weeks with twice-a-week monitoring.

Table 104–4. SEQUENTIAL CHANGES OF DOPPLER STUDIES IN DECOMPENSATING FETAL GROWTH RESTRICTION

Initial changes	Decreased amniotic fluid index Increased uterine artery resistance with EDV
Early changes (in 50% 2–3 weeks before nonreactive FHR)	Decreased MCA resistance (brain sparing) Absent uterine artery EDV
Late changes (~6 days before nonreactive FHR)	Increased resistance in DV-reversed EDV in uterine artery
Very late changes (in 70%, 24 hours before changes in BPP)	Reversed flow in DV (absent or reversed a-wave in DV) and pulsatile flow in umbilical vein

BPP, biophysical profile; DV, ductus venosus; EDV, end-diastolic flow; FHR, fetal heart rate; MCA, middle cerebral artery.

3. **Stage III (fetal deterioration, low suspicion of fetal acidosis):** There is a reversal of EDV in the UA or DV PI >95th percentile. Risks of stillbirth and neurologic handicap are increased. Delivery should be around 32 weeks.
4. **Stage IV (fetal acidosis):** Spontaneous fetal decelerations, reduced variability or reversal of atrial flow on DV. Imminent risk of fetal demise. Deliver immediately.

E. **Neonatal assessment**
   1. **Reduced birthweight for gestational age.** This is the simplest method of diagnosing FGR. However, this method tends to misdiagnose constitutionally small infants.
   2. **Physical appearance.** When infants with congenital malformation syndromes and infections are excluded, the remaining groups of FGR infants have a characteristic physical appearance. These infants, in general, are thin with loose, peeling skin because of loss of subcutaneous tissue, a scaphoid abdomen, and a disproportionately large head.
   3. **Appropriate growth charts should be used.** Several standardized growth charts are available to assess intrauterine and postnatal growth. Fetal growth charts are now available (Chapter 6). Additional postnatal growth charts based on Centers for Disease Control and Prevention (CDC) and WHO data from birth to 36 months can be found at the CDC website: http://www.cdc.gov/growthcharts/ (accessed September 18, 2018).
   4. **Ponderal index.** The **ponderal index** is one of the anthropometric methods used to diagnose impaired fetal growth, especially to assess asymmetrical fetal growth restriction. It can be used to identify infants whose soft tissue mass is below normal for the stage of skeletal development. The higher the score, the higher the level of body fat. Ponderal index is recorded as a number in g/cm^3, but there are also percentile curves for ponderal index. Normal ponderal index is GA dependent, but is generally 2.2 to 3.0 g/cm^3. A ponderal index of <2 or <10% is abnormal and suggests asymmetrical FGR. Infants with constitutional or symmetric FGR typically have a normal ponderal index. Infants with asymmetric FGR have a low ponderal index. The formula for ponderal index is:

$$\text{Ponderal index in } g/cm^3 = [\text{weight (in g)} \times 100] \div [\text{length (in cm)}]^3$$

   5. **Ballard score.** Gestational age can also be assessed by means of the Ballard scoring system. This examination is accurate within 2 weeks of gestation in infants weighing <999 g at birth and is most accurate at 30 to 42 hours of age. (See Chapter 6.)

F. Neonatal complications of fetal growth restriction
   1. Hypoxia
      a. Perinatal asphyxia. FGR fetuses are at risk of hypoxia-ischemia at birth because they tolerate the stress of labor poorly. A large proportion of stillborn infants had FGR in utero.
      b. Persistent pulmonary hypertension. Many FGR infants are subjected to chronic intrauterine hypoxia, which results in abnormal thickening of the smooth muscles of the small pulmonary arterioles. This, in turn, reduces pulmonary blood flow and results in varying degrees of pulmonary artery hypertension. FGR infants are particularly at risk for persistent pulmonary hypertension.
      c. Respiratory distress syndrome. It is controversial whether FGR results in accelerated fetal pulmonary maturation due to chronic intrauterine stress. Respiratory distress syndrome may be seen less frequently in FGR infants; however, these infants are at higher risk of pulmonary morbidities such as bronchopulmonary dysplasia compared to appropriately grown infants.
      d. Meconium aspiration. Postterm FGR infants are particularly at risk for meconium aspiration.
      e. Patent ductus arteriosus. Conflicting data suggest that hemodynamically significant patent ductus arteriosus (PDA) may be bigger and occur earlier in FGR infants compared to AGA infants; nevertheless, spontaneous closure of PDA is more frequent in FGR infants with <1000 g birthweight. FGR infants with PDA are at greater risk for pulmonary hemorrhage, intraventricular hemorrhage (IVH), necrotizing enterocolitis (NEC), and renal failure.
   2. Hypothermia. Thermoregulation is compromised in FGR infants because of diminished subcutaneous fat insulation. Infants with FGR secondary to fetal malnutrition late in gestation tend to be thin as a result of the loss of subcutaneous fat.
   3. Metabolic
      a. Hypoglycemia. Carbohydrate metabolism is seriously disturbed, and FGR infants are highly susceptible to hypoglycemia as a consequence of diminished glycogen reserves and decreased capacity for gluconeogenesis. Oxidation of free fatty acids and triglycerides is reduced in FGR infants, which limits alternate fuel sources. Hyperinsulinism, excess sensitivity to insulin, and deficient catecholamine release during hypoglycemia suggest abnormalities of counterregulatory hormonal mechanisms during periods of hypoglycemia in FGR infants. Hypothermia may potentiate the problem of hypoglycemia as well.
      b. Hyperglycemia. FGR infants may have low insulin secretion, resulting in hyperglycemia.
      c. Hypocalcemia. Hypocalcemia may occur in asphyxiated FGR infants.
      d. Liver disease. FGR infants are at greater risk for developing cholestasis associated with parenteral nutrition. There is also an increased risk of non–fatty liver disease in children born SGA.
      e. Other. Hypertriglyceridemia, increased sympathetic tone, and reduced concentrations of IGF-1 have been associated with increased aortic intimal thickness in FGR infants.
   4. Hematologic disorders. Hyperviscosity and polycythemia may result from increased erythropoietin levels secondary to fetal hypoxia associated with FGR. Thrombocytopenia, neutropenia, and altered coagulation profile are also seen. Polycythemia may also contribute to hypoglycemia and lead to cerebral injury. There is an increased number of nucleated red cells secondary to extramedullary hematopoiesis. Persistent elevation of nucleated red cell counts is associated with worse prognosis.
   5. Altered immunity. FGR infants have decreased immunoglobulin G levels. In addition, the thymus is reduced in size by 50%, and peripheral blood

lymphocytes are decreased. Reduction in total white cell count, neutrophils, monocyte and lymphocyte subpopulations, and thrombocytopenia may occur, and selective suppression of helper and cytotoxic T cells can be seen.

6. **Others.** FGR infants are at increased risk of developing NEC, particularly when associated with an absent or reversed end-diastolic flow in UA Doppler. Preterm FGR infants are also at increased risk of pulmonary hemorrhage, chronic lung disease, more severe IVH, and renal failure.

VII. **Management.** Optimal management of the FGR fetus requires accurate identification of the fetus at risk of adverse outcome, prevention of stillbirth, and appropriate timing of delivery. Antenatal diagnosis is the key to proper management of FGR that allows for appropriate surveillance until delivery.

A. **History of risk factors.** The presence of maternal risk factors should alert the obstetrician to the likelihood of fetal growth retardation. Ultrasonography confirms the diagnosis. Correctable causes of impaired fetal growth warrant immediate attention.

B. **Delivery and resuscitation.** The optimal timing for delivery of FGR infants is still debated, but Doppler measurements provide an important tool for monitoring fetal well-being. Staging of FGR helps in both monitoring and optimizing the time of delivery (see Section VI.D and Table 104–3). FGR infants have a 2- to 3-fold increased risk of preterm delivery when fetal growth standards are used for diagnosis, and preterm delivery increases risks of mortality when delivered before 30 weeks. Outcomes are more favorable with cesarean delivery because the FGR fetus tolerates the stress of labor poorly. Skilled resuscitation should be available because perinatal depression is common.

C. **Prevention of heat loss.** Meticulous care should be taken to conserve body heat (see Chapter 8).

D. **Hypoglycemia.** Close monitoring of blood glucose levels is essential for all FGR infants. Hypoglycemia should be treated promptly with parenteral dextrose and early feeding (see Chapter 67).

E. **Hematologic disorders.** A central hematocrit reading should be obtained to detect polycythemia.

F. **Congenital infection.** FGR infants should be examined for congenital malformations or signs of congenital infections. Many intrauterine infections are clinically silent, and screening for these should be done routinely in FGR infants. At our institution, we consider evaluation for cytomegalovirus in FGR neonates without an underlying etiology. The placenta should be sent for histologic examination, and CPM should be sought.

G. **Genetic anomalies.** Screening for genetic anomalies should be done as indicated by the physical examination.

VIII. **Prognosis.** Mortality increases with decreasing gestational age when FGR is also present. Mortality decreases by 48% for each week that the fetus remains in utero before 30 weeks' gestation. At 24 to 26 weeks' gestation, survival is around 50% (EFW 500 g or ~26 weeks) and intact survival is approximately 20%. Survival improves by approximately 2% per day spent in utero. Intact survival between 26 and 28 weeks only improves to around 30%; survival improves to >90% by 32 weeks. Neonatal morbidities can be minimized by delivering at 38 weeks in late-onset FGR. Neurodevelopmental morbidities are seen 5 to 10 times more often in FGR infants compared with AGA infants and depend not only on the cause of FGR but also on the adverse events in the neonatal course (eg, perinatal depression or hypoglycemia). Many studies reveal evidence of minimal brain dysfunction, including hyperactivity, short attention span, and learning problems. Preterm FGR infants also show alterations in early neurobehavioral functions, such as attention-interaction capacity and cognitive and memory dysfunction, that persist. Increased risk of cerebral palsy, a wide spectrum of learning disabilities, mental retardation, pervasive developmental disorders, and neuropsychiatric disorders are seen in later years. The risk of morbidities is higher in term FGR infants. FGR infants who have normal Doppler studies have better outcomes than those with abnormal antenatal Doppler studies. Even mild FGR increases the risk of mortality and long-term development.

A. **Symmetric versus asymmetric fetal growth restriction.** Infants with symmetric FGR caused by decreased growth potential generally have a poor outcome. The recent PORTO study evaluated 1200 consecutive ultrasound-dated singleton pregnancies with gestational age between 24 0/7 and 36 6/7 weeks and an EFW <10th percentile (fetuses with major structural and/or chromosomal abnormalities were excluded) and used abnormal CPR as a proxy for brain sparing. The study found an almost 11-fold higher risk of adverse outcomes (a composite of IVH, periventricular leukomalacia, hypoxic ischemic encephalopathy, NEC, bronchopulmonary dysplasia, sepsis, and death) in those with asymmetric FGR. Conversely, smaller head circumference is also associated with cognitive, psychomotor, and behavioral delays that persist into adolescence.

B. **Preterm fetal growth-restricted** infants have a higher incidence of abnormalities than the general population because they are subjected to the risks of prematurity in addition to the risks of FGR. Outcomes are significantly worse for children whose brain growth failure occurred before 26 weeks' gestation. Gestational age may be a more important predictor of developmental outcomes than FGR, particularly before 32 to 34 weeks. Moreover, neuroimaging studies using magnetic resonance imaging show that preterm FGR infants have a high incidence of white matter loss, reduced myelination in the internal capsule, and decreased cortical gray matter volume by as much as 28%. The total brain volume is also reduced by 10% when compared with AGA infants, particularly in the hippocampal, parietal, and parietooccipital areas. Preterm FGR infants exhibit an increased prevalence of elevated fasting glucose and metabolic syndrome in childhood and adolescence.

C. **Chromosomal disorders.** FGR infants with major chromosomal disorders have a 100% incidence of disability.

D. **Congenital infections.** Infants with congenital rubella or cytomegalovirus infection with microcephaly have a poor outcome, with a disability rate >50%.

E. **Learning ability.** The school performance of FGR infants is significantly influenced by social class; children from higher social classes score better on achievement tests.

F. **Catch-up growth.** Most children who were born SGA have adequate catch-up growth without pharmacologic intervention. However, for a minority, **growth hormone** therapy (started before 8 years of age and continued for >7 years) can augment growth parameters.

G. **Metabolic syndrome in adulthood.** Epidemiologic evidence indicates that obesity, type 2 diabetes, hypertension, and cardiovascular diseases are more common among adults who were FGR at birth.

H. **Risk for recurrence of fetal growth restriction in subsequent pregnancies** depends on the underlying etiology for FGR. Previous history of FGR, preeclampsia, placental abruption or infarction, and acquired or inherited thrombophilias increase the risk of FGR in the subsequent pregnancies. The placental pathologic examination should be attempted in all FGR infants because the risk of FGR in subsequent pregnancies is very high (eg, the risk of recurrence is 50%–100% with fibrin deposition). In selected cases, folic acid, aspirin, and supplementation with L-arginine to improve placental blood flow may improve outcomes. Aspirin supplementation started before 16 weeks decreases FGR and preeclampsia, preferably taken in the evening due to concerns for effect on maternal circadian rhythm and renin activity. Benefits have, however, not been noted with use of low molecular weight heparin. Ongoing studies for preventing FGR include phosphodiesterase-5 inhibitors (eg, sildenafil), melatonin, N-acetylcysteine, statins, and nitric oxide donors.

I. **Fetal growth restriction and stillbirth.** FGR is an important predictor of unexplained stillbirths. Greater than 50% of stillborn fetuses without congenital anomalies are FGR. Maternal obesity increases the risk of concomitant FGR and stillbirth.

105 Magnesium Disorders (Hypomagnesemia, Hypermagnesemia)

Abnormalities of magnesium (Mg^{2+}) and calcium (Ca^{2+}) metabolism are commonly seen in the neonatal intensive care unit. Calcium disturbances may be mirrored by magnesium, as seen in hypocalcemia with hypomagnesemia or hypercalcemia with hypermagnesemia. Infants of diabetic mothers and infants with fetal growth restriction may present with hypocalcemia, hypomagnesemia, or both. Abnormalities in serum values for Ca^{2+} and Mg^{2+} are of concern in any infant and warrant further investigation.

I. **Hypomagnesemia**
   A. **Definition.** Normal serum levels for Mg^{2+} are typically 0.6 to 1.0 mmol/L (1.6–2.4 mg/dL). Hypomagnesemia is usually seen as any value <0.66 mmol/L (1.6 mg/dL); however, clinical signs do not manifest until levels drop below 0.5 mmol/L (1.2 mg/dL).
   B. **Incidence.** True overall incidence in neonates is not well documented and remains to be determined; however, neonates appear to be more predisposed than other groups of patients, and the most frequent occurrence tends to follow that of those infants with hypocalcemia.
   C. **Pathophysiology.** Mg^{2+} is a key trace element for maintaining skeletal integrity, and it acts as a catalyst for intracellular enzymes for adenosine triphosphate (ATP) activation in skeletal and myocardial contractility. It has an important role in different processes related to cell physiology, hormonal and metabolic pathways, nerve conduction, and blood coagulation. It is also integral to protein synthesis, vitamin D metabolism, parathyroid function, and calcium homeostasis.
   D. **Risk factors**
      1. **Hypocalcemia**
      2. **Preterm and late-preterm infants**
      3. **Inadequate intake of magnesium**
      4. **Infant of diabetic mother,** reflecting maternal Mg^{2+} deficiency secondary to gestational diabetes
      5. **Fetal growth restriction,** especially if mother had preeclampsia
      6. **Inherited renal wasting** (eg, Gitelman syndrome, Na^+/K-ATPase mutation)
      7. **Hypoparathyroidism**
      8. **Associated hypocalciuria and nephrocalcinosis**
      9. **Magnesuria secondary to furosemide or gentamicin administration**
      10. **Citrated blood exchange transfusions**
   E. **Clinical presentation**
      1. **Similar to hypocalcemia** (see Chapter 91) (eg, jitteriness, apnea, feeding intolerance) and may also present as seizures.
      2. **Clinical signs may be masked as hypocalcemia.** If symptoms persist after adequate calcium gluconate therapy, hypomagnesemia should be considered.
   F. **Diagnosis.** Laboratory testing to establish serum levels.
      1. **Serum magnesium level.** Normal values are 0.6 to 1.0 mmol/L (1.6–2.4 mg/dL), although it may vary minimally with gestational age. Twin gestation, multiple births, or vaginal delivery may result in lower levels of Mg^{2+}. It is important to note that most methods to assess Mg^{2+} levels measure total Mg^{2+} concentration, whereas only free Mg^{2+} is biologically active and almost 30% is inactive and bound to albumin.
      2. **Total and ionized calcium levels.** Usually hypomagnesemia is associated with hypocalcemia, but hypercalcemia may inhibit magnesium reabsorption in the distal loop of Henle and can cause hypomagnesemia as well.

G. **Prevention.** Adequate intake of magnesium should be assured in parenteral and enteral nutrition to prevent hypomagnesemia (recommend 8–15 mg/kg/d).

H. **Management. Acute hypomagnesemia should be treated with intravenous magnesium sulfate** (see Chapter 155 for specific dosing guidelines). Infusion must be monitored closely for cardiac arrhythmias and hypotension. Maintenance Mg^{2+} can be administered by parenteral nutrition solutions or by oral feeds with a 5-fold dilution of Mg^{2+} salt solution. Mg^{2+} infusion should be used cautiously if the infant has impaired renal function due to its accumulated toxicity.

I. **Prognosis.** Hypomagnesemia generally has a good outcome if diagnosed promptly and treated adequately. The exception is a clinical presentation that includes seizures associated with hypomagnesemia and asphyxia.

II. **Hypermagnesemia**

A. **Definition.** Reference levels of serum magnesium signifying hypermagnesemia vary from >1.15 mmol/L (2.3 mg/dL) to >1.5 mmol/L (3.0 mg/dL).

B. **Incidence.** Largely unknown; however, it occurs more frequently in infants whose mothers have been treated with magnesium sulfate. Otherwise, it occurs rarely in healthy newborns. Randomized trials and 2 meta-analyses performed during the past decade concluded that there is enough evidence to support the use of maternal magnesium sulfate for reducing cerebral palsy in preterm infants. The American College of Obstetricians and Gynecologists and Australian national guidelines have recommended the prenatal administration of magnesium sulfate as neuroprotection for <32 weeks' gestational age preterm infants. **This new trend of magnesium sulfate use may increase the incidence of hypermagnesemia in preterm infants being admitted to neonatal units and may need to be monitored.**

C. **Pathophysiology.** Increased serum Mg^{2+} levels depress the central nervous system, impair electrical conduction, and decrease skeletal muscle contractility. Antenatal magnesium sulfate administration to mothers before preterm delivery is associated with a decreased incidence of cerebral palsy in preterm infants. The precise mechanism by which magnesium sulfate exerts a neuroprotective benefit is not known, but it is speculated that it possesses anti-inflammatory and anti-excitotoxic effects while also improving cerebral blood flow and stabilizing fluctuations in blood pressure in the newborn. Magnesium may serve as an N-methyl-D-aspartate receptor antagonist, membrane stabilizer, and vasodilator.

D. **Risk factors**

1. **Increased maternal serum levels** following magnesium sulfate therapy for pregnancy-related hypertension, preeclampsia, and neonatal neuroprotection before preterm delivery.

2. **Excessive magnesium sulfate administration** to an infant with hypomagnesemia (iatrogenic medication error) or following administration of Mg^{2+}-containing antacids, especially if dehydrated. Excess magnesium in total parenteral nutrition (TPN) is a common cause.

E. **Clinical presentation.** Severity of symptoms and signs of hypermagnesemia may not correlate with serum Mg^{2+} levels. Symptoms may mimic hypercalcemia.

1. **Hypotonia, hypotension, hyporeflexia, seizures**

2. **Respiratory depression, hypoventilation, apnea**

3. **Bradycardia, hypotension, cardiac arrest with toxic Mg^{2+} levels (ie, >7.5 mmol/L)**

4. **Poor suck, feeding intolerance, decreased gastrointestinal motility, increased gastric aspirates,** abdominal distention, and delayed meconium passage

5. **Meconium plug syndrome, intestinal perforation**

6. **Urinary retention**

F. **Diagnosis**

1. **Laboratory studies**

a. **Serum magnesium.** Normal levels are 0.6 to 1.0 mmol/L (1.6–2.4 mg/dL).

b. **Serum calcium.** Always determine both total and ionized calcium levels with Mg^{2+} abnormalities.

      2. **Electrocardiogram** may reveal a prolonged PR interval, increased QRS interval, prolonged QT interval, and atrioventricular block.

G. **Management**

      1. **Identify and remove the source of excess magnesium** (eg, TPN, antacids).

      2. **Urinary excretion** is the only mechanism for decreasing serum Mg^{2+} levels.

      3. **Maintain intravenous hydration** if the patient is symptomatic.

      4. **Furosemide diuresis** may facilitate magnesium excretion, but close monitoring of electrolytes is needed, and its effect is not well studied.

      5. **Monitor serum electrolytes,** urine output, and acid-base status.

      6. **With acute signs such as seizures or electrocardiogram changes,** give intravenous calcium gluconate in doses as for hypocalcemia.

      7. **Avoid aminoglycosides** because they may potentiate the neuromuscular manifestations of hypermagnesemia.

      8. **Respiratory support** may be needed in severely affected infants (hypoventilation, apnea).

      9. **Exchange transfusion** has been used. Dialysis is uncommon in neonates.

H. **Prognosis is good following treatment,** especially if normal renal function has been preserved. In general, antenatal use of magnesium sulfate is safe for preterm infants during the postnatal period, but it needs to be further studied and monitored.

106 Meconium Aspiration

I. **Definition.** Meconium is the first intestinal discharge of the newborn infant. In addition to epithelial cells, fetal hair, mucus, and bile, meconium also contains a number of proinflammatory components. With the passage of meconium in utero, the **meconium-stained amniotic fluid (MSAF)** may be aspirated. The presence of MSAF in the trachea can cause airway obstruction. With aspiration below the vocal cords, further obstruction, air trapping, and an inflammatory response can result in severe respiratory distress. Hallmarks include early onset of respiratory distress in an infant with MSAF who presents with poor lung compliance, hypoxemia, and a characteristic lung radiograph.

II. **Incidence.** The incidence of **MSAF** varies from 8% to 20% of all deliveries. With improved perinatal care, the incidence has decreased. The incidence of MSAF increases from 1.6% at 34 to 37 weeks to 30% at ≥42 weeks. Of infants born through MSAF, approximately 5% go on to develop meconium aspiration syndrome (**MAS**). MAS primarily affects **term and postmature infants**. The intrauterine passage of meconium by infants <34 weeks' gestation is very unusual and may represent bilious reflux secondary to intestinal obstruction, not MAS.

III. **Pathophysiology**

A. **In utero passage of meconium** depends on hormonal and parasympathetic neural maturation. The exact mechanisms for in utero passage of meconium remain unclear, but fetal distress, vagal stimulation, and placental dysfunction are probable factors.

B. **Aspiration of meconium.** After intrauterine passage of meconium, deep irregular respiration or gasping, associated with fetal hypoxia, can cause aspiration of the MSAF. Early consequences of meconium aspiration include airway obstruction, decreased lung compliance, and increased expiratory large airway resistance.

      1. **Airway obstruction.** Thick MSAF can result in acute upper airway obstruction. As the aspirated meconium progresses distally, total and partial airway obstruction may occur. Partial airway obstruction can result in a ball-valve phenomenon

leading to air trapping and alveolar hyperexpansion with a subsequent 20% to 50% risk of air leak. Total obstruction may lead to asymmetric areas of atelectasis, resulting in hypoxia and increased pulmonary vascular resistance (PVR).

2. **Chemical pneumonitis.** With distal progression of meconium, chemical pneumonitis develops, which causes bronchiolar edema and narrowing of the small airways, all leading to increased hypercarbia and hypoxemia.

3. **Inflammatory mediators.** Intrapulmonary meconium triggers the release of a number of proinflammatory cytokines that lead to further airway edema, apoptosis, hypoxia, and increased PVR. Endogenous production of phospholipase A_2, identified in the lungs of infants with MAS, is associated with upregulation of inflammatory mediators, direct injury to the alveolar cell membrane, airway constriction, and surfactant catabolism.

4. **Surfactant dysfunction.** The free fatty acids in meconium can strip surfactant from the surface of the alveoli. Meconium also impacts surfactant production and clearance by affecting phosphatidylcholine metabolism.

5. **Persistent pulmonary hypertension.** A third of infants with meconium aspiration develop **persistent pulmonary hypertension of the newborn (PPHN)**. Meconium aspiration alone may result in a delay of the normal decline in PVR. Additional increases in PVR are multifactorial. PVR increases as a direct result of alveolar hypoxia, acidosis, and lung hyperinflation. PVR increases in areas of obstruction with alveolar hypoxia. The increase in PVR may lead to atrial and ductal right-to-left shunting and further hypoxemia.

IV. **Risk factors.** A number of factors have been associated with the development of MAS. Risk factors that have held statistical significance across a number of trials include thick MSAF, low 5-minute Apgar scores, and evidence of fetal distress. Ethnic groups including African Americans, Africans, Pacific Islanders, and indigenous Australians have an increased risk.

V. **Clinical presentation.** The presentation of an infant who has aspirated MSAF is variable, ranging from mild to profound respiratory distress.

A. **General features**

1. **Infant.** Infants with MAS often exhibit signs of postmaturity. Respiratory distress is evident at birth or in the transition period. Respiratory depression, poor respiratory effort, and decreased tone are often accompanied by perinatal asphyxia. Meconium-stained skin is proportional to the length of exposure and meconium concentration. Fifteen minutes of exposure to thick MSAF or 1 hour to lightly stained fluid will begin to stain the umbilical cord. Yellow staining of the newborn's nails requires 4 to 6 hours; staining of the vernix caseosa takes approximately 12 hours.

2. **Amniotic fluid.** The meconium present in amniotic fluid varies in appearance and viscosity, ranging from a thin green-stained fluid to a thick "pea soup" consistency. The majority of infants who develop MAS have a history of thick MSAF.

B. **Airway obstruction.** Large amounts of thick MSAF, if not removed, can result in an acute large airway obstruction. These infants may be apneic or have gasping respirations, cyanosis, and poor air exchange. As the meconium is driven down to more distal airways, the smaller airways are affected, resulting in air trapping and scattered atelectasis.

C. **Respiratory distress.** The infant who has aspirated meconium into the distal airways but does not have total airway obstruction manifests signs of respiratory distress secondary to increased airway resistance, decreased compliance, and air trapping (ie, **tachypnea, nasal flaring, intercostal retractions, increased anteroposterior diameter of the chest,** and **cyanosis**). Air trapping can lead to air leak syndromes. Some infants **may have a delayed presentation,** with only mild initial respiratory distress that worsens hours after delivery as atelectasis, surfactant inactivation, and chemical pneumonitis develop. *Note:* Most infants with MSAF appear normal at birth with no signs of respiratory distress.

VI. Diagnosis

A. Laboratory studies. Arterial blood gas results characteristically reveal hypoxemia. In mild cases, hyperventilation may result in respiratory alkalosis. Infants with severe disease usually have a respiratory acidosis due to airway obstruction, atelectasis, and pneumonitis. With concomitant perinatal asphyxia, combined respiratory and metabolic acidosis is present.

B. Imaging studies

1. **Chest radiographs** typically reveal hyperinflation of the lung fields and flattened diaphragms. There are coarse, irregular patchy infiltrates. A pneumothorax or pneumomediastinum may be present. The severity of radiographic findings does not always correlate with the clinical disease. (See Figure 12–17.)

2. **Point-of-care lung ultrasonography** can be used to diagnose MAS. The most specific finding in MAS was a large consolidation area with irregular edges with air bronchograms (100% of cases). Other findings include pleural line anomalies and disappearance of A lines (100% of cases), alveolar-interstitial syndrome or B line in the nonconsolidation area (100%), atelectasis (16%), and pleural effusion (~14%).

C. Cardiac echocardiogram. Pulmonary hypertension and subsequent hypoxemia from right-to-left atrial and ductal shunt are frequently associated findings in infants with meconium aspiration pneumonia.

D. Placental evaluation. Funisitis (inflammation of the connective tissue of the umbilical cord) occurs prenatally in MAS, and the stage of funisitis and chorionic vascular muscle necrosis may be a marker for MAS and predict the severity of MAS.

VII. Management

A. Prenatal management. The key to management of meconium aspiration lies in prevention of fetal distress during the prenatal period.

1. **Identification of high-risk pregnancies.** The approach to prevention begins with recognition of predisposing maternal factors that may result in fetal hypoxia during labor. Risk of MAS is highest in infants with gestational ages >41 weeks. Thus, induction as early as 41 weeks may help prevent meconium aspiration.

2. **Monitoring.** During labor, any sign of fetal distress (eg, appearance of meconium-stained fluid, loss of beat-to-beat variability, fetal tachycardia, or deceleration patterns) warrants assessment of fetal well-being. If the assessment identifies a compromised fetus, corrective measures should be undertaken or the infant should be delivered in a timely manner.

3. **Amnioinfusion.** The efficiency of amnioinfusion (instilling isotonic fluid into the amniotic cavity) in altering the risk or severity of meconium aspiration has not been demonstrated except in settings with limited perinatal surveillance. In this setting, amnioinfusion is associated with substantial improvements in perinatal outcomes. A Cochrane 2014 review notes that amnioinfusion for MSAF is associated with substantive improvements in perinatal outcome only in settings where perinatal surveillance is limited. The American Congress of Obstetricians and Gynecologists (2016) states that "routine prophylactic amnioinfusion is not recommended for dilution of meconium-stained amniotic fluid. It should only be done in the setting of additional clinical trials." It is recommended in the treatment of repetitive variable decelerations, whether or not there is MSAF.

B. Delivery room management. As outlined in Chapter 3, a skilled resuscitation team must be present in all deliveries of infants with MSAF. Management depends on whether the infant is vigorous or nonvigorous.

1. **Vigorous infants.** The appropriate intervention for **vigorous infants** (spontaneous respirations and movements, a heart rate >100 beats/min, flexed extremities) with MASF of any consistency should be limited to routine care. The infant can stay with the mother to receive the initial steps of newborn care. Use a bulb syringe to clear meconium-stained secretions from the mouth and then the nose.

2. **Nonvigorous infants.** Those **nonvigorous infants** who have depressed/inadequate respirations or poor muscle tone should be brought to the radiant warmer. Use a bulb syringe to clear meconium-stained secretions from the mouth and then the nose, and perform the initial steps of newborn care. If the infant is not breathing or the heart rate is <100 beats/min, proceed with positive-pressure ventilation. If the infant does not improve, chest movement does not occur, and the endotracheal tube (ETT) has been verified as properly placed, then meconium may be obstructing the airway. At this time, use a suction catheter through the ETT (see Table 33–1). If this does not work, clear the airway by connecting the ETT to a meconium trap aspirator attached to wall suction at a pressure of 80 to 100 mm Hg. Repeat the suctioning until the airway is cleared. Positive-pressure ventilation should be avoided, if possible, until tracheal suctioning is accomplished.

C. **Management of the newborn with meconium aspiration.** Infants with meconium below the vocal cords are at risk for pulmonary hypertension, air leak syndromes, and pneumonitis and must be observed closely for signs of respiratory distress. Observation in the special care nursery or neonatal intensive care unit for infants with MSAF who have any signs of respiratory distress in the delivery room is recommended for a minimum of 4 to 6 hours.

1. **General management.** Infants who have aspirated meconium and require resuscitation often develop metabolic abnormalities such as hypoxia, acidosis, hypoglycemia, and hypocalcemia. Because these patients may have suffered perinatal asphyxia, surveillance for any end-organ damage is essential.

   a. **Maintain a neutral thermal environment.**
   b. **Minimal handling protocol to avoid agitation.**
   c. **Maintain adequate blood pressure and perfusion.** Volume expansion may be necessary with normal saline or packed red blood as well as vasopressor support such as dopamine. Maintaining a hematocrit >40% to 45% will optimize tissue oxygen delivery.
   d. **Correct any metabolic abnormalities** such as hypoglycemia, hypocalcemia, or metabolic acidosis.
   e. **Sedation may be needed in infants on mechanical ventilation.** Intravenous morphine (loading dose 100–150 mcg/kg over 1 hour, continuous infusion of 10–20 mcg/kg/h) and fentanyl (1–5 mcg/kg/h) can be used. A neuromuscular blocker (eg, pancuronium, 0.1 mg/kg push per dose) can be used.

2. **Respiratory management**

   a. **Pulmonary toilet.** If suctioning the trachea does not result in clearing of secretions, it may be advisable to leave an ETT in place in symptomatic infants for pulmonary toilet. Chest physiotherapy every 30 minutes to 1 hour, as tolerated, will aid in clearing the airway (*controversial*). Chest physiotherapy is contraindicated in labile infants when associated PPHN is suspected. Some neonatologists avoid chest physiotherapy in all infants because of possible PPHN.
   b. **Arterial blood gas levels.** On admission to the neonatal intensive care unit, obtain blood gas measurements to assess ventilatory compromise and supplemental oxygen requirements. If the patient requires >0.4 FiO_2 or demonstrates pronounced lability, an arterial catheter for frequent sampling should be inserted.
   c. **Oxygen monitoring.** A pulse oximeter provides information regarding the severity of the infant's respiratory status. Comparing oxygen saturation values from a pulse oximeter on the right arm to those placed on the lower extremities may help identify infants with right-to-left ductal shunting secondary to MAS-associated pulmonary hypertension.
   d. **A chest radiograph** should be obtained after delivery if the infant is in distress. It may also help determine which patients will experience respiratory distress. However, radiographs often poorly correlate with the clinical presentation.

e. **Antibiotic coverage.** MAS alone is not an indication for antibiotic therapy. However, meconium does inhibit the normally bacteriostatic quality of amniotic fluid. Due to the difficulty of radiographically differentiating MAS from pneumonia, infants with infiltrates on a chest radiograph should be started on broad-spectrum antibiotics (ampicillin and gentamicin; for dosages, see Chapter 155) after appropriate cultures have been obtained. A Cochrane review (2017) found no differences in infection rates (sepsis risk) following antibiotic treatment among neonates exposed to meconium (with MAS and those born through meconium-stained fluid). Another study stated that antibiotics did not show any benefits in infants with MAS with no evidence of sepsis.

f. **Supplemental oxygen.** A major goal is to prevent episodes of alveolar hypoxia leading to hypoxic pulmonary vasoconstriction and the development of PPHN. Supplemental oxygen is provided "generously" to maintain the arterial oxygen tension at least in the range of 80 to 90 mm Hg. Some clinicians may elect to maintain PaO_2 at a higher level (95%–98%) because the risk of retinopathy should be negligible among full-term infants. The same goal of preventing alveolar hypoxia requires cautious weaning from oxygen therapy. Many of the patients are very labile. Weaning from oxygen should be done slowly, sometimes at a pace of 1% at a time. The prevention of alveolar hypoxia includes a high index of suspicion for the diagnosis of air leak as well as efforts to minimize handling of the infant.

g. **Continuous positive airway pressure (CPAP)** can be used to improve oxygenation if the FiO_2 exceeds 40%. If hyperinflation is present, use CPAP cautiously since it can make air trapping worse.

h. **Mechanical ventilation.** Patients with severe disease who are in impending respiratory failure with hypercapnia and persistent hypoxemia require mechanical ventilation. Infants with severe hypoxemia (PaO_2 <50 mm Hg), hypercarbia ($PaCO_2$ >60 mm Hg), or acidosis (pH <7.25) with FiO_2 >0.6 should be intubated and ventilated.

   i. **Specific ventilatory strategies.** Ventilation must be tailored to the individual patient and depends on the presence or absence of PPHN. Volume-targeted ventilation may decrease lung overdistension. The use of a relatively short inspiratory time may further limit potential air trapping. Modes of ventilation that allow the infant to regulate the frequency and degree of mechanical assistance (assist/control or pressure support ventilation) may be preferable. Infants with MAS typically require higher tidal volumes and overall higher minute ventilation than those with respiratory distress syndrome.

   ii. **Pulmonary complications.** For any unexplained deterioration of clinical status, the possibility of a **pneumothorax** or **pneumomediastinum** should be considered and appropriate evaluation undertaken. The need to use high mean airway pressures to maintain adequate oxygenation and ventilation with concomitant atelectasis and air trapping furthers the risk of air leak. The approach to ventilation must be directed at preventing hypoxemia and providing adequate ventilation at the lowest mean airway pressure possible to reduce the risk of catastrophic air leak.

   iii. **High-frequency ventilation.** Randomized controlled trials supporting the use of high-frequency ventilation (HFV) specifically for MAS are lacking. Other prospective studies have demonstrated that HFV can be an effective modality. HFV at 10 Hz may provide improved ventilation and lower the risk of air trapping. Both high-frequency jet ventilation and high-frequency oscillatory ventilation are efficacious in infants in whom adequate ventilation cannot be maintained on conventional ventilation without using excessive ventilatory pressures. HFV has also been used to maximize the beneficial effects of inhaled nitric oxide (see Chapter 9).

    iv. **Heliox ventilation.** In a limited study, the use of heliox was associated with improved oxygenation but failed to demonstrate significant improvement in other outcomes, including oxygenation index, survival, or degree of respiratory support, beyond the reduction in FiO_2.

    i. **Surfactant.** A number of randomized controlled trials have shown that infants with severe MAS who require mechanical ventilation and have radiologic evidence of parenchymal lung disease are likely to benefit from early surfactant therapy via bolus or lavage. Doses may exceed those used for preterm infants with respiratory distress syndrome. Because of the potential for concomitant pulmonary hypertension, close observation is required to prevent the consequences of transient airway obstruction that may develop during the tracheal instillation of surfactant. Analysis of clinical trials has failed to show an impact on survival but has shown a reduction in the duration of mechanical ventilation and hospital stay. Surfactant lavage has also been shown to decrease systemic proinflammatory cytokines that normally accompany MAS. A Cochrane review (2014) reports that in term and late preterm infants with MAS, surfactant administration may decrease the severity of respiratory illness and decrease the number of infants with progressive respiratory failure requiring support with extracorporeal life support (ECLS). **The Committee on Fetus and Newborn of the American Academy of Pediatrics recommends** that rescue surfactant can be considered in infants with hypoxic respiratory failure caused by surfactant deficiency from meconium aspiration, with recent data supporting that surfactant, either as lavage or bolus, decreased the duration of mechanical ventilation and hospital stay and that surfactant as a bolus decreased the need for ECLS.

    j. **Inhaled nitric oxide.** Pulmonary hypertension commonly affects infants with severe MAS. This can be effectively treated by inhaled nitric oxide (see Chapter 115). In an update of an earlier Cochrane System Review, data suggest that in settings without access to nitric oxide or HFV, **sildenafil** has been shown to be effective in reducing PVR, improving oxygenation, and decreasing mortality. In infants who do not respond to inhaled nitric oxide therapy, sildenafil, milrinone, and dipyridamole may be tried.

    k. **Extracorporeal life support (ECLS).** The use of inhaled nitric oxide and surfactant therapy has decreased the number of infants who go on to require ECLS. Compared with other population subsets that require ECLS, infants with meconium aspiration have a high survival rate (93%–100%). (See Chapter 20.) Venovenous ECLS is as reliable as venoarterial ECLS in infants with MAS with refractory respiratory failure who require ECLS.

    l. **Steroids.** Limited human trials are conflicting in regard to the potential benefit, and there are not sufficient data to warrant the use of steroids. Some human trials suggest that steroid therapy for MAS may be harmful. Until sufficient data are available, steroids should not be employed for MAS.

    m. **New therapies being studied.** Antioxidants such as N-acetylcysteine given intravenously improved lung functions and decreased meconium-induced inflammation and oxidative lung injury in the animal model of MAS and may enhance the therapeutic outcome of MAS. N-acetylcysteine with surfactant worked better than either treatment alone. Protease inhibitors (fetal pancreatic enzymes) may be useful in the treatment or prophylaxis of MAS.

3. **Persistent pulmonary hypertension.** Meconium aspiration is the most common respiratory disorder associated with PPHN and occurs in approximately 40% of cases. (See Chapter 115.)

D. **Prognosis.** Complications are common. New modalities of therapy such as exogenous surfactant, HFV, inhaled nitric oxide, and ECLS have reduced the mortality to <5%. In patients surviving severe meconium aspiration, bronchopulmonary dysplasia/chronic lung disease may result from prolonged mechanical ventilation. MAS is associated with neurodevelopmental sequelae, including global developmental delay, cerebral palsy, and autism, and therefore warrants long-term follow-up. Infants with a high aspartate aminotransferase levels have a poorer neurodevelopmental outcome.

107 Multiple Gestation

I. **Definition.** A multiple gestation occurs when >1 fetus is carried during a pregnancy.
II. **Incidence.** As of 2017, the overall rate of twin births was 33.3 in 1000 live births, and the rate of triplet or other higher order multiple births was 101.6 in 100,000 live births in the United States. Between 1980 and 2009, the twinning rate climbed 76% (18.9–32.2 per 100 live births) and has slowly increased since. The rate of triplet births escalated more rapidly, increasing 400% during the 1980s and 1990s, with a peak in 1998. The rate of triplets and higher order multiple births has dropped 46% from the 1998 peak to present. The incidence of multiple gestation pregnancies is probably underestimated. Fewer than half of twin pregnancies diagnosed by ultrasonography during the first trimester are delivered as twins, a phenomenon that has been termed *vanishing twin.* Two gestational sacs can be identified with ultrasonography by 6 weeks' gestation. In addition, routine screening for maternal α-fetoprotein (AFP) may identify pregnancies with multiple gestations at an early gestational age. About a third of twins in the United States are monozygotic. The incidence of monozygotic twinning is constant at 3 to 5 per 1000 pregnancies, whereas the rate for dizygotic twinning varies from 4 to 50 per 1000 pregnancies.
III. **Pathophysiology.** Placental classification and determination of zygosity are important in the pathophysiology of twins.
   A. **Classification.** Placental examination affords a unique opportunity to identify two-thirds to three-fourths of monozygotic twins at birth.
      1. **Twin placentation is classified according to the placental disk** (single, fused, or separate), number of chorions (monochorionic or dichorionic), and number of amnions (monoamniotic or diamniotic) (Figure 107–1).
      2. **Heterosexual (assuredly dizygotic) twins** always have a dichorionic placenta.
      3. **Monochorionic twins** are always of the same sex. All monochorionic twins are believed to be monozygotic. In 70% of monozygotic twin pregnancies, the placentas are monochorionic, and the possibility exists for commingling of the fetal circulations. Less than 1% of twin pregnancies are monoamniotic.
   B. **Placental complications.** Twin gestations are associated with an increased frequency of anomalies of the placenta and adnexa, for example, a single umbilical artery or velamentous or marginal cord insertion (6–9 times more common with twin gestation). The cord is more susceptible to trauma from twisting. The vessels near the insertion are often unprotected by Wharton jelly and are especially prone to thrombosis when compression or twisting occurs. Intrapartum fetal distress from cord compression and fetal hemorrhage from associated vasa previa are potential problems with velamentous insertion of the cord.

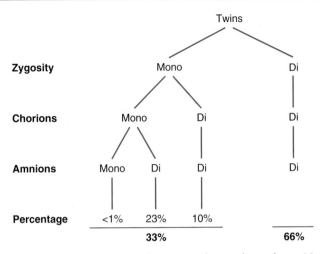

FIGURE 107–1. Percentage distribution of twins according to placental type. Mono, monoamniotic; Di, diamniotic.

C. **Determination of zygosity.** The most efficient way to identify zygosity is as follows:
1. **Gender examination.** Male-female pairs are dizygotic. The dichorionic placenta may be separate or fused.
2. **Placental examination.** Twins with a monochorionic placenta (monoamniotic or diamniotic) are monozygotic. Care should be taken not to confuse apposed fused placentas for a single chorion. If doubt exists on a gross inspection of the dividing membranes, a transverse section should be studied. The zygosity of twins of the same sex with dichorionic membranes cannot be immediately known. Genetic studies are needed (eg, blood typing, human leukocyte antigen typing, DNA markers, and chromosome marking) to determine zygosity.
IV. **Risk factors.** Use of assisted reproductive technology is a risk factor for multiple births, but the risk of higher order multiple gestation pregnancies associated with assisted reproductive technology has dropped steadily over the past decade. The incidence of dizygotic twinning increases with a family history of twins, maternal age (peak at 35–39 years), previous twin gestation, increasing parity, maternal height, fecundity, social class, frequency of coitus, and exposure to exogenous gonadotropins, clomiphene, or in vitro fertilization. The risk of twinning decreases with undernourishment. Ethnic background (African Americans > Caucasians > Asians) is a preconception risk factor for naturally conceived multiple gestation births.
V. **Clinical presentation.** Twins are more likely to have prematurity, fetal growth restriction, congenital anomalies, and twin-twin transfusion.
A. **Prematurity and uteroplacental insufficiency** are the major contributors to perinatal complications. In 2015, 1% of singletons, 10% of twins, and 36% of triplets had birthweights of <1500 g.
B. **Fetal growth restriction (intrauterine growth restriction).** The incidence of low birthweight in twins is approximately 50% to 60%, a figure that is 5 to 7 times higher than the incidence of low birthweight in singletons. In general, the more fetuses in a gestation, the smaller is their weight for gestational age (Figure 107–2). Twins tend to grow at normal rates up to about 30 to 34 weeks' gestation when they reach a combined weight of 4 kg. Thereafter, they grow more slowly. Two-thirds of twins show some signs of growth restriction at birth.

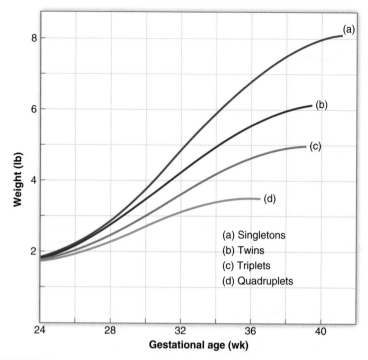

FIGURE 107–2. Growth curve showing the mean weights of infants from single and multiple pregnancies by gestational age. (*Modified with permission from McKeown T, Record RG: Observations on foetal growth in multiple pregnancy in man,* J Endocrinol. *1952 Oct;8(4):386-401.*)

C. **Uteroplacental insufficiency.** The incidence of acute and chronic uteroplacental insufficiency is increased in multiple gestations. Five-minute Apgar scores of 0 to 3 are reported for 5% to 10% of twin gestations. These low scores may relate to acute stresses of labor, cord prolapse (1%–5%), or trauma during delivery superimposed on chronic uteroplacental insufficiency.

D. **Congenital anomalies.** Birth defects are 2 to 3 times more common in monozygotic twins than in singletons or dizygotic twins, who have a 2% to 3% incidence of major defects diagnosed at birth. Three mechanisms are postulated for the increased frequency of structural defects in monozygotic twins: deformations caused by intrauterine space constraint, disruption of normal blood flow secondary to placental vascular anastomoses, and defects in morphogenesis. Such defects are usually discordant in monozygotic twins; however, in purely genetic conditions (eg, chromosomal abnormalities or single-gene defects), concordance would be the rule. Twins conceived by in vitro fertilization have twice the risk of major congenital anomalies compared with twins conceived naturally.

1. **Anomalies unique to multiple pregnancies.** Certain anomalies, such as conjoined twins and acardia, are unique to multiple pregnancies.

2. **Deformations.** Twins are more likely to suffer from intrauterine crowding and restriction of movement, leading to synostosis, torticollis, facial palsy, positional foot defects, and other defects.

3. **Vascular disruptions.** Disruptions related to monozygotic vascular shunts may result in birth defects. Acardia occurs from an artery-to-artery placental shunt, in which reverse flow leads to the development of an amorphous recipient twin. In utero death of a co-twin may result in a thromboembolic phenomenon, including disseminated intravascular coagulation, cutis aplasia, porencephaly or hydranencephaly, limb reduction defects, intestinal atresias, or gastroschisis.

E. **Twin-twin transfusion syndrome**

1. **Vascular anastomoses.** Almost all monochorionic placentas demonstrate vascular anastomoses, whereas dichorionic placentas rarely do. Vascular anastomoses may be superficial direct communications easily visible on inspection between arteries (most common) or veins (uncommon), deep connections from arteries to veins via villi, or combinations of superficial and deep connections.

2. **Incidence.** Despite the high frequency of vascular anastomosis in monochorionic placentation, the twin-twin transfusion syndrome is relatively uncommon (~15% of monochorionic gestations).

3. **Clinical manifestations.** Clinically, the twin-twin transfusion syndrome is diagnosed when twins have a hemoglobin difference of >5 g/dL and is due to artery-to-vein anastomoses.

   a. **The donor twin** tends to be pale and have a low birthweight, oligohydramnios, anemia, hypoglycemia, decreased organ mass, hypovolemia, and amnion nodosum. Donor twins often require volume expansion, red blood cell transfusion, or both.

   b. **The recipient twin** is frequently plethoric and has a high birthweight, polyhydramnios, polycythemia or hyperviscosity, increased organ mass, hypervolemia, and hyperbilirubinemia. Recipient twins often require partial exchange transfusion.

   c. **Infants born with twin-twin transfusion syndrome** have an increased risk of being diagnosed with antenatally acquired severe cerebral lesions and are at an increased risk of neurodevelopmental sequelae, even when treatment is initiated antenatally. Antenatal treatment with fetoscopic selective laser coagulation may reduce the risk of death or long-term impairment.

   d. **Very low birthweight infants** who are multiple births may have an increased risk of mortality and intraventricular hemorrhage compared with singletons.

VI. **Diagnosis.** Multiple gestation is usually diagnosed prenatally by ultrasound as early as 5 weeks (can see gestational sacs) and by an increased AFP (in twin pregnancies, the average AFP is double that found in a singleton pregnancy).

VII. **Management**

A. **Site of delivery.** When a complicated twin gestation has been identified, delivery should ideally be conducted at a high-risk perinatal center with experienced pediatric delivery teams in attendance.

B. **Physical examination.** Infants should be examined for evidence of fetal growth restriction, congenital anomalies, and twin-twin transfusion syndrome. Central hematocrits should be obtained in both infants. When 1 of the infants has a congenital anomaly, the other twin is at increased risk for complications. In particular, death of 1 fetus puts the others at risk for fetal disseminated intravascular coagulation.

C. **Complications in newborn period.** The second-born twin is more likely to develop respiratory distress syndrome and bronchopulmonary dysplasia and to die.

D. **Co-bedding of multiples.** Although co-bedding multiples was once common practice, the safety or the benefit of this practice has not been established, and the practice is discouraged.

E. **Risks beyond the neonatal period**
  1. **Catch-up growth.** In monozygotic twins, birthweight differences may be as much as 20%, but the lighter twin has a remarkable ability to make up intrauterine growth deficits.
  2. **Social problems.** Parents of multiple births may have an increased level of stress and may respond differently to their children compared with singletons. Counseling for parents of twins may be invaluable.

VIII. **Prognosis**
  A. **Twins.** The perinatal death rate for twins may be higher in the second twin, especially if the second twin is smaller. Delivery may be considered at 37 weeks to minimize the risk of stillbirth in dichorionic twins. Between 2005 and 2013, survival improved in periviable twins (23–24 weeks), whereas composite morbidity in surviving twins increased in this population.
    1. **Monoamniotic twins.** Monoamniotic twins have the highest mortality rate among the different types of twins, largely because of cord entanglement.
    2. **Monozygotic twins.** Monozygotic twins have a perinatal mortality and morbidity rate that is 2 to 3 times that of dizygotic twins. There is insufficient evidence, however, to recommend elective delivery prior to 36 weeks.
    3. **Fetal death in twins.** When the cause of death is intrinsic to 1 dichorionic fetus and does not threaten the other fetus, complications are rare. Hazardous intrauterine environments threaten both twins, whether monochorionic or dichorionic. With monochorionic placentas, the incidence of major complications or death in the surviving twin is approximately 50%.
  B. **Triplets.** The neonatal mortality rate for triplets is 18.8%, and the perinatal mortality rate is 25.5%. The risk of death or neurodevelopmental impairment has been shown to be increased in extremely low birthweight triplets and other higher order multiples compared to singletons (adjusted odds, 1.7; 95% confidence interval, 1.3–2.2).

108 Myasthenia Gravis (Transient Neonatal)

I. **Definition. Myasthenia gravis (MG)** is an autoimmune disease where antibodies attack and destroy nerve muscle connections that affect neuromuscular function. MG presents with skeletal muscle weakness and progressive fatigability that increases with activity and improves with rest. MG has multiple subgroups, but 3 distinct forms are seen in children: **transient neonatal MG (TNMG), juvenile MG**, and **congenital MG** (now known as congenital myasthenic syndromes).
  A. **Transient neonatal myasthenia gravis** is the **most common form of MG in the neonate** and will be discussed here. It is seen in neonates born to mothers with active MG (most common), but it can occur in infants of mothers who are in remission. This occurs when maternal AChR antibodies passively cross from the mother through the placenta into the fetus, resulting in destruction of fetal AChRs. Only some infants born to mothers with MG develop TNMG. It is transient, and the condition only lasts a few weeks.
  B. **Juvenile myasthenia gravis** is rare and presents in late infancy and adolescence, typically in female, usually before 19 years of age, is not transient, has no genetic component, and has a clear autoimmune component.
  C. **Congenital myasthenic syndromes** are very rare causes of neuromuscular junction failure in neonates (reported incidence of approximately 600 families with affected

individuals) that are not related to maternal disease. Common examples include primary AChR deficiency (MC), RAPSN mutations, DOK7 mutations, and COLQ mutations. It is almost always a permanent disorder without remission. Characteristics include a positive family history, inherited in an autosomal recessive pattern, usually manifest in infancy or early childhood with variable degrees of weakness that fluctuates, are caused by genetic defects (specific mutations) in components of the neuromuscular junction (presynaptic, synaptic, and postsynaptic), and has no autoimmune component. Weakness in the ocular and bulbar muscles typically occurs in these infants. Ptosis is more common in these infants than in infants with TNMG. Infants can have feeding difficulties, delay in crawling and walking. Note that life-threatening episodes of apnea can occur in these infants.

II. **Incidence.** The annual incidence of MG is 8 to 10 cases per million; the prevalence is 150 to 250 cases per million. **TNMG occurs in 10% to 20% of infants born to mothers with MG.** There is no race or sex preference and no correlation between maternal disease severity or maternal antibody level and risk of TNMG in the neonate. Occasionally an infant with TNMG is born to a mother with asymptomatically elevated AChR antibody levels. The risk of recurrence in subsequent pregnancies is 75%.

III. **Pathophysiology.** MG is an autoimmune disease that affects acetylcholine neurotransmission at the neuromuscular junction. Immunoglobulin G autoantibodies bind to the AChR (75%–85%), muscle-specific kinase (1%–10%), or lipoprotein receptor–related peptide 4 (1%–3%), preventing the nerve impulse from activating the muscle. Other autoantibodies may also play a role in disease severity. Antibody binding to these proteins directly blocks acetylcholine, accelerates receptor degradation, and induces the lysis of the postsynaptic membrane through induction of the complement system. **TNMG is caused by transplacental passage of maternal antibodies to the fetus.** Antibodies can be directed against the fetal AChR (present until 30 weeks' gestation) or the adult receptor. Higher maternal antibody titers directed against the fetal AChR have been shown to increase the risk and severity of TNMG and may lead to fetal AChR inactivation syndrome. α-Fetoprotein inhibits this binding and may be partly responsible for the unpredictable nature of maternal disease and development of TNMG.

IV. **Risk factors.** Mother with MG, mothers who have already had a child affected by TNMG (75% risk of recurrence in second child), higher levels of maternal autoantibodies. Infants of mothers with MG who had their thymus gland surgically removed are at a lower risk of developing TNMG.

V. **Clinical presentation.** Two clinical presentations exist, typical and atypical. Infants with **typical TNMG** will have **poor sucking, swallowing and respiratory difficulties, lethargy, generalized weakness, and hypotonia**. They present within a few hours of birth (usually 3–72 hours). If the diaphragm or intercostals are affected, they may have mild respiratory distress. In severe cases, mechanical ventilation may be necessary. Other signs include weak cry, facial diplegia or paresis, ptosis, ophthalmoparesis, and swallowing difficulties. Deep tendon reflexes will be present. **Atypical presentations** can include arthrogryposis, pulmonary hypoplasia, and fetal or neonatal death if not adequately supported. Severe cases can present with fetal manifestations of arthrogryposis multiplex congenita and polyhydramnios. Infants can also present with hypertrophic pyloric stenosis. Prematurity is seen in one-third of cases, and mothers may report decreased fetal movement and polyhydramnios. Symptoms begin within 24 hours of life in 75% of patients with TNMG, and nearly all present by 3 days of age. Infants whose mothers have been taking anticholinesterase agents tend to present later than infants whose mothers have not been treated. Infants born to mothers with seronegative maternal ocular MG also tend to present later.

VI. **Diagnosis.** A symptomatic infant born to a mother with MG is classic for TNMG. Antibody titers and pharmacologic challenge tests confirm the diagnosis. **Other disorders of the neuromuscular junction that present with similar symptoms include** congenital myasthenic syndromes, hypermagnesemia, aminoglycoside toxicity, and infant botulism.

A. **Antibody titers.** Commercial assays are available to test for autoantibodies of the AChR, muscle-specific kinase, or lipoprotein receptor–related peptide 4. Required blood volume for testing should be considered. If mother's status is unknown, she should be tested first. There have been antibody-negative cases, but these are less common with the evolution of cell-based assays for antibody detection.

B. **Anticholinesterase agents.** Symptomatic improvement after the administration of an anticholinesterase agent confirms the diagnosis. Improvement is defined as the reversal of definite neurologic impairments (usually sucking or swallowing difficulties) or a decrease in ventilatory requirements. Observing for changes in hypotonia or spontaneous motor activity is not as accurate, particularly in premature infants, infants with hypoxic ischemic encephalopathy, or those with intraventricular hemorrhage. Atropine may be required to help manage the muscarinic side effects (ie, diarrhea and salivation) of the drug.

1. **Neostigmine methylsulfate.** A single 0.15 mg/kg dose administered intramuscularly (IM) or subcutaneously. In a positive test, neurologic improvement is seen 10 to 15 minutes after administration and persists for 1 to 3 hours. Muscarinic side effects, in particular tracheal secretions, can be problematic. False-negative results have been reported. Intravenous (IV) administration in the neonate can cause fatal ventricular fibrillation and should not be done.

2. **Edrophonium chloride.** A single 0.15 mg/kg dose IM or subcutaneously or 0.1 mg/kg IV. Positive effects are seen within 3 minutes (IV) or 3 to 5 minutes (IM or subcutaneously) and last for 10 to 15 minutes. Muscarinic side effects are not as severe as with neostigmine. Edrophonium can rarely cause respiratory arrest (especially in larger doses). False-negative results are reported particularly in premature infants.

C. **Electromyography.** Repetitive nerve stimulation can be used for diagnosis when pharmacologic testing has yielded equivocal results. May be useful in patients with prematurity or intrapartum asphyxia where the response to an anticholinesterase inhibitor is questionable and also provides a quantitative assessment of neuromuscular function. The amplitude of the fifth evoked muscle action potential is compared with the first before and after an anticholinesterase agent is administered. The test is considered positive when the fifth action potential has decreased by at least 10% and is restored to normal after anticholinesterase treatment.

VII. **Management.** Due to the unpredictable nature of TNMG, delivery should always occur at a tertiary center. Asymptomatic infants born to mothers with MG should be observed in the hospital for 1 week.

A. **Supportive care.** The primary TNMG strategy is to provide supportive care as antibody levels gradually decline and the symptoms resolve. In 20% of patients, symptoms are mild, requiring only small, frequent oral feedings and close observation. In 80% of patients, greater support is required, including gavage feeds, respiratory support, and/or anticholinesterase medications.

B. **Anticholinesterase treatment.** Neostigmine methylsulfate, 0.05 to 0.15 mg/kg (up to 0.1 mg) IM or subcutaneously every 4 to 6 hours administered 30 minutes before feeding, or neostigmine bromide, 0.5 mg/kg (up to 1 mg) orally or nasogastrically every 4 to 6 hours administered 1 to 2 hours before feeding, is the treatment of choice. Doses may be titrated gradually until sucking and swallowing are reestablished. As the dose is increased, careful monitoring for side effects (eg, diarrhea, increased secretions, muscle fasciculations) must occur. As symptoms improve, the dose can be decreased. When symptoms are no longer present and/or when repetitive nerve stimulation is normal, the medication can slowly be discontinued. For patients presenting with moderate or severe symptoms, 50% will require anticholinesterase treatment for 1 to 2 weeks, 30% will require treatment for 3 to 4 weeks, and 20% will need >5 weeks of therapy.

C. **Ephedrine.** Treatment with ephedrine has been used when other medications have failed. Ephedrine may improve muscle weakness and fatigue, but more studies are needed. A Cochrane review found no randomized controlled trials on ephedrine in the treatment of neonatal MG.

D. **Other.** Exchange transfusion and IV immunoglobulin have been used with some benefit in the few infants who are resistant to anticholinesterase therapy. Adults with MG (including pregnant women) are currently being managed with a variety of other treatments including steroids, immunosuppressants, immunomodulators, chemotherapeutics, thymectomy, and plasmapheresis, and their potential effects on the fetus and neonate should be considered.

E. **Caution with medications.** Many medications interfere with the neuromuscular junction and may worsen MG or be associated with an exacerbation. Medications that should be avoided include antibiotics (aminoglycosides, tobramycin, macrolides, clindamycin, ampicillin [safe but some cases of respiratory depression reported]), high-dose steroids, β-blockers, neuromuscular blocking agents, antiarrhythmic medications, some anticonvulsants, and ophthalmologic medications (Timolol).

VIII. **Prognosis.** TNMG can be life-threatening if not identified and treated promptly, but for the majority of infants, it is a transient illness with no lasting effects. Symptoms last for an average of 18 days (5 days to 4 weeks), and full recovery is seen in 90% of patients by 2 months of age. The remaining 10% of patients recover by 4 months. In rare cases, symptoms persist and can lead to permanent disability including persistent myopathy, multiple joint contractures, dysarthria, velopharyngeal incompetence, mild learning disabilities, and hearing impairment. Rarely, persistent myopathic sequelae (usually facial and bulbar myopathy) have been reported following TNMG and can be caused by maternal antibodies against the AChR-γ subunit. **Fetal AChR inactivation syndrome (FARIS)** should be considered in this group of infants, especially those with marked dysarthria and velopharyngeal incompetence. Treatment with albuterol was beneficial in 1 child with this disorder. Infants with TNMG should be followed up for subtle myopathic signs and potential complications.

109 Necrotizing Enterocolitis

I. **Definition. Necrotizing enterocolitis (NEC)** is an ischemic and inflammatory necrosis of the bowel primarily affecting premature neonates after the initiation of enteral feeding.

II. **Incidence.** NEC develops in 4% to 10% of infants weighing <1500 g, with the highest incidence in the most premature infants. About 10% of NEC cases occur in term infants, many of whom have preexisting medical conditions.

III. **Pathophysiology.** Multifactorial theory has been suggested in which several risk factors, including prematurity, formula feeds, ischemia, and altered intestinal microbiota, interact to initiate mucosal damage via a final common pathway involving activation of the inflammatory cascade. A recently proposed unifying hypothesis suggests that the premature intestine exists in a hyperreactive state with higher expression of toll-like receptor-4 (TLR-4). Activation of TLR-4 by lipopolysaccharide from colonizing gram-negative bacteria leads to inflammation, impaired healing (impaired crypt stem cell function), and apoptosis of enterocytes. Translocation of bacteria leads to TLR-4 activation on the endothelium of the bowel mesentery, leading to intestinal ischemia via decreased production of endothelial nitric oxide. This and other described pathways (eg, those involving platelet-activating factor [PAF]) may lead to intestinal necrosis. The process can be exacerbated by an upregulation of proinflammatory T-helper cells and activation of intestinal macrophages.

IV. **Risk factors**

   A. **Prematurity.** There is an inverse relationship between gestational age (GA), birth weight, and risk for developing NEC. Although most preterm infants develop NEC at postmenstrual age (PMA) of 30 to 32 weeks, various factors resulting from premature birth places them at increased risk for NEC. These may involve immature mucosal (mucin) barrier, mucosal enzymes, and various gastrointestinal (GI) hormones, as well as immature bowel motility and function. Premature infants have immature local host defenses and may have an imbalance between pro- and anti-inflammatory factors, and thus have increased activation of inflammatory mediators and decreased inactivation of specific mediators such as PAF, which have been linked to NEC. Abnormal TLR-4 signaling in the premature intestine and increased activation of nuclear factor-κB (NFKB) may play a role in the pathogenesis of NEC. An inability to effectively regulate the intestinal microcirculation and differences in bacterial colonization may also make preterm infants more susceptible to NEC.

   B. **Abnormal intestinal microbiome.** Microbial colonization of the intestine starts in utero and is dependent on the mode of delivery, level of maturity, and exposure to antibiotics. During the first week of life in healthy infants, the intestinal microbiome changes to a preponderance of organisms (eg, *Bifidobacterium longum* subspecies *infantis* and lactobacilli) capable of consuming human milk oligosaccharides (HMO). These normal microbiota play a symbiotic role with the intestine through toll-like receptors by regulating the expression of genes involved in intestinal physiology, postnatal maturation and function (eg, barrier, digestion, angiogenesis, and production of immunoglobulin A [IgA]), and protection against more pathologic organisms. Exposure to prolonged antibiotic courses (>5 days) or increased use of H$_2$ blockers can lead to colonization with gram-negative bacteria (intestinal dysbiosis), which promotes inflammation and apoptosis by signaling pathways such as NFKB. Abundance of proteobacteria (gram-negative facultative bacteria such as *Escherichia coli* and *Klebsiella*) and underrepresentation of obligate anaerobic bacteria such as Firmicutes and Bacteroidetes in infants' intestines has been noted before NEC develops. Although several bacteria and viruses have been implicated in NEC, blood cultures are positive in only 20% to 30% of cases.

   C. **Enteral feedings.** NEC is rare in unfed infants, and 90% to 95% infants with NEC have received at least 1 enteral feed. Enteral feeding provides necessary substrate for proliferation of enteric pathogens. Hyperosmolar formulas/medications may alter mucosal permeability and cause mucosal damage. Short-chain fatty acids, produced as a result of colonic fermentation, may add to the damage.

   Breast milk significantly lowers risk of NEC. Mammalian breast milk is a biologic fluid that has been highly conserved for millions of years to provide survival advantage to the newborn. It contains immune cells, growth factors (eg, epidermal growth factor), anti-inflammatory factors (eg, interleukin [IL]-10), secretory IgA, lactoferrin, and live bacteria. It also contains HMOs that have no nutritive value for the infant but can be consumed by bacteria such as *B infantis* and help protect and develop the neonatal GI tract. Additionally, breast milk inactivates PAF as well as inhibits TLR-4 signaling. In 1 study, receiving a diet of >50% breast milk in the first 14 days of life resulted in an 83% reduction in the incidence of NEC.

   D. **Intestinal ischemia.** During periods of hypoxia/ischemia, blood is diverted away from the splanchnic circulation (diving reflex). This is usually followed by reperfusion, which may lead to oxidant damage and bowel injury. Imbalance between vascular dilator (eg, endothelial nitric oxide) and constrictor (eg, endothelin-1) molecules leads to defective splanchnic blood flow autoregulation and may contribute to injury. Infants who subsequently develop NEC have been shown (by Doppler flow) to have higher flow resistance in the superior mesenteric artery on the first day of life. Infants with a symptomatic patent ductus arteriosus are at higher risk for NEC possibly due to intestinal ischemia associated with aortopulmonary shunt and diastolic steal. A diminished blood supply to the gut in infants exposed to maternal cocaine (and other vasoconstrictive drugs) may also increase the risk for NEC. Most term infants who develop NEC have predisposing conditions associated with hypoxia/ischemia including congenital heart disease (eg, hypoplastic left heart syndrome), polycythemia/hyperviscosity, and birth asphyxia.

E. **Other factors.** A recent study has found an association between **maternal cigarette smoking** during pregnancy and development of NEC in the newborn infant. The underlying mechanism may be the effect of nicotine on blood vessel development in the fetal GI tract. A significant association between **red blood cell transfusion** and NEC has been reported in some retrospective studies, with about 25% to 35% of NEC cases occurring within 48 hours of packed red blood cell (PRBC) transfusions. However, 3 randomized controlled trials performed to date comparing liberal versus restrictive blood transfusion parameters have not shown a causative relationship. A recent prospective, multicenter observational cohort study found that, among very low birthweight infants, severe anemia, but not PRBC transfusion, was associated with an increased risk of NEC. It is possible that anemia may place significant stress on the intestine, leading to reperfusion-type injury following transfusion. H_2-**receptor antagonists**, which are inhibitors of gastric acid production, increase the gastric pH, which may enhance pathogenic bacterial growth and increase the risk of NEC. Finally, a **genetic predisposition**, through variation in pattern recognition receptors such as TLR-4 and NFKB, can lead to unregulated inflammation and NEC. In addition, immune-modulating single nucleotide polymorphisms involving certain cytokines (eg, IL-6) and growth factors (eg, transforming growth factor-β1) have been associated with severe NEC. Similarly, alterations in antioxidants, vascular endothelial growth factor, arginine, and nitric oxide may also increase the risk for developing NEC.

V. **Clinical presentation.** Although term infants who develop NEC are often diagnosed in the first week of life, most premature infants who develop NEC are older than 14 days or at 30 to 32 weeks' PMA. Most of them are healthy, feeding well, and growing. The early clinical presentation may include feeding intolerance, increased gastric residuals, and blood in stools. Specific abdominal signs include abdominal distension, tenderness, abdominal skin discoloration, and bilious drainage from nasogastric tube. Systemic symptoms are nonspecific (similar to those of neonatal sepsis) and include increased apnea/bradycardia episodes, temperature instability, hypotension, and circulatory shock. The clinical course of NEC is variable. Although about 30% may have a mild presentation that responds to medical treatment, about 7% may have a fulminant course with rapid progression to NEC totalis, septic shock, severe metabolic acidosis, and death. The **modified Bell's staging criteria** are often used to classify NEC according to clinical and radiographic presentations and are broken down into 3 stages.

A. **Stage I: Suspected necrotizing enterocolitis.** Characterized by nonspecific systemic signs, such as temperature instability, apnea, and lethargy. Abdominal signs include increased gastric residuals, abdominal distention, emesis, and heme-positive stool. Abdominal radiographs may be normal or show dilation of the bowel loops consistent with mild ileus. There is disagreement among experts in the field regarding whether or not the entity described as Bell stage I is actually NEC.

B. **Stage II: Proven necrotizing enterocolitis.** Includes symptoms and signs of stage I plus absent bowel sounds with abdominal tenderness. Some infants have cellulitis of the abdominal wall or a mass in the right lower quadrant. Other findings include mild metabolic acidosis and thrombocytopenia (stage IIb). Radiographic signs include pneumatosis intestinalis with or without portal venous gas (PVG). (See Figures 12–26 and 12–27.)

C. **Stage III: Advanced necrotizing enterocolitis.** Findings include severe respiratory and metabolic acidosis, respiratory failure, hypotension, oliguria, shock, neutropenia, and disseminated intravascular coagulation (DIC). The abdomen is tense and discolored with spreading erythema, edema, and induration (signs of peritonitis). The hallmark radiographic sign is pneumoperitoneum (free air; see Figure 12–25).

VI. **Diagnosis.** NEC is a tentative diagnosis in any infant presenting with the triad of feeding intolerance, abdominal distension, and grossly bloody stools.

A. **Laboratory studies.** These tests should be performed and repeated as necessary:

1. **Complete blood count with differential.** The white blood cell count is frequently either elevated with increased left shift or depressed with low neutrophil count (neutropenia). Thrombocytopenia is often seen.

2. **C-reactive protein (CRP)** correlates with the inflammatory response. Because initial CRP may be normal, serial CRP levels done at 12- to 24-hour intervals are more useful. Markers of inflammation, such as tumor necrosis factor-α, Il-6, IL-8, fecal calprotectin levels, and urine intestinal fatty acid-binding proteins, have been suggested as screening tools but have not gained widespread use.

3. **Blood culture** for aerobes, anaerobes, and fungi (*Candida* species) is indicated.

4. **Stool cultures** for rotavirus and enteroviruses may be useful when there is clustering of cases within a single unit.

5. **Electrolyte panel** may show hyponatremia and hyperkalemia.

6. **Arterial blood gas measurements** often show metabolic or combined acidosis.

7. **Coagulation studies** include prothrombin time (PT), partial thromboplastin time (PTT), fibrinogen, and fibrin degradation products (FDP and D-dimer). An elevated PT, PTT, and FDP indicate DIC, a frequent complication of severe NEC.

B. **Imaging and other studies**

1. **Radiographs of the abdomen (supine with left lateral decubitus or cross-table views)**

a. **Suspicious for necrotizing enterocolitis.** Abnormal bowel gas pattern, ileus, dilated or thickened bowel loops.

b. **Confirmatory for necrotizing enterocolitis.** Pneumatosis intestinalis, PVG (in the absence of umbilical venous catheter (see Figures 12–26 and 12–27), and free air (pneumoperitoneum). Left lateral decubitus or cross-table views are very helpful in confirming free peritoneal air. Serial radiographic studies of the abdomen should be obtained every 6 to 8 hours in the presence of pneumatosis intestinalis or PVG to look for pneumoperitoneum because these infants are at risk for bowel perforation within 48 to 72 hours of disease onset.

2. **Abdominal ultrasound.** May be useful in the presence of nonspecific clinical and radiologic findings (gasless abdomen) or in infants with NEC not responding to medical management. Ultrasound (US) can detect intramural intestinal gas (pneumatosis) and intermittent gas bubbles in the liver parenchyma and the portal venous system. In addition, focal fluid collections, bowel wall thickness, and bowel motility can be viewed in real time. Color Doppler US is useful in detecting bowel necrosis and mesenteric flow. Point-of-care US is currently being evaluated and offers some promise for the future. See Chapter 44.

3. **Mesenteric oxygen saturation.** Recent studies have shown the possibility of using near-infrared spectroscopy to detect mesenteric oxygen saturations. This provides hope of early detection and real-time noninvasive monitoring for mesenteric bowel perfusion in infants at risk for NEC. This technique is still experimental.

VII. **Differential diagnosis.** The differential diagnosis of NEC includes other conditions that cause rectal bleeding, abdominal distension, gastric retention, or intestinal perforation. These include infectious enteritis, spontaneous intestinal perforation (see Chapter 121), anal fissure, neonatal appendicitis, neonatal sepsis (presents similar to stage I NEC), and cow's milk protein allergy.

VIII. **Management.** The goal is to provide bowel rest and prevent progression of disease to intestinal perforation, septic peritonitis, and shock.

A. **Medical management**

1. **Nil per os (NPO)** to allow GI rest for 7 to 14 days (shorter course for stage I NEC). Total parenteral nutrition (TPN) to provide basic nutritional needs.

2. **Gastric decompression** with large-bore orogastric tube (Replogle) at low intermittent or continuous suctioning.
3. **Close monitoring** of vital signs and abdominal circumference. Check all gastric aspirates and stools for blood.
4. **Respiratory support.** Provide optimal respiratory support to maintain acceptable blood gas parameters. Progressive abdominal distension causing loss of lung volume may increase need for positive-pressure ventilation.
5. **Circulatory support.** There may be excessive third spacing of fluid, which requires effective volume replacement. Inotropic support may be needed to maintain normal blood pressure. Maintain urine output of 1 to 3 mL/kg/h. Remove potassium from intravenous fluids in the presence of hyperkalemia or anuria.
6. **Laboratory monitoring.** Check complete blood count and electrolyte panel every 12 to 24 hours until stable. Obtain blood and urine culture prior to starting antibiotics.
7. **Antibiotic therapy.** Treat with parenteral antibiotics for 10 to 14 days. Antibiotic regimen should cover pathogens that cause late-onset sepsis in premature infants. Add anaerobic coverage if bowel necrosis or perforation is suspected. Reasonable antibiotic regimens include the following:
   a. **Ampicillin (or vancomycin, in the presence of central line)**, gentamicin, and clindamycin (or metronidazole).
   b. **Vancomycin (in the presence of central line)** and piperacillin/tazobactam.
8. **Monitoring for bleeding and disseminated intravascular coagulation.** Infants in stage II and III may develop DIC and require fresh frozen plasma and cryoprecipitate. PRBC and platelet transfusions may also be needed.
9. **Surgical consultation** is needed for confirmed stage II and III NEC, especially when the condition is rapidly progressing or there is evidence of GI perforation.
B. **Surgical management.** Goal is to prevent enteric spillage and resect necrotic intestine while preserving as much of viable intestine as possible. A pneumoperitoneum is the only absolute indication for surgical intervention but is present in only half of the infants with intestinal perforation and necrosis at time of surgery. Relative indications for surgery include PVG, abdominal wall edema and cellulitis (indicating peritonitis), fixed dilated intestinal segment by x-ray (sentinel loop), tender abdominal mass, and clinical deterioration refractory to medical management. Biochemical markers such as thrombocytopenia, elevated CRP, fecal calprotectin, intestinal fatty acid binding protein, and elevated IL-6 and IL-8 levels have been suggested as markers to predict surgical NEC, but their practical clinical application remains questionable.
   1. **Exploratory laparotomy.** This involves examining the bowel and resecting the necrotic segments. A portion of viable bowel is used to create an enterostomy and mucous fistula. Reanastomosis takes place after 8 to 12 weeks. If NEC only involves a short segment of bowel with limited resection, primary anastomosis is used by some surgeons; this avoids complications associated with ileostomy and need for second reanastomosis surgery. In situations of widespread intestinal necrosis, the abdomen may be closed after placement of a drain and reexplored later. A poor prognosis is associated with severe short bowel syndrome, and foregoing further treatment may be considered.
   2. **Peritoneal drain placement.** A small transverse incision is made at McBurney's point. Abdominal layers are bluntly dissected, and a Penrose drain is threaded into the abdomen and secured.
      Two multicenter trials have shown that use of a peritoneal drain (PD) and laparotomy in infants with bowel perforation have similar mortality, need for TPN, and length of hospital stay. Secondary laparotomy after PD has varied from 38% in the study by Moss et al to 74% in that by Rees et al, without affecting survival. PD is a relatively simple procedure and can be done with local anesthesia

at the bedside. Hence, it is often used as a temporizing procedure in critically sick infants. However, PD has been questioned by Rees et al because they have shown lack of improvement in physiologic measurements following PD and the majority of infants required definitive laparotomy later. Currently, the optimal surgical management for infants with bowel perforation remains *controversial*. The Necrotizing Enterocolitis Surgery Trial (NEST), which is evaluating survival without neurodevelopmental impairment at 18 to 22 months for infants undergoing laparotomy or PD for NEC or intestinal perforation, is currently underway (ClinicalTrials.gov identifier: NCT01029353).

IX. **Prevention**

A. **Human milk has been shown to prevent NEC.** Although a mother's own milk is ideal, a meta-analysis of 9 randomized clinical trials of donor human milk versus formula suggests that human milk was beneficial; infants randomized to formula had a 2.8 times increased risk of NEC. The rate of NEC was also shown to be lower in infants receiving human milk fortifier compared to those receiving bovine milk–based fortifier.

B. **Use of standardized feeding regimens with initial period of trophic feeds** has been shown to decrease the incidence of NEC. A cautious approach to feeding in high-risk infants with circulatory compromise or congenital heart disease or those receiving PRBC transfusions is recommended.

C. **Probiotics.** Probiotics are live nonpathogenic microbial preparations that colonize the healthy intestine. They have the potential to prevent NEC by promoting colonization of the gut with beneficial organisms, preventing colonization by pathogens and improving the maturity and function of gut mucosal barrier and modulation of the immune system. Probiotics have been studied extensively to prevent NEC; the largest clinical trial to date of 1315 preterm infants (GA 23–30 weeks) demonstrated no difference in the incidence of Bell stage II or III NEC between patients randomly assigned to receive the probiotic *Bifidobacterium breve* BBG-001 compared with the placebo group (9% vs 10%). A recent meta-analysis, which included 38 trials (total of 10,520 preterm infants), showed a significant reduction of NEC (relative risk [RR], 0.43; confidence interval [CI], 33–0.56) and mortality (RR, 0.79; CI, 0.68–0.93) with no significant change in incidence of culture-proven sepsis (RR, 0.88; CI, 0.77–1). However, this benefit was not seen in the most premature infants with birthweight <1 kg. Because probiotics are considered nutritional supplements and not "drugs," they are not controlled by the US Food and Drug Administration. As such, there are no established regimens of optimal strain and dosing and no quality control regulations to ensure consistency and safety of these products; therefore, they cannot be recommended at this time. In addition, there have been some case reports of bacteremia from the probiotic strain used and 1 case of fatal mucormycosis in a preterm infant exposed to probiotics.

D. **Prebiotics, or nutrients that enhance the growth of beneficial microbes,** have been proposed as a preventive strategy. These include oligosaccharides, inulin, galactose, fructose, lactose, and others. Although prebiotics enhance the proliferation of endogenous flora, their efficacy in prevention of NEC is unclear.

E. **Avoidance of prolonged empiric antibiotic use.** Antibiotics alter the gut flora, promoting growth of pathogens, and should be avoided in premature infants. This is supported by a retrospective study that showed that extremely low birthweight infants receiving an initial antibiotic course of >5 days had an increased risk of NEC or death. The association was confirmed in a recent systematic review and meta-analysis.

F. **Avoidance of H_2 blockers.** Innate GI immunity provided by gastric acid may be important in preventing the cascade of infectious and inflammatory events leading to NEC. A large retrospective study from the National Institute of Child Health and Human Development (NICHD) Neonatal Research Network showed that infants with NEC were more likely to have received H_2 blockers compared to matched controls (odds ratio, 1.71; CI, 1.34–2.19). Therefore, routine use of H_2 blockers in premature infants should be avoided.

X. **Complications**

   A. **Recurrence of NEC** may occur in about 5% to 10% of cases.

   B. **Colonic strictures** may occur in 10% to 20% cases and present with recurrent abdominal distension and persisting feeding intolerance. Contrast radiographic studies are usually diagnostic. The most common site for stricture formation is the colonic splenic flexure.

   C. **Short bowel syndrome** may develop in infants undergoing extensive resection of bowel (occurs in 9% of surgical NEC cases). The traditional limits of intestinal length for successful survival (at least 20 cm of viable small bowel remaining with an intact ileocecal valve, or 40 cm viable remaining small bowel with loss of ileocecal valve) are now being challenged with improvements in short bowel management by multidisciplinary teams. Fewer infants are now being referred for intestinal transplant after the use of intestinal lengthening procedures such as serial transverse enteroplasty and improved TPN and infection prevention strategies. Intestinal (with or without liver) transplant remains an option for some of these infants.

   D. **Total parenteral nutrition–associated liver disease** occurs more frequently in infants with surgical therapy for NEC.

XI. **Prognosis.** Risk of mortality is 20% to 30%; the mortality is higher with lower GA and surgical interventions. Infants with surgical NEC have been shown to have significant growth and neurodevelopmental impairment. They are at risk for developing periventricular leukomalacia, cerebral palsy, deafness, and blindness. In a report from NICHD, only half the infants with surgical NEC survived. Among the survivors, 56.7% had neurodevelopmental impairment (cerebral palsy, mental development index <70, physical development index <70, blindness, or deafness). Overall, mortality or neurodevelopmental impairment was present in 82.3% of infants in this high-risk group.

110 Neonatal Encephalopathy

I. **Definition**

   A. **Neonatal encephalopathy (NE)** is a clinically defined syndrome of disturbed neurologic function in the earliest days of life in infants born ≥35 weeks' gestation, demonstrated by an altered level of consciousness or seizures and frequently associated with depressed respiratory drive, hypotonia, and depressed or absent reflexes. NE may result from a metabolic disorder, infection, drug exposure, **hypoxic ischemic encephalopathy (HIE)**, or neonatal stroke. NE is the preferred terminology to describe a depressed newborn from any cause at the time of birth.

   B. **Perinatal asphyxia** is a condition of impaired blood gas exchange that, if persistent, leads to progressive hypoxemia and hypercapnia. HIE, which is a subset of NE, can result from perinatal asphyxia whereby inadequate oxygen delivery to the brain leads to compromised brain metabolism

   C. **The likelihood that acute intrapartum or peripartum hypoxia-ischemia (HI)** may have contributed to NE is based on the following factors identified by the American College of Obstetricians and Gynecologists (ACOG) task force on NE:

      1. **Neonatal signs**

         a. **Apgar score <5 at 5 minutes and 10 minutes.**

         b. **Fetal umbilical artery acidemia** pH <7 and base deficit >12 mmol/L or both.

      c. **Neuroimaging evidence of acute brain injury** seen on brain magnetic resonance imaging (MRI) or magnetic resonance spectroscopy consistent with HI.

      d. **Presence of multisystem organ failure** consistent with HIE.

    2. **Type and timing of contributing factors**

      a. **A sentinel hypoxic or ischemic event** occurring immediately before or during labor and delivery.

      b. **Fetal heart rate monitor patterns** consistent with an acute peripartum or intrapartum event.

      c. **Timing and type of brain injury patterns** based on imaging studies consistent with an etiology of an acute peripartum or intrapartum event.

      d. **No evidence of other proximal or distal factors** that could be contributing factors.

    3. **Developmental outcome**

      a. **Developmental outcome is spastic quadriplegia or dyskinetic cerebral palsy.** Other subtypes of cerebral palsy (CP) and other developmental abnormalities are not specific to acute intrapartum HIE.

II. **Incidence.** NE occurs in 3.0 per 1000 live term births and leads to death in 15% to 20% of cases and permanent neurologic deficits in 25% of infants. It is estimated that 70% of cases of NE are due to events that arise before onset of labor, 20% are due to intrapartum events, and 10% are due to postnatal complications. Several case-control studies suggest that a combination of antepartum and intrapartum events is involved in moderate to severe NE. HIE has an incidence of 1.5 per 1000 live births. The worldwide prevalence of CP is 2 to 3 per 1000 live births. Intrapartum hypoxia-acidemia accounts for only approximately 10% to 20% of CP cases.

III. **Pathophysiology**

  A. **Hypoxic ischemic injury.** A reduction in oxygen delivery precipitates an immediate drop in cellular high-energy phosphate levels, which is termed a **primary energy failure**. Lactic acid accumulation leads to cellular swelling via failure of membrane ion pump. Calcium influx releases glutamate and ultimately leads to an excitotoxic cycle resulting in free radical and nitric oxide production, lipid peroxidation of cell membranes, and necrotic cell death. If cerebral blood flow is restored with resuscitation, partial restoration of energy sources can occur during the **reperfusion period**. A **latent phase** follows with varying duration based on the severity of the insult. Within 6 to 48 hours after the initial insult, the latent phase can progress to a **secondary energy failure**, which is characterized by inflammation, oxidative and free radical damage, and neuronal death via **apoptosis**. The severity of the insult determines the extent of brain injury. Current neuroprotective therapies are designed to intervene within the latent phase before the onset of secondary energy failure.

  B. **Adaptive responses of the fetus or newborn to asphyxia.** The fetus and neonate are much more resistant to asphyxia than adults. In response to asphyxia, the mature fetus uses the "diving reflex" physiology to redistribute cardiac output to the heart, brain, and adrenals to ensure adequate oxygen and substrate delivery to these vital organs. Autoregulation of cerebral blood flow becomes disrupted and the cerebral circulation becomes pressure passive; this increases the risk for cerebral ischemia with systemic hypotension and cerebral hemorrhage with systemic hypertension. Cerebrovascular hemorrhage may occur upon reperfusion of the ischemic areas of the brain. However, when there has been prolonged and severe asphyxia, local tissue recirculation may not be restored because of collapsed capillaries in the presence of severe cytotoxic edema.

  C. **Neuropathology.** Neuropathologic injury from HIE includes the following classic patterns. Different combinations of injury can result based on duration and severity of the injury.

    1. **Selective neuronal necrosis** is the most common type of brain injury and can present in 3 patterns: diffuse, cortical–deep nuclear, and deep nuclear–brainstem.

2. **Parasagittal cerebral injury** occurs in the end-arterial watershed area of the parieto-occipital cortex and subcortical white matter.

3. **Periventricular leukomalacia (PVL)** is necrosis and gliosis of periventricular white matter. Although more common in preterm infants, it can be seen in term infants with HIE. PVL involving the pyramidal tracts usually results in spastic diplegic or quadriplegic CP.

4. **Focal ischemic necrosis** refers to arterial stroke along the vascular distribution of cerebral arteries.

5. **Porencephaly, hydrocephalus, hydranencephaly, and multicystic encephalomalacia** may follow focal and multifocal ischemic cortical necrosis, PVL, or intraparenchymal hemorrhage.

6. **Brainstem damage** is seen in the most severe cases of HI brain injury and results in permanent respiratory impairment.

IV. **Risk factors.** The following risk factors have been established for HIE, but the timing of fetal hypoxia may be difficult to establish.

   A. **Preconception risk factors** include maternal age ≥35 years, family history of seizures or neurologic disease, and infertility treatment.

   B. **Antepartum risk factors** include maternal thyroid disease, diabetes, severe preeclampsia, multiple gestation, genetic abnormalities, fetal growth restriction, maternal trauma, and antepartum hemorrhage.

   C. **Intrapartum risk factors** include sentinel events such as placental abruption, umbilical cord prolapse, uterine rupture, fetomaternal hemorrhage, and shoulder dystocia, as well as other intrapartum risk factors such as maternal fever with or without chorioamnionitis. Case-control studies have suggested an interaction between brain injury due to inflammation and HI.

   D. **Postnatal risk factors** include postnatal injury secondary to cardiorespiratory failure, congenital heart disease, and neurologic abnormalities.

V. **Clinical presentation.** HIE can result in central nervous system (CNS) injury alone, CNS and other end-organ damage, isolated non-CNS organ injury, or no end-organ damage.

   A. **Central nervous system injury in severe cases of hypoxic ischemic encephalopathy manifest with variable clinical signs that evolve over time:**

   1. **Birth to 12 hours.** Deep stupor or coma, respiratory failure or periodic breathing, diffuse hypotonia with minimal movement, intact pupillary and oculomotor responses. Term infants may have subtle or focal clonic seizures by 6 to 12 hours, whereas preterm infants can present with generalized tonic seizures and posturing.

   2. **12 to 24 hours.** The level of alertness can appear to improve in less critical cases of brain injury, but severe seizures, marked jitteriness, and apnea can also emerge. Term infants can present with weakness of the proximal upper limbs, whereas preterm infants have lower extremity weakness.

   3. **24 to 72 hours.** The consciousness level worsens, leading to deep stupor or coma and respiratory arrest. Pupillary and oculomotor disturbances are now present due to brainstem involvement. Death due to HIE most often occurs at a median age of 2 days.

   4. **After 72 hours.** Mild to moderate stupor may persist, but the overall level of alertness improves. Diffuse hypotonia may persist, or hypertonia can become evident. Feeding difficulties become obvious due to abnormal sucking, swallowing, and tongue movements.

   B. **Non–central nervous system multiorgan dysfunction can present as follows:**

   1. **Renal.** Acute tubular necrosis (ATN) and syndrome of inappropriate antidiuretic hormone (SIADH) are common.

   2. **Pulmonary.** Respiratory failure may result from poor central drive, persistent pulmonary hypertension, and meconium aspiration.

   3. **Cardiac.** Myocardial dysfunction and congestive heart failure may result in arrhythmias and hypotension.

   4. **Hepatic dysfunction** may manifest as transaminitis, coagulopathy, and hypoglycemia.
   5. **Hematologic.** Thrombocytopenia and leukopenia may occur due to hypoxic marrow suppression. An increased release of nucleated red blood cells may occur as well.
   6. **Gastrointestinal.** Paralytic ileus or necrotizing enterocolitis may occur due to mesenteric hypoperfusion.
   7. **Metabolic.** Acidosis (elevated lactate), hypoglycemia, hypocalcemia, and hyponatremia may be seen.

VI. **Diagnosis**
   A. **Maternal data**
      1. **History.** A thorough maternal history (prior pregnancy loss, thyroid disease, fever, drug use, infection) and family history (thromboembolic disorders, seizure disorder) can help identify causes of NE other than HIE.
      2. **Fetal heart rate patterns.** Per ACOG guidelines, a fetal heart rate (FHR) pattern suggestive of previous fetal injury is a category II tracing lasting 60 minutes$\geq$ that is identified on initial presentation with persistently minimal or absent variability and lacking accelerations. A category I tracing on presentation that converts to a category III tracing is **suggestive** of an HI event. Additional FHR patterns that **may suggest** intrapartum timing of an HI event include a category I tracing that evolves into tachycardia with recurrent decelerations or persistent minimal variability with recurrent decelerations. (FHR categories are discussed in Chapter 1.)
      3. **Umbilical cord blood gases.** Per ACOG guidelines, the probability but not the timing of an intrapartum hypoxic event leading to NE may be suggested by metabolic acidosis in umbilical cord gases. Fetal umbilical artery pH ≤ 7.0, base deficit ≥ 12 mmol/L, or both increase the probability of NE having an intrapartum hypoxic component. For cord arterial pH >7.20, NE is unlikely to be a result of intrapartum hypoxia.
      4. **Placental pathology.** Important information regarding the etiology of NE may be gleaned from abnormalities seen on the maternal or fetal side of the placenta. Pathologic umbilical cord lesions, such as velamentous or marginal cord insertion or cord hematoma or tears, may indicate a disruption in the fetal vascular supply. Chorioamnionitis and funisitis may indicate an infectious etiology of NE, whereas fetal thrombotic vasculopathy can point to a genetic coagulopathic disorder. While placental findings should be taken in context of the clinical scenario, findings favoring acute in utero compromise include acute villous edema, acute intravillous hemorrhage, acute retroplacental hemorrhage, and acute meconium staining.
   B. **Neonatal data**
      1. **Apgar scores.** Although most infants with a low Apgar score will not develop CP, a low Apgar score at 5 minutes and 10 minutes confers an increased relative risk of CP. Per ACOG, if the 5-minute Apgar score is ≥ 7, peripartum HI is unlikely to be a major contributor to NE.
      2. **Physical examination.** The classification of HIE into clinical stages based on severity is determined by the **Sarnat scale and its modified versions**.
         a. **Stage 1 (mild).** Hyperalert, normal activity, normal muscle tone, weak suck, strong Moro, mydriasis, tachycardia, and absence of seizures.
         b. **Stage 2 (moderate).** Lethargic or obtunded, decreased activity, hypotonia, strong distal flexion, weak or absent suck, weak Moro, miosis, bradycardia, and focal or multifocal seizures are common.
         c. **Stage 3 (severe).** Stupor or coma, absent activity, flaccid muscle tone, intermittent decerebration, absent suck, absent Moro, poor pupillary light response with fixed, dilated pupils, variable heart rate, and frequent prolonged seizures.

3. **Laboratory studies.** Complete blood count with differential, blood culture, serum electrolytes, glucose, lactate, blood urea nitrogen, creatinine, cardiac enzymes, liver enzymes, a coagulation panel, and blood gases should be obtained at time of admission and serially monitored as indicated. Further metabolic workup including ammonia, urine ketones, plasma amino acids, urine amino acids, urine organic acids, and acylcarnitine profile may be indicated in the workup of NE not consistent with HIE.

4. **Imaging other than cranium.** An echocardiogram can be obtained to evaluate cardiac ventricular function, presence of tricuspid regurgitation, and right to left shunting via foramen ovale and patent ductus arteriosus. Renal and hepatic ultrasounds may provide further information regarding end-organ damage.

5. **Conventional electroencephalogram.** Along with evaluation of seizure burden, interpretation of electroencephalography (EEG) background includes the following variables.

   a. **Amplitude.** Refers to the voltage measured from peak to peak of the waveform. Amplitude decreases with increasing gestational age. Abnormalities can include an isoelectric EEG (maximally depressed or flat) or low voltage.

   b. **Symmetry.** Refers to the symmetry of activity arising from both hemispheres. Asymmetry can indicate a stroke or structural lesion.

   c. **Continuity.** Refers to a tracing with relatively constant and consistent amplitude. Discontinuity refers to high-amplitude bursts that alternate with periods of low amplitude. Continuity increases with increasing gestational age.

   d. **Sleep-wake state.** Refers to the pattern of EEG alterations among different behavioral states. The presence of sleep-wake cycling (SWC), as expected in a normal EEG, may be poorly defined or absent in a neonate affected by HIE. SWC is also gestational age dependent.

6. **Amplitude-integrated EEG.** This mode of monitoring uses a bedside cerebral function monitor, which records and amplitude integrates a single- or double-channel EEG from biparietal electrodes. Amplitude-integrated EEG (aEEG) has the advantage over conventional EEG of not requiring extensive formal training for interpretation. Studies have shown aEEG to be useful in predicting long-term neurodevelopmental outcomes in infants with HIE. The following is 1 classification scheme suggested to describe aEEG findings.

   a. **Continuous normal voltage.** Continuous activity with lower margin (minimum amplitude) above 5 µV and upper margin (maximum amplitude) above 10 µV.

   b. **Discontinuous normal voltage.** Discontinuous background with lower margin below 5 µV and upper margin above 10 µV.

   c. **Burst suppression.** Discontinuous background with lower margins below 10 µV with occasional bursts with amplitude >25 µV.

   d. **Continuous extremely low voltage.** Continuous background pattern of very low voltage (around or below 5 µV). Occasional spikes are seen over 10 µV.

   e. **Isoelectric or flat tracing.** Primarily inactive (isoelectric) background below 5 µV; prominent spikes are likely due to patient movements/artifacts.

   Computer-based automated quantitative EEG power analysis is an emerging field that may play a role in identifying and managing seizures and predicting outcome in neonate with HIE.

7. **Magnetic resonance imaging of the brain.** The pattern of brain involvement, rather than the severity of injury, determines neurodevelopment outcomes of infants with HIE.

   a. **Watershed predominant pattern.** Results from partial prolonged HIE injury and affects the vascular watershed area in the white matter.

   b. **Basal ganglia/thalamus predominant pattern.** Results from acute profound HIE and affects deep gray nuclei and perirolandic cortex. The total cortex can be involved in severe HIE. This pattern is associated with severe cognitive and motor deficiencies, including CP.

   c. **Additional injuries.** Involvement of the cortical gray matter can be seen in severe HIE. This pattern is associated with cognitive impairment. Hemorrhages, focal-multifocal white matter injury, and global brain injury can also occur.

8. **Magnetic resonance spectroscopy.** Magnetic resonance spectroscopy is used to evaluate cerebral metabolic abnormalities after HIE. The best predictors of neurodevelopmental outcomes are the ratio of lactate to N-acetyl aspartate (NAA) and the absolute concentration of NAA.

9. **Diffusion-weighted imaging and diffusion tensor imaging.** Diffusion-weighted imaging (DWI) relies on water molecule diffusion in the brain to provide image contrast. DWI allows quantification of lesions by measuring the apparent diffusion coefficient and fractional anisotropy. Diffusion tensor imaging (DTI) measures the magnitude and directionality of water molecule diffusion. The time-dependent nature of apparent diffusion coefficient contributes to its poor predictive value for neurodevelopment. Fractional anisotropy calculated from DTI data has been associated with neurodevelopment outcomes in infants with HIE.

10. **Near-infrared spectroscopy (NIRS)** provides a noninvasive method of monitoring cerebral hemodynamics and oxygenation. Measurement of cerebral perfusion by NIRS has been correlated with brain MRI findings in HIE infants.

11. **Biomarkers.** Early biochemical markers of perinatal brain damage include the following: absolute nucleated red blood cells, S100B (cytosolic calcium-binding protein), adrenomedullin, erythropoietin (EPO), activin A (growth and differentiation factor), neuron-specific enolase, oxidative stress markers, glial fibrillary acidic protein, and creatine kinase BB, among others.

VII. **Management.** The management of infants with HIE begins with the identification of perinatal patients at a high risk for asphyxia and optimal resuscitation in the delivery room. Because many cases of HIE are unanticipated and unpreventable, clinical care mostly focuses on providing supportive care to prevent further exacerbation of injury and specific neuroprotective therapies targeted at the therapeutic window prior to the onset of irreversible secondary energy failure. The ethical and medicolegal aspects of care also need to be considered.

A. **Supportive care**

   1. **Resuscitation.** The 2015 Neonatal Resuscitation Program guidelines recommend initiating resuscitation of newborn ≥35 weeks with 21% oxygen with a targeted preductal saturation of 60% to 65% by 1 minute of life and 80% to 85% by 5 minutes of life. When chest compressions are indicated, after optimal ventilation has been established, oxygen concentration should be increased to 100% and weaned as soon as the heart rate recovers.

   2. **Ventilation.** Assisted ventilation may be required to maintain Pco_2 within the physiologic range. While hypercarbia exacerbates cerebral intracellular acidosis and impairs cerebrovascular autoregulation, hypocarbia decreases cerebral blood flow and is associated with poor outcomes in neonates with HIE. It is unclear whether hypocarbia is a risk factor or an early marker for poor neurodevelopmental outcome.

   3. **Perfusion.** Mean arterial blood pressure should be maintained in the normotensive range. Due to the loss of cerebrovascular autoregulation, volume expanders and inotropic support should be used cautiously to avoid rapid shifts between systemic hypotension and hypertension. Blood pressure management needs to be individualized based on the presence of comorbidities such as pulmonary hypertension and myocardial dysfunction.

4. **Acid-base status.** The base deficit is thought to increase in the first 30 minutes of life due to an initial washout effect secondary to improved perfusion and transient increase in lactic acid levels. In most infants, acidosis normalizes by 4 hours of life regardless of bicarbonate therapy. The rate of recovery from acidosis is reflective of HIE severity but not duration and is not predictive of outcomes. **Sodium bicarbonate therapy is not recommended** as it causes a concomitant rise in intracellular Pco_2 levels, negating any changes in pH, and is associated with increased rates of intraventricular hemorrhage and mortality. An inborn error of metabolism must be considered if the degree and duration of acidosis seem out of proportion to the history and presentation.

5. **Fluid status.** Initial fluid restriction is recommended as HIE infants are predisposed to a fluid overload state from renal failure secondary to ATN and SIADH. The avoidance of volume overload helps avert cerebral edema. Subsequence fluid management is based on clinical status including renal function, urine output, and electrolytes.

6. **Blood glucose.** The maintenance of normoglycemia plays a vital role in determining neurologic outcome after an HI event. Both hypoglycemia and hyperglycemia in infants with moderate to severe HIE are independently associated with unfavorable outcome.

7. **Temperature.** Hyperthermia for infants with HIE has been associated with adverse outcomes and should be avoided in the delivery room.

8. **Infection.** Evaluate for sepsis with use of antibiotics (not gentamicin) as NE may be the result of infection.

9. **Seizures.** Seizure activity is both a consequence and determinant of brain injury regardless of the primary neurologic insult. Seizures are frequently unrecognized or subclinical (electrographic). Jitteriness, tremors, and benign sleep myoclonus may be misdiagnosed as seizures. Continuous monitoring of EEG allows for timely treatment of subclinical seizures. Phenobarbital is the main antiepileptic drug (AED) used. A 2016 Cochrane review showed prophylactic barbiturate therapy to result in a reduction in seizure burden but no reduction in mortality; insufficient data regarding long-term outcome were provided. Other AEDs used include levetiracetam, phenytoin (and fosphenytoin), benzodiazepines, and lidocaine. AED levels in asphyxiated infants should be carefully monitored due to impaired hepatic and renal clearance.

B. **Neuroprotective strategies**

1. **Hypothermia.** Therapeutic hypothermia attenuates secondary energy failure by decreasing cerebral metabolism, inflammation, excitotoxicity, oxidative damage, and cellular apoptosis. A 2013 Cochrane review of 11 trials of both whole-body and selective cooling showed that hypothermia therapy initiated within 6 hours of birth for infants with moderate or severe encephalopathy reduced mortality and neurodevelopmental disability. **Hypothermia therapy is the standard of care for newborns with moderate to severe HIE,** and timely identification and referral to cooling centers is crucial. Whole-body cooling can be safely and effectively done during neonatal transport. Hypothermia protocols and recommended temperature regulation prior to admission (eg, passive cooling or active cooling on transport) are institution specific and must be clarified with the accepting facility at the time of referral. A recent trial looking at longer (120 hours vs 72 hours) and/or deeper (32°C vs 33.5°C) cooling, either alone or combined, did not reduce neonatal deaths, and the trial was closed early for safety concerns. The time to initiate cooling has been correlated with outcomes. A multicenter National Institute of Child Health and Human Development (NICHD) trial evaluating the effectiveness of whole-body cooling initiated between 6 and 24 hours of age and continued for 96 hours in infants with HIE was recently published; it showed the primary outcome (death or disability) at 18 to 22 months to be present in 19 (24.4%) of 78 hypothermic

infants and 22 (27.9%) of 79 noncooled infants (absolute difference, 3.5%; 95% confidence interval, –1% to 17%). Using Bayesian analysis, the authors concluded that hypothermia initiated at 6 to 24 hours after birth may have benefit, but there is uncertainty in its effectiveness. An NICHD trial to assess the safety and effectiveness of whole-body hypothermia for preterm infants 33 to 35 weeks' gestation is currently underway. Therapeutic hypothermia is currently not recommended for infants with mild encephalopathy, but some studies are investigating this area as well.

2. **Pharmacotherapy.** Multiple drugs are currently being studied to augment neuroprotection in infants with HIE. Demand for combination therapies stems from the realization that 45% of infants with HIE treated with hypothermia alone have adverse outcome. EPO provides neuroprotection via its anti-inflammatory and antiapoptotic effect on neural cells and promotion of neural regeneration. A phase II clinical trial showed that high doses of EPO given with hypothermia for HIE reduced MRI brain injury and improved 1-year motor function. An upcoming large phase III trial is underway to determine if EPO and hypothermia can improve long-term outcome. Trials using darbepoetin as an adjunctive therapy to hypothermia are also in process. Allopurinol, a free radical scavenger, has been shown to provide long-term neuroprotection in some studies. Melatonin has antioxidant and anti-inflammatory properties and has been shown to be neuroprotective in a pilot study. Xenon is an inhaled anesthetic that inhibits excitatory amino acid release. A trial of total-body hypothermia plus xenon did not demonstrate an enhanced neuroprotective effect. Agents such as deferoxamine and N-acetyl-L-cysteine have been studied in animal models but not human trials. Stem cell therapy is also an area of interest.

C. **Ethics.** Families are often unprepared to deal with the complexities of HIE. Direct and timely communication between the medical team and the neonate's family is therefore essential to foster shared decision making with difficult medical and emotional decisions such as discontinuation of artificial life support. A multidisciplinary team approach is essential, as severely depressed infants may have multiple complex medical needs. A neurology consult is helpful to provide parents with important prognostic information based on the infant's neurologic assessment. A palliative care consult may offer families support while optimizing the quality of the life for the infant. Therapeutic hypothermia has been shown to significantly reduce death without an increase in survivors with disability. Withdrawal of artificial support and allowing natural death can be addressed with families during hypothermia in profoundly affected infants.

D. **Medicolegal aspects**

1. **Obstetric care.** Fetal status must be assessed with electronic fetal monitoring at the time of maternal admission to identify and categorize risk for intrapartum fetal distress. A reactive FHR pattern is a reliable sign of fetal well-being, whereas a nonreactive pattern indicates a higher probability of intrapartum fetal distress and adverse fetal outcome. The early recognition of FHR patterns that are associated with fetal academia and HI with timely intervention may potentially alleviate brain injury. However, FHR patterns may reflect preexisting or underlying neurologic impairment originating prior to the perinatal period. Caution must be used in identifying a specific event as the cause for an adverse outcome, as the baseline fetal brain status is often unknown.

2. **Neonatal care.** Many cases of NE are unanticipated, and an experienced resuscitation team may not always be readily available. In an anticipated high-risk birth, clear communication between members of the obstetric and neonatal teams prior to delivery is imperative. The resuscitation team must be thoroughly prepared for the potential for vigorous resuscitation per current Neonatal Resuscitation Program guidelines. Careful attention must be paid to avoiding hyperthermia, hypoglycemia, hypotension, and hypocarbia in the

postresuscitation stabilization period. Early referral for evaluation for hypothermia therapy is crucial, as transport and admission to the tertiary center is ideally achieved within 6 hours after birth. Documentation of the resuscitation and stabilization process as well as informed consent for transport are important parts of the medical record.

VIII. **Prognosis.** The presence of NE is considered an essential etiologic link between perinatal events and permanent brain damage. Mild cases of neonatal HIE have a favorable outcome, whereas severe cases have a high rate of mortality and neurodevelopmental disability. Despite the use of therapeutic hypothermia, the mortality rate and the composite outcome of death or major disability remain high. Findings of persistent severe HIE at 72 hours and an abnormal neurologic exam at discharge are associated with a greater risk of death or disability. The discharge exam also improves the predictive ability of the initial stage of encephalopathy at <6 hours for death or disability. Other findings associated with an increased risk of death or disability include hypertonia, fisted hand, abnormal movements, absent gag reflex, asymmetric tonic neck reflex, and need for gavage tube/gastrostomy feeds at time of discharge. EEG and aEEG play an important part in predicting outcomes. A persistently abnormal aEEG at 48 hours or more is associated with an adverse neurodevelopmental outcome. Infants with high seizure burden and moderate to severe injury on MRI (basal ganglia, thalamus, and posterior limb of the internal capsule) are at greatest risk of abnormal outcome. Diffusion-weighted MRI in the first week of life has the highest specificity, whereas T1/T2-weighted MRI in the first 2 weeks of life has the highest sensitivity. Basal ganglia or thalamic lactate/NAA ratio is a predictor for adverse neurodevelopmental outcome. Visual evoked potentials may also provide prognostic information. Reassuring prognostic factors include early return of SWC with normalization of background EEG, normal MRI, oral feeding, and normal neurologic examination at discharge.

111 Neural Tube Defects

I. **Definitions. Neural tube defects (NTDs) are malformations of the developing brain and spinal cord.** In normal development, the closure of the neural tube occurs over a 4- to 6-day period with completion around the 29th day postconception, often before a woman has realized that she is pregnant. Most current hypotheses consider NTDs to be defects from failure of a neural tube closure rather than the reopening of a previously closed tube. The nomenclature for NTDs is not standardized; frequently used terms are as follows:

A. **Anencephaly.** The defective closure of the upper or rostral end of the anterior neural tube. Hemorrhagic and degenerated neural tissue is exposed through an uncovered cranial opening extending from the lamina terminalis to the foramen magnum. Infants with anencephaly have a typical appearance with prominent eyes when viewed face on. **Craniorachischisis totalis** (a neural platelike structure without skeletal or dermal covering resulting from complete failure of neural tube closure) and **myeloschisis** or **rachischisis** (in which the spinal cord is exposed posteriorly without skeletal or dermal covering because of failure of posterior neural tube closure) are other, less frequent open lesions.

B. **Encephalocele.** Herniation of brain tissue outside the cranial cavity resulting from a mesodermal defect occurring at or shortly after anterior neural tube closure; usually a closed lesion. Approximately 80% of encephaloceles occur in the occipital region.

C. **Myelomeningocele.** Often also referred to as **spina bifida** (protrusion of the spinal cord into a sac on the back through a deficient axial skeleton with variable dermal covering). Considering that, strictly speaking, "spina bifida" only describes the bony defect, the term **spinal dysraphism** is considered more accurate by some. More than 80% of defects in this category occur in the lumbar region, and approximately 80% are not covered by skin. In contrast to myelomeningoceles, **meningoceles** (closed lesions involving the meninges only) usually do not result in neurologic deficits.

D. **Spina bifida occulta and occult spinal dysraphism.** Disorders of the caudal neural tube that are covered by skin (skin dimples or only very small skin lesions are present). These dysraphic disturbances range from cystic dilation of the central canal (**myelocystocele**), over bifida spinal cords with or without a separating bony, cartilaginous, or fibrous septum (**diastematomyelia** or **diplomyelia**), to a **tethered cord with a dermal sinus** or other visible changes such as hair tufts, lipomas, or hemangiomas. The term *spina bifida occulta* is used incorrectly when it is applied to an incomplete ossification of the posterior vertebral arch, a frequent and insignificant finding that is neither clinically nor developmentally related to NTDs.

II. **Incidence.** Ninety-five percent of children with NTDs are born to couples with no family history of such defects.

A. **Statistics related to neural tube defects are to be interpreted with caution** and in the context of population, location, and time because occurrence of NTDs is affected by many epidemiologic and medical factors (see later sections).

B. **The overall worldwide incidence** has been quoted as approximately 1 in 1000 live births. Folic acid supplementation and clinical practice (eg, termination of pregnancy) have affected the incidence at birth; differences between countries are significant (see Section II.H).

C. **Spina bifida occulta, myelomeningocele, and anencephaly are the more frequently encountered NTDs.**

D. **At early embryonic stages, the incidence of neural tube defects is as high as 2.5%;** many abort spontaneously.

E. **The Centers for Disease Control and Prevention report that approximately 1500 infants with spina bifida are born in the United States per year.** The prevalence has decreased with folic acid food fortification (initiated in 1998) from 7.92 per 10,000 in 1996 (year of birth) to 4.61 per 10,000 in 2006. In 2016, it was estimated that in the United States alone, 600 to 700 babies are born without spina bifida per year as a result of folic acid fortification.

F. **Medical costs are significant.** Lifetime cost of NTDs are significant. In 2017, lifetime cost (for a US patient) was estimated at $791,900, or $577,000 excluding caregiving cost.

G. **Countries that have implemented mandatory fortification programs have reported a 20% to 50% reduction in incidence and subsequent decreases in prevalence of neural tube defects.** In the United States, a 19% reduction in the birth prevalence of NTDs was reported after fortification of the food supply.

H. **Geographic variation, sex, race, and social class**

1. **The incidence is higher in females versus males.**

2. **The risk is higher in Eastern Europeans, Hispanics, and in those from parts of Asia (northern China).** The risk is lower in Africans Americans, Africans, those from other regions of Asia, Pacific Islanders, and Ashkenazi Jews (compared to whites of European descent).

3. **Some populations with frequent consanguineous matings have an increased risk.**

4. **The risk is increased in infants of particularly young or particularly older mothers of lower socioeconomic class.** This increase may be related to nutritional factors.

III. **Pathophysiology.** The causes of NTDs seem to be multifactorial in most cases of anencephaly, encephalocele, myelomeningocele, and meningocele. Interactions between genetic and environmental factors result in disturbance of normal development. Recognized causes or contributing factors include the following:

A. **Nutritional and vitamin deficiencies.** Main concern: folate deficiency; other deficiencies linked to NTDs: vitamin B12 and zinc. *Note:* Folate occurs naturally; folic acid is the synthesized supplement.

B. **Chromosome abnormalities.** Include trisomies 13 and 18, triploidy, unbalanced translocations, and ring chromosomes.

C. **Genetic syndromes.** NTDs have been observed as part of a variety of syndromes, some with Mendelian inheritance patterns. A typical example is **Meckel-Gruber syndrome** (autosomal recessive), which presents with encephalocele, microcephaly, polydactyly, cystic dysplastic kidneys, and other anomalies of the urogenital system. Genetic references and databases list >50 syndromes associated with NTDs in the differential diagnosis. Recent advances into the understanding of neurodevelopment emphasize the importance of intact folate metabolism, primary cilia function and intact signaling pathways for normal development.

D. **Teratogens. Nitrates** (cured meat, blighted potatoes, salicylates, and hard water), **antifolates** (aminopterin, methotrexate, phenytoin, phenobarbital, primidone, carbamazepine, and valproic acid), **thalidomide**, and **abnormal glucose homeostasis in diabetic mothers** have all been implicated to contribute to the occurrence of NTDs. The role of other potential causes of NTD remains *controversial*; a potential interference with normal neurodevelopment has been discussed for a variety of exposures, including (but not limited to) **lead, glycol, clomiphene, hazardous waste**, and **maternal hyperthermia**.

E. **Other causes.** An overall increase in birth defects has been reported in infants of teenage mothers (<20 years old) compared with those mothers in the 25- to 29-year age range. The relative risk of nervous system defects in infants of teen mothers is 3.4 times that for children of 25- to 29-year-old mothers. Although a low body mass index does not increase the risk for NTDs, obesity does. The parents' ages are not related to the occurrence of NTDs per se; the risk for twins maybe higher.

IV. **Risk factors**

A. **Considering pathophysiology and introduction of folic acid food fortification,** the main clinically relevant risk groups are currently the following:

1. **Women with insulin-dependent diabetes mellitus** (the risk appears to be influenced by the level of control).

2. **Women with seizure disorders** who are being treated with valproic acid or carbamazepine.

3. **Women with a family history of neural tube defects.**

B. **The recurrence risk is as follows:**

1. **Two to three percent with 1 affected sibling.** Some types of NTDs may be folic acid resistant, and even with folic acid treatment, a residual risk of approximately 1% remains.

2. **Approximately 4% to 6% with 2 affected siblings.** Higher if other associated findings suggest a syndrome/condition with possible Mendelian inheritance.

V. **Clinical presentation.** Clinical presentations of the most severe NTDs are the obvious cranial defect in anencephaly and open spinal defects of the thoracic and/or lumbar spine with open spinal NTDs, both with exposure of neural tissue. NTDs with an intact skin cover may show an obvious mass (eg, an occipital encephalocele) or be more subtle. Subtle findings include bulging of the skin cover over the occipital or spinal defect, small openings sometimes missed on initial examination, dimples, or hair patches. See Section I for definitions and description of the different NTDs.

VI. Diagnosis
  A. **Prenatal screen using maternal serum α-fetoprotein at 14 to 16 weeks' gestation.** Elevated levels (>2.5 multiples of the mean, which are adjusted to gestational age) are indicative of open NTDs at a sensitivity of 90% to 100%, a specificity of 96%, and a negative predictive value of 99% to 100% but a low positive predictive value.
  B. **Prenatal diagnosis.** Documentation of an elevated maternal serum α-fetoprotein (AFP) is followed by:
    1. **Genetic counseling.** The patient should receive counseling regarding the risk of NTDs and other conditions with elevated AFP (gastroschisis or other conditions leading to fetal skin defects) in her fetus. The possibility of false-positive results (imprecise dates or twin pregnancies) should be considered; further evaluation (see following text) should be discussed, and nondirective counseling regarding treatment options should be provided.
    2. **Detailed fetal ultrasonography with anomaly screening.** In skilled hands, a detailed ultrasonogram (now often enhanced by 3-dimensional images) is extremely sensitive and specific for detection of NTDs. Sonographic determination of the level of the lesion is useful in predicting the ambulatory potential of fetuses with NTDs. Ultrasonography is also done to rule out other major congenital defects and is now often aided by fetal magnetic resonance imaging (MRI).
    3. **Measurement of the amniotic fluid α-fetoprotein and acetylcholinesterase.** Amniocentesis is usually done between 16 and 18 weeks' gestation. The detection rate for anencephaly and open spina bifida is 100% when results of amniotic fluid acetylcholinesterase and AFP are combined, with a false-positive rate of only 0.04%. If indicated, cells for a karyotype or microarray analysis can also be obtained.
  C. **Postnatal diagnosis.** Physical examination, imaging (as discussed for each NTD), and, if not done prenatally, genetic testing (karyotype, microarray or genome sequencing) as indicated.
VII. Management
  A. **Prevention of neural tube defections**
    1. **The British Medical Research Council** demonstrated in 1991 that high-dose folic acid (4 mg/d) reduced the recurrence risk of NTDs by 72%.
    2. **Multiple guidelines addressing supplementation have been published by a number of public health agencies and professional organizations.** Most address folic acid and/or prenatal vitamin supplementation for women capable of becoming pregnant and higher dose folic acid for women with a history of NTDs:
      a. **All women of childbearing age who are capable of becoming pregnant should consume a daily supplement containing 0.4 to 0.8 mg of folic acid.** This recommendation was most recently reaffirmed by the US Preventative Services Task Force (2017).
      b. **Women with a previous pregnancy resulting in a fetus affected by a neural tube defect should consume 4 mg of folic acid daily.** This was most recently affirmed in a policy statement by the American College of Medical Genetics (2011).
      c. **Ideally, folic acid should be taken before conception and at least through the first few months of gestation.**
    3. **Sources of folate and folic acid**
      a. **Dietary.** The average US diet used to contain about 0.2 mg of folate, which is less bioavailable than folic acid. Folate intake of 0.4 mg/d can be achieved through careful selection of folate-rich foods (spinach and other leafy green vegetables, dried beans, peas, liver, and citrus fruits). **Since January 1998, enriched grains (including flour, bread, rolls, cornmeal, pasta, and rice) in**

the United States are fortified with folic acid by order of the US Food and Drug Administration. Some countries have opted against food fortification due to concerns about adverse effects (masking of vitamin B12 deficiency, potential promotion of tumor growth) and issues relating to freedom of choice.

   b. **Supplementation.** Folic acid is available over the counter and by prescription. Prenatal vitamins also contain folic acid. Multiple sources are available to provide educational material: March of Dimes (www.marchofdimes.com; accessed September 20, 2018), Centers for Disease Control and Prevention (www.cdc.gov; accessed September 20, 2018), American Academy of Pediatrics via their Healthy Children Website (www.healthchildren.org; accessed September 20, 2018), and American College of Obstetrics and Gynecology (www.acog.org; accessed September 20, 2018).

4. **Current epidemiologic, biochemical, and genetic evidence** suggests that some NTDs are not primarily due to folate insufficiency but rather arise from changes in the metabolism of folate and possibly vitamin B12 in predisposed women. The mechanisms may also involve homocysteine metabolism. Polymorphisms of methylene tetrahydrofolate reductase and other genes encoding proteins involved in folate metabolism may be associated with an increased frequency of NTDs. Due to the homocysteine-lowering effect of folic acid, **supplementation may also reduce the risk for cardiovascular disease.** Some studies suggest that **folate and vitamin supplementation may also reduce the risk for other birth defects** (including congenital heart defects, orofacial clefts, urinary tract and limb defects, or even occurrence of trisomy 21). Other reports suggest an inverse association between folate intake and breast cancer, childhood neuroblastoma, and acute lymphoblastic leukemia. Promotion of tumor growth and the obscuring of vitamin B12 deficiency have been discussed as **potential adverse effects** of folate supplementation.

B. **Specific management**

1. **Anencephaly**

   a. **Approximately 75% of anencephalic infants are stillborn.** Live-born infants die within the first 2 weeks after birth.

   b. **Considering the lethality of anencephaly, palliative care is given.** Support services for the family, including social work and genetic and general counseling, are essential. Ethically *controversial* issues regarding the extent of care and other issues (eg, organ donation) may require involvement of other support systems (eg, ethics committees, support groups, or religious guidance—if desired by the family).

2. **Encephalocele**

   a. **Physical examination and initial management.** In addition to the general principles of neonatal resuscitation, an especially careful physical examination is indicated to assess the NTD and detect any **associated malformations.** We recommend that the child be given nothing by mouth until the **consultations** by subspecialties such as neurosurgery are obtained and a treatment plan has been formulated. **Imaging studies** (ultrasonography and MRI) should be arranged as indicated. If not done prenatally, genetic evaluation and testing (karyotype, microarray, and/or genome sequencing) should be initiated if indicated.

   b. **Neurosurgical intervention.** May be indicated to prevent ulceration and infection, except in cases with massive lesions and marked microcephaly where the decision might be for comfort care only. The encephalocele and its contents are often excised because the brain tissue within is frequently infarcted and distorted. Surgery may be deferred, depending on the size, skin coverage, and location. **Ventriculoperitoneal (VP) shunt** placement may be required because as many as 50% of cases have secondary hydrocephalus.

   c. **Counseling and long-term outcome.** A multidisciplinary approach is necessary to counsel the family regarding recurrence risk, long-term outcome, and follow-up. For family support and other resources, see Section VII.B.3.j. The degree of **deficits** is determined mainly by the extent of herniation and location; 1 or both cerebral hemispheres, the cerebellum, and even the brainstem can be involved. **Visual deficits** are common with occipital encephaloceles. **Motor and intellectual deficits** are found in approximately 50% of patients.

3. **Myelomeningocele.** Traditionally, postnatal surgery and management by a multidisciplinary team are the treatment for myelomeningocele. A multidisciplinary team approach, including a neonatologist, neurosurgeon, geneticist, genetic counselor, urologist, orthopedic surgeon, social worker, physiotherapist, and primary care physician, is necessary. The Management of Myelomeningocele Study (MOMS) was published in 2011 and found that prenatal surgery for myelomeningocele reduced the need for placement of a cerebrospinal fluid shunt and improved motor outcomes at 30 months but was associated with maternal and fetal risks. A Cochrane review in 2014 assessed evidence to be insufficient to recommend in utero repair for unborn babies with spina bifida; several centers in the United States continue to perform fetal surgery, and the MOMS study is ongoing.

a. **Physical examination.** Initial care as per Section VII.B.2.a; physical examination should include careful evaluation for other malformations (see Section III.C). See Table 111–1 for correlations between the level of a

Table 111–1. **CORRELATION OF THE LEVEL OF MYELOMENINGOCELE WITH LEVELS OF CUTANEOUS SENSATION, SPHINCTER FUNCTION, REFLEXES, AND POTENTIAL FOR AMBULATION**

Level of Lesion	Innervation	Cutaneous Sensation (Pinprick)	Sphincter Function	Reflexes	Ambulation Potential
Thoracolumbar	T12–L2	Groin (L1) Anterior upper thigh (L2)	—	—	Nonfunctional ambulation: Wheelchair, standing frame, full-leg orthosis
Lumbar	L3–L4	Anterior lower thigh and knee (L3) Medial leg (L4)	—	Knee jerk	Mainly household ambulation: May ambulate with orthosis and crutches
Lumbosacral	L5–S1	Lateral leg and medial foot (L5) Sole of foot (S1)	—	Ankle jerk	Usually household and community ambulation: May ambulate with or without short leg orthosis
Sacral	S2–S4	Posterior leg and thigh (S2) Medial buttock (S4) Middle of buttock (S3)	Bladder and rectal function	Anal wink	Community ambulation without orthosis

myelomeningocele and cutaneous sensation, sphincter function, reflexes, and potential for ambulation. Voluntary muscle movements may be difficult to elicit in newborns with myelomeningocele, and examination may be distorted initially by reversible spinal cord dysfunction above the level of the actual defect induced by exposure of the open cord.

    i. **Extent of neurologic dysfunction** tends to correlate with the level of the spinal cord lesion.

    ii. **Paraplegia** typically below the level of the defect.

    iii. **The presence of the anal wink and anal sphincter tone** suggests functioning sacral spinal segments and is prognostically important. In one study, 90% of patients with a positive anocutaneous reflex were determined to be "dry" on a regimen of intermittent catheterization as opposed to 50% of those with a negative reflex.

  b. **Initial management of the spinal lesion.**

    i. **There are institutional differences on how to cover the lesion,** and provision of a **sterile cover** can be achieved by several means. Some surgeons request that the infant be placed in a sterile plastic bag; others prefer application of plastic wrap to cover the lesion. Contact with gauze or other material that could adhere to the tissue and result in mechanical damage when removed is to be avoided. It is advisable to try to keep the defective area moist while avoiding bacterial contamination. If tolerated, the patient should be positioned on the side; fecal contamination should be avoided as much as possible.

    ii. **Be aware that a high rate of latex allergies** is reported in patients with NTDs. All patients with myelodysplasia should be considered at risk for anaphylaxis and other allergic complications. **Latex avoidance** is practiced as a preventive protocol. One study showed that after 6 years of a latex-free environment, the prevalence of latex sensitization fell from 26.7% to 4.5% of children with spina bifida. For information about latex allergy see American Latex Allergy Association (https://www.allergyhome.org/blogger/the-american-latex-allergy-association-and-latex-allergy/).

    iii. **In most centers, patients are started on antibiotics and given nothing by mouth.**

  c. **Surgical management.** Usually closure of the back lesion is done within 48 to 72 hours to prevent infection and further loss of function.

  d. **Hydrocephalus.** Common and often **noncommunicative** secondary to associated **Arnold-Chiari malformation** of the foramen magnum and upper cervical canal (usually type II) with resultant downward displacement of the medulla, pons, and cerebellum and obstruction of cerebrospinal fluid flow.

    i. **The risk of hydrocephalus** is 95% for infants with thoracolumbar, lumbar, and lumbosacral lesions and 63% for those with occipital, cervical, thoracic, or sacral lesions.

    ii. **In some cases, hydrocephalus may not be evident** until after closure of the myelomeningocele, and placement of a **VP shunt** may be required at a later date.

    iii. **Aggressive treatment with early ventriculoperitoneal shunt placement may improve cognitive function,** but cognitive function may also be affected by developmental abnormalities of the brain.

    iv. **Serial ultrasound scans are necessary to monitor the degree of hydrocephalus** because ventricular dilation may occur without rapid head growth or signs of increased intracranial pressure. The hydrocephalus often becomes clinically overt 2 to 3 weeks after birth.

    e. **Urinary tract dysfunction.** One of the major causes of morbidity and mortality after the first year of life.

        i. **More than 85% of myelomeningoceles located above S2 are associated with neurogenic bladder dysfunction, urinary incontinence, and ureteral reflux.** Poor bladder emptying immediately after NTD closure may be temporary ("spinal shock"), and improvement of bladder function may be observed up to 6 weeks after repair.

        ii. **Without proper management, hydronephrosis** may develop, with progressive scarring and destruction of the kidneys.

        iii. **Renal ultrasonography and a voiding cystourethrogram** may identify patients who may benefit from anticholinergic medication, clean and intermittent catheterization, prophylactic antibiotics, or early surgical intervention.

        iv. **Other associated renal anomalies** may be present in patients with NTDs, including renal agenesis, horseshoe kidneys, and ureteral duplications.

    f. **Bowel dysfunction.** A high percentage (>90% reported) of spina bifida patients have a neurogenic bowel that may result in fecal incontinence requiring diet modification, stool softeners, laxatives, or even surgical interventions.

    g. **Orthopedic issues**

        i. **With impairment of lower extremity innervation,** the risk of atrophy is high.

        ii. **Deformities of the foot, knee, hip, and spine** are common as a result of muscle imbalance, abnormal in utero positioning, or teratologic factors.

        iii. **Hip dislocation or subluxation** may occur and is usually evident within the first year of life; common in patients with midlumbar myelomeningocele.

        iv. **Treatment of orthopedic abnormalities** should be instituted as soon as there is sufficient healing of the back wound.

        v. **Physical therapists** assist with proper positioning of the extremities to minimize contractures and to maximize function.

    h. **Endocrine dysfunction.** NTDs can adversely affect the hypothalamic-pituitary axis. Precocious puberty and growth hormone deficiency (30%–70%) have been noted in children with NTDs.

    i. **Outcome of aggressive therapy**

        i. **The overall mortality rate** is now <15% by 3 to 7 years of age; 1-year survival of infants with spina bifida has been reported as high as 87.2%. Factors associated with increased mortality are low birthweight and high lesions.

        ii. **Infants with sacral lesions** have essentially no mortality.

        iii. **The outcome in regard to the highest potential for ambulation** depends largely on the level of the original lesion (see Table 111–1) and is modified by the orthopedic treatment and potential complications.

        iv. **Children with lumbar myelomeningocele score within the normal range on intelligence and achievement tests,** but deficits, possibly progressive, for performance intelligence quotient (IQ), arithmetic achievement, and visuomotor integration have been reported; reading and spelling may be less affected.

        v. **An intelligence quotient >80** is found in essentially all patients with lesions below S1; approximately 50% of survivors with thoracolumbar lesions have an IQ >80.

        vi. **Cognitive function** is improved in the presence of favorable socioeconomic and environmental factors.

    j. **Family support groups, educational material, and other resources.** Educational material and further information may be found at the following sites: March of Dimes (www.marchofdimes.com); Spina Bifida Association of America (www.spinabifidaassociation.org); International

Federation for Spina Bifida and Hydrocephalus (based in Europe; www .ifglobal.org). For information about latex allergy see American Latex Allergy Association (https://www.allergyhome.org/blogger/the-american-latex-allergy-association-and-latex-allergy/).

4. **Spina bifida occulta**
   a. **Neonatal features.** The presence of spina bifida occulta is suggested by overlying abnormal collections of hair, hemangiomas, pigmented macules, aplasia cutis congenita, skin tags, subcutaneous masses, and cutaneous tracts, usually in the lumbosacral area. Shallow sacral dimples are common and less of a concern.
   b. **If undetected in the neonatal period,** clinical presentation later in infancy may include delayed development of sphincter control, delayed walking, foot deformities, and/or recurrent meningitis. Sudden symptoms may represent vascular insufficiency produced by tension on a **tethered cord**, angulation of the cord around fibrous or related structures, or cord compression from a mass or cyst.
   c. **Diagnosis**
      i. **Ultrasonography is useful for screening.** Note that the acoustic window used to diagnose a tethered cord closes at 3 to 6 months.
      ii. **Magnetic resonance imaging** provides superior anatomic details; contrast is usually not needed.
   d. **Early surgical correction of a tethered cord** may be necessary to avoid the onset of symptoms. A timely surgical release and spinal cord decompression in patients developing symptoms may completely or partially reverse recently acquired deficits.

VIII. **Prognosis.** See individual topics in management section.

112 Orthopedic and Musculoskeletal Problems

Orthopedic problems are common in neonates. The problems can be isolated deformities or part of a generalized disorder. Usually these deformities are obvious, but a comprehensive musculoskeletal examination is the key for diagnosis of associated generalized disorders. This chapter provides an overview of the common problems encountered in the neonatal intensive care unit. **Many images of these neonatal orthopedic and musculoskeletal conditions, designated by [✿], can be found online** by visiting our website www.neonatologybook.com and clicking on the image tab.

I. **Spine problems**
   A. **Scoliosis**
      1. **Definition.** Scoliosis is a lateral deviation of the spine that is >10 degrees and typically includes the rotation and sagittal deformity. Scoliosis is classified into several types including idiopathic, congenital, and neuromuscular.
         a. **Infantile idiopathic scoliosis** is more common in boys and in Europe than North America. It is an uncommon scoliosis and thought to be related to infant positioning. Most children are diagnosed within the first 6 months of life and have left-sided thoracic curves. Plagiocephaly is a common association. The natural history is *controversial*, but these curves can improve

spontaneously. Radiographic measures described by Mehta have been used to predict the likelihood of progression. Neuro-axis abnormalities have been noted in >20% of these children, and a magnetic resonance image (MRI) of the spine is recommended for children with curves measuring 20 degrees or more. Casting and bracing have been successful treatment modalities in this condition. Occasionally surgical treatment is required, and the instrumentation is typically a growing rod.

    b. **Congenital scoliosis** is caused by anomalies in the growing vertebra. The etiology is unknown, but studies have indicated that carbon monoxide exposure may be a factor, and recent genetic studies suggest a possible congenital basis.

    The neuro-axis, vertebral column, and organ systems develop at similar periods in utero. Neuro-axis abnormalities can occur in up to a third of these children, 20% will have a genitourinary abnormality, and 20% will have a cardiac abnormality. The classification consists of 2 basic abnormalities: defects of vertebral formation and defects of vertebral segmentation. The hemivertebrae is an example of a defect in formation, while defects of segmentation include block vertebra and unilateral bars (this is where 1 side of 2 vertebrae are connected, leading to a growth tether).

    Progression of the deformity is typically due to an unbalanced growth and can be highly variable. A hemivertebrae with normal growth caudally and cranially can progress significantly. The unilateral bar is the most common cause of congenital scoliosis and can result in significant deformity, particularly if there are hemivertebrae associated.

  2. **Treatment.** Bracing is usually not a successful treatment regimen. Surgical management may be indicated for progressive curves. It may consist of a vertebral resection and spine realignment or a fusion to prevent further progression.

B. **Spina bifida.** [☼] See also Chapter 111.

  1. **Definition.** This group of disorders is characterized by congenital malformation of the spinal cord and vertebral column. Whereas the etiology of spina bifida is unknown, inadequate maternal intake of folic acid, gestational diabetes, and history of previously affected siblings with the same partner are contributory factors. There are 2 types:

    a. **Spina bifida occulta** is a defective formation of the posterior elements with intact skin and normal meninges and spinal cord.

    b. **Spina bifida cystica** is open skin with abnormal meninges and spinal cord. Spina bifida cystica is further subdivided into 3 types:

      i. **Meningocele.** The meningeal cyst herniates through a defect of the posterior elements of the spine but without the spinal cord or roots.

      ii. **Myelocele.** All the neural tissues are exposed without overlying tissues.

      iii. **Myelomeningocele.** This is the most common type (90%). The spinal cord and the nerve roots protrude outside the spinal canal through a defect in the posterior arch along with the meninges (dura, arachnoid). Other abnormalities of the spinal cord often occur with the myelomeningocele, including duplication of the cord (**diplomyelia**) and vertebral bony anomalies, such as defects in segmentation and failure of fusion of vertebral bodies, which cause congenital scoliosis, kyphosis, and kyphoscoliosis.

  2. **Diagnosis.** The diagnosis can be made prenatally by elevated maternal serum α-fetoprotein or by ultrasound, or postnatally by the presence of the lesion in the neonate's back. **A tuft of hair over the neonate's lumbosacral spine or skin dimple may be a sign of underlying anomalies.** Associated conditions are hydrocephalus, Arnold-Chiari malformation, congenital spinal deformity, and tethered cord syndrome. Ambulation is usually lost in upper thoracic or high lumbar lesions and is often preserved in lower lumbar and sacral lesions.

3. **Treatment.** Surgical repair is usually indicated within 48 hours after birth. If hydrocephalus is present, a shunt is required.

C. **Torticollis**

1. **Definition.** A lateral tilt of the neck and head typically due to a tight sternocleidomastoid muscle. The head and neck tilt toward the involved side, and the chin is turned toward the contralateral side. The most common causes are:

   a. **Congenital muscular torticollis.** [✿] Fibrosis of the sternomastoid muscle, which may be due to a localized compartment syndrome or uterine packing problems.

   b. **Vertebral anomalies.** Klippel-Feil syndrome (congenital anomalies of the cervical spine) or congenital occipitocervical anomalies.

2. **Diagnosis.** The diagnosis can be made with the observation of the typical deformity as well as palpation of a tight sternocleidomastoid muscle. A palpable mass in the muscle may appear in the postnatal period and resolve later on. Examination of the neonate for other congenital anomalies (developmental dysplasia of hip [DDH], metatarsus adductus) is essential. Radiographs of the cervical spine should be done to rule out any vertebral anomalies when there is no response to stretching exercises of the sternomastoid. Complications include plagiocephaly with facial asymmetry and restriction of neck movement.

3. **Treatment.** Stretching exercises are successful in 90% of the cases. Surgical correction may be considered in resistant cases after 1 year of age.

II. **Upper limb and hand anomalies**

A. **Radial club hand**

1. **Definition.** Radial club hand is a longitudinal partial or complete deficiency of the radius. The typical deformity is radial deviation of the wrist and hand with or without thumb hypoplasia. The ulna is usually short and deformed. It may be associated with thrombocytopenia (TAR [thrombocytopenia with absent radius] syndrome), Fanconi anemia, Holt-Oram syndrome, Nager syndrome, VATER/ VACTERL (*v*ertebral defects, *a*nal atresia, *t*racheoesophageal fistula, and *r*adial or *r*enal dysplasia/*v*ertebral defects, *a*nal atresia, *c*ardiac malformations, *t*racheoesophageal fistula, *r*enal dysplasia, and *l*imb abnormalities) association, and other skeletal and cardiac abnormalities.

2. **Treatment.** Splinting, stretching, physical therapy, and surgery.

B. **Below-elbow amputation (congenital amputation)**

1. **Definition.** Below-elbow amputation is a transverse deficiency resulting in the complete absence of the forearm just below the elbow. It is the most common form of congenital amputation (1 in 20,000 newborns has a transverse forearm deficiency). The hand or its remnants can be attached to the proximal forearm. Commonly, it is unilateral with no genetic basis or known cause.

2. **Treatment.** There is no treatment required, although prosthesis fitting may be useful.

C. **Polydactyly**

1. **Definition.** Polydactyly is duplication of 1 or more fingers. It is most common among African Americans. It may be associated with Ellis-van Creveld syndrome or chromosomal anomalies.

   a. **Ulnar polydactyly, postaxial type.** [✿] It may affect the little finger. It has an autosomal dominant inheritance with variable penetration.

   b. **Central polydactyly.** It affects the central 3 fingers (central polydactyly). It typically has autosomal dominant inheritance.

   c. **Thumb polydactyly, preaxial type.** [✿] It affects the thumb.

2. **Treatment.** Surgical reconstruction is often indicated.

D. **Macrodactyly**

1. **Definition.** Macrodactyly is an abnormal enlargement of the digits due to an osseous and/or soft tissue enlargement. Generalized enlargement may be due to a complex vascular malformation or neurofibromatosis. Klippel-Trenaunay-Weber

syndrome (triad of port-wine stain, varicose veins, and bony and soft tissue hypertrophy involving an extremity) and Proteus syndrome are rare syndromes associated with macrodactyly. There are 2 varieties of macrodactyly: 1 presents as a large digit at birth, which grows at a normal growth rate, and in the other, the digit is normal at birth and then grows at a faster rate subsequently.

2. **Treatment.** Surgical reconstruction is usually indicated.

E. **Syndactyly**

1. **Definition.** Syndactyly [✿] is congenital webbing between the fingers. The fusion may be complete if it extends to the fingertips or complex if it involves the bony elements of the adjacent digits. It may be an isolated anomaly or associated with chromosomal or genetic disorders (eg, trisomies 21, 13, 18; Silver syndrome; Prader-Willi syndrome; or focal dermal hypoplasia). It is more common in boys, often with bilateral involvement. Also, it is more common in the ring and middle fingers than the index finger and thumb.

2. **Treatment.** Surgical reconstruction is often indicated in the first year of life to allow for development of hand function.

III. **Hip disorders**

A. **Developmental dysplasia of the hip.** [✿] (See also Chapter 7.) A wide spectrum of hip abnormalities ranging from hip instability to frank dislocation. In certain cultures, newborn cradling may be an etiologic factor in DDH (eg, American Indians' use of the cradleboard with the hip extended and adducted). Hip examinations usually demonstrate hip instability. The following tests are used for clinical screening of the neonates:

1. **Ortolani test** (reduction test for the dislocated hip). [✿] The child should be positioned supine with both the knees and hips flexed 90 degrees. The test is then performed with 1 hand stabilizing the pelvis and the other hand with the thumb over the hip adductors and the index finger over the greater trochanter. The hip is slowly abducted, so the dislocated femoral head slips toward the acetabulum, creating reduction (audible and palpable). The positive Ortolani test is a sign of dislocated hip.

2. **Barlow test** (provocative test for the dislocatable hip). [✿] The child is positioned as for the **Ortolani test**. The hip is mildly adducted and pressure is applied posteriorly. If the femoral head slips over the posterior rim of the acetabulum and slides back again into the acetabulum when the pressure is released, this is considered Barlow positive, which means the hip is dislocatable.

3. **Hip ultrasound examination** is indicated for screening of high-risk neonates (Table 112–1), although some clinical communities do ultrasound screening of all children. **Pavlik harness** is the treatment of choice for neonates with dislocated hips (positive Ortolani test). In the majority of Barlow-positive neonates, the hips stabilize in the postnatal period. Neonates with a positive Barlow test should have a repeat clinical and ultrasound examination after 4 weeks. If the hip is not stable at that time, a Pavlik harness should be used. Surgical treatment is rarely indicated in the postnatal period [✿].

B. **Surveillance versus screening.** Surveillance is suggested to replace the term *screening* because it means "close monitoring of someone or something to avoid adverse outcome." In clinical practice, this means periodic physical examinations during the well-child visits. Surveillance should be done until the age of 6 to 9 months. These exams should be supplemented with ultrasound or pelvis x-rays according to the child's age.

C. **Treatment.** Evidence supports screening and treatment of a hip dislocation (positive Ortolani test). It also supports observing instability (positive Barlow test) and mild early forms of dysplasia. The goal is to diagnose hip dislocation/subluxation by 6 months of age by doing periodic physical examinations and selective ultrasonography or radiography, with consultation with pediatric radiology and/or orthopedics.

Table 112–1. RISK FACTORS FOR DEVELOPMENTAL DYSPLASIA OF THE HIP (THE RISK FACTORS HAVE ADDITIVE EFFECT)

Important risk factors:
- Breech presentation
- Female gender
- Incorrect lower extremity swaddling
- Family history of DDH
- Second infant of identical twin if the other had DDH (40% risk), nonidentical twin (3% risk)

Other suggested factors (not found to increase the risk of nonsyndromic DDH):
- First-born infant
- Torticollis
- Foot abnormalities
- Oligohydramnios

DDH, developmental dysplasia of the hip.

1. **Observation** for early milder forms of dysplasia and instability (as seen in positive Barlow test). Observation involves periodic reexamination and possible repeat imaging by a pediatrician or orthopedist. If those infants with a positive Barlow test continue to show clinical instability, they need to be referred to an orthopedist. The majority of hip anomalies seen on ultrasound at 6 weeks to 4 months of age will resolve without treatment. There are no specific recommendations on whether to observe or treat these minor ultrasound findings (minor variations in the alpha and beta angles and subluxation with stress maneuvers).

2. **Treatment for hip dislocation (positive Ortolani test)** is recommended, and it is not an emergency. These infants can follow up with an orthopedist within several weeks of discharge. Hip-abduction braces are usually recommended and do not have to be initiated in the hospital. Use of "triple diapers" (theoretically prevents hip adduction) is not recommended with presumed DDH.

3. **Practice safe swaddling. Avoid traditional/tight swaddling.** Safe swaddling is hip-healthy swaddling (allows for hip motion, hip flexion and abduction, and knee flexion), avoids the forced position of hip extension and adduction, and decreases the risk of DDH.

IV. **Lower extremity disorders**
   A. **Proximal focal femoral deficiency [✿]**
      1. **Definition.** Proximal focal femoral deficiency (PFFD) is a congenital anomaly of the proximal femur and pelvis resulting in a short femur and hip deformity. There is no known genetic etiology. The femoral segment is short, abducted, flexed, and externally rotated. There may be genu valgum and anterior cruciate ligament deficiency of the knee joint. The deformity is bilateral in 15% of cases. Fibular hemimelia may be associated with PFFD.
      2. **Treatment.** Either reconstruction (limb lengthening and realignment) or amputation.
   B. **Fibular hemimelia [✿]**
      1. **Definition.** This is characterized by congenital complete or partial absence of the fibula. There is no known genetic etiology. The tibia is short with a valgus and procurvatum deformity. There is often a skin dimple at the apex of the deformity. Fibular hemimelia is frequently associated with foot deformities with or without deletion of the lateral foot rays. Equinovalgus foot deformity is the most common associated foot deformity.
      2. **Treatment.** Depends on the foot deformity and degree of limb length discrepancy (LLD). The surgical options are limb reconstruction (lengthening and realignment) or amputation of the deformed foot and fitting of a prosthesis.

C. **Tibial hemimelia** [✿]
1. **Definition.** This is a congenital partial or complete absence of the tibia. The infant usually presents with a short extremity with a rigid equinovarus, supinated foot deformity. [✿] Preaxial polydactyly is a relatively common associated anomaly. Other congenital anomalies may be associated with tibial hemimelia, such as congenital cardiac anomalies and/or spine deformities. It is one of the few congenital limb deformities that have a genetic etiology and is seen with syndromes associated with ectrodactyly (cleft hand and foot deformity).
2. **Treatment.** The surgical options are either reconstruction or knee disarticulation.
D. **Posteromedial bowing of the tibia**
1. **Definition.** This is a benign condition characterized by a posteromedial bowing of the tibia. It is associated with a calcaneovalgus foot deformity and LLD. The condition should be differentiated from anterolateral bowing of the tibia (associated with congenital pseudarthrosis of the tibia and neurofibromatosis) and from fibular hemimelia.
2. **Treatment.** The natural history is complete resolution of the tibial deformity, although LLD may be significant.
E. **Hyperextension deformity of the knee (congenital knee dislocation)**
1. **Definition.** It is a rare deformity and varies from a simple hyperextension of the knee to a frank anterior dislocation of the tibia on the femur. It is seen as an isolated deformity and may be associated with other conditions (eg, Larsen syndrome). There is a loss of ability to flex the knee actively or passively. Radiographs are helpful to make the diagnosis and to differentiate simple hyperextension deformities from congenital knee dislocation.
2. **Treatment.** Mild cases respond to serial manipulation and casting. Surgery may be required in severe cases.
V. **Foot disorders.** Foot disorders are common and require careful assessment for proper diagnosis. Examples of common foot disorders are noted in the following text and in Table 112–2.
A. **Syndactyly**
1. **Definition.** Syndactyly is congenital webbing between toes. There are usually no functional problems associated with foot syndactyly. The fusion may be complete if it extends to the toenails or complex if it involves the bony elements of the adjacent digits. It may be associated with polydactyly.
2. **Treatment.** Surgical release is rarely indicated for foot syndactyly.
B. **Cleft foot** [✿]
1. **Definition.** Cleft foot is due to an absence of the central 2 or 3 rays of the foot. The cone-shaped cleft of the forefoot tapers proximally. Autosomal inheritance is common in bilateral cases and uncommon in unilateral cases. In bilateral cases, the hand may be affected as well.
2. **Treatment.** Surgery may be indicated to improve shoe fitting.
C. **Macrodactyly** [✿]
1. **Definition.** This is an uncommon deformity due to an enlargement of both soft tissue and osseous elements of the toes; it may affect the great toes or lesser toes. The hand may be affected as well.
2. **Treatment.** Debulking (excision of bone and soft tissues) procedures are usually indicated.
D. **Constriction band (amniotic band) syndrome**
1. **Definition.** This syndrome is due to a tight band around the extremity. It can present in different forms: congenital amputations, acrosyndactyly, clubfoot, and craniofacial defects such as cleft palate (see Figure 93–1).
2. **Treatment.** A surgical release of the tight band. The band may cause acute vascular compromise, and emergency surgical release of the band may be indicated to preserve the neonate's limb.

Table 112–2. DIFFERENTIAL DIAGNOSIS OF COMMON NEONATAL AND NEWBORN FOOT DISORDERS

Foot Deformity	HF	FF	Missing Rays	Flexibility	Treatment	Comments
FH (fibular hemimelia) [☼]	Equinovalgus	Normal or adductus	Lateral rays may be missing	Flexible or rigid	Amputation vs reconstruction	Tibia is short and deformed
CF (clubfoot) [☼]	Equinovarus	1. Adductus, cavus, supination				May be associated with DDH or spine anomalies
	Posterior crease	2. Transverse crease of the midfoot crossing longitudinal arch	No	Rigid	Serial casting	Genetic factors may have role Prenatal diagnosis at 16–20 weeks
VT (vertical talus) [☼]	Equinovalgus	Adductus	No	Very rigid	Serial casting and surgery	Isolated deformity 50% Spina bifida 50% bilateral
MA (metatarsus adductus) [☼]	Normal	Adductus	No	Flexible	No treatment vs serial casting	Associated with DDH or spine anomalies Related to intrauterine packing
CV (calcaneovalgus foot) [☼]	Equinovalgus	Normal	No	Flexible	No treatment vs stretching	May be associated with posteromedial bowing tibia

[☼] Images can be found at www.neonatologybook.com.
Adductus, medial deviation of metatarsus; cavus, increased medial longitudinal arch of the foot; DDH, developmental dysplasia of the hip; equinus, limited ankle dorsiflexion; FF, forefoot; HF, hindfoot; valgus, eversion deformity; varus, inversion deformity.

E. **Polydactyly** [☼]

1. **Definition.** Polydactyly is characterized by duplication of 1 or more toes. Pre-axial polydactyly refers to a duplication of the great toe; postaxial is a duplication of the fifth toe (the most common type—80%). It is less common in central toes. It is more common in African American children. Fifty percent are bilateral, and 30% of patients have a positive family history. There is an autosomal dominant inheritance with variable expressivity. Foot polydactyly is commonly an isolated deformity but may be associated with other syndromes such as **Ellis-van Creveld syndrome** or trisomy 13. The diagnosis is usually obvious, and radiographs are essential to detect the type of polydactyly (which bony structures are duplicated). Preaxial polydactyly may be associated with tibial hemimelia.

2. **Treatment.** Amputation of the extra digit is the treatment of choice.

VI. **Arthrogryposis multiplex congenita** [☼]

A. **Definition.** It is a syndrome characterized by multiple (at least 2 or more) joint contractures in multiple body areas (literally the word means "curved joints"). The specific etiology is still unknown. Reduced fetal movement is an etiologic factor. The typical newborn has all the extremities affected. The typical joint contractures are internally rotated shoulders, elbow extension, a pronated forearm, and flexion contractures of the wrist and fingers. Lower extremity contractures include flexion and external contracture of the hip, or the hip may be extended and dislocated. The knee may be extended or flexed, and severe foot deformities are common.

1. **Treatment.** Stretching and splinting are the treatments of choice in early life to avoid fixed deformities.

VII. **Birth trauma.** Orthopedic injuries or fractures that occur during birth (Table 112–3). Recent reports suggested the use of ultrasound for fracture diagnosis to minimize the risk of radiation exposure. Ultrasound is comparable to x-ray for the detection of fractures and should be used first. It is simple, readily available, and not expensive for detection of birth-related injuries, especially around unossified epiphysis.

A. **Clavicular fractures**

1. **Definition.** Clavicular fractures are the most common birth fractures in neonates. These typically occur during delivery with shoulder dystocia or complete extension of the arm in breech presentations or in large infants. The neonate may have minimal symptoms or signs, and the diagnosis may be retrospective with palpation of the callus in the second week of life. The neonate may be irritable with tenderness over the clavicle; there may also be loss of motion of the affected arm, an asymmetric Moro reflex, and pseudo-paralysis. **The radiograph is diagnostic with the fracture at the junction between the middle and outer thirds.** The condition should be differentiated from a humerus fracture or brachial plexus injury. Prognosis is very benign.

2. **Treatment.** Treatment is immobilization with pinning of the sleeve of the shirt to the chest of the neonate's clothes for 7 to 10 days.

Table 112–3. **RISK FACTORS FOR ORTHOPEDIC-RELATED BIRTH INJURIES**[a]

Oversized infants >4 kg
Premature infants <37 weeks (due to their fragile bones, which can be easily fractured)
Shoulder dystocia with difficult labor
Cephalopelvic disproportions
Prolonged labor

[a]Birth fractures rarely occur below the elbow or below the knee.

B. **Humeral and femoral fractures**
   1. **Definition.** These fractures are less common than the clavicle fracture. **Both are associated with prolonged labor, extension of the injured extremity during breech presentation, rapid extraction of the infant during fetal distress, and forceps delivery.** The fracture usually occurs through the diaphysis (femur; less commonly the humerus) or through the growth plate (proximal or distal humerus, distal femur). The neonate usually has pain, limitation of movements, pseudo-paralysis, tenderness, and crepitus at the fractured ends. Periarticular fractures can be easily overlooked. The diagnosis is made by radiograph.
   2. **Treatment.** Immobilization of the limb with splints for 3 weeks is satisfactory, and the prognosis is excellent. There is a remarkable remodeling potential and rarely residual shortening or angulation.
C. **Brachial plexus injuries**
   1. **Definition.** Stretching of the cervical nerve roots during delivery results in brachial plexus injuries. **The condition is usually associated with oversized neonates with a vertex presentation and shoulder dystocia, or after a breech presentation.** The fifth and sixth cervical nerve roots are commonly affected and result in **Erb palsy.** The arm is adducted and internally rotated with elbow extension and forearm pronation with normal hand function. The extremity sensation is intact, and the Moro reflex and biceps reflex are usually absent in the affected limb. If the lower cervical and first thoracic roots are affected, it is called **Klumpke paralysis.** There is a loss of the grasp response of the hand with forearm paralysis, and both are poor prognostic signs. Examination of the other extremities is essential to exclude neonatal quadriplegia. Occasionally, it may be bilateral, especially with breech deliveries. Full muscle testing is essential 48 hours after delivery. **Horner syndrome (eg, decreased pupil size, a drooping eyelid) is usually present on the affected side.** Recovery may occur within 48 hours or it can take up to 6 months. Imaging studies include plain radiograph, computed tomographic myelography, and MRI. Nerve conduction studies may be helpful to differentiate between root avulsion versus neurapraxia. For upper plexus injuries, the biceps function is a marker of spontaneous recovery. A preserved biceps function has a better prognosis. The prognosis depends on the type of injury to nerve roots (neurapraxia, axonotmesis, or neurotmesis) and the extent of nerve involvement and degree of recovery after initial palsy.
   2. **Treatment.** Surgery is rarely indicated in neonates. Surgical options include a microsurgical repair, tendon transfers to replace the weak muscles, or humeral osteotomy to correct the residual deformities in untreated cases.
VIII. **Orthopedic infections (osteomyelitis).** [✿] Prematurity, skin infections, and a complicated delivery are known risk factors for osteomyelitis. Hematogenous spread is the most common route of spread. The organisms may gain access to the circulation through venous or umbilical catheters, intravenous feeding lines, or invasive monitoring. The infection usually starts in the metaphysis of long bones. Because the nutrient vessels cross the growth plate to supply the epiphysis, septic thrombophlebitis of these vessels can lead to a growth plate injury and growth disturbances later in life. The thin cortex and periosteum of the neonate's bones are poor barriers for infection spread, allowing an infection to be easily spread to the adjacent tissues. When the metaphysis of long tubular bones is intracapsular, these infections usually result in septic arthritis (hip joint, shoulder joints). The osteomyelitis in premature infants or severely ill full-term infants tends to be multifocal with or without septic arthritis (usually 2 or 3 sites). **The most common organism is *Staphylococcus aureus;* the least common organism is group B streptococci, although other organisms may be isolated.** Diagnosis may be difficult due to a lack of symptoms and signs, especially in mild cases, but limitation of movements or pseudo-paralysis and/or local swelling should be taken seriously. Less common presentations are pain on passive motion and abnormal posture of the limb. Once the sepsis is suspected, joint or bone aspiration is indicated to confirm the

diagnosis. Laboratory tests include a complete blood count, erythrocyte sedimentation rate, C-reactive protein, and blood culture. Other diagnostic tools include a plain radiograph (usually normal or might only show a soft tissue swelling), ultrasound, bone scan, or MRI. Surgical drainage is indicated when an abscess is formed. The common sites are hip, shoulder, and knee joints. It is considered a surgical emergency to avoid the long-term results of infection.

113 Osteopenia of Prematurity (Metabolic Bone Disease)

I.   **Definition.** Prematurity affects bone mineralization and bone mineral content (BMC). **Metabolic bone disease (MBD)** of prematurity is a term currently used more often compared with osteopenia of prematurity. MBD is best defined as a decrease in BMC relative to expected level of mineralization for gestational age (GA) with **biochemical** and **radiologic** features. Normal bone is formed by the deposition of minerals, predominantly calcium (Ca^{2+}) and phosphorus (P), onto an organic matrix (osteoid) secreted by the osteoblasts. Osteoclasts play an important role in bone resorption and remodeling. Although osteopenia and rickets result in decreased bone mineralization and may have similar clinical findings, they are not identical processes and thus the term *rickets of prematurity* is not used in this chapter. Osteopenia or MBD is principally a result of inadequate Ca^{2+} and P intake to meet bone growth demands. Rickets, however, is principally due to vitamin D deficiency; vitamin D supplementation alone will not resolve either osteopenia or rickets. Both disease processes involve the utilization of Ca^{2+}, P, and vitamin D.

   A.   **Osteopenia** refers to a decrease in the amount of organic bone matrix (osteoid) due to a decrease in the thickness or number of trabeculae and/or decreased thickness of the bone cortex. These can be due to either insufficient deposition or increased resorption of the organic bone matrix. Bone mineral density is the amount of minerals per square centimeter of bone (measured as T-scores [the number of standard deviations (SDs) above or below the mean of a healthy adult of the same sex] or Z-scores [the number of SDs above or below the mean compared with someone with the same age, gender, weight, and ethnicity]). Osteopenia is defined as bone density with as a score of –1 to –2.5.

   B.   **Osteomalacia** refers to the lack of *mineralization* of the organic bone matrix resulting in accumulation of nonmineralized osteoid and softening of bones. *When involving the growth plate*, it results in **rickets**. Bone density and BMC are both decreased.

   C.   **Osteoporosis.** Refers to a decrease in bone mineral density (T-scores) <2.5 standard deviations from the norm (adults). There is no accepted definition of osteoporosis in infants.

II. **Incidence.** The current incidence of MBD in very low birthweight (VLBW; <1500 g) infants is unknown because there is no universal consensus on its definition and no large population-based or network-based studies have addressed this issue. However, due to improvements in nutritional management such as initiation of early feedings, changes in nutritional formulas, and initiation of early parenteral nutrition, the current incidence of MBD may be decreasing. MBD is now more commonly seen in extremely low birthweight (ELBW; <1000 g) infants and those with chronic illnesses such as bronchopulmonary dysplasia/chronic lung disease and necrotizing enterocolitis.

Previous studies have reported osteopenia to occur in 23% of VLBW infants and in 55% to 60% of ELBW infants. A more recent prospective study found mild MBD (alkaline phosphatase [ALP] >500 IU/L and P ≥4.5 mg/dL) in 13.7% and severe MBD (ALP >500 IU/L and P <4.5 mg/dL) in 3.3% of VLBW infants. Fractures have been reported previously in up to 10% of VLBW infants but are likely to be less common now. A recent multicenter retrospective study from England found evidence of rib fractures in approximately 2% of ex-preterm infants (median GA at birth, 26 weeks; median corrected GA at time of chest radiograph, 39 weeks).

III. **Pathophysiology.** Intrauterine bone formation occurs either as endochondral ossification (axial and appendicular skeleton) with the deposition of an osteoid matrix with a cartilaginous core or as membranous matrix without the cartilaginous precursors (skull, maxilla, mandible). Several vitamins (A, C, D), cytokines, minerals (Ca^{2+}, P), and hormones (thyroid hormone, estrogen, calcitonin, growth hormone, parathyroid hormone [PTH]–related peptide) play important roles in fetal bone growth. The placenta is essential to fetal nutrient and mineral accretion. Conditions that affect placental sufficiency directly impact fetal mineral accretion.

A. **An increase in trabecular thickness and bone volume occurs faster in utero compared with ex utero.** After birth, bone growth is secondary to cyclical bone formation and resorption. In the first year, bone growth occurs by increases in length and diameter but with a decrease in cortical thickness; however, there is an overall 3-fold increase in bone strength. This adaptation occurs earlier in preterm infants than in term infants. Mineral retention is affected more than linear growth, contributing to a reduction in bone density following preterm birth. In preterm infants, the BMC remains lower at term-equivalent than for full-term infants.

B. **Approximately 99% of body calcium and 80% of phosphorus is in the skeleton at a term birth, and nearly 80% of this transfer occurs between 25 weeks' gestation and term.** Fetal accretion rate for Ca^{2+} (120 mg/k/d) and P cannot be met ex utero. Further, inadequate intake (Ca^{2+} and P) in the face of increased growth demands results in nutrient deficiency.

C. **Genetics and bone disease.** In adults and in VLBW infants, osteoporosis is associated with polymorphisms involving *VDR*, *ER*, and *COLIA1* genes. In VLBW infants, homozygous allelic variants of ERα genotype with a low number of thymidine-adenine repeats [(TA)n] were correlated with high urinary pyridinoline crosslink levels (indicating increased bone resorption) and with the development of MBD. The locus interaction between *VDR* and *COLIA1* was found to be protective in the development of bone disease.

IV. **Risk factors**

A. **Fetal and neonatal causes**

1. **Prematurity and low birthweight.** Preterm birth interrupts placental transfer of minerals to the newborn resulting in Ca^{2+} and P deficiency. Physiologic adaption following preterm birth also increases bone reabsorption. **The frequency of MBD is inversely related to GA and birthweight.** Both conditions predispose these infants to mineral deficiencies in the face of increased nutritional and growth requirements.

2. **Feeding practices.** Delayed enteral feeding, prolonged use of parenteral nutrition, use of unfortified human milk, enteral feeding restrictions, and malabsorption states can result in mineral deficiencies. Chronic metabolic acidosis increases bone reabsorption. A recent multicenter study found that **widespread hypophosphatemia and MBD were associated with elemental formula (Neocate)** use in infants; presumably due to impaired bioavailability of formula P.

3. **Human milk** is low in P, and donor milk content is even lower compared with preterm maternal milk. Prolonged use can result in low serum P levels and decreased incorporation into the organic bone matrix. Unfortified human milk cannot match the mineral accretion that can be achieved across the placenta.

   4. **Drugs.** Corticosteroids, furosemide, and methylxanthines are commonly used in preterm infants and cause mobilization of Ca^{2+} from the bone, resulting in decreased BMC.
   5. **Lack of mechanical stimulation.** Bone growth requires mechanical stimulation that is interrupted by preterm birth, illness, sedation, and paralysis. Neurologically impaired infants with spina bifida or arthrogryposis with limited mobility have poor bone growth.
   6. **Vitamin D.** Preterm infants can absorb vitamin D and convert 25-OH to 1,25-dihydroxy vitamin D. Vitamin D is also converted to 1,25-dihydrocholecalciferol in the placenta, which is important in the transfer of P to the fetus. Generally, **MBD of prematurity is not secondary to vitamin D deficiency.** Postnatal vitamin D deficiency may occur in breast-fed infants without fortification due to low levels (25–50 IU/L) in breast milk. Other causes of vitamin D deficiency in preterm infants include the following:
      a. **Renal (osteodystrophy) disorders.**
      b. **Drugs such as phenytoin and phenobarbital** increase vitamin D metabolism.
      c. **Pseudo–vitamin D deficiency** (absence of 1-α hydroxylase enzyme that converts 25-OH to 1,25-dihydroxy vitamin D [type I] or tissue resistance to 1,25-dihydroxy vitamin D [type II]).
   7. **Aluminum contamination of parenteral nutrition.**
   8. **Malabsorption of vitamin D and calcium** can occur in infants with prolonged cholestasis and short gut syndrome.
B. **Maternal factors**
   1. **Maternal deficiency of vitamin D results in low fetal levels.** Maternal vitamin D deficiency in Europe, particularly in the winter, is associated with a low total BMC and a decreased intrauterine long bone growth. Maternal vitamin D status may also influence head circumference (at 3–6 months) and BMC at 9 years of age.
   2. **Maternal smoking, thin body habitus,** low Ca^{2+} intake, and increased physical activity in the third trimester result in a decreased BMC in the fetus.
   3. **Exposure to high doses of magnesium** in utero, preeclampsia, chorioamnionitis, and placental infections are associated with osteopenia.
   4. **Higher incidence of postnatal rickets** is seen in infants with **fetal growth restriction** (chronic damage to the placenta may alter P transport).
   5. **Placental hormones including estrogen** and PTH and PTH-related protein also play a role.
V. **Clinical presentation.** Clinically, osteopenia manifests between 6 and 12 weeks of age and is usually asymptomatic; however, signs may include the following:
   A. **Severe manifestations**
      1. **Poor weight gain and growth failure.**
      2. **Rickets-like findings** may include growth retardation, frontal bossing, craniotabes, prominence of the costochondral junction (rachitic rosary), and epiphyseal widening.
      3. **Fractures** may manifest as pain on handling.
      4. **Respiratory difficulties** or failure to wean off ventilator support due to poor chest wall compliance.
   B. **Consequences of osteopenia.** Osteopenia can result in myopia of prematurity due to alterations in the shape of the skull. In childhood, infants remain thinner and shorter with a decreased total BMC and density. Increased urinary Ca^{2+} excretion has also been reported.
VI. **Diagnosis**
   A. **Radiographs.** Osteopenia may be been subjectively on radiographs obtained for other indications. Objective changes are not seen until a 20% to 40% decrease in bone mineralization occurs. Thin "washed-out" bones, cupping, fraying, and rarefaction of the end of long bones may occur. Subperiosteal new bone formation

and fractures may also be visible. Serial radiographs in 3 to 4 weeks may be useful for follow-up. A radiologic scoring system has also been developed but is not well validated.

B. **Screening.** The American Academy of Pediatrics Committee on Nutrition (AAP-CON) recommends screening all VLBW infants for MBD with serum P and ALP starting at 4 to 5 weeks of age and biweekly thereafter until stable and down trending ALP. Other high-risk infants (eg, prolonged total parenteral nutrition use [>4 weeks], cholestasis, exposure to chronic steroids or diuretics, unable to reach full fortified enteral feeds by 4 weeks, elemental formula feeding) should be screened as well.

C. **Biochemical markers of bone turnover**
   1. **Markers of bone activity**
      a. **Calcium levels** usually remain normal until late in the course.
      b. **Phosphorous.** Serum P levels are low (<4 mg/dL) in this disease. Low P levels have low sensitivity but high specificity. Low levels of inorganic phosphate <1.8 mmol/L with elevated ALP may be more specific for diagnosing inadequate intake. Phosphate deficiency may be the earliest sign of poor mineralization. Some experts also recommend measuring urine P and calculating tubular reabsorption of phosphate, which is elevated (>95%) in MBD.
      c. **Alkaline phosphatase.** Serum ALP is the sum of 3 isoforms (liver, intestine, and bone). The bone isoform contributes to the largest proportion (90%). ALP in infants can be up to 5 times the normal adult values. Elevated levels can be due to both osteoblastic and osteoclastic activity. The use of bone-specific isoform has not been found to improve sensitivity for predicting the development of osteopenia. Serial monitoring of ALP may be helpful in diagnosing osteopenia, with levels >500 IU/L suggestive in ELBW infants. ALP is also negatively correlated with P levels in MBD.
         i. **Elevated levels of alkaline phosphatase** can be seen with normal growth, healing rickets, fractures, or copper deficiency.
         ii. **Low levels of alkaline phosphatase are seen with zinc deficiency,** severe malnutrition, and congenital hypophosphatasia.
         iii. **Isolated elevation in alkaline phosphatase** without Ca^{2+} and P derangements may occur with transient hyperphosphatasemia of infancy.
         iv. **Elevated alkaline phosphatase >900 IU/L and low phosphorous** (<4.6 mg/dL) have high sensitivity (100%) but low specificity (70%) for diagnosing low bone density. **Very high levels (>1200 IU/L) have been associated with short stature in childhood.**
      d. **Parathyroid hormone** may be an early marker with better sensitivity than ALP in screening for MBD. In 1 study, at 3 weeks of chronologic age, a PTH level >180 mg/dL^{-1} or a P level <4.6 pg/mL^{-1} yielded a sensitivity of 100% and specificity of 94% for severe MBD.
      e. **1,25-Dihydroxy vitamin D levels** are elevated with osteopenia. Routine measurement of vitamin D or its metabolites is not recommended.
      f. **Osteocalcin (marker for osteoblastic activity)** may be elevated.
   2. **Markers of bone resorption**
      a. **Urinary calcium and phosphorous.** Extreme prematurity is associated with a low P threshold and an increased excretion even with low serum P levels. High tubular resorption of P suggests inadequate intake. Urinary Ca^{2+} excretion >1.2 mmol/L and inorganic phosphate at >0.4 mmol/L suggest a high bone mineral accretion.
      b. **Crosslinked carboxy-terminal telopeptide of type I collagen,** urinary pyridinium crosslink products, crosslinked *N*-telopeptides of type I collagen, and pyridinoline crosslinks of collagen are markers for bone resorption but are in limited clinical use.

3. **Bone mineral density.** Reference values for bone mineral densities in healthy preterm infants with normal ALP levels have been developed that correlate with dual-energy x-ray absorptiometry (DEXA). A normal bone mineral density >0.068 g/cm^2 has a high negative predictive value for developing MBD.

D. **Ultrasound.** A quantitative ultrasound, using a broadband ultrasound measurement, speed of sound (SOS), or bone transmission time, has been used. However, SOS cannot be used as surrogate for DEXA.

   1. **Advantages.** Ultrasound offers several advantages, including easy accessibility and lack of exposure to ionizing radiation. It uses peripheral sites such as the calcaneus and tibia. It measures both qualitative and quantitative bone properties, such as bone mineralization and cortical thickness, respectively, in addition to bone mass (osteopenia), elasticity, and microarchitecture.

   2. **Speed of sound is most commonly used.** The SOS decreases in preterm infants from birth to term (corrected age) and is suggestive of decreased BMC. Inverse correlation between tibial SOS at birth and serum ALP has also been noted. Higher Ca^{2+} intake may inversely affect the decline in SOS noted after preterm birth.

E. **Dual-energy x-ray absorptiometry.** It is the gold standard used to assess both bone size and bone mineral status and can predict risk of fractures in newborn infants. Normative data and guidelines for use in infants are lacking, making interpretation of results difficult. Disadvantages also include expense, radiation, and possible need for sedation.

VII. **Management**

A. **Feeding and nutritional practices.** Establishment of early enteral feeding, decreasing length of parenteral nutrition, fortification of human milk, and using specialized preterm formula can limit osteopenia. Postdischarge use of specially designed preterm or transitional formulas (see also Chapter 11 on nutrition) and human milk fortification promotes mineralization. AAP-CON recommends Ca^{2+} (150–220 mg/kg/d) and P (75–140 mg/kg/d) supplementation to achieve adequate *retention* levels. This is usually achieved by feeding preterm formula/fortified human milk at 160 mL/kg/d. Calcium gluconate and sodium or potassium phosphate supplements are suitable choices for infants who require intravenous administration. Occasionally, additional enteral supplements are needed based on P and ALP level. Care should be taken to avoid adding them directly to milk to prevent precipitation. Adequate vitamin D intake is also essential.

B. **Vitamin D.** Vitamin D sufficiency in mothers is important to prevent deficiency in the fetus. Requirements have been reported to vary between 150 and 1000 IU/d of vitamin D. AAP-CON recommends that infants should receive 200 to 400 IU/d of vitamin D.

C. **Physical activity/stimulation.** Mechanical stimulation by passive exercises to improve bone mineralization has yielded conflicting outcomes. Improved weight gain and length but not head circumference have been reported with some improvements in BMC, bone length, and bone area in individual studies. A recent Cochrane review concluded that current evidence does not justify the standard use of physical activity programs in preterm infants.

D. **Minimize use of furosemide and corticosteroids.** The use of thiazide diuretics, although of theoretical advantage, has not been shown to prevent osteopenia.

E. **Malabsorption.** Infants at risk of cholestasis and malabsorption may benefit from additional supplementation with fat-soluble vitamins and use of a specialized formula to facilitate fat absorption.

VIII. **Prognosis.** MBD appears to be decreasing with improved prevention and treatment practices. BMC remains 25% to 70% lower at term in the extremely premature infants. Catch-up mineralization occurs by 6 months of age. Long-term follow-up suggests that bone growth and adult height may also be impacted in these infants.

114 Patent Ductus Arteriosus

I. **Definition.** The ductus arteriosus is a large vessel that connects the main pulmonary trunk (or proximal left pulmonary artery) with the descending aorta, some 5 to 10 mm distal to the origin of the left subclavian artery. In the fetus, it serves to shunt blood away from the lungs and is essential (closure in utero may lead to fetal demise or pulmonary hypertension). In full-term healthy newborns, functional closure of the ductus occurs rapidly after birth. Final functional closure occurs in almost half of full-term infants by 24 hours of age, in 90% by 48 hours, and in all by 96 hours after birth. **Patent ductus arteriosus (PDA) refers to the failure of the closure process and continued patency of this fetal channel.**

II. **Incidence.** The incidence varies according to means of diagnosis (eg, clinical signs vs echocardiography).

   A. **Factors associated with increased incidence of patent ductus arteriosus**

      1. **Prematurity.** The incidence is inversely related to gestational age. PDA is found in approximately 45% of infants <1750 g; in infants weighing <1000 g, the incidence is closer to 80%.

      2. **Respiratory distress syndrome and surfactant treatment.** The presence of respiratory distress syndrome (RDS) is associated with an increased incidence of a PDA, and this is correlated with the severity of RDS. After surfactant treatment, there is an increased risk of a clinically symptomatic PDA; moreover, surfactant may lead to an earlier clinical presentation of a PDA.

      3. **Fluid administration.** An increased intravenous fluid load in the first few days of life is associated with an increased incidence of PDA.

      4. **Asphyxia.**

      5. **Congenital syndromes.** PDA is present in 60% to 70% of infants with congenital rubella syndrome. Trisomy 13, trisomy 18, Rubinstein-Taybi syndrome, and XXXXX (penta-X) syndrome are associated with an increased incidence of PDA.

      6. **High altitude.** Infants born at a high altitude have an increased incidence of PDA.

      7. **Congenital heart disease.** A PDA may occur as part of a congenital heart disease (eg, coarctation, pulmonary atresia with intact septum, transposition of the great vessels, or total anomalous pulmonary venous return).

   B. **Factors associated with a decreased incidence of patent ductus arteriosus**

      1. **Antenatal steroid administration**

      2. **Fetal growth restriction**

      3. **Prolonged rupture of membranes**

III. **Pathophysiology.** In the fetus, the ductus is essential to divert blood flow from the high-resistance pulmonary circulation to the descending aorta. After birth, functional closure of the ductus occurs within hours (but up to 3–4 days). The patency of the ductus depends on the balance between the various constricting effects (eg, of oxygen) and the relaxing effects of various substances (most importantly, the prostaglandin E family). The effects of oxygen and prostaglandins vary at different gestational ages. Oxygen has less of a constricting effect with decreasing gestational age. However, the sensitivity of the ductus to the relaxing effects of prostaglandin E_2 is greatest in immature animals (and decreases with advancing gestational age). In term infants, responsiveness is lost shortly after birth, but this does not occur in the immature ductus. Indomethacin constricts the immature ductus more than it does in the close-to-term ductus.

    The magnitude and direction of the ductus shunt are related to the vessel size (diameter and length), the pressure difference between the aorta and the pulmonary artery, and the ratio between the systemic and pulmonary vascular resistances. The clinical features associated with a left-to-right ductal shunt depend on the magnitude of the shunt and the ability of the infant to handle the extra volume load. Left ventricular output is increased by the extra volume return. The increase in pulmonary venous return causes an increase in ventricular diastolic volume (preload). Left ventricular dilation will result, with an increase in left ventricular end-diastolic pressure and a secondary increase in left atrial pressure. This may eventually result in left heart failure with pulmonary edema. Eventually, these changes may lead to right ventricular failure. With a PDA, there is also a redistribution of systemic blood flow secondary to retrograde aortic flow (ductal steal, or "run off"). Renal and mesenteric blood flows are thus reduced, as is cerebral blood flow.

IV. **Risk factors.** See Section II.

V. **Clinical presentation.** The initial presentation may be at birth but is usually on days 1 to 4 of life. The cardiopulmonary signs and symptoms are as follows:

    A. **Heart murmur.** The murmur is usually systolic and heard best in the second or third intercostal space at the left sternal border. The murmur may also be continuous and sometimes heard only intermittently. Frequently, it may be necessary to disconnect the infant from mechanical ventilation to appreciate the murmur.

    B. **Hyperactive precordium.** The increased left ventricular stroke volume may result in a hyperactive precordium.

    C. **Bounding peripheral pulses and increased pulse pressure.** The increased stroke volume with diastolic runoff through the PDA may lead to these signs.

    D. **Hypotension.** A PDA is associated with a decreased mean arterial blood pressure. In some infants (particularly those of extremely low birthweight), hypotension may be the earliest clinical manifestation of a PDA, sometimes without a murmur (ie, the "silent" PDA).

    E. **Respiratory deterioration.** Respiratory deterioration after an initial improvement in a small premature infant with RDS should arouse suspicion of a PDA. The deterioration may be gradual (days) or brisk (hours) but is usually not sudden (as in pneumothorax). PDA may similarly complicate the respiratory course of chronic lung disease.

    F. **Other signs.** These may include tachypnea, crackles, or apneic spells. If the PDA is untreated, the left-to-right shunt may lead to heart failure with frank pulmonary edema and hepatomegaly.

VI. **Diagnosis**

    A. **Echocardiography.** Two-dimensional echocardiography combined with Doppler ultrasonography is by far the most sensitive means of diagnosing a PDA. The ductus can be directly visualized, and the direction of flow may be demonstrated. In addition, echocardiography can assess the secondary effects of the PDA (eg, left atrial and ventricular size) and contractility. The echocardiogram will also rule out alternative or additional cardiac diagnoses.

    B. **Imaging studies.** On initial presentation, the chest film may be unremarkable, especially if the PDA has occurred against a background of preexisting RDS. Later, pulmonary plethora and increased interstitial fluid may be noted with subsequent florid pulmonary edema. True cardiomegaly is usually a later sign.

VII. **Management**

    A. **Ventilatory support.** Respiratory distress secondary to a PDA may require intubation and mechanical ventilation. If the infant is already ventilated, the PDA may lead to increased ventilatory requirements. These should be determined by blood gases. Increasing positive end-expiratory pressure is helpful in controlling pulmonary edema.

    B. **Fluid restriction.** Decreasing fluid intake as far as possible decreases the PDA shunt as well as the accumulation of fluid in the lungs. Increased fluid intake in the first few weeks of life is associated with an increased risk of patency of the ductus in premature infants with RDS.

    C. **Increasing hematocrit.** Increasing the hematocrit (Hct) above 40% to 45% will decrease the left-to-right shunt. Frequently, an increase in Hct abates some of the signs of the PDA (eg, the murmur may disappear).

D. **Indomethacin.** A prostaglandin synthetase inhibitor that has proved to be effective in promoting ductal closure. Its effectiveness is limited to premature infants and also decreases with increasing postnatal age; thus, it has limited efficacy beyond 3 to 4 weeks of age, even in premature infants. There are essentially 3 approaches to administering indomethacin for ductal closure in premature infants: **prophylactic, early symptomatic, and late symptomatic.** *Note:* There are minor variations in dosage regimens, and what follows are guidelines. Pharmacologic information on indomethacin can be found in Chapter 155.

1. **Prophylactic indomethacin.** A dose of 0.1 mg/kg/dose is given intravenously (infused over 20 minutes) every 24 hours from the first day of life for 6 days. In this regimen, indomethacin is given prophylactically to all infants <1250 g birthweight who have received surfactant for RDS (before any clinical signs suggestive of PDA). It would also be appropriate to limit this regimen to infants with RDS who are <1000 g birthweight. Clinical trials have shown that this treatment is safe and effective in reducing the incidence of symptomatic PDA in these infants. The major drawback is that up to 40% of these infants probably would never have had a symptomatic PDA and hence did not require treatment.

2. **Early symptomatic indomethacin.** Infants are given indomethacin, 0.2 mg/kg intravenously (infused over 20 minutes). Second and third doses are given 12 and 36 hours after the first dose. The second and third doses are 0.1 mg/kg/dose if the infant is <1250 g birthweight and <7 days old. If the infant is either >7 days old or >1250 g, the second and third doses are also 0.2 mg/kg/dose. Indomethacin is given if there is any clinical sign of a PDA (eg, a murmur) and before there are signs of overt failure. This is usually on days 2 to 4 of life.

3. **Late symptomatic indomethacin.** Infants are given indomethacin when signs of congestive failure appear (usually at 7–10 days). Dosage is as described in Section VII.D.2. The problem with this approach is that if indomethacin fails to constrict the ductus significantly, there is less opportunity for a second trial of indomethacin, and the infant is more likely to require surgery.

4. **Ductus reopening and indomethacin failure.** In 20% to 30% of infants, the ductus reopens after the first course of indomethacin. In such cases, a second course of indomethacin may be worthwhile because a significant proportion of these infants have their PDA closed with this course. The ductus is more likely to reopen in infants of very low gestational age and in those who had received a greater amount of fluids previously. Infection and necrotizing enterocolitis (NEC) are also risk factors for ductus reopening (and may be contraindications for indomethacin).

5. **Complications of indomethacin**

   a. **Renal effects.** Indomethacin causes a transient decrease in the glomerular filtration rate and urine output. In such cases, fluid intake should be reduced to correct for the decreased urine output, which should improve with time (usually within 24 hours).

   b. **Gastrointestinal bleeding.** Stools may be heme positive after indomethacin. This is transient and usually of no clinical significance. Indomethacin is a mesenteric vasoconstrictor, but the PDA itself also decreases mesenteric blood flow. In most trials of indomethacin, there was no increased incidence of NEC.

   c. **Spontaneous intestinal perforation.** Indomethacin exposure has been associated with spontaneous intestinal perforation, especially when the drug was given early or when given together with postnatal corticosteroids. Caution is warranted, although none of the randomized trials comparing indomethacin with placebo have shown this finding.

     d. Platelet function. Indomethacin impairs platelet function for 7 to 9 days regardless of platelet number. In the various trials of indomethacin, there is no increased incidence of intraventricular hemorrhage (IVH) associated with the drug, and there is no evidence that it extends the degree of preexisting IVH. Nevertheless, it may be unwise to impose additional platelet dysfunction in infants who are also significantly thrombocytopenic.

   6. **Indomethacin contraindications**

     a. Serum creatinine >1.7 mg/dL.

     b. Frank renal or gastrointestinal bleeding or generalized coagulopathy.

     c. Necrotizing enterocolitis.

     d. Sepsis. All anti-inflammatory drugs should be withheld if there is sepsis. Indomethacin may be given once sepsis is controlled.

E. Ibuprofen. Another nonselective cyclooxygenase inhibitor that closes the ductus in animals. Clinical studies have shown that ibuprofen is as effective as indomethacin for the treatment of PDA in preterm infants. It has an advantage in that it does not reduce mesenteric and renal blood flow as much as indomethacin and is associated with fewer renal side effects. Urine output is higher and serum creatinine is lower in infants treated with ibuprofen compared with those treated with indomethacin. However, in trials comparing indomethacin with ibuprofen, no differences were found in incidence of significant clinical side effects (eg, NEC, renal failure, IVH). Choice of 1 drug over the other is largely a matter of institutional preference and may be often based on physiologic rather than clinical considerations. The dose used is an initial dose of 10 mg/kg followed by 2 doses of 5 mg/kg each after 24 and 48 hours if treatment is given in the first week of life. Due to change in pharmacokinetics, dosages of 18 mg/kg, 9 mg/kg, and 9 mg/kg at 24-hour intervals have been recommended when given in the second week of life.

F. Acetaminophen (Paracetamol) acts by inhibiting prostaglandin synthetase at its peroxidase segment, thereby reducing the production of prostaglandin E_2. It is unknown whether this is the only mechanism whereby acetaminophen affects the PDA. However, a number of recent studies, both observational and randomized controlled, have shown that acetaminophen has a success rate comparable to that of ibuprofen in closing the PDA. Although the optimal dosage has yet to be ascertained, a common protocol for intravenous acetaminophen is a loading dose of 20 mg/kg followed by doses of 10 mg/kg every 6 hours for a duration of 3 days. Dosage may be continued for a further 3 days if the PDA remains open. For extremely premature babies (<28 weeks), it may be prudent to increase the interval between doses to 8 to 12 hours. For older neonates, dosages of 15 mg/kg have also been suggested. Acetaminophen can also be given orally, and in that form, dosage of 15 mg/kg/dose given every 6 to 8 hours has been used. Case series have suggested that acetaminophen may be useful in some cases where the postnatal age may mitigate against the success rate of indomethacin or ibuprofen or in cases where there is contraindication to their use. The primary concern in using acetaminophen in premature neonates is the potential for hepatic dysfunction. Although current data suggest that the drug is safe, there are still insufficient data, especially in extremely low birthweight neonates, and it may be prudent to monitor liver enzymes.

G. Surgery. Surgery should be performed in patients with a hemodynamically significant PDA in whom medical treatment has failed or in whom there is a contraindication to the use of indomethacin. Surgical mortality is low (<1%). However, some observational studies have suggested that surgical ligation is associated with an increased risk of chronic lung disease and neurodevelopmental/neurosensory impairment in extremely premature infants. It is not clear whether this association is causal or whether the need for ligation served as a marker for a higher risk subgroup of patients. However, a recent large observational study has suggested that surgical ligation of the PDA does not carry an additional burden of mortality or morbidity.

H. **Patent ductus arteriosus in the full-term infant.** PDA accounts for approximately 10% of all congenital heart disease in full-term infants. The PDA in a full-term infant is structurally different, which may explain why it does not respond appropriately to the various stimuli for closure. Indomethacin is usually ineffective. The infant should be monitored carefully, and surgical ligation should be considered at the earliest signs of significant congestion. Even without signs of failure, the PDA should be ligated before 1 year of age to prevent endocarditis and pulmonary hypertension.

I. **Should the ductus be treated?** (*Controversial*) The issues of when and whether to treat the PDA in the preterm infant are matters of ongoing controversy. There is no doubt that there is an association between the PDA and various morbidities of the premature infant. However, there is a debate about whether this relationship is a causal one and hence whether treatment is likely to be of benefit. Numerous controlled trials have failed to show clinical benefit to the pharmacologic closure of the symptomatic PDA in terms of duration of mechanical ventilation, incidence of bronchopulmonary dysplasia/chronic lung disease, NEC, retinopathy of prematurity, or length of hospitalization. Early pharmacologic closure is, unsurprisingly, associated with a decreased need for later surgical ligation (and hence surgical morbidities). Meta-analyses have confirmed these findings. The only beneficial effect of very early prophylactic treatment with indomethacin appears to be a reduction in the incidence of severe pulmonary hemorrhage and of severe IVH, and even this does not necessarily translate into improved long-term neurodevelopmental outcome. Hence, there has been an increasing trend, over the past few years, to leave many cases of PDA untreated in the neonatal period and during the neonatal intensive care unit stay. However, a differing overview and analysis of the clinical trials carried out to date and controlled observational data have suggested that prolonged exposure to a large PDA is associated with a prolonged need for supplemental oxygen or mechanical ventilation. In addition, studies in premature baboons have shown diminished alveolar development and impaired pulmonary mechanics in animals exposed to a moderate PDA for 14 days. The impaired alveolarization and pulmonary mechanics were attenuated by pharmacologic closure of the PDA (but not by surgical ligation). It is thus possible that the adverse effects of the ductus would be primarily seen in those infants destined to have either a PDA with a sizable shunt and/or prolonged exposure to significant ductal patency. Thus, only a subgroup of neonates may require treatment. Various attempts to identify such a select subgroup of high-risk neonates who might benefit from treatment have been made using a variety of clinical and echocardiographic criteria or biochemical ones (eg, B-type natriuretic peptide). However, no outcomes-based randomized controlled trials have been done to demonstrate improved outcomes with selective treatment based on these criteria.

J. **Feeding infants with patent ductus arteriosus (or on treatment)** (*controversial*). Given the physiologic effects of the PDA, and medications used to treat it, on intestinal blood flow, there is no consensus regarding whether feedings should be withheld or continued in the presence of a PDA or during its treatment. Data are lacking, and there is wide variability in clinical practice.

VIII. **Prognosis.** Prognosis is excellent in infants who only have a PDA. Studies show that premature infants <30 weeks have a spontaneous closure of the PDA 72% of the time. Conservative treatment (with medication) has a closure rate of approximately 94%.

115 Persistent Pulmonary Hypertension of the Newborn

I. **Definition. Persistent pulmonary hypertension of the newborn (PPHN)** is a condition characterized by marked pulmonary hypertension resulting from elevated pulmonary vascular resistance (PVR) and altered pulmonary vasoreactivity, leading to right-to-left extrapulmonary shunting of blood across the foramen ovale and the ductus arteriosus, if it is patent. It is associated with a wide array of cardiopulmonary disorders that may also cause intrapulmonary shunting. When this disorder is of unknown cause and is the primary cause of cardiopulmonary distress, it is often called idiopathic PPHN or persistent fetal circulation.

II. **Incidence:** 2 to 6 per 1000 live births.

III. **Pathophysiology.** PPHN may be the result of underdevelopment of the lung together with its vascular bed (eg, congenital diaphragmatic hernia and hypoplastic lungs), maladaptation of the pulmonary vascular bed to the transition occurring around the time of birth (eg, various conditions of perinatal stress, hemorrhage, aspiration, hypoxia, and hypoglycemia), and maldevelopment of the pulmonary vascular bed in utero from a known or unknown cause. It is convenient to think in terms of this basic pathologic classification. However, the clinical manifestations of PPHN are often not attributable to a single physiologic or structural entity, and many disorders exhibit >1 underlying pathology. Often, even when there is evidence of perinatal or postnatal stress (eg, meconium aspiration), the underlying cause of PPHN had been secondary to an in utero process of some duration.

Preacinar arteries are already present in the lungs by 16 weeks' gestation; thereafter, respiratory units are added with further growth of the appropriate arteries. Muscularization, differentiation, and growth of the peripheral pulmonary arteries are influenced by numerous trophic factors (eg, fibroblast growth factors) and by changes that occur in the connective tissue matrix. The lungs of infants with PPHN contain many undilated precapillary arteries, and pulmonary arterial medial thickness is increased. There may be extension of muscle in small and peripheral arteries that are normally nonmuscular. After a few days, there is already evidence of structural remodeling with connective tissue deposition.

In the fetus, PVR is high, and only 5% to 10% of the combined cardiac output flows into the lungs, with most of the right ventricular output crossing the ductus arteriosus to the aorta. After birth, with expansion of the lungs, there is a sharp drop in PVR, and pulmonary blood flow increases approximately 10-fold. The factors responsible for maintaining high PVR in the fetus and for effecting the acute reduction in PVR that occurs after birth are incompletely understood. Fetal and neonatal pulmonary vascular tone is modulated through a balance between vasoconstrictive and vasodilatory stimuli. Vasoconstrictive stimuli include various products of arachidonic acid metabolism (eg, thromboxane) and the endothelins (ETs). The hemodynamic effects of the ETs are mediated by at least 2 receptors: ET-A and ET-B. The fetal lung also produces a number of cyclooxygenase-dependent metabolites that function as pulmonary vasodilators (eg, prostaglandin [PG] I_2, PGE_1, and PGE_2). It has also become clear that the endothelium (and its interaction with vascular smooth muscle cells) plays a crucial role in regulating pulmonary vascular tone. Nitric oxide (NO), a potent vasodilator, is synthesized from L-arginine by endothelial NO synthase. NO stimulates soluble guanylate cyclase, which produces cyclic guanosine monophosphate (cGMP) and causes vasodilation. cGMP, in turn, is hydrolyzed by cyclic nucleotide phosphodiesterases (PDEs), and manipulation of these controls the intensity and duration of cGMP action. Various isoenzymes of

PDE have been identified, and inhibition of PDE type 5 (PDE5; by, eg, sildenafil) causes pulmonary vasodilation.

In summary, for successful pulmonary circulatory transition to occur, various mechanical, physiologic, and biochemical factors, which maintain high fetal PVR, must be eliminated or reversed. Major events are the replacement of the fluid-filled lung of the fetus with the air-filled postnatal lung, the increase in oxygen tension, and the increase in pulmonary blood flow (which increases shear stress and thereby increases NO). At the same time, changes occur in the synthesis and release of various biochemical modulators of vascular tone, and there are interactions between the mechanical and biochemical events surrounding birth. Disturbances in this cascade of events may lead to PPHN. At the same time, manipulation of these pathways enables us to treat it.

IV. **Risk factors.** The following factors or conditions may be associated with PPHN:
   A. **Lung disease.** Meconium aspiration, respiratory distress syndrome (RDS), pneumonia, pulmonary hypoplasia, cystic lung disease (including congenital cystic adenomatoid malformation and congenital lobar emphysema), diaphragmatic hernia, and congenital alveolar capillary dysplasia.
   B. **Systemic disorders.** Polycythemia, hypoglycemia, hypoxia, acidosis, hypocalcemia, hypothermia, and sepsis.
   C. **Congenital heart disease.** Particularly, total anomalous venous return, hypoplastic left heart syndrome, transient tricuspid insufficiency (transient myocardial ischemia), coarctation of the aorta, critical aortic stenosis, endocardial cushion defects, Ebstein anomaly, transposition of the great arteries, endocardial fibroelastosis, and cerebral venous malformations.
   D. **Perinatal factors.** Asphyxia, perinatal hypoxia, and maternal ingestion of aspirin or indomethacin.
   E. **Miscellaneous.** Central nervous system disorders, neuromuscular disease, and upper airway obstruction. Although still contentious, some observational studies have suggested that the use of selective serotonin reuptake inhibitors during the last half of pregnancy may be associated with PPHN in the newborn.
V. **Clinical presentation.** The primary finding is respiratory distress with cyanosis (confirmed by demonstrating hypoxemia). This may occur despite adequate ventilation. Other clinical findings are highly variable and depend on the severity, stage, and other associated disorders (particularly pulmonary and cardiac diseases).
   A. **Respiratory.** Initial respiratory symptoms may be limited to tachypnea, and onset may be at birth or within 4 to 8 hours of age. In addition, in an infant with pulmonary disease, PPHN should be suspected as a complicating factor when there is marked lability in oxygenation. These infants may have significant decreases in pulse oximetry readings with routine nursing care or minor stress (eg, movement or noise). Furthermore, a minor decrease in inspired oxygen concentration may lead to a surprisingly large decrease in arterial oxygenation (eg, the alveolar-to-arterial oxygen gradient [AaDO$_2$] changes more rapidly and is more labile than that seen in the normal course of progression of uncomplicated RDS or other pulmonary disease).
   B. **Cardiac signs.** Physical findings may include a prominent right ventricular impulse, a single second heart sound, and a murmur of tricuspid insufficiency. In extreme cases, there may be hepatomegaly and signs of heart failure.
   C. **Imaging.** The chest film may show either cardiomegaly or a normal-sized heart. If there is no associated pulmonary disease, the film may show normal or diminished pulmonary vascularity. If there is also a parenchymal lung disorder, the degree of hypoxemia may be out of proportion to the radiographic measure of severity of the pulmonary disease.
VI. **Diagnosis. PPHN is essentially a diagnosis of exclusion.**
   A. **Differential oximeter readings.** In the presence of right-to-left shunting of blood via the patent ductus arteriosus, the partial pressure of oxygen (PaO$_2$) in preductal blood (eg, from the right radial artery) is higher than that in the postductal

blood (obtained from left radial, umbilical, or tibial arteries). Hence, simultaneous preductal and postductal monitoring of oxygen saturation is a useful indicator of right-to-left shunting at the ductal level. However, it is important to note that PPHN cannot be excluded if no difference is found because the right-to-left shunting may be predominantly at the atrial level (or the ductus may not be patent at all). A difference >5% between preductal and postductal oxygen saturations is considered indicative of a right-to-left ductal shunt. A difference >10 to 15 mm Hg between preductal and postductal PaO_2 is also considered suggestive of a right-to-left ductal shunt. Preductal and postductal oxygenation should be assessed simultaneously.

   B. **Hyperventilation test.** (See pages 489 and 490.) PPHN should be considered if marked improvement in oxygenation (>30 mm Hg increase in PaO_2) is noted on hyperventilating the infant (lowering arterial partial pressure of carbon dioxide [$PaCO_2$] and increasing pH). When a "critical" pH value is reached (often ~7.55 or greater), PVR decreases, there is less right-to-left shunting, and Pao_2 increases. This test may differentiate PPHN from cyanotic congenital heart disease. Little or no response is expected in infants with the latter diagnoses. It has been suggested that infants subjected to this test should be hyperventilated for 10 minutes. Prolonged hyperventilation is not recommended, however, particularly in premature infants (see later discussion).

   C. **Imaging.** Clear lung fields or only minor disease in the face of severe hypoxemia is strongly suggestive of PPHN, if cyanotic congenital heart disease has been ruled out. In an infant with significant pulmonary parenchymal disease, a chest film is of little help in diagnosing PPHN (although it is indicated for other reasons). In an infant with rapidly worsening oxygenation, the major value of a chest film is in the exclusion of alternative diagnosis (eg, pneumothorax or pneumopericardium).

   D. **Echocardiography.** Often essential in distinguishing cyanotic congenital heart disease from PPHN because the latter is frequently a diagnosis of exclusion. Furthermore, whereas all the other previously mentioned signs and tests are suggestive, echocardiography (together with Doppler studies) can provide confirmatory evidence that is often diagnostic. The first question that needs to be answered is whether the heart is structurally normal. Then the pulmonary artery pressure can be assessed indirectly by measuring the velocity of the tricuspid regurgitant jet when present. A flattened interventricular septum or one that is bowing into the left ventricle also supports the diagnosis of PPHN. Similarly, information about right-to-left shunting at the atrial and ductal levels supports the diagnosis of PPHN. Echocardiography can also be used to assess ventricular output and contractility (both of which may be depressed in infants with PPHN).

VII. **Management**

   A. **Prevention.** Adequate resuscitation and support from birth may presumably prevent or ameliorate, to some degree, PPHN when it may occur superimposed on a preexisting condition. An example is adequate and timely ventilation of an asphyxiated infant with appropriate attention to temperature control.

   B. **General management.** Infants with PPHN clearly require careful and intensive monitoring. Fluid management is important because hypovolemia aggravates the right-to-left shunt. However, once normovolemia can be assumed, there is no known benefit to be gained from repeated administration of either colloids or crystalloids. Normal serum glucose and calcium should be maintained because hypoglycemia and hypocalcemia aggravate PPHN. Temperature control is also crucial. Significant acidosis should be avoided. It is useful to use 2 pulse oximeters: 1 preductal and 1 postductal.

   C. **Minimal handling.** Because infants with PPHN are extremely labile with significant deterioration after seemingly "minor" stimuli, this aspect of care deserves special mention. Endotracheal tube suctioning, in particular, should be performed only if indicated and not as a matter of routine. Noise level and physical manipulation should be kept to a minimum.

D. **Mechanical ventilation.** Often needed to ensure adequate oxygenation and should first be attempted using "conventional" ventilation. The goal is to maintain adequate and stable oxygenation using the lowest possible mean airway pressures. The lowest possible positive end-expiratory pressure should also be sought. However, atelectasis should be avoided because it may aggravate pulmonary hypertension (PH) and also impair effective delivery of inhaled NO (iNO) to the lungs. Hyperventilation should be avoided, and as a guide, $PaCO_2$ values should be kept >30 mm Hg if possible; levels of 40 to 50 mm Hg, or even higher, are also acceptable if there is no associated compromise in oxygenation. Initially, it would be wise to ventilate with 100% inspired oxygen concentration. Weaning should be gradual and in small steps. In infants who cannot be adequately oxygenated with conventional ventilation, high-frequency oscillatory ventilation (HFOV) should be considered early. In the presence of parenchymal lung disease, infants treated with HFOV combined with iNO were less likely to be referred for ECLS than those treated with either therapy alone.

E. **Surfactant.** In infants with RDS, administration of surfactant is associated with a fall in PVR. Surfactant may also be of benefit in various other pulmonary disorders (eg, meconium aspiration), although it is unknown whether its actions in these disorders are related to a reduction in PVR. There is evidence for surfactant deficiency in some patients with PPHN.

F. **Pressor agents.** Some infants with PPHN have reduced cardiac output. In addition, increasing systemic blood pressure reduces the right-to-left shunt. Hence, at least a normal blood pressure should be maintained, and some recommend maintaining blood pressure of >40 mm Hg. **Dopamine is the most commonly used drug for this purpose.** Dobutamine has the disadvantage, in this context, that, although it may improve cardiac output, it has less of a pressor effect than dopamine. **Milrinone**, a type 3 PDE inhibitor, is also sometimes employed to improve cardiac output. Milrinone reduces PH in experimental animal models, and a few small case series have reported on its beneficial effects in neonates with PPHN. However, the use of milrinone has been associated with occasional cases of systemic hypotension in adults and of higher heart rates in neonates. Hence, more data are needed before widespread use of milrinone can be recommended.

G. **Sedation.** The lability of these infants has been mentioned previously, and hence, sedation is commonly used. Pentobarbital (1–5 mg/kg) or midazolam (0.1 mg/kg) is frequently used, and analgesia with morphine (0.05–0.2 mg/kg) is also used.

H. **Inhaled nitric oxide.** See also Chapters 9 and 155.
   1. **Background.** Controlled clinical trials have shown that NO, when given by inhalation, reduces PVR and improves oxygenation and outcomes in a significant proportion of term and near-term neonates with PPHN. The administration of iNO to infants with PPHN reduces the number requiring ECLS without increasing morbidity at 2 years of age. In another large multicenter trial, iNO was demonstrated to reduce both the need for ECLS and the incidence of bronchopulmonary dysplasia (BPD)/chronic lung disease (CLD). Oxygenation can also improve during iNO therapy via mechanisms additional to its effect of reducing extrapulmonary right-to-left shunting. iNO can also improve oxygenation by redirecting blood from poorly aerated or diseased lung regions to better aerated distal air spaces (which are better exposed to the inhaled drug), thereby improving ventilation-perfusion mismatching. Although the benefits of iNO have been demonstrated in full- and near-term neonates with PH, iNO treatment of preterm infants was controversial until recently. In preterm neonates, the hope was that iNO would decrease the incidence of BPD/CLD and, possibly, mitigate other morbidities. However, results of clinical trials have shown that the universal (ie, nonselective) administration of iNO to premature neonates with RDS does not confer such benefits. However, there is substantial evidence that the selective administration of iNO to those premature babies who have both RDS and PH

does improve survival and reduce morbidity. Hence, iNO is commonly used for this indication in premature babies and has been shown to be safe.

2. **Physiology.** NO is a colorless gas with a half-life of seconds. Exogenous iNO diffuses from alveoli to pulmonary vascular smooth muscle and produces vasodilation. Excess NO diffuses into the bloodstream, where it is rapidly inactivated by binding to hemoglobin and subsequent metabolism to nitrates and nitrites. This rapid inactivation thereby limits its action to the pulmonary vasculature. Dosage of iNO is measured as ppm (parts per million) of gas.

3. **Toxicity.** NO reacts with oxygen to form other oxides of nitrogen and, in particular, NO_2 (nitrogen dioxide). The latter may produce toxic effects and hence must be removed from the respiratory circuit (which can be done by using an adsorbent). When NO combines with hemoglobin, it forms methemoglobin, and this is also of potential concern. In the several large trials that have been completed, methemoglobinemia has not been a significant complication at NO doses <20 ppm. The rate of accumulation of methemoglobin depends on both the dose and duration of NO administration. Even when using doses >20 ppm, clinically significant methemoglobinemia does not appear to be a frequent complication. NO inhibits platelet adhesion to endothelium. Hence another potential complication is the prolongation of bleeding time described at NO doses of 30 to 300 ppm. NO may also have an adverse effect on surfactant function, but this appears to require much higher doses than those relevant in clinical applications. On the contrary, low-dose NO also has antioxidant effects, and these may be potentially beneficial. Because of these potential complications, when administering NO, NO_2 levels should be monitored. In addition, blood methemoglobin concentration should be measured. Follow-up studies in infants receiving iNO have not shown any adverse effects.

4. **Dosage and administration.** Available evidence supports the use of doses of iNO beginning at 20 ppm. Among infants with a positive response to iNO, the response time is rapid. There is no agreement, however, about the duration of treatment and criteria for discontinuation; these vary and often reflect institutional preferences. Thus, some recommend weaning once PaO_2 is >50 mm Hg; others suggest an oxygenation index <10 as an indication for weaning. Moreover, no evidence suggests the superiority of one weaning regimen over another. However, some observations are available to assist in weaning considerations. One point is, however, beyond contention: weaning should be done under careful and intensive monitoring of each step. Particular note should be made of the observation that sudden discontinuation of iNO can be associated with "rebound" PH (see Section VII.H.4.b).

a. **Initial dose.** Start treatment with iNO at 20 ppm. Little is to be gained by administering higher doses because, at most, only a few patients will respond to these higher doses after not having responded to a dose of 20 ppm. Higher doses may significantly increase the rate of methemoglobinemia. Also, initial treatment with subtherapeutic low-dose iNO may diminish the subsequent response to iNO at 20 ppm. Among infants with a positive response to iNO, the response time is rapid.

b. **Weaning.** Wean inspired oxygen concentration until fraction of inspired oxygen (FiO_2) is <0.6. Then start weaning iNO concentrations in steps of 5 ppm until iNO is 5 ppm. Weaning may be initiated as early as 4 to 6 hours after starting treatment, or later, and should be attempted at least once per day, but may be done as frequently as every 30 minutes. Hemodynamic stability and adequate oxygenation should be monitored closely 30 to 60 minutes after each weaning step. Significant deterioration should be an indication for reversing the previous weaning step. Once iNO is at 5 ppm, weaning should be continued at a slower pace, in steps of 1 ppm, until iNO is 1 ppm. Once the patient has demonstrated stability at iNO of 1 ppm for a few hours, iNO may be discontinued. Some decline in oxygen saturation should be anticipated, and an increase of 10% to 20% in required inspired oxygen concentration may be considered reasonable when discontinuing iNO and need not be an indication for reinstating therapy. However, if an FiO_2 >0.75 is required to maintain adequate oxygenation, the patient may benefit from being placed back on iNO. *Caution:* Although there are various weaning regimens of iNO, evidence suggests that iNO should be discontinued from a dose of 1 ppm and not from a higher one. The rate of success is higher when discontinuation is done from a dose of 1 ppm than from 5 ppm or higher. Moreover, the phenomenon of rebound PH should be kept in mind after discontinuation of iNO. Sudden discontinuation of iNO can be associated with rebound PH, and this rebound can be severe and may occur even in infants who had initially failed to respond to iNO treatment when it was initiated. Clinical observations have suggested that the risk of rebound PH following discontinuation of iNO may be reduced if treatment with sildenafil is started a few hours prior to the discontinuation of iNO (see Section VII.I). We should emphasize that this protocol is merely a suggestion and is compatible with data derived from trials and experience with the use of iNO. Many other regimens would be just as reasonable.

5. **Failure to respond to inhaled nitric oxide or the need for prolonged administration.** Patients not responding to iNO or those in whom iNO cannot be weaned after 5 days of treatment merit a reevaluation. Effective therapy requires adequate lung inflation, and an infant who fails to respond should be evaluated by chest radiograph for airway obstruction and atelectasis. Lung volume recruitment strategies may be required, as may surfactant treatment in appropriate circumstances. Pressor support or volume administration may be required because impaired cardiac output may render iNO treatment ineffective. An echocardiogram is warranted to rule out cardiac anomalies that may have been missed and to assess cardiac function. Consideration should be directed toward lung diseases that respond poorly to iNO, such as alveolar-capillary dysplasia or those associated with pulmonary hypoplasia. Fewer than 35% of infants with congenital diaphragmatic hernia respond to iNO or survive without ECLS.

I. **Sildenafil.** PDE5 is abundantly expressed in lung tissue and degrades cGMP. Sildenafil, a PDE5 inhibitor, prolongs the half-life of cGMP and would be expected to enhance the actions of both endogenous and exogenous NO. A few small randomized trials, in addition to observational studies, in infants have shown its effectiveness in treating PH. It has been successful in treating PH in infants after cardiac surgery, and case series have shown it to be useful in attenuating the rebound PH after withdrawal of iNO. In some patients, sildenafil may confer benefit additional to that obtained by iNO alone. In some units, sildenafil is given prophylactically before the final step in weaning off iNO. Patients treated with sildenafil have not shown an increased propensity for systemic hypotension. Concern has been raised about possible adverse effects of this drug in those infants at risk for retinopathy of prematurity, although the putative association has been questioned. Larger trials will be required to address issues of risk and benefits. Although an intravenous (IV) preparation is available, the drug is mostly given enterally. Reported enteral dosages vary and range from 2 to 3 mg/kg/d divided 3 to 4 times daily, which may be increased up to a total maximum of 8 mg/kg/d. Dosage for the IV preparation is 50% that of the enteral, or it may be given as a (IV) loading dose of 0.4 mg/kg (given over 3 hours) followed by a maintenance infusion of 1.6 mg/kg/d (approximately 0.07 mg/kg/h). *Caution:* In 2012, the US Food and Drug Administration (FDA) issued a recommendation against the use of sildenafil in children aged 1 to 17 years. The basis for this recommendation has been strongly contested (even though it does not apply to those under 1 year of age), and with the same data, the European Medicines Agency approved sildenafil for use in the pediatric age group. In 2014, the FDA issued a clarification, stating that there may be situations in which the risk-benefit profile of sildenafil may be acceptable in individual children. Sildenafil remains one of the most commonly used medications in neonates and infants with PH, although appropriate monitoring is advised and further studies are needed, in particular with prolonged usage in this age group.

J. **Prostacyclin.** Prostacyclin (PGI_2) is a short-acting, potent vasodilator of both the pulmonary and systemic circulations. The greatest experience of its use is as a continuous IV infusion of epoprostenol. Trials in adults and older children with PH have shown an improvement in symptoms and mortality. However, epoprostenol treatment is associated with various limitations. The drug has a very short half-life and requires continuous infusion, preferably through a central vein (to minimize risk of systemic hypotension). There are special storage requirements, and side effects include, as mentioned, systemic hypotension. The data in neonates are sparse and consist of a few case reports and small series of the drug's successful use in this patient population, including some patients who had failed to respond to iNO. Reported dosages have varied between 4 and 40 ng/kg/min IV, and it is suggested that a low starting dose be initiated, with increasing dosage rate being titrated according to response. Higher doses are associated with increased risk of systemic hypotension, and blood pressure should be monitored. There are also reports of the IV preparation being aerosolized and administered by continuous inhalation at a dose of 50 to 100 ng/kg/min. Treprostinil is a stable prostacyclin analog with longer half-life that can be administered by oral, subcutaneous, or IV routes, but data are limited in infants.

K. **Inhaled/nebulized prostaglandin I_2 (iloprost).** This is a stable PGI_2 analogue with a longer half-life, and it acts by stimulating adenyl cyclase and increasing cyclic adenosine monophosphate. It is gaining wider acceptance due to its selective pulmonary vasodilation without decreasing systemic blood pressure. Randomized trials in adults have shown its effectiveness and safety, but the pediatric and neonatal literature consists of a few case series and case reports, some including infants who were resistant to treatment with iNO. No systemic vascular effects were noted. Dosage varies between reports but is mostly in the range of 0.25 to 2.5 mcg/kg per inhalation, with inhalations being given over 5 to 10 minutes every 2 to 4 hours.

L. **Bosentan.** ET-1 is a potent vasoconstrictor and is increased in newborns with PPHN. Bosentan is an ET receptor antagonist that improves hemodynamics and quality of life in adults with PH. Up to 10% of patients are affected by liver toxicity. Bosentan improved hemodynamics in a study of its use in pediatric patients with PH. Its use also enabled a reduction of the epoprostenol dose. While case series have reported on the successful use of bosentan, controlled trials have shown conflicting results, and further studies are needed to identify patients who may benefit from this drug, especially in combination with other medications used to treat PH in neonates and infants. Dosage is started at 1 mg/kg twice daily and may be advanced to 2 mg/kg twice daily. Liver enzymes should be monitored.

M. **Paralyzing agents.** The use of these agents is *controversial*. Their use has been advocated in infants who have not responded to sedation and are still labile or who appear to "fight" the ventilator. In a retrospective survey, the use of paralysis was associated with increased mortality, although a causal relation cannot be inferred. Pancuronium is the drug most commonly used, although it may increase PVR to some extent and worsen ventilation-perfusion mismatch. Vecuronium (0.1 mg/kg) has also been used.

N. **Alkalinization.** In the past, it had been noted that hyperventilation, with the resulting hypocapnia, improved oxygenation secondary to pulmonary vasodilation. Subsequently, it was shown, in animal studies, that the beneficial effect of hypocapnia was actually a result of the increased pH rather than of the low $PaCO_2$ values achieved. Furthermore, follow-up of infants with PPHN had suggested that hypocapnia was related to poor neurodevelopmental outcome (especially sensorineural hearing loss). Hypocapnia is known to reduce cerebral blood flow. The use of alkalinization is ***controversial***, and there are no adequately controlled trials on its use to alleviate PPHN. If alkalinization is employed, it may be advisable to increase pH using an infusion of sodium bicarbonate (0.5–1 mEq/kg/h) if possible. Serum sodium should be monitored to avoid hypernatremia. Improvement in oxygenation has been anecdotally reported with arterial pH of 7.50 to 7.55 (sometimes levels as high as 7.65 are required).

O. **Magnesium sulfate.** Magnesium causes vasodilation by antagonizing calcium ion entry into smooth muscle cells. A few small observational studies have suggested that magnesium sulfate ($MgSO_4$) may effectively treat PPHN, but the evidence is conflicting, and there is some risk of systemic hypotension. The dose reported is a loading dosage of 200 mg/kg followed by an infusion of 20 to 150 mg/kg/h (the drug is given IV). Two small trials in neonates with PPHN have shown that sildenafil and iNO are each superior to IV $MgSO_4$.

P. **Adenosine.** Adenosine causes vasodilation by stimulation of adenosine receptors on endothelial cells and release of endothelial NO. A small randomized trial reported the effectiveness of adenosine infusion (25–50 mcg/kg/min) in treating PPHN in term babies. Subsequently, a few further cases have been published. Despite initial favorable data, the drug has not attracted attention, and its use awaits further clinical trials.

Q. **Extracorporeal life support.** (See Chapter 20.) ECLS may be indicated for term or near-term infants with PPHN who fail to respond to conventional therapy and who meet ECLS entry criteria. The survival rate with ECLS is reportedly >80%, although only the most severely afflicted infants are referred for this treatment.

VIII. **Pulmonary hypertension in bronchopulmonary dysplasia/chronic lung disease.** A significant number of cases of BPD/CLD exhibit pulmonary hypertension (PH). The pulmonary circulation in BPD/CLD exhibits elevated PVR and increased vasoreactivity, vascular remodeling, and decreased and disrupted growth. The disruption in angiogenesis also impairs alveolarization, and furthermore, there is formation of bronchial and other systemic-to-pulmonary collateral vessels. The presence of PH complicating the course of BPD/CLD is associated with significantly increased mortality and morbidity. The rationale for aggressively diagnosing and treating PH complicating BPD/CLD is the hope that it would affect the increased mortality. Which patients with BPD/CLD should be screened for the presence of PH? There are no data to indicate an optimal approach, but a few guidelines have been suggested. Patients still requiring ventilatory assistance or significant supplemental oxygen at 36 weeks' postconceptional age might benefit from an echocardiographic evaluation. Some suggest echocardiographic screening at an earlier stage (as early as 1–2 months of age if baby is still on mechanical ventilation). Furthermore, infants with severe respiratory disease that fails to improve, those with respiratory disease out of proportion to the expected course or radiologic findings, those with recurrent and persistent cyanotic spells or respiratory deteriorations, and those with repeated need for diuretic administration might also benefit from screening for PH. Screening for PH in patients with BPD/CLD may require serial interval echocardiograms. The echocardiographic evaluation of PH is far from perfect, and certain patients may require cardiac catheterization for diagnosis of PH and to assess its severity and response to treatment. Serial measurements of brain natriuretic peptide (BNP) or N-terminal pro-BNP may help in the assessment of cardiac performance in the context of BPD and PH. BNP and N-terminal pro-BNP are released by the myocardium in response to stretch, although they are not specific for PH. However, serial assays may augment echocardiographic findings and may be useful in monitoring disease progression or improvement. The therapeutic options most commonly used in patients with BPD and PH are iNO, sildenafil, and bosentan. However, treatment of PH should always occur in a context whereby attempts have been made to optimize ventilatory support and complicating factors (eg, reflux and aspirations) have been considered and treated, if necessary.

IX. **Prognosis.** The overall survival rate is >70% to 75%. However, there is a marked difference in survival and long-term outcome according to the cause of the PPHN. More than 80% of term or near-term neonates with PPHN are expected to have an essentially normal neurodevelopmental outcome. Abnormal long-term outcome in PPHN survivors (and a high incidence of sensorineural hearing loss) has been reported to correlate with duration of hyperventilation. However, the relationship may not be causal because prolonged hyperventilation may simply be a marker for the severity of PPHN and hypoxic insult. Full-term survivors of idiopathic PPHN usually have no residual lung or heart disease. However, low birthweight infants with PPHN accompanying severe RDS have a much higher rate of mortality, and there are few data on the long-term outcome of the survivors. These babies are at higher risk of developing BPD and subsequently requiring more prolonged therapy for PH. In some cases, treatment for PH may be required after discharge from the neonatal intensive care unit, and these patients then require close cardiac supervision as outpatients. PH may be exacerbated during episodes of viral respiratory diseases.

116 Polycythemia and Hyperviscosity

I. **Definitions.** Polycythemia is an increased total red blood cell (RBC) mass. Polycythemic hyperviscosity is an increased viscosity of the blood resulting from, or associated with, increased numbers of RBCs.

   A. **Polycythemia of the newborn.** Defined empirically as a central venous hematocrit >65%.

   B. **Hyperviscosity.** Defined as a viscosity >14 centipoises (cP) at a shear rate of 11.5/s and is measured by a viscometer. Viscosity is the measure of a fluid's resistance to being deformed. It is defined as the **shear stress** (refers to frictional forces within a fluid) divided by the **shear rate** (a measure of flow velocity). In neonates, the major determinant of total blood viscosity is hematocrit, with plasma viscosity playing a minor role. The relationship between hematocrit and blood viscosity is exponential. Hyperviscosity is the cause of clinical symptoms in infants presumed to be symptomatic from polycythemia.

II. **Incidence**

   A. **Polycythemia** occurs in 1% to 4% of the general newborn population. Half of these patients are symptomatic, although it is not at all certain whether their symptoms are caused by polycythemia.

   B. **Hyperviscosity without polycythemia** occurs in 1% of normal (nonpolycythemic) newborns. In infants with a hematocrit of 60% to 64%, a fourth will have hyperviscosity.

III. **Pathophysiology.** Polycythemia and hyperviscosity are associated with presumed alteration in organ blood flow. In general, there is a decrease in organ blood flow due to changes in red cell mass, arterial oxygen content, and/or viscosity. The decrease in cerebral blood flow and cardiac output may represent a physiologic response to an increase in arterial oxygen content rather than ischemia. Many infants with polycythemia have a reduced plasma volume, which may lead to hypoglycemia (12%–40% of the infants) as glucose is present in the plasma fraction of the blood. Whole blood glucose concentration might be significantly reduced even when the plasma concentration is normal. Clinical signs attributed to polycythemia may result from coexisting perinatal circumstances in the presence or absence of hyperviscosity.

The frictional forces identified within whole blood and their relative contributions to hyperviscosity in the newborn include the following:

A. **Hematocrit. An increase in the hematocrit is the most important single factor contributing to hyperviscosity in the neonate.** An increased hematocrit results from either an absolute increase in circulating RBC volume or a decrease in plasma volume.

B. **Plasma viscosity.** A direct linear relationship exists between plasma viscosity and the concentration of plasma proteins, particularly those of high molecular weight, such as fibrinogen. Term infants and, to a greater degree, preterm infants have low plasma fibrinogen levels compared with adults. Consequently, except for the rare case of primary hyperfibrinogenemia, plasma viscosity does not contribute to an increased whole-blood viscosity in the neonate.

C. **Red blood cell aggregation.** Occurs only in areas of low blood flow and is usually limited to the venous microcirculation. Because fibrinogen levels are typically low in term and preterm infants, RBC aggregation does not contribute significantly to whole blood viscosity in newborn infants. There is some concern that the use of adult fresh-frozen plasma for partial exchange transfusion in neonates might critically alter the concentration of fibrinogen and paradoxically raise whole blood viscosity within the microcirculation.

D. **Deformability of red blood cell membrane.** RBC deformability is increased in preterm neonates as compared with term neonates and in term neonates as compared with adults. The increase in deformability is presumed to reduce blood viscosity and to reduce the likelihood that polycythemia will cause hyperviscosity. Because infants of diabetic mothers are thought to have RBCs with reduced deformability, hyperviscosity may be more likely at polycythemic hematocrit levels than in unaffected neonates.

IV. **Risk factors**

A. **Conditions that alter incidence**

1. **Altitude.** There is an absolute increase in RBC mass as part of physiologic adaptation to high altitude.

2. **Neonatal age.** The normal pattern of fluid shifts during the first 6 hours of life is away from the intravascular compartment. The period of maximum physiologic increase in the hematocrit occurs at 2 to 4 hours of age.

3. **Obstetric factors.** A delay in cord clamping or milking of the umbilical cord results in a higher incidence of polycythemia. However, the subsequent development of symptomatic polycythemia or severe hyperbilirubinemia is rare.

4. **High-risk delivery.** A high-risk delivery is associated with an increased incidence of polycythemia, particularly if precipitous or uncontrolled.

B. **Perinatal processes**

1. **Enhanced fetal erythropoiesis.** Elevated erythropoietin levels result from a direct stimulus, usually related to fetal hypoxia, or from an altered regulation of erythropoietin production.

   a. **Placental insufficiency**

      i. **Maternal hypertensive disease (preeclampsia/eclampsia) or primary renovascular disease**

      ii. **Abruptio placentae (chronic recurrent)**

      iii. **Postmaturity**

      iv. **Maternal cyanotic congenital heart disease**

      v. **Intrauterine growth restriction**

      vi. **Maternal cigarette smoking**

   b. **Endocrine disorders.** Increased oxygen consumption is the suggested mechanism by which hyperinsulinism or hyperthyroxinemia creates fetal hypoxemia and stimulates erythropoietin production.

      i. **Infant of a diabetic mother (>40% incidence of polycythemia)**

      ii. **Infant of a mother with gestational diabetes (>30% incidence of polycythemia)**

          iii. **Congenital thyrotoxicosis**
          iv. **Congenital adrenal hyperplasia**
          v. **Beckwith-Wiedemann syndrome (secondary hyperinsulinism)**
      c. **Genetic trisomies.** Trisomies 13, 18, and 21.
  2. **Hypertransfusion.** Conditions that enhance placental transfusion at birth may create hypervolemic normocythemia, which evolves into hypervolemic polycythemia as the normal pattern of fluid shift occurs. A larger transfusion may create hypervolemic polycythemia at birth, with signs present in the infant. Conditions associated with hypertransfusion include the following:
      a. **Delay in cord clamping.** Placental vessels contain up to a third of the fetal blood volume, half of which is returned to the infant within 1 minute after birth Definition of delayed cord clamping is variable, and ranges from 30 seconds to up to 5 minutes. The risks associated with delayed cord clamping are probably negligible compared with the benefits, which include, in term infants, reduction in the rate of iron deficiency in the first 2 years of life and, in preterm infants, decreased postnatal need for blood transfusions, inotrope support, and incidence of intraventricular hemorrhage and necrotizing enterocolitis. Representative blood volumes for term infants with a variable delay in cord clamping are as follows:
          i. **15-second delay: 75 to 78 mL/kg**
          ii. **60-second delay: 80 to 87 mL/kg**
          iii. **120-second delay: 83 to 93 mL/kg**
      b. **Gravity.** Positioning the infant below the placental bed (>10 cm below the placenta) may enhance placental transfusion via the umbilical vein. Elevation of the infant >50 cm above the placenta may decrease the placental transfusion. Soon after the birth, under the influence of maternal uterotonics, placing the baby on the mother's abdomen or chest at term vaginal birth had no impact on the volume of placental transfusion and infants can be safely placed on their mothers' chest.
      c. **Twin–twin transfusion.** Interfetal transfusion (**parabiosis syndrome**) is observed in monochorionic twin pregnancy with an incidence of 15%. The recipient twin, on the venous side of the anastomosis, becomes polycythemic, and the donor, on the arterial side, becomes anemic. Simultaneous venous hematocrits obtained after delivery usually differ by >12% to 15%.
V. **Clinical presentation.** Clinical signs observed in polycythemia are often nonspecific. The conditions listed next may occur independently of polycythemia or hyperviscosity and must be considered in the differential diagnosis.
  A. **Central nervous system.** There may be an altered state of consciousness, including lethargy and decreased activity, hyperirritability, muscle hypotonia, vasomotor instability, and vomiting. Seizures, thromboses, and cerebral infarction are extraordinarily rare.
  B. **Cardiopulmonary system.** Respiratory distress and tachycardia may be present. Congestive heart failure with cardiomegaly may be seen but is rarely clinically prominent. Pulmonary hypertension may occur but is not usually severe unless other predisposing factors are present.
  C. **Gastrointestinal tract.** Feeding intolerance occurs occasionally. Necrotizing enterocolitis has been reported but rarely without other factors (eg, intrauterine growth restriction), which casts doubt on the primary cause.
  D. **Genitourinary tract.** Oliguria, acute renal failure/acute kidney injury, renal vein thrombosis, or priapism may occur.
  E. **Metabolic disorders.** Hypoglycemia, hypocalcemia, or hypomagnesemia may be seen.
  F. **Hematologic disorders.** There may be hyperbilirubinemia, thrombocytopenia, or reticulocytosis (with enhanced erythropoiesis only).
VI. **Diagnosis**
  A. **Venous (not capillary) hematocrit.** Polycythemia is present when the central venous hematocrit is >65%.

B. **The following screening studies may be used:**
1. **A cord blood hematocrit >56% suggests polycythemia.**
2. **A warmed capillary hematocrit >65% suggests polycythemia.**
VII. **Management.** (See also Chapter 76 for polycythemia management.) Clinical management of the polycythemic infant is more expectant now than 2 decades ago. Studies and reviews have created much doubt about any long-term benefits of partial (isovolumetric) exchange transfusion (PET). Consequently, PET should probably be performed only in infants in whom significant morbidity is in question.
   A. **Asymptomatic infants.** Only expectant observation is required for virtually all asymptomatic infants. The possible exception is an infant with a central venous hematocrit of >75%, but even in this group, the risks of central catheter insertion probably outweigh the benefits of PET.
   B. **Symptomatic infants.** When the central venous hematocrit is >65%, PET with normal saline may ameliorate acute signs of polycythemia or hyperviscosity. However, whether treatment of a self-limited problem justifies the risks of central catheter insertion and an exchange procedure is debatable. PET procedures using peripheral vessels may be preferred to avoid the complications related to the central catheter insertion. For the procedure for partial exchange transfusion, see Chapter 34.
VIII. **Prognosis.** The long-term outcome of infants with polycythemia or hyperviscosity and response to PET is as follows:
   A. **A causal relationship may exist** between PET (through an umbilical vessel) and an increase in gastrointestinal tract disorders such as necrotizing enterocolitis.
   B. **Most randomized controlled prospective studies** of polycythemic and hyperviscous infants indicate that PET does not eliminate the risk of neurologic sequelae.
   C. **Infants with "asymptomatic" polycythemia** have an increased risk for neurologic sequelae, but normocythemic controls with the same perinatal histories have a similarly increased risk.
   D. **The efficacy of partial exchange transfusion among infants with "symptomatic" polycythemia** remains unclear at this time.

117 Respiratory Distress Syndrome

I. **Definition. Respiratory distress syndrome (RDS) was previously called hyaline membrane disease (HMD).** The Vermont Oxford Network definition for RDS requires that babies have:
   A. **An arterial oxygen tension (PaO_2) <50 mm Hg and central cyanosis in room air,** a requirement for supplemental oxygen to maintain PaO_2 >50 mm Hg, or a requirement for supplemental oxygen to maintain a pulse oximeter saturation >85%.
   B. **A characteristic chest radiographic appearance** (uniform reticulogranular pattern to lung fields and air bronchogram) within the first 24 hours of life. The clinical course of the disease has been changed because of advances in treatment practices, including the use of early continuous positive airway pressure (CPAP).
II. **Incidence.** Incidence of RDS is about 85% at 28 weeks' gestation and increases to 95% at 24 weeks' gestation. However, by using early CPAP, approximately 50% of babies born at 26 to 29 weeks' gestation can be managed without intubation or surfactant. The survival from RDS is generally >90%.

III. **Pathophysiology.** Surfactant deficiency is the primary cause of RDS, often complicated by an overly compliant chest wall. Both factors lead to progressive atelectasis and failure to develop an effective functional residual capacity (FRC). Surfactant is produced by airway epithelial cells called type II pneumocytes. Surfactant synthesis begins at 24 to 28 weeks' gestation. Type II cells are sensitive to and decreased by perinatal asphyxial insults. The maturation of these cells is delayed in the presence of fetal hyperinsulinemia. The maturity of type II cells is enhanced by the administration of antenatal corticosteroids and by chronic intrauterine stress such as pregnancy-induced hypertension and intrauterine growth restriction. Surfactant, composed chiefly of phospholipid (75%) and protein (10%), is produced and stored in the lamellar bodies of type II pneumocytes. This lipoprotein is released into the airways, where it functions to decrease surface tension and maintain alveolar expansion at physiologic pressures.

A. **Lack of surfactant.** In the absence of surfactant, the small airspaces collapse; each expiration results in progressive atelectasis. Exudative proteinaceous material and epithelial debris, resulting from progressive cellular damage, collect in the airway and directly decrease total lung capacity. In pathologic specimens, this material stains typically as eosinophilic hyaline membranes lining the alveolar spaces and extending into small airways.

B. **Presence of an overly compliant chest wall.** In the presence of a chest wall with weak structural support secondary to prematurity, the large negative pressures generated to open the collapsed airways cause retraction and deformation of the chest wall instead of inflation of the lungs.

C. **Decreased intrathoracic pressure.** The infant with RDS who is <30 weeks' gestational age often has immediate respiratory failure because of an inability to generate the intrathoracic pressure necessary to inflate the lungs without surfactant.

D. **Shunting.** The presence or absence of a cardiovascular shunt through a patent ductus arteriosus (PDA) and/or foramen ovale may change the course of the disease. Shortly after birth, the predominant shunting is right to left across the foramen ovale into the left atrium, which may result in worsening hypoxemia. After 18 to 24 hours, left-to-right shunting through the PDA may become predominant as a result of falling pulmonary vascular resistance, leading to pulmonary edema and impaired alveolar gas exchange. Unfortunately, this usually occurs when the infant is starting to recover from RDS and can be aggravated by surfactant replacement therapy.

IV. **Risk factors.** Table 117–1 lists factors that increase or decrease the risk of RDS.

Table 117–1. RISK FACTORS THAT INCREASE OR DECREASE THE RISK OF RESPIRATORY DISTRESS SYNDROME

Increased Risk	Decreased Risk
Prematurity	Prolonged rupture of membranes
Male sex	Intrauterine infection
Familial predisposition	Female sex
Cesarean delivery without labor	Vaginal delivery
Perinatal asphyxia	Narcotic/cocaine use
Multiple gestation	Corticosteroids
Maternal diabetes	Thyroid hormone
European descent	Tocolytic agents
Mutation in single *ABCA3* gene	African descent

V. **Clinical presentation**

    A. **History.** The infant is often preterm or has a history of perinatal asphyxia. Infants have at birth some respiratory difficulty, which becomes progressively more severe. The classic worsening of the atelectasis seen on chest radiograph and increasing oxygen requirement for these infants have been greatly modified by exogenous surfactant therapy and effective ventilatory support.

    B. **Physical examination.** The infant with RDS exhibits tachypnea, grunting, nasal flaring, and retractions of the chest wall, and may have cyanosis in room air. Grunting occurs when the infant partially closes the vocal cords to prolong expiration and develop or maintain some FRC. This actually improves alveolar ventilation. The retractions occur and increase as the infant is forced to develop high transpulmonary pressure to reinflate atelectatic air spaces.

VI. **Diagnosis**

    A. **Chest radiograph.** An anteroposterior chest radiograph should be obtained for all infants with respiratory distress of any duration. The typical radiographic finding of RDS is a uniform reticulogranular pattern, referred to as a ground-glass appearance, accompanied by peripheral air bronchograms (see Figure 12–16). Sequential radiographs may later reveal air leaks secondary to mechanical ventilatory support as well as the onset of changes compatible with bronchopulmonary dysplasia/chronic lung disease (BPD/CLD) (see Figure 12–20).

    B. **Point-of-care lung ultrasonography showing** lung consolidation, pleural line abnormalities, and A-line disappearance provides a sensitivity and specificity of 100% for the diagnosis of neonatal RDS. However, some acute complications secondary to air leak syndrome (eg, pneumomediastinum, interstitial emphysema, pneumopericardium) cannot easily be discovered by using ultrasound (see also Chapter 44).

    C. **Laboratory studies**

        1. **Blood gas sampling** is essential in the management of RDS. Although there is no consensus, most neonatologists agree that arterial oxygen tensions of 50 to 70 mm Hg and arterial carbon dioxide tensions of 45 to 60 mm Hg are acceptable. Most would maintain the pH at or above 7.22 and the arterial oxygen saturation at 90% to 94%. Continuous transcutaneous oxygen and carbon dioxide monitoring and/or oxygen saturation monitoring are valuable in the treatment of these infants.

        2. **Sepsis workup.** A partial sepsis workup, including complete blood cell count and blood culture, should be considered for each infant with RDS because early-onset sepsis (eg, infection with group B *Streptococcus*) can be indistinguishable from RDS on clinical grounds alone.

        3. **Serum glucose levels** must be monitored closely to assess the adequacy of dextrose infusion. Hypoglycemia alone can lead to tachypnea and respiratory distress.

        4. **Serum electrolyte levels and calcium** should be monitored for management of parenteral fluids. Hypocalcemia can contribute to more respiratory symptoms and is common in sick, nonfed, preterm, or asphyxiated infants. Hyponatremia can occur.

    D. **Echocardiography** is used to confirm the diagnosis of PDA and in the evaluation of an infant with hypoxemia and respiratory distress. A significant congenital heart disease can also be excluded.

    E. **Respiratory severity score.** Some facilities in low-resource settings use the respiratory severity score (RSS) designed by Silverman and Andersen to quantify respiratory distress among neonates. The RSS is objective, easy to learn, quick to perform, and requires no expensive equipment. It is rated by giving scores from 0 to 2 from upper chest movement, lower chest retractions, xiphoid retractions, nares dilatation, and expiratory grunting. Details can be found in *Journal of Perinatology* (2018;38:505-511). The RSS can be used for predicting the need for escalation of respiratory support and can help facilitate transfer decision making to higher resourced facilities. Scores ≥5 have been the most useful cutoff point for transfer, although the sensitivity of the score is decreased in patients with a higher score.

VII. **Management.** Listed below are guidelines for the management of RDS. Note that there are specific European Consensus Guidelines that were updated in 2019 by Sweet et al (*Neonatology*, 2019;115(4):432-451).

  A. **Prevention**

   1. **Antenatal corticosteroids.** Treatment with antenatal corticosteroids is associated with an overall reduction in neonatal death, RDS, intraventricular hemorrhage (IVH), necrotizing enterocolitis (NEC), respiratory support, intensive care admissions, and systemic infections in the first 48 hours of life. Guidelines from the American College of Obstetricians and Gynecologists (ACOG) and the European consensus, which differ in recommendations, are listed in Table 117–2. The optimal treatment to delivery interval is >24 and <7 days after the steroid treatment.

   a. **Repeated courses of corticosteroids.** Because of short-term benefits for babies with less respiratory distress and fewer serious health problems in the

Table 117–2. AMERICAN COLLEGE OF OBSTETRICIANS AND GYNECOLOGISTS (ACOG) AND EUROPEAN CONSENSUS ON RECOMMENDATIONS FOR ANTENATAL CORTICOSTEROID TREATMENT

ACOG	European Consensus
Give a course of antenatal corticosteroids to pregnant women (including rupture of membranes [ROM] and multiple gestation) 24 0/7 to 33 6/7 weeks' gestation who are at risk of preterm delivery within 7 days. Consider a course of antenatal corticosteroids to pregnant women (including ROM and multiple gestation) at 23 0/7 weeks' gestation who are at risk of preterm delivery within 7 days, based on the family's decision on resuscitation.	Offer a single course of prenatal corticosteroids to all women at risk of preterm delivery, before 34 weeks' gestation, for whom the pregnancy is considered potentially viable, ideally 24 hours before birth.
Give a single dose of betamethasone to pregnant women 34 0/7 to 36 6/7 weeks' gestation who are at risk of preterm delivery within 7 days who have not received a prior dose of antenatal corticosteroids.	It is appropriate to give a repeat course of antenatal steroids in threatened preterm delivery before 32 weeks' gestation, if the first course was given at least 1 to 2 weeks earlier.
Consider a course of antenatal corticosteroids for pregnant women in the periviable period (defined as 20 0/7 to 25 6/7 weeks' gestation) who are at risk of preterm delivery within 7 days, depending on the family's decision on resuscitation.	
>2 repeat courses are not recommended.	
Consider a repeat course of antenatal corticosteroids to a pregnant woman <34 0/7 weeks' gestation who are at risk of preterm delivery within 7 days and whose prior course was >14 days before. Rescue course prior to 7 days can be given if necessary due to the clinical picture.	
Controversial as to whether to give a repeat/rescue course for preterm/prelabor ROM.	

Data from Committee on Obstetric Practice. Committee Opinion No. 713: Antenatal Corticosteroid Therapy for Fetal Maturation, *Obstet Gynecol.* 2017 Aug;130(2):e102-e109; Sweet D, Carnielli V, Greisen G, et al: European consensus guidelines on the management of neonatal respiratory distress syndrome in preterm infants: 2016 update. *Neonatology.* 2017;111(2):107-125.

first weeks after birth, a repeated course should be considered if the risk of preterm delivery persists or recurs 7 to 14 days after having received the previous course (ie, when the delivery is expected to occur within the following 7 days). Weekly repeated courses are, however, not recommended.

b. **The recommended regimen** consists of the administration to the mother of 2 doses of betamethasone 12 mg given intramuscularly 24 hours apart. Dexamethasone is not recommended because of increased risk for cystic periventricular leukomalacia among very premature infants exposed to the drug prenatally. The ACOG recommendations differ from the European guidelines; see Table 117–2.

2. **Ambroxol.** There is insufficient scientific evidence either to support or discourage the use of ambroxol in pregnant women at risk of preterm birth for preventing neonatal RDS.

3. **Preventive measures** to improve the survival of infants at risk for RDS include **antenatal ultrasonography** for accurate assessment of gestational age and fetal well-being, **continuous fetal monitoring** to document fetal well-being during labor or to signal the need for intervention when fetal distress is discovered, and **tocolytic agents** that prevent and treat preterm labor. **Assessment of fetal lung maturity** before delivery (lecithin-to-sphingomyelin ratio and phosphatidylglycerol or amniotic fluid lamellar bodies; see Chapter 1) might be of help in determining the timing of some late preterm or early term deliveries. Testing is not commonly used because mature test results do not guarantee good neonatal outcomes.

B. **Delivery room management.** In spontaneously breathing babies, stabilize with CPAP via mask or nasal prongs. Gentle positive-pressure lung inflations should be used for persistently apneic or bradycardic infants. Intubation should be reserved for babies who have not responded to positive-pressure ventilation via face mask. Babies who require intubation for stabilization should be given surfactant (see later in chapter).

C. **Respiratory support**

1. **Continuous positive airway pressure and nasal synchronized intermittent mandatory ventilation.** Nasal CPAP (nCPAP) or nasopharyngeal CPAP (NPC-PAP) providing a pressure of 5 to 6 cm H_2O can be used early to delay or prevent the need for endotracheal intubation and mechanical ventilation. CPAP treatment is recommended to be started from birth in all infants at risk of RDS, such as those born at <30 weeks' gestation. In this way many, infants with RDS can be managed without surfactant replacement. By not using surfactant, however, the risk of pneumothorax is increased. Use of nCPAP or NPCPAP on extubation after mechanical ventilation decreases the chance of reintubation **Nasal synchronized intermittent mandatory ventilation (SIMV)** is a potentially useful way of augmenting nCPAP. The ability to synchronize the ventilator breaths with the infant's own respiratory cycle has made this mode of ventilation feasible. Nasal SIMV has reduced the incidence of symptoms of extubation failure when compared with nCPAP. Short binasal prongs should be used instead of a single prong.

2. **Humidified high-flow nasal cannula system.** This has been introduced as a way to provide positive distending pressure, even comparable to nCPAP, to a neonate with respiratory distress. It aims to maximize patient tolerance by using heated, humidified gas of usually 4.0 to 8.0 L/min flow. It has shown similar efficacy and safety compared with nCPAP and bilevel positive airway pressure (BiPAP) as a primary treatment of moderate RDS in preterm infants >28 weeks' gestational age. Further studies are underway.

3. **Endotracheal intubation and mechanical ventilation** are mainstays of therapy for infants with RDS in whom apnea or hypoxemia with respiratory acidosis develops.

a. **Mechanical ventilation** (MV) modes include conventional modes, such as intermittent positive-pressure ventilation (IPPV), and high-frequency oscillatory ventilation (HFOV). Ventilators with the capacity to synchronize respiratory effort may generate less inadvertent airway pressure and lessen barotrauma. Ventilator settings should be adjusted frequently to maintain the lowest possible pressures and inspired oxygen concentrations in an attempt to minimize damage to parenchymal tissue. Volume-targeted ventilation allows patient-adjusted variability in tidal volumes and weaning from ventilator in accordance with the improving lung compliance.

  i. **High frequency oscillatory ventilation** may be beneficial as a rescue therapy in infants with respiratory failure on IPPV. A recent meta-analysis of randomized controlled trials showed a decreased risk of BPD in infants treated with HFOV compared to those treated with pressure-limited ventilation. In contrast, an increased risk of pulmonary air leaks was shown in the HFOV-treated cases. One randomized controlled trial has reported a better lung function at 11 to 14 years of age in HFOV-treated patients compared to those treated with conventional ventilation. Instead, no differences in neurodevelopmental outcomes have been detected in follow-up studies.

  ii. **Weaning from mechanical ventilation** should be started as soon as satisfactory gas exchange is achieved. Modest hypercarbia can be allowed, if the pH can be maintained above 7.22, in order to facilitate weaning. **Caffeine** should be routinely used for very preterm neonates with RDS to augment extubation.

  iii. **Inhaled nitric oxide (iNO)** has been used mostly off label in extremely premature neonates with RDS. It should not be used in preterm infants with RDS unless there is pulmonary hypertension or hypoplasia. A recent study shows that it does not improve survival, and infants treated with iNO without evidence of PPHN actually had an increased mortality.

D. **Surfactant replacement.** (See also Chapter 9.) Now considered a standard of care in the treatment of intubated infants with RDS.

  1. **Prophylactic versus selective use.** Systematic reviews of >30 randomized trials demonstrate that surfactant, whether used prophylactically in the delivery room or in the treatment of established disease, leads to a significant decrease in the risk of pneumothorax and death. These benefits were observed in both the trials of natural surfactant extracts and synthetic surfactants. According to the recent evidence, prophylactic surfactant replacement to prevent RDS is not recommended in infants receiving noninvasive respiratory support for stabilization in the delivery room. Instead, early CPAP after birth and early selective surfactant treatment in infants with signs of RDS are recommended. However, surfactant is needed in infants who require delivery room intubation for stabilization. Surfactant should be given as early as possible during the course of RDS. Infants of ≤26 weeks' gestation should be treated when they need >30% inspired oxygen to maintain oxygen saturation in the normal range. The treatment threshold for infants of >26 weeks' gestational age is recommended to be an inspired oxygen requirement of >40%.

  2. **Surfactant preparations.** Natural (derived from animal lungs) surfactant preparations are better than synthetic (protein-free) preparations at reducing pulmonary air leaks (Table 117–3). Synthetic surfactants containing surfactant protein B and protein C analogs are currently studied in clinical trials. Currently, natural surfactants are the treatment of choice. Trials comparing natural bovine surfactants, whether given prophylactically or as rescue therapy, have shown similar outcomes. Trials comparing bovine- and porcine-derived surfactants have shown a more rapid improvement in oxygenation in the latter. A better survival has been demonstrated using a 200-mg/kg dose of poractant alfa compared with 100 mg/kg of beractant or 100 mg/kg of poractant alfa for treatment of moderate to severe RDS.

Table 117–3. **SURFACTANT PREPARATIONS**

Generic/Trade Name	Source	Manufacturer	Dose (volume)
Beractant/ Survanta	Bovine	Ross Laboratories (United States)	100 mg/kg/dose (4 mL/kg) Prophylaxis[a]: 100 mg within 15 min of birth; up to 4 doses during the first 48 h of life; maximum frequency, every 6 h Treatment[a]: 100 mg within 8 h of birth; up to 4 doses during the first 48 h of life; maximum frequency, every 6 h
Bovactant/ Alveofact	Bovine	Lyomark (Germany)	50 mg/kg/dose (1.2 mL/kg) (European approval)
Poractant alfa/ Curosurf	Porcine	Chiesi Farmaceutici (Italy) Chiesi (United States)	100–200 mg/kg/dose (1.5–3.0 mL/kg) Prophylaxis[b]: 1.25–2.5 mL/kg once within 15 min of birth; additional doses only if infant requires mechanical ventilation/ supplemental oxygen Treatment[b]: initial 2.5 mL/kg, then 1.25 mL/kg every 12 h × 2 as needed (5 mL/kg total dose); additional doses only if infant continues to require mechanical ventilation/supplemental oxygen
Calfactant/ Infasurf	Bovine	ONY (United States)	105 mg/kg/dose (3 mL/kg) Prophylaxis: 3 mL/kg body weight within 30 min of birth; then as needed every 12 h for a total of up to 3 doses Treatment: same as prophylaxis

Note: Lucinatant (Surfaxin) has been discontinued.
[a]Each dose is given as 4 quarter doses, with body in different positions to assure adequate distribution and with 30 seconds of ventilation between positions.
[b]Each dose given as 2 half doses, with body in different positions to assure adequate distribution.

3. **Administration techniques.** Surfactant is administered when the infant is lying supine. Positional maneuvers are not indicated. MV can be avoided by using the **INSURE (intubate-surfactant-extubate) to CPAP technique** when surfactant is administered. This has reduced the need for MV and development of BPD/CLD in randomized trials. Immediate (or early) extubation to noninvasive respiratory support (CPAP or nasal IPPV) following surfactant administration should be considered in otherwise stabile infants. Recently, even less invasive techniques for surfactant treatment have been developed, aiming for total avoidance of endotracheal intubation and MV. The LISA (less invasive surfactant administration) method uses a thin flexible catheter (5-F end-hole catheter), which is inserted into the trachea using Magill forceps. Surfactant is administered while the spontaneously breathing infant is on nasal CPAP. The MIST (minimally invasive surfactant treatment) method is a similar strategy, where a thin but stiff vascular catheter is inserted into trachea under direct laryngoscopy while the baby is on nCPAP.

4. **Repeated doses.** A second and sometimes a third dose of surfactant should be administered in cases with ongoing evidence of RDS (ie, persistent need of MV

and oxygen supplementation). Using a larger dose (200 mg/kg) of poractant alfa has reduced the need of subsequent doses. Multiple INSURE treatments have been successful without worsening outcomes. The addition of budesonide to natural surfactant preparations may also decrease lung inflammation in ventilated preterm babies and reduce the risk of BPD, although this will need further verification by randomized multicenter trials.

E. **Inhaled nitric oxide** therapy is not recommended for the routine treatment of RDS in premature neonates. However, persistent pulmonary hypertension of the newborn often occurs concurrently with RDS in very preterm infants. iNO therapy can improve oxygenation in such cases.

F. **Fluid and nutritional support.** In the very ill infant, it is possible to maintain nutritional support with parenteral nutrition for an extended period. Full parenteral nutrition and minimal enteral feeding can be initiated on the first day of life. Careful fluid balance should, however, be maintained. The specific needs of preterm and term infants are becoming better understood, and the nutrient preparations available reflect this understanding (see Chapters 10 and 11). Use of diuretics is not recommended in this patient group.

G. **Antibiotic therapy.** Antibiotics that cover the most common neonatal infections are usually begun initially.

H. **Caffeine.** Should be initiated for all premature infants at high risk of MV, such as those with birthweight of 1250 g who are on CPAP treatment. It should also be used in order to facilitate weaning from MV.

I. **Sedation.** Commonly used to control ventilation in these sick infants. **Morphine and fentanyl** may be used for analgesia as well as sedation, preferably by using validated pain scoring systems. Minimal handling to avoid pain is an important means to decrease need for pain management in ventilated infants. Routine sedation is usually not needed in babies, who are stabile on ventilation. Opioids have neither decreased mortality rates and duration of MV nor improved short-term and long-term neurodevelopmental outcomes in neonates receiving MV in meta-analyses. Instead, the number of days to reach full enteral feeding has been increased in opioid-treated infants. Advantages of treatment include improved ventilator synchrony and pulmonary function, especially in infants who "fight" against the ventilator. Adverse effects of medication, especially opioids, including hypotension with morphine and chest wall rigidity with fentanyl, should be kept in mind. Tolerance, dependence, and withdrawal occur. Muscle paralysis with **pancuronium** for infants with RDS remains *controversial*. Sedation of infants with fluctuating cerebral blood flow velocity theoretically decreases the risk of IVH. (See also Chapter 81.)

J. **Complications.** Pulmonary air leaks, such as pneumothorax, pneumomediastinum, pneumopericardium, and pulmonary interstitial emphysema, as well as pulmonary hemorrhage, may occur (see Chapter 87). Chronic complications include respiratory problems such as BPD/CLD (see Chapter 90) and tracheal stenosis.

VIII. **Prognosis.** Although the survival of infants with RDS has improved greatly, the survival with or without respiratory and neurologic sequelae is highly dependent on birthweight and gestational age. Major morbidity (BPD/CLD, NEC, and severe IVH) and poor postnatal growth remain high for the smallest infants.

118 Retinopathy of Prematurity

I. **Definitions**
   A. **Retinopathy of prematurity** is a disorder resulting from the disruption of the normal development of retinal vasculature. Vasoconstriction and obliteration of the advancing capillary bed are followed in succession by neovascularization extending into the vitreous, retinal edema, retinal hemorrhages, fibrosis, and traction on, and eventual detachment of, the retina. In most cases, the process is reversed before fibrosis occurs. Because it is found chiefly in premature infants, it is called *retinopathy of prematurity (ROP)*. **Advanced stages may lead to blindness.**
   B. **Retrolental fibroplasia.** ROP was previously termed *retrolental fibroplasia (RLF)*. The condition was first described in its most advanced form, after extensive fibrosis had already occurred behind the lens.
   C. **Cicatricial retinopathy of prematurity.** The term *cicatricial ROP* refers to fibrotic disease.

II. **Incidence.** Overall, approximately 65% of infants weighing <1251 g develop some form of ROP. Approximately 2% of infants weighing 1000 to 1250 g develop threshold stage 3+ disease eligible for treatment, and approximately 16% of infants weighing <750 g do so. Three large National Institutes of Health–sponsored studies have supported these numbers: the Cryotherapy for Retinopathy of Prematurity (CRYO-ROP) study in 1986 to 1987, the Early Treatment for Retinopathy of Prematurity study (ETROP) in 2000 to 2002, and the Telemedicine Approaches for the Evaluation of Acute-Phase Retinopathy of Prematurity (e-ROP) from 2011 to 2013. These numbers have stayed consistent over almost 3 decades of study, although the incidence and survival of low birthweight infants have increased. This suggests that the overall care of these infants has improved. **Threshold disease occurred at a median postconceptional age of 36 to 37 weeks, regardless of gestational age at birth or chronologic age.** Of note, the International NO-ROP Group in 2005 suggested that severe ROP in larger infants is an emerging worldwide issue. Care and survival of these premature infants are improving, whereas specialized treatment for ROP is not yet as prevalent, making ROP a significant long-term morbidity in these patients.

III. **Pathophysiology**
   A. **Historical perspective.** RLF was first described by Terry in the 1940s and was associated with the use of oxygen in newborn infants by Patz in 1984. The **first epidemic**, estimated to be responsible for 30% of cases of blindness in preschool children by the end of the 1940s, occurred during a period of relatively liberal oxygen administration. After this association was recognized, oxygen use in nurseries was curtailed. Although the incidence of RLF fell, mortality rates in newborn infants increased. In the 1960s, improved oxygen monitoring techniques made possible the cautious reintroduction of oxygen into the nursery. Despite improved oxygen monitoring, however, a **second epidemic** of RLF (ROP) appeared in the late 1970s and was associated with the increased survival of very low birthweight infants.
   B. **Normal embryology of the eye.** In the normally developing retina, there are no retinal vessels until approximately 16 weeks' gestation. Until then, oxygen diffuses from the underlying choroidal circulation. At 16 weeks, in response to a stimulus (experimental evidence suggests relative hypoxia stimulating the release of angiogenic factors as the retina thickens), cells derived from mesenchyme traveling in the nerve fiber layer emanate from the optic nerve head. These cells are the precursors of the retinal vascular system. A fine capillary network advances through the retina to the ora serrata, or retinal edge. More mature vessels form behind this advancing network. Vascularization on the nasal side of the ora serrata is complete at approximately 8 months' gestation and at term on the temporal side. Regulation

of this process involves various factors including vascular endothelial growth factor (VEGF) and insulin-like growth factor 1 (IGF-1) working in combination. Once the retinal vasculature is completely vascularized, it is no longer susceptible to insults of the type that lead to ROP.

   C. **Causes.** There appear to be 2 phases in the development of ROP.

      1. **Early vasoconstriction and obliteration of the capillary network** occurs in response to high oxygen concentrations or another vascular insult. Concentrations of IGF-1 are low in the very low birthweight infant in the early postnatal period as maternal levels are no longer available. Experimental evidence in the mouse model suggests that low IGF-1 contributes to the lack of retinal blood vessel formation in early ROP.

      2. **Vasoproliferation** follows the period of high oxygen exposure or insult, in response to angiogenic factors such as VEGF released by the hypoxic retina. Recent data suggest that VEGF only leads to angiogenesis in the presence of adequate tissue concentrations of IGF-1. When endogenous IGF-1 levels rise in the maturing at-risk premature infant, vasoproliferation is triggered in the presence of VEGF. Considerable evidence has been developed to support this hypothesis. Further research will surely elucidate other modulators of this process.

IV. Risk factors. The association of ROP with oxygen alone is not so clear. Transient hyperoxemia alone is not sufficient. Many other factors, such as extreme prematurity, apnea, sepsis, hyper- and hypocapnia, intraventricular hemorrhage, anemia, exchange transfusion, hypoxia, lactic acidosis, and possibly erythropoietin, which is angiogenic, have been implicated. Experimental studies have focused chiefly on the role of oxygen. Oxygen monitoring is an important part of the care of the premature infant, although **extreme prematurity is known to be the significant risk factor**. Data from Wu et al have shown that postnatal weight gain also significantly affects the development of ROP.

V. Clinical presentation. Several methods of classification of ROP have been used. Here the **International Classification of ROP** is described.

   A. **Stage 1.** A thin demarcation line develops between the vascularized region of the retina and the avascular zone.

   B. **Stage 2.** This line develops into a ridge protruding into the vitreous.

   C. **Stage 3.** Extraretinal fibrovascular proliferation occurs with the ridge. Neovascular tufts may be found just posterior to the ridge (Figure 118–1).

   D. **Stage 4.** Fibrosis and scarring occur as the neovascularization extends into the vitreous. Traction occurs on the retina, resulting in partial retinal detachment.

   E. **Stage 5.** Complete retinal detachment.

   F. **Plus disease (eg, stage 3+).** This occurs when vessels posterior of the posterior pole become dilated and tortuous. **Plus disease has become a primary factor in treatment decisions.**

   G. **Pre-plus disease.** Dilation and tortuosity of posterior pole vessels in zone 1; less severe than plus disease.

   H. **Aggressive posterior retinopathy of prematurity.** Rapidly progressive ROP primarily in zone I. **Requires immediate treatment.**

   I. **Zones.** The retina is divided into circumferential **zones I, II, and III** to designate how far from the posterior pole disease is present. The most severe disease is any stage with plus disease close to the posterior pole, in zone I. The least severe is disease in the temporal peripheral retina, in zone III. No treatment is necessary for peripheral zone III disease, as it regresses spontaneously.

VI. Diagnosis. Ophthalmoscopic examination by an experienced examiner usually confirms the diagnosis. **Binocular indirect ophthalmoscopy (BIO)** is generally used. Increasingly, fundus photography of the posterior retina with remote interpretation of the images is being used for screening in areas where no ophthalmologist is available. Validated through e-ROP, this technique is limited in that it does not permit adequate assessment of ROP in the retinal periphery. BIO must be employed to determine when screening can be discontinued.

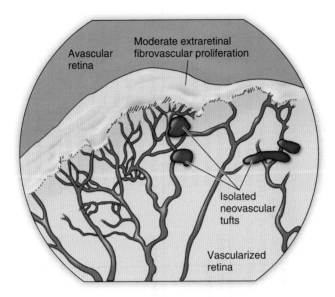

FIGURE 118–1. Schematic drawing of moderate stage 3 retinopathy of prematurity. Optic nerve head is shown at the bottom, and periphery of the retina is at the top.

For BIO to be performed, dilation drops must be administered prior to examination. Protocols vary depending on the institution and the location throughout the world, but in general, cyclopentolate (0.2% or 0.5%) and phenylephrine (1% or 2.5%) are used at the lowest concentration deemed reasonable to achieve sufficient examination of the peripheral retina. (See Table 118–1 for a full list of medications used and their side effects.) Just prior to examination, proparacaine drops are also often administered to provide topical anesthesia. The American Academy of Pediatrics (AAP) pain management recommendations from 2006, reaffirmed in 2010, state that retinal examinations are painful, and pain relief measures should be used. They further state that a reasonable approach would be to administer local anesthetic eye drops, pacifiers, and oral sucrose. A 2013 joint statement by the AAP, the American Association for Pediatric Ophthalmology and Strabismus, and the American Academy of Ophthalmology provided updated recommendations for ROP screening examinations in premature infants.

A. **Infants weighing ≤1500 g or ≤30 weeks' gestation** and those weighing >1500 g or >30 weeks' gestation with an unstable clinical course should have dilated eye examinations starting at 4 to 6 weeks of age or 31 to 33 weeks' postmenstrual age. Examinations should continue every 2 to 3 weeks until retinal vascular maturity is reached, if no disease is present.

B. **Infants with retinopathy of prematurity or very immature vessels** should be examined every 1 to 2 weeks until vessels are mature or the risk of disease requiring treatment has passed. Those at greatest risk should be examined every week.

VII. **Management.** Disease that requires treatment was defined by the ETROP study and includes zone I ROP of any stage with plus disease, zone I ROP stage 3 with no plus disease, and zone II ROP stage 2 or 3 with plus disease. The possible interventions are as follows:

A. **Circumferential cryopexy.** Proven to be an effective treatment for progressive disease, this approach prevents further ROP progression by destroying cells that

Table 118–1. COMMON OCULAR AGENTS USED FOR RETINOPATHY OF PREMATURITY EVALUATION IN NEONATES (ANESTHETIC AND MYDRIATIC AGENTS; EXCLUDES ANTIBIOTICS)

Medication	Form	Concentration	Frequency	Class	Indication	Side Effects
Proparacaine	Ophthalmic solution	0.50%	1 time[a]	Anesthetic	Topical anesthesia prior to dilation eye drops	Conjunctival hemorrhage, corneal erosion, cycloplegia (rare), passive conjunctival congestion
Cyclopentolate	Ophthalmic solution	0.2%, 0.5%, 1%, 2%	1 time[a]	Anticholinergic	Mydriasis induction, cycloplegia	Blurred vision, burning sensation in eye, photophobia, conjunctivitis, raised intraocular pressure, tachyarrhythmia, vasodilatation, ataxia, confusion, seizure, psychotic disorder
Phenylephrine hydrochloride	Ophthalmic solution	1%, 2.5%	1 time[a]	Adrenergic alkylarylamine	Mydriasis induction	Eye irritation, nasal congestion, sneezing. *Note:* Topical instillation of phenylephrine 10% ophthalmic solution has resulted in rare occurrences of tachycardia, ventricular arrythmias, myocardial infarction, subarachnoid hemorrhage, and rupture of aneurysms. Phenylephrine 10% is not used routinely in neonates.
Tropicamide	Ophthalmic solution	0.5%, 1%	1 time[a]	Anticholinergic	Mydriasis induction, cycloplegia	Blurred vision, burning sensation in eye, photophobia, raised intraocular pressure

[a]May repeat 1–2 times after 5–10 minutes, if needed, for additional dilation.

may be releasing angiogenic factors. Results of the Cryotherapy for Retinopathy of Prematurity (CRYO-ROP) study indicate that cryopexy carried out at stage 3+ can reduce the incidence of severe visual impairment by approximately 50% if performed within 72 hours of detecting threshold disease. Ten-year follow-up shows significant improvement in visual acuity of treated versus control eyes. It is imperative that an ophthalmologist skilled in cryopexy performs the procedure.

B. **Laser photocoagulation.** This technique is equally effective yet safer than cryopexy, and it has become **the treatment of choice.** In 1994, the Laser ROP Study Group conducted a meta-analysis of 4 laser ROP trials. Treatment was based on the same criteria used in the CRYO-ROP trial. Recognizing the limitations of a meta-analysis, the study group concluded that laser therapy is at least as effective as cryotherapy for ROP, despite a small risk of cataract formation. Ten-year follow-up of a small group of patients suggested better outcomes with laser photocoagulation. The ETROP study (2002) demonstrated improved outcomes with treatment at any stage when plus disease is present. AAP pain recommendations from 2006, reaffirmed in 2010, state that retinal surgery should be considered major surgery, and effective opiate-based pain relief should be provided while monitoring the infant with an appropriate pain assessment scale.

C. **Oxygen for treatment of retinopathy of prematurity.** In an attempt to reduce angiogenic factors from the hypoxic retina and to prevent the progression of ROP, oxygen therapy was administered in a large collaborative trial, the Supplemental Therapeutic Oxygen for Prethreshold Retinopathy of Prematurity (STOP-ROP) study. Oxygen saturations were targeted at 96% to 99% in the treatment group and 89% to 94% in the conventional group once prethreshold ROP was diagnosed. No significant difference was seen in the rate of progression to threshold disease between the 2 groups, although there was a significant increase in bronchopulmonary dysplasia/chronic lung disease in the high-saturation group. The appropriate saturation ranges remain *controversial* and under study, although most neonatal intensive care units keep infants <1250 g at saturations <95% when on supplemental oxygen.

D. **Intravitreal injection of anti–vascular endothelial growth factor therapy.** Given the contribution of VEGF to the pathophysiology of ROP, recent studies have explored the use of intravitreal injection of anti-VEGF agents as an alternative to traditional ablative therapies. In 2011, Mintz-Hittner et al published their results for the Bevacizumab Eliminates the Angiogenic Threat of Retinopathy of Prematurity BEAT-ROP collaborative trial in which infants with stage 3+ ROP were randomly assigned to intravitreal bevacizumab monotherapy versus laser therapy. A significant benefit for zone 1 ROP (the most difficult to treat conventionally) was demonstrated. The time to recurrence of ROP after bevacizumab was much later, however, than after laser photocoagulation (~16 weeks vs ~6 weeks), necessitating longer follow-up time to ensure no recurrence of ROP requiring treatment. Further studies are being conducted to determine if lower concentrations of bevacizumab will be equally effective at treating ROP with less risk of systemic suppression of VEGF. In addition, treatment with other anti-VEGF agents is being explored.

E. **Insulin-like growth factor 1 supplementation.** A recent multicenter phase II study investigated the administration of mecasermin rinfabate in 121 infants of 23 to 27 weeks' gestation until 30 weeks' gestation in an effort to prevent ROP. The study found no change in the incidence of ROP, although the rates of intraventricular hemorrhage and bronchopulmonary dysplasia were significantly decreased. Further study is needed to elucidate the possible prevention of ROP through IGF-1 supplementation.

F. **Dietary supplementation of omega-3 polyunsaturated fatty acids.** The balance of omega-3 and omega-6 polyunsaturated fatty acids in the retina affects cell survival. Studies in the mouse model have shown a protective effect of omega-3 supplementation.

G. **Vitamin E.** The administration of pharmacologic doses of vitamin E for ROP has been studied with no proof of clear benefit. Reported side effects include sepsis, necrotizing enterocolitis, and intraventricular hemorrhage. Even so, maintenance of normal serum vitamin E levels is a prudent management objective. (For doses, see Chapter 155.)

H. **Retinal reattachment surgery.** Stage 4 and 5 disease has been treated surgically with vitrectomy and scleral buckle with some anatomic success. Visual prognosis, however, remains guarded to poor in these patients.

I. **Follow-up eye examinations.** Advocated every 1 to 2 years for infants with fully regressed ROP and every 6 to 12 months for those with cicatricial ROP. Premature infants are at risk for myopia even in the absence of ROP and should have an eye examination by 6 months of age.

VIII. **Prognosis.** Ninety percent of cases of stage 1 and stage 2 disease regress spontaneously. Approximately 50% of cases of stage 3+ disease regress spontaneously. Of those that do progress to stage 3+, the incidence of unfavorable structural outcomes can be reduced by approximately 50% and unfavorable visual outcomes by approximately 30% if circumferential cryopexy is carried out by a skilled ophthalmologist. Laser photocoagulation appears equally and possibly more effective than cryopexy and is now the procedure of choice in the United States. Sequelae of regressed disease such as myopia, strabismus, amblyopia, glaucoma, and late detachment require regular follow-up.

119 Rh Incompatibility

I. **Definition.** Rh incompatibility is a condition that occurs during pregnancy when a mother with Rh-negative blood [who is previously sensitized to the Rh(D) antigen] is exposed to her fetus who is Rh-positive leading to the development of Rh antibodies and resulting in fetal isoimmune hemolytic anemia of variable severity. The onset of clinical disease begins in utero as the result of active placental transfer of maternal immunoglobulin (Ig)G-Rh antibody. It is manifested as a partially compensated, moderate to severe hemolytic anemia at birth, with unconjugated hyperbilirubinemia developing in the early neonatal period.

II. **Incidence.** Historically, Rh hemolytic disease of the newborn accounted for up to a third of symptomatic cases seen and was associated with detectable antibody in approximately 15% of Rh-incompatible mothers. **The use of Rh immunoglobulin (RhoGAM) prophylaxis has reduced the incidence of Rh sensitization to <1% of Rh-incompatible pregnancies.** In developing countries without prophylaxis, stillbirth still occurs in 14% of affected pregnancies, and 50% of pregnancies survivors either die in the neonatal period or develop cerebral injury. Other alloimmune antibodies have become relatively more important as a cause of hemolysis. Anti-c, Kell (K and k), Duffy (Fya), Kidd (Jka and Jkb), MNS (M, N, S, and s), and less commonly anti-C and anti-E may cause severe hemolytic disease of the newborn.

III. **Pathophysiology.** Initial exposure of the mother to the Rh antigen occurs most often during parturition, miscarriage, abortion, and ectopic pregnancy. Invasive investigative procedures such as amniocentesis, chorionic villus sampling, and fetal blood sampling also increase the risk of fetal transplacental hemorrhage and alloimmunization. Recognition of the antigen by the immune system ensues after initial exposure, and reexposure to the Rh antigen induces a maternal anamnestic response and elevation of specific IgG-Rh antibody. Active placental transport of this antibody and immune attachment to the Rh-antigenic sites on the fetal erythrocyte are followed by extravascular hemolysis of erythrocytes within the fetal liver and spleen. The rate of the hemolytic process is proportionate in part to the levels of the maternal antibody titer but is more accurately reflected in the antepartum period by elevation of the amniotic fluid bilirubin concentration and in the postpartum period by the rate of rise of unconjugated bilirubin. In contrast to ABO incompatibility, the greater antigenicity and density of the Rh-antigen loci on the fetal erythrocyte facilitates progressive, rapid clearance of fetal erythrocytes from the circulation. A demonstrable phase of spherocytosis will be absent. Compensatory reticulocytosis and shortening of the erythrocyte generation time, if unable to match the often high rate of hemolysis in utero, result in anemia in the newborn infant and a risk of multiple systemic complications.

IV. **Risk factors**
   A. **Birth order.** The first-born infant is at minimum risk (<1%) unless sensitization has occurred previously. Once sensitization has occurred, subsequent pregnancies are at a progressive increased risk for fetal disease.
   B. **Fetomaternal hemorrhage.** The volume of fetal erythrocytes entering the maternal circulation correlates with the risk of sensitization. The risk is approximately 8% with each pregnancy but ranges from 3% to 65%, depending on the volume of fetal blood (3% with 0.1 mL compared with 22% with >0.1 mL) that passes into the maternal circulation.
   C. **ABO incompatibility.** Coexistent incompatibility for either the A or B blood group antigen reduces the risk of maternal Rh sensitization to 1.5% to 3.0%. Rapid immune clearance of these fetal erythrocytes after their entry into the maternal circulation exerts a partial protective effect. It confers no protection once sensitization has occurred.
   D. **Obstetric factors.** Cesarean delivery or trauma to the placental bed during the third stage of labor increases the risk of significant fetomaternal transfusion and subsequent maternal sensitization.
   E. **Gender.** Male infants are reported to have an increased risk of more severe disease than females, although the basis for this observation is unclear.
   F. **Ethnicity.** Approximately 15% of whites are Rh negative compared with 7% of blacks and almost 0% of Asiatic Chinese and Japanese. The risk to the fetus varies accordingly.

V. **Clinical presentation**
   A. **Symptoms and signs**
      1. **Jaundice.** Unconjugated hyperbilirubinemia is the most common presenting neonatal sign of Rh disease, usually appearing within the first 24 hours of life.
      2. **Anemia.** Low cord blood hemoglobin at birth reflects the relative severity of the hemolytic process in utero and is present in approximately 50% of cases.
      3. **Hepatosplenomegaly.** Enlargement of the liver and spleen is seen in severe hemolysis, sometimes occurring in association with ascites, with an increased risk for splenic rupture.
      4. **Hydrops fetalis.** Severe Rh disease has a historical association with hydrops fetalis and at one time was its most common cause. Clinical features in the fetus include progressive hypoalbuminemia with ascites, pleural effusion, or both; severe chronic anemia with secondary hypoxemia; and cardiac failure. There is an increased risk of late fetal death, stillbirth, and intolerance of active labor. The neonate frequently has generalized edema, notably of the scalp, which can be detected by antepartum ultrasonography; cardiopulmonary distress often involving pulmonary edema and severe surfactant deficiency; congestive heart failure; hypotension and peripheral perfusion defects; cardiac rhythm disturbances; and severe anemia with secondary hypoxemia and metabolic acidosis. Currently, nonimmune conditions are more commonly associated with hydrops fetalis. Secondary involvement of other organ systems may result in hypoglycemia or thrombocytopenic purpura.

VI. **Diagnosis.** Obligatory screening in an infant with unconjugated hyperbilirubinemia includes the following studies:

A. **Blood type and Rh type (mother and infant).** The Rhesus (Rh) factor is an inherited protein found on the surface of red blood cells (RBCs). If the RBCs have the protein, then one is Rh-positive; if the RBCs lack the protein, then one is Rh-negative. Obtaining the blood type and Rh type establish the likelihood of Rh incompatibility and exclude the diagnosis if the infant is Rh negative, with 1 exception (see direct antiglobulin test [direct Coombs test], Section VI.C). This can be done prenatally by detection of cell-free fetal DNA of the *RHD* gene in the maternal blood.

B. **Reticulocyte count.** Elevated reticulocyte levels, adjusted for the degree of anemia and gestational age in preterm infants, reflect the degree of compensation and support a diagnosis of an ongoing hemolytic process. Normal values are 4% to 5% for term infants and 6% to 10% for preterm infants (30–36 weeks' gestational age). In symptomatic Rh disease, expected values are 10% to 40%.

C. **Direct antiglobulin test (direct Coombs test).** A strongly positive direct Coombs test indicates that fetal RBCs are coated with antibodies and is diagnostic of Rh incompatibility in the presence of the appropriate setup and an elevated reticulocyte count. If Rh immunoglobulin was given at 28 weeks' gestation, subsequent passive transfer of antibody will result in a false-positive direct Coombs test without associated reticulocytosis. Very rarely, a strongly positive direct Coombs test is associated with a falsely Rh-negative infant when all fetal RBC Rh-antigenic sites are covered by a high titer of maternal antibodies.

D. **Blood smear.** Polychromasia and normoblastosis proportionate to the reticulocyte count are typically present. Spherocytes are not usually present. The nucleated RBC count is often >10 per 100 white blood cells.

E. **Bilirubin levels.** Progressive elevation of unconjugated bilirubin on serial testing provides an index of the severity of the hemolytic process. An elevated direct fraction is most likely to be secondary to a laboratory artifact in the first 3 days of life and should not be subtracted from the total bilirubin when making management decisions. In the most severely affected infants, particularly those who are hydropic, the intense extramedullary erythropoiesis may cause hepatocellular dysfunction and biliary canalicular obstruction with significant elevated direct bilirubin by 5 to 6 days of age (inspissated bile syndrome).

F. **Bilirubin-binding capacity tests.** Correlation between measurements of serum albumin, free bilirubin, bilirubin saturation index, and reserve binding capacity and outcome has been variable. The role of these values in directing the management of patients remains unclear.

G. **Glucose and blood gas levels.** These should be monitored closely.

H. **Supplementary laboratory studies.** Supportive diagnostic studies may be required when the basis of the hemolytic process remains unclear.

1. **Indirect antiglobulin titer (indirect Coombs test).** This test detects the presence of antibodies in the maternal serum. Rh-positive RBCs are incubated with the serum being tested for the presence of anti-D. If present, the RBCs now coated with anti-D are agglutinated by an antihuman globulin serum reflecting a positive indirect antiglobulin (Coombs) test result. The reciprocal of the highest dilution of maternal serum that produces agglutination is the indirect antiglobulin titer.

2. **Carbon monoxide.** The severity of Rh disease may be determined by measurement of endogenous carbon monoxide (CO) production. When heme is catabolized to bilirubin, CO is produced in equimolar amounts. Hemoglobin binds the CO to form carboxyhemoglobin (COHb) and then is finally excreted in the breath. COHb levels are increased in neonates with hemolysis. COHb levels >1.4% have been correlated with an increased need for exchange transfusion.

VII. **Management**
  A. **Antepartum treatment.** Verification of the Rh-negative status at the first prenatal visit may be obtained by the following measures:
    1. **Maternal antibody titer.** Once an IgG-Rh antibody has been identified, it is important to determine the titer. Serial antibody titer determinations are required every 1 to 4 weeks (depending on the gestational age) during pregnancy. Invasive fetal testing becomes indicated when the titer is above a critical level, usually between 1:8 and 1:16. A negative antibody screen (indirect Coombs test) signifies absence of sensitization. This test should be repeated at 28 to 34 weeks' gestation.
    2. **RhoGAM.** Current obstetric guidelines suggest giving immunoprophylaxis at 28 weeks' gestation in the absence of sensitization.
    3. **Amniocentesis.** If maternal antibody titers indicate a risk of fetal death (usual range, 1:16–1:32), amniocentesis may be performed to assess fetal Rh genotype and assess severity. Fetal Rh genotype determination can also be made from fetal cell-free DNA found in maternal plasma. To reasonably predict the risk of moderate to severe fetal disease, serial determinations of amniotic fluid bilirubin levels present photometrically at 450 nm (ΔOD_{450}) are plotted on standard graphs according to gestational age (known as the **Liley curve**). Readings falling into very high zone II or zone III indicate that hydrops will develop within 7 to 10 days. Zone I indicate no fetal hemolytic disease or no anemia.
    4. **Ultrasonography.** As a screening study in pregnancies at risk, serial fetal ultrasound examinations allow detection of scalp edema, ascites, or other signs of developing hydrops fetalis. Serial peak systolic middle cerebral artery velocity can reliably detect moderate and severe fetal anemia and thus is now replacing the more invasive and less predictive ΔOD_{450} analysis for fetal anemia monitoring.
    5. **Intrauterine transfusion.** Based on the studies just mentioned, intrauterine transfusion may be indicated because of possible fetal demise or the presence of fetal hydrops. This procedure must be performed by an experienced team. The goal is maintenance of effective erythrocyte mass within the fetal circulation and maintenance of the pregnancy until there is a reasonable chance for successful extrauterine survival of the infant.
    6. **Glucocorticoids.** If premature delivery is anticipated, glucocorticoids should be given to accelerate fetal lung maturation and reduce the risk of intraventricular hemorrhage.
    7. **Reduction of maternal antibody level.** Intensive maternal plasma exchange and high-dose intravenous immunoglobulins (IVIGs) have been reported to be of value in the severely alloimmunized pregnant woman to reduce circulating maternal antibodies levels by >50%.
  B. **Postpartum treatment**
    1. **Resuscitation.** Moderately to severely anemic infants with or without hydropic features are at risk for high-output cardiac failure, hypoxemia secondary to decreased oxygen-carrying capacity or surfactant deficiency, and hypoglycemia. These infants may require immediate single-volume exchange blood transfusion at delivery to improve oxygen-carrying capacity, mechanical support of ventilation, and an extended period of monitoring for hypoglycemia.
    2. **Cord blood studies.** A cord blood bilirubin level >4 mg/dL, a cord hemoglobin <12 g/dL, or both usually suggests moderate to severe disease. The cord blood is used for these and initial screening studies, including blood typing, Rh typing, and Coombs test.
    3. **Serial unconjugated bilirubin studies.** Determination of the rate of increase in unconjugated bilirubin levels provides an index of the severity of the hemolytic process and the need for exchange transfusion. Commonly used guidelines include a rise of >0.5 mg/dL/h or >5 mg/dL over 24 hours within the first 2 days

of life or projection of a serum level that will exceed a predetermined "exchange level" for a given infant (usually 20 mg/dL in term infants).

4. **Phototherapy.** In severe Rh hemolytic disease, phototherapy is used only as an adjunct to exchange transfusion. Phototherapy decreases bilirubin levels and reduces the number of total exchange transfusions required. See Chapters 63 and 99 for phototherapy details.

5. **Exchange transfusion.** For the procedure, see Chapter 34. Exchange transfusion is indicated if the unconjugated bilirubin level is likely to reach a predetermined "exchange level" for that patient. Optimally, exchange transfusion is done well before this exchange level is reached to minimize the risk of entry of unconjugated bilirubin into the central nervous system. Consideration should be given to irradiation of blood before the transfusion is given, particularly in preterm infants or infants expected to require multiple transfusions, to reduce the risk of graft-versus-host disease. The process removes 70% to 90% of the fetal red cells, but only 25% of the total bilirubin because most of the bilirubin is in the extravascular space. A rapid rebound of serum bilirubin is common after reequilibration, and thus, additional exchange transfusions may be required.

6. **Heme oxygenase inhibitors (stannsoporfin).** See Chapter 85 on ABO incompatibility. Tin (Sn) porphyrin is an inhibitor of heme oxygenase, the enzyme that allows the production of bilirubin from heme.

7. **Intravenous immunoglobulin.** By blocking neonatal reticuloendothelial Fc receptors, and thus decreasing hemolysis of the antibody-coated RBCs, high-dose IVIG (1 g/kg over 4 hours) reduces serum bilirubin levels and the need for blood exchange transfusion with ABO or Rh hemolytic diseases. (See Chapter 85.) Caution should be used when considering treatment with IVIG because there are emerging reports of increased incidence of necrotizing enterocolitis in term and late preterm infants with hemolytic disease of the newborn and isoimmune neonatal thrombocytopenia who were treated with IVIG.

C. **RhoGAM prophylaxis.** Most cases of incompatibility involve the D antigen. RhoGAM given at 28 weeks' gestation, within 72 hours of suspected Rh-antigen exposure, or both reduces the risk of sensitization to <1%; the recommended dosage (300 mcg) should be well in excess of the amount of Rh antigen transfused (300 mcg for every 25 mL of fetal blood in maternal circulation). The amount of fetal blood entering the maternal circulation may be estimated using the Kleihauer-Betke acid elution technique (pages 819 and 820) during the immediate postpartum period.

D. **Hydrops fetalis.** Skilled resuscitation and anticipation of selective systemic complications may prevent early neonatal death.

1. **Isovolumetric partial exchange transfusion with type O Rh-negative packed erythrocytes.** Raises the hematocrit and improves the oxygen-carrying capacity (see Chapter 34).

2. **Central arterial and venous catheterization.** May be performed to provide the following measures:
   a. **Isovolumetric exchange transfusion.**
   b. **Monitoring of arterial blood gas levels** and central venous and systemic blood pressures.
   c. **Monitoring of fluid and electrolyte balance,** particularly renal and hepatic function, calcium-to-phosphorus ratio, and serum albumin levels, as well as appropriate hematologic studies and serum bilirubin levels.

3. **Positive-pressure mechanical ventilation.** This measure may include increased levels of positive end-expiratory pressure, if pulmonary edema is present, as a means of stabilizing alveolar ventilation. Treatment with exogenous surfactant may be considered in particular when the infant is judged to be not fully mature.

4. **Therapeutic thoracentesis or paracentesis** may be performed to remove fluid that may further compromise respiratory effort. Excessive removal of ascitic fluid may lead to systemic hypotension. (See Chapters 31 and 40.)

5. **Volume expanders** may be necessary, in addition to erythrocytes, to improve peripheral perfusion defects. This should be done with caution because most hydropic infants are hypotensive or poorly perfused because of hypoxic heart failure rather than hypovolemia, or both.

6. **Drug treatment.** Includes diuretics for pulmonary edema and pressor agents such as dopamine (for dosing, see Chapter 155). Diuretics that contain a sulfonamide group (such as furosemide) should be avoided.

7. **Electrocardiography or echocardiography.** May be used to determine whether cardiac abnormalities are present.

VIII. **Prognosis.** Prenatal mortality for infants at risk of anti-D Rh isoimmunization is currently approximately 1.5% and has decreased significantly over the past 2 decades. Antenatal immune prophylaxis and improved management techniques, including amniotic fluid spectrophotometry, intrauterine transfusion, and advances in neonatal intensive care, have been largely responsible for this reduction. Isolated cases of severe isoimmunization still occur because of isoimmunization by other than anti-D antibody or failure to receive immune prophylaxis and may exhibit the full spectrum of disease, including an increased risk of stillbirths and early neonatal morbidity and mortality.

120 Seizures

I. **Definition.** A seizure is defined clinically as a paroxysmal alteration in neurologic function (ie, behavioral, motor, or autonomic function). (See also Chapter 82 for on-call management of seizures).

II. **Incidence.** Neonatal seizures are relatively common and occur in 2 to 3 neonates per 1000 births of all neonates; the incidence is more common in premature infants, with an occurrence in up to 130 per 1000.

III. **Pathophysiology.** The neurons within the central nervous system (CNS) undergo depolarization as a result of inward migration of sodium. Repolarization occurs via efflux of potassium. A seizure occurs when there is excessive depolarization, resulting in excessive synchronous electrical discharge. Volpe (2001) proposed the following 4 possible reasons for excessive depolarization: failure of the sodium-potassium pump because of a disturbance in energy production, a relative excess of excitatory versus inhibitory neurotransmitters, a relative deficiency of inhibitory versus excitatory neurotransmitters, and alteration in the neuronal membrane, causing inhibition of sodium movement. The basic mechanisms of neonatal seizures, however, are unknown.

IV. **Etiology.** There are numerous causes of neonatal seizures, but relatively few account for most cases. Therefore, only common causes of seizures are discussed here. See Table 120–1 for a more extensive list of causes.

A. **Perinatal asphyxia** is the most common cause of neonatal seizures. Hypoxic ischemic encephalopathy (HIE) is seen in approximately 1 to 2 per 1000 live births. In fact, about two-thirds of cases of neonatal seizures are due to HIE. These occur within the first 24 hours of life in most cases. In premature infants, seizures are of the generalized tonic type, whereas in full-term infants they are of the multifocal clonic type. Accompanying subtle seizures are usually present in both types.

B. **Intracranial hemorrhage**
1. **In primary subarachnoid hemorrhage,** convulsions often occur on the second postnatal day, and the infant appears quite well during the interictal period.

Table 120–1. CAUSES OF NEONATAL SEIZURES

Perinatal asphyxia/hypoxic ischemic encephalopathy

Intracranial hemorrhage: Subarachnoid hemorrhage; intraventricular hemorrhage; subdural hemorrhage; parenchymal hemorrhage

Acute metabolic abnormalities: Hypoglycemia; hypocalcemia; hyponatremia; hypernatremia; hypomagnesemia

Inborn errors of metabolism: Amino acid disorders; urea cycle abnormalities; organic acidemias; mitochondrial disorders; peroxisomal disturbances; pyridoxine dependency; pyridoxal phosphate–dependent seizures; folinic acid responsive seizures; multiple carboxylase deficiency; others

Congenital malformations: Lissencephaly; focal cortical dysplasia; schizencephaly; hydranencephaly; hemimegalencephaly

Infections: Meningitis; encephalitis; cerebral abscess

Congenital infections: Syphilis; cytomegalovirus infections; toxoplasmosis; herpes simplex; rubella; coxsackie B virus; Zika

Drug withdrawal

Toxin exposure (particularly local anesthetics)

Neonatal epilepsy syndromes: Self-limited (benign) familial neonatal epilepsy; early myoclonic encephalopathy; early infantile epileptic encephalopathy (Ohtahara syndrome)

Miscellaneous: Zellweger syndrome; tuberous sclerosis; polycythemia with hyperviscosity; bilirubin encephalopathy; ECLS-related seizures; congenital heart disease; congenital hypothyroidism

ECLS, extracorporeal life support.

    2. **Periventricular or intraventricular hemorrhage** arising from the subependymal germinal matrix in preterm neonates is accompanied by subtle seizures, decerebrate posturing, or generalized tonic seizures, depending on the severity of the hemorrhage.

    3. **Subdural hemorrhage** over the cerebral convexities leads to focal seizures and focal cerebral signs. It is usually secondary to trauma.

C. **Metabolic disturbances**

    1. **Hypoglycemia** is frequently seen in infants with intrauterine growth retardation and in infants of diabetic mothers. The duration of hypoglycemia and the time lapse before initiation of treatment determine the occurrence of seizures.

    2. **Hypocalcemia** has been noted in low birthweight infants, infants of diabetic mothers, asphyxiated infants, infants with DiGeorge syndrome, and infants born to mothers with hyperparathyroidism. Hypomagnesemia is a frequent accompanying problem.

    3. **Hyponatremia** occurs because of improper fluid management or as a result of the syndrome of inappropriate antidiuretic hormone.

    4. **Hypernatremia** is seen with dehydration as a result of inadequate intake in breast-fed infants or incorrect dilution of concentrated formula.

    5. **Other metabolic disorders**

       a. **Pyridoxine dependency.** Leads to seizures resistant to anticonvulsants. Infants with this disorder experience intrauterine convulsions.

       b. **Amino acid disorders.** Seizures in infants with amino acid disturbances are invariably accompanied by other neurologic manifestations. Hyperammonemia and acidosis are commonly present in amino acid disorders.

D. **Infections.** Intracranial infection secondary to bacterial or nonbacterial agents may be acquired by the neonate in utero, during delivery, or in the immediate perinatal period.

  1. **Bacterial infection.** Meningitis resulting from group B *Streptococcus*, *Escherichia coli*, or *Listeria monocytogenes* infection is accompanied by seizures during the first week of life.

  2. **Nonbacterial infection.** Nonbacterial causes such as toxoplasmosis and infection with herpes simplex, cytomegalovirus, rubella, and coxsackie B viruses lead to intracranial infection and seizures.

E. **Drug withdrawal.** Three categories of drugs used by the mother lead to passive addiction and drug withdrawal (sometimes accompanied by seizures) in the infant. These are **analgesics**, such as heroin, methadone, and others; **sedative-hypnotics**, such as secobarbital; and **alcohol**.

F. **Toxins.** Inadvertent injection of local anesthetics into the fetus at the time of delivery (paracervical, pudendal, or saddle block anesthesia) may cause seizures. Mothers often notice the absence of pain relief during delivery.

G. **Congenital/developmental abnormalities of the brain.** Often the infant has obvious anomalies of the face or head if developmental abnormalities are present. Most common are lissencephaly and holoprosencephaly.

H. **Neonatal cerebral infarction (perinatal stroke).** A common cause of seizures in full-term infants (1 in 2300–5000). Usually presents with focal seizures with cerebral artery or vein infarction.

V. **Clinical presentation.** It is important to understand that **seizures in the neonate are different from those seen in older children.** The differences are perhaps due to the neuroanatomic and neurophysiologic developmental status of the newborn infant. In the neonatal brain, glial proliferation, neuronal migration, establishment of axonal and dendritic contacts, and myelin deposition are incomplete. Clinical seizures may occur without any electrographic correlation and vice versa (electroclinical dissociation). Approximately 80% of electroencephalogram (EEG)-documented seizures are not accompanied by observable clinical seizures. **Four types of seizures**, based on clinical presentation, are recognized: **subtle, clonic, tonic, and myoclonic.**

A. **Subtle seizures** are more common in premature infants than in full-term infants. They consist of tonic horizontal deviation of the eyes with or without jerking; eyelid blinking or fluttering; sucking, smacking, or drooling; "swimming," "rowing," or "pedaling" movements; and apneic spells. In premature infants, apnea is less likely to be a manifestation of seizures.

B. **Clonic seizures** are more common in full-term infants than in premature infants and are commonly associated with an EEG seizure. There are 2 types of clonic seizures:

  1. **Focal seizures.** Well-localized, rhythmic, slow jerking movements involving the face and upper or lower extremities on 1 side of the body or the neck or trunk on 1 side of the body.

  2. **Multifocal seizures.** Several body parts seize in a sequential, non-jacksonian fashion (eg, left arm jerking followed by right leg jerking).

C. **Tonic seizures** occur primarily in premature infants. Two types of tonic seizures are seen.

  1. **Focal seizures.** Sustained posturing of a limb, asymmetric posturing of the trunk or neck, or both. These are commonly associated with an EEG seizure.

  2. **Generalized seizures.** Most commonly, these occur with a tonic extension of both upper and lower extremities (as in decerebrate posturing) but may also present with tonic flexion of the upper extremities with extension of the lower extremities (as in decorticate posturing). It is uncommon to see EEG seizure disorders.

    D. **Myoclonic seizures** are seen in both full-term and premature infants and are characterized by single or multiple synchronous jerks. Three types of myoclonic seizures are seen.

      1. **Focal seizures.** Typically involve the flexor muscles of an upper extremity and are not commonly associated with EEG seizure activity.

      2. **Multifocal seizures.** Exhibit asynchronous twitching of several parts of the body and are not commonly associated with EEG seizure activity.

      3. **Generalized seizures.** Present with bilateral jerks of flexion of the upper and sometimes the lower extremities. They are more commonly associated with EEG seizure activity. ***Note:*** It is important to distinguish **jitteriness** from **seizures**. Jitteriness is accompanied by neither abnormal gaze nor eye movements, nor by autonomic changes. It is highly stimulus sensitive; tremor is the dominant movement, and it can be stopped by gentle flexion.

VI. Diagnosis

    A. **History.** Although it is often difficult to obtain a thorough history in infants transported to tertiary care facilities from other hospitals, the physician must make a concerted effort to elicit pertinent historical data.

      1. **Family history.** A positive family history of neonatal seizures is usually obtained in cases of metabolic errors and benign familial neonatal convulsions.

      2. **Maternal drug history.** This is critical in cases of narcotic withdrawal syndrome.

      3. **Delivery.** Details of the delivery provide information regarding maternal analgesia, the mode and nature of delivery, the fetal intrapartum status, and the resuscitative measures used. Information regarding maternal infections during pregnancy points toward an infectious basis for seizures in an infant.

    B. **Physical examination**

      1. **Physical examination.** A thorough general physical examination (including measurement of head circumference and careful attention to any dysmorphic features) should precede a well-planned neurologic examination. Determine the following:

        a. **Gestational age**

        b. **Blood pressure**

        c. **Presence of skin lesions**

        d. **Presence of hepatosplenomegaly**

      2. **Neurologic evaluation.** A neurologic evaluation should include assessment of the level of alertness, cranial nerves, motor function, primary neonatal reflexes, and sensory function. Some of the specific features to look for are the size and "feel" of the fontanelle, retinal hemorrhages, chorioretinitis, pupillary size and reaction to light, extraocular movements, changes in muscle tone, and status of primary reflexes.

      3. **Notation of the seizure pattern.** When seizures are observed, they should be described in detail, including the site of onset, spread, nature, duration, and level of consciousness. Recognition of subtle seizures requires special attention.

    C. **Laboratory studies.** In selecting and prioritizing laboratory tests, use the information obtained by history taking and physical examination and look for common and treatable causes.

      1. **Complete blood count and differential.** To rule out infection and polycythemia.

      2. **Biochemistry.** Estimations of serum glucose, calcium, sodium, blood urea nitrogen, and magnesium and blood gas levels must be performed.

      3. **Spinal fluid examination.** Evaluation of the cerebrospinal fluid (CSF) is essential because the consequences of delayed treatment or nontreatment of bacterial meningitis are grave. CSF polymerase chain reaction (PCR) should be performed for herpes simplex virus if suspected. A low CSF glucose and normal blood glucose indicate meningitis or glucose transporter defect. An increase in CSF glycine concentration together with an increased CSF-to-plasma glycine ratio suggests glycine encephalopathy, and elevated CSF lactate suggests a mitochondrial disorder.

4. **Inborn errors of metabolism.** (See also Chapter 100.) With a family history of neonatal convulsions, a peculiar odor about the infant, milk intolerance, acidosis, alkalosis, or seizures not responsive to anticonvulsants, other metabolic causes should be investigated.

    a. **Blood ammonia levels** should be checked.

    b. **Amino acids** should be measured in urine and plasma. The urine should be tested for reducing substances and organic acids.

        i. **Urea cycle disorders.** Respiratory alkalosis is seen as a result of direct stimulation of the respiratory center by ammonia.

D. **Imaging and other studies**

1. **Ultrasonography of the head.** Performed to rule out intraventricular hemorrhage (IVH) or periventricular hemorrhage.

2. **Computed tomography scanning of the head.** Computed tomography scanning is helpful in looking for evidence of infarction, hemorrhage, calcification, and cerebral malformations. It is useful in term infants with seizures, especially when seizures are asymmetric. Be mindful of heavy doses of radiation and avoid repeating unless absolutely essential.

3. **Magnetic resonance imaging.** Magnetic resonance imaging (MRI) is the study of choice and can detect congenital abnormalities of brain such as lissencephaly, pachygyria, and polymicrogyria, along with IVH with infarct and HIE. A cranial MRI is the most sensitive test to determine the etiology of seizures in the neonate. It is difficult to do in an unstable infant.

4. **Electroencephalography.** EEGs obtained during a seizure are abnormal. Interictal EEGs may be normal. However, an order to obtain an ictal EEG should not delay other diagnostic and therapeutic steps. The diagnostic value of an EEG is greater when it is obtained in the first few days because diagnostic patterns indicative of unfavorable prognosis disappear thereafter. EEG is valuable in confirming the presence of seizures when manifestations are subtle, when neuromuscular paralyzing agents have been given, and in defining the interictal background features. EEGs are of prognostic significance in full-term infants with recognized seizures. Video EEG monitoring can be done when infrequent seizures occur. Continuous EEG monitoring with **amplitude-integrated EEG (aEEG)** has improved seizure detection and is useful in full-term infants with hypoxia-ischemia.

VII. **Management.** Optimal treatment for neonatal seizures is *controversial* and highly variable between centers, especially concerning the use of anticonvulsants. Airway, breathing, and circulation should be assessed. Intubation and mechanical ventilation may be necessary to maintain oxygenation and ventilation. In all neonates with seizures, hypoglycemia should be ruled out and treated if present, before antiepileptic drug treatment is considered.

A. **Hypoglycemia.** Hypoglycemic infants with seizures should receive 10% dextrose in water, 2 to 4 mL/kg intravenously (IV), followed by 6 to 8 mg/kg/min by continuous infusion. (See Chapter 67.)

B. **Hypocalcemia.** Treated with slow IV infusion of calcium gluconate (for dosage and other information, see Chapter 91). If serum magnesium levels are low (<1.52 mEq/L), magnesium sulfate should be given. (See Chapter 105.)

C. **Anticonvulsant therapy.** (See also Table 82–1.) Conventional anticonvulsant treatment is used when no underlying metabolic cause is found. Loading doses of phenobarbital and phenytoin control 85% of neonatal seizures.

1. **Phenobarbital** is usually (for dosage and other pharmacologic information, see Chapter 155) the initial drug of choice in most centers. Neither gestational age nor birthweight seems to influence the loading or maintenance dose of phenobarbital. Gilman et al (1989) found that sequentially administered phenobarbital controlled seizures in term and preterm newborns in 77% of cases. If seizures are not controlled at a serum phenobarbital level of 40 mcg/mL, administer a second agent (eg, phenytoin [Dilantin]).

2. **Phenytoin (Dilantin)** is usually used as second-line treatment for refractory seizures by many practitioners. Fosphenytoin may be a preferred form as it is associated with fewer side effects than phenytoin (less hypotension, fewer cardiac abnormalities, and less soft tissue injury). (For dosage and other pharmacologic information, see Chapter 155.)

3. **Levetiracetam in neonatal seizures.** Over the past decade, there is an increasing interest in levetiracetam usage in neonatal seizures. It has been used off-label by pediatric neurologists for treating neonatal seizures for many years. According to the current research, it has a good safety profile, good efficacy, and favorable pharmacokinetics and seems to be a promising agent for seizure control in neonates. Loading dose is 20 mg/kg, and maintenance dose is 10 to 80 mg/kg/d in 2 divided doses.

4. **If seizures still persist, then the next anticonvulsant usually given is a benzodiazepine.** Midazolam is a short-acting benzodiazepine that can be given by a continuous infusion. IV dose is 0.1 mg/kg, then 0.1 to 0.4 mg/kg/h.

5. **Topiramate.** Although the research is limited, topiramate has been used as an add-on agent for refractory neonatal seizures and has been found to be effective. Furthermore, the benefit of topiramate lies in the fact that it is neuroprotective in hypoxic injury. Bumetanide is another novel neuroprotective agent that has been tried in refractory seizures.

6. **If seizures are still present, then 3 disorders need to be ruled out before more medications are given:**

   a. **Pyridoxine-dependent seizures.** A trial of pyridoxine (vitamin B6), 50 to 100 mg, given IV with EEG monitoring is now recommended. With pyridoxine dependency, the seizures stop quickly after the medication is given. The administration should be continued, as stoppage leads to recurrence of seizures, requiring reinstitution.

   b. **Folinic acid–responsive seizures.** Obtain CSF neurotransmitter studies. Then folinic acid is given at 2.5 mg twice daily (up to 4 mg/kg/d initially) in 2 doses. After 24 hours of treatment, seizures may stop. Folinic acid can be given for 48 hours as a trial.

   c. **DeVivo syndrome (glucose transporter deficiency).** Treatment is a ketogenic diet.

7. **If seizures still persist.** The following salvage drugs may be used depending on institutional preference: pentobarbital 10 mg/kg IV, then 1 mg/kg/h; thiopental 10 mg/kg IV (not available in United States), then 2 to 4 mg/kg/h; clonazepam 0.1 mg/kg orally; and valproic acid 10 to 25 mg/kg, then 20 mg/kg/d in 3 doses.

8. **Duration of anticonvulsant therapy.** The optimal duration of anticonvulsant therapy has not been established. Anticonvulsants may have to be continued when seizures are due to abnormality of the brain. Although International League Against Epilepsy guidelines recommend stopping anticonvulsants if seizure free for >3 days in neonates with normal neurologic examination and/or normal EEG, most neonatologists taper after seizures have been absent for 2 weeks.

VIII. **Prognosis.** The most reliable early predictors of later neurologic outcomes are the underlying etiology of the seizures and specific EEG background patterns. In infants with transient or metabolic disorders that can be corrected, the outcome is usually favorable. In infants with CNS infections, HIE, or brain malformations, the outcome is not as favorable. Background EEG activity is significantly and independently related to the neurodevelopment outcome. The type of seizure can also dictate outcome. An abnormal neurologic examination appears to be related to an adverse outcome. Prognosis is usually better for term infants than preterm infants.

121 Spontaneous Intestinal Perforation

I. **Definition.** A **spontaneous intestinal perforation (SIP)** is a **single intestinal perforation typically involving the antimesenteric border of distal ileum** and usually occurs in extremely premature infants in the first 1 to 2 weeks of life. These infants, typically, have not been fed (or have received minimum feeds). If laparotomy is performed, a focal hemorrhagic necrosis with well-defined margins is observed, in contrast to ischemic and coagulative necrosis seen in necrotizing enterocolitis (NEC). The bowel proximal and distal to the perforation appears normal.

II. **Incidence.** Two to three percent in very low birthweight (VLBW, birthweight <1500 g) infants and approximately 5% in extremely low birthweight (ELBW, birthweight <1000 g) infants.

III. **Risk factors.** Prematurity is the only well-established risk factor for SIP. Several antenatal and postnatal risk factors have been identified based on case series and datasets. These include placental chorioamnionitis, maternal antibiotics, male gender, inotropic agents, lack of initiation of feeding, severe intraventricular hemorrhage (IVH) (≥ grade 3), early administration of glucocorticoids (both dexamethasone and hydrocortisone), and early use of indomethacin to treat symptomatic patent ductus arteriosus. The risk is greater when there is combined exposure to indomethacin and either elevated endogenous cortisol levels or administration of exogenous glucocorticoids in the first 3 days of life.

IV. **Pathogenesis.** SIP histopathology is characterized by preservation of the mucosal villus architecture and thinning of muscularis propria. Although some cases of SIP (especially in larger infants) can be associated with congenital deficits in the muscularis layer of the bowel, theories have been developed for the unique association of SIP with perinatal stress and postnatal early steroids and indomethacin exposure. The following sequence of events has been proposed: Early postnatal steroids promote mucosal growth at the expense of bowel wall integrity with thinning/necrosis of the submucosal layer (skewed trophism). Indomethacin, in combination with steroids, causes a transient ileus due to depletion of nitric oxide synthase. Swallowing of air and return of bowel motility at about 7 days of age leads to increased intraluminal pressure resulting in bowel perforation. Infection may have a role in the pathogenesis; *Candida, Staphylococcus epidermidis,* and cytomegalovirus have been isolated from peritoneal fluid and surgical intestinal specimens of infants with SIP.

V. **Presentation.** These infants present suddenly with abdominal distension, bluish discoloration of the abdomen, hypotension, and metabolic acidosis. The bluish discoloration may extend into the groin and, in males, the scrotum. According to a large case series, 2 distinct groups have been described based on age of presentation: early SIP (0–3 days) and late SIP (7–10 days). Early SIP infants were larger (median birth weight of 1.4 kg) and less likely to have received antenatal glucocorticoids, indomethacin, surfactant, or mechanical ventilation compared with infants in the late SIP group (median birth weight of 775 g).

VI. **Diagnosis.**
   A. **Clinical diagnosis.** This is based on sudden presentation with abdominal distension and bluish discoloration of abdominal wall, often associated with hypotension and clinical deterioration. Three features are helpful in distinguishing SIP from NEC with perforation:
   1. **Early presentation,** usually in the first 1 to 2 weeks of life.
   2. **Physical findings** of abdominal distension and bluish discoloration of abdominal wall, and occasionally the scrotum in male infants. Abdominal wall erythema, crepitus, and induration (typical in NEC) are characteristically absent.
   3. **Free air with absence of pneumatosis or portal venous gas** on abdominal radiograph.

B. **Laboratory studies**
1. **Complete blood count with differential.** May show elevated or depressed white blood cell count (with occasional left shift and increased immature forms). Low platelet count may be seen as well.
2. **Disseminated intravascular coagulation panel.** Prothrombin time, partial thromboplastin time, fibrinogen degradation products, and fibrinogen level need to be corrected when abnormal and infant needs surgical intervention.
3. **Blood culture.** *Candida albicans* and *S epidermidis* have been cultured from blood or peritoneal fluid in infants with SIP. It is unknown whether the infections with these organisms precede or are a result of bowel perforation.
4. **Electrolyte panel.** May show hyponatremia and hyperkalemia.
5. **Blood gas analysis.** May show respiratory and/or metabolic acidosis.
C. **Imaging and other studies**
1. **Supine and lateral decubitus or cross-table lateral radiographs of the abdomen.** Typically show pneumoperitoneum (free air); however, a gasless abdomen may be seen as well. Specific radiographic findings associated with NEC are not observed in patients with SIP, such as pneumatosis intestinalis, portal venous air, thickening of the intestinal wall, and fixed dilated small bowel loops.
2. **Ultrasound of the abdomen** can be used in infants with gasless abdomen. Presence of echogenic free fluid is predictive of SIP.
VII. **Management**
A. **Medical management**
1. **Nothing by mouth** to allow gastrointestinal rest for 7 to 14 days. Total parenteral nutrition to provide basic nutritional needs.
2. **Gastric decompression** with a large-bore oro- or nasogastric tube at low intermittent or continuous suctioning.
3. **Respiratory support.** Provide optimal respiratory support to maintain acceptable blood gas parameters.
4. **Circulatory support.** There may be third spacing of fluid, which requires effective volume replacement. Ionotropic support may be needed to maintain normal blood pressure. Monitor intake/output and maintain urine output of 1 to 3 mL/kg/h.
5. **Antibiotic therapy.** Treat with parenteral antibiotics for 7 to 10 days. Antibiotic regimen to cover pathogens including *S epidermidis* and *Candida*, along with effective gram-positive, gram-negative, and anaerobic coverage. See doses in Chapter 155. Recommendations are to **start fluconazole** and 1 of the following antibiotic regimens:
   a. **Vancomycin, gentamicin, and clindamycin (or metronidazole)**
   b. **Vancomycin and piperacillin/tazobactam**
B. **Surgical management.** The optimal surgical management of SIP continues to be *controversial*. The traditional approach has been exploratory laparotomy with bowel resection; however, an alternate option is primary peritoneal drainage (PPD). The prospective randomized trials by Moss et al and Rees et al included infants with NEC or SIP, and both studies showed similar clinical outcomes using the 2 surgical techniques. The concern, expressed more in the latter study, was the high number of infants requiring secondary laparotomies for failure of clinical improvement or later development of bowel obstruction. In another retrospective study that looked exclusively at SIP, PPD was the definitive treatment in 75% of the cases. Peritoneal drain is an attractive option for very unstable low birthweight infants since it can be done with relative ease at the bedside using local anesthesia.
1. **Laparotomy with primary repair.** An abdominal incision is made and the bowel is explored. The segment of the bowel with perforation is resected and followed by end-to-end anastomosis of the bowel loops or creation of an ileostomy and distal mucous fistula. Reanastomosis is usually undertaken after 8 to 12 weeks. Surgical outcomes are not affected by infant's weight at time of enterostomy reversal.

      2. **Peritoneal drain placement.** After making a small transverse incision at McBurney's point (two-thirds of the distance from the umbilicus to the anterior superior iliac crest in the right lower quadrant), a Penrose drain is placed. The drain is removed when there is no meconium or intestinal drainage. After return of bowel function, feeds are started or a contrast enema is done to ensure patency of intestine.

VIII. **Prognosis.** SIP in the ELBW infants is associated with high morbidity and mortality. Review of a large database (Vermont Oxford Network) has shown a mortality of 19% in VLBW infants with SIP (compared to 5% in controls and 38% for infants with surgical NEC). Review of ELBW infants registered in the National Institute of Child Health and Human Development Neonatal Research Network (NICHD-NRN) showed mortality before discharge of 39% in SIP cases compared with 54% in surgical NEC cases and 22% in cases without either NEC or SIP. Infants with SIP are at risk for developing bronchopulmonary dysplasia, late-onset sepsis, severe IVH, cystic periventricular leukomalacia, and growth failure. Patients with SIP and NEC appear to have similar risks for either death or neurodevelopmental impairment. In the NICHD-NRN study, death or neurologic impairment occurred in 82%, 79%, and 53% of patients with surgical NEC, patients with SIP, and those without NEC or SIP, respectively. It remains ***controversial*** whether some of the neurodevelopmental outcome is related to surgical technique (drain vs laparotomy), and results from the multicenter Necrotizing Enterocolitis Surgery Trial (ongoing) are awaited.

IX. **Prevention.** Caution regarding early use of indomethacin (within first week of life), especially in infants who may be stressed with endogenously elevated cortisol levels. Avoid combined use of indomethacin and hydrocortisone in preterm infants. Closely monitor ELBW infants for any signs of SIP.

122 Surgical Diseases of the Newborn: Abdominal Masses

I. **Introduction. Abdominal masses may be found on initial newborn exam but are increasingly identified on prenatal ultrasound.** They can arise from peritoneal viscera (solid organs, mesentery, and GI tract) as well as retroperitoneum (kidneys and adrenal glands). Other causes can include obstruction of the urinary system or reproductive organs which can present as an abdominal or pelvic mass. Ovarian cysts are common in the neonatal period.

II. **Gastrointestinal masses**

    A. **Intestinal duplications and mesenteric cysts**

        1. Majority of congenital gastrointestinal masses.

        2. Present with obstruction or palpable mass, or remain asymptomatic.

        3. Ultrasound shows simple, smooth, cystic lesion.

        4. Treatment is surgical resection.

    B. **Meconium cysts**

        1. Associated with in utero perforation.

        2. See Chapter 72.

III. **Hepatic masses**

    A. **Smaller masses are usually found incidentally.** Larger masses may present with hepatomegaly or palpable right upper quadrant lesion. Evaluation begins with ultrasound, followed by cross-sectional imaging (MRI or CT scan) for better definition, diagnosis, and surgical planning.

B. Cystic lesions
  1. Hepatic cysts
    a. **Benign lesions;** occur in 2.5% of newborns.
    b. **Majority are asymptomatic.**
    c. **May be complicated by infection or rapid growth,** resulting in abdominal pain and compressive symptoms.
    d. **Resection** reserved for symptomatic lesions.
    e. **Multiple cysts** may be associated with polycystic liver and kidney disease.
  2. Choledochal cysts (biliary cysts)
    a. **Originate from bile ducts,** resulting in abnormal dilation of biliary tree with an incidence of 1 in 100,000 to 150,000. There is a male-to-female ratio of 1:4.
    b. **Present with cholangitis or biliary obstruction,** but may remain insidious. May cause direct (conjugated) hyperbilirubinemia with jaundice. Management is discussed further in Chapter 62.
    c. **Surgical resection recommended** due to 30% lifetime risk of cholangiocarcinoma.
C. Solid lesions
  1. Hemangioendotheliomas
    a. **Most common benign hepatic neoplasm in children.**
    b. **When large, may result in consumptive coagulopathy and thrombocytopenia (Kasabach-Merritt syndrome)** and high output heart failure.
    c. **Majority undergo spontaneous regression** with treatment reserved for symptomatic lesions.
    d. **Systemic therapy with interferon, corticosteroids, or vincristine may be attempted.** Angioembolization, segmental resection, and liver transplantation have been described for refractory neoplasms.
  2. Hamartoma
    a. **Is the second most common benign liver neoplasm in the pediatric age group.** Larger lesions can cause neonatal respiratory distress and/or circulatory complications relating to intra-abdominal space-occupying lesion.
    b. **Imaging shows multiseptated lesions** with a cystic component and minimal vascularity.
    c. **Liver function studies and α-fetoprotein** are typically normal.
    d. **Excision or marsupialization** may be pursued.
  3. Hepatoblastoma
    a. **Most common hepatic malignancy in neonates.**
    b. **Premature very low birthweight infants are at higher risk.** Associated conditions can include Beckwith-Wiedemann syndrome, hemihypertrophy, and thrombocytosis.
    c. **Diagnosis made with imaging and elevated serum α-fetoprotein.**
    d. **Biopsy** may be needed to guide chemotherapeutic protocols for lesions that are not immediately resectable.
    e. **Cisplatin and doxorubicin and surgical resection** remain the mainstay of therapy, resulting in improved cure rates.
    f. **Hepatic transplantation** is indicated for unresectable lesions and associated with improved survival.
IV. Renal masses
  A. **Majority of neonatal abdominal masses arise from kidney.**
  B. **May be unilateral or bilateral, and solid or cystic.**
  C. **Physical exam and ultrasound** are often sufficient to make diagnosis and assess for other intra-abdominal anomalies. Further assessment is made in conjunction with pediatric surgery, urology, and nephrology. Additional evaluation may be needed depending on the lesion, including MRI, CT scan, renal scan, voiding cystourethrogram and pyelography, venography, and arteriography.

D. Ureteropelvic junction obstruction
  1. **Most common etiology of newborn obstructive uropathy,** which may present as a palpable unilateral or bilateral flank mass, associated with hydronephrosis. It is much more common in girls.
  2. **Associated conditions** can include congenital heart disease, imperforate anus, contralateral multicystic kidney, VATER/VACTERL (*v*ertebral anomalies, *a*nal atresia, *t*racheo*e*sophageal fistula, and *r*adial or *r*enal dysplasia, limb abnormalities) association, and esophageal atresia.
  3. **Other lesions to consider in the differential diagnosis** include severe vesicoureteral reflux and bladder outlet obstruction due to posterior urethral valves (males). Renal ultrasound is diagnostic.
  4. **Prophylactic antibiotic therapy** is used in the setting of moderate-to-severe dilatation.
  5. **Obstructive uropathy** may be suitable for in utero intervention in selected centers. In newborn period, urinary diversion may be needed if kidney remains viable. Nonfunctional kidney is best removed.
E. Cystic renal disease
  1. Multicystic dysplastic kidney disease
    a. More common and usually unilateral.
    b. Diagnosis made with ultrasound. Renal scan often obtained to ascertain function of contralateral kidney.
    c. Affected kidney will often involute, obviating need for further intervention. Nephrectomy may be warranted for resultant hypertension.
  2. Infantile polycystic kidney disease
    a. Also known as autosomal dominant polycystic kidney disease.
    b. Involves both kidneys and carries a grim prognosis, unless renal replacement can be instituted in anticipation of renal transplant.
F. Renal vein thrombosis
  1. Typically presents within first days of life with hematuria and 1 or more flank masses.
  2. Maternal diabetes and dehydration are risk factors.
  3. Conservative management is generally recommended and is outlined in Chapter 92.
G. Wilms tumor
  1. Represents the most common form of kidney cancer in childhood and can present in the newborn period. See Chapter 126.
V. Ovarian masses
  A. Simple ovarian cyst
    1. Frequent cause of palpable mass in females.
    2. Relatively mobile, smooth-walled lesion, which may spontaneously regress as maternal hormonal effects wane after delivery.
    3. Not associated with malignancy.
    4. Smaller lesions (≤5 cm) are followed to assure regression.
    5. Larger lesions may benefit from percutaneous aspiration.
    6. Torsion may occur, necessitating a surgical intervention.
    7. Surgical goals are simple cystectomy with preservation of ovarian tissue.

123 Surgical Diseases of the Newborn: Abdominal Wall Defects

I. Gastroschisis
   A. Definition
      1. Full-thickness abdominal wall defect, occurring to the right of the intact umbilical cord, leaving exposed viscera to herniate into amniotic fluid. Ruptured omphalocele may mimic gastroschisis but the omphalocele defect in the abdominal wall is at the umbilicus.
      2. Defect measures 2 to 4 cm. Stomach, bowel, and occasionally gonads are visible. Solid organs (liver and spleen) remain intraperitoneal. (Figure 123–1).
   B. Incidence
      1. Rare malformation but incidence remains on the rise.
      2. Latest estimates range between 1.5 and 5 per 10,000 births.
   C. Pathophysiology
      1. Defect occurs sporadically, but familial clusters suggest genetic component.
      2. Improper involution of right umbilical vein and other vascular accidents have been implicated in pathogenesis, as have environmental influences, vasoactive drugs, and nutritional deficiencies.
   D. Clinical presentation
      1. The infant is born with varying amounts of herniated intestine.
      2. Prenatal exposure to amniotic fluid results in intestinal edema, induration, and foreshortened mesentery.

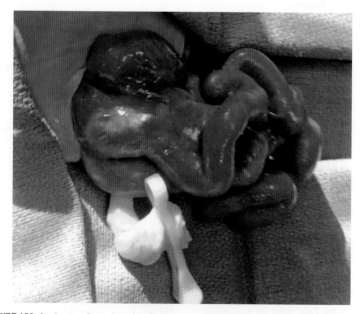

FIGURE 123–1. Gastroschisis. (*Used with permission from Drs. Ana Ruzic and John Draus.*)

3. **Inflammatory peel covers the bowel,** leading to intestinal dysmotility and delayed feeding tolerance.
4. **Up to 10% have an intestinal atresia,** and all are malrotated. Other congenital anomalies are rare.
E. Diagnosis
   1. **Usually identified on prenatal ultrasound** and readily apparent at birth.
   2. **Ruptured omphalocele may mimic gastroschisis,** and the 2 conditions must be distinguished to optimize care.
F. Management
   1. General considerations
      a. **Prenatal diagnosis affords prenatal counseling and planned delivery at a center capable of providing definitive care.**
      b. **Safety has been established for both vaginal and cesarean deliveries.**
      c. **Some centers advocate elective, late preterm delivery,** with data favoring earlier time to feeds and decreased length of stay, presumably due to decreased inflammatory effects on the bowel. This practice remains controversial.
   2. Specific measures
      a. Care in the delivery room
         i. **The exposed bowel is at risk for injury, hypoperfusion, and fluid and heat loss.** The baby's abdomen and legs should be placed in a plastic bag. Alternatively, the viscera may be covered with saline-soaked gauze and wrapped in cellophane.
         ii. **While awaiting surgical evaluation, the newborn is laid on either flank** to minimize occlusion of the narrow mesentery.
         iii. **Orogastric tube should be placed.**
      b. Fluid resuscitation
         i. **Due to exposed viscera, insensible losses begin at birth and remain significant until abdominal domain is restored.**
         ii. **Prompt venous access and fluid resuscitation are needed to replace losses** leading to further bowel compromise. Delay in care worsens the shock state.
      c. **Thermoregulation.** Hypothermia risk due to evaporative losses occurs rapidly. Immediate measures are needed to restore and maintain normal temperature.
      d. **Prophylactic antibiotics. Broad-spectrum antibiotics** are generally recommended, due to unavoidable seeding of the peritoneum during delivery and handling of the defect. Prolonged use is discouraged.
G. Surgical management
   1. **Surgical options** include primary closure (when possible) or placement of silastic silo with staged reduction (Figure 123–2).
   2. **Operative decision** is guided by bowel appearance, defect size, and baby's general condition. Primary reduction is contraindicated with respiratory distress syndrome, lung hypoplasia, or concern for compartment syndrome.
H. Nutrition
   1. **Gastroschisis places the newborn in a catabolic state,** necessitating early focus on nutrition.
   2. **Intestinal dysmotility leads to delayed tolerance of enteral feeds,** necessitating total parenteral nutrition and early central venous access.
   3. **Aggressive feeding strategies** may lead to necrotizing enterocolitis.
II. Omphalocele
   A. Definition
      1. **Central abdominal wall defect at the base of the umbilical cord,** covered by a protective sac made of amnion, Wharton's jelly, and peritoneum. Antenatal rupture is possible and should be differentiated from a gastroschisis. A normal cord inserts into the sac (Figure 123–3).

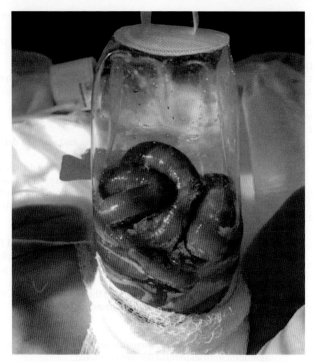

FIGURE 123–2. Gastroschisis with a protective silastic silo in place. (*Used with permission from Drs. Ana Ruzic and John Draus.*)

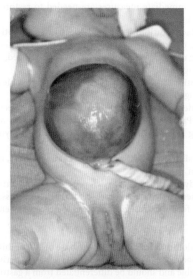

FIGURE 123–3. Omphalocele. (*Used with permission from Drs. Ana Ruzic and John Draus.*)

      2. Other congenital anomalies are present in up to 80% of patients and are more likely with smaller defects.

      3. Latest incidence estimate is 1 in 3000 births.

      4. Incidence decreases over the course of gestation, secondary to fetal demise or termination of pregnancy.

  B. Clinical presentation

      1. Prenatal diagnosis is common based on maternal ultrasound, prompting multidisciplinary counseling and investigation into associated anomalies. Cardiac, pulmonary, renal, central nervous system, and chromosomal anomalies can occur. Cardiopulmonary defects drive the ultimate prognosis.

      2. From 10% to 12% occur within a syndrome, including Beckwith-Wiedemann, pentalogy of Cantrell, and bladder exstrophy.

  C. Diagnosis

      1. Small omphalocele (<5 cm) contains intestine only.

      2. Giant omphalocele with liver herniation results in significant loss of abdominal domain, presenting a treatment challenge.

      3. Ruptured omphalocele may be confused with gastroschisis, but the location of the umbilical cord helps clarify the diagnosis.

      4. Echocardiography and renal and sacral ultrasound are performed to assess for other anomalies.

  D. Management

      1. Unless ruptured, most require no immediate surgical intervention. A ruptured omphalocele resembles gastroschisis and is managed similarly.

      2. Initial priorities focus on cardiac and pulmonary stabilization. Mechanical ventilation may be needed. Fluid management is more judicious, particularly in cases of complex cardiac disease.

      3. Once the baby is stabilized, most small defects (2–4 cm) can be repaired primarily.

      4. When primary repair is not possible, the sac must be kept intact, allowing for slow, staged reduction, and regain of abdominal domain. Escharotic agents are applied to protect and thicken the sac, ultimately resulting in epithelialization. The defect is slowly reduced with a compressive dressing until final closure. This may take years for large defects.

III. Umbilical cord hernia

  A. Typically an isolated entity; may be mistaken for small omphalocele.

  B. The defect is small (<2 cm), and carries no risk of associated anomalies.

  C. Umbilical cord is anatomically normal, but may be associated with a persistent omphalomesenteric remnant.

  D. Usually observed.

IV. Umbilical hernia

  A. Skin-covered defect in the umbilical fascia with associated protrusion of intra-abdominal contents.

  B. Physical examination establishes the diagnosis.

  C. Most remain asymptomatic in early childhood, allowing for expectant management. Operative closure is rarely warranted, and the majority undergo spontaneous closure. If persistent after 4 years, herniorrhaphy should be considered.

V. Inguinal hernia and hydrocele

  A. Definitions

      1. Processus vaginalis (PV) connects the peritoneal cavity with the inguinal canal. Following testicular descent, PV slowly obliterates. A patent PV may result in inguinal hernia, hydrocele, or both.

      2. With inguinal hernia, the processus vaginalis opening is large enough to allow herniation of abdominal viscera into inguinal canal.

      3. With hydrocele, the narrow processus vaginalis allows peritoneal fluid to accumulate along its path. May be communicating (if PV remains patent) or noncommunicating (if PV obliterates and fluid is trapped distally).

B. **Diagnosis**
1. **Inguinal hernia presents as a bulge along the inguinal canal** and, less commonly, in the scrotum.
2. **Hydroceles are found in the groin or scrotum, usually transilluminate, and often cannot be reduced.**
C. **Management**
1. **Inguinal hernias carry 5% to 15% risk of incarceration** during first year of life, necessitating repair once infant's general condition permits.
2. **Hydroceles frequently resolve without intervention** as PV slowly obliterates. Repair is advised if still present after 6 to 12 months.

---

124 Surgical Diseases of the Newborn: Alimentary Tract Obstruction

I. **Esophageal atresia**
  A. **Definitions**
    1. **Type C esophageal atresia is the most common type,** accounting for up to 85% of cases. It consists of proximal esophageal atresia with distal tracheoesophageal fistula.
    2. **Type A esophageal atresia is the second most common type,** accounting for about 10% of cases. This is a pure esophageal atresia without fistula.
    3. **Other forms of esophageal atresia are less common.**
  B. **Pathophysiology**
    1. **Embryologic failure** of migration and separation of longitudinal tracheoesophageal fold. Normally, folding results in larynx and trachea anteriorly and esophagus posteriorly.
  C. **Clinical presentation**
    1. **Polyhydramnios** due to proximal esophageal obstruction; fetus cannot swallow amniotic fluid.
    2. **Neonates display feeding intolerance, excess salivation, and respiratory distress** from aspiration of feeds.
    3. **In type C, gastric distention may cause respiratory compromise,** and gastric reflux into airway may cause chemical pneumonitis and pneumonia.
  D. **Diagnosis**
    1. **Prenatal ultrasound** may show small or absent gastric bubble if pure esophageal atresia.
    2. **Inability to pass an orogastric tube.** The chest radiograph shows an orogastric tube in the proximal esophagus. Air below the diaphragm confirms presence of a distal fistula.
    3. **VATER/VACTERL association** (*v*ertebral defects, *a*nal atresia, *t*racheoesophageal fistula, and *r*adial or *r*enal dysplasia/*v*ertebral defects, *a*nal atresia, *c*ardiac malformations, *t*racheoesophageal fistula, *r*enal dysplasia, and *l*imb abnormalities) workup necessary.
  E. **Management**
    1. **Preoperative optimization is focused on minimizing risk of aspiration and gastric distention.**
      a. **Place Replogle tube in proximal esophageal pouch** to evacuate oral secretions.
      b. **Keep baby in upright position** (45 degrees) to lessen risk of reflux and aspiration.

    c. If possible, avoid positive-pressure ventilation.

    d. If mechanical ventilation is necessary, low tidal volumes and inspiratory pressures are preferable. In select babies, high-frequency oscillatory ventilation may provide gentler ventilation.

    e. Broad-spectrum antibiotics should be administered.

    f. VATER/VACTERL association workup should be performed. This includes an echocardiogram prior to surgery to assess for cardiac and aortic arch anomalies.

  2. Goals of operative therapy are to ligate fistula and establish esophageal continuity if possible.

    a. Repair via open or thoracoscopic techniques.

    b. If long-gap esophageal atresia (>3 vertebral bodies) is present, one may not be able to perform immediate esophageal anastomosis and a gastrostomy tube should be placed.

    c. If defect cannot be bridged with native esophagus, use of gastric or intestinal conduits may be necessary.

II. **Duodenal obstruction**

  A. **Definition.** Duodenal luminal obstruction can be classified as complete or partial; as pre- or postampullary; and as caused by intrinsic or extrinsic problems.

  B. **Pathophysiology**

    1. Intrinsic obstruction results from either failure of endodermal proliferation or luminal recanalization.

    2. Atresia may occur in the setting of external compression, such as annular pancreas.

  C. **Internal duodenal obstruction**

    1. Results from classic atresia with resultant stenosis or complete obstruction.

    2. Frequently associated with trisomy 21 (33%).

  D. **External duodenal obstruction**

    1. Annular pancreas. Occurs secondary to incomplete rotation of ventral pancreatic bud, resulting in ring of pancreatic tissue that encircles second portion of duodenum. Results in either complete or partial obstruction.

    2. Malrotation. Abnormal midgut rotation and fixation causing complete or partial duodenal obstruction. Abnormal peritoneal attachments (Ladd bands) extrinsically compress duodenum. The **narrow vascular pedicle** (superior mesenteric artery) can cause ischemia of the entire midgut due to the volvulus.

  E. **Clinical presentation**

    1. General

      a. Neonates with duodenal obstruction present with bilious emesis, unless obstruction is proximal to ampulla.

      b. Abdominal distention is not common.

      c. Polyhydramnios may be evident on prenatal exam.

    2. Duodenal atresia. Down syndrome, esophageal atresia, and imperforate anus are associated with duodenal atresia. **Classic double-bubble sign** may be seen prenatally and confirmed with abdominal radiograph at delivery.

    3. Midgut volvulus. **Presents with bilious vomiting** in an otherwise well baby, and represents a true surgical emergency. Incidence highest in first few weeks of life and remains elevated for first year. If care is delayed or diagnosis unrecognized, infant can develop peritonitis and shock secondary to irreversible intestinal ischemia.

  F. **Diagnosis**

    1. In a stable infant, upper gastrointestinal imaging is diagnostic, but imaging should not delay definitive care of critically ill baby.

    2. If prenatal history suggests duodenal atresia, air may be injected via orogastric tube, looking for the double-bubble sign.

    3. Exact cause of obstruction may not be apparent until laparotomy, but prompt exploration is needed if diagnosis is unclear or malrotation is suspected.

G. **Management**
1. **In cases of atresia or annular pancreas, gastric decompression with an orogastric tube allows for "elective" surgical correction.**
2. **Insensible fluid losses may be high,** particularly with postampullary lesions, and need to be replaced with isotonic fluids.
3. **Malrotation necessitates prompt surgical evaluation, and volvulus mandates emergent laparotomy.** Fluid resuscitation and antibiotics are started while the operating room is mobilized.

III. **Proximal intestinal obstruction**
A. **Definition. Proximal intestinal obstruction occurs at level of jejunum,** most often from segmental atresia.
B. **Pathophysiology. Jejunal atresia** usually results from an in utero vascular accident with possible loss of significant portion of bowel, leading to short gut syndrome.
C. **Clinical presentation. Bilious emesis** is seen with minimal abdominal distention.
D. **Diagnosis**
1. **Abdominal radiograph shows dilated small bowel loops with no distal gas, and contrast enema shows microcolon.**
2. **May be difficult to distinguish from midgut volvulus,** necessitating early surgical evaluation.
E. **Management**
1. **Surgical correction consists of resection and/or tapering of dilated proximal bowel with enteroenterostomy.**
2. **Multiple atresias** may be present.
3. **Outcome** is determined by length and motility of the remaining bowel.

IV. **Distal intestinal obstruction**
A. **Definition.** Distal intestinal obstruction occurs in either small bowel (distal jejunum and ileum) or colon. It may be a physical obstruction (meconium disease or atresia) or functional obstruction (small left colon syndrome or Hirschsprung disease).
1. **Jejunal/ileal atresia.** Can be found at a single site or multiple sites, and it occurs as result of fetal vascular accident or complication of meconium ileus.
2. **Meconium ileus** is due to inspissated, thick meconium in distal bowel, often in setting of cystic fibrosis. It can be further classified as simple or complicated.
   a. **Complicated meconium ileus** results from compromise of bowel viability, either prenatally or postnatally, due to perforation, volvulus, or atresia.
   b. **Cystic fibrosis testing** with newborn screening and sweat chloride measurement is essential.
3. **Meconium peritonitis** is seen in cases of prenatal bowel perforation, most commonly resulting in atresia. Radiographs typically show peritoneal calcifications. If the perforation becomes walled off, it can develop into a large meconium cyst. Babies with meconium peritonitis have a surgically hostile abdomen and complications similar to meconium ileus.
4. **Colonic atresia is a rare cause of intestinal obstruction,** likely due to compression of mesocolon, resulting in vascular compromise. It is often associated with **choledochal (biliary) cysts and Hirschsprung disease**.
5. **Meconium plug syndrome** is a colonic obstruction due inspissated meconium. Usually associated with Hirschsprung disease.
6. **Hypoplastic left colon syndrome** is frequently found in babies of diabetic mothers.
7. **Hirschsprung disease** is a congenital aganglionic megacolon. It results from failure of ganglion cells to migrate distally, rendering the bowel contracted and aperistaltic. The rectosigmoid colon is most commonly affected, but more proximal pathology is possible.

B. **Clinical presentation** is usually abdominal distension, failure to pass meconium, and bilious emesis, which may be delayed by 1 to 2 days.

C. Diagnosis

1. **Plain abdominal radiographs** show multiple dilated loops of bowel and paucity of rectal air.

2. **Site of obstruction is better ascertained with a contrast enema,** which may be therapeutic in cases of meconium plug syndrome, simple meconium ileus, and small left colon syndrome.

3. **Contrast enema shows microcolon** in babies with distal small bowel atresias or complicated meconium ileus. May define transition zone in Hirschsprung disease.

4. **Suction rectal biopsy** shows absence or paucity of ganglion cells and hypertrophic nerves in Hirschsprung disease.

D. Management (see also Chapter 72)

1. **Nonoperative management**

   a. **Meconium plug syndrome,** small left colon syndrome, and simple meconium ileus may be treated with the contrast enema alone. May need to be repeated until meconium is evacuated and peristalsis returns.

   b. **If ongoing stimulation is needed, Hirschsprung disease should be considered** and biopsy performed.

   c. **Water soluble contrast enemas** may be useful to clear residual contents in meconium ileus.

E. **Surgical therapy**

1. **Urgent surgical intervention** required for atresias and complicated meconium ileus.

2. **Hirschsprung disease is always treated surgically,** and exploration may be needed if diagnostic dilemma persists.

3. **Laparoscopic, open, and transanal pull-through procedures are all used for Hirschsprung disease** and can be undertaken during the neonatal period or several weeks later. If early surgery is contraindicated and colon cannot be decompressed with rectal irrigations, colostomy may be needed.

V. **Imperforate anus**

A. Definition

1. **Absence or improper location of the anal opening.**

2. **Anal canal and sphincter complex are present,** but muscles may be attenuated.

3. **In absence of normal anal opening,** rectum tapers into fistula that may communicate with genitourinary tract in boys and reproductive tract in girls.

4. **Modern classification guided by location of fistula:**

   a. **Imperforate anus with perineal fistula** carries best prognosis, with continence rates >95%.

   b. **Imperforate anus with rectourethral, rectobladder, or rectovaginal fistula (high imperforate anus)** has lower continence rates, but still relatively good outcomes with appropriate bowel management.

   c. **Imperforate anus without fistula may be associated with Down syndrome.**

B. Diagnosis

1. **Perineal inspection** and calibration of any opening that drains meconium.

2. **All patients should have radiographic studies of lumbosacral spine** and urinary tract due to high incidence of associated anomalies.

3. **Spinal ultrasound and magnetic resonance imaging** to evaluate for tethered cord.

4. **VATER/VACTERL association** workup.

C. Management

1. **Neonatal surgical intervention** consists of colostomy for high anomalies and perineal anoplasty or fistula dilation for low lesions.

2. **If level is unknown,** divided colostomy is created and anatomy is delineated with a contrast study at later date.

VI. Necrotizing enterocolitis. Necrotizing enterocolitis (NEC) is caused by a combination of mucosal injury, relative hypoxia, and infection of intestinal wall. In most centers, **NEC is the most common indication** for abdominal operation in neonates. Surgery is indicated for pneumoperitoneum or sepsis with poor source control. **Peritoneal drain placement** and/or celiotomy with bowel resection may be necessary. (See details in Chapter 109.)

125 Surgical Diseases of the Newborn: Diseases of the Airway, Tracheobronchial Tree, and Lungs

I. **Overview of airway problems in the newborn.** Any newborn experiencing feeding problems, repeated aspiration, and respiratory distress should have a complete evaluation of the airway. Temporary or permanent feeding difficulty may be caused by congenital infections, maternal drug use, hypoxia, or some type of birth trauma. A variety of surgical diseases (intrinsic airway abnormalities such as vocal cord paralysis or laryngomalacia), choanal atresia, laryngotracheal esophageal cleft, tracheoesophageal fistula, cricopharyngeal spasm, syndromic anomalies, and others should be included in the differential diagnosis of these patients. Respiratory distress in the absence of feeding can also be caused by intrinsic and extrinsic pulmonary issues.

II. **Intrinsic abnormalities of the airway**
   A. **There are 4 common intrinsic upper airway diseases in the newborn.**
      1. **Laryngomalacia** is due to delayed development of supraglottic pharynx.
      2. **Congenital vocal cord paralysis** can be congenital or acquired (birth trauma, patent ductus arteriosus ligation) and unilateral or bilateral.
      3. **Subglottic web** is a congenital short segment obstruction that may be partial or complete.
      4. **Hemangioma** is a vascular malformation that can occur below the glottis, engorge, and obstruct with agitation.
   B. **Clinical presentation.** Varies from mild respiratory stridor to complete airway obstruction.
   C. **Diagnosis.** Airway endoscopy with careful visual inspection.
   D. **Management**
      1. **Individualized based on pathology and endoscopic findings.**
      2. **Some problems (laryngomalacia)** may be outgrown and require supportive care only.
      3. **Other lesions (subglottic webs and hemangiomas)** may require endoscopic resection or laser therapy.
III. **Choanal atresia**
   A. **Definition**
      1. **Choanal atresia is congenital blockage of posterior nares** caused by persistence of the bony septum (90%) or soft tissue membrane (10%). It can be associated with Treacher Collins, Tessier, and CHARGE (coloboma, central nervous system abnormalities, heart defects, atresia of the choanae, restricted growth and/or development, genital abnormalities, and ear anomalies) syndromes.

   B. Pathophysiology
      1. **Neonates are obligate nose breathers.**
      2. **True choanal atresia is complete and bilateral** and causes immediate respiratory distress in the newborn.
      3. **Unilateral defects** may be well tolerated and often go unnoticed.
   C. Clinical presentation
      1. **Respiratory distress** resulting from partial or complete upper airway obstruction.
      2. **Cyanosis in an infant while breast feeding** is another presentation.
   D. Diagnosis. Inability to pass catheter into nasopharynx via either nostril.
   E. Management
      1. **Stimulating baby to cry** will initiate mouth breathing and temporarily improve respiratory status.
      2. **Insertion of oral airway.**
      3. **Definitive management** requires resection of soft tissue or bony septum.
IV. **Pierre Robin syndrome/sequence**
   A. Definition
      1. **Pierre Robin syndrome/sequence** is a set of anomalies including mandibular hypoplasia (micrognathia) and a tongue that is placed further back than normal (glossoptosis) in association with cleft palate.
      2. **Other associated syndromes** include Stickler, velocardiofacial, craniofacial microsomia, and Treacher Collins syndromes.
   B. Pathophysiology. **Airway obstruction** produced by posterior displacement of the tongue associated with small mandible. Feeding difficulty is also usually present.
   C. Clinical presentation. **Severity of symptoms varies,** but most neonates manifest high-grade partial upper airway obstruction.
   D. Management
      1. **Infants with mild involvement** can be placed in prone position and fed using special **Breck nipple**. Over next few weeks to months, the mandible grows, and the degree of airway obstruction subsides.
      2. **If there is continuing evidence of breathing difficulty** and desaturation, a nasopharyngeal tube is indicated. Attention to feeding and weight gain is important. Some babies need nasogastric tube feeding to maintain weight and grow.
      3. **More severe cases** require mandibular distraction or other procedures to hold tongue in anterior position. Tracheostomy is generally a last resort.
V. **Laryngotracheal esophageal cleft**
   A. Definition
      1. **Laryngotracheal esophageal cleft** is a rare congenital anomaly with incomplete separation of larynx (and sometimes trachea) from the esophagus, resulting in a common channel (1 in 10,000–20,000 live births).
      2. **Communication** may be short or may extend almost entire length of trachea.
      3. **Increased incidence of laryngeal cleft** is seen with Pallister-Hall and Opitz-Frias syndromes.
      4. **Gastrointestinal, genitourinary, and cardiovascular anomalies** may be seen in the laryngeal cleft patient.
   B. Pathophysiology. Persistent communication between larynx (and occasionally trachea) and esophagus results in recurring symptoms of aspiration and respiratory distress with feeding.
   C. Clinical presentation. Respiratory distress during feeding. Stridor, choking, cyanosis, and regurgitation are typically seen.
   D. Diagnosis. Contrast swallow may suggest the anomaly. Endoscopy is essential to establish diagnosis and delineate extent of defect.
   E. Management. Surgical correction is difficult and often unsuccessful. There is an overall mortality rate of 46% due to laryngeal cleft and associated anomalies.

VI. **Vascular ring**
   A. **Definition. Vascular ring** describes a variety of anomalies of the aortic arch and its branches that create a "ring" of vessels around the trachea and esophagus.
   B. **Pathophysiology.** Partial obstruction of trachea, esophagus, or both may result from extrinsic compression by encircling vessels.
   C. **Clinical presentation**
      1. Dysphagia and/or stridor are common.
      2. Airway compromise is rarely severe.
   D. **Diagnosis**
      1. Contrast esophagram identifies esophageal narrowing in the region of aortic arch.
      2. Computed tomography angiography or magnetic resonance angiography better defines anatomy and assists in surgical planning.
   E. **Management.** Surgical division of vascular ring.
VII. **H-type tracheoesophageal fistula (type E)**
   A. **Definition**
      1. H-type tracheoesophageal fistula (type E TEF) is an uncommon type of TEF, accounting for about 5% of all TEFs.
      2. There is no esophageal atresia, but fistula connects proximal esophagus to airway.
   B. **Pathophysiology.** Similar to other types of esophageal atresia (see Chapter 124).
   C. **Clinical presentation**
      1. Symptoms depend on fistula diameter. Babies are typically asymptomatic until feeds are started.
      2. If tracheoesophageal fistula is small, "silent" aspiration occurs, leading to recurrent pneumonitis and aspiration pneumonia.
      3. Large fistulas present with choking and cyanotic spells while feeding.
   D. **Diagnosis**
      1. Contrast esophagram may show fistula.
      2. Bronchoscopy identifies tracheal side of fistula, allowing for passage of small catheter from trachea into the esophagus.
      3. Esophagoscopy is then performed.
   E. **Management.** Surgical ligation of fistula.
VIII. **Congenital lobar emphysema**
   A. **Definition**
      1. Congenital lobar emphysema (congenital alveolar overdistension/infantile lobar emphysema) generally affects entire lobe with hyperexpansion of small airways and expiratory air trapping.
      2. More common in upper lung segments.
      3. Cause of congenital lobar emphysema is obstruction of the developing airway with air trapping.
   B. **Pathophysiology.** As amount of air entrapped increases, normal lung is increasingly compressed, leading to mass effect and respiratory compromise.
   C. **Clinical presentation**
      1. Small cysts may cause few or no symptoms.
      2. Giant cysts may cause significant respiratory distress with mediastinal shift and compromise of contralateral lung.
   D. **Diagnosis**
      1. Cyst is usually seen on chest radiographs and may be confused with tension pneumothorax.
      2. Chest computed tomography is often useful for better definition and surgical planning.
   E. **Management**
      1. Small asymptomatic lesions can be observed.
      2. Symptomatic lesions can be temporarily managed by selective intubation of contralateral lung. Ultimately, these lesions need to be resected. Lobectomy is the operation of choice.

IX. Cystic pulmonary airway malformations
- A. Definition
  1. **Cystic pulmonary airway malformations** were formerly known as cystic adenomatoid malformations.
  2. **Lobar lesions** that may involve >1 lung segment.
  3. **Cystic changes occur within the lobe** with presence of microcysts, macrocysts, or both, and they communicate with normal tracheobronchial tree.
- B. Pathophysiology
  1. **Severity of symptoms** is related to amount of lung involved and degree to which normal lung is compressed.
  2. **Rarely, large cysts may be confused with congenital diaphragmatic hernia.**
- C. Clinical presentation
  1. **Small lesions** are asymptomatic.
  2. **Large lesions** may cause respiratory distress, lung hypoplasia of contralateral lung, and pulmonary hypertension.
- D. Diagnosis
  1. **Chest radiograph** may show multiple discrete air bubbles, occasionally with air-fluid levels, involving a region of the lung.
  2. **Cross-sectional imaging (computed tomography)** is obtained for operative planning around 6 months of age or sooner if more urgent resection is needed.
- E. Management
  1. **Surgical resection** of involved lobe of lung is advised.
  2. **Preferably delayed until 3 to 6 months of age,** when thoracoscopic resection can be attempted.
  3. **Some advocate observation of asymptomatic lesions,** but many recommend resection, given risk of infection and malignant transformation.

X. Pulmonary sequestration
- A. Definition
  1. **Pulmonary sequestration** is when nonfunctioning lung tissue is separated from main tracheobronchial tree.
  2. **Intralobar and extralobar forms.**
  3. **Have a systemic (rather than pulmonary) blood supply.**
- B. Pathophysiology
  1. **Usually not recognized in the neonate.** Intralobar sequestrations are found after frequent recurrent infections.
  2. **Extralobar sequestrations are often an incidental finding** and are often associated with diaphragmatic hernia and other lung malformations (congenital cystic adenomatoid malformation and bronchogenic cysts), pectus excavatum, pericardial problems, and duplication cysts.
- C. **Clinical presentation.** Lung mass is found with or without frequent recurrent infections.
- D. **Diagnosis.** Chest radiograph and computed tomography scan.
- E. **Management.** Intralobar masses are usually surgically resected due to the risk of recurrent infections. Extralobular pulmonary sequestration sites can be resected or, in some cases, embolized.

XI. Congenital diaphragmatic hernia
- A. Definition
  1. **Congenital diaphragmatic hernia** is most commonly due to a patent pleuroperitoneal canal through foramen of Bochdalek (95%).
  2. **Central, anterior defect** (Morgagni hernia) is less common and usually not associated with lung hypoplasia.
- B. Pathophysiology
  1. Prenatal
     a. **Abnormal communication** allows herniation of intestine into pleural space.

      b. **Compression of ipsilateral lung results in hypoplasia,** which may be bilateral if degree of compression is significant.

      c. **If liver herniates, there is higher incidence of pulmonary hypoplasia,** leading to chronic lung disease and fixed pulmonary hypertension.

   2. **Postnatal**

      a. **Pulmonary parenchymal insufficiency** in an abnormally small functional lung mass.

      b. **Infants with congenital diaphragmatic hernia** are predisposed to fixed and reactive pulmonary hypertension.

C. Clinical presentation

   1. **Most infants exhibit significant respiratory distress** within first few hours of life.

   2. **Delivery should occur in tertiary center** with experience in congenital diaphragmatic hernia physiology and immediate ECLS access if needed.

D. Diagnosis

   1. **Prenatal diagnosis** can be made by ultrasonography.

   2. **At birth, infants tend to have scaphoid abdomen** with diminished breath sounds on ipsilateral side; heart sounds shifted to contralateral side.

   3. **Diagnosis established by chest radiograph.**

E. Management

   1. **Intubation and positive-pressure ventilation** may reduce some hernia contents and allow for lung recruitment.

   2. **Orogastric tube is placed** to lessen gaseous distention of stomach and bowel.

   3. **Venous and arterial lines needed for resuscitation and monitoring.** Pre- and postductal saturations are measured (pulse oximeter screen).

   4. **Gentle lung ventilation is essential.** Barotrauma should be avoided. Permissive hypercapnia is allowed as long as it does not worsen acidosis.

   5. **Inhaled and systemic pulmonary arterial vasodilators** may be needed to assist with pulmonary hypertension. Surfactant may be administered.

   6. **Surgical correction is delayed until the baby stabilizes,** which may require initiation of ECLS.

   7. **Clinical practice guidelines for optimal neonatal treatment of CDH.** Canada and Europe have published standardized clinical practice guidelines. See references below for guidelines:

     • **Canada:** The Canadian Congenital Diaphragmatic Hernia Collaborative, Puligandla PS, Skarsgard ED, et al. Diagnosis and management of congenital diaphragmatic hernia: a clinical practice guideline. *CMAJ.* 2018;190(4): E103–E112.

     • **Europe:** Snoek KG, Reiss IK, Greenough A, et al. Standardized postnatal management of infants with congenital diaphragmatic hernia in Europe: The CDH EURO Consortium Consensus - 2015 update. *Neonatology.* 2016;110(1): 66-74.

F. Prognosis. Review of Extracorporeal Life Support Organization and congenital diaphragmatic hernia database shows mortality rates of approximately 50%.

126 Surgical Diseases of the Newborn: Retroperitoneal Tumors

I. Neuroblastoma
   A. Definition
      1. Primitive malignant neoplasm that arises from neural crest tissue.
      2. Usually located in adrenal gland but can occur anywhere neural crest cells migrate.
      3. Most common extracranial solid malignancy of childhood.
      4. Incidence of 1 per 100,000 children in the United States.
   B. Clinical presentation. Typically presents as firm, fixed, irregular mass extending obliquely from costal margin, occasionally across midline, and into lower abdomen.
   C. Diagnosis
      1. Laboratory studies
         a. Twenty-four–hour urine collection should be analyzed for vanillylmandelic acid and other catecholamine metabolites.
         b. Elevated lactate dehydrogenase is associated with poor prognosis.
      2. Radiologic studies
         a. Plain abdominal radiograph may reveal calcifications within tumor.
         b. Computed tomography scan typically shows extrinsic compression and inferolateral displacement of kidney.
         c. Metastatic evaluation involves bone marrow aspiration and biopsy, bone scan, chest radiograph, and chest computed tomography (CT) scan.
   D. Management
      1. Treatment based on tumor stage. Two staging systems are used:
         a. International Neuroblastoma Risk Group Staging System (INRGSS). Uses image-defined risk factors to determine suitability for surgery.
         b. International Neuroblastoma Staging System (INSS). Takes into account the surgical staging.
      2. Complete surgical resection remains best hope for cure.
      3. Infants with type 4S disease ("special" neuroblastoma) are typically younger than 1 year old and may undergo spontaneous regression. Planned therapy should consider this well-recognized, but poorly understood, fact.
      4. Advanced tumors require multimodality therapy with surgery, radiation, and chemotherapy, but this is uncommon in neonates.
II. Congenital mesoblastic nephroma
   A. Definition
      1. Embryonic solid renal tissue that is not usually malignant.
      2. Most common renal tumor in neonates and young infants.
      3. Pathologically divided into 3 groups: classic, cellular, and mixed.
   B. Clinical presentation
      1. Can be identified on prenatal ultrasound.
      2. More commonly, palpable mass found on abdominal exam.
      3. Paraneoplastic syndromes (hypertension or hypercalcemia) are possible.
   C. Diagnosis
      1. Physical examination
         a. Mass found on examination in newborn period or becomes apparent in first few months of life.

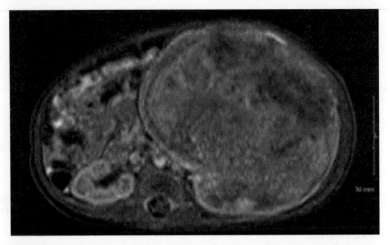

FIGURE 126–1. Congenital mesoblastic nephroma. (*Used with permission from Drs. Ana Ruzic and John Draus.*)

    2. **Radiologic studies** (Figure 126–1)
      a. **Ultrasonography** obtained when a solid mass is identified.
      b. **Cross-sectional imaging** needed to assess tumor origin, local extension, and impact on surrounding structures (magnetic resonance imaging/CT scan).
  D. **Management**
    1. **Nephrectomy and lymph node sampling** to assess for rare malignant degeneration.
    2. **Classic form** effectively treated with complete resection.
    3. **Cellular form** has propensity to recur locally or metastasize.
III. **Wilms tumor (nephroblastoma)**
  A. **Definition**
    1. **Embryonal renal neoplasm** with blastemic, stromal, and epithelial cell types. Histology can be either favorable or unfavorable (anaplastic).
    2. **Usually unilateral renal involvement**, but may be bilateral (5%).
  B. **Clinical presentation.** Palpable abdominal mass extending from below costal margin is usual presentation.
  C. **Risk factors.** Aniridia, hemihypertrophy, certain genitourinary anomalies, and family history of nephroblastoma are well recognized.
  D. **Diagnosis**
    1. **Ultrasonography generally followed by computed tomography scan**, which reveals intrinsic distortion of caliceal system of involved kidney.
    2. **Possibility of tumor thrombus** in renal vein and inferior vena cava should be evaluated.
  E. **Management**
    1. **Children's Oncology Group** staging system is used most often.
    2. **Unilateral renal involvement**
      a. **Radical nephrectomy** with lymph node sampling.
      b. **Surgical staging** determines the need for radiotherapy and chemotherapy.
    3. **Bilateral renal involvement**
      a. **Treatment highly individualized.**
      b. **Neoadjuvant therapy followed by nephron-sparing resection** may be attempted.

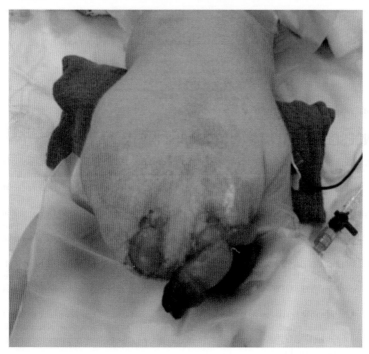

FIGURE 126–2. Sacrococcygeal teratoma. (*Used with permission from Drs. Ana Ruzic and John Draus.*)

IV. Teratoma
  A. Definition
    1. Neoplasm containing elements derived from all 3 germ cell layers: endoderm, mesoderm, and ectoderm. Mainly isolated lesions and may occur anywhere in the body.
    2. Primarily sacrococcygeal teratomas are seen in neonates, followed in frequency by the anterior mediastinum (Figure 126–2).
  B. Clinical presentation
    1. Usually evident as large external mass in sacrococcygeal area.
    2. Occasionally, may be presacral and retroperitoneal in location or may present as abdominal mass.
  C. Diagnosis
    1. Most sacrococcygeal teratomas identified on prenatal ultrasound.
    2. Digital rectal examination of presacral space is important.
    3. α-Fetoprotein levels should be assayed.
  D. Management
    1. Prompt surgical excision is required.
    2. Incidence of malignant tumors increases with age.

127 Surgical Diseases of the Newborn: Urologic Disorders

Renal masses are discussed in Chapter 126.

UNDESCENDED TESTIS (CRYPTORCHIDISM)

I. **Definition.** Undescended testis (UDT), or cryptorchidism, refers to the absence of the testis within the scrotum and is the most common congenital anomaly of the male genitalia. The incidence is 1% to 4% in full-term neonates and up to 45% in preterm neonates; 10% to 25% of patients with UDT at birth have bilateral cryptorchidism.

II. **Clinical presentation.** UDT is diagnosed by physical exam. A UDT may be nonpalpable or palpable. Other exam findings may include ipsilateral hypoplastic scrotum, inguinal hernia, and hydrocele. UDT can be an isolated finding or occur as part of a syndrome (eg, disorder of sexual differentiation, Eagle-Barrett syndrome, bladder exstrophy).

III. **Diagnosis.** Begin the exam with the patient in a supine position and legs abducted. Sweep a hand lateral to medial from the anterior superior iliac spine toward the ipsilateral scrotum. If the UDT is palpable, note the location, size, mobility, and consistency of the testis. The contralateral testis and penis should be examined as well.

   A. **Palpable testis.** A palpable testis is a testis that can be felt on exam within the inguinal canal, upper scrotum, perineum, or an ectopic location. Neonates with palpable UDT should be reexamined as they grow to ensure proper descent by age 6 months.

   B. **Nonpalpable testis.** If the testis cannot be palpated on exam, it may be intra-abdominal, absent, or atrophic (vanishing testis or testicular regression). If both testes are nonpalpable, urgent evaluation for congenital adrenal hyperplasia (CAH) in a genetic female or other disorder of sexual differentiation (DSD) is warranted.

IV. **Management.** Spontaneous descent of the testis can occur within the first 3 to 6 months of life. After age 6 months corrected for gestational age, surgery is recommended for a UDT. Inguinal or scrotal orchiopexy is done for palpable testes. Diagnostic laparoscopy and potential laparoscopic orchiopexy are standard of care for nonpalpable testes. Imaging studies are not recommended to help locate nonpalpable undescended testes, as they usually do not alter management recommendations. Neonates with hypospadias and UDT should undergo urgent evaluation for underlying genetic or endocrine anomaly such as CAH or other DSD. CAH with salt wasting can be life threatening.

SCROTAL AND TESTICULAR MASSES

I. **Definition and clinical presentation.** The differential diagnosis of neonatal scrotal masses includes the following:

   A. **Hydrocele.** Characterized by transilluminating fluid within the scrotum, which often has a bluish tint. Communicating hydroceles are contiguous with the peritoneal cavity via a patent processus vaginalis and present with size fluctuation in the scrotum. Simple hydroceles are confined to the tunica vaginalis and present as painless scrotal enlargement that does not fluctuate in size.

   B. **Inguinal hernia.** Protrusion of intra-abdominal contents through a patent processus vaginalis (ie, indirect inguinal hernia). These are usually painless and present with intermittent inguinal or scrotal bulge. They may become painful if contents within the hernia become incarcerated.

   C. **Perinatal testicular torsion.** Testicular torsion is defined as twisting of the spermatic cord with severe reduction of testicular blood flow. This can occur prenatally, during delivery, or postnatally. It presents with enlarged, hardened, discolored hemiscrotum with or without scrotal swelling.

   D. **Testicular tumor.** Rare in neonates. Presents as a painless, firm mass. Tumors reported in infants <1 month old include yolk sac tumors, gonadal stromal tumors, granulosa cell tumors, and others in case reports. Note that a common tumor marker, α-fetoprotein, can remain elevated for 6 to 8 months postpartum.

   E. **Rare lesions** include teratomas, supernumerary testis (polyorchidism), splenogonadal fusion, and adrenal rests.

  II. **Diagnosis.** Diagnosis is based on history and physical exam. Scrotal ultrasound with Doppler studies can diagnose testicular torsion or suspected tumor.

 III. **Management**

   A. **Most simple hydroceles** resolve spontaneously within the first year of life and should be observed.

   B. **Communicating hydroceles and inguinal hernias** should be repaired when diagnosed in order to prevent incarceration of intra-abdominal contents.

   C. **Timing of repair for perinatal torsion** is controversial. If the infant is hemodynamically stable, he should undergo emergent scrotal exploration and contralateral orchiopexy. This is especially the case if there is an acute change in the scrotal exam after a previously normal scrotal exam was documented.

   D. **If a testicular tumor is suspected,** orchiectomy via an inguinal approach should be done. In selected cases, testis-sparing surgery is appropriate because many tumors are not malignant.

HYPOSPADIAS

  I. **Definition.** Hypospadias is characterized by altered development of the ventral urethra, ventral (downward) penile curvature, and dorsal hooded prepuce with deficient ventral foreskin. It occurs in about 1 in 200 to 300 live births.

  II. **Clinical presentation/diagnosis.** The urethral abnormality is usually noted on physical exam. In most cases, the urethral meatus is on the distal third of the penile shaft. Moderate or severe cases include cases where the meatus is more proximal on the penile shaft, scrotum, or perineum. In general, the more proximal the location of the urethral meatus, the more severe is the degree of curvature. Megameatus with an intact prepuce is an uncommon variant and is usually found at the time of circumcision.

 III. **Management.** Surgical correction of hypospadias is ideally done between 6 and 18 months of age. Because the foreskin is sometimes used for surgical repair, **a neonatal circumcision should not be done**. If the infant with hypospadias also has a UDT and in cases of severe penoscrotal hypospadias, an evaluation for DSD is warranted.

EPISPADIAS-EXSTROPHY COMPLEX

  I. **Definition.** Epispadias-exstrophy complex is a spectrum of genitourinary malformations ranging from isolated epispadias (least severe) to cloacal exstrophy (most severe).

   A. **Isolated epispadias** ranges from a mild defect of the dorsal urethra at the glans penis to a penopubic variant with complete incontinence. Incidence is about 1 in 117,000 males.

   B. **Classic bladder exstrophy** occurs in 1 in 10,000 to 50,000 live births. It is defined by incomplete formation of the anterior abdominal wall, bladder, and dorsal phallus due to altered development of the cloacal membrane. Male-to-female ratio is 3:1 to 6:1 (Figure 127–1).

   C. **Cloacal exstrophy** includes the features of bladder exstrophy in addition to altered hindgut development and presence of an omphalocele.

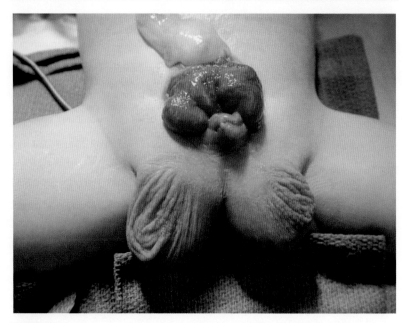

FIGURE 127–1. Exstrophy, bladder (classic exstrophy). In this newborn, the bladder is exposed on the abdominal wall. The penis is short and broad with a bivalved urethra and bifid scrotum.

II. **Clinical presentation**
   A. **Epispadias is usually diagnosed at birth on physical exam.** Males have an incomplete dorsal urethra, incomplete glans fusion, exposed urethral plate, and dorsal penile curvature. Females present with bifid clitoris and anteriorly positioned vagina.
   B. **Bladder exstrophy** may be identified prenatally or at birth. In addition to epispadias findings, there is a large abdominal wall defect and visible bladder plate.
   C. **Cloacal exstrophy** can present on prenatal ultrasound as absence of a full bladder, infraumbilical abdominal wall defect, or omphalocele. On exam, an open bladder plate is divided by hindgut structures, and the omphalocele extends superiorly. Genital malformations are similar to bladder exstrophy but more severe.

III. **Diagnosis**
   A. **Most abnormalities are easily visible at birth.** In bladder exstrophy, the pelvic bones are externally rotated with a wide pubic diastasis and anterior displacement of the anus.
   B. **Cloacal exstrophy** is associated with renal abnormalities, müllerian fusion anomalies, intestinal anomalies, hip or limb defects, and neural tube defects. Renal and spinal ultrasound and skeletal imaging should be done.

IV. **Management**
   A. **In epispadias, surgical correction of the urethra and penile curvature is done electively between 6 and 18 months of age.** The bladder neck and continence mechanism repair are delayed until 4 to 5 years of age.
   B. **In bladder and cloacal exstrophy, the bladder plate must be protected with a thin plastic nonadherent covering.** Do not use saline-soaked gauze. Timing and method of closure in bladder exstrophy are variable across institutions. Most children will require multiple surgeries to correct the defects.

C. **Cloacal exstrophy repair requires multiple staged procedures.** First, the bladder plate and omphalocele are repaired. Subsequent procedures address the hindgut and genital malformations.
D. **Latex precautions** should be instituted as there is a high incidence of latex sensitization in these patients.

PRUNE BELLY (EAGLE-BARRETT OR TRIAD) SYNDROME

I. **Definition.** Prune belly syndrome is characterized by the triad of dilation of the urinary tract resulting in renal dysplasia, deficient abdominal wall musculature, and bilateral intra-abdominal undescended testes.
II. **Clinical presentation.** The term *prune belly* refers to the classic wrinkled appearance of the abdominal wall with bulging flanks due to abnormal abdominal musculature. Presentation ranges in severity with the degree of renal dysplasia as the single most important factor in determining the severity of the disease. The most severe cases present with oligohydramnios, renal insufficiency, and pulmonary hypoplasia.
III. **Diagnosis.** While prenatal imaging may reveal urinary tract anomalies, diagnosis is based on physical exam, noting the appearance of the abdominal wall and bilateral nonpalpable undescended testes. Renal ultrasound and voiding cystourethrogram (VCUG) are the first imaging studies done to evaluate the urinary tract abnormalities.
IV. **Management.** Initial evaluation should consist of renal function assessment, optimizing pulmonary function, and management of the urinary tract. Antibiotic prophylaxis against urinary tract infection should be started. Most patients undergo elective surgical repair of the abdominal wall defect and bilateral orchiopexy. More extensive surgical decompression of the urinary tract is controversial.

POSTERIOR URETHRAL VALVES

I. **Definition.** Posterior urethral valves (PUVs) are aberrant obstructive folds of tissue in the male urethra just proximal to the external urethral sphincter. PUVs result in bladder outlet obstruction and subsequent urinary tract dysfunction. The incidence is approximately 1 in 5000 live births.
II. **Clinical presentation.** There is wide variation in the presentation of a male child with a PUV, ranging from mild bladder outlet obstruction to severe obstructive uropathy, renal insufficiency, and pulmonary hypoplasia.
III. **Diagnosis.** Most cases present prenatally with hydronephrosis and enlarged bladder with or without oligohydramnios. Postnatally, a VCUG is the gold standard for diagnosis; classic findings are a thickened bladder wall, dilated prostatic urethra, and decreased urethral caliber distal to the obstruction.
IV. **Management.** Placement of an indwelling urethral catheter to decompress the urinary tract allows time to stabilize the neonate postnatally. When the patient is hemodynamically stable, cystoscopic ablation of the PUV is performed. Serial chemistries will allow determination of renal function, and a nadir serum creatinine of <0.8 mg/dL in the first year of life suggests better long-term prognosis. Lifelong urologic follow-up is needed.

HYDRONEPHROSIS (URINARY TRACT DILATION)

I. **Definition.** Hydronephrosis refers to dilation of the renal pelvis and calyces on imaging studies. The underlying causes of urinary tract dilation (UTD) vary from obstructive lesions to vesicoureteral reflux or other etiology. The Urinary Tract Dilation Classification System is used to determine risk of postnatal uropathy.

II. **Clinical presentation.** Prenatal UTD occurs in 1% to 2% of all pregnancies. Prenatal ultrasound is the most common way to identify UTD. In some patients, hydronephrosis will be detected after a urinary tract infection or as an incidental finding on imaging for another anomaly. Severe dilation, bilateral hydronephrosis, and oligohydramnios are all suggestive of a significant urinary tract obstruction.

III. **Diagnosis.** Based on the UTD classification, the anterior-posterior renal pelvis diameter, calyceal dilation, renal parenchymal thickness and appearance, ureter and bladder appearance, and presence of unexplained oligohydramnios are all key factors to note on fetal ultrasound. Postnatally, a renal and bladder ultrasound should be performed 24 to 48 hours after birth, especially when bladder outlet obstruction is suspected (eg, in males with bilateral hydronephrosis). Based on the postnatal ultrasound findings, other studies such as VCUG or diuretic renogram can be done to diagnose the underlying cause of UTD. The differential diagnosis of UTD can vary based on the timing of the imaging study and the age of the infant. These may include ureteropelvic junction obstruction, vesicoureteral reflux, posterior urethral valves, prune belly syndrome, megaureter, duplicated collecting system, ureterocele, ectopic ureter, and a variety of cystic renal diseases.

IV. **Management.** A normal postnatal ultrasound precludes the need for additional studies unless the patient develops symptoms such as urinary tract infection. Specific management is dictated by the underlying cause of hydronephrosis. Prophylactic antibiotic use for infants with hydronephrosis is highly variable and ***controversial***. In our practice, it is usually reserved for patients with severe hydronephrosis, hydroureter, or vesicoureteral reflux.

128 Thrombocytopenia and Platelet Dysfunction

I. **Definition.** Thrombocytopenia is defined as a platelet count <150,000/μL and is further classified as **mild** (100,000–149,000/μL), **moderate** (50,000–99,000/μL), or **severe** (<50,000/μL).

II. **Incidence.** Thrombocytopenia is more common in preterm (20%–30%) than term (<1%) infants. **It is the most common hematologic abnormality among sick newborn infants in the neonatal intensive care unit (NICU).** Pseudothrombocytopenia (lab error due to clumping) accounts for 15% of all isolated thrombocytopenia.

III. **Pathophysiology**
  A. **Normal platelets.** Similar to older children and adults, the platelet life span in neonates is 7 to 10 days, and the mean platelet count is >200,000/μL.
  B. **Etiology of thrombocytopenia.** See Figure 128–1.
    1. **Maternal disorders causing thrombocytopenia in infant**
      a. **Chronic intrauterine hypoxia** is the most frequent cause of thrombocytopenia in preterm neonates in the first 72 hours of life. This is seen in cases of placenta insufficiency such as diabetes and pregnancy-induced hypertension.
      b. **Preeclampsia** (in particular with HELLP syndrome [*h*emolysis, *e*levated *l*iver enzymes, *l*ow *p*latelet count]). Thrombocytopenia is present at birth, is usually associated with neutropenia, and should recover by the second week of life.
      c. **Maternal medications** (eg, heparin, quinine, hydralazine, tolbutamide, and thiazide diuretics).

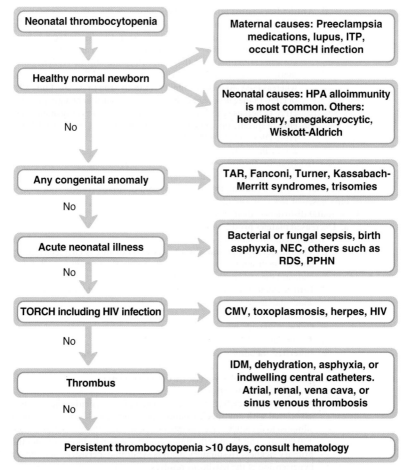

FIGURE 128–1. Algorithm for the evaluation of neonatal thrombocytopenia. CMV, cytomegalovirus; HIV, human immunodeficiency virus; HPA, human platelet antigen; IDM, infant of diabetic mother; ITP, idiopathic thrombocytopenic purpura; NEC, necrotizing enterocolitis; PPHN, persistent pulmonary hypertension of the newborn; RDS, respiratory distress syndrome; TAR, thrombocytopenia and absent radius; TORCH, *t*oxoplasmosis, *o*ther infections, *r*ubella, *c*ytomegalovirus, and *h*erpes simplex virus.

    d. Infections (eg, TORCH [*t*oxoplasmosis, *o*ther infections, *r*ubella, *c*ytomegalovirus, and *h*erpes simplex virus] infections, bacterial or viral infections). Not a component of perinatal Zika infection.
    e. Disseminated intravascular coagulation.
    f. Antiplatelet antibodies
      i. Antibodies against maternal and fetal platelets (autoimmune thrombocytopenia)
        (a) Idiopathic thrombocytopenic purpura
        (b) Drug-induced thrombocytopenia
        (c) Systemic lupus erythematosus

      ii. **Antibodies against fetal platelets** (isoimmune thrombocytopenia)

         (a) **Neonatal alloimmune thrombocytopenia** is the most common cause of severe thrombocytopenia, seen mostly in term infants <72 hours of age. It is due to an incompatibility in human platelet antigen (HPA) between the newborn infant and its HPA-negative mother. HPA-1a is the most common incompatibility in Caucasians, whereas HPA-4b incompatibility is mostly seen in Asians. Only 10% of HPA-1a–negative women become sensitized after being exposed to HPA-1a because this immunologic response occurs only in the presence of specific human leukocyte antigens (HLAs) such as HLA-B8, HLA-DR3, and HLA-DR52a. HLA antibodies, although common, do not by themselves cause significant thrombocytopenia.

         (b) **Immune thrombocytopenia** can be found in some cases of hemolytic disease of the newborn.

  2. **Placental disorders causing thrombocytopenia in infant (rare):** Chorioangioma, vascular thrombi, and placental abruption.

  3. **Neonatal disorders causing thrombocytopenia**

    a. **Decreased platelet production**

      i. **Isolated.** No identified cause.

      ii. **Thrombocytopenia and absent radius syndrome** is characterized by normal neutrophil and red blood cell counts; absent radii, usually bilateral; and the presence of a normal thumb.

      iii. **Fanconi anemia** is characterized by pancytopenia and the presence of an abnormal (hypoplastic or aplastic) thumb.

      iv. **Rubella syndrome.**

      v. **Congenital leukemia.**

      vi. **Trisomies 13, 18, or 21 or Turner syndrome.**

      vii. **Inherited metabolic disorders** include methylmalonic, propionic, and isovaleric acidemia; ketotic glycinemia.

      viii. **Congenital amegakaryocytic thrombocytopenia.**

    b. **Increased platelet destruction**

      i. **Many "sick" newborns develop thrombocytopenia that is not associated with any specific pathologic state.** About 20% of newborns admitted to the NICU have thrombocytopenia, and 20% of those counts are <50,000/μL. This form of thrombocytopenia generally improves after the primary sickness (respiratory distress syndrome, persistent pulmonary hypertension of the newborn) resolves.

      ii. **Pathologic states associated with thrombocytopenia**

         (a) **Sepsis.** Bacterial and *Candida* species.

         (b) **Congenital infections.** TORCH infections, especially cytomegalovirus (CMV). Neonates with human immunodeficiency virus (HIV) and *Enterovirus* frequently have thrombocytopenia.

         (c) **Thrombosis** (major blood vessels, intracardiac).

         (d) **Disseminated intravascular coagulation.**

         (e) **Intrauterine growth restriction.**

         (f) **Birth asphyxia.**

         (g) **Necrotizing enterocolitis or bowel ischemia.**

         (h) **Platelet destruction** associated with giant hemangioma (Kasabach-Merritt syndrome).

C. **Platelet dysfunction**

  1. **Drug-induced platelet dysfunction**

    a. **Maternal use of aspirin**

    b. **Indomethacin**

  2. **Metabolic disorders**

    a. **Phototherapy-induced metabolic abnormalities**

        b. Acidosis

        c. Fatty acid deficiency

        d. Maternal diabetes

    3. Inherited thrombasthenia (Glanzmann disease)

IV. Risk factors. Low birthweight; low gestational age; small for gestational age; hypoxia at birth (Apgar score <5 at 5 minutes); umbilical line placement; respiratory assistance; phototherapy; respiratory distress syndrome; sepsis, especially by fungal infection; meconium aspiration; necrotizing enterocolitis; mother with idiopathic thrombocytopenic purpura (ITP); preterm infants of hypertensive mothers.

V. Clinical presentation. Other coagulation disorders are discussed in Chapter 92.

    A. Symptoms and signs. Summarized in Figure 128–1.

        1. Generalized superficial petechiae are often present, particularly in response to minor trauma or pressure or increased venous pressure. Platelet counts are usually <60,000/μL. *Note:* Petechiae are common in normal infants and tend to be clustered on the head and upper chest, do not recur, and are associated with normal platelet counts. They are a result of a transient increase in venous pressure during birth.

        2. Gastrointestinal bleeding, mucosal bleeding, or spontaneous hemorrhage in other sites may occur with platelet counts <20,000/μL.

        3. Intracranial hemorrhage may occur with severe thrombocytopenia.

        4. Large ecchymosis and muscle hemorrhages are more likely to be due to coagulation disturbances than to platelet disturbances.

    B. History

        1. Family history of thrombocytopenia (hereditary) or a history of intracranial hemorrhage in a sibling (alloimmune or ITP).

        2. Maternal diabetes.

        3. A history of any infection should be noted.

        4. Previous episodes of bleeding may have occurred.

        5. Presence of intravascular catheter

    C. Placental examination. The placenta should be carefully examined for evidence of chorioangioma, thrombi, or abruptio placentae.

    D. Physical examination

        1. Petechiae and bleeding sites should be noted.

        2. Physical malformations may be present. Thrombocytopenia and absent radius syndrome, rubella syndrome, giant hemangioma, or trisomy syndromes.

        3. Hepatosplenomegaly may be caused by viral or bacterial infection or congenital leukemia.

VI. Diagnosis

    A. Laboratory studies

        1. For all newborns

            a. Pseudothrombocytopenia. Isolated thrombocytopenia diagnosed from a capillary sample should be confirmed by a repeated count from a venous sample and processed immediately. In addition, careful examination of peripheral blood smear can identify clumping on the original specimen.

            b. Complete blood count and differential.

            c. Blood typing.

        2. For healthy newborns without congenital anomalies

            a. Coombs test.

            b. Maternal sample for rapid HPA-1a (PlA1) phenotyping plus screen for anti-HPA alloantibodies. **Platelet antibody results are usually available within 24 hours.** These antibodies are detected in 90% of sensitized mothers.

            c. Maternal, paternal, and infant genotyping of HPA-1 to HPA-5 and HPA-15 is required for diagnosis and for matching platelet donors.

            d. TORCH evaluation and rapid human immunodeficiency virus test. Most are available as prenatal universal screen in the United States, except for toxoplasmosis and CMV.

e. **Test for maternal thrombocytopenia.** A low maternal count suggests autoimmune thrombocytopenia or inherited thrombocytopenia (X-linked recessive thrombocytopenia or autosomal dominant thrombocytopenia).

f. **In cases of unexplained and severe thrombocytopenia, a bone marrow study is indicated.** However, because of its technical difficulties in neonates, new blood tests are being developed to evaluate platelet production. Many have shown promising results (serum thrombopoietin concentrations, megakaryocyte progenitors, reticulated platelet percentages [RP%], and glycocalicin concentrations). An immature platelet fraction test is similar to RP% and readily available in automated cell counters. Bone marrow studies are still indicated in selected few patients (marrow cellularity or megakaryocyte morphology).

3. **For healthy newborns with congenital anomalies**

a. **Chromosome analysis for trisomies and Turner syndrome.**

b. **Diepoxybutane/mitomycin C stress test** to establish DNA breakage in peripheral blood lymphocytes.

4. **For "sick" newborns**

a. **Differential of white blood count,** serum C-reactive protein, and bacterial and fungal blood cultures.

b. **TORCH panel.** (See Chapter 148.) Culture of CMV from urine samples and other viruses if indicated (coxsackie, echovirus).

c. **Coagulation studies.** Prothrombin time, activated partial thromboplastin time, fibrinogen, and D-dimer level.

VII. **Management**

A. **Obstetric management of maternal autoimmune thrombocytopenia**

1. **The occurrence of fetal hemorrhage (in utero) is very rare** compared with the risk of such hemorrhage in alloimmune thrombocytopenia (10%).

2. **Treatment is aimed at prevention** of an intracranial hemorrhage during vaginal delivery.

3. **There is an increased risk of severe neonatal thrombocytopenia and intracranial hemorrhage** if antibody is present in the maternal plasma or if fetal scalp platelet counts are <50,000/μL.

4. **Cesarean delivery may be indicated.**

B. **Management of maternal alloimmune thrombocytopenia**

1. **After a pregnancy has been affected by alloimmune thrombocytopenia,** the proportion of subsequent pregnancies affected mostly depends on the father's genotype. If the father is heterozygous (HPA-1a/HPA-1b), the risk is 50%, and the risk is close to 100% if he is homozygous (HPA-1a/HPA-1a). The history of intracranial hemorrhage in a previous sibling is predictive of the presence of severe thrombocytopenia for the next fetus. In subsequent pregnancies, administering corticosteroids and intravenous immunoglobulin (IVIG) during the third trimester coupled with transfusions of platelets to the fetus using ultrasound-guided intraumbilical cord infusion has been advocated.

2. **Instrumental vaginal delivery, fetal scalp electrodes,** and fetal scalp blood sampling should be avoided. Vaginal delivery is allowed when fetal platelet count is known to be >50,000/μL and presentation and labor are normal. Otherwise cesarean delivery is indicated.

C. **Treatment of infants with thrombocytopenia**

1. **Treat the underlying cause (eg, sepsis).** If drugs are the cause, stop their administration.

2. **Platelet transfusions**

a. **Indications**

i. **Platelets must be given urgently** if active bleeding is occurring with any degree of thrombocytopenia or if there is no active bleeding but platelet counts are <20,000/μL.

      ii. **Platelet transfusion is recommended for premature infants** with a greater risk of hemorrhage (those who are sick or in the first week of life) if the platelet count is between 20,000/μL and 50,000/μL.

      iii. **Platelets are administered for major surgical interventions** if count is <100,000/μL.

    b. **Management.** Request for 10 to 20 mL/kg of leukocyte-reduced/poor, irradiated, random donor platelets. Platelet count should be repeated 1 hour after transfusion and is expected to increase to >100,000/μL. Failure to achieve or sustain a rise in platelet count suggests a destructive process. Washed and irradiated maternal platelets or platelets from an HPA-compatible donor (in general HPA-1a–negative platelets) need to be used for infants with alloimmune thrombocytopenia. **When not available, a random donor platelet transfusion combined with IVIG may achieve a transient rise.**

    c. **Harmful effects related to platelet transfusions have been raised,** such as an increased incidence of bacterial infection and an exacerbation of inflammatory injury. In addition, mortality rate in thrombocytopenic NICU patients who received platelet transfusions increased dramatically with the increase in the number of platelet transfusions.

  3. **Intravenous immunoglobulin.** A dose of 400 mg/kg/d for 3 to 5 consecutive days or a single dose of 1000 mg/kg on 2 consecutive days is given for immune thrombocytopenia.

  4. **Prednisone.** A dose of 2 mg/kg/d may also be beneficial in immune thrombocytopenia.

VIII. **Prognosis.** Etiology of the thrombocytopenia dictates the outcome and prognosis.

129 Thyroid Disorders

Disorders of thyroid function in neonates often present a diagnostic dilemma. The initial clinical signs and symptoms are often subtle or misleading. A good understanding of the unique thyroid physiology, assessment of thyroid function, and a sense of urgency are necessary to recognize, diagnose, and treat thyroid disorders early. As an example, congenital hypothyroidism can cause neurologic intellectual development issues unless thyroid therapy is initiated within 2 weeks of birth.

GENERAL CONSIDERATIONS

  I. **Fetal and neonatal thyroid function**

    A. **Embryogenesis.** Thyroid gland forms from invagination of foregut endoderm at the floor of the pharynx beginning in the third week of gestation, with thyroglobulin synthesis detected by 4 to 6 weeks, thyrotropin-releasing hormone (TRH) synthesis by 6 to 8 weeks, and iodine trapping by 8 to 10 weeks through 12 weeks of gestation. At that time, thyroxine (T_4), triiodothyronine (T_3), and thyroid-stimulating hormone (TSH) secretion can be detected. Thyroid activity remains low until midgestation and then increases slowly until term.

    B. **Thyroid hormones** undergo rapid and dramatic changes in the immediate postnatal period.

      1. **An acute release of thyroid-stimulating hormone occurs within minutes after birth.** Peak values of 60 to 80 mU/L are seen at 30 to 90 minutes attributed to exposure of the infant to a colder postnatal environment, clamping of the cord, and the stress of delivery. Levels decrease to <10 mU/L by the end of the first postnatal week.

2. **Stimulated by the thyroid-stimulating hormone surge, thyroxine, free thyroxine, and triiodothyronine rapidly increase,** reaching peak levels by 24 to 36 hours. TSH level decreases slowly over the first 2 weeks of life to values slightly higher than what are found typically in adults.

C. **Thyroid function in the premature infant.** Similar changes in TSH, T_4, and T_3 are seen in premature infants; however, absolute values are lower in proportion to the gestational age and birthweight. TSH levels return to normal by 5 to 10 days of life.

II. **Physiologic action of thyroid hormones.** Thyroid hormones have profound effects on growth and neurologic development. They also influence oxygen consumption, thermogenesis, and the metabolic rate of many organs. Maternal T_4 is critical for normal central nervous system maturation in the fetus.

III. **Biochemical steps involved in thyroid hormone synthesis.** Thyroid hormone production involves the steps of iodide transport/trapping, thyroglobulin synthesis, organification of iodide, monoiodotyrosine and diiodotyrosine coupling, thyroglobulin endocytosis, proteolysis, and release. In addition, T_4 is converted to T_3 in peripheral tissue.

IV. **Maternal thyroid disease and pregnancy outcome.** Maternal thyroid diseases (hypo- and hyperthyroidism) are associated with increased risk for pregnancy complications including miscarriage, preeclampsia, placental abruption, preterm birth, and cesarean section. Maternal symptoms of autoimmune thyroid diseases tend to improve during pregnancy. Maintaining euthyroidism and achieving a serum total T_4 in the upper limit of normal throughout pregnancy is key to reducing the risk of maternal, fetal, and newborn complications.

V. **Assessment of thyroid function.** Thyroid tests are intended to measure the level of thyroid activity and to identify the cause of thyroid dysfunction.

A. **Thyroxine concentration** is important in the evaluation of thyroid function. More than 99% of T_4 is bound to thyroid hormone–binding proteins. Therefore, changes in these proteins may affect T_4 levels. Serum levels for term newborn infants range between 6.4 and 23.2 mcg/dL.

B. **Free thyroxine** reflects the availability of thyroid hormone to enter tissues. Serum levels vary widely by gestational age; term newborn infant levels (2.0–5.3 ng/dL) are higher than those of infants who are 25 to 30 weeks' gestation (0.6–3.3 ng/dL).

C. **Thyroid-stimulating hormone measurement** is valuable in evaluating thyroid disorders, particularly primary hyperthyroidism. Serum levels over all gestational ages of 25 to 42 weeks range from 2.5 to 18.0 mU/L. Levels should drop to <10 mU/L by 1 month of age.

D. **Triiodothyronine concentration** is useful in the diagnosis and treatment of hyperthyroidism. Serum levels of T_3 are very low in the fetus and cord blood (20–75 ng/dL). Shortly after birth, levels exceed 100 to approximately 400 ng/dL. In hyperthyroid states, levels may exceed 400 ng/dL. In sick preterm infants, a very low T_3 (hypothyroid range) may signal the **euthyroid sick syndrome,** also known as the **nonthyroidal illness syndrome.**

E. **Thyroid-binding globulin** can be measured directly by radioimmunoassay.

F. **The thyrotropin-releasing hormone stimulation test** assesses pituitary and thyroid responsiveness and differentiates between secondary and tertiary hypothyroidism.

G. **Thyroid imaging**
1. **Thyroid scanning** with iodine-123 (preferred isotope) is used to identify functional thyroid tissue.
2. **Color Doppler ultrasonography** has shown improved sensitivity in detecting ectopic thyroid tissue in recent studies.

CONGENITAL HYPOTHYROIDISM

I. **Definition.** Congenital hypothyroidism (CH) is defined as a significant decrease in, or the absence of, thyroid function at or shortly after birth. Unrecognized CH leads to intellectual disability.

II. **Incidence.** The overall incidence is 1 in 2000 to 3000 live newborn infants. Sporadic cases account for 85% of patients, whereas 15% are hereditary. The incidence of CH is higher in Hispanic individuals and lower in blacks. There is a 2:1 female-to-male ratio. In addition, there is an increased risk in infants with Down syndrome.

III. **Pathophysiology**
   A. **Primary hypothyroidism**
      1. **Developmental defects** such as ectopic thyroid (most common), thyroid hypoplasia, or agenesis. In a minority of cases (2%–5%), a mutation may be present in 1 of several genes involved in thyroid gland formation, including the TSH receptor (TSHR) or the transcription factors PAX8, NKX2-1, or FOXE1.
      2. **Inborn errors of thyroid hormone synthesis** including total and partial iodide organification defects.
      3. **Maternal exposure** to radioiodine, propylthiouracil (PTU), or methimazole (MMI) during pregnancy.
      4. **Iodine deficiency** (endemic cretinism).
   B. **Secondary hypothyroidism.** TSH deficiency.
   C. **Tertiary hypothyroidism.** Thyrotropin-releasing hormone (TRH) deficiency.
   D. **Hypopituitary hypothyroidism.** Associated with other hormonal deficiencies.

IV. **Risk factors.** Genetic or family history, birth defects, female sex, and gestational age >40 weeks.

V. **Clinical presentation**
   A. **Antenatal diagnosis** is suspected when goiter is incidentally discovered during fetal ultrasound, with a family history of dyshormonogenesis, or with known defects of genes involved in thyroid function or development. Cordocentesis or percutaneous umbilical blood sampling, rather than amniocentesis, should be the reference method for assessing fetal thyroid function but should only be performed if prenatal intervention is considered. In a euthyroid pregnant woman, a large goiter in the fetus with progressive hydramnios and a risk of premature labor and delivery and/or concerns about tracheal occlusion are criteria in favor of fetal treatment in utero. Interventions such as intra-amniotic levothyroxine (L-T_4) injection may be considered only by a multidisciplinary specialist team.
   B. **Postnatal.** Symptoms are usually absent at birth; however, subtle signs may be detected during the first few weeks of life. Obtain a serum free T_4 and TSH for any clinical signs, even if the newborn screening is negative. CH can occur even after a normal newborn screening.
      1. **Early manifestations.** Signs at birth include prolonged gestation, large size for gestational age, large fontanelle, and respiratory distress syndrome. Manifestations as early as 2 weeks include hypotonia, umbilical hernia, lethargy, constipation hypothermia, prolonged jaundice, and feeding difficulty.
      2. **Late manifestation.** Classic features usually appear after 6 weeks and include puffy eyelids, coarse hair, large tongue, myxedema, and hoarse cry. Late manifestations in borderline hypothyroidism detected in screening programs can present as significant hearing impairment with speech delay.

VI. **Diagnosis**
   A. **Screening**
      1. **Methods.** The screening strategies include primary TSH with backup T_4 (may miss thyroid-binding globulin [TBG] deficiency, hypothalamic-pituitary hypothyroidism, and hypothyroxinemia with delayed TSH elevation), primary T_4 with backup TSH (will miss delayed TSH elevation with initial normal T_4), and **primary T_4 and TSH (considered the ideal screening approach)**. In other countries such as the Netherlands, the measurement of T_4/TBG ratio in newborns with low T_4 and nonelevated TSH levels and TRH stimulation tests are used to identify central CH.

2. **Timing.** The ideal time for screening is 48 hours to 4 days of age. Infants discharged before 48 hours should be screened before discharge; however, this increases the number of false-positive TSH elevations. A repeat test at 2 to 6 weeks identifies approximately 10% of cases.

3. **American Academy of Pediatrics recommended screening.**
   a. **Term delivery in hospital.** Filter paper blood spot collection at 2 to 4 days of age or at discharge.
   b. **Neonatal intensive care unit/preterm birth/home birth.** Within 7 days of birth.
   c. **Mother on thyroid medication/family history of CH.** Screen cord blood.

4. A strategy of second screening (2–4 weeks of age) should be considered for the following conditions: preterm neonates; low birthweight and very low birthweight neonates; ill and preterm newborns admitted to neonatal intensive care units; specimen collection within the first 24 hours of life; and multiple births (particularly same-sex twins).

5. **Results.** Accurate screening results depend on good quality of blood spots. A low T_4 level and TSH concentrations >40 mU/L are indicative of CH. Normal TSH at 2 to 12 weeks is 9.1 mU/L. The update of newborn screening and therapy for CH (June 2006, reaffirmed December 2011) by the American Academy of Pediatrics, American Thyroid Association, and Lawson Wilkins Pediatric Endocrine Society provides a useful algorithm (Figure 129–1). The European Society for Pediatric Endocrinology Consensus Guidelines on Screening, Diagnosis and Management of Congenital Hypothyroidism (Léger et al; February 2014) also has an updated guideline.

B. **Diagnostic studies**
   1. **Serum for confirmatory measurements of T_4 and TSH concentrations.** If an abnormality of TBG is suspected, free T_4 (FT_4) and TBG concentrations should also be evaluated.
   2. **Ultrasonography** is used to separate a structural defect from a normal or enlarged gland.
   3. **Thyroid scan (scintigraphy) with radioactive iodine or technetium** remains the most accurate diagnostic modality to determine the cause of CH.
   4. **Knee radiographs** may be used to assess the severity of intrauterine hypothyroidism by the presence or absence of femoral and tibial epiphyses.
   5. **Genetic testing and counseling** are indicated with inborn errors of thyroid hormone synthesis and when a mutation in 1 of genes involved in thyroid gland formation is suspected.

VII. **Management**
   A. **Consultation with a pediatric endocrinologist** is recommended.
   B. **Goal of therapy** is to ensure normal growth and development, normalize TSH, and maintain T_4 or FT_4 in upper half of reference range.
   C. **Treatment.** L-T_4 is the treatment of choice. L-T_4 treatment should be initiated as soon as possible and no later than 2 weeks after birth or immediately after confirmatory serum test results in infants in whom CH is detected by a second screening test. The average L-T_4 starting dose is 10 to 15 mcg/kg/d orally. Customization of the doses based on underlying cause and severity may result in more rapid normalization of values of TSH and T_4. The pill, universally available, should be crushed and suspended in breast milk, formula, or water. **Care should be taken to avoid concomitant administration of soy, fiber, or iron.** In Europe, liquid preparations with 5 mcg/drop concentrations are approved. The goal of therapy is to maintain T_4 concentration in the upper normal range (total T_4: 10–16 mcg/dL; FT_4: 1.4–2.3 ng/dL) with low-normal serum TSH (0.5–2 mU/L).
   D. **Follow-up.** Clinical evaluation, including assessment of growth and development, should be performed every few months during the first 3 years of life. Infants with CH are at risk of other congenital anomalies. Cardiovascular anomalies, including pulmonary stenosis, atrial septal defect, and ventricular septal defect, are the

most common. Infants need to undergo frequent laboratory and clinical evaluations of thyroid function, growth, and development to ensure optimal T_4 dosage and adherence to their therapy regimen. **Serum T_4 and TSH measurements should be performed as follows:**

1. At 2 and 4 weeks after initiation of L-T_4 therapy.
2. Every 1 to 2 months during the first 6 months of life.
3. Every 3 to 4 months between 6 months and 3 years.
4. Every 6 to 12 months until growth is completed.
5. More frequent intervals with dose change, abnormal values, and compliance concerns.
6. Monitoring more intensely during puberty is recommended to prevent unwanted cardiovascular dysfunction.

VIII. Assess permanence of congenital hypothyroidism
    A. If initial thyroid scan shows an ectopic or absent gland, CH is a permanent condition.
    B. If initial thyroid-stimulating hormone is <50 mU/L and there is no increase in TSH after newborn period, then a trial off therapy at 3 years of age may be considered.
    C. If thyroid-stimulating hormone increases off therapy, consider CH as a permanent condition.

IX. **Prognosis.** CH can adversely influence growth, intelligence, cardiovascular function, and quality of life in the long term. The more severe the thyroid dysfunction at diagnosis, the lower is the performance intelligence quotient (IQ) later in life. Early initiation of therapy within the first 2 weeks of life, at doses of 10 to 15 mcg/kg of L-T_4, and subsequent management through puberty may help to mitigate these deficits and promote optimal somatic growth.

NEONATAL THYROTOXICOSIS

I. **Definition.** Neonatal thyrotoxicosis is defined as a hypermetabolic state resulting from excessive thyroid hormone activity in the newborn.

II. **Incidence.** This is a rare disorder, occurring in only approximately 1 of 70 thyrotoxic pregnancies (autoimmune disease). The incidence of maternal thyrotoxicosis in pregnancy is 1 to 2 per 1000 pregnancies.

III. **Pathophysiology**
    A. **Usually results from transplacental passage of TSH receptor antibodies** from a mother with current or past history of Graves disease or Hashimoto thyroiditis.
    B. **Nonimmune hyperthyroidism** has been identified as a result of activating mutations in the TSH receptor gene, stimulatory G protein in McCune-Albright syndrome, thyroid hormone resistance due to mutation in thyroid hormone receptor gene, or excessive iodine use.

IV. **Risk factors.** Mother with active or inactive Graves' disease or Hashimoto thyroiditis.

V. **Clinical presentation.** Both stillbirths and preterm births are increased. Fetal hyperthyroidism due to Graves disease may be seen during the third trimester. Signs include fetal tachycardia, heart failure with nonimmune hydrops, intrauterine growth retardation, preterm birth, advanced skeletal maturation, and craniosynostosis. In symptomatic cases, fetal hyperthyroidism may be treated by administering antithyroid drugs to the mother. **Postnatal signs** are usually apparent within hours after birth to the first 10 days of life. Delayed presentation up to 45 days may occur in the presence of coexisting maternal blocking and stimulating antibodies. Thyrotoxic signs include irritability, tachycardia, dysrhythmia, hepatomegaly, small-for-gestational age, poor weight gain, hypertension, flushing, tremor, and thrombocytopenia. A goiter is usually present and may be large enough to cause tracheal compression. Eye signs such as lid retraction and exophthalmos, as well as premature bone ossification and craniosynostosis, may also be present.

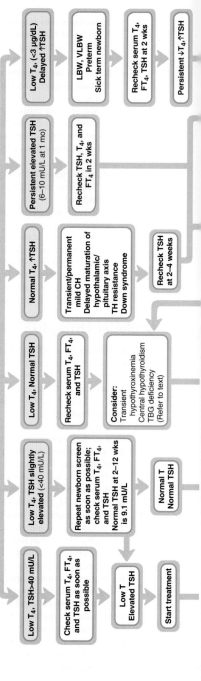

When to Screen
- Normal hospital delivery at term—Filter-paper collection ideally at 2–4 d of age or at time of discharge
- NICU/preterm home birth—Within 7 d of birth
- Maternal history of thyroid medication/family history of CH—Cord blood for screening

Type of Screening

Primary TSH, Backup T₄
- May miss—TBG deficiency
  - Hypothalamic-pituitary hypothyroidism
  - Hypothyroxinemia with delayed TSH elevation
- For better sensitivity—Use sensitive TSH assay and
  - Age-adjusted TSH cutoff (20–25 mU/L at 24 h of age)

Primary T₄, Backup TSH
- Will miss delayed TSH elevation with initial normal T₄

Primary T₄ and TSH
- Ideal screening approach

TIMELY FOLLOW-UP AND TRANSMISSION OF RESULTS (refer to text)

Interpretation of Results

Low T₄, TSH>40 mU/L → Check serum T₄, FT₄, and TSH as soon as possible → Low T Elevated TSH → Start treatment

Low T₄, TSH slightly elevated (<40 mU/L) → Repeat newborn screen as soon as possible; check serum T₄, FT₄, and TSH Normal TSH at 2–12 wks is 9.1 mU/L → Normal T Normal TSH

Low T₄, Normal TSH → Recheck serum T₄, FT₄, and TSH → Consider: Transient hypothyroxinemia, Central hypothyroidism, TBG deficiency (Refer to text)

Normal T₄, ↑TSH → Transient/permanent mild CH, Delayed maturation of hypothalamic/pituitary axis, TH resistance, Down syndrome → Recheck TSH at 2–4 weeks

Persistent elevated TSH (6–10 mU/L at 1 mo) → Recheck TSH, T₄, and FT₄ in 2 wks

Low T₄ (<3 µg/dL), Delayed ↑TSH → LBW, VLBW, Preterm, Sick term newborn → Recheck serum T₄, FT₄, TSH at 2 wks → Persistent ↓T₄,↑TSH

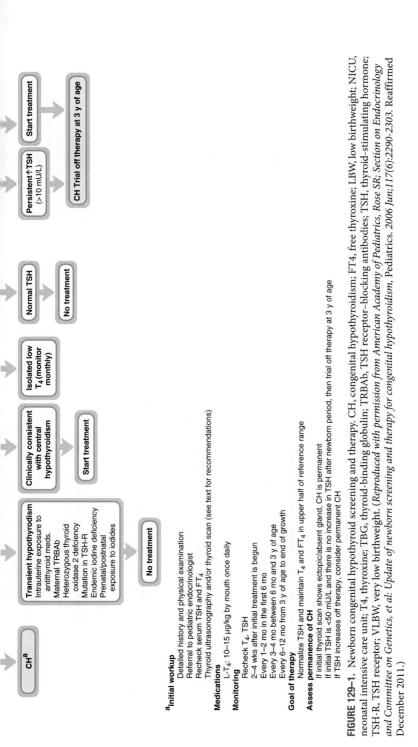

FIGURE 129–1. Newborn congenital hypothyroid screening and therapy. CH, congenital hypothyroidism; FT4, free thyroxine; LBW, low birthweight; NICU, neonatal intensive care unit; T4, thyroxine; TBG, thyroid-binding globulin; TRBAb, TSH receptor–blocking antibodies; TSH, thyroid-stimulating hormone; TSH-R, TSH receptor; VLBW, very low birthweight. (*Reproduced with permission from American Academy of Pediatrics, Rose SR; Section on Endocrinology and Committee on Genetics, et al: Update of newborn screening and therapy for congenital hypothyroidism, Pediatrics. 2006 Jun;117(6):2290-2303. Reaffirmed December 2011.*)

Positive or unknown maternal TSH receptor antibody (TRAb) level in 2nd or 3rd trimester in setting of maternal Graves' disease

↓

High risk neonate

↓

1. Determine TRAb in cord blood, if assay available

↓

TRAb levels not available or TRAb positive

↓

Newborn day of life 1:
• History + physical exam
• TRAb if assay available and *not* done in cord blood

↓

Newborn day of life 3–5:
• History + physical exam
• FT4 + TSH level: **if abnormal, see section 2 below**
• TRAb if assay available and *not* done in cord blood/post birth

↓

Newborn day of life 10–14:
• History + physical exam
• FT4 + TSH level: **if abnormal, see section 2 below**
• TRAb if assay available and *not* done in cord blood/post birth

↓

In case of negative cord/infant TRAb levels: low risk newborn: no specific follow-up needed

In case of unknown or positive TRAb levels, an asymptomatic newborn and normal thyroid function test: continue clinical follow-up with general practitioner or pediatrician at age 4 weeks and age 2–3 months

---

Negative maternal TSH receptor antibody (TRAb) level in 2nd or 3rd trimester

↓

Low-risk newborn No specific follow-up needed

Clinical manifestations:
- Irritability
- Increased appetite
- Poor weight gain
- Feeding difficulties
- Diarrhea
- Flushing/sweating

Possible findings on examination:
- Tachycardia
- Tachypnea/respiratory distress
- Hypertension
- Hyperthermia
- Goiter
- Small fontanelle
- Stare and/or eyelid retraction
- Warm, moist skin

Criteria for admission:
- Need for β-blockers
- Hemodynamic instability
- Arrhythmias, heart failure
- Tracheal compression due to goiter

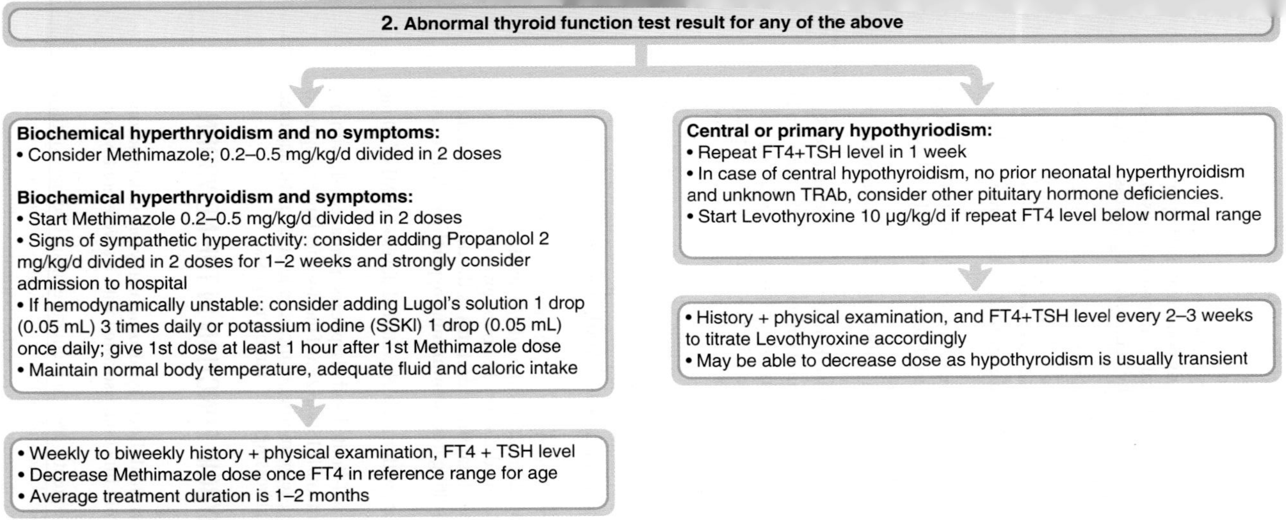

2. Abnormal thyroid function test result for any of the above

Biochemical hyperthyroidism and no symptoms:
- Consider Methimazole; 0.2–0.5 mg/kg/d divided in 2 doses

Biochemical hyperthyroidism and symptoms:
- Start Methimazole 0.2–0.5 mg/kg/d divided in 2 doses
- Signs of sympathetic hyperactivity: consider adding Propanolol 2 mg/kg/d divided in 2 doses for 1–2 weeks and strongly consider admission to hospital
- If hemodynamically unstable: consider adding Lugol's solution 1 drop (0.05 mL) 3 times daily or potassium iodine (SSKI) 1 drop (0.05 mL) once daily; give 1st dose at least 1 hour after 1st Methimazole dose
- Maintain normal body temperature, adequate fluid and caloric intake

- Weekly to biweekly history + physical examination, FT4 + TSH level
- Decrease Methimazole dose once FT4 in reference range for age
- Average treatment duration is 1–2 months

Central or primary hypothyriodism:
- Repeat FT4+TSH level in 1 week
- In case of central hypothyroidism, no prior neonatal hyperthyroidism and unknown TRAb, consider other pituitary hormone deficiencies.
- Start Levothyroxine 10 μg/kg/d if repeat FT4 level below normal range

- History + physical examination, and FT4+TSH level every 2–3 weeks to titrate Levothyroxine accordingly
- May be able to decrease dose as hypothyroidism is usually transient

FIGURE 129-2. Management algorithm for neonates born to mothers with Graves disease. FT₄, free thyroxine; TSH, thyroid-stimulating hormone. (*Reproduced with permission from van der Kaay DC, Wasserman JD2, Palmert MR: Management of Neonates Born to Mothers With Graves' Disease, Pediatrics. 2016 Apr;137(4). pii: e20151878.*)

VI. **Diagnosis**

    A. **History and physical examination.** A maternal past history of thyrotoxicosis and presence of maternal thyroid-stimulating antibodies in the last trimester correlate well with the development of neonatal thyrotoxicosis. Determining maternal TSH receptor antibody levels at 20 to 24 weeks' gestation is recommended. At birth, the infant may be euthyroid or even hypothyroid by laboratory values; however, para-doxically, the presence of goiter may be the only abnormal finding in addition to the clinical features of thyrotoxicosis on physical examination, as discussed earlier.

    B. **Laboratory studies.** Diagnosis is confirmed by demonstrating increased levels of T_4, FT_4, and T_3 with suppressed levels of TSH.

VII. **Management.** Although the disorder is usually self-limited, therapy depends on the severity of the symptoms, and thyrotoxicosis is a life-threatening emergency in its most severe form. Care should be exercised not to induce hypothyroidism with excessive medication. Figure 129–2 represents a useful management algorithm proposed by van der Kaay et al.

    A. **Asymptomatic biochemical hyperthyroidism.** Consider MMI 0.2 to 0.5 mg/kg/d in 2 divided doses. Close observation is required. Therapy may not be necessary if FT_4 elevation and/or TSH suppression are mild.

    B. **Symptomatic biochemical hyperthyroidism.** Administer 1 or more of the following medications:

        1. **Methimazole is the drug of choice.** It blocks thyroid hormone synthesis. Start with 0.2 to 0.5 mg/kg/d in 2 divided doses until euthyroid, then the dose can be reduced by 30% to 60%. PTU blocks synthesis and peripheral T_4 to T_3 conversion and may be used instead of MMI. Initial dose is 5 to 10 mg/kg/d in 3 divided doses, then the dose can be reduced by 30% to 60%. Use with caution due to risk of liver toxicity.

        2. **Propranolol** is used to control tachycardia, 2 mg/kg/d in 2 to 3 divided doses. Diuretics and digitalis may be needed to treat congestive heart failure.

        3. **Oral iodine.** Lugol's solution or saturated solution of potassium iodide, 1 drop (0.05 mL) every 8 hours, in conjunction with MMI. Give the first dose 1 hour after the first MMI dose.

        4. **Corticosteroids** inhibit thyroid hormone secretion and inhibit conversion of T_4 to T_3. Use either **hydrocortisone** 2.5 to 10 mg/kg/d divided every 8 hours or **prednisolone** 1 to 2 mg/kg/d divided every 12 hours; give only in severe cases.

    C. **Thyroid gland ablation or near-total thyroidectomy** is the definitive treatment of permanent thyrotoxicosis resulting from **nonimmune hyperthyroidism** caused by activating mutations.

    D. **Breastfeeding** is regarded as safe with maximal maternal doses of MMI of 20 mg or PTU of 450 mg.

VIII. **Prognosis.** The disorder is usually self-limited and disappears spontaneously within 2 to 4 months. Mortality in affected infants is 15% to 25% if the disorder is not recognized and treated properly. Potential long-term morbidity includes hyperactivity, impaired intellect, advanced bone age, frontal bossing, and craniosynostosis.

TRANSIENT DISORDERS OF THYROID FUNCTION IN THE NEWBORN

I. **EUTHYROID SICK SYNDROME**

    A. **Definition.** Also called **nonthyroidal illness syndrome,** euthyroid sick syndrome is a transient alteration in thyroid function associated with a severe nonthyroidal illness.

    B. **Incidence.** The syndrome is frequently seen in premature infants because of their increased susceptibility to neonatal morbidity. Preterm infants with respiratory distress syndrome have been the most frequently reported patients with this disorder.

    C. **Diagnosis.** A low T_3 level is usually present, associated with low or normal T_4 and normal TSH. Infants are euthyroid (normal TSH).

D. **Treatment.** Treatment has not been shown to be beneficial. Abnormal thyroid functions return to normal as the sick infant improves. However, preterm infants at risk should be monitored by serial determinations of FT_4 and TSH, and treatment should be initiated if there is progressive increase in TSH and decrease in FT_4. Treatment should be initiated if the illness state is expected to be persistent and TSH remains elevated for a month or longer.

II. **TRANSIENT HYPOTHYROXINEMIA OF PREMATURITY**

A. **Definition.** Low thyroid levels without elevated TSH, but not as low as CH.

B. **Incidence.** Almost all preterm infants have some degree of hypothyroxinemia (>50% have T_4 levels <6.5 mcg/dL).

C. **Pathophysiology.** The condition is presumed to be related to immaturity of the hypothalamic-pituitary-thyroid axis that cannot compensate for the loss of maternal thyroid hormone.

D. **Diagnosis.** The biochemical profile of transient hypothyroxinemia in premature infants (before 30–32 weeks' gestation) comprises low T_4 and FT_4 levels with normal or low TSH levels. Treatment with $L-T_4$ causes further drop in TSH levels.

E. **Treatment.** Therapy has not been consistently effective in improving neurologic outcome or reducing morbidity. Therapy is only recommended when low T_4 is accompanied by TSH elevation.

130 Transient Tachypnea of the Newborn

I. **Definition. Transient tachypnea of the newborn (TTN) is a benign self-limited respiratory distress syndrome of term and late preterm infants related to delayed clearance of lung liquid.** The distress appears shortly after birth and usually resolves within 3 to 5 days. **Synonymous terms** include wet lung syndrome, type II respiratory distress syndrome (RDS), transient RDS, neonatal retained fluid syndrome, and benign unexplained respiratory distress in the newborn.

II. **Incidence.** It is the most common perinatal respiratory disorder, responsible for 40% of respiratory distress after birth. Incidence varies in the literature from 4 to 11 cases per 1000 singleton live births.

III. **Pathophysiology.** A delayed resorption of liquid from the lungs is believed to be the central mechanism for TTN. The lung liquid inhibits gas exchange, leading to an increased work of breathing. Tachypnea develops to compensate for that. Hypoxia develops because of poorly ventilated alveoli. The following factors are involved:

A. **Elevated airway liquid volumes**

1. **Inactivated/immature amiloride-sensitive sodium channels.** During gestation, the pulmonary epithelium actively secretes fluid and chloride into the air spaces. **During labor,** a surge of fetal catecholamines (adrenaline, glucocorticoids) is released, and the lung switches from active chloride and fluid secretion to active sodium absorption. However, when sodium channels are inactivated or ineffective during labor, this will result in a larger volume of lung liquid at birth, leading to reduced postnatal respiratory function. Infants born by elective cesarean section have a higher risk of TTN as they are not exposed to the stress (catecholamines) during labor.

Whatever mechanism is responsible for the liquid remaining in the lung, at birth, the transpulmonary pressure created during inspiration is largely responsible for the direct lung aeration and clearance of lung liquid

(seconds). The pressure moves the column of liquid distally toward the alveolus, where it is transferred passively through the membrane into the interstitium. Then the liquid in the interstitium is slowly absorbed by the lymph and blood vessels (hours), leading temporarily to positive pressure in the interstitium. The role of the activated sodium transport from alveolus to interstitium after birth is to prevent the liquid from going back into the alveolus as a consequence of the positive pressure in the interstitium.

2. **Uterine contractions.** Infants delivered by elective cesarean section miss the lung liquid efflux via the trachea by high transpulmonary pressures caused by uterine contractions. Infants delivered by cesarean and breech deliveries miss the fetal trunk flexion when the head goes through the birth canal first, which increases abdominal pressure, elevates the diaphragm, and increases transpulmonary pressure, thereby forcing liquid out via the nose and mouth.

Both mechanisms will lead to larger airway liquid volumes at birth that must be accommodated within the lung tissue following lung aeration, resulting in higher interstitial pressures and a greater likelihood of liquid flooding back into the airways when the lungs are at functional residual capacity (FRC). The elevated airway liquid volumes will affect respiratory structure and function, resulting in lower FRCs and a reduced ability of the lung to aerate efficiently.

B. **Pulmonary immaturity.** One study noted that a mild degree of pulmonary immaturity is a central factor in the cause of TTN. The authors found a mature lecithin-sphingomyelin ratio but negative phosphatidylglycerol (the presence of phosphatidylglycerol indicates completed lung maturation) in infants with TTN. Infants who were closer to 36 weeks' gestation than 38 weeks' gestation had an increased risk of TTN. One study demonstrated that a **relative surfactant deficiency** may play a role in prolonged TTN. Surfactant deficiency leads to an increased surface tension and lowers the compliance of the lung. A layer of surfactant also plays a role in preventing lung liquid from going back to the alveoli. A recent study suggested that TTN is associated with surfactant dysfunction by showing that infants with TTN delivered by cesarean section had low stable microbubble counts in oral aspirates at birth.

C. **Genetic predisposition.** Because of familial clustering of some cases, there is speculation that there may be a genetic predisposition.

1. Some propose that there may be a genetic predisposition for β-adrenergic hyporesponsiveness and that this plays a role in TTN.
2. Polymorphisms in the β-adrenergic receptor (ADRB)-encoding genes, β_1 Gly-49 homozygosity and TACC haplotype of *ADRB2* gene, may predispose to TTN.
3. Maternal and fetal mutated alleles of the *PROGINS* progesterone receptor polymorphism reduce the risk for TTN.

IV. **Risk factors**

A. **Cesarean delivery** (with or without labor). Labor prior to a cesarean delivery is not protective for TTN. General anesthesia resulted in higher rates of TTN compared with spinal anesthesia in elective cesarean sections.
B. **Male gender.**
C. **Prematurity/late preterm.**
D. **Macrosomia** (birthweight ≥4500 g).
E. **Multiple gestations.**
F. **Prolonged labor with long intervals.**
G. **Negative amniotic fluid phosphatidylglycerol.**
H. **Perinatal/birth asphyxia.**
I. **Fluid overload in the mother,** especially with oxytocin infusion.
J. **Family history of asthma** (especially history in the mother).
K. **Breech delivery.**

    L. **Infant of a diabetic mother (2–3 times more common).** Reasons could be the increased rate of cesarean sections in this group or the decreased fluid clearance in the diabetic fetal lung.

    M. **Infant of drug-dependent mother** (narcotics).

    N. **Exposure to β-mimetic agents.**

    O. **Precipitous delivery** (rapid vaginal delivery)/absence of exposure to labor.

    P. **Urban location.**

    Q. **Nulliparity.**

    R. **History of infertility therapy.**

    S. **Augmentation of labor/vacuum/forceps delivery.**

    T. **Low Apgar score (<7) at 1 and 5 minutes.** A low Apgar at 1 minute was associated the most with TTN.

    U. **Absence of premature rupture of membranes.**

    V. **Hypothyroxinemia in the infant.**

    W. **Maternal epilepsy**

  V. **Increased risk of prolonged transient tachypnea of the newborn/increased severity of transient tachypnea of the newborn**

    A. **Grunting, maximum respiratory rate >90 breaths/min, and a fraction of inspired oxygen >0.40** within 6 hours of life were associated with an increase in prolonged TTN.

    B. **Peak respiratory rate in the first 36 hours of life >90 breaths/min** caused a 7-fold increased risk of prolonged tachypnea. The group with prolonged tachypnea had longer hospitalization and antibiotic treatment. The white blood cell count and hematocrit levels were lower in the group with prolonged tachypnea than the group with tachypnea that lasted <72 hours.

    C. **Absence of labor contractions or reduced labor duration** is associated with a more severe course of TTN at term, requiring longer oxygen supplementation.

    D. **Long-distance land-based transport in neonates with transient tachypnea of the newborn.** These infants required increased respiratory support in the neonatal intensive care unit (NICU), and incidence of pulmonary air leak syndrome was higher.

  VI. **Clinical presentation.** The infant is usually near term, term, or large and premature. Tachypnea (>60 breaths/min and as high as 100–120 breaths/min) occurs shortly after delivery or within the first 6 hours of delivery. The infant may also have grunting (persistent grunting after birth), nasal flaring, minimal rib retractions, and varying degrees of cyanosis (uncommon, usually mild hypoxemia responsive to oxygen). The infant often appears to have the classic "barrel chest" secondary to the increased anteroposterior diameter (hyperinflation). One can hear crackles on auscultation, and the liver and spleen are palpable because of the hyperinflation. There are usually no signs of sepsis. Some infants may have edema and a mild ileus on physical examination. One can also see tachycardia with usually a normal blood pressure. The infant is neurologically normal and has no signs of sepsis. **Some clinicians differentiate between transitional delay, transient tachypnea, and prolonged tachypnea.**

    A. **Transitional delay.** Tachypnea right after birth for usually <6 hours (but can be 2–12 hours). Grunting can occur right after birth with transitional delay and usually subsides by 2 hours (93%). Transitional delay usually subsides within 6 hours, and infants are able to feed orally.

    B. **Transient tachypnea of the newborn.** Tachypnea that lasts from after birth to usually <72 hours. It typically resolves by 12 to 24 hours. One study found that 74% of infants had resolution of their symptoms by 48 hours.

    C. **Prolonged transient tachypnea of the newborn.** Some infants have prolonged tachypnea, lasting >72 hours. Some have classified this as prolonged tachypnea of the newborn. Infants with prolonged TTN were found to have an increased asymmetric dimethylarginine (ADMA) level. ADMA may decrease nitric oxide synthesis, causing an increase in pulmonary artery pressure and thereby causing the tachypnea to last longer.

VII. **Diagnosis.** TTN is a clinical diagnosis based on clinical and radiologic findings.
   A. **Laboratory studies**
      1. **Prenatal testing**
         a. **A mature lecithin-sphingomyelin ratio** with the presence of phosphatidyl-glycerol in the amniotic fluid may help rule out RDS. This test is no longer commonly performed.
         b. **Quantitative ultrasound texture analysis of the fetal lung (quantusFLM; Transmural Biotech)** is able to predict fetal lung maturity with an accuracy comparable to amniotic fluid tests. It can predict respiratory morbidity (RDS or TTN) with an accuracy of 86.5%.
      2. **Amniotic fluid sampling at delivery. Amniotic lamellar body counts** can predict the occurrence of TTN. The count is lower than in controls and higher than in infants with RDS.
      3. **Postnatal testing**
         a. **Arterial blood gas on room air** shows some degree of mild to moderate hypoxemia. Arterial partial pressure of carbon dioxide is usually normal because of the tachypnea. Hypercapnia/hypercarbia, if it exists, is usually mild (partial pressure of carbon dioxide >55 mm Hg), and a mild respiratory acidosis can be seen, but if it worsens, it can be a sign of fatigue and impending respiratory failure or complication such as a pneumothorax. If there is a severe respiratory alkalosis, consider hyperammonemia.
         b. **Pulse oximetry should be monitored continuously.**
         c. **Complete blood count with differential** is normal in TTN but should be obtained if an infectious process is being considered. The hematocrit will also rule out polycythemia.
      4. **Other promising tests that may aid in the diagnosis but are usually not needed. Plasma endothelin-1 levels** may be higher in RDS compared with those in TTN. This test may prove useful in differentiating RDS from TTN. **Interleukin-6 (IL-6)** may distinguish proven and clinical sepsis from TTN. This may make it possible to avoid antibiotics in this group of infants. **Serum atrial natriuretic peptide levels** were lower in infants with TTN than in normal infants in one study. **Ischemia-modified albumin levels** can be used to predict TTN and severity because they are significantly higher in infants diagnosed with TTN. The **fetal pulmonary artery acceleration to ejection time ratio** seems to be promising to predict or rule out TTN.
   B. **Imaging and other studies**
      1. **Chest radiograph.** (See example in Figures 12–19A and B.) The chest radiograph is the diagnostic standard. The typical findings in TTN are as follows:
         a. **Hyperexpansion (hyperinflation)** of the lungs is a hallmark of TTN. Hyperaeration with wide intercostal spaces is secondary to partial airway obstruction from fluid in the interstitium.
         b. **Prominent perihilar markings or streaking is generally symmetrical** and is due to engorgement of pulmonary vessels and periarterial lymphatics.
         c. **Occasionally mild to moderate cardiomegaly.** May be secondary to myocardial insufficiency from hypoxemia, perinatal asphyxia, or abnormal pulmonary vascular transition.
         d. **Depression (flattening) of the diaphragm** is best seen on a lateral view of the chest.
         e. **Fluid in the minor fissures** and perhaps fluid in the pleural space (pleural effusions) and laminar effusions.
         f. **Prominent pulmonary vascular markings.** "Fuzzy vessels," a sunburst pattern, peripheral air trapping resulting in increased lung volumes.
         g. **Air leaks** are rarely seen.
         h. **There should be no areas of consolidation.**

2. **Lung ultrasonography.** In recent studies, lung ultrasound has been a promising technique in diagnosing lung disease (RDS and TTN) and differentiating between the 2 conditions in infants. Reviews suggest that it is an accurate and reliable tool for diagnosing TTN. The use of ultrasound has many advantages, including the following: It is noninvasive, has no radiation, and can be done at the bedside but does require properly trained staff with available equipment. Findings vary but may include double lung point (seen more often in less severe TTN), interstitial lung syndrome, pleural line abnormalities (disappearance or thickening, partial or total disappearance of A lines, pleural effusion), and white lung (seen more often in severe TTN).

C. **Other tests for transient tachypnea of the newborn**

1. **Hyperoxia test.** Infants who are hypoxic on room air should have an evaluation to rule out congenital heart disease. A hyperoxia test can be done, but many institutions are doing away with this test because of the concern of using 100% oxygen in preterm infants. An echocardiogram should be done to rule out congenital heart disease. See pages 489 and 490 for more information on the hyperoxia test.

2. **Echocardiography.** One study found that infants with TTN had significantly more structural cardiac lesions. Echocardiogram is recommended in infants with persistent tachypnea or persistent or severe hypoxia to rule out congenital cardiac anomalies.

D. **Confirm the diagnosis.** As noted, TTN is a clinical diagnosis and often a **diagnosis of exclusion**, and other causes of tachypnea (especially pathologic causes) should be excluded first. There are many causes of tachypnea, and usually the history, physical examination, and initial radiograph will help to narrow down the differential. If still uncertain, the clinical course can help guide you. **An infant who does not improve, who worsens, whose radiograph pattern changes, who requires mechanical ventilation, who is on a high concentration of oxygen, and who is not following the typical pattern should alert the provider that the diagnosis may not be TTN.**

1. **Causes of tachypnea are extensive in the newborn.** Use the mnemonic **TRACHEAS** to help remember some of the causes of tachypnea in a newborn: **T:** TTN; **R:** RDS, respiratory infections (pneumonia); **A:** aspiration syndromes (meconium, blood, or amniotic fluid); **C:** congenital malformations, congenital cyanotic heart disease; **H:** hyperventilation (cerebral), hypoplastic lungs, hypertension (persistent pulmonary); **E:** edema (pulmonary); **A:** air leaks and acidosis; **S:** some other causes (sepsis, metabolic disorders, polycythemia).

2. **Respiratory distress syndrome and respiratory infections.** (See also Chapter 117.)

a. **Respiratory distress syndrome.** Approximately 77% of infants with TTN are clinically misdiagnosed with RDS. The infant with RDS is normally premature (<34 weeks), requires higher respiratory support, and has a characteristic radiograph (typical RDS reticulogranular pattern with air bronchograms) and underexpansion (atelectasis) of the lungs.

b. **Respiratory infections (pneumonia).** If the infant has pneumonia, the prenatal history usually suggests infection. There may be maternal intraamniotic infection, premature rupture of membranes, and fever. The blood cell count may show evidence of infection (neutropenia or leukocytosis with abnormal numbers of immature cells). The urine antigen test may be positive if the infant has group B streptococcal infection. Pneumonia may mimic the x-ray findings of TTN (hyperaeration, pleural effusions). It is best to give broad-spectrum antibiotics if there is any suspicion or evidence of infection as they can be discontinued if the cultures are negative in 36 to 48 hours.

3. **Aspiration syndromes (meconium, blood, or amniotic fluid).** Infants with meconium aspiration syndrome (most common syndrome) are usually fully mature or postmature. Blood and amniotic fluid can also be aspirated. All of these aspiration syndromes can present at birth or several hours after birth. Infants usually have more severe respiratory distress and require more oxygen than in TTN. The x-ray can be similar to that in TTN but usually has perihilar infiltrates/opacities. TTN can have patchy opacities from fluid in the alveoli. The blood gases usually show more hypoxemia, hypercapnia, and acidosis.

4. **Congenital conditions**
   a. **Congenital diaphragmatic hernia, congenital pulmonary airway malformations).** These can present with respiratory distress, and a chest x-ray will help make the diagnosis.
   b. **Congenital cyanotic heart disease.** Infants with hypoplastic right and left heart syndromes, tetralogy of Fallot, and transposition of the great arteries can all present after birth with cyanosis, usually with few respiratory symptoms, but they can have tachypnea. Cardiomegaly and vascular engorgement can be seen from congestive heart failure on chest x-ray, which can be similar to perihilar streaking of retained fluid seen in transient tachypnea. The hyperoxia test, pulse oximetry screening, and echocardiogram should be done to rule out heart disease (see pages 489 and 490).

5. **Hyperventilation**
   a. **Cerebral hyperventilation.** This disorder is seen when central nervous system lesions (eg, subarachnoid hemorrhage, meningitis, hypoxic ischemic encephalopathy) cause overstimulation of the respiratory center, resulting in tachypnea. Arterial blood gas measurements show respiratory alkalosis. Chest x-ray may show cardiomegaly and normal lungs. Infants with severe hyperammonemia can have hyperventilation secondary to cerebral edema, which causes a respiratory alkalosis.
   b. **Primary pulmonary hypoplasia** can cause persistent tachypnea.
   c. **Persistent pulmonary hypertension can cause** tachypnea. See Chapter 115.

6. **Edema (pulmonary)** secondary to a patent ductus arteriosus (left-to-right shunt with failure, anomalous venous drainage).

7. **Air leaks and acidosis**
   a. **Air leaks (pneumothorax, pneumomediastinum).** Chest transillumination and a chest x-ray should be obtained.
   b. **Metabolic acidosis.** Infants respond to metabolic acidosis with tachypnea to compensate. With a simple metabolic acidosis, there is a decrease in bicarbonate, and the respiratory rate is increased, which results in a decrease in partial pressure of carbon dioxide, which raises the pH toward normal. Rule out causes of metabolic acidosis (see Chapter 51).

8. **Some other causes**
   a. **Sepsis.** Infants with sepsis can have metabolic acidosis and shock and can thus have tachypnea (clinical response to an infectious insult), but it usually takes time to develop.
   b. **Metabolic disorders.** Infants with hypothermia, hyperthermia, or hypoglycemia may have tachypnea.
   c. **Polycythemia and hyperviscosity.** This syndrome may present with tachypnea with or without cyanosis.
   d. **Very rare causes of full term neonatal respiratory distress** include congenital surfactant dysfunction and primary ciliary dyskinesia, both of which are inherited primary lung diseases. Consider primary ciliary dyskinesia in a term neonate with unexplained respiratory distress with lobar collapse, situs inversus, and/or prolonged oxygen therapy need >2 days. Congenital surfactant deficiency presents like RDS in term infants and the CXR can be consistent with TTN.

VIII. **Management**
  A. **Preventive**
    1. **Limit cesarean sections** and, if necessary, plan the elective cesarean section at a gestational age of 39 weeks or later, which may decrease the frequency of TTN. Labor prior to cesarean section did not prevent TTN. Vaginal birth appears to be protective against TTN (even after 37 weeks of gestation). Spinal anesthesia is better than general anesthesia for elective cesarean section for avoidance of TTN.
    2. **Establish fetal maturity** prior to elective cesarean section, although this is not commonly done. See Chapter 1.
    3. **Antenatal betamethasone prior to elective cesarean section at term** reduced the incidence of respiratory morbidity in infants (reduced TTN rate from 4% of elective cesarean sections to 2.1%). The steroids encourage the expression of the epithelial channel gene and allow the lung to switch from fluid secretion to fluid absorption. It induces lung Na^+ reabsorption by increasing the number and activity of channels even in hypoxia. In addition, antenatal glucocorticoids induce maturation of the surfactant system.
    4. **Prevent low Apgar scores.** A low Apgar score at <1 minute is strongly associated with TTN. Improved obstetric surveillance may decrease low Apgar scores.
    5. **Prophylactic continuous positive airway pressure in the delivery room** *(controversial, not standard of care).* One earlier study did not show any adverse or beneficial effects of prophylactic continuous positive airway pressure (CPAP) in the delivery room to prevent TTN. Two more recent studies showed that it decreased the rate of TTN (not statistically significant) and the rate of NICU admission in newborns delivered by elective cesarean section and that it decreased the duration and severity of respiratory distress in infants with TTN. Some studies have shown an increased risk of pneumothoraces with CPAP use in the delivery room in early term neonates.
  B. **General. Management is mostly supportive.**
    1. **Oxygenation and ventilation.** Initial management consists of providing adequate oxygenation. Start with **extra oxygen via hood or nasal cannula** and deliver enough to maintain normal arterial saturation. If there is an increased work of breathing and the oxygen need is >30%, then nasal **CPAP** is an effective alternative treatment. CPAP gives a continuous positive pressure on the airways, helping to oppose the reentry of liquid and maintaining FRC. **Intubation** criteria vary by center, but a common practice is to intubate when the oxygen need is >40% when on a CPAP of 8 cm H_2O.
    2. **Surfactant.** If the infant requires intubation, other diseases should be considered, but administration of exogenous surfactant promotes a dramatic clinical response in infants with TTN needing intubation and mechanical ventilation, underlining the role of surfactant deficiency in severe TTN.
    3. **Maintain a neutral thermal environment.**
    4. **Antibiotics.** Most infants are initially treated with broad-spectrum antibiotics (usually ampicillin and gentamicin) for 36 to 48 hours until the diagnosis of sepsis or pneumonia is excluded *(controversial).* In a randomized controlled trial of restrictive fluid management in TTN, all 73 infants with TTN were not treated with antibiotics and none of the infants manifested neonatal pneumonia or bacteremia. A combined strategy technique (perinatal risk factors, clinical signs, and laboratory tests for infection) to decide whether antibiotics are necessary may be able to decrease the use of antibiotics in this group.
    5. **Feeding.** Because of the risk of aspiration, an infant should not be fed by mouth if the respiratory rate is >60 breaths/min. If the respiratory rate is <60 breaths/min, oral feeding is permissible. If the rate is 60 to 80 breaths/min, feeding should be by nasogastric tube. If the rate is >80 breaths/min, intravenous nutrition is indicated.
    6. **Fluid and electrolytes** should be monitored and hydration maintained. Fluid management is *controversial.* A small randomized trial of restrictive fluid

management in infants with severe TTN showed a reduced duration of respiratory support and reduced hospitalization cost. However, the control group in this trial received a more liberal fluid intake than currently recommended, and although significant, the differences were small.

7. **Diuretics are not recommended.** Diuretics have been used in practice in some centers with the rationale of accelerating lung liquid absorption with an immediate diuresis-independent lung liquid resorption and a delayed increase in urine output. Furosemide also causes pulmonary vasodilatation, leading to an improved ventilation/perfusion match. However, trials investigating the oral or aerosolized administration of furosemide in infants with TTN have shown no differences in the course of disease. A Cochrane review (2015) noted that neither oral nor intravenous furosemide provided any benefit for the management of TTN and therefore cannot be recommended.

8. **Dopamine treatment.** Low-dose dopamine (3 mcg/kg/min) has been used to increase renal perfusion, and moderate doses (5 mcg/kg/min) may stimulate the clearance of pulmonary edema. One study of low- and moderate-dose dopamine did not improve the outcome of TTN.

9. **Inhaled epinephrine.** Infants with TTN have low levels of epinephrine, and epinephrine helps to mediate fetal lung fluid absorption. However, a recent meta-analysis demonstrated that there is insufficient evidence to determine the safety and efficacy of inhaled racemic epinephrine in the management of TTN.

10. **β_2-Agonist salbutamol.** Stimulation of β-adrenergic receptors with salbutamol upregulates the activity of the sodium channels. However, a recent meta-analysis demonstrated that there is insufficient evidence to determine the safety and efficacy of salbutamol in the management of TTN. A pilot study showed there was no beneficial effect of early inhaled steroids in TTN.

IX. **Prognosis**

A. **Transient tachypnea of the newborn is usually self-limited** and usually lasts only 2 to 5 days.

B. **Asthma/wheezing syndromes.** Asthma is a multifactorial disease. Recent studies have revealed that TTN is associated with the development of wheezing syndromes (bronchiolitis, acute bronchitis, chronic bronchitis, asthma, or prescription for asthma medication) in early childhood and subsequent diagnosis of childhood asthma. The risk of TTN is increased in babies born to mothers with asthma. In 1 study, the risk was found to be greatest in males of nonwhite race whose mothers lived at an urban address and did not have asthma. Some believe TTN may be a marker for deficient pulmonary function, increasing the (inherited) susceptibility to the development of asthma. Liem et al proposed that environmental and genetic interactions predispose these infants to asthma.

C. **Increased risk of RSV hospitalization during the first year of life.** The rate of RSV hospitalization is higher in children with TTN compared to children without a TTN diagnosis.

D. **Complications (rare).** If these occur, it is best to reevaluate the infant.

1. **Some infants can develop prolonged tachypnea (>72 hours) and can progress to respiratory failure** (hypoxia, respiratory fatigue with acidosis) and require intubation and mechanical ventilation.

2. **Although rare, a few infants may develop air leaks (usually a pneumothorax or pneumomediastinum).** There is a higher risk of air leak if the infant is on CPAP. Familial neonatal pneumothorax has been associated with TTN in siblings of 2 families.

3. **Some may develop pulmonary hypertension with right-to-left shunting** across the ductus arteriosus or foramen ovale. This may be present because of possible elevation in the pulmonary vascular resistance associated with retained fetal lung fluid and hyperinflation of the lungs and require extracorporeal membrane oxygenation/extracorporeal life support. (See Chapter 20.)

131 Chlamydial Infection

I. **Definition.** *Chlamydia trachomatis* is an obligate, intracellular, small, gram-negative bacterium that possesses a cell wall, contains DNA and RNA, and can be inactivated by several antimicrobial agents. It is the most common cause of sexually transmitted genital infections. It may cause urethritis, cervicitis, and salpingitis in the mother. In the infant, it can cause conjunctivitis and pneumonia.

II. **Incidence.** The prevalence of *C trachomatis* in pregnant women varies from 2% to 20%. The risk of infection to infants born to infected mothers is high; conjunctivitis occurs in 20% to 50% and pneumonia in 5% to 30%. The nasopharynx is the anatomic site most commonly infected. In the Netherlands, where prenatal screening is not routine, 1 study showed *C trachomatis* to be responsible for 64% of all cases of neonatal conjunctivitis.

III. **Pathophysiology.** *C trachomatis* serovariants B and D through K cause the sexually transmitted form of the disease and the associated neonatal infection. They frequently cause a subclinical infection in the mother. The infant acquires infection during vaginal delivery through an infected cervix. Infection after cesarean delivery is rare and usually occurs with early rupture of amniotic membranes; however, infection associated with intact membranes has been reported. Population-based studies suggest that maternal *C trachomatis* infection is associated with an increased risk of preterm delivery and premature rupture of membranes.

IV. **Risk factors.** Risk is inversely proportional to gestational age. Risk factors include vaginal delivery of an infant with an infected mother and early or prolonged rupture of the amniotic membranes.

V. **Clinical presentation**
   A. **Conjunctivitis.** See Chapter 58.
   B. **Pneumonia.** This is one of the most common forms of pneumonia in the first 3 months of life. The respiratory tract may be directly infected during delivery. Approximately half of infants presenting with pneumonia have concurrent or previous conjunctivitis. Pneumonia usually presents at 2 to 19 weeks of life. The infants experience a gradual increase in symptoms over several weeks. Initially, there is often a period of 1 to 2 weeks of mucoid rhinorrhea followed by cough and increasing respiratory rate. More than 95% of cases are afebrile. The cough is characteristic, paroxysmal, and staccato, and it interferes with sleeping and eating. Approximately a third of infants have otitis media. Preterm infants may present with apneic spells. *C trachomatis* has been isolated from tracheal secretions of preterm infants with pneumonia in the first week after birth.
   C. **Asymptomatic infection** of the nasopharynx, conjunctivae, vagina, and rectum can be acquired at birth. Nasopharyngeal cultures have been observed to remain positive for as long as 28 months in infants with infection acquired at birth.

VI. **Diagnosis**
   A. **Laboratory studies**
      1. **Tissue culture.** Because chlamydiae are obligate intracellular organisms, culture specimens must contain epithelial cells. **Culture of the organism** is the **gold standard** for diagnosing neonatal conjunctivitis and pneumonia. The specificity and sensitivity of culture are nearly 100% with adequate sampling and transport. Material should be obtained from the tarsal conjunctiva (for conjunctivitis) or from nasopharyngeal aspiration or deep suctioning of the trachea (for suspected pneumonia).

2. **Nucleic acid amplification tests.** These tests use methods to amplify *C trachomatis* DNA or RNA sequences. Currently available tests are polymerase chain reaction (Amplicor), transcription-mediated amplification (Aptima Combo 2), and strand displacement amplification (ProbeTec). These tests are approved by the US Food and Drug Administration (FDA) to be used in adults and have largely replaced tissue culture as the diagnostic method of choice; limited data in infants suggest that nucleic acid amplification tests are more sensitive than culture.
3. **Antigen detection tests.** Include direct fluorescent antibody (**DFA**) and enzyme immunoassay tests. These tests appear to be sensitive and specific when used with conjunctival specimens, but the sensitivity with nasopharyngeal samples is poor. DFA is the only culture-independent method that is FDA approved for the detection of chlamydia from conjunctival swab specimens.
4. **Serum antichlamydial antibody (immunoglobulin M) concentration.** Difficult to determine and not widely available. In children with pneumonia, a titer >1:32 is diagnostic of infection.
5. **Other tests.** In cases of pneumonia, the white blood cell count is normal, but there is **eosinophilia** in 70% of cases. Blood gas measurements show mild to moderate hypoxemia.
   B. **Imaging and other studies.** In cases of pneumonia, the chest radiograph may reveal hyperexpansion of the lungs, with bilateral diffuse interstitial or alveolar infiltrates.
VII. **Management.** Isolation precautions for all infectious diseases, including maternal and neonatal precautions, breast feeding, and visiting issues, can be found in Appendix F.
   A. **Prevention.** Identification and treatment of infected pregnant mothers can reduce the risk of preterm birth and prevent disease in the infant. The US Centers for Disease Control and Prevention recommend that all pregnant women be screened for chlamydia at the first prenatal visit. Women under age 25 and those at increased risk for chlamydial infection should have repeat testing in the third trimester. Pregnant women diagnosed with a chlamydial infection during the first trimester should receive a test to document chlamydial eradication 3 to 4 weeks after treatment and should be tested 3 months after treatment as well as in the third trimester. Infants born to mothers known to have untreated chlamydial infection should be monitored clinically. Prophylactic antimicrobial treatment is not recommended because the efficacy of such therapy is unknown. In addition, erythromycin, the agent most commonly used, is associated with significant risk for **infantile hypertrophic pyloric stenosis (IHPS)**.
   B. **Chlamydial conjunctivitis or pneumonia.** Treated with oral erythromycin base or ethylsuccinate (50 mg/kg/d in 4 divided doses) for 14 days or with azithromycin (20 mg/kg as a single daily dose) for 3 days. Topical therapy for conjunctivitis is ineffective and unnecessary. Treatment not only shortens the clinical course but also decreases the duration of nasopharyngeal shedding. Because the efficacy of erythromycin (and azithromycin) is only about 80% for both of these conditions, a second course may be required, and follow-up of infants is recommended. The mother and her sexual partner(s) should be evaluated and treated. **IHPS** may occur when infants are treated with erythromycin in the first 2 weeks of life. The risk of IHPS after treatment with other macrolides (eg, azithromycin and clarithromycin) is unknown, although IHPS has been reported after use of azithromycin. Because confirmation of erythromycin as a contributor to cases of IHPS will require additional investigation and because alternative therapies are not as well studied, the American Academy of Pediatrics continues to recommend erythromycin to treat neonatal chlamydia infection. Parents should be informed about the signs and potential risks of developing IHPS. Cases of IHPS after the use of oral erythromycin or azithromycin should be reported to MedWatch, the FDA Safety Information and Adverse Event Reporting Program. No isolation measures are necessary.

VIII. **Prognosis.** Infants who are diagnosed and treated early generally recover. Experimental studies suggest that neonatal chlamydial pneumonia, especially in preterm neonates, may cause airway hyperreactivity and respiratory dysfunction that continues into adulthood.

132 Cytomegalovirus

I. **Definition.** Human cytomegalovirus (CMV), also known as human herpesvirus 5, is a DNA virus and a member of the herpesvirus family (Herpesviridae).

II. **Incidence. CMV is the most common cause of congenital infection** in the United States and occurs in approximately 0.5% to 1.3% of all live births. This results in approximately 40,000 new cases in the United States per year.

III. **Pathophysiology.** CMV is highly species specific, and only human CMV has been shown to infect humans and cause disease. CMV is a ubiquitous virus that is transmitted in secretions, including saliva, tears, semen, urine, cervical secretions, blood (white blood cells), and breast milk. The seroprevalence increases with age and is influenced by many factors, such as hygienic circumstances, socioeconomic factors, breast feeding, and sexual contacts. In addition to **transplacental infection,** CMV may also be transmitted to the infant **intrapartum** (through exposure to CMV in cervical secretions), via **breast milk,** and via **blood transfusion.** CMV infection acquired during delivery or via breast milk is often asymptomatic in full-term infants with no effect on future neurodevelopmental outcome; however, a sepsis-like illness has been described in premature infants.

In developed countries, CMV seroprevalence varies inversely with socioeconomic status, with 40% to 80% of women of childbearing age in the United States having serologic evidence of past CMV infection. Seroconversion and initial infection can occur around the time of puberty, and shedding of the virus may continue for a long time. CMV can also become latent in white blood cells and reactivate periodically. In addition, a seropositive individual can be infected by a different strain of CMV. Reactivation and reinfection are grouped as a "nonprimary" infection.

CMV is capable of penetrating the placental barrier as well as the blood–brain barrier. During early pregnancy, CMV has a **teratogenic potential** in the fetus. CMV infections may result in neuronal migration disturbances in the brain. Both **primary** and **nonprimary** maternal CMV infection can lead to transmission of the virus to the fetus. When primary maternal infection occurs during pregnancy, the virus is transmitted to the fetus in approximately 35% of cases. The rate of fetal transmission appears to increase with advancing gestation; however, infection in early pregnancy causes more severe fetal infection with significant central nervous system (CNS) sequelae compared to infection acquired later. During nonprimary infection, transmission rate is low (only 0.2% to 1.8%), except for human immunodeficiency virus (HIV)-infected women, who show higher transmission despite receiving antiretroviral prophylaxis. Even though the risk for congenital infection is high after primary maternal infection, nonprimary infection is responsible for 75% of the overall burden of congenital CMV disease.

More than 85% of infants born with congenital CMV have a subclinical infection. Symptomatic infants are usually born to women with a primary infection. When the placenta becomes infected with CMV after a primary maternal infection, its ability to provide oxygen and nutrients to the developing fetus becomes impaired. This leads to placental enlargement due to viral **placentitis and revascularization**. Although not completely elucidated, placental tissue damage occurs due to direct tissue injury by persistent CMV replication, ischemic tissue damage due to vasculitis with viral infection of endothelial cells, and tissue damage by immune complex deposition. Eventual fetal viremia leads to fetal multiorgan involvement. The primary target organs are the CNS, eyes, liver, lungs, and kidneys. Characteristic histopathologic features include focal necrosis, inflammatory response, formation of enlarged cells with intranuclear inclusions (cytomegalic cells), and the production of multinucleated giant cells.

IV. **Risk factors.** CMV infection in neonates is associated with nonwhite race, lower socioeconomic status, drug abuse, and neonatal intensive care unit admittance. Premature infants are more often affected than full-term infants. Transfusion with unscreened blood is an additional risk factor for neonatal disease. Risk factors for primary CMV infection during pregnancy include prolonged exposure to young children (daycare workers, multiparous women) and sexual contact (young maternal age, greater numbers of sexual partners, abnormal cervical cytology, and having a sexually transmitted infection during pregnancy).

V. **Clinical presentation**

A. **Prenatal presentation.** Pregnant women who acquire primary CMV may develop a mononucleosis-like illness with mild hepatitis (<25% of the time). Maternal screening is currently not recommended routinely. Fetal anomalies consistent with congenital CMV infection that can be detected on prenatal ultrasound examination include fetal growth restriction, cerebral periventricular echogenicity or calcifications, cerebral ventriculomegaly, microcephaly, polymicrogyria, cerebellar hypoplasia, hyperechogenic fetal bowel, hepatosplenomegaly, hepatic calcifications, amniotic fluid abnormalities, ascites and/or pleural effusion, and placental enlargement. Prenatal magnetic resonance imaging (MRI), especially to evaluate brain anomalies, is increasingly being used. Amniocentesis to perform polymerase chain reaction (PCR) for CMV DNA in amniotic fluid is the preferred diagnostic approach for identifying an infected fetus. Amniocentesis is most sensitive when done after 21 weeks of gestation and after 6 weeks from maternal infection/exposure.

B. **Postnatal presentation**

1. **Subclinical infection.** Occurs in 85% to 90% of cases. Despite being asymptomatic at birth, these infants are at risk for **sensorineural hearing loss (SNHL)** during the first 6 years of life. Universal CMV screening at birth is not recommended in the United States at this time; however, some authorities suggest a targeted approach that focuses on newborns who fail their universal hearing screening.

2. **Low birthweight.** Maternal CMV infection is associated with low birthweight and small for gestational age infants, even when the infant is not infected.

3. **Classic cytomegalovirus inclusion disease.** Occurs in 10% to 15% of the cases and consists of fetal growth restriction, hepatosplenomegaly with jaundice, transaminitis, thrombocytopenia with or without purpura, and severe CNS involvement. CNS complications include microcephaly, intracerebral calcifications (most characteristically in the subependymal periventricular area), chorioretinitis, and progressive SNHL. Other symptoms include hemolytic anemia and pneumonitis. The most severely affected infants have a mortality rate of approximately 30%. Deaths are usually due to hepatic dysfunction, bleeding, disseminated intravascular coagulation, or secondary bacterial infection.

4. **Late sequelae.** SNHL occurs in 33% to 50% of symptomatic and in 10% to 15% of asymptomatic infants. CMV-related SNHL may be present at birth or occur later in childhood. Approximately 55% and 75% of symptomatic and

asymptomatic infants, respectively, who ultimately develop congenital CMV-associated SNHL will not have hearing loss detectable within the first month of life. Therefore, repeated auditory evaluation during the first 6 years of life is strongly recommended. Visual impairment and strabismus are common in children with clinically symptomatic CMV infection. Visual complications usually occur secondary to chorioretinitis, pigmentary retinitis, macular scarring, optic atrophy, and central cortical defects.

VI. **Diagnosis**
   A. **Laboratory studies**
      1. **Culture for demonstration of the virus.** The **gold standard** for the diagnosis of congenital CMV is **urine** or **saliva** culture obtained **before 3 weeks of age**. Most urine specimens from infants with congenital CMV are positive within 48 to 72 hours, especially if shell vial tissue culture techniques are used. Shell vial assay detects CMV-induced antigens by monoclonal antibodies, allowing for identification of the virus within 48 hours compared with the standard tissue culture, which takes 2 to 4 weeks.
      2. **Polymerase chain reaction.** PCR for CMV DNA is as sensitive as a urine or saliva culture for the detection of CMV infection. Studies evaluating saliva for rapid detection of CMV (PCR or shell vial assay) have shown it to be at least as sensitive as urine for detecting congenital CMV infection, although there is risk of contamination of the saliva sample with retained breast milk in the mouth of the newborn. PCR has been used successfully in retrospective diagnosis of congenital CMV beyond 3 weeks of age through CMV DNA analysis of dried blood spots (Guthrie cards). The sensitivity of CMV DNA detection by PCR assay of dried blood spots is low, limiting use of this type of specimen for widespread screening for congenital CMV. A positive PCR assay result from a neonatal dried blood spot confirms congenital infection, but a negative result does not rule it out.
      3. **Serologic tests.** Serologic tests based on the detection of immunoglobulin M (IgM) should not be used to diagnose congenital CMV because they are less sensitive and more subject to false-positive results than culture or PCR. Only 70% of neonates infected with congenital CMV have IgM antibodies at birth.
      4. **Other laboratory tests.** Other lab tests that are indicated in the workup include complete blood count, liver function tests, coagulation panel and cerebrospinal fluid analysis, culture, and PCR.
   B. **Imaging and other studies.** Ultrasound or computed tomography scans of the head may demonstrate characteristic periventricular calcifications in addition to other abnormalities (see prenatal presentation earlier). Brain MRI is preferred over other modalities because it is likely to identify most of the brain anomalies associated with congenital CMV.
VII. **Management**
   A. **Prevention and treatment of maternal infection during pregnancy.** These include changes in hygienic behavior for seronegative pregnant women, administration of CMV hyperimmune globulin (CMV-HIG) to pregnant women with a primary infection, administration of antiviral therapy to women with primary infection, and administration of vaccines to girls or women well before or during pregnancy. With regard to **hygienic** measures, epidemiologic studies have shown that instructing mothers who are pregnant on frequent hand washing; wearing gloves for specific childcare tasks; avoiding kissing children under age 6 on the mouth or cheek; not sharing food, drinks, or oral utensils (eg, fork, spoon, toothbrush, pacifier) with young children; and cleaning toys, countertops, and other surfaces that come into contact with children's urine or saliva reduces their chances of acquiring congenital CMV infection. **CMV-HIG** given to women with primary congenital infection before 20 weeks' gestation has shown

promise in reducing congenital CMV infection in the fetus in observational and small randomized trials; however, the benefits need to be confirmed in large randomized controlled studies (a trial is underway by the National Institute of Child Health and Human Development; trial identifier NCT01376778; available at https://clinicaltrials.gov; accessed February 11, 2018). Use of **antiviral therapy** for the infected pregnant woman has been studied recently in a multicenter, open-label, phase II trial using high-dose (8 g daily) oral valacyclovir in women carrying CMV-infected fetuses with measurable extracerebral or mild cerebral ultrasound findings starting at a median gestational age of 25 weeks until delivery. The study found that the use of valacyclovir increased the proportion of asymptomatic neonates from 43% without treatment to 82% with treatment. The benefit of valacyclovir needs to be confirmed in large randomized trials before it can be recommended. The most effective preventive strategy is developing a **vaccine** against CMV. A vaccine targeted toward CMV envelope glycoprotein B, an antigen that typically induces a serum antibody response, was tested in phase II clinical trials in adult women as well as adolescent girls. This vaccine has been shown to be immunogenic with an acceptable risk profile with the potential to decrease incident cases of maternal and congenital CMV infection. Phase III trials are underway.

B. **Prevention of cytomegalovirus transmission in the neonatal intensive care unit.** Neonatal intensive care unit infants requiring packed red cell transfusion should be transfused from CMV antibody-negative donors, and the blood should be filtered to remove white blood cells. Pasteurization or freezing of donated human milk can decrease the likelihood of CMV transmission. Short-term pasteurization (72°C for 5 seconds) of milk appears to inactivate CMV; this short-term pasteurization is less harmful to the beneficial constituents of human milk compared to Holder pasteurization. If pasteurization is not available, freezing milk at −20°C for 24 hours will decrease viral titers but does not eliminate CMV reliably. Breast feeding is recommended for CMV antibody–positive mothers as benefits outweigh risks of potential postnatal CMV infection.

C. **Antiviral agents.** Neonates with symptomatic congenital CMV disease with or without CNS involvement have improved audiologic and neurodevelopmental outcomes at 2 years of age when treated with oral **valganciclovir** (a prodrug for ganciclovir) at 16 mg/kg/dose, given orally twice a day for 6 months. The dose should be adjusted each month to account for weight gain. If the infant is unable to absorb the medication due to gastrointestinal illness (eg, necrotizing enterocolitis), intravenous **ganciclovir** at 6 mg/kg/dose is an alternative. Significant neutropenia occurs in 20% of infants treated with oral valganciclovir and in 67% of infants treated with ganciclovir. Absolute neutrophil counts should be performed weekly for 6 weeks, then at 8 weeks, and then monthly for the duration of antiviral treatment; serum aminotransferase concentration should be measured monthly during treatment. Some authorities also recommend monitoring viral load (CMV DNA PCR in the blood) to document response to therapy and check for ganciclovir resistance. Antiviral therapy should be limited to patients with symptomatic congenital CMV disease who are able to start treatment within the first month of life. Preterm infants with perinatally or nosocomially acquired CMV infection can have significant symptomatic disease with end-organ dysfunction (eg, pneumonitis, hepatitis, thrombocytopenia). Antiviral treatment has not been studied in this population; however, these patients are reasonable candidates for oral valganciclovir or intravenous ganciclovir treatment for 2 to 4 weeks, depending on responsiveness of symptoms. The antivirals **foscarnet** and **cidofovir** are reserved for cases of refractory CMV disease, ganciclovir resistance, ganciclovir toxicity, and co-infection with adenovirus. Infants with asymptomatic congenital CMV infection should not receive antiviral treatment.

VIII. **Prognosis.** Congenital CMV is the leading cause of nonhereditary SNHL. Overall mortality rate among infants with congenital CMV infection is approximately 4% to 8% within the first year of life. For symptomatic infants with fulminant disease at birth, mortality is up to 30%, and late complications including intellectual or developmental impairment, progressive hearing loss, and spasticity develop in 70% to 80% of cases. Visual impairment develops in 10% to 20% of symptomatic newborns. With asymptomatic, congenitally infected infants, the prognosis is uncertain, but they are at risk for SNHL (up to 20% by 6 years of age).

133 Dengue Infection, Neonatal

I. **Definition.** Dengue fever (DF) is a worldwide infection caused by 4 related RNA viruses of the genus *Flavivirus*, dengue viruses (DENV) DENV-1, DENV-2, DENV-3, and DENV-4. DENV is primarily transmitted to humans through the bite of infected *Aedes aegypti* (and less commonly *Aedes albopictus* or *Aedes polynesiensis*) mosquitoes. DENV causes asymptomatic infection, DF, or a severe syndrome (dengue hemorrhagic fever [DHF]/dengue shock syndrome [DSS]). The latter is characterized by systemic capillary leakage, thrombocytopenia, and hypovolemic shock.

II. **Incidence.** Dengue is a major public health problem in the tropics and subtropics; an estimated 50 to 100 million dengue cases occur annually in more than 100 countries, and 40% of the world's population lives in areas with DENV transmission. In the United States, dengue is endemic in Puerto Rico, the Virgin Islands, and American Samoa. Additionally, limited outbreaks with local DENV transmission have occurred in Texas, Hawaii, and Florida in the past decade, but no neonatal cases have been reported from the United States. Millions of US travelers, including children, are at risk. Neonatal dengue has been described in case reports and case series from outside the United States; therefore, its true incidence worldwide is unknown.

III. **Pathophysiology.** Viremia is usually detected about 6 to 18 hours before the onset of symptoms and ends as the fever resolves. Both innate and adaptive immune responses seem to play a role in the clearance of infection. Infection with 1 of the 4 DENVs (primary infection) provides long-lasting immunity to infection with a virus of the same serotype; however, immunity to the other dengue serotypes is transient. Individuals can subsequently be infected with another dengue serotype (secondary infection), often with more severe manifestations. DHF can develop with any of the 4 DENVs, but the risk is highest with DENV-2. DHF can usually be distinguished from DF as it progresses through 3 predictable pathophysiologic phases:

   A. **Febrile phase:** Viremia-driven high fevers.

   B. **Critical/plasma leak phase:** Sudden onset of varying degrees of plasma leak into the pleural and abdominal cavities. This phase probably occurs due to endothelial cell dysfunction rather than injury.

   C. **Convalescence or reabsorption phase:** Sudden arrest of plasma leak with concomitant reabsorption of extravasated plasma and fluids.

   Neonates can be infected through mosquito bites but also as a vertical infection from the mother. The highest risk period is when the mother becomes acutely ill with dengue at or near the time of delivery. It has been hypothesized that there is an insufficient level of protective maternal antibodies (immunoglobulin [Ig] G) transferred to the fetus, and therefore, the newborn can manifest serious disease. Endothelial damage and plasma leakage may enable the virus an easy access across the placental barrier.

Dengue virus has been identified in the breast milk of viremic mothers, and postnatal transmission through breast feeding has been documented, albeit this is rare. Blood-borne transmission is possible through exposure to infected blood during the viremic phase; however, it is not known how common this mode of transmission is because blood donations are not systematically screened for DENV.

IV. **Risk factors.** Maternal DF, especially during late pregnancy, places the fetus/baby at risk. To date, there are no reports of congenital malformations from DF when mothers are infected in the first trimester.

V. **Clinical presentation**

    A. **Neonatal consequences of maternal dengue fever.** Neonatal dengue has been described in case reports and case series. It typically results from hematogenous spread during the maternal viremic stage, especially if the mother is symptomatic during the last 5 to 8 days of pregnancy. Transmission rate can be as high as 90%. The incubation period is 3 to 8 days. The neonate may stay asymptomatic with only laboratory evidence of infection (positive serology, leukopenia, or thrombocytopenia). Symptomatic neonates may have a high fever that can be biphasic, lethargy, anorexia, abdominal pain, diarrhea, vomiting, hepatomegaly, and purpuric rash. **Severe dengue symptoms can occur by day 5 when fever ceases**, with easy bruising, severe thrombocytopenia (<30,000 platelets/mm^3), and evidence of plasma leakage–induced hypovolemia, hepatomegaly, and circulatory disturbances. **Shock can happen in severe dengue after defervescence** and includes rapid/weak pulse and narrow pulse pressure. Fortunately, this situation is rarely seen during the neonatal period.

    B. **Consequences of dengue to the pregnant women and adverse pregnancy outcomes.** Severe bleeding may complicate delivery and/or surgical procedures performed on pregnant patients with dengue **during the critical phase** (ie, the period coinciding with marked thrombocytopenia with or without plasma leak). DF does not warrant termination of pregnancy. Even though earlier reports and a meta-analysis suggested an increased risk of adverse pregnancy outcome with DF, a recently updated meta-analysis did not suggest an increased risk of premature birth, low birthweight, miscarriage, or stillbirth with maternal DF. DENV is not teratogenic.

VI. **Diagnosis**

    A. **Laboratory studies**

        1. **Nonspecific findings:** Include increased hematocrit of 20% from baseline (hemoconcentration during capillary leak phase), leukopenia/neutropenia, thrombocytopenia, hyponatremia, hypoalbuminemia, transaminitis, cholestasis, and abnormal coagulation studies (elevated prothrombin and activated partial thromboplastin time).

        2. **Diagnostic tests:** DENV infection can be confirmed by detection of DENV RNA via reverse transcriptase–polymerase chain reaction (**RT-PCR**) assay or detection of DENV nonstructural protein 1 antigen (**NS-1**) by immunoassay and testing for anti-DENV IgM or IgG antibodies by enzyme immunoassay (**EIA**). RT-PCR or NS-1 can be done from the beginning of the febrile phase until day 7 to 10 after illness onset, but anti-DENV IgM antibodies are not detectable until at least 5 days after illness onset. A 4-fold or greater increase in anti-DENV IgG antibody titers between the acute (≤5 days after onset of symptoms) and convalescent (>15 days after onset of symptoms) samples confirms recent infection as well.

    B. **Imaging and other studies.** Chest radiographs and ultrasound can show pleural effusion, ascites, hepatomegaly and gallbladder edema.

VII. **Management.** Treatment is symptomatic with an antipyretic such as acetaminophen. Ibuprofen, aspirin, and other nonsteroidal anti-inflammatory drugs are contraindicated due to hemorrhagic predisposition. **Hemodynamics must be monitored closely when fever resolves (by day 5–7 of illness), because shock can abruptly develop.**

Heart rate, capillary refill time, blood pressure, weight, and serum electrolytes should be checked once or twice a day. Intravenous fluids (colloids and crystalloid) must be prescribed as soon as possible, starting typically with normal saline (0.9% sodium chloride) boluses of 10 to 20 mL/kg to restore perfusion. Total daily fluid intake may vary between 150 and 200 mL/kg/d. Furthermore, extra intravenous sodium chloride may be indicated if shock or hyponatremia (<130 mEq/L) develops. In cases of **severe thrombocytopenia (<30,000/mm³) or serious bleeding**, platelet transfusion is prescribed. **Albumin transfusion** (1 g/kg every 6–12 hours for 2–4 doses) may be indicated with severe hypoalbuminemia (<2 g/dL) or when pleural or peritoneal fluid effusion is present. Prior to establishing the diagnosis in neonates, antibiotics (amoxicillin, cefotaxime, or gentamicin) are empirically prescribed given the high risk of bacterial sepsis at this age. Breast feeding is encouraged despite the minimal risk of transmission via breast milk.

VIII. **Prognosis.** Neonatal dengue can be potentially lethal. Affected newborns should be carefully observed for a minimum of a 2-week period before discharge. Vigilant monitoring and proper hydration often lead to an uneventful recovery. However, poor outcome may occur; a recent study from India that involved 16 women diagnosed with DF (3 had DSS and 8 had DHF) showed that bleeding manifestations occurred in 7 women, and there were 3 maternal deaths. Perinatal complications from the study included 3 intrauterine deaths, 6 nursery admissions, and 1 neonatal death.

IX. **Prevention.** Methods for prevention of dengue infection in endemic areas include mosquito control and vaccine development. Mosquito control is effective but difficult to sustain. Several DENV vaccines are in development, and 1 became commercially available recently; it is licensed in several countries in Latin America and Southeast Asia. It gained the US Food and Drug Administration approval in May 2019. CYD-TDV (Dengvaxia) is a prophylactic, tetravalent, live attenuated viral vaccine administered to individuals age 9 to 45 years (age 9–16 years in the US) who have laboratory-confirmed previous dengue infection and living in dengue-endemic areas. Unfortunately, it is contraindicated in pregnant women because it is a live virus; however, the limited data collected during the clinical trials on inadvertent immunization of pregnant women have yielded no evidence of harm to the fetus or pregnant woman.

134 Enteroviruses and Parechoviruses

I. **Definition.** Enteroviruses (EVs) and parechoviruses (HPeVs) are a large group of viral pathogens represented by 2 different genera of the family Picornaviridae. They are all made of a single strand of RNA in a capsid of individually distinct polypeptides. The capsid proteins impart antigenicity and facilitate transfer of RNA into the cells of newly infected hosts.

A. **Enteroviruses.** The genus of EVs traditionally consisted of 5 groups, each with a well-known human pathogenicity: coxsackie A viruses, coxsackie B virus, echoviruses, EVs 68 to 71, and poliovirus. The new classification (based on viral genomic structure) groups nonpolio EVs into 4 species: human EV types A, B, C, and D. Although they were reclassified, many authorities continue to use their original names.

B. **Parechoviruses.** The genus of HPeVs is made up of at least 16 types. HPeV1 and HPeV2 previously were classified as echoviruses 22 and 23, respectively. HPeVs (especially HPeV3) have been implicated in severe neonatal diseases including sepsis, hepatitis and coagulopathy, and/or meningoencephalitis with long-term sequelae. Interestingly, severe central nervous system (CNS) disease is associated with normal inflammatory markers and **little or no cerebrospinal fluid (CSF) pleocytosis** in the majority of cases.

II. Incidence

    A. Enteroviruses. EVs have worldwide distribution and produce human illness of varying severity, from mild coryza to life-threatening multisystem disease. The diseases have some seasonal variation with increased incidence during summer and fall in temperate zones, but there is little seasonal variation in tropical areas.

        Enteroviral infections are spread by fecal–oral and respiratory routes and in neonates transplacentally, perinatally, and possibly via breast feeding. Incubation periods are typically 3 to 6 days. All subgroups of EVs are linked to nursery and neonatal intensive care unit (NICU) outbreaks. Enteroviral infections are not reportable nationally, and the current incidence of EV illness among neonates is unknown. However, there is a National Enterovirus Surveillance System (NESS), which is a passive surveillance system that has been collecting laboratory data on types of EV and HPeV in the United States since the 1960s. During 2009 to 2013, 2724 specimens representing 2532 patients tested positive for EV and HPeV were reported to NESS; 39% were from children <1 year of age, and coxsackie A6 virus (CVA6) was the most reported type overall. The most common serotypes associated with neonatal infections are EV6, EV9, and EV11 and CVB2, CVB4, and CVB5. In 2014, EVD68 caused a nationwide outbreak, with many patients admitted to intensive care units for respiratory symptoms.

    B. Parechoviruses. During NESS 2009 to 2013 surveillance, HPeV3 was the most common isolate of that genus (12.3%) and was identified as an important cause of neonatal sepsis. A report from Edinburgh, Scotland, for EV surveillance from 2006 to 2010 revealed an incidence of 2.8% for HPeV, but for infants <3 months of age, HPeV3 was also the predominant isolate (22%–25%). A recent study from Ireland found an HPeV infection rate of 13% in infants being tested for late-onset neonatal sepsis.

III. Pathophysiology

    A. Enteroviruses. EVs manifest disease in nearly all body systems. Paradoxically, signs of disease can range from mild to life threatening within the same serotype. Host susceptibility (including absence of serotype-specific maternal neutralizing antibody) seems to be the most important predisposing factor. For the great majority of children and adults, enteroviral illnesses are mild, but for the neonate, EVs can cause serious multiorgan dysfunction and death (sepsis-like illness, meningoencephalitis myocarditis, hepatitis, coagulopathy, and pneumonitis). Some human EVs are more pathogenic than others. Examples of the more serious serotypes include echovirus 11, CVB3, CVA9, CVB1, and EV71.

        1. Echovirus 11. This has been particularly associated with neonatal death. Pathologic findings include extensive hepatic necrosis with adrenal hemorrhage and acute tubular necrosis.

        2. Coxsackievirus B3. Neonatal infections have been marked by hepatitis, disseminated intravascular infection, fever, thrombocytopenia, and intracranial hemorrhage. CVB3 has also been closely associated with antenatal maternal infection and positive virus cultures from placenta, cord, and infant tissues at death, suggesting probable transplacental infection.

        3. Coxsackievirus B1. Until recently, this has been a fairly uncommon strain. In 2006, for the first time, CVB1 became the most commonly reported EV and remained so through 2008. In 2007, there was a significant increase in neonatal disease, including fever, hepatitis, coagulopathy, meningitis, respiratory distress, and myocarditis; in 4 of 5 cases of neonatal death, mothers had chorioamnionitis or febrile illness near the time of delivery.

4. **Enterovirus 71.** This serotype has evolved as a unique cause of epidemic paralysis, with localized and regional outbreaks. Infants and young children are at risk of brainstem encephalitis associated with high mortality related to rapid cardiovascular collapse and pulmonary edema.

5. **Enterovirus D68.** This strain caused a severe outbreak in 2014 associated with severe respiratory illnesses in infants and children. Nine children died. In addition, a polio-like acute neurologic syndrome was reported in a few cases.

B. **Parechovirus.** HPeVs are now recognized as agents for nursery outbreaks of diarrhea coupled with respiratory illnesses. Several cases of more severe illness have been reported, including meningoencephalitis, neonatal sepsis-like disease, hepatitis, and coagulopathy. Other conditions have included myocarditis and conjunctivitis. HPeVs are implicated in other conditions such as hemorrhage hepatitis syndrome, necrotizing enterocolitis, myocarditis, herpangina, and other febrile illness.

1. **Human *Parechovirus* type 1 (previously echovirus 21).** Most common HPeV identified. HPeV1 may cause asymptomatic infection or mild gastrointestinal (GI) or respiratory symptoms. Very rarely, it can cause myocarditis and CNS involvement (encephalitis and paralysis).

2. **Human *Parechovirus* type 3** is probably the most serious type and is associated with seizures and destructive periventricular white matter lesions in preterm and term infants. Usually, the CSF is unremarkable, but HPeV3 RNA can be amplified from CSF and nasopharyngeal and rectal swabs. It can also be associated with sepsis-like illness and hepatitis.

IV. **Risk factors**

A. **Infants born to mothers** who have symptoms of EV/HPeV around the time of the delivery have a higher chance of being infected. The outcome of neonatal infection is strongly influenced by the presence or absence of passively acquired maternal neutralizing antibodies.

B. **Risk of severe infection** is higher if the infant is infected during the first 2 weeks of life.

V. **Clinical presentations.** HPeV infections may mimic EV infections. When evaluating an infant clinically, it is not possible to distinguish neonatal HPeV from an EV infection.

A. **Enteroviruses.** The clinical presentations of EV diseases are varied and overlap with the many subspecies and serotypes. In neonates, the signs that suggest an enteroviral outbreak in a nursery might include a cluster of infants with similar findings of coryza, morbilliform rash, low-grade fever, or diarrhea. A sepsis-like illness is frequently ascribed to enteroviral infection. Sepsis evaluation is often negative, but findings of lethargy, poor feeding, and fever are hallmarks suggesting sepsis. It can also cause hepatitis, coagulopathy, pneumonia, meningoencephalitis, and myocarditis. Hemophagocytic lymphohistiocytosis and severe enteroviral infection can be difficult to distinguish based on clinical presentation and CSF findings.

B. **Parechoviruses.** May mimic the presentation of EVs. The majority of infants with HPeV1 and HPeV2 have mild GI and respiratory syndromes. HPeV3 has been associated with severe neonatal infections, including CNS involvement. Symptoms include irritability, fever, seizures, and a nonspecific rash. **CSF pleocytosis is characteristically lacking in most cases.** Infants with HPeV may present with an acute distended abdomen accompanied by an erythematous rash, low C-reactive protein, and low lymphocyte count, and HPeV has been associated with small clusters of patients with necrotizing enterocolitis.

VI. **Diagnosis**

    A. **Enteroviruses.** Reverse transcriptase–polymerase chain reaction (RT-PCR) is the main diagnostic modality; it is readily available in commercial laboratories but lacks specificity for serotyping. Advanced RT-PCR techniques are required to further identify most EV subspecies. **RT-PCR is both more rapid and more sensitive than cell culture.** Some serotypes (EV71 neurologic disease) are difficult to isolate from CSF (even with CSF pleocytosis) but can be readily isolated from either throat or rectal swab. Cell culture was the standard method for isolation and diagnosis, but specific serotype identification requires time-consuming and expensive neutralization assays or genomic sequencing. Several serotypes cannot be grown effectively in culture. Specimens for cell culture or RT-PCR assays should include CSF, blood, urine, nasal swabs, throat swabs, and stool specimens. Positive RT-PCR tests from stool are supportive but less definitive, because detection may represent prolonged carriage from a previous infection. In countries where oral poliovirus vaccine (OPV) is used, OPV viruses are widely transmitted and may produce false-positive results in cell culture and some RT-PCR assays.

    B. **Parechoviruses.** Current EV RT-PCR does not detect HPeV infection because of the genetic differences between the 2 viruses. The best diagnostic tests are PCR primers that have been developed by the Centers for Disease Control and Prevention that detect all known parechoviruses, some of which are commercially available now. White matter injury has been visualized with a cranial ultrasound and magnetic resonance imaging with diffusion-weighted imaging in infants with HPeV3 encephalitis. Many of the HPeVs do not grow well in cell culture. A direct PCR of stool samples can be obtained. **Most neonates with HPeV3 encephalitis have no CSF pleocytosis and can be diagnosed only with CSF PCR.**

VII. **Management.** Specific therapy for human EVs or HPeVs is limited. Intravenous immunoglobulin (IVIG) may be beneficial for life-threatening neonatal EV infections, severe organ-specific disease (myocarditis, chronic meningoencephalitis), CNS infection with EV71, or in immunocompromised patients to prevent chronic CNS infections. Prophylactic IVIG has been shown to help control hospital outbreaks. High-titer EV71 immunoglobulin is evaluated in epidemic disease areas. Pleconaril, an orally administered capsid inhibitor, has been studied in EV infections recently. In a trial of 61 neonates with suspected EV disease who were randomly assigned to 7 days of pleconaril or placebo, there was a trend toward more rapid viral clearance and lower overall mortality among pleconaril-treated infants (23% vs 44% with placebo); more studies are needed before pleconaril can be recommended. Overall care involves supportive measures, contact isolation in addition to standard precautions, cohorting infected infants in the nurseries to control outbreaks, and close observation for organ-specific disease (eg, meningitis, myocarditis). If fulminant hepatic disease is present, oral neomycin therapy to minimize gut flora may be beneficial. Extracorporeal life support may be indicated for neonatal collapse caused by EV myocarditis.

VIII. **Prevention.** Simple hygienic measures, such as hand washing, are important to prevent the spread of EVs and HPeVs. IVIG is used to stop outbreaks in NICUs. Three inactivated EVA71 vaccines are licensed in China; these have demonstrated high efficacy in randomized clinical trials against the predominant C4 genotype circulating in that country.

IX. **Prognosis.** The illness is mild and recoverable in most cases. Mortality is increased with the more severe forms of the infection (hepatitis, coagulopathy, and encephalitis). Infants with encephalitis and white matter abnormalities on magnetic resonance imaging (especially CVB3 and HPeV3) are at risk for cerebral palsy and neurodevelopmental impairment.

135 Gonorrhea

I. **Definition.** Gonorrhea is a sexually transmitted disease caused by a bacterial infection with *Neisseria gonorrhoeae* (a gram-negative oxidase-positive diplococcus) with possible serious consequences if spread to the newborn.

II. **Incidence.** In 2017, the Centers for Disease Control and Prevention reported the rate of gonorrhea in the United States at approximately 171.9 gonorrhea cases per 100,000 population. The incidence is highest in females 15 to 24 years of age. If routine ophthalmic prophylaxis was not used, it is estimated that 30% to 40% of newborn infants born to infected mothers would become infected.

III. **Pathophysiology.** *N gonorrhoeae* primarily affects the endocervical canal of the mother. The infant may become infected during passage through an infected cervical canal or by contact with contaminated amniotic fluid if rupture of membranes has occurred. Co-infection with *Chlamydia trachomatis* is frequent, and human immunodeficiency virus (HIV) transmission is enhanced in the presence of gonorrhea. Untreated maternal gonococcal disease is associated with increased risk of preterm delivery and small for gestational age infants.

IV. **Clinical presentations**

A. **Ophthalmia neonatorum (neonatal conjunctivitis).** The most common clinical manifestation of neonatal disease (~80% of the cases). This occurs in 1% to 2% of infants born to mothers with gonococcal infection despite appropriate eye prophylaxis. For a description of this disease, see Chapter 58.

B. **Gonococcal arthritis.** The onset of gonococcal arthritis can occur at any time from 2 to 21 days after delivery. It is secondary to gonococcemia. The source of bacteremia has been attributed to infection of the mouth, nares, and umbilicus. Multiple joints usually are affected, with the most common sites being the knees and ankles. The infant may present with mild or moderate symptoms.

C. **Sepsis and meningitis.** See Chapters 146 and 140, respectively.

D. **Scalp abscess.** Usually secondary to intrauterine fetal monitoring.

E. **Other localized infections.** Gonococcal infections involving mucous membranes such as the pharynx, vagina, urethra, and anus have been described.

V. **Diagnosis**

A. **Gram stain and culture.** Gram stain of any exudate should be performed. Material may be obtained by swabbing the eye, pharynx, or anorectal areas. Blood should be obtained for culture. Fluid should be aspirated from an affected joint and Gram stain and culture obtained (in case of arthritis). Gonococcal cultures from nonsterile sites (eg, the pharynx, rectum, and vagina) should be done using selective media.

B. **Lumbar puncture with spinal fluid studies.** Cell count, protein, glucose, culture, and Gram stain should be ordered to rule out bacterial meningitis.

VI. **Management.** Isolation precautions for all infectious diseases, including maternal and neonatal precautions, breast feeding, and visiting issues, can be found in Appendix F.

A. **Hospitalization.** Infants with clinical evidence of ophthalmia neonatorum, scalp abscess, or disseminated infection should be hospitalized. Complete sepsis evaluation including lumbar puncture should be performed. Tests for concomitant *C trachomatis,* congenital syphilis, and HIV infection should be done. Results of the maternal tests for hepatitis B surface antigen should be confirmed.

B. **Antibiotic therapy**

1. **Known exposure at birth (maternal infection) but asymptomatic.** Because of the serious nature of neonatal disease, it is recommended that exposed infants receive a single injection of ceftriaxone (25–50 mg/kg; maximum 125 mg). The mother and her sexual partner(s) should be evaluated (and treated) for other sexually transmitted infections, including HIV.

2. **Ophthalmia neonatorum (and other localized infections).** Treatment is ceftriaxone (25–50 mg/kg; maximum 125 mg) intravenously or intramuscularly in a single dose. Do not use ceftriaxone in neonates who have hyperbilirubinemia, especially those born preterm or in neonates (28 days of age or younger) receiving or expected to receive calcium containing IV products. Alternative treatment is cefotaxime as a single dose (100 mg/kg). Infants should have their eyes irrigated with saline immediately and at frequent intervals until the discharge is eliminated. Topical antibiotics are inadequate and unnecessary with systemic therapy. Infants with conjunctivitis should be hospitalized and evaluated as described earlier. Treatment of ophthalmia neonatorum may need to be continued beyond the single treatment dose until systemic infection has been ruled out.

3. **Disseminated infections and scalp abscesses. For arthritis, septicemia or abscesses:** Ceftriaxone (25–50 mg/kg/d as single daily dose) or cefotaxime (25 mg/kg every 12 hours) for 7 days. **For meningitis:** Ceftriaxone or cefotaxime for 10 to 14 days. Use cefotaxime if the infant has hyperbilirubinemia or if he or she is receiving calcium-containing intravenous fluids.

C. **Isolation.** All infants with gonococcal infection should be placed in contact isolation until effective parenteral antimicrobial therapy has been given for 24 hours. See Appendix F.

VII. **Prognosis.** Excellent if treatment is started early.

136 Hepatitis

Neonatal hepatitis is an inflammation of the liver tissue in a newborn infant and may be caused by many infectious and noninfectious agents. Typically, viral hepatitis refers to several clinically similar diseases that differ in cause and epidemiology. These include hepatitis A, B, C, D (delta), and E. Chronic lifelong infection has only been documented with hepatitis B and hepatitis C viruses.

The differential diagnosis of newborn liver disease includes idiopathic neonatal hepatitis (giant cell), biliary atresia, metabolic disorders, antitrypsin deficiency, cystic fibrosis, iron storage disease, and other infectious agents that cause hepatocellular injury (eg, cytomegalovirus [CMV], herpes simplex, rubella, varicella, toxoplasmosis, *Listeria monocytogenes*, syphilis, and tuberculosis, as well as bacterial sepsis, which can cause nonspecific hepatic dysfunction). Table 136–1 outlines various hepatitis panel tests useful in the management of this disease. Isolation precautions for all infectious diseases, including maternal and neonatal precautions, breast feeding, and visiting issues, can be found in Appendix F. This chapter will go over neonatal hepatitis caused by Hepatitis A, B, C, D, and E.

HEPATITIS A

I. **Definition.** Hepatitis A is also known as **infectious hepatitis** and is caused by a non-enveloped 27-nM RNA virus that is a member of the Picornaviridae family (hepatitis A virus [HAV]). It is transmitted by the fecal–oral route. A high concentration of the virus is found in stools of infected persons, especially during the late incubation and early symptomatic phases. Children, especially neonates, may excrete HAV for a more prolonged period than has been noted in adults. HAV RNA is detected in neonatal stool samples for 4 to 5 months in 23% of infants diagnosed with HAV infection. Incubation period is 15 to 50 days. There is no chronic carrier state.

Table 136–1. HEPATITIS TESTING

Specific Test	Description
HAV	Etiologic agent of "infectious" hepatitis
Anti-HAV	Detectable at onset of symptoms; lifetime persistence
Anti-HAV-IgM	Indicates recent infection with HAV; positive up to 4–6 months after infection
Anti-HAV-IgG	Signifies previous HAV infection; confers immunity
HBV	Etiologic agent of "serum" hepatitis
HBsAg	Detectable in serum; earliest indicator of acute infection or indicative of chronic infection if present >6 months
Anti-HBs	Indicates past infection with and immunity to HBV, passive antibody from HBIG, or immune response from HBV vaccine
HBeAg	Correlates with HBV replication; high-titer HBV in serum signifies high infectivity; persistence for 6–8 weeks suggests a chronic carrier state
Anti-HBe	Presence in carrier of HBsAg suggests a lower titer of HBV and lower risk of transmitting HBV
HBcAg	No commercial test available; found only in liver tissue
Anti-HBc	Identifies people with acute, resolved, or chronic HBV infection (not present after immunization); high titer indicates active HBV infection; low titer presents in chronic infection
Anti-HBc-IgM	Recent infection with HBV positive for 4–6 months after infection; detectable in "window" period after surface antigen disappears
Anti-HBc-IgG	Appears later and may persist for years if viral replication continues
HCV	Etiologic agent of hepatitis C
Anti-HCV	Serologic determinant of hepatitis C infection
HDV	Etiologic agent for delta hepatitis
anti-HDV IgG	Serologic determinant of delta hepatitis infection
HEV	Hepatitis E virus, a common cause of infectious hepatitis worldwide
anti-HEV IgG	Serologic determinant of HEV infection

anti-HAV, antibody to HAV (IgM and IgG subclasses); anti-HAV-IgG, IgG class antibody to HAV; anti-HAV-IgM, IgM class antibody to HAV; anti-HBc, antibody to HBcAg; anti-HBc-IgG, IgG class antibody to HBcAg; anti-HBc-IgM, IGM class antibody to HBcAg; anti-HBe, antibody to HBeAg; anti-HBs, antibody to HBsAg; anti-HCV, antibody to hepatitis C; anti-HDV-IgG, IgG class antibody to HDV; anti-HEV-IgG, IgG class antibody to HEV; HBeAg, hepatitis B e antigen; HBcAg, hepatitis B core antigen; HBsAg, hepatitis B surface antigen; HBV, hepatitis B virus; HCV, hepatitis C virus; HDV, hepatitis D virus; HEV, hepatitis E virus; IgM and IgG, immunoglobulins M and G.

II. **Incidence.** The true incidence of HAV infection in neonates is unknown. The overall incidence of HAV infection in the US population decreased significantly after the introduction of HAV vaccine (26,150 cases per year from 1980–1999 to 1390 cases per year in 2015; ~0.4/100,000).

III. **Pathophysiology.** In addition to fecal–oral transmission, parenteral transmission is possible via blood transfusion. HAV infection in pregnancy, especially in the second or third trimester, is associated with increased risk of preterm labor. Maternal–infant transmission appears to be very rare; however, both intrauterine and perinatal transmissions have been documented in case reports. The risk of transmission is limited because the period of viremia is short, and fecal contamination does not occur at the time of delivery. Occasional outbreaks of HAV infection in neonatal intensive care units (NICUs) have been reported, presumably from neonates infected through transfused blood who subsequently transmitted HAV to other neonates and staff. Severe disease in an otherwise healthy infant is rare.

IV. **Risk factors.** The newborn infant born to an infected mother whose symptoms began between 2 weeks before and 1 week after delivery is at risk. Risk factors for postnatal acquisition of HAV include poor hygiene, poor sanitation, contact with an infected individual (which can be nosocomial), and recent travel to a developing country where the disease is endemic.

V. **Clinical presentation.** Most infected infants (>80%) are asymptomatic, with mild abnormalities of liver function.

VI. **Diagnosis**

   A. **Immunoglobulin M antibody to hepatitis A virus.** Present during the acute or early convalescent phase of disease. In most cases, it becomes detectable 5 to 10 days after exposure and can persist for up to 6 months after infection. Occasionally, false-positive results may occur; in addition, anti-HAV immunoglobulin (Ig) M is detectable in up to 20% of vaccine recipients when measured 2 weeks after hepatitis A immunization. **Anti-HAV IgG** appears in the convalescent phase, remains detectable, and confers immunity. Research laboratories also can detect virus in blood or stool by means of reverse transcriptase–polymerase chain reaction (RT-PCR).

   B. **Liver function tests.** Characteristically, the transaminases (alanine aminotransferase [ALT] and aspartate aminotransferase [AST]) and serum bilirubin levels (total and direct) are elevated, whereas the alkaline phosphatase level is normal.

VII. **Management**

   A. **Intramuscular immunoglobulin.** A dose of 0.02 mL/kg should be given to the newborn whose mother's symptoms began between 2 weeks before and 1 week after delivery. If an outbreak of hepatitis A is documented in the nursery, postexposure prophylaxis with intramuscular immunoglobulin should be given to susceptible healthcare workers as well as exposed neonates who may have close contact with infectious secretions. Intramuscular immunoglobulin offers >85% protection against symptomatic infection.

   B. **Hepatitis A virus vaccine.** Two inactivated HAV vaccines, Havrix and Vaqta, are available in the United States. They are recommended for all children (1–18 years old). Their protective efficacy in preventing clinical HAV infection is 94% to 100%.

   C. **Isolation.** The infant should be isolated with enteric precautions.

   D. **Breast feeding.** Not contraindicated.

VIII. **Prognosis** for HAV-infected infants is favorable. Less than 20% are clinically symptomatic after infection. Chronic carrier state does not exist.

HEPATITIS B

I. **Definition.** Hepatitis B (**serum hepatitis**) is caused by a DNA-containing, 42-nM-diameter hepadnavirus (hepatitis B virus [HBV]). Important components of the viral particle include an outer lipoprotein envelope containing HBsAg and an inner nucleocapsid consisting of hepatitis B core antigen (HBc). HBV has a long incubation period (45–160 days) after exposure.

II. **Incidence.** Each year in the United States, approximately 20,000 infants are born to HBV-infected pregnant women, and without immunoprophylaxis, approximately 5500 would become chronically infected. As a result of universal immunization against HBV, the incidence of acute HBV infection among US children decreased by 98% between 1990 and 2014.

III. **Pathophysiology.** Transmission in the fetus and newborn has been suggested by the following mechanisms:

   A. **Transplacental transmission** is either during pregnancy or at the time of delivery secondary to placental leaks. This is rare and accounts for <2% of neonatal infections.

   B. **Intrapartum transmission** occurs by exposure to HBV in amniotic fluid, vaginal secretions, or maternal blood; accounts for 90% of neonatal infections. Vaginal delivery appears to increase the risk compared with cesarean section.

   C. **Postnatal transmission.** By blood transfusion and other unknown mechanisms. Breast feeding is not a risk factor for postnatal transmission.

   D. **Father-to-child transmission** of HBV can rarely occur through the germ cells to the offspring or postnatal intimate contact. The germline route is considered an intrauterine infection.

IV. **Risk factors**

   A. **Factors associated with higher rates of hepatitis B virus transmission to neonates** include the following:

      1. **The presence of hepatitis B e antigen and absence of anti–hepatitis B e antigen in maternal serum:** Attack rates of 70% to 90%, with up to 90% of these infants becoming chronic carriers. In hepatitis B e antigen (HBeAg)-negative and hepatitis B surface antigen (HBsAg)-positive mothers, the transmission rate is 5% to 20%; however, those infants are at risk for acute hepatitis and acute fulminant hepatitis.

      2. **Asian racial origin,** particularly Chinese, with attack rates of 40% to 70%.

      3. **Maternal acute hepatitis in the third trimester or immediately postpartum** (70% attack rate).

      4. **High maternal Hepatitis B DNA level.**

      5. **Vaginal delivery.**

      6. **Antigenemia present in older siblings.**

V. **Clinical presentation.** Maternal HBV infection has not been associated with abortion, stillbirth, or congenital malformations. Prematurity has occurred, especially with acute hepatitis during pregnancy. Fetuses or newborns exposed to HBV present a wide spectrum of disease, but most (>90%) will become chronic carriers. Because of the long incubation period, symptoms do not occur in the neonatal period. Even after the neonatal period, infants are rarely ill; jaundice appears <3% of the time. They typically have normal ALT concentrations and minimal or mild liver histologic abnormalities, with detectable HBeAg and high HBV DNA concentrations (≥20,000 IU/mL) for years to decades after initial infection ("immune-tolerant phase"). Various clinical presentations include the following:

   A. **Mild transient acute infection.**

   B. **Chronic active hepatitis with or without cirrhosis.**

   C. **Chronic persistent hepatitis.**

   D. **Chronic asymptomatic hepatitis B surface antigen carriage.**

   E. **Fulminant fatal hepatitis B (rare).**

   F. **Hepatocellular carcinoma in older children and young adults (rare).**

VI. **Diagnosis**

   A. **Differential diagnosis.** Major diseases to consider include biliary atresia and acute hepatitis secondary to other viruses (eg, HAV, CMV, rubella, and herpes simplex virus).

   B. **Liver function tests.** ALT and AST levels may be increased before the rise in bilirubin levels.

   C. **Hepatitis panel testing.** See Table 136–1.

      1. **Mother.** Test for HBsAg, HBeAg, anti-HBe, and anti-HBc.

      2. **Infant.** Test for HBsAg and anti-HBc IgM. Anti-HBc IgM is highly specific for establishing the diagnosis of acute infection and is the only marker of acute infection during the "window" period. Most infants demonstrate HBsAg

antigenemia by 6 months of age, with peak acquisition at 3 to 4 months. Nucleic acid amplification testing (NAAT), gene amplification techniques (eg, polymerase chain reaction assay, branched DNA methods), and hybridization assays are available to detect and quantify HBV DNA. Cord blood is not a reliable indicator of neonatal infection because contamination could have occurred with antigen-positive maternal blood or vaginal secretions and possible noninfectious antigenemia from the mother. Transient HBsAg antigenemia can occur following receipt of hepatitis B (HB) vaccine, with HBsAg being detected as early as 24 hours after and up to 2 to 3 weeks following administration of the vaccine.

VII. Management

A. Hepatitis B surface antigen–positive mother. If the mother is HBsAg positive, regardless of the status of her HBe antigen or antibody, the infant should be given hepatitis B immune globulin (HBIG), 0.5 mL intramuscularly, within 12 hours after delivery. In addition, HB vaccine is given at birth (within 12 hours), at 1 month, and at 6 months of age. If the first dose is given simultaneously with HBIG, it should be administered at a separate site, preferably in the opposite leg. **For preterm infants weighing <2 kg, this initial dose of vaccine should not be counted in the required 3-dose schedule,** and the subsequent 3 doses should be initiated when the infant is 30 days old. HBIG and HB vaccine do not interfere with routine childhood immunizations. No specific antiviral therapy exists for acute HBV infection in infants <3 months age; however, the US Food and Drug Administration (FDA) licensed lamivudine (≥3 months of age) and interferon (≥1 year of age) as treatment of chronic HBV in children. The goal of treatment is to prevent progression to cirrhosis, hepatic failure, and hepatocellular carcinoma (HCC). Current indications for treatment of chronic HBV infection include evidence of ongoing HBV viral replication, as indicated by the presence for longer than 6 months of serum HBV DNA >20,000 IU/mL without HBeAg positivity, >2000 IU/mL with HBeAg positivity, and elevated serum ALT concentrations for longer than 6 months or evidence of chronic hepatitis on liver biopsy. Consultation with an infectious disease specialist is recommended for clinical monitoring and treatment.

B. Infant born to mother whose hepatitis B surface antigen status is unknown. Test the mother as soon as possible. While awaiting the results, give the infant HBV vaccine within 12 hours of birth. If the mother is found to be HBsAg positive, the infant should receive HBIG (0.5 mL) as soon as feasible (within 7 days) of birth. If the infant's **birthweight is <2000 g** and the maternal HBsAg status cannot be determined within the initial 12 hours after birth, HBIG should be given as well as HB vaccine.

C. Infant born to hepatitis B surface antigen–negative mother. For all infants with birth weight ≥2000 g, administer HB vaccine as a universal routine prophylaxis within 24 hours of birth. Deferral to a time after birth or discharge from the hospital no longer is considered to be an acceptable option, because it might deprive an HBV-exposed infant of timely administration of HBV prophylaxis. For all infants with birthweight <2000 g, administer HB vaccine as a universal routine prophylaxis at 1 month of age or at hospital discharge (whichever is first).

D. Isolation. Precautions are needed in handling blood and secretions.

E. Breast feeding. HBsAg has been detected in breast milk of HBsAg-positive mothers but only with special concentrating techniques. With appropriate immunoprophylaxis (HBIG and HB vaccine), breast feeding of infants of chronic HBV carrier mothers poses no additional risk for the transmission of the HBV. Therefore, breast feeding should be encouraged.

F. Vaccine efficacy. The overall protective efficiency rate in neonates given HB vaccine and HBIG is approximately 95%. The World Health Organization recommends that all countries add HB vaccine to their routine childhood immunization programs. Such programs (in Taiwan) have been shown to lower the incidence of chronic HBsAg carrier state, fulminant hepatic failure, and HCC. Infants born to HBsAg-positive women should be tested for anti-HBs and HBsAg after completion of the immunization (1–2 months after the last vaccine dose) at 9 to 12 months of age, generally at the next well-child visit after completion of the vaccine series. Testing should not be performed before 9 months of age to maximize the likelihood of detecting late-onset HBV infections. HBsAg-negative infants with anti-HBs titers <10 mIU/mL after completing the 3-dose vaccine series should be revaccinated with a single dose of HB vaccine and retested for anti-HBs antibody titers 1 to 2 months later. Infants who have anti-HBs titers ≥10 mIU/mL after this fourth dose of HB vaccine do not need any additional doses of the HB vaccine. Infants who fail to reach anti-HBs titers ≥10 mIU/mL after the fourth dose of HB vaccine should receive 2 additional doses of the HB vaccine followed by retesting for anti-HBs antibody titers 1 to 2 months later.

   G. Prevention of hepatitis B vaccine failure. Failure of combined immunoprophylaxis (HBIG and HB vaccine) occurs in approximately 5% infants born to HBsAg-positive mothers. Often these infants are HBsAg positive at birth, suggesting the infection is already established in utero. Their mothers may have acquired the infection in the third trimester and/or have had a high viral load at time of delivery. Specifically, women with HBV DNA >10^6 to 10^8 IU/mL or who are HBeAg positive have an increased risk of perinatal transmission even if appropriate combined immunoprophylaxis is given to the newborn infant (~15%–30% risk of transmission vs <5% risk of transmission for women with lower HBV DNA or who are HBeAg negative). For these women, antiviral therapy with tenofovir, telbivudine, or lamivudine in the third trimester (in addition to HBIG and HB vaccine to the newborn) may further reduce the transmission rate to 0% to 2%. Telbivudine presents a favorable safety profile during pregnancy.

VIII. Prognosis. The majority of perinatally infected infants remain clinically healthy. Approximately 30% to 50% develop persistently elevated transaminase values on liver function tests. About 5% have moderately severe histopathologic changes on liver biopsy. Late complications such as cirrhosis and HCC are rare.

HEPATITIS C

   I. Definition. Hepatitis C virus (HCV) is a small, single-stranded, enveloped RNA virus that is a member of the Flaviviridae family. At least 6 HCV genotypes exist with multiple subtypes.

   II. Incidence. The pediatric prevalence of HCV is approximately 0.1%. The true incidence of neonatal HCV is unknown. A 3-fold increase in reported cases of acute HCV was seen recently in the United States, mostly attributed to rising rates of injection-drug use such as heroin and oxycodone.

   III. Pathophysiology. HCV is transmitted primarily by parenteral means. Historically, exposure to blood and blood products was the most common source of infection; however, because of screening tests to exclude infectious donors, the risk of HCV is currently estimated to be 1 per 2 million units transfused. The most common route of infection for children is maternal–fetal transmission. Seroprevalence among pregnant women is estimated to be at 1% to 2%. The risk of perinatal transmission averages 5% to 6%, and transmission occurs only from women who are HCV RNA positive at the time of delivery. Infants of HCV-positive mothers are more likely to be low birthweight, to be growth restricted, and to require NICU admission.

   IV. Risk factors
      A. Maternal hepatitis C virus viremia correlates with transmission. However, viremia levels fluctuate over time, and no "safe level" can be defined below which transmission never occurs.

    B. Maternal human immunodeficiency virus–hepatitis C virus coinfection is associated with a 2- to 3-fold increase in risk of transmission. This may be explained, in part, by higher HCV RNA levels resulting from human immunodeficiency virus (HIV)-mediated immunosuppression

    C. Maternal intravenous drug use. Several studies have shown that the maternal history of intravenous drug use increases the risk for perinatal transmission of HCV.

    D. Prolonged rupture of membranes and obstetric procedures. Rupture of membranes >6 hours before delivery and obstetric procedures, such as amniocentesis and scalp electrode monitoring of the fetus during delivery, may increase the risk of HCV transmission. However, **mode of delivery** (eg, cesarean delivery) does not seem to offer any protection except if the mother is co-infected with HIV.

V. Clinical presentation. The average incubation period is about 6 to 7 weeks. Infants with acute hepatitis C typically are asymptomatic, have mildly elevated transaminases, or occasionally have a mild clinical illness. Spontaneous clearance, typically by 3 years of age, occurs in 10% to 20% of the cases. Of the remainder, approximately 70% experience chronic hepatitis (majority asymptomatic), 20% develop cirrhosis, and 1% develop HCC.

VI. Diagnosis of HCV infection in infants can be made by detecting **anti-HCV IgG** in serum after 15 months of age. Testing for anti-HCV IgG earlier may detect maternal transplacentally acquired antibodies (may persist until 18 months of age). For earlier diagnosis, NAAT to detect **HCV RNA** (commercially available and approved by FDA) can be performed as early as 2 months of age. NAATs carry a low sensitivity if used at birth. All children born to HCV-infected women need to be tested with NAAT at 2 to 3 months of age and again at 6 months of age. Two positive tests are highly suggestive of infection. Regardless of NAAT testing, anti-HCV IgG needs to be done after 15 months of age. Assays for anti-HCV IgM are not available. Liver function tests may be elevated and fluctuate widely over time. Neonates diagnosed with HCV infection should also be screened for co-infection with HBV and HIV due to common modes of transmission.

VII. Management

    A. If the mother was infected during the last trimester. The risk of transmission to the infant is highest. Successful treatment of HCV infection (elimination of viremia) significantly reduces the risk of mother-to-infant transmission; however, there are no FDA approved therapies for HCV that can be used during pregnancy. Women with HCV infection should be treated prior to conception if possible, and they should avoid pregnancy for at least 6 months after completing a ribavirin-containing regimen (due to teratogenic effects). Immune globulin prophylaxis is not recommended.

    B. Breast feeding. HCV RNA has been detected in breast milk and colostrum of viremic mothers; however, transmission of HCV by breast feeding has not been documented. According to guidelines of the Centers for Disease Control and Prevention and the American Academy of Pediatrics, asymptomatic maternal HCV infection is not a contraindication to breast feeding. Mothers who are HCV positive and choose to breast feed should consider abstaining if their nipples are cracked or bleeding.

    C. Treatment. Currently, the only FDA-approved treatment for HCV in children 3 to 17 years of age consists of a combination of peginterferon and ribavirin. The treatment of chronic HCV infection is rapidly evolving, and several trials of **direct-acting antiviral agents** such as ledipasvir and sofosbuvir as well as combination drug regimens are being evaluated in several trials. HCV genotyping is useful for guiding the selection and duration of therapy. In 2017, the FDA approved sofosbuvir plus ribavirin and ledipasvir plus sofosbuvir for treatment of HCV infection in children age 12 years and older. There are different protocols that depend on the HCV genotype. These agents permit effective, well-tolerated, all-oral, interferon-free regimens for most patients. No specific therapy is currently recommended for HCV-positive infants; consultation with a pediatric infectious disease specialist should be sought as the field and use of direct-acting antiviral agents is rapidly evolving. All infants with chronic HCV infection should be **immunized against HAV and HBV** because of the very high rate of severe hepatitis if co-infection with HAV or HBV develops. Evidence-based consensus recommendations for management of HCV can be found online (**www.HCVguidelines.org**).

VIII.   **Prognosis.** Approximately 10% to 20% of children with perinatally acquired HCV infection clear the virus during the first 2 years of life; the rest will develop chronic hepatitis. Genotype 3 is associated with better chance of spontaneous clearance. Progression to cirrhosis occurs in 20% of patients with chronic hepatitis, typically over an average of 20 years. Decompensated cirrhosis develops in approximately 2%. Risk factors for end-stage liver disease include perinatal exposure, maternal drug use, and infection with HCV genotype 1a. Children with such features should be considered for early treatment. HCC is rare and occurs almost exclusively in children with additional risk factors such as cirrhosis, co-infection with HBV, and history of childhood leukemia or other malignancy

HEPATITIS D

Hepatitis D virus (HDV), also known as **delta hepatitis**, is a defective RNA virus that cannot survive independently and requires the helper function of HBV DNA. Therefore, it occurs either as coinfection (simultaneous with the initial HBV) or as superinfection (infection in a person already chronically infected with HBV). Acquisition of HDV is by parenteral, percutaneous, or mucous membrane inoculation. The incubation period for HDV superinfection is approximately 2 to 8 weeks. Transmission from mother to newborn infant has been documented but is uncommon. Prevention of HBV infection prevents hepatitis D. There are, however, no available treatments to prevent HDV in HBsAg carriers before or after exposure. Management should be similar to that for HBV infection (see prior discussion). Diagnosis of HDV is based on the detection of antibody to HDV (anti-HDV IgG) by radioimmunoassay or enzyme immunoassay as well as HDV RNA testing (by RT-PCR). HDV status should be assessed in known carriers of HBV because co-infection may lead to acute or fulminant hepatitis or a more rapid progression of chronic hepatitis and development of HCC. HDV is difficult to treat; however, data suggest pegylated interferon-alfa for 1 year may result in up to 40% of patients having a sustained response to therapy.

HEPATITIS E

Hepatitis E virus (HEV) is a nonenveloped, positive-sense, single-stranded RNA virus; it usually causes a self-limiting acute hepatitis similar to HAV. Transmission is by fecal–oral route. Unlike other viral hepatitis, certain HEV genotypes (genotypes 3 and 4) also have zoonotic hosts, such as swine, and can be transmitted by eating undercooked pork. HEV genotypes 1 and 2 exclusively infect humans. Person-to-person transmission appears to be much less efficient than with HAV virus but occurs in sporadic and outbreak settings. HEV also is transmitted through blood product transfusion. HEV is the most common cause of viral hepatitis in the world. Globally, an estimated 20 million HEV infections occur annually, resulting in 3.4 million cases of acute hepatitis and 70,000 deaths. HEV is particularly common in Africa and the Indian subcontinent. In the United States, HEV infection is uncommon and generally occurs in travelers returning from endemic areas or swine workers. However, seroprevalence is higher than expected based on clinical disease (20% of the population have anti-HEV IgG). HEV commonly causes an acute illness with jaundice, malaise, fever, and arthralgia. Hepatitis E is clinically indistinguishable from hepatitis A. It is rarely symptomatic in children <15 years old. There is a very high maternal mortality (10%–25%) when HEV is acquired during pregnancy, especially during the third trimester. Mother-to-infant transmission is high

(50%–100%). Fetal loss or early neonatal mortality is also significant. Commercial kits are available to detect anti-HEV IgG and IgM. Definitive diagnosis may be made by demonstrating viral RNA in serum or stool by RT-PCR. The only treatment is supportive. It is unclear if breast feeding is a potential route of HEV transmission. A recombinant HEV vaccine evaluated in a phase III clinical trial was demonstrated to be effective in preventing disease and is approved for use by the Chinese Food and Drug Administration.

137 Herpes Simplex Viruses

I. **Definition.** Herpes simplex viruses (HSV-1 and HSV-2) are enveloped, double-stranded DNA viruses. They are part of the herpes group, which also includes cytomegalovirus, Epstein-Barr virus, varicella-zoster virus, and human herpes viruses (HHV-6 and HHV-7). HSV infection is among the most prevalent of all viral infections encountered by humans.

II. **Incidence.** The incidence of neonatal HSV infection is estimated to range from 1 in 2000 to 1 in 3000 live births. As of 2014, seroprevalence of HSV-1 and HSV-2 in pregnant women in the United States was approximately 59.3% and 21.1%, respectively.

III. **Pathophysiology.** HSV enters the human host through inoculation of oral, genital, or conjunctival mucosa or breaks in skin, infects the sensory nerve endings, and then passes via retrograde axonal flow to the dorsal root ganglia, where it remains for the life of the host. Two serologic subtypes can be distinguished by antigenic and serologic tests: HSV-1 (usually affects face and skin above the waist) and HSV-2 (genitalia and skin below the waist). Three quarters of neonatal herpes infections are secondary to HSV-2. HSV-1, however, can be the cause of maternal genital herpes infections in 9% of the cases, and its rate appears to be increasing (eg, HSV-1 is the major serotype causing neonatal disease in Australia). HSV infection of the neonate can be acquired at 1 of 3 times: intrauterine, intrapartum, or postnatal. Most infections (85%) are acquired in the **intrapartum** period as ascending infections with ruptured membranes (the period of 4–6 hours is considered a critical period for this to occur) or by delivery through an infected cervix or vagina. An additional 10% of infected neonates acquire the virus **postnatally** (eg, from someone shedding HSV from the mouth who then kisses the infant). The final 5% of neonatal HSV infections occur **in utero**. In utero infection is acquired transplacentally and occurs only in women with primary HSV infection. It is usually associated with placental infarcts and necrotizing funisitis and may result in miscarriage, congenital anomalies, preterm birth, and/or fetal growth restriction. The incubation period is from 2 to 20 days. Three general patterns of neonatal HSV infection are recognized: **disease localized to the skin, eyes, and mouth (SEM)**; **central nervous system (CNS) disease** (with or without SEM involvement); and **disseminated disease** (which also may include signs of the first 2 groups). Maternal infection can be **classified** as either *first-episode* or *recurrent* infections. First-episode infections are further classified as either *primary* or *first-episode nonprimary* based on type-specific serologic testing. *Primary infections* are those in which the mother is experiencing a new infection with either HSV-1 or HSV-2 and has not already been infected with the other virus type. *First-episode nonprimary* infections are those in which the mother has a new infection with 1 virus type, usually HSV-2, but has antibodies to the other virus type, usually HSV-1. Infants born vaginally to mothers with a true primary infection are at highest risk, with a transmission rate of approximately 60%. Those born to a mother with a first-episode nonprimary infection are at a somewhat lower risk of 25%. The lowest risk infants (2%) are those born to mothers with recurrent infections. Maternal antibody is not always protective in the fetus.

IV. **Risk factors.** The risk of genital herpes infection varies with maternal age, socioeconomic status, and number of sexual partners. Only approximately 12% of pregnant women who test seropositive for HSV-2 give a clinical history suggestive of the disease. The first-episode infection may stay "active" with asymptomatic cervical shedding for as long as 2 months. Besides a first-episode infection (primary or nonprimary), additional risk factors for neonatal HSV infection include acquisition of HSV shortly before labor, viral genital shedding in labor, genital shedding of HSV-1 rather than HSV-2, the use of a fetal-scalp electrode, preterm birth, and maternal age <21 years.

V. **Clinical presentation.** Congenital in utero HSV infection is rare and is associated with high rate of fetal demise; it shares clinical features such as microcephaly, hydrocephalus, and chorioretinitis with other congenital infections. In addition, skin ulcerations or scarring and eye damage are commonly noted. The neonatal disease is commonly acquired intrapartum. It may be localized or disseminated. Humoral and cellular immune mechanisms appear important in preventing initial HSV infections or limiting their spread. Infants with disseminated and SEM disease generally present at 10 to 12 days of life, whereas patients with CNS disease usually present at 16 to 19 days of life. More than 20% of infants with disseminated disease and 30% to 40% of infants with encephalitis never have skin vesicles (see Figure 80–10).

A. **Skin, eyes, and mouth disease.** HSV disease localized to the skin, eyes, or oral cavity accounts for approximately 45% of the cases. **Skin lesions** vary from discrete vesicles to large bullous lesions and denuded skin. It typically involves the presenting part (eg, vertex) and sites of skin trauma (eg, scalp electrodes). There is skin involvement in 80% to 85% of SEM cases. **Ulcerative mouth lesions** (~10% of SEM cases) with or without cutaneous involvement can be seen. **Ocular findings** include keratoconjunctivitis and chorioretinitis (see Chapter 58). Without treatment, there is a high risk of progression to encephalitis or disseminated disease.

B. **Disseminated disease** accounts for 25% of neonatal HSV disease and carries the worst prognosis with respect to mortality. Patients commonly present with fever, lethargy, apnea, and a septic shock–like picture, including respiratory collapse (hemorrhagic pneumonitis), liver failure, neutropenia, thrombocytopenia, and disseminated intravascular coagulation (DIC). Approximately half of these cases also have SEM manifestations, and 60% to 75% have CNS involvement. Skin involvement may appear late, but approximately 20% of infants with disseminated disease will not develop any cutaneous vesicles during the course of their illness. Recognition of the disseminated HSV disease is often delayed. It should be suspected in any infant presenting with a sepsis-like picture associated with thrombocytopenia, elevated liver enzymes, consumptive coagulopathy, and cerebrospinal fluid (CSF) pleocytosis.

C. **Central nervous system disease** accounts for approximately 30% of neonatal HSV infection. It may develop as a result of localized retrograde spread from the nasopharynx and olfactory nerves to the brain or through hematogenous spread in neonates with disseminated disease. Clinical manifestations include seizures (focal and generalized), lethargy, irritability, tremors, poor feeding, temperature instability, and a bulging fontanelle. These infants usually present at 16 to 19 days of age, and 30% to 40% have no herpetic skin lesions. CSF findings are variable and typically show a mild pleocytosis, increased protein, and a slightly low glucose. Abnormalities of the CSF may be more pronounced as CNS disease progresses.

VI. **Diagnosis.** Diagnosis of neonatal HSV infection can be challenging, and the diagnosis is often delayed. Early manifestations are subtle and nonspecific (especially for the disseminated form). The maternal history is often not helpful (negative in 80% of the cases).

A. **Laboratory studies**

1. **Surface viral cultures.** Isolation of HSV by culture remains the definitive diagnostic method of documenting infection. Skin or mucous membrane lesions or surfaces (mouth, nasopharynx, conjunctivae, and anus) are scraped and transferred in appropriate viral transport media on ice. Swab specimens from mouth, nasopharynx, conjunctivae, and anus can be obtained with a single swab starting with the eyes and ending with the anus and placed in 1 viral transport media tube. With the exception of CNS involvement, the important information gathered from such cultures is the presence or absence of the replicating virus, rather than its precise location. Preliminary results may become available in 24 to 72 hours. Positive cultures obtained from any of these sites more than 12 to 24 hours after birth indicate viral replication and, therefore, are suggestive of infant infection rather than mere contamination after intrapartum exposure.

2. **Polymerase chain reaction.** Polymerase chain reaction (PCR) is an important tool in the diagnosis of HSV infection. PCR has been used to detect HSV DNA in **CSF** and **blood** specimens. PCR is especially useful for the diagnosis of HSV encephalitis. Overall sensitivities of CSF PCR in neonatal HSV disease have ranged from 75% to 100%, with overall specificities ranging from 71% to 100%. Negative CSF PCR does not exclude the diagnosis of HSV CNS disease; it may be negative early in the course of the disease or if the test is done after antiviral therapy has been given for a few days. PCR is especially important in monitoring therapy of CNS disease, with discontinuation of therapy only when PCR is negative. Blood PCR assay should not supplant surface cultures or be used to classify disease because viremia can be present in any of the 3 forms of disease. The performance of PCR assay on skin and mucosal specimens from neonates has not been studied; if used, surface or skin PCR assays should be performed in addition to (and not instead of) the gold standard surface culture.

3. **Immunologic assays.** Immunologic assays to detect HSV antigen in lesion scrapings, usually using monoclonal anti-HSV antibodies in either an enzyme-linked immunosorbent assay or direct fluorescent antibody staining, are very specific and 80% to 90% sensitive.

4. **Liver function tests.** Measuring serum liver function tests, especially alanine aminotransferase (ALT), is recommended. HSV characteristically invades the liver and causes hepatocellular damage.

5. **Serologic tests.** These are not helpful in the diagnosis of neonatal infection but are helpful in diagnosing and classifying maternal disease (primary vs secondary).

6. **Lumbar puncture** should be performed in all suspected cases including SEM disease. CSF may be normal early in the course of the disease but typically will show a mononuclear cell pleocytosis, normal or moderately low glucose, and mildly elevated protein. Contrary to the historical suggestion, erythrocytes are not notably increased in HSV CNS disease. HSV PCR should always be performed on CSF.

B. **Imaging and other studies**

1. **Brain imaging with computed tomography or preferably magnetic resonance imaging** is recommended in all infants with HSV CNS disease. Findings include parenchymal brain edema or attenuation, hemorrhage, and destructive lesions, especially in the temporal lobe.

2. **Electroencephalogram.** Should be performed in all neonates suspected to have CNS involvement (seizures, abnormal CSF, abnormal neurologic examination). Electroencephalogram is often abnormal very early in the course of the CNS disease; it may show focal or multifocal epileptiform discharges before abnormal changes are detected by computed tomography or magnetic resonance imaging.

VII. Management

A. Antepartum. The history of genital herpes in a pregnant woman or in her partner(s) should be solicited and recorded in the prenatal record. If a positive history is obtained, the following steps may be taken:

1. **Antiviral therapy.** **Acyclovir** or **valacyclovir** may be given to pregnant women who have a primary episode of genital HSV as well as to women with an active infection (primary or secondary) near or at the time of delivery. Multiple trials showed that prophylactic acyclovir beginning at 36 weeks' gestation, given to women who present with a genital HSV lesion anytime during pregnancy, reduces the risk of clinical HSV recurrence at delivery, cesarean delivery, and HSV viral shedding at delivery. Valacyclovir also demonstrated similar results in randomized studies. These studies did not identify any neonatal side effects from maternal suppressive therapy. These infants will need to be monitored closely because the risk of neonatal HSV infection is not totally eliminated. See dosing in Chapter 155.

2. **If there are no visible lesions** at the onset of labor or prodromal symptoms, vaginal delivery is acceptable.

3. **Cesarean delivery is recommended** in women with a history of HSV who have genital HSV lesions or prodromal HSV symptoms at the time of labor. Some experts also recommend cesarean delivery for women who had a primary or nonprimary first episode genital infection during the latter weeks of pregnancy (eg, within 6 weeks of delivery) even with no active genital lesions at the time of labor, due to significant and prolonged viral shedding. Debate exists if membranes have already been ruptured for >4 hours in the presence of active lesion; most experts still recommend cesarean delivery in this situation. All neonates delivered by cesarean section should be monitored closely because neonatal HSV infections have occasionally occurred despite delivery before the membranes rupture.

B. Neonatal treatment

1. **Infants born to mothers with a genital lesion.** The American Academy of Pediatrics has published an algorithm (Figures 137–1 and 137–2) addressing management of asymptomatic neonates following vaginal or cesarean delivery to women with active genital HSV lesions. The algorithm calls for obtaining HSV surface cultures and HSV blood PCR (in addition to CSF cell count, chemistries, and HSV PCR, as well as serum ALT when maternal history for HSV is negative) in all exposed infants at approximately 24 hours of age. Because of the high transmission rate after primary or first episode nonprimary maternal infection (25%–60%), the algorithm recommends preemptive therapy for those exposed infants with acyclovir at 60 mg/kg/d for 10 days. Infants exposed to active lesions with maternal recurrent infection have 2% risk of acquiring the neonatal HSV disease; those infants can be monitored clinically with education of the family about signs and symptoms of the disease and treatment only if the infant becomes symptomatic.

2. **Infants born to mothers with a history of genital herpes but no active genital lesions at delivery.** Should be observed for signs of infection but no surface cultures or parenteral acyclovir is needed. Education of parents and caregivers about the signs and symptoms of neonatal HSV infection during the first 6 weeks of life is prudent.

3. **Pharmacologic therapy for established herpes simplex virus disease.**

   a. Intravenous acyclovir. Neonates with HSV disease should be treated with **intravenous acyclovir at 60 mg/kg/d**, divided every 8 hours (20 mg/kg/dose). The dosing interval of intravenous acyclovir may need to be increased in premature infants, based on their creatinine clearance. Duration of therapy is a minimum of 21 days for patients with disseminated or CNS disease and 14 days for those with SEM disease. All patients with CNS involvement should

Asymptomatic neonate following vaginal or cesarean delivery to mother with visible genital lesions that are characteristic of HSV

Obstetric provider obtains swab of lesion for HSV PCR assay and culture
Type all positive results

Maternal history of genital HSV preceding pregnancy?

No

Send maternal type specific serology for HSV-1 and HSV-2 antibodies, if assays are available at the delivery hospital

At ~24 hours of age* obtain from the neonate:
- HSV surface† cultures (and PCRs if desired)
- HSV blood PCR‡
- CSF cell count, chemistries, and HSV PCR
- Serum ALT

Start IV acyclovir at 60 mg/kg/day in 3 divided doses

Determine Maternal HSV Infection Classification (Table 2)

First-Episode Primary or First-Episode Nonprimary

Recurrent infection

Yes

At ~24 hours of age* obtain from the neonate:
- HSV surface† cultures (and PCRs if desired)
- HSV blood PCR‡

If infant remains asymptomatic, do not start acyclovir

Neonatal surface cultures negative, AND blood and surface PCRs negative

Neonatal surface cultures positive, OR blood and surface PCRs positive

Obtain CSF for cell count, chemistries, and HSV PCR. Send serum ALT. Start IV acyclovir at 60 mg/kg/day in 3 divided doses

Go to Figure 137–2

Educate family on signs and symptoms of neonatal HSV disease and follow closely§

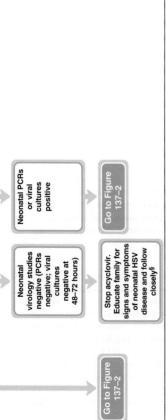

Go to Figure 137–2

Neonatal virology studies negative (PCRs negative; viral cultures negative at 48–72 hours)

Neonatal PCRs or viral cultures positive

Stop acyclovir. Educate family for signs and symptoms of neonatal HSV disease and follow closely§

Go to Figure 137–2

Evaluation and treatment is indicated prior to 24 hours of age if the infant develops signs and symptoms of neonatal HSV disease. In addition, immediate evaluation and treatment may be considered if:
• *There is prolonged rupture of membranes (>4–6 hours)*
• *The infant is premature (≤37 weeks' gestation)*

†*Conjunctivae, mouth, nasopharynx, and rectum, and scalp electrode site, if present.*

‡*HSV blood PCR is not utilized for assignment of disease classification.*

§*Discharge after 48 hours of negative HSV cultures (and negative PCRs) is acceptable if other discharge criteria have been met, there is ready access to medical care, and a person who is able to comply fully with instructions for home observation will be present. If any of these conditions is not met, the infant should be observed in the hospital until HSV cultures are finalized as negative or are negative for 96 hours after being set up in cell culture, whichever is shorter.*

This algorithm should be applied only in facilities where access to PCR and type type-specific serologic testing is readily available and turnaround time for test results is appropriately short. In situations where this is not possible, the approach detailed in the algorithm will have limited and perhaps no applicability.

TABLE 2. Maternal Infection Classification by Genital HSV Viral Type and Maternal Serology[a]

Classification of Maternal Infection	PCR/Culture from Genital Lesion	Maternal HSV-1 and HSV-2 IgG Antibody Status
Documented first-episode primary infection	Positive, either virus	Both negative
Documented first-episode nonprimary infection	Positive for HSV-1	Positive for HSV-2 AND negative for HSV-1
	Positive for HSV-2	Positive for HSV-1 AND negative for HSV-2
Assume first-episode (primary or nonprimary) infection	Positive for HSV-1 OR HSV-2	Not available
	Negative OR not available[b]	Negative for HSV-1 and/or HSV-2 OR not available
Recurrent infection	Positive for HSV-1	Positive for HSV-1
	Positive for HSV-2	Positive for HSV-2

[a]To be used for women without a clinical history of genital herpes.
[b]When a genital lesion is strongly suspicious for HSV, clinical judgment should supersede the virological test results for the conservative purposes of this neonatal management algorithm. Conversely, if in retrospect, the genital lesion was not likely to be caused by HSV and the PCR assay result or culture is negative, departure from the evaluation and management in this conservative algorithm may be warranted.

FIGURE 137–1. Algorithm for the evaluation of asymptomatic neonates following vaginal or cesarean delivery to women with active genital herpes lesions. ALT, alanine aminotransferase; D/C, discontinue; HSV, herpes simplex virus; IV, intravenous; PCR, polymerase chain reaction. (*Reproduced with permission from Kimberlin DW, Baley J; Committee on infectious diseases, et al: Guidance on management of asymptomatic neonates born to women with active genital herpes lesions, Pediatrics. 2013 Feb;131(2):e635-e646.*)

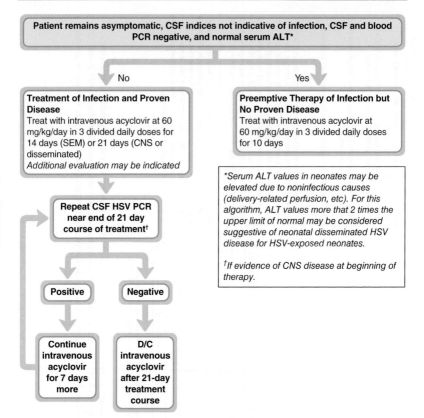

FIGURE 137–2. Algorithm for the treatment of asymptomatic neonates following vaginal or cesarean delivery to women with active genital herpes lesions. ALT, alanine aminotransferase; CNS, central nervous system; CSF, cerebrospinal fluid; D/C, discontinue; HSV, herpes simplex virus; PCR, polymerase chain reaction; SEM, skin, eyes, and mouth. (*Reproduced with permission from Kimberlin DW, Baley J; Committee on infectious diseases, et al: Guidance on management of asymptomatic neonates born to women with active genital herpes lesions,* Pediatrics. *2013 Feb;131(2):e635-e646.*)

have a repeat lumbar puncture near the end of acyclovir therapy to determine whether CSF HSV PCR is negative. Infants who remain PCR positive should receive intravenous acyclovir therapy for another week, with repeat CSF HSV PCR assay performed near the end of the extended treatment period. Parenteral acyclovir therapy should be extended in 1-week intervals until the CSF HSV PCR negativity is achieved. Absolute neutrophil counts should be followed twice weekly during the course of therapy. **If IV acyclovir is not available,** IV ganciclovir is considered a first-line alternative at a dose of 6 mg/kg every 12 hours for infants ≤90 days of age and 5 mg/kg every 12 hours for infants >90 days old.

  b. **Infants with ocular HSV involvement** should receive a topical ophthalmic drug (1% trifluridine, 0.1% iododeoxyuridine, or 0.15% ganciclovir) as well as parenteral acyclovir. An ophthalmologist should be involved in the management.

    c. **Oral acyclovir suppressive therapy** is recommended for 6 months after treatment of acute neonatal HSV disease. In particular, improved neurodevelopmental outcome has been observed with suppressive therapy after HSV CNS disease. Moreover, suppressive therapy has been associated with reduced recurrences of skin lesions after other forms of HSV. The oral acyclovir dose is 300 mg/m^2/dose, 3 times per day for 6 months; the dose should be adjusted each month to account for growth. Absolute neutrophil counts should be assessed at 2 and 4 weeks after initiating suppressive therapy and then monthly during the treatment period.

  C. **Breast feeding.** The infant may breast feed as long as no breast lesions are present on the mother, and the mother should be instructed in good hand washing technique.

  D. **Parents with orolabial herpes.** Parents should wear a mask when handling the newborn and should not kiss or nuzzle the infant.

VIII. **Prognosis.** High-dose acyclovir (60 mg/kg/d) therapy has greatly reduced **mortality** for neonatal HSV infection. Twelve-month mortality has been reduced to 29% for disseminated disease and 4% for CNS disease. Predictors of mortality include disease severity (pneumonia, DIC, seizures, and hepatitis), virus type (HSV-1 in systemic disease, HSV-2 in CNS disease), and prematurity. Systemic infection in premature infants is associated with near 100% mortality. Improvements in **morbidity** rates have not been as dramatic as with mortality. The proportion of survivors of disseminated neonatal HSV disease who have normal neurologic development has increased to 83%. In the case of CNS disease, morbidity in survivors has not changed, with only approximately 30% developing normally by 12 months of age. Seizures at or before the initiation of antiviral therapy and persistently positive CSF PCR after 4 weeks of acyclovir therapy are associated with poor neurodevelopmental outcome. The outcome for infants with SEM disease is excellent, with <2% of acyclovir recipients experiencing developmental delays. Survivors of neonatal HSV infections should undergo **developmental assessments** regularly. Cutaneous recurrences are relatively common (~50%), especially for SEM disease, and those can be reduced by suppressive oral acyclovir therapy.

138 Human Immunodeficiency Virus

I. **Definition.** Two types of human immunodeficiency virus (HIV) cause disease in humans: HIV-1 and HIV-2. These are enveloped RNA cytopathic lentiviruses belonging to the family Retroviridae. Infection is most commonly secondary to HIV-1. HIV-2 is rare in the United States but more common in West Africa. Unless otherwise specified, this chapter addresses HIV-1 infection. HIV results in a broad spectrum of disease, with **acquired immunodeficiency syndrome (AIDS)** representing the most severe end of the clinical spectrum.

II. **Incidence.** The Joint United Nations Program on HIV/AIDS estimated that 36.7 million people worldwide were infected with HIV at the end of 2015. More than 95% of the total cases reside in developing countries. In the same year, an estimated 150,000 children contracted HIV, down from 290,000 in 2010 (down 50%). This drop reflects the fact that access to services for preventing the mother-to-child transmission (MTCT) of HIV has significantly increased. The estimated number of children living with HIV declined to 1.8 million worldwide in 2015. Among infants born in the United States, the overall annual rate of perinatally acquired HIV infections decreased from 3.6 per 100,000 live births in 2008 to 1.8 per 100,000 live births in 2013.

III. **Pathophysiology.** HIV is particularly tropic for CD4⁺ T cells and cells of monocyte or macrophage lineage. After infection of the cell, viral RNA is uncoated and a double-stranded DNA transcript is made (through the activity of a viral enzyme, reverse transcriptase). This DNA then moves to the nucleus and integrates into the host genome DNA where it persists as a provirus. There is eventual destruction of both the cellular and humoral arms of the immune system. In addition, HIV gene products or cytokines elaborated by infected cells may affect macrophage, B-lymphocyte, and T-lymphocyte function. Hypergammaglobulinemia, caused by HIV-induced polyclonal B-cell activation, is often detected in early infancy. Disruption of B-cell function results in poor secondary antibody synthesis and response to vaccination. A small proportion (<10%) of patients will develop panhypogammaglobulinemia. Additionally, profound defects in cell-mediated immunity occur, allowing a predisposition to opportunistic infections such as fungus, *Pneumocystis jirovecii* pneumonia (PCP), and chronic diarrhea. The virus can also invade the central nervous system and produce psychosis and brain atrophy.

IV. **Risk factors**

A. **High-risk mother.** Any infant born to a high-risk mother is at risk. High-risk mothers include intravenous (IV) drug users, hemophiliacs, spouses of hemophiliacs, spouses of bisexual males, those with a history of exchanging sex for money or drugs, sex partners of HIV-infected persons, and those who were diagnosed with sexually transmitted infection during pregnancy. Several mechanisms account for viral transmission, but **maternal plasma HIV RNA level (viral load) is the best single predictor of MTCT risk**. Other risk factors include mode of delivery, duration of rupture of membranes, prematurity and low birthweight, cervical-vaginal viral load, low maternal CD4⁺ cell count, maternal symptomatic HIV disease/AIDS, viral subtype, and host genetic factors. Most MTCT occurs intrapartum, with smaller proportions of transmission occurring in utero and postnatally through breast feeding. Transplacental infection has been proven by evidence of infection in aborted first-trimester fetal tissues as well as isolation of HIV in blood samples obtained within 48 hours of birth. Potential routes of infection include mixture of maternal and fetal blood and infection across the placenta when its integrity is compromised (eg, placentitis [syphilitic] and chorioamnionitis).

B. **Blood transfusion.** Screening of blood donors has reduced but has not totally eliminated the risk. This happens because some newly infected persons are viremic but seronegative for 2 to 4 months and because some rare infected persons remain seronegative. The current risk of transmission of HIV per unit transfused is 1 in 2 million. (See also Chapter 19.)

C. **Breast milk.** Breast feeding is the predominant means of **postnatal HIV transmission to infants** and accounts for an estimated 25% to 45% of all MTCT events in breast-feeding populations. HIV RNA and proviral DNA have been detected in both the cell-free and cellular portions of breast milk. Colostrum viral load appears to be particularly high. Risk from breast milk is highest when maternal primary infection occurs within a few months after delivery, and it correlates with degree of viremia and breast milk HIV DNA/RNA levels. In addition, several studies have noted increased transmission among immunosuppressed women with low CD4 cell counts and in women with mastitis and breast abscesses. In areas where infant formula is accessible, affordable, safe, and sustainable, avoidance of breast feeding has represented 1 of the main components of preventing MTCT. Complete avoidance of breast feeding by HIV-infected women has been recommended by the American Academy of Pediatrics (AAP) and Centers for Disease Control and Prevention (CDC) and remains the only means by which prevention of breast-feeding transmission of HIV can be absolutely ensured. In resource-limited countries where local sanitary conditions are poor and access to infant formulas is limited, the World Health Organization (WHO) guidelines recommend **exclusive** breast feeding in combination with **maternal *and* infant** antiretroviral prophylaxis/therapy (discussed later). Exclusive breast feeding is associated with a lower risk of postnatal transmission compared to mixed breast feeding and formula feeding.

D. **Premastication.** Possible transmission of HIV by caregivers who premasticate food for infants has been described in 3 cases in the United States. HIV-infected caregivers should be asked and counseled not to premasticate food for infants.

V. **Clinical presentation.** Disease progression after vertical HIV infection is highly variable.

A. **Incubation period.** The onset of symptoms is approximately 12 to 18 months of age for untreated, perinatally infected infants in the United States; however, some may become ill in the first few months of life (15%–20%).

B. **Signs and symptoms.** The newborn is usually asymptomatic or may have low birthweight, weight loss, or failure to thrive (if infected in utero). The frequency of different opportunistic pathogens among HIV-infected children decreased significantly with the application and widespread use of **combination antiretroviral therapy (cART)**. In the pre-cART era, serious bacterial infection, herpes zoster, disseminated *Mycobacterium avium* complex (MAC), PCP, and esophageal candidiasis were common. History of a previous AIDS-defining opportunistic infection was a predictor of developing a new infection. In the cART era, descriptions of opportunistic infections among HIV-infected children have been limited because of the substantial decreases in morbidity and mortality among children receiving cART. Nonspecific features of HIV infection include hepatosplenomegaly, lymphadenopathy, and fever. Neurologic disease may be either static (delayed attainment of milestones) or progressive, with impaired brain growth, failure to reach milestones, and progressive motor deficits. Common computed tomography (CT) scan findings include basal ganglia calcification and cortical atrophy. Cardiac abnormalities include pericardial disease, myocardial dysfunction, and dysrhythmias.

VI. **Diagnosis.** Diagnosis is based on suspicion of infection based on epidemiologic risk or clinical presentation and confirmation by different virologic assays in infants <24 months old or serologic tests (enzyme-linked immunosorbent assay [ELISA] or Western blot) if the infant is >24 months old. Historically, 18 months was considered the age at which a positive antibody assay could accurately distinguish between presence of maternal and infant antibodies. However, using medical record data for a cohort of HIV-uninfected infants born from 2000 to 2007, it was demonstrated that clearance of maternal HIV antibodies occurred later than previously reported (14% of infants remained seropositive after 18 months, 4.3% after 21 months, and 1.2% after 24 months).

A. **All other causes of immunodeficiency must be excluded.** These include both primary and secondary immunodeficiency states. Primary immunodeficiency diseases include DiGeorge and Wiskott-Aldrich syndromes, ataxia-telangiectasia, agammaglobulinemia, severe combined immunodeficiency, and neutrophil function abnormalities. Secondary immunodeficiency states include those caused by immunosuppressive therapy, starvation, and lymphoreticular cancer.

B. **Laboratory studies**

1. **Virologic assays.** HIV DNA and RNA polymerase chain reaction (PCR) are considered the gold standard for diagnosis of HIV in infants and children <24 months. With the use of these tests, HIV infection may be diagnosed as early as the first day after birth in some infants and by 1 month of age in most infected infants. The **HIV DNA PCR** assay is the preferred diagnostic tool. Amplification of proviral DNA allows detection of cells that harbor quiescent provirus as well as cells with actively replicating virus. Approximately 30% of infants with perinatal HIV infection have a positive DNA PCR in samples obtained by 48 hours of age. A positive result identifies infants who were infected in utero. The test can routinely detect 1 to 10 DNA copies. The test will be positive in 93% and 95% of all infected infants by 2 weeks and 1 month of age, respectively.

A single HIV DNA PCR assay has a sensitivity of 95% and a specificity of 97% for samples collected from infected children 1 to 36 months of age. **HIV RNA PCR** assays detect plasma (cell-free) viral RNA by PCR amplification. These assays are available as either "standard" or "ultrasensitive," and the lower limit of detection when using the ultrasensitive assays is in the range of 50 to 75 HIV copies per milliliter of plasma. The reported sensitivity for RNA assays ranges from 25% to 40% within the first few days of life to 100% by 6 to 12 weeks of age. HIV RNA assays are commonly used for quantifying "viral load" as 1 predictor of disease progression. They are used in follow-up testing of patients during treatment for HIV infection. The first test result should be confirmed as soon as possible by a repeat virologic test on a second specimen because false-positive results can occur with both RNA and DNA assays. Zidovudine (ZDV) and nevirapine prophylaxis does not appear to alter the diagnostic sensitivity of either HIV DNA or RNA PCR assays. It is also established that HIV DNA PCR but not HIV RNA PCR remains positive even in infected individuals receiving effective therapeutic cART.

Virologic assays should be performed within the first 48 hours after birth, at 14 to 21 days, between 1 and 2 months, and at 4 to 6 months of age. Cord blood should not be used because of the possibility of contamination with maternal blood. A positive virologic test confirmed at 2 weeks of age warrants a change in the recommended ZDV prophylactic monotherapy. HIV infection can be *presumptively* excluded in non–breast-fed infants with 2 or more negative virologic tests, with 1 test obtained at ≥14 days of age and 1 obtained at ≥4 weeks of age; or 1 negative virologic test obtained at ≥8 weeks of age; or 1 negative HIV antibody test obtained at ≥6 months of age. PCP prophylaxis is recommended for infants with indeterminate HIV infection status starting at 4 to 6 weeks of age until they are determined to be HIV uninfected or presumptively uninfected. *Definitive* exclusion of HIV infection in a non–breast-fed infant is based on 2 or more negative virologic tests, with 1 obtained at ≥1 month of age and one at ≥4 months of age; or 2 negative HIV antibody tests from separate specimens obtained at ≥6 months of age (in the absence of hypogammaglobulinemia). For both *presumptive* and *definitive* exclusion of HIV infection, the child must have no other laboratory (eg, no positive virologic test results or low CD4 count/percentage) or clinical evidence of HIV infection and not be breast feeding. Many experts confirm the absence of HIV infection in infants with negative virologic tests by performing an antibody test at 12 to 24 months of age to document seroreversion to HIV antibody–negative status. The p24 antigen assay is less sensitive than DNA or RNA PCR and is generally not recommended. Viral HIV culture is labor intensive and poses a significant biohazard risk; in addition, it is less sensitive, less available, and more expensive than the DNA PCR assay. Definitive HIV culture results may take up to 28 days.

2. **Rapid tests.** A number of rapid tests for detection of HIV antibodies in blood, urine, or oral fluid have been licensed in the United States (www.fda.gov/cber/products/testkits.htm; accessed September 4, 2018). These tests are comparable to enzyme immunoassays (EIAs) in both sensitivity (99.3%–100%) and specificity (98.6%–100%). As with routine EIAs, confirmation of positive results is necessary, but confirmation of a negative result is not. The rapid tests are valuable as a screening tool for pregnant women with no or limited prenatal care or for infants with unknown maternal HIV status. They have the potential to reduce MTCT, with immediate provision of antiretroviral prophylaxis and formula feeding to prevent postnatal transmission. They should be available in all hospitals providing delivery services in the United States. In 2012, a home HIV test (OraQuick In-Home HIV Test, OraSure Technologies, Bethlehem, PA) received US Food and Drug Administration (FDA) approval.

3. **Surrogate markers for disease.** Immunologic abnormalities found in HIV-infected infants include hypergammaglobulinemia, a low CD4$^+$ T-lymphocyte count, or a decreased CD4$^+$ percentage.
C. **Presence of an acquired immunodeficiency virus–defining condition that indicates cellular immunodeficiency.** The most common AIDS-defining conditions observed among American children with vertically acquired HIV infection are PCP, recurrent bacterial infections, wasting syndrome, esophageal candidiasis, HIV encephalopathy, and cytomegalovirus pneumonia, colitis, encephalitis, or retinitis.
VII. **Management.** Isolation precautions for all infectious diseases, including maternal and neonatal precautions, breast feeding, and visiting issues, can be found in Appendix F.
A. **Prevention of mother-to-child transmission in resource-rich settings.** In 2012, the CDC presented a framework for the elimination of MTCT HIV transmission. The framework included prevention of HIV infection in women and girls of childbearing potential, identification of HIV infection among them, assurance of adequate preconception care and family planning services, early identification of HIV infection of pregnant women through universal prenatal screening, provision of adequate prenatal care for women with HIV infection, maximal reduction of maternal viral load through appropriate use of antiretroviral (ARV) drugs, cesarean section (CS) delivery when maternal viral load is not maximally suppressed, provision of neonatal ARV prophylaxis and neonatal replacement feeding, and maternal support for lactation suppression. MTCT can take place in utero, during labor, at delivery, and postnatally through breast feeding; however, most transmissions (50%–80%) are believed to occur around labor and delivery. Before the widespread use of MTCT interventions (described later), transmission rates in the United States ranged from 16% to 30%. More recently, MTCT has dropped to approximately 1% (<0.5% in England).
1. **Identification of human immunodeficiency virus infection in pregnant women and newborns.** The CDC guidelines recommend that HIV screening be included in the routine panel of prenatal screening tests for **all pregnant women**. HIV screening is recommended after the patient is notified that testing will be performed unless the patient declines (opt-out screening). **Separate written consent for HIV testing should not be required.** Repeat screening in the third trimester is recommended in certain jurisdictions with elevated rates of HIV infection. The AAP and American College of Obstetricians and Gynecologists (ACOG) issued similar recommendations supporting routine testing and the opt-out strategy. Most guidelines now state that healthcare providers have a **responsibility** not only to offer, but also **to recommend** antenatal HIV testing. The benefits of antenatal HIV testing extend beyond reducing MTCT and include the opportunity to evaluate the infected woman's health status, to initiate cART if required, and to allow the woman to reduce the risk of transmitting HIV to her sexual partner. For a **newborn infant whose mother's HIV infection status is unknown**, the newborn infant's physician should perform rapid HIV antibody testing on the mother or the infant (with appropriate consent). Test results should be reported to the physician as soon as possible to allow effective ARV prophylaxis, ideally within 12 hours. In some states, rapid testing of the neonate is required by law if the mother refuses HIV testing.
2. **Maternal antiretroviral therapy and perinatal human immunodeficiency virus prophylaxis.** HIV-infected pregnant women should receive cART, both for treatment of the mother's HIV infection and for prevention of MTCT of HIV. Virologic suppression to **undetectable viral load** is the goal. Therapy should be initiated as soon as possible, regardless of plasma HIV RNA copy number or CD4$^+$ cell count, even in the first trimester. One study from France showed that the transmission rate increased from 0.2% for women receiving cART before conception to 0.4%, 0.9%, and 2.2% for women initiating cART in the first, second, and third trimesters, respectively. Ideally, women initiating such a

regimen during pregnancy should be tested for the presence of ARV resistance. For optimal prevention of perinatal HIV transmission, cART should continue intrapartum, and the infant should receive ARV prophylaxis as recommended. Maternal cART is usually composed of 3 drugs from 2 different classes of ARV. **The use of ZDV alone is *not recommended*.** Oral ZDV may be included in the antenatal ARV regimen unless there is severe toxicity or documented resistance. ZDV rapidly crosses the placenta, providing protective drug levels for the fetus. Clinical trial data (including the original ACTG 076 trial published in 1994) clearly demonstrate the efficacy and safety of ZDV in reducing MTCT. HIV-infected women with HIV RNA ≥400 copies/mL (or unknown HIV RNA) near delivery should receive IV ZDV during labor, regardless of antepartum regimen or mode of delivery. A pregnant woman already on cART that does not include ZDV need not have her regimen changed if her viral load is suppressed. The details of what combination drugs to use in pregnancy are outlined by guidelines released by the US Department of Health and Human Services. These guidelines are updated regularly and are available online (http://aidsinfo.nih.gov/ContentFiles/PerinatalGL.pdf; accessed September 4, 2018). Additionally, there is a National Perinatal HIV hotline that can also be accessed at 1-888-448-8765 for questions and guidance. ARV medications are largely safe during pregnancy, even when used in the first trimester. In particular, efavirenz, which was thought to be teratogenic in the past, is not associated with increased risk of neural tube defects according to a registry's data (www.apregistry.com; accessed September 4, 2018) and is considered safe.

3. **Mode of delivery.** Historical data from individual patient meta-analysis and a randomized controlled trial showed that CS performed before labor and rupture of membranes can reduce MTCT by 50% to 80%. However, in women with plasma HIV RNA ≤1000 copies/mL on cART, the overall incidence of transmission of HIV is low regardless of the mode of delivery or duration of membrane rupture, and a further decrease in transmission risk with CS in such women is unclear. In contrast, in women whose viral loads are unknown or remain >1000 copies/mL prior to 38 weeks' gestation (eg, women not taking cART, women presenting late in pregnancy, or women not responding to their current cART regimen), performing CS at 38 weeks is recommended. Elective CS is associated with a higher rate of postpartum complications among HIV-infected women than vaginal delivery; therefore, women with an undetectable viral load should be allowed to have vaginal delivery regardless of the duration of membrane rupture. The use of invasive procedures in labor (eg, amniocentesis, fetal scalp electrodes, operative vaginal delivery, and episiotomy) should be avoided because of the potential risk for enhanced transmission.

4. **Postdelivery.** Amniotic fluid and blood should be cleaned thoroughly. The infant should be isolated with the same precautions as for hepatitis B (blood and secretion precautions). When the mother has received cART regimen during pregnancy with sustained viral suppression, a 4-week ZDV postexposure prophylaxis regimen is recommended in infants ≥35 weeks' gestation. See dose in Chapter 155. However, if the mother did not receive any ARV before onset of labor, ARV was received intrapartum only, cART regimen was received but without sustained viral suppression achieved, or infant is <35 weeks, then a combination ARV prophylaxis regimen is needed for the infant. Currently, this combination regimen consists of 2 drugs: ZDV for 6 weeks and nevirapine for 3 doses during the first week of life (as soon as possible after delivery up to 48 hours of life, 48 hours after first dose, and 96 hours after second dose). Serial virologic studies should be obtained as discussed previously. The HIV-infected mother may be co-infected with other pathogens that can be transmitted from mother to child, such as cytomegalovirus, herpes simplex virus, hepatitis B, hepatitis C, syphilis, toxoplasmosis, or tuberculosis. Infants born to mothers

with such co-infections should undergo appropriate evaluations as indicated to rule out transmission of additional infectious agents. Breast feeding must be discouraged. Both mother and infant should have prescriptions for the HIV drugs when they leave the hospital, and the infant should have an appointment for a postnatal visit at 2 to 4 weeks of age to monitor medication adherence, obtain virologic testing (HIV DNA PCR), and screen the infant for anemia from ZDV.

B. **Prevention of mother-to-child transmission in resource-limited settings.** Similar to CDC, WHO guidelines recommend initiation of cART, if available, for all HIV-infected pregnant or breast-feeding women, regardless of their CD4 cell count, to reduce the risk of MTCT and to treat their own disease. The preferred regimen is a once-daily, fixed-dose combination of tenofovir, lamivudine (or emtricitabine), and efavirenz. Lifelong continuation of cART is recommended for the mother including the whole duration of breast feeding. As for infants, **exclusive breast feeding is recommended**, in addition to oral **ARV prophylaxis**. When infants are born to mothers who had achieved viral suppression on cART or had been regularly taking cART for >4 weeks, ARV prophylaxis for the infant is daily nevirapine for 6 weeks. However, if the infant is born to an HIV-infected mother with a viral load >1000 copies/mL within the 4 weeks prior to delivery, if the mother received no cART or <4 weeks of cART by the time of delivery, or if the mother acquired HIV infection during late pregnancy or breast feeding, then ARV prophylaxis regimen for the infant is daily nevirapine *plus* twice-daily ZDV for 6 weeks, followed by an additional 6 weeks of the same combination regimen or nevirapine alone. If the mother cannot tolerate or declines cART, then the infant should continue nevirapine prophylaxis throughout the duration of breast feeding, until 1 week following breast-feeding cessation.

C. **Treatment of infants with established human immunodeficiency virus infection.** Management of HIV infection is an area of medicine that is changing rapidly. Current treatment recommendations for HIV-infected children are available online (http://aidsinfo.nih.gov; accessed February 20, 2018) and are **continuously updated**. Initiation of cART is recommended for all HIV-infected infants <12 months of age as soon as infection is confirmed, irrespective of clinical symptoms, immune status, or viral load. The principal objectives of therapy are to suppress viral replication maximally, to restore and preserve immune function, to reduce HIV-associated morbidity and mortality, to minimize drug toxicity, to maintain normal growth and development, and to improve quality of life. Aggressive therapy is warranted in the youngest children who are at greatest risk of rapid disease progression. In general, cART with at least 3 drugs from at least 2 classes of ARV is recommended. Drug regimens most often used include 2 nucleoside reverse transcriptase inhibitors plus either a boosted protease inhibitor, a nonnucleoside reverse transcriptase inhibitor, or an integrase strand transfer inhibitor. ARV resistance testing (viral genotyping) is recommended before starting treatment, because infected infants may acquire resistant virus from their mothers.

D. **General supportive care**

1. **Intravenous immunoglobulin.** HIV-infected infants who have recurrent, serious bacterial infections (eg, bacteremia, meningitis, pneumonia) are appropriate candidates for routine intravenous immunoglobulin (IVIG) prophylaxis (400 mg/kg/dose every 28 days). Trimethoprim-sulfamethoxazole prophylaxis may provide comparable protection.

2. **Immunization**

   a. **Active immunization.** All routine infant immunizations should be given to HIV-exposed infants. If HIV infection is confirmed, then guidelines for the HIV-infected child should be followed. Children with HIV infection should be immunized as soon as they are age appropriate with inactivated vaccines. Trivalent inactivated influenza vaccine (TIV) should be given annually. In addition, live virus–containing measles-mumps-rubella (MMR) and varicella vaccines should be given to asymptomatic HIV-infected children without severe immunosuppression (ie, CD4$^+$ T-lymphocyte count >15% for at least 6 months in children 1 through 5 years of age). Severely immunocompromised HIV-infected children should not receive measles virus–containing vaccine because vaccine-related pneumonia has been reported. **The quadrivalent measles-mumps-rubella-varicella vaccine should not be administered to any HIV-infected infants, regardless of degree of immunosuppression because of lack of safety data in this population.** Rotavirus vaccine may be given to HIV-exposed and HIV-infected infants. All HIV-infected children should receive a dose of 23-valent polysaccharide pneumococcal vaccine after 24 months of age, with a minimal interval of 8 weeks since the last conjugate pneumococcal vaccine. Infants and children with HIV infection who are 2 months of age or older should receive an age-appropriate series of the meningococcal ACWY conjugate vaccine. The immunologic response to these vaccines in HIV-infected children may be less robust and less persistent than in immunologically normal children. Members of households in which a child has HIV infection can receive MMR vaccine. Yearly influenza immunization is recommended to all household members 6 months of age or older. Immunization with varicella vaccine of siblings and susceptible adult caregivers of HIV-infected patients is encouraged.

   b. **Passive immunization.** HIV-infected children exposed to measles should receive intramuscular immunoglobulin, with the dose depending on the level of immune suppression. Asymptomatic, mildly or moderately immunocompromised patients should receive intramuscular immunoglobulin at a dose of 0.5 mL/kg (maximum 15 mL), regardless of immunization status. Severely immunocompromised HIV-infected patients should receive IVIG at a dose of 400 mg/kg. In addition, children with HIV infection who sustain wounds classified as **tetanus** prone should receive tetanus immune globulin regardless of immunization status. Finally, for **chickenpox** or shingles exposure, HIV-infected children without a history of previous chickenpox or varicella vaccination should receive varicella-zoster immune globulin (VariZIG), especially when they are moderately or severely immunocompromised, within 10 days after exposure. If VariZIG is not available, IVIG should be given.

3. **Nutrition.** Close nutritional monitoring should be part of the routine care of these children.

4. *Pneumocystis jirovecii* **prophylaxis.** CDC guidelines state that all infants born to HIV-infected women receive prophylaxis for 1 year beginning at 4 to 6 weeks regardless of CD4$^+$ lymphocyte count. If HIV infection is excluded, then prophylaxis can be stopped. The drug of choice for this is trimethoprim-sulfamethoxazole. The need for prophylaxis after 1 year can be determined by the degree of immunosuppression as determined by CD4$^+$ T-lymphocyte count.

5. **Other aspects of supportive care.** Neurodevelopmental supportive services including preschool early intervention programs and school-based developmental disability programs should be offered to all HIV-infected children.

VIII. **Prognosis.** In developed countries, a bimodal pattern of symptomatic HIV infection has been recognized in children who are not treated. Some children become symptomatic quickly and die before 4 years of age, with a median age of death of 11 months (15%–20%, termed *rapid progressors*). The majority (80%–85%) of untreated children, on the other hand, have delayed onset of milder symptoms and survive beyond 5 years of age (termed *slow progressors*). Only a minority of patients remain asymptomatic by 8 years. Clinical and laboratory factors associated with poor prognosis include being born to mothers with low CD4$^+$ counts or high viral load (ie, >100,000 copies/mL), high virus copy number in the cord blood, and early manifestation of symptoms (opportunistic infections, encephalopathy, severe wasting, and hepatosplenomegaly). Use of cART has substantially reduced both mortality and morbidity and improved quality of life in HIV-infected children. Children with HIV infection acquired through blood transfusion tend to have a prolonged asymptomatic period. In the United States, mortality in HIV-infected children has declined from 7.2 per 100 person-years in 1993 to 0.66 per 100 person-years in 2010 to 2014. In resource-limited developing countries, before the use of cART, the prognosis was much worse, with 1 study showing 89% of the infected children dying by 3 years of age, 10% being in HIV disease category B or C, and only approximately 1% remaining without HIV symptoms. With availability of ARVs to some developing countries, the prognosis is significantly improving. Recent studies from South Africa showed that implementation of a national ARV treatment program resulted in 1- and 3-year mortality rates of 4.6% and 7.7%, respectively.

139 Lyme Disease

I. **Definition.** Lyme disease is a zoonotic infection and was first reported in 1977, following an unusual cluster of adults and children with oligoarticular arthritis in a certain neighborhood of Lyme, Connecticut. Subsequently, a multisystem disease was described and attributed to the spirochete *Borrelia burgdorferi*. Lyme disease manifests as a spectrum of skin, musculoskeletal, cardiac, and neurologic findings. It is a vector-borne disease that follows the bite of an *Ixodes* tick, usually the black-legged *Ixodes scapularis*, commonly known as the deer tick. Lyme disease has a worldwide distribution and is known to be endemic in the Americas, Europe, Asia, Africa, and Australia. **Prenatal exposure to *B burgdorferi* and the development of gestational borreliosis can result in maternal Lyme disease with placentitis and possible transplacental infection of the fetus and newborn.**

II. **Incidence.** In 2017, a total of 42,743 cases of Lyme disease were reported and confirmed by the Centers for Disease Control and Prevention with an incidence of 106.6 cases per 100,000 nationwide. No specific data on pregnancy-related Lyme disease is available; however, the number of infected pregnant women in the United States is presumably small. Estimates for active infection after exposure to a deer-tick bite are only 1% to 3%.

III. **Pathophysiology**

  A. **Transmission.** The *Ixodes* tick lives a 2-year life cycle consisting of 3 stages: larval, nymph, and adult. The preferred reservoirs are the white-footed field mouse for the larval and nymph tick and the white-tailed deer for the adult tick. The larval stage emerges from eggs in early summer and feeds on previously infected mice, from which they acquire the *B burgdorferi* spirochete. The infected nymph stage emerges in the next spring and is the most likely source of human infection as its activity corresponds to outdoor human activities in spring and summer. The adult tick may infect before laying eggs in summer and dying soon after.

  B. **Human spirochetemia.** After the tick bite, the incubation period of the spirochetes is 1 to 32 days, with a median of 11 days. The disease is characterized by "early" and "late" manifestations. Early disease occurs in 2 stages (early localized and early disseminated). Spirochete dissemination is presumed to be facilitated by the surface of the organism binding to human plasminogen and subsequently binding to integrins, matrix glycosaminoglycans, and extracellular matrix proteins. These complexes may explain the propensity of the spirochetes to localize to collagen fibrils in the extracellular matrices of the heart, nervous system, and joints. Late Lyme disease occurs months to a year or more after dissemination.

C. Placentitis and transplacental disease. Before 1990, a number of case reports had confirmed the transplacental passage of *B burgdorferi* by identifying spirochetes in placental tissues, umbilical vessels, fetal brain, heart, spleen, kidneys, bone marrow, liver, and adrenal glands. However, several recent clinical, serologic, and epidemiologic studies have failed to confirm a causal association between Lyme disease in pregnancy and adverse fetal outcomes, congenital malformations, or cardiac defects.

IV. **Risk factors.** Maternal Lyme disease is a result of exposure to deer ticks in known endemic areas. If an expectant mother presents with a history of outdoor exposure or has dogs or cats in the home, a known tick embedment, or cutaneous lesions consistent with early disease, **prompt antibiotic therapy lessens the risk for transplacental transmission of spirochetes.** There are no other known predilections to Lyme disease related to pregnancy.

V. **Clinical presentation**
A. **Maternal**
1. **Early localized.** The cutaneous stage begins with a papule at the site of the tick bite, becoming an annular erythematous migrating rash (also known as erythema migrans) with central clearing. Rash may last 3 to 4 weeks and is nonpruritic and painless. The early stage is often accompanied by low-grade fever, evanescent arthralgia, myalgia, fatigue, headache, and neck muscle stiffness.
2. **Early disseminated.** This is most often characterized by multiple erythema migrans several weeks after the tick bite. This stage is accompanied by worsening fatigue, severe malaise, and migratory musculoskeletal pain. Systemic disease affecting target organs becomes more apparent, namely as mono- or pauciarticular arthritis and cardiac manifestations, such as heart block. Nervous system involvement can include lymphocytic meningitis or cranial nerve palsies.
3. **Late Lyme disease.** Months after exposure to disease, arthralgia and pauciarticular arthritis persist and recur. The knees are the most often affected joint with marked swelling, but with pain that is less than that of rheumatoid-type arthritis. On rare occasions, chronic neurologic conditions of encephalopathy, peripheral neuropathy, demyelination, or dementia have been reported.

B. **Neonatal**
1. **No specific clinical presentation of Lyme disease in the newborn has been described as a result of transplacental transmission.** Of importance is the maternal history of disease and whether or not the mother has been adequately treated. Placental pathology in suspected cases may offer information that would prompt testing and perhaps treatment for at-risk neonates. A case of postnatal transmission has been reported recently in a 2-week-old female infant presenting to the emergency department with 5-cm annular area of abdominal wall erythema with central clearing that was confirmed to be neonatal Lyme disease; it developed after a tick bite at 1 week of age. The rash resolved with treatment, and the patient was well at her 3-month well-child visit.
2. **Congenital Lyme disease as a clinical entity has been reviewed and found not to be substantive.** In particular, congenital heart defects have been reviewed in large follow-up studies of mothers with positive *B burgdorferi* serology, and no association was found by multiple researchers. Walsh et al searched the worldwide literature for obstetric associations to Lyme disease and came up with the following conclusions:
a. **Women who are seropositive at conception** have no increased incidence of adverse pregnancy.
b. **Women who develop a confirmed diagnosis** of Lyme disease in pregnancy should receive appropriate antimicrobial treatment.
c. **Women with Lyme disease in pregnancy** and who have been appropriately treated have shown no association with specific adverse fetal outcomes.

VI. **Diagnosis.** Laboratory testing for Lyme disease should be done if careful history taking and physical examination strongly suggest active disease.

    A. **Early localized disease.** Diagnosis is made largely on clinical grounds (history of exposure, rash, and symptoms). Serologic tests are not recommended secondary to late development of antibodies to *B burgdorferi*.

    B. **Early disseminated disease.** Dissemination of the disease is diagnosed clinically as described earlier. If rash is not present, serologic studies should be obtained.

        1. **Enzyme immunoassay.**

        2. **Immunofluorescent antibody assay.**

        3. **If both tests are negative, no further testing is needed, and clinical reevaluation for other conditions is indicated.** Screening tests are known to have high false-positive rates.

        4. **If either is positive, it should be followed by:**

            a. **Western immunoblot standardized for antibodies to *B burgdorferi*.** Subsequently, positive Western blot assays should include specific immunoglobulin (Ig) G and IgM. If the Western blot assays are negative, the false-positive enzyme immunoassay (EIA) or immunofluorescent antibody assay (IFA) testing suggests other spirochetal diseases, such as syphilis, leptospirosis, an intercurrent viral disease (eg, Epstein-Barr), or an autoimmune condition such as lupus erythematosus.

            b. **Late disease.** If late disease is suspected, only a positive IgG immunoblot is needed.

VII. **Management**

    A. **Maternal**

        1. **Early localized disease.** *Note:* Doxycycline is the drug of choice for Lyme disease. It can be used in children of any age. Doxycycline has not been adequately studied during pregnancy to make a recommendation regarding its use in the pregnant woman.

            a. **Amoxicillin**

            b. **Cefuroxime axetil (alternative)**

        2. **Early disseminated or late disease**

            a. **Oral antibiotic therapy is considered adequate.**

            b. **Parenteral antibiotics for a maximum of 4 weeks** are only indicated in patients with symptoms of increased intracranial pressure and pleocytosis in cerebrospinal fluid. Routine lumbar puncture is not recommended.

    B. **Newborn**

        1. **Treat if infant is thought to be symptomatic at birth** especially if mother is confirmed with Lyme disease but has not been adequately or appropriately treated. **Doxycycline is the drug of choice.** Amoxicillin, cefuroxime, and azithromycin (for a patient unable to take a β-lactam or doxycycline) are alternatives. Obtain infectious disease consultation before starting treatment.

        2. **If the infant is asymptomatic at birth,** given low risk for active disease, current recommendations do not call for empirical treatment, especially if the mother was appropriately treated during pregnancy. Placental pathology may offer information helpful in the decision of whether or not to treat; consultation with an infectious disease specialist is recommended.

        3. **Lyme disease is *not* a contraindication for breast feeding.** No evidence is known for the passage of *B burgdorferi* to the infant through breast feeding.

VIII. **Prognosis.** Prompt diagnosis and antibiotic therapy are essential for the pregnant woman; however, there is no evidence that Lyme disease during pregnancy causes harm to the developing fetus.

140 Meningitis

I. **Definition.** Neonatal meningitis is an infection of the meninges and central nervous system (CNS) in the first month of life. This is the most common time of life for meningitis to occur.

II. **Incidence.** The incidence is approximately 0.16 to 0.45 per 1000 live births in developed countries. The incidence may be higher in underdeveloped countries.

III. **Pathophysiology.** In most cases, infection occurs because of hematogenous seeding of the meninges and CNS. After attaching to the endothelium of the cerebral microvasculature and choroid plexus, bacteria can enter the cerebrospinal fluid (CSF) by several mechanisms including transcellular movement across the endothelial cell (eg, *Escherichia coli*), paracellular movement by disruption of intercellular tight junctions, and through transport across the blood–brain barrier within infected phagocytes (so-called "Trojan horse mechanism," eg, *Listeria monocytogenes*). Inflammatory mediators are then released into the CSF in reaction to bacterial products, resulting in meningitis and increased permeability of the blood–brain barrier. In cases of CNS or spinal anomalies (eg, myelomeningocele), there may be direct inoculation by flora on the skin or in the environment. Neonatal meningitis is often accompanied by **ventriculitis**, which makes resolution of infection more difficult. There is also a predilection for **vasculitis**, which may lead to hemorrhage, thrombosis, and infarction. Subdural effusions and brain abscess may also complicate the course.

Most organisms implicated in neonatal sepsis also cause neonatal meningitis. Some have a definite predilection for CNS infection. **Group B *Streptococcus* (GBS)** (especially type III) and the **gram-negative rods** (especially *E coli* with K1 antigen) are the **most common causative agents**. GBS and *E coli* account for approximately two-thirds of all cases of neonatal meningitis. **Galactosemia** should be considered if *E coli* is the causative agent in late-onset meningitis. Multidrug-resistant *E coli* (eg, extended-spectrum β-lactamase producing) is an emerging problem in some neonatal units. Other causative organisms include *L monocytogenes* (serotype IVb), other streptococci (enterococci, *Streptococcus pneumoniae*), other gram-negative enteric bacilli (*Klebsiella*, *Enterobacter*, and *Serratia* spp), and rarely, *Neisseria meningitides*. In the very low birthweight (VLBW) infant, coagulase-negative staphylococci (CONS) need to be considered as causative organisms in bacterial meningitis.

With CNS anomalies involving open defects or indwelling devices (eg, ventriculoperitoneal shunts), staphylococcal disease (*Staphylococcus aureus* and *Staphylococcus epidermidis*) is more common, as is disease caused by other skin flora, including streptococci and diphtheroids. Many unusual organisms, including *Ureaplasma*, fungi, and anaerobes, have been described in case reports of neonatal meningitis.

IV. **Risk factors.** Risk factors for neonatal meningitis are similar for neonatal sepsis and include low birthweight, prematurity, premature or prolonged rupture of membranes, septic or traumatic delivery, fetal hypoxia, maternal peripartum infection, and galactosemia. The characteristics of some bacteria make them more virulent, especially for neonates (eg, capsular polysaccharide of GBS type III, *E coli* K1, and *L monocytogenes* serotype IVb all contain sialic acid in high concentrations). Infants with CNS defects necessitating ventriculoperitoneal shunt procedures also are at increased risk.

V. **Clinical presentation.** The clinical presentation is usually nonspecific and indistinguishable from that caused by sepsis. Meningitis must be excluded in any infant being evaluated for sepsis or infection. **Signs and symptoms of meningitis include** temperature instability (the most common, found in 60% of the cases), lethargy, irritability, poor tone, seizures, feeding intolerance, vomiting, respiratory distress, apnea, or cyanotic episodes. Term infants are more likely to have fever, whereas preterm infants are more likely to have hypothermia. Seizures, often focal, can be the presenting manifestation in up to 50% of the cases. Late manifestations of meningitis include a full or bulging anterior fontanelle and coma. Syndrome of inappropriate antidiuretic hormone may accompany meningitis.

VI. **Diagnosis**

  A. **Laboratory studies.** The clinical presentation of bacterial meningitis in the neonate is nonspecific; therefore, neonates with suspected bacterial meningitis should undergo a full sepsis evaluation including a complete blood count with differential, blood culture, urine culture (if >3–5 days), and lumbar puncture (LP) to obtain CSF for Gram stain, culture, protein, glucose, and cell count. CSF examination is critical in the investigation of possible meningitis and the only way to confirm the diagnosis. Approximately 15% to 50% of all infants with positive CSF cultures for bacteria have negative blood cultures. Conversely, initial CSF findings may be questionable, and a repeat LP 24 to 48 hours later will provide definitive diagnosis (when the meninges are inflamed, the second LP always shows a pleocytosis and other parameters consistent with the diagnosis of meningitis). The technique for obtaining CSF fluid and CSF normal values are discussed in Chapter 38.

  1. **Culture and Gram stain.** A **CSF culture is the gold standard** for the diagnosis of bacterial meningitis. It may be positive in association with a normal or minimally abnormal CSF analysis. However, CSF culture may be negative in some neonates with bacterial meningitis whose LP was delayed until after antibiotic administration (eg, critically ill infants). **Gram-stained smear** can be helpful in making a more rapid definitive diagnosis; however, the absence of organisms on Gram stain does not exclude the diagnosis.

  2. **Cerebrospinal fluid pleocytosis is variable.** There are usually more cells with gram-negative rods than with GBS disease. Normal values range from 0 to 30 white blood cells (WBCs), some of which may be polymorphonuclear cells. Traumatic LP (>500 red cells/mm^3) occurs in up to 40% of the attempts, and adjustment of CSF WBCs down to account for increased red cells does not improve diagnostic utility of the CSF examination. Reactive pleocytosis may be seen secondary to CNS hemorrhage.

  3. **Decreased cerebrospinal fluid glucose.** CSF glucose level must be compared with serum glucose level. Normal CSF values are one-half to two-thirds of serum values. Typically, neonates with meningitis have a CSF glucose level of <20 (preterm) or <30 (term) mg/dL.

  4. **Cerebrospinal fluid protein** is usually elevated (>100 [term] or >150 [preterm] mg/dL), although normal values for infants, especially premature infants, may be much higher than in later life, and the test may be confounded by the presence of blood in the specimen.

  5. **Cerebrospinal fluid biomarkers.** A number of CSF biomarkers have been examined for differentiating bacterial meningitis from viral meningitis and noninfectious origins, with some encouraging results. These CSF biomarkers include tumor necrosis factor-α, interleukin (IL)-1β, IL-6, IL-8, IL-12, IL-17, procalcitonin, and lipocalin, among others. However, the clinical utility of using these markers is currently limited.

  B. **Imaging studies** are recommended to detect the complications of meningitis, especially when the clinical course is complicated. Infection with certain microorganisms such as *Citrobacter koseri*, *Serratia marcescens*, *Proteus mirabilis*, and *Enterobacter sakazakii* predispose for the development of brain abscesses. The most useful and noninvasive method of imaging is **ultrasonography** (especially early in the course when the infant is critically ill), which provides information regarding ventricular size, inflammation (echogenic strands), and the presence of hemorrhage. Contrast-enhanced **computed tomography** (CT) or **magnetic resonance imaging** (MRI) is needed later in the course of the illness; they are useful in detecting cerebral abscesses, areas of infarct or encephalomalacia, and degree of cerebral cortical and white matter atrophy. **MRI is preferred over CT** because it provides better detail, optimizes assessment of injury to white matter, and avoids radiation exposure.

VII. Management. General supportive measures such as ventilation/oxygenation, cardiovascular support, intravenous dextrose, and anticonvulsant therapy are considered essential components of managing the neonate with bacterial meningitis. Isolation precautions for all infectious diseases, including maternal and neonatal precautions, breast feeding, and visiting issues, can be found in Appendix F.

A. Drug therapy. For drug dosages and other pharmacologic information, see Chapter 155. (*Note:* Dosages for ampicillin, nafcillin, and penicillin G are **doubled** when treating meningitis.)

1. **Empirical therapy.** Optimal antibiotic selection depends on culture and sensitivity testing of the causative organisms. **Ampicillin** and **gentamicin** are usually started as empirical therapy for suspected early sepsis. If meningitis is suspected, **cefotaxime** should be added. High rates of ampicillin resistance among *E coli* isolates and a link between maternal intrapartum ampicillin and *E coli* resistance have been well documented in VLBW infants. For hospitalized infants with late-onset presentation, empiric therapy consists of **vancomycin** (to cover gram-positive organisms, especially CONS and *S aureus* [methicillin sensitive and methicillin resistant]) and **gentamicin** with the addition of **cefotaxime** when CSF findings suggest meningitis (extended coverage of gram-negative rods). Lastly, for the infant <60 days who is coming from home to the emergency department, the empiric therapy consists of **ampicillin** and **cefotaxime**. If cefotaxime is unavailable, alternative agents include cefepime or ceftazidime.

2. **Gram-positive meningitis (group B *Streptococcus* and *Listeria*).** Penicillin or ampicillin is the drug of choice. Gentamicin (for **synergism**) can be added until sterility of the bloodstream and CSF has been documented. Monotherapy is continued for 14 days.

3. **Staphylococcal disease.** Because of the increased prevalence of MRSA in the nosocomial setting, **vancomycin** should be substituted for ampicillin as initial coverage. For MSSA, therapy can be switched to nafcillin. If the CSF is persistently positive, consideration should be given to adding rifampin for synergy.

4. **Gram-negative meningitis.** Most clinicians would use **ampicillin plus cefotaxime plus an aminoglycoside** as initial therapy. Further therapy is dictated by sensitivity results. "Double" gram-negative coverage is maintained for 10 days after sterility of CSF. Subsequently, cefotaxime can be continued alone to complete 21 days of therapy. There is an emerging problem with multidrug-resistant enteric microorganisms (especially *E coli*, *Klebsiella pneumoniae*); for this situation, the drug of choice is **meropenem**. (See Chapter 155.) Studies have shown no advantage for intrathecal or intraventricular gentamicin.

5. **Repeat lumbar puncture 48 to 72 hours into antibiotic therapy** is recommended to document CSF sterilization. Persistence of infection may indicate a focus, such as obstructive ventriculitis, subdural empyema, or multiple small-vessel thrombi. Infants with repeat positive CSF cultures after initiation of appropriate antibiotics are at risk for complications as well as a poor outcome. In general, approximately 3 days are required to sterilize the CSF in infants with gram-negative meningitis, whereas in gram-positive meningitis, sterilization usually occurs within 36 to 48 hours. External ventricular drainage may be indicated in certain cases complicated by ventriculitis. Treatment should continue until 14 days after cultures are negative or for 21 days, whichever is longer.

6. **Adjunctive therapy.** Contrary to childhood meningitis, dexamethasone does not seem to improve the outcome of neonatal meningitis. Other therapies focusing on enhancing the immune system in the newborn, such as hematopoietic growth factors or intravenous immune globulins, do not seem to help either.

B. Supportive measures and monitoring for complications. Head circumference should be measured daily, and neurologic examination should be performed frequently. Electroencephalogram (EEG) is important to detect seizures and to assess background cerebral function. Imaging studies (especially MRI) are helpful for prognosis and guiding the length of therapy. Hearing and vision evaluation should be done in all neonates who develop meningitis. All of them should undergo long-term neurodevelopmental follow-up.

VIII. **Prognosis.** The **mortality rate** has decreased recently to 3% to 13%, compared with 25% to 30% from earlier decades. There is a high incidence (~20%–40%) of neurodevelopmental sequelae in survivors, and this figure has not changed much over the years. Major neurologic sequelae include cerebral palsy, hypertonia, hypotonia, shunt-dependent hydrocephalus, blindness, deafness, and mental retardation. Factors predictive of death or serious sequelae include preterm birth, gram-negative etiology (as opposed to gram positive), neutropenia, seizures persisting >72 hours after hospitalization, focal neurologic deficits, initial inotropic support, delayed sterilization of the CSF, low-voltage background on EEG, and parenchymal lesions (abscess, thrombi, infarcts, and encephalomalacia) on neuroimaging studies.

141 Methicillin-Resistant *Staphylococcus aureus* Infections

I. **Definition.** Infection with methicillin-resistant *Staphylococcus aureus* (**MRSA**) (**clustered gram-positive cocci**) causes a variety of localized and invasive purulent infections and toxin-mediated syndromes such as toxic shock syndrome and staphylococcal scalded skin syndrome (SSSS). MRSA infections used to be limited to healthcare facilities and were strictly nosocomial; however, a significant increase in community-acquired MRSA (CA-MRSA) has been seen in the past 10 to 15 years. The separation between healthcare-related MRSA and CA-MRSA is becoming less distinct, as CA-MRSA is becoming more virulent and causing significantly more healthcare-associated infections.

II. **Incidence.** The methicillin-sensitive *S aureus* normally colonizes the nose, umbilicus, and groin area by 1 week of age, with a colonization rate of 30% to 70%. Maternal anogenital colonization with MRSA ranges from 0.5% to 10.4%, with small risk for early-onset disease in the newborn. Case reports have described maternal vertical transmission of MRSA from maternal chorioamnionitis, by nasal colonization, and through breast feeding. Horizontal transmission from siblings and other family members has been documented as well. There are several documented outbreaks of invasive CA-MRSA that developed in healthy newborn infants discharged from normal newborn nurseries as well as neonatal intensive care units (NICUs). **The majority of MRSA infections in the NICU are of late onset.** According to neonatal data reported from the National Nosocomial Infections Surveillance System for the years 1995 to 2004, MRSA accounted for 23% of all hospital-associated *S aureus* infections. The incidence of MRSA infections increased by 308% during the study period (from 0.7 per 100,000 patient-days in 1995 to 3.1 in 2004). In a recent meta-analysis of 18 studies reporting data from 1999 to 2011, the prevalence of MRSA colonization at admission to a NICU or pediatric intensive care unit was 1.9%, and the acquisition rate was 4.1%. Neonates who were admitted to the NICU after discharge from the birth hospitalization were more likely to be colonized than those who had never left the NICU (5.8% vs 0.2%). The risk of MRSA infection during hospitalization is increased 24-fold among colonized versus noncolonized patients. Another study that involved 1320 NICU patients found a MRSA colonization rate of 4% within 7 days of NICU discharge. Hand carriage of MRSA in healthcare personnel working in NICUs is estimated at 8%.

III. **Pathophysiology.** If the newborn infant is exposed to MRSA, whether from the community or the hospital, then he or she will be colonized with more virulent strains that are more likely to cause invasive disease. MRSA has specific virulence factors that make it more invasive than methicillin-sensitive *S aureus*. These include staphylococcal chromosome cassette (SCC) *mecA*, Panton-Valentine leukocidin (PVL), and staphylococcal enterotoxins. The SCC *mecA* has the genes that encode antibiotic resistance. PVL genes lead to the production of cytotoxins that form pores in the cellular membrane and cause tissue necrosis and cell lysis. Exfoliative toxins A and B secreted by *S aureus* are implicated in SSSS.

IV. **Risk factors.** Include overcrowding, inconsistent hand washing, invasive procedures (eg, central lines, endotracheal intubations, nasogastric tubes), prematurity, low birthweight and very low birthweight (VLBW), multiple gestation, the practice of kangaroo (skin-to-skin) mother care, a high MRSA colonization rate, and prolonged hospital stay. Interestingly, a recent study from Brazil showed maternal skin-to-skin contact for 60 minutes twice daily for 7 days between MRSA-colonized NICU infants and their mothers (MRSA negative) resulted in a 53.8% decolonization rate compared to a rate of 22.4% in the control group (risk ratio = 2.27; number needed to treat = 4). The decolonization presumably occurred due to "bacterial interference," through which the mother's sensitive and nonpathogenic bacteria replaced the infant's MRSA.

V. **Clinical presentations.** Invasive MRSA disease is likely to be preceded by colonization (skin, umbilicus, and nasopharynx). The source of the bacteria could be a healthcare worker, another patient, equipment, or a family member.

A. **Bloodstream infections.** These are usually catheter related. Common clinical signs are nonspecific and include apnea or hypoxia, fever, elevated C-reactive protein, and leukocytosis. The infant needs to be examined repeatedly and meticulously for subtle clues of focal infection (eg, phlebitis, pustulosis).

B. **Septic arthritis and osteomyelitis.** *S aureus* is the primary cause of septic arthritis and osteomyelitis in the neonate. Symptoms are nonspecific, such as poor feeding or increased irritability. Signs include soft tissue swelling and erythema.

C. **Endocarditis.** Neonates with congenital heart disease and percutaneous central catheters are at a higher risk for endocarditis.

D. **Skin and soft tissue infections.** *S aureus* is the most common pathogen causing pustulosis and cellulitis in the neonate. MRSA has virulence factors that contribute to the pathogen's ability to damage the neonatal skin that is already compromised.

E. **Conjunctivitis.** See Chapter 58.

F. **Pneumonia.** Pneumonia can be primary or associated with ventilator therapy. The course is frequently complicated by alveolar necrosis, pneumatocele formation, and pleural empyema.

G. **Surgical site infections.**

H. **Meningitis and brain abscesses.** Uncommon but have been reported.

I. **Staphylococcal scalded skin syndrome, also known as Ritter disease** in newborns, is a very rare complication of methicillin-sensitive *S aureus* or MRSA infection. It is characterized by rash all over the body and peeling off of the skin, which resolves without scarring within 10 days of treatment. Epidermolytic lesions in pressure zones, with a positive Nikolsky sign, and palmoplantar exfoliative erythema are characteristic signs of SSSS.

VI. **Diagnosis.** The **gold standard for diagnosing bloodstream infection is a positive blood culture.** Diagnosing arthritis and osteomyelitis can be challenging. In addition to a blood culture, the workup should include a joint aspirate, bone culture (if surgical debridement is done), radiography, and possibly magnetic resonance imaging. Echocardiography (to diagnose endocarditis) is strongly recommended in infants with >1 positive blood culture. For skin and soft tissue infections, incision and drainage, with subsequent Gram stain and culture of aspirated fluid, is recommended. Molecular typing is important in the identification and management of MRSA NICU outbreaks.

VII. **Management**

A. **Eradication of colonization.** Adult intensive care unit studies demonstrated that eradication of MRSA colonization using a combination of 5 days of intranasal mupirocin and 3 daily chlorhexidine baths resulted in reducing MRSA infections. There are no randomized studies in neonates showing similar efficacy; however, mupirocin (+/– chlorhexidine) has been used effectively in controlling outbreaks of MRSA in NICU populations. Mupirocin resistance is an increasing problem; routine mupirocin testing is an important factor for MRSA decolonization strategies. In cases of mupirocin resistance, retapamulin ointment 1% has been used for nasal decolonization.

B. **Antibiotic therapy.** Vancomycin is the first-line therapy for MRSA, and many NICUs with endemic MRSA use vancomycin as an empirical therapy for late-onset sepsis while awaiting culture results. In cases of vancomycin-intermediate *S aureus* (VISA) or vancomycin allergy, linezolid and clindamycin have been used effectively. Daptomycin is another antibiotic that could be used. Treatment duration depends on the specific infection. For **skin and soft tissue infections** and **bacteremia**, a 7- to 10-day course is generally appropriate. In cases of **endocarditis** and **osteomyelitis**, 6 to 8 weeks of treatment are necessary. In patients with **extensive disease with persistently positive blood cultures** despite therapeutic doses of vancomycin, both rifampin and gentamicin can be used for synergy. Mupirocin may be adequate for mild cases of localized neonatal pustulosis in the well-appearing full-term infant.

VIII. **Prevention**

A. **Hand hygiene.** The Centers for Disease Control and Prevention recommend using an alcohol-based hand sanitizer before touching patients, after touching patients, after removing gloves, and after touching the patient care environment and equipment due to the ability of MRSA to survive on inanimate objects. Alcohol-based hand sanitizers greatly improve compliance with hand hygiene policies (see Chapter 25).

B. **Controlling outbreaks (see Table 141–1).** During an outbreak, many measures are instituted concurrently. Hand hygiene should be emphasized to all personnel and visitors. Chlorhexidine 4% may be used for cleansing of the umbilical stump (has been reported to reduce the risk of omphalitis in resource-limited countries). Other measures recommended include reinforcement and monitoring of hand hygiene, alleviating overcrowding and understaffing, colonization surveillance cultures of newborn infants at admission and periodically thereafter, use of contact precautions for colonized or infected infants, and cohorting of colonized or infected infants and their caregivers. For hand hygiene, soaps containing chlorhexidine or alcohol-based hand rubs are preferred during an outbreak. Decolonization of colonized/infected patients with mupirocin and chlorhexidine baths may reduce patient-to-patient transmission. Colonized healthcare professionals epidemiologically implicated in transmission should receive decolonization therapy, but eradication of colonization may not occur. Use of molecular typing is an integral part of control because it can determine the ongoing transmission of a particular clone. Passive protection of neonates by using monoclonal antibodies or pooled human immunoglobulin G has been studied but does not seem to be efficacious. Efforts to develop an effective *S aureus* vaccine are ongoing.

IX. **Outcome.** Mortality from invasive MRSA infection (eg, bacteremia, meningitis) ranges from 11.9% for all NICU patients to 26.1% for VLBW infants. Survivors are at risk for neurodevelopmental impairment.

Table 141–1. GUIDELINES FOR OUTBREAKS OF METHICILLIN-RESISTANT
STAPHYLOCOCCUS AUREUS IN THE NICU

Recommendation Type, Rating Category[a]	Consensus Recommendation
Hand hygiene	
IA	A waterless, alcohol-based hand hygiene product should be made available and easily accessible; soap and water should be used if hands are visibly soiled.
IA	Monitoring of hand hygiene is a key component in preventing MRSA transmission in the NICU. Direct observations of hand hygiene practices on a regular basis, or consistent enforcement of proper hand hygiene (eg, use of a unit guard, providing feedback), contribute to increased rates of compliance.
Cohorting and isolation	
IA	MRSA-positive infants should be placed under contact precautions and cohorted (placed in a designated room or area), as should the supplies used in the care of these infants.
IA	Gloves and gowns should be worn when caring for or visiting infants known or suspected to be MRSA positive.
IA	Masks should be worn for aerosol-generating procedures, such as suctioning. The environment in the area of the infant should be kept clean and neat at all times.
NR/UI	Disposal of infant supplies used in the care of the MRSA-positive cohort should be decided by the institution's infection control experts.
IA	Whenever possible, nurses should be cohorted (designated exclusively) for care of MRSA-positive infants. Other HCWs should also be cohorted to the maximum extent allowed by the institution's resources.
II	If cohorting of nurses is not possible, nurses should care for the noncohorted patients before working with the cohorted neonates, when feasible.
II	The number of people (including HCWs and visitors) who enter a room or area designated for MRSA-positive infants should be limited to the minimum possible.
II	Cohorting of infants should be maintained until the last infected or colonized infant has been discharged from the NICU.
Neonatal surveillance cultures	
IB	Infants in the NICU should be screened periodically to detect MRSA colonization. The frequency of screening should increase (eg, to once per week) when clusters of colonization are detected; after evidence suggests a halt in transmission, it may decrease to a lower frequency (eg, to once per month) until the investigation is over.
IA	Although cultures of swab specimens from multiple body sites, including nares, throat, rectum, and umbilicus, have been used to detect MRSA colonization, culture of nasal or nasopharyngeal specimens alone is sufficiently sensitive to detect MRSA colonization in neonates.

(Continued)

Table 141–1. GUIDELINES FOR OUTBREAKS OF METHICILLIN-RESISTANT *STAPHYLOCOCCUS AUREUS* IN THE NICU (*CONTINUED*)

Recommendation Type, Rating Category[a]	Consensus Recommendation
Screening of health care workers (HCWs)	
IB	Screening of HCWs in response to a cluster of MRSA colonization or infection in the NICU should be performed only to corroborate or refute epidemiologic data that link an HCW to transmission.
Decolonization	
IB	Mupirocin may be used for decolonization of neonates and/or HCWs if deemed necessary by the affected institution (off-label use).
Environmental cultures	
IA	Environmental cultures should be performed in response to a cluster of MRSA colonization or infection in the NICU only to corroborate or refute epidemiologic data that link an environmental source to transmission.
Molecular analysis	
IA	When investigating an outbreak, molecular analysis with pulsed-field gel electrophoresis or a comparable molecular epidemiologic tool should be performed to assess the relatedness of strains found in NICU patients, HCWs, and the environment.
IB	If the hospital cannot perform genotyping in-house, then the isolates should be sent to a suitable laboratory for molecular analysis.
Communication	
II	Open communication between regional NICUs is essential to prevent spread between NICUs at different institutions, particularly when an infant is transferred from one NICU to another.
II	In the intake of a transferred patient, the receiving facility should be able to determine whether the infant has been screened previously for MRSA, and if so, the date, specimen source, and result of the culture.
II	In the intake of a transferred patient, the receiving facility should be able to determine whether the transferring institution currently knows of any MRSA-positive infants in its NICU.
IB	The receiving facility should consider isolation and screening of any infant transferred from another NICU, regardless of the transferring institution's MRSA status.
II	Standardized instruction sheets describing methods to prevent transmission of MRSA should be developed as a resource for parents and visitors of infants in NICUs in which MRSA has been detected.
Regulation	
IA	Overcrowding increases the likelihood of MRSA transmission in the NICU; institutions should adhere to all appropriate licensing requirements.
IA	Agency HCWs should be oriented to and monitored periodically for compliance with the institution's infection control and hand hygiene procedures.

(*Continued*)

Table 141–1. GUIDELINES FOR OUTBREAKS OF METHICILLIN-RESISTANT *STAPHYLOCOCCUS AUREUS* IN THE NICU (*CONTINUED*)

Recommendation Type, Rating Category[a]	Consensus Recommendation
Regulation (*cont.*)	
II	Logs of shifts worked by agency HCWs should be updated frequently to ensure that, in the case of an epidemiologic investigation, transmission links to these staff may be evaluated.
IC	Hospitals must comply with all local and state regulations regarding the reporting of MRSA in NICUs.
Hospital and public health collaboration	
II	Hospital officials should collaborate with state and local public health officials to conduct surveillance for MRSA in NICUs, facilitate inter-institutional communication and coordination of prevention activities, and provide laboratory support to allow detection of shared MRSA clones among NICUs in multiple institutions.

MRSA, methicillin-resistant *Staphylococcus aureus*; NICU, neonatal intensive care unit; HCW, health care worker.

[a]Rating categories are defined as follows. **IA:** Strongly recommended for implementation and strongly supported by well-designed experimental, clinical, or epidemiologic studies. **IB:** Strongly recommended for implementation and supported by some experimental, clinical, or epidemiologic studies and a strong theoretical rationale. **IC:** Required by state or federal regulations, rules, or standards. **II:** Suggested for implementation and supported by suggestive clinical or epidemiologic studies or a theoretical rationale. **NR/UI:** No recommendation or unresolved issue for which evidence is insufficient or no consensus regarding efficacy exists. Definitions from Boyce et al.

Reproduced with permission from Gerber SI, Jones RC, Scott MV, et al: Management of outbreaks of methicillin-resistant *Staphylococcus aureus* infection in the neonatal intensive care unit: a consensus statement, *Infect Control Hosp Epidemiol.* 2006 Feb;27(2):139-145.

142 Parvovirus B19 Infection

I. **Definition.** Human parvovirus B19 (B19V) is a small, single-stranded, nonenveloped DNA virus in the family Parvoviridae, genus *Erythrovirus*.

II. **Incidence.** Infection with B19V is common worldwide. Infection occurs mostly among school-aged children where the major manifestation is **erythema infectiosum** (also called **fifth disease**). Infection in adults can be entirely asymptomatic or may result in **polyarthropathy syndrome** and/or **petechial, papular-purpuric gloves-and-socks syndrome.** The prevalence of immunoglobulin G (IgG) antibodies directed against B19V ranges from 15% to 60% in children 6 to 19 years old. About 35% to 45% of women of childbearing age do not possess protective IgG antibodies against B19V and therefore are susceptible to primary infection. The incidence of acute B19V infection in pregnancy is 3.3% to 3.8%. Annual seroconversion rates in pregnant women in the United States range from 1% to 1.5%. The incubation period is between 4 and 14 days but can be as long as 21 days.

III. **Pathophysiology.** The pathogenesis of B19V infection is related to its tropism for erythroid progenitor cells. Infection and lysis of these cells make **B19V a potent inhibitor of hematopoiesis.** The cellular receptor for B19V is globoside or P-antigen, which is found on erythrocyte progenitor cells, synovium, placental tissue, fetal myocardium, and endothelial cells. The B19V-associated red blood cell aplasia is related to caspase–mediated apoptosis of erythrocyte precursors. Infection with B19V is usually acquired through respiratory droplets, but the virus can also be transmitted by blood or blood products and vertically from mother to fetus. In children and adults, viremia develops 2 days after exposure and reaches its peak at approximately 1 week. During the phase of viral replication and shedding, the patient is generally asymptomatic. When the typical rash (characterized by a "slapped cheek" appearance on the face and a "lace-like" erythematous rash on the trunk and extremities) or arthralgias develop, the patient is no longer infectious to others. Symptoms of the papular-purpuric gloves-and-socks syndrome can occur in association with viremia and before development of antibody response, and affected patients should be considered infectious. Symptoms during pregnancy are nonspecific and include a flulike syndrome with a low-grade fever, sore throat, generalized malaise, and headache. The fetus may become infected during the maternal viremic stage. Because of active erythropoiesis in the fetus with a shortened red cell life span, marked fetal anemia, high-output cardiac failure, and fetal hydrops may develop. Myocarditis, and less often fetal hepatic infection, may contribute to fetal cardiac failure. Teratogenicity from B19V has been described in case reports; also, one study found high prevalence of trisomy in pregnancy loss ascribable to B19V/erythrovirus infection. Despite that, B19V is considered nonteratogenic based on large epidemiologic studies.

IV. **Risk factors.** The risk of acquiring B19V infection during pregnancy is highest in schoolteachers, daycare workers, and women who have school-aged children at home.

V. **Clinical presentation**
   A. **During pregnancy.** The mother may report a history of exposure to a child with **erythema infectiosum**. More commonly, the mother does not recall such exposure and the diagnosis is made based on ultrasound findings. Fortunately, most maternal infections are associated with normal pregnancy outcomes. The overall risk of adverse outcomes after primary infection is probably <10% despite a transplacental transmission rate of 32% to 50%. Adverse outcomes include the following:
      1. **Fetal death.** Infection in the first trimester may result in fetal loss or miscarriage. A large prospective study of B19V infection in pregnant women reported fetal death in 6.3% of pregnancies (up to 10.2% in other smaller studies). All deaths were limited to B19V infections diagnosed in the first half of pregnancy (13% for first-trimester infections, 9% for infections diagnosed between 13 and 20 weeks of gestation). Fetal death in the third trimester is exceedingly rare (<1%), and those fetuses (stillborn) are usually nonhydropic.
      2. **Nonimmune hydrops fetalis.** The observed risk of B19V-induced hydrops fetalis is approximately 4% after maternal infection throughout pregnancy, with a maximum rate of approximately 10% when infection occurs between 9 and 20 weeks' gestation. The median interval between diagnosis of maternal infection and hydrops is 3 weeks. Hydrops can progress rapidly to fetal death (days to weeks) or can resolve spontaneously with an apparently normal infant at delivery. The spontaneous resolution is estimated at 34%. Severe thrombocytopenia can develop in 37% of parvovirus-infected fetuses with hydrops. This can lead to significant blood loss and exsanguination at the time of periumbilical blood sampling (PUBS) or other fetal procedures; for this reason, the platelet count should be determined and platelets should be available for transfusion if needed.
   B. **Neonatal period.** The newborn infant may present with anemia and thrombocytopenia, especially if maternal infection occurred in the third trimester. Few cases of encephalopathy, meningitis, and severe central nervous system abnormalities following intrauterine B19V infection have been reported.

VI. Diagnosis

    A. Laboratory studies

        1. Serologic tests. B19V IgG and IgM antibodies are first ordered when B19V infection is suspected. B19V-specific IgM antibodies become detectable in maternal serum within 7 to 10 days after infection, sharply peak at 10 to 14 days, and then rapidly decrease within 2 or 3 months. IgG antibodies rise considerably more slowly and reach a plateau at 4 weeks after infection. Measurement of maternal IgM is sensitive and detects approximately 90% of patients with clinical B19V infection. However, at the time of clinically overt hydrops fetalis, IgM levels may already have become low or (rarely) even undetectable. In such cases, detection of B19V DNA in maternal blood/serum by polymerase chain reaction (PCR) can be useful. In contrast to maternal testing, serologic examination of fetal and neonatal blood samples is highly unreliable.

        2. Polymerase chain reaction to detect B19V DNA is extremely sensitive. This method is especially useful in patients lacking an adequate antibody-mediated immune response, in immunocompromised individuals, and in fetuses. Using standard procedures, detection of B19V-specific IgM in fetal blood has a sensitivity of 29% compared with almost 100% for PCR. Use of PCR on amniotic fluid is particularly helpful when attempting to determine the cause of hydrops and is the method of choice to diagnose fetal B19V infection. However, low viral DNA levels may persist for years after acute infection in children and adults, and therefore, low-positive PCR results do not prove recent infection. The World Health Organization published a standard for B19V DNA amplification technology so that assay results can be reported in international units per milliliter (IU/mL) to allow for straightforward comparison across assays.

    B. Ultrasound and Doppler velocimetry are very useful noninvasive measures to monitor the pregnant woman who is exposed to B19V. Ultrasound is used to monitor for hydrops and fluid accumulation in fetal body cavities. **Doppler velocimetry is used to detect blood flow pattern in the fetal middle cerebral artery (MCA).** An increase in the MCA peak systolic velocity (MCA-PSV) is a very sensitive measure of fetal anemia.

VII. Management. Isolation precautions for all infectious diseases, including maternal and neonatal precautions, breast feeding, and visiting issues, can be found in Appendix F.

    A. Monitoring of the exposed pregnant woman. Women who have been exposed or symptomatic should be assessed by determining their B19V IgG and IgM status. Blood PCR is recommended when the fetus is hydropic. If the woman is immune to B19V (IgG positive, IgM negative), she can be reassured that recent exposure will not result in adverse consequences in her pregnancy. If there is no immunity to the virus and seroconversion has not taken place after 2 weeks, the woman is not infected but remains at risk. If the woman has been infected with B19V (IgM positive), the fetus should be monitored for the development of hydrops fetalis by ultrasound examination and Doppler assessment of MCA-PSV, preferably weekly until 8 to 10 weeks after exposure.

    B. Intrauterine blood transfusion. If the fetus subsequently develops hydrops and/or anemia (increase in MCA-PSV), PUBS and intrauterine blood transfusion (PUBS-IUT) should be considered. PUBS-IUT is an invasive procedure and carries a complication rate of 2% to 6% but can be lifesaving. It should be considered only for fetuses who are symptomatic. In most cases, 1 transfusion is sufficient for fetal recovery. When preparing for fetal transfusion, both packed red blood cells (PRBCs) and platelets must be available because some fetuses have severe thrombocytopenia in addition to anemia. Platelet transfusion may help if the fetus develops a hemorrhagic complication secondary to the procedure.

    C. Packed red blood cell transfusion. PRBC transfusion may be indicated for the symptomatic anemic newborn patient.

D. **Intravenous immunoglobulin.** Intravenous immunoglobulin (IVIG) has been used to treat acute B19V infection in immunodeficient adults and human immunodeficiency virus–infected children with aplastic crisis. However, there are only limited case reports on its use during pregnancy; as such, the use of IVIG cannot be recommended.

E. **Antiviral agents.** No antiviral agents are effective against B19V.

VIII. **Prognosis.** Mortality with parvovirus-related fetal hydrops is better than the generally reported mortality for nonimmune fetal hydrops (40%–90%). Children who survive fetal hydrops caused by B19V may have an increased risk of neurodevelopmental impairments. However, large population-based studies show B19V infection during pregnancy is not associated with overall morbidity or mortality in infancy and childhood.

143 Pertussis

I. **Definition.** Pertussis (whooping cough) is a highly contagious respiratory tract infection caused by the gram-negative bacteria *Bordetella pertussis*. While children may present with the classic whooping cough, neonates often present with an atypical and severe disease course.

II. **Incidence.** The Centers for Disease Control and Prevention (CDC) reported a national incidence rate of 6.5 cases per 100,000 in 2015, and despite vaccination, the incidence has been rising. The overall pertussis incidence rate among infants <12 months of age is approximately 118 per 100,000 person-years (infants <3 months of age have the highest incidence rate of ~248 per 100,000 person-years). Outbreaks in neonatal units with serious morbidity have been reported.

III. **Pathophysiology.** B pertussis is transmitted via close contact with respiratory secretions or aerosolized respiratory droplets. The source of pertussis infection in infants is unknown in about 50% of cases. In infants with a known origin of infection, the most commonly identified source has now shifted from mothers to siblings.

B pertussis is primarily a toxin-mediated disease. The organism produces multiple virulence factors including pertussis toxin, filamentous hemagglutinin, agglutinogens, adenylate cyclase, pertactin, and tracheal cytotoxin. Pertussis toxin leads to induction of lymphocytosis, and tracheal cytotoxin damages cilia in the respiratory epithelium via a nitric oxide synthase–dependent pathway. Lymphocytosis can lead to aggregation of leukocytes in the pulmonary circulation, causing severe pulmonary hypertension.

IV. **Risk factors.** Infants <6 months of age are at highest risk for severe pertussis and complications or death from pertussis, especially if they are unvaccinated. Other risk factors include prematurity and low birthweight.

V. **Clinical presentation.** The 3 phases of classic pertussis, namely **catarrhal** (1–2 weeks), **paroxysmal** (2–6 weeks), and **convalescent** (2–6 weeks), are not typically observed in young infants. Neonatal cases tend to present with paroxysmal cough, gagging, bradycardia, gasping, apnea (67%), and cyanotic spells, but not fever or tachypnea. They do not have the characteristic "whoop" due to lack of prolonged inspiratory effort at the end of a paroxysm. Infants <6 months of age tend to have a short or absent catarrhal phase. The following complications may be observed in neonates and young infants with pertussis:

A. **Secondary infections.** Pertussis can be complicated by secondary infections such as pneumonia (23%), meningoencephalitis, and otitis media.

    B. Ophthalmologic complications. The forceful coughing paroxysms characteristic of pertussis can result in eye bulging and subconjunctival, scleral, or rarely retinal hemorrhages.

    C. Central nervous system manifestations. Subdural bleeding may result from increased intracranial pressure secondary to the Valsalva effect of paroxysmal coughing. Seizures (2%) are attributed to hypoxemia from apnea or relentless coughing, but may also be due to hyponatremia secondary to pneumonia-induced syndrome of inappropriate antidiuretic hormone secretion. Encephalopathy (<0.5%) can also present with fever, convulsions, focal neurologic signs, and altered mental status.

    D. Respiratory complications. Infants with pertussis are at increased risk for severe pulmonary hypertension due to pulmonary vasoconstriction from hypoxia and acidosis secondary to recurrent prolonged apnea, as well as restriction of pulmonary blood flow from leukocyte aggregates. Neonates with pertussis have a greater need for mechanical ventilation due to frequent apnea, respiratory compromise during paroxysms of coughing, and pulmonary hypertension.

    E. Miscellaneous. The increased intrathoracic and intra-abdominal pressures associated with paroxysmal coughing can result in other physical sequelae such as epistaxis, petechiae, pneumothorax, and umbilical and inguinal hernias. Posttussive emesis can lead to alkalosis, dehydration, and malnutrition.

VI. Diagnosis. Pertussis should be differentiated from other infectious causes of respiratory distress in neonates. Adenoviral infections can produce apnea and intractable coughing but usually present with fever, lethargy, maculopapular rash, pharyngitis, conjunctivitis, and coagulopathy. *Mycoplasma pneumoniae* can present with protracted cough and pneumonia. *Chlamydia trachomatis* infections may present with conjunctivitis, nasal congestion, pneumonia, and a staccato cough in afebrile patients. Respiratory syncytial virus (RSV) can present with apnea and lower respiratory tract infection. Pertussis and RSV, as coexisting infections, are not infrequent. Other viral respiratory pathogens, such as influenza A and B viruses, parainfluenza viruses, rhinovirus, and human metapneumovirus, need to be considered in the differential diagnosis.

    A. Laboratory studies

        1. Complete blood count with differential. Leukocytosis (white blood cell [WBC] count of >20,000 cells/mm³) with lymphocytosis (>50% lymphocytes) is very strongly associated with pertussis. Marked leukocytosis (WBC ≥30,000 cells/mm³) has been associated with increased disease severity (pulmonary hypertension) and death.

        2. Bacterial culture. The gold standard for diagnosis is bacterial culture of a nasopharyngeal specimen placed in a special transport medium (Regan-Lowe). While this method is 100% specific, false-negative cultures can occur if the specimen is obtained >2 weeks after onset of cough or in pretreated or vaccinated patients.

        3. Polymerase chain reaction. Testing for pertussis by polymerase chain reaction (PCR) has increased sensitivity over bacterial culture. PCR is widely used due to its increased sensitivity and rapid turnaround time; however, false-positive cases have been reported. PCR is more reliable during the first 3 weeks of illness.

    B. Imaging studies

        1. Chest radiograph. Infants with uncomplicated pertussis usually have normal findings. Radiographic evidence of pneumonia may be seen in severe or complicated cases.

VII. Management

    A. Antimicrobial therapy. Macrolide antibiotics alleviate disease severity if given during the initial catarrhal stage. Treatment after cough is established does not affect the disease course but is recommended to reduce the risk of contagion. Azithromycin (10 mg/kg/d as a single daily dose for 5 days) is the current drug of choice for treatment and postexposure prophylaxis of pertussis in infants <1 month of age. Azithromycin should be used with caution in people with prolonged QT interval and proarrhythmic conditions. Neonates who receive macrolides (erythromycin and azithromycin, especially during the first 2 weeks of life) should be monitored for the development of infantile hypertrophic pyloric stenosis.

B. Respiratory support

1. **Mechanical ventilation.** Intubation and mechanical ventilation are often necessary due to frequent apnea or respiratory failure.

2. **Airway therapies.** Bronchodilators, inhaled steroids, and cough suppressants are not routinely recommended.

3. **Inhaled nitric oxide.** Vasodilator therapy with inhaled nitric oxide (iNO) does not address the issues of pertussis-associated pulmonary hypertension secondary to leukocyte thrombi in the pulmonary vasculature. Moreover, although there are some published reports of successful resolution of pertussis-related pulmonary hypertension with iNO, recent literature suggests that iNO might actually be detrimental in the setting of pertussis.

4. **Double-volume exchange transfusion** is suggested for high and rapidly rising WBC count and is thought to work by both leukodepletion and removal of the pertussis toxin. In case series, hypoxemia, pulmonary hypertension, and cardiac failure that were unresponsive to other measures improved after exchange transfusion.

5. **Extracorporeal life support (ECLS)** has been used for pertussis cases with refractory respiratory failure and pulmonary hypertension, but the mortality rate is significantly higher than that of infants on ECMO for other reasons.

C. Prevention/control measures

1. **Isolation.** Standard precautions are recommended for the entire course of illness. Droplet precaution is recommended for 5 days after initiation of effective therapy.

2. **Postexposure prophylaxis.** Early chemoprophylaxis (typically with azithromycin for 5 days) is recommended for all household contacts of the index case and other close contacts, including children in childcare, regardless of immunization status. Due to limited efficacy, late chemoprophylaxis (after 21 days) is only recommended for high-risk contacts (pregnant women and young infants or their contacts). The agents, doses, and duration of postexposure prophylaxis (PEP) are the same as for treatment of pertussis. Healthcare facilities should maximize efforts to immunize all healthcare personnel with tetanus, diphtheria, and pertussis (Tdap). PEP is recommended for all healthcare personnel (even if immunized with Tdap) who have been exposed to pertussis and are likely to expose other patients at risk of severe pertussis (eg, hospitalized neonates and pregnant women).

3. **Immunizations.** Six doses of pertussis vaccine are recommended during childhood. Preterm birth is not a contraindication to the pertussis vaccine.

4. **Newborn exposure.** Due to the drastic increase in pertussis cases, the CDC updated vaccine guidelines in 2013 to recommend that a dose of Tdap be administered during each pregnancy regardless of prior Tdap immunizations. Tdap should be administered preferably early in the interval between 27 and 36 weeks' gestation, although Tdap may be administered at any time during pregnancy. Current evidence suggests that immunization early in the interval between 27 and 36 weeks' gestation will maximize passive antibody transfer to the infant; this strategy has been shown to be highly protective against infant pertussis, especially in the first 2 months of life. In addition, the CDC, American Academy of Pediatrics, and American College of Obstetricians and Gynecologists advocate "cocooning" of newborns by providing postpartum immunization to all close contacts of the infant.

VIII. Prognosis. Factors associated with adverse outcomes in infants include low birthweight, younger gestational age, younger age at time of cough onset, higher peak WBC count, intubation, and use of nitric oxide.

144 Respiratory Syncytial Virus

I. **Definition.** Respiratory syncytial virus (RSV) is a large, enveloped, nonsegmented, negative-strand RNA virus of the genus *Pneumovirus* of the family Paramyxoviridae. The virus uses attachment (G) and fusion (F) surface glycoproteins for virus entry. Two major strains (groups A and B) have been identified and often circulate concurrently.

II. **Incidence.** Almost all children are infected at least once by 2 years of age. Humans are the only source of infection. Initial infection occurs most commonly during the child's first year. Reinfection throughout life is common. In the United States, RSV occurs in annual epidemics during winter and early spring (predominantly November through March). Communities in the southern United States, particularly some communities in the state of Florida, tend to experience the earliest onset of RSV activity (as early as July). In the southern hemisphere, wintertime epidemics occur from May to September, with a peak in May, June, or July. RSV is the most common cause of acute lower respiratory tract infection (ALRI) in children <1 year of age. **RSV is associated with up to 120,000 pediatric hospitalizations (1%–3% of children in the first 12 months of life) each year in the United States.** Globally, the annual rate of RSV hospitalization among children <5 years is approximately 4.4 per 1000; hospitalization rates are highest among children <6 months old (2%) and premature infants <1 year old (6.4%). In addition, RSV is a common cause of nosocomial infection in the neonatal intensive care unit (NICU). It can persist on environmental surfaces for several hours and for a half-hour or more on hands. Infection among hospital personnel and others may occur by hand-to-eye or hand-to-nasal epithelium self-inoculation with contaminated secretions.

III. **Pathophysiology.** The disease is generally limited to the respiratory tract. RSV usually is transmitted by direct or close contact with contaminated secretions, which may occur from exposure to large-particle droplets at short distances (typically <6 feet) or from fomites. The inoculation of the virus occurs in nasopharyngeal or ocular mucous membranes after contact with virus-containing secretions or fomites. The virus replicates in the nasopharynx and spreads to the small bronchiolar epithelium, sparing the basal cells. Subsequently, the virus extends to type 1 and 2 alveolar pneumocytes in the lung, presumably by cell-to-cell spread or via aspiration of secretions. In infants, the disease manifests itself as bronchiolitis or pneumonia. In very rare cases, RSV may be recovered from extrapulmonary tissues, such as liver, spinal, or pericardial fluid. Up to 30% of children with RSV bronchiolitis may be **coinfected** with another respiratory tract virus, such as human metapneumovirus, rhinovirus, bocavirus, adenovirus, coronavirus, influenza virus, or parainfluenza virus.

IV. **Risk factors.** Risk factors for RSV ALRI include infants <6 months of age, premature infants born <35 weeks' gestation, infants with underlying lung disease such as chronic lung disease (CLD) of prematurity, infants <2 years of age with heart disease, infants with school-aged siblings, infants who attend daycare, family history of asthma, regular exposure to secondhand smoke or air pollution, multiple birth babies, peak RSV season (fall to end of spring), being male, immunocompromised patients (eg, severe combined immunodeficiency, leukemia, or undergoing organ transplant), <1 month of or no breast feeding, and others sharing the bedroom with the infant. High altitude increases the risk of RSV hospitalization. Children with Down syndrome are at increased risk for severe RSV disease.

V. **Clinical presentation.** The incubation period ranges from 2 to 8 days. RSV usually begins in the nasopharynx with coryza and congestion. During the first 2 to 5 days, it may progress to the lower respiratory tract (20%–30%) with development of cough, dyspnea, and wheezing. RSV is the most common cause of bronchiolitis and pneumonia in infants <2 years old. Lethargy, irritability, and poor feeding are commonly present in young infants. **Apnea** may be the presenting symptom in approximately 20% of infants hospitalized with RSV and may be the cause of sudden, unexpected death. Most previously healthy infants infected with RSV do not require hospitalization. Most RSV hospitalizations occur in the first 3 months of life. RSV infection may predispose to reactive airway disease and recurrent wheezing during the first decade of life; the association between RSV bronchiolitis early in life and subsequent asthma remains poorly understood.

VI. **Diagnosis**
  A. **Enzyme-linked immunosorbent assay and direct fluorescent antibody tests** use antigen capture technology that can be performed in <30 minutes on nasal wash or tracheal aspirate. Their sensitivity is approximately 80%, and specificity is approximately 95% (in comparison with culture). False-positive test results are more likely to occur when the incidence of disease is low. Multiplex assays or viral respiratory panels (which test for multiple respiratory viruses with 1 test) may be preferred in many clinical settings because they are able to identify co-infection. Viral isolation from nasopharyngeal secretions in cell culture requires 1 to 5 days (shell vial techniques can produce results within 24–48 hours). Molecular diagnostic tests using reverse transcriptase–polymerase chain reaction (RT-PCR) are cleared by the US Food and Drug Administration and available widely; they increase RSV detection rates over viral isolation or antigen detection assays. RT-PCR is an alternative to culture for confirming the result of rapid antigen detection assay, which is rarely needed except to mark the start of the RSV season. Additionally, palivizumab exposure (see Section VII on management) may interfere with immunologic-based antigen detection assays (enzyme-linked immunosorbent assay and direct fluorescent antibody) as well cell culture, but it does not interfere with RT-PCR. Diagnostic serology is not helpful in infants because of the passive transplacental transfer of maternal antibody.
  B. **Chest radiograph** usually reveals infiltrates or hyperinflation.
  C. **Blood gas analysis** may show hypoxemia and occasionally hypercarbia. Development of hypercarbia is an ominous sign of impending respiratory failure.

VII. **Management.** Primary treatment of young infants hospitalized with RSV bronchiolitis is supportive and should include hydration, careful assessment of respiratory status, measurement of oxygen saturation, suction of the upper airway, use of a nasal continuous positive airway pressure or high-flow nasal cannula therapy, and if necessary, intubation and mechanical ventilation. Isolation precautions for all infectious diseases, including maternal and neonatal precautions, breast feeding, and visiting issues, can be found in Appendix F.
  A. **Immunization**
    1. **Passive**
      a. **Palivizumab (Synagis)** provides passive immunity. It is a humanized RSV monoclonal antibody administered intramuscularly (15 mg/kg) monthly during RSV season. It is well tolerated with infrequent or minimal side effects. According to the American Academy of Pediatrics guidelines, palivizumab should be considered for:
        i. **Infants with chronic lung disease of prematurity,** defined as having a gestational age <32 weeks, 0 days and a requirement for >21% oxygen for at least the first 28 days after birth. Prophylaxis may be given during the first RSV season (first year of life). During the second year of life, palivizumab is recommended only for CLD infants who continue to require medical support (chronic corticosteroid therapy, diuretic therapy, or supplemental oxygen) during the 6-month period before the start of the second RSV season.
        ii. **Infants with hemodynamically significant congenital heart disease.** Defined as acyanotic heart disease requiring medication to control congestive heart failure (CHF) and that will require cardiac surgical

procedures or as moderate to severe pulmonary hypertension. Decisions regarding palivizumab prophylaxis for infants with cyanotic heart defects in the first year of life may be made in consultation with a pediatric cardiologist. Palivizumab is given to qualifying infants in the first year of life who are born within 12 months of onset of the RSV season. Infants with hemodynamically insignificant congenital heart disease (CHD; eg, secundum atrial septal defect, small ventricular septal defect) should not receive prophylaxis. Infants with lesions adequately corrected by surgery, unless they continue to require medication for CHF, should also not receive palivizumab prophylaxis. Postoperative dose of palivizumab (15 mg/kg) should be considered after cardiac bypass or at the conclusion of extracorporeal membrane oxygenation for infants and children younger than 24 months.

iii. **Preterm infants without chronic lung disease or congenital heart disease.** Palivizumab prophylaxis may be administered to preterm infants born before 29 weeks, 0 days' gestation who are younger than 12 months at the start of the RSV season. For infants born during the RSV season, fewer than 5 monthly doses will be needed (usually until 3 months of age). Infants born at 29 weeks, 0 days' gestation or later are not universally recommended to receive palivizumab prophylaxis unless they qualify under the CLD or CHD criteria provided earlier.

iv. **Infants with congenital abnormalities of the airway or neuromuscular disease.** Palivizumab prophylaxis may be considered for infants who have either significant congenital abnormalities of the airway or a neuromuscular condition that compromises handling of respiratory tract secretions. Infants and young children in this category should receive a maximum of 5 doses of palivizumab during the first year of life.

v. **Immunocompromised children.** Prophylaxis may be considered for children younger than 24 months who will be profoundly immunocompromised during the RSV season (primary immune deficiency or secondary immune deficiency due to solid organ or hematopoietic stem cell transplantation or those receiving chemotherapy).

vi. **Children with cystic fibrosis.** Routine use of palivizumab prophylaxis in patients with cystic fibrosis (CF) is not recommended unless other indications are present. However, an infant with CF with clinical evidence of CLD and/or nutritional compromise in the first year of life may be considered for prophylaxis.

vii. **Special situations.** A lower threshold for administration of palivizumab prophylaxis may be warranted for **Alaska Native and American Indian infants <12 months of age** because of higher rate of RSV hospitalization and the costs associated with transport of such infants from remote locations. If any infant receiving monthly palivizumab prophylaxis experiences a **breakthrough RSV hospitalization**, monthly **prophylaxis should be discontinued** because of the extremely low likelihood of a second RSV hospitalization in the same season (<0.5%). No rigorous data exist to support palivizumab use in controlling **NICU RSV nosocomial outbreaks,** and palivizumab is **not recommended** for this purpose. Infants in the **NICU** who qualify for palivizumab prophylaxis may receive the first dose **48 to 72 hours before discharge** to home or promptly after discharge.

b. **Motavizumab** is another RSV-neutralizing antibody that has undergone clinical trials for RSV prevention, but it is no longer available (the manufacturer discontinued its development for RSV prevention).

2. **Active.** Several promising candidate RSV vaccines (both live attenuated and subunit vaccines from RSV F and G glycoproteins) are currently in development,

both at the preclinical and clinical stages. RSV maternal immunization is a strategy that is being studied for the prevention of RSV in neonates and young infants.

B. **Nebulized hypertonic saline (3%)** may be safe and effective at improving the symptoms of mild to moderate bronchiolitis after 24 hours of use and in reducing hospital length of stay in settings where the duration of stay is likely to exceed 3 days. Hypertonic saline has not been studied in NICU settings.

C. **Ribavirin** has in vitro antiviral activity against RSV, but ribavirin aerosol treatment for RSV is not recommended routinely.

D. **Surfactant.** Two small, randomized studies showed that surfactant therapy improves gas exchange and decreases mechanical ventilation days and intensive care unit stay in infants with severe RSV-induced respiratory failure.

E. **α-Adrenergic and β-adrenergic agents are not recommended** for care of first-time wheezing associated with RSV bronchiolitis based on randomized clinical trial findings.

F. **Antibiotics, theophylline, and corticosteroids** have not been shown to be helpful in the treatment of RSV.

G. **Isolation.** Contact precautions are recommended for the duration of the illness. RSV present in secretions remains viable for up to 6 hours on countertops. Gowns, gloves, and scrupulous hand-washing practices are required. Patients with RSV infection should be cared for in a single room or placed in a cohort. High-risk infants should be kept away from crowds and from situations in which exposure to infected people cannot be controlled. Participation in group childcare should be restricted during the RSV season for high-risk infants whenever feasible.

VIII. **Prognosis.** Globally, RSV is estimated to cause as many as 2.3% of deaths among neonates 0 to 27 days of age and 6.7% of deaths among infants 28 to 364 days of age. In the United States, estimated mortality is approximately 3.1 per 100,000 person-years in children <1 year old, mostly in children born prematurely and those with underlying cardiopulmonary disease or other chronic conditions. In prematurely born infants with CLD who are hospitalized because of RSV in the first 2 years of life, there is a reduced airway caliber at school age. Even in normal infants, RSV infection in the first 3 years of life predisposes them to recurrent wheezing up to 11 years of age. Palivizumab prophylaxis administered to preterm infants does not suppress the onset of atopic asthma but results in a significantly lower incidence of recurrent wheezing during the first 6 years.

145 Rubella

I. **Definition.** Rubella virus is an enveloped, positive-stranded RNA virus classified as a *Rubivirus* in the Togaviridae family. It is capable of causing chronic intrauterine infection and damage to the developing fetus (**congenital rubella syndrome [CRS]**).

II. **Incidence.** The incidence of rubella in the United States has decreased by >99% from the prevaccine era. In 2004, the United States was determined to no longer have endemic rubella, and from 2004 through 2014, 94 cases of rubella and 9 cases of CRS, including 3 cases in 2012, were reported; all of them were associated with individuals outside the United States or from unknown sources. Of childbearing women, 92% are estimated to be seropositive (rubella immune). Endemic transmission of rubella was declared eliminated from the Americas in 2015. However, rubella continues to be endemic in other parts of the world. It is estimated that >100,000 infants worldwide are born with CRS each year.

III. Pathophysiology. Rubella typically has an epidemic seasonal pattern of increased frequency in the spring. In developing countries with no vaccination programs, epidemics have occurred at 4- to 7-year intervals, with major pandemics every 10 to 30 years. Humans are the only known hosts, with an incubation period of 14 to 21 days after contact. Virus is spread by respiratory secretions and also from stool, urine, and cervical secretions. A live virus vaccine has been available since 1969. In places with no vaccination, 15% to 20% of women of childbearing age are susceptible to rubella. There is a high incidence of subclinical infections. Maternal viremia is a prerequisite for placental infection, which may or may not spread to the fetus. Most cases occur after primary disease, although few cases (2%) have been described after reinfection.

Rubella infection can have catastrophic effects on the developing fetus, resulting in spontaneous abortion, fetal infection, stillbirth, or intrauterine growth restriction. The fetal infection rate varies according to the timing of maternal infection during pregnancy. If infection occurs at 1 to 12 weeks and is associated with maternal rash, there is an 81% risk of fetal infection; at 13 to 16 weeks, 54%; at 17 to 22 weeks, 36%; at 23 to 30 weeks, 30%. There is a rise to 60% at 31 to 36 weeks and to 100% in the last month of pregnancy, but late infection is not associated with CRS. No correlation exists between the severity of maternal rubella and teratogenicity. However, the incidence of fetal effects is greater the earlier in gestation that infection occurs, especially at 1 to 12 weeks, when 85% of infected fetuses will have congenital defects. Infection during weeks 13 to 16 results in 35% of fetuses having congenital defects; infection at later gestational ages rarely causes deafness or congenital malformations. Spontaneous abortion may occur in up to 20% of cases when rubella occurs in the first 8 weeks of pregnancy. The disease involves angiopathy as well as cytolytic changes. Other viral effects include chromosome breakage, decreased cell multiplication time, induction of programmed cell death (apoptosis), and mitotic arrest in certain cell types. There is little inflammatory reaction.

IV. Risk factors. Women of childbearing age who are rubella nonimmune or foreign born are at risk.

V. Clinical presentation. Congenital rubella infection has a wide spectrum of presentations, ranging from asymptomatic infection to acute disseminated infection to deficits not evident at birth.

   A. Systemic transient manifestations include low birthweight, hepatosplenomegaly, meningoencephalitis, thrombocytopenia with or without purpura, and bony radiolucencies. These are probably a consequence of extensive viral infection and usually resolve spontaneously within days or weeks. Infants with these abnormalities usually fail to thrive during infancy.

   B. Systemic permanent manifestations include heart defects (eg, patent ductus arteriosus [PDA], pulmonary artery stenosis or hypoplasia), eye defects (eg, cataracts, iris hypoplasia, microphthalmos, and retinopathy), central nervous system (CNS) problems (eg, intellectual disability and psychomotor developmental delay, speech and language delay), microcephaly, and sensorineural deafness (unilateral or bilateral). More than half of children infected during the first 8 weeks of gestation have heart defects; **branch pulmonary artery stenosis** (78%) and **PDA** (62%) are the most common. Of the eye defects, a **"salt and pepper"** retinopathy is the most common. **Cataract** occurs in approximately 30% of cases of CRS (~50% bilateral); rubella virus is recovered in high titer from lens aspirates in children with congenital cataracts for several years. **Deafness** is a major disabling abnormality and may occur alone.

   C. Developmental and late-onset abnormalities. Rubella is a progressive disease due to the persistence of the viral infection and the defective immune response to the virus. Existing manifestations, such as deafness and CNS disease, may progress, and some abnormalities may not be detected until the second year of life or later. These include hearing, developmental and eye defects, diabetes mellitus (DM), thyroid disorders, behavioral and educational difficulties, and progressive panencephalitis. Insulin-dependent DM is the most frequent endocrine abnormality, occurring in approximately 20% of cases.

VI. **Diagnosis.** Timely diagnosis of congenital rubella infection is important both for management of the individual patient and for prevention of secondary infection because these infants may remain infectious for 1 year. The diagnosis may be suspected clinically but needs to be confirmed with laboratory tests. The Centers for Disease Control and Prevention (CDC) has published an elaborate case definition for congenital rubella infection that is updated regularly (https://wwwn.cdc.gov/nndss/conditions/rubella-congenital-syndrome/; accessed September 6, 2018). According to the most recent update available at the time of publication (2010), cases of CRS are classified as suspected, probable, confirmed, or infection only, depending on clinical findings and laboratory criteria for diagnosis.

A. **Centers for Disease Control and Prevention case definition**

1. **Suspected. An infant who has 1 or more of the following findings (but does not meet the criteria for a confirmed or probable case):** cataracts or congenital glaucoma, congenital heart disease (most commonly PDA or peripheral pulmonary artery stenosis), hearing impairment, pigmentary retinopathy, purpura, hepatosplenomegaly, jaundice, microcephaly, developmental delay, meningoencephalitis, or radiolucent bone disease.

2. **Probable. An infant who has at least 2 of the following findings (but does not have laboratory confirmation of rubella infection or a more plausible etiology):** either cataracts or congenital glaucoma or both (counts as 1), congenital heart disease (most commonly PDA or peripheral pulmonary artery stenosis), hearing impairment, or pigmentary retinopathy.

   OR

   An infant who has at least 1 or more of the following (but does not have laboratory confirmation or an alternative more plausible etiology): either cataracts or congenital glaucoma or both (counts as 1), congenital heart disease (PDA or peripheral pulmonary artery stenosis), hearing impairment, or pigmentary retinopathy

   AND

   1 or more of the following of the following: purpura, hepatosplenomegaly, microcephaly, developmental delay, meningoencephalitis, or radiolucent bone disease.

3. **Confirmed. An infant with at least 1 symptom (listed previously) that is clinically consistent with CRS and laboratory evidence of congenital rubella infection as demonstrated by:** isolation of rubella virus, or detection of rubella-specific immunoglobulin (Ig) M antibody, or infant rubella antibody level that persists at a higher level and for a longer period than expected from passive transfer of maternal antibody (ie, rubella titer that does not drop at the expected rate of a 2-fold dilution per month), or a specimen that is polymerase chain reaction (PCR) positive for rubella virus.

4. **Infection only. An infant with laboratory evidence of infection but with no clinical symptoms or signs.** Laboratory evidence is as shown in Section VI.A.3. **If any signs or symptoms are identified later such as hearing loss, then the diagnosis is reclassified as confirmed.**

5. **Congenital rubella syndrome cases are further classified epidemiologically as internationally imported or United States acquired**, according to the source of infection in the mother.

B. **Laboratory studies**

1. **Open cultures.** The virus can be cultured for up to 1 year despite measurable antibody titer. The best specimens for viral recovery are from nasopharyngeal swabs, conjunctival scrapings, urine, and cerebrospinal fluid (CSF), in decreasing order of usefulness.

2. **Serologic studies.** These are the mainstay of rubella diagnosis. CRS is diagnosed by the detection of **rubella-specific IgM in a serum or oral fluid taken before 3 months of age**. IgM testing is less reliable after 3 months of age as levels of

specific IgM decline. However, if sensitive assays are used, specific IgM may be detected in 85% of symptomatic infants at 3 to 6 months and >30% at 6 to 12 months of age. A negative result by IgM-capture enzyme immunosorbent assay in the first 3 months of age virtually excludes congenital infection. It is also possible to make a diagnosis by demonstrating persistence of rubella IgG in sera taken between 6 and 12 months of age. It is difficult to make a serologic diagnosis of congenital rubella after rubella vaccination. Testing of oral fluid samples (IgM, IgG, and PCR) as an alternative to serum has been used and standardized. It offers many advantages for surveillance of CRS in developing countries. A false-positive IgM test result may rarely occur; this is caused by a number of factors including rheumatoid factor, parvovirus IgM, and heterophile antibodies. If false-positive IgM results are suspected, IgG avidity assay in a reference laboratory (eg, CDC) can be used to confirm or refute the diagnosis. IgG avidity and IgG response to the 3 viral structural proteins (E1, E2, and C), reflected by immunoblot fluorescent signals may help to establish the diagnosis of CRS in older school-aged children.

3. **Rubella virus polymerase chain reaction.** CRS may also be diagnosed by detection of viral RNA by nested reverse transcriptase (RT)-PCR in nasopharyngeal swabs, urine, oral fluid, CSF, lens aspirate, and ethylenediaminetetraacetic acid (EDTA)-blood.

4. **Cerebrospinal fluid examination.** This may reveal encephalitis with an increased protein and cell count.

C. **Imaging studies.** Long-bone films may show metaphyseal radiolucencies that correlate with metaphyseal osteoporosis.

VII. **Management.** Prenatal serologic screening for rubella immunity should be undertaken for all pregnant women. Those without antibody concentrations above the standard positive cutoff or those with equivocal test results **should receive rubella vaccine during the immediate postpartum period before discharge**. Cases of CRS (suspected or confirmed) in the United States should be reported to the CDC through local and state health departments. All newborns who fail hearing screening and born to mothers who are rubella nonimmune should undergo evaluation for rubella (measurement of rubella-specific IgM antibodies) and other intrauterine infections. There is no specific treatment for rubella. Long-term follow-up is needed secondary to late-onset symptoms. Prevention consists of vaccination of the susceptible population (especially young children). **Vaccine should not be given to pregnant women.** Pregnancy should be avoided for 28 days after vaccination. Inadvertent vaccination of pregnant women does not cause CRS, although there is a 3% chance of congenital infection. Passive immunization (with immune globulin [IG]) does not prevent rubella infection after exposure and is not recommended. Administration of IG should be considered only if a pregnant woman who has been exposed to rubella will not consider termination of pregnancy under any circumstance. Administration of IG eliminates the value of IgG antibody testing to detect maternal infection; however, IgM antibody can still be used to detect maternal infection after exposure. Children with congenital rubella should be considered contagious until they are at least 1 year of age, unless 2 cultures of clinical specimens (nasopharyngeal and urine cultures) obtained 1 month apart are negative for rubella virus after 3 months of age. Rubella vaccine virus can be isolated from breast milk in lactating women who have received the vaccine. However, **breast feeding is not a contraindication to vaccination** because no evidence indicates that the vaccine virus is in any way harmful to the infant.

VIII. **Prognosis.** Infection in the first or second trimester can cause growth restriction, deafness, and other congenital malformations (CRS, discussed earlier). Congenital rubella is a progressive disease, some of its consequences may not present until the second decade of life (motor and mental retardation, hearing and communication disorders, DM). Natural rubella infection in pregnancy is 1 of the few known causes of autism.

146 Sepsis

Neonatal sepsis is a clinical syndrome of systemic illness accompanied by bacteremia occurring in the first month of life. It can be classified into 2 relatively distinct syndromes based on the age of presentation: early-onset and late-onset sepsis. These 2 entities will be discussed separately.

NEONATAL EARLY ONSET SEPSIS

   I. **Definition.** Early-onset sepsis (EOS) is defined by the Centers for Disease Control and Prevention (CDC) as blood and/or cerebrospinal fluid (CSF) culture–proven infection occurring in the newborn at <7 days of age. For the continuously hospitalized very low birthweight (VLBW; <1500 g) infant, EOS is defined as culture-proven infection occurring at <72 hours of age.
  II. **Incidence.** The overall incidence of EOS in the United States is estimated at 0.77 to 0.98 per 1000 live births. Incidence is strongly influenced by gestational age (GA) at birth. Among infants born at ≥37 weeks' gestation, the incidence is around 0.53 per 1000 live births, whereas in the preterm population, the incidence is 3.7 per 1000 live births (7 times higher), and among VLBW infants, it is approximately 11 per 1000 live births (20 times higher).
 III. **Pathophysiology**
      A. **Infants usually present with a multisystem, sometimes fulminant, illness with prominent respiratory symptoms.** Typically, the infant has acquired the organism during the antepartum or intrapartum period from the maternal genital tract. Several infectious agents, notably treponemes, viruses (eg, herpes simplex virus, enteroviruses, and parechoviruses), *Listeria*, and probably *Candida*, can be acquired transplacentally via hematogenous routes. Acquisition of other organisms is associated with the birth process. With rupture of membranes, vaginal flora or other bacterial pathogens may ascend to reach the amniotic fluid and the fetus. Chorioamnionitis develops, leading to fetal colonization and infection. Aspiration of infected amniotic fluid by the fetus or neonate may play a role in the resultant respiratory symptoms. Finally, the infant may be exposed to vaginal flora as it passes through the birth canal. The primary sites of colonization tend to be the skin, nasopharynx, oropharynx, conjunctiva, and umbilical cord. Trauma to these mucosal surfaces may lead to infection. The disease may present suddenly with a fulminant course that can progress rapidly to septic shock and death.
      B. **Microbiology.** The principal pathogens involved in EOS have tended to change with time. Before 1965, *Staphylococcus aureus* and *Escherichia coli* used to be the most commonly isolated organisms. In the late 1960s and early 1970s, **group B Streptococcus (GBS)** emerged as the most common microorganism. Currently, most centers continue to report GBS as the most common microorganism, even though the incidence has decreased considerably after the widespread adoption of universal antenatal screening for GBS colonization at 35 to 37 weeks' gestation and intrapartum antibiotic prophylaxis (IAP) with penicillin or ampicillin for colonized women. **The incidence of EOS secondary to GBS decreased from 1.7 per 1000 live births in 1993 to 0.22 per 1000 in 2016 (>85% reduction).** The second most common bacteria are gram-negative enteric organisms, especially *E coli*. An increase in the incidence of *E coli* has been noted in EOS in VLBW infants to the extent that *E coli* is currently the predominant microorganism in this group of patients. GBS and *E coli* account for two-thirds of all cases of EOS. Other pathogens causing EOS include *Listeria monocytogenes, S aureus,* enterococci, other gram-negative bacteria (*Klebsiella, Citrobacter, Serratia,* and *Enterobacter*), anaerobes (especially *Bacteroides fraglis*), *Haemophilus influenzae,* and *Streptococcus pneumoniae.*

IV. **Risk factors for neonatal early-onset sepsis**

   A. **Prematurity and low birthweight.** Prematurity (especially if <35 weeks' gestation) is the single most significant factor correlated with sepsis. The risk increases in proportion to the decrease in birthweight and GA.

   B. **Rupture of membranes ≥18 hours.** The risk for proven sepsis increases 10-fold.

   C. **Maternal peripartum infection.** Infections such as **chorioamnionitis** manifesting as **maternal fever**, urinary tract infection (UTI) especially **GBS bacteriuria**, **rectovaginal colonization with GBS**, and perineal colonization with *E coli* are well-recognized risk factors for EOS. Chorioamnionitis is an imprecise and heterogeneous disorder; the National Institute of Child Health and Human Development (NICHD) convened a group of experts in 2015 to a workshop that issued evidence-based recommendations with regard to this issue. The group proposed to replace the term *chorioamnionitis* with a more general descriptive term: "**intrauterine inflammation or infection or both,**" abbreviated as "**triple I.**" However, this terminology has not been widely accepted yet. The American College of Obstetricians and Gynecologists (ACOG) endorsed the recommendations of the NICHD workshop but chose to use the term "intraamniotic infection" instead.

   D. **Previous delivery of a neonate with group B streptococcal disease.**

   E. **Fetal and intrapartum distress.** Infants who had intrapartum fetal tachycardia, meconium-stained amniotic fluid, were born by traumatic delivery, or were severely depressed at birth and required intubation and resuscitation are either infected in utero or at significant risk for EOS.

   F. **Multiple gestation.**

   G. **Metabolic factors.** Hypoxia, acidosis, inherited metabolic disorders (eg, galacto-semia predisposing to *E coli* sepsis), and immune defects (eg, asplenia) are factors that predispose to, as well as increase the severity of, sepsis.

   H. **Other factors.** Males are affected 4 times more often than females, and the possibil-ity of a sex-linked genetic basis for host susceptibility is postulated. **Black African descent** is an independent risk factor for EOS with GBS. Reasons for the dispropor-tionately high disease burden among black populations cannot be fully explained by prematurity or socioeconomic status. However, Black African descent is known to be associated with higher rates of GBS colonization.

V. **Clinical presentation of neonatal early-onset sepsis.** Because the initial diagnosis of sepsis is, by necessity, a clinical one, it is crucial to begin treatment before the results of cultures are available. Clinical signs and symptoms of sepsis are nonspecific, and the differential diagnosis is broad. Some signs are subtle or insidious, and therefore, a high index of suspicion is required to identify and evaluate infected neonates. Clinical signs and symptoms most often mentioned include the following:

   A. **Temperature irregularity.** Hypothermia is more common than fever as a presenting sign for bacterial sepsis in premature infants. Hyperthermia is more common in full-term infants beyond the first 24 hours of life and if viral agents (eg, herpes) are involved.

   B. **Change in behavior.** Lethargy, irritability, seizures, or change in tone.

   C. **Skin.** Poor peripheral perfusion, cyanosis, mottling, pallor, petechiae, rashes, sclerema, and jaundice singularly or in combinations are known signs of sepsis.

   D. **Cardiopulmonary.** Tachypnea, respiratory distress (grunting, flaring, and retrac-tions), apnea within the first 24 hours of birth, tachycardia, and hypotension singu-larly or in combinations should suggest sepsis. Hypotension tends to be a late sign.

   E. **Metabolic.** Metabolic findings include hyperkalemia, hyponatremia, hyperglyce-mia, or metabolic acidosis. There is no evidence that hypoglycemia occurring in isolation is a risk factor or manifestation of EOS.

VI. **Diagnosis**

   A. **Differential diagnosis.** Because signs and symptoms of neonatal sepsis are nonspecific, noninfectious etiologies need to be considered. If the infant is presenting with respiratory symptoms, respiratory distress syndrome, transient tachypnea of the newborn, meconium aspiration, and aspiration pneumonia are considered. If the infant is showing central nervous system (CNS) symptoms, then meningitis, intracranial hemorrhage, drug withdrawal, and inborn errors of metabolism are considered.

B. Laboratory studies

1. **Cultures.** Blood and other normally sterile body fluids (eg, tracheal aspirate and CSF) should be obtained for culture. Body surface cultures are not recommended.

    a. **Blood cultures.** Modern, computer-assisted automated blood culture systems use optimized enriched culture media with antimicrobial neutralization properties; they provide continuous-read detection and are able to identify up to 94% to 96% of all microorganisms by 36 hours of incubation. Results may vary because of a number of factors, including maternal antibiotics administered before birth, organisms that are difficult to grow and isolate (ie, anaerobes), and sampling error with small sample volumes (**the minimum volume for blood culture is 1 mL**). The concerns about low-level bacteremia and the effect of intrapartum antibiotic administration are not substantiated as these systems have been shown to reliably detect bacteremia at a level of 1 to 10 colony-forming units per mL if a minimum blood volume of 1 mL is inoculated. Additionally, several studies have reported no effect of intrapartum antibiotic therapy on time to positivity since the culture media contains antimicrobial neutralization elements that efficiently neutralize β-lactam antibiotic agents as well as gentamicin. One aerobic blood culture is typically obtained in cases of EOS, however, the use of 2 separate culture bottles (1 aerobic and 1 anaerobic) may provide the opportunity to determine if commensal species are true infections by comparing growth in the 2 cultures. In some clinical situations where the infant is critically ill, it may be appropriate to treat for "presumed" sepsis despite negative cultures.

    b. **Lumbar puncture.** Some *controversy* currently exists regarding whether a lumbar puncture (LP) is needed in asymptomatic newborns being worked up for presumptive EOS. Many institutions perform LPs only on infants who are clinically ill, infants who have CNS symptoms such as apnea or seizures, or in cases of documented positive blood cultures or if the decision is made to extend antibiotics beyond 48 hours for presumptive clinical sepsis.

    c. **Urine cultures.** In neonates <24 hours of age, a sterile urine specimen is **not recommended** given that the occurrence of UTIs is exceedingly rare in this age group.

    d. **Tracheal cultures** may be obtained shortly after intubation (within 3 hours) in ill neonates with a clinical picture suggestive of early-onset pneumonia or if the mother developed intraamniotic infection with overwhelming EOS of the newborn. Tracheal aspirates done after several hours or days of intubation are of limited value.

2. **Gram stain.** Gram staining is especially helpful for the study of CSF. Gram-stained smears and cultures of amniotic fluid are helpful in diagnosing intraamniotic infection. A Gram stain of tracheal aspirate can show the infecting microorganism in EOS/pneumonia.

3. **Molecular testing.** Molecular methods for detection of neonatal sepsis in blood include polymerase chain reaction (PCR) and DNA microarray–based methods. Most of these tests hold the promise of rapid detection directly from blood without prior culture combined with high sensitivity and specificity in relation to cultures and with using small volume of blood. A recent Cochrane review that evaluated 35 studies found a summary estimate of sensitivity of 0.90 and specificity of 0.93 and concluded that molecular assays have the advantage of producing rapid results and may perform well as add-on tests.

4. **Other laboratory tests**

    a. **Complete blood count with differential.** These values alone are very non-specific. There are reference values for total white blood cell (WBC) count and absolute neutrophil counts as a function of postnatal age in hours (they peak during the first 12–14 hours of age; see Chapter 78, particularly Tables 78–1 and 78–2). Neutropenia may be a significant finding with an ominous prognosis when associated with EOS. The presence of immature forms is more specific but still rather insensitive. Ratio of immature to total polymorphonuclear cells **(I/T) >0.2** has good predictive value, if present. The diagnostic yield of WBC count improves when testing is done **after 6 hours of age**. A variety of conditions other than sepsis can alter neutrophil counts and ratios, including maternal hypertension and fever, neonatal asphyxia, maternal intrapartum oxytocin, hypoglycemia, stressful labor, meconium aspiration syndrome, pneumothorax, and even prolonged crying. Serial WBC counts obtained several hours apart may be helpful in establishing a trend. **Decreased platelet count** can be associated with EOS; however, this is usually a late sign and very nonspecific.

b. **Acute-phase reactants (APRs).** APRs are complex multifunctional group comprising complement components, coagulation proteins, protease inhibitors, C-reactive protein (CRP), and others that rise in concentration in the serum in response to inflammation. The inflammation may be secondary to infection, trauma, or other processes of cellular destruction. An elevated APR does not distinguish between infectious and noninfectious causes of inflammation. Except for CRP and procalcitonin (PCT), most APRs are not commercially available for routine testing.

   i. **C-reactive protein** is an APR that increases the most in the presence of inflammation caused by infection or tissue injury. The highest concentrations of CRP are reported in patients with bacterial infections, whereas moderate elevations typify chronic inflammatory conditions. Synthesis of CPR by hepatocytes is modulated by cytokines. Interleukin (IL)-1β, IL-6, IL-8, and tumor necrosis factor (TNF) are the most important regulators of CRP synthesis. CRP secretion starts within 4 to 6 hours after the inflammatory stimulus and peaks at approximately 36 to 48 hours. The biologic half-life of CRP is 19 hours, with a 50% reduction daily after the acute-phase stimulus resolves. A single normal value (<1 mg/dL) cannot rule out infection because the sampling may have preceded the rise in CRP; if a single value is obtained, it needs to be done after 18 hours of age. If CRP is obtained, serial determinations are better than a single value. Two normal CRP determinations (8–24 hours after birth and 24 hours later) have been shown to have a negative predictive value of 99.7% for proven neonatal sepsis. CRP elevations in noninfected neonates have been seen with fetal hypoxia, respiratory distress syndrome (RDS), and meconium aspiration; after trauma/surgery; and after immunizations. Serial abnormal CRP values alone should not be used to decide whether to administer antibiotics in the absence of a culture-confirmed infection. A false-positive rate of 8% has been found in healthy neonates. Nonetheless, CRP is a valuable adjunct in the diagnosis of sepsis (ruling it out when serial CRPs are low), monitoring the response to treatment, and guiding duration of treatment.

   ii. **Procalcitonin** is a propeptide of calcitonin that is released by parenchymal cells in response to bacterial toxins. A recent systematic review showed a sensitivity of 0.85 and specificity of 0.54 for detection of neonatal sepsis (EOS and late-onset sepsis [LOS]) at the PCT cutoff of 2.0 to 2.5 ng/mL. A recent multicenter randomized controlled trial showed that PCT seems to have some utility in guiding the duration of antibiotic therapy in neonates with suspected EOS. A physiologic increase in the PCT concentration occurs within the first 24 hours of birth.

   iii. **Cytokines interleukin-6, interleukin-8, and tumor necrosis factor** are produced primarily by activated monocytes and macrophages and are major mediators of the systemic response to infection. Studies have shown that combining cytokines with CRP may be better than using CRP alone.

iv. **Neutrophil surface antigens CD11, CD14, and CD64** are promising markers of early infection that correlate well with CRP but peak earlier. **Presepsin** (soluble CD14 subtype) has attracted recent attention because of its utility as a sepsis marker in adults. Preliminary studies in neonates have shown that most variables commonly affecting CRP and PCT values do not affect presepsin levels, which suggests that presepsin could become an effective sepsis marker in neonates.

C. **Imaging studies.** **Chest radiograph** should be obtained in cases with respiratory symptoms, although it is often impossible to distinguish GBS or *Listeria* pneumonia from uncomplicated RDS. One distinguishing feature is the presence of pleural effusion, which occurs in 67% of cases of pneumonia.

D. **Other studies.** Examination of the placenta and fetal membranes may disclose evidence of chorioamnionitis and thus an increased potential for neonatal infection.

VII. **Management.** Isolation precautions for all infectious diseases, including maternal and neonatal precautions, breast feeding, and visiting issues, can be found in Appendix F. Chapter 78 (on call problem "Post-delivery Antibiotics") discusses which infants should be considered for antibiotics.

A. **Prevention: group B *Streptococcus* prophylaxis.** Because of the widespread use of IAP, EOS secondary to GBS has been reduced by >85%. Fortunately, GBS prevention efforts have not led to an increasing burden of early-onset *E coli* infections. Approximately 20% to 30% of pregnant women are colonized with GBS in the vaginal or rectal area. Consensus guidelines regarding management of GBS were published by the CDC in 1996 and were later revised in 2002 and in 2010. In 2017, representatives from the CDC, AAP, ACOG, and other stakeholder organizations agreed to review and revise the 2010 GBS guidelines. It was decided that the AAP would revise neonatal care recommendations and ACOG would revise obstetric care guidelines. These separate but congruent clinical reports were published in July 2019 and replaced the CDC 2010 GBS perinatal guidelines. They recommend that all pregnant women should be screened at **36 0/7 to 37 6/7 weeks' gestation** for vaginal and rectal GBS colonization. At the time of labor or rupture of membranes, IAP should be given to all pregnant women identified as GBS carriers. Women with GBS isolated from the urine (**GBS bacteriuria, any colony count**) during their current pregnancy should receive IAP because such women usually are heavily colonized with GBS and are at increased risk of delivering an infant with EOS. Women who have **previously given birth to an infant with invasive GBS disease** should receive IAP as well. Additionally, women who were **GBS colonized during a previous pregnancy have a 50% likelihood of GBS carriage in the current pregnancy**, therefore, ACOG guidelines recommend that if a woman with unknown GBS status presents in labor and is known to have had GBS colonization in a previous pregnancy, IAP should be considered for such woman. **Penicillin is the drug of choice**, but ampicillin is an acceptable alternative. First generation cephalosporins (ie, cefazolin) are recommended for women whose reported penicillin allergy indicates a low risk of anaphylaxis or is of uncertain severity. Penicillin allergy skin testing, if available, is safe during pregnancy and can be recommended to "penicillin-allergic" women to ascertain their true risk of anaphylaxis. Clindamycin is the recommended alternative to penicillin only if the GBS isolate is known to be susceptible to clindamycin. Vancomycin is used when there is a high-risk penicillin allergy and when GBS isolate is not susceptible to clindamycin. The risk-based approach is not acceptable except for circumstances in which screening results are not available before labor and delivery. In these circumstances, IAP should be given to women <37 weeks' gestation, those with rupture of membranes ≥18 hours, and women who have a fever ≥38°C (100.4°F). Women with GBS colonization in one pregnancy have an estimated 50% risk of colonization in a subsequent pregnancy, therefore GBS IAP may be considered for such women. The guidelines recognize the availability of commercial **nucleic acid amplification tests (NAAT) such as PCR for rapid detection of GBS**. If available, NAAT intrapartum rectovaginal testing can be performed on women with unknown GBS status and no intrapartum GBS risk factors. IAP should be given if the NAAT testing returns positive or an intrapartum risk factor develops regardless of NAAT results. In addition, the guidelines specifically addressed **threatened preterm labor (PTL) and preterm prelabor rupture of membranes (pPROM) with detailed algorithms**. Briefly, women with threatened PTL or pPROM should be screened for GBS colonization on admission unless a GBS culture was obtained within the preceding 5 weeks. In both of these situations, women should receive GBS prophylaxis (typically for 48 hours) unless the screening results are negative. The recommendations also provide clarification on optimal GBS culturing methods. On the neonatal side, the GBS guidelines (published by AAP) review the epidemiology of neonatal GBS disease and provide specific algorithms for neonatal management based on risk assessment and gestational age (see next sections).

B. **Neonatal risk assessment for infants born at ≥35 weeks' gestation.** The AAP report acknowledges and endorses 3 commonly used approaches to risk assessment among infants born at ≥35 weeks' gestation as follows:

1. **Categorical risk assessment.** This approach uses risk factor (mainly maternal intrapartum fever–oral temperature >38°C) to identify infants at increased risk for EOS due to GBS (Figure 146–1A). Different versions of this approach

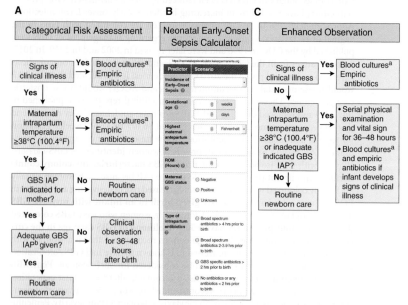

FIGURE 146–1. Options for EOS risk assessment among infants born ≥35 weeks' gestation. (A) Categorical risk assessment. (B) Neonatal Early-Onset Sepsis Calculator. (*The screenshot of the Neonatal Early-Onset Sepsis Calculator [https://neonatalsepsiscalculator.kaiserpermanente .org/] was used with permission from Kaiser-Permanente Division of Research.*) (C) Enhanced observation. ªConsider lumbar puncture and CSF culture before initiation of empiric antibiotics for infants who are at the highest risk of infection, especially those with critical illness. Lumbar puncture should not be performed if the infant's clinical condition would be compromised, and antibiotics should be administered promptly and not deferred because of procedure delays. ᵇAdequate GBS IAP is defined as the administration of penicillin G, ampicillin, or cefazolin ≥4 hours before delivery. (*Reproduced with permission from Puopolo KM, Lynfield R, Cummings JJ, et al: Management of Infants at Risk for Group B Streptococcal Disease, Pediatrics. 2019 Aug;144(2). pii: e20191881.*)

have been published previously including the algorithm published by CDC in 2010. For the purpose of categorical risk assessment, maternal intrapartum temperature >38°C is used as a surrogate for intraamniotic infection (called chorioamnionitis in the 2010 CDC algorithm). The administration of penicillin G, ampicillin, or cefazolin >4 hours before delivery is considered adequate GBS IAP; other antibiotics or other durations of treatment <4 hours are considered inadequate for this approach. It has been recognized that the risk of EOS is highly variable when maternal fever (any degree) is used alone as the principal categorical risk. Other important factors that modify the risk substantially include gestational age, duration of ROM, and timing and content of administered intrapartum antibiotics. Adopting this approach may result in many relatively low risk infants receiving empirical antibiotic treatment unnecessarily, especially if their only risk is exposure to low-grade maternal fever.

2. **Multivariate risk assessment (the Neonatal Early-Onset Sepsis Calculator):** Multivariate risk assessment integrates the individual infant's combination of objective quantifiable risk factors and his/her clinical examination to estimate the individual infant's risk of EOS (including EOS secondary to GBS). Predictive models based on gestational age at birth (weeks and days), highest maternal intrapartum temperature (centigrade or Fahrenheit), maternal GBS colonization status (positive, negative, uncertain), duration of ROM (hours), and type and duration of intrapartum antibiotic therapies (1 of 4 categories) have been developed and validated. The models are available as web-based Neonatal Early-Onset Sepsis Calculator (Figure 146–1B) (**neonatalsepsiscalculator .kaiserpermanente.org**). The calculator begins with the previous probability of EOS (typically of 0.5/1000 in the United States, unless local incidence of EOS is known to differ). When using the calculator, only penicillin, ampicillin, or cefazolin should be considered as "GBS-specific antibiotics." The administration of clindamycin or vancomycin alone for intrapartum GBS prophylaxis for any duration is currently recommended to be entered as "no antibiotics." Entering the data listed above in the calculator produces risk estimate of EOS per 1000 births and recommends further action based on infant's examination ranging from enhanced clinical observation to blood culture and empirical antibiotic therapy. Using the original dataset, if the hypothetical risk of sepsis ranged from 0.65 to 1.54 per 1000 live births (based solely on objective risk factors), 823 well-appearing neonates born to women with maternal fever/possible intraamniotic infection would need treatment to capture the one truly infected neonate (the number needed to treat). Such newborns account for 11% of all live births. For example, if a well-appearing newborn infant is born at 39 2/7 weeks' gestation to a GBS positive mother with maximum intrapartum temperature of 38.5°C (called by obstetricians as chorioamnionitis), with ROM for 18 hours and IAP with Penicillin G, one dose 3 hours prior to delivery, this infant's sepsis risk score is calculated at 1.13. The management of the infant in this scenario would be different if categorical risk assessment is used (blood culture followed by empirical antibiotics) compared to Neonatal Sepsis Calculator (no culture, no antibiotics; vitals every 4 hours for 24 hours). Several retrospective and prospective studies have demonstrated the utility of the sepsis calculator in substantially reducing laboratory testing and exposure to antimicrobial agents (compared to categorical risk strategy) in populations of well-appearing neonates with gestational age ≥35 weeks without missing EOS, provided that these neonates receive continued observation for 48 hours after birth. Centers that opt for this approach will need to develop a structured method for close clinical observation of infants at specific levels of estimated risk.

3. **Risk assessment based on clinical condition (enhanced observation):** This approach relies on clinical signs of illness to identify infants with EOS (including that secondary to GBS) regardless of neonatal or maternal

risk factors (Figure 146–1C). Infants who appear ill at birth and those who develop signs of illness over the first 48 hours after birth are treated empirically with antibiotic agents (after blood culture is obtained). Among term infants, "good clinical condition" at birth is associated with a reduction in risk for EOS of approximately 60% to 70%. Researchers at 1 center in Italy reported a cohort of 7628 term infants who were managed with a categorical approach to risk identification and compared the outcomes with a cohort of 7611 infants who were managed with serial physical examinations every 4 to 6 hours through 48 hours of age. Significant decreases in the use of laboratory tests, blood cultures, and empirical antibiotic agents were observed in the second cohort. Two infants who developed EOS in the second cohort were identified as they developed signs of illness. This approach is embraced by the NICHD workshop on chorioamnionitis. Centers that adopt this approach need to establish processes to ensure serial, structured, documented physical assessments and develop clear criteria for additional evaluation and empirical antibiotic administration. Physicians and families must understand that the identification of initially well-appearing infants who develop clinical illness is not a failure of care, but rather an anticipated outcome of this approach to EOS (including EOS due to GBS). Additionally, it may be reasonable to consider supplementing the structured clinical examination with a limited evaluation (eg, CBC, CRP) at 6 hours of age.

The AAP guidelines stop short of recommending one approach over the other. Instead, they recommend that birth centers consider the development of locally tailored, documented guidelines for EOS risk assessment and clinical management. They also recommend ongoing surveillance once guidelines are implemented.

C. **Neonatal risk assessment for infants born at ≤ 34 6/7 weeks' gestation.** The AAP report on GBS addresses infants born at ≤34 6/7 weeks' gestation at risk for GBS in a similar fashion to infants at risk from all other causes of EOS. It indicates that those infants can be categorized by level of risk for EOS by the circumstances of their preterm birth as follows (Figure 146–2):

1. **Preterm infants at highest risk for EOS.** Infants born preterm because of maternal cervical incompetence, preterm labor, pPROM, clinical concern for intraamniotic infection, and/or acute onset of unexplained nonreassuring fetal status are at the highest risk for EOS. Such neonates should undergo EOS evaluation with a blood culture and empiric antibiotic treatment.

2. **Preterm infants at lowest risk for EOS.** Preterm infants at lowest risk for EOS (including EOS due to GBS) are those born under circumstances that include **all** of these criteria: (1) maternal and/or fetal indications for preterm birth (such as maternal preeclampsia or other noninfectious medical illness, placental insufficiency, or fetal growth restriction), (2) birth by cesarean delivery, and (3) absence of labor, attempts to induce labor, or any ROM before delivery. Acceptable initial approaches to these infants include (1) no laboratory evaluation and no empirical antibiotic therapy or (2) blood culture and clinical monitoring. For infants who do not improve after initial stabilization and/or those who have severe systemic instability, the administration of empirical antibiotics may be reasonable but is not mandatory.

3. **Preterm infants delivered for maternal and/or fetal indications but who are ultimately born by vaginal or cesarean delivery after efforts to induce labor and/or with ROM before delivery.** Those infants are subject to factors associated with the pathogenesis of EOS due to GBS or other bacteria. If the mother has an indication for GBS prophylaxis and appropriate treatment (penicillin, ampicillin, or cefazolin >4 hours before delivery) is not given or if any other concern for infection arises during the process of delivery, the infant should be managed as recommended above for preterm infants at higher risk for EOS

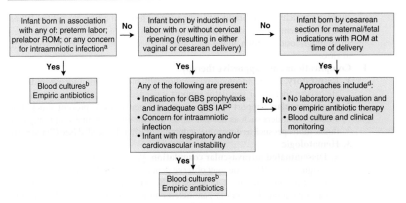

FIGURE 146–2. EOS risk assessment among infants born ≤34 weeks' gestation. [a]Intraamniotic infection should be considered when a pregnant woman presents with unexplained decreased fetal movement and/or there is sudden and unexplained poor fetal testing. [b]Lumbar puncture and CSF culture should be performed before initiation of empiric antibiotics for infants who are at the highest risk of infection unless the procedure would compromise the infant's clinical condition. Antibiotics should be administered promptly and not deferred because of procedural delays. [c]Adequate GBS IAP is defined as the administration of penicillin G, ampicillin, or cefazolin ≥4 hours before delivery. [d]For infants who do not improve after initial stabilization and/or those who have severe systemic instability, the administration of empiric antibiotics may be reasonable but is not mandatory. (*Reproduced with permission from Puopolo KM, Lynfield R, Cummings JJ, et al: Management of Infants at Risk for Group B Streptococcal Disease, Pediatrics. 2019 Aug;144(2). pii: e20191881.*)

(Section VII.C.1). Otherwise, an acceptable approach to these infants is close observation for those infants who are well appearing at birth and to obtain a blood culture and initiate antibiotic therapy for infants with respiratory and/or cardiovascular instability after birth.

D. **Empiric antibiotic therapy.** Treatment for EOS is often begun before a definite causative agent is identified. It usually consists of **ampicillin** and **gentamicin**. (Dosages are presented in Chapter 155.) This empirical regimen covers the most commonly encountered microorganisms, namely GBS and *E coli*, and has proved to be efficacious over the years. Third-generation cephalosporins should be avoided as an empirical therapy for EOS because they are associated with increased risk for antibiotic resistance and invasive fungal infections. Third-generation cephalosporins may be considered for infants suspected to have meningitis or who have renal impairment. According to recent CDC surveillance studies, approximately 1.7% of all *E coli* EOS cases were resistant to both ampicillin and gentamicin; therefore, the empirical addition of broader spectrum antibiotics should be considered in critically ill newborns who deteriorate despite being on ampicillin and gentamicin, or in preterm infants exposed to prolonged antepartum maternal antibiotic treatment. When blood cultures are sterile, antibiotic therapy should be discontinued by 36 to 48 hours of incubation, unless there is clear evidence of site-specific infection or unexplained persistent cardiorespiratory instability. Laboratory test abnormalities alone rarely justify prolonged empirical antibiotic administration, particularly among preterm infants at a lower risk for EOS.

E. **Continuing therapy** is based on culture and sensitivity results, clinical course, and occasionally other serial laboratory studies (eg, CRP and PCT). Monitoring for antibiotic toxicity is important, as is monitoring levels of aminoglycosides. When GBS is documented as the causative agent, penicillin G is the drug of choice; however, an aminoglycoside is often added for a few days because of documented synergism in vitro.

F. **Complications and supportive therapy**
   1. **Respiratory.** Ensure adequate oxygenation with blood gas monitoring, and initiate oxygen therapy or ventilator support if needed.
   2. **Cardiovascular.** Support blood pressure and perfusion to prevent shock. Use volume expanders such as normal saline, and monitor the intake and output of fluids. Inotropes such as dopamine or dobutamine may be needed (see Chapter 70).
   3. **Hematologic**
      a. **Disseminated intravascular coagulation.** With disseminated intravascular coagulation (DIC), one may observe generalized bleeding at puncture sites, the gastrointestinal tract, or CNS. In the skin, large-vessel thrombosis may cause gangrene. Laboratory parameters consistent with DIC include thrombocytopenia, increased prothrombin time, and increased partial thromboplastin time. There is an increase in fibrin split products or d-dimers. Treatment options include fresh-frozen plasma, 10 mL/kg; vitamin K (see Chapter 155); platelet infusion; and possible exchange transfusion (see Chapter 34).
      b. **Neutropenia.** Multiple factors contribute to the increased susceptibility of neonates to infection, including developmental quantitative and qualitative neutrophil defects. Colony-stimulating factors comprise a group of cytokines that are central to the hematopoiesis of blood cells, as well as to the maintenance of homeostasis and overall immune competence. Granulocyte colony-stimulating factor (G-CSF) and granulocyte-macrophage colony-stimulating factor (GM-CSF) have been used in neonates with established sepsis associated with neutropenia, in neutropenic infants without sepsis, and prophylactically in neonates at risk for sepsis. Limited data suggest that colony-stimulating factor administration may reduce mortality when systemic infection is accompanied by severe neutropenia. Intravenous immunoglobulin does not appear useful either as a prophylactic agent or as an adjunct to antibiotic therapy in serious neonatal infection.
   4. **Central nervous system.** Implement seizure control measures using phenobarbital, and monitor for the syndrome of inappropriate antidiuretic hormone (decreased urine output, hyponatremia, decreased serum osmolarity, and increased urine specific gravity and osmolarity).
   5. **Metabolic.** Monitor for and treat hypoglycemia or hyperglycemia. Metabolic acidosis may accompany sepsis and is treated with bicarbonate and fluid replacement.
G. **Future developments.** Intensive research continues in the development of vaccines (especially for GBS). Research is also ongoing into blocking some of the body's own inflammatory mediators that result in significant tissue injury, including endotoxin inhibitors, cytokine inhibitors, nitric oxide synthetase inhibitors, and neutrophil adhesion inhibitors.

VIII. **Prognosis.** With early diagnosis and treatment, most infants will recover and not have long-term complications. However, the mortality rate is still significant for EOS, especially in VLBW infants. For term and late preterm infants, the reported mortality is approximately 3%, whereas EOS mortality for VLBW infants is approximately 16%. Neonatal EOS is a risk factor for long-term neurodevelopmental impairment in premature infants.

NEONATAL LATE-ONSET SEPSIS

I. **Definition.** Neonatal LOS is defined by the CDC as blood and/or CSF culture–proven infection occurring in the newborn after 7 days of age caused by a postnatal acquisition (nosocomial or community sources). For the continuously hospitalized VLBW infant, LOS is defined as culture-proven infection occurring at >72 hours of age.

II. **Incidence of neonatal late-onset sepsis.** The overall incidence of primary sepsis (EOS and LOS) is 1 to 2 per 1000 live births. The incidence of LOS in term infants is hard to know; however, a study that looked at late preterm infants hospitalized in the first 3 months of life identified LOS in 6.3 per 1000 admissions. According to the CDC, late-onset GBS infection rates have remained relatively stable over the past 20 years and are not impacted by intrapartum antibiotics prophylaxis (0.32 per 1000 live births in 2015). Incidence of LOS is much higher for VLBW infants; according to data from the NICHD Neonatal Research Network (NICHD-NRN), the incidence is 32% and appears to be decreasing in recent years (37% in 2005, 27% in 2012).

III. **Pathophysiology of neonatal late-onset sepsis.** LOS is usually more insidious (compared to EOS), but it can be fulminant at times. It is usually not associated with early obstetric complications. In addition to bacteremia, these infants may have an identifiable focus, most often meningitis in addition to sepsis. Bacteria responsible for LOS and meningitis include those acquired after birth from the maternal genital tract (vertical transmission) as well as organisms acquired after birth from human contact or from contaminated equipment/environment (nosocomial). Therefore, horizontal transmission appears to play a significant role in LOS. The reasons for the delay in development of clinical illness, the predilection for CNS disease, and the less severe systemic and cardiorespiratory symptoms are unclear. Transplacental transfer of maternal antibodies (also in breastmilk) to the mother's own vaginal flora may play a role in determining which exposed infants become infected, especially in the case of GBS infections. In case of nosocomial spread, the pathogenesis is related to the underlying illness and debilitation of the infant, the flora in the neonatal intensive care (NICU) environment, and invasive monitoring and other techniques used in the NICU, especially the use of peripherally inserted central catheters (PICCs). Breaks in the natural barrier function of the skin and intestine allow opportunistic organisms to invade and overwhelm the neonate. Infants, especially the premature, have an increased susceptibility to infection because of underlying illnesses and immature immune defenses that are less efficient at localizing and clearing bacterial invasion.

   A. **Microbiology.** The pathogens that cause LOS or nosocomial sepsis tend to vary in each nursery; however, coagulase-negative staphylococci (CONS), especially *Staphylococcus epidermidis*, are the most predominant (53% of cases in NICHD-NRN). Other microorganisms causing LOS include gram-negative rods (including *Pseudomonas, Klebsiella, Serratia, E coli*, and *Proteus*), *S aureus* (both methicillin-susceptible and methicillin-resistant), GBS, and fungal microorganisms.

   B. **Antibiotic resistance.** Antibiotics resistance, especially to Enterobacteriaceae such as *E coli*, is an emerging problem in many NICUs. Multiple mechanisms of resistance may be present simultaneously. Resistance resulting from production of chromosomally encoded or plasmid-derived AmpC β-lactamases or from plasmid-mediated extended-spectrum β-lactamases (ESBLs) occurs primarily in *E coli, Klebsiella* species, and *Enterobacter* species but has been reported in many other gram-negative species. Resistant gram-negative infections have been associated with nursery outbreaks, especially in VLBW infants. Organisms that produce ESBLs typically are resistant to penicillins, cephalosporins, and monobactams and can be resistant to aminoglycosides. Carbapenemase-producing Enterobacteriaceae (CPE) also have emerged, especially *Klebsiella pneumoniae, Pseudomonas aeruginosa*, and *Acinetobacter* species. ESBL- and carbapenemase-producing bacteria often carry additional plasmid-borne genes that encode for high-level resistance to aminoglycosides, fluoroquinolones, and trimethoprim-sulfamethoxazole.

IV. **Risk factors of neonatal late-onset sepsis**

   A. **Prematurity and low birthweight.** Prematurity (<37 weeks' gestation) is the single most significant factor correlated with sepsis. The risk increases in proportion to the decrease in birthweight and GA (GA <25 weeks: 41%; GA 25–28 weeks: 21%; GA 29–32 weeks: 10%). Being small for gestational age increases the risk further.

B. **Invasive procedures/devices.** Intravascular catheterization (PICC and umbilical catheters) and respiratory (endotracheal intubation) or metabolic support (total parenteral nutrition) are important risk factors for LOS. Mechanical ventilation and continuous positive airway pressure have been associated with an increased risk of LOS in VLBW infants.

C. **Risk factors for extended-spectrum β-lactamase infection and carbapenemase-producing Enterobacteriaceae.** Additional risk factors associated with neonatal ESBL infection include prolonged mechanical ventilation, extended hospital stay, use of invasive devices, and use of antimicrobial agents. Infants born to mothers colonized with ESBL-producing *E coli* are themselves at an increased risk of acquiring colonization with ESBL-producing *E coli*.

D. **Other factors.** Bottle feeding (as opposed to breast feeding) predisposes to infection. Black African descent has been found as an independent risk factor for GBS sepsis (both EOS and LOS). Reasons for the disproportionately high disease burden among black populations cannot be fully explained by prematurity or socioeconomic status. NICU staff and family members are often vectors for the spread of microorganisms, primarily as a result of improper or lack of hand washing. The risk of infection correlates with length of stay in the NICU.

V. **Clinical presentation of neonatal late-onset sepsis.** Because the initial diagnosis of sepsis is, by necessity, a clinical one, it is crucial to begin treatment before the results of cultures are available. Clinical signs and symptoms of sepsis are nonspecific, and the differential diagnosis is broad. Some signs are subtle or insidious, and therefore, a high index of suspicion is required to identify and evaluate infected neonates. Clinical signs and symptoms most often mentioned include the following:

A. **Temperature irregularity.** Hypothermia is more common than fever as a presenting sign for bacterial sepsis in premature infants. Hyperthermia is more common in full-term infants beyond the first 24 hours of life and if viral agents (eg, herpes) are involved.

B. **Change in behavior.** Lethargy, irritability, or change in tone.

C. **Skin.** Poor peripheral perfusion, cyanosis, mottling, pallor, petechiae, rashes, sclerema, and jaundice singularly or in combinations are known signs of sepsis.

D. **Feeding problems.** Feeding intolerance, vomiting, diarrhea, or abdominal distention with or without visible bowel loops.

E. **Cardiopulmonary.** Tachypnea, respiratory distress (grunting, flaring, and retractions), new onset of apnea, bradycardia and desaturation episodes (ABD [apnea, bradycardia, desaturation] spells), tachycardia, and hypotension singularly or in combinations should suggest sepsis. Hypotension tends to be a late sign.

Reduced variability and transient decelerations in heart rate (HR) may be present in the hours to days before diagnosis of LOS. These **abnormal HR characteristics (HRC)** in response to systemic infection and inflammation have been characterized mathematically, and the resulting **HRC index** can be computed in real time and displayed continuously at the bedside. Some studies suggest that monitoring the HRC index in high-risk premature infants may result in improved outcomes and decreased mortality (through early warning with diagnosing early sepsis and prompt treatment with antibiotics).

F. **Metabolic.** Metabolic findings include hypoglycemia, hyperglycemia, or metabolic acidosis.

G. **Focal infections.** These may precede or accompany LOS. Look for cellulitis, impetigo, soft tissue abscesses, omphalitis, conjunctivitis, otitis media, meningitis, or osteomyelitis.

VI. **Diagnosis of neonatal late-onset sepsis**

A. **Differential diagnosis.** Because signs and symptoms of neonatal sepsis are nonspecific, noninfectious etiologies need to be considered. If the infant is presenting with cardiorespiratory symptoms, aspiration pneumonia, patent ductus arteriosus, or other congenital heart diseases need to be considered. If the infant is showing CNS symptoms, then intracranial hemorrhage, drug withdrawal, and inborn errors of metabolism are considered. Patients with feeding intolerance and bloody stool may have necrotizing enterocolitis (NEC), gastrointestinal perforation, or obstruction. Some nonbacterial infections such as disseminated herpes simplex virus can be indistinguishable from bacterial sepsis and should be considered in the differential diagnosis, especially if the infant has fever. **Postnatal cytomegalovirus** (acquired through breast milk or blood transfusion) is another agent that is increasingly being recognized as a cause of sepsis-like illness in extremely low birth weight infants beyond the first week of life. Other viral agents that need to be considered include respiratory syncytial virus (RSV) and *Enterovirus/Parechovirus*.

B. Laboratory studies of neonatal late-onset sepsis

1. **Cultures.** Blood and other normally sterile body fluids (urine, spinal fluid, and occasionally tracheal aspirate) should be obtained for culture. Body surface cultures are not recommended unless the infant has pustules or a characteristic rash (eg, candida).

   a. **Blood cultures.** Computer-assisted automated blood culture systems identify up to 94% to 96% of all microorganisms by 36 to 48 hours of incubation. The minimum volume for blood culture is 1 mL (some have suggested weight-based criteria; 1 mL for infants weighing <1.5 kg, 2 mL for infants weighing 1.5–3 kg, and 3 mL for infants >3 kg). **Two blood cultures (1 from PICC and 1 peripheral) are recommended.** In many clinical situations, infants are treated for "presumed" sepsis despite negative cultures, if clinical and laboratory findings are suggestive of infection and no other etiology is found to explain the clinical deterioration.

   b. **Lumbar puncture.** LP should be part of the routine evaluation for LOS. Meningitis is likely to happen without sepsis in VLBW infants, and therefore, LP is mandatory.

   c. **Urine culture** must be obtained as part of evaluation for LOS. Urine specimen should be obtained by either a suprapubic tap (see Chapter 29) or catheterized specimen (see Chapter 30). Bag urine samples should not be used to diagnose UTI in neonates.

   d. **Tracheal cultures** may be considered in intubated neonates with a clinical picture suggestive of pneumonia, especially when the quality and volume of tracheal secretions change substantially. However, it is often hard to differentiate tube colonization from true infection.

2. **Gram stain of various fluids.** Gram staining is especially helpful for the study of CSF. A Gram stain of tracheal aspirate fluid may suggest an inflammatory process if numerous WBCs, together with bacteria, are identified.

3. **Molecular testing.** See prior discussion under EOS of this chapter (page 1177).

4. **Other laboratory tests**

   a. **Complete blood count with differential.** See prior discussion under EOS of this chapter. LOS is associated with both low and high WBC (<1000/mm³ and >50,000/mm³), high absolute neutrophil count (>17,670/mm³), elevated I/T ratio (>0.2), and low platelet count (<50,000/mm³). It is also important to note that neutropenia has been described commonly as an incidental finding in otherwise healthy growing VLBW infants.

   b. **Acute-phase reactants.** See prior discussion under EOS section of this chapter. **Serial CRP determinations** are helpful in ruling out infection when normal (high negative predictive value). **PCT** may be better than CRP in the diagnosis and follow-up of neonatal sepsis secondary to **CONS**.

C. Imaging and other studies

1. **Chest radiograph.** A chest radiograph should be obtained in cases with respiratory symptoms, although it is often difficult to differentiate changes associated with true bacterial pneumonia from those associated with bronchopulmonary dysplasia, simple aspiration, or atelectasis.

2. **Urinary tract imaging.** Imaging with renal ultrasound, renal scan, and possibly voiding cystourethrogram should be considered when UTI accompanies sepsis.

VII. **Management of neonatal late-onset sepsis.** Isolation precautions for all infectious diseases, including maternal and neonatal precautions, breast feeding, and visiting issues, can be found in Appendix F.

A. **Prevention of neonatal nosocomial late-onset sepsis.** A subset of nosocomial sepsis is **central line–associated bloodstream infections (CLABSIs).** Although primary prevention of CLABSI relies on minimizing the use of central lines, novel technologies such as antiseptic- and antimicrobial-impregnated catheters in addition to meticulous care during PICC insertion and maintenance are key factors in preventing CLABSIs. Quality improvement initiatives that focus on adherence to best practices of catheter insertion and maintenance (NICU Central Catheter Bundles) have resulted in widespread reduction in CLABSIs across different NICUs. Some of those bundles were adopted and disseminated through statewide collaboratives such as the California Perinatal Quality Care Collaborative (CPQCC). **Hand hygiene is the single most important strategy** for avoiding transmission of contagions in the NICU. Fresh maternal milk contains a number of substances responsible for innate immune and humoral responses against pathogens; therefore, promotion of **breast feeding** is considered a key step in the prevention of NICU infections. Medical stewardship of antibiotics, steroids, and H_2 blockers is mandatory; indiscriminate use of these agents has been associated with increased nosocomial sepsis. Enhancement of the enteric microbiome composition with the possible use of **probiotics** may restore gut immune function and help prevent NEC and sepsis. In a recent meta-analysis of 37 trials, probiotics were associated with a small, but statistically significant, reduction in the risk of LOS compared with placebo or no treatment. Use of bioactive substances with known anti-infective properties such as **lactoferrin** may be helpful. **A recently published Cochrane review that included 6 trials suggested that lactoferrin supplementation to enteral feeds with or without probiotics may decrease LOS and NEC in preterm infants.** However, no recommendations can be made until ongoing trials that enrolled >6000 preterm neonates are completed. Finally, specific and targeted pharmacologic prophylactic interventions have been used with some success. For example, specific antifungal prophylaxis with fluconazole has been associated with significant reduction in invasive fungal infection; it is recommended in NICUs that experience high rates of invasive candidiasis. However, the use of pagibaximab, a recombinant monoclonal antibody targeting staphylococcal species, does not appear to offer protection against gram-positive CLABSIs in the NICU.

B. **Empiric antibiotic therapy.** Treatment is most often begun before a definite causative agent is identified. In nosocomial sepsis, the flora of the NICU must be considered in choosing antibiotics; however, staphylococcal coverage with **vancomycin plus an aminoglycoside** such as gentamicin or amikacin is usually begun. Some NICUs use a **cefazolin** or **nafcillin** for staphylococcal coverage instead of vancomycin. The empirical treatment for suspected LOS in a neonate admitted from the community is ampicillin and gentamicin; cefotaxime can be added only when there is a concern for meningitis. Dosages are presented in Chapter 155.

C. **Continuing therapy** is based on culture and sensitivity results, clinical course, and other serial laboratory studies (eg, CRP or PCT). If an **ESBL-producing organism**, such as *K pneumoniae*, is suspected or identified, then **carbapenem** is the drug of choice (with aminoglycoside for double coverage). Of the aminoglycosides, **amikacin** retains the most activity against ESBL-producing strains. An aminoglycoside or cefepime can be used if the organism is susceptible, because **cefepime** does not induce chromosomal AmpC enzymes. Monitoring for antibiotic toxicity is important, as well as monitoring levels of aminoglycosides and vancomycin.

D. **Complications and supportive therapy** are reviewed under the EOS section of this chapter (page 1184). In particular, administration of **intravenous immunoglobulin** to neonates with suspected or proven LOS does not result in reduction in mortality during hospital stay or major disability at 2 years of age. Similarly, administration of colony-stimulating factors, namely **G-CSF** and **GM-CSF**, does not result in reduced mortality or better neurodevelopmental outcome at 2 and 5 years. However, there might be a place for using **G-CSF** in cases of severe infection complicated by **severe neutropenia (absolute neutrophil count <500/mm^3)** and/or in the presence of specific hematologic diseases causing severe neutropenia.

E. **Future developments.** Intensive research continues in the development of vaccines as well as synthetic monoclonal antibodies to the specific pathogens causing neonatal LOS. Research is also ongoing into blocking some of the body's own inflammatory mediators that result in significant tissue injury, including endotoxin inhibitors, cytokine inhibitors, nitric oxide synthetase inhibitors, and neutrophil adhesion inhibitors. Finally, recent research is showing prebiotics, probiotics, and lactoferrin to be promising agents in the prevention of LOS and NEC.

VIII. **Prognosis.** Neonatal LOS remains a major cause of death in VLBW infants, with a reported mortality rate of approximately 18%. Mortality due to gram-negative infections is higher than that due to gram-positive infections. Risk factors for LOS mortality include endotracheal intubation, administration of vasopressors, hypoglycemia, thrombocytopenia, and development of NEC. VLBW infants who survive LOS are at risk for long term neurodevelopmental impairment including cerebral palsy.

147 Syphilis

I. **Definition.** Syphilis is a sexually transmitted infection caused by *Treponema pallidum*, which is a thin, motile spirochete that is extremely fastidious, surviving only briefly outside the host. The Centers for Disease Control and Prevention (CDC) issued a case definition of **congenital syphilis (CS)** in 2018 as follows: a condition caused by infection in utero with *T pallidum*. A wide spectrum of severity exists, from inapparent infection to severe cases that are clinically apparent at birth. **Laboratory criteria for diagnosis** entail demonstration of *T pallidum* by: (1) darkfield microscopy of lesions, body fluids, or neonatal nasal discharge; **or** (2) polymerase chain reaction (PCR) or other equivalent direct molecular methods of lesions, neonatal nasal discharge, placenta, umbilical cord, or autopsy material; **or** (3) immunohistochemistry or special stains (eg, silver staining) of specimens from lesions, placenta, umbilical cord, or autopsy material. **Cases are classified as confirmed (by laboratory diagnosis) or probable. Probable CS** is a condition affecting an infant whose mother had untreated or inadequately treated syphilis at delivery, regardless of signs in the infant, *or* an infant or child who has a reactive nontreponemal test for syphilis (Venereal Disease Research Laboratory [VDRL], rapid plasma reagin [RPR], or equivalent serologic methods) *and* any 1 of the following: (1) any evidence of CS on physical examination; (2) any evidence of CS on radiographs of long bones; (3) a reactive cerebrospinal fluid (CSF) VDRL test; (4) an elevated CSF leukocyte (white blood cell [WBC]) count or protein (without other cause) in a nontraumatic lumbar puncture. Suggested parameters for **abnormal CSF WBC and protein** values include the following: during the first 30 days of life, a CSF WBC count of >15 WBC/mm^3 or a CSF protein >120 mg/dL is abnormal; after the first 30 days of life, a CSF WBC count of >5 WBC/mm^3 or a CSF protein >40 mg/dL is abnormal, regardless of CSF serology. **Adequate treatment** is defined as completion of a penicillin-based regimen, in accordance with CDC treatment guidelines, appropriate for stage of infection, initiated ≥30 days before delivery.

II. **Incidence.** According the CDC, from 2013 through 2017, there was a 76% increase in cases of syphilis in the United States (from 17,375 to 30,644 cases). The incidence of CS parallels that of primary and secondary syphilis in the general population. In the United States, in 2016, there were a total of 628 reported cases of CS, including 41 syphilitic stillbirths, with a national rate of 15.7 cases per 100,000 live births. This rate represents an increase of 86.9% relative to 2012. Worldwide, syphilis continues to represent a serious public health problem; a World Health Organization analysis showed that in 2012, an estimated 930,000 maternal syphilis infections caused 350,000 adverse pregnancy outcomes including 143,000 early fetal deaths and stillbirths, 62,000 neonatal deaths, 44,000 preterm or low-weight births, and 102,000 infected infants worldwide. The rate of CS is increased among infants born to mothers with human immunodeficiency virus (HIV) infection.

III. **Pathophysiology.** Treponemes are able to cross the placenta at any time during pregnancy, thereby infecting the fetus. **Syphilis can cause stillbirth (30% to 40% of fetuses with CS are stillborn), preterm delivery, congenital infection, or neonatal death,** depending on the stage of maternal infection and duration of fetal infection before delivery. Untreated infection in the first and second trimesters often leads to significant fetal morbidity, whereas with third-trimester infection, many infants are asymptomatic. The most common cause of fetal death is placental infection associated with decreasing blood flow to the fetus, although direct fetal infection also plays a role. Infection can also be acquired by the neonate via contact with infectious lesions during passage through the birth canal. Kassowitz's law states that the risk of vertical transmission of syphilis from an infected, untreated mother decreases as maternal disease progresses. Thus, transmission ranges from 70% to 90% in primary and secondary syphilis, to 40% for early latent syphilis, and to 8% for late latent disease. CS can cause placentomegaly and congenital hydrops. *T pallidum* is not transferred in breast milk, but transmission may occur if the mother has an infectious lesion (eg, chancre) on her breast.

IV. **Risk factors.** At-risk group include infants whose mothers received no or inadequate treatment (dose was unknown, inadequate, or undocumented), whose mother received a nonpenicillin treatment during pregnancy for syphilis, or whose mother was treated within 30 days of the infant's birth. Infants of high-risk mothers (drug use, especially cocaine use; low socioeconomic levels; HIV infection; teen pregnancy; commercial sex work; and lack of prenatal care) are at increased risk for syphilis. **Lack of early prenatal care is the strongest predictor of CS.**

V. **Clinical presentation.** CS is a multiorgan infection that may cause neurologic or skeletal disabilities or death in the fetus or newborn. However, when mothers with syphilis are treated early in pregnancy, the disease is almost entirely preventable. The risk of fetal infection increases with advancing gestation. Approximately two-thirds of live-born neonates with CS are asymptomatic at birth but have low birthweight. Clinical manifestations after birth are arbitrarily divided into **early CS** (<2 years of age) and **late CS** (>2 years of age).

   A. **Early manifestations** include nasal discharge (snuffles) and maculopapular or vesiculobullous rash that appears on the palms and soles. The rash may be associated with desquamation. Other early stigmata include fever, abnormal bone radiographs, hepatosplenomegaly, petechiae, lymphadenopathy, jaundice, pneumonia, osteochondritis, pseudoparalysis, hemolytic anemia, leukocytosis, thrombocytopenia, and central nervous system (CNS) involvement. Skin lesions and moist nasal secretions in infected babies are highly contagious. However, organisms are rarely found in lesions >24 hours after treatment has begun.

   B. **Late manifestations** develop in untreated infants and are characterized by chronic granulomatous inflammation. The sites most often involved include bones and joints, teeth, eyes, and the nervous system. **Hutchinson triad** (blunted upper incisors, interstitial keratitis, and eighth nerve deafness) and saddle nose are distinct complications. Some of these consequences may not become apparent until many years after birth, such as interstitial keratitis (5–20 years of age) and eighth cranial nerve deafness (10–40 years of age). A poor response to antibiotic treatment is often noted.

VI. Diagnosis. Diagnosis relies on active surveillance and laboratory studies. Maternal testing during pregnancy to treat the mother and identify the at-risk newborn is crucial. Most infants are asymptomatic at birth. Besides testing for syphilis, these infants should be tested for HIV infection as well.

A. Laboratory studies. Patients with congenital or acquired syphilis produce several different antibodies that can be tested in the laboratory. These are grouped as **nonspecific nontreponemal antibody (NTA) tests** and **specific treponemal antibody (STA) tests.** NTA tests (including VDRL, RPR, and automated reagin test) are inexpensive, rapid, and convenient screening tests that may indicate disease activity. These tests measure the antibody directed against lipoidal antigen from *T pallidum*, antibody interaction with host tissues, or both. They are used as initial screening tests and quantitatively to monitor a patient's response to treatment and to detect reinfection and relapse. False-positive reactions can be secondary to autoimmune disease, intravenous drug addiction, aging, pregnancy, and many infections, such as hepatitis, mononucleosis, measles, and endocarditis. The interpretation of NTA and STA tests can be confounded by maternal immunoglobulin (Ig) G antibodies that are passed transplacentally to the fetus.

1. **Nonspecific nontreponemal antibody tests.** The 2 most often used of these nonspecific screening tests are **VDRL** and **RPR.** A titer of at least 2 dilutions (4-fold) higher in the infant than in the mother signifies probable active infection. Titers should be monitored and repeated every 2 to 3 months after therapy. A sustained 4-fold decrease in titer, equivalent to a change of 2 dilutions (eg, from 1:16 to 1:4), of the NTA test result after treatment usually demonstrates adequate therapy, whereas a sustained 4-fold increase in titer (eg, from 1:8 to 1:32) after treatment suggests reinfection or relapse. The NTA test titer usually decreases 4-fold within 6 to 12 months after therapy for primary or secondary syphilis and usually becomes nonreactive within 1 year. **VDRL (not RPR) should be used on CSF.** A normal test result is negative, and any positive test should be followed up with a specific treponemal test. When NTA tests are used to monitor treatment response, the same test (eg, VDRL or RPR) must be used throughout the follow-up period, preferably by the same laboratory, to ensure comparability of results.

2. **Specific treponemal antibody tests.** These tests verify a diagnosis of current or past infection and should be performed if NTA test results are positive. These antibody tests do not correlate with disease activity and are not usually quantified. They are useful for diagnosing a first episode of syphilis and for distinguishing a false-positive result of NTA tests. However, they have limited use for evaluating response to therapy and possible reinfections. Once the STA test is positive, it will stay positive for life. In addition, STA tests are not 100% specific for syphilis; positive reactions variably occur in patients with other spirochetal diseases, such as yaws, pinta, leptospirosis, rat-bite fever, relapsing fever, and Lyme disease. NTA tests can be used to differentiate Lyme disease from syphilis, because the **VDRL test is nonreactive in Lyme disease.** Examples of STA tests include the *T pallidum* particle agglutination (TP-PA) test, *T pallidum* enzyme immunoassay (TP-EIA), *T pallidum* chemiluminescent assay (TP-CIA), and fluorescent treponemal antibody absorption (FTA-ABS) test. ***T pallidum*–specific IgM immunoblot** testing in the newborn is able to identify infants with CS with high sensitivity; however, the test is not commercially available. Recently, some clinical laboratories and blood banks have begun to screen samples using **TP-EIA,** rather than beginning with an NTA test; the reasons for this change in sequence of the screening relate to cost and manpower issues. However, this "reverse sequence screening" approach is associated with high rates of false-positive results, and in 2011, the CDC recommended against adopting it. Despite that, an increasing number of laboratories are adopting it and the Committee on Infectious Diseases of the American Academy of Pediatrics modified its diagnostic algorithm to CS to include the "reverse sequence screening approach" (see Section VII, "Management," and Figure 147–1).

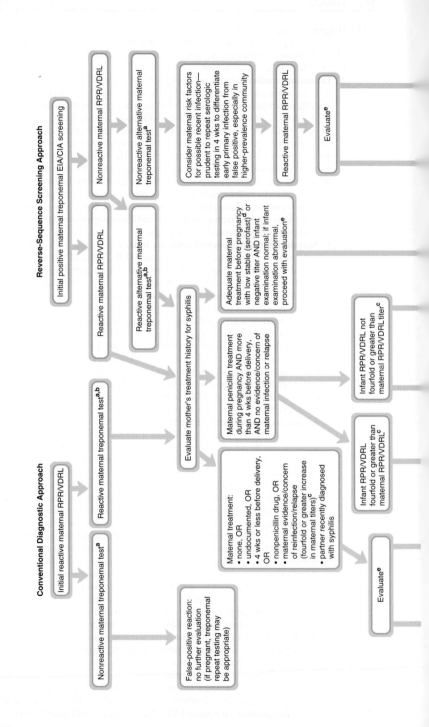

Conventional Diagnostic Approach

Initial reactive maternal treponemal test[a]

Nonreactive maternal treponemal test[a] → Reactive maternal treponemal test[a,b]

False-positive reaction: no further evaluation (if pregnant, treponemal repeat testing may be appropriate)

Evaluate mother's treatment history for syphilis

Maternal treatment:
- none, OR
- undocumented, OR
- 4 wks or less before delivery, OR
- nonpenicillin drug, OR
- maternal evidence/concern of reinfection/relapse (fourfold or greater increase in maternal titers)[c]
- partner recently diagnosed with syphilis

Maternal penicillin treatment during pregnancy AND more than 4 wks before delivery, AND no evidence/concern of maternal infection or relapse

Adequate maternal treatment before pregnancy with low stable (serofast)[d] or negative titer AND infant examination normal; if infant examination abnormal, proceed with evaluation[e]

Infant RPR/VDRL fourfold or greater than maternal RPR/VDRL[c]

Infant RPR/VDRL not fourfold or greater than maternal RPR/VDRL titer[c]

Evaluate[e]

Reverse-Sequence Screening Approach

Initial positive maternal treponemal EIA/CIA screening

Reactive maternal RPR/VDRL → Reactive alternative maternal treponemal test[a,b]

Nonreactive maternal RPR/VDRL → Nonreactive alternative maternal treponemal test[a]

Consider maternal risk factors for possible recent infection—prudent to repeat serologic testing in 4 wks to differentiate early primary infection from false positive, especially in higher-prevalence community

Reactive maternal RPR/VDRL

Evaluate[e]

1192

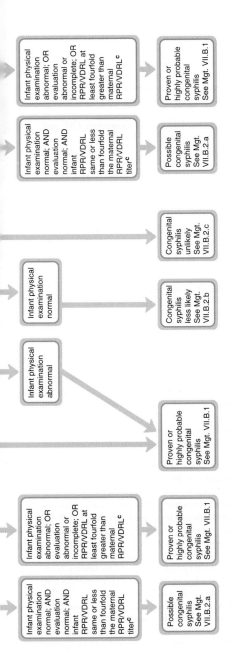

Infant physical examination normal; AND evaluation normal; AND infant RPR/VDRL same or less than fourfold the maternal RPR/VDRL titer[c]

Infant physical examination abnormal; OR evaluation abnormal or incomplete; OR RPR/VDRL at least fourfold greater than maternal RPR/VDRL[c]

Infant physical examination abnormal

Infant physical examination normal

Infant physical examination normal; AND evaluation normal; AND infant RPR/VDRL same or less than fourfold the maternal RPR/VDRL[c]

Infant physical examination abnormal; OR evaluation abnormal or incomplete; OR RPR/VDRL at least fourfold greater than maternal RPR/VDRL[c]

Possible congenital syphilis See Mgt. VII.B.2.a

Proven or highly probable congenital syphilis See Mgt. VII.B.1

Proven or highly probable congenital syphilis See Mgt. VII.B.1

Congenital syphilis less likely See Mgt. VII.B.b

Congenital syphilis unlikely See Mgt. VII.B.2.c

Possible congenital syphilis See Mgt. VII.B.2.a

Proven or highly probable congenital syphilis See Mgt. VII.B.1

RPR indicates rapid plasma reagin; VDRL, Venereal Disease Research Laboratory.

[a] *Treponema pallidum* particle agglutination (TP-PA) (which is the preferred treponemal test), fluorescent treponemal antibody absorption (FTA-ABS), or microhemagglutination test for antibodies to *T pallidum* (MHA-TP).

[b] Test for human immunodeficiency virus (HIV) antibody. Infants of HIV-infected mothers do not require different evaluation or treatment for syphilis.

[c] A fourfold change in titer is the same as a change of 2 dilutions. For example, a titer of 1:64 is fourfold greater than a titer of 1:16, and a titer of 1:4 is fourfold lower than a titer of 1:16. When comparing titers, the same type of nontreponemal test should be used (eg, if the initial test was a RPR, the follow-up test should also be an RPR).

[d] Stable VDRL titers 1:2 or less or RPR 1:4 or less beyond 1 year after successful treatment are considerd low serofast.

[e] Complete blood cell (CBC) and platelet count; cerebrospinal fluid (CSF) examination for cell count, protein, and quantitative VDRL; other tests as clinically indicated (eg, chest radiographs, long-bone radiographs, eye examination, liver function tests, neuroimaging, and auditory brainstem response).

FIGURE 147-1. Algorithm for diagnostic approach of infants born to mothers with reactive serologic tests for syphilis. (*Reproduced with permission from Kimberlin DW, Long SS, Brady MT, et al: Red Book: 2018 Report of the Committee on Infectious Diseases, 31st ed. Elk Grove Village, IL: American Academy of Pediatrics; 2018.*)

3. **Direct identification of *T pallidum*.** Microscopic **darkfield examination** can be performed on appropriate specimens (lesion exudate, nasal discharge, or tissue, such as placenta, umbilical cord, or autopsy specimens) to detect spirochetes. Specimens from mouth lesions can contain nonpathogenic treponemes that can be difficult to distinguish from *T pallidum* by darkfield microscopy. **Direct fluorescent antibody** tests are no longer available in the United States. *T pallidum* can be detected by PCR assay, but clinical diagnostic PCR assays cleared by the US Food and Drug Administration (FDA) are not yet available.

4. **Lumbar puncture.** CNS disease may be detected by examining CSF and finding positive serologic tests (VDRL or FTA-ABS), darkfield examination positive for spirochetes, positive syphilis PCR, elevated monocyte count, or elevated spinal fluid protein levels. VDRL is most commonly used, but some experts recommend the FTA-ABS test as well. FTA-ABS may be more sensitive but less specific than VDRL. Results from the VDRL test should be interpreted cautiously because a negative result on a VDRL test of CSF does not exclude a diagnosis of neurosyphilis. Alternatively, a reactive VDRL test in the CSF of neonates can be the result of nontreponemal IgG antibodies that cross the blood–brain barrier. PCR testing of CSF may prove very useful for the diagnosis of CNS syphilis. The CDC has included age-appropriate definitions of abnormal CSF cell count and protein levels in the 2018 case definition of CS (see Section I).

B. **Histopathologic examination of the placenta and umbilical cord.** The placenta of neonates with CS is often large, thick, and pale. The umbilical cord is edematous and may resemble a "barber's pole" with spiral stripes of red and light blue discoloration alternating with streaks of chalky white. It may be significantly inflamed with micro-abscesses and necrotizing funisitis. The placenta and the cord should be carefully examined with darkfield microscopy and special stains looking for spirochetes.

C. **Imaging studies.** Radiographic abnormalities may be noted in 65% of the cases. These manifestations noted on long bones include periostitis, osteitis, and sclerotic metaphyseal changes. Infants may also present with pseudoparalysis or pathologic fractures.

VII. **Management.** Isolation precautions for all infectious diseases, including maternal and neonatal precautions, breast feeding, and visiting issues, can be found in Appendix F.

A. **Maternal testing during pregnancy.** CDC recommends serologic syphilis testing for all pregnant women at the first prenatal visit. In communities and populations in which the risk for CS is high, serologic testing and a sexual history also should be obtained at 28 to 32 weeks' gestation and at delivery. **Any woman who delivers a stillborn infant after 20 weeks' gestation should be tested for syphilis.** An NTA test (RPR or VDRL) is recommended for screening, followed by a treponemal (eg, TP-PA) test if the screening result is positive. If the reverse-sequence screening algorithm is used, pregnant women with reactive treponemal TP-EIA/TP-CIA screening test results should have confirmatory testing with a quantitative NTA test. If the NTA test result is negative (discordant result), a second treponemal test using a different *T pallidum* antigen should be obtained to determine whether the initial treponemal test result was a false positive. If the second treponemal test result is positive, it may be attributable to a prior infection adequately treated in the past or to untreated syphilis in a late stage. For women treated during pregnancy, follow-up serologic testing is necessary to assess the effectiveness of therapy. Treated pregnant women with syphilis should have quantitative NTA serologic tests repeated at 28 to 32 weeks of gestation, at delivery, and according to recommendations for the stage of disease. Serologic titers may be repeated monthly in women at high risk of reinfection or in geographic areas where the prevalence of syphilis is high. **Rapid** point-of-care prenatal syphilis screening using an immunochromographic strip has been used in several resource-limited countries.

B. **Evaluation and treatment of infants.** No newborn infant should be discharged from the hospital without determination of the mother's serologic status for syphilis at least once during pregnancy and also at delivery in communities and populations in which the risk for CS is high. Testing of umbilical cord blood or an infant serum sample is inadequate for screening, because these can be nonreactive if the mother's serologic test result is of low titer or she was infected late in pregnancy. All infants born to seropositive mothers require a careful examination and a quantitative NTA test. The test performed on the infant should be the same as that performed on the mother to enable comparison of titer results. **The diagnostic and therapeutic approach to infants being evaluated for CS is summarized in Figure 147–1.**

1. **Infants with proven or highly probable congenital syphilis** (abnormal physical examination consistent with CS or a serum quantitative NTA titer that is 4-fold higher than the mother's titer or a positive darkfield microscopy or PCR of a lesion or body fluid). The recommended treatment according to the CDC guidelines is **aqueous crystalline penicillin G** 50,000 U/kg/dose intravenously every 12 hours during the first 7 days of life and every 8 hours thereafter for a total of 10 days (preferred treatment) *or* **procaine penicillin G** 50,000 U/kg/dose intramuscularly (IM) in a single daily dose for 10 days. If >1 day of therapy is missed, the entire course should be restarted. Data are insufficient regarding the use of other antimicrobial agents (eg, ampicillin). A full 10-day course of penicillin is needed, even if ampicillin was initially provided for possible sepsis. These patients always should be treated with penicillin, even if desensitization for penicillin allergy is necessary (extremely rare in the newborn period).

2. **Asymptomatic infants who have normal physical examination and a serum quantitative nonspecific nontreponemal antibody titer ≤4-fold the maternal titer** should be managed according to the status of maternal treatment:

   a. **Maternal treatment *uncertain* (possible congenital syphilis).** The mother was not treated, was inadequately treated, or has no documentation of having received treatment; the mother was treated with erythromycin or other nonpenicillin regimen; or the mother received treatment <4 weeks before delivery. These infants should be fully evaluated and treated as described in Section VII.B.1. Alternatively, **benzathine penicillin G,** 50,000 U/kg as a single **IM** dose, is acceptable provided that all components of the evaluation are obtained and are normal, including normal CSF results, and follow-up is ensured.

   b. **Maternal treatment *during* pregnancy is adequate (congenital syphilis less likely).** (Penicillin therapy given >4 weeks before delivery and the mother has no evidence of reinfection or relapse.) No evaluation is needed; however, a single **IM** dose of **benzathine penicillin G,** 50,000 U/kg, is recommended. Alternatively, infants whose mother's NTA titers decreased at least 4-fold after appropriate therapy for early syphilis or remained stable at low titer (eg, VDRL ≤1:2; RPR ≤1:4) may be followed every 2 to 3 months without treatment until the NTA test becomes nonreactive.

   c. **Maternal treatment *before* pregnancy is adequate, and mother's nonspecific nontreponemal antibody titer remained low and stable before and during pregnancy and at delivery (eg, VDRL <1:2; RPR <1:4; congenital syphilis is unlikely).** No evaluation or therapy is needed for the infant. Infants with reactive NTA tests should be followed serologically to ensure test result returns to negative. Benzathine penicillin G, 50,000 U/kg IM as single dose, can be considered if follow-up is uncertain and infant has a reactive test. Neonates with a negative NTA test result at birth and whose mothers were seroreactive at delivery should be retested at 3 months to rule out serologically negative incubating CS at the time of birth.

C. Isolation procedures. Precautions regarding drainage, secretions, and blood and body fluids are indicated for all infants with suspected or proven CS until therapy has been given for 24 hours.

D. Follow-up care. The infant should have repeated quantitative NTA tests at 3, 6, and 12 months. Most infants will have a negative titer with adequate treatment. A rising titer requires further investigation and retreatment.

VIII. Prognosis. Infants infected early in the pregnancy are usually stillborn. Infants infected in the second and third trimesters are at risk for premature delivery, low birthweight, neonatal death, and symptomatic congenital infection. In the United States, the case fatality rate for CS is 6% to 8%. Late manifestations of CS such as interstitial keratitis and anterior tibial bowing ("saber shins") may occur despite appropriate treatment. Infants infected through the birth canal and treated early have excellent prognosis.

148 TORCH (TORCHZ) Infections

TORCH is an acronym that denotes a chronic nonbacterial perinatal infection. It stands for *t*oxoplasmosis, *o*ther infections, *r*ubella virus, *c*ytomegalovirus (CMV), *h*erpes simplex virus (HSV). The Zika virus (ZIKV) infection during pregnancy results in a congenital infection syndrome in the fetus and the newborn similar to other TORCH infections; manifestations include fetal growth restriction (FGR), microcephaly, craniofacial disproportion, ventriculomegaly, intracranial calcification, optic nerve hypoplasia, and chorioretinal atrophy, among others. Thus, it has been suggested that ZIKV be added to the TORCH acronym to become **TORCHZ.** "Other" infections include syphilis, hepatitis B, coxsackievirus, Epstein-Barr virus, varicella-zoster virus (VZV), *Enterovirus/ Parechovirus*, human immunodeficiency virus (HIV), tuberculosis, and parvovirus B19. HSV disease in the neonate does not fit the pattern of chronic intrauterine infection but is traditionally grouped with TORCH. This group of infections may present in the neonate with similar clinical and laboratory findings (ie, IUGR, hepatosplenomegaly, rash, central nervous system [CNS] manifestations including calcifications, early jaundice, and low platelets), hence the usefulness of the TORCHZ concept. However, because the "*o*ther infections" category of responsible pathogens is growing and becoming diverse, the validity of indiscriminate screening of neonates presenting with findings compatible with congenital infection using "TORCH titers" has been questioned. Additionally, some of this serologic testing yields both false-positive and false-negative results. An alternative approach involves testing of infants with suspected congenital infections for specific pathogens based on their clinical presentation (see Table 148–1 and individual chapters on each pathogen). A high index of suspicion for congenital infection and awareness of the prominent features of the most common congenital infections help to facilitate early diagnosis and possible therapy. Clinicians are getting away from the acronym TORCHZ; therefore, each of these chapters has been separated and listed as a single chapter. See Chapter 149 for toxoplasmosis, Chapter 145 for rubella, Chapter 132 for cytomegalovirus, Chapter 137 for herpes simplex viruses, Chapter 154 for ZIKV, and other disease-specific chapters. See Appendix F for isolation precautions for all infectious diseases, including maternal and neonatal precautions, breast feeding, and visiting issues.

Table 148–1. SIGNS SUGGESTIVE OF A SPECIFIC CONGENITAL INFECTION IN THE NEONATE

Toxoplasmosis	Intracranial calcifications (diffuse), hydrocephalus, chorioretinitis
Syphilis	Snuffles, maculopapular rash (on palms and soles), skeletal abnormalities (osteochondritis and periostitis)
Rubella	Blueberry muffin lesions,[a] eye findings (cataracts, congenital glaucoma, pigmentary retinopathy), congenital heart disease (most commonly patent ductus arteriosus), radiolucent bone disease
Cytomegalovirus	Periventricular intracranial calcifications, microcephaly
Herpes simplex virus	Mucocutaneous vesicles or scarring, conjunctivitis or keratoconjunctivitis, elevated liver transaminases
Zika virus	Microcephaly, craniofacial disproportion, ventriculomegaly, intracranial calcification, optic nerve hypoplasia

[a]See Figure 80–18.

149 Toxoplasmosis

I. **Definition.** Toxoplasmosis is caused by *Toxoplasma gondii*, a protozoan and obligate intracellular parasite capable of causing intrauterine infection (part of TORCH [toxoplasmosis, other, rubella, cytomegalovirus, herpes simplex virus] infections; see Chapter 148).

II. **Incidence.** The incidence of congenital toxoplasmosis (CT) is 0.23 to 0.91 per 10,000 live births based on published data from the New England Newborn Screening Program; the true incidence might be higher, because the sensitivity of the newborn screening test (blot-spot immunoglobulin [Ig] M test) is approximately 50% to 75%, and fetal losses attributable to severe CT are not counted. Seroprevalence of *T gondii* among women of childbearing age (15–44 years) has declined over time (15%, 11%, and 9% in 1988–1994, 1999–2004, and 2009–2010, respectively).

III. **Pathophysiology.** *T gondii* is a coccidian parasite ubiquitous in nature. Members of the feline family are the definitive hosts. The organism exists in 3 forms: **oocyst, tachyzoite,** and **tissue cyst** (bradyzoites). Cats generally acquire the infection by feeding on infected animals such as mice or uncooked household meats. The parasite replicates sexually in the feline intestine. Cats may begin to excrete **oocysts** in their stool for 7 to 14 days after infection. During this phase, the cat can shed millions of oocysts daily for 2 weeks. After excretion, oocysts require a maturation phase (sporulation) of 24 to 48 hours before they become infective by the oral route. Intermediate hosts (sheep, cattle, and pigs) can have tissue cysts within organs and skeletal muscle. These cysts can remain viable for the lifetime of the host. The pregnant woman usually becomes infected by consumption of raw or undercooked meat that contains cysts or by the accidental ingestion of sporulated oocysts from soil or contaminated food. Ingestion of oocysts (and cysts) releases sporozoites that penetrate the gastrointestinal mucosa and later differentiate into **tachyzoites.** Tachyzoites are ovoid unicellular organisms characteristic of the acute infection. Tachyzoites spread throughout the body via the bloodstream and lymphatics. It is during this stage that vertical transmission from mother to the child (MTCT) occurs. In the immunocompetent host, the tachyzoites are sequestered in **tissue cysts** and form bradyzoites. Bradyzoites are indicative of the chronic stage of infection and can persist in the brain, liver, and skeletal tissue for the life of the individual. There are reports of transmission of toxoplasmosis through contaminated municipal water, blood transfusion, organ donation, and occasionally as a result of a laboratory accident.

Acute infection in the pregnant woman is often **subclinical** (90% of the cases). If symptoms are present, they are generally nonspecific: mononucleosis-like illness with fever, painless lymphadenopathy, fatigue, malaise, myalgia, fever, skin rash, and splenomegaly. Placental infection occurs and persists throughout pregnancy. The infection may or may not be transmitted to the fetus. The later in pregnancy that infection is acquired, the more likely is MTCT (**first trimester, 17%; second trimester, 25%; and third trimester, 65% transmission**). In women who are screened routinely during pregnancy and treated once primary infection is diagnosed, the MTCT rate is <5%. Infections transmitted earlier in gestation are likely to cause more severe fetal effects (abortion, stillbirth, or severe disease with teratogenesis). Those transmitted later are more likely to be subclinical. Factors associated with an increased risk of MTCT are as follows: (1) acute *T gondii* infection during pregnancy, (2) immunocompromising conditions, (3) lack of antepartum treatment, (4) high *T gondii* strain virulence, and (5) high parasite load. Infection in the fetus or neonate usually involves the central nervous system (CNS) or the eyes with or without disseminated systemic infection. Approximately 60% to 80% of infants with congenital infection are asymptomatic at birth; however, visual impairment, learning disabilities, or mental impairment becomes apparent in a large percentage of children months to several years later.

IV. **Risk factors.** Epidemiologic risk factors for acquiring toxoplasmosis during pregnancy include eating or contact with raw or undercooked meat, cleaning the cat litter box, eating unwashed raw vegetables or fruits, exposure to soil, and travel outside the United States, Europe, or Canada. Interestingly, cat ownership by itself is not linked to toxoplasmosis (except having ≥3 kittens). One study found that eating raw oysters, clams, or mussels was a novel risk factor for acquiring toxoplasmosis. Premature infants have a higher incidence of CT than term infants (25%–50% of cases in most series).

V. **Clinical presentation**

   A. **Antenatal detection.** Fetuses that are infected early in pregnancy may become symptomatic in utero with abnormalities detected on fetal ultrasound. These include intracranial hyperechogenic foci or calcifications and ventricular dilatation. Other abnormalities include anemia, hydrops, and ascites.

   B. **Subclinical neonatal infection.** Occurs in **60% to 80% of infected newborns**, where no manifestations are found on routine physical examination. These infants are typically identified by routine maternal or newborn screening. When more specific tests are performed (eg, cerebrospinal fluid [CSF] tap, CNS imaging, and retinal eye examinations), up to 40% have abnormalities such as macular retinal scars, focal cerebral calcifications, and elevations of CSF protein and mononuclear cell count. Infants born to mothers known to be infected with both human immunodeficiency virus (HIV) and *T gondii* should be tested for CT. There is an increased risk for intrauterine reinfection after maternal reactivated *T gondii* disease.

   C. **Clinical neonatal disease.** Those with evident clinical disease may have disseminated illness or isolated CNS or ocular disease. Late sequelae are primarily related to ocular or CNS disease. **Obstructive hydrocephalus, chorioretinitis, and diffuse intracranial calcifications** form the **classic triad of toxoplasmosis,** which is found in <10% of the cases. Beside the classic triad, other prominent features in symptomatic infants include abnormalities of CSF (high protein), anemia, seizures, direct hyperbilirubinemia, fever, hepatosplenomegaly, lymphadenopathy, eosinophilia, bleeding diathesis, hypothermia, rash, and pneumonitis. Some of these symptoms may develop in the first few months of life.

   D. Late manifestations may develop in congenitally infected infants, especially in those who do not receive extended antiparasitic therapy. **Chorioretinitis** is the most common late manifestation. The lifetime incidence for untreated infants **approaches 90%,** and the risk extends into adulthood. Treated patients may have episodic recurrences of chorioretinitis. Associated ophthalmologic findings may include microphthalmia, strabismus, cataract, glaucoma, and nystagmus. These complications can lead to vision loss and retinal detachment. Other late CNS manifestations include microcephaly, seizures, motor and cerebellar dysfunction, mental retardation, and sensorineural hearing loss.

VI. Diagnosis. CT should be suspected in infants born to mothers who had primary infection during pregnancy, infants born to women who are immunosuppressed, infants who have suggestive clinical findings, and infants who test positive (toxoplasma IgM) through universal newborn screening (in regions where it is done). Infants suspected of the disease should undergo detailed evaluation that includes eye examination, CNS imaging, spinal tap, and detailed laboratory evaluation. In early 2017, the American Academy of Pediatrics issued an elaborate report discussing the diagnosis, treatment, and prevention of CT in the United States (Maldonado et al. *Pediatrics* 2017;139[2]:e20163860).

   A. Laboratory studies. Laboratory tools for the diagnosis of *T gondii* infection include serologic tests, such as the *Toxoplasma* IgG, IgM, IgA, IgE, or IgG avidity or differential agglutination (AC/HS) tests; polymerase chain reaction (PCR) assays; histologic and cytologic examination of tissue and body fluids; and attempts to isolate the parasite with mice subinoculation (this test is only performed in reference laboratories). Commercial laboratories in the United States usually offer *Toxoplasma* IgG and IgM testing; some of them also offer *Toxoplasma* IgA and IgG avidity tests (approved by the US Food and Drug Administration [FDA] since 2011) and PCR assays. In reference laboratories for toxoplasmosis, like the one at Palo Alto Medical Foundation (Palo Alto Medical Foundation Toxoplasma Serology Laboratory [PAMF-TSL], http://www.pamf.org/serology/; phone: 650-853-4828; fax: 650-614-3292; e-mail: toxolab@pamf.org), panels of serologic tests are offered. The majority of the tests in those panels are not available in nonreference laboratories (NRL), including the *Toxoplasma* IgG dye test, the *Toxoplasma* IgM immunosorbent agglutination assay (ISAGA), the *Toxoplasma* IgE enzyme-linked immunosorbent assay, and the AC/HS differential agglutination test. The reference laboratories offer expert advice on the interpretation of these results.

     1. Diagnosis of *T gondii* infection during pregnancy. When there is clinical suspicion of acute toxoplasmosis during pregnancy, serologic samples should be sent to a reference laboratory to avoid any unnecessary delays in the establishment of diagnosis and initiation of prenatal treatment. Prompt initiation of prenatal treatment has been recently shown to decrease MTCT and ameliorate the severity of clinical manifestations. In a recent publication from PAMF-TSL involving 451 patients with positive toxoplasmosis IgM and IgG from NRL, 335 of patients (74%) had a chronic infection, 100 (22%) had an acute infection, and 7 (2%) were not infected, and for 9 patients (2%), results were indeterminate. Positive *Toxoplasma* IgM and IgG test results obtained at NRLs cannot accurately distinguish between acute and chronic infections. To do so, testing at reference laboratories is required, as mandated by a 1997 letter from the FDA to clinicians and laboratories in the United States.

     2. Prenatal diagnosis of congenital *T gondii* infection in the fetus. CT can occur in 3 ways: (1) transmission of *T gondii* infection to the fetus from a mother who acquired acute primary infection during pregnancy or shortly before conception; (2) reactivation of a *Toxoplasma* infection in an immune woman who became immunocompromised during gestation (eg, due to HIV infection or immunosuppressive medications); and (3) reinfection of a previously immune mother with a new, more virulent strain (eg, after international travel). Amplification of *Toxoplasma* DNA by PCR assay in amniotic fluid sample **(AF PCR) is the**

preferred method to diagnose fetal infection. The sensitivity and negative predictive value (NPV) for AF PCR is influenced by the gestational age at which infection is acquired. NPV of AF PCR assay for early maternal primary infections (first or second trimester) is very high (92%–99%). However, for infections acquired in the third trimester, the NPV is lower. Explanations for poor NPV include a dilution effect attributable to a larger amount of AF in the third trimester and/or maternal treatment before AF PCR testing. Moreover, it probably takes several weeks for the infection to cross the placenta from the mother to the fetus in large enough quantities to spill into the AF. The positive predictive value of an AF PCR at any time during pregnancy is very high (95%–100%). In general, AF PCR assay should be performed at least 4 weeks after acute primary maternal infection and at ≥18 weeks of gestation.

3. **Diagnosis of *T gondii* infection in the infant.** Persistence of positive *Toxoplasma* IgG in the child beyond 12 months of age is considered as the gold standard for the diagnosis of CT. In general, any maternal *Toxoplasma* IgG antibodies transferred transplacentally are expected to decrease by 50% per month after birth and usually disappear by 6 to 12 months of age. Maternal treatment during pregnancy and/or postnatal treatment of the infant could affect the production and kinetics of *Toxoplasma* IgG antibodies in the infant. **A positive *Toxoplasma* IgM ISAGA result (at or after 5 days of age) and/or a positive *Toxoplasma* IgA test result (at or after 10 days of age) are considered diagnostic of CT in infants with a positive *Toxoplasma* IgG.** Because IgM and IgA antibodies do not cross the placenta, they reflect the infant's response to *T gondii* infection. Of note, positive results before 5 or 10 days of age could represent false-positive results from contamination of the infant's blood with maternal blood (maternal–fetal blood leak). Moreover, false-positive *Toxoplasma* IgG and IgM test results can occur after recent transfusion of blood products or receipt of immunoglobulin intravenously. False-negative results occur in 13% of patients with IgM ISAGA, 23% with IgA, and 7% with both IgM and IgA. Infants with negative *Toxoplasma* IgM and IgA antibodies but with positive neonatal *Toxoplasma* IgG, serologic evidence of acute maternal *T gondii* infection during pregnancy, and evidence of clinical manifestations suggestive of CT should be regarded as having CT and treated as such. **Positive PCR assay results from peripheral blood, CSF, urine, or other body fluid in symptomatic patients are also diagnostic of CT.** One study showed that the sensitivity is 29% for blood PCR assay, 46% for CSF PCR assay, and 50% for urine PCR assay. The CSF PCR assay result was positive in 71% of infants with CT and hydrocephalus, in 53% of infants with CT and intracranial calcifications, and in 51% of infants with CT eye disease. Placentas can be examined with PCR assay as well; however, a positive placental PCR assay result may suggest CT but is not diagnostic of CT per se.

B. **Cerebrospinal fluid examination** should be performed in suspected cases. The most characteristic abnormalities are xanthochromia, mononuclear pleocytosis, and a very high protein level (sometimes >1 g/L). Tests for PCR and CSF IgM to toxoplasmosis should also be performed.

C. **Imaging studies. Fetal ultrasound** every month until delivery is recommended in a mother with definite seroconversion during pregnancy. Postnatal imaging studies include:

1. **Computed tomography of the head** should be considered when there is suspicion of CT to evaluate for the presence of intracranial calcifications, ventriculomegaly, hydrocephalus, and other findings. Computed tomography is superior to ultrasound or magnetic resonance imaging in identifying calcifications.

2. **Abdominal ultrasonography** at birth for intrahepatic calcifications and/or hepatosplenomegaly is also indicated.

3. **Long-bone films** may show abnormalities, specifically metaphyseal lucency and irregularity of the line of calcification at the epiphyseal plates without periosteal reaction.

D. **Ophthalmologic examination (preferably by retinal specialist)** characteristically shows chorioretinitis. It may also show other findings such as microphthalmia, cataract, macular scarring, and optic nerve atrophy.

VII. **Management**

A. **Antepartum management of pregnant women.** Initiating treatment of the pregnant woman as soon as possible after seroconversion helps to prevent MTCT. The odds of MTCT decrease by 52% when treatment is promptly initiated within 3 weeks after seroconversion. Additionally, antepartum treatment is associated with lower odds of severe neurologic sequelae in infants with CT. **Spiramycin** is recommended for women who acquire their infection at <18 weeks of pregnancy. It should be continued until delivery to prevent MTCT. Spiramycin is not teratogenic and is available in the United States only through the Investigational New Drug process at the FDA (phone: 301-796-1600). Spiramycin is not recommended when fetal infection is established (it should be stopped if AF PCR or fetal ultrasound is suggestive of CT). For established fetal infections (based on AF PCR or fetal ultrasound), maternal treatment with **pyrimethamine, sulfadiazine, and folinic acid should be instituted** after 18 weeks of gestation. Pyrimethamine is potentially teratogenic and should not be used before the 18th week of pregnancy.

B. **Postnatal management of the infant with congenital toxoplasmosis.** Antiparasitic therapy is indicated for infants in whom a diagnosis of CT is confirmed or probable based on serology, PCR, or clinical symptoms. The typical course consists of **sulfadiazine** (50 mg/kg, twice daily), **pyrimethamine** (2 mg/kg/d for 2 days, then 1 mg/kg/d for 2–6 months, then 1 mg/kg/d 3 times a week), and **folinic acid** (10 mg, 3 times weekly) for a minimum of 12 months. Serial follow-up to gauge the response of the infant to therapy should include neuroradiology, ophthalmologic examinations, and CSF analysis if indicated. Corticosteroids in the form of **prednisone** (1 mg/kg/d in 2 divided doses) should be given when **CSF protein is >1 g/dL and when active chorioretinitis threatens vision.** Prednisone is continued until resolution of CSF protein elevation and active chorioretinitis. Infants treated with pyrimethamine and sulfadiazine require weekly blood counts (complete blood count [CBC] including platelets) and urine microscopy to detect any adverse drug effects. CBC can be spaced to every 2 weeks if counts remain stable.

C. **Prevention**

1. **Primary prevention** should be done through education. Pregnant women should be counseled that toxoplasma infection can be prevented in large part by cooking meat to a safe temperature (152°F); peeling or thoroughly washing fruits and vegetables before eating; avoiding drinking unfiltered water in any setting; cleaning cooking surfaces and utensils after they have contacted raw meat, poultry, seafood, or unwashed fruits or vegetables; avoiding ingestion of raw shellfish such as oysters, clams, and mussels; avoiding ingestion of raw goat milk; avoiding changing cat litter or, if necessary, using gloves, and then washing hands thoroughly; not feeding raw or undercooked meat to cats; and keeping cats inside to prevent acquisition of *Toxoplasma* by eating infected prey.

2. **Secondary prevention.** Only approximately 50% of mothers of infants with CT had clinical symptoms suggestive of acute toxoplasmosis during pregnancy or had reported risk factors for *T gondii* exposure (eg, exposure to undercooked meat or to cat feces). Therefore, only routine serologic screening during pregnancy would have identified the other 50%. Secondary prevention by routine serologic screening of the pregnant woman is done in some countries (France and Austria) but is not widely used in the United States.

VIII. **Prognosis.** Maternal toxoplasmosis acquired during the first and second trimesters is associated with stillbirth (35%) and perinatal death (7%). Infants with CT have a mortality rate as high as 12% and are at risk for many other problems later in life (seizures, visual impairment, learning disabilities, deafness, mental retardation, and spasticity). Adults who were treated as infants for CT appear to have reasonable quality of life and visual function.

150 Tuberculosis

I. **Definition.** Tuberculosis (TB), an infection caused by the organism *Mycobacterium tuberculosis*, can be congenital or acquired in the postnatal period.

II. **Incidence.** The World Health Organization (WHO) estimates an incidence of 10.4 million new TB cases and 1.3 million TB deaths in 2016. Although congenital TB is rare, with about 350 cases reported in the English literature, the mortality rate is as high as 50%.

III. **Pathophysiology.** *M tuberculosis* transmission occurs via inhalation of airborne droplet nuclei, which are carried by alveolar macrophages through the lymphatic system to hilar lymph nodes. The infection can either be contained or lead to primary progressive TB. Infected macrophages interact with T lymphocytes to release cytokines that promote phagocytosis of *M tuberculosis*, leading to granuloma formation within 2 to 8 weeks in most individuals. Young children and immunosuppressed individuals lack host immunity and instead develop active primary progressive disease in the lung parenchyma and hilar lymph nodes. In these individuals, the characteristic fibrous granuloma capsule becomes disrupted, causing liquefactive necrosis of the central caseous material. The necrotic material can then flow into adjacent vasculature and disseminate systemically or to adjacent bronchi and spread externally via respiratory droplets. Immunosuppression and malnutrition are risk factors for reactivation of latent infection.

Vertical transmission causing **congenital TB** can occur due to hematogenous spread via the umbilical vein leading to a primary tuberculous lesion in the liver or lung. Alternatively, fetal aspiration or ingestion of infected amniotic fluid can lead to pulmonary or gastrointestinal TB.

IV. **Risk factors.** The highest risk of transmission to newborns occurs via respiratory transmission from **untreated mothers** during the postnatal period. This is more common than congenital TB, and diagnosis of neonatal TB can lead to identification of previously unrecognized diagnosis of TB in the mother. Maternal extrapulmonary TB, such as miliary TB or tuberculous endometritis, increases the risk of congenital infection. Maternal treatment for 2 to 3 weeks in the antenatal period reduces the risk of postnatal infection. Human immunodeficiency virus (HIV) is a risk factor for maternal TB, which in turn increases the risk of mother-to-child transmission of HIV. Living in endemic areas or crowded conditions also increases the risk of TB.

V. **Clinical presentation**

A. **Pregnancy.** Pregnant women with TB tend to have fewer of the typical symptoms associated with TB. Active TB symptoms and signs include fever, cough, night sweats, anorexia, weight loss, general malaise, and weakness. Extrapulmonary TB can affect the genitourinary tract, bones and joints, meninges, lymph nodes, pleural lining, and peritoneum. Extrapulmonary TB is more common when there is co-infection with HIV. The natural history of TB is thought to be unaffected by pregnancy. Maternal TB, especially extrapulmonary disease, does increase pregnancy and perinatal complications such as preeclampsia, vaginal bleeding, early pregnancy loss, preterm labor, and low birthweight.

B. **Neonatal period.** Congenital TB can mimic neonatal sepsis, or the infant may present in the first 90 days of life with **bronchopneumonia** and/or **hepatosplenomegaly.** Symptoms are usually present by the second or third week of life. As neonates tend to present with atypical signs, the diagnosis of TB must be considered in the differential diagnosis of other congenital infections (syphilis, cytomegalovirus, and toxoplasmosis). Beside bronchopneumonia and/or hepatosplenomegaly, congenital TB can present with fever, lymphadenopathy, abdominal distention, lethargy or irritability, ear discharge, and papular skin lesions. Less common symptoms include vomiting, apnea, cyanosis, jaundice, seizures, and petechiae. Respiratory signs include cough, wheezing, tachypnea, stridor, and crepitation, which is thought to result from obstruction of bronchi by enlarged hilar lymph nodes. Young infants are at increased risk for meningeal involvement and disseminated or miliary TB due to their immature immune systems. Meningeal presentations include meningoencephalitis, basal arachnoiditis, and intracranial tuberculomas. TB of the spine (Pott disease) has also been described in congenital infection. Clinical signs of congenital or postnatally acquired TB are typically occult and delayed in presentation because of the immaturity of the newborn and infant immune system.

VI. Diagnosis

   A. Clinical criteria. Congenital infection is diagnosed if the infant has the primary criterion and meets 1 of the secondary criteria for congenital TB (Cantwell criteria). Otherwise, postnatally acquired TB is diagnosed based on known exposure and a proven tuberculous lesion.

   1. Primary criterion. The infant must have proven tuberculous lesions.

   2. Secondary criteria

   a. Lesions in the first week of life.

   b. A primary hepatic complex or caseating hepatic granulomas.

   c. Tuberculous infection of the placenta or the maternal genital tract.

   d. Exclusion of postnatal transmission by a thorough investigation.

   B. Acid-fast *Bacillus* smear and culture. *M tuberculosis* can be identified by culture from the following specimens: gastric aspirates, sputum, bronchial washings, pleural fluid, cerebrospinal fluid (CSF), urine, or other body fluids. A biopsy specimen can also be obtained from lymph node, pleura, mesentery, liver, bone marrow, or other tissues. **The best specimen in neonates and infants who may have an absent or nonproductive cough is an early-morning gastric aspirate, obtained by a nasogastric tube before feeding.** Aspirates should be collected on 3 separate days. Gastric aspirates usually yield negative acid-fast *Bacillus* (AFB) smears, with an overall diagnostic yield of <50%. Fluorescent staining methods increase the sensitivity of gastric aspirates. The presence of nontuberculous mycobacteria can result in a false-positive smear. Liquid media culture facilitates growth of *M tuberculosis*, which can take between 3 and 6 weeks to grow.

   C. Nucleic acid amplification test. Nucleic acid amplification tests for rapid diagnosis of TB are available but have varying sensitivity and specificity. False-positive and false-negative results have also been reported.

   D. Tuberculin skin testing. A negative tuberculin skin test (TST) result should be considered unreliable in infants <3 months of age. The definition of a **positive** Mantoux skin test is as follows:

   1. Reaction ≥5 mm

   a. Infants in close contact with known or suspected infectious cases of TB.

   b. Infants suspected to have tuberculous disease based on clinical evidence or abnormal chest radiograph.

   c. Infants with an immunosuppressive condition, including HIV, or receiving immunosuppressive therapy.

   2. Reaction ≥10 mm

   a. Age <4 years.

   b. Medical risk factors such as chronic renal failure or malnutrition.

   c. Increased environmental exposure.

   E. Interferon-γ release assays. Interferon-γ release assays (IGRAs) measure interferon-γ production from T lymphocytes in response to antigens specific to *M tuberculosis*. Because these antigens are not found on *Mycobacterium bovis*–bacille Calmette-Guérin (BCG) vaccine or most nontuberculous mycobacteria, IGRAs are more specific tests than the TST, yielding fewer false-positive results. IGRAs may be used in conjunction with TST, but a negative test is unreliable in newborns due to low sensitivity.

F. Chest radiograph. Chest imaging may initially be normal, but most infants present with abnormal findings, including miliary TB, multiple pulmonary nodules, lobar pneumonia, bronchopneumonia, interstitial pneumonia, pleural effusion, and mediastinal adenopathy. The upper lobes and posterior lung segments are thought to be the most common sites for TB in infants.

G. Imaging. Other imaging modalities include abdominal sonography for hepatic involvement and thoracic computed tomography (CT) for adenopathies. Central nervous system (CNS) imaging includes ultrasonography, CT, and magnetic resonance imaging.

H. Laboratory markers. Leukocytosis with neutrophil predominance and elevation of C-reactive protein has been reported in congenital TB due to the inflammatory response associated with *M tuberculosis*. Thrombocytopenia has also been observed, although it is a nonspecific finding.

I. Cerebrospinal fluid. A lumbar puncture should promptly be performed when congenital or postnatally acquired TB is suspected. CSF findings can include lymphocytic pleocytosis, increased protein levels, and decreased CSF–to–serum glucose ratio.

J. Human immunodeficiency virus testing. All individuals with TB should be evaluated for HIV infection due to the increased incidence of TB co-infection.

K. Placental pathology. The placenta may demonstrate evidence of granulomas, and an AFB smear and culture should be sent from placental specimen.

VII. Management

A. Antimicrobial therapy during pregnancy

    1. Latent infection. The Centers for Disease Control and Prevention (CDC) recommends deferring treatment of pregnant women with latent infection until the postpartum period except in high-risk situations. Isoniazid therapy for 9 months should be considered for latent TB (positive TST and normal chest radiographic findings) in pregnant women with HIV, recent contagious contact, and skin test conversion within the prior 2 years. Pyridoxine supplementation should be administered for the duration of pregnancy and breast feeding.

    2. Active infection. The CDC recommends an initial treatment regimen with isoniazid, rifampin, and ethambutol for 2 months, followed by isoniazid and rifampin for a total of 9 months. Isoniazid, rifampin, and ethambutol are considered relatively safe for the fetus. Streptomycin should not be administered to the mother due to ototoxic effects in the fetus. Although pyrazinamide is used in some regimens, its safety during pregnancy has not been established.

B. Antimicrobial therapy during the neonatal period

    1. Active maternal and congenital or neonatal acquired infection. In cases in which the maternal physical examination and chest radiographic findings are diagnostic of active TB, **the infant should be treated promptly with isoniazid, rifampin, pyrazinamide, and an aminoglycoside such as amikacin.** Pyridoxine (to prevent neurotoxicity) supplementation in infants receiving isoniazid therapy is recommended in the following instances: exclusively breast-fed infants, malnourished infants, and those with symptomatic HIV infection. Hepatotoxic effects of isoniazid therapy are rare but can be life threatening.

    2. Active maternal infection without congenital infection. If the mother has active TB disease but the neonate is not affected, isoniazid should be given until 3 or 4 months of age. If a negative TST result is obtained at the end of therapy and the mother demonstrates successful response to therapy, the infant's isoniazid can be discontinued. A positive TST at 3 to 4 months of age necessitates a reevaluation for TB disease in the infant and continued isoniazid therapy for a total of 9 months with monthly evaluation.

    3. Latent maternal infection. Neonatal evaluation and therapy are not required in cases where the mother is asymptomatic and is diagnosed with latent TB infection.

4. **Postnatal tuberculosis infection.** For infants with pulmonary disease, pulmonary disease with hilar adenopathy, and hilar adenopathy disease, a 6-month 4-drug regimen is recommended as follows: isoniazid, rifampin, pyrazinamide, and ethambutol for 2 months followed by isoniazid and rifampin for 4 months. The duration of therapy is extended to 9 months if there is evidence of cavitary pulmonary lesions or sputum culture remains positive after 2 months of therapy. The risks and benefits of using ethambutol in infants need to be considered due to a dose- and duration-dependent risk of optic neuritis. An infectious disease consultation is essential for managing infants who are co-infected with HIV due to drug interactions and overlapping drug toxicities, especially between antiretrovirals and rifampin.

5. **Extrapulmonary tuberculosis.** For tuberculous meningitis, treatment is initiated with isoniazid, rifampin, pyrazinamide, and ethionamide/aminoglycoside. Pyrazinamide is given for a total of 2 months, and isoniazid and rifampin are given for a total of 9 to 12 months. Ethionamide or aminoglycoside is discontinued after drug susceptibility is established. **Corticosteroids** should be added in confirmed cases of TB meningitis as they reduce mortality rates and long-term neurologic impairment. Corticosteroids can also be considered for pleural and pericardial effusions, severe miliary disease, endobronchial disease, and abdominal TB. Surgical therapy for lymphadenitis, bone and joint abscesses, and hydrocephalus complicating CNS disease may be indicated.

C. **Isolation precautions/breast feeding**

1. **Maternal latent infection.** No separation or restrictions on breast feeding are required.

2. **Maternal active disease.** In suspected or proven cases of maternal TB, the mother and infant should be separated pending evaluation and appropriate maternal and infant therapy. Separation is not necessary once the infant begins isoniazid and the mother adheres to treatment, wears a mask, and follows infection control measures. In cases of multidrug-resistant TB or maternal nonadherence to therapy, the infant should be separated, and BCG vaccine should be considered in consultation with an infectious disease specialist. Breast-feeding restrictions can be removed after the mother has been treated appropriately for ≥2 weeks and is not considered contagious.

D. **Hospital control measures.** Restriction to an airborne infection isolation room is indicated in the following cases: neonates with congenital or acquired TB undergoing manipulation of the oropharyngeal airway, infants with cavitary lesions, positive sputum AFB smears, and laryngeal or extensive pulmonary involvement. Nosocomial transmission from infants to healthcare workers and between infants via contaminated respiratory equipment has been reported.

E. **Prevention.** The BCG vaccine contains a live attenuated strain of *M bovis*. The WHO recommends that a single dose of BCG vaccine should be given to all infants soon after birth in countries with a high TB burden. BCG vaccine should not be given to symptomatic HIV-positive or immunosuppressed infants. If the neonate was exposed to smear-positive pulmonary TB shortly after birth, BCG vaccine should be delayed pending completion of isoniazid therapy. The CDC does not recommend routine use of BCG vaccine in the United States due to the low burden of disease and interference of the vaccine with TST reactivity.

VIII. **Prognosis.** Information on prognostic factors is not well defined for infants with either congenital or acquired disease. Survival rate is not influenced by the following factors: specific signs or symptoms, birthweight, the nature or severity of maternal disease, timing of maternal diagnosis, prematurity, hepatic dysfunction, or thrombocytopenia. An improved survival rate has been seen in infants with the following: presentation of symptoms after 3 weeks of age, no CNS TB disease, appropriate anti-TB therapy, higher leukocyte count, and absence of miliary or multiple pulmonary nodules pattern on chest radiograph.

151 *Ureaplasma* Infection

I. **Definition.** *Ureaplasma* belongs to the Mycoplasmataceae family. These are small pleomorphic bacteria that characteristically lack a cell wall. The genus *Ureaplasma* contains 2 species capable of causing human infection, *Ureaplasma urealyticum* and *Ureaplasma parvum.*

II. **Incidence.** *Ureaplasma* species are frequently present in the lower genital tract of sexually active women with a colonization rate ranging between 40% and 80%. Vertical transmission to the newborn is high, especially in premature infants <1000 g birthweight, in whom the transmission rate approaches 90%.

III. **Pathophysiology.** *U urealyticum* has been implicated in a variety of obstetric and neonatal diseases including **preterm labor, preterm premature rupture of membranes (pPROM), chorioamnionitis, postpartum fever and endometritis, congenital pneumonia, bacteremia, meningitis, intraventricular hemorrhage (IVH), necrotizing enterocolitis (NEC), and bronchopulmonary dysplasia (BPD).** The presumed mechanisms of infection include fetal exposure to ascending intrauterine infection, passage through an infected birth canal, and hematogenous dissemination through the placenta into umbilical vessels. This exposure leads to colonization of the skin, mucosal membranes, gastrointestinal and respiratory tract, and sometimes dissemination into the bloodstream and central nervous system (CNS). Phospholipases and cytokines produced through the inflammatory response can trigger uterine contractions and premature birth. *Ureaplasma* infection of the respiratory tract in the newborn promotes a proinflammatory cytokine cascade with increase in tumor necrosis factor-α, interleukin (IL)-1β, and IL-8. These cytokines recruit neutrophils to the lungs and intensify the inflammatory cascade, which damages the premature lung and impairs future alveolar development. The same mechanisms may be involved in *Ureaplasma*-mediated intestinal injury and NEC.

IV. **Risk factors.** *Ureaplasma* colonization is associated with preterm labor, chorioamnionitis, birthweight <1000 g, and gestational age (GA) <30 weeks. Respiratory colonization is inversely related to GA at birth (65% in infants <26 weeks vs 31% in infants ≥26 weeks).

V. **Clinical presentation**

   A. **Preterm labor, preterm premature rupture of membranes, and chorioamnionitis.** *Ureaplasma* can invade the amniotic fluid early in pregnancy and are the single most common organisms that can be isolated from inflamed placentas. *Ureaplasma* can persist in the amniotic fluid subclinically for several weeks. Detection of *Ureaplasma* in second-trimester amniotic fluid by polymerase chain reaction (PCR) correlates with subsequent preterm labor and delivery (58.6% for those with positive PCR vs 4.4% for those with negative results). In addition, *Ureaplasma* cord blood infections (identified by cultures) are far more common in spontaneous than indicated preterm deliveries and are strongly associated with markers of acute placental inflammation. Positive cord cultures are also associated with neonatal systemic inflammatory response syndrome.

   B. **Congenital pneumonia.** Evidence that suggests *Ureaplasma* as a cause of congenital pneumonia includes isolation of the organism in pure culture from amniotic fluid and tracheal aspirate of neonates <24 hours after birth with specific immunoglobulin M (IgM) response in the midst of an acute inflammatory reaction and radiographic changes. These infants develop early interstitial pulmonary infiltrates with cystic/dysplastic changes as early as 7 to 10 days of age.

   C. **Meningitis and intraventricular hemorrhage.** Multiple studies have shown *Ureaplasma* to be isolated from cerebrospinal fluid (CSF) of premature infants with meningitis, IVH, and hydrocephalus. The contribution of *Ureaplasma* to the outcome of these newborns is uncertain.

    D. Association with necrotizing enterocolitis. One study showed that the incidence of NEC was 3.3-fold higher in *Ureaplasma*-positive, ≤28 weeks preterm infants with higher cord blood IL-6 and IL-1β.

    E. Predisposition to bronchopulmonary dysplasia. Multiple cohort studies have linked the development of BPD with colonization of the airways with *Ureaplasma*.

VI. Diagnosis

    A. Laboratory studies

        1. Culture. Specimens for culture require specific transport media with refrigeration at 4°C. Dacron or calcium alginate swabs should be used instead of cotton swabs.

        2. Other tests. Several sensitive PCR assays have been developed, but they are not available routinely. Serologic assays are of limited value.

VII. Management. Standard precautions are recommended.

    A. Treatment of the colonized pregnant mother. Treatment of pregnant women who present with pPROM with a 7-day course of **erythromycin** has been shown to prolong pregnancy, reduce neonatal treatment with surfactant, decrease infant oxygen dependency at ≥28 days of age, and result in fewer major cerebral abnormalities on ultrasonography before discharge. A recent study showed that a single oral dose of **azithromycin** (1 g) is comparable to a 7-day regimen of erythromycin. Those same benefits are not accrued if the mother presents with preterm labor but with intact membranes.

    B. Treatment of the colonized newborn infant is *controversial*. For infants with congenital pneumonia with radiographic evidence of early interstitial pneumonitis and when *Ureaplasma* is the only microorganism isolated from the respiratory tract, some experts recommend treatment with a 3-day course of intravenous azithromycin (20 mg/kg/d). Treatment may also be considered when *Ureaplasma* is isolated from a normally sterile site such as the bloodstream or CSF. Azithromycin has both anti-inflammatory and anti-infective properties; limited evidence suggests that azithromycin significantly reduces the risk of BPD in preterm neonates irrespective of *Ureaplasma* colonization. However, given the limited information on pharmacokinetics and potential harmful effects including risk of pyloric stenosis, its routine use for the prevention of BPD cannot be recommended.

VIII. Prognosis. In utero exposure to *Ureaplasma* is associated with reactive airway disease and wheezing in the first 2 to 3 years of life. It is also associated with adverse neurodevelopmental outcome and cerebral palsy at 2 years of adjusted age in these infants.

152 Urinary Tract Infection

I. Definition. A urinary tract infection (UTI) is the presence of pathogenic bacteria or fungus in the urinary tract. It is the most common bacterial infection in febrile neonates, although it is very uncommon in the first few days of life.

II. Incidence. UTI incidence in all neonates is approximately 0.1% to 2%. However, in preterm and low birthweight infants, the incidence is as high as 20%. In infants younger than 3 months, boys have a higher prevalence of UTI than girls.

III. Pathophysiology. See Table 152–1 for the most common pathogens isolated in neonatal UTI. Nosocomial infections occur more often due to indwelling urinary catheters.

    A. Term infants. Ascending infection through the urethra is the most common source of infection in term infants. *Escherichia coli* is the most common bacterial pathogen, followed by other gram-negative bacilli (*Klebsiella*, *Proteus*, *Enterobacter*).

Table 152–1. COMMON PATHOGENS ISOLATED IN NEONATAL UTI

Organism	Incidence (%)
Gram-negative rods	
E. coli	40–72
Klebsiella spp	7–40
Enterobacter cloacae	3–8
Proteus vulgaris	3
Serratia marcescens	1–7
Pseudomonas aeruginosa	1
Gram-positive cocci	
Enterococcus spp	10–16
Staphylococcus aureus	1–5
Group B streptococcus	1–3
Staphylococcus, coagulase negative	1
Viridans streptococcus	1
Yeast	
Candida spp	25–42

Reproduced with permission from Arshad M, Seed PC: Urinary tract infections in the infant, *Clin Perinatol.* 2015 Mar;42(1):17-28.

    B. Preterm infants. Hematogenous spread of infection plays a bigger role in preterm infants. *Klebsiella* and coagulase-negative *Staphylococcus* are more commonly identified than *E coli*. *Candida* UTIs are also common in this group.

    C. Fungal urinary tract infections. Most often caused by *Candida* species and are more common in nosocomial infections. Fungal UTIs are also more common in extremely low birthweight babies.

IV. Risk factors

    A. Congenital anomalies of the kidney and urinary tract (CAKUT) such as urinary tract dilatation (eg, ureteropelvic junction obstruction, ureterovesical junction obstructions, ureterocele, ectopic ureter), posterior urethral valves, and vesicoureteral reflux can predispose to UTIs.

    B. Alteration in normal bladder function (eg, neurogenic bladder) predisposes the infant to UTI.

    C. Recent urinary tract instrumentation or indwelling catheters are the most common risk factors for nosocomial infections.

    D. Uncircumcised males have a 10-fold increased risk for UTI compared to circumcised males. This is presumably due to increased bacterial adherence to the mucosal surface of the foreskin and bacterial colonization under the foreskin.

    E. Prematurity is a risk factor for UTI because premature infants are relatively immunocompromised compared to term infants. Risk increases with decreasing gestational age and birthweight.

    F. Prolonged unexplained jaundice can be a marker for UTI in infants and warrants screening with a urinalysis and culture. Indirect (unconjugated) hyperbilirubinemia is thought to be secondary to hemolysis caused by *E coli* infection. Direct (conjugated) hyperbilirubinemia-associated UTI is secondary to cholestasis, but the mechanism is not known.

G. **Maternal urinary tract infection during pregnancy and premature rupture of membranes** are potential risk factors for UTI. These were reported in 2 small case series. The increased incidence may be because these mothers harbor pathogens transmitted to the infant during birth.

H. **White race is risk factor for urinary tract infection.** Febrile white infants have a higher probability of being diagnosed with UTI compared to black infants or infants of other ethnic groups. This is especially the case in female white infants. In 1 study, African American infants were much less likely to be diagnosed with UTI than white or Hispanic infants.

V. **Clinical presentation.** Infants may appear acutely toxic, similar to neonatal sepsis, or present with nonspecific findings of fever, lethargy, irritability, poor feeding, vomiting, jaundice secondary to cholestasis, loose stools, or failure to thrive. Fever does not always occur. Newborns with UTI are at higher risk for bacteremia than older infants. Preterm infants have the same signs as term infants but can also have apnea, bradycardia, and hypoxia. Term infants usually present in the second to third week with a UTI.

VI. **Diagnosis**

A. **Laboratory studies**

1. **Urinalysis.** Positive leukocyte esterase suggests inflammation in the urinary tract; it has a sensitivity of 84% and specificity of 78%. Positive nitrite suggests the presence of gram-negative bacteria and is 98% specific; sensitivity is only 50%. Detection of bacteria by microscopy adds specificity to other urine findings. Hemocytometer white blood cell (WBC) counts in the urine specimen may be of value in diagnosing UTI. A recent study stated that a minimum of 3 to 6 WBCs per high-power field depending on urine concentration is required for a presumptive diagnosis of UTI. Although no single finding on urinalysis is diagnostic of UTI, neonates without pyuria or bacteriuria have a very low likelihood of UTI.

2. **Urine culture.** A urine culture is no longer recommended in infants <72 hours of age in an early-onset sepsis workup and is more appropriately done for late-onset sepsis workup.

a. **Suprapubic aspiration and bladder catheterizations** are the only truly reliable methods to obtain urine cultures in neonates (see Chapters 29 and 30). Cultures obtained from a suprapubic bladder aspiration that grow >1000 colony-forming units (CFU)/mL are significant. The optimal definition for UTI from catheter-obtained specimens in neonates has not been established. However, >50,000 CFU/mL or 10,000 to 50,000 CFU/mL with pyuria on the urinalysis are generally accepted definitions.

b. **Clean-catch or collection bag specimens** often are inaccurate due to contamination and are only clinically reliable if the culture demonstrates no growth. **Due to high false-positive rates, this type of collection is not recommended.**

c. **Rapid culture** techniques using reverse transcriptase–polymerase chain reaction and next-generation sequencing to identify organisms are available in many facilities.

3. **Serum tests.** Complete blood count, blood cultures, serum creatinine, C-reactive protein, and erythrocyte sedimentation rate may be clinically useful in guiding management.

4. **Sepsis evaluation** should be done in all infants suspected of a UTI (see Chapter 146). The risk of sepsis is about 4% to 7% in term newborns and young infants and is greater in preterm infants. Blood culture is mandatory in all infants with a suspected UTI and prior to starting antibiotics. The risk of bacterial meningitis is approximately 1% to 3% in infants with a UTI; therefore, the decision to perform a lumbar puncture depends on the severity of illness of the infant.

VII. **Management**

A. **Initial antibiotic treatment.** For the majority of neonatal cases, initial treatment with broad-spectrum intravenous (IV) antibiotics is appropriate (usually ampicillin and gentamicin). It is also important to consider maternal use of antibiotics prior to delivery (which increases the risk of a neonatal UTI with β-lactamase–producing *E coli*) and local antibiotic resistance patterns. Antibiotics can be tailored according to susceptibility testing on urine culture. Ideal duration of therapy is not completely known but is usually 10 to 14 days. For an infant in the hospital who is older than 7 days, consider vancomycin and gentamicin. Oral antibiotics can be initiated for mature infants who are able to tolerate oral intake and who are not ill appearing. A delay in initiation of antibiotic treatment of 72 hours or more was a risk factor for permanent renal scars after the first febrile UTI. There is no difference in renal scarring between oral and IV antibiotic therapy.

B. Imaging after urinary tract infection

1. **Renal ultrasound.** Because of the high rate of congenital anomalies of the kidney and urinary tract, all neonates with a documented UTI should undergo **renal ultrasound**. The timing of this study remains under debate. Hydronephrosis or upper urinary tract dilatation is the most common finding.

2. **Voiding cystourethrogram.** Children younger than 2 months of age and any child with an *abnormal* renal ultrasound should also have a voiding cystourethrogram (VCUG) to look for vesicoureteral reflux, obstructive lesions (eg, ureterocele, posterior urethral valve), or signs of neurogenic bladder. VCUG for children older than 2 months of age with *normal* renal ultrasound after first febrile UTI is controversial and is currently not recommended by the American Academy of Pediatrics (AAP). Any child with a history of >1 febrile UTI should undergo a VCUG.

3. **Watchful waiting without voiding cystourethrogram.** In children 0 to 3 months of age with *E coli* UTI (first, febrile UTI) and normal renal ultrasound, watchful waiting without VCUG can be considered. This is based on evidence that the probability of high-grade vesicoureteral reflux was low in children with *E coli* UTIs and normal renal ultrasounds (1%). The presence of non–*E coli* UTI increased the probability of high-grade vesicoureteral reflux to 26%, and adding an abnormal renal ultrasound further increased the probability to 55%.

4. **Other imaging studies.** Ultrasound of the spine or magnetic resonance imaging (MRI) of the spine may be considered if there is evidence of neurogenic bladder. MRI of the urinary tract is rarely done but can provide excellent anatomic detail of the urinary tract. Diuretic renogram can be done to localize and quantify the degree of urinary tract obstruction.

C. Antibiotic prophylaxis. Use and efficacy of antibiotic prophylaxis are debated subjects in the fields of pediatrics and urology. Although prophylactic antibiotics may reduce the incidence of UTI, they may not reduce the risk of renal scarring. The use of prophylactic antibiotics may also increase the risk of acquiring pathogens with antibiotic resistance. The AAP Red Book states that "data do not support the use of antimicrobial prophylaxis to prevent febrile recurrent UTIs in infants without vesicoureteral reflux." For neonates with vesicoureteral reflux, moderate to severe hydronephrosis, or other abnormalities such as posterior urethral valves, antibiotic prophylaxis should be considered. Amoxicillin (10 mg/kg/d) is the most commonly used. If vesicoureteral reflux is present, prophylaxis is continued. Trimethoprim-sulfamethoxazole is contraindicated because of liver and kidney immaturity in neonates.

D. Circumcision should be considered in uncircumcised males with a history of recurrent UTIs. Newborn circumcision is a common procedure with relatively few associated complications. Pathogenic bacteria may be more adherent to the mucosal surface of the foreskin than the keratinzed surface of the penis after circumcision. In theory, circumcision also reduces the bacterial colonization of the periurethral area, thereby reducing the risk of UTIs. The AAP feels that the potential benefits of male circumcision outweigh the risks; therefore, the procedure should be accessible to families who choose it. There is insufficient evidence to recommend routine circumcision in all newborns. The risks and potential benefits of the procedure should be outlined to parents to help them make an informed decision.

E. **American Academy of Pediatrics Urinary Tract Infection Guidelines.** In 2011, the AAP revised its practice parameters for diagnosis and management of initial UTI in febrile infants and children age 2 to 24 months. This report did not include infants younger than 2 months of age due to insufficient data in this age group. Therefore, there is no consensus on evaluation and management in infants <2 months old.

153 Varicella-Zoster Infections

Varicella-zoster virus (VZV) is a member of the herpesvirus family. Primary maternal VZV infection (chickenpox) can result in fetal or neonatal infection. Other rare complications include spontaneous abortion, fetal demise, and premature delivery. Reactivation infection (zoster, shingles) does not result in fetal infection. Primary maternal VZV infection during the last trimester can cause maternal pneumonia with significant morbidity and mortality. The overall incidence of maternal and neonatal varicella has decreased over the past 15 to 20 years, presumably due to varicella vaccination. Active surveillance among adults has shown that the incidence of varicella declined 74% during 1995 to 2005, despite vaccination rates among adults of only 3%. Herd immunity is the likely explanation for this phenomenon. As of 2013, more than 78% of 13- to 17-year-old adolescents have received 2 doses of varicella vaccine. Varicella immunization is recommended for all nonimmune women as part of prepregnancy and postpartum care. **Varicella vaccine should not be administered to pregnant women**, because the possible effects on fetal development are unknown, although no cases of congenital varicella syndrome or patterns of malformation have been identified after inadvertent immunization of pregnant women. When postpubertal females are immunized, pregnancy should be avoided for at least 1 month after immunization. Reporting of instances of inadvertent immunization to the US Food and Drug Administration with a varicella-zoster–containing vaccine during pregnancy is encouraged (1-877-888-4231).

There are 3 forms of varicella-zoster infections involving the fetus and neonate: **fetal, congenital (early neonatal), and postnatal**.

FETAL VARICELLA SYNDROME

I. **Definition.** VZV is a teratogen that can cross the placenta and cause a pattern of congenital malformations called fetal varicella syndrome (FVS). This form occurs when the mother has her first exposure to VZV during the first half of pregnancy. The syndrome is also recognized in the literature as **congenital varicella syndrome (CVS)**.

II. **Incidence.** Only approximately 5% of women of childbearing age are susceptible to VZV. The incidence of varicella during pregnancy is estimated at 1 to 5 cases per 10,000 pregnancies. The incidence of **embryopathy and fetopathy (FVS)** after maternal varicella infection in the first 20 weeks is 1% to 2%.

III. **Pathophysiology.** Maternal acquisition of the virus probably occurs via respiratory droplets or direct contact with chickenpox or zoster lesions. The virus replicates in the oropharynx, and viremia results, before the onset of rash, with transplacental passage to the fetus. Almost all cases reported have involved exposure between the 8th and 20th weeks of pregnancy. The pathogenesis of FVS may reflect disseminated infection in utero or be a consequence of failure of the virus–host interaction to result in establishment of latency, as normally occurs in postnatal VZV infection. Because VZV is a lymphotropic virus, it has the potential to spread to all fetal organs by the hematogenous route. Pathology specimens from aborted fetuses with VZV infection have shown the virus to be distributed throughout fetal tissues. Microcephaly can be attributed to VZV encephalitis and irreversible damage to the developing brain. Of interest, the virus does not appear to cause intrauterine damage to the lungs or liver in infants with FVS, as it does in perinatal varicella or in other immunocompromised hosts. Fulminant infection involving these organs may result in fetal demise, rather than birth of an infant with FVS. VZV is also a neurotropic virus; many of the defects have been postulated to be a direct result of spinal cord and ganglia infection, which causes destruction of the plexi during embryogenesis, leading to denervation of the limb bud and subsequent hypoplasia. Failure of muscle development has consequences for limb bone formation. The cutaneous defects are also likely to reflect VZV infection of sensory nerves. VZV infection of cells in developing optic tracts also explains the optic atrophy and chorioretinitis. From the pattern of dermatomal distribution of the skin defects seen in FVS, particularly the scarring and limb hypoplasia, it has been suggested that FVS is the result of intrauterine zoster. The extremely short latent period between fetal infection and reactivation, if latency is established at all, is the consequence of the lack of cell-mediated immunity in the fetus before 20 weeks' gestation. Infants exposed to VZV in utero also can develop zoster (shingles) early in life without having had extrauterine varicella (chickenpox).

IV. **Risk factors.** A pregnant woman with no history of varicella infection or vaccination who becomes exposed to VZV between the 8th and 20th weeks of gestation is at risk.

V. **Clinical presentation.** The main symptoms of FVS are:

   A. **Skin lesions (60%–70%).** Cicatricial scars and skin loss.

   B. **Central nervous system defects or disease (60%).** Microcephaly, seizures, encephalitis, cortical atrophy and spinal cord atrophy, mental retardation, and cerebral calcifications.

   C. **Ocular abnormalities (60%).** Microphthalmia, chorioretinitis, cataracts, optic atrophy, nystagmus, and Horner syndrome (ptosis, miosis, and enophthalmos).

   D. **Limb abnormalities, which often include hypoplasia of bone and muscle (50%).**

   E. **Prematurity and intrauterine growth restriction (35%).**

VI. **Diagnosis.** Alkalay et al proposed the following criteria for the diagnosis of FVS in the newborn:

   A. **Appearance of maternal varicella during pregnancy.**

   B. **Presence of congenital skin lesions** in dermatomal distribution and/or neurologic defects, eye disease, or limb hypoplasia.

   C. **Proof of intrauterine varicella-zoster virus infection** by detection of viral DNA in the infant by polymerase chain reaction (PCR), presence of VZV-specific immunoglobulin (Ig) M, persistence of VZV IgG beyond 7 months of age, or appearance of zoster (shingles) during early infancy.

   Prenatal diagnosis is most often done by detailed ultrasound, searching for typical anomalies and VZV-specific PCR in amniotic fluid. At least a 5-week interval is advised between onset of maternal rash and obtaining of the ultrasound. An initial ultrasound is recommended at 17 to 21 weeks of gestation with a follow-up study done 4 to 6 weeks later. The role of prenatal magnetic resonance imaging for assessment of the fetus after maternal varicella is only beginning to be delineated, but it may provide improved specificity, particularly for central nervous system damage.

VII. **Management.** Isolation precautions for all infectious diseases, including maternal and neonatal precautions, breast feeding, and visiting issues, can be found in Appendix F.

   A. **Mother.** If the mother is exposed to VZV infection in the first or second trimester, treat the mother with **varicella-zoster immune globulin (VariZIG)** if her past history of varicella infection or vaccination is negative or uncertain. For dosage, see Chapter 155. **VariZIG** should be given as soon as possible after exposure (preferably within 72 hours, but up to 10 days), and it appears to protect both mother and fetus. If VariZIG is not available, intravenous immunoglobulin (IVIG) can be used. If chickenpox is diagnosed during pregnancy, antiviral therapy with **acyclovir** or **valacyclovir** should be strongly considered. Acyclovir and valacyclovir therapy during pregnancy appears to be safe; it has not been associated with increased congenital abnormalities compared with the general population.

B. **Infant.** Supportive care of the infant is required because there is usually profound neurologic impairment. Acyclovir therapy may be helpful to stop the progression of eye disease or to treat recurrent zoster (shingles), which is common in the first 2 years of life.

C. **Isolation.** Isolation is not necessary.

VIII. **Prognosis.** Approximately 30% of these infants with FVS die in the first months of life, often because of intractable gastroesophageal reflux, severe recurrent aspiration pneumonia, and respiratory failure. Survivors usually suffer profound mental retardation and major neurologic disabilities. These infants are also at risk for developing zoster (shingles) in the first 2 years of life.

CONGENITAL (EARLY NEONATAL) VARICELLA INFECTION

I. **Definition.** This is the form of the disease that occurs when a pregnant woman suffers chickenpox during the last 3 weeks of pregnancy or within the first few days postpartum. Disease begins in the neonate just before delivery or within the first 10 to 12 days of life.

II. **Incidence.** Although the congenital (early neonatal) form is more common than the teratogenic form, it is still rare, with recent estimates of 0.7 per 100,000 live births per annum. The introduction of varicella vaccination in 1995 greatly reduced the incidence of varicella infection in all age groups (herd immunity).

III. **Pathophysiology.** Maternal chickenpox near term or soon after delivery may cause severe or fatal illness in the newborn. Maternal varicella can affect the baby through transplacental viremia, ascending infection during birth, or respiratory droplet/direct contact with infectious lesions after birth. Neonatal chickenpox occurring in the first 10 to 12 days of life is typically caused by intrauterine transmission of VZV (incubation period 10–21 days). Chickenpox after the 12th day of life is most likely acquired by postnatal VZV exposure. If the onset of **maternal disease is between 5 days before delivery or 2 days postpartum**, there is a high attack rate (up to 50%) with significant associated mortality (up to 30%). Those babies present with the classic skin lesions, but can disseminate with pneumonia, hepatitis, meningoencephalitis, and severe coagulopathy (disseminated intravascular coagulation [DIC]) resulting from liver failure and thrombocytopenia. If the maternal rash happens >5 days before delivery, there is enough maternal anti-VZV IgG production with subsequent transplacental transfer to protect the newborn, which results in a milder case of chickenpox.

IV. **Risk factors.** Primarily a mother with chickenpox during the last 3 weeks of pregnancy or within the first few days postpartum. There is a higher risk of mortality if the onset of maternal disease is **5 days before delivery or 2 days postpartum**. Premature infants, especially those <28 weeks, are extremely susceptible.

V. **Clinical presentation** is variable. There may be only mild involvement of the infant, with vesicles on the skin, or the following may be seen:

A. **Skin.** A centripetal rash (beginning on the trunk and spreading to the face and scalp, sparing the extremities) begins as red macules and progresses to vesicles and encrustation. Lesions are more common in the diaper area and skin folds. There may be 2 or 3 lesions or thousands of them. The differential diagnosis includes herpes simplex virus and enterovirus. The main complication is staphylococcal and streptococcal secondary skin infections.

B. **Lungs.** Lung involvement is seen in all fatal cases. It usually appears 2 to 4 days after the onset of the rash but may be seen up to 10 days after. Signs include fever, cyanosis, rales, and hemoptysis. Chest radiograph shows a diffuse nodular-miliary pattern, especially in the perihilar region.

   C. **Other organs.** Focal necrosis may be seen in the liver, adrenals, intestines, kidneys, and thymus. Glomerulonephritis, myocarditis, encephalitis, and cerebellar ataxia are sometimes seen.

VI. **Diagnosis.** The diagnosis of varicella usually is made clinically based on the characteristic appearance of skin lesions.

   A. **Polymerase chain reaction** is the **most sensitive and specific method for detection** of VZV DNA in clinical specimens. This is the diagnostic method of choice for investigation of vesicular fluid or scabs, biopsies, and amniotic fluid. This testing also can be used to distinguish between wild-type and vaccine-strain VZV (genotyping). Viral culture and direct fluorescent antibody assay are less sensitive than PCR and are not usually recommended.

   B. **Serum testing of varicella-zoster virus antibody.** Serologic tests may help to document acute infection in difficult cases. IgM antibody may be detected as soon as 3 days after the appearance of VZV symptoms, but the test may not be reliable.

VII. **Management**

   A. **VariZIG.** Infants of mothers who develop VZV infection (rash) **within 5 days before or 2 days after** delivery should receive 125 U (62.5 U if <2 kg) of **VariZIG** as soon as possible and no later than 10 days. **IVIG** (400 mg/kg) should be used if VariZIG is not available. Infants treated with immune globulins should be placed in strict respiratory isolation for 28 days because immunoglobulin treatment may prolong the incubation period. VariZIG is not expected to reduce the clinical attack rate in treated newborns; however, these infants tend to develop milder infections than the untreated neonates. Prophylactic administration of oral **acyclovir** beginning 7 days after exposure also may prevent or attenuate varicella disease in exposed infants. Infants born to mothers with rash occurring >**5 days before delivery** do not need VZIG, unless they are born at <28 weeks' gestation; it is believed that these infants should have received protective transplacental antibodies.

   B. **Acyclovir therapy** 15 mg/kg/dose every 8 hours for 7 days should be considered for postexposure prophylaxis as well as a treatment in symptomatic neonates.

   C. **Antibiotics.** Use antibiotics if secondary bacterial skin infections occur.

   D. **Breast feeding.** Neither wild-type VZV nor Oka vaccine strain virus has been shown to be transmitted by human milk; expressed/pumped milk from a mother with varicella or zoster can be given to the infant, provided no lesions are on the breast.

VIII. **Prognosis.** If the mother has onset of disease within 5 days before delivery or 2 days after, the infant is exposed with no antibodies and will be at risk for severe disease. Overwhelming sepsis and multiple organ failure can lead to a mortality rate as high as 30%. The usual causes of death are pneumonia, fulminant hepatitis, and DIC. With the use of VariZIG, the mortality rate is reduced to 7%. There is an increased risk of developing zoster (shingles) in the first 2 years of life.

POSTNATAL CHICKENPOX

   I. **Definition.** This form of the disease presents after the 12th day of life. It does not represent transplacental infection from the mother.

   II. **Incidence.** There has been a significant decline in the incidence since the introduction of the varicella vaccine in 1995 (by 90%). The incidence of neonatal varicella in the vaccine era is approximately 0.7 per 100,000 live births.

   III. **Pathophysiology.** Postnatal VZV infection occurs by droplet transmission. This disease is usually mild because of passive protection from maternal antibodies. Placental antibody transfer is lower in preterm infants, which makes them more susceptible compared with term infants. Horizontal transmission in neonatal intensive care units has been well documented. Neonatal vaccine-strain VZV infection after maternal postpartum vaccination has been reported.

IV. Risk factors. Seronegative mother, delivery before 28 weeks, birthweight <1.5 kg, postnatal age >2 months (maternal transplacental immunity has waned), immunocompromised neonates (eg, sepsis, steroids).

V. Clinical presentation. The typical chickenpox rash is seen with centripetal spread, beginning on the trunk and spreading to the face and scalp and sparing the extremities. All stages of the rash may appear at the same time, from red macules to clear vesicles to crusting lesions. Complications of this form of the disease are rare but may include secondary infections and varicella pneumonia. In older children, necrotizing fasciitis secondary to group A streptococcal infections is particularly worrisome and may be associated with ibuprofen use (see Figure 80–11).

VI. Diagnosis. Same as for congenital varicella (see the previous section). Diagnosis is usually made based on clinical grounds.

VII. Management. For the full-term infant in the community setting, the disease is usually mild. Therefore, acyclovir therapy is ***controversial***. For nosocomial chickenpox in the intensive care nursery (exposure):

    A. Varicella-zoster immune globulin. Recommended for all exposed infants of **<28 weeks'** gestational age or weighing **≤1000 g regardless of their mothers' evidence of immunity to varicella**. It is also recommended in older premature infants (28–36 weeks) whose mothers do not have a history of chickenpox or varicella vaccination **(seronegative)**. Some experts recommend administration of VariZIG to term infants who have been exposed to varicella in the first 2 weeks after birth and whose mothers do not have evidence of immunity.

    B. Infants ≥28 weeks' gestation born to seropositive (immune) mothers. These infants should have sufficient transplacental antibodies to protect them from the risk of complications.

    C. Isolation. Exposed infants should be placed in strict isolation (airborne and contact precautions) from 8 until 21 days after the onset of the rash in the index case. Exposed infants who receive VariZIG/IVIG should be in strict respiratory isolation for 28 days.

    D. Breast feeding. Expressed/pumped milk from a mother with varicella or zoster can be given to the infant, provided no lesions are on the breast. Breast feeding is encouraged in infants exposed to or infected with varicella because antibody in breast milk may be protective.

    E. Acyclovir. Recommended for infants who develop breakthrough lesions or prophylactically beginning 7 days after exposure. Therapy should be continued for 7 days (if used prophylactically) or for 48 hours after the last new lesions have appeared.

VIII. Prognosis. This form of the disease is mild, and death is extremely rare. Normal term infants who develop postnatal chickenpox have the same risk of complications of chickenpox as older children. Premature infants are at increased risk for nosocomial acquisition of VZV. The risk of complications for infants <28 weeks who develop postnatal chickenpox is unknown.

154 Zika Virus (Congenital Zika Syndrome)

I. Definition. Congenital Zika syndrome (CZS) is a constellation of central nervous system (CNS), ocular, and neuromuscular abnormalities seen in newborns after in utero exposure to Zika virus, a member of the *Flaviviridae* virus family (which includes dengue, yellow fever, and West Nile viruses).

II. Incidence. As of late August 2017, the Pan American Health Organization reported 48 countries in the Americas with vector-borne transmission of Zika virus and 27 countries and territories in the Americas with confirmed cases of CZS. As of mid-April 2018, the Centers for Disease Control and Prevention (CDC) identified 2328 completed pregnancies in the United States (including the District of Columbia) in women with laboratory evidence of possible Zika virus infection. Of these pregnancies, 115 liveborn neonates and 9 pregnancy losses had documented birth defects. The prevalence of CZS-associated birth defects in infants of women in the US Zika Pregnancy Registry during the first 9 months of 2016 was 58.8 cases per 1000 live births, roughly 20-fold greater than a "pre-Zika" cohort in 2013 to 2014.

III. Pathophysiology. Zika virus is an arbovirus (arthropod-borne virus) first identified in the Zika Forest of Uganda in 1947. Mosquitoes of the *Aedes* genus (specifically, *Aedes aegypti* and *Aedes albopictus*) are the primary arthropod vectors and are endemic to regions of the continental United States and Hawaii, Puerto Rico, and the US Virgin Islands. In urban and suburban areas, the virus is transmitted from human to human via mosquito bites ("blood meals") commonly during daylight hours. Sexual transmission of the virus can occur from an infected person to his or her partner and is of great concern to pregnant women or women attempting to conceive.

Human disease secondary to Zika virus had been noted sporadically worldwide until outbreaks in the State of Yap, Federated States of Micronesia in 2007 and multiple Pacific Islands from 2013 to 2016. In most cases, persons infected with Zika virus are asymptomatic. In symptomatic patients, acute Zika syndrome typically is a mild illness presenting in adults and children roughly 7 to 10 days after exposure with a pruritic, maculopapular rash, a low-grade fever, musculoskeletal discomfort (myalgia/arthritis/arthralgia), extremity edema, conjunctivitis, and headache. Zika infection and Guillain-Barré syndrome, an autoimmune-mediated peripheral neuropathy, first were associated during an outbreak in French Polynesia in 2013 to 2014; a strong link between the virus and the disease was confirmed in a later case-control study in that area.

The first outbreak of Zika infection in the Americas occurred in early 2015 in the Bahia state of Brazil, with an estimated 1.3 million cases throughout the country. Later that year, health officials in Brazil noted an increased incidence of anomalies in babies born in Zika-affected areas. Zika RNA and proteins subsequently were found in fetal and maternal tissues from microcephalic fetuses, infants, and early pregnancy losses of Brazilian mothers with symptoms of acute Zika infection in pregnancy. Additional research has demonstrated that the virus generates a placentitis and has a notable trophism for human neuronal tissue in vitro and in vivo, specifically for neural progenitor cells. Furthermore, clinical, imaging, and autopsy findings in affected fetuses and newborns documented significant cranial, CNS, and ophthalmologic abnormalities. Using criteria for teratogenicity and evidence of causation, the CDC concluded in May 2016 that a causal relationship may be inferred between antenatal maternal Zika virus infection and neonatal microcephaly and other brain anomalies.

IV. Risk factors. Risk factors for Zika virus infection include:

A. Residing in or travel to a Zika-endemic region. As of September 2017, the following countries have been designated by the CDC as areas with risks of acquiring Zika:

1. **Africa:** Angola, Benin, Burkina-Faso, Burundi, Cameroon, Cape Verde, Central African Republic, Chad, Congo (Congo-Brazzaville), Côte d'Ivoire, Democratic Republic of the Congo (Congo-Kinshasa), Equatorial Guinea, Gabon, Gambia, Ghana, Guinea, Guinea-Bissau, Kenya, Liberia, Mali, Niger, Nigeria, Rwanda, Senegal, Sierra Leone, South Sudan, Sudan, Tanzania, Togo, Uganda.

2. **Asia:** Bangladesh, Burma (Myanmar), Cambodia, India, Indonesia, Laos, Malaysia, Maldives, Pakistan, Philippines, Singapore, Thailand, Timor-Leste (East Timor), Vietnam.

3. **The Caribbean:** Anguilla, Antigua and Barbuda, Aruba, The Bahamas, Barbados, Bonaire, British Virgin Islands, Cuba, Curaçao, Dominica, Dominican Republic, Grenada, Haiti, Jamaica, Montserrat, Puerto Rico, Saba, Saint Kitts and Nevis,

Saint Lucia, Saint Martin, Saint Vincent and the Grenadines, Saint Eustatius, Saint Maarten, Trinidad and Tobago, Turks and Caicos Islands, US Virgin Islands.

   4. **Central America:** Belize, Costa Rica, El Salvador, Guatemala, Honduras, Nicaragua, Panama.

   5. **North America:** Mexico.

   6. **The Pacific Islands:** Fiji, Marshall Islands, Micronesia, Palau, Papua New Guinea, Samoa, Solomon Islands, Tonga.

   7. **South America:** Argentina, Bolivia, Brazil, Colombia, Ecuador, French Guiana, Guyana, Paraguay, Peru, Suriname, Venezuela.

   8. **United States travel precautions:** Autochthonous infection (ie, infection caused by endemic mosquitoes) previously was documented in the United States in Miami-Dade County, Florida, and Brownsville, Texas, leading to Zika cautionary (yellow) designations. Pregnant women (or women wishing to conceive) were recommended to limit travel to these areas. As of August 2017, however, the CDC lifted these designations, although people residing in or traveling to these regions should take precautions to minimize the risk of mosquito bites. Up-to-date, worldwide travel recommendations may be obtained from the CDC's Zika virus (cdc.gov/Zika).

   B. **Sex with a person who resides in or has traveled to a Zika-endemic region.** The Zika virus persists in human body fluids, even after resolution of the acute infection. Notably, Zika virus can persist in semen for up to 6 months after infection. Women who wish to conceive or who are pregnant should discuss with their healthcare provider strategies to prevent Zika infection in this manner.

   C. **Blood product transfusion.** To date, 4 suspected cases of transfusion-associated Zika virus transmission have been reported (all in Brazil). As of late 2016, however, blood banks in the United States test all donations for Zika virus or subject the samples to pathogen reduction techniques, with all positive blood products quarantined and removed from the blood supply.

   D. **Breast milk.** Although Zika virus has been isolated from breast milk, cases of Zika transmission via breast feeding have not been reported. In the absence of other contraindications (eg, human immunodeficiency virus infection, medications), women with confirmed, probable, or suspected Zika exposure may breast feed their babies.

V. **Clinical presentation.** The clinical features of CZS are due to direct CNS injury and resultant calvarial abnormalities. These findings initially may be detected on antenatal imaging, recognized at the time of birth, or identified in childhood.

   A. **Microcephaly and brain or spinal cord abnormalities.** CZS has been associated with the fetal brain disruption sequence (FBDS), a constellation of findings including severe microcephaly (occipitofrontal head circumference [OFC] <3 standard deviations below the mean for gestational age), overlapping cranial sutures, occipital prominence, craniofacial disproportion, and excessive scalp skin. In CZS, FBDS theoretically occurs secondary to loss of brain volume after Zika-induced neuronal death and impaired neuronal migration. Specific brain abnormalities include subcortical calcifications (in contrast to periventricular calcifications seen in congenital cytomegalovirus infection), cortical dysgenesis (heterotopias, pachygyria, lissencephaly), cortical thinning, ventriculomegaly, and callosal and cerebellar hypoplasia. Neural tube defects (eg, spina bifida, anencephaly) have been reported among babies in the US Zika Pregnancy Registry, although a causal relationship has not been established. Of note, microcephaly, postnatal hydrocephalus, and developmental delays not noted at birth may develop later as the infant grows (secondary to early neuronal injury).

   B. **Ophthalmologic abnormalities.** As many as half of newborns with CZS and associated microcephaly have eye anomalies. Posterior segment abnormalities are the most common findings, including chorioretinal atrophy, retinal pigment mottling, and optic nerve findings (atrophy/hypoplasia or cupping). Acute chorioretinitis, often seen in other congenital infections (eg, *Toxoplasma*, cytomegalovirus), is not present in neonates with Zika infection. Anterior segment abnormalities in CZS include iris coloboma, microphthalmia, lens subluxation, cataracts, glaucoma, and intraocular calcifications.

C. **Neurologic/neuromuscular abnormalities.** Abnormal neurologic findings in neonates with CZS may include hypotonia or hypertonia, hyperreflexia, seizures (or abnormal electroencephalography without clinical seizures), irritability, extraocular muscle paresis, dysphagia, and developmental delays. Congenital sensorineural hearing loss has been demonstrated, but delayed-onset hearing loss (as seen with congenital cytomegalovirus infection) has not been documented. Congenital neuromuscular abnormalities observed in CZS include contractures of ≥1 joint (arthrogryposis), club foot (talipes equinovarus), diaphragmatic paralysis, and hip and knee dislocation.

D. **Laboratory markers of hepatic involvement** (ie, elevated transaminases) are extremely rare in CZS, unlike in other congenital or perinatally acquired infections (eg, neonatal herpes simplex virus infection). However, autopsies of a small cohort of newborns with CZS demonstrated hepatic (steatosis, hepatocyte necrosis) and genitourinary (cystitis, focal glomerular sclerosis) injury.

VI. **Diagnosis.** Confirmative diagnosis of Zika virus infection in expectant mothers, fetuses, and neonates is challenging due to a paucity of data and a limited number of available tests. Diagnosis of CZS relies on identification of clinical signs and symptoms, laboratory analyses, and imaging modalities in the fetus and newborn in combination with maternal history and testing results. All pregnant women should be asked whether they have had possible Zika virus exposure during pregnancy. For infants with concern for CZS, coordination of care between healthcare facilities, local and regional health departments, and the CDC is important to ensure appropriate procurement and processing of samples and appropriate follow-up of neonates with suspected, probable, or confirmed CZS. See Figure 154–1 for the evaluation of infants with possible congenital Zika virus infection.

A. **Laboratory studies.** Currently available diagnostic tests for Zika virus include molecular nucleic acid amplification tests (NAATs) and serologic assays approved by the US Food and Drug Administration under an Emergency Use Authorization. Samples for neonatal testing should be obtained as early as possible (preferably within the first 2 days of age) because delayed testing may prevent clinicians from distinguishing congenital Zika infection from postnatally acquired Zika infection. **Cord blood should not be used for Zika testing,** because false-positive and/or false-negative results may occur.

1. **Zika nucleic acid amplification testing (NAAT).** Zika virus real-time reverse transcription polymerase chain reaction (rRT-PCR) is used to identify viral RNA. This assay may be used for serum or whole blood; urine; cerebrospinal, seminal, or amniotic fluid; and placental tissue specimens. Zika virus RNA has been detected in serum for up to 2 weeks after acute infection in nonpregnant individuals and up to 62 days in pregnant women. RNA may persist for longer in other specimens and has been documented in seminal fluid months after acute infection. A positive rRT-PCR test result in any specimen indicates active Zika virus infection. However, a negative Zika virus rRT-PCR test does not exclude infection because patient sampling may have occurred outside the acute phase of infection. Zika NAAT testing should be performed in tandem with serologic testing in patients with concern for Zika infection.

2. **Zika serologic testing.** Zika immunoglobulin (Ig) M antibody is the current first-line serologic test in the United States. IgM antibodies may be detectable within days of acute infection and persist for at least 4 months thereafter. However, Zika IgM testing has several limitations. False-negative results may occur if testing occurs outside the window of IgM detection or if the patient failed to generate an IgM antibody response. False-positive or equivocal results may occur in patients who have been infected with other arboviruses (eg, dengue or

chikungunya viruses) or vaccinated against Japanese encephalitis or yellow fever. Presently, there is no approved Zika IgG assay available in the United States. **All positive Zika IgM results should be confirmed with a plaque reduction neutralization test (PRNT),** which measures virus-specific neutralizing antibodies that develop soon after infection and that may persist for years. PRNT testing may help confirm or rule out a prior infection (congenital or postnatal). However, a positive PRNT test alone cannot distinguish timing of infection, and the results of this test must be interpreted within the clinical context of the patient. In low-risk areas, postnatally acquired infections are unlikely; therefore, a positive PRNT test shortly after birth in a neonate is more likely to reflect a congenital infection. In addition, the PRNT assay cannot distinguish between maternal and infant antibodies in specimens collected from infants at or near birth. Because maternal Zika antibodies are expected to become undetectable by 18 months of age, repeat serologic testing in infants beyond this age may aid in confirming or ruling out congenital Zika virus infection.

3. **Interpretation and caveats of neonatal and infant Zika testing.** Interpretation of laboratory testing of neonatal and infant serum, urine, and/or CSF samples for Zika virus, per the CDC, is as follows:

    a. **Nucleic acid amplification test positive, any immunoglobulin M result.** These results are consistent with **confirmed** congenital Zika virus infection in the infant. However, distinguishing congenital and postnatal Zika virus infection may be difficult if the infant is born in an area of ongoing Zika virus transmission and testing is not done soon after birth. If the timing of the infection cannot be determined, the infant should be evaluated as if she or he has a congenital Zika virus infection.

    b. **Nucleic acid amplification test negative, immunoglobulin M nonnegative.** These results are consistent with **probable** congenital Zika virus infection but should be interpreted within the context of timing of infection (or potential infection) in pregnancy, maternal laboratory results, and the infant's PRNT test results and clinical exam. *If the Zika PRNT test is negative, the infant's Zika IgM result likely is a false positive.*

    c. **Nucleic acid amplification test negative, immunoglobulin M negative.** These results are consistent with congenital Zika virus infection being **unlikely,** particularly if specimens collected soon after birth and the clinical evaluation are normal. Again, these results must be interpreted in light of the factors mentioned in **Section VI.A.3.b.** Furthermore, clinicians should remain vigilant for any signs or symptoms of CZS in infancy and childhood.

4. **Other laboratory tests,** including a complete blood count, metabolic panel, hepatic enzymes, and liver function tests, should be sent in children with high suspicion of CZS and may aid in diagnosis or exclusion of other congenital infectious, genetic, or metabolic conditions.

5. **Clinicians also should be aware** that cases of infants with **clinical findings consistent with possible CZS** but with **negative laboratory results** have been reported.

B. **Imaging and other studies**

1. **Ultrasound, computed tomography, or magnetic resonance imaging.** CNS imaging should be performed in all infants with suspicion of CZS within the first month of age. Ultrasound is the most convenient method to assess intracranial anatomy in neonates. Subtle abnormalities may be detected more readily by magnetic resonance imaging (MRI) or computed tomography (CT) scan. Therefore, particularly in children with restrictive anterior fontanelles or whose clinical findings strongly suggest CZS, MRI or CT should be considered.

2. **Ophthalmologic exam.** This should be performed by an ophthalmologist or retinal specialist, with specific attention to the retinae and optic nerves.

Ask about possible Zika virus exposure

Possible Zika virus exposure → **Does infant have findings consistent with CZS?**

If no maternal Zika virus exposure is identified, routine pediatric care is recommended.

Yes

Initial evaluation:
- Standard evaluation[a]
- Zika virus NAAT and IgM testing
- Consider Zika virus NAAT and IgM testing on CSF
- Head ultrasound by age 1 month
- Comprehensive opthalmologic exam by age 1 month
- Automated ABR by age 1 month[b]
- Evaluate for other causes of congenital anomalies

Refer to developmental specialist and early intervention services
Provide family support services
Consider additional consultations with:
- Infectious disease specialist
- Clinical geneticist
- Neurologist
- Other clinical specialists based on clinical findings on infant

No → **Is there laboratory evidence of possible maternal Zika virus infection during pregnancy?**

Laboratory evidence of possible maternal Zika virus infection during pregnancy[c]

Initial evaluation:
- Standard evaluation[a]
- Zika virus NAAT and IgM testing[e]
- Head ultrasound by age 1 month
- Comprehensive opthalmologic exam by age 1 month
- Automated ABR by age 1 month[b]

No laboratory evidence of possible maternal Zika virus infection during pregnancy[d]

Testing and clinical evaluation for congenital Zika virus infection beyond standard evaluation[c] is not routinely recommended. If findings suggestive of CZS are identified at any time, refer to appropriate specialists and evaluate for congenital Zika virus infection.

Is initial evaluation normal?

Yes

No

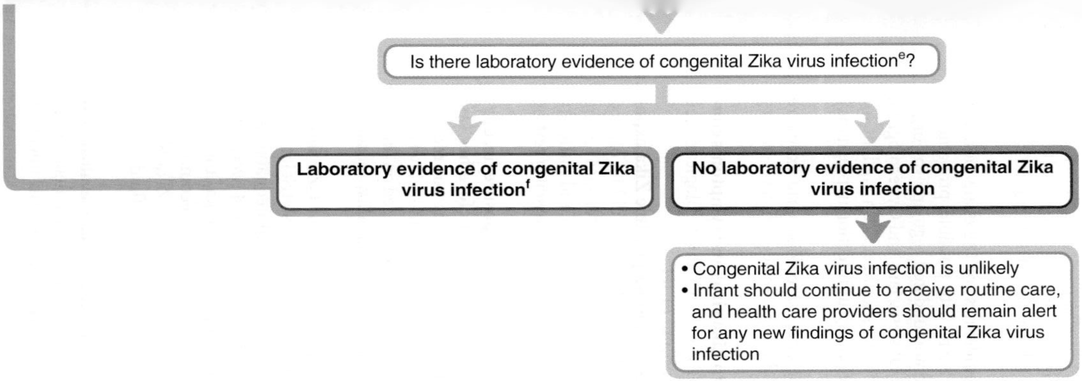

FIGURE 154-1. Recommendations for the evaluation of infants with possible congenital Zika virus infection based on infant clinical findings,[a,b] maternal testing results,[c,d] and infant testing results[e,f] United States October 2017. ABR, auditory brainstem response; CSF, cerebrospinal fluid; CZS, congenital Zika syndrome; IgM, immunoglobulin M; NAAT, nucleic acid amplification test; PRNT, plaque reduction neutralization test. [a]**All infants should receive a standard evaluation at birth** and at each subsequent well-child visit by their healthcare providers including (1) comprehensive physical examination, including growth parameters and (2) age-appropriate vision screening and developmental monitoring and screening using validated tools. Infants should receive a standard newborn hearing screen at birth, preferably using ABR. [b]**Automated ABR by age 1 month if newborn hearing screen passed** but performed with otoacoustic emission methodology. [c]**Laboratory evidence of possible Zika virus infection during pregnancy** is defined as (1) Zika virus infection detected by a Zika virus RNA NAAT on any maternal, placental, or fetal specimen (referred to as NAAT-confirmed), or (2) diagnosis of Zika virus infection, timing of infection cannot be determined or unspecified flavivirus infection, timing of infection cannot be determined by serologic tests on a maternal specimen (ie, positive/equivocal Zika virus IgM and Zika virus PRNT titer ≥10, regardless of dengue virus PRNT value; or negative Zika virus IgM, and positive or equivocal dengue virus IgM, and Zika virus PRNT titer ≥10, regardless of dengue virus PRNT titer). The use of PRNT for confirmation of Zika virus infection, including in pregnant women, is not routinely recommended in Puerto Rico (https://www.cdc.gov/zika/laboratories/lab-guidance.html). [d]**This group includes women who were never tested during pregnancy as well as those whose test result was negative** because of issues related to timing or sensitivity and specificity of the test. Because the latter issues are not easily discerned, all mothers with possible exposure to Zika virus during pregnancy who do not have laboratory evidence of possible Zika virus infection, including those who tested negative with currently available technology, should be considered in this group. [e]**Laboratory testing of infants for Zika virus should be performed as early as possible,** preferably within the first few days after birth, and includes concurrent Zika virus NAAT in infant serum and urine, and Zika virus IgM testing in serum. If CSF is obtained for other purposes, Zika virus NAAT and Zika virus IgM testing should be performed on CSF. [f]**Laboratory evidence of congenital Zika virus infection** includes a positive Zika virus NAAT or a nonnegative Zika virus IgM with confirmatory neutralizing antibody testing, if PRNT confirmation is performed. (*Reproduced with permission from Adebanjo T, Godfred-Cato S, Viens L, et al: Update: Interim Guidance for the Diagnosis, Evaluation, and Management of Infants with Possible Congenital Zika Virus Infection—United States, October 2017, MMWR Morb Mortal Wkly Rep. 2017 Oct 20;66(41):1089-1099.*)

3. **Hearing screening.** In children with laboratory and clinical abnormalities consistent with CZS, automated auditory brainstem response should be performed by 1 month of age if the newborn screening test was passed (via otoacoustic emissions [OAE] testing). Automated auditory brainstem response will detect abnormalities along the auditory brainstem pathway or in the 8 cranial nerves not reflected in OAE testing.

VII. **Management.** During the recent Zika epidemic, guidelines for the evaluation and management of pregnant woman, fetuses, and newborns with possible, probable, or confirmed Zika virus infection have been published and updated regularly (by organizations such as the CDC, the American College of Obstetricians and Gynecologists, and the Society of Maternal-Fetal Medicine). Clinicians should remain vigilant for further updates as more information is learned about Zika virus infection in pregnancy and CZS.

A. **Pregnant women.** All pregnant women should be assessed for Zika virus exposure prior to pregnancy and at each prenatal visit, including a review of travel history (including her partner's history). As of July, 2017:

1. **If a pregnant woman has possible exposure to Zika virus and symptoms consistent with infection,** she should be offered Zika NAAT and serologic testing **immediately and through 12 weeks after symptom onset.**

2. **If a pregnant woman is asymptomatic but has ongoing possible Zika exposure (from residing in or traveling to an at-risk area),** she should be offered NAAT testing at initiation of prenatal care and twice more thereafter. IgM testing in these women is no longer recommended due to limitations of and difficulty in interpreting these tests. *Of note, the optimal timing and frequency of testing asymptomatic women with NAAT only are not known.*

3. **If a pregnant woman is asymptomatic with recent possible exposure (ie, during the pregnancy, 8 weeks before conception, or 6 weeks before her last menstrual period) but no ongoing exposure,** routine testing **is not recommended** but can be considered using a shared decision-making model between the patient and provider. This recommendation may be adapted based on unique factors in the jurisdiction where the woman resides (eg, seasonality, mosquito control factors).

Pregnant women whose fetuses have anomalies concerning for CZS should have NAAT and serologic testing and be referred to a high-risk obstetrician and/or a tertiary care medical center for comprehensive maternal and neonatal care. Previously, the CDC suggested serial ultrasounds roughly every 4 weeks for women exposed in pregnancy and with laboratory evidence of Zika infection; however, there are no data specific to this infection to support this recommendation. If amniocentesis is performed for abnormal prenatal findings, Zika NAAT testing can be considered. However, a negative NAAT on amniotic fluid cannot rule out CZS.

B. **Neonates and infants.** Based on risk and findings of affected neonates evaluated to date, the CDC has recommended the following evaluation and management strategies for newborns and infants born to mothers with possible Zika virus infection during pregnancy:

1. **Infants with clinical findings consistent with congenital Zika syndrome and maternal history with possible Zika virus exposure during pregnancy.** The initial evaluation and subspecialty involvement may be done prior to discharge or within the first month of life as deemed appropriate based on the clinical context, setting, and feasibility of outpatient care. The evaluation should include the following:

a. **A standard evaluation, including a comprehensive physical exam** (with documentation of weight, length, and OFC) and age-appropriate vision, hearing, and developmental surveillance and screening.

b. **Zika virus nucleic acid amplification testing and immunoglobulin M from serum or blood** and NAAT from urine.

    c. **Zika virus nucleic acid amplification testing and immunoglobulin M from cerebrospinal fluid (CSF)** if CSF is obtained for other diagnostic purposes. Clinicians should consider CSF testing if serum and urine Zika results are negative and other explanation for abnormalities are ruled out, given reports of CZS in infants where CSF testing yielded the only positive result. At our institution (Johns Hopkins), due to logistical considerations, we recommend obtaining CSF at initial evaluation if the clinician has a high suspicion of CZS in the patient, especially if the results of serum and urine assays are not available at the time of patient evaluation or discharge.

    d. **Head ultrasound by age 1 month.** Consider additional neuroimaging as discussed earlier.

    e. **Comprehensive ophthalmologic exam by age 1 month of age.**

    f. **Automated auditory brainstem response hearing evaluation by 1 month of age,** even if OAE screening is completed in the newborn nursery or neonatal intensive care unit (NICU).

    g. **Evaluation for other causes of congenital anomalies.**

    h. **Referral to developmental specialists and early intervention service programs** for infants and toddlers.

    i. **Psychosocial support to the family (via social work and/or psychology).**

    j. **Consultation with additional specialists** (as appropriate) based on the patient's clinical findings, including:

        i. **Genetics,** for confirmation of the phenotype and evaluation for chromosomal/genetic/metabolic causes of microcephaly (eg, trisomies).

        ii. **Infectious diseases** for evaluation other congenital infections (eg, rubella, cytomegalovirus) and assistance with Zika diagnosis and testing.

        iii. **Neurology and neuroradiology,** by 1 month of age, for a thorough neurologic examination, consideration of other disorders of neuronal development (eg, intrauterine intracranial hemorrhage, inhalant embryopathy), and guidance regarding additional testing (eg, electroencephalography).

        iv. **Consultations with other pediatric specialists,** including **orthopedics, otolaryngology, pulmonology, gastroenterology, endocrinology,** and **speech and language pathology,** may be appropriate based on clinical findings to assess and manage sequelae of CZS (eg, joint contractures, aspiration risk, feeding problems, hypothalamic-pituitary axis abnormalities). Clinicians and families may wish to pursue palliative care in severely affected children.

2. **Infants without clinical findings consistent with CZS but maternal history of laboratory evidence of possible Zika virus infection during pregnancy.**

    a. **Standard evaluation as noted earlier.**

    b. **Zika virus nucleic acid amplification testing and immunoglobulin M** from serum or blood and NAAT from urine.

    c. **Head ultrasound by age 1 month.** Consider more advanced neuroimaging as discussed earlier.

    d. **Comprehensive ophthalmologic exam by age 1 month,** with follow-up as determined by the ophthalmologist.

    e. **Automated auditory brainstem response hearing evaluation by 1 month of age,** even if OAE screening is completed in the newborn nursery or NICU.

If the infant is found to have abnormalities consistent with CZS at any time (eg, vision impairment, hearing problems, developmental delay, or delayed head growth) *or* the infant remains asymptomatic but has positive Zika testing results (positive NAAT or nonnegative IgM with confirmatory positive PRNT), then the infant should undergo additional evaluations and subspecialist involvement as described in **Section VII.B.1.** If the infant remains asymptomatic and Zika virus testing is negative, CZS is unlikely. The child should continue to receive routine pediatric care, with clinicians remaining vigilant for findings consistent with CZS.

3. **Infants without clinical findings** consistent with CZS and mothers with possible Zika virus exposure in pregnancy but without maternal testing or negative maternal laboratory results.
   a. **A standard evaluation as noted earlier.**
   b. **No additional Zika-specific testing or evaluations.**
   c. **These infants should continue to receive routine pediatric care,** and providers should remain alert to the possibility of CZS and development of its sequelae. In some cases, additional evaluations may be considered depending on the context of the risk of exposure, maternal history, and infant's exam or if abnormalities are identified as the infant grows and develops. Should a child in this category demonstrate abnormalities consistent with CZS, he or she should undergo a complete evaluation as noted in **Section VII.B.1.**

C. **Infants with congenital Zika syndrome or in utero Zika exposure** should receive ongoing pediatric care, including monitoring of growth and development, preventive care, and immunizations in a stable medical home. Subspecialty care and referrals should be based on initial and newly identified medical concerns.

VIII. **Primary prevention.** Primary prevention should focus on educating pregnant and periconceptual women and their partners on reducing exposure to the virus. Mechanisms include avoiding primary acquisition via mosquito bites (by using mosquito nets, insect repellent containing N,N-diethyl-meta-toluamide [DEET], and air conditioning in endemic areas), avoiding exposure (for up to 6 months) to semen of a man infected with Zika virus (via abstinence or barrier contraception), and avoidance or limited travel of women and their male sexual partners to Zika-endemic areas. As of October 2018, a Zika virus vaccine does not exist, although clinical trials are ongoing.

IX. **Prognosis.** CZS is a newly recognized syndrome, but the sequelae in neonates and infants can be striking. Mortality among the initial cohort of Brazilian infants with laboratory confirmed Zika virus infection was 41.1 per 1000 live births. Data from another group of CZS infants during their first year of life show striking decreases in weight, length, and OFC. These children also demonstrated irritability (85.4%), pyramidal and extrapyramidal abnormalities (56.3%), and seizures (50%). Continued surveillance is necessary among infants with documented Zika infection or in utero exposure but without neonatal manifestations of the disease based on experience with other congenital infections (eg, rubella) causing complications later in childhood.

SECTION VIII. **Neonatal Pharmacology**

155 Medications Used in the Neonatal Intensive Care Unit[1]

This section provides a description of medications used in the contemporary care of sick newborn infants. It is not intended to be an exhaustive list of all drugs available for infants, nor is it intended to be an in-depth source of information about neonatal pharmacology. Readers are encouraged to consult with their institutional pharmacists regarding issues of pharmacokinetics, drug interactions, drug elimination and metabolism, and monitoring drug serum levels. Many of these medications may not have formal US Food and Drug Administration (FDA) approval for use in neonates but have become commonly used in this population. The chapter does not provide detailed information about the medication but rather focuses on the use in neonatal population. Information on medications and breast feeding and pregnancy can be found in Chapter 156.

   When the designations of neonate/newborn or infant are used for medication doses, it refers to the following:

Neonate/Newborn: Birth to 28 days postnatal age (PNA).
Infant: >28 days (1 month) to 1 year of age.

ACETAMINOPHEN (APAP) (LIQUIPRIN, TEMPRA, TYLENOL)

INDICATIONS AND USE: Analgesic, antipyretic.
ACTIONS: Analgesic effect—inhibition of prostaglandin synthesis in the central nervous system (CNS) and peripherally, blocking pain impulse generation. Antipyretic effect—inhibition of hypothalamic heat-regulating center.
DOSAGE: oral (PO), per rectum (PR), intravenous (IV).
- **Preterm infants 28 to 32 weeks:** 10 to 12 mg/kg/dose PO every 6 to 8 hours or 20 mg/kg/dose PR every 12 hours. Maximum daily dose: 40 mg/kg. IV: 20 mg/kg IV loading dose; then 7.5 to 10 mg/kg/dose IV every 12 hours. Maximum daily dose: 22.5 mg/kg.
- **Preterm infants 33 to 37 weeks; term neonates <10 days:** 10 to 15 mg/kg/dose PO every 6 hours or 30 mg/kg PR loading dose; then 15 mg/kg/dose every 8 hours. Maximum daily dose: 60 mg/kg. IV: 20 mg/kg IV loading dose; then 7.5 to 10 mg/kg/dose IV every 8 hours. Maximum daily dose: 40 mg/kg.
- **Term infants ≥10 days:** 10 to 15 mg/kg/dose PO every 4 to 6 hours or 30 mg/kg PR loading dose; then 20 mg/kg/dose PR every 6 to 8 hours. Do not exceed 5 doses in 24 hours. Maximum daily dose: 75 mg/kg. IV: 20 mg/kg IV loading dose; then 10 mg/kg/dose IV every 6 hours. Maximum daily dose: 40 mg/kg.

ADVERSE EFFECTS: Rash, blood dyscrasias (neutropenia, leukopenia, and thrombocytopenia), and hepatic necrosis with overdose; renal injury may occur with chronic use.
PHARMACOLOGY: Extensively metabolized by the liver primarily by sulfonation, and by glucuronidation to a much lesser extent. Excretion by the kidney with elimination half-life: term infants—approximately 3 hours, preterm infants >32 weeks—5 hours, and in premature infants <32 weeks—up to 11 hours. Prolonged elimination with liver dysfunction.

---

[1]Edited Black Box "Warnings" are provided for select medications. Readers should review the entire package insert for each medication. Selected common brand names are provided in addition to the generic name. Many of these drugs are available as generic medications.

COMMENTS: Rectal administration may result in inaccurate dosing. Prophylactic use during vaccination may result in potential reduction in antibody response. IV administration in premature infants <32 weeks postmenstrual age has not yet been studied, so some experts do not recommend use in this age group. Beginning 2011 into 2012—transition to 1 pediatric concentration 160 mg/5 mL and elimination of 80 mg/0.8 mL infant drops per FDA recommendations. N-Acetylcysteine is the antidote of choice for acetaminophen poisoning.

ACETAZOLAMIDE (DIAMOX)

INDICATIONS AND USE: Reduce intraocular pressure in glaucoma; an anticonvulsant in refractory neonatal seizures; decrease cerebrospinal fluid (CSF) production in posthemorrhagic hydrocephalus; treatment of renal tubular acidosis.
ACTIONS: Competitive, reversible, carbonic anhydrase inhibitor; increases renal excretion of sodium, potassium, bicarbonate, and water, resulting in the production of acidosis. Decreases the production of aqueous humor and reduces abnormal discharge from CNS neurons.
DOSAGE: IV, PO.
- **Glaucoma:** 8 to 30 mg/kg/day PO divided every 8 hours or IV 20 to 40 mg/kg/day divided every 6 hours; maximum 1 g/day.
- **Anticonvulsant:** 4 to 16 mg/kg/day PO divided every 6 to 8 hours not to exceed 30 mg/kg/day or 1 g/day.
- **Alkalinize urine:** 5 mg/kg/dose PO 2 to 3 times over 24 hours.
- **Decrease CSF production:** 5 mg/kg/dose IV/PO every 6 hours; increased by 25 mg/kg/day to a maximum of 100 mg/kg/day. Furosemide has been used in combination.

ADVERSE EFFECTS: Gastrointestinal irritation, transient hypokalemia, hyperchloremic metabolic acidosis, growth retardation, bone marrow suppression, thrombocytopenia, hemolytic anemia, pancytopenia, agranulocytosis, leukopenia, drowsiness, and paresthesia.
PHARMACOLOGY: Unchanged in urine. Half-life is 4 to 10 hours.
COMMENTS: Currently, rarely used in neonates; a 1998 study failed to show efficacy in slowing the progression of posthemorrhagic hydrocephalus in neonates and infants. In neonates, use is limited to the treatment of glaucoma. Used as an adjunct to other medications in refractory seizures. Tolerance to diuretic effect may occur with long-term use. Oral solution may be compounded by using tablets.

ACYCLOVIR (ZOVIRAX)

ACTION AND SPECTRUM: Treatment and prophylaxis of herpes simplex virus (HSV-1 and HSV-2) infections, herpes simplex encephalitis, herpes zoster infections, and varicella-zoster infections.
DOSAGE: PO, IV.
Herpes simplex (based on American Academy of Pediatrics [AAP] *Red Book*, 2018–2021):
- **Neonatal:** 20 mg/kg/dose IV every 8 hours for 14 to 21 days. Treat CNS infections for 21 days (more than 21 days if CSF PCR remains positive) and all other infections for 14 days. Reduce dosing interval to every 12 hours in neonates <30 weeks' gestational age.
- **Dosing in renal impairment:**
  - **Serum creatinine 0.8 to 1.1 mg/dL:** 20 mg/kg IV every 12 hours.
  - **Serum creatinine 1.2 to 1.5 mg/dL:** 20 mg/kg IV every 24 hours.
  - **Serum creatinine >1.5 mg/dL:** 10 mg/kg IV every 24 hours.

Herpes simplex: chronic suppression following any herpes simplex infection
- 300 mg/m^2/dose PO every 8 hours for 6 months.

Herpes zoster (shingles):
- **Infants and children:** 10 mg/kg/dose IV every 8 hours for 7 to 10 days. In immunocompromised host, the acquired immunodeficiency syndrome (AIDS) information guidelines recommend duration of therapy of 10 to 14 days.

Varicella-zoster (chickenpox) in immunocompromised host:
- **Infants <2 years:** 10 mg/kg/dose IV every 8 hours for 7 to 10 days.

ADVERSE EFFECTS: Generally well tolerated. Thrombophlebitis and inflammation of injection site. Acute renal failure/acute kidney injury, increased blood urea nitrogen (BUN) and serum creatinine, nephrotoxicity. Increased liver transaminases. Neutropenia, thrombocytopenia, anemia, thrombocytosis, leukocytosis, and neutrophilia. Neutropenia may necessitate reduction in dose or treatment with granulocyte colony-stimulating factor (G-CSF) if absolute neutrophil count (ANC) remains <500/mm^3. Adequate hydration and infusion rate of at least 1 hour reduces risk of transient renal impairment and crystalluria.

PHARMACOLOGY: Inhibits DNA synthesis and viral replication. Oral absorption is 15% to 30%, CSF concentrations are 50% of serum, and primarily excreted by the kidneys.

COMMENTS: Infuse over at least 1 hour; concentration <7 mg/mL, 5 mg/mL is preferred. Do not refrigerate. Monitor complete blood cell count (CBC) and renal and liver function.

ACYCLOVIR OPHTHALMIC

See Chapter 58.

ADENOSINE (ADENOCARD)

INDICATIONS AND USE: Acute treatment of sustained paroxysmal supraventricular tachycardia for conversion to normal sinus rhythm.

ACTIONS: A purine nucleoside that slows conduction time through the atrioventricular (AV) node and interrupts reentry pathways through the AV node to restore normal sinus rhythm. Effects are mediated by depression of calcium slow-channel conduction, an increase in potassium conductance, and possibly indirect antiadrenergic effects.

DOSAGE: IV.

- 0.05 to 0.1 mg/kg by rapid IV push over 1 to 2 seconds. Repeat bolus doses at 2-minute intervals by increasing increments of 0.05 to 0.1 mg/kg until sinus rhythm is achieved or until a maximum single dose of 0.3 mg/kg is reached. Infuse as close as possible to the patient's heart and immediately flush IV with saline to ensure dose enters circulation. For doses <0.2 mL, prepare dilution using normal saline (NS) to final concentration of 300 mcg/mL.

ADVERSE EFFECTS: Contraindicated in heart block. Transient arrhythmias, flushing, dyspnea, and hypotension. May cause bronchoconstriction; use with caution in patients with history of bronchospasm.

PHARMACOLOGY: Rapid onset of action; half-life is <10 seconds; duration is 20 to 30 seconds.

COMMENTS: Methylxanthines (caffeine and theophylline) are competitive antagonists; larger adenosine doses may be required.

ALBUMIN, HUMAN

INDICATIONS AND USE: Treatment of hypovolemia, maintenance of cardiac output in shock, plasma volume expansion, hypoproteinemia associated with generalized edema or decreased intravascular volume; acute nephrotic syndrome in premature infants. Not recommended for initial volume expansion; use isotonic crystalloid solutions—0.9% sodium chloride or lactated Ringer's (per Pediatric Advanced Life Support [PALS] and Neonatal Resuscitation Program [NRP] guidelines).

ACTIONS: Increases intravascular oncotic pressure, which results in a mobilization of fluid from the interstitial spaces into the intravascular space.

DOSAGE: IV.

- **Neonates, infants, and children:** 0.5 to 1 g/kg IV (or 10–20 mL/kg of 5% IV bolus) repeated as necessary. Maximum: 6 g/kg/day. Five percent solutions should be used in hypovolemic or intravascularly depleted patients; 25% solutions should be used in cases of fluid or sodium restriction.
- **Hypoproteinemia in neonates:** Dose may be added to hyperalimentation solutions; however, may increase potential for growth of bacteria or fungi.

ADVERSE EFFECTS: Rapid infusion may cause vascular overload and precipitation of congestive heart failure or pulmonary edema. The 25% solution should be used with extreme caution in premature neonates due to increased risk of intraventricular hemorrhage.

PHARMACOLOGY: Duration of volume expansion is approximately 24 hours.

COMMENTS: Refer to individual product information for use of correct in-line IV filter. A 5% concentration is osmotically equivalent to equal volume of plasma, and 25% concentration is osmotically equivalent to 5 times its volume of plasma. If unavailable, 5% solutions can be prepared by diluting the 25% solution with normal saline (NS) or 5% dextrose in water (D5W). Do not use sterile water to prepare dilution; this may cause hypotonic-associated hemolysis, which can be fatal.

ALBUTEROL (PROVENTIL, VENTOLIN)

INDICATIONS AND USE: Prevention and treatment of bronchospasm; bronchodilator in respiratory distress syndrome (RDS) and bronchopulmonary dysplasia/chronic lung disease (BPD/CLD). Used for treatment of hyperkalemia.

ACTIONS: Primarily β_2-adrenergic stimulation (bronchodilation and vasodilation) with minor β_1 stimulation (increased myocardial contractility and conduction).

DOSAGE: Inhalation, nebulization.

- **Nebulization:** 1.25 to 2.5 mg/dose every 2 to 6 hours as needed.
- **Inhalation:** Metered dose inhaler 90 mcg/spray: 1 to 2 puffs every 2 to 6 hours as needed.

ADVERSE EFFECTS: Tachycardia, tremors, CNS stimulation, hypokalemia, hyperglycemia, and hypertension.

COMMENTS: Duration of action is approximately 2 to 5 hours. Titrate dose according to the effect on heart rate and improvement in respiratory symptoms. Albuterol should not be used as the sole agent for treating severe hyperkalemia.

ALPROSTADIL (PROSTAGLANDIN E₁) (PROSTIN VR)

> **WARNING:** Apnea is experienced by about 10% to 12% of neonates with congenital heart defects treated with alprostadil injection, US Pharmacopeia (USP). Apnea is most often seen in neonates weighing <2 kg at birth and usually appears during the first hour of drug infusion. Therefore, respiratory status should be monitored throughout treatment, and alprostadil should be used where ventilatory assistance is immediately available.

INDICATIONS AND USE: Any clinical condition in which blood flow must be maintained through the ductus arteriosus to sustain either pulmonary or systemic circulation until corrective or palliative surgery can be performed. Examples are pulmonary atresia, pulmonary stenosis, tricuspid atresia, transposition of the great arteries, aortic arch interruption, coarctation of the aorta, and severe tetralogy of Fallot (TOF).

ACTIONS: Causes vasodilation of all vascular smooth muscle including the ductus arteriosus.

DOSAGE: IV.

- **Initial:** 0.05 to 0.1 mcg/kg/min by continuous infusion. Gradually titrate to maintain acceptable oxygen levels without adverse effects. Use the lowest rate to maintain improved oxygenation response.
- **Maintenance:** 0.01 to 0.4 mcg/kg/min. Higher doses may be required in patients receiving ECLS.

ADVERSE EFFECTS: See Black Box warning. May cause gastric outlet obstruction and reversible cortical proliferation of the long bones after prolonged treatment. Hypotension, cutaneous vasodilation, bradycardia, inhibits platelet aggregation, hypoventilation, seizure-like activity, jitteriness, temperature elevation, hypocalcemia, hypoglycemia.

COMMENTS: Decreased response after 96 hours of infusion. Maximal improvement in PaO₂, usually within 30 minutes in cyanotic infants and 1.5 to 3 hours in acyanotic infants. Use cautiously in infants with bleeding tendencies.

ALTEPLASE, RECOMBINANT (ACTIVASE, CATHFLO ACTIVASE, TISSUE PLASMINOGEN ACTIVATOR [tPA])

INDICATIONS AND USE: Used to restore patency of occluded central venous catheters and for the dissolution of large-vessel thrombus (systemic use). (See also Chapters 84 and 92.)

ACTIONS: Alteplase is a thrombolytic. It enhances conversion of plasminogen to plasmin, which then cleaves fibrin, fibrinogen, factor V, and factor VIII, resulting in clot dissolution.

DOSAGE: IV.

Occluded central venous catheter:

- **Manufacturer's recommendations (CathFlo, Activase):** PNA ≥14 days, use 1 mg/mL; instill a volume equal to 110% of the internal lumen volume; do not exceed 2 mg in 2 mL; leave in lumen for up to 2 hours and then aspirate out of catheter. May repeat process if lumen is still occluded. Check the catheter product literature or manufacturer for catheter volume.
- *Chest,* 2008 dosing recommendations (Monagle et al, 2008): 0.5 mg diluted in a volume of normal saline (NS) equal to the catheter lumen internal volume; instill over 1 to 2 minutes; dwell time is 1 to 2 hours. Aspirate solution from catheter and then flush catheter with NS.

Dissolution of large-vessel thrombus (systemic use):

- **Dose is *controversial,*** and optimal dose has not been established. May consider fresh-frozen plasma (FFP) prior to administration of alteplase. *Chest,* 2012 recommends use only when major vessel occlusion is causing critical compromise of organs or limbs.
- *Chest,* 2012 recommendations (Monagle et al, 2012): 0.1 to 0.6 mg/kg/h for 6 hours. Dose must be titrated to effect; some patients require longer or shorter duration of therapy.

ADVERSE EFFECTS: The risk of complications increases at rates >0.4 mg/kg/h. Systemic use is not recommended with preexisting intraventricular hemorrhage or cerebral ischemic changes. Bleeding from venipuncture sites may occur. During the treatment of occluded central venous catheter, bleeding may occur if excess alteplase is inadvertently injected into the systemic circulation. Excessive pressure during instillation may force clot into systemic circulation.

COMMENTS: Increases risk of bleeding in infants concurrently on heparin, warfarin, or indomethacin. Monitor prothrombin time (PT), activated partial thromboplastin time (aPTT), fibrinogen, and fibrin split products prior to the initiation of therapy and at least daily through the duration of therapy. Fibrinogen levels should be maintained >100 mg/dL and platelets >50,000/mm^3.

AMIKACIN SULFATE (AMIKIN)

> **WARNING:** May cause neurotoxicity, nephrotoxicity, and/or neuromuscular blockade and respiratory paralysis. Avoid concomitant use with potent diuretics since diuretics themselves may cause ototoxicity and may enhance aminoglycoside toxicity. Avoid concomitant or sequential use of other neurotoxic and/or nephrotoxic drugs (eg, amphotericin B, colistin, polymyxin B, vancomycin, other aminoglycosides).

ACTION AND SPECTRUM: Active against gram-negative bacteria, including most *Pseudomonas, Klebsiella, Enterobacter, Proteus, Escherichia coli,* and *Serratia* spp. No activity against anaerobic organisms. Reserve for treatment of gram-negative organisms resistant to gentamicin and tobramycin. Treatment of susceptible mycobacterial organisms.

DOSAGE: Intramuscular (IM), IV. Infuse over 30 minutes. Dosage should be monitored and adjusted by use of pharmacokinetics. Initial empirical dosing based on body weight (*Red Book,* 2018–2021):

- **Neonates ≤28 PNA:**
- **GA <30 weeks:**
  - **PNA ≤14 days:** 15 mg/kg every 48 hours.
  - **PNA >14 days:** 15 mg/kg every 24 hours.

- **GA 30–34 weeks:**
  - **PNA ≤14 days:** 15 mg/kg every 36 hours.
  - **PNA >14 days:** 15 mg/kg every 24 hours.
- **GA ≥35 weeks:**
  - **PNA ≤7 days:** 15 mg/kg every 24 hours.
  - **PNA >7 days:** 18 mg/kg every 24 hours.
- **Infants and children:** 15 to 22.5 mg/kg/day divided in 2 to 3 doses or 1 dose; some patients may require higher doses (eg, cystis fibrosis).
- **Treatment of nontuberculous mycobacterial infection:** 15 to 30 mg/kg/day divided every 12 to 24 hours as a part of a multidrug regimen.
- **Meningitis:**
  - **PNA ≤7 days:** 15 to 20 mg/kg/day divided every 12 hours.
  - **PNA >7 days:** 20 to 30 mg/kg/day divided every 8 hours.

PHARMACOLOGY: Displays concentration-dependent killing; bactericidal activity. Renal elimination (glomerular filtration); half-life is 4 to 8 hours; volume of distribution is 0.6 L/kg.

ADVERSE EFFECTS: Possible nephrotoxicity and ototoxicity. Toxicities may be potentiated when used with furosemide or vancomycin, and neuromuscular blockade is increased if used with pancuronium or with coexisting hypermagnesemia.

COMMENTS: Monitor serum levels when treating >48 hours, in patients with decreased or changing renal function, with signs of nephrotoxicity or ototoxicity, with concomitant use of other nephrotoxic agents, and in patients who may require higher doses. Adjust the dosage according to serum peak and trough levels. Desired serum neonate concentration 24 to 40 mg/L (peak), <7 mg/L (trough) for neonates ≤28 postnatal days of age. Nephrotoxicity is associated with serum trough concentrations >10 mcg/mL; ototoxicity, with serum peak concentrations >35 to 40 mg/mL (more cochlear damage than vestibular).

AMINOPHYLLINE/THEOPHYLLINE

INDICATIONS AND USE: To reduce frequency and severity of apnea of prematurity, following extubation or during alprostadil administration. A bronchodilator in the treatment of bronchopulmonary dysplasia/chronic lung disease. Caffeine is more effective and safer for the treatment of apnea of prematurity. Caffeine also has the advantage of once-a-day dosing. Aminophylline/theophylline has greater bronchodilator effects.

ACTIONS: Theophylline (the active component of aminophylline) causes relaxation of bronchial smooth muscle; increases the force of contraction of the diaphragmatic muscles; dilates the pulmonary, coronary, and renal arteries; causes mild diuretic action; causes increased sensitivity of the CNS medullary respiratory centers to carbon dioxide; stimulates central respiratory drive and peripheral chemoreceptors; and increases sensitivity to catecholamines, resulting in increased cardiac output and improved oxygenation. Aminophylline is approximately 80% theophylline. Neonates have a unique ability to convert theophylline to caffeine in a ratio of 1:0.3. Caffeine may account for as much as 50% of the theophylline level.

DOSAGE: PO, IV.

- **IV loading dose:** 5 to 8 mg/kg, slowly over 30 minutes. IV maintenance dosage is 2 to 6 mg/kg/day divided every 8 to 12 hours starting 8 to 12 hours after loading dose.
- **PO (use immediate-release dosage form) loading dose:** Same as IV. PO maintenance dose as theophylline is 2 to 6 mg/kg/day divided every 6 to 8 hours. Older infants may need higher doses as clearance rate increases with increased PNA, possibly up to 25 to 30 mg/kg/day.

ADVERSE EFFECTS: Hyperglycemia, dehydration, diuresis, and feeding intolerance. CNS effects include jitteriness, hyperreflexia, and seizures. Most common side effects are cardiovascular with tachycardia (heart rate ≥180 beats/min) and other tachyarrhythmias.

COMMENTS: Therapeutic levels: apnea 6 to 12 mcg/mL; bronchospasm 5 to 15 mcg/mL. Toxicity usually >20 mcg/mL. Monitor serum levels at a peak 1 hour after IV dosing or 1 hours after PO dosing. Take trough levels 30 minutes before next dose. Serum levels should be monitored any time toxicity is suspected or when apneic episodes are increased. Steady state expected to be reached after 48 to 72 hours of therapy.

AMIODARONE (CORDARONE)

INDICATIONS AND USE: Treatment of resistant life-threatening ventricular arrhythmias unresponsive to other agents; prevention and suppression of supraventricular arrhythmias (especially those associated with Wolff-Parkinson-White syndrome) and postoperative junctional ectopic tachycardia.

ACTIONS: An iodinated benzofuran that prolongs the action potential and increases the effective refractory period. It decreases afterload (causes peripheral and coronary vasodilation), and demonstrates α- and β-blocking properties and calcium channel inhibition. It slows the heart rate (decreases atrioventricular node and sinus node conduction–negative inotropic effects).

DOSAGE: IV. Limited data are available. Generally not first line due to high incidence of adverse effects. Recommend consultation with pediatric cardiologist prior to use.

- **IV loading dose:** 5 mg/kg over 60 minutes; do not exceed 0.25 mg/kg/min unless clinically indicated; central venous access is recommended. May repeat dose up to total loading dose of 15 mg/kg/day.
- **Continuous IV infusion:** 5 mcg/kg/min gradually increasing as needed to 15 mcg/kg/min.
- **PO loading dose:** 10 to 20 mg/kg/day divided into 2 doses per day for 7 to 10 days or until adequate control of arrhythmia is achieved or significant adverse effects occur. Reduce dose to 5 to 10 mg/kg/day given once daily for several weeks. Attempt to reduce dose to lowest possible without the recurrence of arrhythmia: 2.5 mg/kg/day.

ADVERSE EFFECTS: Bradycardia and hypotension (may be related to rate of infusion), proarrhythmias (including torsade de pointes), heart block, congestive heart failure (CHF), and paroxysmal ventricular tachycardia. Amiodarone may cause hypothyroidism or hyperthyroidism (may partially inhibit the peripheral conversion of thyroxine [T_4] to triiodothyronine [T_3]; serum T_4, and reverse T_3 concentrations may be increased, and serum T_3 may be decreased). Amiodarone hydrochloride contains 37% iodine by weight and is a potential source of iodine; approximately 3 mg of inorganic iodine/100 mg of amiodarone is released into the circulation. Elevated liver enzymes, elevated bilirubin. Phlebitis and local injection site irritation: avoid concentrations >2.5 mg/mL, administer through central vein.

PHARMACOLOGY: Adult data: onset of oral antiarrhythmic effects may take up to 3 to 6 weeks. Duration of antiarrhythmic effects may persist for 30 to 90 days or longer following discontinuation of therapy. Protein binding: 96%. Metabolized in liver.

COMMENTS: Potential drug interactions may occur. Amiodarone inhibits certain cytochrome P450 enzymes and may increase serum levels of digoxin, flecainide, lidocaine, theophylline, procainamide, quinidine, warfarin, and phenytoin. To avoid toxicities with these agents, dosage reduction and serum concentration monitoring is recommended. Dosage reductions of 30% to 50% have been recommended. Concurrent administration of amiodarone with β-blockers, digoxin, or calcium channel blockers may result in bradycardia, sinus arrest, and heart block.

AMPHOTERICIN B (AMPHOCIN); AMPHOTERICIN B, LIPOSOMAL (AMBISOME); AMPHOTERICIN B LIPID COMPLEX (ABELCET)

ACTION AND SPECTRUM: Antifungal agent that acts by binding to sterols and disrupting the fungal cell membrane permeability. Broad spectrum of activity against *Candida* spp. and other fungi.

DOSAGE: IV, intrathecal, intraventricular.

Conventional amphotericin B (amphotericin B deoxycholate):
- **IV:** 1 to 1.5 mg/kg IV every 24 hours for 2 to 6 weeks or longer, but a lower dose may suffice. Infuse over 2 to 6 hours, but infusion over 1 to 2 hours may be used if tolerated. Use a 0.1 mg/mL concentration in 5% dextrose in water (D5W), D10W, or D20W. May use maximum concentration of 0.25 mg/mL for infusion through central venous catheter. Incompatible with sodium chloride.

- **Intrathecal or intraventricular:** Reconstitute with sterile water at 0.25 mg/mL; dilute with CSF and reinfuse. Usual dose: 25 to 100 mcg every 48 to 72 hours; increase to 1000 mcg as tolerated.
- **Irrigation, bladder:** 50 mcg/mL solution, administered as continuous irrigation or as intermittent irrigation 3 times per day with a 60- to 90-minute dwell time.

Liposomal amphotericin B:
- Concentrates in liver and spleen, but penetrates the CNS, kidneys, urinary tract, and eyes less than conventional amphotericin B. Used when refractory to or intolerant of conventional amphotericin B.
- 5 to 7 mg/kg/dose IV infused over 2 hours. May be diluted with D5W, D10W, D20W, or D25W to a final concentration of 1 to 2 mg/mL; concentrations of 0.2 to 0.5 mg/mL may be needed to provide sufficient volume for infusion.

Amphotericin B lipid complex:
- Used when refractory to or intolerant of conventional amphotericin B. Less nephrotoxic.
- 3 to 5 mg/kg/dose IV every 24 hours infused over 2 hours. Dilute with D5W, D10W, or D15W to final concentration of 1 mg/mL; a maximum concentration of 2 mg/mL. Manufacturer recommends that an in-line filter should *not* be used.

PHARMACOKINETICS: Slow renal excretion.

ADVERSE EFFECTS: Fewer adverse effects in neonates as compared to adults. May cause fever, chills, vomiting, thrombophlebitis at injection sites, renal tubular acidosis, renal failure, hypomagnesemia, hypokalemia, bone marrow suppression with reversible decline in hematocrit, hypotension, hypertension, wheezing, and hypoxemia.

COMMENTS: Protect the solution from light. Monitor serum potassium, magnesium, blood urea nitrogen (BUN), creatinine, and urine output at least every other day until the dosage is stabilized, then every week. Monitor complete blood cell count (CBC) and liver function every week. Discontinue if BUN is >40 mg/dL, serum creatinine is >3 mg/dL, or liver function tests are abnormal.

AMPICILLIN (POLYCILLIN, OTHERS)

ACTION AND SPECTRUM: Semisynthetic penicillinase-sensitive penicillin that is bactericidal and acts by inhibiting the late stages of cell wall synthesis. Treatment of susceptible bacterial infections caused by streptococci, pneumococci, enterococci, non–penicillinase-producing staphylococci, *Listeria*, meningococci; some strains of *Haemophilus influenzae*, *Proteus mirabilis*, *Salmonella*, *Shigella*, *Escherichia coli*, *Enterobacter*, and *Klebsiella*; used in combination with an aminoglycoside or cefotaxime in neonates for prevention and treatment of infections due to group B streptococci, *Listeria*, and *E coli*.

DOSAGE: IM, IV (WEIGHT-DIRECTED DOSING [BRADLEY, 2019]).

Body weight ≤2 kg:
- **PNA ≤7 days:** 50 mg/kg/dose every 12 hours.
- **PNA 8 to 28 days:** 75 mg/kg/dose every 12 hours.
- **PNA 29 to 60 days:** 50 mg/kg/dose every 6 hours.

Body weight >2 kg:
- **PNA ≤28 days:** 50 mg/kg/dose every 8 hours.
- **PNA 29 to 60 days:** 50 mg/kg/dose every 6 hours.

Group B streptococcal meningitis:
- **PNA ≤7 days:** 200 to 300 mg/kg/day IV divided every 6 to 8 hours.
- **PNA >7 days:** 300 mg/kg/day IV divided every 6 hours.

Infants and children:
- 100 to 200 mg/kg/day IM, IV divided every 6 hours. Maximum dose: 4000 mg/day.
- **Meningitis:** 200 to 400 mg/kg/day IM, IV divided every 6 hours. Maximum dose: 12 g/day.

ADVERSE EFFECTS: Hypersensitivity, rash, abdominal discomfort, nausea, vomiting, diarrhea, hemolytic anemia, thrombocytopenia, neutropenia, prolongation of bleeding time, interstitial nephritis, and eosinophilia. Large doses may cause CNS excitation or seizures.

AMPICILLIN SODIUM/SULBACTAM SODIUM (UNASYN)

ACTION AND SPECTRUM: Combination β-lactamase inhibitor and β-lactam. The bactericidal spectrum of ampicillin that is extended by the addition of sulbactam, a β-lactamase inhibitor; includes organisms producing β-lactamases such as *Staphylococcus aureus, Haemophilus influenzae, Escherichia coli, Klebsiella, Acinetobacter, Enterobacter,* and anaerobes.

DOSAGE: IV, IM. Dose based on ampicillin component.

Preterm infants and neonates during the first week of life (0–7 days):
- 100 mg ampicillin/kg/day IM/IV divided every 12 hours.

Neonates >7 days:
- 100 mg ampicillin/kg/day IM/IV divided every 6 to 8 hours.

Infants ≥1 month:
- 100 to 200 mg ampicillin/kg/day IM/IV divided every 6 hours. Maximum dose: 1000 mg ampicillin/dose.

Severe infection:
- 200 to 300 mg ampicillin/kg/day IM/IV divided every 6 hours. Maximum dose: 2000 mg ampicillin/dose.

ADVERSE EFFECTS: Elevated blood urea nitrogen (BUN) and serum creatinine. See Ampicillin.

COMMENTS: Modify dosage in patients with renal impairment.

ANAKINRA (KINERET)

INDICATIONS AND USE: Neonatal-onset multisystem inflammatory disease or chronic infantile neurologic, cutaneous, and articular syndrome.

ACTIONS: Interleukin-1 (IL-1) receptor antagonist.

DOSAGE: Subcutaneous.
- **Initial:** 1 to 2 mg/kg daily in 1 to 2 divided doses.
- **Usual maintenance dose:** 3 to 4 mg/kg daily; maximum dose 8 mg/kg/day.

ADVERSE EFFECTS: Skin rash, vomiting, injection site reaction, upper respiratory tract infection, thrombocytopenia.

PHARMACOLOGY: Half-life elimination 4 to 6 hours; time to peak 3 to 7 hours.

COMMENTS: Monitor complete blood count (CBC) with differential, liver function tests, and renal function at baseline. Monitor CBC with differential every 3 months for up to 1 year.

ARGININE HCL (R-GENE)

INDICATIONS AND USE: Treatment of severe metabolic alkalosis after other treatment has failed, pituitary function test (stimulant for the release of growth hormone), and treatment of certain neonatal-onset urea cycle disorders. Limited data available on potential role for necrotizing enterocolitis prevention.

ACTIONS: Corrects severe hypochloremic metabolic alkalosis resulting from the high chloride content of arginine. Arginine stimulates pituitary release of growth hormone and prolactin and the pancreatic release of glucagon and insulin.

DOSAGE: IV.

Metabolic alkalosis in infants and children:
- Arginine HCl dose (mEq) = $0.5 \times$ weight (kg) $\times [HCO_3^- - 24]$, where HCO_3^- = the patient's serum bicarbonate concentration in mEq/L; give one-half to two-thirds of calculated dose and reevaluate.

Correct hypochloremia in infants and children:
- Arginine HCl dose (mEq) = $0.2 \times$ weight (kg) $\times [103 - Cl^-]$, where Cl^- = the patient's serum chloride concentration in mEq/L; give one-half to two-thirds of the calculated dose, then reevaluate.
- IV: May use undiluted (irritating to tissues) or dilute with normal saline (NS) or dextrose. Administer through a central line. Infuse over at least 30 minutes or over 24 hours in maintenance IV. Maximum: 1 g/kg/h (= 10 mL/kg/h of 10% solution). PO: May use the injectable form, diluted.

Pituitary function test:
- IV 500 mg/kg (= 5 mL/kg of the 10% solution) infused IV over 30 minutes. (Use only IV, not PO administration, for this test.) Maximum dose: 30 g dose.

Urea cycle disorders:
- Consult specialists in metabolic disorders if a urea cycle disorder is suspected.

Necrotizing enterocolitis prevention:
- 261 mg/kg/day added to enteral or parenteral nutrition beginning on day 2 to 5 of life and continuing for 28 consecutive days.

ADVERSE EFFECTS: Not a first-line treatment for metabolic alkalosis and should never be used as initial therapy; try sodium, potassium, or ammonium chlorides first. May be toxic in infants with arginase deficiency. Do not use in patients sensitive to arginine HCl or in those with hepatic or renal failure. May cause hyperchloremic metabolic acidosis; elevated gastrin, glucagon, and growth hormone; flushing and gastrointestinal upset with rapid IV administration; hyperglycemia, hypoglycemia, hyperkalemia; tissue necrosis on extravasation, vein irritation; allergic reactions; elevated blood urea nitrogen (BUN) and creatinine.

COMMENTS: Monitor IV site, blood glucose, chloride, and blood pressure. If intact pituitary function, human growth hormone levels should rise after arginine administration to 10 to 30 ng/mL.

ASFOTASE ALFA (STRENSIQ)

INDICATIONS AND USE: Perinatal/infantile- and juvenile-onset hypophosphatasia.

ACTIONS: Human recombinant tissue-nonspecific alkaline phosphatase–Fc–deca-aspartate fusion protein with enzymatic activity that promotes bone mineralization in patients with hypophosphatasia.

DOSAGE: Subcutaneous.
- 6 mg/kg/wk administered as either 2 mg/kg/dose 3 times weekly or 1 mg/kg/dose 6 times weekly. Maximum total weekly dose: 9 mg/kg/wk.

ADVERSE EFFECTS: Ectopic calcification, injection site reactions, hypocalcemia.

PHARMACOLOGY: Onset of action in reducing plasma tissue-nonspecific alkaline phosphatase (TNSALP) takes 6 to 12 weeks of treatment. Elimination half-life approximately 5 days.

COMMENTS: Round patient weight to the nearest kilogram when determining dose. Do not administer the 80 mg/0.8 mL concentration to neonates.

ATROPINE SULFATE

INDICATIONS AND USE: Sinus bradycardia, in conjunction with neostigmine for the reversal of nondepolarizing neuromuscular blockade. Used preoperatively to inhibit salivation and reduce excessive secretions of the respiratory tract.

ACTIONS: A competitive antagonist of acetylcholine at parasympathetic sites in smooth muscle, cardiac muscle, and various glandular cells, leading to increased heart rate, increased cardiac output, reduced gastrointestinal (GI) motility and tone, urinary retention, cycloplegia, and decreased salivation and sweating.

DOSAGE: IM, IV, endotracheal tube (ETT), PO.

Bradycardia in infants and children:
- **IV, intraosseous (IO):** 0.02 mg/kg/dose; may repeat once in 3 to 5 minutes; reserve use for those patients unresponsive to improved oxygenation and epinephrine. **No longer part of American Heart Association neonatal resuscitation algorithm.**

Preanesthetic:
- **Infants <5 kg:** 0.02 mg/kg/dose IV, IM, subcutaneous 30 to 60 minutes preoperatively, then every 4 to 6 hours as needed.
- **Infants >5 kg:** 0.01 to 0.02 mg/kg/dose IV, IM, subcutaneous 30 to 60 minutes preoperatively, then every 4 to 6 hours as needed. Maximum single dose: 0.4 mg.

Reversal of neuromuscular blockade:
- Neostigmine 0.06 mg/kg/dose with atropine 0.02 mg/kg/dose.

Intubation, nonemergent (preferred vagolytic):
- 0.02 mg/kg/dose IM, IV.

ETT:
- 0.04 to 0.06 mg/kg/dose; may repeat once if needed. Flush with 3 to 5 mL normal saline (NS) based on patient size.

ADVERSE EFFECTS: Xerostomia, mydriasis, tachycardia, palpitations, constipation, urinary retention, ataxia, tremor, hyperthermia, and swelling. Toxic effects are especially likely in children receiving low doses.

COMMENTS: Avoid use in patients with thyrotoxicosis, tachycardia secondary to cardiac insufficiency, and obstructive GI disease. In low doses, it may cause paradoxical bradycardia secondary to its central actions. Monitor heart rate, blood pressure, and pulse.

AZITHROMYCIN

ACTION AND SPECTRUM: Treatment of upper respiratory tract infections due to *Haemophilus influenzae, Moraxella catarrhalis, Streptococcus pyogenes, Chlamydophila pneumoniae, Mycoplasma pneumoniae, Streptococcus pneumoniae, Chlamydia trachomatis, Neisseria gonorrhoeae, Staphylococcus aureus, Mycobacterium avium* complex, *Chlamydophila psittaci*, and *Mycoplasma hominis*. Has also been used for treatment of pertussis.

DOSAGE: PO, IV.

Infants <6 months:
- **Pertussis:** 10 mg/kg/dose PO, IV once daily for 5 days (based on AAP *Red Book*, 2018–2021). Azithromycin is drug of choice for age <1 month because of idiopathic hypertrophic pyloric stenosis with erythromycin.
- **Chlamydial conjunctivitis or chlamydial pneumonia:** 20 mg/kg PO once daily for 3 days.

Children ≥6 months:
- **Respiratory tract infections:** 10 mg/kg on day 1 (maximum dose 500 mg) followed by 5 mg/kg/day (maximum dose 250 mg) once daily on days 2 to 5.
- **Pertussis:** 10 mg/kg on day 1 (maximum dose 500 mg) followed by 5 mg/kg/day (maximum dose 250 mg) once daily on days 2 to 5 (based on AAP *Red Book*, 2018–2021).

ADVERSE EFFECTS: Diarrhea, vomiting, irritability, rash, fever.

PHARMACOLOGY: Macrolide antibiotic; elimination half-life of approximately 55 hours in infants and children.

COMMENTS: Limited data in neonates. Monitor liver function tests and white blood cell count, and monitor infants for diarrhea.

AZTREONAM (AZACTAM)

ACTION AND SPECTRUM: Monobactam antibiotic that is bactericidal against most Enterobacteriaceae, *Pseudomonas aeruginosa, Escherichia coli, Klebsiella pneumoniae, Proteus mirabilis, Serratia, Haemophilus influenzae*, and *Citrobacter* spp., but essentially no activity against grampositive aerobic or anaerobic bacteria.

DOSAGE: IV, IM.

Body weight <1 kg:
- **PNA ≤14 days:** 30 mg/kg/dose every 12 hours.
- **PNA 15 to 28 days:** 30 mg/kg/dose every 8 hours to 12 hours.

Body weight 1 to 2 kg:
- **PNA ≤7 days:** 30 mg/kg/dose every 12 hours.
- **PNA 8 to 28 days:** 30 mg/kg/dose every 8 to 12 hours.

Body weight >2 kg:
- **PNA ≤7 days:** 30 mg/kg/dose every 8 hours.
- **PNA 8 to 28 days:** 30 mg/kg/dose every 6 hours.

Children >1 month:
- 90 to 120 mg/kg/day divided every 6 to 8 hours.

ADVERSE EFFECTS: Diarrhea, nausea, vomiting, rash, hypoglycemia, irritation at the infusion site. May cause transient eosinophilia, leukopenia, thrombocytopenia, hypoglycemia, and elevated liver enzymes.

PHARMACOLOGY: Renal elimination as unchanged drug. Half-life is 3 to 9 hours in neonates. Widely distributed into body tissues, CSF, bronchial secretions, peritoneal fluid, bile, bone.

COMMENTS: Demonstrates synergistic activity with aminoglycosides against most strains of *P aeruginosa*, many strains of Enterobacteriaceae, and other gram-negative aerobic bacilli.

BACITRACIN OPHTHALMIC

See Chapter 58.

BERACTANT (SURVANTA)

INDICATIONS AND USE: Prevention and treatment of respiratory distress syndrome in preterm infants. Also has been used for treatment of meconium aspiration syndrome in term and near-term infants.

ACTIONS: A natural bovine lung extract containing phospholipids, neutral lipids, fatty acids, and surfactant-associated proteins to which dipalmitoylphosphatidylcholine (DPPC), palmitic acid, and tripalmitin are added to mimic the surface tension–lowering properties of natural lung surfactant. Surfactant lowers surface tension on alveolar surfaces during respiration and stabilizes the alveoli against collapse.

DOSAGE: ETT.

- 4 mL/kg (100 mg of phospholipids/kg) birthweight. Divide dose into 4 aliquots, repositioning the infant with each dose. Inject each aliquot gently into the catheter over 2 to 3 seconds. Ventilate the infant after each one-quarter dose for at least 30 seconds or until stable. Four doses of 4 mL/kg can be given in the first 48 hours of life, no more frequently than every 6 hours. Wean ventilator settings rapidly after administration.

ADVERSE EFFECTS: Most adverse effects are associated while administering beractant to the infant: transient bradycardia, oxygen desaturation, ETT reflux, pallor, vasoconstriction, hypotension, endotracheal blockage, hypertension, hypocarbia, hypercarbia, and apnea. Pulmonary hemorrhage has been reported, especially in very low birthweight infants.

BUMETANIDE (BUMEX)

> **WARNING:** Bumetanide is a potent diuretic that, if given in excessive amounts, can lead to a profound diuresis with water and electrolyte depletion. Therefore, careful medical supervision is required, and dose and dosage schedule have to be adjusted to the individual patient's needs.

INDICATIONS AND USE: A potent loop diuretic used for the management of edema associated with congenital heart disease, congestive heart failure, and hepatic or renal disease.

ACTIONS: Inhibition of sodium and chloride in the ascending loop of Henle and proximal renal tubule. Urinary excretion of sodium, chloride, potassium, hydrogen, calcium, magnesium, ammonium, phosphate, and bicarbonate increases with bumetanide-induced diuresis. Renal blood flow increases substantially as a result of renovascular dilation and increases prostaglandin secretion.

DOSAGE: IV, IM, PO.

- **Preterm neonates:** 0.01 to 0.05 mg/kg/dose every 24 to 48 hours.
- **Term neonates:** 0.01 to 0.05 mg/kg/dose every 12 to 24 hours.
- **Infants and children:** 0.015 mg/kg/dose up to 0.1 mg/kg/dose every 6 to 24 hours (maximum dose is 10 mg/day).

Neonatal seizures, refractory (emerging therapy to be given concurrently with phenobarbital):

- 0.05 to 0.3 mg/kg/dose every 12 hours for 4 doses.

ADVERSE EFFECTS: Hypokalemia, hypochloremia, hyponatremia, metabolic alkalosis, and hypotension. Potentially ototoxic but less so than furosemide.

COMMENTS: Patients refractory to furosemide may respond to bumetanide for diuretic therapy. Although patients may respond differently, bumetanide is approximately 40 times more potent on a milligram-per-milligram basis than furosemide. Follow electrolytes and serum creatinine.

CAFFEINE CITRATE

INDICATIONS AND USE: Treatment of apnea of prematurity; postextubation and postanesthesia apnea.

ACTIONS: Similar to other methylxanthine drugs (eg, aminophylline and theophylline). Caffeine appears to be more active on and less toxic to the CNS and the respiratory system. Proposed mechanisms of action include increased production of cyclic adenosine monophosphate (cAMP) alterations of intracellular calcium concentrations. Stimulates the CNS, which increases the medullary respiratory center sensitivity to carbon dioxide, stimulates central inspiratory drive, and improves diaphragmatic contractility. Caffeine exerts a positive inotropic effect on the myocardium, increases renal blood flow and glomerular filtration rate, and stimulates glycogenolysis and lipolysis.

DOSAGE: IV, PO.
- **Loading dose:** 20 to 40 mg/kg of caffeine citrate IV or PO (equivalent to 10–20 mg of caffeine base).
- **Maintenance:** 5 to 20 mg/kg/day caffeine citrate IV or PO every 24 hours, starting 24 hours after loading dose (equivalent to 2.5–10 mg of caffeine base).

ADVERSE EFFECTS: Nausea, vomiting, gastric irritation, agitation, tachycardia (if heart rate >180 beats/min, may consider holding dose), and diuresis. Symptoms of overdosage include arrhythmias and tonic-clonic seizures.

PHARMACOLOGY: Therapeutic serum trough levels 8 to 20 mcg/mL; potential toxicity >20 mcg/mL; severe toxicity is with levels >50 mcg/mL. Draw trough on day 5 of treatment. The serum half-life in neonates ranges from 40 to 230 hours and decreases with increased PNA; in infants >9 months, half-life is approximately 5 hours. Half-life is prolonged with cholestasis. FDA approved in infants with gestational age of 28 to <33 weeks.

CALCIUM CHLORIDE (VARIOUS)

INDICATIONS AND USE: Acute treatment of symptomatic hypocalcemia, treatment of hypermagnesemia, cardiac disturbances of hyperkalemia, hypocalcemia, or calcium channel blocker toxicity and prevention of hypocalcemia.

ACTIONS: Calcium is essential for the functional integrity of the nervous, muscular, skeletal, and cardiac systems and for clotting function.

DOSAGE: IV. Dosage expressed in milligrams of calcium chloride.
- **Acute treatment of symptomatic hypocalcemia:** 10 to 20 mg/kg/dose, dilute in appropriate fluid and infuse IV over 10 minutes. May repeat every 4 to 6 hours as needed.
- **Cardiac arrest in the presence of hyperkalemia or hypocalcemia, magnesium toxicity, or calcium antagonist toxicity:** 20 mg/kg/dose IV, IO every 10 minutes as needed. If effective, consider IV infusion 20 to 50 mg/kg/h.
- **Tetany:** IV: 10 mg/kg over 5 to 10 minutes; may repeat after 6 hours or follow with an infusion with a maximum dose of 200 mg/kg/day.

ADVERSE EFFECTS: Arrhythmias (in particular, bradycardia) and deterioration of cardiovascular function; may potentiate digoxin-related arrhythmias; may increase risk of metabolic acidosis. Calcium chloride is contraindicated in ventricular fibrillation or hypercalcemia. Extravasation may cause severe tissue damage (sloughing and necrosis).

COMMENTS: Supplied as a 10% solution (10 mL) (equivalent to elemental calcium 27 mg [1.36 mEq]/mL). Chloride salt is preferred to the gluconate form in cardiac arrest because it may be more bioavailable. Calcium chloride precipitates when mixed with sodium bicarbonate.

Warning: Multiple salt forms of calcium exist; when ordering and administering calcium, incorrect selection or substitution of one salt for another without proper dosage adjustment may result in serious over- or underdosing. There is a 3-fold difference in the primary cation concentration between calcium chloride (1 g = 13.6 mEq [270 mg] of elemental Ca^{2+}) and calcium gluconate (1 g = 4.65 mEq [90 mg] of elemental Ca^{2+}).

CALCIUM GLUCONATE

INDICATIONS AND USE: Treatment and prevention of hypocalcemia and prevention of hypocalcemia during exchange transfusion.

ACTIONS: See Calcium Chloride. Calcium gluconate must be metabolized to release calcium ion.

DOSAGE: IV, PO (dosage expressed in milligrams of calcium gluconate).

- **Acute treatment of symptomatic hypocalcemia:** 100 to 200 mg/kg/dose IV diluted in appropriate fluid and administered over 10 to 30 minutes.
- **Maintenance IV:** 200 to 800 mg/kg/day divided every 6 hours or as infusion; maximum rate: 50 to 100 mg/min of calcium gluconate. Continuous infusion is more efficacious than intermittent infusion due to less renal calcium loss.
- **Maintenance PO:** 200 to 800 mg/kg/day divided every 6 hours, mixed in feedings. The 10% calcium gluconate injection may be administered orally in young pediatric patients.
- **Cardiac arrest in the presence of hyperkalemia or hypocalcemia, magnesium toxicity, or calcium antagonist toxicity:** 60 to 100 mg/kg/dose IV, IO every 10 minutes as needed.
- **Exchange transfusion:** 100 mg calcium gluconate/100 mL of citrated blood exchanged infused IV over 10 minutes.

ADVERSE EFFECTS: See Calcium Chloride. Oral administration may cause gastrointestinal irritation; dilute and use with caution in infants at risk for necrotizing enterocolitis.

CALFACTANT (INFASURF)

INDICATIONS AND USE: Prevention and treatment of neonatal respiratory distress syndrome (RDS). FDA approved in premature infants <29 weeks' gestational age.

ACTIONS: Natural, preservative-free calf lung extract that contains phospholipids, neutral lipids, fatty acids, and surfactant-associated proteins B and C. Each milliliter of calfactant contains 35 mg of total phospholipids and 0.65 mg of proteins (0.26 mg of protein B). Calfactant decreases the surface tension on alveolar surfaces, stabilizing the alveoli and preventing collapse. This results in improved ventilation, lung compliance, and gas exchange.

DOSAGE: ETT.

- **RDS:** As soon as possible after birth, give 3 mL/kg/dose, divided into two 1.5 mL/kg aliquots. After the instillation of each aliquot, position infant either on the right or left side. Ventilation is continued during administration over 20 to 30 seconds. The 2 aliquots should be separated by a pause to evaluate respiratory status and reposition the patient.
- The initial dose may be followed by 3 subsequent doses of 3 mL/kg/dose at 12-hour intervals, if necessary.

ADVERSE EFFECTS: Bradycardia, cyanosis, airway obstruction, pneumothorax, pulmonary hemorrhage, and apnea. Most adverse effects occur during administration of dose.

COMMENTS: Following administration, lung compliance and oxygenation often rapidly improve. Patients should be closely monitored, and appropriate changes in ventilatory support should be made as clinically indicated.

CAPTOPRIL (CAPOTEN)

INDICATIONS AND USE: Moderate to severe congestive heart failure (reduction of afterload) and hypertension.

ACTIONS: Competitive inhibitor of angiotensin-converting enzyme. Causes a decrease in angiotensin II and aldosterone levels; increases plasma and tissue renin activity; decreases systemic vascular resistance without reflex tachycardia and augmentation of cardiac output.

DOSAGE: PO.

- **Premature and term neonates, PNA ≤7 days:** Initial dose: 0.01 mg/kg/dose every 8 to 12 hours; titrate dose and interval based on response.
- **Term neonates, PNA >7 days:** Initial dose: 0.05 to 0.1 mg/kg/dose every 8 to 24 hours; titrate dose up to maximum 0.5 mg/kg/dose given every 6 to 24 hours.
- **Infants:**
  - **Hypertension:** Initial dose: 0.15 to 0.3 mg/kg/dose; titrate dose up to 6 mg/kg/day divided in 1 to 4 doses.
  - **Heart failure:** Initial dose: 0.3 to 2.5 mg/kg/day divided every 8 to 12 hours.

ADVERSE EFFECTS: Hypotension, rash, fever, eosinophilia, angioedema, neutropenia, gastrointestinal disturbances, and hyperkalemia. Significant decreases in cerebral and renal blood flow have occurred in premature infants who have chronic hypertension and received higher doses (0.15–0.3 mg/kg/dose); may result in neurologic complications including seizures, apnea and lethargy, and oliguria.

COMMENTS: Administer 1 hour before or 2 hours after feedings if possible; food decreases absorption. Contraindicated in patients with bilateral renovascular disease. Use with caution in patients with low renal perfusion pressure. Reduce the dose with renal impairment and in sodium- and water-depleted patients (use with caution if on concurrent diuretic therapy).

CARBAMAZEPINE (TEGRETOL)

> **WARNING:** Serious dermatologic reactions associated with HLA-B1502 allele (mostly Asian ancestry). Aplastic anemia and agranulocytosis have been reported. Monitor complete blood count (CBC), platelets, and differential prior to and during therapy; discontinue if significant bone marrow suppression occurs.

INDICATIONS AND USE: Anticonvulsant. Treatment of partial (especially complex partial), primary generalized tonic-clonic seizures and mixed partial or generalized seizures.

ACTIONS: Decrease synaptic transmission, limits influx of sodium ions across cell membrane.

DOSAGE: PO.

- 10 to 20 mg/kg/day of oral suspension, initially divided 4 times a day; may increase weekly to optimal response, then to a maximum of 35 mg/kg/day. Administer daily dose in 3 to 4 divided doses with feedings.

ADVERSE EFFECTS: Nausea, vomiting, leukopenia, thrombocytopenia, aplastic anemia and agranulocytosis, congestive heart failure, heart block, dystonia, drowsiness, behavioral changes, syndrome of inappropriate antidiuretic hormone secretion, hyponatremia, hepatitis and cholestasis, rash and Stevens-Johnson syndrome, urine retention, azotemia, oliguria, and anuria. Monitor CBC, liver function, blood urea nitrogen, serum iron, and urinalysis; perform periodic eye examination. Do not discontinue abruptly because seizures may result in epileptic patients.

PHARMACOLOGY: Metabolized in liver by cytochrome P450 3A4. Induces liver enzymes and increases its own metabolism. Half-life in neonates is 8 to 28 hours. Therapeutic range is 4 to 12 mcg/mL. If used in combination with other anticonvulsants, therapeutic range is 4 to 8 mcg/mL.

COMMENTS: Avoid switching between Tegretol and generic carbamazepine; changes in serum concentration and seizure activity may result; monitor serum concentrations. Interactions are numerous. Erythromycin, isoniazid, and cimetidine may inhibit hepatic metabolism of carbamazepine, resulting in increased carbamazepine serum concentrations. Concurrent phenobarbital may lower carbamazepine serum levels. Carbamazepine may induce metabolism of warfarin, phenytoin, theophylline, benzodiazepines, and corticosteroids.

CASPOFUNGIN

ACTION AND SPECTRUM: Treatment of invasive aspergillosis that is refractory to other antifungal agents or in patients intolerant of other agents; infections caused by susceptible *Candida* species.

DOSAGE: IV.

- **Preterm neonates—infants <3 months:** 25 mg/m^2 (or equivalent to ~2 mg/kg)/dose IV every 24 hours; infuse over at least 1 hour via syringe pump.
- **Infants ≥3 months:** Initial dose of 70 mg/m^2/dose IV followed by 50 mg/m^2/dose IV every 24 hours starting on day 2. May increase to 70 mg/m^2/dose IV every 24 hours if clinical response is inadequate. Maximum dose is 70 mg/day.
- **Length of therapy:** At least 14 days after last positive culture.

ADVERSE EFFECTS: Hypokalemia, hypercalcemia, elevated liver enzymes, thrombocytopenia, direct hyperbilirubinemia, thrombophlebitis, hypotension, fever, and rash.

PHARMACOLOGY: An echinocandin acts by inhibiting the synthesis of β-(1,3)-D-glucan, an important component of the fungal cell wall. Fungicidal against *Candida* species and fungistatic against *Aspergillus*. Metabolized by the liver, not cytochrome P450 enzymes; results in fewer drug–drug interactions than the azole class of antifungal agents. Serum concentrations of caspofungin may be lower if concomitant therapy with dexamethasone, phenytoin, carbamazepine, nevirapine, and rifampin. Caspofungin clearance is induced and higher doses may be required: 70 mg/m^2/dose.

COMMENTS: *Note:* Dosing information based on very limited pharmacokinetic data of 18 neonates and infants (Saez-Liorens, 2009). Do not use diluents containing dextrose for reconstitution. Maximum concentration not to exceed 0.5 mg/mL.

CEFAZOLIN SODIUM (ANCEF, KEFZOL)

ACTION AND SPECTRUM: First-generation cephalosporin; a broad-spectrum semisynthetic β-lactam antibiotic with bactericidal activity. Activity against susceptible gram-positive cocci (except enterococci), including penicillinase-producing staphylococci; some gram-negative coverage of susceptible *Escherichia coli*, *Klebsiella*, and *Proteus*. Primarily used in neonates for urinary tract infections, perioperative prophylaxis, and soft tissue infections.

DOSAGE: IV.

Neonates:

- **Body weight ≤2 kg:**
  - **PNA ≤7 days:** 25 mg/kg/dose every 12 hours.
  - **PNA >7 days:** 25 mg/kg/dose every 8 hours.
- **Body weight >2 kg:**
  - **PNA ≤7 days:** 50 mg/kg/dose every 12 hours.
  - **PNA >7 days:** 50 mg/kg/dose every 8 hours.

Infants and children:

- 50 to 150 mg/kg/day divided every 8 hours; maximum dose: 6 g/day.

ADVERSE EFFECTS: Infrequent; fever, rash, and urticaria. May cause eosinophilia, leukopenia, neutropenia, and thrombocytopenia. Excessive dosage (especially in renal impairment) may result in CNS irritation with seizure activity.

PHARMACOLOGY: 70% to 80% excreted unchanged in urine. Half-life is 3 to 5 hours in neonates.

COMMENTS: Dosage reduction is required in moderate to severe renal failure.

CEFEPIME

ACTION AND SPECTRUM: Fourth-generation cephalosporin used for treatment of infections caused by susceptible gram-negative bacteria: *Escherichia coli*, *Haemophilus influenzae*, *Enterobacter*, *Klebsiella*, *Providencia*, *Serratia*, *Proteus*, *Morganella*, *Neisseria*, *Pseudomonas aeruginosa*, *Acinetobacter*, and *Citrobacter*. Treatment of infections caused by susceptible gram-positive bacteria: *Staphylococcus aureus*, *Streptococcus pyogenes*, *Streptococcus pneumoniae*, and *Streptococcus agalactiae*.

DOSAGE: IV.

- **Body weight <1 kg:**
  - **PNA (PNA) <14 days:** 50 mg/kg/dose IV every 12 hours.
  - **PNA ≥14 days:** 50 mg/kg/dose every 8 hours.

- **Body weight 1 to 2 kg:**
  - **PNA <8 days:** 50 mg/kg/dose every 12 hours.
  - **PNA ≥8 days:** 50 mg/kg/dose every 8 hours.
- **Body weight >2 kg:** 50 mg/kg/dose every 8 hours.
- *Red Book* **2018–2021 dose:**
  - **GA <36 wks:** 30 mg/kg every 12 hours.
  - **GA ≥36 weeks:** 50 mg/kg every 12 hours (may give 30 mg/kg every 12 hours if target pathogen MIC <8 mg/L).

ADVERSE EFFECTS: Rash, elevated hepatic transaminase enzymes, prothrombin time (PT), partial thromboplastin time (PTT), thrombocytopenia, leukopenia, neutropenia, eosinophilia, and hypophosphatemia.

PHARMACOLOGY: Distributes well into body tissues and fluids. Low protein binding; primarily excreted in urine unchanged.

COMMENTS: Manufacturer does not recommend use for treatment of serious infections due to *H influenzae* type b for suspected meningitis.

CEFOTAXIME SODIUM (CLAFORAN)

ACTION AND SPECTRUM: Third-generation cephalosporin with bactericidal activity against susceptible gram-negative organisms (except *Pseudomonas*), including *Escherichia coli*, *Enterobacter*, *Klebsiella*, *Haemophilus influenzae* (including ampicillin-resistant strains), *Proteus*, *Serratia*, *Neisseria gonorrhoeae*, and *Neisseria meningitidis*. Generally poor activity against gram-positive aerobic organisms.

DOSAGE: IV, IM.

- **Body weight <1 kg:**
  - **PNA ≤14 days:** 50 mg/kg/dose every 12 hours.
  - **PNA 15 to 28 days:** 50 mg/kg/dose every 8 to 12 hours.
- **Body weight 1 to 2 kg:**
  - **PNA ≤7 days:** 50 mg/kg/dose every 12 hours.
  - **PNA 8 to 28 days:** 50 mg/kg/dose every 8 to 12 hours.
- **Body weight >2 kg:**
  - **PNA ≤7 days:** 50 mg/kg/dose every 12 hours.
  - **PNA 8 to 28 days:** 50 mg/kg/dose every 8 hours.

Infants and children ≥1 month:

- **Body weight <50 kg:** 100 to 225 mg/kg/day divided every 6 to 8 hours. Maximum daily dose: 12 g/day.

Meningitis:

- **PNA ≤7 days and ≥2 kg:** 100 to 150 mg/kg/day divided every 8 to 12 hours.
- **PNA >7 days and ≥2 kg:** 150 to 200 mg/kg/day divided every 6 to 8 hours.
- **Infants >1 month:** 225 to 300 mg/kg/day divided every 6 to 8 hours. Maximum dose: 2000 mg.

Disseminated gonococcal infection, disseminated/scalp abscesses:

- The Centers for Disease Control and Prevention recommends cefotaxime as an alternative to ceftriaxone in the treatment of disseminated gonococcal infection and gonococcal scalp abscesses in newborns. The dose of cefotaxime is 25 mg/kg/dose every 12 hours IM or IV for 7 days; duration is 10 to 14 days for meningitis.

Gonococcal ophthalmia prophylaxis in newborns of mothers with gonorrhea at delivery:

- 100 mg/kg IV or IM as a single dose (topical antibiotic therapy alone is inadequate).

ADVERSE EFFECTS: Arrhythmias; transient neutropenia, thrombocytopenia, eosinophilia, leukopenia; transient hepatic and renal dysfunction.

PHARMACOLOGY: Excreted principally unchanged in the urine (~60%). Half-life in neonates is 1 to 4 hours.

COMMENTS: Reserved for suspected or documented gram-negative meningitis or sepsis. When used as empiric therapy, combine with ampicillin or penicillin to provide gram-positive coverage (ie, group B streptococci, pneumococci, and *Listeria monocytogenes*). Third-generation cephalosporins induce the emergence of multidrug-resistant bacteria or fungal infection when used excessively and without proper clinical indications. Cefotaxime is currently unavailable in the United States due to manufacturing issues.

CEFOXITIN (MEFOXIN)

ACTIONS AND SPECTRUM: Second-generation cephalosporin used for infections from gram-negative enteric organisms *Escherichia coli*, *Klebsiella*, and *Proteus*; active against many strains of *Neisseria gonorrhoeae*, ampicillin-resistant *Haemophilus influenzae*, and anaerobic bacteria, including *Bacteroides* species of the gastrointestinal (GI) tract.

DOSAGE: IV.

Neonates:
- 90 to 100 mg/kg/day divided every 8 hours.

Infants ≥3 months and children:
- **Mild-moderate infection:** 80 mg/kg/day divided every 6 to 8 hours.
- **Severe infection:** 160 mg/kg/day divided every 6 hours. Maximum dose: 12 g/day.
- **Surgical prophylaxis:** 30 to 40 mg/kg 30 to 60 minutes prior to incision, followed by 30 to 40 mg/kg every 6 hours for up to 24 hours. Maximum dose: 2000 mg/dose.

PHARMACOLOGY: Highly protein bound and renally excreted essentially unchanged (85%).

ADVERSE EFFECTS: Usually well tolerated. May cause diarrhea, rash, thrombophlebitis; transient leukopenia, thrombocytopenia, neutropenia, anemia, and eosinophilia; and transient elevation of blood urea nitrogen, serum creatinine, and liver enzymes.

COMMENTS: Not inactivated by β-lactamase. Has poor CNS penetration. The safety and efficacy in infants <3 months have not been established.

CEFTAZIDIME (FORTAZ, TAZIDIME)

ACTION AND SPECTRUM: Third-generation cephalosporin with bactericidal activity against gram-negative aerobic bacteria, including *Neisseria*, *Haemophilus influenzae*, some Enterobacteriaceae, and *Pseudomonas*. Pseudomonal infections in patients at risk of developing aminoglycoside-induced nephrotoxicity and/or ototoxicity. Poor gram-positive activity. Aminoglycosides act synergistically with ceftazidime.

DOSAGE: IV.
- **Body weight <1 kg:**
  - **PNA ≤14 days:** 50 mg/kg/dose every 12 hours.
  - **PNA 15 to 28 days:** 50 mg/kg/dose every 8 to 12 hours.
- **Body weight 1 to 2 kg:**
  - **PNA ≤7 days:** 50 mg/kg/dose every 12 hours.
  - **PNA 8 to 28 days:** 50 mg/kg/dose every 8 to 12 hours.
- **Body weight >2 kg:**
  - **PNA ≤7 days:** 50 mg/kg/dose every 12 hours.
  - **PNA 8 to 28 days:** 50 mg/kg/dose every 8 hours.

Infants and children ≥1 month:
- 100 to 200 mg/kg/day divided every 8 hours; maximum dose: 6 g/day.

Meningitis:
- **PNA ≤7 days and ≥2 kg:** 100 to 150 mg/kg/day divided every 8 to 12 hours.
- **PNA >7 days and ≥2 kg:** 150 mg/kg/day divided every 8 hours.
- **Infants >1 month:** 150 mg/kg/day divided every 8 hours; maximum dose: 6 g/day.

ADVERSE EFFECTS: Infrequent except for fever, rash, urticaria. May cause transient leukopenia, neutropenia, thrombocytopenia, and hemolytic anemia; transient elevation in liver enzymes, hyperbilirubinemia, and transient elevation of blood urea nitrogen and serum creatinine.

PHARMACOLOGY: Renally excreted 80% to 90% unchanged. Half-life is 2.2 to 4.7 hours; penetrates well into CSF.

CEFTRIAXONE SODIUM (ROCEPHIN)

ACTION AND SPECTRUM: Third-generation cephalosporin with activity against gram-negative aerobic bacteria, *Haemophilus influenzae*, Enterobacteriaceae, and *Neisseria*, and activity against gram-positive cocci, methicillin-susceptible *Staphylococcus*, and *Streptococcus*. No activity against *Pseudomonas aeruginosa, Chlamydia trachomatis,* methicillin-resistant staphylococci, and enterococci.

DOSAGE: IV, IM.

Meningitis:
- **PNA <14 days:** 50 mg/kg/day every 24 hours.
- **PNA ≥14 days:**
  - **≤2 kg:** 50 mg/kg/day every 24 hours.
  - **>2 kg:** 80 to 100 mg/kg/day every 24 hours.

Gonococcal prophylaxis:
- 25 to 50 mg/kg as a single dose. Maximum dose: 125 mg/dose.

Gonococcal infection:
- 25 to 50 mg/kg/dose every 24 hours for 7 days; up to 10 to 14 days if meningitis is documented. Maximum dose: 125 mg/dose. (*Note:* Use cefotaxime in place of ceftriaxone in hyperbilirubinemic neonates.)

Ophthalmia neonatorum:
- 25 to 50 mg/kg as a single dose. Maximum dose: 125 mg/dose.

Infants and children:
- 50 to 100 mg/kg/day divided every 12 to 24 hours.

Meningitis:
- 80 to 100 mg/kg/day divided every 12 to 24 hours; loading dose of 75 mg/kg may be administered at the start of therapy. Maximum dose: 4 g/day.

ADVERSE EFFECTS: Diarrhea, cholelithiasis, gallbladder sludging. May also cause neutropenia, eosinophilia, hemolytic anemia, increased prothrombin times, rash, thrombophlebitis, elevated liver enzymes, jaundice, hyperbilirubinemia; use with caution in infants with hyperbilirubinemia.

PHARMACOLOGY: Biliary and renal excretion. Half-life is 5 to 19 hours.

COMMENTS: *Warning:* Use extreme caution in neonates due to risk of hyperbilirubinemia. Ceftriaxone use is contraindicated in hyperbilirubinemic neonates and neonates <41 weeks' postmenstrual age. Ceftriaxone is incompatible with calcium-containing solutions. Calcium-containing solutions or products must not be administered within 48 hours of the ceftriaxone dose due to the fatal reaction involving calcium-ceftriaxone precipitates in the lungs and kidneys of neonates. Dosage reduction is required only in patients with both renal and hepatic dysfunction.

CEFUROXIME SODIUM (KEFUROX, ZINACEF)

ACTION AND SPECTRUM: Second-generation cephalosporin with activity against susceptible staphylococci, group B streptococci, pneumococci, *Haemophilus influenzae* (type A and B), *Escherichia coli, Enterobacter,* and *Klebsiella.*

DOSAGE: IM, IV.
- **Meningitis:** Not recommended due to reports of treatment failures and slower bacteriologic response time.
- **Body weight <1 kg:**
  - **PNA ≤14 days:** 50 mg/kg/dose every 12 hours.
  - **PNA 15 to 28 days:** 50 mg/kg/dose every 8 to 12 hours.
- **Body weight 1 to 2 kg:**
  - **PNA ≤7 days:** 50 mg/kg/dose every 12 hours.
  - **PNA 8 to 28 days:** 50 mg/kg/dose every 8 to 12 hours.
- **Body weight >2 kg:**
  - **PNA ≤7 days:** 50 mg/kg/dose every 12 hours.
  - **PNA 8 to 28 days:** 50 mg/kg/dose every 8 hours.
- **Infants and children:**
  - **IV, IM:** 75 to 200 mg/kg/day divided every 8 hours. Maximum dose: 1500 mg/dose.
  - **PO:** 20 to 30 mg/kg/day divided every 12 hours. Maximum dose: 500 mg/dose.

ADVERSE EFFECTS: Fever, seizures, rash, thrombophlebitis, diarrhea, hemolytic anemia, transient neutropenia and leukopenia, eosinophilia, increased prothrombin time. Transient elevation in liver enzymes, hepatitis, and cholestasis; elevation in blood urea nitrogen and serum creatinine.

PHARMACOLOGY: Primarily excreted unchanged in the urine. Half-life is approximately 5.8 hours in infants <3 days old and 1.4 to 3.8 hours in infants ≥8 days of age.

COMMENTS: Decrease the dosage in renal failure. Limited experience in neonates. Safety and efficacy in infants <3 months of age have not been established.

CHLORAL HYDRATE (NOCTEC)

INDICATIONS AND USE: Short-term sedative and hypnotic; CNS depressant.

DOSAGE: PO, PR. Use the lowest effective dose.

- **Usual dose:** 25 to 50 mg/kg/dose PO or PR every 6 to 8 hours as needed.
- **Sedation prior to electroencephalography and other procedures:** 25 to 75 mg/kg/dose once PO or PR. Typical dose: 50 mg/kg/dose once; repeat 25 mg/kg/dose once if needed. Maximum total dose: 100 mg/kg or 1 g total for infants.

ADVERSE EFFECTS: Gastrointestinal irritation resulting in nausea, vomiting, and diarrhea; paradoxical excitation; and respiratory depression, particularly if administered with opiates and barbiturates. May cause direct hyperbilirubinemia with chronic use (active metabolite 2,2,2-trichloroethanol [TCE]); competes with bilirubin for glucuronide conjugation in the liver); overdose can be lethal.

COMMENTS: Contraindicated with marked renal or hepatic impairment. Syrup may contain sodium benzoate; benzoic acid (benzoate) is a metabolite of benzyl alcohol, which can be toxic and fatal in neonates.

CHLORAMPHENICOL (CHLOROMYCETIN)

> **WARNING:** Serious and fatal blood dyscrasias (aplastic anemia, hypoplastic anemia, thrombocytopenia, and granulocytopenia) have occurred after both short-term and prolonged therapy; do not use for minor infections or when less potentially toxic agents are effective. Monitor complete blood count (CBC) frequently in all patients.

ACTION AND SPECTRUM: Broad-spectrum bacteriostatic agent, reserved for serious infections due to organisms resistant to other less toxic agent such as *Haemophilus influenzae*, *Neisseria meningitides*, and *Escherichia coli*; *Klebsiella*, *Serratia*, *Enterobacter*, *Salmonella*, *Shigella*, *Neisseria gonorrhoeae*, staphylococci, *Streptococcus pneumoniae*, and *Bacteroides*; active against many vancomycin-resistant enterococci.

DOSAGE: IV.

Neonates:

- **Meningitis:**
  - **PNA ≤7 days:** 25 mg/kg/dose IV every 24 hours.
  - **PNA 8 to 28 days:** 25 mg/kg/dose every 12 hours or 50 mg/kg/dose every 24 hours.
- **Severe infection: age-based dosing**
  - **PNA ≤7 days:** 25 mg/kg/dose IV every 24 hours; or loading dose of 20 mg/kg followed 12 hours later by 12.5 mg/kg/dose IV every 12 hours.
  - **PNA >7 days:** 25 mg/kg/dose IV every 12 hours; or 12.5 mg/kg/dose IV every 6 hours.

Infants and children:

- **Meningitis:** 75 to 100 mg/kg/day IV divided every 6 hours.
- **Other infections:** 50 to 100 mg/kg/day IV divided every 6 hours. Maximum daily dose 4 g/day.

ADVERSE EFFECTS: Idiosyncratic reactions result in aplastic anemia (irreversible and rare), reversible bone marrow suppression (dose related), allergy (rash and fever), diarrhea, vomiting, stomatitis, glossitis, fungal overgrowth, "gray baby" syndrome (early signs are hyperammonemia and unexplained metabolic acidosis; other signs are abdominal distention, hypotonia, gray skin color, and cardiorespiratory collapse), and cardiotoxicity due to left ventricular dysfunction. Use with extreme caution in neonates.

PHARMACOLOGY: Metabolized by hepatic glucuronyl transferase. Half-life is 10 to 24 hours in neonates.

COMMENTS: Must monitor serum levels. Desired peak is 15 to 25 mcg/mL; levels >50 mcg/mL are strongly associated with "gray baby" syndrome. Trough 5 to 15 mcg/mL. Draw peak concentrations 30 minutes to 1.5 hours after completion of IV dose; trough immediately before next dose. Monitor CBC with differential, platelet count, and reticulocyte count every 3 days.

CHLORAMPHENICOL OPHTHALMIC

See Chapter 58.

CHLOROTHIAZIDE (DIURIL)

INDICATIONS AND USE: Mild to moderate edema, hypertension, central diabetes insipidus of infancy, and hyperinsulinemia.

ACTIONS: Thiazide diuretic; inhibits sodium reabsorption in the distal renal tubules. Sodium, potassium, bicarbonate, magnesium, phosphate, and chloride excretion are increased, whereas calcium excretion is decreased.

DOSAGE: PO, IV. *Note:* IV dosage in infants and children has not been established. IV doses in infants and children are based on anecdotal reports. The IV dosing regimens have been extrapolated from oral dosing regimens considering only 10% to 20% of an oral dose is absorbed.

Neonates:
- **Edema, heart failure, bronchopulmonary dysplasia:**
  - **Oral:** 20 to 40 mg/kg/day PO divided every 12 hours; maximum 375 mg/day.
  - **IV:** 5 to 10 mg/kg/day IV divided every 12 hours; doses up to 20 mg/kg/day have been used.
- **Hyperinsulinemia hypoglycemia, congenital hyperinsulinemia:**
  - **Oral:** 7 to 10 mg/kg/day PO divided every 12 hours in combination with diazoxide.
- **Diabetes insipidus (central):**
  - **Oral:** 10 mg/kg/day PO divided every 12 hours; may titrate dose to target urine osmolality of 100 to 150 mOsm/L.

Infants <6 months:
- **Oral:** 10 to 30 mg/kg/day PO in divided doses once or twice daily.

Infants >6 months and children:
- **Oral:** 10 to 20 mg/kg/day PO divided once or twice daily; maximum 1 g/day in children ≥2 years.
- **IV:** 5 to 10 mg/kg/day IV divided once or twice daily; doses up to 20 mg/kg/day have been used. Maximum dose 500 mg.

ADVERSE EFFECTS: Hypokalemia, hypercalcemia, hypochloremic alkalosis, dehydration and prerenal azotemia, hyperuricemia, hyperglycemia, hypermagnesemia, hyperlipidemia, Stevens-Johnson syndrome, aplastic anemia, thrombocytopenia, hypotension, respiratory distress.

PHARMACOLOGY: Duration of action for oral is 6 to 12 hours and onset of action is within 2 hours. Duration of action for IV is about 2 hours and onset of action is 15 minutes.

COMMENTS: Do not use in patients with anuria or severe hepatic dysfunction.

CHOLESTYRAMINE RESIN (QUESTRAN)

INDICATIONS AND USE: Diaper dermatitis and as a skin protectant around enterostomy fistula sites.

ACTION: Cholestyramine resin binds to bile acids in the intestine, forms a nonabsorbable complex preventing the reabsorption and enterohepatic recirculation of bile salts, and releases chloride ions in the process.

DOSAGE: Topical.
- Apply to affected area with each diaper change.

ADVERSE EFFECTS: Constipation. High doses can cause hyperchloremic acidosis and increase urinary calcium excretion. Adverse effects seen when medication taken orally.

PHARMACOLOGY: Not absorbed; excreted in the feces.
COMMENTS: Not commercially available. Extemporaneous compound ointment or paste in Aquaphor; usual concentration 5% to 10%.

CHOLIC ACID (CHOLBAM)

INDICATIONS AND USE: Bile acid synthesis disorders.
ACTIONS: Cholic acid enhances bile flow and provides the physiologic feedback inhibition of bile acid synthesis to maintain bile acid homeostasis.
DOSAGE: PO.
• **Neonates ≥3 weeks, infants, and children:** 10 to 15 mg/kg/day divided once or twice daily.
ADVERSE EFFECTS: Increased serum bilirubin, increased serum transaminases, cholestasis, jaundice.
PHARMACOLOGY: Hepatic metabolism, absorbed by passive diffusion along the gastrointestinal tract.
COMMENTS: Patients with concomitant familial hypertriglyceridemia may have poor absorption.

CIMETIDINE (TAGAMET)

INDICATIONS AND USE: Prevention and treatment of duodenal and gastric ulcers, gastroesophageal reflux, esophagitis, and hypersecretory conditions.
ACTIONS: A histamine (H_2)-receptor antagonist; competitively inhibits the action of histamine on the gastric parietal cells, decreasing gastric acid secretion.
DOSAGE: PO.
• **Neonates:** 5 to 10 mg/kg/day PO divided every 6 to 12 hours.
• **Infants:** 20 to 40 mg/kg/day PO divided every 6 to 8 hours. Maximum dose: 400 mg/dose.
ADVERSE EFFECTS: CNS toxicity such as agitation and alterations in consciousness, neutropenia, agranulocytosis, thrombocytopenia, antiandrogenic effects; elevated aspartate aminotransferase (AST), alanine aminotransferase (ALT), and creatinine levels.
PHARMACOLOGY: Cimetidine reduces the hepatic metabolism of drugs metabolized by the cytochrome P450 pathway, which may result in decreased elimination of diazepam, theophylline, phenytoin, propranolol, and carbamazepine. Doses of these drugs may need to be decreased.
COMMENTS: Limited use in neonates due to association of H_2 blocker use and increased incidence of necrotizing enterocolitis, mortality, and infection in very low birthweight neonates receiving ranitidine.

CIPROFLOXACIN OPHTHALMIC

See Chapter 58.

CISATRACURIUM (NIMBEX)

HIGH-ALERT MEDICATION: To be administered only by experienced clinicians or adequately trained individuals supervised by an experienced clinician familiar with the use and actions, characteristics, and complications of neuromuscular-blocking agents.
INDICATIONS AND USE: Skeletal muscle relaxation during surgery; increases pulmonary compliance during assisted mechanical ventilation and facilitates endotracheal intubation.
ACTIONS: Nondepolarizing neuromuscular-blocking agent that produces skeletal muscle paralysis by blocking acetylcholine binding at the receptor at the myoneural junction.
DOSAGE: IV.
Infants and children <2 years:
• 0.15 mg/kg/dose; repeat every hour as needed; may be administered as a continuous infusion at 1 to 4 mcg/kg/min (0.06–0.24 mg/kg/h).
ADVERSE EFFECTS: May cause hypoxemia with inadequate mechanical ventilation; bronchospasm, apnea, arrhythmias, tachycardia, hypotension, hypertension, excessive salivation. Potentiation of neuromuscular blockade may result from aminoglycosides, electrolyte abnormalities, severe

hyponatremia, severe hypocalcemia, severe hypokalemia, hypermagnesemia, neuromuscular diseases, acidosis, renal failure, and hepatic failure. Antagonism of neuromuscular blockade may result from alkalosis, hypercalcemia, hyperkalemia, and epinephrine.

PHARMACOLOGY: Onset of action is 2 to 3 minutes with a duration that varies with dose and age.

COMMENTS: When used with narcotics, decreases in heart rate and blood pressure have been observed.

CITRATE AND CITRIC ACIDS SOLUTIONS (ORACIT, OTHERS)

INDICATIONS AND USE: Treatment of metabolic acidosis or as a urinary alkalinizing agent for conditions that require the maintenance of alkaline urine.

ACTIONS: Sodium and potassium citrate salts are capable of buffering gastric acidity (pH >2.5) and are metabolized to bicarbonate to act as systemic alkalinizers.

DOSAGE: PO.
- 2 to 3 mEq/kg/day of bicarbonate in divided doses 3 to 4 times per day with water.

ADVERSE EFFECTS: Metabolic alkalosis, hypernatremia (if sodium salt used), hypocalcemia, hyperkalemia (if potassium salt used), diarrhea, nausea, vomiting.

COMMENTS: Supplied as oral solutions: Sodium citrate–citric acid solution contains 1 mEq of sodium and 1 mEq of potassium and 2 mEq of bicarbonate equivalents per milliliter; potassium citrate–citric acid oral solution contains 2 mEq of potassium and 2 mEq of bicarbonate equivalents per milliliter. Conversion to bicarbonate may be impaired in patients with hepatic failure. Polycitra: only generic available (citric acid 334 mg, sodium citrate 500 mg, and potassium citrate 550 mg/5 mL). Oracit: available in brand and generic formulations (different concentrations).

CLINDAMYCIN (CLEOCIN)

ACTION AND SPECTRUM: Bacteriostatic agent active against most aerobic gram-positive staphylococci and streptococci (except enterococci); *Fusobacterium*, *Bacteroides* spp., *Actinomyces*, and certain anaerobic gram-positive organisms.

DOSAGE: IM, IV, PO.
Neonates:
- **Body weight <1 kg:**
  - **PNA ≤14 days:** 5 mg/kg/dose every 12 hours.
  - **PNA 15 to 28 days:** 5 mg/kg/dose every 8 hours.
- **Body weight 1 to 2 kg:**
  - **PNA ≤7 days:** 5 mg/kg/dose every 12 hours.
  - **PNA 8 to 28 days:** 5 mg/kg/dose every 8 hours.
- **Body weight >2 kg:**
  - **PNA ≤7 days:** 5 mg/kg/dose every 8 hours.
  - **PNA 8 to 28 days:** 5 mg/kg/dose every 6 hours.

Infants and children:
- **IM/IV:** 20 to 40 mg/kg/day divided every 6 to 8 hours; doses as high as 4.8 g/day have been given IV in life-threatening situations; general maximum: 2.7 g/day.
- **PO:** 10 to 30 mg/kg/day PO divided every 6 to 8 hours; maximum dose: 1.8 g/day.

ADVERSE EFFECTS: Diarrhea, colitis, pseudomembranous colitis rash, pruritus, neutropenia, granulocytopenia and thrombocytopenia, hypersensitivity reactions, and elevated liver enzymes. Sterile abscess formation at the IM injection site.

PHARMACOLOGY: Primarily hepatic metabolism, highly protein bound.

COMMENTS: Does not cross the blood–brain barrier; therefore, do not use to treat meningitis.

CLONAZEPAM (KLONOPIN)

INDICATIONS AND USE: For the treatment of petit mal, Lennox-Gastaut, infantile spasms, and akinetic and myoclonic seizures, either as a single agent or as adjunctive therapy.

ACTIONS: Depresses all levels of the CNS, including the limbic and reticular formation, by binding to the benzodiazepine site on the γ-aminobutyric acid (GABA) receptor complex; suppresses the spike-and-wave discharge in absence seizures by depressing nerve transmission in the motor cortex.

DOSAGE: PO.

Seizure disorders

- **Infants and children <10 years or 30 kg.**
- **Initial daily dose:** 0.01 to 0.03 mg/kg/day PO (maximum 0.05 mg/kg/day) given in 2 to 3 divided doses; increase by no more than 0.5 mg every third day until seizures are controlled or adverse effects occur.
- **Maintenance:** 0.1 to 0.2 mg/kg/day PO divided into 3 doses; do not exceed 0.2 mg/kg/day.

ADVERSE EFFECTS: Hypotension, drowsiness, hypotonia, thrombocytopenia, anemia, leukopenia, eosinophilia, tremor, choreiform movements, bronchial hypersecretion, respiratory depression.

PHARMACOLOGY: Cytochrome P450 isoenzyme CYP3A3/4 substrate. CNS depressants increase sedation; phenytoin, carbamazepine, rifampin, and barbiturates increase clonazepam clearance; drugs that inhibit cytochrome P450 isoenzyme CYP3A3/4 may increase levels and effects of clonazepam (monitor for altered benzodiazepine response); concurrent use with valproic acid may result in absence status.

COMMENTS: Caution in patients with chronic respiratory disease, hepatic disease, or impaired renal function. Abrupt discontinuation of clonazepam may precipitate withdrawal symptoms, status epilepticus, or seizures. (Withdraw gradually when discontinuing therapy in children. Safely reduce by ≤0.04 mg/kg/wk and discontinue when the daily dose is ≤0.04 mg/kg/day.) Worsening of seizures may occur when clonazepam is administered to patients with multiple seizure types.

CLONIDINE (CATAPRES; CATAPRES-TTS)

INDICATIONS AND USE: Adjunctive treatment of neonatal abstinence syndrome (NAS) and iatrogenic narcotic dependency.

ACTIONS: Stimulates CNS α_2-adrenergic receptors, which results in decreased sympathetic outflow, peripheral vascular resistance, systolic and diastolic blood pressure, and heart rate. Clonidine reduces circulating plasma renin levels.

DOSAGE: PO.

Neonatal abstinence syndrome (opioid withdrawal):

- **Preterm neonate <35 weeks' gestation:** 0.5 to 1 mcg/kg/dose PO every 6 hours. Taper dose when stabilized by 0.25 mcg/kg/dose PO every 6 hours (Leikin et al, 2009).
- **Neonate ≥35 weeks' gestation:** 0.5 to 1 mcg/kg/dose PO every 4 to 6 hours in combination with diluted opium tincture. A randomized, controlled, comparative trial in 80 neonates (gestational age: ≥35 weeks) with NAS demonstrated a decreased length of therapy and opioid doses in the combination treatment (clonidine plus diluted opium tincture) as compared to diluted tincture of opium alone (Agthe et al, 2009).
- **Alternate dosing:** Initial dose of 0.5 to 1 mcg/kg/dose every 3 to 6 hours; maximum dose 1 mcg/kg/dose every 3 hours (AAP Clinical Report—Neonatal Drug Withdrawal, reaffirmed February 2016).

ADVERSE EFFECTS: Very few side effects reported when used to treat NAS. Observe for hypotension and bradycardia and avoid abrupt discontinuation.

COMMENTS: More experience is needed before clonidine is routinely used to treat opioid withdrawal in infants. Compounded oral suspensions may be available in multiple concentrations. Precautions should be taken to verify and avoid confusion between different concentrations.

COSYNTROPIN (CORTROSYN)

INDICATIONS AND USE: Aid in the diagnosis of adrenocortical insufficiency; used in the diagnosis of congenital adrenal hyperplasia.

ACTIONS: Stimulates the adrenal cortex to secrete cortisol (hydrocortisone and cortisone), androgenic substances, and a small amount of aldosterone.

DOSAGE: IM/IV. Diagnostic test doses.

Adrenocortical insufficiency:

- **Preterm neonates:** Not well defined; 0.1 mcg/kg, 0.2 mcg/kg, 1 mcg/kg, and 3.5 mcg/kg have been used.
- **Neonates:** 15 mcg/kg (1 dose only).
- **Infants and children ≤2 years:** 0.125 mg or 15 mcg/kg; maximum dose 0.125 mg.

Congenital adrenal hyperplasia evaluation:

- 125 to 250 mcg.

ADVERSE EFFECTS: Bradycardia, hypertension, skin rash, urticaria at injection site.

COMMENTS: Plasma cortisol concentrations should be measured immediately before and exactly 30 minutes after administration of cosyntropin; dose should be given in early morning; 0.25 mg of cosyntropin = 25 USP units of corticotropin.

CYCLOPENTOLATE

INDICATIONS AND USE: For diagnostic and therapeutic ophthalmologic procedures that require mydriasis and cycloplegia.

ACTIONS: Causes pupillary dilatation by inhibition of the cholinergic response of the ciliary body muscle and sphincter muscle of iris.

DOSAGE: Ocular.

- 1 to 2 drops into the eye 10 to 30 minutes prior to procedure; usually used in conjunction with phenylephrine 2.5%. The 0.5% concentration is recommended for neonates.

ADVERSE EFFECTS: Tachycardia, vasodilatation, restlessness, delayed gastric emptying, urinary retention.

PHARMACOLOGY: Maximal effect occurs 30 to 60 minutes after administration, with pharmacologic effects lasting 6 to 24 hours.

COMMENTS: Consider holding feeds for 4 hours after procedure.

DEXAMETHASONE (DECADRON)

INDICATIONS: Treatment of airway edema prior to extubation. Used in infants with bronchopulmonary dysplasia/chronic lung disease to facilitate weaning from the ventilator.

ACTIONS: Long-acting, potent glucocorticoid without mineralocorticoid properties; prevents or suppresses inflammatory and immune responses in pharmacologic doses. Inhibits leukocyte infiltration at site of inflammation, interferes in function of mediators of inflammatory response, and suppresses humoral immune responses. May reduce edema and scar tissue formation; reversal of increased capillary permeability and general suppression in immune response.

DOSAGE: IV, PO.

Neonates:

- **Airway edema or extubation:** Usual dose: 0.25 mg/kg/dose IV given approximately 4 hours prior to scheduled extubation and then every 8 hours for 3 doses total. Range: 0.25 to 0.5 mg/kg/dose for 1 to 3 doses. Maximum dose: 1.5 mg/kg/day. *Note:* A longer duration of therapy may be needed with more severe cases.
- **Bronchopulmonary dysplasia/chronic lung disease (facilitate ventilator weaning):**
  - **Numerous dosing schedules proposed:** Range: 0.5 to 0.6 mg/kg/day given in divided doses PO or IV every 12 hours for 3 to 7 days, then taper over 1 to 6 weeks.
  - **DART trial protocol (Doyle et al, 2006):** 0.075 mg/kg/dose every 12 hours for 3 days, 0.05 mg/kg/dose every 12 hours for 3 days, 0.025 mg/kg/dose every 12 hours for 2 days, 0.01 mg/kg/dose every 12 hours for 2 days. Total dose 0.89 mg/kg over 10 days.

ADVERSE EFFECTS: With long-term use, increased susceptibility to infection, osteoporosis, growth retardation, hyperglycemia, fluid and electrolyte disturbances, cataracts, myopathy, gastrointestinal perforation and hemorrhage, hypertension, and acute adrenal insufficiency.

Dexamethasone use for low birthweight infants has come under close scrutiny because of increasing numbers of reports indicating neurodevelopmental compromise (see Comments). **COMMENTS:** Please review the important statement from the American Academy of Pediatrics Committee on Fetus and Newborn (2002, reaffirmed 2014). High-dose dexamethasone (~0.5 mg/kg/day) is associated with adverse neurodevelopmental outcomes without additional clinical benefit over lower doses.

DEXTROSE (GLUCOSE [ORAL GEL])

INDICATIONS AND USE: Hypoglycemia, hyperkalemia (used in combination with regular insulin).
ACTIONS: Restores low blood glucose levels; stimulates transient uptake of potassium into the cells.
DOSAGE: IV, buccal, IO.
For hypoglycemia:
- **Intravenous:** 0.2 g/kg/dose (2 mL/kg/dose of dextrose 10% in water [D10W]) followed by continuous IV infusion rate of 5 to 8 mg/kg/min. If plasma glucose remains low, increase infusion in 2 mg/kg/min increments. If rates >12 to 14 mg/kg/min are needed, further workup may be necessary.
- **Buccal:** (Dextrose gel 40%) 0.2 g/kg/dose (0.5 mL/kg of 40% dextrose gel); dry mouth with gauze and massage into the buccal mucosa, dividing the dose between the 2 sides of the mucosa. If still hypoglycemic after 30 minutes or if it recurs later, give a repeat dose. Maximum of 6 doses over 48 hours. Should also offer a bottle at time of treatment.
- **Pediatric Advanced Life Support guidelines:** IV, IO: 0.5 to 1 g/kg/dose (5–10 mL/kg/dose of D10W).

For hyperkalemia:
- Recommended 4 g of dextrose for every 1 unit of insulin; 0.4 g/kg/dose (4 mL/kg/dose of D10W) in combination with regular insulin.

COMMENTS: Dextrose is an IV vesicant at concentrations ≥10%; avoid extravasation. Rapid administration of hypertonic solutions may cause shifts in electrolytes, particularly potassium and sodium; in very low birthweight infants, increased serum osmolarity creates risk for intracerebral hemorrhage.

DIAZEPAM (VALIUM)

INDICATIONS: Alternative choice to lorazepam for status epilepticus. Treatment of seizures refractory to other combined anticonvulsant agents. Reduces anxiety, and can use for preoperative or preprocedural sedation.
ACTIONS: Exact action is unknown; acts as a CNS depressant. Like other benzodiazepines, diazepam increases the activity of the inhibitory neurotransmitter γ-aminobutyric acid (GABA) by binding the benzodiazepine receptor sites in the CNS.
DOSAGE: IV, PO.
Status epilepticus:
- **Neonates:** 0.1 to 0.3 mg/kg/dose IV given over 3 to 5 minutes, every 15 to 30 minutes to a maximum total dose of 2 mg. (Not recommended as first line; injection contains benzoic acid, benzyl alcohol, and sodium benzoate.)
- **Infants >30 days and children <5 years:** 0.1 to 0.3 mg/kg/dose given over 3 to 5 minutes, every 5 to 10 minutes to a maximum total dose of 10 mg, or 0.2 to 0.5 mg/dose every 2 to 5 minutes to a maximum total dose of 5 mg; repeat in 2 to 4 hours as needed.

ADVERSE EFFECTS: May cause rash, vasodilation, bradycardia, respiratory arrest, and hypotension. Use with caution in patients receiving other CNS depressants; may have additive CNS and respiratory depressant effects.
COMMENTS: Observe for and be prepared to manage respiratory arrest. Rapid IV push may cause sudden respiratory depression, apnea, or hypotension. Use of the rectal gel formulation in infants <6 months is not recommended; for use in children <2 years, the safety and efficacy

have not been studied; contains benzoic acid, benzyl alcohol, ethanol 10%, propylene glycol, and sodium benzoate.

DIAZOXIDE (PROGLYCEM)

INDICATIONS AND USE: Persistent hyperinsulinemic neonatal hypoglycemia (oral).

ACTIONS: Nondiuretic thiazide with antihypertensive and hyperglycemic effects. Inhibits the release of insulin from the pancreas and reduces total peripheral vascular resistance by direct relaxation of arteriolar smooth muscle, which results in a decrease in blood pressure and reflex increase in heart rate and cardiac output.

DOSAGE: PO.

Hyperinsulinemic hypoglycemia:

- **Neonates:** Initial: 10 mg/kg/day PO in divided doses every 8 hours; usual range: 5 to 15 mg/kg/day in divided doses every 8 to 12 hours.
- **Infants:** Initial: 10 mg/kg/day in divided doses every 8 hours; usual range: 5 to 20 mg/kg/day in divided doses every 8 hours (Hussain et al, 2004; Kapoor et al, 2009).

ADVERSE EFFECTS: Tachycardia; sodium and fluid retention is common; congestive heart failure may cause bilirubin displacement from albumin, hypotension, hyperglycemia, hyperuricemia, rash, fever, leukopenia, thrombocytopenia, and ketosis.

COMMENTS: Oral solution contains propylene glycol and sodium benzoate.

DIGIBIND (DIGOXIN IMMUNE FAB)

INDICATIONS AND USE: Treatment of potentially life-threatening digoxin or digitoxin toxicity in carefully selected patients; use in life-threatening ventricular arrhythmias secondary to digoxin, acute digoxin ingestion (ie, >0.1 mg/kg or >4 mg in children), and hyperkalemia (serum potassium >6 mEq/L) in the setting of digoxin toxicity.

ACTIONS: Binds with molecules of free (unbound) digoxin or digitoxin and then is removed from the body by renal excretion.

DOSAGE: IV.

Dose determination:

- Determine the dose by determining the total body-loading dose (TBL) of digoxin using either method 1 or method 2.
  - **Method 1:** An approximation of the amount ingested:
    - TBL of digoxin (in mg) = Concentration (in ng/mL) × 5.6 × body weight (in kg)/1000 or TBL = mg of digoxin ingested (as tablets or elixir) × 0.8.
    - Dose of Digibind (in mg) IV = TBL × 76.
    - Dose of digoxin immune Fab (Digibind) (number of vials) IV = TBL/0.5.
  - **Method 2:** A postdistribution serum digoxin concentration determination (Table 155–1).
    - Digoxin immune Fab dose (mg) = [(serum digoxin concentration [ng/mL] × weight [kg])/100] × 40 mg/vial
    - Digoxin immune Fab dose (vials) = (serum digoxin concentration [ng/mL] × weight [kg])/100

Acute digoxin toxicity:

- **Ingestion of known amount of digoxin:** Each vial (38 mg) IV binds approximately 0.5 mg digoxin. Bioavailability of digoxin is 0.8 for 0.25-mg tablets *or* 1 for 0.2-mg Lanoxicaps.
- **Use the following formula:** Dose (in vials) = digoxin ingested (mg) × bioavailability/0.5 mg of digoxin bound/vial.

Chronic digoxin toxicity:

- **Infants and small children:** Single vial (38 mg) IV initially.
- **Or use the following formula:** Number of vials needed = (serum digoxin concentration in ng/mL) × (weight in kg)/100, then dose (in mg) = number of vials × 38 mg/vial.

ADVERSE EFFECTS: Caution in renal or cardiac failure; allergic reactions possible; epinephrine should be immediately available; patients may deteriorate due to withdrawal of digoxin and

Table 155–1. DOSE ESTIMATES OF DIGOXIN IMMUNE FAB BASED ON SERUM ON DIGOXIN CONCENTRATION

Patient Weight 1 kg and Serum Digoxin Concentration	Patient Weight 3 kg and Serum Digoxin Concentration	Patient Weight 5 kg and Serum Digoxin Concentration
1 ng/mL: 0.4 mg	1 ng/mL: 1 mg	1 ng/mL: 2 mg
2 ng/mL: 1 mg	2 ng/mL: 2–2.5 mg	2 ng/mL: 4 mg
4 ng/mL: 1.5 mg	4 ng/mL: 5 mg	4 ng/mL: 8 mg
8 ng/mL: 3 mg	8 ng/mL: 9–10 mg	8 ng/mL: 15–16 mg
12 ng/mL: 5 mg	12 ng/mL: 14 mg	12 ng/mL: 23–24 mg
16 ng/mL: 6–6.5 mg	16 ng/mL: 18–19 mg	16 ng/mL: 30–32 mg
20 ng/mL: 8 mg	20 ng/mL: 23–24 mg	20 ng/mL: 38–40 mg

may require IV inotropic support (eg, dobutamine) or vasodilators. Hypokalemia reported following reversal of digitalis intoxication; monitor serum potassium levels.

PHARMACOLOGY: Volume of distribution: 0.3 L/kg; half-life: 15 to 20 hours; renal impairment prolongs the half-life of both agents. Improvement in signs and symptoms occurs within 20 to 90 minutes following IV infusion.

DIGOXIN (LANOXIN)

INDICATIONS AND USE: Treatment of congestive heart failure, atrial fibrillation or flutter, and supraventricular tachycardia.

ACTIONS: Exerts a positive inotropic effect (increased myocardial contractility). Its negative chronotropic effects (antiarrhythmic actions/decrease in heart rate) are due to the slowing of conduction through the sinoatrial (SA) and atrioventricular (AV) nodes caused by vagal stimulation.

DOSAGE: IV, PO. Total digitalizing dose (TDD) to be divided one-half, one-fourth, and one-fourth every 8 hours. *Note:* Oral doses (elixir) are approximately 25% higher than IV doses listed in the following.

Preterm neonates:
- **TDD:** 15 to 25 mcg/kg IV or 20 to 30 mcg/kg PO.
- **Daily maintenance:** 4 to 6 mcg/kg/day IV divided every 12 hours or 5 to 7.5 mcg/kg/day PO divided every 12 hours.

Full-term neonates:
- **TDD:** 20 to 30 mcg/kg IV, 25 to 35 mcg/kg PO.
- **Daily maintenance:** 5 to 8 mcg/kg/day IV divided every 12 hours or 8 to 10 mcg/kg/day PO divided every 12 hours.

1 month to 2 years:
- **TDD:** 30 to 50 mcg/kg IV or 35 to 60 PO mcg/kg.
- **Daily maintenance:** 7.5 to 12 mcg/kg/day IV divided every 12 hours or 10 to 15 mcg/kg/day PO divided every 12 hours.

ADVERSE EFFECTS: Sinus bradycardia may be a sign of digoxin toxicity. Any dysrhythmias (paroxysmal ventricular contractions, bradycardia, tachycardia) in a child on digoxin should be considered as digoxin toxicity. The gastrointestinal and CNS symptoms are not frequently seen in children. To manage toxicity, see Digibind.

COMMENTS: Therapeutic levels: 0.5 to 2.0 ng/mL. Considerable overlap exists between toxic and therapeutic serum levels. Digoxin-like immunoreactive substance (DLIS) may cross-react with digoxin immunoassay and falsely increases serum concentrations; DLIS has been found in neonates. Use with caution and reduce dosage in patients with renal impairment; use with caution in patients with sinus nodal disease (may worsen condition). Correct electrolyte disturbances, especially hypokalemia or hypomagnesemia, prior to use and throughout therapy. Hypercalcemia may increase the risk of digoxin toxicity. Contraindicated in second- and third-degree block, idiopathic hypertrophic subaortic stenosis, and atrial flutter or fibrillation with slow ventricular rates.

DOBUTAMINE HCL (DOBUTREX)

INDICATIONS AND USE: To increase cardiac output during states of depressed contractility, such as septic shock, organic heart disease, or cardiac surgical procedures. Treat hypotension and hypoperfusion related to myocardial dysfunction.

ACTIONS: A direct β_1-agonist that increases myocardial contractility, oxygen delivery, and oxygen consumption; actions on β_2- and α-adrenergic receptors are much less marked than those of dopamine. Unlike dopamine, dobutamine does not cause release of endogenous norepinephrine, nor does it have any effect on dopaminergic receptors.

DOSAGE: IV.

- 2 to 20 mcg/kg/min by continuous infusion; titrate gradually to desired response. Maximum: 20 mcg/kg/min.

ADVERSE EFFECTS: Tachycardia and arrhythmias at higher doses, hypotension if patient is hypovolemic, ectopic heartbeats, and elevated blood pressure.

PHARMACOLOGY: Has more prominent effect on cardiac output than dopamine and less effect on blood pressure. Onset of action 1 to 2 minutes; peak effect in 10 minutes. Serum half-life is several minutes. Metabolized in liver and renally excreted.

COMMENTS: Correct hypovolemia prior to initiation of therapy; contraindicated in idiopathic subaortic stenosis and atrial fibrillation. Correct electrolyte abnormalities and monitor throughout therapy to minimize risk of arrhythmias (especially potassium and magnesium).

DOPAMINE HCL

INDICATIONS AND USE: To increase cardiac output, blood pressure, renal perfusion, and glomerular filtration rate (low dosages), which persists despite volume resuscitation.

ACTIONS: Actions are dose dependent. Low doses act directly on dopaminergic receptors to produce renal and mesenteric vasodilation. In moderate doses, β_1-adrenergic effects become prominent, resulting in a positive inotropic effect on the myocardium. High doses stimulate α-adrenergic receptors, producing increased peripheral resistance (vasoconstriction and increased blood pressure) and renal vasoconstriction.

DOSAGE: IV. *Note:* Dose-effect relationship is speculative in neonates.

Continuous IV infusion:

- 1 to 20 mcg/kg/min; titrate to desired response.
- **Low:** 1 to 5 mcg/kg/min may increase renal perfusion and urine output.
- **Moderate:** 5 to 15 mcg/kg/min facilitates increased cardiac output, renal blood flow, heart rate, cardiac contractility, blood pressure.
- **High:** >15 mcg/kg/min causes systemic vasoconstriction and blood pressure.

ADVERSE EFFECTS: Dopamine may cause ectopic heartbeats, tachycardia, ventricular arrhythmias, hypertension, and azotemia. Gangrene of the extremities has occurred with high doses over prolonged periods. **Extravasation may cause tissue necrosis and sloughing of surrounding tissues; if this occurs,** infiltrate area with a small amount (1 mL) of phentolamine, made by diluting 5 to 10 mg in 10 to 15 mL of preservative-free normal saline (NS); do not exceed 0.1 mg/kg or 2.5 mg total for neonates and 0.1 to 0.2 mg/kg or 5 mg total for infants (see Chapter 42).

PHARMACOLOGY: Rapidly metabolized; serum half-life 2 to 5 minutes, variable clearance. Individual developmental differences in endogenous norepinephrine stores; α-adrenergic, β-adrenergic, and dopaminergic receptor function and the ability of the neonatal heart to increase stroke volume will affect response to different dopamine doses.

COMMENTS: Administration of phenytoin IV to patients receiving dopamine may result in severe hypotension and bradycardia; therefore, use with extreme caution. Do not infuse through umbilical arterial catheter or other arterial catheter.

DORNASE ALPHA

INDICATIONS AND USE: Reduce frequency of pulmonary infections and improve pulmonary function in cystic fibrosis patients; treatment of atelectasis as a result of mucous plugging that has failed to respond to conventional therapies.

ACTIONS: Selectively cleaves DNA, resulting in a reduction of the viscosity of mucus in pulmonary secretions.

DOSAGE:
- 2.5 mg/day administered through selected nebulizers

ADVERSE EFFECTS: Airway obstruction secondary to mobilization of secretions in airway, desaturations, fever, cough, dyspnea, wheezing.

PHARMACOLOGY: Recombinant human DNA enzyme; hydrolyzes DNA released by degenerating leukocytes from purulent pulmonary secretions resulting in decreased viscosity.

COMMENTS: Not formally approved for use in infants and children ≤5 years of age; however, studies with small numbers of children as young as 3 months have shown efficacy and similar side effect profile with slightly increased frequency of cough and rhinitis reported in children <5 years old.

DOXAPRAM HCL (DOPRAM)

INDICATIONS AND USE: Apnea of prematurity unresponsive to methylxanthine therapy.

ACTIONS: Stimulates respiration through action on central respiratory centers and reflex stimulation of carotid, aortic, or other peripheral chemoreceptors; decreases PCO_2 and increases minute ventilation and tidal volume without changing respiratory rate or inspiratory and expiratory times.

DOSAGE: IV.
- **Loading dose:** 2.5 to 3 mg/kg IV over 30 minutes followed by maintenance dose.
- **Continuous IV infusion:** 0.5 to 1.5 mg/kg/h (maximum 2.5 mg/kg/h); decrease the infusion rate when control of apnea is achieved.

ADVERSE EFFECTS: Hypertension, QT prolongation with heart block, tachycardia, skeletal muscle hyperactivity, abdominal distention, increased gastric residuals, bloody stools, necrotizing enterocolitis, vomiting, jitteriness, hyperglycemia, and glycosuria.

PHARMACOLOGY: Therapeutic range: 1.5 to 3 mcg/mL (toxicity seen typically at >4–5 mcg/mL). Onset of respiratory stimulation is 20 to 40 seconds; maximum effect is 1 to 2 minutes; duration is 5 to 12 minutes.

COMMENTS: Use cautiously in premature neonates because of its side effects. Avoid use during the first few days of life, when hypertensive episodes may be associated with increased risk of intraventricular hemorrhage; contraindicated in cardiovascular and seizure disorders. Potential adverse effects on mental development have been reported (Lando, 2005; Sreenan, 2001). Doxapram contains benzyl alcohol.

ENALAPRIL (PO)/ENALAPRILAT (IV) (VASOTEC)

INDICATIONS AND USE: Treatment of moderate to severe hypertension and heart failure by reducing left ventricular preload and afterload.

ACTIONS: An angiotensin-converting enzyme inhibitor that acts by inhibiting the conversion of angiotensin I to angiotensin II and results in lower levels of angiotensin II, which causes an increase in plasma renin activity and a reduction in aldosterone secretion and the breakdown of bradykinin, causing vasodilation. Enalapril increases sodium loss, fluid loss, and serum potassium.

DOSAGE: IV, PO.
- **IV:** 5 to 10 mcg/kg/dose every 8 to 24 hours. Maximum dose: 1.25 mg/dose. The frequency depends on blood pressure response. Monitor patient closely.
- **PO:** Initial: 0.04 to 0.3 mg/kg/dose every 12 to 24 hours; initiate at the lower end of the range and titrate to effect as required every few days;

ADVERSE EFFECTS: Hypotension, hyperkalemia, decreased renal function, oliguria, cough, anemia, neutropenia, and angioedema.

PHARMACOLOGY: Onset of action after oral dose is 1 to 2 hours. The duration of action is variable (12–24 hours).

COMMENTS: Use with extreme caution in renal dysfunction; reduce dose. Use a low initial dose to avoid a profound drop in blood pressure, especially in patients on diuretics who are hyponatremic or hypovolemic. Monitor blood pressure hourly for the first 12 hours. Note that the IV dose is much smaller than the PO dose; use caution to adjust the dose when changing route of administration.

ENOXAPARIN (LOVENOX)

INDICATIONS AND USE: Prophylaxis and treatment of thromboembolic disorders. (See Chapter 92.)
ACTIONS: Low molecular weight heparin that potentiates the action of antithrombin III and inactivates coagulation factor Xa and factor IIa (thrombin).
DOSAGE: Subcutaneous.
Initial treatment:
- **Infants <2 months:** 1.5 mg/kg subcutaneous every 12 hours.
- **Infants >2 months and children ≤18 years:** 1 mg/kg subcutaneous every 12 hours.
- **Maintenance:** Adjust dose to maintain antifactor Xa level between 0.5 and 1.0 units/mL. It may take several days to reach target range. Preterm infants may require higher doses to maintain antifactor Xa levels in target range: mean dose of 2 mg/kg every 12 hours, range of 0.8 to 3 mg/kg every 12 hours.

Initial prophylaxis:
- **Infants <2 months:** 0.75 mg/kg subcutaneous every 12 hours.
- **Infants >2 months and children ≤18 years:** 0.5 mg/kg subcutaneous every 12 hours.
- **Maintenance:** Adjust to maintain antifactor Xa level between 0.1 and 0.3 units/mL.

ADVERSE EFFECTS: Bleeding, intracranial hemorrhage, thrombocytopenia (incidence of heparin-induced thrombocytopenia is less than that with heparin therapy). Hematoma, irritation, ecchymosis, and erythema can occur at the injection site.

PHARMACOLOGY: Measure antifactor Xa levels 4 to 6 hours after a dose. After target level is reached, dosage adjustments may be required once or twice a month. Preterm infants and infants with hepatic or renal dysfunction may require more frequent adjustments.

COMMENTS: Compared with standard heparin, enoxaparin has much less activity against thrombin. Low antithrombin plasma concentration reduces the efficacy in neonates. Enoxaparin is less likely to cause thrombocytopenia and osteoporosis.

EPINEPHRINE

INDICATIONS AND USE: Bradycardia, cardiac arrest, cardiogenic shock, anaphylactic reactions, and bronchospasm.
ACTIONS: Acts directly on both α- and β-adrenergic receptors; β₂ effects predominate at lower doses. Exerts both positive chronotropic and inotropic effects on the heart, and relaxes bronchial smooth muscle. The α-adrenergic stimulation increases systolic blood pressure and constricts renal blood vessels.
DOSAGE: IV, ETT.
- **IV bolus:** (0.1 mg/mL) 0.01 to 0.03 mg/kg (0.1–0.3 mL/kg) every 3 to 5 minutes, as needed. Follow administration with a flush of 0.5 to 1 mL of normal saline (NS).

- **IV infusion:** Initial rate: 0.05 to 0.3 mcg/kg/min; titrate to desired response to a maximum of 1 mcg/kg/min.
- **Endotracheal:** 0.05 to 0.1 mg/kg (0.5–1 mL/kg of 0.1 mg/mL solution) every 3 to 5 minutes until IV access is established or return of spontaneous circulation; immediately followed by 1 mL of NS.
- **Nebulization:** 0.25 to 0.5 mL of 2.25% racemic epinephrine diluted in 2 to 3 mL of NS.

ADVERSE EFFECTS: Hypertension, tachycardia, nausea, pallor, tremor, cardiac arrhythmias, increased myocardial oxygen consumption, and decreased renal and splanchnic blood flow.

ERYTHROMYCIN

ACTION AND SPECTRUM: Macrolide antibiotic; bactericidal or bacteriostatic depending on the tissue concentration of drug and the microorganism. Spectrum of activity is broad and includes susceptible streptococci and staphylococci; also *Mycoplasma, Legionella*, pertussis, *Chlamydia*, and *Campylobacter* gastroenteritis.

DOSAGE: PO, IV, ocular.

Neonates:
- **Oral ethylsuccinate form, PNA:**
- **Body weight <1 kg:**
  - **PNA ≤14 days:** 10 mg/kg/dose PO every 12 hours.
  - **PNA 15 to 28 days:** 10 mg/kg/dose PO every 8 hours.
- **Body weight ≥1 kg**
  - **PNA ≤7 days:** 10 mg/kg/dose PO every 12 hours.
  - **PNA 8 to 28 days:** 10 mg/kg/dose PO every 8 hours.
- **IV lactobionate form:** 5 to 10 mg/kg/dose every 6 hours for severe infections or when PO route is unavailable.
- **Chlamydial conjunctivitis or pneumonia:** Oral: ethylsuccinate 50 mg/kg/day divided every 6 hours for 14 days (based on AAP *Red Book*, 2018–2021).
- **Pertussis; treatment or postexposure prophylaxis:** Oral: ethylsuccinate 10 mg/kg/dose every 6 hours for 14 days (AAP *Red Book*, 2018–2021).

Infants and children:
- **Oral base and ethylsuccinate:** 30 to 50 mg/kg/day PO divided every 6 to 8 hours; do not exceed 2 g/day (as base) or 3.2 g/day (as ethylsuccinate). *Note:* 200 mg erythromycin ethylsuccinate produces the same serum levels as 125 mg erythromycin base due to absorptive differences.
- **IV lactobionate:** 15 to 20 mg/kg/day IV divided every 6 hours, not to exceed 4 g/day.
- **Stearate:** 30 to 50 mg/kg/day PO divided every 6 hours; maximum 2 g/day.
- *Chlamydia trachomatis:* Infants and children <45 kg: 50 mg/kg/day PO divided every 6 hours for 14 days; maximum 2 g/day.
- **Pertussis treatment or postexposure prophylaxis:** Ethylsuccinate: 40 mg/kg/day divided every 6 hours for 14 days. *Note:* Azithromycin considered first-line agent in infants <1 month of age; erythromycin is associated with infantile hypertrophic pyloric stenosis in neonates (based on AAP *Red Book*. 2018–2021).
- **Ophthalmic prophylaxis:** 0.5- to 1-cm ribbon in each eye once. (See also Chapter 58.)
- **Ophthalmic for acute infection:** 0.5- to 1-cm ribbon in each eye every 6 hours. (See also Chapter 58.)
- **Gastrointestinal motility disorders:** 1.5 to 10 mg/kg/dose PO every 6 to 8 hours, 30 minutes before feedings; in neonates up to 2 weeks old, exposure to high doses (30–50 mg/kg/day) for ≥14 days has been associated with a 10-fold increase in the risk of hypertrophic pyloric stenosis. May be given IV 1 to 3 mg/kg infused over 60 minutes, but PO is preferred route.

ADVERSE EFFECTS: Infantile hypertrophic pyloric stenosis, stomatitis, epigastric distress, transient cholestatic hepatitis, and allergic reactions occur rarely. Cardiac toxicity requiring cardiopulmonary resuscitation may occur with IV erythromycin; reduce risk of arrhythmias by slowly infusing over 1 hour.

PHARMACOLOGY: Hepatic metabolism, excreted via the bile and kidneys. Half-life is 1.5 to 3 hours (prolonged in renal failure). May cause increased serum levels of theophylline, digoxin, and carbamazepine.
COMMENTS: Parenteral forms are painful and irritating; dilute to 5 mg/mL and infuse >60 minutes. Do not use IM.

ERYTHROPOIETIN/EPOETIN ALFA (EPOGEN, PROCRIT) [EPO, REPO]

> **WARNING:** ESAs increase the risk of death, myocardial infarction, stroke, venous thromboembolism, thrombosis of vascular access and tumor progression or recurrence.

INDICATIONS AND USE: To stimulate erythropoiesis and decrease the need for erythrocyte transfusions (rEpo) in preterm infants; treatment of anemia of prematurity.
ACTIONS: Epoetin alfa (EPO) induces erythropoiesis by stimulating division and differentiation of committed erythroid progenitor cells; induces release of reticulocytes from the bone marrow into the bloodstream where they mature to erythrocytes (dose-response relationship).
DOSAGE: Subcutaneous, IV.
- **Anemia of prematurity:** 200 to 400 units/kg/dose, 3 to 5 times per week, for 2 to 6 weeks. Total dose per week: 150 to 1500 units/kg/wk. Short course: 250 units/kg/dose 3 times weekly × 10 doses.
- **Neuroprotective/hypoxic ischemia encephalopathy:**
  - **Low dose:** 300 or 500 units/kg/dose every other day for 2 weeks beginning within first 48 hours of life
  - **High dose:** 1000 or 2500 units/kg/dose once daily for 3 to 5 days beginning within 24 hours of life

ADVERSE EFFECTS: May cause hypertension, edema, fever, rash, possible seizures, transient early thrombocytosis and late neutropenia, polycythemia, and local skin reaction at injection site.
PHARMACOLOGY: Noticeable effects on hematocrit and reticulocyte counts occur within 2 weeks. Half-life in neonates: subcutaneous: 7.6 to 19.4 hours.
COMMENTS: Supplement with oral iron therapy 3 to 8 mg/kg/day; optimal response is achieved when iron stores are adequate. EPO should be used in conjunction with restrictive transfusion guidelines and minimizing of phlebotomy losses. EPO is not a substitute for emergency blood transfusion. Do not use in patients with uncontrolled hypertension.

ESMOLOL

INDICATIONS AND USE: Treatment of supraventricular tachycardia (SVT); acute management of postoperative tachycardia and hypertension.
ACTIONS: Competitively blocks response to β_1-adrenergic stimulation with little or no effect on β_2-receptors except at high doses.
DOSAGE: IV.
Neonatal (limited data available):
- **SVT:** 100 mcg/kg/min by continuous infusion; adjust dose based on individual clinical response and tolerance. Increase by 50 to 100 mcg/kg/min every 5 minutes until ventricular rate is controlled.
- **Postoperative tachycardia and hypertension:**
  - **≤7 days:** 50 mcg/kg/min by continuous infusion; increase by 25 to 50 mcg/kg/min every 20 minutes until target blood pressure is reached.
  - **8 to 28 days:** 75 mcg/kg/min by continuous infusion; increase by 50 mcg/kg/min every 20 minutes until target blood pressure is reached.
- **Maximum dosage:** 1000 mcg/kg/min.
Infants and children (limited data available):
- **SVT:** 100 to 500 mcg/kg over 1 minute; initial rate 25 to 100 mcg/kg/min; titrate infusion rate by 25 to 50 mcg/kg/min every 5 to 10 minutes until ventricular rate is controlled.

- **Postoperative tachycardia and hypertension:** Loading dose of 100 to 500 mcg/kg/min over 1 minute followed by continuous infusion of 100 to 500 mcg/kg/min; titrate infusion rate by 50 mcg/kg/min every 10 minutes until target blood pressure is reached.
- **Maximum dose:** 1000 mcg/kg/min.

ADVERSE EFFECTS: Hypotension and bradycardia at higher doses; peripheral ischemia, agitation, local induration, inflammation phlebitis, and skin necrosis after extravasation.

PHARMACOLOGY: Ultra-short-acting β_1-selective blocking agent with half-life of 2.8 to 4.5 minutes and duration of action of 10 to 30 minutes. Onset of action ranges from 2 to 10 minutes; shorter if loading dose is given.

COMMENTS: Monitor IV site for infiltration, especially with the use of concentrations >10 mg/mL.

ETHACRYNIC ACID (EDECRIN)

> **WARNING:** Ethacrynic acid is a potent diuretic that, if given in excessive amounts, may lead to profound diuresis with water and electrolyte depletion. Therefore, careful medical supervision is required, and dose and dose schedule must be adjusted to the individual patient's needs.

INDICATIONS AND USE: Reserved for use only when other diuretics have failed to produce effective diuresis due to toxicities.

ACTIONS: Loop diuretic that inhibits reabsorption of sodium and chloride in ascending loop of Henle and distal tubules, resulting in increased excretion of water, sodium, chloride, magnesium, and calcium. The inhibition of sodium reabsorption is greater than that of other diuretics. Also, there is not a direct effect on the pulmonary vasculature, as seen with furosemide.

DOSAGE: IV, PO.
- **IV:** 0.5 to 1 mg/kg/dose. Repeat doses are not routinely recommended; however, if indicated, repeat doses every 8 to 12 hours.
- **PO:** 1 mg/kg/dose once daily; increase at intervals of 2 to 3 days to a maximum of 3 mg/kg/day.

ADVERSE EFFECTS: Inject IV dose slowly over several minutes; may cause hypotension, dehydration, electrolyte depletion, diarrhea, gastrointestinal bleeding, hearing loss, rash, local irritation and pain, hematuria, and, rarely, hypoglycemia and neutropenia.

COMMENTS: Close medical supervision and dose evaluation are required; may increase risk of gastric hemorrhage associated with corticosteroid treatment.

FAMOTIDINE (PEPCID)

> **Caution:** Use of proton pump inhibitors and H2 blockers have been associated with an increased risk for developing acute gastroenteritis and community-acquired pneumonia in children (Canani, 2006). A cohort analysis with over 11,000 neonates reported an increased incidence of NEC in VLBW neonates associated with H2 blockers use (Guillet, 2006). An approximate six-fold increase in mortality, NEC, and infection (ie, sepsis, pneumonia, UTI) was reported in patients receiving ranitidine in a cohort analysis of 274 VLBW neonates (Terrin, 2012).

INDICATIONS AND USE: Prevention and short-term treatment of gastroesophageal reflux disease (GERD), stress, gastric and duodenal ulcers, and gastrointestinal (GI) hemorrhage.

ACTIONS: Inhibits gastric acid secretion by reversible, competitive antagonism of histamine on the H_2 receptor of the gastric parietal cells.

DOSAGE: IV, PO (neonatal dosing).
- **Stress ulcer prophylaxis/gastric acid suppression:** IV 0.25 to 0.5 mg/kg/dose every 24 hours via slow IV push.
- **GERD/gastric acid suppression:** PO 0.5 mg/kg/dose once daily; may increase to 1 mg/kg/dose once daily if ineffective with lower dose.

ADVERSE EFFECTS: Hypotension and cardiac arrhythmias with rapid IV administration; agitation, constipation, diarrhea, necrotizing enterocolitis (very low birthweight neonates), vomiting, tachycardia, thrombocytopenia, elevated liver enzymes, and cholestatic jaundice.
PHARMACOLOGY: Onset of GI effect is within 1 hour. Duration is 10 to 12 hours. Elimination with IV administration is 65% to 70% unchanged in urine versus 25% to 30% unchanged in urine with PO administration.
COMMENTS: Limited experience in infants and children. Famotidine does not inhibit cytochrome P450. Prolonged treatment (ie, ≥2 years) may result in vitamin B12 deficiency due to dietary vitamin B12 malabsorption (Lam et al, 2013). Dosing adjustment is recommended in patients with moderate to severe renal impairment.

FENTANYL (SUBLIMAZE)

INDICATIONS AND USE: Analgesia, anesthesia, and sedation.
ACTIONS: A synthetic opiate agonist that binds to the opioid μ-receptors within the CNS, increases the pain threshold, alters pain reception, and inhibits ascending pain pathway. Acts similarly to morphine and meperidine but without the cardiovascular effects of those drugs and with shorter respiratory depressant effects.
DOSAGE: IV.
Neonates:
- **Analgesia:** World Health Organization Guidelines for Pediatric Pain (2012).
  - **Intermittent doses:** Slow IV push: 1 to 2 mcg/kg/dose and may repeat every 2 to 4 hours as needed.
  - **Continuous infusion:** Initial 1 to 2 mcg/kg IV bolus, followed by 0.5 to 1 mcg/kg/h. May titrate up to 3 mcg/kg/h.

Continuous analgesia/sedation in mechanically ventilated patient: Initial 1 to 2 mcg/kg IV bolus, followed by 0.5 to 1 mcg/kg/h; titrate to effect.
Continuous sedation/analgesia during extracorporeal life support (ECLS): Initial IV bolus: 5 to 10 mcg/kg slow IV push over 10 minutes, then 1 to 5 mcg/kg/h; titrate to effect; tolerance may develop; higher doses (up to 20 mcg/kg/h) may be needed by day 6 of ECLS.
Endotracheal intubation: Slow IV push: 1 to 4 mcg/kg.
ADVERSE EFFECTS: CNS and respiratory depression (US boxed warning); hypotension, bradycardia; seizures; skeletal muscle and chest wall rigidity with reduced pulmonary compliance, apnea, and laryngospasm, which is reversible with naloxone. Tolerance and withdrawal symptoms reported with continuous use. Urinary retention, gastrointestinal symptoms, and biliary spasms may occur.
PHARMACOLOGY: Metabolized in liver by CYP3A4 enzyme and excreted primarily by kidneys as inactive metabolites. Clearance may be significantly correlated to birthweight and gestational age in newborn infants. Liver failure prolongs serum half-life; 79% to 87% protein bound; highly lipid soluble. The volume of distribution and half-life are highly variable.
COMMENTS: Synthetic opioid narcotic analgesic that is 50 to 100 times more potent on a weight basis than morphine. Concurrent ventilatory assistance is suggested with its use. Tachyphylaxis occurs after several days of therapy. Adheres to ECLS filter membranes; may have to adjust the dose. Neonates who receive a total fentanyl dose >1.6 mg/kg or continuous infusion duration >5 days have increased risk of developing opioid withdrawal symptoms. Infants and children age 1 week to 22 months who receive a total dose of 1.5 mg/kg or duration >5 days have a 50% chance of developing opioid withdrawal; those receiving a total dose >2.5 mg/kg or duration of infusion >9 days have a 100% chance of developing withdrawal.

FERROUS SULFATE (20% ELEMENTAL IRON)

INDICATIONS AND USE: Treatment and prevention of iron deficiency anemia; supplemental therapy for patients receiving epoetin alfa.

ACTIONS: Iron is required for production of heme proteins. Iron is released from the plasma to replenish the depleted stores in the bone marrow where it is incorporated into hemoglobin.

DOSAGE: PO. Recommendations of the American Academy of Pediatrics (AAP) for treatment and prevention of iron deficiency in breastfed infants; dosages are for **elemental iron.**

- **Term infants:** 1 mg/kg/day divided every 12 to 24 hours. Begin at 4 months of age.
- **Preterm infants:** 2 to 4 mg/kg/day divided every 12 to 24 hours. Begin therapy by 1 month of age after vitamin E level are restored.
- **Iron deficiency anemia:** 4 to 6 mg/kg/day in 3 divided doses.
- **Iron supplementation with erythropoietin:** 6 mg/kg/day in 1 or 2 divided doses.

ADVERSE EFFECTS: Gastrointestinal irritation (vomiting, diarrhea, constipation, and darkened stool color).

COMMENTS: The use of iron-fortified formulas during the first year of life usually prevents iron deficiency anemia in both preterm and term infants. Iron-fortified formulas can be fed safely to preterm infants. Of the ferrous salts available (sulfate, fumarate, and gluconate), sulfate is preferred. *Note :* Multiple concentrations of ferrous sulfate oral liquid exist. Caution parents to guard against iron poisoning from accidental ingestion. Antidote is chelation with deferoxamine; consult specialized references and regional poison control center for further information.

FILGRASTIM (GRANULOCYTE COLONY-STIMULATING FACTOR [G-CSF])

INDICATIONS AND USE: For the reduction of neutropenia in neonates with sepsis or congenital neutropenia.

ACTIONS: Stimulates the production, maturation, and activation of neutrophil granulocytes and activates neutrophils to enhance both their migration and cytotoxicity.

DOSAGE: IV or subcutaneous.

- **Neutropenia with sepsis:** 10 mcg/kg/day in 1 or 2 divided doses for 3 to 14 days with 3-day regimen being the most used.
- **Neutropenia, infection prophylaxis:** 5 to 10 mcg/kg/day once daily for 3 to 5 days.
- **Neutropenia, congenital:** Subcutaneous with initial dose at 5 mcg/kg/day, then 10 mcg/kg/day. May titrate up by 10 mcg/kg/day every 2 weeks to maintain goal absolute neutrophil count (ANC) with maximum dose at 120 mcg/kg/day. Reduce to the lowest effective dose if ANC >5000/mm^3.

ADVERSE EFFECTS: Thrombocytopenia, anemia, leukocytosis, increase in serum alkaline phosphatase, and transient decrease in blood pressure.

PHARMACOLOGY: There is an immediate transient leukopenia with nadir occurring 5 to 15 minutes after an IV dose or 30 to 60 minutes after a subcutaneous dose followed by a sustained elevation in neutrophil levels within the first 24 hours, which plateaus in 3 to 5 days. Following discontinuation of granulocyte colony-stimulating factor, ANC decreases by 50% within 2 days and returns to pretreatment levels within 1 week; WBC counts return to normal range in 4 to 7 days.

FLECAINIDE

> **WARNING:** Should only be used for sustained, life-threatening arrhythmias that have not responded to conventional therapies.

INDICATIONS AND USE: Prevention and treatment of sustained, life-threatening ventricular arrhythmias; prophylaxis of paroxysmal atrial flutter and fibrillation and supraventricular tachycardia. Contraindicated in patients with structural heart disease.

ACTIONS: Class 1C antiarrhythmic that slows conduction throughout the myocardium, with the greatest effect on the His-Purkinje system.

DOSAGE: PO.

- **Supraventricular tachycardia:** Initial dose 2 mg/kg/day divided into 2 doses; titrate dose based on response up to 8 mg/kg/day divided into 2 doses.
- **Arrhythmias:** Initial dose: 1 to 3 mg/kg/day divided into 2 or 3 doses; maintenance dose of 3 to 6 mg/kg/day up to 8 mg/kg/day divided into 2 or 3 doses. Titrate dose based on response. Higher doses have been associated with increased risk of proarrhythmias.

ADVERSE EFFECTS: May cause new or worsening ventricular arrhythmias, heart block, bradycardia, torsade de pointes, dizziness, blurred vision, headache, blood dyscrasias, and hepatic dysfunction.

PHARMACOLOGY: Demonstrates both local anesthetic and moderate negative inotropic effects. Reduction in conduction throughout the myocardium results in increased PR, QRS, and QT intervals. Infant formula and milk products may inhibit absorption. Elimination half-life in children <1 year of age is approximately 11 to 12 hours, and in newborns and after maternal administration, it is approximately 29 hours. Half-life is increased with congestive heart failure or renal impairment.

COMMENTS: Therapeutic trough concentration: 0.2 to 1 mcg/mL. Obtain serum concentration at steady state (at least 5 doses administered) after initiation or dose adjustment. Milk consumption can interfere with drug absorption, and monitoring of serum trough levels during major changes in dietary milk intake is recommended.

FLUCONAZOLE (DIFLUCAN)

INDICATIONS AND USE: Antifungal agent for treatment of susceptible fungal infections including oropharyngeal and esophageal candidiasis; treatment of systemic candidal infections including urinary tract infection, peritonitis, cystitis, and pneumonia. There continues to be an increased number of strains of *Candida* isolated with decreased susceptibility to fluconazole. Fluconazole is more active against *Candida albicans* than other *Candida* strains such as *Candida parapsilosis*, *Candida glabrata*, and *Candida tropicalis*; alternative to amphotericin B in patients with preexisting renal impairment or when requiring concomitant therapy with other potentially nephrotoxic drugs.

ACTIONS: Interferes with fungal cytochrome P450 and sterol C-14 α-demethylation, resulting in a fungistatic effect.

DOSAGE: IV, PO.

Treatment for systemic invasive candidiasis:

- **PNA <8 days:** 12 to 25 mg/kg IV loading dose, then 12 mg/kg IV/PO every 48 hours.
- **PNA ≥8 days:** 12 to 25 mg/kg IV loading dose, then 12 mg/kg IV/PO every 24 hours.

Treatment for oral thrush/esophageal disease in term neonates:

- **PNA ≤14 days:** 6 mg/kg loading dose, then 3 mg/kg IV/PO every 24 to 72 hours for a minimum of 14 to 21 days, depending on indication and clinical response.
- **PNA >14 days:** 6 mg/kg loading dose, then 3 mg/kg IV/PO every 24 hours for a minimum of 14 to 21 days, depending on indication and clinical response.

Cryptococcal meningitis:

- **PNA >14 days:** 12 mg/kg loading dose, then 6 to 12 mg/kg IV/PO every 24 hours for a minimum of 10 weeks after the first negative CSF culture.

Candidiasis prophylaxis (IV/PO):

- **<30 weeks' gestation and PNA at the time of therapy initiation:**
  - **PNA <7 days:** 3 or 6 mg/kg/dose IV twice weekly for 6 weeks is recommended in extremely low birthweight infants at increased risk of invasive fungal infection (eg, nurseries with >10% of invasive candidiasis) per Infectious Diseases Society of America clinical practice guideline 2016 update. Dose of 6 mg/kg may be used if targeting *Candida* strains with higher minimal inhibitory concentrations >2 mcg/mL.
  - **PNA ≥7 to 42 days:** 3 mg/kg/dose every 24 hours or 6 mg/kg/dose every 72 hours.
  - **PNA >42 days:** 6 mg/kg/dose every 48 hours.
- **30 to 40 weeks' gestation:** 6 mg/kg/dose every 48 hours.

ADVERSE EFFECTS: Usually well tolerated. Vomiting, diarrhea, rash, and elevations in liver transaminases. Eosinophilia, leukopenia, thrombocytopenia, neutropenia.

PHARMACOLOGY: Good oral bioavailability; absorption not affected by food, with peak serum concentrations achieved in 1 to 2 hours; good penetration into tissues and body fluids including CSF. Less than 12% protein bound; primarily excreted unchanged in urine.

COMMENTS: Reduce dose in renal dysfunction. Use caution in preexisting renal dysfunction. Monitor liver function tests. Cimetidine and rifampin decrease fluconazole levels. Hydrochlorothiazide increases fluconazole area under the curve. Fluconazole interferes with the metabolism of barbiturates, theophylline, midazolam, phenytoin, and zidovudine. Contraindicated in patients receiving cisapride.

FLUCYTOSINE (ANCOBON)

> **WARNING:** Use with extreme caution in renally impaired patients and monitor closely for hematologic, renal, and hepatic toxicity.

ACTION AND SPECTRUM: Antifungal agent that penetrates fungal cells and is converted to fluorouracil, which competes with uracil interfering with fungal RNA and protein synthesis. Used in combination with amphotericin B in the treatment of serious *Candida* or cryptococcal pulmonary or urinary tract infections, sepsis, meningitis, or endocarditis (resistance emerges if flucytosine is used as a single agent); used in combination with another antifungal agent for treatment of chromomycosis and aspergillosis.

DOSAGE: PO. Monitoring of serum drug levels is highly recommended.
- **Neonates:**
  - **General dosing:**
    - **Weight <1 kg and postnatal age ≤14 days:** 75 mg/kg/day divided in 3 doses.
    - **Weight <1 kg and postnatal age 15 to 28 days:** 75 mg/kg/day divided in 4 doses.
    - **Weight 1 to 2 kg and postnatal age ≤7 days:** 75 mg/kg/day divided in 3 doses.
    - **Weight 1 to 2 kg and postnatal age 8 to 28 days:** 75 mg/kg/day divided in 4 doses.
    - **Weight >2 kg and postnatal age ≤60 days:** 75 mg/kg/day divided in 4 doses.
- **Candidal meningitis:** 75 to 100 mg/kg/day divided in 3 to 4 doses in combination with amphotericin B.
- **Infants and children:** 50 to 150 mg/kg/day PO divided every 6 hours.
- **Renal impairment:** Use lower initial dose.
  - **Creatinine clearance 30 to 50 mL/min/1.73 m²:** Usual dose every 8 hours.
  - **Creatinine clearance 10 to 29 mL/min/1.72 m²:** Usual dose every 12 hours.
  - **Creatinine clearance <10 mL/min/1.72 m²:** Usual dose every 24 hours.

ADVERSE EFFECTS: Vomiting, diarrhea, rash, anemia, leukopenia, thrombocytopenia, elevated liver enzymes and bilirubin, increased blood urea nitrogen and creatinine, renal failure, CNS disturbances and cardiotoxicity.

PHARMACOLOGY: Obtain peak level 2 hours after dose and desired peak serum concentration: 50 to 100 mcg/mL or obtain trough level just prior to dose and desired trough serum concentration: 25 to 50 mcg/mL. Half-life, neonates: 4 to 34 hours. Renal elimination.

COMMENTS: Toxicities related to serum concentration >100 mcg/mL and usually reversible when drug is discontinued or dose is reduced. Amphotericin B may increase toxicity by decreasing renal excretion. Liquid formulation of flucytosine is not commercially available.

FLUDROCORTISONE

INDICATIONS AND USE: Used for partial replacement therapy for adrenocortical insufficiency and used in conjunction with hydrocortisone in patients with salt-losing forms of congenital adrenogenital syndrome.

ACTIONS: Fludrocortisone is a potent mineralocorticoid with glucocorticoid activity that acts on the renal distal tubules to enhance loss of potassium and hydrogen ion and increase reabsorption of sodium with subsequent water retention.

DOSAGE: PO.

Congenital adrenal hyperplasia (salt losers):

- **Neonates:** Maintenance: 0.05 to 0.2 mg/day in 1 to 2 divided doses in combination with sodium supplementation.
- **Infants/children:** Maintenance: 0.05 to 0.3 mg/day in 1 to 2 divided doses with or without concurrent glucocorticoid and sodium supplementation (American Academy of Pediatrics, Section on Endocrinology and Committee on Genetics, 2000).

ADVERSE EFFECTS: Hypertension, congestive heart failure, abdominal distention, seizure, hypokalemia, growth suppression, hyperglycemia, salt and water retention, edema, hypothalamic-pituitary-adrenal suppression, osteoporosis, and muscle weakness resulting from excessive potassium loss. Monitor serum electrolytes (particularly sodium and potassium).

COMMENTS: Fludrocortisone 0.1 mg has a sodium retention activity equal to deoxycorticosterone acetate 1 mg. May administer with feeds.

FLUMAZENIL

> **WARNING:** Flumazenil has been associated with the occurrence of seizures. These are most frequent in patients who have been on benzodiazepines for long-term sedation or in overdose cases where patients are showing signs of serious cyclic antidepressant overdose. Individualize the dosage of flumazenil injection and be prepared to manage seizures.

INDICATIONS AND USE: Reversal of benzodiazepine sedative effect; management of benzodiazepine overdose.

ACTIONS: Competitive inhibition of effects of benzodiazepines on the γ-aminobutyric acid (GABA)/benzodiazepine receptor complex and does not reverse opioids effects.

DOSAGE: IV.

- **Intermittent dosing:** 0.01 mg/kg up to a maximum of 0.2 mg IV over 15 seconds; may repeat after 45 seconds and then every minute until patient is awake. The maximum total cumulative dose is 0.05 mg/kg or 1 mg, whichever is lower.
- **Continuous IV infusion:** 0.005 to 0.01 mg/kg/h (as an alternative to repeat bolus doses).
- **Benzodiazepine-induced myoclonus:** 0.0078 mg/kg/dose for 1 dose.

ADVERSE EFFECTS: Very limited data in neonates; hypotension, arrhythmias reported in adults. Use with caution in patients with preexisting seizure disorders. May precipitate acute withdrawal in patients with long-term benzodiazepine exposure.

PHARMACOLOGY: Highly lipid soluble. In children, peak concentration is achieved in 3 minutes and half-life is 20 to 75 minutes. There are very limited data in neonates.

COMMENTS: Administer IV through a large vein to minimize pain on injection and phlebitis. Monitor injection site for extravasation.

FOLIC ACID

INDICATIONS AND USE: Treatment of anemia due to nutritional deficit, prematurity, megaloblastic anemia, or macrocytic anemia.

ACTIONS: Required for formation of a number of coenzymes in many metabolic systems, specifically for purine and pyrimidine synthesis, nucleoprotein synthesis, and maintenance of erythropoiesis. Also stimulates white blood cell and platelet production in folate deficiency anemia.

DOSAGE: PO, IM, IV, subcutaneous.

Recommended daily allowance (Vanek, 2012):

- **Premature neonates:** 25 to 50 mcg/kg/day PO or 56 mcg/kg/day IV via parental nutrition.
- **Full-term neonates:** 65 mcg/day PO or 140 mcg/day IV via parental nutrition.
- **Neonates to 6 months:** 25 to 35 mcg/day PO.

Folic acid deficiency (PO, IM, IV, subcutaneous):

- **Infants:** 0.1 mg/day.
- **Children <4 years:** Up to 0.3 mg/day.

ADVERSE EFFECTS: Generally well tolerated.

PHARMACOLOGY: Absorbed in the proximal portion of small intestine; metabolized in the liver and renally eliminated.

FOLINIC ACID/LEUCOVORIN CALCIUM

CAUTION: May be confused with folic acid.

INDICATIONS: Adjunctive treatment with sulfadiazine and pyrimethamine to prevent hematologic toxicity; antidote for folic acid antagonist overdosage; treatment of folinic acid–responsive seizures and treatment of megaloblastic anemias secondary to folic acid deficiency.

ACTIONS: Folinic acid is a derivative of tetrahydrofolic acid, a reduced form of folic acid; enables purine and thymidine synthesis; required for normal erythropoiesis.

DOSAGE: PO, IV.

Folic acid antagonist overdosage (eg, pyrimethamine, trimethoprim):

- 5 to 15 mg PO/IV per day for 3 days or until blood counts are normal.

Adjunctive treatment with sulfadiazine to prevent pyrimethamine hematologic toxicity: For congenital toxoplasmosis:

- **Human immunodeficiency virus (HIV) exposed or positive:**
  - **Neonates, infants, and children:** 10 mg IM/PO with each pyrimethamine dose for 12 months.
  - **Non–HIV exposed or positive:**
  - **Neonates, infants, and children:** 10 mg IM/PO 3 times weekly for 12 months.

Folinic acid–dependent seizures (limited data):

- 2.5 to 5 mg PO twice a day; may titrate dose up to 8 mg/kg/day (ie, 25 mg PO 3 times a day), as reported in a small case series.

ADVERSE EFFECT: Thrombocytosis, erythema, and wheezing.

PHARMACOLOGY: Onset of action following oral dose is within 30 minutes; IV administration is within 5 minutes. Metabolism: Folinic acid is rapidly converted to 5-methyl-tetrahydrofolate, an active metabolite, in the intestinal mucosa and liver.

FOSPHENYTOIN (CEREBYX)

INDICATIONS AND USE: Management of generalized convulsive status epilepticus; used for short-term parenteral administration of phenytoin, prevention and management of seizures.

ACTIONS AND SPECTRUM: Fosphenytoin is a water-soluble prodrug of phenytoin that is rapidly converted by phosphatases in blood and tissues.

DOSAGE: IM, IV (fosphenytoin 1 mg phenytoin equivalent [PE] = phenytoin 1 mg).

- **Loading dose:** 15 to 20 mg PE/kg IM or IV infusion over at least 10 minutes.
- **Maintenance dose:** 4 to 10 mg PE/kg/day divided every 12 hours IM or IV over at least 10 minutes. Start maintenance dose ≥12 hours after loading dose.

ADVERSE EFFECTS: Hypotension (with rapid IV administration), vasodilation, tachycardia, bradycardia, drowsiness, anemia, thrombocytopenia, and fever.

PHARMACOLOGY: Conversion to phenytoin half-life is approximately 7 minutes. Fosphenytoin is highly protein bound. (Caution in neonates with hyperbilirubinemia: Both fosphenytoin and bilirubin displace phenytoin from protein-binding sites, which results in increased serum-free phenytoin concentrations.)

COMMENTS: Dilute with 5% dextrose in water (D5W) or normal saline (NS) to 1.5 to 25 mg PE/mL. Maximum rate of infusion is 2 mg PE/kg/min. Flush IV with saline before and after administration. Monitor blood pressure during infusion. Wait at least 2 hours after end of the loading dose infusion prior to drawing a serum phenytoin concentration.

FUROSEMIDE (LASIX)

INDICATIONS AND USE: Fluid overload, pulmonary edema, congestive heart failure, and hypertension.

ACTIONS: Inhibits reabsorption of sodium and chloride in the ascending limb of the loop of Henle and proximal and distal rental tubules. Furosemide-induced diuresis results in enhanced excretion of sodium, chloride, potassium, calcium, magnesium, bicarbonate, ammonium, hydrogen, and possibly phosphate. Nondiuretic effects include decreased pulmonary transvascular fluid filtration and improved pulmonary function.

DOSAGE: PO, IM, IV.

Neonates, premature:
- **PO:** 1 to 2 mg/kg/dose 1 to 2 times a day as initial dose has been used, and increase slowly if needed; highly variable oral bioavailability.
- **IV or IM:** 1 to 2 mg/kg/dose every 12 to 24 hours.

Infants and children:
- **Oral:** 2 mg/kg PO once daily; if effective, may increase in increments of 1 to 2 mg/kg/dose every 6 to 8 hours; not to exceed 6 mg/kg/dose. In most cases, it is unnecessary to exceed individual doses of 4 mg/kg or a dosing frequency of once or twice daily.
- **IM, IV:** 1 to 2 mg/kg/dose every 6 to 12 hours.
- **Continuous infusion:** 0.05 to 0.2 mg/kg/h; titrate in 0.1 mg/kg/h increments every 12 to 24 hours to a maximum infusion rate of 0.4 mg/kg/h.

ADVERSE EFFECTS: Hypokalemia, hypocalcemia, hyponatremia, hypercalciuria; and with prolonged use, nephrocalcinosis and hypochloremic metabolic alkalosis. Ototoxicity is possible, especially in association with concurrent use of aminoglycosides.

PHARMACOLOGY: Onset of action: oral within 30 to 60 minutes; IV 5 minutes. Duration of action: oral dose is 6 to 8 hours; IV dose is 2 hours.

GANCICLOVIR (CYTOVENE IV)

INDICATIONS AND USE: Symptomatic congenital cytomegalovirus (CMV) infection for the prevention of progressive hearing loss and decreased developmental delay.

ACTIONS AND SPECTRUM: An acyclic nucleoside structurally related to acyclovir, possesses antiviral activity against herpes viruses. Ganciclovir is a prodrug that is phosphorylated to a substrate that inhibits viral DNA synthesis by competitive inhibition of viral DNA polymerases and incorporation into viral DNA, resulting in eventual termination of viral DNA elongation. Ganciclovir is preferentially metabolized in virus-infected cells.

DOSAGE: IV.
- **Neonates:** 6 mg/kg/dose every 12 hours IV, infused over 1 hour. Treat for a minimum of 6 weeks. Reduce dose by half for significant neutropenia (<500 cells/mm^3).

ADVERSE EFFECTS: Edema, arrhythmias, hypertension, seizures, sedation, vomiting, diarrhea, neutropenia, thrombocytopenia, leukopenia, anemia, eosinophilia, elevated liver enzymes, phlebitis, retinal detachment in patients with CMV retinitis, hematuria, elevated blood urea nitrogen and serum creatinine, and dyspnea.

PHARMACOLOGY: Oral bioavailability is poor. Renal excretion is the major route of elimination; primarily excreted unchanged in the urine via glomerular filtration and active tubular secretion.

COMMENTS: Handle and dispose according to guidelines issued for cytotoxic drugs; avoid direct contact of skin or mucous membranes with the powder contained in capsules or the IV solution. Dosage adjustment or interruption of ganciclovir therapy may be necessary in patients with neutropenia and/or thrombocytopenia and patients with impaired renal function.

GANCICLOVIR OPHTHALMIC

See Chapter 58.

GENTAMICIN OPHTHALMIC

See Chapter 58.

GENTAMICIN SULFATE

ACTION AND SPECTRUM: Aminoglycoside with bactericidal activity by binding to 30S ribosomal subunit interfering with bacterial protein synthesis. It is active against gram-negative aerobic bacteria, including most *Pseudomonas*, *Proteus*, and *Serratia*. Some activity against coagulase-positive staphylococci, but ineffective against anaerobes and streptococci.

DOSAGE: IV, IM, intrathecal, intraventricular. Base the initial dose on body weight, then monitor levels and adjust using pharmacokinetics. Many dosing strategies exist such as extended interval, age based, weight based, and traditional.

Age based:
- **≤30 weeks' gestational age:**
  - **PNA ≤14 days:** 5 mg/kg/dose IV/IM every 48 hours.
  - **PNA ≥15 days:** 5 mg/kg/dose IV/IM every 36 hours.
- **30 to 34 weeks' gestational age:**
  - **PNA ≤10 days:** 4.5 mg/kg/dose IV/IM every 36 hours.
  - **PNA ≥11 days:** 5 mg/kg/dose IV/IM every 36 hours.
- **≥35 weeks' gestational age:**
  - **PNA ≤7 days:** 4 mg/kg/dose IV/IM every 24 hours.
  - **PNA ≥8 days:** 5 mg/kg/dose IV/IM every 24 hours.

Intrathecal or intraventricular (use preservative-free):
- **Newborns:** 1 mg/day.
- **Infants >3 months and children:** 1 to 2 mg/day.

Ophthalmic solution: 1 drop into each eye every 4 hours.
Ophthalmic ointment: Apply 2 to 3 times a day.

ADVERSE EFFECTS: Ototoxicity (may be associated with high serum aminoglycoside concentrations persisting for prolonged periods) with tinnitus, hearing loss; early toxicity usually affects high-pitched sound; nephrotoxicity (high trough levels) with proteinuria, elevated serum creatinine, oliguria, and macular rash.

PHARMACOLOGY: Renal excretion by glomerular filtration. Half-life is 3 to 11.5 hours initially. Volume of distribution is increased in neonates and with fever, edema, ascites, and fluid overload.

COMMENTS: Desired serum peak is 4 to 12 mcg/mL (sample obtained 30 minutes after infusion has been completed), and desired serum trough is 0.5 to 2 mcg/mL (sample obtained 30 minutes prior to next dose). Obtain serum levels if treating for >48 hours or patient has declining renal function. Monitor serum creatinine. Aminoglycosides should not be used alone against gram-positive pathogens.

GLUCAGON

INDICATIONS AND USE: Management of severe hypoglycemia unresponsive to routine treatment.
ACTIONS: Glucagon, a hormone produced by the alpha cells of the pancreas, stimulates synthesis of cyclic adenosine monophosphate, hepatic glycogenolysis, and gluconeogenesis, causing an increase in blood glucose levels; it inhibits small bowel motility and gastric acid secretion and produces both positive inotropic and chronotropic effects.

DOSAGE: IV, IM, subcutaneous.

Persistent hypoglycemia:
- 0.02 to 0.2 mg/kg/dose IV, IM, subcutaneous; may repeat in 20 minutes as needed. Maximum single dose: 1 mg.
- **Continuous infusion:** Initial: 0.01 to 0.02 mg/kg/h or 0.5 to 1 mg infused over 24 hours.

Congenital hyperinsulinism; hyperinsulinemic hypoglycemia:
- **Continuous IV infusion:** 0.005 to 0.02 mg/kg/h.

ADVERSE EFFECTS: Tachycardia, hypertension, hypotension up to 2 hours after GI procedure, thrombocytopenia, nausea, and vomiting.

COMMENTS: Do not delay initiation of glucose infusion while observing for glucagon effect.

HEPARIN SODIUM

INDICATIONS AND USE: Prophylaxis and treatment of thromboembolic disorders, anticoagulant for dialysis and extracorporeal procedures and to maintain patency of arterial or venous catheters. (See Chapter 84.)

ACTIONS: Activates antithrombin III (heparin cofactor) and inactivates coagulation factors IX, X, XI, and XII and thrombin, inhibiting the conversion of fibrinogen to fibrin. Heparin also stimulates release of lipoprotein lipase (lipoprotein lipase hydrolyzes triglycerides to glycerol and free fatty acids).

DOSAGE: IV.

Treatment of thrombosis:

- **Loading dose:** 75 units/kg as IV bolus given over 10 minutes, followed by 28 units/kg/h as continuous infusion; adjust dose to maintain an anti-Xa activity of 0.35 to 0.7 units/mL.

Maintain catheter patency:

- **Heparinized fluid** with a usual final concentration of 0.5 to 1 unit/mL; may use concentration as low as 0.25 unit/mL.

Line flushing:

- **Daily flushes of heparin to maintain patency of central catheters:** a dose of 10 units/mL is commonly used for younger infants (eg, <10 kg); 100 units/mL is used for older infants and children with central line access or infusion port devices. May need to flush every 6 to 8 hours for some catheters.

ADVERSE REACTIONS: Heparin-induced thrombocytopenia, bleeding tendency, hemorrhage, fever, rash, and abnormal liver function tests. Follow platelet counts every 2 to 3 days.

PHARMACOLOGY: Clearance in neonates is more rapid than in children or adults; half-life is dose dependent, but the average is 1 to 2 hours.

COMMENTS: Antidote: protamine sulfate; refer to monograph for dosing.

HEPATITIS B IMMUNE GLOBULIN (HBIG; HYPERHEP B S/D, HEPAGAM B)

INDICATIONS AND USE: Provide prophylactic passive immunity to hepatitis B infection following perinatal, sexual, household or bloodborne exposure.

ACTIONS: Passive immunization agent. Immune serum provides protection against the hepatitis B virus by directly providing specific immunoglobulin G to hepatitis B surface antigen (HBsAg). The duration of immunity is short (3–6 months).

DOSAGE: IM.

Neonates born to HBsAg-positive mothers:

- 0.5 mL as soon after birth as possible (within 12 hours; efficacy decreases significantly if treatment is delayed >48 hours); hepatitis B vaccine series to begin at the same time; if this series is delayed for as long as 3 months, the HBIG dose may be repeated.

Neonates born to mothers with unknown HBsAg status at birth:

- **Birthweight <2 kg:** 0.5 mL within 12 hours of birth (along with hepatitis B vaccine) if unable to determine maternal HBsAg status within 12 hours.
- **Birthweight ≥2 kg:** 0.5 mL within 7 days of birth while awaiting maternal HBsAg result.

ADVERSE EFFECTS: Swelling, warmth, erythema, and soreness at the injection site. Rash, fever, and urticaria are rare.

COMMENTS: Administer with caution in patients with immunoglobulin A deficiency, thrombocytopenia, or coagulopathy. Do not administer IV. Do not administer hepatitis vaccine and HBIG in same syringe because vaccine will be neutralized. However, they can be given concurrently at separate sites.

HEPATITIS B VACCINE (RECOMBIVAX HB, ENGERIX-B)

INDICATIONS AND USE: Immunization against infection caused by all known subtypes of hepatitis B virus in individuals considered at high risk of potential exposure to hepatitis B virus.

ACTIONS: Promotes immunity to hepatitis B virus by inducing the production of specific antibodies to the virus.

DOSAGE: IM. Recommended schedule: 0.5 mL/dose in 3 total doses.

Infants born to hepatitis B surface antigen (HBsAg)-positive mothers:

- **First dose within the first 12 hours of life, even if premature** and regardless of birthweight (hepatitis immune globulin should also be administered at the same time/different site);

second dose at 1 to 2 months of age; and third dose at 6 months of age. Check anti-HBs and HBsAg at 9 to 15 months of age. If anti-HBs and HBsAg are negative, reimmunize with 3 doses 2 months apart and reassess. *Note:* Premature infants <2000 g should receive 4 total doses at 0, 1, 2 to 3, and 6 to 7 months of chronological age.

Infants born to HBsAg-negative mothers:
- **First dose prior to discharge**; however, the first dose may be given at 1 to 2 months of age. Another dose is given 1 to 2 months later, and a final dose at 6 months of age. A total of 4 doses of vaccine may be given if a "birth dose" is administered and a combination vaccine is used to complete the series. *Note:* Premature infants <2000 g may have the initial dose deferred to up to 30 days of chronological age.

Infants born to mothers whose HBsAg status is unknown at birth:
- **First dose within 12 hours of birth even if premature, regardless of birthweight**; second dose following 1 to 2 months later; the third dose at 6 months of age; if the mother's blood HBsAg test is positive, the infant should receive hepatitis immune globulin as soon as possible (no later than age 1 week). Due to possible decreased immunogenicity, premature neonates <2 kg who received an initial dose within 12 hours of birth should receive 4 total doses at 0, 1, 2 to 3, and 6 to 7 months of chronological age.

ADVERSE EFFECTS: Swelling, warmth, erythema, soreness at the injection site, and, rarely, vomiting, rash, and low-grade fever.

COMMENTS: Do not give IV or intradermally.

HYALURONIDASE (HYLENEX, AMPHADASE, VITRASE)

INDICATIONS AND USE: Treatment of extravasation injuries.

ACTIONS: An enzyme that temporarily hydrolyzes hyaluronic acid (1 of the chief components of tissue cement) and thereby allows the infiltrated drug or solution to be absorbed over a larger surface area. This speeds absorption and reduces tissue contact time with the irritant substance.

DOSAGE: Subcutaneous, intradermal.
- Using a 25- or 26-gauge needle, inject 5 separate 0.2-mL injections of 150 units/mL solution around the periphery of the extravasation site. Change the needle after each injection. Elevate the extremity. Do not apply heat. Repeat as needed. Some use 5 separate 0.2-mL subcutaneous injections of 15 units/mL dilution.

ADVERSE EFFECTS: Usually well tolerated. Urticaria occurs rarely. Administer hyaluronidase within 1 hour of the extravasation, if possible. Reduction in swelling can be observed within 15 to 30 minutes after administration.

HYDRALAZINE HCL (APRESOLINE HCL)

INDICATIONS AND USE: For the management of moderate to severe hypertension and as an afterload-reducing agent to treat congestive heart failure.

ACTIONS: Causes direct relaxation of smooth muscle in the arteriolar resistance vessels; decreases systemic vascular resistance and increases cardiac output; increases renal, coronary, cerebral, and splanchnic blood flow.

DOSAGE: IM, IV, PO.
- **IM or IV:** 0.1 to 0.5 mg/kg/dose every 6 to 8 hours (maximum 2 mg/kg/dose). In case of hypertensive emergency/urgency in infants, may administer initial dose of 0.1 to 0.2 mg/kg/dose every 4 to 6 hours as needed and increase up to 0.6 mg/kg/dose or 20 mg/dose as required.
- **PO:** 0.25 to 1 mg/kg/dose every 6 to 8 hours; increase over 3 to 4 weeks to maximum of 7.5 mg/kg/day in infants.

ADVERSE EFFECTS: Most frequent are tachycardia and hypotension; most serious is a reversible lupus-like syndrome. Tachyphylaxis often occurs on chronic therapy. Gastrointestinal bleeding, diarrhea, anemia, leukopenia, agranulocytosis, and purpura have also been reported.

COMMENTS: Contraindicated in mitral valve rheumatic heart disease or coronary artery disease. Due to concern for reflex tachycardia, concurrent use of β-blocker is recommended in heart failure patients.

HYDROCHLOROTHIAZIDE (MICROZIDE)

INDICATIONS AND USE: Mild to moderate edema and hypertension, bronchopulmonary dysplasia, idiopathic hypercalciuria, congenital nephrogenic diabetes insipidus.

ACTIONS: Inhibits reabsorption of sodium in the distal tubules, resulting in increased excretion of sodium and water as well as potassium, hydrogen, magnesium, and bicarbonate ions.

DOSAGE: PO.

Neonates:
- 2 to 4 mg/kg/day divided in 2 doses.

Edema:
- **Infants <6 months:** 1 to 3 mg/kg/day in 2 divided doses; maximum dose 37.5 mg/day.
- **Infants ≥6 months and children<2 years:** 1 to 2 mg/kg/day in 1 to 2 divided doses; maximum dose 37.5 mg/day.

Hypertension:
- **Infants and children<2 years:** Initially, administer 1 mg/kg/day once daily; increase to maximum of 3 mg/kg/day if needed; not to exceed 50 mg/day.

ADVERSE EFFECTS: Hypokalemia, hyperglycemia, hyperuricemia, hypochloremic metabolic alkalosis.

PHARMACOLOGY: Onset of action (infants) approximately 2 to 6 hours with a duration of 8 hours. Half-life is roughly 6 to 15 hours. Drug is renally eliminated.

HYDROCORTISONE, SYSTEMIC

INDICATIONS AND USE: Management of acute adrenal insufficiency, congenital adrenal hyperplasia, and vasopressor-resistant hypotension. Adjunctive treatment for persistent hypoglycemia.

ACTIONS: The short-acting adrenal corticosteroid that possesses glucocorticoid activity, anti-inflammatory activity, and minimal mineralocorticoid effects; most effects probably result from modification of enzyme activity, thus affecting almost all body systems. Promotes protein catabolism, gluconeogenesis, renal excretion of calcium, capillary wall permeability and stability, and red blood cell production; suppresses immune and inflammatory responses.

DOSAGE: IV, IM, PO.

Acute adrenal insufficiency/adrenal crisis:
- 2 to 3 mg/kg IV bolus (maximum at 100 mg/dose), then 1 to 5 mg/kg/dose IV every 6 hours.

Congenital adrenal hyperplasia (AAP recommendations):
- **Initial:** 10 to 20 mg/m²/day PO in 3 divided doses.
- **Usual requirement for infants:** 2.5 to 5 mg 3 times per day using tablet formulation.

Physiologic replacement:
- **PO:** 8 to 12 mg/m²/day divided every 8 hours.

Stress doses (treatment-resistant hypotension; shock):
- **IV:** 50 to 100 mg/m²/day IV divided into 2 to 4 doses; alternatively, 1 mg/kg/dose IV every 8 hours or 2 mg/kg IV bolus followed by 1 mg/kg/dose IV every 12 hours.

Refractory hypoglycemia (refractory to continuous glucose infusion rates >12–15 mg/kg/min):
- **IV, PO:** 5 mg/kg/day divided every 8 to 12 hours or 1 to 2 mg/kg/dose IV every 6 hours. Consider consultation with pediatric endocrinologist for treatment guidance.

ADVERSE EFFECTS: Hypertension, hypothalamic-pituitary-adrenal axis suppression, hypokalemia, hyperglycemia, growth suppression, sodium and water retention, decreased bone mineral density, and immunosuppression.

COMMENTS: *Note:* Morning dose should be administered as early as possible; tablets may result in more reliable serum concentrations than oral liquid formulation; individualize dose by monitoring growth, hormone levels, and bone age; mineralocorticoid (eg, fludrocortisone) and sodium supplement may be required in salt losers.

HYDROXYCHLOROQUINE (PLAQUENIL)

ACTION AND SPECTRUM: Interferes with digestive vacuole function within sensitive malarial parasites by increasing the pH and interfering with lysosomal degradation of hemoglobin. Suppression or treatment of acute attacks of malaria.

DOSAGE: All doses below are expressed as hydroxychloroquine sulfate; hydroxychloroquine sulfate 200 mg is equivalent to 155 mg of hydroxychloroquine base and 250 mg of chloroquine phosphate.

Malaria:

- **Treatment:** 13 mg/kg/dose PO (maximum initial dose 800 mg) followed by 6.5 mg/kg/dose at 6, 24, and 48 hours after initial dose (maximum per dose 400 mg).
- **Prophylaxis:** 6.5 mg/kg/dose once weekly on the same day each week (maximum per dose 400 mg); begin 1 to 2 weeks before exposure and continue for at least 4 weeks after leaving endemic area. If initiation of prophylaxis is delayed (ie, 2 weeks of therapy not competed prior to the exposure), the manufacturer recommends doubling the initial dose to 13 mg/kg/dose and administering in 2 divided doses 6 hours apart (maximum per dose 400 mg); continue for 8 weeks after leaving endemic area.

ADVERSE EFFECTS: Cardiomyopathy, QT interval prolongation, dermatitis, erythema, bone marrow suppression (anemia, leukopenia, thrombocytopenia), hypoglycemia, proximal myopathy or neuromyopathy, visual disturbances, acute hepatic insufficiency, renal toxicity. Use with caution in patients with glucose-6-phosphate dehydrogenase deficiency due to a potential for hemolytic anemia.

COMMENTS: A 25 mg/mL hydroxychloroquine sulfate oral suspension may be made with tablets. With a towel moistened with alcohol, remove the coating from 15 200-mg hydroxychloroquine sulfate tablets. Crush tablets in a mortar and reduce to a fine powder. Add 15 mL of Ora-Plus and mix to a uniform paste; add an additional 45 mL of vehicle and mix until uniform. Mix while adding sterile water for irrigation in incremental proportions to almost 120 mL; transfer to a calibrated bottle, rinse mortar with sterile water, and add sufficient quantity of sterile water to make 120 mL. Label "shake well." A 30-day expiration date is recommended, although stability testing has not been performed.

IBUPROFEN (MOTRIN, OTHERS)

INDICATIONS AND USE: Treatment of mild to moderate pain, fever, and inflammatory diseases. Oral ibuprofen may be a safe alternative for patent ductus arteriosus (PDA) closure as shown in recent studies, but larger studies are needed.

ACTIONS: Decreases prostaglandin synthesis by reversibly inhibiting the activities of cyclooxygenase-1 and -2 enzymes.

DOSAGE: PO.

Infants and children:

- **Analgesic:** 4 to 10 mg/kg/dose PO every 6 to 8 hours; maximum daily dose is 40 mg/kg/day.
- **Antipyretic:** (>6 months) 5 to 10 mg/kg/dose PO every 6 to 8 hours; maximum daily dose is 40 mg/kg/day or 2400 mg/day.
- **PDA closure:** 10 mg/kg for the first dose, followed by 2 doses of 5 mg/kg at 24 and 48 hours after the first dose. Use birthweight to calculate all doses.

ADVERSE EFFECTS: Edema, hypertension, fluid retention, hyperkalemia, gastrointestinal (GI) bleed, GI perforation, neutropenia, anemia, inhibition of platelet aggregation, elevated liver enzymes, acute renal failure/acute kidney injury.

PHARMACOLOGY: Highly protein bound (>95%). Hepatic metabolism via oxidation. Primarily renally excreted.

COMMENTS: To reduce the risk of adverse cardiovascular and GI effects, use the lowest effective dose for the shortest time period. May increase risk of GI irritation, ulceration, bleeding, and perforation; may compromise existing renal function; use with caution in patients with decreased liver function.

IBUPROFEN LYSINE (NEOPROFEN)

INDICATIONS AND USE: Pharmacologic closure of patent ductus arteriosus. Not indicated for intraventricular hemorrhage prophylaxis.

ACTIONS: Nonsteroidal anti-inflammatory drug with analgesic and antipyretic properties. Action is principally by inhibition of prostaglandin synthesis, thus inhibiting cyclooxygenase, an enzyme that catalyzes the formation of prostaglandin precursors (endoperoxides) from arachidonic acid.

DOSAGE: IV (use birthweight for all dosing calculation).

- **Standard-dose regimen (manufacturer's labeling):** 10 mg/kg for the initial dose, followed by 2 doses of 5 mg/kg at 24- and 48-hour intervals after the first dose.
- **High-dose regimen (limited data):** 20 mg/kg for the initial dose, followed by 2 doses of 10 mg/kg at 24- and 48-hour intervals after the first dose. Of note, high-dose regimen was found to have a higher rate of PDA closure without additional side effects (Dani, 2012; Meißner, 2012).

ADVERSE EFFECTS: Anemia, fluid retention, edema, tachycardia, hepatic dysfunction, decrease in urine output, elevated blood urea nitrogen and serum creatinine (renal effects are less severe and less frequent than those with indomethacin); may inhibit platelet aggregation; monitor for signs of bleeding. Use with caution in infants when total bilirubin is elevated (ibuprofen may displace bilirubin from albumin-binding sites). Feeding intolerance, gastrointestinal irritation, ileus.

COMMENTS: Contraindicated in preterm neonates with infection, active bleeding, thrombocytopenia or coagulation defects, necrotizing enterocolitis, significant renal dysfunction, and congenital heart disease with ductal-dependent systemic blood flow. Withhold subsequent dose(s) in patients who became anuric or with urinary output <0.6 mL/kg/h until renal function is normalized.

IMIPENEM/CILASTATIN (PRIMAXIN IV)

ACTION AND SPECTRUM: Treatment of non-CNS infections caused by documented multidrug-resistant gram-negative organisms in children.

DOSAGE: IV. (Dosing based on imipenem component.)

Neonates (AAP *Red Book*, 2018–2021):

- **PNA ≤7 days:** 25 mg/kg every 12 hours.
- **PNA >7 to 28 days:** 25 mg/kg every 8 hours.

Infants >28 days and children:

- 60 to 100 mg/kg/day divided every 6 hours; maximum dose 4 g/day.

ADVERSE EFFECTS: Irritation, pain, phlebitis at injection site, elevated liver transaminases; urine discoloration, decreased in hematocrit, elevated serum creatinine, diarrhea, and seizures in patients with meningitis.

PHARMACOLOGY: Broad-spectrum carbapenem combines with cilastatin (renal dipeptidase inhibitor that prevents renal metabolism of imipenem). Inhibits cell wall biosynthesis. Half-life is prolonged with renal insufficiency.

COMMENTS: Dosing adjustment is recommended in patients with renal impairment. Caution use in preterm infants due to risk of cilastatin accumulation and possible seizures.

IMMUNE GLOBULIN, INTRAVENOUS (IVIG; VARIOUS)

INDICATIONS AND USE: Neonatal alloimmune thrombocytopenia, isoimmune hemolytic disease, adjuvant treatment of fulminant neonatal sepsis (***controversial***) and immunodeficiency syndromes.

ACTIONS: The pooled, heterogeneous immunoglobulin G (IgG) present in IVIG provides a plethora of antibodies capable of opsonization and neutralization of many toxins and microbes, as well as complement activation. Although the amount of each IgG subclass in the parenteral products is similar to that of human plasma, the titers against specific antigens vary from manufacturer to manufacturer. The passive immunity imparted by IVIG is capable of attenuating or preventing infectious diseases or deleterious reactions from toxins,

Mycoplasma, parasites, bacteria, and viruses. IVIG is thought to promote blockade of Fc receptors in macrophages (preventing phagocytosis of circulating opsonized platelets or cells tagged with autoantibodies).

DOSAGE: IV.

- **Usual dosage:** 400 to 1000 mg/kg/dose infused over 2 to 6 hours daily for 2 to 5 days (total dose of 2000 mg/kg). Many different products available; consult specific product insert for dosing details.

ADVERSE EFFECTS: Hypotension, transient tachycardia, and anaphylaxis. If either occurs, the rate of infusion should be decreased or stopped until resolved, then resumed at a slower rate as tolerated. Contraindicated in IgA deficiency (except with the use of Gammagard S/D or Polygam S/D).

PHARMACOLOGY: Initial response seen in 1 to 3 days with peak response between 2 and 7 days in the treatment of immune thrombocytopenia. Immune effect is expected to last for 3 to 4 weeks.

INDOMETHACIN, IV

INDICATIONS AND USE: Pharmacologic closure of patent ductus arteriosus (PDA). May provide prophylaxis for intraventricular hemorrhage (IVH) in low birthweight infants.

ACTIONS: Nonsteroidal anti-inflammatory drug with analgesic and antipyretic properties. Inhibits prostaglandin synthesis by decreasing cyclooxygenase activity, an enzyme that catalyzes the formation of prostaglandin precursors (endoperoxides) from arachidonic acid. Decreases cerebral blood flow.

DOSAGE: IV.

PDA:

- **Initially,** 0.2 mg/kg IV, followed by 2 doses depending on PNA:
  - **PNA at first dose <48 hours:** 0.1 mg/kg at 12- to 24-hour intervals.
  - **PNA at first dose 2 to 7 days:** 0.2 mg/kg at 12- to 24-hour intervals.
  - **PNA at first dose >7 days:** 0.25 mg/kg at 12- to 24-hour intervals.
- **Dosing interval:**
  - **12-hour dosing** interval if urine output is >1 mL/kg/h after prior dose.
  - **24-hour dosing** interval if urine output is <1 mL/kg/h but >0.6 mL/kg/h.
  - **Hold dose if patient has oliguria** (urine output <0.6 mL/kg/h) or anuria.

IVH prophylaxis: 0.1 mg/kg/dose IV every 24 hours for 3 doses; give first dose at 6 to 12 hours of age.

ADVERSE EFFECTS: May cause decreased platelet aggregation, transient oliguria (decreased glomerular filtration rate), increased serum creatinine, and increased serum concentration of renally excreted drugs such as gentamicin. May also cause hyponatremia, hyperkalemia, and hypoglycemia. Gastrointestinal perforations are known to occur if used concurrently with corticosteroids.

COMMENTS: Contraindicated in premature neonates with necrotizing enterocolitis, severe renal impairment (urine output <0.6 mL/kg/h or creatinine ≥1.8 mg/dL), thrombocytopenia, or active bleeding or if there has been intraventricular bleeding within the preceding 7 days (*controversial*). Do not administer via umbilical catheter or intra-arterially.

INSULIN, REGULAR

INDICATIONS AND USE: Hyperglycemia, acute management of hyperkalemia, and increasing caloric intake in infants with glucose intolerance on parenteral nutrition.

ACTIONS: Hormone derived from the β cells of the pancreas and the principal hormone required for glucose utilization. In skeletal and cardiac muscle and adipose tissue, insulin facilitates transport of glucose into these cells. Insulin stimulates lipogenesis and protein synthesis and inhibits lipolysis and release of free fatty acids from adipose cells. Promotes intracellular shift of potassium and magnesium.

DOSAGE: IV.

Hyperglycemia (Cloherty et al, 2012):

- **Continuous IV infusion:** 0.01 to 0.2 units/kg/h (titrate in 0.01 unit/kg/h increments with blood glucose monitoring every 30 minutes until stable, then every 4–6 hours).
- **Intermittent:** 0.05 to 0.1 unit/kg/dose infused over 15 minutes every 4 to 6 hours as needed; monitor blood glucose 30 minutes to 1 hour after doses.

Hyperkalemia:

- **Continuous IV infusion:** 0.05 to 0.1 unit/kg/h in combination with a continuous infusion of 0.2 to 0.4 g/kg/h of dextrose. Adjust infusion rates based on serum glucose and potassium concentrations.
- **Intermittent:** 0.1 unit/kg given IV in combination with 400 mg/kg glucose.

ADVERSE EFFECTS: Hypoglycemia (may cause coma and severe CNS injury), hyperglycemic rebound (Somogyi effect), hypokalemia, urticaria, and anaphylaxis.

COMMENTS: To minimize adsorption of insulin to plastic IV solution bag or tubing: If new tubing is not needed, wait a minimum of 30 minutes between the preparation of the solution and the initiation of the infusion. If new tubing is needed, after receiving the insulin continuous infusion solution, the administration set should be attached to the IV container and the line should be flushed with the insulin solution; wait 30 minutes, then flush the line again with the insulin solution prior to initiating the infusion. Because of adsorption, the actual amount of insulin being administered could be substantially less than the apparent amount. Therefore, adjustment of the insulin drip rate should be based on the effect and not solely on the apparent insulin dose.

IODODEOXYURIDINE OPHTHALMIC

See Chapter 58.

IPRATROPIUM BROMIDE (ATROVENT)

INDICATIONS AND USE: Bronchodilator for adjunctive treatment of acute bronchospasm.

ACTIONS: Anticholinergic drug that acts by antagonizing the action of acetylcholine at the parasympathetic receptor sites, thereby producing bronchodilation.

DOSAGE: Inhalation.

- **Neonates:** 25 mcg/kg/dose nebulized every 8 hours.
- **Infants:** 125 to 250 mcg/dose nebulized every 8 hours. Dilute to 3 mL with normal saline or concurrent albuterol.
- **Metered inhaler:** 2 to 4 puffs as needed every 6 to 8 hours.

ADVERSE EFFECTS: Rebound airway hyperresponsiveness after discontinuation. Nervousness, dizziness, nausea, blurred vision, dry mouth, exacerbation of symptoms, airway irritation, cough, palpitations, rash, and urinary retention. Use with caution in narrow-angle glaucoma or bladder neck obstruction.

COMMENTS: Compatible when admixed with albuterol if given within 1 hour. Bronchodilator effect may be potentiated when given with β_2-agonist (ie, albuterol).

IRON DEXTRAN

INDICATIONS AND USE: Used to treat iron deficiency anemia, as an iron supplement for infants on epoetin, and for infants on long-term parenteral nutrition (PN). Oral iron is much safer than the parenteral form; the parenteral form is usually reserved for patients who cannot take oral iron.

ACTIONS: Iron is a component in the formation of hemoglobin, and adequate amounts are necessary for erythropoiesis and oxygen transport capacity of blood.

DOSAGE: IV. *Note:* Multiple parenteral iron forms exist.

Total replacement dosage of iron dextran for iron deficiency anemia:

- Dose (mL) = 0.0442 × LBW (kg) × (Hbn – Hbo) + [0.26 × LBW (kg)]
  - LBW = lean body weight
  - Hbn = desired hemoglobin (g/dL) = 12 if <15 kg or 14.8 if >15 kg
  - Hbo = measured hemoglobin (g/dL)

Total iron replacement dosage for acute blood loss (assumes 1 mL of normocytic, normochromic red cells = 1 mg elemental iron):
- Iron dextran (mL) = 0.02 × blood loss (mL) × hematocrit (expressed as a decimal fraction)

Anemia of prematurity:
- 0.2 to 1 mg/kg/day IV or 20 mg/kg/wk with epoetin alfa therapy.

PN addition:
- Admixed in the PN solution (solution must contain at least 2% amino acids): 0.4 to 1 mg/kg/day (or 3–5 mg/kg as a single weekly dose).

ADVERSE EFFECTS: Iron accumulation in patients with serious liver dysfunction; anaphylaxis, fever, and arthralgia. IV use: Pain and redness at IV site, rash, shivering; hypotension and flushing with rapid infusion.

ISONIAZID (INH)

INDICATIONS AND USE: Treatment of susceptible *Mycobacterium* spp. (eg, *Mycobacterium tuberculosis*, *Mycobacterium kansasii*, and *Mycobacterium avium*) and for prophylaxis for individuals exposed to tuberculosis.

ACTION AND SPECTRUM: Antimycobacterial agent that is bactericidal for both extracellular and intracellular organisms. Inhibits mycolic acid synthesis resulting in disruption of the bacterial cell wall.

DOSAGE: PO.
- **Perinatal tuberculosis:** 10 to 15 mg/kg/day PO divided every 12 hours with rifampin (see Rifampin for dosage) for 3 to 12 months. If skin test conversion is positive, treat with 10 to 15 mg/kg/day PO every 24 hours for 9 to 12 months.

ADVERSE EFFECTS: Peripheral neuropathy, seizures, encephalopathy, blood dyscrasias, nausea, vomiting, and diarrhea (associated with administration of syrup formulation) and hypersensitivity reactions. May be hepatotoxic; follow liver function tests at regular intervals during treatment.

ISOPROTERENOL (ISUPREL, OTHERS)

INDICATIONS AND USE: Low cardiac output or vasoconstrictive shock states, cardiac arrest, ventricular arrhythmias resulting from atrioventricular block.

ACTIONS: Stimulates both β_1- and β_2-adrenergic receptors with minimal or no effect on α-receptors in therapeutic doses. Relaxes bronchial smooth muscle, cardiac stimulation (inotropic and chronotropic), and peripheral vasodilation (reduces cardiac afterload).

DOSAGE: IV.
- 0.05 to 0.5 mcg/kg/minute IV continuous infusion; maximum dose is 2 mcg/kg/minute. Correct acidosis before initiating therapy.

ADVERSE EFFECTS: Tremor, vomiting, hypertension, tachycardia, cardiac arrhythmias, hypotension, and hypoglycemia.

COMMENTS: Contraindicated in hypertension, hyperthyroidism, tachycardia caused by digoxin toxicity, and preexisting cardiac arrhythmias. Increases cardiac oxygen consumption disproportional to the increase in cardiac oxygen output. Not considered an inotropic agent of choice.

KETAMINE HYDROCHLORIDE (KETALAR)

INDICATIONS AND USE: Ketamine is a rapid-acting general anesthetic agent for short diagnostic and minor surgical procedures that do not require skeletal muscle relaxation.

ACTIONS: Produces dissociative anesthesia by direct action on the cortex and limbic system; does not usually impair pharyngeal or laryngeal reflexes. Induces coma, analgesia, and amnesia. Increases cerebral blood flow and cerebral oxygen consumption; improves pulmonary compliance and relieves bronchospasm.

DOSAGE: IV, IM, PO.
- **IV: 0.5 to 2 mg/kg/dose;** use smaller doses (0.5–1 mg/kg) for sedation for minor procedures.
- **Usual induction dose: 1 to 2 mg/kg IV.** Reduce dose in hepatic dysfunction.

ADVERSE EFFECTS: Avoid use of ketamine in patients with increased intracranial pressure, increased cerebral blood flow, increased CSF pressure, increased cerebral metabolism, or if a significant elevation in blood pressure may present a risk to the patient. Elevated blood pressure (frequent), tachycardia, arrhythmia, hypotension, bradycardia, increased cerebral blood flow, and decreased cardiac output may occur. Respiratory depression and apnea after rapid IV administration of high doses; laryngospasm; and hypersalivation. Increased airway resistance, cough reflex may be depressed, decreased bronchospasm. Nystagmus and increased intraocular pressure. Emergence reactions (psychic disturbances such as hallucinations and delirium lasting up to 24 hours). Minimize by reducing verbal, tactile, and visual simulation in the recovery period. These occur less commonly in pediatric patients than in adults. Severe reactions can be treated with a benzodiazepine. Increased muscle tone that may resemble seizures and extensor spasm with opisthotonos may occur in infants receiving high, repeated doses. Rash as well as pain and redness at the IM injection site.

PHARMACOLOGY: IV acts in 30 seconds and lasts 5 to 10 minutes. Amnesia lasts for 1 to 2 hours. Concurrent narcotics or barbiturates prolong recovery time.

COMMENTS: Pretreatment with a benzodiazepine 15 minutes before ketamine may reduce side effects such as psychic disturbances, increased intracranial pressure and cerebral blood flow, tachycardia, and jerking movements. Monitor heart rate, respiratory rate, blood pressure, and pulse oximetry. Observe for CNS side effects during the recovery period. Have equipment for resuscitation available.

KETOCONAZOLE (NIZORAL)

> **WARNING:** Ketoconazole has been associated with hepatic toxicity. Coadministration of cisapride or astemizole with ketoconazole is contraindicated. Serious cardiovascular adverse events have occurred.

INDICATIONS AND USE: Synthetic broad spectrum antifungal.

ACTION AND SPECTRUM: An antifungal agent that acts by disrupting cell membranes. Fungicidal against susceptible candidiasis, blastomycosis, coccidioidomycosis, histoplasmosis, paracoccidioidomycosis, chronic mucocutaneous candidiasis, as well as certain recalcitrant cutaneous dermatophytoses (FDA approved in those ≥2 years of age).

DOSAGE: PO.

- 3.3 to 6.6 mg/kg/day PO once daily with food to decrease nausea and vomiting; administer 2 hours prior to antacids, proton pump inhibitors, or H_2-receptor antagonists to prevent decreased ketoconazole absorption; shake suspension well before use.

ADVERSE EFFECTS: Gastric distress is the most common side effect. Check periodic liver function tests; caution in patients with impaired hepatic function; high doses of ketoconazole may depress adrenocortical function and decrease serum testosterone concentrations.

PHARMACOLOGY: Hepatic metabolism. Penetration into CSF is poor.

COMMENTS: Not indicated for treatment of fungal meningitis. Minimum period of treatment for candidiasis is 1 to 2 weeks, but duration should be based on clinical response. Limited experience in neonates.

LABETALOL

INDICATIONS AND USE: Treatment of mild to severe hypertension. IV form for hypertensive emergencies.

ACTIONS: Dose-related decrease in blood pressure through α-, β_1-, and β_2-adrenergic receptor blockade without causing significant reflex tachycardia or a decrease in heart rate. Reduces elevated renin levels.

DOSAGE: PO, IV. Limited experience in neonates; labetalol should be initiated cautiously; carefully monitor blood pressure, heart rate, and electrocardiogram, and adjust the dose accordingly. Use the lowest effective dose.

IV intermittent bolus:

- 0.2 to 0.5 mg/kg/dose over 2 to 3 minutes every 4 to 6 hours with a range of 0.2 to 1 mg/kg/dose has been suggested; maximum dose 20 mg/dose.

Treatment of pediatric hypertensive emergencies:
- **Continuous IV infusion:** 0.4 to 1 mg/kg/h, with a maximum of 3 mg/kg/h.
- **Alternate dosing:** Bolus 0.2 to 1 mg/kg followed by a continuous infusion of 0.25 to 1.5 mg/kg/h.

Oral:
- **Initial:** 1 to 2 mg/kg/day in 2 divided doses. Maximum dose 10 to 20 mg/kg/day.

ADVERSE EFFECTS: Orthostatic hypotension, bronchospasm, nasal congestion, edema, congestive heart failure, bradycardia, myopathy, and rash. Intensifies atrioventricular block. Reversible hepatic dysfunction (rare).

PHARMACOLOGY: Peak effect with PO is 1 to 4 hours after the dose, while peak effect with IV is 5 to 15 minutes. Metabolized in the liver by glucuronidation. Oral labetalol has a bioavailability of only 25% because of extensive first-pass effect. Oral absorption is improved by taking with food. Concomitant oral cimetidine may increase the bioavailability of oral labetalol.

COMMENTS: Do not discontinue chronic labetalol abruptly; taper over 1 to 2 weeks. Contraindicated in patients with asthma, overt cardiac failure, heart block, cardiogenic shock, or severe bradycardia. May cause a paradoxical increase in blood pressure in patients with pheochromocytoma. Use with caution in hepatic dysfunction. Incompatible with sodium bicarbonate.

LAMIVUDINE (EPIVIR, EPIVIR HBV)

WARNING: Risk of lactic acidosis, exacerbations of hepatitis B upon discontinuation of epivir-HBV®, and risk of HIV-1 resistance if epivir-HBV is used in patients with unrecognized or untreated HIV-1.

ACTION AND SPECTRUM: Antiretroviral agent that inhibits reverse transcription by viral DNA chain termination. Used for the prevention of mother-to-child transmission of human immunodeficiency virus (HIV); treatment of HIV infection.

DOSAGE: PO. Use in combination with other antiretroviral agents—regimen containing 3 antiretroviral agents is strongly recommended.

Prevention of maternal-to-child HIV transmission:
- 2 mg/kg/dose every 12 hours for 7 days; given from birth to 1 week of age. Given to neonate in combination with nevirapine and 6 weeks of zidovudine in certain maternal situations, such as no treatment prior to labor or during labor, only intrapartum therapy; inadequate viral suppression at time of delivery or known drug-resistant virus.

Treatment of HIV infection:
- **Neonates <30 days:** 2 mg/kg/dose every 12 hours.
- **Infants 1 to 3 months:** 4 mg/kg/dose every 12 hours.
- **Infants >3 months and children <16 years:** 4 mg/kg/dose every 12 hours; maximum dose 150 mg every 12 hours.

ADVERSE EFFECTS: Very limited data in neonates; Black Box warning of lactic acidosis and severe hepatomegaly in adults; some fatal cases.

PHARMACOLOGY: Synthetic nucleoside analog that is converted to active metabolite; oral solution is well absorbed with 66% bioavailability. Resistance develops rapidly with monotherapy.

COMMENTS: Blood levels/effects may be increased by ganciclovir, valganciclovir, ribavirin, and trimethoprim.

LANSOPRAZOLE (PREVACID)

INDICATIONS AND USE: Short-term treatment of gastroesophageal reflux disease (GERD); erosive esophagitis.

ACTIONS: Suppression of gastric acid secretion by selective inhibition of parietal cell membrane enzyme hydrogen-potassium adenosine triphosphatase (ATPase) or proton pump.

DOSAGE: PO.

Neonatal:
- **0.2 to 0.3 mg/kg/dose once daily** (Zhang et al, 2008) based on pharmacokinetic data; patients <10 weeks of age have decreased clearance.

- **Alternate dosing has been used**: 0.5 to 1 mg/kg/dose once daily (Springer, 2008).

Infants >4 weeks:

- 1 to 1.5 mg/kg/dose once daily (Springer, 2008).

Infants ≥10 weeks:

- 1 to 2 mg/kg/dose once daily (Orenstein et al, 2009; Springer, 2008; Zhang et al, 2008).

ADVERSE EFFECTS: Limited data; proteinuria, abdominal pain, mild elevation of serum transaminases.

PHARMACOLOGY: Degrades in acid pH of stomach; extensively metabolized in liver by CYP2C19 and CYP3A4; the absorption of weakly acidic drugs such as digoxin and furosemide is increased, and absorption of weakly basic drugs is inhibited.

COMMENTS: Recent clinical trial (Orenstein et al, 2009) did not demonstrate efficacy in the treatment of GERD in patients <12 months of age, and the use in this patient population is ***controversial***.

LEVETIRACETAM (KEPPRA)

INDICATIONS AND USE: Adjunctive therapy in the treatment of partial-onset seizures in patients 1 month of age and older. It is only approved for use in combination with other seizure medications.

ACTIONS: Mechanism of action unknown; studies suggest that ≥1 of the following central pharmacologic effects may be involved: inhibition of voltage-dependent N-type calcium channels; blockade of γ-aminobutyric acid (GABA)-ergic inhibitory transmission through displacement of negative modulators; reversal of the inhibition of glycine currents; reduction of delayed rectifier potassium current; and/or binding to synaptic proteins that modulate neurotransmitter release.

DOSAGE: IV, PO. (***Note:*** When switching from PO to IV formulation, the total daily dose should be the same.)

Neonatal dosing:

- **Initial dose:** 10 mg/kg/day IV given in 2 divided doses; may increase over 3 days to 30 mg/kg/day, if tolerated, to maximum of 45 to 60 mg/kg/day. Loading doses of 20 to 30 mg/kg have been used. (Dosing information is from studies with very small sample size.)
- **Oral:** 10 mg/kg/day PO in 1 to 2 divided doses; increase daily by 10 mg/kg to 30 mg/kg/day (maximum dose used: 60 mg/kg/day).

Infant (FDA approved):

- **1 month to <6 months:** 7 mg/kg twice daily; increase in increments of 7 mg/kg twice daily every 2 weeks to recommended dose of 21 mg/kg twice daily.

ADVERSE EFFECTS: Somnolence, nervousness. Use with caution in patients with renal dysfunction; decrease dose.

PHARMACOLOGY: Oral absorption is rapid and complete; oral bioavailability 100%.

COMMENTS: Do not abruptly discontinue therapy; gradually decrease dose to reduce risk of increased seizure activity.

LEVOTHYROXINE SODIUM (T₄) (SYNTHROID, LEVOXYL, OTHERS)

INDICATIONS AND USE: Replacement or supplemental therapy in congenital or acquired hypothyroidism.

ACTIONS: The exact mechanism of action is unknown; however, it is believed the thyroid hormone exerts its many metabolic effects through control of DNA transcription and protein synthesis. Thyroid hormones increase the metabolic rate of body tissues, noted by increases in oxygen consumption; respiratory rate; body temperature; cardiac output; heart rate; blood volume; rates of fat, protein, and carbohydrate metabolism; and enzyme system activity, growth, and maturation. Thyroid hormones are very important in CNS development. Deficiency in infants results in growth retardation and failure of brain growth and development.

DOSAGE: PO, IV, IM (use 50%–75% of the oral dose).

- **0 to 3 months:** 10 to 15 mcg/kg PO; if the infant is at risk for development of cardiac failure, use a lower starting dose, approximately 25 mcg/day; if the initial serum thyroxine is very low (<5 mcg/dL), begin treatment at a higher dosage, approximately 50 mcg/day.

- **>3 to 6 months:** 8 to 10 mcg/kg or 25 to 50 mcg PO.
- **>6 to 12 months:** 6 to 8 mcg/kg or 50 to 75 mcg PO.
- **Alternate dosing:** 8 to 10 mcg/kg/day PO for infants from birth to 1 year.

ADVERSE EFFECTS: Adverse effects are usually due to excessive dose. If the following occur, discontinue and reinstitute at a lower dose: tachycardia, cardiac arrhythmias, tremors, diarrhea, weight loss, and fever.

PHARMACOLOGY: Onset of action—PO: 3 to 5 days; IV: 6 to 8 hours. Maximum effect occurs in 4 to 6 weeks. Protein binding >99%.

LIDOCAINE (XYLOCAINE, OTHERS)

INDICATIONS AND USE: IV lidocaine is used almost exclusively for the short-term control of ventricular arrhythmias (premature beats, tachycardia, and fibrillation) or for prophylactic treatment of such arrhythmias. Also used as a local anesthetic or for the treatment of severe recurrent or prolonged seizures that fail to respond to first-line therapies.

ACTIONS: Class IB antiarrhythmic agent; suppresses spontaneous depolarization of the ventricles during diastole by a direct action on the tissues; blocks both the initiation and conduction of nerve impulses by decreasing the neuronal membrane's permeability to sodium ions; inhibits depolarization and results in blockade of conduction.

DOSAGE: IV, ETT.

Antiarrhythmic:

- **Initial:** 0.5 to 1 mg/kg/dose as IV bolus over 5 minutes. May repeat dose every 10 minutes as necessary to control arrhythmia; maximum total bolus dose is 5 mg/kg.
- **Maintenance IV infusion:** 10 to 50 mcg/kg/min. Use lowest possible dose for preterm infants.
- **Endotracheal:** 2 to 3 mg/kg; flush with 5 mL of normal saline and follow with 5 assisted manual ventilations.

Anticonvulsant in term, normothermic neonates:

- **Loading dose** of 2 mg/kg IV over 10 minutes, immediately followed by
- **Maintenance infusion** of 6 mg/kg/h for 6 hours, then 4 mg/kg/h for 12 hours, then 2 mg/kg/h for 12 hours.

ADVERSE EFFECTS: Drowsiness, dizziness, tremulousness, paresthesias, muscle twitching, seizures, and coma; respiratory depression and/or arrest. Hypotension and heart block can occur.

PHARMACOLOGY: Onset of action 1 to 2 minutes after IV bolus; half-life in neonates is 3 hours; primarily metabolized by the liver.

COMMENTS: Therapeutic levels: 1.5 to 5 mcg/mL; toxic levels >6 mcg/mL. Adjust dosage in liver failure. Contraindicated in sinoatrial or atrioventricular nodal block and Wolff-Parkinson-White syndrome. Avoid using with epinephrine.

LIDOCAINE/PRILOCAINE CREAM (EMLA)

INDICATIONS AND USE: Topical anesthetic for use on intact skin for minor procedures such as insertion of intravenous catheters, venipuncture, and lumbar puncture in infants ≥37 weeks' gestational age.

ACTIONS: EMLA (eutectic mixture of local anesthetics) contains 2 local anesthetics: lidocaine and prilocaine. Local anesthetics inhibit conduction of nerve impulses from sensory nerves by changing the cell membrane's permeability to ions.

DOSAGE: Topical.

Maximum EMLA dose, application area, and application time:

- **0 to 3 months or <5 kg:** Maximum 1 g over 10 cm^2 for 1 hour.
- **3 to 12 months and >5 kg:** Maximum 2 g over 20 cm^2 for 4 hours.
- **1 to 6 years and >10 kg:** Maximum 10 g over 100 cm^2 for 4 hours.

ADVERSE EFFECTS: Not for use on mucous membranes or for ophthalmic use. May cause methemoglobinemia. Not for use in infants <37 weeks' gestational age or infants <12 months old receiving concurrent methemoglobin-inducing agents (sulfonamides, acetaminophen, nitroprusside, nitric oxide, phenobarbital, phenytoin). Reduce amounts if infant has hepatic and/or renal dysfunction.

COMMENT: Do not rub into skin; cover with occlusive dressing.

LINEZOLID (ZYVOX)

ACTIONS AND SPECTRUM: Oxazolidinone agent for treatment of pneumonia; complicated and uncomplicated skin and soft tissue infections; bacteremia caused by susceptible vancomycin-resistant *Enterococcus faecium* (VREF), *Enterococcus faecalis*, *Streptococcus pneumoniae* including multidrug-resistant strains, *Staphylococcus aureus* including methicillin-resistant *S aureus* (MRSA), *Streptococcus pyogenes*, or *Streptococcus agalactiae*. **Note:** There have been reports of VREF and MRSA developing resistance to linezolid during its clinical use.

DOSAGE: PO, IV.

Neonates 0 to 4 weeks and <1.2 kg:

- **PO, IV:** 10 mg/kg/dose every 8 to 12 hours. (**Note:** Use every 12 hours in patients <34 weeks' gestation and <1 week of age.)

Neonates <7 days and ≥1.2 kg:

- **PO, IV:** 10 mg/kg/dose every 8 to 12 hours. (**Note:** Use every 12 hours in patients <34 weeks' gestation and <1 week of age.)

Neonates ≥7 days and ≥1.2 kg (infants and children):

- **PO, IV:** 10 mg/kg/dose every 8 hours.

Complicated skin and skin structure infections and nosocomial or community-acquired pneumonia including concurrent bacteremia: Treat for 10 to 14 days.

VREF: Treat for 14 to 28 days.

ADVERSE EFFECTS: Thrombocytopenia, anemia, leukopenia, and pancytopenia have been reported in patients receiving linezolid—may be dependent on duration of therapy (generally >2 weeks of treatment); monitor patient's complete blood cell count weekly during linezolid therapy; discontinuation of therapy may be required in patients who develop or have worsening myelosuppression. *Clostridium difficile*–associated colitis has been reported; fluid and electrolyte management, protein supplementation, antibiotic treatment, and surgical evaluation may be indicated. Peripheral and optic neuropathy with vision loss has been reported primarily in patients treated for >28 days with linezolid. Cases of lactic acidosis in which patients experienced repeated episodes of nausea and vomiting, acidosis, and low bicarbonate levels have been reported. Elevated transaminases, rash, and diarrhea.

PHARMACOLOGY: Orally well absorbed; low protein binding; metabolized in the liver.

COMMENTS: Therapeutic linezolid concentrations inconsistently achieved in the CSF of pediatric patients with ventriculoperitoneal shunts; not recommended for the empiric treatment of pediatric CNS infections. Not approved for the treatment of catheter-related bloodstream, catheter-site, or gram-negative infections. Linezolid is a reversible, nonselective inhibitor of monoamine oxidase: enhanced vasopressor effects if used with sympathomimetic agents such as dopamine, epinephrine; myelosuppressive drugs (may increase risk of myelosuppression with linezolid).

LORAZEPAM (ATIVAN)

INDICATIONS AND USE: Treatment of status epilepticus resistant to conventional anticonvulsant therapy; sedation.

ACTIONS: A benzodiazepine that binds to the γ-aminobutyric acid (GABA) receptor complex and facilitates the inhibitory effect of GABA on the CNS.

DOSAGE: IV.

Status epilepticus:

- **Neonates:** 0.05 mg/kg/dose IV over 2 to 5 minutes. If no response after 10 to 15 minutes, repeat the dose; dilute with an equal volume of sterile water, normal saline (NS), or 5% dextrose in water (D5W).
- **Infants and children:** 0.05 to 0.1 mg/kg slow IV over 2 to 5 minutes; do not exceed 4 mg per single dose; may repeat second dose of 0.05 mg/kg slow IV in 10 to 15 minutes if needed; dilute with an equal volume of sterile water, NS, or D5W.

Sedation, anxiety:

- 0.02 to 0.1 mg/kg/dose IV or PO every 4 to 8 hours as needed; not to exceed 2 mg/dose.

ADVERSE EFFECTS: May cause respiratory depression, apnea, hypotension, bradycardia, cardiac arrest, and seizure-like activity. Paradoxical CNS stimulation may occur, usually early in therapy. Some preterm infants may exhibit myoclonic activity; discontinue if any CNS effect occurs. Overdose may be reversed using flumazenil (Romazicon), 5 to 10 mcg/kg/dose IV. Reversal agent may trigger seizures.

COMMENTS: *Note:* IV preparations contain benzyl alcohol, propylene glycol, and polyethylene glycol. Contraindicated for infants with preexisting CNS, hepatic, or renal disease.

MAGNESIUM SULFATE

INDICATIONS AND USE: Treatment and prevention of hypomagnesemia and refractory hypocalcemia.

ACTIONS: Magnesium is an important cofactor in many enzymatic reactions. In the CNS, magnesium prevents or controls seizures by blocking neuromuscular transmission and decreasing the amount of acetylcholine liberated. It also has a depressant effect on the CNS. In the heart, magnesium acts as a calcium channel blocker and acts on cardiac muscle to slow sinoatrial nodal impulse formation and prolong conduction time. Magnesium is necessary for the maintenance of serum potassium and calcium levels through its effect on the renal tubule.

DOSAGE: IV, IM (1 g of magnesium sulfate = 98.6 mg elemental magnesium = 8.12 mEq magnesium).

Hypomagnesemia:

- **Neonates:** 25 to 50 mg/kg/dose (0.2–0.4 mEq/kg/dose) IV every 8 to 12 hours for 2 to 3 doses until magnesium level is normal or symptoms resolve.
- **Maintenance:** 0.25 to 0.5 mEq/kg every 24 hours IV (add to infusion or give IV).
- **Children:** 25 to 50 mg/kg/dose (0.2–0.4 mEq/kg/dose) IM/IV every 4 to 6 hours for 3 to 4 doses; maximum single dose 2000 mg (16 mEq).

ADVERSE EFFECTS: Primarily related to magnesium serum level; hypotension, bradycardia, flushing, depression of reflexes, depressed cardiac function, and CNS and respiratory depression.

COMMENTS: Contraindicated in renal failure. Monitor serum magnesium, calcium, and phosphate levels. For intermittent infusion: dilute to a concentration of 0.5 mEq/mL (60 mg/mL) of magnesium sulfate; maximum concentration 1.6 mEq/mL (200 mg/mL) of magnesium sulfate; infuse magnesium sulfate over 2 to 4 hours and do not exceed 1 mEq/kg/h.

MEROPENEM (MERREM IV)

ACTIONS AND SPECTRUM: Broad-spectrum carbapenem that penetrates well into CSF and most body tissues; specifically active against pneumococcal and *Pseudomonas* meningitis, extended-spectrum β-lactamase–producing *Klebsiella pneumoniae*. Treatment of serious infections caused by multidrug-resistant gram-negative organisms and gram-positive aerobic and anaerobic pathogens susceptible to meropenem.

DOSAGE: IV.

Neonatal sepsis:

- **Gestational age <32 weeks and ≤14 days postnatal:** 20 mg/kg/dose IV every 12 hours; >14 days postnatal, dosing interval is every 8 hours.
- **Gestational age ≥32 weeks and ≤7 days postnatal:** 20 mg/kg/dose IV every 12 hours; >7 days postnatal, dosing interval is every 8 hours.

Neonatal meningitis caused by *Pseudomonas* species:

- **All ages:** 40 mg/kg/dose IV every 8 hours.

Children ≥3 months:

- **Complicated skin and skin structure infection:** 10 mg/kg/dose IV every 8 hours; maximum dose 500 mg.
- **Intra-abdominal infection:** 20 mg/kg/dose IV every 8 hours; maximum dose 1 g.
- **Meningitis:** 40 mg/kg/dose IV every 8 hours; maximum dose 2 g.

ADVERSE EFFECTS: Gastrointestinal effects such as diarrhea, vomiting, and rarely pseudomembranous colitis; fungal infections are a risk. Thrombocytosis and eosinophilia have been noted. Monitoring liver enzymes is recommended. Some cautionary reports have noted seizure-like episodes in a few preterm infants.

COMMENT: Serum half-life of meropenem is relatively short in infants (≤3 hours).

METHADONE HCL (DOLOPHINE)

> **WARNING:** Deaths have been reported during initiation of methadone treatment for opioid dependence. Respiratory depression is the chief hazard associated with methadone hydrochloride administration. Cases of QT interval prolongation and serious arrhythmia (torsade de pointes) have been observed.

INDICATIONS AND USE: Long-acting narcotic analgesic used for the treatment of neonatal abstinence syndrome and opioid dependence.
ACTIONS: CNS opiate receptor agonist resulting in analgesia and sedation; produces generalized CNS depression.
DOSAGE: PO, IV.
Neonatal abstinence syndrome:
- 0.05 to 0.2 mg/kg/dose PO/IV every 12 to 24 hours or 0.5 mg/kg/day divided every 8 hours. Individualize dose and tapering schedule to control symptoms of withdrawal; usually taper dose by 10% to 20% per week over 1 to 1.5 months. *Note:* Due to long elimination half-life, tapering is difficult; consider alternate agent like morphine.
ADVERSE EFFECTS: Respiratory depression, gastric residuals, abdominal distension, constipation, hypotension, bradycardia, prolongation of QT interval, torsade de pointes, CNS depression, sedation, increased intracranial pressure, urinary tract spasm, urine retention, biliary tract spasm, and dependence with prolonged use.
COMMENTS: *Caution:* Methadone may accumulate; reassess for the need to adjust the dose downward after 3 to 5 days to avoid overdose. Smaller doses or less frequent administration may be required in renal and hepatic dysfunction. Rifampin and phenytoin increase metabolism of methadone and may precipitate withdrawal symptoms. Methadone 10 mg IM = morphine 10 mg IM.

METOCLOPRAMIDE HCL (REGLAN)

> **WARNING:** Tardive dyskinesia may occur with metoclopramide use, and the risk increases with duration of treatment and total cumulative dose. Discontinue therapy immediately in patients who develop signs and symptoms of tardive dyskinesia. Symptoms may improve or resolve after drug is discontinued. Avoid treatment with metoclopramide for longer than 12 weeks due to increased risk of developing tardive dyskinesia.

INDICATIONS AND USE: In neonates and infants, the drug is used to facilitate gastric emptying and gastrointestinal (GI) motility. May improve feeding intolerance and gastroesophageal reflux.
ACTIONS: Dopamine receptor antagonist acting on the CNS. Metoclopramide improves GI motility by releasing acetylcholine from the myenteric plexus, resulting in contraction of the smooth muscle. Metoclopramide's effects on the GI tract include the following: increased resting esophageal sphincter tone, improved gastric tone and peristalsis, relaxed pyloric sphincter, and augmented duodenal peristalsis, which leads to increased gastric emptying and a decrease in the transit time through the duodenum, jejunum, and ileum.
DOSAGE: PO, IM, IV.
Gastroesophageal reflux:
- **Neonates:** 0.1 to 0.15 mg/kg/dose PO/IM/IV every 6 hours, 30 minutes before feedings.
- **Infants and children:** 0.4 to 0.8 mg/kg/day PO/IM/IV divided into 4 doses.
ADVERSE EFFECTS: CNS effects include restlessness, drowsiness, and fatigue. Extrapyramidal reactions may occur, generally manifested as acute dystonic reactions within the initial 24 to 48 hours of use (increased with higher doses). May cause tardive dyskinesia, which is often irreversible; duration of treatment and total cumulative dose are associated with an increased risk.
COMMENTS: Therapy durations >12 weeks should be avoided (except in rare cases where benefit exceeds risk). Contraindicated with bowel obstruction and seizure disorders.

METRONIDAZOLE (FLAGYL)

ACTION AND SPECTRUM: Treatment of meningitis, ventriculitis, and endocarditis due to *Bacteroides fragilis* and other anaerobes that are resistant to penicillin; serious intra-abdominal infections; treatment of *Clostridium difficile* colitis.

DOSAGE: PO, IV.

Neonates, susceptible infections:

- **Loading dose:** 15 mg/kg
- **Maintenance dose:**
  - **≤2 kg:**
    - **PNA ≤28 days:** 7.5 mg/kg/dose every 12 hours.
    - **PNA 29 to 60 days:** 10 mg/kg/dose every 8 hours.
  - **>2 kg:**
    - **PNA ≤7 days:** 7.5 mg/kg/dose every 8 hours.
    - **PNA ≥8 days:** 10 mg/kg/dose every 8 hours.

Infants and children:

- **Anaerobic infections:** 30 mg/kg/day PO/IV in divided doses every 6 hours; maximum dose 4 g/day.
- **C difficile diarrhea:** 30 mg/kg/day PO divided every 6 hours for at least 10 days; do not exceed 2 g/day.

ADVERSE EFFECTS: Occasional vomiting, diarrhea, insomnia, irritability, seizures, rash, discoloration of urine (dark or reddish brown), phlebitis at the injection site, and (rarely) leukopenia.

PHARMACOLOGY: Hepatic metabolism with final excretion via the urine and feces. Large volume of distribution (penetrates into all body tissues and fluids).

COMMENTS: Effectively penetrates the CSF (indicated for meningitis). *Note:* Some centers use metronidazole for empiric coverage with ampicillin and gentamicin for necrotizing enterocolitis (NEC). Use of metronidazole in NEC remains *controversial*.

MICAFUNGIN (MYCAMINE)

ACTION AND SPECTRUM: Treatment of fungal septicemia, peritonitis, and disseminated infections due to *Candida* species, including *Candida albicans* and non-albicans species—*Candida krusei, Candida glabrata, Candida tropicalis,* and *Candida parapsilosis.*

DOSAGE: IV.

Neonates:

- **<1 kg:** 10 mg/kg/dose every 24 hours; doses as high as 15 mg/kg/dose have been used in extremely low birthweight neonates.
- **≥1 kg:** 7 mg/kg/dose every 24 hours.

Infants and children:

- 2 to 4 mg/kg/dose every 24 hours.

ADVERSE EFFECTS: Limited data in neonates; in adults—vomiting, diarrhea, hypokalemia, thrombocytopenia.

PHARMACOLOGY: Echinocandin agent with broad-spectrum fungicidal activity. The volume of distribution in extremely premature infants is very high; therefore, higher doses are required. Highly protein bound to albumin but does not displace bilirubin. Metabolized in the liver.

COMMENTS: Infuse over at least 1 hour. Not FDA approved for use in children, and data are limited.

MIDAZOLAM HCL (VERSED)

> **WARNING:** Intravenous midazolam has been associated with respiratory depression and respiratory arrest, especially when used for sedation in noncritical care settings. In some cases where this was not recognized promptly and treated effectively, death or hypoxic encephalopathy has resulted.

INDICATIONS AND USE: Anxiolytic and antiepileptic agent. Used as a sedative before procedures and given IV continuously to sedate intubated patients.

ACTIONS: Short-acting benzodiazepine; depresses CNS by binding to the benzodiazepine site on the γ-aminobutyric acid (GABA) receptor complex and increasing GABA, which is a major inhibitory neurotransmitter in the brain.

DOSAGE: IM, IV, PO, intranasal, sublingual.

Intermittent:
- 0.05 to 0.15 mg/kg/dose IV/IM over at least 5 minutes every 2 to 4 hours as needed.

Continuous infusion:
- **<32 weeks:** Initial 0.03 mg/kg/h (0.5 mcg/kg/min).
- **>32 weeks:** Initial 0.06 mg/kg/h (1 mcg/kg/min).
- **Dosage ranges from 0.01 to 0.06 mg/kg/h.** May need to increase dose after several days due to tolerance or increased clearance. *Note:* Do not use IV loading doses in neonates; for faster sedation effect, infuse the continuous infusion at a faster rate for the first several hours; use the smallest dose possible.

Antiepileptic:
- **Loading dose:** 0.06 to 0.15 mg/kg/dose IV followed by a continuous infusion of 0.06 to 0.4 mg/kg/h (1–7 mcg/kg/min). Start with lower end of dosing range.

Oral sedation:
- 0.25 to 0.5 mg/kg/dose using oral syrup.

Intranasal:
- 0.2 to 0.3 mg/kg/dose using 5-mg/mL injectable form; may repeat in 5 to 15 minutes.

Sublingual:
- 0.2 mg/kg/dose using 5-mg/mL injectable form mixed with small amount of flavored syrup.

ADVERSE EFFECTS: Respiratory depression and cardiac arrest with excessive doses or rapid IV infusions. May cause hypotension and bradycardia. Myoclonic activity and other seizure-like activity have been reported in preterm infants.

COMMENT: Infuse IV slowly. Benzodiazepine withdrawal may occur if abruptly discontinued in patients receiving prolonged IV continuous infusions; doses should be tapered slowly with prolonged use. Contraindicated if preexisting CNS depression.

MILRINONE (PRIMACOR)

INDICATIONS AND USE: Short-term (<72 hours) treatment of acute low cardiac output due to septic shock or following cardiac surgery.

ACTIONS AND SPECTRUM: Inhibits phosphodiesterase III (PDE III), which increases cyclic adenosine monophosphate and potentiates the delivery of calcium to myocardial contractile systems; results in a positive inotropic effect. Inhibition of PDE III in vascular tissue results in relaxation of vascular muscle and vasodilatation. Unlike catecholamines, milrinone does not increase myocardial oxygen consumption.

DOSAGE: IV, intraosseous.

Neonates, infants, and children: A limited number of studies have used different dosing schemes. Further pharmacodynamic studies are needed to define pediatric milrinone guidelines. Several centers use the following guidelines:
- **Loading dose:** 50 mcg/kg over 15 minutes followed by a continuous infusion of 0.5 mcg/kg/min; range: 0.25 to 0.75 mcg/kg/min; titrate to effect.
- **IV, IO (Pediatric Advanced Life Support Guidelines, 2019):** Loading dose 50 mcg/kg over 10 to 60 minutes followed by a continuous infusion of 0.25 to 0.75 mcg/kg/min; titrate dose to effect.

ADVERSE EFFECTS: Hypokalemia, thrombocytopenia, abnormal liver function tests, ventricular arrhythmias, and hypotension.

PHARMACOLOGY: Excreted in urine as unchanged drug (83%) and glucuronide metabolite (12%). With renal impairment, half-life is prolonged and clearance is decreased.

COMMENTS: Use with caution and modify dosage in patients with impaired renal function; adequate intravascular volume is necessary prior to initiating therapy. Omit bolus dose to reduce risk of hypotension.

MORPHINE SULFATE (VARIOUS)

INDICATIONS AND USE: Analgesia, preoperative sedation, supplement to anesthesia, treatment of opioid withdrawal, and relief of dyspnea associated with pulmonary edema.

ACTIONS: A pure opioid agonist, selective to the μ-receptor in the CNS. The interaction with these opioid receptors results in effects that mimic the actions of enkephalins, β-endorphin, and other exogenous ligands.

DOSAGE: IM, IV, PO, subcutaneous.

Neonates (use preservative-free form):

- **Initial:** 0.05 mg/kg IM, IV, subcutaneous every 4 to 8 hours; titrate carefully to effect; maximum dose 0.1 mg/kg/dose.
- **Continuous infusion:** Initial: 0.01 mg/kg/h (10 mcg/kg/h); do not exceed infusion rates of 0.015 to 0.02 mg/kg/h due to decreased elimination, increased CNS sensitivity, and adverse effects; may need to use slightly higher doses, especially in neonates who develop tolerance.
- **International evidence-based group for neonatal pain recommendations (Anand et al, 2001):**
  - **Intermittent dose:** 0.05 to 0.1 mg/kg/dose.
- **Continuous infusion:** Range: 0.01 to 0.03 mg/kg/h.
  - **Neonatal narcotic abstinence:** 0.03 to 0.1 mg/kg/dose PO every 3 to 4 hours. Taper dose by 10% to 20% every 2 to 3 days based on abstinence scoring.

Infants and children:

- **Oral:** 0.2 to 0.5 mg/kg/dose every 4 to 6 hours as needed.

ADVERSE EFFECTS: Dose-dependent side effects include miosis, respiratory depression, drowsiness, bradycardia, and hypotension. Constipation, sedation, gastrointestinal upset, urinary retention, histamine release, and sweating may occur. Causes physiologic dependence; taper the dose gradually after long-term use to avoid withdrawal.

PHARMACOLOGY: Metabolized in the liver via glucuronide conjugation to morphine-6-glucuronide (active) and morphine-3-glucuronide (inactive). Morphine is 20% to 40% bioavailable when administered orally. Metabolites are renally excreted.

COMMENTS: When changing routes of administration in chronically treated patients, oral doses are approximately 3 to 5 times the parenteral dose.

MOXIFLOXACIN OPHTHALMIC

See Chapter 58.

MUPIROCIN (BACTROBAN)

INDICATIONS AND USE: Topical treatment of impetigo resulting from *Staphylococcus aureus* (including methicillin-resistant strains), β-hemolytic *Streptococcus*, and *Streptococcus pyogenes*. Used for minor bacterial skin infections resulting from susceptible organisms and eradication of *S aureus* from nasal and perineal carriage sites.

ACTIONS: Inhibits protein and RNA synthesis by binding to bacterial isoleucyl-tRNA synthetase.

DOSAGE: Intranasal, topical.

Intranasal:

- Apply sparingly 2 to 3 times a day for 5 to 14 days. Reevaluate in 5 days if no response.

Topical:

- **Cream:** Apply small amount 3 times a day for 10 days.
- **Ointment:** Apply a small amount 3 to 5 times a day for 5 to 14 days.

ADVERSE EFFECTS: Burning, rash, erythema, and pruritus.

COMMENTS: Use with caution in burn patients and patients with impaired renal function. Avoid contact with eyes; not for ophthalmic use. When applied to extensive open wounds or burns, the possibility of absorption of the polyethylene glycol vehicle, resulting in serious renal toxicity, should be considered.

NAFCILLIN SODIUM

ACTION AND SPECTRUM: Semisynthetic penicillinase-resistant penicillin with bactericidal activity against susceptible bacteria; treatment of bacterial infections such as osteomyelitis, septicemia, endocarditis, and CNS infections due to susceptible penicillinase-producing strains of *Staphylococcus*.

DOSAGE: IM, IV. Consider higher doses when treating CNS infections.

Neonates:
- **0 to 14 days and <1 kg:** 50 mg/kg/day IM/IV in divided doses every 12 hours.
- **≤7 days:**
  - **1 to 2 kg:** 50 mg/kg/day IM/IV in divided doses every 12 hours.
  - **>2 kg:** 75 mg/kg/day IM/IV in divided doses every 8 hours.
- **>7 days:**
  - **1 to 2 kg:** 75 mg/kg/day IM/IV in divided doses every 8 hours.
  - **>2 kg:** 100 mg/kg/day IM/IV in divided doses every 6 hours.

Meningitis:
- **0 to 7 days:** 75 mg/kg/day IM/IV in divided doses every 8 to 12 hours.
- **>7 days:** 100 to 150 mg/kg/day in divided doses every 6 to 8 hours.

Infants and children:
- **Mild to moderate infections:** 100 to 150 mg/kg/day IM/IV in divided doses every 6 hours; maximum dose 4 g/day.
- **Severe infections:** 150 to 200 mg/kg/day IM/IV in divided doses every 4 to 6 hours; maximum dose 12 g/day.

ADVERSE EFFECTS: Thrombophlebitis, hypersensitivity, granulocytopenia, and agranulocytosis. Severe tissue injury after IV extravasation.

PHARMACOLOGY: Hepatic metabolism, undergoes enterohepatic recirculation; concentrated in bile. Has better CNS penetration than methicillin.

COMMENTS: Avoid IM use if possible.

NALOXONE HCL (EVIZIO, NARCAN)

INDICATIONS AND USE: Narcotic antagonist that reverses CNS and respiratory depression in suspected narcotic overdose; neonatal opiate depression.

ACTIONS: An opiate antagonist that competes with and displaces narcotics at narcotic receptor sites. It has little to no agonistic activity.

DOSAGE: IV. May be given IM if perfusion is adequate. Also ETT, intranasal.

Opioid intoxication:
- **Usual dose:** 0.1 mg/kg IV/IO and may repeat every 2 to 3 minutes as needed; repeat doses may be required every 20 to 60 minutes if duration of action of narcotic is longer than naloxone.
- **ETT:** Optimal dose unknown; current recommendation is 2 to 3 times the IV dose.
- **IM:** 0.4 mg as a single dose, may repeat every 2 to 3 minutes as needed; absorption may be delayed or erratic.
- **Intranasal:** 4 mg nasal spray as a single dose, may repeat every 2 to 3 minutes in alternating nostrils as needed; absorption may be delayed or erratic.

Alternative dosing to reverse opioid-induced depression: 0.01 mg/kg and repeat every 2 to 3 minutes as needed.

ADVERSE EFFECTS: Hypertension, hypotension, tachycardia, ventricular arrhythmias, hyperreflexia, withdrawal syndrome, seizure, and excessive crying.

PHARMACOLOGY: Onset of action is within 1 to 2 minutes after IV injection, 2 to 5 minutes after IM injection, and 8 to 15 minutes after intranasal inhalation. Duration of action is generally 30 to 60 minutes. Bioavailability of intranasal naloxone is only 43 to 54% when compared to IM route.

COMMENTS: Avoid use in infants of narcotic-addicted mothers and infants with physical dependence to opiates (may precipitate acute withdrawal syndrome). IV/IO administration preferred to allow dosing according to weight and titration to effect. Infants must be monitored for reappearance of respiratory depression and the need for repeated doses. Naloxone is not recommended as part of initial resuscitation in the delivery room for newborns with respiratory depression.

NEOMYCIN OPHTHALMIC

See Chapter 58.

NEOMYCIN SULFATE

ACTION AND SPECTRUM: Aminoglycoside indicated in the treatment of diarrhea resulting from enteropathogenic *Escherichia coli* and as preoperative prophylaxis before intestinal surgery; an adjunct therapy in hepatic encephalopathy. Neomycin is inactive against anaerobic organisms.
DOSAGE: PO.
• 50 to 100 mg/kg/day PO divided every 6 to 8 hours.
ADVERSE EFFECTS: Diarrhea, colitis, and malabsorption; nephrotoxicity and ototoxicity.
PHARMACOLOGY: Renal excretion if systemic absorption occurs. Poorly absorbed from the gastrointestinal tract if administered orally; 97% of unchanged drug in the feces.

NEOSTIGMINE METHYLSULFATE (BLOXIVERZ)

INDICATIONS AND USE: Improvement of muscle strength in the treatment of myasthenia gravis; may be used to reverse nondepolarizing neuromuscular-blocking agents.
ACTIONS: Neostigmine competitively inhibits hydrolysis of acetylcholine by acetylcholinesterase, facilitating transmission of impulses across the myoneural junction and producing cholinergic activity.
DOSAGE: IV, IM, subcutaneous.
Myasthenia gravis:
• **Diagnostic testing:** 0.025 to 0.04 mg/kg/dose IM once. (Discontinue all cholinesterase medications at least 8 hours before; atropine should be administered IV immediately prior to or IM 30 minutes before neostigmine.)
• **Treatment:** 0.01 to 0.04 mg/kg/dose IM, IV, or subcutaneous every 2 to 6 hours as needed or 1 mg PO given 2 hours prior to feeding.
Reversal of nondepolarizing neuromuscular blockade:
• 0.03 to 0.07 mg/kg/dose; recommend lower dose for agents with shorter half-lives and higher dose for agents with lower half-lives. (Use with atropine: 0.01 to 0.04 mg/kg, or 0.4 mg of atropine for each 1 mg of neostigmine.)
ADVERSE EFFECTS: Cholinergic crisis, which may include bronchospasm, increased bronchial secretions and salivation, vomiting, diarrhea, bradycardia, respiratory depression, and seizures.
COMMENTS: Does not antagonize and may prolong the phase I block of depolarizing muscle.

NEVIRAPINE (VIRAMUNE)

> **WARNING:** Reports of fatal hepatotoxicity even after short-term use; severe life-threatening skin reactions (Stevens-Johnson, toxic epidermal necrolysis, and allergic reactions); monitor closely during first 8 weeks of treatment.

ACTION AND SPECTRUM: Nonnucleoside antiretroviral agent that inhibits human immunodeficiency virus (HIV) type 1 replication by selectively interfering with viral reverse transcriptase. Acts synergistically with zidovudine. Used for the prevention of maternal-fetal HIV transmission and HIV treatment. FDA approved in ages ≥15 days, although recommended as preferred agent in infants from birth to 14 days of age per guidelines.
DOSAGE: PO (based on **aidsinfo.nih.gov/guidelines**, 2019).
Prevention of maternal-fetal HIV transmission:
• **Three doses given in the first week of life as follows:** First dose within 48 hours of birth, second dose 48 hours after first dose, and third dose 96 hours after second dose. Give in combination with **zidovudine.** Used in select situations such as infants born to HIV-infected mothers with no antiretroviral therapy prior to labor or during labor; infants born to mothers with only intrapartum therapy; infants born to mothers with suboptimal viral suppression at delivery; or infants born to mothers with known antiretroviral drug–resistant virus.

- **Birthweight 1.5 to 2 kg:** 8 mg/dose PO.
- **Birthweight >2 kg:** 12 mg/dose PO.

Treatment of HIV infection (in combination with other antiretroviral agents): Consultation with infectious disease expert is recommended.

ADVERSE EFFECTS: Limited data in neonates; rash, elevated liver enzymes, hepatotoxicity, liver failure, cholestatic hepatitis, hepatic necrosis, jaundice.

PHARMACOLOGY: Metabolized by cytochrome P450 isoenzymes 3A4 and 2B6 and has potential for drug interactions; more rapidly metabolized in pediatric patients. It does not require intracellular phosphorylation for antiviral activity.

COMMENTS: Please note manufacturers' Black Box warning regarding severe life-threatening and fatal skin reactions and hepatotoxicity. If administering with a dosing cup, rinse cup with water and also administer rinse.

NICARDIPINE (CARDENE IV)

INDICATIONS AND USE: Short-term treatment of severe hypertension.

ACTIONS: Inhibits calcium ions from entering select voltage-sensitive channels in vascular smooth muscle and myocardium during depolarization; produces relaxation of coronary vascular smooth muscle and coronary vasodilatation.

DOSAGE: IV.

Neonates:

- **Initial dose**: 0.5 mcg/kg/min by continuous infusion. Titrate to desired response; blood pressure will decrease within minutes of starting infusion. Maintenance doses of 0.5 to 2 mcg/kg/min.

Infants and children:

- **Initial dose:** 0.5 to 1 mcg/kg/min by continuous infusion. Titrate increasing rate of infusion every 15 to 30 minutes to a maximum dose of 4 to 5 mcg/kg/min.

ADVERSE EFFECTS: Hypotension, tachycardia, peripheral edema, hypokalemia.

PHARMACOLOGY: Extensively metabolized by the liver and is highly protein bound. Experience in neonates is very limited, and there are no pharmacokinetic data.

COMMENTS: Use with caution in the presence of cardiac, renal, and hepatic disease.

NITRIC OXIDE (INOMAX FOR INHALATION; INHALED NITRIC OXIDE [INO])

INDICATIONS AND USE: iNO is indicated for the treatment of term and near-term (≥34 weeks) neonates with hypoxic respiratory failure associated with clinical or echocardiographic evidence of persistent pulmonary hypertension of the newborn.

ACTIONS: iNO is a selective pulmonary vasodilator without significant effects on the systemic circulation that decreases extrapulmonary right-to-left shunting. Nitric oxide relaxes vascular smooth muscle by binding to the heme moiety of cytosolic guanylate cyclase, activating guanylate cyclase, and increasing intracellular levels of cyclic guanosine 3'5'-monophosphate, which leads to vasodilation and an increase in the partial pressure of arterial oxygen.

DOSAGE: Inhalation.

Term infants or >34 weeks' gestation:

- **Begin at 20 ppm.** Reduce dose to lowest possible level. Doses >20 ppm are usually not used due to increased risk of methemoglobinemia and elevated nitric dioxide (NO_2). Maintain treatment up to 14 days or until the underlying oxygen desaturation has resolved and the infant is ready to be weaned from iNO. Abrupt discontinuation may lead to worsening hypotension, oxygenation, and increasing pulmonary artery pressure; clinical trials suggest weaning by 5 to 10 ppm every 4 hours until the patient is stable at 5 ppm, then decreasing by 1 ppm every 4 hours until discontinued. Further diagnostic testing should be sought for infants who are unable to be weaned off iNO after 4 days of therapy.

ADVERSE EFFECTS: Do not use in neonates dependent on right-to-left shunting of blood. Direct pulmonary injury from excess levels of NO_2 and ambient air contamination may occur. May cause methemoglobinemia and elevated NO_2. Risk of adverse effects increases when iNO is given at doses >20 ppm. Conflicting data have been published on whether or not iNO inhibits platelet aggregation and prolongs bleeding time. Monitor methemoglobin levels, iNO, NO_2, and oxygen levels. iNO therapy should be directed by physicians qualified by education and experience in its use and offered only at centers that are qualified to provide multisystem support, generally including on-site ECLS capability or with a collaborating ECLS center. Consult the manufacturer's product literature and specialized references for complete information on the use of iNO.

NITROPRUSSIDE SODIUM (NIPRIDE RTU, NITROPRESS)

> **WARNING:** Nitroprusside is not suitable for direct injection and must be further diluted in sterile 5% dextrose in water (D5W) before infusion. Nitroprusside can cause precipitous decreases in blood pressure. In patients not properly monitored, these decreases can lead to irreversible ischemic injuries or death. Nitroprusside can give rise to cyanide ion, which can reach toxic, potentially lethal levels. If blood pressure has not been adequately controlled after 10 minutes of infusion at the maximum rate, stop the infusion. Review package insert before administration.

INDICATIONS AND USE: Severe hypertension and hypertension crisis; acute reduction of afterload in patients with refractory congestive heart failure.

ACTIONS: Direct-acting vasodilator (arterial and venous) that reduces peripheral vascular resistance (afterload). Venous return is reduced (preload); increases cardiac output by decreasing afterload.

DOSAGE: IV. Infuse through a large vein.
- **Initial:** 0.25 to 0.5 mcg/kg/min; titrate dose every 20 minutes to the desired response.
- **Usual dose:** 3 mcg/kg/min; rarely need >4 mcg/kg/min; maximum dose 8 to 10 mcg/kg/min.

ADVERSE EFFECTS: Generally related to a very rapid reduction in blood pressure. Thiocyanate may accumulate, especially in patients receiving high doses or those who have impaired renal function. Cyanide toxicity can develop abruptly if large doses are administered rapidly. Cyanide causes early persistent acidosis. Thiocyanate toxicity appears at plasma levels of approximately 35 to 100 mcg/mL; levels >200 mcg/mL are associated with death. Thiocyanate levels should be monitored in any patient receiving ≥3 mcg/kg/min of nitroprusside or prolonged infusion (>3 days), especially those with renal impairment. Toxicity is treated with IV sodium thiosulfate.

PHARMACOLOGY: Acts within seconds to lower blood pressure; when discontinued, the effect dissipates within minutes. Rapidly metabolized to thiocyanate, which is eliminated by the kidneys.

COMMENTS: Contraindicated with decreased cerebral perfusion, hypertension secondary to arteriovenous shunts, or coarctation of the aorta. May add sodium thiosulfate to infusion solution at a 10:1 ratio to minimize thiocyanate toxicity; however, this has not been studied. Protect from light.

NOREPINEPHRINE BITARTRATE (LEVARTERENOL BITARTRATE) (LEVOPHED)

> **WARNING:** Antidote for extravasation ischemia. To prevent sloughing and necrosis, the area should be infiltrated as soon as possible with saline solution containing phentolamine, an adrenergic blocking agent (see Comments).

INDICATIONS AND USE: Treatment of shock, which persists after adequate fluid volume replacement; severe hypotension; cardiogenic shock.

ACTIONS: Stimulates β_1-adrenergic receptors and α-adrenergic receptors, causing increased contractility and heart rate as well as vasoconstriction, resulting in an increase in systemic blood pressure and coronary blood flow; clinically, α-adrenergic effects (vasoconstriction) are greater than β_1-adrenergic effects (inotropic and chronotropic effects).

DOSAGE: IV.
- 0.02 to 0.1 mcg/kg/min initially, titrated to desired perfusion; maximum dose 2 mcg/kg/min.

ADVERSE EFFECTS: Respiratory distress, arrhythmias, bradycardia or tachycardia, hypertension, chest pain, headache, and vomiting. Organ ischemia (due to vasoconstriction of renal and mesenteric arteries).

COMMENTS: Ischemic necrosis may occur after extravasation. Administer phentolamine, 0.1 to 0.2 mg/kg subcutaneous, infiltrated into the area of extravasation within 12 hours to minimize damage. (See Chapter 42.)

NUSINERSEN (SPINRAZA)

INDICATIONS AND USE: Treatment of spinal muscular atrophy (SMA).

ACTIONS: Treats SMA caused by mutations in chromosome 5q that lead to survival motor neuron (SMN) protein deficiency by binding to a specific sequence in the mRNA transcript and increasing production of SMN protein.

DOSAGE: Intrathecal
- **Loading dose:** 12 mg once every 14 days for 3 doses; then 12 mg once 30 days after the third dose.
- **Maintenance dose:** 12 mg once every 4 months.

ADVERSE EFFECTS: Feeding difficulties, dysphagia, headache, back pain, constipation, otic infection, aspiration, severe dyspnea.

COMMENTS: Allow to warm to room temperature before use. Prior to administration, remove 5 mL of CSF. Administer as an intrathecal bolus injection over 1 to 3 minutes using spinal anesthesia needle; do not administer in areas with signs of infection or inflammation.

NYSTATIN

ACTION AND SPECTRUM: May be fungistatic or fungicidal, which acts by binding to sterols and disrupting fungal cell membranes. Treatment of susceptible cutaneous, mucocutaneous, and oral cavity fungal infections normally caused by the *Candida* species.

DOSAGE: PO, topical.

ORAL THRUSH:
- **Therapeutic:** Continue for 3 days after symptoms have resolved.
  - **Neonates:** 1 to 4 mL (100,000–400,000 units) divided to each side of the mouth 4 times a day after feedings.
  - **Infants:** 2 to 4 mL (100,000–400,000 units) divided to each side of mouth 4 times a day after feedings.
- **Prophylaxis:** 1 mL (100,000 units) divided to each side of mouth or 1 mL orally or via oral gavage tube 3 to 4 times a day.

Diaper rash:
- Topical cream/ointment/powder applied 3 to 4 times a day for 7 to 10 days.

ADVERSE EFFECTS: Side effects are uncommon but may cause diarrhea, local irritation, contact dermatitis, rash, pruritus, and Stevens-Johnson syndrome.

PHARMACOLOGY: Poorly absorbed orally. Most is passed unchanged in the stool.

OCTREOTIDE (SANDOSTATIN)

INDICATIONS AND USE: Short-term management of persistent hyperinsulinemic hypoglycemia of the newborn. Useful in the management of chylothorax. Chyle accumulation usually decreases after 24 hours of continuous infusion. Has also been used to treat hypersecretory diarrhea and fistulas in infants. Significant reductions in stool or ileal output were achieved with this drug.

ACTIONS: A synthetic polypeptide that mimics natural somatostatin by inhibiting serotonin release and the secretion of gastrin, vasoactive intestinal peptide, insulin, glucagon, secretin, motilin, thyrotropin, and cholecystokinin; reduces splanchnic blood flow, decreases gastrointestinal motility, and inhibits intestinal secretion of water and electrolytes.

DOSAGE: IV, subcutaneous.

Persistent hyperinsulinemic hypoglycemia of infancy:

- **Initial dose:** 2 to 10 mcg/kg/day subcutaneous divided every 6 to 8 hours; titrate based on response up to 40 mcg/kg/day divided every 6 to 8 hours. Adjust to maintain symptomatic control.

Diarrhea:

- 1 to 10 mcg/kg/dose IV/subcutaneous given every 12 hours. Adjust the dose to maintain symptomatic control.

Chylothorax:

- 0.5 to 4 mcg/kg/h IV continuous infusion; titrate dose to response; case reports of effective dosage ranging between 0.3 and 10 mcg/kg/h; treatment duration is usually 1 to 3 weeks but may vary with clinical response.

ADVERSE EFFECTS: Possible growth retardation during long-term treatment, flushing, hypertension, insomnia, fever, chills, seizures, Bell palsy, hair loss, bruising, rash, hypoglycemia, hyperglycemia, galactorrhea, hypothyroidism, diarrhea, abdominal distention, vomiting, constipation, hepatitis, jaundice, local injection site pain, thrombophlebitis, muscle weakness, increased creatine kinase, muscle spasm, tremor, oliguria, shortness of breath, and rhinorrhea.

PHARMACOLOGY: Duration of action (subcutaneous) is 6 to 12 hours with immediate-release formulation; excreted unchanged in the urine.

COMMENTS: Tachyphylaxis may occur.

OMEPRAZOLE (PRILOSEC)

INDICATIONS AND USE: Short-term (<8 weeks) treatment of reflux esophagitis, duodenal ulcer refractory to conventional therapy.

ACTIONS: Inhibits gastric acid secretion by inactivating the parietal cell membrane enzyme (H^+/K^+)-adenosine triphosphatase (ATPase) or proton pump.

DOSAGE: PO.

- **Neonates:** 0.5 to 1.5 mg/kg once daily in the morning.
- **1 month to 2 years:** 0.7 mg/kg once daily; increase to 3 mg/kg once daily if necessary (maximum dose 20 mg).

ADVERSE EFFECTS: Mild elevation of liver enzymes, diarrhea (*Clostridium difficile*–associated diarrhea), and increased risk of bone fractures (decreased bone mineral density).

PHARMACOLOGY: Cytochrome P450 isoenzyme CYP1A2 inducer; isoenzyme CYP2C8, CYP2C18, CYP2C19, and CYP3A3/4 substrate; isoenzyme CYP2C9, CYP3A3/4, CYP2C8, and CYP2C19 inhibitor. Maximum secretory inhibition is 4 days. Extensive first-pass metabolism in the liver. Bioavailability: 30% to 40%; improves slightly with repeated administration.

ADVERSE EFFECTS: Mild elevation of liver enzymes, diarrhea.

COMMENTS: Lack of data regarding the safety of long-term use in children. Oral delayed-release suspension available.

OPIUM TINCTURE

HIGH-ALERT MEDICATION: May also be confused with camphorated tincture of opium (Paregoric). Opium tincture is 25 times as potent as paregoric. Avoid the use of the abbreviation "DTO."

INDICATIONS AND USE: A 25-fold dilution with water (final concentration 0.4 mg/mL) can be used to treat neonatal abstinence syndrome (opiate withdrawal).

ACTIONS: Contains many narcotic alkaloids including morphine; inhibition of gastrointestinal (GI) motility due to morphine content; decreases digestive secretions; increases GI muscle tone.

DOSAGE: PO.

Neonates (full-term):

- **Neonatal abstinence syndrome (opiate withdrawal):** Use a 25-fold dilution with water of opium tincture (final concentration 0.4 mg/mL morphine).
  - **Initial dose:** Give 0.04 mg/kg/dose of a 0.4 mg/mL solution with feedings every 3 to 4 hours; increase as needed by 0.04 mg/kg/dose of a 0.4 mg/mL solution every 3 to 4 hours until withdrawal symptoms are controlled.

- **Usual dose:** 0.08 to 0.2 mg/dose of a 0.4 mg/mL solution given every 3 to 4 hours; it is rare to exceed 0.28 mg/dose of a 0.4 mg/mL solution; stabilize withdrawal symptoms for 3 to 5 days, then gradually decrease the dosage (keeping the same dosage interval) over a 2- to 4-week period.

ADVERSE EFFECTS: Hypotension, bradycardia, peripheral vasodilation, CNS depression, drowsiness, sedation, urinary retention, constipation, respiratory depression, and histamine release.

PHARMACOLOGY: Metabolized in liver and eliminated in urine and bile.

COMMENTS: Observe for excessive sedation and respiratory depression. Do not abruptly discontinue. Monitor for the resolution of withdrawal symptoms (eg, irritability, high-pitched cry, stuffy nose, rhinorrhea, vomiting, poor feeding, diarrhea, sneezing, yawning) and signs of overtreatment (eg, bradycardia, lethargy, hypotonia, irregular respirations, respiratory depression). An abstinence scoring system (eg, Finnegan abstinence scoring system) should be used to more objectively assess neonatal opiate withdrawal symptoms and the need for dosage adjustment (see Chapter 102). Use 25-fold dilution with water for the treatment of neonatal abstinence syndrome.

OXACILLIN SODIUM

ACTION AND SPECTRUM: Semisynthetic penicillinase-resistant penicillin; bactericidal activity used for the treatment of bacterial infections such as osteomyelitis, septicemia, endocarditis, and CNS infections due to susceptible penicillinase-producing strains of *Staphylococcus*.

DOSAGE: IM, IV.

Neonates:

- **0 to 14 days and <1 kg:** 50 mg/kg/day IM/IV in divided doses every 12 hours.
- **>14 days and <1 kg:** 75 mg/kg/day IM/IV in divided doses every 8 hours.
- **≤7 days and 1 to 2 kg:** 50 mg/kg/day IM/IV in divided doses every 12 hours.
- **≤7 days and >2 kg:** 75 mg/kg/day IM/IV in divided doses every 8 hours.
- **>7 days and 1 to 2 kg:** 75 mg/kg/day IM/IV in divided doses every 8 hours.
- **>7 days and >2 kg:** 100 mg/kg/day IM/IV in divided doses every 6 hours.

Meningitis:

- **0 to 7 days:** 75 mg/kg/day IM/IV in divided doses every 8 to 12 hours.
- **>7 days:** 150 to 200 mg/kg/day in divided doses every 6 to 8 hours.

Infants and children:

- **Mild to moderate infections:** 100 to 150 mg/kg/day IM/IV in divided doses every 6 hours; maximum 4 g/day.
- **Severe infections:** 150 to 200 mg/kg/day IM/IV in divided doses every 4 to 6 hours; maximum 12 g/day.

ADVERSE EFFECTS: Hypersensitivity reactions (rash), thrombophlebitis, mild leukopenia, acute interstitial nephritis, hematuria, azotemia, and elevation in aspartate aminotransferase. *Clostridium difficile* colitis has been reported.

PHARMACOLOGY: Metabolized chiefly in the liver and excreted in bile; dosage modification required in patients with renal impairment.

COMMENTS: Avoid IM injection.

PALIVIZUMAB (SYNAGIS)

INDICATIONS AND USE: Immunoprophylaxis against severe respiratory syncytial virus (RSV) lower respiratory tract infections in high-risk infants and children. The American Academy of Pediatrics recommends RSV prophylaxis with palivizumab during RSV season for:

- **Infants ≤12 months of age** who were born at gestational age ≤28 weeks and 6 days.
- **Infants ≤12 months of age** with congenital airway abnormality or neuromuscular disorder that decreases the ability to manage airway secretions.
- **Infants and children ≤24 months of age** with chronic lung disease (CLD) necessitating medical therapy within 6 months of age prior to the beginning of RSV season.

- **Infants and children ≤24 months** with congenital heart disease and 1 of the following:
  - Receiving medication to treat congestive heart failure
  - Moderate to severe pulmonary hypertension
  - Cyanotic heart disease
  - Cardiac transplantation during RSV season
- **Infants and children ≤24 months of age** who are immunocompromised due to chemotherapy or other conditions during RSV season.
- **Infants and children ≤12 months of age** who have cystic fibrosis (CF) and evidence of CLD or nutritional compromise with weight for length <10th percentile.
- **Infants and children ≤24 months of age** who have CF and have previous manifestations of severe lung disease.
  - Previous hospitalization for pulmonary exacerbation in the first year of life
  - Abnormalities on chest radiography or chest computed tomography that persist when stable

ACTION: Humanized monoclonal antibody directed to an epitope in the A-antigenic site of the respiratory syncytial virus F protein, resulting in neutralizing and fusion-inhibitory activity against RSV.

DOSAGE: IM.

- **15 mg/kg/dose IM once a month during the RSV season**. The first dose should be administered before the start of the RSV season; clinicians may administer up to a maximum of 5 monthly doses during the RSV season to infants who qualify for prophylaxis. Qualifying infants born during the RSV season will require fewer doses.

ADVERSE EFFECTS: Upper respiratory tract infection, otitis media, fever, and rhinitis. Rash, injection site reaction, erythema, induration. Rare cases of anaphylaxis (<1 case/100,000 patients) and severe hypersensitivity reactions (<1 case/1000 patients) have been reported.

PHARMACOLOGY: The mean half-life of palivizumab is approximately 20 days and adequate antibody titers are maintained for 30 days. Time to achieve adequate serum antibody titers is 48 hours.

COMMENTS: Palivizumab is not indicated for the treatment of RSV infections. Palivizumab does not interfere with the response to routine childhood vaccines and therefore may be administered concurrently. Qualifying infants who have had a cardiopulmonary bypass procedure or ECLS should receive a dose as soon as possible after conclusion, even if <1 month from previous dose. Hospitalized neonates should receive their first dose 48 to 72 hours before discharge or promptly after discharge. If hospitalization occurs for breakthrough RSV infection, monthly prophylaxis should be discontinued for the remainder of that season.

PANCURONIUM BROMIDE

HIGH-ALERT MEDICATION: To be administered only by experienced clinicians or adequately trained individuals supervised by an experienced clinician familiar with the use and actions, characteristics, and complications of neuromuscular-blocking agents.

INDICATIONS AND USE: Skeletal muscle relaxation during surgery; increases pulmonary compliance during assisted mechanical ventilation and facilitates endotracheal intubation.

ACTIONS: Nondepolarizing neuromuscular-blocking agent that produces skeletal muscle paralysis by blocking acetylcholine binding at the receptor at the myoneural junction. Pancuronium may cause an increase in heart rate and changes in blood pressure.

DOSAGE: IV.

Neonates and infants:

- *Note:* Neonates are especially sensitive to nondepolarizing neuromuscular-blocking agents, such as pancuronium, during the first month of life. It is recommended that a test dose of 0.02 mg/kg be given first to measure responsiveness.
- 0.05 to 0.1 mg/kg IV as needed, maximum of 0.15 mg/kg/dose; or as continuous IV infusion 0.02 to 0.04 mg/kg/h or 0.4 to 0.6 mcg/kg/min.

ADVERSE EFFECTS: May cause hypoxemia with inadequate mechanical ventilation. Apnea, arrhythmias, tachycardia, hypertension, hypotension, excessive salivation, and bronchospasm may occur. Potentiation of neuromuscular blockade may result from aminoglycosides, electrolyte abnormalities, severe hyponatremia, severe hypocalcemia, severe hypokalemia, hypermagnesemia, neuromuscular diseases, acidosis, renal failure, and hepatic failure. Antagonism of neuromuscular blockade may result from alkalosis, hypercalcemia, hyperkalemia, and epinephrine.

PHARMACOLOGY: The onset of action is generally 2 to 5 minutes, with duration of action of approximately 24 to 60 minutes, but is variable and may be prolonged in neonates.

COMMENTS: Neonates are particularly sensitive to its actions; prolonged paralysis may be noted. Ventilation must be supported during neuromuscular blockade. Neostigmine and atropine are used for reversal. Sensation remains intact; analgesia should be used with painful procedures.

PAPAVERINE HCL

INDICATIONS AND USE: Reduce peripheral arterial spasms in efforts to prolong arterial catheter patency.

ACTIONS: Directly relaxes vascular smooth muscle and results in vasodilation.

DOSAGE: IV.

Peripheral arterial catheter patency in full-term neonates:

- Add 30 mg of preservative-free papaverine to 250 mL of arterial catheter solution (normal saline [NS] or ½ NS) that contains heparin 1 unit/mL; infuse at a rate of ≤1 mL/h. Not recommended for use in preterm neonates <3 weeks of age due to potential risk of developing or extending an intracranial hemorrhage.

COMMENTS: IV infusion should be performed under a physician's supervision because arrhythmias and fatal apnea may result from rapid injection. *Note:* Not FDA approved for use in children. Limited experience in neonates.

PENICILLIN G (AQUEOUS), PARENTERAL

ACTION AND SPECTRUM: Treatment of infection due to gram-positive cocci (except *Staphylococcus aureus*), including all susceptible strains of streptococci (nonenterococcal). However, penicillin G–resistant *Streptococcus pneumoniae* strains have been isolated. Gram-positive bacilli are usually sensitive to penicillin G (*Clostridium tetani*, *Corynebacterium diphtheriae*). Penicillin G is effective for some gram-negative organisms including *Neisseria meningitides*, *Haemophilus influenzae*, and *Neisseria gonorrhoeae*. The Enterobacteriaceae are resistant to penicillin G therapy, and resistance of many gram-negative organisms such as *Escherichia coli* is a result of the ability to produce β-lactamase. Used for the treatment of congenital syphilis.

DOSAGE: IM, IV.

Neonates PNA ≤7 days and ≥1 kg *or* ≤14 days and <1 kg:

- 50,000 to 100,000 units/kg/day IM/IV in divided doses every 12 hours.

Neonates PNA >7 days and ≥1 kg *or* >14 days and <1 kg:

- 75,000 to 150,000 units/kg/day IM/IV in divided doses every 8 hours.

Group B streptococcal meningitis:

- **Neonates PNA ≤7 days:** 250,000 to 450,000 units/kg/day IM/IV in divided doses every 8 hours.
- **Neonates PNA >7 days:** 450,000 to 500,000 units/kg/day IM/IV in divided doses every 6 hours.

Other susceptible organism meningitis:

- **Neonates PNA ≤7 days:** 150,000 units/kg/day IM/IV in divided doses every 8 to 12 hours.
- **Neonates PNA >7 days:** 200,000 units/kg/day IM/IV in divided doses every 6 to 8 hours.

Congenital syphilis:

- **Neonates PNA ≤7 days:** 100,000 units/kg/day IM/IV in divided doses every 12 hours for a total of 10 days.
- **Neonates PNA >7 days:** 150,000 units/kg/day IM/IV in divided doses every 8 hours for a total of 10 days.

Infants and children:
- **Usual dose:** 100,000 to 250,000 units/kg/day IM/IV in divided doses every 4 to 6 hours.
- **Severe infections:** 250,000 to 400,000 units/kg/day IM/IV in divided doses every 4 to 6 hours; maximum dose 24 million units/day.

ADVERSE EFFECTS: Allergic reactions, rash, fever, alterations in bowel flora, *Candida* superinfection, diarrhea, and hemolytic anemia. Acute interstitial nephritis. Bone marrow suppression with granulocytopenia. Very large doses may cause seizures. Rapid IV push of potassium penicillin G may cause cardiac arrhythmias and arrest because of the potassium component. Infuse slowly over 30 minutes.

PHARMACOLOGY: Penetration across the blood–brain barrier is poor with normal meninges; excreted in urine mainly by tubular secretion.

COMMENTS: Good activity against anaerobes. Drug of choice for tetanus neonatorum.

PENICILLIN G BENZATHINE (BICILLIN L-A)

ACTION AND SPECTRUM: See Penicillin G (Aqueous), Parenteral. Treatment of asymptomatic congenital syphilis.

DOSAGE: IM.
- **Asymptomatic congenital syphilis:** Single dose of 50,000 units/kg IM.

ADVERSE EFFECTS: See Penicillin G (Aqueous).

PHARMACOLOGY: Renally excreted over a prolonged interval owing to slow absorption from the injection site.

COMMENTS: See Penicillin G (Aqueous). Not often used. For IM injection only.

PENICILLIN G PROCAINE

ACTION AND SPECTRUM: See Penicillin G (Aqueous), Parenteral. Treatment of symptomatic or asymptomatic congenital syphilis.

DOSAGE: IM.
- 50,000 units/kg/dose IM every 24 hours for 10 days; if >1 day of therapy is missed, the entire course should be restarted.

ADVERSE EFFECTS: See Penicillin G (Aqueous), Parenteral. May also cause sterile abscess formation at the injection site. Contains 120 mg of procaine per 300,000 units, which may cause allergic reactions, myocardial depression, or systemic vasodilation. There is cause for much greater concern about these effects in the neonate than in older patients, and therefore, it is not recommended for use in neonates.

COMMENTS: Not often used.

PENTOBARBITAL SODIUM (NEMBUTAL)

INDICATIONS AND USE: Sedative/hypnotic. Used for agitation, for preprocedure sedation, or as an anticonvulsant.

ACTIONS: Short-acting barbiturate.

DOSAGE: IV.

Procedural sedation:
- 1 to 3 mg/kg/dose IV slow push <50 mg/min; additional doses of 1 to 2 mg/kg may be given every 3 to 5 minutes to desired effect. Total dose: 1 to 6 mg/kg, maximum of 100 mg to desired effect.

Hypnotic:
- 2 to 6 mg/kg/dose IM. Maximum 100 mg/dose.

Status epilepticus refractory to standard therapy:
- Loading dose 5 mg/kg IV; maintenance infusion 1 mg/kg/h, may increase up to 3 mg/kg/h. Intubation is required. Adjust dose based on hemodynamics, seizure activity, and electroencephalogram.

ADVERSE EFFECTS: Observe the IV site closely during administration for extravasation injury. Tolerance and physical dependence may occur with continued use. May cause somnolence, bradycardia, rash, pain on IM injection (solutions are highly alkaline), thrombophlebitis, osteomalacia from prolonged use (rare), and excitability.

COMMENTS: Rapid IV administration may cause respiratory depression, apnea, laryngospasm, bronchospasm, and hypotension; administer over 10 to 30 minutes.

PHENOBARBITAL

INDICATIONS AND USE: Treatment of neonatal seizures; used to treat neonatal abstinence symptoms; may also be used for prevention and treatment of neonatal hyperbilirubinemia and lowering of bilirubin in chronic cholestasis.

ACTIONS: Anticonvulsant activity by increasing the threshold for electrical stimulation of the motor cortex and depresses CNS activity by binding to barbiturate site at γ-aminobutyric acid (GABA) receptor complex, enhancing GABA activity.

DOSAGE: PO, IV.

Anticonvulsant, status epilepticus, neonates and infants:
- **Loading dose:** 15 to 20 mg/kg IV in a single dose. *Note:* In select patients, may repeat additional 5 to 10 mg/kg dose every 15 to 20 minutes until seizure controlled or a total dose of 40 mg/kg; be prepared to provide respiratory support.
- **Maintenance:** Begin 12 to 24 hours after loading dose:
  - **Neonates:** 3 to 4 mg/kg/day PO/IV given in 1 to 2 divided doses; assess serum concentrations; increase to 5 mg/kg/day if needed.
  - **Infants:** 5 to 6 mg/kg/day PO/IV in 1 to 2 divided doses.

Hyperbilirubinemia: Doses of 3 to 8 mg/kg/day PO in 2 to 3 divided doses up to 12 mg/kg/day have been used; dose not clearly established and not recommended due to sedation and other adverse effects.

Neonatal abstinence syndrome: 2 to 8 mg/kg/day PO in 2 to 4 divided doses. Monitor serum concentrations coincident to abstinence scores. Loading dose is optional: 16 mg/kg IV as a single dose or PO in divided into 2 doses.

ADVERSE EFFECTS: Sedation, lethargy, paradoxical excitement, hypotension, gastrointestinal distress, ataxia, rash, and phlebitis (pH of IV solution is 10). Drug accumulation may occur if treating concurrently with phenytoin. Monitor drug levels. Respiratory depression can occur at levels exceeding 60 mcg/mL or with rapid IV administration.

PHARMACOLOGY: Initial half-life in neonates is 40 to 200 hours or longer, gradually declining to about 20 to 100 hours at 3 to 4 weeks of age. Reduction in serum bilirubin levels is attributed to increased levels of glucuronyl transferase; stimulates bile flow and increases the concentration of the Y-binding protein involved in the uptake of bilirubin by hepatocytes. Observed reductions usually require 2 to 3 days of treatment.

COMMENTS: Contraindicated if porphyria suspected. Maintenance serum levels usually fall between 15 and 40 mcg/mL. Abrupt withdrawal may precipitate status epilepticus. Do not inject IV faster than 1 mg/kg/min, with a maximum of 30 mg/min for infants and children.

PHENTOLAMINE MESYLATE INJECTION

INDICATIONS AND USE: Treatment of extravasation from IV α-adrenergic drugs (dobutamine, dopamine, epinephrine, norepinephrine, or phenylephrine). Helps prevent dermal necrosis and sloughing. (See also Chapter 42.)

ACTIONS: Phentolamine blocks α-adrenergic receptors and reverses the severe vasoconstriction from the extravasation of α-adrenergic drugs.

DOSAGE: Subcutaneous.

Neonate:
- Infiltrate area with small amount of solution (~1 mL given in 0.1- to 0.2-mL aliquots) made by diluting 2.5 to 5 mg in 10 mL of preservative-free normal saline (NS); treat within

12 hours of extravasation. Total dose required depends on size of extravasation; should not exceed 0.1 mg/kg or 2.5 mg maximum.

Infants and children:
- Infiltrate area with small amount of solution (~1 mL) made by diluting 5 to 10 mg in 10 mL of preservative-free NS; treat within 12 hours of extravasation. Total dose required depends on size of extravasation; should not exceed 0.1 to 0.2 mg/kg or 5 mg maximum.

ADVERSE EFFECTS: Hypotension, tachycardia, cardiac arrhythmias, and flushing.

PHENYLEPHRINE OPHTHALMIC

INDICATIONS AND USE: A mydriatic for ophthalmic procedures. (See also Chapter 58.)

ACTIONS: α-Adrenergic stimulation and weak β-adrenergic activity. Causes pupils to contract by activation of dilator muscle of the pupil. Causes vasoconstriction of the arterioles of the nasal mucosa and conjunctiva; produces systemic arterial vasoconstriction.

DOSAGE: Ophthalmologic.
- **Neonates:** Use combination products containing 1% phenylephrine to minimize increase in blood pressure.
- **Infants <1 year:** Instill 1 drop of 2.5% solution 15 to 30 minutes before ophthalmic procedure.
- **Children:** Instill 1 drop of 2.5% or 10% solution 15 to 30 minutes before ophthalmic procedure; may repeat in 10 to 60 minutes as needed.

ADVERSE EFFECTS: Arrhythmias, hypertension, lacrimation, respiratory distress.

PHARMACOLOGY: Mydriasis within 15 to 30 minutes of instillation; duration of mydriasis is 1 to 2 hours. Complete time to recovery is 3 to 8 hours.

COMMENTS: Apply pressure to the lacrimal sac during and for 2 minutes after instillation to minimize systemic absorption.

PHENYTOIN (DILANTIN)

INDICATIONS AND USE: Management of generalized convulsive status epilepticus; prevention and management of seizures.

ACTIONS: Stabilizes neuronal membranes and decreases seizure activity by increasing efflux or decreasing influx of sodium ions across cell membranes in the motor cortex during generation of nerve impulses.

DOSAGE: PO, IV. Phenytoin should be administered IV directly into a large vein through a large-gauge needle or IV catheter. IV injections should be followed by normal saline (NS) flushes through the same needle or IV catheter to avoid local irritation of the vein. Highly unstable in any IV solution; an in-line 0.22-micron filter is recommended due to potential for precipitation. Avoid infusion through central line due to risk of precipitation. Avoid IM use due to erratic absorption, pain on injection, and precipitation of drug at injection site. pH: 10.0 to 12.3.
- **Loading dose:** 15 to 20 mg/kg IV at a rate not to exceed 0.5 to 1 mg/kg/min or 50 mg/min, whichever is slower.
- **Maintenance:** 12 hours after loading dose, 4 to 8 mg/kg/day PO/IV divided every 12 hours; some patients may require dosing every 8 hours.

ADVERSE EFFECTS: Local tissue damage if extravasation occurs. High serum levels can precipitate seizures. Other CNS complications include drowsiness, lethargy, ataxia, and nystagmus. Cardiovascular effects include arrhythmias, hypotension, and cardiovascular collapse with too rapid an infusion. Reactions also include hypersensitivity rash or Stevens-Johnson syndrome. Other complications include hepatic dysfunction, pancreatic dysfunction with hyperglycemia and hypoinsulinemia, and blood dyscrasias.

PHARMACOLOGY: Bilirubin displaces phenytoin from albumin-binding sites, thereby increasing unbound drug levels and complicating dosage to serum level interpretations. Half-life from 7 to 42 hours in newborns postnatal age <7 days. Neonates absorb phenytoin poorly from gastrointestinal tract; separate tube feedings and oral phenytoin by 2 hours.

COMMENTS: Therapeutic levels 8 to 20 mcg/mL for total phenytoin, 1 to 2.5 mcg/mL for free phenytoin; lower end of therapeutic range preferred for preterm infants. Multiple drug interactions include corticosteroids, carbamazepine, cimetidine, digoxin, furosemide, phenobarbital, and heparin (especially in central lines causing precipitation). Available as an oral suspension.

PHOSPHATE (POTASSIUM AND SODIUM PHOSPHATE, NEUTRA-PHOS)

INDICATIONS AND USE: Treatment of hypophosphatemia, provision of maintenance phosphorus in parenteral nutrition solutions, and treatment of nutritional rickets of prematurity.

ACTIONS: Phosphorus is an intracellular ion required for formation of energy-transfer enzymes such as adenosine diphosphate and adenosine triphosphate. Phosphorus is also needed for bone metabolism and mineralization.

DOSAGE: IV, PO.

Treatment of hypophosphatemia:

- 0.15 to 0.33 mmol/kg/dose IV over 6 hours, with repeat doses to maintain serum phosphorus >2 mg/dL. Potassium or sodium phosphate should be diluted in IV fluids and infused at a rate not faster than 0.2 mmol/kg/h.

Maintenance in hyperalimentation:

- 0.5 to 2 mmol/kg/day. May use parenteral solution for oral dose; give in divided doses and dilute in feedings.

ADVERSE EFFECTS: Hyperphosphatemia, hypocalcemia, and hypotension. Gastrointestinal discomfort may occur with oral administration. Rapid IV bolus of potassium phosphates can cause cardiac arrhythmias.

COMMENTS: Injection, sodium phosphates: 3 mmol of elemental phosphorus/mL and 4 mEq of sodium/mL; and potassium phosphates: 3 mmol of elemental phosphorus/mL and 4.4 mEq of potassium/mL. The amount of sodium and potassium must be considered when ordering phosphate. The most reliable method of ordering IV phosphate is by millimoles; then specify the potassium or sodium salt.

PIPERACILLIN-TAZOBACTAM (ZOSYN)

ACTION AND SPECTRUM: Treatment of sepsis, intra-abdominal infections, infections involving the skin and skin structure, lower respiratory tract, and urinary tract infections caused by β-lactamase–producing strains that are susceptible, including *Staphylococcus aureus, Haemophilus influenzae, Bacteroides fragilis, Klebsiella, Pseudomonas, Proteus mirabilis, Escherichia coli*, and *Acinetobacter*.

DOSAGE: IV. Each 3.375-g vial of piperacillin-tazobactam contains 3 g of piperacillin and 0.375 g of tazobactam sodium in an 8:1 ratio. Dosing recommendations are based on the piperacillin component.

Neonates PNA ≤7 days and ≥1 kg *or* ≤14 days and <1 kg:

- 200 mg piperacillin/kg/day divided every 12 hours.

Neonates PNA >7 days and ≥1 kg *or* >14 days and <1 kg:

- 300 mg piperacillin/kg/day divided every 8 hours.

Alternative dosing for neonates PNA >7 days and ≥2 kg:

- 320 mg piperacillin/kg/day divided every 6 hours.

Infants <2 months of age: IV: 320 mg of piperacillin/kg/day in divided doses every 6 hours.

Infants 2 to 9 months: IV: 240 mg of piperacillin/kg/day in divided doses every 8 hours.

Infants and children >9 months: IV: 300 mg of piperacillin component/kg/day in divided doses every 8 hours.

Higher doses have been used for serious pseudomonal infections: 300 to 400 mg of piperacillin/kg/day in divided doses every 6 hours; maximum dose 16 g of piperacillin/day.

ADVERSE EFFECTS: Elevations in blood urea nitrogen, serum creatinine; interstitial nephritis, renal failure; leukopenia, thrombocytopenia, neutropenia, decrease in hemoglobin/hematocrit, eosinophilia, elevations in aspartate aminotransferase and alanine aminotransferase, hyperbilirubinemia, cholestatic jaundice, hypokalemia.

PHARMACOLOGY: Widely distributed into tissues and body fluids including lungs, intestinal mucosa, interstitial fluid, gallbladder, and bile; penetration into CSF is poor when meninges are not inflamed.

COMMENTS: When used to treat hospital-acquired pneumonia caused by *Pseudomonas aeruginosa,* consider the addition of an aminoglycoside.

PNEUMOCOCCAL 13-VALENT CONJUGATE VACCINE (PREVNAR 13)

INDICATIONS AND USE: For active immunization of infants and toddlers against *Streptococcus pneumoniae* invasive disease caused by the 13 capsular serotypes in the vaccine for all children 2 to 23 months of age. It is also recommended for certain children 24 to 59 months of age. *S pneumoniae* causes invasive infections such as bacteremia and meningitis, pneumonia, otitis media, and sinusitis (see Advisory Committee on Immunization Practices [ACIP] guidelines for the most current recommendations).

ACTIONS: A vaccine of saccharides of the capsular antigens of *S pneumoniae* serotypes 1, 3, 4, 5, 6A, 6B, 7F, 9V, 14, 18C, 19A, 19F, and 23F conjugated to diphtheria CRM197 protein. CRM197 protein is a nontoxic variant of diphtheria toxin.

DOSAGE: IM. According to ACIP, doses administered ≤4 days before minimal interval or age are considered valid.

- 0.5 mL/dose as a single dose IM at 2, 4, 6, and 12 to 15 months of age. Shake well before administration. Refer to the current American Academy of Pediatrics (AAP)/ACIP immunization recommendations. The schedule usually begins at 2 months of age, but starting at 6 weeks of age is acceptable. Three doses of 0.5 mL each are ideally given at approximately 2-month intervals, but a dosing interval of 4 to 8 weeks is acceptable, followed by a fourth dose of 0.5 mL at 12 to 15 months of age. Give the fourth dose at least 8 weeks after the third dose.

ADVERSE EFFECTS: Decreased appetite, drowsiness, irritability, fever, and injection site local tenderness, redness, and edema. Not a treatment of active infection. Do not give if patient is hypersensitive to any component of the vaccine. Use of this vaccine does not replace the use of the 23-valent pneumococcal polysaccharide vaccine in children ≥24 months old with sickle cell disease, chronic illness, asplenia, or human immunodeficiency virus, or those who are immunocompromised. May be administered simultaneously with other vaccines as part of the routine immunization schedule.

POLYMYXIN B OPHTHALMIC

See Chapter 58.

PORACTANT ALFA (CUROSURF)

INDICATIONS AND USE: Treatment of neonatal respiratory distress syndrome (RDS).

ACTIONS: An extract of natural porcine lung surfactant, contains phospholipids, neutral lipids, fatty acids, and surfactant-associated proteins B and C. It replaces deficient or ineffective endogenous lung surfactant in neonates with RDS; surfactant prevents the alveoli from collapsing during expiration by lowering surface tension between air and alveolar surfaces.

DOSAGE: ETT.

- **Initial 2.5 mL/kg (200 mg/kg/dose) intratracheally,** divided into 2 aliquots, followed by up to 2 doses of 1.25 mL/kg (100 mg/kg/dose) administered at 12-hour intervals as needed to infants who continue to require mechanical ventilation and oxygen supplementation. Administer intratracheally through a side port adapter or through a 5-F feeding catheter inserted into the endotracheal tube. Allow to warm to room temperature prior to administration. Do not shake or swirl vial to resuspend particles. Inspect for discoloration; normal color is creamy white. Discard unused drug.

ADVERSE EFFECTS: Transient bradycardia, hypotension, endotracheal tube blockage, and oxygen desaturation. Pulmonary hemorrhage has been reported.

COMMENTS: Following administration, lung compliance and oxygenation often improve rapidly. Patients should be closely monitored and appropriate changes in ventilation support should be made as clinically indicated.

POTASSIUM ACETATE

INDICATIONS AND USE: Treatment and prevention of hypokalemia in clinical situations where the use of chloride is not desirable, or correction of metabolic acidosis through the conversion of acetate to bicarbonate.

ACTIONS: Potassium acetate is metabolized to bicarbonate on an equimolar basis, which neutralizes hydrogen ion concentration and raises the blood and urine pH. Potassium is the major intracellular cation. Potassium is essential for maintaining intracellular tonicity; transmission of nerve impulses; contraction of cardiac, skeletal, and smooth muscle; and maintenance of normal renal function.

DOSAGE: IV.

- **Normal daily requirement (based on mEq of potassium):** 2 to 6 mEq/kg/day. Dose should be added to maintenance IV fluids.
- **Intermittent IV administration for severe hypokalemia (based on mEq of potassium):** 0.5 to 1 mEq/kg/dose, infused at a rate of ≤0.5 mEq/kg/h, not to exceed 1 mEq/kg/h or 40 mEq/h.

ADVERSE EFFECTS: Hyperkalemia, metabolic acidosis. Avoid rapid IV injection. Excessive dose or rate of infusion may cause cardiac arrhythmias (peaked T waves, widened QRS, flattened P waves, bradycardia, and heart block), respiratory paralysis, and hypotension. Monitor renal function, urine output, and serum potassium levels; hyperkalemia may result with renal dysfunction.

PHARMACOLOGY: 1 mEq of acetate is equivalent to the alkalinizing effect of 1 mEq of bicarbonate.

COMMENTS: Continuous monitoring should be used for the infusion of intermittent doses >0.5 mEq/kg/h. Do *not* administer undiluted or IV push. Potassium must be diluted prior to IV administration. Maximum recommended concentration is 80 mEq/L for peripheral line and 150 mEq/L for a central line.

POTASSIUM CHLORIDE (KCL)

INDICATIONS AND USE: Treatment of hypokalemia and as a supplement to maintain adequate serum potassium levels. Also corrects hypochloremia.

ACTIONS: Potassium is the major intracellular cation. Potassium is essential for maintaining intracellular tonicity; transmission of nerve impulses; contraction of cardiac, skeletal, and smooth muscle; and maintenance of normal renal function.

DOSAGE: IV, PO. Monitor serum potassium levels and adjust dose as needed.

Acute treatment of hypokalemia:

- 0.5 to 1 mEq/kg/dose IV over 1 hour. Maximum dose/rate: 1 mEq/kg/h or 40 mEq/h. Same equation from sodium bicarbonate is used for potassium acetate.

Maintenance:

- 2 to 6 mEq/kg/day (usually 2–3 mEq/kg/day) diluted in 24-hour maintenance IV solution. Higher doses are often required in infants receiving diuretics.

Oral supplementation:

- 2 to 6 mEq/kg/day (usually 2–3 mEq/kg/day) in divided doses and diluted with feedings. The injectable form of the drug may be given in divided doses PO and diluted in the infant's formula.

ADVERSE EFFECTS: Avoid rapid IV injection. Excessive dose or rate of infusion may cause cardiac arrhythmias (peaked T waves, widened QRS, flattened P waves, bradycardia, and heart block), respiratory paralysis, and hypotension. Monitor renal function, urine output, and serum potassium levels; hyperkalemia may result with renal dysfunction.

COMMENTS: Hyperkalemia, metabolic acidosis. Continuous monitoring should be used for the infusion of intermittent doses >0.5 mEq/kg/h. Do *not* administer undiluted or IV push. Potassium must be diluted prior to IV administration. It is best for the concentration of infusion to depend on the patient's condition and specific institution policy. Commonly used infusion dose in neonatal intensive care units has been 20 mEq/L (range 20–60 mEq/L) for

peripheral line and 80 mEq/L (range 80–150 mEq/L) for central line. These higher concentrations should be reserved for specific clinical situations and only with electrocardiographic
monitoring.

POVIDONE-IODINE OPHTHALMIC

See Chapter 58.

PREDNISONE

INDICATIONS AND USE: Used chiefly as an anti-inflammatory or immunosuppressive agent.
Prednisone is an intermediate-acting glucocorticoid that has 4 times the anti-inflammatory
potency of hydrocortisone and half the mineralocorticoid potency.
DOSAGE: PO.
- 0.25 to 2 mg/kg/day as a single daily dose or divided every 6 to 12 hours. Many different
dosing regimens have been used.
ADVERSE EFFECTS: Hypertension, leukocytosis, psychiatric disturbance, seizure, skin atrophy, hypokalemia, diabetes mellitus, fluid retention, growth suppression, hypothyroidism, sodium retention, peptic ulcer, osteoporosis, myopathy, glaucoma, cataracts, impaired wound healing, increased
aspartate aminotransferase and alanine aminotransferase, increased susceptibility to infection.
Withdraw the dose gradually after prolonged therapy to prevent acute adrenal insufficiency.

PROCAINAMIDE HCL

> **WARNING:** The prolonged administration of procainamide often leads to the develop-
> ment of a positive antinuclear antibody (ANA) test, with or without symptoms of a lupus
> erythematosus–like syndrome. If a positive ANA titer develops, the benefit versus risks
> of continued procainamide therapy should be assessed. Potentially fatal blood dyscrasias
> (agranulocytosis) have occurred with therapeutic doses; weekly monitoring is recom-
> mended during the first 3 months of therapy and periodically thereafter.

INDICATIONS AND USE: Treatment of ventricular tachycardia, premature ventricular contractions, paroxysmal atrial tachycardia, and atrial fibrillation; to prevent recurrence of ventric-
ular tachycardia, paroxysmal supraventricular tachycardia, and atrial fibrillation or flutter.
Note: Due to proarrhythmic effects, use should be reserved for life-threatening arrhythmias.
ACTIONS: Class I antiarrhythmic agent that increases the effective refractory period of the
atria and ventricles of the heart. Partially metabolized by the liver to the active metabolite
N-acetylprocainamide (NAPA).
DOSAGE: IV. Consider consult with pediatric cardiologist prior to use.
- **Initial bolus dose (monitor electrocardiogram, heart rate, and blood pressure):** 7 to
10 mg/kg (dilute to 20 mg/mL) IV over 10 to 60 minutes, then infusion of 20 to 80 mcg/kg/
min (dilute to 2–4 mg/dL in dextrose 5% in water [D5W]); maximum dose is 2 g/day. Use
lowest dose in preterm neonates.
ADVERSE EFFECTS: Toxic effects if given rapidly IV, including asystole, myocardial depression,
ventricular fibrillation, hypotension, and reversible lupus-like syndrome. May cause nausea,
vomiting, diarrhea, anorexia, skin rash, tachycardia, agranulocytosis, and hepatic toxicity.
Potentially fatal blood dyscrasias have occurred with therapeutic doses.
PHARMACOLOGY: Therapeutic levels—Procainamide: 4 to 10 mcg/mL, toxicity with levels
>10 mcg/mL; NAPA: 6 to 20 mcg/mL, toxicity with levels >30 mcg/mL. Draw 6 to 12 hours
after start of IV infusion.
COMMENTS: Contraindicated in second- or third-degree heart block, bundle branch block,
digitalis intoxication, and allergy to procaine. Do not use in atrial fibrillation or flutter
until the ventricular rate is adequately controlled to avoid a possible paradoxical increase
in ventricular rate. Do not administer with amiodarone; may cause severe hypotension
and prolongation of QT interval.

PROPARACAINE OPHTHALMIC

See Chapter 58.

PROPRANOLOL (HEMANGEOL, INDERAL)

INDICATIONS AND USE: Hypertension; supraventricular tachycardia, especially if associated with Wolff-Parkinson-White syndrome; tachyarrhythmias; and tetralogy of Fallot spells. Adjunctive therapy for neonatal thyrotoxicosis. Treatment of infantile hemangiomas.

ACTIONS: Nonselective β-adrenergic blocking agent that inhibits adrenergic stimuli by competitively blocking β-adrenergic receptors within the myocardium and bronchial and vascular smooth muscle. Propranolol decreases heart rate, myocardial contractility, blood pressure, and myocardial oxygen demand.

DOSAGE: IV, PO.

Arrhythmias:

- **IV:** 0.01 to 0.15 mg/kg/dose IV as slow push over 10 minutes; may repeat every 6 to 8 hours as needed; maximum dose 1 mg (infants) and 3 mg (children).
- **PO:** 0.25 to 1 mg/kg/dose PO every 6 to 8 hours.

Hypertension:

- **PO:** 0.25 to 0.5 mg/kg/dose PO every 8 hours. Increase slowly as needed to 5 mg/kg/day.

Tetralogy spells:

- **IV:** 0.015 to 0.02 mg/kg/dose IV over 10 minutes; titrate to effect, up to 0.1 to 0.2 mg/kg/dose. Some centers use 0.15 to 0.25 mg/kg/dose slow IV; may repeat in 15 minutes; maximum initial dose is 1 mg.
- **Oral palliation:** Initial: 0.25 mg/kg/dose every 6 hours; if ineffective within first week, may increase by 1 mg/kg/day every 24 hours to maximum of 5 mg/kg/day; if patient is refractory, may increase slowly to a maximum of 10 to 15 mg/kg/day but must carefully monitor heart rate, heart size, and cardiac contractility.

Thyrotoxicosis:

- 0.5 to 2 mg/kg/day PO in divided doses every 6 to 12 hours; occasionally higher doses may be required.

ADVERSE EFFECTS: Generally dose-related hypotension and related to β-adrenergic blockage; nausea, vomiting, bronchospasm, increased airway resistance, heart block, depressed myocardial contractility, hypoglycemia.

COMMENTS: Contraindicated in obstructive pulmonary disease, asthma, heart failure, shock, second- or third-degree heart block, and hypoglycemia. Use with caution in renal or hepatic failure. Do not use in neonates with chronic lung disease because bronchoconstriction may occur.

PROTAMINE SULFATE

> **WARNING:** Severe hypersensitivity reaction with hypotension, cardiovascular collapse, pulmonary edema, and pulmonary vasoconstriction/hypertension possible. Risk factors: high dose/overdose, repeat doses, rapid administration, prior protamine use, current or prior protamine-containing products (neutral protamine Hagedorn [NPH; isophane] or protamine zinc insulin, some β-blockers), severe left ventricular dysfunction, abnormal pulmonary hemodynamics. Vasopressors and resuscitation equipment must be available in case of reaction.

INDICATIONS AND USE: Treatment of heparin overdose; neutralize heparin during surgery.

ACTIONS: Combines with heparin, forming a stable salt complex and neutralizing the anticoagulation activity of both drugs. Effect on heparin is rapid (~5 minutes) and persists for approximately 2 hours.

DOSAGE: IV.

Heparin overdosage:

- Blood heparin concentrations decrease rapidly after heparin administration is stopped; adjust the protamine dosage depending on the duration of time since heparin administration as follows:
  - **Time since last heparin <30 minutes:** 1 mg neutralizes 100 units heparin.
  - **Time since last heparin 30 to 60 minutes:** 0.5 to 0.75 mg neutralizes 100 units heparin.
  - **Time since last heparin >60 to 120 minutes:** 0.375 to 0.5 mg neutralizes 100 units heparin.
  - **Time since last heparin >120 minutes:** 0.25 to 0.375 mg protamine neutralizes 100 units heparin.

Low molecular weight heparin (LMWH) overdosage:

- If most recent LMWH dose has been administered within the past 8 hours, use 1 mg protamine/1 mg LMWH; a second dose of 0.5 mg protamine/1 mg LMWH may be given if activated partial thromboplastin time remains prolonged 2 to 4 hours after the first dose.

ADVERSE EFFECTS: May cause hypotension, bradycardia, dyspnea, and anaphylaxis. Excessive administration beyond that needed to reverse a heparin effect may cause bleeding as a paradoxical coagulopathy.

PYRIDOXINE (VITAMIN B6)

INDICATIONS AND USE: Treatment of pyridoxine-dependent seizures; to prevent or treat vitamin B6 deficiency; treatment of drug-induced deficiency or acute intoxication of isoniazid or hydralazine.

ACTIONS: Vitamin B6 is essential in the synthesis of γ-aminobutyric acid (GABA), an inhibitory neurotransmitter in the CNS; GABA increases the seizure threshold. Pyridoxine is also required for heme synthesis and protein, carbohydrate, and fat metabolism.

DOSAGE: PO, IV.

Pyridoxine-dependent seizures:

- 50 to 100 mg IV single test dose, followed by a 30-minute observation period. If a response is seen, begin maintenance of 50 to 100 mg PO daily; range: 10 to 200 mg.

Adequate intake: 0.1 mg/day PO (0.01 mg/kg/day).

ADVERSE REACTIONS: Sensory neuropathy (after chronic administration of large doses), seizures (following IV administration of very large doses), acidosis, nausea, decreased serum folic acid concentration, respiratory distress.

PYRIMETHAMINE (DARAPRIM)

ACTION AND SPECTRUM: Inhibits parasitic dihydrofolate reductase resulting in inhibition of tetrahydrofolic acid synthesis. Used in combination with sulfadiazine for treatment of toxoplasmosis.

DOSAGE: PO.

Newborns and infants:

- **Toxoplasmosis:** 2 mg/kg/day once daily for 2 days, then 1 mg/kg/day once daily together with sulfadiazine for 2 to 6 months, followed by 1 mg/kg/day 3 times weekly with sulfadiazine. Total treatment duration of 12 months. Oral leucovorin (folinic acid) 5 to 10 mg 3 times per week should be administered throughout course to prevent hematologic toxicity.

Infants and children ≥1 month of age:

- **Prophylaxis for first episode of *Toxoplasma gondii*:** 1 mg/kg/day (maximum 25 mg/day) once daily with dapsone plus oral folinic acid (5 mg every 3 days).
- **Prophylaxis for recurrence of *T gondii*:** 1 mg/kg/day (maximum 25 mg/day) once daily given with sulfadiazine or clindamycin plus oral folinic acid (5 mg every 3 days).

ADVERSE EFFECTS: Anorexia, vomiting, hematuria, megaloblastic anemia, leukopenia, thrombocytopenia, pancytopenia, atrophic glossitis, rash, seizures, and cardiac arrhythmia.

COMMENTS: Administer with feedings if vomiting persists. Upon discontinuation of pyrimethamine, leucovorin should be continued for another week (due to long half-life of pyrimethamine). Dose reduction is necessary in hepatic dysfunction. Although an FDA-labeled indication, use of pyrimethamine for prophylaxis or treatment of malaria is not routinely recommended due to reports of resistance.

RANITIDINE (ZANTAC)

INDICATIONS AND USE: Short-term treatment of duodenal and gastric ulcers, gastroesophageal reflux disease (GERD), upper gastrointestinal bleed, and hypersecretory conditions.
ACTIONS: Histamine (H_2)-receptor antagonist; competitively inhibits the action of histamine on the gastric parietal cells; inhibits gastric acid secretion.
DOSAGE: PO, IV.
IV dosing:
- **Loading dose:** 1.5 mg/kg/dose IV, then maintenance 12 hours later. Maintenance 1 to 2 mg/kg/day divided every 12 hours IV.
- **Continuous infusion:** 1.5 mg/kg/dose loading dose, then 0.04 to 0.08 mg/kg/h infusion (or 1 to 2 mg/kg/day).
Oral dosing:
- **Neonatal:** 2 to 6 mg/kg/day PO divided every 8 to 12 hours.
- **Infants >1 month:** GERD: 4 to 10 mg/kg/day PO divided twice daily.
Gastric/duodenal ulcer:
- **Treatment:** 4 to 8 mg/kg/day PO divided twice daily.
- **Maintenance:** 2 to 4 mg/kg/day PO once daily.
ADVERSE EFFECTS: Constipation, abdominal discomfort, sedation, malaise, leukopenia, thrombocytopenia, elevated serum creatinine, bradycardia, and tachycardia.
COMMENTS: Use of H_2 blockers in preterm infants is associated with increased risk for necrotizing enterocolitis, late-onset sepsis, and fungal sepsis. Routine use of gastric acid suppression in neonates should be avoided. Dose adjustment needed in renal dysfunction. May add the daily dose to the total parenteral nutrition regimen and infuse over 24 hours to avoid the need for intermittent dosing.

RIFAMPIN

ACTION AND SPECTRUM: Broad-spectrum antibiotic with bacteriostatic activity against mycobacteria, *Neisseria meningitidis*, and gram-positive cocci; used to eliminate meningococci from asymptomatic carriers; for prophylaxis in contacts of patients with *Haemophilus influenzae* type B infection; management of active tuberculosis (TB) in combination with other agents; and used in combination with other antibiotics for the treatment of staphylococcal infections.
DOSAGE: PO, IV.
Synergy for staphylococcal infections:
- **Neonates:** 5 to 20 mg/kg/day PO/IV in divided doses every 12 hours with other antibiotics.
H influenzae prophylaxis:
- **Neonates <1 month:** 10 mg/kg/day PO/IV every 24 hours for 4 days.
- **Infants and children:** 20 mg/kg/day PO every 24 hours for 4 days, not to exceed 600 mg/dose.
Nasal carriers of *Staphylococcus aureus*:
- **Children:** 15 mg/kg/day PO/IV divided every 12 hours for 5 to 10 days, not to exceed 600 mg/dose in combination with at least 1 other systemic antistaphylococcal antibiotic. Not recommended for first-line therapy.
Meningococcal prophylaxis:
- **Neonates <1 month:** 10 mg/kg/day PO/IV in divided doses every 12 hours for 2 days.
- **Infants and children:** 20 mg/kg/day PO in divided doses every 12 hours for 2 days, not to exceed 600 mg/dose.

TB:

- **Active infection:** A 4-drug regimen (isoniazid, rifampin, pyrazinamide, and ethambutol) is preferred for the initial, empiric treatment of TB. Alter therapy regimen when drug susceptibility results are available.
- **Infants and children:** 10 to 20 mg/kg/day PO/IV every 24 hours, not to exceed 600 mg/dose.

ADVERSE EFFECTS: Anorexia, vomiting, and diarrhea; rash, pruritus, and eosinophilia; drowsiness, ataxia, blood dyscrasias (leukopenia, thrombocytopenia, and hemolytic anemia), hepatitis (rare), and elevation of serum urea nitrogen and uric acid levels. Causes red-orange discoloration of body fluids.

PHARMACOLOGY: Highly lipophilic; crosses the blood–brain barrier and is widely distributed into body tissues and fluids; hepatic metabolism; undergoes enterohepatic recycling. Half-life is approximately 1 to 3 hours.

COMMENTS: Rifampin should always be used in combination with other agents; if used as monotherapy, resistance develops rapidly. Administer by slow IV infusion over 30 minutes to 3 hours at 6 mg/mL concentration. Extravasation may cause local irritation and inflammation. Administer oral doses on an empty stomach and avoid acid suppressive medications. Shake oral suspension well or may mix content of capsule with applesauce. *Note:* A potent enzyme inducer of hepatic metabolism. Patients receiving digoxin, phenytoin, phenobarbital, or theophylline may have a substantial decrease in the serum concentration of these drugs after starting rifampin. Careful monitoring of serum drug concentrations is necessary.

ROCURONIUM

HIGH-ALERT MEDICATION: To be administered only by experienced clinicians or adequately trained individuals supervised by an experienced clinician familiar with the use and actions, characteristics, and complications of neuromuscular-blocking agents.

INDICATIONS AND USE: Skeletal muscle relaxation during surgery; increases pulmonary compliance during assisted mechanical ventilation and facilitates endotracheal intubation.

ACTIONS: Nondepolarizing neuromuscular-blocking agent that produces skeletal muscle paralysis by blocking acetylcholine binding at the receptor at the myoneural junction.

DOSAGE: IV.

- 0.6 to 1.2 mg/kg/dose IV push over 5 to 10 seconds for tracheal intubation (not recommended for rapid sequence intubation in pediatrics).

ADVERSE EFFECTS: May cause hypoxemia with inadequate mechanical ventilation. Apnea, arrhythmias, tachycardia, hypertension, hypotension, excessive salivation, and bronchospasm may occur. Potentiation of neuromuscular blockade may result from aminoglycosides, electrolyte abnormalities, severe hyponatremia, severe hypocalcemia, severe hypokalemia, hypermagnesemia, neuromuscular diseases, acidosis, renal failure, and hepatic failure. Antagonism of neuromuscular blockade may result from alkalosis, hypercalcemia, hyperkalemia, and epinephrine.

PHARMACOLOGY: Onset of clinical effect is within 30 second to 2 minutes, and the duration of effect ranges from 20 minutes to 2 hours.

COMMENTS: Adequate sedation/analgesia should be provided with the use of rocuronium.

SILDENAFIL (VIAGRA, REVATIO)

INDICATIONS AND USE: (Revatio) Treatment of persistent pulmonary hypertension of the newborn refractory to treatment with inhaled nitric oxide; to facilitate weaning from nitric oxide (by attenuating rebound effects after discontinuing inhaled nitric oxide); secondary pulmonary hypertension following cardiac surgery.

ACTIONS: Selective phosphodiesterase type 5 (PDE-5) inhibitor found in the pulmonary vascular smooth muscle, vascular and visceral smooth muscle, corpus cavernosum, and platelets, and is responsible for the degradation of cyclic guanosine monophosphate (cGMP). Normally, nitric oxide activates the enzyme guanylate cyclase, which increases the levels of cGMP; cGMP produces smooth muscle relaxation. Inhibition of PDE-5 by sildenafil increases the cellular levels of cGMP that potentiate vascular smooth muscle relaxation, particularly in the lung where there are high PDE-5 concentrations. Sildenafil causes vasodilation in the pulmonary vasculature and, to a lesser extent, in the systemic circulation.

DOSAGE: PO, IV. Limited pediatric information exists; most pediatric literature consists of case reports or small studies, and a wide range of doses have been used; further studies are needed.

PO dosing (suspension available):
- **Full-term neonates:** 0.3 to 2 mg/kg/dose PO every 6 to 24 hours. Usual range: 0.5 to 3 mg/kg/dose every 6 to 12 hours.
- **Infants and children:** Initial: 0.25 to 0.5 mg/kg/dose PO every 6 to 8 hours; increase if needed and tolerated to 1 mg/kg/dose every 6 to 8 hours; doses as high as 2 mg/kg/dose every 6 to 8 hours have been used in several case reports.

IV dosing:
- **Neonates >34 weeks' gestation and <72 hours:** Loading dose of 0.4 mg/kg over 3 hours followed by continuous infusion of 1.6 mg/kg/day or 0.067 mg/kg/h for up to 7 days.

ADVERSE EFFECTS: Use in neonatal and pediatric patients should be limited and considered experimental; chronic use is not recommended due to a dose-dependent increased mortality risk observed in trials. The safety and efficacy in pediatric patients have not been established. There is short-term concern for worsening oxygenation and systemic hypotension, and concern for increased risk of retinopathy of prematurity and platelet dysfunction.

PHARMACOLOGY: Metabolism is via the liver via cytochrome P450 isoenzyme CYP3A4 (major) and CYP2C9 (minor). Major metabolite is formed via the *N*-demethylation pathway and has 50% of the activity of sildenafil.

COMMENTS: Significant increases in sildenafil concentrations may occur when used concurrently with CYP3A4 inhibitors such as azole antifungal agents, cimetidine, and erythromycin. Concurrent use with heparin may have an additive effect on bleeding time.

SODIUM ACETATE

INDICATIONS AND USE: Correction of metabolic acidosis through the conversion of acetate to bicarbonate; sodium replacement.

ACTIONS: Sodium acetate is metabolized to bicarbonate on an equimolar basis, which neutralizes hydrogen ion concentration and raises the blood and urine pH. Sodium is the primary extracellular cation.

DOSAGE: IV. If sodium acetate is desired over sodium bicarbonate (dosing and same equation used for sodium acetate as sodium bicarbonate; see Sodium Bicarbonate).
- **Neonates, infants, and children:** IV 2 to 5 mEq/kg/day, maintenance sodium requirements.

ADVERSE EFFECTS: Hypernatremia, hypokalemic metabolic alkalosis, hypocalcemia, edema.

COMMENTS: Use with caution with hepatic failure, congestive heart failure.

SODIUM BICARBONATE

INDICATIONS AND USE: Management of metabolic acidosis; alkalinization of urine; stabilization of acid-base status in cardiac arrest; and treatment of life-threatening hyperkalemia or management of overdose of certain drugs.

ACTIONS: Alkalinizing agent that dissociates to provide bicarbonate ion, which neutralizes hydrogen ions and raises the pH of the blood and urine.

DOSAGE: IV.

Initial dose: 1 to 2 mEq/kg; can be given in either of the following 2 ways:
- Slow IV over 30 minutes using 4.2% (0.5 mEq/mL) sodium bicarbonate solution.
- Further dilute in dextrose solution to a maximum concentration of 0.5 mEq/mL and infuse over 2 hours at a maximum rate of 1 mEq/kg/h.

Blood gas–directed dosing (the following equations provide an estimated replacement dose):

$$HCO_3^- \ (mEq) = 0.3 \times weight \ (kg) \times base \ deficit \ (mEq/L)$$

or

$$HCO_3^- \ (mEq) = 0.5 \times weight \ (kg) \times [24 \ a \ serum \ HCO_3^- \ (mEq/L)]$$

- Administer half of the calculated dose initially, and then reassess clinical status, serum bicarbonate, and pH. Give remaining half dose as infusion over the next 24 hours if needed.

ADVERSE EFFECTS: Rapid correction of metabolic acidosis with sodium bicarbonate can lead to intraventricular hemorrhage, hyperosmolality, metabolic alkalosis, hypernatremia, hypokalemia, and hypocalcemia.

COMMENTS: Use with close monitoring of arterial blood pH. Use only when adequate ventilation is confirmed. Routine use in cardiac arrest is not recommended. Avoid extravasation; tissue necrosis can occur due to the hypertonicity of sodium bicarbonate. For direct IV administration: in neonates and infants, use the 0.5 mEq/mL solution or dilute the 1 mEq/mL solution 1:1 with sterile water for injection; administer slowly, maximum rate in neonates and infants: 10 mEq/min; for infusion, dilute to a maximum concentration of 0.5 mEq/mL in dextrose solution and infuse over 2 hours at a maximum rate of 1 mEq/kg/h.

SODIUM CHLORIDE

INDICATIONS AND USE: Hyponatremia.
DOSAGE: IV. Dosage is dependent on clinical condition and fluid, electrolyte, and acid-base balance of neonate.
- **Sodium chloride 0.9% isotonic solution** or **3% hypertonic solution** depending on clinical severity and etiology.

$$Dose \ (mEq \ sodium) = [desired \ serum \ sodium \ (mEq/L) - actual \ serum \ sodium \ (mEq/L)] \times 0.6 \times weight \ (kg)$$

- Use 125 mEq/L as the desired serum sodium for acute correction with a serum correction rate of <0.5 mEq/L/h; goal serum correction rate ≤8 to 10 mEq/L/day. [To determine dose in "mL" using 3% NaCl: Calculated dose in mEq of Na using equation above divided by 0.513; infuse NO faster than 1 mEq/kg/h via CENTRAL LINE ONLY.]

ADVERSE EFFECTS: Extravasation of hypertonic saline (>0.9%) is a vesicant; sodium toxicity with osmotic demyelination syndrome for rapid or overcorrection of serum sodium levels, transient hypotension, cardiac failure, electrolyte disturbances.
PHARMACOLOGY: Normal saline (0.9%) = 154 mEq/L; hypertonic saline (3%) = 513 mEq/L, 1027 mOsm/L.
COMMENTS: Hypertonic saline should be used with caution and only for severe cases of hyponatremia with a serum sodium <120 mEq/L and patient experiencing symptoms. Central line administration is preferred for hypertonic saline (>0.9%).

SODIUM POLYSTYRENE SULFONATE

INDICATIONS AND USE: Treatment of hyperkalemia.
ACTIONS: Cation exchange resin that removes potassium by exchanging sodium ions for potassium ions in the intestine before the resin is passed from the body.
DOSAGE: PO, PR (1 g of resin will exchange 1 mEq of sodium for 1 mEq of potassium).
- **Infants and children:** 1 g/kg/dose every 6 hours PO or every 2 to 6 hours PR.
ADVERSE EFFECTS: Large doses may cause fecal impaction, ischemic colitis, or intestinal perforation. Hypokalemia, hypocalcemia, hypomagnesemia, and sodium retention may occur.

COMMENTS: Due to complications of hypernatremia and necrotizing enterocolitis, **use in neonates is not usually recommended. Contraindicated in neonates via oral route or those with reduced gut motility or obstructive bowel disease.** Small amounts of magnesium and calcium may also be lost in binding. When using the powder for oral administration, dilute in 3 to 4 mL of fluid per gram of resin; 10% sorbitol, water, or syrup may be used as diluent. When using powder for rectal administration, dilute in water or 25% sorbitol at a concentration of 0.3 to 0.5 g/mL; retain enema in colon for at least 30 to 60 minutes or several hours, and follow with a cleansing enema of non–sodium-containing solution.

SOTALOL (BETAPACE, SORINE, SOTYLIZE)

INDICATIONS AND USE: Treatment of supraventricular tachycardia and maintenance of normal sinus rhythm in patients with symptomatic atrial fibrillation or flutter.

ACTIONS: Dose-related decrease in blood pressure through β_1- and β_2-adrenergic receptor blockade without causing significant reflex tachycardia or a decrease in heart rate.

DOSAGE: PO.

- **PNA ≥3 days:** 30 mg/m^2/dose PO every 8 hours; dose should be reduced by an age-related factor obtained from a graph available within the package insert. Dose should be adjusted based on individual response and tolerance with continuous electrocardiogram monitoring.
- **Alternative dosing (limited data available):** 2 mg/kg/day PO divided every 8 hours; increase dose gradually by increments of 1 to 2 mg/kg/day a minimum of 3 days between titrations. Proposed target dose: 4 mg/kg/day PO divided every 8 hours; it is not necessary to achieve target dose if desired clinical effect has been achieved at a lower dosage.

ADVERSE EFFECTS: Hypotension and bradycardia at higher doses, congestive heart failure; edema, diaphoresis, dyspnea, increased liver enzymes, thrombocytopenia, inflammation phlebitis. Prolonged QT$_c$ interval ≥500 ms, reduce dose or discontinue sotalol.

PHARMACOLOGY: Larger drug exposure (area under the curve) and greater pharmacologic effects were observed in studies in smaller subjects (body surface area <0.33 m^2). Time to reach steady state in a neonate may be ≥1 week. Half-life elimination in neonates and infants is 7.5 to 8.5 hours.

COMMENTS: Baseline QT$_c$ interval must be determined prior to initiation. Contraindicated in patients with asthma, overt cardiac failure, heart block, cardiogenic shock, or severe bradycardia. May cause a paradoxical increase in blood pressure in patients with pheochromocytoma. Use with caution in renal dysfunction.

SPIRONOLACTONE (ALDACTONE, CAROSPIR)

> **WARNING:** Aldactone has been shown to be tumorigenic in chronic animal studies. Unnecessary use of this drug should be avoided.

INDICATIONS AND USE: Primarily used in conjunction with other diuretics for the treatment of hypertension, congestive heart failure, and edema with prolonged diuretic therapy.

ACTIONS: Competes with aldosterone for receptor sites in the distal renal tubules; increases sodium chloride and water excretion while conserving potassium and hydrogen ions; it also may block the effect of aldosterone on arteriolar smooth muscle.

DOSAGE: PO. Commercially available suspension (25 mg/5 mL) is not therapeutically equivalent to the tablets; pediatric dosing is based on experience with tablets and extemporaneously compounded suspension.

- 1 to 3 mg/kg/day PO divided every 12 to 24 hours.

ADVERSE EFFECTS: Hyperkalemia, dehydration, hyponatremia, hyperchloremic metabolic acidosis, rash, vomiting, diarrhea, hepatotoxicity, and gynecomastia in males.

COMMENTS: Contraindicated in hyperkalemia, anuria, and rapidly deteriorating renal function. Monitor potassium closely when giving potassium supplements.

SUCROSE (SWEET-EASE, TOOTSWEET)

INDICATIONS AND USE: Mild analgesia in neonates during minor procedures, such as heel stick, eye examination for retinopathy of prematurity, circumcision, immunization, venipuncture, endotracheal tube intubation and suctioning, nasogastric tube insertion, or IM or subcutaneous injection. (See also Chapters 15 and 81.)

ACTIONS: Exact mechanism of action is unknown; sucrose may induce endogenous opioid release.

DOSAGE: PO. May be administered directly into baby's mouth or via a pacifier dipped into solution.

- **Neonates:** 0.1 to 0.5 mL of 24% solution placed on the tongue or buccal surface 2 minutes prior to procedure.
- **Infants:** 2 mL of 24% solution.

ADVERSE EFFECTS: Avoid in patients with gastrointestinal tract abnormalities—use only in patients with functioning gastrointestinal tract; necrotizing enterocolitis has not been reported with sucrose administration. Avoid use in patients at risk for aspiration. Do not use in patients requiring ongoing analgesia.

PHARMACOLOGY: Time to maximum effect is 2 minutes; duration of effect is 3 to 10 minutes.

COMMENTS: Sucrose 24% solution has an osmolarity of 1000 mOsmol/L.

SULFACETAMIDE OPHTHALMIC

See Chapter 58.

SULFACETAMIDE SODIUM

ACTION AND SPECTRUM: Interferes with bacterial growth by inhibiting bacterial folic acid synthesis. Used for the treatment and prophylaxis of conjunctivitis caused by susceptible strains of gram-positive and gram-negative bacteria such as *Staphylococcus aureus, Streptococcus pneumoniae, Haemophilus influenzae,* and *Moraxella.*

DOSAGE: Ocular.

- Instill 1 to 2 drops into each eye every 2 to 3 hours initially, then increase the time interval as the condition responds; apply ointment to each eye every 3 to 4 hours and at bedtime; treatment duration is usually 7 to 10 days.

ADVERSE EFFECTS: May cause burning and stinging sensation of eyes, increased sensitivity to light, blurred vision, and pruritus.

COMMENTS: Contraindicated in infants <2 months of age or with hypersensitivity to sulfonamides.

SULFADIAZINE

ACTION AND SPECTRUM: Interferes with bacterial growth by inhibiting bacterial folic acid synthesis. Used for adjunctive treatment of *Toxoplasma gondii* in combination with pyrimethamine.

DOSAGE: PO. See also Pyrimethamine (page 1302) for dosing information.

Congenital toxoplasmosis:

- **Newborns and infants:** 100 mg/kg/day PO divided every 12 hours for 12 months in conjunction with pyrimethamine and supplemental leucovorin.

Acquired toxoplasmosis:

- **Infants ≥2 months and children:** 100 to 200 mg/kg/day PO divided every 4 to 6 hours in conjunction with pyrimethamine (maximum dose 6000 mg/day) and supplemental leucovorin.

ADVERSE EFFECTS: Hypersensitivity (fever, rash, hepatitis, vasculitis, and lupus-like syndrome), neutropenia, agranulocytosis, thrombocytopenia, aplastic anemia, Stevens-Johnson syndrome, and crystalluria (keep urine alkaline, maintain adequate hydration and high urine output). Kernicterus may occur.

COMMENTS: Avoid use in neonates, except for treatment of congenital toxoplasmosis. Concurrent leucovorin (oral folinic acid) supplementation is necessary to prevent folic acid deficiency.

Caution in patients with glucose-6-phosphate dehydrogenase deficiency. Contraindicated with hypersensitivity to sulfonamides.

TETRACYCLINE OPHTHALMIC

See Chapter 58.

TOBRAMYCIN OPHTHALMIC

See Chapter 58.

TOBRAMYCIN SULFATE

ACTION AND SPECTRUM: Aminoglycoside antibiotic used for documented or suspected infections caused by susceptible gram-negative bacilli including *Pseudomonas aeruginosa* and nonpseudomonal enteric bacillus infection, which is more sensitive to tobramycin than gentamicin based on susceptibility tests; usually used in combination with a β-lactam antibiotic.
DOSAGE: IV, IM, ocular, inhalation. Base the initial dose on body weight, then monitor levels and adjust using pharmacokinetics. Many dosing strategies exist such as extended interval, age based, weight based, and traditional. Monitor serum levels after 2 days of therapy.
Age based:
- **≤29 weeks' gestational age (GA):**
  - **0 to 7 days:** 5 mg/kg/dose IV/IM every 48 hours.
  - **8 to 28 days:** 4 mg/kg/dose IV/IM every 36 hours.
  - **≥29 days:** 4 mg/kg/dose IV/IM every 24 hours.
- **30 to 34 weeks' GA:**
  - **0 to 7 days:** 4.5 mg/kg/dose IV/IM every 36 hours.
  - **>7 days:** 4 mg/kg/dose IV/IM every 24 hours.
- **>35 weeks GA:** 4 mg/kg/dose IV/IM every 36 hours.
Infants and children: 2.5 mg/kg/dose IM/IV every 8 hours.
Ophthalmic:
- Instill 1 to 2 drops into each eye every 4 hours or more often if infection is severe, or apply a small amount of ointment into each eye 2 to 3 times per day or, for severe infections, every 3 to 4 hours.
Inhalation:
- 150 mg twice daily nebulized has been used for difficult-to-manage neonatal intensive care unit patients.
ADVERSE EFFECTS: Ototoxicity (may be associated with high serum aminoglycoside concentrations persisting for prolonged periods) with tinnitus, hearing loss; early toxicity usually affects high-pitched sound; nephrotoxicity (high trough levels) with proteinuria, elevated serum creatinine, oliguria, and macular rash.
COMMENTS: Reserve for cases resistant to gentamicin. Obtain serum peak and trough concentrations at about the third maintenance dose. Desired peak is 4 to 12 mcg/mL (sample 30 minutes after the infusion is complete); desired trough is 0.5 to 2 mcg/mL (sample 30 minutes to just before the next dose).

TOPIRAMATE (TOPAMAX)

INDICATIONS AND USE: Treatment of refractory neonatal seizures; infantile spasms; neuroprotectant following anoxic injury (with cooling).
ACTIONS: Combination of potential mechanisms: blocks neuronal voltage-dependent sodium channels, enhances γ-aminobutyric acid activity, antagonizes glutamate receptors, and weakly inhibits carbonic anhydrase.
DOSAGE: PO. Very limited data.
Infantile spasms: Initial: 1 to 3 mg/kg/day in 1 to 2 divided doses, titrate every 3 to 7 days in increments of 1 to 3 mg/kg/day as tolerated until seizures are controlled; reported range 4 to 27 mg/kg/day.

Neonatal seizures, refractory: 5 to 10 mg/kg/day PO in 1 to 2 divided doses.

Neuroprotectant following anoxic injury: 5 mg/kg/dose PO on day 1, followed by 3 mg/kg/dose PO on days 2 and 3.

ADVERSE EFFECTS: Cognitive dysfunction, somnolence, fatigue, hyperammonemia, encephalopathy, metabolic acidosis (increased with diarrhea, hepatic impairment, renal dysfunction, ketogenic diet, or surgery), oligohydrosis, hyperthermia, increased intraocular pressure, renal calculus, reduction in growth.

PHARMACOLOGY: Percentage of dose metabolized in liver and clearance are increased in patients receiving enzyme inducers; hypothermia significantly decreases elimination rate. Dosing adjustment may be required in renal and hepatic impairment. Immediate-release preparations are bioequivalent.

COMMENTS: Pediatric patients <24 months of age may be at increased risk for topiramate-associated hyperammonemia, especially when used concurrently with valproic acid. Sprinkle capsules may be opened and mixed in a small amount of soft food (applesauce, pudding, yogurt) to be swallowed immediately; do not chew or store for later use. Abrupt discontinuation may increase seizure frequency.

TRIFLURIDINE OPHTHALMIC

See Chapter 58.

TROPICAMIDE OPHTHALMIC

INDICATIONS AND USE: Mydriasis and cycloplegia for diagnostic and therapeutic ophthalmic procedures. (See also Chapter 58.)

ACTIONS: Anticholinergic activity produces pupillary dilation.

DOSAGE: Ocular.

- One drop of 0.5% ophthalmic solution instilled into eye at least 15 minutes prior to procedure. Apply pressure to lacrimal sac during and for 2 minutes after instillation to reduce systemic absorption.

ADVERSE EFFECTS: Blurred vision, photophobia, stinging of the eyes, tachycardia, vasodilatation, restlessness, decreased gastrointestinal motility, xerostomia, urinary retention.

PHARMACOLOGY: Onset of mydriasis is 5 to 20 minutes; cycloplegia 20 to 40 minutes.

COMMENTS: Consider holding feeds for 4 hours after procedure.

URSODIOL (ACTIGALL)

INDICATIONS AND USE: Facilitate bile excretion in infants with biliary atresia; treatment of cholestasis secondary to parenteral nutrition; improve the hepatic metabolism of essential fatty acids in patients with cystic fibrosis.

ACTIONS: A hydrophobic bile acid that decreases the cholesterol content of bile and bile stones by reducing the secretion of cholesterol from the liver and decreases the fractional reabsorption of cholesterol by the intestines.

DOSAGE: PO.

Biliary atresia:

- **Neonates and infants:** 10 to 20 mg/kg/day PO in 2 to 3 divided doses.

Total parenteral nutrition–induced cholestasis:

- **Infants and children:** 30 mg/kg/day PO in 3 divided doses.

Improvement in the hepatic metabolism of essential fatty acids in cystic fibrosis:

- **Infants and children:** 20 mg/kg/day PO in 2 divided doses.

ADVERSE EFFECTS: Rash, diarrhea, biliary pain, constipation, stomatitis, flatulence, nausea, vomiting, abdominal pain, elevated liver enzymes.

PHARMACOLOGY: Absorbed well orally. During metabolism, the drug undergoes extensive enterohepatic recycling; following hepatic conjugation and biliary secretion, the drug is hydrolyzed to the unconjugated form and is recycled or transformed to lithocholic acid by colonic microbial flora.

COMMENTS: Use with caution in patients with nonvisualizing gallbladder and patients with chronic liver disease.

VALGANCICLOVIR (VALCYTE)

> **WARNING:** Valganciclovir may cause severe neutropenia, anemia, thrombocytopenia, pancytopenia, and bone marrow failure.

ACTION AND SPECTRUM: Prodrug of ganciclovir that is converted to ganciclovir by the liver and intestinal esterases. Used to treat symptomatic congenital cytomegalovirus infection.
DOSAGE: PO.
- 16 mg/kg/dose PO every 12 hours for 6 months. Use commercially available product only.

ADVERSE EFFECTS: Neutropenia is frequent; if absolute neutrophil count (ANC) is <500 cells/mm^3, hold dose until ANC is >750 cells/mm^3. If ANC falls below 750 cells/mm^3, reduce dose by 50%; if ANC falls again to below 500 cells/mm^3, discontinue drug. Also, granulocytopenia, anemia, thrombocytopenia; acute renal failure/acute kidney injury, dysuria, increased serum creatinine; hyperglycemia, hyper-/hypokalemia, hypocalcemia, hypomagnesemia, hypophosphatemia, and edema.

PHARMACOLOGY: Excreted primarily as ganciclovir by the kidney; elimination half-life is 3 hours; dosing adjustment necessary with renal impairment.

VANCOMYCIN HCL

ACTION AND SPECTRUM: Bactericidal action through inhibition of cell wall synthesis by blocking glycopeptide polymerization with activity against most gram-positive cocci and bacilli, including streptococci, staphylococci (including methicillin-resistant staphylococci), clostridia (including *Clostridium difficile*), *Corynebacterium*, and *Listeria monocytogenes*. Bacteriostatic against enterococci.
DOSAGE: PO, IV, intrathecal, intraventricular.
Neonates:
- **PNA <7 days:**
  - **<1.2 kg:** 15 mg/kg/day IV every 24 hours.
  - **1.2 to 2 kg:** 10 to 15 mg/kg/dose IV every 12 to 18 hours.
  - **>2 kg:** 10 to 15 mg/kg/dose IV every 8 to 12 hours.
- **PNA ≥7 days:**
  - **<1.2 kg:** 15 mg/kg/day IV every 24 hours.
  - **1.2 to 2 kg:** 10 to 15 mg/kg/dose IV every 8 to 12 hours.
  - **>2 kg:** 10 to 15 mg/kg/dose IV every 6 to 8 hours.

Infants >1 month and children:
- 40 to 45 mg/kg/day IV in divided doses every 6 to 8 hours.

Intrathecal/intraventricular: Use a preservative-free preparation.
- **Neonates:** 5 to 10 mg/day.

Serious infection or organisms with a minimum inhibitory concentration (MIC) = 1 mcg/mL:
- **Initial:** 15 to 20 mg/kg/dose IV every 6 to 8 hours.
- **Methicillin-resistant *Staphylococcus aureus* (MRSA) infections/bacteremia:** 15 mg/kg/dose IV every 6 hours for 2 to 6 weeks depending on severity.
- **Complicated skin and skin structure infections:** Treat for 7 to 14 days.
- **Meningitis:** Treat for 2 weeks (± rifampin).
- **Osteomyelitis:** Treat for minimum of 4 to 6 weeks.
- **Pneumonia:** Treat for 7 to 21 days.

Antibiotic-associated pseudomembranous colitis:
- (*Note:* Metronidazole is the drug of initial choice based on 2018–2021 AAP *Red Book* recommendations.) Children: 30 mg/kg/day PO in divided doses every 6 hours for 10 days, not to exceed 2 g/day.

ADVERSE EFFECTS: Allergy (rash and fever), ototoxicity (with prolonged peak >40 mcg/mL), nephrotoxicity (higher incidence with trough >10 mcg/mL), and thrombophlebitis at the site of injection. Rapid infusion may cause rash, chills, and fever ("red man" syndrome), mimicking anaphylactic reaction. Apnea and bradycardia without other signs of red man syndrome have also been associated with rapid infusion. Infuse dose over at least 60 minutes.

PHARMACOLOGY: Renally excreted. Half-life is 6 to 10 hours.

COMMENTS: Peak drawn 60 minutes after completion of infusion, goal range 25 to 40 mcg/mL; 30 to 40 mcg/mL recommended when treating meningitis. Trough level drawn 30 minutes prior to scheduled dose, goal range 10 to 15 mcg/mL; experts recommend 15 to 20 mcg/mL for organisms with an MIC ≥1 mcg/mL when treating MRSA pneumonia, endocarditis, or bone/joint infections. Draw serum peak and trough levels around the fourth maintenance dose. Monitor serum creatinine, blood urea nitrogen, and urine output. If staphylococci exhibit tolerance to the drug, combine with an aminoglycoside, with or without rifampin. Oral doses are poorly absorbed.

VANCOMYCIN OPHTHALMIC

See Chapter 58.

VARICELLA-ZOSTER IMMUNE GLOBULIN (VARIZIG)

INDICATIONS AND USE: For protection of infants of mothers with onset of varicella-zoster infections (chickenpox) within 5 days before or 48 hours after delivery of postnatally exposed preterm infants ≤1 kg or <28 weeks' gestation regardless of maternal history, and of postnatally exposed premature infants ≥28 weeks' gestation whose mothers have no evidence of immunity.

ACTIONS: Passive immunity through infusion of immunoglobulin G antibodies. Protection lasts 1 month or longer and does not reduce the incidence, but acts to decrease the risk of complications.

DOSAGE: IM.
- **≤2 kg:** 62.5 units.
- **2.1 to <10 kg:** 125 units

ADVERSE EFFECTS: Pain, erythema, swelling, rash at the site of injection, and, rarely, anaphylaxis.

COMMENTS: Best results are achieved if given within 96 hours after exposure. VZIG was discontinued in the United States in 2006. It is currently available as VariZIG under an Investigational New Drug Application Expanded Access protocol. Inventory for anticipated patients may be obtained by contacting FFF Enterprises at 800-843-7477. Additional information may be found at: http://www.fffenterprises.com/products/varizig.html.

VASOPRESSIN

INDICATIONS AND USE: Treatment of diabetes insipidus, vasoconstriction to increase blood pressure in patients with vasodilatory shock who remain hypotensive despite fluids and catecholamines, systemic hypotension, and persistent pulmonary hypertension in neonates.

ACTIONS: Stimulates a family of arginine vasopressin receptors, oxytocin receptors, and purinergic receptors; increases systemic vascular resistance and mean arterial blood pressure; in response to these effects, a decrease in heart rate and cardiac output may be seen; increases water permeability at the renal tubule, resulting in decreased urine volume and increased osmolality.

DOSAGE: IV. Units of measure vary by indication and age (eg, milliunits/kg/h, units/kg/h, milliunits/kg/min, units/kg/min, units/h, units/min); extra precautions should be taken.

Cardiac surgery: Continuous IV infusion 0.3 to 0.5 milliunits/kg/min, titrated to hemodynamic goals.

Diabetes insipidus: Variable dosage; titrate based on serum and urine osmolality in addition to fluid balance and urine output. *Central diabetes insipidus*: Continuous IV infusion 0.5 milliunits/kg/h; titrate in increments of 0.5 milliunits/kg/h every 10 minutes to target urine output (approximately <2 mL/kg/h).

Hypotension: Very limited data; continuous IV infusion 0.17 to 0.67 milliunits/kg/min (0.01–0.04 units/kg/h); dosing initiated at low end of range and titrated at 20-minute intervals.
Persistent pulmonary hypertension of the newborn: Very limited data; continuous IV infusion 0.1 milliunits/kg/min; increase by 0.1 milliunits/kg/min every hour as needed for clinical response to maximum dose of 1.2 milliunits/kg/min.
Shock, refractory hypotension unresponsive to fluid resuscitation and catecholamines: Continuous IV infusion 0.17 to 10 milliunits/kg/min (0.01–0.6 units/kg/h); dosing initiated at the lower end of the range and titrated to effect.
ADVERSE EFFECTS: Hyponatremia, atrial fibrillation, bradycardia, low cardiac output, right heart failure, peripheral vasoconstriction and limb ischemia, water intoxication, mesenteric ischemia, increased serum bilirubin, renal insufficiency, bronchoconstriction.
PHARMACOLOGY: Rapid vasopressor effect when administered IV; peak effect occurs within 15 minutes of initiation of continuous infusion.
COMMENTS: Vesicant; infusion through central line is highly recommended. Monitor blood pressure, heart rate, fluid intake and output, urine specific gravity, and urine and serum osmolality.

VECURONIUM BROMIDE

> **WARNING:** This drug should be administered by adequately trained individuals familiar with its actions, characteristics, and hazards.

INDICATIONS AND USE: Skeletal muscle relaxation during surgery; increases pulmonary compliance during assisted mechanical ventilation and facilitates endotracheal intubation.
ACTIONS: Nondepolarizing neuromuscular-blocking agent that produces skeletal muscle paralysis by blocking acetylcholine binding at the receptor at the myoneural junction.
DOSAGE: IV.
Neonates:
• 0.1 mg/kg/dose, then maintenance 0.03 to 0.15 mg/kg IV push every 1 to 2 hours as needed.
Infants >7 weeks:
• 0.1 mg/kg/dose, repeat every hour as needed; may be administered as a continuous infusion at 0.8 to 1.7 mcg/kg/min (0.05–0.1 mg/kg/h).
ADVERSE EFFECTS: May cause hypoxemia with inadequate mechanical ventilation; bronchospasm, apnea, arrhythmias, tachycardia, hypotension, hypertension, and excessive salivation may occur. Potentiation of neuromuscular blockade may result from aminoglycosides, electrolyte abnormalities, severe hyponatremia, severe hypocalcemia, severe hypokalemia, hypermagnesemia, neuromuscular diseases, acidosis, renal failure, and hepatic failure. Antagonism of neuromuscular blockade may result from alkalosis, hypercalcemia, hyperkalemia, and epinephrine.
PHARMACOLOGY: Onset of action is 2.5 to 3 minutes, with a duration that varies with dose and age. Elimination is reduced with hepatic dysfunction.
COMMENTS: Causes less tachycardia than pancuronium bromide. When used with narcotics, decreases in heart rate and blood pressure have been observed. Adequate sedation/analgesia should be provided with the use of vecuronium. Must be reconstituted prior to administration; for neonates, reconstitute with sterile water for injection instead of provided diluent.

VIDARABINE OPHTHALMIC

See Chapter 58.

VITAMIN A

INDICATIONS AND USE: Treatment and prevention of vitamin A deficiency; to reduce the risk of chronic lung disease in high-risk premature neonates with vitamin A deficiency.
ACTIONS: Vitamin A is required for growth and bone development, vision, reproduction, and differentiation and maintenance of epithelial tissue. The pulmonary histopathologic changes

seen in patients with bronchopulmonary dysplasia/chronic lung disease are similar to those seen with vitamin A deficiency. Retinol metabolites exhibit potent and site-specific effects on gene expression as well as lung growth and development.

DOSAGE: PO, IM.

Prevention of bronchopulmonary dysplasia/chronic lung disease in premature infants:
- 5000 units IM 3 times a week for 4 weeks; start within first 4 days of life.

Prophylactic therapy for children at risk for developing deficiency:
- **Infants age 6 months to 1 year:** 100,000 units PO every 4 to 6 months.

Adequate intake:
- **1 to <6 months:** 400 mcg/day (1330 units).
- **6 to <12 months:** 500 mcg/day (1670 units).

ADVERSE EFFECTS: Concomitant use with glucocorticoids should be avoided, as it significantly raises plasma vitamin A concentrations; seen only with doses that exceed physiologic replacement. Monitor for signs of toxicity: full fontanel, lethargy, irritability, hepatosplenomegaly, edema, and mucocutaneous lesions. Avoid products containing benzyl alcohol in neonates.

VITAMIN D3 (CHOLECALCIFEROL)

INDICATIONS AND USE: Prevention and treatment of vitamin D deficiency and/or rickets; dietary supplement.

ACTIONS: Stimulates calcium and phosphate absorption from the small intestine; promotes secretion of calcium from bone to blood; promotes renal tubule phosphate resorption; acts on osteoblasts to stimulate skeletal growth and on the parathyroid glands to suppress parathyroid hormone synthesis and secretion.

DOSAGE: PO.

Prevention of vitamin D deficiency:
- **Premature infants:** <1.5 kg 200 international units per day; >1.5 kg 200 international units per day; increase to 400 international units per day when tolerating full enteral nutrition.
- **Breast-fed neonates (fully or partially):** 400 international units per day beginning in first few days of life. Continue supplementation until infant is weaned to ≥1000 mL/day or 1 quart per day of vitamin D–fortified formula or whole milk (after 12 months of age).
- **Formula-fed neonates ingesting <1000 mL of vitamin D–fortified formula:** 400 international units per day.

Treatment of vitamin D deficiency and/or rickets:
- 2000 international units per day for 2 to 3 months together with calcium and phosphorus supplementation; once radiologic evidence of healing is observed, decrease to 400 to 1000 international units per day.

ADVERSE EFFECTS: Hypercalcemia, azotemia, vomiting, and nephrocalcinosis.

PHARMACOLOGY: 25(OH)-D concentration >250 nmol/L may be associated with risk of vitamin D intoxication.

COMMENTS: For detailed information, see the 2008 American Academy of Pediatrics (AAP) statement, *Prevention of Rickets and Vitamin D Deficiency in Infants, Children and Adolescents* (Wagner et al, 2008) and the 2013 AAP statement, *Calcium and Vitamin D Requirements of Enterally Fed Preterm Infants* (Abrams et al, 2013). Excessive doses may lead to hypervitaminosis D, manifested by hypercalcemia and its associated complications. (See also Chapter 91.)

VITAMIN E (DL-α-TOCOPHEROL ACETATE)

INDICATIONS AND USE: Treatment or prevention of vitamin E deficiency.

ACTIONS: Antioxidant that prevents oxidation of vitamins A and C; protects polyunsaturated fatty acids in membranes from attack by free radicals and protects red blood cells against hemolysis by oxidizing agents.

DOSAGE: PO.
Prevention of vitamin E deficiency:
- **Premature or low birthweight neonates:** 5 units PO per day diluted with feedings. Do not give simultaneously with iron; will decrease iron absorption.

Vitamin E deficiency:
- 25 to 50 units PO per day.

COMMENTS: Physiologic serum vitamin E levels are 0.8 to 3.5 mg/dL. Serum levels should be monitored when pharmacologic doses of vitamin E are administered. Liquid preparation is very hyperosmolar (3620 mOsmol/kg H_2O) and should be diluted (1 mg of DL-α-tocopherol acetate = 1 unit), large dosage has been associated with necrotizing enterocolitis.

VITAMIN K1 (PHYTONADIONE)

INDICATIONS AND USE: Prevention and treatment of hemorrhagic disease of the newborn and vitamin K deficiency.

ACTIONS: Required for the synthesis of blood coagulation factors II, VII, IX, and X. Because vitamin K1 may require 3 hours or more to stop active bleeding, fresh-frozen plasma, 10 mL/kg, may be necessary when bleeding is severe. The drug has no antagonistic effects against heparin.

DOSAGE: PO, IM, IV.
Neonatal hemorrhagic disease: For prophylaxis, administer within 1 hour of birth.
- **Term neonate prevention:** 1 mg IM at birth.
- **Preterm infant <32 weeks' gestation, prevention:**
  - **Birthweight <1000 g:** 0.3 to 0.5 mg/kg IM at birth.
  - **Birthweight ≥1000 g:** 0.5 to 1 mg IM at birth.
- **Treatment:** 1 to 2 mg IM per day.

Vitamin K deficiency (drugs, malabsorption, or decreased synthesis of vitamin K):
- **Infants and children:** 2.5 to 5 mg PO per day or 1 to 2 mg subcutaneous, IM, IV, as a single dose.

Oral anticoagulant overdose:
- 0.5 to 2 mg/dose subcutaneous, IV every 12 hours as needed. (Monitor the serial prothrombin time and partial thromboplastin time for response.)

ADVERSE EFFECTS: Relatively nontoxic. Hemolytic anemia and kernicterus have been reported in neonates given greater than recommended dose. Severe hypersensitivity or anaphylactic reactions have been associated with IV administration of vitamin K1. Efficacy of treatment with vitamin K1 is decreased in patients with liver disease.

ZIDOVUDINE (AZT, ZDV; RETROVIR)

> **WARNING:** Zidovudine may cause hematologic toxicity including severe neutropenia and anemia. Lactic acidosis and severe hepatomegaly with steatosis have been reported with nucleoside analogs. Prolonged use has been associated with symptomatic myopathy and myositis.

INDICATIONS AND USE: Chemoprophylaxis to reduce perinatal human immunodeficiency virus (HIV) transmission; prophylactic treatment of neonates born to HIV-infected mothers; treatment of HIV infection in combination with other antiretroviral agents.

ACTIONS: Nucleoside reverse transcriptase inhibitor that inhibits HIV viral polymerases and DNA replication.

DOSAGE: IV, PO (aidsinfo.nih.gov/guidelines, 2017).
Prevention of maternal–fetal HIV transmission and treatment of HIV infection:
- Dosing should begin as soon as possible after birth (by 6–12 hours after delivery) and continue for the first 4 to 6 weeks of life. Use IV route only until oral therapy can be

administered. For infants unable to tolerate oral agents, the IV dose should be 75% of the oral dose while maintaining the same dosing interval. Syrup available 50 mg/5 mL

- **<30 weeks' gestation:** 2 mg/kg/dose PO every 12 hours; or if unable to tolerate oral medications, 1.5 mg/kg/dose IV every 12 hours. Advance to every 3 mg/kg PO every 12 hours at 4 weeks' PNA. Advance to 12 mg/kg PO every 12 hours at 8 weeks' PNA.
- **≥30 to <35 weeks' gestation:** 2 mg/kg/dose PO every 12 hours; or if unable to tolerate oral medications, 1.5 mg/kg/dose IV every 12 hours. Advance to 3 mg/kg PO every 12 hours at 2 weeks' PNA. Advance to 12 mg/kg PO every 12 hours at 6 weeks' PNA.
- **≥35 weeks' gestation:** 4 mg/kg/dose PO twice daily; or if unable to tolerate oral medications, 3 mg/kg/dose IV every 12 hours. Advance to 12 mg/kg PO every 12 hours at 4 weeks' PNA.

ADVERSE EFFECTS: The most frequent are granulocytopenia and severe anemia. Others include thrombocytopenia, leukopenia, diarrhea, fever, seizures, insomnia, cholestatic hepatitis, and lactic acidosis.

COMMENTS: Use with caution in patients with impaired hepatic function, bone marrow compromise, or folic acid or vitamin B12 deficiency.

INTERACTIONS: Concurrent acetaminophen, probenecid, cimetidine, indomethacin, morphine, and benzodiazepines may increase toxicity as a result of decreased glucuronidation or reduced renal excretion of zidovudine. Concomitant acyclovir may cause neurotoxicity; ganciclovir and flucytosine may cause severe hematologic toxicity as a result of synergistic myelosuppression. Ribavirin and zidovudine are antagonistic and should not be used concurrently.

156 Effects of Drugs and Substances on Lactation and Infants

The chapter provides some summary data on some of the medications and substances that may be taken by the mother during pregnancy and/or breast feeding. **Regardless of the designated risk category or presumed safety, no drug or substance should be used during pregnancy and/or breast feeding unless it is clearly needed and the potential benefits clearly outweigh the risks.** The table lists the generic medication name and, in parentheses, the US Food and Drug Administration (FDA) fetal risk category followed by the breast-feeding compatibility. At the present time, there is no formally FDA-sanctioned breast-feeding category, and the system used here is discussed later. Lastly, any reported effects on lactation or on infant effects based on breast milk consumption are noted. The editorial board has made an attempt to summarize the data based on the best information available for an individual agent where sources disagree. These data are subject to change as new information becomes available. The reader is advised to consult the FDA (www.fda.gov) and manufacturer's website for the latest information concerning risks of these medications. The FDA developed a revised labeling that replaces the old 5-letter (A, B, C, D, X) system with more helpful information about a medication's risks to the expectant mother, the developing fetus, and the breast-fed infant. The labeling changes went into effect on June 30, 2015, for all new drugs, which will use the new format immediately, whereas labeling for prescription drugs approved on or after June 30, 2001, will be phased in gradually. Lactation will include (1) risk summary; (2) clinical considerations; and (3) data. This project will take several years to complete. Labeling for over-the-counter (OTC) medicines will not change.

US FDA FETAL RISK CATEGORIES

CATEGORY A

Adequate studies in pregnant women have not demonstrated a risk to the fetus in the first trimester of pregnancy; there is no evidence of risk in the last 2 trimesters.

CATEGORY B

Animal studies have not demonstrated a risk to the fetus, but there are no adequate studies in pregnant women.

or

Animal studies have shown an adverse effect, but adequate studies in pregnant women have not demonstrated a risk to the fetus during the first trimester of pregnancy, and there is no evidence of risk in the last 2 trimesters.

CATEGORY C

Animal studies have shown an adverse effect on the fetus, but there are no adequate studies in humans. The benefits from the use of the drug in pregnant women may be acceptable despite its potential risks.

or

There are no animal reproduction studies and no adequate studies in humans.

CATEGORY D

There is evidence of human fetal risk, but the potential benefits from the use of the drug in pregnant women may be acceptable despite its potential risks.

CATEGORY X

Studies in animals or humans or adverse reaction reports, or both, have demonstrated fetal abnormalities. The risk of use in pregnant women clearly outweighs any possible benefit.

BREAST-FEEDING COMPATIBILITY

As noted, no formal system exists for categorizing drugs or substances and their effect on breast feeding, lactation, and effects on the infant. The following system is used in this book:
CATEGORY (+): Generally compatible with breast feeding.
CATEGORY (−): Avoid with breast feeding. Toxicity can be seen.
CATEGORY (CI): Contraindicated.

Drug (FDA Fetal Risk Category/ Breast-Feeding Compatibility)	Effect on Lactation and Adverse Effects on Infant
Abacavir (C/−)	CDC recommends HIV-infected mothers in developed countries to not breast feed.
Acarbose (B/−)	No human lactation data available. Avoid breast feeding until safety data available.
Acebutolol (B/−)	AAP recommends to use cautiously due to adverse effects of hypotension, cyanosis, and bradycardia related to β-blockade.
Acetaminophen (B/+)	AAP classifies acetaminophen as compatible with breast feeding.
Acetylcysteine (B/+)	No human lactation data available. Probably compatible.

(Continued)

Drug (FDA Fetal Risk Category/ Breast-Feeding Compatibility)	Effect on Lactation and Adverse Effects on Infant
Acitretin (X/CI)	Because of the teratogenicity of acitretin, a program called PPET (Pregnancy Prevention Is Essential with Treatment) has been developed to educate women of childbearing potential and their healthcare providers about the serious risks associated with acitretin and to help prevent pregnancies from occurring with the use of this drug and for 3 years after its discontinuation.
Acyclovir (B/+)	AAP classifies acyclovir as compatible with breast feeding; breast-feeding mothers with herpetic lesions near or on the breast should avoid breast feeding.
Adalimumab (C/+)	Excreted into breast milk in low concentrations. Effects on nursing infant unknown.
Adenosine (C/+)	IV drug, used in acute care situations, short half-life.
Ado-trastuzumab emtansine (X/CI)	No human lactation data available. Due to potential for serious adverse effects, breast feeding not recommended during treatment and for 7 months following the last dose.
Albendazole (C/+)	Probably compatible with a single oral dose. Low oral bioavailability suggests excretion into breast milk not clinically significant. Avoid ingestion with high-fat meal.
Albiglutide (C/−)	No human lactation data available. Manufacturer recommends a decision be made to continue nursing or discontinue the drug, taking into account the importance of treatment to the mother.
Albuterol (C/+)	Monitor nursing infant for agitation and spitting up. Use inhaled form to decrease maternal absorption. Generally considered acceptable in breast-feeding women when used in usual doses.
Alendronate (C/+)	Probably compatible. Low plasma concentrations and rapid plasma clearance suggest minimal amounts excreted into breast milk. Consider monitoring the infant's serum calcium during the first 2 months postpartum.
Alfentanil (C/−)	Used epidurally or intravenously during labor or for a short time immediately postpartum would not be expected to cause adverse effects. Opioid therapy should be avoided in breast-feeding mothers due to potential for apnea and sedation in the infant.
Allopurinol (C/+)	Allopurinol and its metabolite are excreted into human milk. AAP classifies allopurinol as compatible with breast feeding.
Almotriptan (C/+)	No human lactation data available. Low molecular weight of drug suggests excretion into breast milk but effect on nursing infant is unknown.
Alogliptin (C/−)	No human lactation data available. Low molecular weight of drug suggests excretion into breast milk, but effect on nursing infant is unknown. Alternative agents are preferred.
Alprazolam (D/−)	Excreted into breast milk. Because of the potent effects on neurodevelopment, probable withdrawal, lethargy, and weight loss in infant, use should be avoided during breast feeding.
Amantadine (C/CI)	Excreted into breast milk in low concentrations. Not recommended due to potential for urinary retention, vomiting, and skin rash.

(Continued)

Drug (FDA Fetal Risk Category/ Breast-Feeding Compatibility)	Effect on Lactation and Adverse Effects on Infant
Amikacin (D/−)	Low concentrations in breast milk because of poor oral absorption. Risk for modification of bowel flora.
Amiloride (B/+)	Excreted into breast milk of lactating rats at higher concentrations than in blood. No human lactation data available. Probably compatible.
Amiodarone (C/−)	Long half-life, iodine-containing molecule, neonates should be monitored for thyroid disorders and cardiac arrhythmias with in utero exposure.
Amitriptyline (C/−)	Milk/plasma ratio of 1.0. AAP classifies amitriptyline effect on breast feeding as unknown but may be of concern.
Amlodipine (C/+)	No human lactation data available. Low molecular weight suggests excretion into breast milk. Effects on nursing infant are unknown. Probably compatible.
Amoxapine (C/−)	Active metabolites in milk. AAP classifies amoxapine effect on breast feeding as unknown but may be of concern.
Amoxicillin (B/+)	Monitor nursing infant for diarrhea, rash, and somnolence. Potential for allergic sensitization and modification of bowel flora. AAP classifies amoxicillin as compatible with breast feeding.
Amphetamine (C/Cl)	AAP classifies amphetamine as contraindicated during breast feeding. Monitor nursing infant for irritability and poor sleeping pattern.
Amphotericin B (B/+)	No human lactation data available. Probably compatible.
Amphotericin B lipid complex (B/+)	No human lactation data available. Probably compatible.
Ampicillin (B/+)	Monitor nursing infant for diarrhea. Potential for allergic sensitization and modification of bowel flora. AAP classifies ampicillin as compatible with breast feeding.
Anakinra (B/−)	No human lactation data available. Recommended to avoid in breast feeding.
Aripiprazole (C/−)	Mixed data concerning concentrations in breast milk. Potential for toxicity. The low molecular weight of the drug combined with the prolonged half-life and the active metabolite suggest that 1 or both will be excreted into breast milk. However, the extensive protein binding should limit the excretion. If mother breast feeds while taking drug, observe nursing infant for potent CNS effects, orthostatic hypotension, seizures, dysphasia, nausea, and vomiting. Long-term evaluation is warranted.
Aspirin (C, D/−)	May affect platelet function; monitor nursing infant for hemolysis or bleeding. Increased risk with high doses used for rheumatoid arthritis (3–5 g/day). Metabolic acidosis may occur. Theoretical risk of Reye syndrome. AAP recommends to use cautiously due to potential adverse effects.
Atazanavir (B/Cl)	CDC recommends HIV-infected mothers in developed countries to not breast feed.
Atenolol (D/−)	AAP recommends to use cautiously due to adverse effects of hypotension, cyanosis, and bradycardia; suggested to avoid water-soluble, low-protein-bound, renally excreted β-blockers during lactation.

(Continued)

Drug (FDA Fetal Risk Category/ Breast-Feeding Compatibility)	Effect on Lactation and Adverse Effects on Infant
Atorvastatin (X/CI)	Some excretion into breast milk is expected; therefore, the potential for adverse effects in nursing infants exists and breast feeding should be avoided.
Atropine (C/+)	Mixed data concerning passage into breast milk. AAP classifies atropine as compatible with breast feeding.
Azathioprine (D/−)	Theoretical concerns of potential for toxicity with the active metabolites of the drug. May be considered acceptable; monitor complete blood count with differential and liver function tests.
Azithromycin (B/+)	Accumulates in breast milk. Macrolide antibiotics may be associated with risk of infantile hypertrophic pyloric stenosis; potential for modification of bowel flora. Recommended agent for various infections.
Aztreonam (B/+)	Excreted into breast milk in low amounts, due to acidic nature of the drug and low lipid solubility. Oral absorption is poor, and systemic effects in nursing infants are unlikely. AAP classifies aztreonam as compatible with breast feeding.
Bacitracin (C/+)	No human lactation data available. Topical use compatible.
Baclofen (C/+)	Limited human lactation data available. AAP classifies baclofen as compatible with breast feeding.
Beclomethasone (C/+)	Limited human lactation data available. May be excreted into breast milk. Use of inhaled corticosteroids is considered acceptable during breast feeding.
Belladonna (C/−)	No human lactation data available. Due to narrow therapeutic index and viable potency, use should be avoided during lactation.
Benazepril (C 1st tri; D 2nd, 3rd tri/+)	Limited human lactation data available. Some excretion into breast milk is expected; not expected to cause adverse effects on nursing infants.
Benztropine (C/−)	No human lactation data available. Probably compatible.
Betamethasone (C, D/+)	No human lactation data available. Molecular weight suggests excretion into breast milk. Best avoided in favor of a shorter acting and better studied alternative due to potency and low protein binding.
Bethanechol (C/−)	Limited human lactation data available. Low molecular weight suggests excretion into breast milk. Abdominal pain and diarrhea reported in nursing infant exposed to bethanechol.
Bisacodyl (C/+)	Not absorbed from the gastrointestinal tract; active metabolite is not detectable in breast milk. Probably compatible.
Bismuth subsalicylate (C/−)	AAP recommends to use cautiously due to adverse effects because of potential for adverse effects from salicylates. Should be avoided because of systemic absorption.
Bisoprolol (C/−)	No human lactation data available. AAP recommends to use cautiously due to adverse effects of hypotension, cyanosis, and bradycardia related to β-blockade.
Botulinum toxin type A (C/+)	No human lactation data available. Probably compatible. Toxin not expected to appear in circulation and therefore will not appear in breast milk.

(Continued)

Drug (FDA Fetal Risk Category/ Breast-Feeding Compatibility)	Effect on Lactation and Adverse Effects on Infant
Brompheniramine (C/+)	Monitor nursing infant for agitation, poor sleeping pattern, and feeding problems. AAP classifies brompheniramine as usually compatible with breast feeding.
Budesonide (oral/inhaler/nasal) (B, inhaler; C, oral/+)	Systemic bioavailability of inhaled budesonide is low, so the actual amount in breast milk may also be low. Use of inhaled corticosteroids is considered acceptable during breast feeding.
Bumetanide (C/+)	No human lactation data available. Probably compatible. Diuretics may suppress lactation.
Buprenorphine (C/−)	Excreted into breast milk. When used to treat opioid addiction, most guidelines allow breast feeding as long as the infant is tolerant to the dose and other contraindications do not exist. Monitor for drowsiness, adequate weight gain, and developmental milestones; observe infants for withdrawal signs if breast feeding is stopped abruptly.
Bupropion (B/−)	Excreted into breast milk. Seizures and sleep disturbances have been reported; monitor for changes in sleep, feeding patterns, and behavior. AAP classifies the effect of bupropion on breast feeding as unknown but may be of concern.
Buspirone (B/−)	Limited human lactation data available. Buspirone and its metabolites are excreted into the milk of lactating rats. Potential exists for CNS impairment in nursing infant. AAP classifies the effect of buspirone on breast feeding as unknown but may be of concern because of effects on the developing brain that may not be known until later in life.
Butorphanol (C/+)	Limited human lactation data available. Excreted into breast milk at levels that are probably not clinically significant. AAP classifies butorphanol as usually compatible with breast feeding. Opioid therapy should be avoided in breast-feeding mothers due to potential for apnea and sedation in the infant.
Caffeine (C/+)	Monitor nursing infant for irritability and poor sleeping pattern. AAP classifies caffeine as usually compatible with breast-feeding with moderate intake (2–3 cups/day).
Calcifediol (C/+)	Low molecular weight of drug suggests excretion into breast milk but effect on nursing infant is unknown.
Calcitonin—salmon (C/+)	Calcitonin is a normal component of human milk; exogenous administration may inhibit lactation.
Calcitriol (C/+)	High-dose supplementation in mothers can lead to elevated levels of vitamin D2 in breast milk and subsequently lead to hypercalcemia in breast-fed infants. Caution is advised.
Canagliflozin (D, −)	No human lactation data available. Alternative agents are preferred.
Candesartan (C 1st tri; D 2nd, 3rd tri/+)	No human lactation data available. Low molecular weight suggests that the drug would be excreted into breast milk. Effects on the nursing infant are unknown.
Captopril (C 1st tri; D 2nd, 3rd tri/+)	Excreted into breast milk in low concentrations. Available data showed no effects on nursing infants. AAP classifies captopril as compatible with breast feeding.

(Continued)

Drug (FDA Fetal Risk Category/ Breast-Feeding Compatibility)	Effect on Lactation and Adverse Effects on Infant
Carbamazepine (D/+)	Monitor for sedation, poor sucking, and potential for withdrawal. Risk of bone marrow suppression if taken chronically; recommend monitoring complete blood count and liver enzymes. AAP classifies carbamazepine as compatible with breast feeding.
Carbidopa/levodopa (C/+)	Excreted into breast milk in low concentrations. Effects on nursing infant unknown.
Carisoprodol (C/+)	Limited human lactation data available. Probably compatible. Observe nursing infant for sedation and other behavioral changes.
Carvedilol (C/−)	AAP recommends to use cautiously due to adverse effects of hypotension, cyanosis, and bradycardia related to β-blockade.
Cascara sagrada (C/+)	Limited human lactation data available. Probably compatible. Observe nursing infant for diarrhea.
Cefaclor (B/+)	Excreted into breast milk in low concentrations. Potential for allergic sensitization and modification of bowel flora. AAP classifies other cephalosporins as compatible with breast feeding.
Cefadroxil (B/+)	Excreted into breast milk in low concentrations. Potential for allergic sensitization and modification of bowel flora. AAP classifies cephalosporins as compatible with breast feeding.
Cefazolin (B/+)	Excreted into breast milk in low concentrations. Potential for allergic sensitization and modification of bowel flora. AAP classifies cephalosporins as compatible with breast feeding.
Cefdinir (B/+)	Probably excreted into breast milk in low concentrations. Potential for allergic sensitization and modification of bowel flora. AAP classifies other cephalosporins as compatible with breast feeding.
Cefepime (B/+)	Excreted into breast milk in low concentrations. Potential for allergic sensitization and modification of bowel flora. AAP classifies other cephalosporins as compatible with breast feeding.
Cefixime (B/+)	Probably excreted into breast milk in low concentrations. Potential for allergic sensitization and modification of bowel flora. AAP classifies other cephalosporins as compatible with breast feeding.
Cefotaxime (B/+)	Excreted into breast milk in low concentrations. Potential for allergic sensitization and modification of bowel flora. AAP classifies cephalosporins as compatible with breast feeding.
Cefotetan (B/+)	Excreted into breast milk in low concentrations. Potential for allergic sensitization and modification of bowel flora. AAP classifies other cephalosporins as compatible with breast feeding.
Cefoxitin (B/+)	Excreted into breast milk in low concentrations. Potential for allergic sensitization and modification of bowel flora. AAP classifies cephalosporins as compatible with breast feeding.

(Continued)

Drug (FDA Fetal Risk Category/ Breast-Feeding Compatibility)	Effect on Lactation and Adverse Effects on Infant
Ceftazidime (B/+)	Excreted into breast milk in low concentrations; not absorbed when given orally. Potential for allergic sensitization and modification of bowel flora. AAP classifies cephalosporins as compatible with breast feeding.
Ceftolozane/tazobactam (B/+)	Excreted into breast milk in low concentrations. Potential for allergic sensitization and modification of bowel flora.
Ceftriaxone (B/+)	Excreted into breast milk in low concentrations. Potential for allergic sensitization and modification of bowel flora. AAP classifies cephalosporins as compatible with breast feeding.
Cefuroxime (B/+)	Excreted into breast milk in low concentrations. Potential for allergic sensitization and modification of bowel flora. AAP classifies other cephalosporins as compatible with breast feeding.
Celecoxib (C 1st, 2nd tri; D 3rd tri/−)	Excreted into breast milk. Safest course of action is to avoid use during breast feeding.
Cephalexin (B/+)	Excreted into breast milk in low concentrations. Potential for allergic sensitization and modification of bowel flora. AAP classifies other cephalosporins as compatible with breast feeding.
Cetirizine (B/+)	Manufacturer states drug excreted into breast milk. Effects on nursing infant unknown but observe for sedation, irritability, or jitteriness.
Chloral hydrate (C/+)	Monitor nursing infant for sedation and rash. AAP classifies chloral hydrate as compatible with breast feeding.
Chlordiazepoxide (D/−)	No human lactation data available. Low molecular weight suggests excretion into breast milk should be expected. Other benzodiazepines have produced adverse effects in nursing infants. Use should be avoided during breast feeding.
Chlorhexidine (B/+)	No reports of excretion into breast milk available. Oral rinse is not intended to be swallowed. Rinse nipples if chlorhexidine is used to cleanse them. Probably compatible.
Chloroquine (C/+)	Insufficient amounts excreted in breast milk to provide adequate protection against malaria. AAP classifies chloroquine as compatible with breast feeding.
Chlorothiazide (C/+)	Diuretics may suppress lactation, especially in the first month. Adverse effects have not been reported, but infant's electrolytes and platelets should be monitored. AAP classifies chlorothizide as compatible with breast feeding.
Chlorpheniramine (B/+)	Effects on nursing infant unknown, but observe for sedation, irritability, or jitteriness. Second-generation antihistamines are preferred.
Chlorpromazine (C/−)	Excreted into breast milk in low amounts. Observe nursing infant for sedation. AAP classifies the effect of chlorpromazine on breast feeding as unknown but may be of concern due to potential drowsiness and lethargy in addition to galactorrhea in adults.

(Continued)

Drug (FDA Fetal Risk Category/ Breast-Feeding Compatibility)	Effect on Lactation and Adverse Effects on Infant
Cholecalciferol (C, D/+)	Excreted into breast milk in limited amounts. The Committee on Nutrition of the AAP recommends vitamin D supplementation in breast-fed infants if maternal intake is low or exposure to ultraviolet light is insufficient. AAP classifies cholecalciferol as compatible with breast feeding. Monitor serum calcium levels of nursing infant if mother is taking pharmacologic doses of vitamin D.
Cholestyramine (C/+)	Nonabsorbable resin. No human lactation data available. Drug binds fat-soluble vitamins, and prolonged use may result in deficiencies of these vitamins in mother and nursing infant.
Cimetidine (B/+)	Use with caution. May suppress gastric acidity in infant, inhibit drug metabolism, and cause CNS stimulation. AAP classifies cimetidine as compatible with breast feeding.
Ciprofloxacin (C/+)	Data are limited and the amount of drug in breast milk does not appear to represent significant risk to nursing infant. Potential for modification of bowel flora. AAP classifies ciprofloxacin as compatible with breast feeding. However, the manufacturer recommends that mother should wait 48 hours after last dose before breast feeding.
Citalopram (C/−)	Doses >20 mg/day or concurrent use of other sedative agents may increase risk of adverse effects to nursing infants. Observe for excessive somnolence, changes in sleep, decreased feeding, and weight loss. Long-term effects on neurobehavioral development are unknown. AAP classifies effect of SSRIs on breast feeding as unknown but may be of concern. However, if required by the mother, it is not a reason to discontinue breast feeding.
Clarithromycin (C/+)	Excreted into breast milk. Macrolide antibiotics may be associated with risk of infantile hypertrophic pyloric stenosis; potential for modification of bowel flora, rash, diarrhea, and loss of appetite.
Clavulanate (B/+)	No human lactation data available. Molecular weight suggests excretion into breast milk. Effects of lactamase inhibitors on nursing infants are unknown.
Clindamycin (B/+)	Excreted into breast milk. Potential for allergic sensitization and modification of bowel flora. Monitor for bloody stools associated with colitis. AAP classifies clindamycin as compatible with breast feeding.
Clonazepam (D/−)	Long half-life may cause accumulation in a breast-feeding infant. If chronic use of a benzodiazepine is needed, other shorter acting agents preferred. Monitor nursing infant for decreased feeding and respiratory and CNS depression.
Clonidine (C/+)	Excreted in breast milk. Hypotension was not observed in nursing infants, although clonidine was found in the serum of these nursing infants. Long-term significance of this exposure is unknown; other agents may be preferred.

(Continued)

Drug (FDA Fetal Risk Category/ Breast-Feeding Compatibility)	Effect on Lactation and Adverse Effects on Infant
Clopidogrel (B/+)	No human lactation data available. Low molecular weight suggests excretion into breast milk. Effects on nursing infants are unknown. Manufacturer recommends a decision be made to continue nursing or discontinue the drug, taking into account the importance of treatment to the mother.
Clotrimazole (B/+)	Absorption from skin and vagina is minimal. Unlikely that the levels of this antifungal agent appear in breast milk.
Clozapine (B/−)	Concentrated in breast milk. Avoid breast feeding. AAP classifies clozapine as a drug for which the effect on the nursing infant is unknown but may be of concern.
Cobicistat (C/CI)	CDC recommends HIV-infected mothers in developed countries to not breast feed.
Cocaine (C/CI)	Causes cocaine intoxication in infant from maternal intranasal use (hypertension, tachycardia, mydriasis, and apnea) and from topical use on mother's nipples (apnea and seizures). AAP classifies cocaine as contraindicated during breast feeding.
Codeine (C, D/−)	Codeine and active metabolite, morphine, are present in breast milk; concentrations are dependent on CYD2D6 metabolism. Short term therapy (1–2 days) with close monitoring is compatible, however long term therapy is not compatible with breast feeding. May suppress lactation. Opioid therapy should be avoided in breast-feeding mothers due to potential for apnea and sedation in the infant.
Colchicine (C/+)	Excreted into breast milk. No adverse effects on nursing infants have been observed. Waiting 8 hours after dose to breast feed or taking the dose after breast feeding minimizes exposure of nursing infant. AAP classifies colchicine as compatible with breast feeding.
Cortisone (C, D/+)	Corticosteroids are excreted in breast milk. Monitor for growth suppression, interference with endogenous production. Unlikely that it poses risk to nursing infant.
Cromolyn sodium (B/+)	No human lactation data available. Maternal levels are likely to be low; considered to be compatible with breast feeding.
Cyclobenzaprine (B/−)	No reports of excretion into breast milk available. Low molecular weight suggests excretion into breast milk.
Dactinomycin (D 1st tri; C 2nd, 3rd tri/−)	No human lactation data available. Despite the high molecular weight, women receiving the drug should avoid breast feeding because of the potential risk of severe adverse effects.
Dalbavancin (C/−)	No human lactation data available. Drug has a long half-life and caution should be exercised when used among nursing women.
Dalteparin (B/+)	No human lactation data available. Based on the molecular weight and because the drug would be inactivated in the GI tract, the risk to the nursing infant would be negligible.
Dapagliflozin (C/−)	No human lactation data available. Avoid breast feeding until safety data available.
Darbepoetin alfa (C/+)	No human lactation data available. Passage into breast milk is not expected. Risk to nursing infant appears to be negligible.

(Continued)

Drug (FDA Fetal Risk Category/ Breast-Feeding Compatibility)	Effect on Lactation and Adverse Effects on Infant
Deferasirox (C/−)	No human lactation data available. Molecular weight and long elimination half-life suggest excretion into breast milk. Amount of oral absorption in infants unknown; in adults, oral bioavailability is 70%. With the potential to deplete infant's iron stores, breast feeding should be avoided during therapy.
Deferoxamine (C/+)	No human lactation data available. Molecular weight is low enough for some excretion into breast milk to be expected. Effects, if any, on nursing infant are unknown.
Delafloxacin (C/−)	No human lactation data available. Avoid breast feeding until safety data available.
Delavirdine (C/CI)	No human lactation data available. Molecular weight suggests excretion into breast milk should be expected. Effect on nursing infant is unknown. CDC recommends HIV-infected mothers in developed countries to not breast feed.
Desloratadine (C/+)	No human lactation data available. Desloratadine and loratadine are excreted into breast milk. Probably compatible.
Dexamethasone (C, D/+)	No human lactation data available. Excretion into breast milk should be expected. Probably compatible.
Dextroamphetamine (C/−)	May cause infant stimulation. Nonmedical use is considered contraindicated in breast feeding.
Dextromethorphan (C/+)	No human lactation data available. Low molecular weight suggests excretion into breast milk. Probably compatible. Use alcohol-free preparation.
Diatrizoate (C/+)	In 1 study, not detected in breast milk. Probably compatible.
Diazepam (D/−)	May cause infant sedation. May accumulate in breast-fed infants.
Diclofenac (C/D ≥30 weeks' gestation/+)	No human lactation data available. Manufacturer states that the drug is excreted into breast milk. Short half-life in adults. Probably compatible.
Dicloxacillin (B/+)	No human lactation data. However, other penicillins are excreted into breast milk in low concentrations. Adverse effects rare. The bowel flora of nursing infants may be altered, and there is the potential for interference with the interpretation of an infectious workup. Observe nursing infants for possible allergic reaction.
Didanosine (B/CI)	No human lactation data available. Molecular weight suggests excretion into breast milk should be expected. Effect on nursing infant is unknown. CDC recommends HIV-infected mothers in developed countries to not breast feed.
Digoxin (C/+)	Excreted into breast milk in small amounts. Monitor nursing infant for spitting up, diarrhea, and heart rate changes. Compatible with breast feeding.
Dihydroergotamine (X/CI)	No human lactation data available. Molecular weight and long half-life suggest excretion into breast milk, but high protein binding will limit this. Concern for symptoms of ergotism: vomiting, diarrhea, and convulsions in nursing infants. Breast feeding is contraindicated.
Diltiazem (C/+)	Excreted into breast milk. Two nursing infants were not affected. Probably compatible.

(Continued)

Drug (FDA Fetal Risk Category/ Breast-Feeding Compatibility)	Effect on Lactation and Adverse Effects on Infant
Dimenhydrinate (B/+)	No human lactation data available. Molecular weight suggests excretion into breast milk should be expected. Probably compatible. Caution: newborns and premature infants have increased sensitivity to antihistamines.
Diphenhydramine (B/+)	Excreted into breast milk, but levels are thought not to be in sufficiently high amounts to affect the nursing infant. Monitor the nursing infant for agitation, poor sleeping pattern, and feeding problems. Probably compatible.
Diphenoxylate (C/−)	Active metabolite probably excreted into breast milk. Potential toxicity.
Diphtheria and tetanus vaccine (C/+)	No human lactation data. Probably compatible.
Dipyridamole (B/+)	Excreted into breast milk. Effect unknown on nursing infant. Probably compatible.
Docusate (calcium, potassium, sodium) (C/+)	Probably compatible. Monitor nursing infant for diarrhea.
Dolasetron (B/+)	No human lactation data available. Low molecular weight of drug suggests excretion into breast milk should be expected. Effects on nursing infant are unknown.
Dolutegravir (B/CI)	No human lactation data available. CDC recommends HIV-infected mothers in developed countries to not breast feed.
Dornase alfa (B/+)	No human lactation data available. Inhaled drug does not increase endogenous serum concentration of DNase. Not expected to be excreted into breast milk. Negligible risk to nursing infant.
Doxycycline (D/+)	Excreted into breast milk in low concentrations. Theoretical dental staining and inhibition of bone growth are remote. The bowel flora of nursing infants may be altered and there is the potential for interference with the interpretation of an infectious workup. Observe nursing infants for possible allergic reaction. AAP classifies doxycycline as compatible with breast feeding.
Doxylamine (C/−)	No human lactation data available. Low molecular weight suggests excretion into breast milk should be expected. Effects on nursing infant unknown. Potential effects include sedation, excitement, and irritability. Avoid breast feeding.
Dulaglutide (C/−)	No human lactation data available. Avoid breast feeding until safety data available.
Echinacea (C/−)	Avoid use during breast feeding.
Edoxaban (C/−)	No human lactation data available. Avoid breast feeding until safety data available.
Efavirenz (C/CI)	No human lactation data available. Molecular weight suggests excretion into breast milk should be expected. Effect on nursing infant is unknown. CDC recommends HIV-infected mothers in developed countries to not breast feed.
Eletriptan (C/+)	Excreted into breast milk. Effects of exposure to nursing infants are unknown, but low concentration not thought to be significant. Compatible with breast feeding.

(Continued)

Drug (FDA Fetal Risk Category/ Breast-Feeding Compatibility)	Effect on Lactation and Adverse Effects on Infant
Empagliflozin (C/–)	No human lactation data available. Avoid breast feeding until safety data available.
Emtricitabine (B/CI)	No human lactation data available. Molecular weight, low plasma protein binding, and long half-life suggest excretion into breast milk should be expected. Effect on nursing infant is unknown. CDC recommends HIV-infected mothers in developed countries to not breast feed.
Enalapril (C 1st tri; D 2nd, 3rd tri/+)	Enalapril and enalaprilat are excreted into breast milk in small amounts such that risk to nursing infant appears negligible/ clinically insignificant. AAP classifies enalapril as compatible with breast feeding.
Enfuvirtide (B/CI)	No human lactation data available. Molecular weight and high plasma protein binding should inhibit but not prevent excretion into breast milk. Effect on nursing infant is unknown. CDC recommends HIV-infected mothers in developed countries to not breast feed.
Enoxaparin (B/+)	No human lactation data available. Based on high molecular weight and probable inactivation by GI tract, the passage of drug into breast milk and its risk to nursing infant is considered negligible.
Entecavir (C/CI HIV; C/hepatitis B)	No human lactation data available. Molecular weight and half-life suggest the drug should be excreted into breast milk. Effects on nursing infants are unknown. Infants of HBsAg-positive or HBeAg-positive mothers should receive HBIG at birth and hepatitis B vaccine soon after birth. Then breast feeding is permitted. Breast feeding is contraindicated in HIV-1 positive mothers in the United States.
Ephedrine (C/–)	Limited human lactation data available. Observe nursing infant for irritability, excessive crying, and disturbed sleeping patterns. Avoiding breast feeding is recommended.
Epoetin alfa (C/+)	No human lactation data available. Excretion into breast milk is not expected and drug would be digested in GI tract. No risk to nursing infant expected.
Epoprostenol (B/+)	No human lactation data available. Based on its rapid degradation, a physiologic pH, and the GI tract, the amount of drug the nursing infant would be exposed to would not be clinically significant.
Eprosartan (C 1st tri; D 2nd, 3rd tri/+)	No human lactation data available. Expect excretion into breast milk. Effects on nursing infant are unknown. AAP classifies ACE inhibitors, a similar class of agents, as compatible with breast feeding.
Ergotamine (X/CI)	Causes vomiting, diarrhea, and convulsions in the nursing infant. May hinder lactation. Breast feeding is contraindicated.
Ertapenem (B/+)	Excreted into breast milk in low concentrations. Effects on nursing infant unknown but probably are not clinically significant. The bowel flora of nursing infants may be altered, and there is the potential for interference with the interpretation of an infectious workup. Observe nursing infants for possible allergic reaction. Probably compatible with breast feeding.

(Continued)

Drug (FDA Fetal Risk Category/ Breast-Feeding Compatibility)	Effect on Lactation and Adverse Effects on Infant
Erythromycin (B/+)	Excreted into breast milk in low concentrations. No reports of adverse effects in nursing infants. The bowel flora of nursing infants may be altered, and there is potential for interference with the interpretation of an infectious workup. Observe nursing infants for possible allergic reaction. AAP classifies erythromycin as compatible with breast feeding.
Escitalopram (C/−)	No human lactation data available. Expect excretion into breast milk. Effects on nursing infant unknown. Adverse effects have been seen with similar agent (citalopram), expect similar effects. Closely monitor nursing infants. AAP classifies other SSRIs as drugs for which effect on nursing infants is unknown but may be of concern.
Eslicarbazepine (C/+)	No human lactation data available. Expect excretion into breast milk. Closely monitor nursing infants for common side effects reported in adults.
Esomeprazole (B/−)	No human lactation data available. Expect excretion into breast milk. Effects on nursing infant unknown. Potential for toxic effects: headache, diarrhea and abdominal pain, and suppression of gastric acid secretion. Half-life is short, 1–1.5 hours. Waiting 5–7.5 hours after dose should eliminate 97% of drug from plasma.
Estrogens, conjugated (X/+)	No adverse effects in nursing infants reported. May decrease milk volume and nitrogen and protein content.
Etelcalcetide (C/−)	No human lactation data available. Avoid breast feeding until safety data available.
Ethambutol (C/+)	Excreted into breast milk. AAP classifies ethambutol as compatible with breast feeding.
Ethanol (X/−)	Passes freely into breast milk in levels similar to those in maternal serum. Because of risk of toxicity in nursing infant, safest course is to hold breast-feeding for 1–2 hours for each ounce of alcohol consumed.
Ethinyl estradiol (X/+)	No adverse effects in nursing infants reported. Expect trace amount in breast milk. May decrease milk volume and nitrogen and protein content. Monitor weight gain of infant, and use lowest dose.
Evolocumab (B/−)	No human lactation data available. Avoid breast feeding until safety data available.
Famciclovir (B/−)	No human lactation data available. Expect excretion into breast milk. Avoid breast feeding.
Famotidine (B/+)	Excreted into breast milk but to lesser extent than cimetidine and ranitidine. Effects on nursing infant are unknown. Potential risk for adverse effects; however, AAP classifies cimetidine as compatible with breast feeding. Famotidine may be preferred over other H$_2$ blockers because of lesser amount in breast milk.
Ferric citrate (B/−)	No human lactation data available. Avoid breast feeding until safety data available.
Flecainide (C/+)	Excreted into breast milk but effects on nursing infant are unknown. Probably not toxic. AAP classifies flecainide as compatible with breast feeding.

(Continued)

Drug (FDA Fetal Risk Category/ Breast-Feeding Compatibility)	Effect on Lactation and Adverse Effects on Infant
Fluconazole (C for single dose, D/+)	Excreted into breast milk. No drug-associated toxicity has been reported. AAP classifies fluconazole as compatible with breast feeding.
Flucytosine (C/−)	No human lactation data available. Because of potential serious adverse effects in nursing infant, breast feeding should be avoided.
Fluoxetine (C 1st, 2nd tri; D 3rd tri/−)	Excreted into breast milk. Long-term effects on neurobehavioral development from exposure to potent serotonin reuptake blocker during period of rapid CNS development have not been adequately studied. Manufacturer recommends breast feeding should be avoided during fluoxetine therapy. AAP indicates that effects on nursing infant are unknown but may be of concern. Maternal benefits may outweigh risks to nursing infant if treating postpartum depression. Colic, irritability, sleep disorders, and poor weight gain may occur.
Fondaparinux (B/+)	No human lactation data available. Excretion into breast milk should be expected. Effects on nursing infants unknown but not thought to be clinically significant.
Fosamprenavir (C/CI)	No human lactation data available. Molecular weight suggests excretion into breast milk should be expected. Effect on nursing infant is unknown. CDC recommends HIV-infected mothers in developed countries to not breast feed.
Furosemide (C/+)	Excreted into breast milk. No reports of adverse effects in a nursing infant. Probably compatible.
Gabapentin (C/+)	No human lactation data available. Probably compatible. Low molecular weight of drug suggests excretion into breast milk but effect on nursing infant is unknown.
Gadopentetate dimeglumine (MRI contrast) (C/+)	Excreted into breast milk in small amounts. Very little is absorbed systemically. AAP classifies gadopentetate dimeglumine as compatible with breast feeding.
Ganciclovir (D 1st tri; C 2nd, 3rd tri/−)	No human lactation data available. Potential for serious toxicity in nursing infant. Avoid breast feeding.
Gentamicin (C/+)	Small amounts excreted into breast milk and absorbed by nursing infants. Observe infant for bloody stools and diarrhea. AAP classifies as compatible with breast feeding.
Ginkgo biloba (C/−)	No human lactation data available. Herbal product that is not standardized and may contain other compounds. Safest course is to avoid breast feeding.
Ginseng (B/−)	No human lactation data available. Herbal product that is not standardized and may contain other compounds. Safest course is to avoid breast feeding.
Glimepiride (C/+)	No human lactation data available. Molecular weight suggests excretion into breast milk should be expected. Risk of neonatal hypoglycemia. Breast-feeding women should consider insulin instead.
Glipizide (C/+)	Minimal to nondetectable levels in breast milk. Normal glucose levels in nursing infants.

(Continued)

Drug (FDA Fetal Risk Category/ Breast-Feeding Compatibility)	Effect on Lactation and Adverse Effects on Infant
Glucosamine (C/+)	No human lactation data available. Molecular weight and prolonged plasma protein elimination half-life suggest excretion into breast milk should be expected. Unbound drug is undetectable in plasma; therefore, little if any drug will be excreted into milk. Probably compatible.
Glutamine (C/−)	No human lactation data available. Avoid breast feeding until safety data available.
Glyburide (C/+)	Nondetectable levels in breast milk. Normal glucose levels in nursing infants. Probably compatible.
Guaifenesin (C/+)	No human lactation data available. Probably compatible.
Haemophilus b conjugate vaccine (C/+)	Compatible with breast feeding.
Haloperidol (C/−)	Excreted into breast milk. Use may be of concern. Effects on nursing infant unknown. Possible decline in developmental score.
Heparin (C/+)	Not excreted into breast milk.
Hepatitis A vaccine (C/+)	No human lactation data available. Probably compatible.
Hepatitis B vaccine (C/+)	No human lactation data available. Probably compatible.
Heroin (D/CI)	Crosses into breast milk in sufficient amounts to cause addiction in nursing infant. Breast feeding is contraindicated.
Human papillomavirus vaccine (B/+)	Compatible with breast feeding.
Hydralazine (C/+)	Excreted into breast milk. No adverse effects noted in nursing infants. AAP hydralazine classifies as compatible with breast feeding.
Hydrochlorothiazide (B/+)	May suppress lactation, especially in the first month of lactation. Adverse effects have not been reported, but infant's electrolytes and platelets should be monitored.
Hydrocodone (C, D/+)	No human lactation data available. Molecular weight suggests excretion into breast milk should be expected. Observe nursing infant for GI effects, sedation, and changes in feeding patterns.
Hydrocortisone (C, D/+)	No human lactation data available. Unlikely that it poses risk to nursing infant. Compatible with breast feeding.
Hydromorphone (B, D/+)	Excreted into breast milk. Monitor nursing infant for sedation. Milk ejection reflex (letdown) may be inhibited.
Hydroxychloroquine (C/+)	Excreted into breast milk. Slow elimination rate. Breast feeding during daily therapy should be done with caution. Once-weekly doses significantly reduce amount of drug exposure to nursing infant. AAP classifies hydroxychloroquine as compatible with breast feeding. Amount in breast milk is not adequate to provide malaria protection for infant.
Hydroxyzine (C/+)	No human lactation data available. Molecular weight suggests excretion into breast milk should be expected. Effects on nursing infant unknown.
Ibuprofen (B 2nd tri; D 1st, 3rd tri/+)	Excreted into breast milk. Amount of drug available to nursing infant is minimal. AAP classifies ibuprofen as compatible with breast feeding.

(Continued)

Drug (FDA Fetal Risk Category/ Breast-Feeding Compatibility)	Effect on Lactation and Adverse Effects on Infant
Imipenem-cilastatin (C/+)	Small amounts excreted into breast milk in amounts comparable to other lactam antibiotics. Effects on nursing infant are unknown.
Indinavir (C/CI)	No human lactation data available. Molecular weight suggests excretion into breast milk should be expected. Effect on nursing infant is unknown. CDC recommends HIV-infected mothers in developed countries to not breast feed.
Indomethacin (C <30 weeks' gestation, D ≥30 weeks' gestation/+)	Excreted into breast milk. One case report of seizure in nursing infant. AAP classifies indomethacin as compatible with breast feeding.
Infliximab (B/+)	Excreted into breast milk in trace amount. Compatible with breast feeding.
Influenza vaccine (B/+)	Live attenuated influenza vaccine is not recommended during pregnancy. Maternal vaccination is compatible with breast feeding.
Iodine (D/+)	May cause fetal goiter or hyperthyroidism. APP classifies iodine as compatible with breast feeding.
Isavuconazonium (C/−)	No human lactation data available. Avoid breast feeding until safety data available.
Isoniazid (C/+)	Isoniazid and its metabolite are excreted into breast milk. Monitor nursing infant for signs and symptoms of peripheral neuritis or hepatitis. Pyridoxine supplementation should be considered in both mother and infants. AAP classifies isoniazid as compatible with breast feeding.
Ivacaftor (B/−)	No human lactation data available. Molecular weight and long half-life suggest excretion into breast milk should be expected. Effects on nursing infant are unknown. Avoid breast feeding until safety data available.
Ivermectin (C/+)	Excreted into breast milk but no human lactation data available. Low drug levels in milk probably not a risk to nursing infant. AAP classifies ivermectin as compatible with breast feeding.
Kaolin/pectin (C/+)	No effect on nursing infant.
Ketamine (B/+)	Should be undetectable in maternal plasma ~11 hours after dose. Breast feeding after this time should not expose the nursing infant to drug.
Ketoconazole (C/+)	Excreted into breast milk. Effects of exposure to nursing infants are unknown but not thought to be significant. AAP classifies ketoconazole as compatible with breast feeding.
Ketorolac (C; D if used in 3rd tri or near delivery/+)	Excreted into breast milk in amounts that are considered clinically insignificant. AAP classifies ketoralac as compatible with breast feeding.
Labetalol (C/+)	Monitor nursing infant for hypotension and bradycardia. AAP classifies labetalol as compatible with breast feeding.
Lactulose (B/+)	No human lactation data. Probably compatible.
Lamivudine (C/CI)	Excreted into breast milk. Effect on nursing infant is unknown. CDC recommends HIV-infected mothers in developed countries to not breast feed.

(Continued)

Drug (FDA Fetal Risk Category/ Breast-Feeding Compatibility)	Effect on Lactation and Adverse Effects on Infant
Lamotrigine (C/–)	May be of concern. Consider monitoring infant's serum lamotrigine concentration.
Lansoprazole (B/–)	No human lactation data available. Excretion into breast milk is expected. Potential effects on nursing infant include carcinogenicity (animal data) and suppression of gastric acid secretion. Avoid breast feeding.
Levetiracetam (C/+)	No human lactation data available. Low molecular weight and protein binding suggest excretion into breast milk should be expected. Effects on nursing infant are unknown. AAP classifies levetiracetam as compatible with breast feeding.
Levofloxacin (C/+)	Excreted into breast milk. Effects on nursing infants are unknown. AAP classifies levofloxacin as compatible with breast-feeding.
Levomilnacipran (C/–)	No human lactation data available. Avoid breast feeding until safety data available.
Levothyroxine (A/+)	Probably does not interfere with neonatal thyroid screening.
Lindane (C/+)	No human lactation data available. Excreted into breast milk. Small amounts ingested by nursing infant are probably clinically insignificant. Waiting 4 days after discontinuing lotion should prevent exposure to nursing infant.
Linezolid (C/–)	No human lactation data available. Excretion into breast milk is expected. Effects on nursing infant unknown. Potential effects: myelosuppression and reversible thrombocytopenia. Avoid breast feeding.
Liraglutide (C/–)	No human lactation data available. Avoid breast feeding until safety data available.
Lisinopril (C 1st tri; D 2nd, 3rd tri/+)	No human lactation data available. Excretion into breast milk should be expected. AAP classifies lisinopril as compatible with breast feeding.
Lithium (D/–)	Milk levels average 40% of maternal serum concentration. Monitor nursing infant for cyanosis, hypotonia, bradycardia, and other lithium toxicities.
Loperamide (B/+)	No human lactation data available. AAP classifies loperamide as compatible with breast feeding.
Lopinavir (C/Cl)	No human lactation data available. Molecular weight and lipid solubility suggest excretion into breast milk should be expected; however, extensive plasma protein binding should limit this. Effect on nursing infant is unknown. CDC recommends HIV-infected mothers in developed countries to not breast feed.
Loratadine (B/+)	Loratadine and its metabolite are excreted into breast milk. Probably little clinical risk to nursing infant. AAP classifies loratadine as compatible with breast feeding.
Lorazepam (D/–)	Excretion into breast milk in small amount. Monitor nursing infant for sedation, especially if exposure is prolonged.
Losartan (C 1st tri; D 2nd, 3rd tri/+)	No human lactation data available. Excretion into breast milk is expected. Effects of exposure to nursing infant are unknown. AAP considers losartan compatible with breast feeding.

(Continued)

Drug (FDA Fetal Risk Category/ Breast-Feeding Compatibility)	Effect on Lactation and Adverse Effects on Infant
Macitentan (X/CI)	No human lactation data available. Molecular weight and half-life suggest excretion into breast milk, but high protein binding affinity may limit the amount. Monitor nursing infants for anemia, influenza, and urinary tract infections.
Measles vaccine (X, C/+)	Compatible with breast feeding.
Meclizine (B/+)	No human lactation data available. Molecular weight suggests excretion into breast milk should be expected. Probably compatible. Caution: newborns and premature infants have increased sensitivity to antihistamines. Prolonged use may decrease milk supply.
Medroxyprogesterone (D/+)	AAP classifies medroxyprogesterone as compatible with breast feeding.
Meloxicam (C 1st tri; D 2nd, 3rd tri/+)	No human lactation data available. Molecular weight would suggest excretion into breast milk. Probably compatible.
Meningococcal vaccine (B/+)	No human lactation data available. Probably compatible. ACIP recommends deferring meningococcal B vaccine in breast-feeding women unless the woman is at increased risk for meningococcal disease.
Meperidine (C, D/+)	Monitor nursing infant for sedation. Milk ejection reflex (letdown) may be inhibited. AAP classifies meperidine as compatible with breast feeding.
Meropenem (B/+)	No human lactation data available. Probably compatible. Expect excretion into breast milk. Potential effects on nursing infant are unknown.
Mesalamine (B/−)	Small amount excreted into breast milk. Risk of adverse effect (diarrhea) in nursing infant. AAP classifies mesalamine as a drug that should be used with caution during breast feeding because there is potential for toxicity.
Metformin (B/+)	Excreted into breast milk. Nursing infants had normal blood glucose levels.
Methadone (C, D/+)	Generally compatible with breast feeding. Monitor nursing infant for sedation, depression, and withdrawal on cessation of methadone treatment. AAP classifies methadone as compatible with breast feeding.
Methamphetamine (C/CI)	AAP classifies amphetamines as contraindicated during breast feeding. Monitor nursing infant for irritability and poor sleeping pattern.
Methimazole (D/+)	Potential for interfering with thyroid function. AAP classifies methimazole as compatible with breast feeding.
Methocarbamol (C/+)	Probably compatible. Any amount of drug excreted into breast milk probably not clinically significant.
Methyldopa (B/C/+)	Risk of hemolysis and increased liver enzymes. AAP classifies methyldopa as compatible with breast feeding.
Methylphenidate (C/−)	Excreted into breast milk. Potential toxicity will probably occur in 1st month of life. Observe nursing infant for signs and symptoms of CNS stimulation: decreased appetite, insomnia, and irritability.
Metoclopramide (B/−)	Increases milk production. Effects on nursing infant unknown but may be of concern because it is a dopaminergic-blocking agent.

(Continued)

Drug (FDA Fetal Risk Category/ Breast-Feeding Compatibility)	Effect on Lactation and Adverse Effects on Infant
Metolazone (B/+)	May suppress lactation, especially in the first month of lactation. Probably compatible. Adverse effects have not been reported, but infant's electrolytes and platelets should be monitored.
Metoprolol (C/−)	Monitor nursing infant for bradycardia and hypotension.
Metronidazole (D 1st tri; B 2nd, 3rd tri/−)	Discontinue during breast feeding. Do not nurse until 12–24 hours after discontinuing to allow excretion of drug.
Miltefosine (D/CI)	No human lactation data available. Molecular weight suggests excretion into breast milk, but high protein binding may limit amount in milk.
Minocycline (D/+)	Excreted into breast milk in low concentrations. Theoretical dental staining and inhibition of bone growth are remote. The bowel flora of nursing infants may be altered, and there is the potential for interference with the interpretation of an infectious workup. Observe nursing infants for possible allergic reaction. Compatible with breast feeding.
Mipomersen (B/−)	No human lactation data available. Molecular weight and protein binding suggest excretion into breast milk will be limited. Potential for disruption of infant lipid metabolism. Monitor nursing infant for flulike symptoms and elevated liver transaminases.
Mirtazapine (C/−)	Excreted into breast milk. Monitor infant for potential sedation and weight gain. Long-term effects on neurobehavioral development unknown. AAP classifies other antidepressants as drugs for which effect on nursing infant is unknown but may be of concern.
Montelukast (B/+)	Monitor nursing infant for sedation. Milk ejection reflex (letdown) may be inhibited.
Morphine (C/−)	Excreted into breast milk. Monitor infant for sedation, apnea and bradycardia, and cyanosis. AAP classifies morphine as compatible with breast feeding. Long-term effects on neurobehavioral development are unknown.
Mumps vaccine (C/+)	No human lactation data. Probably compatible.
Nafcillin (B/+)	No human lactation data. Refer to Penicillin.
Nalbuphine (B/+)	Monitor newborn for respiratory depression and bradycardia if used during labor. No human lactation data available. Probably compatible. Expect small amount of drug to be excreted into breast milk. Amounts are clinically insignificant.
Naloxegol (C/+)	No human lactation data available. Molecular weight and protein binding suggest excretion into breast milk is likely. Probably compatible.
Naloxone (B, C/+)	No human lactation data available. Probably compatible.
Naltrexone (C/+)	No human lactation data available. Expect excretion into breast milk. Probably compatible. Effects on nursing infant are unknown. Potential adverse effects of drug: alteration of opioid receptors in the brain; altered levels of some hormones of hypothalamic, pituitary, adrenal, and gonadal origin.

(Continued)

Drug (FDA Fetal Risk Category/ Breast-Feeding Compatibility)	Effect on Lactation and Adverse Effects on Infant
Naproxen (C/+)	Passes into breast milk in very small quantities. Effects on nursing infant are unknown. AAP classifies naproxen as compatible with breast feeding.
Naratriptan (C/+)	No human lactation data available. Excretion into breast milk should be expected. Probably compatible. Effects on nursing infant are unknown.
Nelfinavir (B/CI)	No human lactation data available. Molecular weight suggests excretion into breast milk should be expected. Effect on nursing infant is unknown. CDC recommends HIV-infected mothers in developed countries to not breast feed.
Netupitant and palonosetron (C/+)	No human lactation data available. Molecular weight and protein binding suggest excretion into breast milk is likely. Probably compatible.
Nevirapine (C/CI)	Excreted into breast milk. CDC recommends HIV-infected mothers in developed countries to not breast feed.
Nicotine (transdermal, others) (D/−)	May be of concern. Excessive amounts may cause diarrhea, vomiting, tachycardia, irritability, decreased milk production, and decreased weight gain.
Nifedipine (C/+)	Manufacturer states significant amounts of drug excreted into breast milk. No human lactation data available. AAP classifies nifedipine as compatible with breast feeding.
Nimodipine (C/+)	Excreted in breast milk. Limited data suggest that milk is excreted in likely clinically insignificant amounts. Probably compatible.
Nitrofurantoin (B/+)	Excreted in breast milk in small amounts. Monitor nursing infants with G6PD deficiency for hemolytic anemia. AAP classifies nitrofurantoin as compatible with breast feeding.
Nortriptyline (C/−)	Excreted into breast milk in low concentrations. No adverse effects noted in breast-feeding infants. Long-term effects of chronic exposure to antidepressants in nursing infants are unknown with concern for effects on the infant's neurobehavioral development. AAP classifies nortriptyline as a drug for which effect on nursing infant is unknown but may be of concern.
Nystatin (C/+)	Poorly absorbed if at all. Excretion into breast milk would not occur.
Olanzapine (C/−)	Sedation has occurred in nursing infants. Decreasing dose may eliminate this problem but may affect control of mother's disease. Avoid use during breast feeding.
Olodaterol (C/+)	No human lactation data available. Molecular weight suggests excretion into breast milk is likely, but low systemic absorption. Probably compatible.
Olsalazine (C/−)	Active metabolite, 5-aminosalicylic acid (mesalamine), is excreted into human milk. Diarrhea reported in nursing infant of mother receiving mesalamine.
Omeprazole (C/−)	Limited human lactation data available. Excretion into breast milk is expected. Effects on nursing infant are unknown. Use during breast feeding should be avoided. Concern for suppression of gastric acid secretion and carcinogenicity observed in animals.

(Continued)

Drug (FDA Fetal Risk Category/ Breast-Feeding Compatibility)	Effect on Lactation and Adverse Effects on Infant
Ondansetron (B/+)	No human lactation data available. Expect excretion into breast milk. Probably compatible. Effects on nursing infant are unknown.
Oral contraceptives (all classes) (X/+)	Causes dose-dependent suppression of lactation. Decreased weight gain, milk production, and nitrogen and protein content of human milk have been associated with this drug. Changes probably only significant in malnourished mothers. Use lowest dose possible. AAP classifies oral contraceptives as compatible with breast feeding.
Oritavancin (C/+)	No human lactation data available. Limited oral bioavailability would suggest low risk of toxicity to nursing infant. Probably compatible.
Orlistat (X/+)	No human lactation data available. Limited systemic bioavailability would suggest that it would not appear in breast milk.
Oseltamivir (C/+)	No human lactation data available. Molecular weight suggests excretion into breast milk should be expected. Effect on nursing infant is unknown.
Oxacillin (B/+)	Excreted into breast milk in low concentrations. Adverse effects rare. The bowel flora of nursing infants may be altered, and there is the potential for interference with the interpretation of an infectious workup. Observe nursing infants for possible allergic reaction.
Oxcarbazepine (C/+)	One report of use during human lactation. No adverse effects reported. Monitor infant for poor suckling, vomiting, and sedation. AAP classifies carbamazepine as compatible with breast feeding; oxcarbazepine can be also considered compatible.
Oxycodone (B/−)	Monitor nursing infant for drowsiness, sedation, feeding difficulties, or limpness. Withdrawal symptoms may occur when maternal use or breast feeding is discontinued.
Pamidronate (D/+)	No human lactation data available. Molecular weight, prolonged half-life, and lack of metabolism suggest drug will be excreted into breast milk. Considering the bioavailability, the amount absorbed by the nursing infant will be clinically insignificant. Probably compatible.
Pantoprazole (C/+)	Excreted into breast milk in small amounts. Has potential for suppression of gastric acid secretion in nursing infant, but overall risk of toxicities is low.
Paregoric (C/+)	Probably excreted into breast milk. Limited human lactation data available. Probably compatible. Refer to morphine.
Paroxetine (D, X/−)	Effect on nursing infant is unknown but may be of concern. Monitor infant for insomnia, lethargy, poor weight gain, and changes in feeding pattern.
Pasireotide (C/−)	No human lactation data available. Molecular weight and protein binding suggest excretion in breast milk. Potential adverse reactions include diarrhea, nausea, hyperglycemia, and cholelithiasis. Recommended to avoid breast feeding due to potential toxicity.

(Continued)

Drug (FDA Fetal Risk Category/ Breast-Feeding Compatibility)	Effect on Lactation and Adverse Effects on Infant
Penicillin G (all forms) (B/+)	All antibiotics are excreted in breast milk in limited amounts. Monitor nursing infant for rash, diarrhea, and spitting up. The bowel flora of nursing infants may be altered, and there is the potential for interference with the interpretation of an infectious workup.
Pentamidine (C/CI)	No human lactation data available. Systemic concentrations reached with aerosolized drug are very low. Breast milk levels would be nil.
Pentobarbital (D/−)	Excreted into breast milk. Effects on nursing infant are unknown.
Permethrin (B/+)	No human lactation data available. Little if any drug expected to be excreted into breast milk. CDC considers permethrin or pyrethrins with piperonyl butoxide treatment of choice for pubic lice during lactation.
Phenobarbital (D/−)	Monitor nursing infant for sucking problems, sedation, rashes, and withdrawal. AAP classifies phenobarbital as a drug that has caused major adverse effects in some nursing infants. Use caution if breast feeding.
Phenytoin (D/+)	Monitor nursing infant for methemoglobinuria (rare), drowsiness, and decreased suckling. Keep maternal phenytoin in therapeutic range. AAP classifies phenytoin as compatible with breast feeding.
Pirfenidone (C/+)	No human lactation data available. Molecular weight and protein binding suggest excretion into breast milk is likely. Probably compatible.
Piroxicam (C/+)	Excreted into breast milk in amounts that probably do not present a risk to nursing infant. AAP classifies piroxicam as compatible with breast feeding.
Pneumococcal vaccine (C/+)	No human lactation data available. Probably compatible.
Poliovirus inactivated vaccine (C/+)	No human lactation data available. Probably compatible.
Pravastatin (X/CI)	No human lactation data available. Excreted into breast milk. Because of the potential for adverse effects in the nursing infant, avoid use during lactation.
Prednisolone (C, D/+)	Trace amounts have been measured in breast milk. Concentration did not pose clinically significant risk to nursing infant. AAP classifies prednisolone as compatible with breast feeding.
Prednisone (C, D/+)	Trace amounts have been measured in breast milk. Concentration did not pose clinically significant risk to nursing infant. AAP classifies prednisone as compatible with breast feeding.
Pregabalin (C/−)	No human lactation data available. Expect excretion into breast milk. Effects on nursing infants are unknown. Monitor nursing infant for dizziness, somnolence, blurred vision, peripheral edema, myopathy, and decreased platelet count. Avoid use during breast feeding.
Probenecid (C/+)	Excreted into breast milk. Toxicity observed probably related to concurrent antibiotic administered. Probably compatible. Observe nursing infant for diarrhea.

(Continued)

Drug (FDA Fetal Risk Category/ Breast-Feeding Compatibility)	Effect on Lactation and Adverse Effects on Infant
Procainamide (C/+)	Excreted in and accumulates in milk. AAP classifies procainamide as compatible with breast feeding. Long-term effects of exposure in nursing infants are unknown.
Prochlorperazine (C/−)	Other phenothiazines excreted into breast milk, so prochlorperazine excretion expected. Sedation in nursing infant a possible side effect.
Propranolol (C/−)	Excreted into breast milk. Monitor nursing infant for hypotension and bradycardia. AAP classifies propranolol as compatible with breast feeding.
Propylthiouracil (D/+)	Excreted into breast milk. Monitor thyroid function of infant periodically. AAP classifies propylthiouracil as compatible with breast feeding.
Prothrombin complex concentrate (C/−)	No human lactation data available. Manufacturer recommends to only use if clearly needed.
Pseudoephedrine (C/+)	Excreted into breast milk. Monitor nursing infant for agitation. AAP classifies pseudoephedrine as compatible with breast feeding.
Pyrazinamide (C/+)	Excreted into breast milk in small amounts. Probably compatible. Monitor infant for signs of toxicity such as jaundice, fever, decreased appetite, nausea, vomiting, thrombocytopenia, or rash.
Pyrimethamine (C/+)	Excreted into breast milk. AAP classifies pyrimethamine as compatible with breast feeding.
Quetiapine (C/−)	Excreted into breast milk. No reports of adverse effects in nursing infants. Long-term effects of this exposure are unknown. Manufacturer recommends avoiding breast feeding.
Quinidine (C/+)	Excreted into breast milk. Monitor nursing infant for rash, anemia, and arrhythmias. Risk of optic neuritis with chronic use. AAP classifies quinidine as compatible with breast feeding.
Quinine (C/+)	Excreted into breast milk. No adverse effects reported in nursing infants. G6PD should be ruled out in infants at risk for the disease. AAP classifies quinine as compatible with breast feeding.
Quinupristin/dalfopristin (B/−)	No human lactation data available. Large molecular size and weakly acidic nature make it unlikely to be excreted into breast milk. Caution: may alter the bowel flora of nursing infants. There is the potential for the development of resistant strains of VRE. Breast feeding is not recommended.
Rabies immune globulin (C/+)	No human lactation data available. Probably compatible.
Ranitidine (B/+)	Excreted into breast milk. Effects on nursing infant are unknown. Decreases gastric acidity but effect on nursing infant has not been studied. AAP classifies similar agent (cimetidine) as compatible with breast feeding.
Remifentanil (C/+)	No human lactation data available. Expect excretion into breast milk. Very short half-life. Other narcotic agents are classified as compatible with breast feeding by AAP.

(Continued)

Drug (FDA Fetal Risk Category/ Breast-Feeding Compatibility)	Effect on Lactation and Adverse Effects on Infant
Rifabutin (B/CI)	No human lactation data available. Excretion into breast milk expected. Milk may be stained brown-orange color. Effects on nursing infants are unknown, but serious toxicities (leukopenia, neutropenia, rash) are potential adverse effects. Contraindicated if nursing mother is HIV-1 positive.
Rifampin (C/+)	Excreted into breast milk in amounts that pose very little risk to nursing infants. No adverse effects reported. AAP classifies rifampin as compatible with breast feeding.
Rifapentine (C/+)	No human lactation data available. Expect excretion into breast milk. May cause red-orange discoloration of breast milk. Effects on nursing infants are unknown. AAP classifies rifampin, a similar agent, as compatible with breast feeding.
Rifaximin (C/+)	No human lactation data available. Expect excretion into breast milk but in very small amounts due to limited systemic absorption. Effects on nursing infants are unknown but probably not clinically significant.
Riociguat (X/−)	No human lactation data available. Expect excretion into breast milk. Effects on nursing infant unknown, but nursing infant should be monitored for diarrhea, vomiting, hypotension, GERD, and constipation.
Risperidone (C/−)	Excreted into breast milk. AAP classifies other antipsychotic drugs for which the effects on nursing infants are unknown but may be of concern, especially with long-term use. Could possibly alter short- and long-term CNS function.
Ritonavir (B/CI)	No human lactation data available. Molecular weight suggests excretion into breast milk should be expected. Effect on nursing infant is unknown. CDC recommends HIV-infected mothers in developed countries to not breast feed.
Rizatriptan (C/+)	No human lactation data available. Expect excretion into breast milk. Effects on nursing infants are unknown. Probably compatible.
Rubella vaccine (C/+)	Compatible with breast feeding. ACOG and CDC recommend vaccination of susceptible women in immediate postpartum period.
Salmeterol (C/+)	No human lactation data available. Expect excretion into breast milk, but maternal plasma levels after inhaled dose are very low to undetectable. It is unlikely that clinically significant amounts would appear in breast milk. Probably compatible.
Saquinavir (B/CI)	No human lactation data available. Molecular weight suggests excretion into breast milk should be expected. Effect on nursing infant is unknown. CDC recommends HIV-infected mothers in developed countries to not breast feed.
Scopolamine (C/+)	No human lactation data available. Excreted into breast milk. AAP classifies scopolamine as compatible with breast feeding.
Secobarbital (D/+)	Excreted into breast milk. Amount and effects on nursing infants are unknown. AAP classifies secobarbital as compatible with breast feeding.

(Continued)

Drug (FDA Fetal Risk Category/ Breast-Feeding Compatibility)	Effect on Lactation and Adverse Effects on Infant
Senna (C/+)	Observe nursing infant for diarrhea. AAP classifies senna as compatible with breast feeding.
Sertraline (C/−)	AAP classifies sertraline as a drug for which the effect on nursing infant is unknown but may be of concern. Concentrated in human milk.
Simeprevir (C/−)	No human lactation data available. Molecular weight and elimination half-life suggest excretion into milk is likely, but high protein binding may limit amount excreted. Monitor nursing infants for rash, myalgia, and dyspnea.
Simvastatin (X/CI)	No human lactation data available. Expect excretion into breast milk. Because of the potential for adverse effects in the nursing infant, avoid use during lactation.
Smallpox vaccine (D, X/CI)	CDC recommends breast-feeding women should not routinely be vaccinated; however, if nursing woman is exposed to smallpox or monkeypox, she should be vaccinated and stop breast feeding.
Sofosbuvir (B, X/+)	No human lactation data available. Molecular weight and protein binding suggest it is likely excreted into milk. Potentially toxic if used in combination with ribavirin. Probably compatible otherwise.
Sotalol (B/−)	Milk levels 3–5 times maternal serum levels. Could cause bradycardia and hypotension. Long-term effects unknown.
Spironolactone (C/+)	Unknown if spironolactone is excreted into breast milk, but metabolite is found in breast milk—probably insignificant amount. Effects on nursing infants unknown. AAP classifies spironolactone as compatible with breast feeding.
SSKI (potassium iodide) (D/+)	The significance to nursing infant of chronic ingestion of higher levels of iodine unknown. AAP recognizes maternal use of iodides during lactation may affect infant's thyroid activity by producing elevated iodine levels in breast milk; it classifies as compatible with breast feeding. Consider monitoring infant's thyroid function.
St. John's wort (C/−)	Unknown if any of the constituents and possible contaminants are excreted into breast milk or if exposure represents risk to nursing infant.
Stavudine (C/CI)	No human lactation data available. Molecular weight suggests excretion into breast milk should be expected. Effect on nursing infant is unknown. CDC recommends HIV-infected mothers in developed countries to not breast feed.
Sucralfate (B/+)	Minimal, if any, drug expected to be excreted into breast milk because only small amounts systemically absorbed.
Sulbactam (B/+)	Excretion into breast milk expected. Effects on nursing infants are unknown. The bowel flora of nursing infants may be altered, and there is the potential for interference with the interpretation of an infectious workup. Observe nursing infants for possible allergic reaction. AAP classifies sulbactam as compatible with breast feeding.
Sulfamethoxazole (C/−)	Excreted into breast milk in low concentrations. Avoid in ill, stressed, or preterm infants and those with hyperbilirubinemia or G6PD deficiency.

(Continued)

Drug (FDA Fetal Risk Category/ Breast-Feeding Compatibility)	Effect on Lactation and Adverse Effects on Infant
Sulfasalazine (B, D/−)	Excreted into breast milk. May cause diarrhea in nursing infants. AAP classifies sulfasalazine as a drug that has been associated with significant effects on some nursing infants and should be given to nursing mother with caution.
Sulindac (C/−)	No human lactation data available. Because of prolonged half-life, use safer alternatives such as diclofenac, fenoprofen, flurbiprofen, ibuprofen, ketoprofen, ketorolac, or tolmetin during breast feeding.
Sumatriptan (C/+)	Excreted into breast milk. Absorption from GI tract is inhibited, so amount reaching nursing infant is probably negligible. AAP classifies sumatriptan as compatible with breast feeding.
Suvorexant (C/+)	No human lactation data available. Molecular weight suggests excretion into breast milk, but high protein binding likely limits the amount in milk. Probably compatible.
Tavaborole (C/+)	No human lactation data available. Probably compatible.
Tedizolid (C/+)	No human lactation data available. Molecular weight suggests that excretion into breast milk should be expected, but high protein binding may limit the amount in milk. Probably compatible.
Telavancin (C/−)	No human lactation data available. High fat solubility suggests some excretion into milk. Monitor nursing infant for diarrhea, vomiting, and foamy urine.
Telmisartan (C 1st tri; D 2nd, 3rd tri/+)	No human lactation data available. Molecular weight suggests that excretion into breast milk should be expected. Effects on nursing infant are unknown. AAP classifies the closely related ACE inhibitors as compatible with breast feeding.
Temazepam (X/−)	Excreted into breast milk. Observe nursing infant for sedation and poor feeding. AAP classifies temazepam as a drug for which the effect on nursing infants is unknown but may be of concern.
Tenofovir (B/CI)	No human lactation data available. Molecular weight suggests excretion into breast milk should be expected. Effect on nursing infant is unknown. CDC recommends HIV-infected mothers in developed countries to not breast feed.
Terbutaline (C/+)	Excreted into breast milk. Monitor nursing infant for agitation and spitting up. Use inhaled form to decrease maternal absorption if available. AAP classifies terbutaline as compatible with breast feeding.
Tetanus/diphtheria toxoids and acellular pertussis vaccine (B, C/+)	No human lactation data available. Compatible with breast feeding.
Tetracycline (D 1st tri; CI 2nd, 3rd tri/+)	Excreted into breast milk in low concentrations. Theoretical dental staining and inhibition of bone growth are remote. The bowel flora of nursing infants may be altered, and there is the potential for interference with the interpretation of an infectious workup. Observe nursing infants for possible allergic reaction. AAP classifies tetracycline as compatible with breast feeding.
THC (marijuana) (X/CI)	Excreted into breast milk. AAP classifies marijuana as a drug that should not be used during breast feeding.

(Continued)

Drug (FDA Fetal Risk Category/ Breast-Feeding Compatibility)	Effect on Lactation and Adverse Effects on Infant
Theophylline (C/+)	Excreted into breast milk. AAP classifies theophylline as compatible with breast feeding. Monitor nursing infant for irritability.
Tobramycin (C, D/+)	Excreted into breast milk. No adverse effects reported, and because of poor oral absorption, ototoxicity risk is low. The bowel flora of nursing infants may be altered, and there is the potential for interference with the interpretation of an infectious workup. Observe nursing infants for possible allergic reaction. Compatible with breast feeding.
Topiramate (D/−)	Excreted into breast milk. No adverse effects noted in limited number of exposed nursing infants. However, potential for adverse effects: fatigue, somnolence, ataxia, purpura, epistaxis, infections (viral and pneumonia), anorexia, and weight loss. Observe nursing infants for signs of toxicity.
Tramadol (C/CI)	Tramadol and active metabolite, M1 (O-desmethyl tramadol), are present in breast milk; concentrations are dependent on CYP2D6 metabolism. Effects on nursing infants unknown. Opioid therapy should be avoided in breast-feeding mothers due to potential for apnea and sedation in the infant.
Trazodone (C/−)	Excreted in breast milk. AAP classifies trazadone as a drug for which the effects on the nursing infant are unknown but may be of concern.
Tretinoin (systemic) (CI 1st tri; D 2nd, 3rd tri/+)	Vitamin A and probably tretinoin are natural constituents of breast milk. No human lactation data available on amounts excreted into breast milk after doses for treatment of promyelocytic leukemia or risk to nursing infant. Probably compatible.
Trimethoprim/sulfamethoxazole (D/−)	Excreted into breast milk in low concentrations. Considered negligible risk to nursing infant. Monitor for jaundice, hemolysis, and GI disturbance. The bowel flora may be altered. Avoid in ill, stressed, or preterm infants and those with hyperbilirubinemia or G6PD deficiency.
Valacyclovir (B/+)	Lack of adverse effects seen with acyclovir, the primary metabolite of valacyclovir. Considered compatible with breast feeding; breast-feeding mothers with herpetic lesions near or on the breast should avoid breast feeding.
Valganciclovir (C/CI)	Active metabolite, ganciclovir, has the potential to cause serious toxicity. CDC recommends HIV-infected mothers in developed countries to not breast feed. Breast feeding contraindicated.
Valproic acid (D, X for migraine prophylaxis/+)	Generally compatible with breast feeding per AAP but carries risk of fatal hepatotoxicity.
Valsartan (C 1st tri; D 2nd, 3rd tri/+)	No human lactation data available. Low molecular weight suggests that the drug would be excreted into breast milk. Effects on nursing infant are unknown.
Vancomycin (B/+)	Excreted into breast milk. Effects on nursing infant are unknown, but vancomycin is poorly absorbed from GI tract. Potential for allergic sensitization and modification of bowel flora. AAP classifies cephalosporins as compatible with breast feeding. Compatible with breast feeding.

(Continued)

Drug (FDA Fetal Risk Category/ Breast-Feeding Compatibility)	Effect on Lactation and Adverse Effects on Infant
Varicella vaccine (D/+)	CDC and AAP classify as compatible with breast feeding.
Vedolizumab (B/−)	No human lactation data available. Effect on nursing infant is unknown.
Velpatasvir (C/−)	No human lactation data available. Potentially toxic if used in combination with ribavirin. Effects on nursing infants are unknown.
Venlafaxine (C/−)	Excreted into breast milk. Observe for excessive somnolence, changes in sleep, decreased feeding, and weight loss. Long-term effects on neurobehavioral development are unknown. AAP classifies effect of SNRIs on breast feeding as unknown but may be of concern. However, if required by the mother, it is not a reason to discontinue breast feeding.
Verapamil (C/+)	Excreted into breast milk. Limited human lactation data available. AAP classifies verapamil as compatible with breast feeding.
Voriconazole (D/−)	No human lactation data available. Low molecular weight suggests excretion into breast milk. Potential for toxicity in neonatal period. Manufacturer recommends a decision be made to continue nursing or discontinue the drug, taking into account the importance of treatment to the mother.
Voxilaprevir (C/−)	No human lactation data available. Potentially toxic if used in combination with ribavirin. Effects on nursing infants are unknown.
Warfarin (X/+)	Maternal warfarin therapy does not appear to pose a significant risk to normal full-term infants; monitor for bleeding or bruising. American College of Chest Physicians (ACCP) classifies as compatible with breast feeding; other oral anticoagulants are contraindicated in lactating women.
Zanamivir (C/+)	No human lactation data available. Low molecular weight and pharmacokinetics of drug suggest it will be excreted into breast milk. Effects on nursing infants are unknown, but risk of harm is low.
Zidovudine (C/CI)	CDC recommends HIV-infected mothers in developed countries to not breast feed.
Zolmitriptan (C/+)	No human lactation data available. Molecular weight and low protein binding suggest drug and its active metabolite will be excreted into breast milk. Effects on nursing infant are unknown.
Zolpidem (C/+)	Excreted into breast milk in small amounts, which would indicate few adverse effects, if any, would occur in nursing infant. Observe for increased sedation, lethargy, and changes in feeding habits. AAP classifies zolpidem as compatible with breast feeding.

AAP, American Academy of Pediatrics; ACE, angiotensin-converting enzyme; ACIP, Advisory Committee on Immunization Practices; ACOG, American Congress of Obstetricians and Gynecologists; CDC, Centers for Disease Control and Prevention; CI, contraindicated; CNS, central nervous system; FDA, US Food and Drug Administration; G6PD, glucose-6-phosphate dehydrogenase; GERD, gastroesophageal reflux disease; GI, gastrointestinal; HBeAg, hepatitis B e antigen; HBIG, hepatitis B immune globulin; HBsAg, hepatitis B surface antigen; HIV, human immunodeficiency virus; IV, intravenous; SNRI, serotonin and norepinephrine reuptake inhibitor; SSRIs, selective serotonin reuptake inhibitors; tri, trimester; VRE, vancomycin-resistant enterococci.

Appendix A. Abbreviations

2,4-DNPH	2,4-Dinitrophenylhydrazine	**aEEG**	Amplitude-integrated electroencephalography
3-MCC	3-Methylcrotonyl-CoA carboxylase		
17-OHP	17-Hydroxyprogesterone	**AEP**	Auditory evoked potential
A1AT or AAT	α_1-Antitrypsin	**AFB**	Acid-fast *Bacillus*
		AFI	Amniotic fluid index
AaDO$_2$	Alveolar-to-arterial oxygen gradient	**AFP**	α-Fetoprotein
A/a gradient	Alveolar/arterial gradient	**AF PCR**	Amniotic fluid polymerase chain reaction
AAOS	American Academy of Orthopedic Surgeons	**AGA**	Appropriate for gestational age
		AGS	Adrenogenital syndrome
AAP	American Academy of Pediatrics	**AHA**	American Heart Association; α-hydroxy acids
AAP-CON	The American Academy of Pediatrics Committee on Nutrition		
		AHT	Abusive head trauma
a/A ratio	Arterial/alveolar oxygen ratio	**AI**	Aortic insufficiency
AATD	α_1-Antitrypsin deficiency	**AIDS**	Acquired immunodeficiency syndrome
A's and B's	Apnea and bradycardia		
		AIS	Amniotic infection syndrome; arterial ischemic stroke
ABC	Airway, breathing, circulation		
ABR	Auditory brainstem response	**AIT**	Alloimmune thrombocytopenia
ABS	Amniotic band syndrome	**ALARA**	As low as reasonably achievable
A/C	Assist/control	**ALGS**	Alagille syndrome
ACAAI	American College of Allergy, Asthma, and Immunology	**ALP**	Alkaline phosphatase
		ALRI	Acute lower respiratory tract infection
ACE	Angiotensin-converting enzyme		
ACF	Asymmetric crying face	**ALT**	Alanine aminotransferase
aCGH	Array comparative genomic hybridization	**ALTE**	Apparent life-threatening event
		AM	Morning
AChR	Acetylcholine receptor	**AMC**	Arthrogryposis multiplex congenita
ACIP	Advisory Committee on Immunization Practices	**ANC**	Absolute neutrophil count
		Ao	Aortic
ACLS	Advanced Cardiac Life Support	**AoI**	Aortic isthmus
ACMG	American College of Medical Genetics and Genomics	**AOI**	Apnea of infancy
		AOP	Apnea of prematurity
ACOG	American College of Obstetricians and Gynecologists	**AP**	Anteroposterior
		Apgar	Appearance, pulse, grimace, activity, respirations
ACT	Activated clotting time; activated coagulation time		
		API	Anal position index
ACTH	Adrenocorticotropic hormone	**ApoA-1**	Apolipoprotein A1
ADH	Antidiuretic hormone	**APR**	Acute-phase reactants
ADHD	Attention deficit hyperactivity disorder	**aPTT**	Activated partial thromboplastin time
		AR	Autosomal recessive
ADMA	Asymmetric dimethylarginine	**ARA/AA**	Arachidonic acid
AE	Adverse effects	**ARC**	AIDS-related complex
AED	Automatic external defibrillator; antiepileptic drug	**ARC syndrome**	Arthrogryposis–renal dysfunction–cholestasis
AEDV	Absent end-diastolic velocity		

ARD	Antibiotic removal device; antiretroviral drug	**BIND**	Bilirubin-induced neurologic dysfunction
ARDS	Acute respiratory distress syndrome	**BIO**	Binocular indirect ophthalmoscopy
AREDFV	Absent or reversed end-diastolic flow velocity	**BIOT**	Biotinidase deficiency
ARF/AKI	Acute renal failure/acute kidney injury	**BKT**	β-Ketothiolase deficiency
ARHB	Age-related/height-based	**BLP**	BabyLance preemie
ARM	Anorectal manometry	**BLS**	Basic Life Support
ART	Assisted reproductive technology; antiretroviral therapy	**BM**	Breast milk
ARV	Antiretroviral	**BMC**	Bone mineral content
AS	Aortic stenosis	**BMI**	Body mass index
ASA	Argininosuccinic aciduria; American Society of Anesthesiologists	**BNP**	B-type (or brain) natriuretic peptide
ASAP	As soon as possible	**BNSM**	Benign neonatal sleep myoclonus
ASD	Atrial septal defect	**BOHB**	β-Hydroxybutyrate
ASH	Asymmetric septal hypertrophy	**BOLD**	Blood oxygen level dependent
ASPEN	American Society for Parenteral and Enteral Nutrition	**BP**	Blood pressure
AST	Aspartate aminotransferase	**BPD**	Biparietal diameter
ATN	Acute tubular necrosis	**BPD/CLD**	Bronchopulmonary dysplasia/chronic lung disease
ATP	Adenosine triphosphate	**bpm**	Breaths per minute
ATTEND	Attunement, trust, touch, egalitarianism, nuance, and death education	**BPP**	Biophysical profile
AV	Atrioventricular; arteriovenous	**BPPT**	Benign pneumoperitoneum
A-VO₂	Arteriovenous oxygen difference	**BPSN**	Bernese Pain Scale for Neonates
B19V	Parvovirus B19	**BRUE**	Brief resolved unexplained event
B/A	Bilirubin-to-albumin ratio	**BSEP**	Bile salt export pump
BA	Biliary atresia	**BUN**	Blood urea nitrogen
BAEP	Brainstem auditory evoked potential	**BW**	Birthweight; body weight
BAER	Brainstem audiometric evoked response	**BWS**	Beckwith-Wiedemann syndrome
BAS	Balloon atrial septostomy	**c̄**	With (from the Latin word cum)
BASDs	Bile acid synthesis disorders	**C**	Cervical; centigrade
BBS	Bronze baby syndrome	**CA**	Community acquired
BCAA	Branched-chain amino acids	**CAGE**	Cerebral arterial gas embolism
BCG	Bacille Calmette-Guérin	**CAH**	Congenital adrenal hyperplasia
BD	Base deficit	**CAKUT**	Congenital anomalies of the kidney and urinary tract
BE	Base excess	**CAM**	Complementary and alternative medicine; chorioamnionitis
BEAT-ROP	Bevacizumab Eliminates the Angiogenic Threat of Retinopathy of Prematurity	**CA-MRSA**	Community-acquired methicillin-resistant *Staphylococcus aureus*
BF	Breast feeding	**CANMWG**	Chicago Area Neonatal MRSA Working Group
BG	Babygram (radiograph that includes the chest and abdomen)	**CAP**	Caffeine for Apnea of Prematurity
β-hCG	β-Human chorionic gonadotropin	**cART**	Combination antiretroviral therapy
BIA	Bacterial inhibition assay	**CAVSD**	Complete atrioventricular septal defect
bid	Twice daily	**CBC**	Complete blood count
BIIP	Behavioral Indicators of Infant Pain	**CBF**	Cerebral blood flow
		CBG	Capillary blood gases
		CBS	Capillary blood sampling
		CC	Congenital chylothorax
		CCAM	Congenital cystic adenomatoid malformation
		CCHB	Congenital complete heart block

CCHD	Critical congenital heart disease	CNS	Central nervous system; Crigler-Najjar syndrome
CCHS	Congenital central hypoventilation syndrome	CO	Cardiac output; carbon monoxide
CDC	Centers for Disease Control and Prevention	CO_2	Carbon dioxide
		COA	Coarctation of aorta
CDH	Congenital diaphragmatic hernia	CoA	Coenzyme A
CDG	Congenital disorders of glycosylation	COFN	Committee on Fetus and Newborn
		COHb	Carboxyhemoglobin
CDT	Catheter-directed thrombolysis	CONS	Coagulase-negative staphylococci
cEEG	Continuous conventional electroencephalogram	cP	Centipoises
		CPAM	Cystic pulmonary airway malformation
CF	Cystic fibrosis; clubfoot		
CFM	Cerebral function monitor	CPAP	Continuous positive airway pressure
CFRD	Cystic fibrosis–related diabetes		
CFU	Colony-forming units	CPD	Citrate phosphate dextrose
CGH	Comparative genomic hybridization	CPDA-1	Citrate phosphate dextrose-adenine
cGMP	Cyclic guanosine monophosphate		
CGMS	Continuous glucose monitoring system	CPE	Carbapenemase-producing Enterobacteriaceae
CH	Congenital hydrocephalus; congenital hypothyroidism	CPIP	Chronic pulmonary insufficiency of prematurity
CHARGE	**C**oloboma of the eye, **c**ranial nerve defects, **h**eart defects, **a**tresia of the choanae, **r**estricted growth and/or development, **g**enital abnormalities, and **e**ar anomalies and sensorineural hearing loss.	CPM	Confined placental mosaicism
		CPQCC	California Perinatal Quality Care Collaborative
		CPR	Cardiopulmonary resuscitation; cerebroplacental ratio
		CPS	Carbamoyl phosphate synthetase
		CRI	Catheter-related infection
CHD	Congenital hip dislocation; congenital heart disease	CRIES	**C**rying, **r**equires increased oxygen administration, **i**ncreased vital signs, **e**xpression, **s**leeplessness
CHF	Congestive heart failure		
CHG	Chlorhexidine gluconate	CRL	Crown-rump length
CHI	Congenital hyperinsulinism	CRMS	Cystic fibrosis transmembrane conductance regulator (CFTR)–related metabolic syndrome
CHIME	Collaborative Home Infant Monitoring Evaluation		
CHYLD	Children with Hypoglycemia and Their Later Development	CRP	C-reactive protein
		CRS	Congenital rubella syndrome
CI	Cardiac index; confidence interval	CRT	Capillary refill time; catheter-related thrombosis
CICU	Cardiac intensive care unit		
CID	Cytomegalic inclusion disease	CRYO-ROP	Cryotherapy for Retinopathy of Prematurity
CIE	Counter immunoelectrophoresis		
CIS	Cold injury syndrome	C-section	Cesarean section
CITI/ CTLN1	Citrullinemia type 1	CS	Congenital syphilis; cesarean section
CLABSI	Central line–associated blood-stream infections	CSE	Combined spinal epidural
		CSF	Cerebrospinal fluid
cm	Centimeter	CSII	Continuous subcutaneous insulin infusion
CMA	Chromosomal microarray analysis		
CMTC	Cutis marmorata telangiectatica congenita	CST	Contraction stress test
		CSTS	Car seat tolerance screening
CMV	Cytomegalovirus	CSVT	Cerebral sinovenous thrombosis
CNLDO	Congenital nasolacrimal duct obstruction	CT	Congenital toxoplasmosis; computed tomography

CTA	Computed tomography angiography	DICOM	Digital Imaging and Communications in Medicine
CTD	Carnitine transport defect		
CTG	Cardiotocography	DISIDA	Diisopropyl iminodiacetic acid
CUD	Carnitine uptake defect/carnitine transport defect	dL	Deciliter
		DLIM	Depressor labii inferioris muscle
CULLP	Congenital unilateral lower lip palsy	DLIS	Digoxin-like immunoreactive substance
cUS/CUS	Cranial ultrasound		
CVA	Coxsackievirus A, cerebrovascular accident	DM	Diabetes mellitus
		DMSA	Dimercaptosuccinic acid
CVAD	Central venous access device	DNR	Do not resuscitate
CVB	Coxsackievirus B	DOA	Dead on arrival
CVB3	Coxsackievirus B3	DOAC	Direct oral anticoagulants
CVC	Central venous catheters	DOCA	Deoxycorticosterone acetate
CVH	Combined ventricular hypertrophy	DORA	Directory of rare analyses
CVI	Cortical visual impairment	DP	Dorsalis pedis
CVL	Central venous line	DPT	Diphtheria-pertussis-tetanus
CVP	Central venous pressure	DRIFT	Drainage, irrigation, and fibrinolytic therapy
CVS	Chorionic villus sampling; congenital varicella syndrome		
		DS	Double strength
CXR	Chest x-ray	DSD	Disorder of sex development
CysC	Cystatin C	DSS	Dengue shock syndrome
CZS	Congenital Zika syndrome	DTaP	Diphtheria and tetanus toxoids with acellular pertussis
d	Day		
D25	25% dextrose solution	DTI	Diffusion tensor imaging
D5W	5% dextrose in water	DTO	Deodorized tincture of opium/diluted tincture of opium (do not use this abbreviation, write out drug name)
D10W	10% dextrose in water		
DAOM	Depressor anguli oris muscle		
DAT	Direct antibody test (Coombs test)		
DBP	Diastolic blood pressure	DTPA	Diethylenetriamine penta-acetic acid
DC	Direct current; differential cyanosis		
D/C	Discharge or discontinue	DTR	Deep tendon reflexes
DCC	Delayed cord clamping	DTwP	Diphtheria and tetanus toxoids with the whole-cell pertussis vaccine
DDAVP	Desmopressin acetate		
DDH	Developmental dysplasia of hip	DV	Ductus venosus
DDST	Denver Developmental Screening Test	DVET	Double-volume exchange transfusion
		DVSNI	Distress Scale for Ventilated Newborn Infants
DDx/DD	Differential diagnosis		
DEET	N,N-Diethyl-meta-toluamide	DVT	Deep venous thrombosis
DEND	Developmental delay, epilepsy, neonatal diabetes	DWI	Diffusion-weighted imaging
		DW-MRI	Diffusion-weighted magnetic resonance imaging
DENV	Dengue virus		
DES	Diethylstilbestrol	Dx	Diagnosis
DEX/DEXA	Dual-energy x-ray absorptiometry	DXA	Dual energy x-ray absorptiometry
DF	Dengue fever	DXM	Dexamethasone
DFA	Direct fluorescent antibody	DZ	Disease
DHA	Docosahexaenoic acid	EA	Esophageal atresia
DHF	Dengue hemorrhagic fever	EBL	Estimated blood loss
DHM	Donor human milk	EBV	Epstein-Barr virus
DHT	Dihydrotestosterone	ECF	Extracellular fluid
DI	Drug interactions; diabetes insipidus	ECG	Electrocardiogram
		ECHO	Echocardiography
DIC	Disseminated intravascular coagulation	ECLS	Extracorporeal life support
		ECM	External cardiac massage

ECMO	Extracorporeal membrane oxygenation	ETCO$_2$	End-tidal carbon dioxide (concentration)
ECP	Eosinophil cationic protein	ETROP	Early Treatment for Retinopathy of Prematurity
ECPR	Extracorporeal cardiopulmonary resuscitation	ETT	Endotracheal tube
ECS	Elective cesarean section	EUGR	Extrauterine growth restriction
ECW	Extracellular water	EV	Enterovirus
EDC	Estimated date of confinement	F	French scale (1 F = 1/3 mm)
EDTA	Ethylenediaminetetraacetic acid	FAH	Fumarylacetoacetate hydrolase
EDV	End-diastolic velocity	FANS	Faceless Acute Neonatal Pain Scale
EEG	Electroencephalogram	FAO	Fatty acid oxidation
EFA	Essential fatty acid	FAOD	Fatty acid oxidation disorders
EFM	Electronic fetal monitoring	FAS	Fetal alcohol syndrome
EFW	Estimated fetal weight	FBDS	Fetal brain disruption sequence
EHDI	Early Hearing Detection and Intervention	FBG	Fetal blood gas
		FBS	Fasting blood sugar; fetal blood sampling
EHEC	Enterohemorrhagic Escherichia coli	FD	Forceps delivery
EHMF	Enfamil human milk fortifier		
EHR	Electronic health records	FDA	Food and Drug Administration
EIA	Enzyme immunoassay	FDP	Fibrin degradation products
ELBW	Extremely low birthweight	Fe	Iron
ELISA	Enzyme-linked immunosorbent assay	FE	Fractional excretion
		FE$_{Na}$	Fractional excretion of sodium
ELSO	Extracorporeal Life Support Organization	FE$_{Urea}$	Fractional excretion of urea
		FF	Forefoot
EMA	Ethylmalonic encephalopathy; European Medicines Agency	FFA	Free fatty acid
		FFP	Fresh-frozen plasma
EME	Early myoclonic encephalopathy	FFTS	Feto-fetal (twin) transfusion syndrome
EMG	Electromyogram		
EMLA	Eutectic mixture of lidocaine and prilocaine	FGR	Fetal growth restriction
		FH	Fibular hemimelia
EMR	Electronic medical records	FHR	Fetal heart rate
EMS	Emergency medical services	FHT	Fetal heart tone
EN	Enteral nutrition	FiO$_2$	Fraction of inspired oxygen
ENNS	Early Neonatal Neurobehavioral Scale	FIRS	Fetal inflammatory response syndrome
ENT	Ear, nose, throat		
EOS	Early-onset sepsis	FISH	Fluorescence in situ hybridization
EPO	Erythropoietin	FLM	Fetal lung maturity
ERCP	Endoscopic retrograde cholangiopancreatography	FMH	Fetomaternal hemorrhage
		fMRI	Functional magnetic resonance imaging
e-ROP	Telemedicine Approaches for the Evaluation of Acute-Phase Retinopathy of Prematurity		
		FMVS	Federal Motor Vehicle Safety Standards
ESBL	Extended-spectrum β-lactamase	FOBT	Fecal occult blood testing
ESPGHAN	European Society for Paediatric Gastroenterology, Hepatology, and Nutrition	FOCUS	Focused cardiac ultrasound
		FPIES	Food protein-induced enterocolitis syndrome
ESR	Erythrocyte sedimentation rate	FRC	Functional residual capacity
ESRD	End-stage renal disease	FSH	Follicle-stimulating hormone
ET	Ejection time; exchange transfusion; endothelin	FSP	Fibrin split products
		FTA-ABS	Fluorescent treponemal antibody absorption
ETCOc	End-tidal carbon monoxide (concentration)	FTCT	Father-to-child transmission

FTT	Failure to thrive	GxPx0000	First zero, full term; second zero, premature; third zero, abortion; fourth zero, living children
F/U	Follow-up		
FUO	Fever of unknown origin		
F-V	Flow-volume	G6PD	Glucose-6-phosphate dehydrogenase
FVC	Forced vital capacity		
FVS	Fetal varicella syndrome	GROW	Gestation-related optimal growth
FVZS	Fetal varicella-zoster syndrome	GSD	Glycogen synthase deficiency
Fx	Fracture	Gt/gtt	Drop, drops (from the Latin)
Fxn	Function	GT	Gastrostomy tubes
g	Gram	GTT	Glucose tolerance test
G	Gravida	GU	Genitourinary
G6PD	Glucose-6-phosphate dehydrogenase	GVHD	Graft-versus-host disease
		HAA	Hepatitis-associated antigen
GA	Gestational age; general anesthesia	HAART	Highly active antiretroviral therapy
GA I	Glutaric acidemia type I	HADH	3-Hydroxyacyl-CoA dehydrogenase
GABA	γ-Aminobutyric acid	HAND	Helping After Neonatal Death
GALD	Gestational alloimmune liver disease	HAV	Hepatitis A virus
		HB	Hepatitis B
GALE	Galactose epimerase	HBcAg	Hepatitis B core antigen
GALK	Galactokinase	HBeAg	Hepatitis B e antigen
GALT	Galactose-1-phosphate uridylyltransferase	HBIG	Hepatitis B immune globulin
		HBOT	Hyperbaric oxygen therapy
GBCA	Gadolinium-based contrast agent	HBP	High blood pressure
GBS	Group B *Streptococcus*	HBsAg	Hepatitis B surface antigen
GBV-C	Hepatitis G virus (GB virus type C)	Hb SS	Sickle cell disease/sickle cell anemia
GC	Gas chromatography		
GCK	Glucokinase	HBV	Hepatitis B virus
GCN	Giant congenital nevi	HBW	High birthweight
G-CSF	Granulocyte colony-stimulating factor	HC	Head circumference
		hCG	Human chorionic gonadotropin
GDM	Gestational diabetes mellitus	HCl	Hydrochloride
GE	Gastroesophageal	HCM	Hypertrophic cardiomyopathy
GER	Gastroesophageal reflux	HCO_3	Bicarbonate
GERD	Gastroesophageal reflux disease	Hct	Hematocrit
GFR	Glomerular filtration rate	HCTZ	Hydrochlorothiazide
GGT	γ-Glutamyl transferase	HCV	Hepatitis C virus
GGTP	γ-Glutamyl transpeptidase	HCW	Health care worker
GH	Growth hormone	HCY	Homocystinuria
GI	Gastrointestinal	HD	Hirschsprung disease
GINA	Genetic Information Nondiscrimination Act	HDFN/HDN	Hemolytic disease of the fetus and newborn
GIR	Glucose infusion rate	HDV	Hepatitis D virus
GLUT	Glucose transporter	HE	Hereditary elliptocytosis
GM-CSF	Granulocyte-macrophage colony-stimulating factor	HEENT	Head, eyes, ears, nose, and throat
		HELLP	Hemolysis, elevated liver enzymes, and low platelet count
GM/IVH	Germinal matrix/intraventricular hemorrhage	HETP	Head elevated tilt position
GxPxAbxLCx	Shorthand for gravida (number of pregnancies)/para (number of deliveries)/number of abortions/ number of living children (subscript variables represent numbers of each)	HEV	Hepatitis E virus, human enterovirus
		HF	Hind foot
		HFJV	High-frequency jet ventilation
		HFNC	High-flow nasal cannula
		HFO	High-frequency oscillation

HFOV	High-frequency oscillatory ventilation	**IAT**	Indirect antiglobulin technique
HFPPV	High-frequency positive-pressure ventilation	**iCa**	Ionized calcium
		ICH	Intracranial hemorrhage
		ICN	Intensive care nursery
HFV	High-frequency ventilation	**ICP**	Intracranial pressure
Hgb	Hemoglobin	**ICPH**	Intracerebellar parenchymal hemorrhage
HGV	Hepatitis G virus		
HHH	Hyperornithinemia/ hyperammonemia/ homocitrullinemia	**ICS**	Intercostal space
		ICU	Intensive care unit
		ICW	Intracellular water
HHS	Department of Health and Human Services	**I&D**	Incision and drainage
		ID	Internal diameter
HHV	Human herpes virus	**IDAM**	Infant of drug-abusing mother
HI	Hypoxia-ischemia	**IDDM**	Insulin-dependent diabetes mellitus
HI/HA	Hyperinsulinism/hyperammonemia syndrome	**IDM**	Infant of diabetic mother
		I:E	Inspiratory-to-expiratory ratio
Hib vaccine	*Haemophilus influenzae* type b vaccine	**IEM**	Inborn error of metabolism
		IFA	Immunofluorescent antibody assay
HIDA	Hepatobiliary iminodiacetic acid	**Ig**	Immunoglobulin
HIE	Hypoxic ischemic encephalopathy	**IG**	Immune globulin
HIG	Hyperimmune globulin	**I/G**	Insulin-to-glucose ratio
HIV	Human immunodeficiency virus	**IgA**	Immunoglobulin A
HLA	Human leukocyte antigen	**IgE**	Immunoglobulin E
HLHS	Hypoplastic left heart syndrome	**IGF**	Insulin-like growth factor
HM	Human milk	**IGRA**	Interferon-γ release assays
HMBANA	Human Milk Banking Association of North America	**IHPS**	Idiopathic/infantile hypertrophic pyloric stenosis
HMD	Hyaline membrane disease	**IL**	Interleukin
HMG	3-Hydroxy-3-methylglutaryl CoA lyase	**ILAE**	International League Against Epilepsy
HMO	Human milk oligosaccharides	**ILCOR**	International Consensus on Cardio-pulmonary Resuscitation
H/O	History of		
H&P	History and physical examination	**IM**	Intramuscular
HPA	Human platelet antigen	**IMV**	Intermittent mandatory ventilation
HPeV	Human *Parechovirus*	**IND**	Investigational new drug
HPF	High-power field	**INF**	Intravenous nutritional feedings
HPI	History of present illness	**iNO**	Inhaled nitric oxide
HPLC	High-performance liquid chromatography	**INR**	International normalized ratio
		INRGSS	International Neuroblastoma Risk Group Staging System
HPS	Hypertrophic pyloric stenosis	**INSS**	International Neuroblastoma Staging System
HR	Heart rate		
HRC	Heart rate characteristics	**INSURE**	Intubation-surfactant-extubation
HS	Hereditary spherocytosis	**I&O**	Intake and output
HSM	Hepatosplenomegaly	**IO**	Intraosseous
HSV	Herpes simplex virus	**IOI**	Intraosseous infusion
H/t	Head-to-trunk ratio	**IOR**	Intraosseous route
HT	Healing touch	**IPPB**	Intermittent positive-pressure breathing
HTLV	Human T-cell lymphotropic virus		
HTN	Hypertension	**IPPV**	Intermediate positive-pressure ventilation
Hx	History		
Hz	Hertz	**IPV**	Inactivated poliovirus vaccine
IAA	Interrupted aortic arch	**IQ**	Intelligence quotient
IAP	Intrapartum antibiotic prophylaxis		

IRT	Immunoreactive trypsinogen	**LC**	Living children
ISAGA	Immunosorbent agglutination assay	**LCAD**	Long-chain acyl-CoA
ISAM	Infant of substance-abusing mother		dehydrogenase
ISG	Immune serum globulin	**LCHAD**	Long-chain 3-hydroxyacyl-CoA
ISSD	Infantile free sialic acid storage		dehydrogenase deficiency
	disorder	**LCMN**	Large congenital melanocytic nevus
IT	Intrathecal; inspiratory time	**LCPUFAs**	Long-chain polyunsaturated fatty
I:T	Ratio of immature to total neutrophils		acids
ITP	Idiopathic thrombocytopenic purpura	**LDH**	Lactate dehydrogenase
IU	International unit (on do not use list;	**LEDs**	Light-emitting diodes
	use "units")	**LFT**	Liver function tests
IUGR	Intrauterine growth restriction	**LGA**	Large for gestational age
IUT	Intrauterine transfusion	**LH**	Luteinizing hormone
IV	Intravenous	**LISA**	Less invasive surfactant
IVA	Isovaleric acidemia		administration
IVC	Inferior vena cava; intravenous	**LLD**	Limb length discrepancy
	cholangiogram	**LLL**	Left lower lobe
IVH	Intraventricular hemorrhage	**LLQ**	Left lower quadrant
IVIG	Intravenous immunoglobulin	**LMA**	Laryngeal mask airway
IVP	Intravenous pyelogram; intravenous	**LMP**	Last menstrual period
	push	**LMPT**	Late and moderately preterm
IWL	Insensible water loss	**LMWH**	Low molecular weight heparin
JEB	Junctional epidermolysis bullosa	**L.M.X.4**	Lidocaine 4%
JODM	Juvenile-onset diabetes mellitus	**LOH**	Loss of heterozygosity
K/K⁺	Potassium	**LOS**	Late-onset sepsis
KC	Kangaroo care	**LOWS**	Low-osmolality water soluble
kcal	Kilocalorie	**LP**	Lumbar puncture
KDIGO	Kidney Disease: Improving Global	**LPS**	Lipopolysaccharide
	Outcomes	**LR**	Lactated Ringer's solution
kg	Kilogram	**L-S ratio**	Lecithin-to-sphingomyelin ratio
KHPE	Kasai hepatic portoenterostomy	**L-T₄**	Levothyroxine
KIM-1	Kidney injury molecule-1	**LV**	Left ventricle
KMC	Kangaroo mother care	**LVH**	Left ventricular hypertrophy
KOH	Potassium hydroxide	**LVO**	Left ventricular output
KSD	Kernicterus spectrum disorder	**LVOTO**	Left ventricular outflow tract
KSHV	Kaposi sarcoma–associated herpes		obstruction
	virus	**M/m**	Molar; meter
KU	Klobusitzky unit	**MA**	Metatarsus adductus
KUB	Kidneys, ureter, bladder	**MAC**	Minimum alveolar concentration;
L	Liter		*Mycobacterium avium* complex
L3–L4	Third lumbar to fourth lumbar	**MAP**	Mean arterial pressure; mean
	vertebra space		airway pressure
LA	Left atrium; lactic acidosis	**MAS**	Meconium aspiration syndrome
LAD	Left axis deviation; left atrial diam-	**Max**	Maximum
	eter; left anterior descending	**MBC**	Minimum bactericidal
LAE	Left atrial enlargement		concentration
LAH	Left atrial hypertrophy	**MBD**	Metabolic bone disease
LANE	Mnemonic for medications accept-	**MC**	Most common
	able through an endotracheal	**MCA**	Multiple congenital anomaly;
	tube (**l**idocaine, **a**tropine,		middle cerebral artery
	naloxone, **e**pinephrine)	**MCAD**	Medium-chain acyl-CoA
LBBB	Left bundle branch block		dehydrogenase
LBC	Lamellar body count	**MCA-PSV**	Middle cerebral artery peak systolic
LBW	Low birthweight		velocity

MCD	Multiple carboxylase deficiency
MCH	Mean cell hemoglobin
MCHC	Mean cell hemoglobin concentration
MCPs	Medical Command Physicians
MCT	Medium-chain triglyceride
MCV	Mean cell volume; mean corpuscular volume
MDCT	Multidetector computed tomography
MDI	Metered dose inhaler
MDR3	Multidrug resistance protein 3
M.E.N.D.	Mommies Enduring Neonatal Death
mEq	Milliequivalent
Mg/Mg²⁺	Magnesium
MG	Myasthenia gravis
MgSO₄	Magnesium sulfate
MH-TPA	Micro hemagglutination assay for *Treponema pallidum*
MI	Myocardial infarction; mitral insufficiency; meconium ileus
MIC	Minimum inhibitory concentration
min	Minute
MIST	Minimally invasive surfactant treatment
mL	Milliliter
mm	Millimeter
MMA	Methylmalonic acidemia
MMI	Methimazole
MMR	Measles-mumps-rubella (vaccine)
MN	Micronucleus
MOMS	Management of Myelomeningocele Study
mOsm	Milliosmole
MPH	Massive pulmonary hemorrhage
MPS-I	Mucopolysaccharidosis type I
MPS-II	Mucopolysaccharidosis type II
MR	Mitral regurgitation (insufficiency)
MRA	Magnetic resonance arteriography
MRCP	Magnetic resonance cholangiopancreatography
mrem	Millirem
MRI	Magnetic resonance imaging
MRS	Magnetic resonance spectroscopy
MRSA	Methicillin-resistant *Staphylococcus aureus*
MRV	Magnetic resonance venography
MS	Mitral stenosis; mass spectrometry **(MS for morphine sulfate, magnesium sulfate: on do not use list**; better to write these out as they can be confused for one another)**

MS/MS	Tandem mass spectrometry
MSAF	Meconium-stained amniotic fluid
MSAFP	Maternal serum α-fetoprotein
MSSA	Methicillin-susceptible *Staphylococcus aureus*
MSUD	Maple syrup urine disease
MTCT	Mother-to-child transmission
MV	Minute volume; multiple vitamin; mechanical ventilation
MVI	Multiple vitamin infusion
MVP	Maximum vertical pocket; mitral valve prolapse
MZ	Monozygotic
N/A	Not applicable
Na/Na²⁺	Sodium
NAA	Nucleic acid amplification; *N*-acetyl aspartate
NAAT	Nucleic acid amplification testing
NACS	Neurologic and adaptive capacity score
NAIT	Neonatal alloimmune thrombocytopenia
NANN	National Association of Neonatal Nurses
NAPA	*N*-Acetylprocainamide
NAS	Neonatal abstinence syndrome
NASPGHAN	North American Society for Pediatric Gastroenterology, Hepatology, and Nutrition
NAVEL	Mnemonic for groin anatomy (nerve, artery, vein, empty space, lymphatic)
NBAS	Neonatal behavior assessment scale
NBS	New Ballard score; newborn screening
NBW	Normal birthweight
NCBI	National Center for Biotechnology and Information
nCPAP	Nasal continuous positive airway pressure
NCV	Nerve conduction velocity
NDM	Neonatal diabetes mellitus
NE	Norepinephrine; neonatal encephalopathy
NEAL	Mnemonic for endotracheal tube–administered medications (**n**aloxone, **e**pinephrine, **a**tropine, and **l**idocaine)
NEC	Necrotizing enterocolitis
NEMU	Nose/ear/mid-umbilicus
NEOCLOT	NEOnatal Central Venous Line Observational Study on Thrombosis

NESS	National Enterovirus Surveillance System	**NPV**	Negative predictive value
NETS	Neonatal emergency transport services	**NRL**	Nonreference laboratories
		NRN	Neonatal Research Network
		NRP	Neonatal Resuscitation Program
NEX	Nose to the ear to the xiphoid	**NS**	Normal saline
NFCS	Neonatal Facial Coding System	**NS1**	Nonstructural protein 1
NFKB	Nuclear factor-kappa B	**NSAID**	Nonsteroidal anti-inflammatory drug
NG	Nasogastric		
NGAL	Neutrophil gelatinase–associated lipocalin	**NSR**	Normal sinus rhythm
		NST	Nonstress test
NGO	Nitroglycerine ointment	**NSVD**	Normal spontaneous vaginal delivery
NGS	Next-generation sequencing		
NHLBI	National Heart, Lung, and Blood Institute	**NT**	Nasotracheal; (fetal) nuchal translucency
NICHD	National Institute of Child Health and Human Development	**NTA**	Nontreponemal antibody (test)
		NTB	Necrotizing tracheobronchitis
NICHD-NRN	National Institute of Child Health and Human Development Neonatal Research Network	**NTBC**	2-(2-Nitro-4-trifluorome-thylbenzoyl)-1, 3-cyclohexanedione
NICU	Neonatal intensive care unit	**NTDs**	Neural tube defects
NIDCAP	Newborn Individualized Developmental Care and Assessment Program	**NTE**	Neutral thermal environment
		NTEC	Neonatal transient eosinophilic colitis
NIPPV	Nasal intermittent positive-pressure ventilation	**NTG**	Nitroglycerin
		NTL	Nasal tragus length
NIPS	Neonatal Infant Pain Scale	**NTT**	Nontreponemal test
NIPT	Noninvasive prenatal testing	**NVP**	Nevirapine
NIRS	Near-infrared spectroscopy	O_2	Oxygen
NISCH	Neonatal ichthyosis and sclerosing cholangitis	**OA**	Organic aciduria/acidemia
		OAE	Otoacoustic emission
NIV	Noninvasive ventilation	**OB**	Obstetrics
NKA	No known allergies	**OCP**	Oral contraceptive pill
NKDA	No known drug allergy	**OCT**	Oxytocin challenge test
NKH	Nonketotic hyperglycinemia	**OD**	Outer diameter
NI	Normal	**OFC**	Occipital frontal circumference
NLDO	Nasolacrimal duct obstruction	**OG**	Orogastric
NMR	Nuclear magnetic resonance	**OI**	Oxygenation index
NNP	Neonatal nurse practitioner	**OM**	Otitis media
NNS	Nonnutritive sucking	**OMIM**	Online Mendelian Inheritance in Man
NNTs	Neonatal teams		
NO	Nitric oxide	**ON**	Ophthalmia neonatorum
NO_2	Nitric dioxide	**OPHTH**	Ophthalmic
NOHK	Nonoliguric hyperkalemia	**OPV**	Oral poliovirus vaccine
NORD	National Organization for Rare Disorders	**OR**	Operating room
		OSA	Obstructive sleep apnea
NP	Nasopharyngeal; neonatal pneumothorax; nurse practitioner	**Osm**	Osmolality
		OTC	Over the counter (nonpre-scription drug); ornithine transcarbamylase
N-PASS	Neonatal Pain, Agitation, and Sedation Scale		
NPCPAP	Nasopharyngeal continuous positive airway pressure	**OU**	Both eyes (from the Latin *oculus unitas*)
		OWB	Oscillating waterbed
NPO	Nothing by mouth	**oz**	Ounce

P	Para (the number of viable [>20 weeks] births); phosphorus	**PEEP**	Positive end-expiratory pressure
PA	Pulmonary artery; posteroanterior; pulmonary atresia; propionic acidemia	**PEP**	Postexposure prophylaxis
		PES	Pediatric Endocrine Society
		PET	Partial exchange transfusion
PAC	Premature atrial contraction	**PetCO$_2$**	Partial pressure of end-tidal carbon dioxide
PaCO$_2$	Partial pressure of carbon dioxide, arterial	**PETS**	Pediatric emergency transport service
PAF	Platelet-activating factor	**PF**	Purpura fulminans
PAHO	Pan American Health Organization	**PF24**	Plasma frozen 24
PAIN	Pain Assessment in Neonates	**PFC**	Persistent fetal circulation
PAL	Pacifier-Activated Lullaby	**PFFD**	Proximal focal femoral deficiency
PALS	Pediatric Advanced Life Support	**pfHb**	Plasma free hemoglobin
PAMF-TSL	Palo Alto Medical Foundation Toxoplasma Serology Laboratory	**PFIC**	Progressive familial intrahepatic cholestasis
PaO$_2$	Partial pressure of oxygen	**PFO**	Patent foramen ovale
PAP	Pulmonary artery pressure	**PFT**	Pulmonary function test
PAPP-A	Pregnancy-associated plasma protein A	**PG**	Phosphatidylglycerol
		PGDM	Pregestational diabetes mellitus
PAPVR	Partial anomalies pulmonary venous return	**PGE**	Prostaglandin E
		PGE$_1$	Prostaglandin E$_1$
PAT	Paroxysmal atrial tachycardia; Pain Assessment Tool	**PGE$_2$**	Prostaglandin E$_2$
		PGI$_2$	Prostaglandin I$_2$ or prostacyclin
PB	Periodic breathing; preterm baby	**PH**	Pulmonary hemorrhage; pulmonary hypertension
PBF	Pulmonary blood flow		
PBLC	Premature birth living child	**Phe**	Phenylalanine
PBP	Perinatal bereavement program	**PHH**	Posthemorrhagic hydrocephalus
PCA	Postconceptional age; primary cutaneous aspergillosis	**PHN**	Pulmonary hypertension
		PHS	Polycythemia hyperviscosity syndrome
PCC	Prothrombin complex concentrate		
PCE	Pericardial effusion	**PI**	Pulsatility index
PCEP	Perinatal Continuing Education Program	**PICC**	Peripherally inserted central catheter
PCG	Pneumocardiogram	**PICU**	Pediatric intensive care unit
PCN	Penicillin	**PID**	Pelvic inflammatory disease
PCP	*Pneumocystis jiroveci* pneumonia; phencyclidine	**PIE**	Pulmonary interstitial emphysema
		PIH	Postinfectious hydrocephalus
PCR	Polymerase chain reaction	**PIP**	Peak inspiratory pressure
PCT	Procalcitonin	**PIPP-R**	Premature Infant Pain Profile–Revised
PCVC	Percutaneous central venous catheter		
		PIV	Peripheral intravenous
PCWP	Pulmonary capillary wedge pressure	**PIVKA-II**	Protein induced by vitamin K absence-II
PD	Peritoneal drainage; peritoneal drain	**PKU**	Phenylketonuria
		PLAST	Percussion, lavage, suction, turn
PDA	Patent ductus arteriosus	**PLV**	Partial liquid ventilation; pressure-limited ventilation
PDE	Phosphodiesterase; pyridoxine-dependent epilepsy		
		PM	At night; pneumomediastinum
PDH	Pyruvate dehydrogenase	**PMA**	Postmenstrual age
PDHM	Pasteurized donor human milk	**PMH**	Past medical history
PE	Pleural effusion; physical examination; pulmonary embolus	**PMN**	Polymorphonuclear neutrophil
		PN	Parenteral nutrition
PEA	Pulseless electrical activity	**PNA**	Postnatal age

PNAC	Parenteral nutrition–associated conjugated hyperbilirubinemia	**PUFA**	Polyunsaturated fatty acids
PNALD	Parenteral nutrition–associated liver disease	**PUV**	Posterior urethral valves
		P-V	Pressure volume
PNCV	Peripheral nerve conduction velocity	**PV**	Processus vaginalis
		PVC	Premature ventricular contraction; polyvinyl chloride
PNDM	Permanent neonatal diabetes mellitus	**PVD**	Posthemorrhagic ventricular dilation
PO	By mouth	**PVET**	Peripheral vessel exchange transfusion
POCUS	Point-of-care ultrasound		
POSNA	Pediatric Orthopedic Society of North America	**PVG**	Portal venous gas
		PVH	Periventricular hemorrhage
P&PD	Percussion and postural drainage	**PVHI**	Periventricular hemorrhagic infarction
PP	Pneumoperitoneum		
PPC	Pediatric palliative care	**PV-IVH/**	Periventricular (hemorrhage)–
PPD	Purified protein derivative; primary peritoneal drainage	**PIVH/**	intraventricular hemorrhage
		PVH-IVH	
PPE	Personal protective equipment	**PVL**	Periventricular leukomalacia; Panton-Valentine leukocidin
PPH/PPHN	Persistent pulmonary hypertension/ persistent pulmonary hyperten-sion of the newborn	**PVR**	Pulmonary vascular resistance
		PVS	Percussion, vibration, and suction-ing; pulmonary vein stenosis; pulmonary valve stenosis
PPI	Proton pump inhibitor		
ppm	Parts per million	**PVT**	Portal vein thrombosis
PPN	Peripheral parenteral nutrition	**q**	Every (from the Latin *quaque*)
pProm, PPROM	Preterm premature rupture of membranes	**qd**	Everyday (on do not use list; better to write daily)
PPS	Peripheral pulmonic stenosis	**qXh**	Every X hours
PPV	Positive-pressure ventilation	**qid**	Four times daily
PR	Per rectum	**qod**	Every other day (from Latin *quaque otram diem*; on do not use list; better to write out every other day)
PRAE	Perioperative respiratory adverse events		
PRBC	Packed red blood cells		
PRN	As needed (from the Latin *pro re nata*)	**Quad screen**	Quadruple screen test (maternal serum α-fetoprotein, human chorionic gonadotropin, estriol, inhibin A)
PRNT	Plaque reduction neutralization test		
PRO	Prolinemia	**RA**	Right atrium
PROM	Premature rupture of membranes	**RAD**	Right axis deviation
PROP	Propionic acidemia	**RAE**	Right atrial enlargement
PS	Pulmonary stenosis; pressure support	**RAH**	Right atrial hypertrophy
		RAST	Radioallergosorbent test
PSV	Peak systolic velocity	**RAT**	Renal artery thrombosis; right atrial thrombosis
PT	Prothrombin time		
PTB	Preterm birth	**RBBB**	Right bundle branch block
PTH	Parathyroid hormone	**RBC**	Red blood cell
PTL	Preterm labor	**RBL**	Rhythm, Breath, and Lullaby Inter-national training
PTNB	Preterm newborn		
PTT	Partial thromboplastin time	**RCT**	Randomized controlled trial
PTTN	Prolonged transient tachypnea of the newborn	**RDA**	Recommended dietary allowance
		RDC	Reversed differential cyanosis
PTU	Propylthiouracil	**RDS**	Respiratory distress syndrome
PTX	Pneumothorax	**REDV**	Reversed end-diastolic velocity
PUBS	Percutaneous umbilical blood sampling	**RFI**	Renal failure index

RFM	Respiratory function monitor
rFVIIa	Recombinant factor VIIa
Rh	Rhesus factor
rhAPC	Recombinant human activated protein C
rhEPO	Recombinant human erythropoietin
RI	Resistance index; reflux index
RIA	Radioimmunoassay
RIVUR	Randomized intervention for children with vesicoureteral reflux
RL	Ringer's lactate
RLF	Retrolental fibroplasia; retained lung fluid
RLL	Right lower lobe
RLQ	Right lower quadrant
RML	Right middle lobe
RN	Registered nurse
R/O	Rule out
ROM	Range of motion; rupture of membranes
ROP	Retinopathy of prematurity
ROS	Review of systems
RP%	Reticulated platelet percentages
RPR	Rapid plasma reagin
RR	Relative risk
rRT-PCR	Real-time reverse transcriptase polymerase chain reaction
RSI	Rapid sequence intubation; rectosigmoid index
rSo$_2$	Regional hemoglobin oxygen saturation
RSS	Respiratory severity score
RSV	Respiratory syncytial virus
RT	Rubella titer; respiratory therapy; radiation therapy
RTA	Renal tubular acidosis
rTPA	Recombinant tissue plasminogen activator
RT-PCR	Reverse transcriptase–polymerase chain reaction
RTU	Ready to use
RUL	Right upper lobe
RUQ	Right upper quadrant
RUSP	Recommended Uniform Screening Panel
RV	Right ventricle; residual volume
RVH	Right ventricular hypertrophy
RVT	Renal vein thrombosis
Rx	Treatment
Rxn	Reaction
SA	Sinoatrial
SAAG	Serum-to-ascites albumin gradient

SAE	Serious adverse event
SAH	Subarachnoid hemorrhage
SaO$_2$	Measurement of arterial oxygen saturation
SBA	Suprapubic bladder aspiration
sBPD	Severe bronchopulmonary dysplasia
SBL	Soy bean lipid
SBP	Systolic blood pressure
SC	Subcutaneous
SCAD	Short-chain acyl-CoA dehydrogenase deficiency
SCC	Staphylococcal cassette chromosome
SCFN	Subcutaneous fat necrosis
SCID	Severe combined immune deficiency
SCM	Sternocleidomastoid muscle
SCr	Serum creatinine
SD	Standard deviation
SDA	Strand displacement amplification
SDH	Subdural hemorrhage
SEH	Subependymal hemorrhage
SEM	Systolic ejection murmur; skin, eyes, and mouth
SEP	Somatosensory evoked potential
SFH	Symphysis–fundal height
SGA	Small for gestational age
SGOT	Serum glutamic oxaloacetic transaminase
SGPT	Serum glutamic pyruvic transaminase
SHC	Selective head cooling
SHMF	Similac human milk fortifier
SIADH	Syndrome of inappropriate antidiuretic hormone
SIDS	Sudden infant death syndrome
SIMV	Synchronized intermittent mandatory ventilation
SIP	Spontaneous intestinal perforation
SIPI	Idiopathic spontaneous intestinal perforation
SIRS	Systemic inflammatory response syndrome
SK	Streptokinase
SLE	Systemic lupus erythematosus
SMX	Sulfamethoxazole
Sn	Tin
SNAP II	Score for Neonatal Acute Physiology II
SNC	Selective neonatal chemoprophylaxis
SNHL	Sensorineural hearing loss

SNIPPV	Synchronized nasal intermittent positive-pressure ventilation	**TAPVC**	Total anomalous pulmonary venous connection
SnMP	Tin mesoporphyrin	**TAR**	Thrombocytopenia and absent radius (syndrome)
SNP	Single nucleotide polymorphism		
SOAP	Mnemonic for subjective (S), objective (O), assessment (A), plan (P)	**TB**	Tuberculosis
		TBG	Thyroid-binding globulin
SOB	Shortness of breath	**TBL**	Total body-loading dose
SOS	Speed of sound	**TBLC**	Term birth, living child
S/P	Status post	**TBW**	Total body water
SpO$_2$	Oxygen saturation measured by pulse oximetry	**tCa**	Total serum calcium
		TcB	Transcutaneous bilirubinometry
SQ	Subcutaneous	**TcPCO$_2$**	Transcutaneous carbon dioxide tension
SS	Sensorial stimulation		
SSC	Skin-to-skin contact	**TcPO$_2$**	Transcutaneous oxygen tension
SSEP	Somatosensory evoked potential	**TD**	Transdermal
SSKI	Saturated solution of potassium iodide	**Tdap**	Tetanus, diphtheria, and pertussis
		TDxFLM II	TDx fetal lung maturity assay
SSRI	Selective serotonin reuptake inhibitors	**TE**	Tracheoesophageal; thromboembolism
SSSS	Staphylococcal scalded skin syndrome	**TEF**	Tracheoesophageal fistula
		TEG	Thromboelastography
STA	Specific treponemal antibody	**TENS**	Transcutaneous electric nerve stimulation
S.T.A.B.L.E.	Sugar, temperature, airway, blood pressure, lab work, and emotional support		
		TEWL	Transepidermal water loss
		TFP	Trifunctional protein deficiency
STAT	Immediately	**TFT**	Thyroid function test
STD/STI	Sexually transmitted disease/sexually transmitted infection	**TGA**	Transposition of the great arteries
		TGV	Transposition of the great vessels
STL/SL	Sternal length	**T&H**	Type and hold
STOP-ROP	Supplemental Therapeutic Oxygen for Prethreshold Retinopathy of Prematurity	**TH**	Therapeutic hypothermia
		THAM	Tris-hydroxymethyl aminomethane (trometamol)
S-U	Shoulder to umbilicus	**THAN**	Transient hyperammonemia of the newborn
SUN	Scale for Use in Newborns		
Supp	Supplement; suppository	**Ti**	Inspiratory time
Susp	Suspension	**TI**	Tricuspid incompetence (regurgitation)
SVC	Superior vena cava		
SVD	Spontaneous vaginal delivery	**tid**	Three times daily (from the Latin *ter in die*)
SvO$_2$	Venous oxygen saturation		
SVR	Systemic vascular resistance	**TIPP**	Trial of indomethacin prophylaxis in preterm infants
SVT	Supraventricular tachycardia		
SWC	Sleep-wake cycle	**TIV**	Trivalent inactivated influenza vaccine
SWI	Sterile water for injection		
Sx	Symptom	**TJP**	Tight-junction protein
Sz	Seizure	**TLC**	Total lung capacity
T	Testosterone	**TLV**	Total liquid ventilation
T$_4$	Thyroxine	**TLR-4**	Toll-like receptor-4
T1DM	Type 1 diabetes mellitus	**TM**	Tympanic membrane
T2DM	Type 2 diabetes mellitus	**TMA**	Transcription-mediated amplification
TA	Tricuspid atresia; truncus arteriosus		
TAC	Truncus arteriosus communis	**TNDM**	Transient neonatal diabetes mellitus
TA-GVHD	Transfusion-associated graft-versus-host disease		
		TNF	Tumor necrosis factor

TNMG	Transient neonatal myasthenia gravis		**UCM**	Umbilical cord milking
TNPM	Transient neonatal pustular melanosis		**UDCA**	Ursodeoxycholic acid
			UDPGT	Uridine diphosphate glucuronyl transferase
TOF	Tetralogy of Fallot		**UDT**	Undescended testis
TORCH	Toxoplasmosis, other, rubella, cytomegalovirus, and herpes simplex virus		**UFH**	Unfractionated heparin
			UGI	Upper gastrointestinal
			UK	Urokinase
TORCHZ	Toxoplasmosis, other, rubella, cytomegalovirus, herpes simplex virus, and Zika virus		**ULN**	Upper limits of normal
			UNFH	Unfractionated heparin
			UPD	Uniparental disomy
TOW	Term optimal weight		**UPEP**	Urine protein electrophoresis
TOXO	Toxoplasmosis		**UPI**	Uteroplacental insufficiency
tPA	Tissue plasminogen activator		**UPJ**	Ureteropelvic junction
TP-CIA	*Treponema pallidum* chemiluminescent assay		**URI**	Upper respiratory infection
			US	Ultrasound
TP-EIA	*Treponema pallidum* enzyme immunoassay		**USP**	U.S. Pharmacopeia
			USPSTF	US Preventive Services Task Force
TP-PA	*Treponema pallidum* particle agglutination		**UtA**	Uterine artery
			UTD	Urinary tract dilation
TPN	Total parenteral nutrition		**UTI**	Urinary tract infection
TPR	Total peripheral resistance		**UV**	Umbilical vein
TPO	Thrombopoietin		**UVC**	Umbilical vein catheter
TR	Tricuspid regurgitation		**VA**	Venoarterial
TRAGI	Transfusion-related acute gut injury		**VA-ECLS**	Venoarterial extracorporeal life support
TRALI	Transfusion-related acute lung injury			
			VariZIG	Varicella-zoster immune globulin
TREC	T-cell receptor excision circles		**VATER/**	Vertebral anomalies, anal atresia,
TRH	Thyrotropin-releasing hormone		**VACTERL**	tracheoesophageal fistula, and radial or renal dysplasia/vertebral defects, anal atresia, cardiac defects, tracheoesophageal fistula, renal and radial abnormalities, and limb abnormalities
TS	Tricuspid stenosis			
TSB	Total serum bilirubin			
TSH	Thyroid-stimulating hormone			
TSHR	Thyroid-stimulating hormone receptor			
			VBG	Venous blood gas
TSOACs	Target-specific oral anticoagulants		**VC**	Vital capacity
TSP	*Toxoplasma* serologic profile; 3-stair position		**VCUG**	Voiding cystourethrogram
			VDRL	Venereal Disease Research Laboratory
TST	Tuberculin skin testing			
TT	Thrombin time; therapeutic touch		**VE**	Vacuum extraction
TTN/TTNB	Transient tachypnea of the newborn		**VEEG**	Video electroencephalogram
TTTS	Twin-twin (feto-fetal) transfusion syndrome		**VEGF**	Vascular endothelial growth factor
			VEP	Visual evoked potential
TTV	Transfusion-transmitted virus		**VER**	Visual evoked response
TV	Tidal volume		**VF**	Ventricular fibrillation
TYR1	Tyrosinemia type 1		**VHBW**	Very high birthweight
U	Unit(s) (**on do not use list;** dangerous abbreviation; write out "unit")		**VISA**	Vancomycin-intermediate *Staphylococcus aureus*
			VKDB	Vitamin K deficiency bleeding
UA	Umbilical artery		**VLBW**	Very low birthweight
U/A	Urinalysis		**VLCAD**	Very long-chain acyl-CoA dehydrogenase deficiency
UBTS	Unit-based teams			
UAC	Umbilical artery catheter		**VLCFA**	Very-long-chain fatty acids
UC	Umbilical cord			

VM	Ventriculomegaly	**vWD**	von Willebrand disease
VMA	Vanillylmandelic acid	**vWF**	von Willebrand factor
V/P	Ventilation perfusion	**VZV**	Varicella-zoster virus
VP	Ventriculoperitoneal	**VZIG**	Varicella-zoster immune globulin
V/Q	Ventilation-perfusion	**WAGR**	Wilms tumor, aniridia, genitourinary
VRE	Vancomycin-resistant *Enterococcus*		anomalies, and intellectual
VREF	Vancomycin-resistant *Enterococcus*		disability
	faecium	**WBC**	White blood cell; whole-body
VRSA	Vancomycin-resistant		cooling
	Staphylococcus aureus	**WES**	Whole-exosome sequencing
VSD	Ventricular septal defect	**W/O**	Without
VSS	Vital signs stable	**WF**	White female
VST	Venous sinus thrombosis	**WGS**	Whole-genome sequencing
VT	Ventricular tachycardia; vertical	**WHO**	World Health Organization
	talus	**WM**	White male
V$_T$	Tidal volume (size of breath)	**WNL, wnl**	Within normal limits
VTV	Volume-targeted ventilation	**WNV**	West Nile virus
VUE	Villitis of unknown etiology	**WPW**	Wolff-Parkinson-White syndrome
VUR	Vesicoureteral reflux	**X-ALD**	X-Linked adrenoleukodystrophy
VUS	Variant of uncertain significance	**XR**	Extended release
VV	Venovenous	**ZDV**	Zidovudine
VV-ECLS	Venovenous extracorporeal life	**ZIKV**	Zika virus
	support	**ZnMP**	Zinc mesoporphyrin

Appendix B. Apgar Score/Expanded Apgar Score

APGAR SCORE

The original Apgar score was devised by Virginia Apgar, MD, an anesthesiologist, in 1952 who invented a scoring system to assess the clinical status of the newborn infant and the need for medical intervention to establish breathing at 1 minute of age. It was presented at a national anesthesiology meeting in 1952. She published the results in 1953 in a paper titled, "A Proposal for a New Method of Evaluation of the Newborn Infant," the purpose of which was to establish a grading system of newborns to be used as a basis to discuss and compare results of obstetric practices, different types of maternal pain relief, and the effects of resuscitation techniques. It was "a simple clear classification or grading of newborns consisting of five signs" that did not require special equipment, were determined easily, did not interfere with the care of the newborn, and could be taught without difficulty. She chose heart rate, respiratory effort, reflex irritability, muscle tone, and color. The most important sign was the heart rate, followed by respiratory rate, and the least important sign was the color of the newborn. A rating of 0, 1, or 2 was given for each sign at 60 seconds after delivery (after the complete birth of the baby and the time of maximal clinical depression after birth). Two subsequent studies were done (1952–1956 and 1959–1966), and the 5-minute Apgar score was added because neonatal mortality strongly correlated with it. In 1962, a "back acronym" (APGAR) was created from Dr. Apgar's last name by 2 pediatricians to help teach the 5 signs of the Apgar score: **A:** appearance (color); **P:** pulse; **G:** grimace (response to stimulation); **A:** activity (tone); **R:** respiration.

EXPANDED APGAR SCORE

In 2015, the American Academy of Pediatrics (AAP) and American College of Obstetricians and Gynecologists (ACOG) published a statement that included the second edition of the Neonatal Encephalopathy and Neurologic Outcome about the purpose of the Apgar score because many were using the score inappropriately. They recommended the new expanded Apgar score (Figure B–1). It has the same 5 signs as the original Apgar score but includes reporting a score also at 10, 15, and 20 minutes (10-, 15-, and 20-minute assessment is recommended by the American Heart Association [AHA] if the 5-minute Apgar score is <7) with added room to record (by a checkmark) if any of the following are used: oxygen, positive-pressure ventilation/nasal continuous positive airway pressure, endotracheal tube, chest compressions, and epinephrine. This new score accounts for resuscitative interventions. The definitions from the Neonatal Encephalopathy and Neurologic Outcome report that are recommended for the 5-minute Apgar score for term and late preterm infants are as follows: score of **7 to 10, reassuring**; score of **4 to 6, moderately abnormal**; and score of **0 to 3, low**. The AAP and ACOG recommend an umbilical arterial blood gas sample from a clamped section of the umbilical cord and possibly submitting the placenta for examination by pathology if the infant has an Apgar score of 5 at <5 minutes. Below is a summary of what the Apgar score does and does not do based on the AAP 2015 Policy Statement and the ACOG Task Force on Neonatal Encephalopathy.

What the Apgar Score Does

1. The Apgar score is an acceptable method for reporting the condition of a newborn immediately after birth and the response to resuscitation if necessary. It is affected by multiple factors including normal transition variations, gestational age, maternal medications, maternal sedation, maternal anesthesia, type of delivery, multiple births, maternal infection, resuscitation, neurologic and cardiorespiratory diseases, trauma, any congenital abnormality, and variability in the observer who is scoring the newborn.
2. A low 5-minute score (0–3) strongly correlates with neonatal mortality (report was in large populations). In the Neonatal Encephalopathy and Neurologic Outcome report, an Apgar score of 0 to 3 at ≥5 minutes was felt to be a nonspecific sign of illness. It does not predict neurologic dysfunction in the future. A low 1-minute score does not correlate or predict the outcome of an infant.
3. An Apgar score <5 at 5 and 10 minutes increases the relative risk of cerebral palsy. The majority of infants with a low 5-minute Apgar score do not develop cerebral palsy.
4. If the Apgar score is <3 at 10, 15, and 20 minutes, the population risk of a poor neurologic outcome is increased.
5. If the Apgar score is 0 after 10 minutes of age (no heart rate detectable for 10 minutes), it might be appropriate to discontinue resuscitation of the infant. This decision of stopping or continuing resuscitation should be individualized. A score of 0 at 10 minutes is a strong predictor of mortality and serious morbidity in term and late preterm infants.
6. Low Apgar scores are inversely related to birthweight.
7. A difference in the score from 1 minute to 5 minutes can be useful as an index to the response to resuscitation.
8. If the Apgar score is ≥7 at 5 minutes and the infant has neonatal encephalopathy, it is probably not due to hypoxia-ischemia in the peripartum period.

What the Apgar Score Does Not Do

1. During resuscitation of an infant, the Apgar score is not as accurate as if performed in an infant who was not resuscitated. There are no standards for assigning and reporting an Apgar score if the infant has been resuscitated.

Apgar Score

Gestational age _____ weeks

Sign	0	1	2	1 minute	5 minute	10 minute	15 minute	20 minute
Color	Blue or Pale	Acrocyanotic	Completely Pink					
Heart rate	Absent	<100 minute	>100 minute					
Reflex irritability	No Response	Grimace	Cry or Active Withdrawal					
Muscle tone	Limp	Some Flexion	Active Motion					
Respiration	Absent	Weak Cry; Hypoventilation	Good, Crying					
			Total					

Resuscitation

Minutes	1	5	10	15	20
Oxygen					
PPV/NCPAP					
ETT					
Chest Compressions					
Epinephrine					

Comments:

FIGURE B–1. Expanded Apgar score reporting form. Scores should be recorded in the appropriate place at specific time intervals. The additional resuscitative measures (if appropriate) are recorded at the same time that the score is reported by using a checkmark in the appropriate box. The comment box is used to list other factors, including maternal medications and/or the response to resuscitation between the recorded times of scoring. ETT, endotracheal tube; PPV/NCPAP, positive pressure ventilation/nasal continuous positive airway pressure. (*Based on data from American Academy of Pediatrics Committee on Fetus and Newborn, American College of Obstetricians and Gynecologists Committee on Obstetric Practice. The Apgar score. Pediatrics. 2015;136:819–822.*)

2. It does not tell you if you need to resuscitate the infant. If an infant needs resuscitation, it should be started before the 1 minute of age score. The score also does not tell you what resuscitation steps are necessary and when to use them.
3. The Apgar score does not predict an infant's morbidity, mortality, or neurologic outcome.
4. The Apgar score does not diagnose, define, measure, or provide evidence of asphyxia.

Appendix C. Blood Pressure Determinations

Table C–1. BLOOD PRESSURE MEASUREMENTS (MM HG) IN PRETERM AND FULL-TERM NEONATES (DAYS 1–7 AND DAY 30)

Postnatal Day	Gestational Age (Noncritically ILL Infants)			
	≤28 Weeks	29–32 Weeks	33–36 Weeks	37 Weeks
1	**Systolic:** 38–46 **Diastolic:** 23–29 **Mean:** 29–35	**Systolic:** 42–52 **Diastolic:** 26–38 **Mean:** 33–43	**Systolic:** 51–61 **Diastolic:** 32–40 **Mean:** 39–47	**Systolic:** 57–69 **Diastolic:** 35–45 **Mean:** 44–52
2	**Systolic:** 38–46 **Diastolic:** 24–32 **Mean:** 29–37	**Systolic:** 46–56 **Diastolic:** 29–39 **Mean:** 35–45	**Systolic:** 54–62 **Diastolic:** 34–42 **Mean:** 42–48	**Systolic:** 58–70 **Diastolic:** 36–46 **Mean:** 46–54
3	**Systolic:** 40–48 **Diastolic:** 25–33 **Mean:** 30–38	**Systolic:** 47–59 **Diastolic:** 30–35 **Mean:** 37–47	**Systolic:** 54–64 **Diastolic:** 35–43 **Mean:** 42–50	**Systolic:** 58–71 **Diastolic:** 37–47 **Mean:** 46–54
4	**Systolic:** 41–49 **Diastolic:** 26–36 **Mean:** 31–41	**Systolic:** 50–62 **Diastolic:** 32–42 **Mean:** 39–49	**Systolic:** 56–66 **Diastolic:** 36–44 **Mean:** 44–50	**Systolic:** 61–73 **Diastolic:** 38–48 **Mean:** 46–56
5	**Systolic:** 42–50 **Diastolic:** 27–37 **Mean:** 32–42	**Systolic:** 51–65 **Diastolic:** 33–43 **Mean:** 40–50	**Systolic:** 57–67 **Diastolic:** 37–45 **Mean:** 44–52	**Systolic:** 62–74 **Diastolic:** 39–49 **Mean:** 47–57
6	**Systolic:** 44–52 **Diastolic:** 30–38 **Mean:** 35–43	**Systolic:** 52–66 **Diastolic:** 35–45 **Mean:** 41–51	**Systolic:** 59–69 **Diastolic:** 37–45 **Mean:** 45–53	**Systolic:** 64–76 **Diastolic:** 40–50 **Mean:** 48–58
7	**Systolic:** 47–53 **Diastolic:** 31–39 **Mean:** 37–45	**Systolic:** 53–67 **Diastolic:** 36–44 **Mean:** 43–51	**Systolic:** 60–70 **Diastolic:** 37–45 **Mean:** 45–53	**Systolic:** 66–76 **Diastolic:** 40–50 **Mean:** 50–58
30	**Systolic:** 59–65 **Diastolic:** 35–49 **Mean:** 42–56	**Systolic:** 67–75 **Diastolic:** 43–53 **Mean:** 52–60	**Systolic:** 68–76 **Diastolic:** 45–55 **Mean:** 53–60	**Systolic:** 72–82 **Diastolic:** 46–54 **Mean:** 55–63

Data from Pejovic B, Peco-Antic A, Marinkovic-Eric J. Blood pressure in non-critically ill preterm and full-term neonates. *Pediatr Nephrol.* 2007;22:249-257.

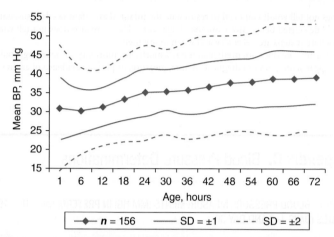

FIGURE C–1. Mean blood pressure (BP) of all infants 401 to 1000 g during the first 72 hours of life. SD, standard deviation. (*Reproduced, with permission, from Fanaroff JM, Wilson-Costello DE, Newman NS, Montpetite MM, Fanaroff AA. Treated hypotension is associated with neonatal morbidity and hearing loss in extremely low birth weight infants. Pediatrics. 2006;117;1131-1135.*)

Appendix D. Chartwork

Many hospitals are now using electronic medical records (EMR) or electronic health records (EHR). These are often in a preformatted template to be completed electronically. Because there are many different formats, there is no all-inclusive EMR example. The following section provides an overview of the basic history, progress note, admission orders, and discharge summary. Chapter 7 outlines the newborn physical examination.

ADMISSION HISTORY

A. **Identification.** State the name, age, sex, and weight of the infant. Include whether the patient or mother was transported from another facility or whether the infant was born at home or within the hospital.

Infant James, a 3-hour-old 1800-g white male, is an inborn patient from Baltimore, Maryland.

B. **Chief complaint.** The major problems of the patient are usually listed in the order of severity of disease process or occurrence.

1. *Respiratory distress syndrome*
2. *Suspected neonatal sepsis*
3. *Premature birth living child (PBLC)*

C. **Referring physician.** Include the name, address, and telephone number of the referring physician.

Dr. Macaca Mulatta, Benjamin Franklin Medical Center, Chadds Ford, PA; (946) 854-8881.

D. **History of present illness.** The history of present illness (HPI) is more helpful if it is divided into 4 separate paragraphs.

    1. **Initial statement.** This part of the HPI includes the patient's name, gestational age, birthweight, sex, age of the mother, and the number of times she has been pregnant along with the number of her living children.

    2. **Prenatal history.** Discuss the maternal prenatal care and record the number of prenatal clinic visits. Include any medications the mother was taking, any pertinent prenatal tests done, and the results.

    3. **Labor and delivery.** Include a detailed history of the labor and delivery: type of delivery, type of anesthesia, any medication used, and any fetal monitoring (including results).

    4. **Infant history.** Discuss the initial condition of the infant and the need for resuscitation, and write a detailed description of what occurred. Include the Apgar scores and discuss when the infant became symptomatic or when problems were first noted.

        Infant James is an 1800-g white male delivered to a 19-year-old G_2 now P_2, LC_2 married white female.

        The mother had excellent prenatal care. She had her first prenatal visit at approximately 8 weeks' gestation and then saw her obstetrician routinely. She was on no medications, and she does not have any history of alcohol or cigarette abuse.

        She had rupture of membranes (ROM) at 33 weeks with some mild contractions. At that time, she was seen by her obstetrician, who confirmed the premature ROM. She was admitted to the hospital and started on tocolytic treatment in an attempt to stop the labor. Vaginal–rectal swab for group B Streptococcus (GBS) cultures was obtained. Intravenous (IV) penicillin was initiated. Because of a positive GBS culture, penicillin was continued during tocolysis. External fetal monitoring had been normal until 4 hours after the tocolytic therapy, at which time it showed persistent late decelerations. At this point, an emergency cesarean delivery was performed. General anesthesia was used, and the infant was delivered within 6 minutes.

        The infant was delivered depressed at birth, with a 1-minute Apgar score of 4. He required positive-pressure ventilation with 30% oxygen. No medications were needed. The 5-minute Apgar was 7. The infant appeared poorly perfused and had poor color without oxygen. He was stabilized and transported on oxygen to the neonatal intensive care unit.

E. **Family history.** The family history should include any previous complicated births and their history, miscarriages, neonatal deaths, or premature births. Also include any major family medical problems (eg, hemophilia, sickle cell disease).

    Mrs. James had 1 prior uncomplicated vaginal delivery that went to term. There is a history of myelodysplasia in infant James's maternal first cousin.

F. **Social history.** In the social history, include a brief statement discussing the parent's age, marital status, siblings, occupation, and where they are from.

    The parents live in Chadds Ford, Pennsylvania. The mother is a 19-year-old mushroom farm worker and cares for their 2-year-old daughter; the father is 24 years old and works in the local museum as a custodial worker.

G. **Physical examination.** See Chapter 7.

H. **Laboratory data.** List the admission laboratory and radiology results.

I. **Assessment.** State your evaluation of the infant's problems. It can include a list of suspected and potential problems as well as a differential diagnosis.

    1. *Respiratory distress syndrome:* Because the infant is premature, respiratory distress syndrome must be considered. Pneumonia is also a likely cause because of the maternal history of suspected chorioamnionitis.

    2. *Suspected neonatal sepsis:* Because of the positive GBS culture and the premature onset of labor, there is an increased septic risk in this infant. Certain pathogens need to be ruled out. GBS is the most common pathogen in this age group, but Listeria monocytogenes and gram-negative pathogens should be considered.

    3. *Premature birth living child:* The infant is at 33 weeks' gestation by Ballard examination.

J. **Plan.** Include the therapeutic and diagnostic plans for the infant. (See section titled "Admission Orders.")

PROGRESS NOTES

The most commonly used format for daily progress notes is the *SOAP* method. *SOAP* is an acronym; *S* = subjective, *O* = objective, *A* = assessment, and *P* = plan. Each problem should be discussed in this format. First, state the problems you are to discuss in the order of severity or occurrence and assign a number to them. Then discuss each problem in the *SOAP* format as outlined next.

A. **Subjective (S).** Include an overall subjective view of the patient by the physician.
B. **Objective (O).** Include data that can be objectively gathered, usually in 3 areas:
    1. **Vital signs (temperature, respiratory rate, pulse, blood pressure).**
    2. **Pertinent physical examination.**
    3. **Laboratory data and other test results.**
C. **Assessment (A).** Include evaluation of the preceding data.
D. **Plan (P).** Discuss the medication changes, laboratory orders, and any other new orders as well as the treatment plan.
E. **Example.** The following is an example of part of a progress note using the SOAP format.

> ***Problem 1. Respiratory distress syndrome.***
> *S:* Infant James is now 4 days old and doing much better. He has been able to wean down to 30% oxygen with good arterial gases.
> *O:* Vital signs: temperature 98.7°F, respirations 52, pulse 140, blood pressure 55/35.
> Physical examination: The peripheral perfusion appears good with no obvious cyanosis. There is no grunting or nasal flaring, but the infant has mild substernal and intercostal retractions. The chest sounds slightly wet. Laboratory data and other test results: Arterial blood gases on 30% oxygen—pH 7.32, CO_2 48, O_2 67, 97% saturation. Chest radiograph shows mild haziness in both lung fields.
> *A:* Infant James has resolving mild respiratory distress syndrome.
> *P:* The plan is to wean the oxygen as long as his arterial PaO_2 is maintained between >55 and 70 mm Hg.
> ***Problem 2. Suspected neonatal sepsis—Follow with SOAP note.***
> ***Problem 3. Premature birth living child (PBLC)—Follow with SOAP note.***

ADMISSION ORDERS

The following format is useful for writing admission orders. It involves the mnemonic *A.D.C. VAN DISSEL:* Admit, Diagnosis, Condition, Vital signs, Activity, Nursing procedures, Diet, Input and output, Specific drugs, Symptomatic drugs, Extras, and Laboratory data. Most centers now have online physician ordering templates.

A. **Admit.** Specify the location of the patient (neonatal intensive care unit, newborn nursery) and the attending physician in charge and the house officer along with their paging/phone numbers.
B. **Diagnosis.** List the admitting diagnoses.
    1. *Respiratory distress syndrome*
    2. *Suspected neonatal sepsis*
    3. *Premature birth living child*
C. **Condition.** Note whether the patient is in stable or critical condition.
D. **Vital signs.** State the desired frequency of monitoring of vital signs. Specify rectal or axillary temperature. Rectal temperature is usually done initially to obtain a core temperature and also to rule out imperforate anus. Then, monitor axillary temperature. Other parameters include blood pressure, pulse, and respiratory rate. Weight, length, and head circumference should also be obtained on admission.
E. **Activity.** All are at bed rest, but one can specify "minimal stress or hands-off protocol" here. This notation is used for infants who react poorly to stress by dropping their oxygenation, as in patients with persistent pulmonary hypertension. At most centers, it means to handle the infant as little as possible and record all vital signs off the monitor.

F. **Nursing procedure.** Respiratory care (ventilator settings, chest percussion and postural drainage orders, endotracheal suctioning with frequency). Also require that a daily weight and head circumference be recorded. The frequency of Dextrostix (or Chemstrip-bG) testing is included in this section because it is a bedside procedure.

G. **Diet.** All infants admitted to the neonatal intensive care unit are usually made NPO (nothing by mouth) for at least 6 to 24 hours until they are accessed and stabilized. When appropriate, write specific diet orders.

H. **Input and output.** Request that the nursing staff record accurate input and output (I&O) of each infant. This record is especially important for infants on IV fluids and those just starting oral feedings. Specify how often you want the urine tested for specific gravity and glucose.

I. **Specific drugs.** State drugs to be administered, giving specific dosages and routes of administration. It is useful to also include the milligrams-per-kilogram-per-day dose of the drug to allow cross-checking and verification of the dose ordered. An example is as follows:

Ampicillin 45 mg IV every 12 hours (50 mg/kg/d divided every 12 hours).

For all infants, order the following medications at the time of admission.

1. Vitamin K (see Chapter 155) is given to prevent vitamin K deficiency disease.

2. Erythromycin eye drops (see Chapter 155) are given to prevent gonococcal ophthalmia.

J. **Symptomatic drugs.** These drugs are not routinely used in a neonatal intensive care unit and would include such items as pain and sleep medications.

K. **Extras.** Any other orders required but not included previously, such as roentgenography, electrocardiography, and ultrasonography.

L. **Laboratory data.** Include laboratory data drawn on admission, plus routine laboratory orders with frequency (eg, arterial blood gases every 2 hours, sodium and potassium bid).

DISCHARGE SUMMARY

The following information is written at the time of discharge and provides a summary of the infant's illness and hospital stay.

A. **Date of admission.**

B. **Date of discharge.**

C. **Admitting diagnosis.**

D. **Discharge diagnosis.** List in order of occurrence or severity.

E. **Attending physician and service caring for the patient.**

F. **Referring physician and address.**

G. **Procedures.** Include all invasive procedures.

H. **Brief history, physical examination, and laboratory data on admission.** Use the admission history, physical examination, and laboratory data as a guide.

I. **Hospital course.** The easiest way to approach this section of the discharge summary is to discuss each problem in paragraph form.

J. **Condition at discharge.** A complete physical examination is done at the time of discharge and included in this section. It is important to include the discharge weight, head circumference, and length so that growth can be assessed at the time of the patient's initial checkup. Also include the type and amount of formula the patient is on and any pertinent discharge laboratory values.

K. **Discharge medications.** Include the name(s) of medication(s), the dosage(s), and length of treatment. If the patient is being sent home on an apnea monitor, it is helpful to include the monitor settings and the planned course of treatment.

L. **Disposition.** Note where the patient is being sent (outside hospital, home, foster home).

M. **Discharge instructions and follow-up.** Include instructions to the parents on medications and when the patient is to return to the clinic (and exact location). It is helpful to indicate tests that need to be done on follow-up and any results that need to be rechecked (eg, bilirubin, repeat phenylketonuria screen).

N. **Problem list.** Same list as the discharge diagnosis list.

Appendix E. Immunization Guidelines

For most up to date changes, see https://www.cdc.gov/vaccines/schedules/downloads/child/0-18yrs-child-combined-schedule.pdf (accessed October 24, 2018). This table is approved by the Centers for Disease Control and Prevention, American Academy of Pediatrics (AAP), American Academy of Family Physicians, and American College of Obstetricians and Gynecologists.

IMMUNIZATIONS FOR TERM INFANTS

Term infants follow the recommended immunization schedule for persons aged 0 to 15 months, then 18 months to 18 years (http://www.immunize.org/cdc/schedules/cdc-child-iz-schedule; accessed October 24, 2018).

IMMUNIZATIONS FOR PRETERM INFANTS

Misconceptions about the safety and efficacy of vaccinations for preterm infants have led to delays in immunization for these infants. It is important that preterm infants with prolonged hospital stays begin necessary immunizations prior to neonatal intensive care unit (NICU) discharge to allow development of early protection from infectious agents prevalent in the community, especially pertussis. The AAP current recommendations can be summarized as follows:

- "Infants born preterm (at less than 37 weeks of gestation) or of low birthweight (less than 2500 g) [who are clinically stable] should, with few exceptions, receive all routinely recommended childhood vaccines at the same chronologic age as term infants," even if they are still hospitalized.
- "The same volume of vaccine used for term infants is appropriate for medically stable preterm infants."
- "The choice of needle lengths used for IM [intramuscular] vaccine administration is determined by available muscle mass of the preterm or low birth weight infant" (Table E–1).
- "Medically stable preterm infants who remain in the hospital at 2 months of chronologic age should receive all inactivated vaccines recommended at that age."
- All vaccines required at 2 months of age can be given simultaneously to preterm or low birthweight infants, except oral rotavirus vaccine, which should be given at discharge.
- Limit the number of injections at 2 months of age by giving combination vaccines. If there are limited injection sites, give the vaccines at different times, separated by 2-week intervals.

Refer to Table E–2 for immunizations for preterm infants.

Table E–1. SITE AND NEEDLE LENGTH BY AGE FOR INTRAMUSCULAR IMMUNIZATION

Age Group	Needle Length, inches (mm)[a]	Suggested Injection Site
Newborns (preterm and term) and infants <1 month of age	⅝–1 (16–25 mm)[b]	Anterolateral thigh muscle
Term infants, 1–12 months of age	⅝–1 (16–25 mm)	Anterolateral thigh muscle

[a]Assumes that needle is inserted fully.
[b]If the skin is stretched tightly and subcutaneous tissues are not bunched.
Based on *Red Book* recommendation (2018–2021).

Effectiveness of Immunizations

For the majority of premature infants, their protective antibody responses to immunizations are comparable to those seen in term infants. Although some studies have shown decreased immunity from vaccines in preterm infants weighing <1500 g and born at <29 weeks of gestation, the vast majority of preterm infants, including those receiving steroids for chronic lung disease, will produce sufficient immunity from vaccines to prevent disease.

Immunization Pain Management

Injection pain is often a source of concern among parents and hospital staff. Needle size is addressed earlier. Many simple pain management strategies are effective, particularly breast feeding, feeding sugar solutions, and applying topical anesthetics. Aspiration before injection is not recommended because it may cause more pain, and is not necessary because the anatomy of the injection site does not have any large blood vessel. For term newborns, infants, and children, the application of EMLA (lidocaine 2.5%/prilocaine 2.5%) approximately 60 minutes prior to the administration of vaccinations is an effective pain management strategy. However, the use of acetaminophen prior to vaccinations is not recommended due to possible loss in vaccine effectiveness. Acetaminophen can be used after immunizations to treat pain or fever.

A Cochrane review from 2015 evaluated several studies to determine whether needle size used for administration of vaccinations in healthy infants could reduce pain and local inflammation, while maintaining immunogenicity. In 3 studies, which including >1000 healthy infants, infants were vaccinated in the thigh with 25-gauge/25-mm needles (narrow, long needles), 23-gauge/25-mm needles (wide, long needles), or 25-gauge/16-mm needles (narrow, short needles). Using the World Health Organization guidelines, the needles were inserted at a 90-degree angle into the skin and pushed down into the muscle of the thigh. Using 25-mm needles (either 23 or 25 gauge) for intramuscular vaccination procedures in the anterolateral thigh of infants seemed to reduce the occurrence of local reactions while achieving a comparable immune response to 25-gauge/16-mm needles. Although this review was limited by its use of combination vaccines including diphtheria (D), tetanus (T), whooping cough (pertussis), and *Haemophilus influenzae* type b disease (Hib), it suggests that reducing pain with smaller, narrower needles maintains immunogenicity and reduces local inflammation. The current AAP recommendations for injection site and needle length are included in Table E–1.

Complications of Immunization

Adverse events have been reported after vaccine administration and historically have led to concern, limiting immunization of premature infants. Adverse events may be caused by the vaccine or may occur by chance after immunization. Any event that is considered **serious** or **unexpected** and possibly related to the vaccination should be reported. Serious adverse events include: **apnea, anaphylaxis, abscess formation, encephalitis, acute flaccid paralysis, fever (>40.5°C), persistent screaming, severe local reactions, and seizures.**

Preterm infants are not at higher risk for these types of adverse reactions as compared with term infants. Premature infants generally tolerate immunizations as well as term infants and experience fewer febrile and local reactions to immunizations because of their more immature immune systems. However, **apnea following immunizations** has been observed in infants with previous apneic spells, particularly within the 24 hours prior to immunizations, and those with younger gestational age or weight <2000 g at the time of immunization and a 12-hour Score for Neonatal Acute Physiology II >10. If these infants are hospitalized at the time of immunization, they should be monitored for 48 hours after immunization. Contraindications to immunizations are the same for all infants and include a significant febrile illness, active seizure disorder or encephalopathy, or any known allergies to the vaccine components (eg, eggs).

An increased incidence of apnea with or without bradycardia after immunization with whole-cell DTP was recognized in extremely low birthweight infants <1000 g but has not been reported with DTaP. Cardiorespiratory events (apnea and bradycardia with desaturations) can be seen in preterm infants given combination DTaP, inactivated polio, hepatitis B, and Hib conjugate vaccines but are not reported to have a detrimental effect on the clinical course of immunized infants according to the AAP *Red Book*. A 2008 retrospective study of >16,000 premature infants showed that specific events could not be associated with specific vaccinations; no difference in the frequency of apnea was observed after either pertussis-containing or non–pertussis-containing vaccines. Thus, the incidence of apnea in this age group is more likely to be related to a generalized inflammatory response, rather than a response to the specific vaccine antigens.

Table E–2. IMMUNIZATIONS FOR PRETERM INFANTS

Age	Infection Prevented	Recommended Vaccine
Birth	Hepatitis B[a]	**Mother HBsAg positive:** Give to all newborns regardless of BW both hepatitis B vaccine and 0.5 mL of HBIG at separate anatomic sites within 12 hours of birth. **Mother HBsAg negative:** **BW ≥2000 g:** Give hepatitis B vaccine as routine prophylaxis to all medically stable infants within 24 hours of birth. **BW <2000 g:** Give hepatitis B vaccine as routine prophylaxis at 1 month of age chronologically or at hospital discharge (whichever occurs first). **Mother HBsAg unknown:** Give hepatitis B vaccine within 12 hours of birth to all newborns regardless of BW. **For HBIG:** **BW ≥2000 g:** Give HBIG within 7 days of birth if maternal status is confirmed positive, or by 7 days of life or at hospital discharge (whichever is first) if maternal status remains unknown. **BW <2000 g:** Give 0.5 mL of HBIG within 12 hours of birth unless maternal status is confirmed negative by that time.
1–2 months	Hepatitis B[a]	Give the second dose of hepatitis B vaccine at 1–2 months of age.
2 months[c]	Diphtheria, tetanus, pertussis *Haemophilus influenzae* type b Inactivated poliovirus Pneumococcal conjugate Rotavirus[d]	DTaP[b] Hib IPV PCV13 Rotavirus vaccine can be given to preterm (clinically stable)/term infants as follows: between 6 weeks and 14 weeks, 6 days of chronologic age, with first dose given **at hospital discharge**, or after discharge—series should not be started after 15 weeks, 0 days of age.

(Continued)

Table E–2. **IMMUNIZATIONS FOR PRETERM INFANTS (*CONTINUED*)**

Age	Infection Prevented	Recommended Vaccine
	Meningococcal vaccine (Menveo)	Only for anatomic/functional asplenia, sickle cell disease, HIV infection, persistent complement component deficiency, or infants who live or travel in countries where meningococcal disease is hyperendemic or epidemic. Give at 2, 4, 6, and 12 months of age.
4 months	All of those listed for 2 months	All of those listed for 2 months except hepatitis B: If using monovalent hepatitis B, no vaccine at 4 months. If using a combination vaccine with hepatitis B, then acceptable to have baby receive a total of 4 doses of hepatitis B vaccine.
6 months	All of those listed for 1–2 and 2 months	All listed for 1–2 and 2 months, except: If Pedvax-HIB is administered at 2 and 4 months, a dose at 6 months for Hib not necessary. Only RotaTeq vaccine given at 6 months.
	Influenza vaccine	Inactivated influenza vaccine: 2 doses beginning at 6 months of age, with second dose 1 month later.
	MMR (only international travel)	For international travel only, give 1 dose before departure.
	Hepatitis A vaccination	For infants traveling to countries with high or intermediate endemic hepatitis A.
Hospital discharge	RSV[e]	Appropriately selected preterm infants may benefit from immunoprophylaxis with palivizumab beginning at hospital discharge and then monthly during RSV season. Refer to yearly regional recommendations for guidelines

BW, birthweight; HBIG, hepatitis B immune globulin; HBsAg, hepatitis B surface antigen; MMR, measles, mumps, rubella; RSV, respiratory syncytial virus.

[a]Only monovalent (single-antigen) hepatitis B vaccine should be used for the dose at birth and any dose given before 6 weeks of age.

[b]Whenever possible, the same brand of DTaP should be used at 2, 4, and 6 months.

[c]Combination vaccines can be given starting at 2 months of age to minimize the number of injections.

[d]Do not use rotavirus if there is a history of intussusception or severe combined immune deficiency. Use precautions when giving rotavirus if the infant has any moderate to severe illness, manifestations of altered immunocompetence, preexisting chronic intestinal tract disease, or bladder exstrophy or spina bifida. Rotavirus can be given the same time as other vaccines or any time a blood product is given. If the infant vomits, regurgitates, or spits up during or after the dose, do not repeat it. Rotarix is a 2-dose series at 2 and 4 months. RotaTeq is a 3-dose series at 2, 4, and 6 months.

[e]RSV eligibility includes: Preterm infants with chronic lung disease (CLD) of prematurity (GA <32 weeks, 0 days, and a requirement for >21% oxygen for at least the first 28 days after birth); infants with acyanotic heart disease on medication to control congestive heart failure who require cardiac surgical procedures; infants with moderate to severe pulmonary hypertension; and preterm infants without CLD or CHD if born at <29 weeks, 0 days of gestation.

Based on Kimberlin DW, Long SS, eds. *Red Book: 2018–2021 Report of the Committee on Infectious Diseases.* 31st ed. Elk Grove Village, IL: American Academy of Pediatrics; 2018–2021.

Special Circumstances

There are few data regarding the immunologic responses of extremely preterm infants receiving steroids for the treatment of bronchopulmonary dysplasia/chronic lung disease (BPD/CLD). Therefore, live vaccines should not be administered to babies receiving prednisolone (2 mg/kg/d for >1 week or 1 mg/kg/d for >1 month) or the equivalent dose of dexamethasone. Live vaccines should not be administered while babies are hospitalized in the NICU.

Premature infants >6 months but <2 years of age with a history of BPD/CLD or reactive airway disease should be considered for vaccination against influenza.

Select premature infants are eligible to receive prophylaxis against the respiratory syncytial virus (RSV) as a monthly injection given during RSV season. Eligibility requirements can change yearly. It is recommended that physicians use local references at the beginning of the RSV season for guidance on dosing.

Immunization for Perinatal Hepatitis B Infection

The AAP recently released an updated policy statement for elimination of perinatal hepatitis B infection. Unfortunately, when infants become infected and are not adequately treated, 90% will go on to develop chronic hepatitis B infection. Further, one-quarter of those infants will die of hepatocellular carcinoma or liver cirrhosis. Hepatitis B vaccination is highly effective when given appropriately; hepatitis B vaccine alone is 75% to 95% effective in preventing perinatal hepatitis B transmission if administered within 24 hours of birth. In addition, when postexposure prophylaxis of both hepatitis B vaccine and hepatitis B immune globulin (HBIG) is given correctly and is followed by completion of the infant hepatitis B immunization series, perinatal infection rates can drop below 1%.

Appendix F. Isolation Guidelines

The following table, Table F–1 Transmission-Based Precautions for Perinatal/Neonatal Patients, in conjunction with Standard Precautions (see Chapter 25), is based on current knowledge and practices in the fields of epidemiology, pediatrics, and perinatology. Published resource references are listed immediately after the table. Always follow local guidelines where they exist.

INSTRUCTIONS FOR USING PRECAUTIONS FOR PERINATAL/NEONATAL PATIENTS (TABLE F–1)

- Each disease is considered individually so that only precautions indicated to interrupt transmission for that disease are recommended.
- The column "Maternal Precautions" describes the precautions to be used by staff providing care to the mother.
- The column "Neonatal Precautions" describes the precautions to be used by staff, patients, or visitors in contact with the neonate.
- Staff should assess the mother's ability to wash hands correctly and comply with precautions when determining the appropriateness of permitting rooming in.
- Precautions should be initiated for suspected as well as confirmed infectious diseases/conditions.

Table F–1. TRANSMISSION-BASED PRECAUTIONS FOR PERINATAL/NEONATAL PATIENTS

Infection/Disease	Maternal Precautions	Neonatal Precautions	Room-In	Mother May Visit in Nursery	Breast Feeding	Additional Considerations
AIDS/HIV positive	Standard	Standard Bathe baby ASAP when stable	Yes	Yes	No HIV may be transmitted through breast milk.	Recommend tuberculosis testing for mother. Due to constant HIV antiretroviral (ARV) treatment option changes, consult with neonatology expert and refer to http://aidsinfo.nih.gov for current ARV treatment options. Follow your local public health department reporting requirements.
Chickenpox (see Varicella)						
Chlamydia trachomatis	Standard	Standard	Yes	Yes	Yes	Topical prophylaxis is ineffective for *Chlamydia* ophthalmic disease. Treatment for *Chlamydia:* Even though infants born to mothers with untreated chlamydial infections are at high risk of infection; prophylaxis is not indicated. The recommended treatment of choice for conjunctivitis and pneumonia is oral erythromycin base or ethylsuccinate (50 mg/kg/d in 4 divided doses daily) for 14 days or azithromycin (20 mg/kg as single dose) for 3 days. Due to 80% treatment efficacy, a second course may be required (*see Red Book*, 2018–2021).
Cytomegalovirus (CMV)	Standard	Standard	Yes	Yes	Yes	No additional precautions for pregnant healthcare workers.

(Continued)

Table F-1. TRANSMISSION-BASED PRECAUTIONS FOR PERINATAL/NEONATAL PATIENTS (*CONTINUED*)

Infection/Disease	Maternal Precautions	Neonatal Precautions	Room-In	Mother May Visit in Nursery	Breast Feeding	Additional Considerations
Gastroenteritis	Contact precautions for diapered or incontinent persons for the duration of illness or to control outbreaks for gastroenteritis caused by infectious agents such as *Clostridium difficile*	Contact precautions for the duration of illness to control outbreaks for gastroenteritis/diarrhea caused by infectious agents such as *C difficile*	Yes	Yes	Yes	The most effective method to remove *C difficile* spores from contaminated hands is through meticulous hand hygiene with soap and water. Alcohol-based hand hygiene products do not inactivate *C difficile* spores. Because *C difficile* spores are difficult to kill, most surface disinfectants are ineffective. When outbreaks of *C difficile* diarrhea are not controlled by other measures, it is recommended to use a disinfectant with sporicidal activity (eg, hypochlorite).
Gonococcal ophthalmia neonatorum	Standard	Standard	Yes After 24 hours of maternal treatment with antibiotics	Yes After 24 hours of maternal treatment with antibiotics	Yes After 24 hours of maternal treatment with antibiotics	In addition to antimicrobial therapy, treatment should include eye irrigations with saline solution immediately after birth and frequently until discharge stops. (See Chapter 58.)
Group B streptococcal infections	Standard	Standard	Yes	Yes	Yes	In case of a nursery outbreak, cohorting of ill and colonized infants and use of contact precautions are recommended,
Hepatitis A, B, C	Standard	Standard (special attention to wear gloves when removing maternal blood at the time of birth)	Yes	Yes	Yes	Early hepatitis B immunization is recommended for all medically stable infants with birthweight >2 kg, regardless of maternal status. The AAP recommends

						that infants born to HBsAg-positive mothers, including preterm and low birth-weight infants, receive the initial dose of hepatitis B vaccine within 12 hours of birth. Report to health department.
Herpes simplex virus (HSV) **Neonatal infection or positive culture in absence of disease**	Contact (gown and gloves) for active HSV lesions during labor, delivery, and the postpartum period.	Contact (gown and gloves) during incubation for infants born to women with active HSV lesions	Yes If baby is at low risk of infection	Yes	Yes If no vesicular herpetic lesion in the breast area and all active skin lesions are covered.	Women with primary HSV infections are more likely to shed the virus and transmit the virus to their newborn infant. The AAP published two algorithms for the evaluation and treatment of asymptomatic neonates following vaginal or cesarean delivery to women with active genital HSV lesions (see Figures 137–1 and 137–2).
Lice (see Pediculosis)						
Measles (rubeola)	Airborne N-95 masks for those susceptible. Labor, delivery, and postpartum recovery should take place in a private room with negative-pressure, nonrecirculating air with door closed. If mother is transferred to the delivery room for the actual delivery, she should wear surgical mask during transfer and delivery.	Standard and airborne For 4 days after the onset of rash in otherwise healthy patients and for duration of illness in immunocompromised patients. Exposed susceptible patients need to be placed in airborne precautions from day 5 after first day of exposure until day 21 after last exposure.	No	No	No Until mother is noncontagious	Contagious during prodrome and for 4 days after onset of rash. Healthcare personnel who may come in contact with patients with measles should have evidence of immunity to measles through their vaccine records. Follow your local health department reporting requirements.

(Continued)

Table F-1. TRANSMISSION-BASED PRECAUTIONS FOR PERINATAL/NEONATAL PATIENTS (*CONTINUED*)

Infection/Disease	Maternal Precautions	Neonatal Precautions	Room-In	Mother May Visit in Nursery	Breast Feeding	Additional Considerations
Methicillin-resistant *Staphylococcus aureus* (MRSA), methicillin-sensitive *S aureus* (MSSA), vancomycin-intermediate susceptible *S aureus* (VISA), and vancomycin-resistant *S aureus* (VRSA)	Contact Gown and gloves	Contact Gown and gloves. For patients with pneumonia, droplet precautions are recommended for the first 24 hours of antimicrobial therapy. Droplet precautions should be maintained throughout the illness for MSSA or MRSA tracheitis with a tracheostomy tube in place. For VISA/VRSA, in addition to contact precautions, wear mask/eye protection or face shield when performing procedures that can generate splash/splatter contaminated materials (eg, wound drainage, blood, bodily fluids, secretions).	Yes	Yes Follow contact precautions	Yes	Apply contact precautions for active infections only. More evidence is needed for recommendations on isolation precautions for patients with known colonization. CDC has issued specific infection control recommendations for VISA and VRSA (http://www.cdc.gov/hai/pdfs/VRSA-Investigation-Guide-05_12_2015.pdf). Follow your local public health department reporting and discharging requirements.
Mumps (infectious parotitis)	Standard and droplet Masks within 3 ft of patient. Private room.	Standard and droplet until 5 days after onset of parotid swelling	No	No	No Until mother is noncontagious	Contagious for 5 days after onset of swelling. Follow your local health department reporting requirements.

Pediculosis (lice)	Contact For 24 hours after effective treatment, gown and gloves	Contact For 24 hours after effective treatment, gown and gloves	Yes	Yes	Yes	Exposed individuals and household contacts should be examined and treated if infected. Bedmates of infested people should also receive prophylactic treatment. Instruct mother to clean breasts before feeding if medication is applied to that area. Stress good hand hygiene with special attention to area under fingernails.
Pertussis (whooping cough)	Standard and droplet for duration of illness as clinically determined by the MD	Standard and droplet for 5 days after initiation of effective therapy and up to 21 days after onset of cough if no treatment given	No	No	No Until mother is noncontagious	Contagious for 5 days after start of effective therapy. Treatment with antimicrobial agents if available for newborns <1 and 2 months of age if the risk of developing severe pertussis and life-threatening complications outweighs the potential risk of developing infantile hypertrophic pyloric stenosis. See *Red Book*, 2018. Follow local public health department reporting requirements.
Respiratory syncytial virus (RSV)	Standard plus contact for duration of illness, including patients treated with ribavirin	Standard and contact for duration of illness including patients treated with ribavirin	Yes	Yes May visit private room or cohort	Yes	Parent education is essential to avoid transmission of the virus. The importance of hand hygiene should be emphasized in all settings. Prophylaxis to prevent RSV in newborns at increased risk for severe disease, particularly those with bronchopulmonary dysplasia/chronic lung disease receiving medical management on a long-term basis, is available. Refer to *Perinatal Guidelines* (AAP/ACOG, 2012) and the *Red Book* (2018). Contagious for duration of illness.

(Continued)

Table F–1. TRANSMISSION-BASED PRECAUTIONS FOR PERINATAL/NEONATAL PATIENTS (*CONTINUED*)

Infection/Disease	Maternal Precautions	Neonatal Precautions	Room-In	Mother May Visit in Nursery	Breast Feeding	Additional Considerations
Rubella (German measles) Postnatal	Standard and droplet	Standard and droplet for 7 days after onset of the rash. Contact precautions indicated if suspected congenital rubella until 1 year of age, unless 2 cultures or clinical specimens obtained 1 month apart after 3 months are negative for the rubella virus.	Yes	No	No	Contagious for 7 days after onset of rash. Susceptible persons should stay out of room, if possible.
Rubella (German measles) Maternal	Masks within 3 ft of patient. Private room; masks for those susceptible.					Follow your local health department reporting requirements.
Rubella (German measles) Congenital		Contact Gown and gloves	Yes	Yes	Yes	Contagious until at least 1 year of age, unless 2 cultures or clinical specimens obtained 1 month apart after 3 months of age are negative for rubella virus. Susceptible persons should stay out of room, if possible. Report to health department.
Scabies	Contact For 24 hours after treatment, gown and gloves.	Contact For 24 hours after treatment, gown and gloves.	Yes	Yes	Yes	Treatment of exposed individuals and household contacts is recommended. Instruct mother to clean breasts before feeding if medication is applied to that area. Stress good hand hygiene.

1378

Syphilis	Standard. Gloves should be worn when caring for patients with congenital, primary, and secondary syphilis with skin or mucous membrane lesions until 24 hours of treatment have been completed.	Yes	Yes	Yes	Treatment for congenital syphilis is available for infants in the first month of life (see *Red Book*, 2018–2021). Follow your local health department reporting requirements.
Tuberculosis (TB) Mother with recent positive purified protein derivative (PPD) and no evidence of active TB.	Standard	Yes	Yes	Yes	If the mother is asymptomatic, no separation is required. The newborn infant needs no special evaluation or therapy.
TB Mother with minimal disease or disease has been treated for ≥2 weeks and is determined by pulmonary or infectious disease specialist to be noncontagious at delivery.	Standard	Yes	Yes	Yes	Management of the newborn infant suspected of congenital TB is based on categorization of the maternal infection. See testing and treatment in the *Red Book*, 2018–2021. Follow your local health department requirements.

(Continued)

Table F–1. TRANSMISSION-BASED PRECAUTIONS FOR PERINATAL/NEONATAL PATIENTS (*CONTINUED*)

Infection/Disease	Maternal Precautions	Neonatal Precautions	Room-In	Mother May Visit in Nursery	Breast Feeding	Additional Considerations
TB **Mother with current pulmonary or laryngeal active TB and suspected of being contagious at time of delivery.**	Airborne N95 respirator for healthcare workers. Labor, delivery, and postpartum care in private room with negative-pressure, nonrecirculating air with door closed. If mother is transferred to the delivery room for the actual delivery, she should wear transfer mask during transfer and delivery.	Standard. Airborne precautions for neonates with congenital TB during procedures involving the oropharyngeal airway (eg, intubation) until effective therapy has been initiated, sputum smears are negative, and cough has been abated.	No Until mother is determined to be noncontagious	No Until mother is determined to be noncontagious	No Until mother is determined to be noncontagious	Management of the newborn infant suspected of congenital TB is based on categorization of the maternal infection. See testing and treatment in the *Red Book*, 2018–2021. Follow your local health department reporting requirements. Report to health department.
TB **Mother has extrapulmonary spread of TB (eg, miliary, bone,**	Standard	Standard	No Until mother is determined to be noncontagious	No Until mother is determined to be noncontagious	No Until mother is determined to be noncontagious	Management of the newborn infant suspected of congenital TB is based on categorization of the maternal infection. See testing and treatment in the *Red Book*, 2018–2021. Report to health department.

Condition	Type of precaution	Precautions					Comments
Varicella (chickenpox) or herpes zoster in immunocompromised mother or if disseminated maternal infection	Airborne/contact	Labor, delivery, and postpartum care in private room with negative-pressure, nonrecirculating air with door closed. If mother is transferred to the delivery room for the actual delivery, she should wear mask during transfer and delivery. Airborne and contact for neonates born to mothers with varicella; neonates should be placed on airborne and contact precautions from birth until 21 days or from birth or until 28 days of age if VariZIG or IGIV was administered. Mother and infant should be isolated separately until the mother's vesicles have dried.	Until mother's lesions have crusted	No Until mother's lesions have crusted	No Until mother's lesions have crusted	No Until mother's lesions have crusted	Consider immunologic titer for neonates <28 weeks' gestational age.
Varicella—newborn or exposure to varicella	Airborne and contact	Masks for those susceptible. Private room with negative-pressure, non-recirculating air with door closed. From 8 until 21 days after exposure and until 28 days if VariZIG or IVIG given.	Yes	Yes May visit private room or cohort	Yes Unless mother has lesions		Hospitalized patients should be discharged prior to the 10th day after exposure, if possible. Infants with varicella embryopathy do not required isolation if they do not have active lesions.

AAP, American Academy of Pediatrics; ACOG, American College of Obstetricians and Gynecologists; AIDS, acquired immunodeficiency syndrome; CDC, Centers for Disease Control and Prevention; HBsAg, hepatitis B surface antigen; HIV, human immunodeficiency virus; IVIG, intravenous immune globulin; MD, physician. Modified and adapted from guidelines issued by Kaiser Permanente Hospital, Fontana, CA.

Appendix G. Temperature Conversion Table

Celsius	Fahrenheit	Celsius	Fahrenheit
34.0	93.2	37.6	99.6
34.2	93.6	37.8	100.0
34.4	93.9	38.0	100.4
34.6	94.3	38.2	100.7
34.8	94.6	38.4	101.1
35.0	95.0	38.6	101.4
35.2	95.4	38.8	101.8
35.4	95.7	39.0	102.2
35.6	96.1	39.2	102.5
35.8	96.4	39.4	102.9
36.0	96.8	39.6	103.2
36.2	97.1	39.8	103.6
36.4	97.5	40.0	104.0
36.6	97.8	40.2	104.3
36.8	98.2	40.4	104.7
37.0	98.6	40.6	105.1
37.2	98.9	40.8	105.4
37.4	99.3	41.0	105.8

Celsius = (Fahrenheit − 32) × 5/9.
Fahrenheit = (Celsius × 9/5) + 32.

Appendix H. Weight Conversion Table[a]

Ounces	1 lb	2 lb	3 lb	4 lb	5 lb	6 lb	7 lb	8 lb
				Grams				
0	454	907	1361	1814	2268	2722	3175	3629
1	482	936	1389	1843	2296	2750	3204	3657
2	510	964	1418	1871	2325	2778	3232	3686
3	539	992	1446	1899	2353	2807	3260	3714
4	567	1021	1474	1928	2381	2835	3289	3742
5	595	1049	1503	1956	2410	2863	3317	3771
6	624	1077	1531	1985	2438	2892	3345	3799
7	652	1106	1559	2013	2466	2920	3374	3827
8	680	1134	1588	2041	2495	2948	3402	3856
9	709	1162	1616	2070	2523	2977	3430	3884
10	737	1191	1644	2098	2552	3005	3459	3912
11	765	1219	1673	2126	2580	3033	3487	3941
12	794	1247	1701	2155	2608	3062	3515	3969
13	822	1276	1729	2183	2637	3090	3544	3997
14	851	1304	1758	2211	2665	3119	3572	4026
15	879	1332	1786	2240	2693	3147	3600	4054

[a]Values represent weight in grams.
To convert from kilograms to pounds, multiply kilograms by 2.2.
To convert from pounds to grams, multiply pounds by 454.

Index

Entries denoted by *f* and *t* indicate figures and tables, respectively.